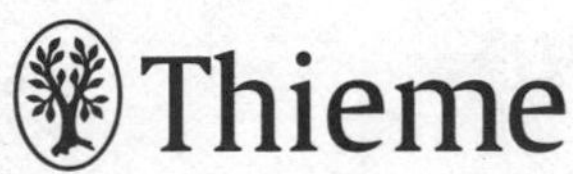

Handbook of Neurosurgery

Mark S. Greenberg, MD
Associate Professor
Department of Neurosurgery and Brain Repair
University of South Florida
Tampa, Florida

Eighth Edition

179 illustrations

Thieme
New York • Stuttgart • Delhi • Rio de Janeiro

Executive Editor: Timothy Hiscock
Managing Editor: Sarah E. Landis
Director, Editorial Services: Mary Jo Casey
Editorial Assistant: Naamah Schwartz
Production Editor: Torsten Scheihagen
International Production Director: Andreas Schabert
Vice President, Editorial and E-Product Development: Vera Spillner
Director, Clinical Solutions: Michael Wachinger
International Marketing Director: Fiona Henderson
International Sales Director: Louisa Turrell
Director of Sales, North America: Mike Roseman
Senior Vice President and Chief Operating Officer: Sarah Vanderbilt
President: Brian D. Scanlan
Printer: Transcontinental Printing
Cover Illustrator: Jennifer Pryll

Library of Congress Cataloging-in-Publication Data
Names: Greenberg, Mark S., M.D., author.
Title: Handbook of neurosurgery / Mark S. Greenberg.
Description: Eighth edition. | New York : Thieme, [2016] | Preceded by Handbook of neurosurgery / editor, Mark S. Greenberg. 7th ed. 2010. | Includes bibliographical references and index.
Identifiers: LCCN 2015051094| ISBN 9781626232419 | ISBN 9781626232426 (e-book)
Subjects: | MESH: Nervous System Diseases–surgery | Neurosurgical Procedures | Handbooks
Classification: LCC RD593 | NLM WL 39 | DDC 617.4/8–dc23 LC record available at http://lccn.loc.gov/2015051094

Thieme Publishers New York
333 Seventh Avenue, New York, NY 10001 USA
+1 800 782 3488 customerservive@thieme.com
www.thieme.com

Thieme Publishers Stuttgart
Rüdigerstrasse 14, 70469 Stuttgart, Germany
+49 [0]711 8931 421
customerservice@thieme.com

Thieme Publishers Delhi
A-12, Second Floor, Sector-2, Noida-201301
Uttar Pradesh, India
+91 120 45 566 00
customerservice@thieme.in

Thieme Publishers Rio de Janeiro,
Thieme Publicações Ltda.
Edifício Rodolpho de Paoli, 25º andar
Av. Nilo Peçanha, 50 – Sala 2508
Rio de Janeiro 20020-906, Brasil
+55 21 3172 2297

Typesetting: DiTech Process Solutions

Printed in Canada

ISBN 978-1-62623-241-9 1 2 3 4 5 6

Also available as an e-book:
eISBN 978-1-62623-242-6

First edition, 1990
Second edition, 1991
Third edition, 1994
Fourth edition, 1997
Fifth edition, 2001
Sixth edition, 2006
Seventh edition, 2010

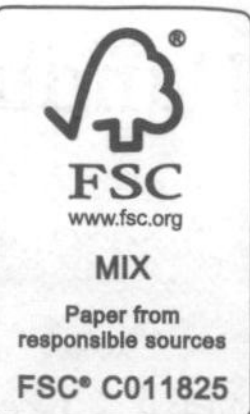

Important note: Medicine is an ever-changing science undergoing continual development. Research and clinical experience are continually expanding our knowledge, in particular our knowledge of proper treatment and drug therapy. Insofar as this book mentions any dosage or application, readers may rest assured that the authors, editors, and publishers have made every effort to ensure that such references are in accordance with **the state of knowledge at the time of production of the book.**

Nevertheless, this does not involve, imply, or express any guarantee or responsibility on the part of the publishers in respect to any dosage instructions and forms of applications stated in the book. **Every user is requested to examine carefully** the manufacturers' leaflets accompanying each drug and to check, if necessary in consultation with a physician or specialist, whether the dosage schedules mentioned therein or the contraindications stated by the manufacturers differ from the statements made in the present book. Such examination is particularly important with drugs that are either rarely used or have been newly released on the market. Every dosage schedule or every form of application used is entirely at the user's own risk and responsibility. The authors and publishers request every user to report to the publishers any discrepancies or inaccuracies noticed. If errors in this work are found after publication, errata will be posted at www.thieme.com on the product description page.

Some of the product names, patents, and registered designs referred to in this book are in fact registered trademarks or proprietary names even though specific reference to this fact is not always made in the text. Therefore, the appearance of a name without designation as proprietary is not to be construed as a representation by the publisher that it is in the public domain.

Dedication

The eighth edition of the Handbook of Neurosurgery *is dedicated to my wonderful wife, Debbie. She inspires me to be the best I can be.*

This book is also dedicated to "Duke" (August Henry Wagner III), beloved uncle of contributor Jayson Sack, who suffered a fatal aneurysmal subarachnoid hemorrhage as this book was going to press. His selfless life was an inspiration to Jayson and his family. He will be missed and never forgotten.

Contributors

Naomi A. Abel, MD
Assistant Professor
Department of Neurosurgery and Brain Repair
University of South Florida Morsani College of Medicine
Tampa, Florida
Failure of carpal tunnel and ulnar nerve surgery
Electrodiagnostics (EDX)

Siviero Agazzi, MD, MBA
Associate Professor
Department of Neurosurgery and Brain Repair
University of South Florida Morsani College of Medicine
Tampa, Florida
Vestibular schwannomas

Amir Ahmadian, MD
Attending physician
Neurosurgery of West Florida
Hudson, Florida
Adult spinal deformity
*Cavernous malformations**

Norberto Andaluz, MD
Associate Professor
Department of Neurosurgery
University of Cincinnati College of Medicine
Cincinnati VA Medical Center
Cincinnati, Ohio
*Carotid stenosis and endarterectomy**
*Emergency carotid endarterectomy**
*Totally occluded carotid artery**

Ramsey Ashour, MD
Complex cranial fellow
Department of Neurosurgery and Brain Repair
University of South Florida Morsani College of Medicine
Tampa, Florida
Dural arteriovenous fistulae

Ali A. Baaj, MD
Assistant Professor
Department of Neurological Surgery
Weill Cornell Medical College
New York Presbyterian Hospital
New York, New York
*Moyamoya disease**

Konrad Bach, MD
Research Associate
University of South Florida Morsani College of Medicine
Tampa, Florida
Ankylosing spondylitis

Clayton Bauer, MD, PhD
Resident physician
Department of Neurosurgery and Brain Repair
University of South Florida Morsani College of Medicine
Tampa, Florida
Status epilepticus

Joshua M. Beckman, MD
Resident physician
Department of Neurosurgery and Brain Repair
University of South Florida Morsani College of Medicine
Tampa, Florida
Concussion (mTBI)

Adarsh Bhimraj, MD
Attending physician
Section Head, Neuroinfections
Cleveland Clinic
Cleveland, Ohio
EVD-related infections

Elias Dakwar, MD
Assistant Professor
Department of Neurosurgery and Brain Repair
University of South Florida Morsani College of Medicine
Tampa, Florida
CSF Fistulas

Angela Downes, MD
Fellow, Neurocritical Care
Department of Neurosurgery
University of Colorado
Denver, Colorado
Stereotactic radiosurgery
*Spontaneous subdural hematoma**

Melissa Giarratano, PharmD, BCPS
Clinical Pharmacist – Neurosciences
Tampa General Hospital
Tampa, Florida
Antibiotics

Alexander Haas, MD
Resident physician
Department of Neurosurgery and Brain Repair
University of South Florida Morsani College of Medicine
Tampa, Florida
Colloid cysts

Ghaith Habboub, MD
Resident physician
Neurological Institute
Cleveland Clinic
Cleveland, Ohio
EVD-related infections

Shannon Hann, MD
Resident physician
Department of Neurological Surgery
Thomas Jefferson University
Philadelphia, Pennsylvania
*Neurocutaneous melanosis**

Shah-Naz H. Khan, MD, FRCS(C), FAANS
Chair and Director
Institute of General and Endovascular Neurosurgery
Clinical Assistant Professor
Department of Surgery
Michigan State University
Flint, Michigan
Endovascular neurosurgery

Tsz Y. Lau, MD
Assistant Professor
Department of Neurosurgery and Brain Repair
University of South Florida Morsani College of Medicine
Tampa, Florida
Subarachnoid hemorrhage

Shih-Sing Liu, MD
Assistant Professor
Department of Neurosurgery and Brain Repair
University of South Florida Morsani College of Medicine
Tampa, Florida
Jugular foramen
Anticoagulation & antiplatelet therapy

Wai-man Liu, MBBS, FRCS, FHKAM
Chief of Service, Honorary Associate Professor
Division of Neurosurgery, Department of Surgery
Li Ka Shing Faculty of Medicine
The University of Hong Kong
Pokfulam, Hong Kong
Astrocytoma

Jotham Manwaring, MD
Attending physician
Southern Utah Neurosciences Institute
St. George, Utah
Third ventriculostomy (ETV)
*X-linked hydrocephalus**

Carlos R. Martinez, MD, FACR
Professor of Radiology
USF College of Medicine
Assistant Chief of Radiology
Bay Pines VA Hospital
Tampa, Florida
Intracranial hypotension

Meleine Martinez-Sosa, MD
Resident physician
Department of Neurosurgery and Brain Repair
University of South Florida Morsani College of Medicine
Tampa, Florida
Intracranial hypotension

Timothy D. Miller Jr., MD
Resident physician
Division of Neurosurgery
Duke University School of Medicine
Durham, North Carolina
Cerebral vasospasm

Jose Montero, MD
Associate Professor
Department of Internal Medicine
University of South Florida Morsani College of Medicine
Tampa, Florida
Antibiotics

Jason Paluzzi, MD
Resident physician
Department of Neurosurgery and Brain Repair
University of South Florida Morsani College of Medicine
Tampa, Florida
Wilbrand's knee

Michael S. Park, MD
Resident physician
Department of Neurosurgery and Brain Repair
University of South Florida Morsani College of Medicine
Tampa, Florida
Carotid endarterectomy vs. stenting

Glen A. Pollock, MD
Attending physician
Raleigh Neurosurgical Clinic
Raleigh, North Carolina
*PRES**

Kan-suen Jenny Pu, BSC, MBBS, FHKAM, FRCSHK, FRCS (Surgical Neurology)
Division of Neurosurgery, Department of Surgery
Li Ka Shing Faculty of Medicine
The University of Hong Kong
Pokfulam, Hong Kong
Astrocytoma

Edwin Ramos, MD
Assistant Professor
Department of Surgery
The University of Chicago Medicine
Chicago, Illinois
*Hypothalamic hamartomas**

Stephen Reintjes, MD
Resident physician
Department of Neurosurgery and Brain Repair
University of South Florida Morsani College of Medicine
Tampa, Florida
Anticoagulation & antiplatelet therapy

Jayson Sack, MD
Resident physician
Division of Neurosurgery
University of California, San Diego
San Diego, California
Subarachnoid hemorrhage

Stephen Sandwell, MD
Resident physician
Department of Neurosurgery
University of Rochester
Rochester, New York
Central neurocytoma

Joseph Serrone, MD
Attending physician
Virginia Mason Hospital and Seattle Medical Center
Seattle, Washington
*Pleomorphic xanthoastrocytomas**

Sananthan Sivakanthan
Medical student
University of South Florida Morsani College of Medicine
Tampa, Florida
Jugular foramen

L. Brannon Thomas, MD, PhD
Attending physician
James A. Haley Veterans Administration Hospital
University Community Hospital
Tampa, Florida
Neuropathology

Fernando L. Vale, MD
Professor and Vice-Chairman
Department of Neurosurgery and Brain Repair
University of South Florida Morsani College of Medicine
Tampa, Florida
Seizure surgery

Jamie J. Van Gompel, MD
Assistant Professor
Department of Neurosurgery
Mayo Clinic
Rochester, Minnesota
Esthesioneuroblastomas

Juan S. Uribe, MD
Associate Professor
Director, Spine Section
Department of Neurosurgery and Brain Repair
University of South Florida Morsani College of Medicine
Tampa, Florida
Transpsoas approach
*Lhermitte-Duclos disease**
*Bone graft materials**
*New spine fusion techniques**

Rohit Vasan, MD
Attending physician
Department of Neurosurgery and Brain Repair
University of South Florida Morsani College of Medicine
Tampa, Florida
*Syncope**

Charles E. Wright, MD
Medical Director
LifeLink of Florida
Tampa, Florida
Brain death & organ donation

Chun-Po Yen, MD
Fellow
Department of Neurosurgery and Brain Repair
University of South Florida Morsani College of Medicine
Tampa, Florida
Transpsoas approach
Stereotactic radiosurgery

Ashraf Samy Youssef, MD, PhD
Visiting Associate Professor
Director of Skull Base Surgery
Department of Neurosurgery
University of Colorado School of Medicine
Denver, Colorado
*Management of pineal region tumors**

****Originally contributed to the Handbook of Neurosurgery, seventh edition***

Preface

Shortly after finishing my residency training in 1989, in a time long before the internet, I wrote the first edition of the *Handbook of Neurosurgery* with the intent to make practical, actionable neurosurgical information accessible at the fingertips of the practitioner.

Over the years, I used desktop publishing technology to expand the scope of the book, and to incorporate diagrams and literature references. I always wanted to make the book "academic" by presenting data that backed up the assertions. My goal was to never publish a cookbook.

Without advertising, I relied solely on word-of-mouth to promote the book. I believed in the same thing that Edwin Land must have when he said, "Marketing is what you do when your product is no good." I had a test run of 600 copies of the book printed at a small vanity press in Ann Arbor, and sold copies to individuals by mail. My big break came when the medical bookstore at the State University of New York in Syracuse purchased 6 copies to put on their shelves. After that, I regularly packaged 5 or 6 books in a box destined for various bookstores and dropped them off at the loading dock on my way to the O.R. in the morning. After a time, the major medical book distributors in the country began ordering cases of books and my garage became a shipping department. (I still have the pallet jack that I used to unload the delivery trucks.) Then, somehow, international orders began to arrive.

I was finally able to get out of the packing and transporting business when I partnered with Thieme Medical Publishers in 2001. At that time the internet was just becoming "a thing," and while it was a great way to make connections, the information explosion was still to come. The goal of the book regardless was still the same—to make useful information readily available.

By the time the 6th edition was published in 2006, the process I used to produce the book was becoming more difficult. The page layout software that had been my workhorse for over 10 years was no longer supported, and the developers of the reference manager I utilized had changed their focus and the product was now compatible primarily with word processors (which were poorly suited for complex multi-chapter books like this one). As a result, I was forced to use an obsolete PowerPC computer and had to hack the chapter files in order to trick the reference manager to work with them! After the 7th edition was completed, I could see no way forward with this approach. I never imagined that desktop publishing was going to atrophy and fall victim to the same fate that would later come to claim print newspapers. With the availability of the world wide web, the internet was quickly becoming the chief means of accessing information on demand.

The birth of this 8th edition of the handbook that you are now reading was a particularly difficult one. Thanks to the people at Thieme, the material was painstakingly converted from the defunct software platform to a contemporary format that will facilitate continued updates and availability in digital media. This time-consuming and labor-intensive process included porting thousands of cross references, index entries, and literature citations.

Interestingly, the objectives of the handbook have also gone through a transformation. It is challenging to distill what all of those objectives are, but I believe that it is important to present material in a framework that can serve as a foundation for studying the field of neurosurgery. This book is intended to be a place that brings together the important information that is increasingly scattered across the literature and the web (for instance, practice guidelines for disparate subjects like spinal cord injury, stroke, aneurysms...) that might not necessarily be encountered unless one is actively seeking it out.

My goal with the book has always been to present information succinctly and clearly. To that end, this edition is a completely restructured version of the *Handbook of Neurosurgery*, presenting the entire content in a collection of more than 100 well-ordered chapters of comparable length and format while retaining the wealth of crosslinks and references the book is known for. This new organization was designed to make the content more easily digestible and accessible – for both browsing the print book and navigating any electronic version.

With its new structure and format, as well as revised and updated content, I hope I have provided readers with an even more valuable resource in this 8th edition of the *Handbook of Neurosurgery*.

Acknowledgments

I would like to thank all of those who participated in the preparation of this edition. Thanks to the many contributors who helped with the material, and the people known and not known to me at Thieme Medical Publishers. To Brian Scanlan, President of Thieme Medical Publishers, for making the resources available to save the book from disappearing entirely. To Sarah Landis and Torsten Scheihagen for their editorial help. And the deepest debt of gratitude to Dr. Michael Wachinger, Thieme's Director of Clinical Solutions, who personally spent countless hours and a number of transatlantic trips, guiding the restructuring of the information into a more accessible and logical framework, and ensuring that the content was preserved in the software transfer.

Thanks also to my colleagues and the residents in the neurosurgery program at the University of South Florida from whom I learn every day. Special thanks to our chairman, Dr. Harry van Loveren, for his advice, calm leadership and for inspiring excellence in neurosurgery.

Abbreviations and Symbols

Abbreviations used only locally are defined in that section using boldface type. Numbers following entries below indicate the page number for the relevant section.

Abbreviations	
a.	artery (aa. = arteries)
AA	anaplastic astrocytoma (p. 616)
ABC	aneurysmal bone cyst (p. 784)
Abx.	antibiotics
AC	arachnoid cyst (p. 248)
ACA	anterior cerebral artery
ACAS	asymptomatic carotid artery stenosis (p. 1275) *or* Asymptomatic Carotid Atherosclerosis Study (p. 1276)
ACDF	anterior cervical discectomy & fusion (p. 1072)
ACE	angiotensin-converting enzyme
ACh	acetylcholine (neurotransmitter)
AChA	anterior choroidal artery
ACoA	anterior communicating artery
ACTH	adrenocorticotropic hormone (corticotropin) (p. 151)
AD	autosomal dominant
ADH	antidiuretic hormone (p. 151)
ADI	atlantodental interval (p. 213)
ADPKD	autosomal dominant polycystic kidney disease (p. 1193)
ADQ	abductor digiti quinti (or minimi)
AED	anti-epileptic drug (anticonvulsant) (p. 443)
AFP	alpha-fetoprotein (p. 600)
Ag	antigen
AHCPR	Agency for Health Care Policy and Research (of the U. S. Public Health Service)
AICA	anterior inferior cerebellar artery (p. 83)
AIDP	acute inflammatory demyelinating polyradiculoneuropathy (p. 185)
AIDS	acquired immunodeficiency syndrome (p. 329)
AIN	anterior interosseous neuropathy (p. 518)
AD	autosomal dominant (inheritance)
AFO	ankle-foot-orthosis (p. 537)
AKA	also known as
ALIF	anterior lumbar interbody fusion (p. 1493)
ALARA	As Low As Reasonably Achievable (p. 224)

A-line	arterial line
ALL	anterior longitudinal ligament
ALS	amyotrophic lateral sclerosis (p. 1086)
AMS	acute mountain sickness (p. 848)
AN	acoustic neuroma (p. 670)
ANA	antinuclear antibodies
AOD	atlantooccipital dislocation (p. 963)
AOI	atlantooccipital interval (p. 964)
AP	antero-posterior
APAG	antipseudomonal aminoglycoside
APAP	acetaminophen (p. 137)
APD	afferent pupillary defect (p. 562)
APTT	(or PTT) activated partial thromboplastin time
ARDS	adult respiratory distress syndrome
ASA	American Society of Anesthesiologists *or* aspirin (acetylsalicylic acid)
ASAP	as soon as possible
ASD	antisiphon device
AT	anterior tibialis (tibialis anterior)
AT/RT	atypical teratoid/rhabdoid tumor (p. 666)
ASHD	atherosclerotic heart disease
AVM	arteriovenous malformation (p. 1238)
AVP	arginine vasopressin (p. 151)
β-hCG	beta-human chorionic gonadotropin (p. 600)
BA	basilar artery
BBB	blood-brain barrier (p. 90)
BC	basal cisterns (p. 921)
BCP	birth control pills (oral contraceptives)
BCVI	blunt cerebrovascular injury (p. 849)
BG	basal ganglia
BI	basilar impression/invagination (p. 217)
BMD	bone mineral density (p. 1009)
BMP	bone morphogenic protein (p. 1439)
BOB	benign osteoblastoma (p. 792)
BP	blood pressure
BR	bed rest (activity restriction)
BSF	basal skull fracture (p. 884)

BSG	brainstem glioma (p. 633)
Ca	cancer
CA	cavernous angioma (p. 1247)
CAA	cerebral amyloid angiopathy (p. 1334)
CABG	coronary artery bypass graft
CAD	coronary artery disease
CAT	(or CT) computerized (axial) tomography
CBF	cerebral blood flow (p. 1264)
CBV	cerebral blood volume
CBZ	carbamazepine (p. 449)
CCB	calcium-channel blocker
CCF	carotid-cavernous (sinus) fistula (p. 1256)
CCHD	congenital cyanotic heart disease
CD	Cushing's disease (p. 723)
CEA	carotid endarterectomy (p. 1290) *or* carcinoembryonic antigen (p. 601)
CECT	contrast enhanced CT
cf	(Latin: confer) compare
cGy	centi-Gray (1cGy = 1 rad)
CHF	congestive heart failure
CI	confidence interval (statistics)
CIDP	chronic inflammatory demyelinating polyradiculoneuropathy (p. 186)
CIP	critical illness polyneuropathy (p. 542)
CJD	Creutzfeldt-Jakob disease (p. 367)
CM	cavernous malformation (p. 1247)
CMAP	compound motor action potential (EMG)
$CMRO_2$	cerebral metabolic rate of oxygen consumption (p. 1265)
CMT	Charcot-Marie-Tooth (p. 541)
CMV	cytomegalovirus
CNL	chemonucleolysis
CNS	central nervous system
cCO	continuous cardiac output
CO	cardiac output *or* carbon monoxide (p. 208)
CPA	cerebellopontine angle
CPM	central pontine myelinolysis (p. 115)
CPN	common peroneal nerve (p. 535)
CPP	cerebral perfusion pressure (p. 856)

Cr. N.	cranial nerve(s)
CRH	corticotropin-releasing hormone (p. 151)
CRP	C-reactive protein
CRPS	complex regional pain syndrome (p. 497)
CSM	cervical spondylotic myelopathy (p. 1084)
CSO	craniosynostosis (p. 252)
CSW	cerebral salt wasting (p. 118)
CTA	CT angiogram (p. 227)
CTP	CT perfusion (p. 228)
CTS	carpal tunnel syndrome (p. 519)
CVA	cerebrovascular accident (stroke) (p. 1264)
CVP	central venous pressure
CVVT	cerebrovascular venous thrombosis (p. 1308)
CVR	cerebrovascular resistance (p. 1264)
CVS	cerebral vasospasm (p. 1178)
CXR	chest x-ray
DACA	distal anterior cerebral artery
DAI	diffuse axonal injury (p. 848)
DBM	demineralized bone matrix (p. 1439)
D/C	discontinue
DDAVP	1-deamino-8-D-arginine vasopressin (desmopressin) (p. 125)
DDx	differential diagnosis (p. 1395)
DBS	deep brain stimulation (p. 1524)
DI	diabetes insipidus (p. 120)
DIND	delayed ischemic neurologic deficit (p. 1179)
DIG	desmoplastic infantile astrocytoma and ganglioglioma (p. 645)
DISH	diffuse idiopathic skeletal hyperostosis (p. 1129)
DKA	diabetic keto-acidosis
DLC	disco-ligamentous complex (p. 986)
DLIF	direct lateral lumbar interbody fusion (p. 1498)
DOC	drug of choice
DM	diabetes mellitus
DMZ	dexamethasone
DNT	(or DNET) dysembryoplastic neuroepithelial tumors (p. 646)
DOE	dyspnea on exertion
DOMS	delayed onset muscle soreness (p. 1101)

DPL	diagnostic peritoneal lavage
DREZ	dorsal root entry zone lesion (p. 1550)
DSA	digital subtraction angiogram
DSD	degenerative spine disease (p. 1096)
DST	dural sinus thrombosis (p. 1308)
DTs	delirium tremens (p. 206)
DTT	diffusion tensor tractography MRI (p. 234)
DVT	deep-vein thrombosis (p. 167)
DWI	(or DWMRI) diffusion-weighted imaging (MRI) (p. 232)
EAC	external auditory canal
EAM	external auditory meatus
EAST	Eastern Association for the Surgery of Trauma
EBRT	external beam radiation therapy
EBV	Epstein-Barr Virus
ECM	erythema chronicum migrans (p. 334)
EDC	electrolytically detachable coils
EDH	epidural hematoma (p. 892)
EHL	extensor hallicus longus
ELISA	enzyme-linked immunosorbent assay
ELST	endolymphatic sac tumors (p. 705)
EM	electron microscope (microscopy)
ENG	electronystagmography (p. 674)
ENT	ear, nose and throat (otolaryngology)
EOM	extra-ocular muscles (p. 565)
EOO	external oculomotor ophthalmoplegia
ESR	erythrocyte sedimentation rate
EST	endodermal sinus tumor (p. 660)
EtOH	ethyl alcohol (ethanol)
ET tube	endotracheal tube
ETV	endoscopic third ventriculostomy (p. 415)
EVD	external ventricular drain (ventriculostomy)
FCU	flexor carpi ulnaris
FDP	flexor digitorum profundus
FIM	Functional Independence Measure (p. 1362)
FLAIR	fluid-attenuated inversion recovery (on MRI) (p. 229)
FM	face mask

FMD	fibromuscular dysplasia (p. 200)
FSH	follicle stimulating hormone (p. 151)
F/U	follow-up
FUO	fever of unknown origin
GABA	gamma-aminobutyric acid
GBM	glioblastoma (multiforme) (p. 616)
GBS	Guillain-Barré syndrome (p. 184)
GCA	giant cell arteritis (p. 195)
GCS	Glasgow coma scale (p. 296)
GCT	granular cell tumor (p. 727) *or* germ cell tumor (p. 659)
GD	Graves' disease
GFAP	glial fibrillary acidic protein (p. 598)
GGT	gamma glutamyl transpeptidase
GH	growth hormone (p. 151)
GH-RH	growth hormone releasing hormone (p. 151)
GMH	germinal matrix hemorrhage (p. 1346)
GNR	gram negative rods
GnRH	gonadotropin-releasing hormone (p. 151)
GSW	gunshot wound
GTC	generalized tonic-clonic (seizure)
H/A	headache (p. 174)
H&H	Hunt and Hess (SAH grade) (p. 1162)
H&P	history and physical exam
HBsAg	hepatitis B surface antigen
HCD	herniated cervical disc (p. 1069)
hCG	human chorionic gonadotropin (p. 600)
HCP	hydrocephalus (p. 394)
HDT	hyperdynamic therapy (p. 1186)
HGB	hemangioblastoma (p. 701)
Hgb-A1C	hemoglobin A1C
hGH	human growth hormone
HH	hypothalamic hamartomas (p. 261) *or* homonymous hemianopsia
HHT	hereditary hemorrhagic telangiectasia (p. 1246)
HIV	human immunodeficiency virus
HLD	herniated lumbar disc (p. 1046)
HLA	human leukocyte antigen

H.O.	house officer
HNP	herniated nucleus pulposus (herniated disc) (p. 1046)
HNPP	hereditary neuropathy with liability to pressure palsies (p. 541)
HOB	head of bed
HPA	hypothalamic-pituitary-adrenal axis
HSE	herpes simplex encephalitis (p. 364)
HTN	hypertension
IAC	internal auditory canal
IASDH	infantile acute subdural hematoma (p. 898)
ICA	internal carotid artery
ICG	indocyanine green
ICH	intracerebral hemorrhage (p. 1330)
IC-HTN	intracranial hypertension (increased ICP)
ICP	intracranial pressure (p. 856)
ICU	intensive care unit
IDDM	insulin-dependent diabetes mellitus
IDET	intradiscal endothermal therapy (p. 1053)
IEP	immune electrophoresis
IG	image guidance (intra-operative)
IGF-1	insulin-like growth factor-1 (AKA somatomedin-C) (p. 151)
IIH	idiopathic intracranial hypertension (pseudotumor cerebri) (p. 766)
IIHWOP	idiopathic intracranial hypertension without papilledema (p. 768)
IJV	internal jugular vein
IMRT	intensity modulated radiation therapy
INO	internuclear ophthalmoplegia (p. 565)
INR	international normalized ratio (p. 164)
IPS	inferior petrosal sinus
IPA	idiopathic paralysis agitans (Parkinson's disease) (p. 176)
ISAT	International Subarachnoid Hemorrhage Aneurysm Trial (p. 1195)
IT	intrathecal
ITB	intrathecal baclofen (p. 1531)
IVC	intraventricular catheter *or* inferior vena cava
IVH	intraventricular hemorrhage (p. 1386)
IVP	intravenous push (medication route) *or* intravenous pyelogram (x-ray study)
JPS	joint position sense
LBP	low back pain (p. 1024)

LDD	Lhermitte-Duclos disease (p. 647)
LE	lower extremity
LFTs	liver function tests
LGG	low-grade glioma
LH	luteinizing hormone (p. 151)
LH-RH	luteinizing hormone releasing hormone (p. 151)
LMD	low molecular weight dextran
LMN	lower motor neuron (p. 504)
LMW	low-molecular-weight (e.g. heparins)
LOC	loss of consciousness
LOH	loss of heterozygosity
LP	lumbar puncture (p. 1504)
LSO	lumbo-sacral orthosis
MAC	mycobacterium avian complex (p. 354)
MAOI	monoamine oxidase inhibitor
MAP	mean arterial pressure
MAST®	military anti-shock trousers
MB	medulloblastoma (p. 664)
MBEN	medulloblastoma with extensive nodularity (p. 665)
MBI	modified Barthel index (▶ Table 88.6)
MBS	medulloblastoma (p. 664)
MCA	middle cerebral artery
mcg	(or μg) microgram
MCP	mean carotid pressure *or* metacarpal phalangeal
MDCTA	multidetector CT angiography
MDMA	methylenedioxymethamphetamine (p. 177)
mg	milligram
MI	myocardial infarction
MIB-1	monoclonal anti-Ki-67 antibody (p. 599)
MIC	minimum inhibitory concentration (for antibiotics)
MID	multi-infarct dementia
MISS	minimally invasive spine surgery
mJOA	modified Japanese Orthopedic Association scale (p. 1086)
MLF	medial longitudinal fasciculus
MLS	midline shift (p. 921)
MM	myelomeningocele (p. 265) *or* multiple myeloma (p. 714)

MMD	moyamoya disease (p. 1313)
MMN	multifocal motor neuropathy (p. 1410)
MMPI	Minnesota Multiphasic Personality Inventory
mos	months
MPTP	1-methyl-4-phenyl-1,2,3,6-tetrahydropyridine (p. 177)
MRA	MRI angiogram (p. 232)
MRS	MRI spectroscopy (p. 233)
MRSA	methicillin resistant *staphylococcus aureus*
MS	microsurgery *or* multiple sclerosis (p. 179)
MSO_4	morphine sulfate
MTP	metatarsal phalangeal
MTT	meant transit time (on CT perfusion) (p. 228)
MUAP	motor unit action potential (p. 243)
MVA	motor vehicle accident
MVD	microvascular decompression (p. 488)
MW	molecular weight
n.	nerve (nn. = nerves)
Na	(or Na^+) sodium
N_2O	nitrous oxide (p. 105)
NAA	N-acetyl aspartate (p. 233)
NAP	nerve action potential (p. 509)
NASCET	North American Symptomatic Carotid Endarterectomy Trial (p. 1290)
NB	(Latin: *nota bene*) note well
NC	nasal cannula
NCCN	National Comprehensive Cancer Network
NCD	neurocutaneous disorders (p. 603)
NCV	nerve conduction velocity
NEC	neurenteric cyst (p. 290) *or* necrotizing enterocolitis
NEXUS	National Emergency X-Radiography Utilization Study (p. 953)
NF	(or NFT) neurofibromatosis (p. 603)
NF1	neurofibromatosis type 1 (p. 604)
NF2	neurofibromatosis type 2 (p. 605)
NG tube	nasogastric tube
NGGCT	non-germinomatous germ cell tumors (p. 659)
NIHSS	NIH Stroke Scale (p. 1282)
NMBA	neuromuscular blocking agent (p. 134)

NMO	neuromyelitis optica (Devic disease) (p. 1409)
NPH	normal pressure hydrocephalus (p. 403)
NPS	neuropathic pain syndrome (p. 476)
NS	normal saline
NSAID	non-steroidal anti-inflammatory drug (p. 137)
NSCLC	non-small-cell cancer of the lung (p. 803)
NSF	nephrogenic systemic fibrosis (p. 231)
NSM	neurogenic stunned myocardium (p. 1177)
N/V	nausea and vomiting
NVB	neurovascular bundle
OAD	occipital atlantal dislocation, see atlantooccipital dislocation (p. 963)
OALL	ossification of the anterior longitudinal ligament (p. 1129)
OC	occipital condyle
OCB	oligoclonal bands (in CSF) (p. 181)
OCF	occipital condyle fracture (p. 885)
ODG	oligodendroglioma (p. 638)
OEF	oxygen extraction fraction
OFC	occipital-frontal (head) circumference
OGST	oral glucose suppression test (for growth hormone) (p. 736)
OMO	open-mouth odontoid (C-spine x-ray view)
OMP	oculomotor (third nerve) palsy
ONSF	optic nerve sheath fenestration (p. 772)
OP	opening pressure (on LP) (p. 1505)
OPLL	ossification of the posterior longitudinal ligament (p. 1127)
ORIF	open reduction/internal fixation
OS	overall survival
OTC	over the counter (i.e. without prescription)
PACU	post-anesthesia care unit (AKA recovery room, PAR)
PADI	posterior atlantodental interval (p. 213)
PAN	poly- (or peri-) arteritis nodosa (p. 199)
PBPP	perinatal brachial plexus palsy (p. 552)
$P_{Bt}O_2$	brain tissue oxygen tension (p. 865)
PC	pineal cyst (p. 658)
PCA	pilocytic astrocytoma (p. 629) *or* posterior cerebral artery
PCB	pneumatic compression boot
PCC	prothrombin complex concentrate (p. 166)

PCI	prophylactic cranial irradiation
PCN	penicillin
PCNSL	primary CNS lymphoma (p. 710)
P-comm	posterior communicating artery
PCV	procarbazine, CCNU, & vincristine (chemotherapy)
PCWP	pulmonary capillary wedge pressure
PDA	patent ductus arteriosus
PDN	painful diabetic neuropathy (p. 476)
PDR	Physicians Desk Reference®
peds	pediatrics (infants & children)
PEEK	poly-ether-ether-ketone (graft material)
PET	positron emission tomography (scan)
p-fossa	posterior fossa
PFS	progression-free survival
PFT	pulmonary function test
PHN	postherpetic neuralgia (p. 493)
PHT	phenytoin (Dilantin®) (p. 446)
PICA	posterior inferior cerebellar artery (p. 82)
PIF	prolactin release inhibitory factor (p. 151)
PIN	posterior interosseous neuropathy (p. 532)
PION	posterior ischemic optic neuropathy (p. 1056)
PIVH	periventricular-intraventricular hemorrhage (p. 1346)
PLAP	placental alkaline phosphatase (p. 660)
PLEDs	periodic lateralizing epileptiform discharges
PLIF	posterior lumbar interbody fusion
PM	pars marginalis (p. 60)
PMA	progressive muscular atrophy (p. 183) *or* pilomyxoid astrocytoma (p. 632)
PMH	pure motor hemiparesis
PML	progressive multifocal leukoencephalopathy (p. 329)
PMMA	polymethylmethacrylate (methylmethacrylate)
PMR	polymyalgia rheumatica (p. 198)
PMV	pontomesencephalic vein
PNET	primitive neuroectodermal tumor (p. 663)
POD	post-operative day
PPV	positive predictive value: in unselected patients who test positive, PPV is the probability that the patient has the disease
PR	per rectum

PRES	posterior reversible encephalopathy syndrome (p. 194)
PRF	prolactin releasing factor (p. 151)
PRIF	prolactin (releasing) inhibitory factor (p. 151)
PRN	as needed
PRSP	penicillinase resistant synthetic PCN
PSNP	progressive supra-nuclear palsy (p. 178)
PSR	percutaneous stereotactic rhizotomy (for trigeminal neuralgia) (p. 483)
PSW	positive sharp waves (on EMG) (p. 242)
pt	patient
PT	physical therapy *or* prothrombin time
PTC	pituicytoma (p. 728)
PTR	percutaneous trigeminal rhizotomy
PTT	(or APTT) partial thromboplastin time
PUD	peptic ulcer disease
PVP	percutaneous vertebroplasty (p. 1011)
PWI	perfusion-weighted imaging (MRI) (p. 233)
PXA	pleomorphic xanthoastrocytoma (p. 635)
q	(Latin: *quaque*) every (medication dosing)
RA	rheumatoid arthritis
RAPD	relative afferent pupillary defect (p. 562)
RASS	Richmond agitation-sedation scale (p. 132)
RCVS	reversible cerebral vasoconstrictive syndrome (p. 1158)
rem	roentgen-equivalent man
REZ	root entry zone
RFR	radiofrequency rhizotomy (p. 483)
rFVIIa	recombinant (activated) factor VII
RH	recurrent artery of Heubner
rhBMP	recombinant human BMP (p. 1439)
R/O	rule out
ROM	range of motion
RPA	recursive partitioning analysis
RPDB	randomized prospective double-blind
RPLS	reversible posterior leukoencephalopathy syndrome; see posterior reversible encephalopathy syndrome (p. 194)
RPNB	randomized prospective non-blinded
RTOG	Radiation Therapy Oncology Group
RTP	return to play (sports)

rt-PA	recombinant tissue plasminogen activator (AKA tissue plasminogen activator)
RTX	(or XRT) radiation therapy (p. 1560)
S/S	signs and symptoms
SAH	subarachnoid hemorrhage (p. 1191)
SBE	subacute bacterial endocarditis
SBO	spina bifida occulta (p. 265)
SBP	systolic blood pressure
SCA	superior cerebellar artery
SCLC	small-cell lung cancer (p. 802)
SCD	sequential compression device
SCI	spinal cord injury (p. 943)
SCM	sternocleidomastoid (muscle)
SD	standard deviation
SDE	subdural empyema (p. 327)
SDH	subdural hematoma (p. 895)
SE	status epilepticus (for seizures) (p. 468)
SEA	spinal epidural abscess (p. 349)
SEP	(or SSEP) somatosensory evoked potential
SG	specific gravity
SIAD	syndrome of inappropriate antidiuresis (p. 112)
SIADH	syndrome of inappropriate antidiuretic hormone (ADH) secretion (p. 114)
SIDS	sudden infant death syndrome
SIH	spontaneous intracranial hypotension (p. 389)
SIRS	septic inflammatory response syndrome
$SjVO_2$	jugular venous oxygen saturation (p. 865)
SLAD	surgical laser aiming device
SLE	systemic lupus erythematosus
SLIC	subaxial injury classification (p. 986)
SMC	spinal meningeal cyst (p. 1142)
SMT	spinal manipulation therapy (p. 1034)
SNAP	sensory nerve action potential (EMG) (p. 243)
SNUC	sinonasal undifferentiated carcinoma (p. 1387)
SOMI	sternal-occipital-mandibular immobilizer (p. 935)
SON	supraorbital neuralgia (p. 491)
S/P	status-post
SPAM	subacute progressive ascending myelopathy (p. 1019)

SPECT	single positron emission computed tomography (scan)
SPEP	serum protein electrophoresis
sPNET	supratentorial primitive neuroectodermal tumor (p. 666)
SQ	subcutaneous injection
SRS	stereotactic radiosurgery (p. 1564)
SRT	stereotactic radiotherapy (p. 1564)
SSEP	(or SEP) somatosensory evoked potential
SSPE	subacute sclerosing panencephalitis (p. 238)
SSRI	selective serotonin reuptake inhibitors
SSS	superior sagittal sinus
STA	superficial temporal artery
STICH	Surgical Trial in Intracerebral Haemorrhage (p. 1343)
STIR	short tau inversion recover (MRI image)
STN	subthalamic nucleus
STSG	Spine Trauma Study Group
SUNCT	short-lasting unilateral neuralgiform H/A with conjunctival injection and tearing (p. 478)
SVC	superior vena cava
SVM	spinal vascular malformations (p. 1140)
SVR	systemic venous resistance
SVT	supraventricular tachycardia
Sz.	seizure (p. 440)
T1WI	T1 weighted image (on MRI) (p. 228)
T2WI	T2 weighted image (on MRI) (p. 229)
TAL	transverse atlantal ligament (p. 70)
TBA	total bilateral adrenalectomy (p. 743)
TBI	traumatic brain injury
TCA	tricyclic antidepressants
TCD	transcranial doppler (p. 1182)
TDL	tumefactive demyelinating lesions (p. 181)
TE	time to echo (on MRI) (p. 228)
TEE	transesophageal echocardiogram
TEN	toxic epidermal necrolysis
TENS	transcutaneous electrical nerve stimulation
TGN	trigeminal neuralgia (p. 479)
T-H lines	Taylor-Haughton lines (p. 61)
TIA	transient ischemic attack (p. 1264)

TICH	traumatic intracerebral hemorrhage (hemorrhagic contusion) (p. 891)
TIVA	total intravenous anesthesia
TLIF	transforaminal lumbar interbody fusion (p. 1497)
TLISS	thoracolumbar injury severity score (p. 1006)
TLJ	thoracolumbar junction
TLSO	thoracolumbar-sacral orthosis
TM	tympanic membrane
TMB	transient monocular blindness (amaurosis fugax) (p. 1271)
t-PA	tissue plasminogen activator
TR	time to repetition (on MRI) (p. 228)
TRH	thyrotropin releasing hormone; AKA TSH-RH (p. 151)
TS	transverse sinus
TSC	tuberous sclerosis complex (p. 606)
TSH	thyroid-stimulating hormone (thyrotropin) (p. 151)
TSV	thalamostriate vein
TTP	thrombotic thrombocytopenic purpura
TVO	transient visual obscurations (p. 768)
Tx.	treatment
UBOs	unidentified bright objects (on MRI)
UE	upper extremity
UMN	upper motor neuron (p. 504)
UTI	urinary tract infection
URI	upper respiratory tract infection
U/S	ultrasound
VA	vertebral artery *or* ventriculoatrial
VB	vertebral body
VBI	vertebrobasilar insufficiency (p. 1305)
VEMP	vestibular evoked myogenic potential (p. 675)
VHL	von Hippel-Lindau (disease) (p. 703)
VMA	vanillylmandelic acid
VP	ventriculoperitoneal
VS	vestibular schwannoma (p. 670)
VZV	(herpes) varicella zoster virus
WBC	white blood cell (count)
WBXRT	whole brain radiation therapy (p. 810)
WFNS	World Federation of Neurosurgical Societies (grading SAH) (p. 1163)

WHO	World Health Organization. For tumor grading, e.g. WHO II indicates WHO grade II
wks	weeks
WNL	within normal limits
w/o	without
WRS	word recognition score (p. 673)
W/U	work-up (evaluation)
XLIF	extreme lateral lumbar interbody fusion (p. 1498)
XRT	(or RTX) radiation therapy (p. 1560)
Symbols	
℞	prescribing information
→	causes or leads to
Δ	change
✔	check (e.g. lab or exam item to check)
↑	increased
↓	decreased
≈	approximately
↯	innervates (nerve distribution)
⇒	vascular supply
↳	a branch of the preceding nerve
✱	crucial point
✖	caution; possible danger; negative factor…
Σ	summary
∴	therefore
Instrumentation: the following shorthand allows rapid identification of metrics for spinal instrumentation:	
ENTRY	screw entry site
TRAJ	screw trajectory
TARGET	object to aim for
SCREWS	typical screw specifications

Conventions

► **Box types.** The *Handbook of Neurosurgery* uses the following seven box types:

Drug info

Drug description & dosage.

Key concepts

Foundational knowledge in brief.

Practice guideline

Evidence-based guidelines. See below (in this section) for definitions. For a listing of evidence-based guidelines contained in this book, see the index under "Practice guideline."

Booking the case

These sections appear under certain specific operations to help when scheduling that surgery. Default information appears below (in this section), for example, a specific type of anesthesia will only be mentioned if something other than general anesthesia is typically used. A list of operations addressed by this means can be found in the index under "Booking the case."

Σ

Summarizing or synthesizing information from the associated text.

Side information

E.g., Greenberg IMHO.

Signs / symptoms

A description of signs and symptoms.

► **Cross references.** Cross references: the terms "see below" and "see above" are normally used when the referenced item is on the same page, or at most on the following (or preceding) page. When further excursions are needed, the page number will usually be included.

► **Default values.** These details are not repeated in each section or "Booking the case" box.

1. position: (depends on the operation)
2. pre-op:
   a) NPO after midnight the night before except meds with sips of water
   b) antithrombotics: discontinue Coumadin® ≥ 3 days prior to surgery, Plavix® 5–7 d pre-op, aspirin 7–10 d pre-op, other NSAIDs 5 d pre-op

3. cardiology/medical clearance as needed
4. anesthesia: default = general anesthesia, unless otherwise specified
5. equipment: special devices such as ultrasonic aspirator, image guidance…
6. instrumentation: standard surgical instrument trays for a specific operation are assumed. Special instrumentation resident in the hospital will be listed
7. implants: this usually requires scheduling with a vendor (manufacturers representative/distributor) to provide
8. neuromonitoring will be listed if typically used
9. post-op: default care is on the ward (ICU is typically needed after craniotomy)
10. blood availability: specified if recommended
11. consent (these items use lay terms for the patient – not all-inclusive):
    ✱ **Disclaimers**: *informed consent* for surgery requires disclosure of risks and benefits that would substantively affect a normal person's decision to have the operation. It cannot and should not attempt to include every possibility. The items listed in this section are included as memory joggers for some items for various procedures, but are not meant to be all inclusive. The omission of information from this memory aid is not to be construed as implying that the omitted item is not important or should not be mentioned.
    a) procedure: the typical operation and some possible common contingencies
    b) alternatives: non-surgical (AKA "conservative") treatment is almost always an option
    c) complications:
       - risks of general anesthesia include: heart attack, stroke, pneumonia
       - infection: a risk with any invasive procedure
       - usual **craniotomy** complications include: bleeding intra-op and postop, seizure, stroke, coma, death, hydrocephalus, meningitis, and neurologic deficit related to the area of surgery including (for applicable locations): paralysis, language or sensory disturbances, coordination impairment…
       - usual **spine surgery** complications include: injury to nerve or spinal cord with possible numbness, weakness or paralysis, failure of the operation to achieve the desired result, dural opening which may cause a CSF leak which occasionally needs to be surgical repair. Hardware complications (when used) include: breakage, pull-out, malposition. Although a rare complication, it is serious enough that it bears mentioning in cases positioned prone with possible significant blood loss (> 2 L): blindness (due to PION (p. 1056))

▶ **Evidence-Based Medicine: Definitions.** These definitions are referred to in the "Practice guideline" boxes.

Strength of recommendation		Description
Level I, II, III[a]	Level A, B, C, D[b]	
Level I High degree of clinical certainty	Level A	Based on consistent Class I evidence (well-designed, prospective randomized controlled studies)
	Level B	Single Class I study or consistent Class II evidence or strong Class II evidence especially when circumstances preclude randomized clinical trials
Level II Moderate degree of clinical certainty	Level C	Usually derived from Class II evidence (one or more well-designed comparative clinical studies or less well-designed randomized studies) or a preponderance of Class III evidence
Level III Unclear clinical certainty	Level D	Generally based on Class III evidence (case series, historical controls, case reports and expert opinion). Useful for educational purposes and to guide future research

[a] as used in the Guidelines for the Management of Severe Traumatic Brain Injury, 3rd edition (Brain Trauma Foundation: Introduction. J Neurotrauma 24, Suppl 1: S1–2, 2007).
[b] as used in the Guidelines for the Surgical Management of Cervical Degenerative Disease (Matz P G, et al.: Introduction and methodology. J Neurosurg: Spine 11 (2): 101–3, 2009).

Contents

Anatomy and Physiology

General and Neurology

Infection

Hydrocephalus and Cerebrospinal Fluid (CSF)

Seizures

Pain

Peripheral Nerves

Spine and Spinal Cord

Vascular Malformations

Stroke and Occlusive Cerebrovascular Disease

Outcome Assessment

Differential Diagnosis

Procedures, Interventions, Operations

Part I

Anatomy and Physiology

1 Gross Anatomy, Cranial and Spine

1.1 Cortical surface anatomy

1.1.1 Lateral cortical surface

▶ Fig. 1.1. For abbreviations, see ▶ Table 1.1 and ▶ Table 1.2. The middle frontal gyrus (MFG) is usually more sinuous than the IFG or SFG, and it often connects to the pre-central gyrus via a thin isthmus.[1] The central sulcus joins the Sylvian fissure in only 2% of cases (i.e. in 98% of cases there is a "subcentral" gyrus). The intraparietal sulcus (ips) separates the superior and inferior parietal lobules. The IPL is composed primarily of the AG and SMG. The Sylvian fissure terminates in the SMG (Brodmann's area 40). The superior temporal sulcus terminates in the AG.

1.1.2 Brodmann's areas

▶ Fig. 1.1 also identifies the clinically significant areas of Brodmann's (Br.) map of the cytoarchitectonic fields of the human brain. Functional significance of these areas is as follows:

1. Br. areas 3, 1, 2: primary somatosensory cortex
2. Br. areas 41 & 42: primary auditory areas (transverse gyri of Heschl)
3. Br. area 4: precentral gyrus, primary motor cortex (AKA "motor strip"). Large concentration of giant pyramidal cells of Betz
4. Br. area 6: premotor area or supplemental motor area. Immediately anterior to motor strip, it plays a role in contralateral motor programming
5. Br. area 44: (dominant hemisphere) Broca's area (motor speech)
6. Br. area 17: primary visual cortex

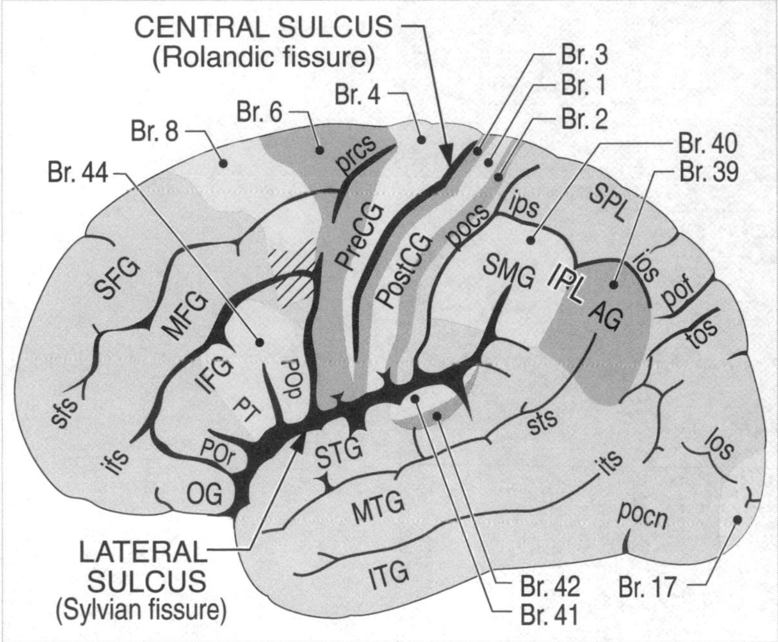

Fig. 1.1 Left lateral cerebral cortical surface anatomy.
Br. = Brodmann's area (shaded). See ▶ Table 1.1 and ▶ Table 1.2 for abbreviations (lowercase = sulci, UPPERCASE = gyri).

Table 1.1 Cerebral sulci (abbreviations)

Abbreviation	Sulcus
cins	cingulate sulcus
cs	central sulcus
ips-ios	intraparietal-intraoccipital sulcus
los	lateral occipital sulcus
pM	pars marginalis
pocn	pre-occipital notch
pocs	post-central sulcus
pof	parieto-occipital fissure
pos	parieto-occipital sulcus
prcs	pre-central sulcus
sfs, ifs	superior, inferior frontal sulcus
sps	superior parietal sulcus
sts, its	superior, inferior temporal sulcus
tos	trans occipital sulcus

Table 1.2 Cerebral gyri and lobules (abbreviations)

Abbreviation	Gyrus / lobule
AG	angular gyrus
CinG	cingulate gyrus
Cu	cuneus
LG	lingual gyrus
MFG, SFG	middle & superior frontal gyrus
OG	orbital gyrus
PCu	precuneous
PreCG, PostCG	pre- and post-central gyrus
PL	paracentral lobule (upper SFG and PreCG and PostCG)
IFG • POp • PT • POr	inferior frontal gyrus • pars opercularis • pars triangularis • pars orbitalis
STG, MTG, ITG	superior, middle & inferior temporal gyrus
SPL, IPL	superior & inferior parietal lobule
SMG	supramarginal gyrus

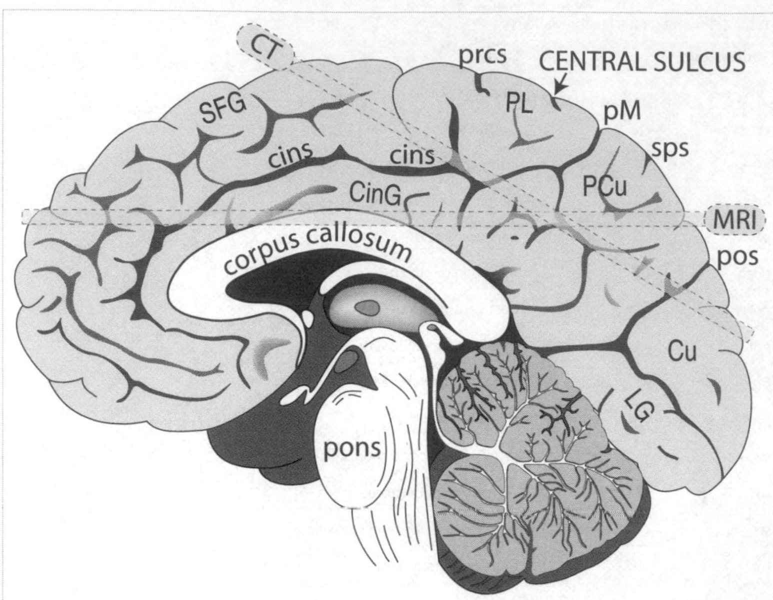

Fig. 1.2 Medial aspect of the right hemisphere.
"CT" & "MRI" bars depict typical axial slice orientation for CT & MRI scans. See ▶ Table 1.1 and ▶ Table 1.2 for abbreviations.

7. Wernicke's area (language): in the dominant hemisphere, most of Br. area 40 and a portion of Br. area 39 (may also include ≈ posterior third of STG)
8. the striped portion of Br. area 8 in ▶ Fig. 1.1 (frontal eye field) initiates voluntary eye movements to the opposite direction

Brodmann's area 44, Wernicke's area: Language function cannot be reliably localized on anatomic grounds due to individual variability in its exact location; in order to perform maximal brain resections with minimal risk of aphasia, techniques such as intra-operative brain mapping[2] or looking for phase reversal on intraoperative cortical SSEP[3] should be employed.

1.1.3 Medial surface

▶ Fig. 1.2. The cingulate sulcus terminates posteriorly in the pars marginalis (pM) (plural: partes marginales). On axial imaging, the pMs: are visible on 95% of CTs and 91% of MRIs,[4] are usually the most prominent of the paired grooves straddling the midline, and they extend a greater distance into the hemispheres.[4] On axial CT, the pM is located slightly posterior to the widest biparietal diameter[4]; on the typically more horizontally oriented MRI slices the pM assumes a more posterior position. The pMs curve posteriorly in lower slices and anteriorly in higher slices (here, the paired pMs form the "pars bracket" – a characteristic "handlebar" configuration straddling the midline).

1.2 Central sulcus on axial imaging

See ▶ Fig. 1.3. Identification of the central sulcus is important to localize the motor strip (contained in the PreCG). The central sulcus (CS) is visible on 93% of CTs and 100% of MRIs.[4] It curves posteriorly as it approaches the interhemispheric fissure (IHF), and often terminates in the paracentral lobule, just anterior to the pars marginalis (pM) within the pars bracket (see above)[4] (i.e. the CS often does not reach the midline).

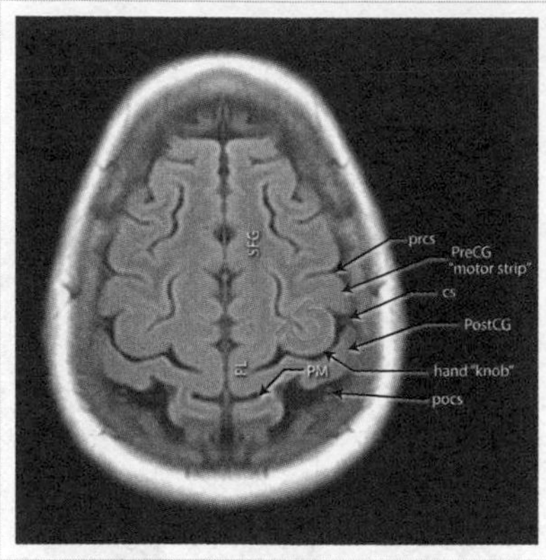

Fig. 1.3 Retouched axial FLAIR MRI with labels for gyri/sulci shown in the left hemisphere, and an unlabeled mirror image shown as the right hemisphere for reference. The inverted Ω illustrates the hand "knob" (see text).
See ▶ Table 1.1 and ▶ Table 1.2 for abbreviations.

Pointers:

- parieto-occipital sulcus (pos) (or fissure): more prominent over the medial surface, and on axial imaging is longer, more complex, and more posterior than the pars marginalis[5]
- post-central sulcus (pocs): usually bifurcates and forms an arc or parenthesis ("lazy-Y") cupping the pM. The anterior limb does not enter the pM-bracket and the posterior limb curves behind the pM to enter the IHF

Hand "Knob": The alpha motor neurons for hand motor function are located in the superior aspect of the prefrontal gyrus.[6] On axial imaging, this appears as a knob-like protrusion (shaped like an inverted greek letter omega Ω) of the precentral gyrus projecting posterolaterally into the central sulcus[7] ▶ Fig. 1.3. On sagittal imaging it has a posteriorly projecting hook-like appearance and is even with the posterior limit of the Sylvian fissure.[7]

1.3 Surface anatomy of the cranium

1.3.1 Craniometric points

See ▶ Fig. 1.4.

Pterion: region where the following bones are approximated: frontal, parietal, temporal and sphenoid (greater wing). Estimated as 2 finger-breadths above the zygomatic arch, and a thumb's breadth behind the frontal process of the zygomatic bone (blue circle in ▶ Fig. 1.4).

Asterion: junction of lambdoid, occipitomastoid and parietomastoid sutures. Usually lies within a few millimeters of the posterior-inferior edge of the junction of the transverse and sigmoid sinuses (not always reliable[8] – may overlie either sinus).

Vertex: the topmost point of the skull.

Lambda: junction of the lambdoid and sagittal sutures.

Stephanion: junction of coronal suture and superior temporal line.

Glabella: the most forward projecting point of the forehead at the level of the supraorbital ridge in the midline.

Opisthion: the posterior margin of the foramen magnum in the midline.

Bregma: the junction of the coronal and sagittal sutures.

Sagittal suture: midline suture from coronal suture to lambdoid suture. Although often assumed to overlie the superior sagittal sinus (SSS), the SSS lies to the right of the sagittal suture in the majority of specimens[9] (but never by > 11 mm).

The most anterior mastoid point lies just in front of the sigmoid sinus.[10]

1.3.2 Relation of skull markings to cerebral anatomy – Taylor-Haughton lines

Taylor-Haughton (T-H) lines can be constructed on an angiogram, CT scout film, or skull x-ray, and can then be reconstructed on the patient in the O.R. based on visible external landmarks.[11] T-H lines are shown as dashed lines in ▶ Fig. 1.5.

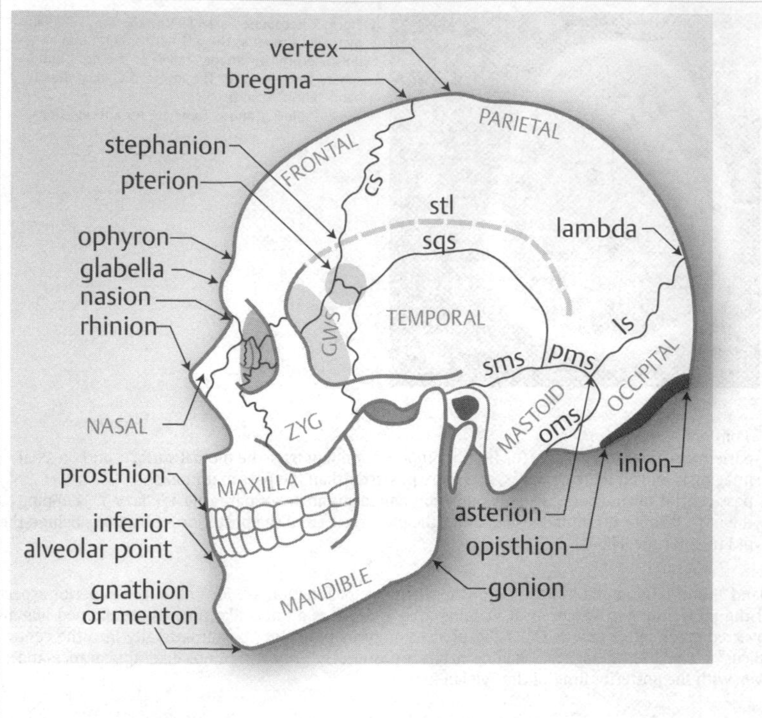

Fig. 1.4 Craniometric points & cranial sutures.
Named bones appear in all upper case letters.
Abbreviations: GWS = greater wing of sphenoid bone, NAS = nasal bone, stl = superior temporal line, ZYG = zygomatic.
Sutures: cs = coronal, ls = lambdoid, oms = occipitomastoid, pms = parietomastoid, sms = squamomastoid, sqs = squamosal

1. Frankfurt plane, AKA baseline: line from inferior margin of orbit through the *upper* margin of the external auditory meatus (EAM) (as distinguished from Reid's base line: from inferior orbital margin through the center of the EAM)[12(p 313)]
2. the distance from the nasion to the inion is measured across the top of the calvaria and is divided into quarters (can be done simply with a piece of tape which is then folded in half twice)
3. posterior ear line: perpendicular to the baseline through the mastoid process
4. condylar line: perpendicular to the baseline through the mandibular condyle
5. T-H lines can then be used to approximate the sylvian fissure (see below) and the motor cortex (also see below)

Sylvian fissure AKA lateral fissure

Approximated by a line connecting the lateral canthus to the point 3/4 of the way posterior along the arc running over convexity from nasion to inion (T-H lines).

Angular gyrus

Located just above the pinna, important on the dominant hemisphere as part of Wernicke's area. Note: there is significant individual variability in the location.[2]

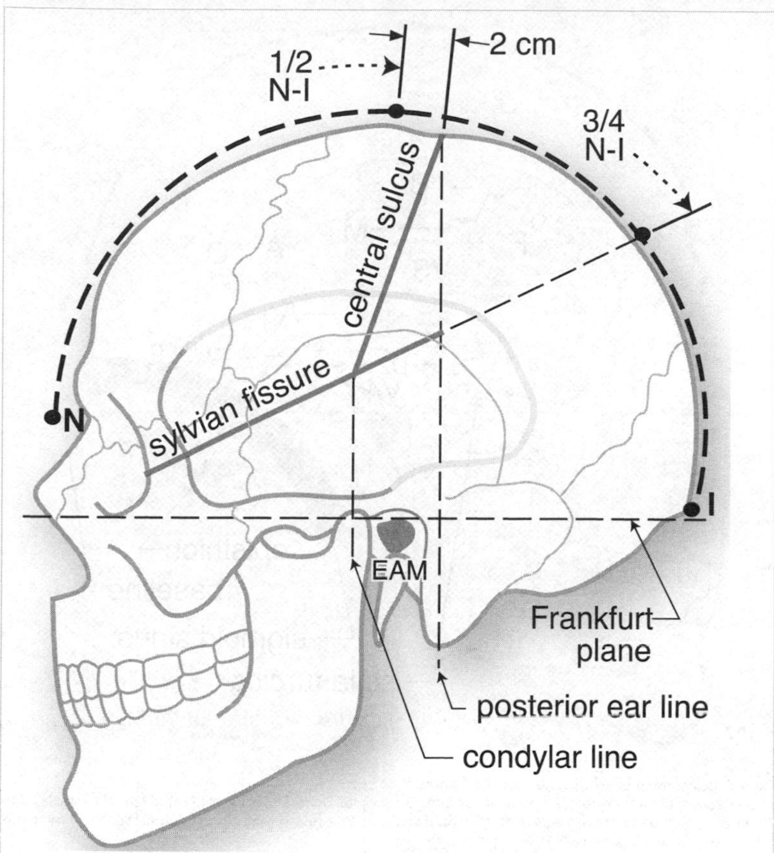

Fig. 1.5 Taylor-Haughton lines and other localizing methods

Angular artery

Located 6 cm above the EAM.

Motor cortex

Numerous methods utilize external landmarks to locate the motor strip (pre-central gyrus) or the *central sulcus* (Rolandic fissure) which separates motor strip anteriorly from primary sensory cortex posteriorly. These are just approximations since individual variability causes the motor strip to lie anywhere from 4 to 5.4 cm behind the coronal suture.[13] The central sulcus cannot even be reliably identified visually at surgery.[14]

1. method 1: the superior aspect of the motor cortex is almost straight up from the EAM near the midline
2. method 2[15]: the central sulcus is approximated by connecting:
   a) the point 2 cm posterior to the midposition of the arc extending from nasion to inion (illustrated in ▶ Fig. 1.5), to
   b) the point 5 cm straight up from the EAM

1

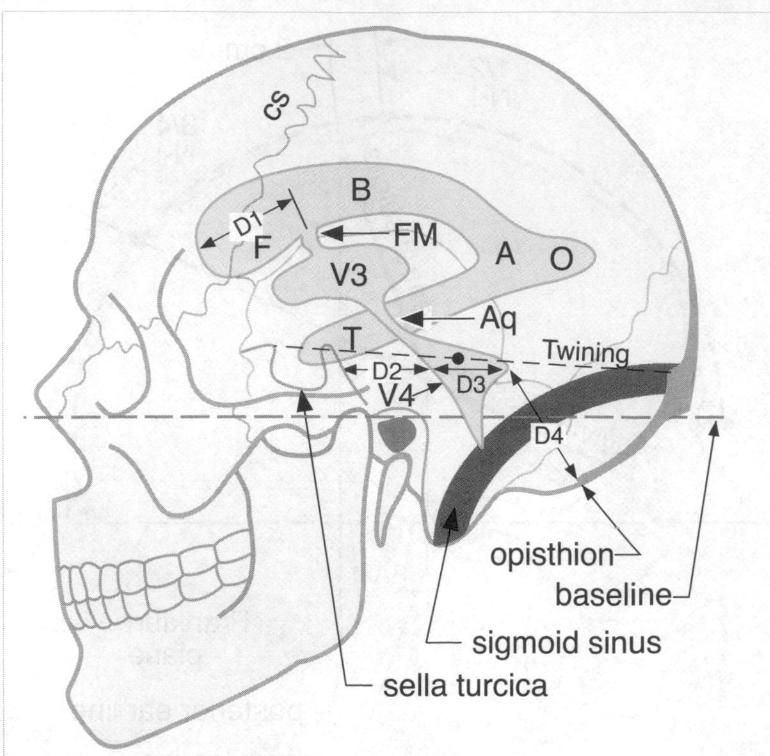

Fig. 1.6 Relationship of ventricles to skull landmarks
Abbreviations: (F = frontal horn, B = body, A = atrium, O = occipital horn, T = temporal horn) of lateral ventricle. FM = foramen of Monro. Aq = sylvian aqueduct. V3 = third ventricle. V4 = fourth ventricle. cs = coronal suture. Dimensions D1–4 see ▶ Table 1.3

3. method 3: using T-H lines, the central sulcus is approximated by connecting:
   a) the point where the "posterior ear line" intersects the circumference of the skull (▶ Fig. 1.5; usually about 1 cm behind the vertex, and 3–4 cm behind the coronal suture), to
   b) the point where the "condylar line" intersects the line representing the sylvian fissure
4. method 4: a line drawn 45° to Reid's base line starting at the pterion points in the *direction* of the motor strip[16(p 584–5)]

1.3.3 Relationship of ventricles to skull

▶ Fig. 1.6 shows the relationship of non-hydrocephalic ventricles to the skull in the lateral view. Some dimensions of interest are shown in ▶ Table 1.3.[17]

In the non-hydrocephalic adult, the lateral ventricles lie 4–5 cm below the outer skull surface. The center of the body of the lateral ventricle sits in the midpupillary line, and the frontal horn is intersected by a line passing perpendicular to the calvaria along this line.[18] The anterior horns extend 1–2 cm anterior to the coronal suture.

Average length of third ventricle≈ 2.8 cm.

The midpoint of Twining's line (• in ▶ Fig. 1.6) should lie within the 4th ventricle.

Table 1.3 Dimensions from ▶ Fig. 1.6

Dimension (▶ Fig. 1.6)	Description	Lower limit (mm)	Average (mm)	Upper limit (mm)
D1	length of frontal horn anterior to FM		25	
D2	distance from clivus to floor of 4th ventricle at level of fastigium[a]	33.3	36.1	40.0
D3	length of 4th ventricle at level of fastigium[a]	10.0	14.6	19.0
D4	distance from fastigium[a] to opisthion	30.0	32.6	40.0
[a]the fastigium is the apex of the 4th ventricle within the cerebellum				

Table 1.4 Cervical levels[19]

Level	Landmark
C1–2	angle of mandible
C3–4	1 cm above thyroid cartilage (≈ hyoid bone)
C4–5	level of thyroid cartilage
C5–6	crico-thyroid membrane
C6	carotid tubercle
C6–7	cricoid cartilage

1.4 Surface landmarks of spine levels

Estimates of cervical levels for anterior cervical spine surgery may be made using the landmarks shown in ▶ Table 1.4. Intra-operative C-spine x-rays are essential to verify these estimates.

The scapular spine is located at about T2–3.

The inferior scapular pole is ≈ T6 posteriorly.

Intercristal line: a line drawn between the highest point of the iliac crests across the back will cross the midline either at the interspace between the L4 and L5 spinous processes, or at the L4 spinous process itself.

1.5 Cranial foramina and their contents

1.5.1 Summary

Table 1.5 Cranial foramina and their contents[a]

Foramen	Contents
nasal slits	anterior ethmoidal nn., a. & v
superior orbital fissure	Cr. Nn. III, IV, VI, all 3 branches of V1 (ophthalmic division divides into nasociliary, frontal, and lacrimal nerves); superior ophthalmic vv.; recurrent meningeal br. from lacrimal a.; orbital branch of middle meningeal a.; sympathetic filaments from ICA plexus
inferior orbital fissure	Cr. N. V-2 (maxillary div.), zygomatic n.; filaments from pterygopalatine branch of maxillary n.; infraorbital a. & v.; v. between inferior ophthalmic v. & pterygoid venous plexus
foramen lacerum	usually nothing (ICA *traverses* the upper portion but doesn't enter, 30% have vidian a.)
carotid canal	internal carotid a., ascending sympathetic nerves

Table 1.5 continued

Foramen	Contents
incisive foramen	descending septal a.; nasopalatine nn.
greater palatine foramen	greater palatine n., a., & v.
lesser palatine foramen	lesser palatine nn.
internal acoustic meatus	Cr. N. VII (facial); Cr. N. VIII (stato-acoustic) – see text & ▶ Fig. 1.7
hypoglossal canal	Cr. N. XII (hypoglossal); a meningeal branch of the ascending pharyngeal a.
foramen magnum	spinal cord (medulla oblongata); Cr. N. XI (spinal accessory nn.) *entering* the skull; vertebral aa.; anterior & posterior spinal arteries
foramen cecum	occasional small vein
cribriform plate	olfactory nn.
optic canal	Cr. N. II (optic); ophthalmic a.
foramen rotundum	Cr. N. V2 (maxillary div.), a. of foramen rotundum
foramen ovale	Cr. N. V3 (mandibular div.) + portio minor (motor for CrN V)
foramen spinosum	middle meningeal a. & v.
jugular foramen	internal jugular v. (beginning); Cr. Nn. IX, X, XI
stylomastoid foramen	Cr. N. VII (facial); stylomastoid a.
condyloid foramen	v. from transverse sinus
mastoid foramen	v. to mastoid sinus; branch of occipital a. to dura mater

[a]Abbreviations: a. = artery, aa. = arteries, v. = vein, vv. = veins, n. = nerve, nn. = nerves, br. = branch, Cr. N. = cranial nerve, fmn. = foramen, div. = division

1.5.2 Porus acusticus

AKA internal auditory canal (▶ Fig. 1.7)

The filaments of the acoustic portion of VIII penetrate tiny openings of the lamina cribrosa of the cochlear area.[20]

Transverse crest: separates superior vestibular area and facial canal (above) from the inferior vestibular area and cochlear area (below).[20]

Vertical crest (AKA Bill's bar – named after Dr. William House): separates the meatus to the facial canal anteriorly (containing VII and nervus intermedius) from the vestibular area posteriorly (containing the superior division of vestibular nerve). Bill's bar is deeper in the IAC than the transverse crest.

The "5 nerves" of the IAC:

1. facial nerve (VII) (mnemonic: "7-up" as VII is in superior portion)
2. nervus intermedius: the somatic sensory branch of the facial nerve primarily innervating mechanoreceptors of the hair follicles on the inner surface of the pinna and deep mechanoreceptors of nasal and buccal cavities and chemoreceptors in the taste buds on the anterior 2/3 of the tongue
3. acoustic portion of the VIII nerve (mnemonic: "Coke down" for cochlear portion)
4. superior branch of vestibular nerve: passes through the superior vestibular area to terminate in the utricle and in the ampullæ of the superior and lateral semicircular canals (mnemonic superior = LSU (Lateral & Superior semicircular canals and the Utricule))
5. inferior branch of vestibular nerve: passes through inferior vestibular area to terminate in the saccule

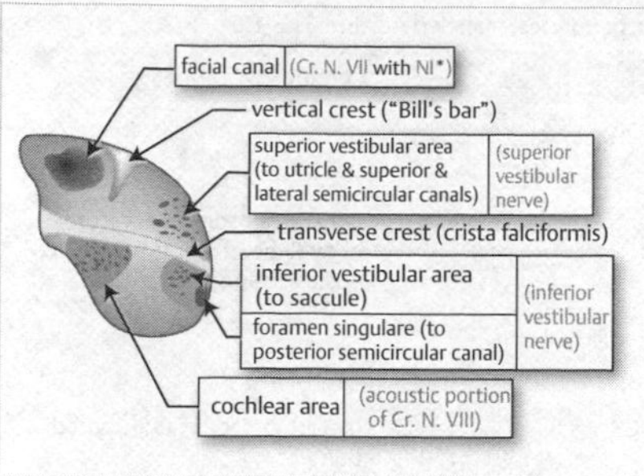

Fig. 1.7 Right internal auditory canal (porus acusticus) & nerves
* NI = nervus intermedius

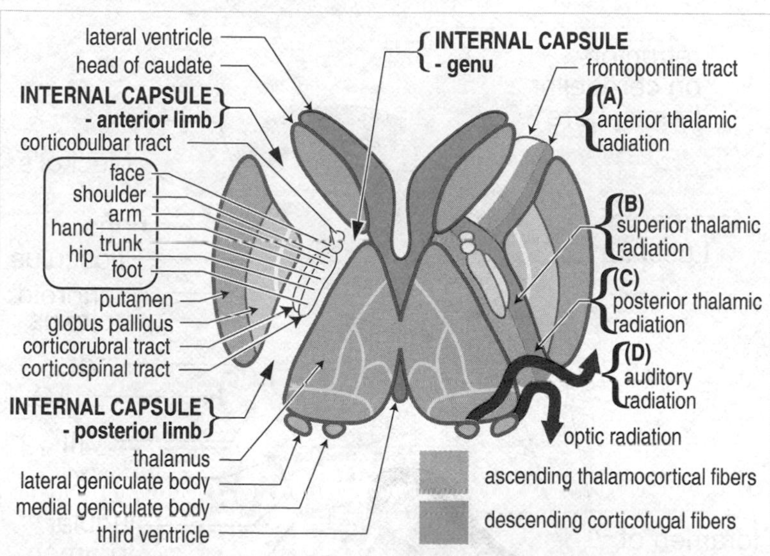

Fig. 1.8 Internal capsule schematic diagram (left side shows tracts, right side shows radiations)

1.6 Internal capsule

1.6.1 Architectural anatomy

For a schematic diagram, ▶ Fig. 1.8; ▶ Table 1.6 delineates the thalamic subradiations.

Most IC lesions are caused by vascular accidents (thrombosis or hemorrhage).

1.6.2 Vascular supply of the internal capsule (IC)

1. anterior choroidal: ⇒ all of retrolenticular part (includes optic radiation) and ventral part of posterior limb of IC
2. lateral striate branches (AKA capsular branches) of middle cerebral artery: ⇒ most of anterior AND posterior limbs of IC
3. genu usually receives some direct branches of the internal carotid artery

1.7 Cerebellopontine angle anatomy

For normal anatomy of right cerebellopontine angle, see ▶ Fig. 1.9.

Table 1.6 Four Thalamic "subradiations" (AKA thalamic peduncles) , labeled A-D in ► Fig. 1.8

Radiation	Connection			Comments
anterior (A)	medial & anterior thalamic nucleus	↔	frontal lobe	
superior (B)	rolandic areas	↔	ventral thalamic nuclei	general sensory fibers from body & head to terminate in postcentral gyrus (areas 3,1,2)
posterior (C)	occipital & posterior parietal	↔	caudal thalamus	
inferior (D)	transverse temporal gyrus of Heschl	↔	MGB	(small) includes auditory radiation

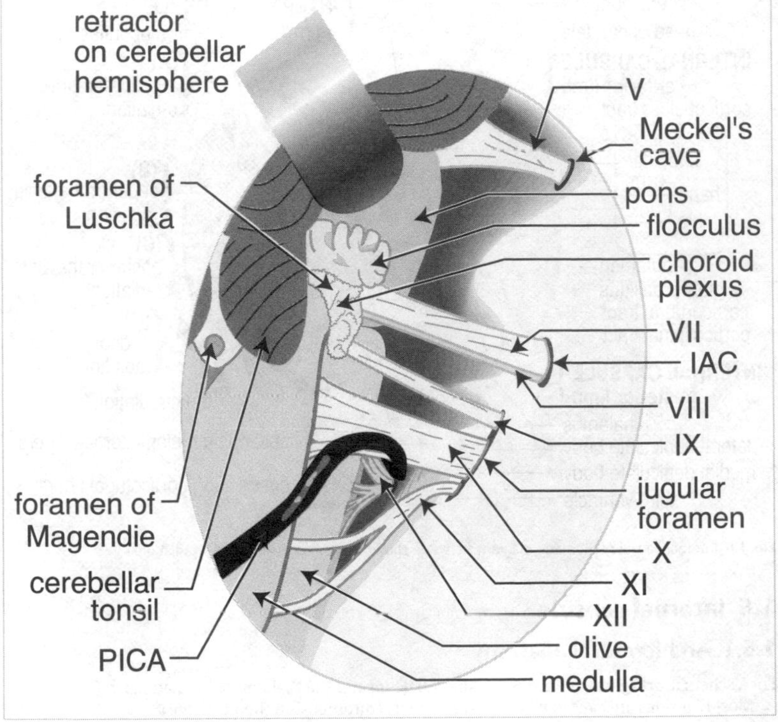

Fig. 1.9 Normal anatomy of right cerebellopontine angle viewed from behind (as in a suboccipital approach)[20]

1.8 Occipitoatlantoaxial-complex anatomy

► **Ligaments of the occipitoatlantoaxial complex.** Stability of the occipitoatlantal joint is primarily due to ligaments, with little contribution from bony articulations and joint capsules (see ► Fig. 1.10, ► Fig. 1.11, ► Fig. 1.12):

1. ligaments that connect the atlas to the occiput:
   a) anterior atlanto-occipital membrane: cephalad extension of the anterior longitudinal ligament. Extends from anterior margin of foramen magnum (FM) to anterior arch of C1

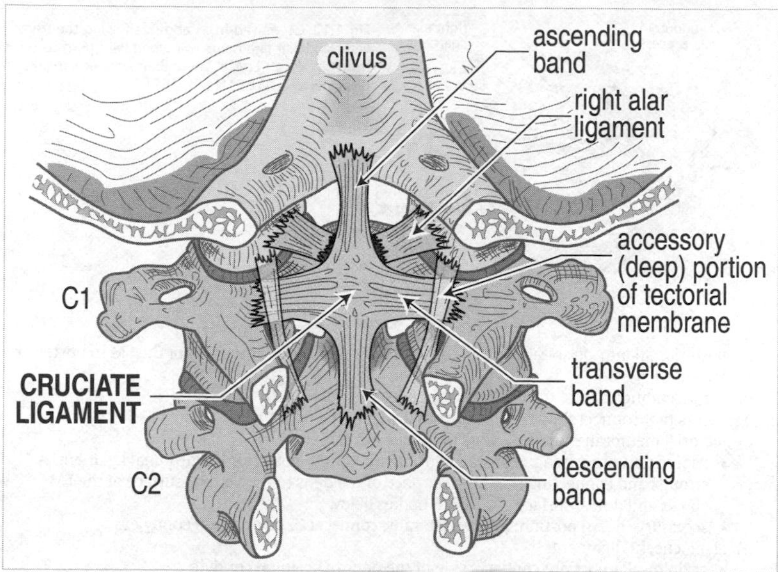

Fig. 1.10 Sagittal view of the ligaments of the craniovertebral junction (Modified with permission from "In Vitro Cervical Spine Biomechanical Testing" BNI Quarterly, Vol.9, No. 4, 1993)

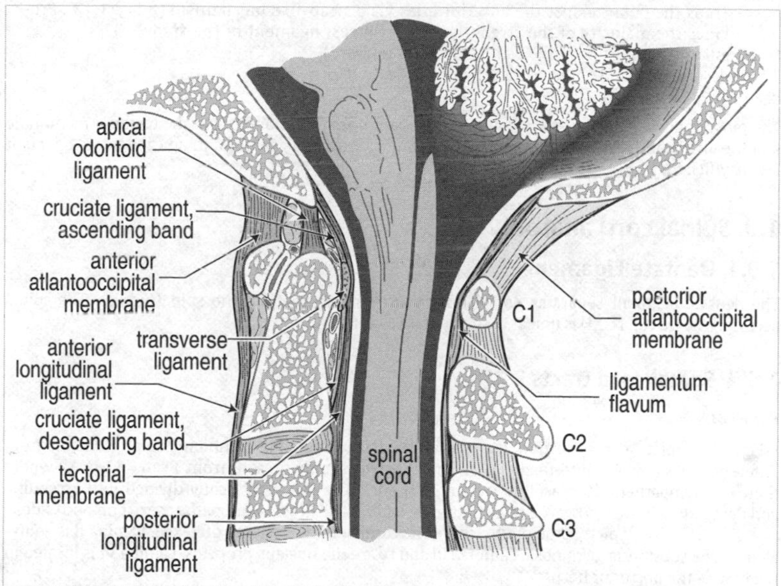

Fig. 1.11 Dorsal view of the cruciate and alar ligaments
Viewed with tectorial membrane removed. (Modified with permission from "In Vitro Cervical Spine Biomechanical Testing" BNI Quarterly, Vol.9, No. 4, 1993)

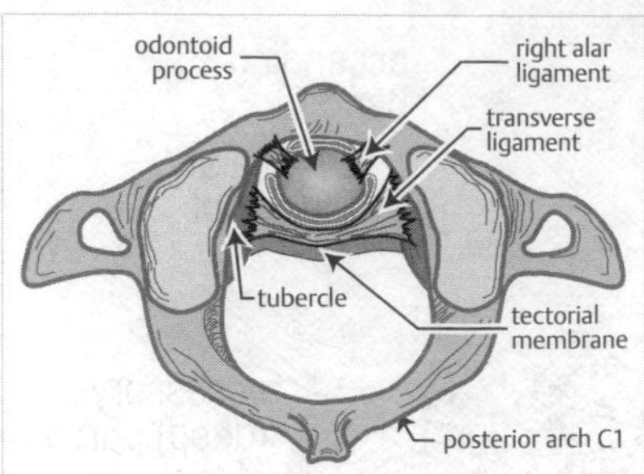

Fig. 1.12 C1 viewed from above, showing the transverse and alar ligaments (Modified with permission from "In Vitro Cervical Spine Biomechanical Testing" BNI Quarterly, Vol.9, No. 4, 199)

   b) posterior atlanto-occipital mem-brane: connects the posterior margin of the FM to posterior arch of C1
   c) the ascending band of the cruciate ligament
2. ligaments that connect the axis (viz. the odontoid) to the occiput:
   a) tectorial membrane: some authors distinguish 2 components
      - superficial component: cephalad continuation of the posterior longitudinal ligament. A strong band connecting the dorsal surface of the dens to the ventral surface of the FM above, and dorsal surface of C2 & C3 bodies below
      - accessory (deep) portion: located laterally, connects C2 to occipital condyles
   b) alar ("check") ligaments[21]
      - occipito-alar portion: connects side of the dens to occipital condyle
      - atlanto-alar portion: connects side of the dens to the lateral mass of C1
   c) apical odontoid ligament: connects tip of dens to the FM. Little mechanical strength
3. ligaments that connect the axis to the atlas:
   a) transverse (atlantoaxial) ligament: the horizontal component of the cruciate ligament. Traps the dens against the anterior atlas via a strap-like mechanism (▶ Fig. 1.12). Provides the majority of the strength ("the strongest ligament of the spine"[22])
   b) atlanto-alar portion of the alar ligaments (see above)
   c) descending band of the cruciate ligament

The most important structures in maintaining atlanto-occipital stability are the tectorial membrane and the alar ligaments. Without these, the remaining cruciate ligament and apical dentate ligament are insufficient.

1.9 Spinal cord anatomy

1.9.1 Dentate Ligament

The dentate ligament separates dorsal from ventral nerve roots in the spinal nerves. The spinal accessory nerve (Cr. N. XI) is dorsal to the dentate ligament.

1.9.2 Spinal cord tracts

Anatomy

▶ Fig. 1.13 depicts a cross-section of a typical spinal cord segment, combining some elements from different levels (e.g. the intermediolateral grey nucleus is only present from T1 to ≈ L1 or L2 where there are sympathetic (thoracolumbar outflow) nuclei). It is schematically divided into ascending and descending halves, however, in actuality, ascending and descending paths coexist on both sides.

▶ Fig. 1.13 also depicts some of the laminae according to the scheme of Rexed. Lamina II is equivalent to the substantia gelatinosa. Laminae III and IV are the nucleus proprius. Lamina VI is located in the base of the posterior horn.

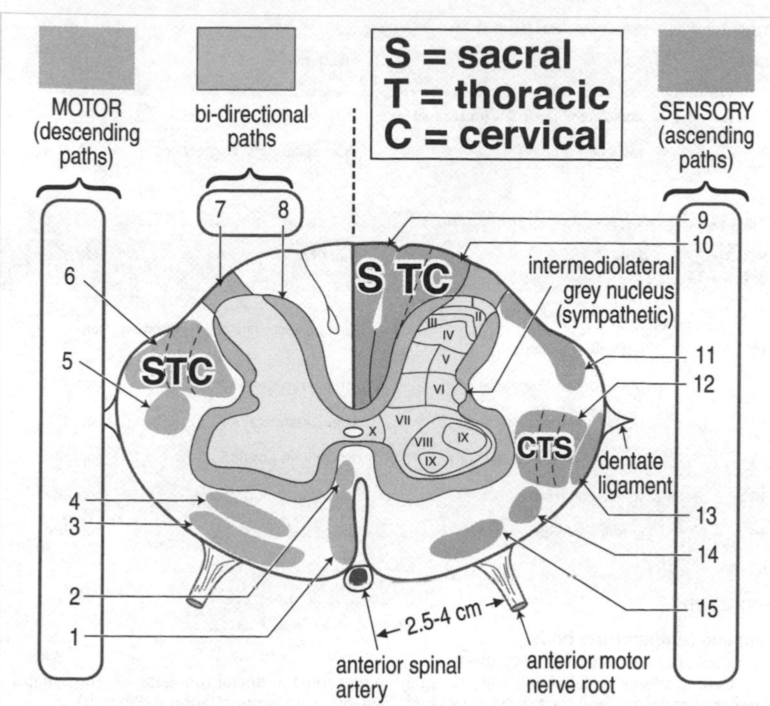

Fig. 1.13 Schematic cross-section of cervical spinal cord. See ▶ Table 1.7, ▶ Table 1.8 and ▶ Table 1.9 for path names.

Table 1.7 Descending (motor) tracts (↓) in ▶ Fig 1.13

Number (▶ Fig. 1.13)	Path	Function	Side of *body*
1	anterior corticospinal tract	skilled movement[a]	opposite
2	medial longitudinal fasciculus	?	same
3	vestibulospinal tract	facilitates extensor muscle tone	same
4	medullary (ventrolateral) reticulospinal tract	automatic respirations?	same
5	rubrospinal tract	flexor muscle tone	same
6	lateral corticospinal (pyramidal) tract	skilled movement	same

[a]The terminal fibers of this uncrossed tract usually cross in the anterior white commissure to synapse on alpha motor neurons or on internuncial neurons. It is true that some of these fibers do stay on the same side, but it is felt to be a minority. Also, the anterior corticospinal tract is easily identified only in the cervical and upper thoracic regions.

Table 1.8 Bi-directional tracts in ▶ Fig. 1.13

Number (▶ Fig. 1.13)	Path	Function
7	dorsolateral fasciculus (of Lissauer)	
8	fasciculus proprius	short spinospinal connections

Table 1.9 Ascending (sensory) tracts (↑) in ▶ Fig. 1.13

Number (▶ Fig. 1.13)	Path	Function	Side of *body*
9	fasciculus gracilis	joint position, fine touch, vibration	same
10	fasciculus cuneatus		
11	posterior spinocerebellar tract	stretch receptors	same
12	lateral spinothalamic tract	pain & temperature	opposite
13	anterior spinocerebellar tract	whole limb position	opposite
14	spinotectal tract	unknown, ? nociceptive	opposite
15	anterior spinothalamic tract	light touch	opposite

Sensation

Pain and temperature: body

Receptors: free nerve endings (probable).

1st order neuron: small, finely myelinated afferents; soma in dorsal root ganglion (no synapse). Enter cord at dorsolateral tract (zone of Lissauer). Synapse: substantia gelatinosa (Rexed II).

2nd order neuron axon cross obliquely in the anterior white commissure ascending ≈ 1–3 segments while crossing to enter the lateral spinothalamic tract.

Synapse: VPL thalamus. 3rd order neurons pass through IC to postcentral gyrus (Brodmann's areas 3, 1, 2).

Fine touch, deep pressure and proprioception: body

Fine touch AKA discriminative touch. Receptors: Meissner's & pacinian corpuscles, Merkel's disks, free nerve endings.

1st order neuron: heavily myelinated afferents; soma in dorsal root ganglion (no synapse). Short branches synapse in nucleus proprius (Rexed III & IV) of posterior gray; long fibers enter the ipsilateral posterior columns without synapsing (below T6: fasciculus gracilis; above T6: fasciculus cuneatus).

Synapse: nucleus gracilis/cuneatus (respectively), just above pyramidal decussation. 2nd order neuron axons form internal arcuate fibers, decussate in lower medulla as medial lemniscus.

Synapse: VPL thalamus. 3rd order neurons pass through IC primarily to postcentral gyrus.

Light (crude) touch: body

Receptors: as fine touch (see above), also peritrichial arborizations.

1st order neuron: large, heavily myelinated afferents (Type II); soma in dorsal root ganglion (no synapse). Some ascend uncrossed in post. columns (with fine touch); most synapse in Rexed VI & VII.

2nd order neuron axons cross in anterior white commissure (a few don't cross); enter anterior spinothalamic tract.

Synapse: VPL thalamus. 3rd order neurons pass through IC primarily to postcentral gyrus.

1.9.3 Dermatomes and sensory nerves

Dermatomes are ares of the body where sensation is subserved by a single nerve root.

Peripheral nerves generally receive contributions from more than one dermatome.

Lesions in peripheral nerves and lesions in nerve roots may sometimes be distinguished in part by the pattern of sensory loss. A classic example is splitting of the ring finger in median nerve or ulnar nerve lesions, which does not occur in C8 nerve root injuries.

▶ Fig. 1.14 shows anterior and posterior view, each schematically separated into sensory dermatomes (segmental) and peripheral sensory nerve distribution.

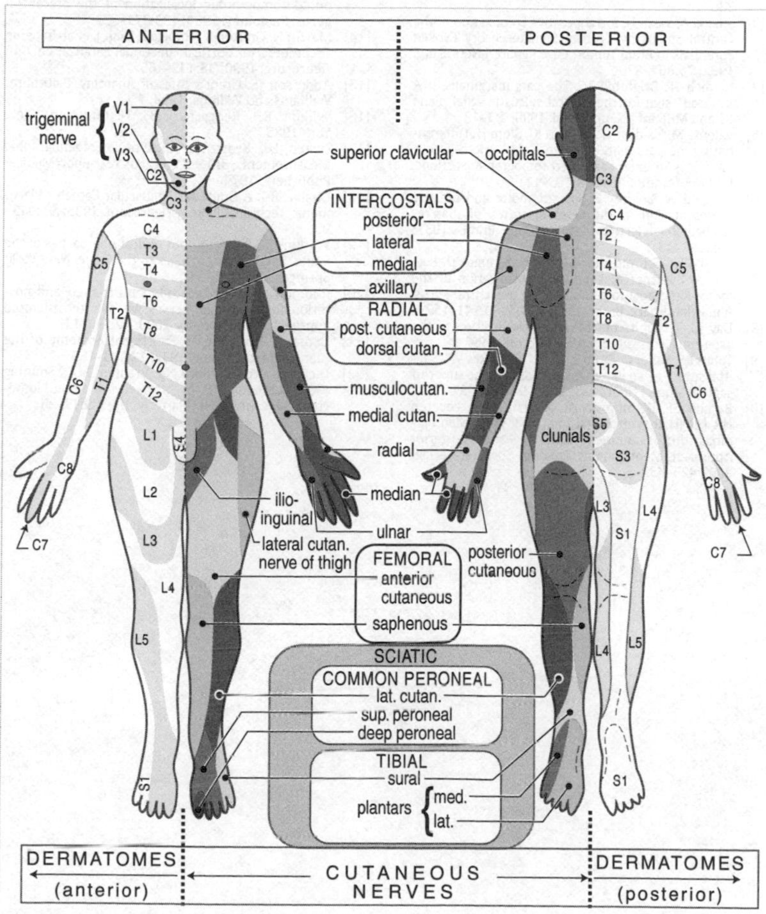

Fig. 1.14 Dermatomal and sensory nerve distribution (Redrawn from "Introduction to Basic Neurology", by Harry D. Patton, John W. Sundsten, Wayne E. Crill and Phillip D. Swanson, © 1976, pp 173, W. B. Saunders Co., Philadelphia, PA, with permission)

References

[1] Naidich TP. MR Imaging of Brain Surface Anatomy. Neuroradiology. 1991; 33:S95–S99

[2] Ojemann G, Ojemann J, Lettich E, Berger M. Cortical Language Localization in Left, Dominant Hemisphere. An Electrical Stimulation Mapping Investigation in 117 Patients. J Neurosurg. 1989; 71:316–326

[3] Suzuki A, Yasui N. Intraoperative Localization of the Central Sulcus by Cortical Somatosensory Evoked Potentials in Brain Tumor: Case Report. J Neurosurg. 1992; 76:867–870

[4] Naidich TP, Brightbill TC. The pars marginalis, I: A "bracket" sign for the central sulcus in axial plane CT and MRI. Int J Neuroradiol. 1996; 2:3–19

[5] Valente M, Naidich TP, Abrams KJ, Blum JT. Differentiating the pars marginalis from the parieto-occipital sulcus in axial computed tomography sections. Int J Neuroradiol. 1998; 4:105–111

[6] Penfield W, Boldrey E. Somatic motor and sensory representation in the cerebral cortex of man as studied by electrical stimulation. Brain. 1937; 60:389–443

[7] Yousry TA, Schmid UD, Alkadhi H, Schmidt D, Peraud A, Buettner A, Winkler P. Localization of the motor hand area to a knob on the precentral gyrus. A new landmark. Brain. 1997; 120 (Pt 1):141–157

[8] Day JD, Tschabitscher M. Anatomic position of the asterion. Neurosurgery. 1998; 42:198–199

[9] Tubbs RS, Salter G, Elton S, Grabb PA, Oakes WJ. Sagittal suture as an external landmark for the superior sagittal sinus. J Neurosurg. 2001; 94:985–987

[10] Barnett SL, D'Ambrosio AL, Agazzi S, van Loveren HR, Lee JH. In: Petroclival and Upper Clival Meningiomas III: Combined Anterior and Posterior Approach. Meningiomas. London: Springer-Verlag; 2009:425–432

[11] Willis WD, Grossman RG. In: The Brain and Its Environment. Medical Neurobiology. 3rd ed. St. Louis: C V Mosby; 1981:192–193

[12] Warwick R, Williams PL. Gray's Anatomy. Philadelphia 1973

[13] Kido DK, LeMay M, Levinson AW, Benson WE. Computed tomographic localization of the precentral gyrus. Radiology. 1980; 135:373–377

[14] Martin N, Grafton S, Viñuela F, Dion J, et al. Imaging Techniques for Cortical Functional Localization. Clin Neurosurg. 1990; 38:132–165

[15] Anderson JE. Grant's Atlas of Anatomy. Baltimore: Williams and Wilkins; 1978; 7

[16] Wilkins RH, Rengachary SS. Neurosurgery. New York 1985

[17] Lusted LB, Keats TE. Atlas of Roentgenographic Measurement. 3rd ed. Chicago: Year Book Medical Publishers; 1972

[18] Ghajar JBG. A Guide for Ventricular Catheter Placement: Technical Note. J Neurosurg. 1985; 63:985–986

[19] Watkins RG. In: Anterior Cervical Approaches to the Spine. Surgical Approaches to the Spine. New York: Springer-Verlag; 1983:1–6

[20] Rhoton AL, Jr. The cerebellopontine angle and posterior fossa cranial nerves by the retrosigmoid approach. Neurosurgery. 2000; 47:S93–129

[21] Dvorak J, Panjabi MM. Functional Anatomy of the Alar Ligaments. Spine. 1987; 12:183–189

[22] Dickman CA, Crawford NR, Brantley AGU, Sonntag VKH, Koeneman JB. In vitro cervical spine biomechanical testing. BNI Quarterly. 1993; 9:17–26

2 Vascular Anatomy

2.1 Cerebral vascular territories

▶ Fig. 2.1 depicts approximate vascular distributions of the major cerebral arteries. There is considerable variability of the major arteries[1] as well as the central distribution. The lenticulostriates may have origins off of different segments of the middle or anterior cerebral artery). Recurrent artery of Heubner (RAH) (AKA medial striate artery) origin: junction of the ACA and a-comm in 62.3%, proximal A2 in 23.3%, A1 in 14.3%.[2]

2.2 Cerebral arterial anatomy

2.2.1 General information

The symbol "⇒" is used to denote a region supplied by the indicated artery. See Angiography (cerebral) (p. 236) for angiographic diagrams of the following anatomy.

2.2.2 Circle of Willis

See ▶ Fig. 2.2. A balanced configuration of the Circle of Willis is present in only 18% of the population. Hypoplasia of 1 or both p-comms occurs in 22–32%, absent or hypoplastic A1 segments occurs in 25%.

Key point: the anterior cerebral arteries pass over the superior surface of the optic chiasm.

2.2.3 Anatomical segments of intracranial cerebral arteries

1. carotid artery: the traditional numbering system[3] was from rostral to caudal (counter to the direction of flow, and to the numbering scheme of the other arteries). A number of systems have been described to addresses this inconsistency and also to identify anatomically important segments of the ICA that were not originally delineated (e.g. see ▶ Table 2.1 [4]). Also see below for more detail

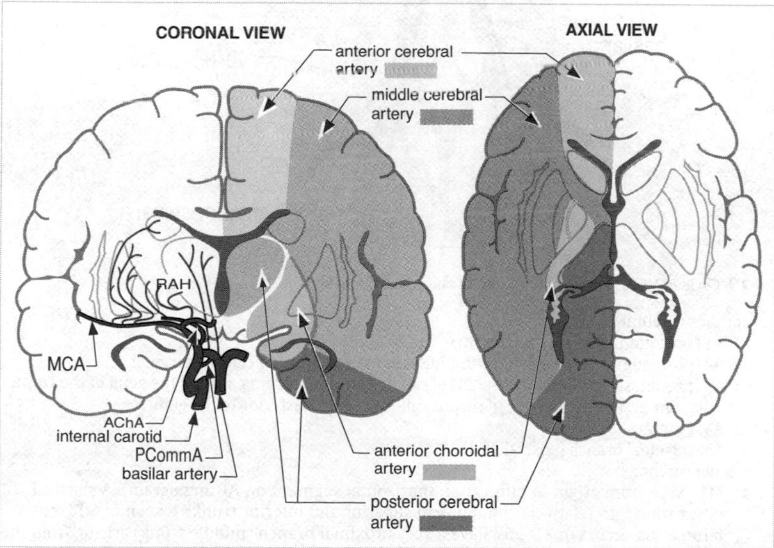

Fig. 2.1 Vascular territories of the cerebral hemispheres. RAH = recurrent artery of Heubner.

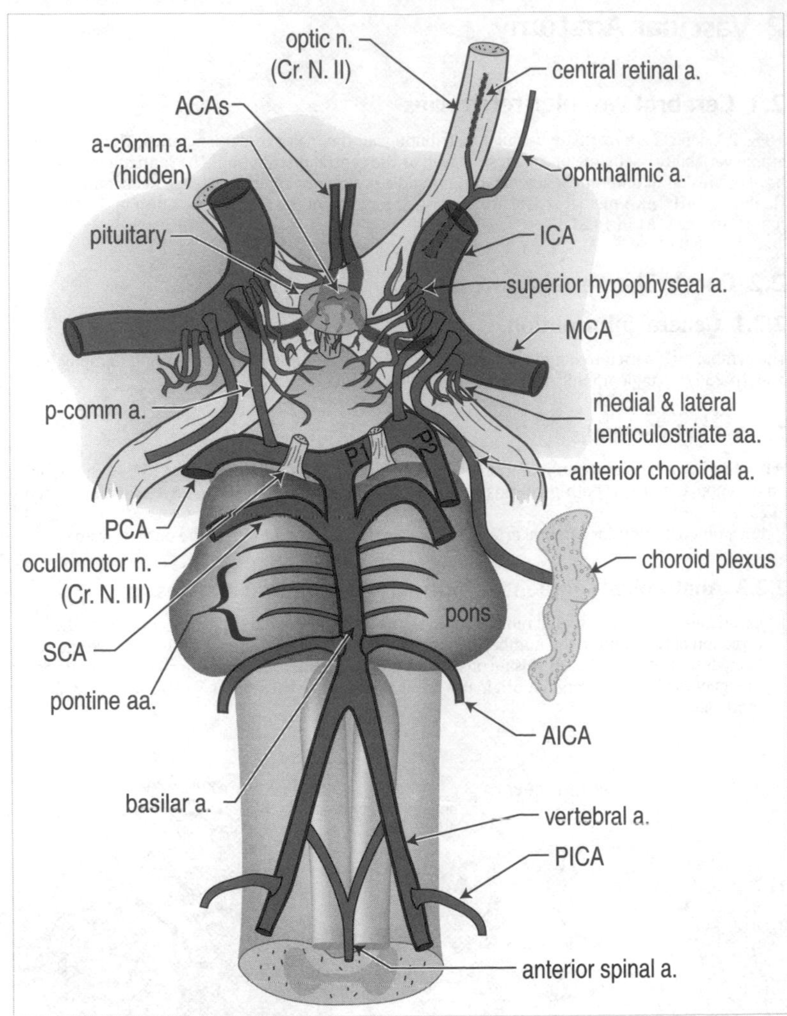

Fig. 2.2 Circle of Willis viewed from in front of and below the brain

2. anterior cerebral[5]:
   a) A1 (precommunicating): ACA from origin to ACoA
   b) A2 (postcommunicating): ACA from ACoA to branch-point of callosomarginal
   c) A3 (precallosal): from branch-point of callosomarginal curving around the genu of the corpus callosum to superior surface of corpus callosum 3 cm posterior to the genu
   d) A4: (supracallosal)
   e) A5: terminal branch (postcallosal)
3. middle cerebral[6]:
   a) M1: MCA from origin to bifurcation (horizontal segment on AP angiogram). A classical bifurcation into relatively symmetrical superior and inferior trunks is seen in 50%, no bifurcation occurs in 2%, 25% have a very proximal branch (middle trunk) arising from the superior (15%) or the inferior (10%) trunk creating a "pseudo-trifurcation", a pseudo-tetrafurcation occurs in 5%

Table 2.1 Segments of the ICA

Cincinnati system	System of Fischer
C1 (cervical)	Not described
C2 (petrous)	
C3 (lacerum)	C5
C4 (cavernous)	C4 + part of C5
C5 (clinoid)	C3
C6 (ophthalmic)	C2
C7 (communicating)	C1

- lateral fronto-orbital and prefrontal branches arise from M1 or superior M2 trunk
- precentral, central, anterior and posterior parietal arteries arise from a superior (60%) or middle (25%) or inferior (15%) trunk
- the superior M2 trunk does not give any branches to the temporal lobe

b) M2: MCA trunks from bifurcation to emergence from Sylvian fissure
c) M3–4: distal branches
d) M5: terminal branch

4. posterior cerebral (PCA) (several nomenclature schemes exist[5,7]):
   a) P1: PCA from the origin to posterior communicating artery (AKA mesencephalic, precommunicating, circular, peduncular, basilar…). The long and short circumflex and thalamoperforating arteries arise from P1
   b) P2: PCA from origin of p-comm to the origin of inferior temporal arteries (AKA ambient, postcommunicating, perimesencephalic), P2 traverses the ambient cistern, Hippocampal, anterior temporal, peduncular perforating and medial posterior choroidal arteries arise from P2
   c) P3: PCA from the origin of the inferior temporal branches to the origin of the terminal branches (AKA quadrigeminal segment). P3 traverses the quadrigeminal cistern
   d) P4: segment after the origin of the parieto-occipital and calcarine arteries, includes the cortical branches of the PCA

2.2.4 Anterior circulation

Anatomic variants

Bovine circulation: the common carotids arise from a common trunk off the aorta.

External carotid

1. superior thyroid a.: 1st anterior branch
2. ascending pharyngeal a.
   a) neuromeningeal trunk of the ascending pharyngeal a.: supplies IX, X & XI (important when embolizing glomus tumors, 20% of lower cranial nerve palsy if this branch is occluded)
   b) pharyngeal branch: usually the primary feeder for jugular foramen tumors (essentially the *only* cause of hypertrophy of the ascending pharyngeal a.)
3. lingual a.
4. facial a.: branches anastamose with ophthalmic a.; important in collateral flow with ICA occlusion (p. 1265)
5. occipital a. ⇒ posterior scalp
6. posterior auricular
7. superficial temporal
   a) frontal branch
   b) parietal branch
8. (internal) maxillary a. – initially within parotid gland
   a) middle meningeal a.
      - anterior branch
      - posterior branch

b) accessory meningeal
c) inferior alveolar
d) infra-orbital
e) others: distal branches of which may anastomose with branches of ophthalmic artery in the orbit

Internal carotid artery (ICA)

Lies posterior & medial to the external carotid (ECA).

Segments of the ICA and its branches

See ▶ Fig. 2.3 for branches, and reference.[4]

1. C1 (cervical): begins in neck at carotid bifurcation where the common carotid artery divides into internal and external carotids. Travels in carotid sheath with IJV and vagal nerve, encircled with postganglionic sympathetic nerves (PGSN). C1 ends where the ICA enters carotid canal of petrous bone. *No branches*
2. C2 (petrous): still surrounded by PGSNs. Ends at the posterior edge of the foramen lacerum (f-Lac) (inferomedial to the edge of the Gasserian ganglion in Meckel's cave). Three divisions:

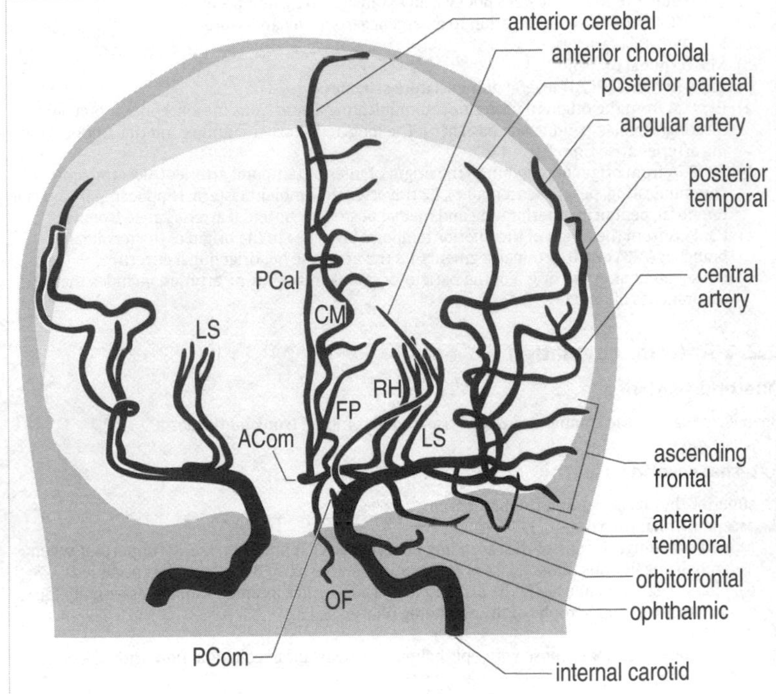

Fig. 2.3 Internal carotid arteriogram (AP view).
ACom: anterior communicating artery
CM: callosomarginal artery
FP: frontopolar artery
LS: lenticulostriate arteries
OF: orbitofrontal artery
PCal: pericallosal artery
PCom: posterior communicating artery
RH: recurrent artery of Heubner (Reprinted courtesy of Eastman Kodak Company)

a) vertical segment: ICA ascends then bends as the...
b) posterior loop: anterior to cochlea, bends antero-medially becoming the...
c) horizontal segment: deep and medial to greater and lesser superficial petrosal nerves, anterior to tympanic membrane (TM)

3. C3 (lacerum): the ICA passes over (but not through) the f-Lac forming the lateral loop. Ascends in the canalicular portion of the f-Lac to juxtasellar position, piercing the dura as it passes the petrolingual ligament to become the cavernous segment. Branches (usually not visible angiographically):
   a) caroticotympanic (inconsistent) ⇒ tympanic cavity
   b) pterygoid (vidian) branch: passes through foramen lacerum, present in only 30%, may continue as artery of pterygoid canal
4. C4 (cavernous): covered by vascular membrane lining sinus, still surrounded by PGSNs. Passes anteriorly then supero-medially, bends posteriorly (medial loop of ICA), travels horizontally, and bends anteriorly (part of anterior loop of ICA) to anterior clinoid process. Ends at the proximal dural ring (incompletely encircles ICA). Many branches, main ones include:
   a) meningohypophyseal trunk (MHT) (largest & most proximal). 2 causes of a prominent MHT: 1) tumor (usually petroclival meningioma – see below), 2) dural AVM (p. 1251)
      - a. of tentorium (AKA artery of Bernasconi & Cassinari): the blood supply of petroclival meningiomas
      - dorsal meningeal a. (AKA dorsal clival a.)
      - inferior hypophyseal a. (⇒ posterior lobe of pituitary): post-partum occlusion causes pituitary infarcts (Sheehan's necrosis), however, DI is rare because the stalk is spared
   b) anterior meningeal a.
   c) a. to inferior portion of cavernous sinus (present in 80%)
   d) capsular aa. of McConnell (in 30%): supply the capsule of the pituitary[8]
5. C5 (clinoid): begins at proximal dural ring, ends at distal dural ring (which completely encircles ICA) where the ICA becomes intradural
6. C6 (ophthalmic): begins at distal dural ring, ends just proximal to p-comm. Branches:
   a) ophthalmic a.: the origin from the ICA is distal to the cavernous sinus in 89% (intracavernous in 8%, the ophthalmic artery is absent in 3%[9]) and can vary from 5 mm anterior to 7 mm posterior to the anterior clinoid.[8] Passes through the optic canal into the orbit (the intracranial course is very short, usually 1–2 mm[8]). Has a characteristic bayonet-like "kink" on lateral angiogram
   b) superior hypophyseal a. branches ⇒ anterior lobe of pituitary & stalk (1st branch of supraclinoid ICA)
7. C7 (communicating): begins just proximal to p-comm origin, travels between Cr. N. II & III, terminates just below anterior perforated substance where it bifurcates into the ACA & MCA
   a) posterior communicating a. (p-comm)
      - few anterior thalamoperforators (⇒ optic tract, chiasm & posterior hypothalamus): below
      - plexal segment: enters supracornual recess of temporal horn, ⇒ only this portion of choroid plexus
      - cisternal segment: passes through crural cistern
   b) anterior choroidal artery[10]: takeoff 2–4 mm distal to p-comm ⇒ (variable) portion of optic tract, medial globus pallidus, genu of internal capsule (IC) (in 50%), inferior half of posterior limb of IC, uncus, retrolenticular fibers (optic radiation), lateral geniculate body; for occlusion syndromes (p. 1265)
8. "Carotid siphon": not a segment, but a region incorporating the cavernous, ophthalmic and communicating segments. Begins at the posterior bend of the cavernous ICA, and ends at the ICA bifurcation

Differentiating p-comm from ACh on arteriogram

1. p-comm origin is proximal to that of the anterior choroidal artery (ACh)
2. p-comm is usually larger than ACh
3. p-comm usually goes up or down a little, then straight back & usually bifurcates
4. ACh usually has a superior "hump" (plexal point) where it pass through the choroidal fissure to enter the ventricle

Anterior cerebral artery (ACA)

Passes between Cr. N. II and anterior perforated substance. See ▶ Fig. 2.4. Branches:

1. recurrent artery (of Heubner): typically arises from the area of the A1/A2 junction. Various statistics can be found in the literature regarding the percentage that arise from distal A1 vs. proximal A2.[11] It most important to be mindful that the takeoff is variable, e.g. when treating aneurysms (one of the larger medial lenticulostriates, remainder of lenticulostriates may arise from this artery) ⇒ head of caudate, putamen, and anterior internal capsule
2. medial orbitofrontal artery
3. frontopolar artery
4. callosomarginal
   a) internal frontal branches
      - anterior
      - middle
      - posterior
   b) paracentral artery
5. pericallosal artery (continuation of ACA)
   a) superior internal parietal (precuneate) artery
   b) inferior internal parietal artery

Anatomic variants

Hypoid: having only one anterior cerebral artery (as in a horse).

Middle cerebral artery (MCA)

See ▶ Fig. 2.5 and anatomy (p. 76). Branches vary widely, 10 common ones:

1. medial (3–6 per side) and lateral lenticulostriate arteries
2. anterior temporal
3. posterior temporal
4. lateral orbitofrontal
5. ascending frontal (candelabra)
6. precentral (prerolandic)
7. central (rolandic)
8. anterior parietal (postrolandic)
9. posterior parietal
10. angular

Posterior circulation

Anatomic variants

Fetal circulation: 15–35% of patients supply their posterior cerebral artery on one or both sides primarily from the carotid (via p-comm) instead of via the vertebrobasilar system.

Vertebral artery (VA)

The VA is the first and usually the largest branch of the subclavian artery. Variant: the left VA arises off the aortic arch in ≈ 4%. Diameter ≈ 3 mm. Mean blood flow ≈ 150 ml/min. The *left* VA is dominant in 60%. The right VA will be hypoplastic in 10%, and the left will be hypoplastic in 5%. The VA is atretic and does not communicate with the BA on the left in 3%, and on the right in 2% (the VA may terminate in PICA).

Four segments:

- V1 prevertebral: from subclavian artery, courses superiorly and posteriorly and enters the foramen transversarium, usually of the 6th vertebral body
- V2 ascends vertically within the transverse foramina of the cervical vertebrae surrounded by sympathetic fibers (from the stellate ganglion) and a venous plexus. It is situated *anterior* to the cervical roots. It turns laterally to enter the foramen within the transverse process of the axis
- V3 exits the foramen of the axis and curves posteriorly and medially in a groove on the upper surface of the atlas and enters the foramen magnum
- V4 pierces the dura (location somewhat variable) and immediately enters the subarachnoid space. Joins the contralateral VA at the vertebral confluens located at the lower pontine border to form the basilar artery (BA)

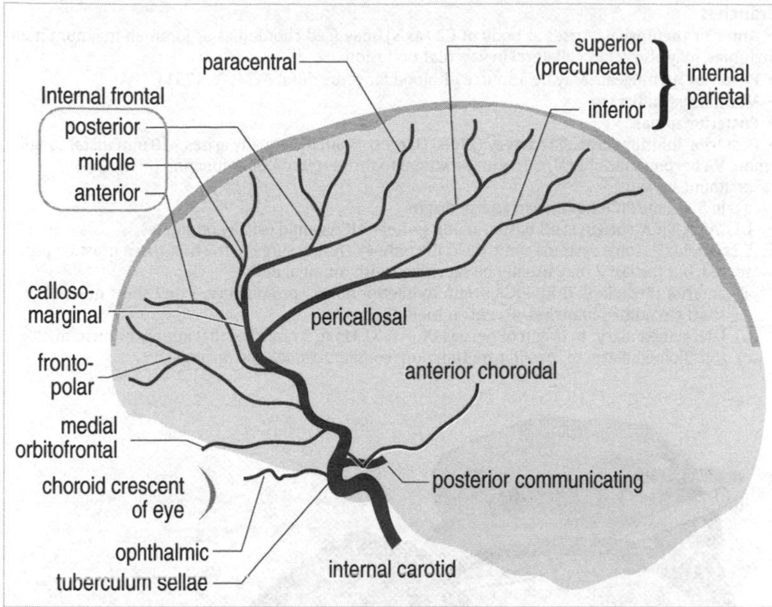

Fig. 2.4 Anterior cerebral arteriogram (lateral view) (Reprinted courtesy of Eastman Kodak Company)

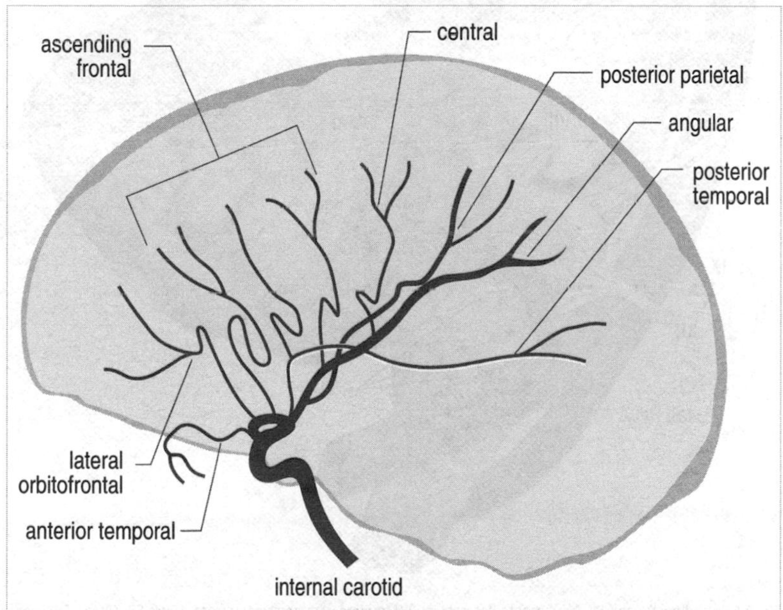

Fig. 2.5 Middle cerebral arteriogram (lateral view) (Reprinted courtesy of Eastman Kodak Company)

Branches

► **Anterior meningeal.** Arises at body of C2 (axis), may feed chordomas or foramen magnum meningiomas, may also act as collateral in vascular occlusion

► **Posterior meningeal.** May be a source of blood for some dural AVMs (p. 1251)

► **Medullary (bulbar) aa**

► **Posterior spinal**

► **Posterior inferior cerebellar artery (PICA) (largest branch).** Usually arises ≈10 mm distal to point where VA becomes intradural, ≈ 15 mm proximal to the vertebrobasilar junction (► Fig. 2.6)

1. anatomic variants:
   a) in 5–8% the PICA has an extradural origin
   b) "AICA-PICA": origin is off basilar trunk (where AICA would usually originate)
2. 5 segments[12] (some systems some describe only 4). During surgery, the first three must be preserved, but the last 2 may usually be sacrificed with minimal deficit[13]:
   a) anterior medullary: from PICA origin to inferior olivary prominence. 1 or 2 short medullary short circumflex branches ⇒ ventral medulla
   b) lateral medullary: to origin of nerves IX, X & XI. Up to 5 branches that supply brainstem
   c) tonsillomedullary: to tonsillar midportion (contains *caudal loop* on angio)

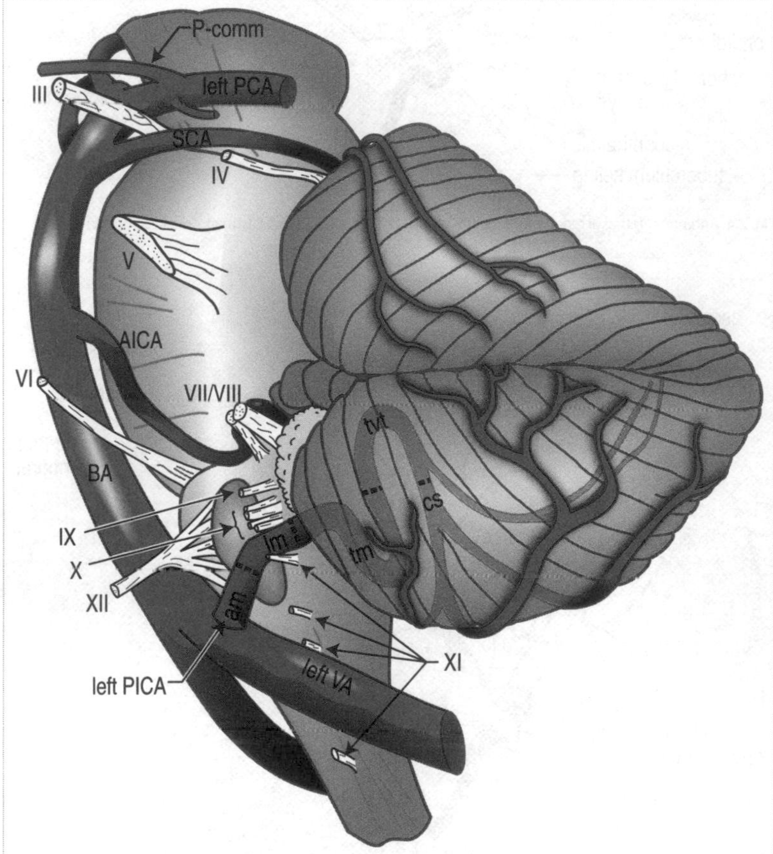

Fig. 2.6 Intradural VA and PICA segments (lateral view) (Modified with permission from: Lewis SB, Chang DJ, Peace DA, Lafrentz PJ, Day AL. Distal posterior inferior cerebellar artery aneurysms: clinical features and management. J Neurosurg 2002;97(4):756-66)

d) telovelotonsillar (supratonsillar): ascends in tonsillomedullary fissure (contains *cranial loop* on angio)
e) cortical segments
3. 3 branches
a) choroidal a. (BRANCH 1) arises from cranial loop (*choroidal point*), ⇒ choroid plexus of 4th ventricle
b) terminal branches:
- tonsillohemispheric (BRANCH 2)
- inferior vermian (BRANCH 3) inferior inflection = *copular point* on angio

▶ **Anterior spinal**

Basilar artery (BA)

Formed by the junction of the 2 vertebral arteries. Branches:
1. anterior inferior cerebellar artery (AICA): from lower part of BA, runs posterolaterally anterior to VI, VII & VIII. Often gives off a loop that runs into the IAC and gives off the labyrinthine artery and then emerges to supply the anterolateral inferior cerebellum and then anastomoses with PICA
2. internal auditory (labyrinthine)
3. pontine branches
4. superior cerebellar a. (SCA)
a) sup. vermian
5. posterior cerebral: joined by p-comms ≈ 1 cm from origin (the p-comm is the major origin of the PCA in 15% and is termed "fetal" circulation, bilateral in 2%).
3 segments (named for surrounding cistern) and their branches:
a) peduncular segment (P1)
- mesencephalic perforating aa. (⇒ tectum, cerebral peduncles, and these nuclei: Edinger-Westphal, oculomotor and trochlear)
- interpeduncular thalamoperforators (1st of 2 groups of posterior thalamoperforating aa.)
- medial post. choroidal (most from P1 or P2)
- "artery of Percheron": a rare anatomic variant[14] in which a solitary arterial trunk arising from the proximal segment of one PCA supplies the paramedian thalami and rostral midbrain bilaterally
b) ambient segment (P2)
- lateral post. choroidal (most from P2)
- thalamogeniculate thalamoperforators (2nd of 2 groups of posterior thalamoperforating aa.) ⇒ geniculate bodies + pulvinar
- anterior temporal (anastamoses with anterior temporal br. of MCA)
- posterior temporal
- parieto-occipital
- calcarine
c) quadrigeminal segment (P3)
- quadrigeminal & geniculate branches ⇒ quadrigeminal plate
- post. pericallosal (splenial) (anastomoses with pericallosal of ACA)

Posterior cerebral artery (PCA)

See ▶ Fig. 2.7.

Carotid-vertebrobasilar anastomoses

P-comm artery: the "normal" (most common) anastomosis.

Persistent fetal anastamoses[15] (▶ Fig. 2.8) result from failure to involute as the VAs and p-comms develop (order of involution: otic, hypoglossal, primitive trigeminal, proatlantal). Most are asymptomatic. However, some may be associated with vascular anomalies such as aneurysms or AVMs, and occasionally cranial nerve symptoms (e.g. trigeminal neuralgia with PPTA) can occur.

Four types (from cranial to caudal – the 1st 3 are named for the associated cranial nerve):
1. persistent primitive trigeminal artery (PPTA): seen in ≈ 0.6% of cerebral angiograms. The most common of the persistent fetal anastomoses (83%). May be associated with trigeminal neuralgia (p. 479). Connects the cavernous carotid to the basilar artery. Arises from the ICA proximal to the origin of the meningohypophyseal trunk (50% go through sella, 50% exit the cavernous sinus & course with the trigeminal nerve) and connects to the upper basilar artery between AICA & SCA. The VAs may be small. Saltzman type 1 variant: the p-comms are hypoplastic and the PPTA provides significant blood supply to the distributions of the distal BA, PCA and the SCAs (the basilar

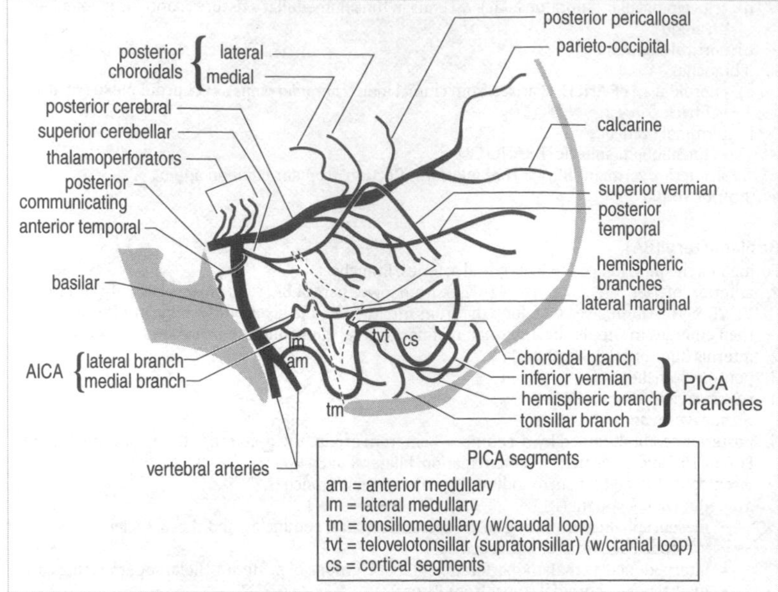

Fig. 2.7 Vertebrobasilar arteriogram (lateral view) (Reprinted courtesy of Eastman Kodak Company)

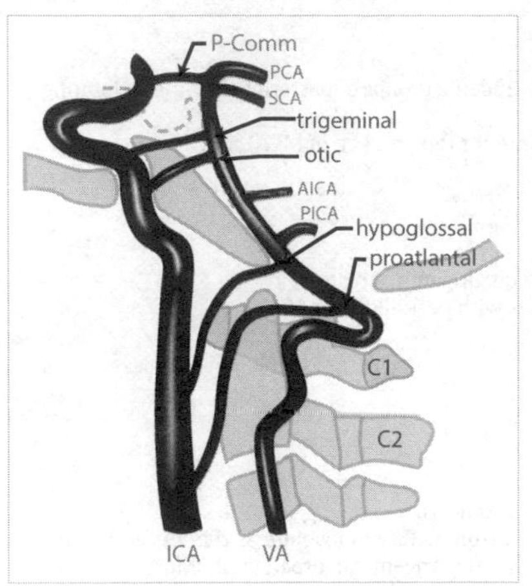

Fig. 2.8 Carotid-vertebrobasilar anastomoses

artery is often hypoplastic). Saltzman type 2: p-comm supplies PCA. Saltzman type 3: PPTA joins the SCA (instead of the BA). It is critical to recognize a PPTA before doing a Wada test (p. 1553) because of the risk anesthetizing the brainstem, and in doing transsphenoidal surgery because of risk of arterial injury. May rarely be an explanation of posterior fossa symptoms in a patient with carotid disease

2. otic: the first to involute, and the rarest to persist (8 cases reported). Passes through IAC to connect petrous carotid to basilar artery
3. hypoglossal: connects petrous or distal cervical ICA (origin usually between C1-C3) to VA. Traverses the hypoglossal canal. Does not cross foramen magnum

4. proatlantal intersegmental: connects cervical ICA to VA. May arise from: bifurcation of common carotid, ECA, or ICA from C2-C4. Anastomosis with VA in suboccipital region. 50% have hypoplastic proximal VA. 40 cases reported

2.3 Cerebral venous anatomy

2.3.1 Supratentorial venous system

Major veins and tributaries

See ▶ Fig. 2.9 for angiogram and branches.

The left and right internal jugular veins (IJVs) are the major source of outflow of blood from the intracranial compartment. The *right* IJV is usually dominant. Other sources of outflow include orbital veins and the venous plexuses around the vertebral arteries. Diploic and scalp veins may act as collateral pathways, e.g. with superior sagittal sinus obstruction.[16] The following outline traces the venous drainage back from the IJVs.

Inferior petrosal sinus

Terminates (i.e. drains to) ≤ 1 cm of junction of sigmoid and transverse sinuses.

Sigmoid sinus

superior petrosal sinus

Drains to IJV near junction with sigmoid sinus

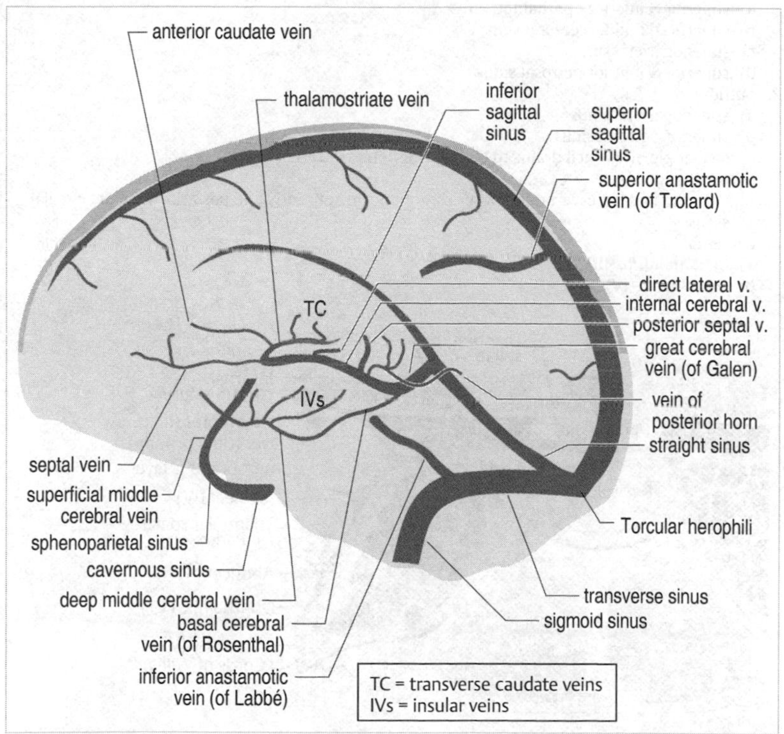

Fig. 2.9 Internal carotid venogram (lateral view) (Reprinted courtesy of Eastman Kodak Company)

Transverse sinus
R > L in 65%.

► **V. of Labbe.** (Inferior anastomotic v.)

► **Confluens of sinuses.** (Torcular herophili)

1. occipital sinus
2. superior sagittal sinus
   a) v. of Trolard (superior anastomotic v.): the prominent superficial vein on the ***non-dominant*** side (Labbé is more prominent on the dominant side)
   b) cortical veins
3. straight sinus
   a) inferior sagittal sinus
   b) great cerebral v. (of Galen)
      - pre-central cerebellar v.
      - basal vein of Rosenthal
      - internal cerebral v.: joined at the foramen of Monro (venous angle) by:
        anterior septal v.
        thalamostriate v.

Cavernous sinus

Originally named for its superficial resemblance to the corpora cavernosa. Although classical teaching depicts the cavernous sinus as a large venous space with multiple trabeculations, injection studies[17] and surgical experience[18] instead supports the concept of the cavernous sinus as a plexus of veins. It is highly variable between individuals and from side-to-side. ► Fig. 2.10 is an oversimplified schematic of one section through the right cavernous sinus.

1. inflowing veins:
   a) superior & inferior ophthalmic veins
   b) superficial middle cerebral veins
   c) sphenoparietal sinus
   d) superior & inferior petrosal sinus
2. outflow:
   a) sphenoparietal sinus
   b) superior petrosal sinus
   c) basilar plexus (which drains to the inferior petrosal sinus)
   d) pterygoid plexus
   e) the right and left cavernous sinuses communicate anteriorly and posteriorly via the circular sinus
3. contents[19]
   a) Oculomotor n. (III)
   b) Trochlear n. (IV)

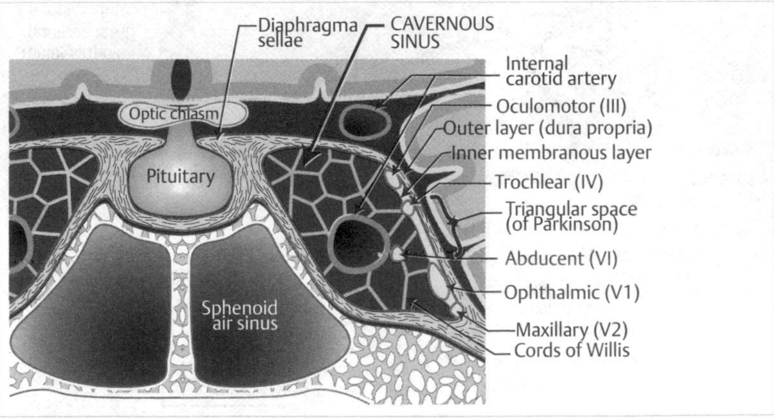

Fig. 2.10 Right cavernous sinus (coronal section)

c) Ophthalmic division of trigeminal (V1)
d) Maxillary division of trigeminal (V2): the only nerve of the cavernous sinus that doesn't exit the skull through the superior orbital fissure (it exits through foramen rotundum)
e) Carotid artery (ICA). 3 segments within the cavernous sinus
  • posterior ascending segment: immediately after ICA enters the sinus
  • horizontal segment: after ICA turns anteriorly (the longest segment of the intracavernous ICA)
  • anterior ascending segment: ICA turns superiorly
f) Abducens n. (VI): the only nerve NOT attached to lateral dural wall, sometimes referred to as the only cranial nerve inside the cavernous sinus

4. triangular space (of Parkinson): superior border formed by Cr. N. III & IV, and the lower margin formed by V1 & VI (a landmark for surgical entrance to the cavernous sinus)[20,21 (p 3007)]

2.3.2 Posterior fossa venous anatomy

See ▸ Fig. 2.11.

2.4 Spinal cord vasculature

See ▸ Fig. 2.12.

Although a radicular artery from the aorta accompanies the nerve root at many levels, most of these contribute little flow to the spinal cord itself. The anterior spinal artery is formed from the junction of two branches, each from one of the vertebral arteries. Major contributors of blood supply to the anterior spinal cord is from 6–8 radicular arteries at the following levels ("radiculomedullary arteries", the levels listed are fairly consistent, but the side varies[22 (p 1180–1)]):

1. C3 – arises from vertebral artery
2. C6 and C8 (≈ 10% of population lack an anterior radicular artery in lower cervical spine[23])
   a) C6 – usually arises from deep cervical artery
   b) C8 – usually from costocervical trunk
3. T4 or T5
4. artery of Adamkiewicz AKA arteria radicularis anterior magna
   a) the main arterial supply for the spinal cord from ≈ T8 to the conus
   b) located on the left in 80%[24]
   c) situated between T9 & L2 in 85% (between T9 & T12 in 75%); in remaining 15% between T5 & T8 (in these latter cases, there may be a supplemental radicular artery further down)

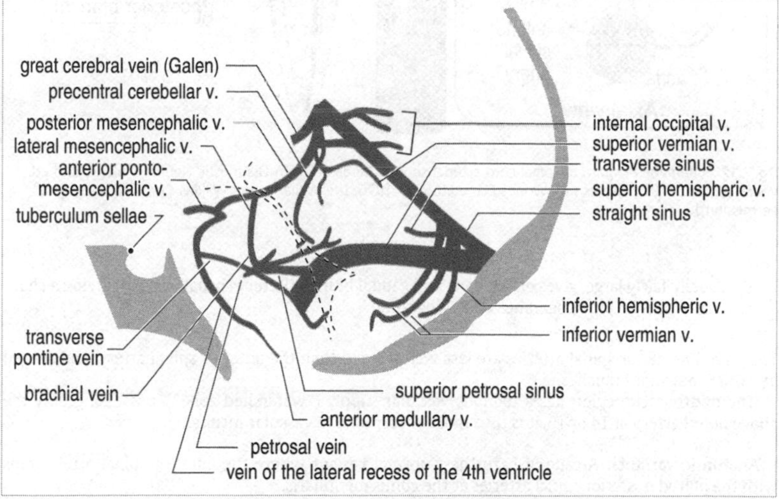

Fig. 2.11 Vertebrobasilar venogram (lateral view) (Reprinted courtesy of Eastman Kodak Company)

2

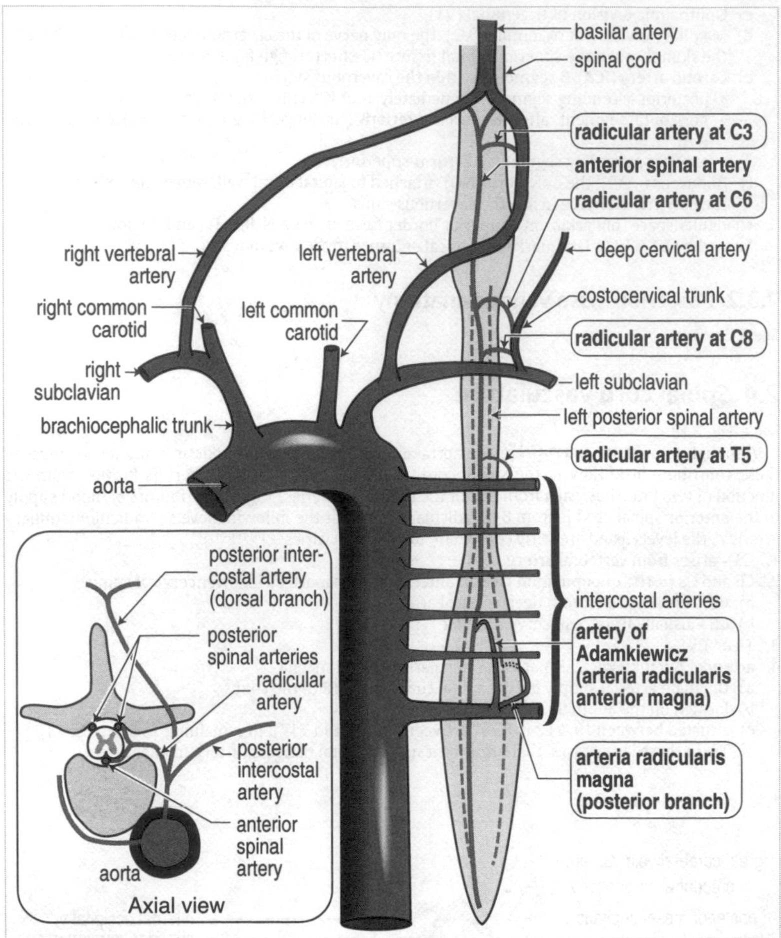

Fig. 2.12 Schematic diagram of spinal cord arterial supply (Modified from Diagnostic Neuroradiology, 2nd ed., Volume II, pp. 1181, Taveras J M, Woods EH, editors, © 1976, the Williams and Wilkins Co., Baltimore, with permission))

d) usually fairly large, gives off cephalic and caudal branch (latter is usually larger) giving a characteristic hair-pin appearance on angiography

The paired posterior spinal arteries are less well defined than the anterior spinal artery, and are fed by 10–23 radicular branches.

The midthoracic region has a tenuous vascular supply ("watershed zone"), possessing only the above noted artery at T4 or T5. It is thus more susceptible to vascular insults.

▶ **Anatomic variants.** Arcade of Lazorthes: normal variant where the anterior spinal artery joins with the paired posterior spinal arteries at the conus medullaris.

References

[1] van der Zwan A, Hillen B, Tulleken CAF, Dujovny M, Dragovic L. Variability of the Territories of the Major Cerebral Arteries. J Neurosurg. 1992; 77:927–940

[2] Loukas M, Louis RG, Jr, Childs RS. Anatomical examination of the recurrent artery of Heubner. Clin Anat. 2006; 19:25–31

[3] Fischer E. Die Lageabweichungen der Vorderen Hirnarterie im Gefässbild. Zentralbl Neurochir. 1938; 3:300–313

[4] Bouthillier A, van Loveren HR, Keller JT. Segments of the internal carotid artery: A new classification. Neurosurgery. 1996; 38:425–433

[5] Krayenbühl HA, Yasargil MG. Cerebral Angiography. 2nd ed. London: Butterworths; 1968:80–81

[6] Krayenbühl H, Yasargil MG, Huber P. In: Rontgenanatomie und Topographie der Hirngefasse. Zerebrale Angiographie fur Klinik und Praxis. Stuttgart: Georg Thieme Verlag; 1979:38–246

[7] Ecker A, Riemenschneider PA. Angiographic Localization of Intracranial Masses. Springfield, Illinois: Charles C. Thomas; 1955

[8] Gibo H, Lenkey C, Rhoton AL. Microsurgical Anatomy of the Supraclinoid Portion of the Internal Carotid Artery. J Neurosurg. 1981; 55:560–574

[9] Renn WH, Rhoton AL. Microsurgical Anatomy of the Sellar Region. J Neurosurg. 1975; 43:288–298

[10] Rhoton AL, Jr. The supratentorial arteries. Neurosurgery. 2002; 51:S53–120

[11] Anatomical examination of the recurrent artery of Heubner. Clin Anat. 2006; 19:25–31

[12] Lister JR, Rhoton AL, Matsushima T, et al. Microsurgical Anatomy of the Posterior Inferior Cerebellar Artery. Neurosurgery. 1982; 10:170–199

[13] Getch CC, O'Shaughnessy BA, Bendok BR, Parkinson RJ, Batjer HH. Surgical management of intracranial aneurysms involving the posterior inferior cerebellar artery. Contemp Neurosurg. 2004; 26:1–7

[14] Percheron G. The anatomy of the arterial supply of the human thalamus and its use for the interpretation of the thalamic vascular pathology. Z Neurol. 1973; 205:1–13

[15] Luh GY, Dean BL, Tomsick TA, Wallace RC. The persistent fetal carotid-vertebrobasilar anastomoses. AJR Am J Roentgenol. 1999; 172:1427–1432

[16] Schmidek HH, Auer LM, Kapp JP. The Cerebral Venous System. Neurosurgery. 1985; 17:663–678

[17] Taptas JN. The So-Called Cavernous Sinus: A Review of the Controversy and Its Implications for Neurosurgeons. Neurosurgery. 1982; 11:712–717

[18] Sekhar LN, Schramm VL. In: Operative Management of Tumors Involving the Cavernous Sinus. Tumors of the Cranial Base: Diagnosis and Treatment. Mount Krisco: Futura Publishing; 1987:393–419

[19] Umansky F, Nathan H. The Lateral Wall of the Cavernous Sinus: with Special Reference to the Nerves Related to It. J Neurosurg. 1982; 56:228–234

[20] van Loveren HR, Keller JT, El-Kalliny M, Scodary DJ, Tew JM. The Dolenc Technique for Cavernous Sinus Exploration (Cadaveric Prosection). J Neurosurg. 1991; 74:837–844

[21] Youmans JR. Neurological Surgery. Philadelphia 1982

[22] Taveras JM, Wood EH. Diagnostic Neuroradiology. 2nd ed. Baltimore: Williams and Wilkins; 1976

[23] Turnbull IM, Breig A, Hassler O. Blood Supply of the Cervical Spinal Cord in Man. A Microangiographic Cadaver Study. J Neurosurg. 1966; 24:951–965

[24] El-Kalliny M, Tew JM, van Loveren H, Dunsker S. Surgical approaches to thoracic disk herniations. Acta Neurochir. 1991; 111:22–32

3 Neurophysiology and Regional Brain Syndromes

3.1 Neurophysiology

3.1.1 Blood-brain barrier

General information

The passage of water-soluble substances from the blood to the CNS is limited by tight junctions (zonulae occludentes) which are found between cerebral capillary endothelial cells, limiting penetration of the cerebral parenchyma (blood-brain barrier, BBB), as well as between choroid plexus epithelial cells (blood-CSF barrier).[1] A number of specialized mediated transport systems allow transmission of, among other things, glucose and certain amino acids (especially precursors to neurotransmitters).

The efficacy of the BBB is compromised in certain pathological states (e.g. tumor, infection, trauma, stroke, hepatic encephalopathy...), and can also be manipulated pharmacologically (e.g. hypertonic mannitol increases the permeability, whereas steroids reduce the penetration of small hydrophilic molecules).

The BBB is absent in the following areas: choroid plexus, hypophysis, tuber cinereum, area postrema, pineal and preoptic recess.

Means of assessing the integrity of the BBB:

- visible dyes: Evan's blue, fluorescein
- radioopaque dyes (imaged with CT scan[2]): iodine (protein bound contrast agent)
- paramagnetic (imaged on MRI): gadolinium (protein-bound contrast agent)
- microscopic: horseradish peroxidase
- radiolabeled: albumin, sucrose

Cerebral edema and the blood brain barrier

Three basic types of cerebral edema; diffusion-weighted MRI (p. 232) may be able to differentiate:

1. cytotoxic: BBB is closed, therefore no protein extravasation, therefore no enhancement on CT or MRI. Cells swell then shrink. Seen e.g. in head injury
2. vasogenic: BBB disrupted. Protein (serum) leaks out of vascular system, and therefore may enhance on imaging. Extracellular space (ECS) expands. Cells are stable. Responds to corticosteroids (e.g. dexamethasone). Seen e.g. surrounding metastatic brain tumor
3. ischemic: a combination of the above. BBB closed initially, but then may open. ECS shrinks then expands. Fluid extravasates late. May cause delayed deterioration following intracerebral hemorrhage (p. 1337).

3.1.2 Babinski sign and Hoffmann sign

Introduction

Although the Babinski sign is regarded as the most famous sign in neurology, there is still disagreement over what constitutes a normal response and when abnormal responses should occur.[3] The following represents one interpretation.

The plantar reflex (PR) (AKA Babinski sign after Joseph François Félix Babinski (1857–1932) a French neurologist of Polish descent) is a primitive reflex, present in infancy, consisting of extension of the great toe in response to a noxious stimulus applied to the foot. The small toes may fan, but this is not a consistent nor clinically important component. The PR disappears usually at ≈ 10 months age (range: 6 mos to 12 yrs), presumably under inhibitory control as myelination of the CNS occurs, and the normal response then converts to plantarflexion of the great toe. An upper motor neuron (UMN) lesion anywhere along the pyramidal (corticospinal) tract from the motor strip down to ≈ L4 will result in a loss of inhibition, and the PR will be "unmasked" producing extension of the great toe. With such an UMN lesion, there may also be exaggeration of flexor synergy resulting in dorsiflexion of the ankle, and flexion of the knee and hip (AKA triple flexor response) in addition to extension of the great toe.

Neuroanatomy

The afferent limb of the reflex originates in cutaneous receptors restricted to the first sacral dermatome (*S1*) and travels proximally via the tibial nerve. The spinal cord segments involved in the reflex-arc lie within *L4-S2*. The efferent limb to the toe extensors travels via the *peroneal nerve*.

Differential diagnosis

Etiologies

Lesions producing a PR need not be structural, but may be functional and reversible. The roster of possible etiologies is extensive, some are listed in ► Table 3.1.

Eliciting the PR, and variations

The optimal stimulus consists of stimulation of the lateral plantar surface and transverse arch in a single movement lasting 5–6 seconds.[4] Other means for applying noxious stimuli may also elicit the plantar reflex (even outside the S1 dermatome, although these do not produce toe flexion in normals). Described maneuvers include: Chaddock (scratch the lateral foot; positive in 3% where plantar stimulation was negative), Schaeffer (pinch the Achilles tendon), Oppenheim (slide knuckles down shin), Gordon (momentarily squeeze lower gastrocnemius), Bing (light pinpricks on dorsolateral foot), Gonda or Stronsky (pull the 4th or 5th toe down and out and allow it to snap back).

Hoffman's (or Hoffmann's or Hoffmann) sign

Attributed to Johann Hoffmann, a German neurologist practicing in the late 1800. May signify a similar UMN interruption to the upper extremities. Elicited by flicking downward on the nail of the middle or ring finger: a positive (pathologic) response consists of involuntary flexion of the adjacent fingers and/or thumb (may be weakly present in normals).[5] Differs from the plantar reflex since it is monosynaptic (synapse in Rexed lamina IX).

Can sometimes be seen as normal in young individual with diffusely brisk reflexes & positive jaw jerk, usually symmetric. When present pathologically, represents disinhibition of a C8 reflex, ∴ indicates lesion above C8.

Hoffmann sign was observed in 68% of patients operated for cervical spondylotic myelopathy.[5] In 11 patients presenting with lumbar symptoms but no myelopathy, a bilateral Hoffman sign was associated with occult cervical spinal cord compression in 10 (91%).[5] The Hoffmann test has a sensitivity of 33-68%, specificity of 59-78%, a positive predictive value of 26-62% and negative predictive value of 67-75%.[6]

3.1.3 Bladder neurophysiology

Central pathways

The primary coordinating center for bladder function resides within the nucleus locus coeruleus of the pons. This center synchronizes bladder contraction with relaxation of the urethral sphincter during voiding.[7]

Voluntary cortical control primarily involves inhibition of the pontine reflex, and originates in the anteromedial portion of the frontal lobes and in the genu of the corpus callosum. In an uninhibited bladder (e.g. infancy) the pontine voiding center functions without cortical inhibition and the detrusor muscle contracts when the bladder reaches a critical capacity. Voluntary suppression from the cortex via the pyramidal tract may contract the external sphincter and may also inhibit detrusor contraction. Cortical lesions in this location → urgency incontinence with inability to suppress the micturition reflex.[8 (p 1031)]

Efferents to the bladder travel in the dorsal portion of the lateral columns of the spinal cord (shaded areas in ► Fig. 3.1).

Table 3.1 Differential diagnosis of the plantar reflex (PR)

Etiologies
• spinal cord injuries[a] • cervical spinal myelopathy • lesions in motor strip or internal capsule (stroke, tumor, contusion...) • subdural or epidural hematoma • hydranencephaly • toxic-metabolic coma • seizures • trauma • TIAs • hemiplegic migraine • motor neuron disease (ALS)
[a]in spinal cord injuries, the PR may initially be absent during the period of spinal "shock" (p. 931)

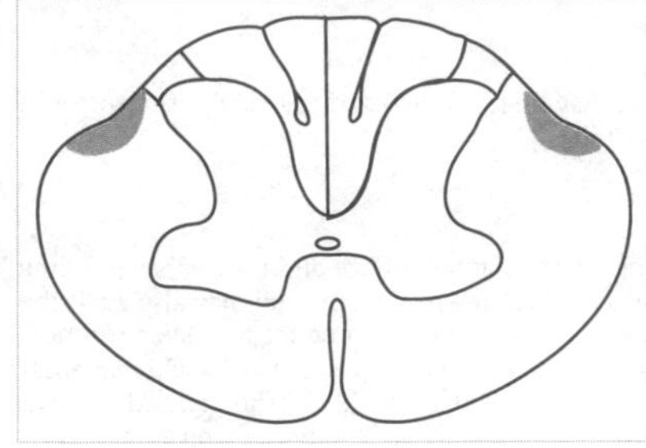

Fig. 3.1 Location of spinal cord bladder efferents (shaded)

Motor

There are two sphincters that prevent the flow of urine from the bladder: internal (autonomic, involuntary control), and external (striated muscle, voluntary control).

Parasympathetics (PSN)

The detrusor muscle of the bladder contracts and the internal sphincter relaxes under PSN stimulation. PSN preganglionic cell bodies reside in the intermediolateral grey of spinal cord segments *S2–4*. Fibers exit as ventral nerve roots and travel via pelvic splanchnic nerves (nervi erigentes) to terminate on ganglia within the wall of the detrusor muscle in the body and dome of the bladder.

Somatic nerves

Somatic voluntary control descends in the pyramidal tract to synapse on motor nerves in S2–4, and then travels via the pudendal nerve to the external sphincter. This sphincter may be voluntarily contracted, but relaxes reflexly with opening of the internal sphincter at the initiation of micturition. Primarily maintains continence during ↑ vesical pressure (e.g. valsalva).

Sympathetics

Sympathetic cell bodies lie within the intermediolateral gray column of lumbar spinal cord from segments T12 – L2. Preganglionic axons pass through the sympathetic chain (without synapsing) to the inferior mesenteric ganglion. Postganglionic fibers pass through the inferior hypogastric plexus to the bladder wall and internal sphincter. Sympathetics heavily innervate the bladder neck and trigone. Sympathetics have little effect on bladder motor activity, but alpha adrenergic stimulation results in bladder neck closure which is necessary for bladder filling.

Pelvic nerve stimulation → increased sympathetic tone → detrusor relaxation & increased bladder neck tone (allowing larger volume to be accommodated).

Sensory

Less well understood than motor innervation. Bladder wall stretch receptors sense bladder filling and send afferent signals via pelvic, pudendal and hypogastric nerves to spinal cord segments T10-L2 & S2–4. Fibers ascend primarily in the spinothalamic tract.

Urinary bladder dysfunction

The term neurogenic bladder describes bladder dysfunction due to lesions within the central or peripheral nervous systems. Some use the term synonymously with detrusor areflexia.

Dorsal (sensory) roots lesions interrupt the afferent limb, producing an atonic bladder that fills until dribbling and overflow incontinence occur. No sensation of bladder fullness is appreciated. Voluntary voiding is still possible, but is usually incomplete.

Detrusor hyperreflexia

Can result from interruption of efferents anywhere from cortex to sacral cord. When a critical volume is attained, reflex bladder emptying occurs. Clinically associated with frequent, uncontrollable, precipitous voiding. Cerebral lesions include: stroke, head injury, brain tumors, hydrocephalus, Parkinson's disease, various dementias, and MS. Cord lesions include anything that causes myelopathy (p. 1407).

Detrusor areflexia

Clinically correlates with difficulty initiating micturition, interrupted flow, and significant residual urine. Incontinence may result from over-distention of the bladder (overflow incontinence), or may be associated with absence of sphincter tone. Etiologies include: chronic infection, long-term bladder catheterization, certain drugs (especially phenothiazines), injury or tumor of the cauda equina or conus medullaris, myelomeningocele, and diabetes mellitus (autonomic neuropathy).

Specific injuries affecting the bladder

In general, regarding discrete neurologic lesions affecting the bladder[9]:

1. supraspinal (lesions above the brain stem): loss of centrally mediated inhibition of the pontine voiding reflex. Usually produces involuntary bladder contractions with smooth and striated sphincter synergy, often with preserved sensation and voluntary striated sphincter function. Symptoms: urinary frequency or urgency, urgency incontinence, and nocturia.[7] If sensory pathways are interrupted, unconscious incontinence occurs (incontinence of the unawares type). Since muscles are coordinated, normal bladder pressures are maintained and there is low risk of high-pressure related renal dysfunction. Voluntary bladder emptying is usually maintained, and timed voiding together with anticholinergic medications (see below) are used in management. Areflexia may sometimes occur
2. complete (or near complete) spinal cord lesions:
   a) suprasacral (lesion *above* the S2 spinal *cord* level, which is ≈ T12/L1 vertebral body level in an adult): the sacral voiding center is located in the conus medullaris. Etiologies: spinal cord injuries, tumors, transverse myelitis.
      - Initially following spinal cord injury, there may be spinal shock. During spinal shock (p. 931), the bladder is acontractile and areflexic (detrusor areflexia); sphincter tone usually persists and urinary retention is the rule (urinary incontinence generally does not occur except with overdistention)
      - After spinal shocksubsides, most develop *detrusor hyperreflexia* → involuntary bladder contractions without sensation (automatic bladder), smooth sphincter synergy, but striated dyssynergy (involuntary contraction of the external sphincter during voiding which produces a functional outlet obstruction with poor emptying and high vesical pressures). Bladder fills and empties spontaneously (or in response to lower extremity cutaneous stimulation). Bladder compliance is often reduced. Managed by intermittent catheterizations + anticholinergics
   b) infrasacral lesions (lesion below the S2 spinal cord level): includes injury to conus medullaris, cauda equina or peripheral nerves (formerly referred to as lower motor neuron lesions). Etiologies: large HLD, trauma with compromise of spinal canal. Usually develop detrusor areflexia, and do not have involuntary bladder contractions. Reduced urinary flow rate or retention results, and voluntary voiding may be lost. Overflow incontinence develops. There may be reduced compliance during filling, and paralysis of the smooth sphincter (the neurologic basis of this has not been settled, and may be due to sympathetic or PSN involvement). Usually associated with loss of bulbocavernosus and anal wink reflex (preserved in suprasacral lesions, except when spinal shock is present (p. 931)) and perineal sensory loss
3. interruption of the peripheral reflex arc: may produce disturbances similar to low spinal cord injury with detrusor areflexia, low compliance and inability to relax the striated sphincter
4. herniated lumbar disc (p. 1046): most consist initially of difficulty voiding, straining, or urinary retention. Later, irritative symptoms may develop
5. spinal stenosis (lumbar or cervical): urologic symptoms vary, and depend on the spinal level(s) involved and the type of involvement (e.g. in cervical spinal stenosis, detrusor hyperactivity or underactivity may occur depending on whether the involvement of the micturition neural axis is compression of the inhibitory reticulospinal tracts or myelopathy involving the posterior funiculus)
6. cauda equina syndrome (p. 1050): usually produces urinary retention, although sometimes incontinence may occur (some cases are overflow incontinence)
7. peripheral neuropathies: such as with diabetes, usually produce impaired detrusor activity
8. neurospinal dysraphism: most myelodysplastic patients have an areflexic bladder with an open bladder neck. The bladder usually fills until the resting residual fixed external sphincter pressure is exceeded and the leakage occurs

9. multiple sclerosis: 50–90% of patients develop voiding symptoms at some time. The demyelination primarily involves the posterior and lateral columns of the cervical spinal cord. Detrusor hyperreflexia is the most common urodynamic abnormality (in 50–99% of cases), with bladder areflexia being less common (5–20%)

Urinary retention

Etiologies of urinary retention:

1. bladder outlet obstruction (a brief differential diagnosis list is presented here)
   a) urethral stricture: retention tends to be progressive over time
   b) prostatic enlargement in males:
      - benign prostatic hypertrophy (BPH) & prostate cancer: retention tends to be progressive over time
      - acute prostatitis: onset of retention may be *sudden*
      - rare: extruded prostatic stone
   c) women may develop a cystocele which can produce a urethral kink
   d) rare: urethral cancer
2. detrusor areflexia (p. 93) or hypotonia
   a) spinal cord injury
   b) cauda equina syndrome (p. 1050)
   c) chronic infection
   d) long-term bladder catheterization
   e) certain drugs (narcotics, phenothiazines)
   f) injury of the cauda equina or conus medullaris, or of the spinal cord at or below the sacrum
      - trauma
      - tumor
      - myelomeningocele
   g) diabetes mellitus (autonomic neuropathy)
   h) herpes zoster at the level of the sacral dorsal root ganglia[9 (p 967)]
   i) incomplete opening of the bladder neck during voiding: occurs almost exclusively in young and middle-aged males with longstanding obstructive and irritative symptoms[9 (p 968)]
   j) initially following severe bladder over distention or with chronic distention and decompression from any of the above
3. postoperative retention: well-recognized but poorly understood. More common after lower urinary tract, perineal, gynecologic and anorectal operations. Anesthesia and analgesia may contribute to a number of factors[9 (p 969)]
4. psychogenic

Evaluation of bladder function

Urodynamics

Usually combined with x-ray (cystometrogram (CMG))or fluoro (videourodynamics). Measures intravesicular pressures during retrograde bladder filling through a urethral catheter, usually combined with sphincter electromyography. Presence or absence (detrusor areflexia, see below) of detrusor reflex is detected. If present, procedure is repeated, asking patient to suppress the urge to void. Inability to suppress is called an uninhibited detrusor reflex (AKA detrusor hyperreflexia, see above).

Sphincter electromyography (EMG)

Either via needle electrodes, or with externally mounted surface electrodes. Voluntary sphincter contraction tests intactness of supraspinal innervation. When combined with CMG, detects electrical activity in sphincters during associated phases of detrusor contraction.

Voiding cystourethrogram and intravenous pyelography (IVP)

Voiding cystourethrogram (VCUG) detects urethral pathology (diverticula, strictures…), abnormalities of bladder (diverticula, detrusor trabeculations associated with longstanding contractions against high resistance…), and vesical-ureteral reflux.

3

Pharmacologic Treatment

Goals are to preserve renal function (which usually involves prevention of UTIs, renal calculi, and ureteral reflux due to high intravesicular pressures) and optimization of urinary continence. Patients with inadequate emptying or increased bladder pressure are often managed by intermittent catheterizations and anticholinergics (see below). Anticholinergics and behavioral therapy are used for patients with maintained voluntary bladder emptying with urinary frequency or urgency incontinence.

The majority of the neurologic involvement in bladder contraction is ACh-mediated stimulation of postganglionic parasympathetic muscarinic cholinergic receptors on bladder smooth muscle.

Detrusor hyperreflexia

The following are all synthetic anticholinergics that block postganglionic synapses (muscarinic action) without blocking skeletal neuromuscular or autonomic ganglia (nicotinic junctions). This increases the volume at which automatic (reflex) contraction occurs in the neurogenic (uninhibited) bladder, effectively increasing bladder capacity. These agents increase the threshold at which involuntary bladder contraction occurs, but they do not increase the warning time and they do not increase the ability to suppress contraction, therefore, urgency and incontinence will still occur unless treatment is combined with a regimen of timed voiding.[9(p 972)]

All are contraindicated in glaucoma as the anticholinergic effects include mydriasis. Overdosage results in the classic anticholinergic symptoms ("red as a beet, hot as a stove, dry as a rock, mad as a hatter"). Use is often limited by side effects such as dry mouth.

Drug info: Oxybutynin (Ditropan®)

Probably the most widely prescribed agent. Combines anticholinergic activity with independent musculotropic relaxant effect and local anesthetic activity.

℞ Adults: usual dose is 5 mg BID-TID (maximum 4 times daily). ℞ Peds: not recommended for age < 5 years; usual dose is 5 mg BID (maximum 5 mg TID). **Supplied:** 5 mg tablets, 5 mg/5 ml syrup.

Drug info: Tolterodine (Detrol®)

Milder side effects than oxybutynin, but may also be less effective.[10]

℞ 2 mg PO BID. Can be lowered to 1 mg PO BID in some patients. **Supplied:** 1 & 2 mg tablets. Detrol® LA 2 & 4 mg capsule

Drug info: Flavoxate HCl (Urispas®)

Weak anticholinergic. Direct smooth muscle inhibitor. Few reported side effects. Some studies have shown no benefit in the elderly population.[9(p 974)]

℞ Adult: 100–200 mg PO TID-QID.

Drug info: Imipramine HCl (Tofranil®)

A tricyclic antidepressant. Mechanism of beneficial effect is controversial. Does possess some anticholinergic activity as well as other porperties.[9(p 977)] Appears to decrease bladder contractility and increase outlet resistance.

3

Detrusor areflexia

Drug info: Bethanechol (Urecholine®)

A parasympathomimetic agent, primarily muscarinic with little nicotinic activity; related to acetylcholine but not destroyed by cholinesterase. Increases the tone of the detrusor muscle, aiding bladder emptying. Also increases gastric motility. Sub-Q administration produces a more intense effect on the bladder than PO. Always have atropine available when giving by sub-Q route. Effects occur within 30–90 minutes after PO dose, and within 15 minutes of sub-Q dose.

Indicated for acute post-op non-obstructive urinary retention and for neurogenic atony due to spinal cord injury or dysfunction.

Side effects: sweating and diarrhea are not uncommon but of little danger. Can precipitate severe bronchospasm in asthmatics. Nausea may be reduced by giving with an empty stomach. Atropine is a specific antidote for overdosage (atropine sub-Q: 0.6 mg in adults, or 0.01 mg/kg in children < 12 yrs).

℞ Start with 5–10 mg PO, and increase hourly until desired effect obtained or 50 mg given. Then, continue minimum effective dosage TID-QID (usual: 10–50 mg PO TID-QID). Sub-Q (have atropine available): 0.5–1 ml, repeat q 15 mins until desired response or 4 doses given; continue minimal effective dose TID-QID. **Supplied:** 5, 10, 25 & 50 mg tabs. Injection: 5.15 mg/ml (for sub-Q use only).

Bladder management after cauda equina compression

In situations where there is urinary retention with some prospect of return of function (e.g. following surgery for acute cauda equina compression) the following bladder management regimen may be employed:

- teach the patient or a family member to perform clean intermittent catheterizations (CIC), if CICs can be done:
  - have them monitor post-void residuals (PVR)
  - start tamsulosin (Flomax®) 0.4 mg PO q d (see below)
  - if PVRs ever fall to < 75 cc, discontinue CICs
- if CICs cannot be performed, manage with an indwelling Foley catheter for a week, and check the PVR after that time
- if after 1 week the PVR is ≥ 75 cc, D/C tamsulosin if used, and refer the patient to a urologist for urodynamics (urodynamics earlier than this time will usually not result in a change in management)

Drug info: Tamsulosin (Flomax®)

A prostate $alpha_{1A}$adrenoreceptor antagonist. Used to treat voiding difficulties resulting from outlet obstruction due to benign prostatic hypertrophy (BPH). Has been shown to have some effectiveness in women via other mechanisms. Similar to terazosin (Hytrin®) and doxazosin (Cardura®), but has an advantage for acute relief because the dose of tamsulosin does not need to be gradually ramped up (it can be started at the therapeutic dose). It takes at least 5–7 days to work.

Side effects : very few. Rhinitis, retrograde or diminished ejaculation, or postural hypotension may occur.[11]

℞: 0.4 mg PO q d (usually given 30 minutes after the same meal each day). If there is no response by 2–4 weeks, a dose of 0.8 mg PO q d can be tried.[11]

3.2 Regional brain syndromes

This section serves to briefly describe typical syndrome associated with lesions in various areas of the brain. Unless otherwise noted, lesions considered are *destructive*.

3.2.1 Overview

1. frontal lobe
   a) unilateral injury:
      - may produce few clinical findings except with very large lesions
      - bilateral or large unilateral lesions: apathy, abulia

- the frontal eye field (for contralateral gaze) is located in the posterior frontal lobe (Br. area 8, shown as the striped area in ▶ Fig. 1.1). Destructive lesions impair gaze to the contralateral side (patient looks *towards* the side of the lesion), whereas irritative lesions (i.e. seizures) cause the center to activate, producing contralateral gaze (patient looks *away* from the side of the lesion). See also **Extraocular muscle (EOM) system** (p.565) for more details.

b) bilateral injury: may produce apathy, abulia
c) olfactory groove region: may produce Foster Kennedy syndrome (see below)
d) prefrontal lobes control "executive function": planning, prioritizing, organizing thoughts, suppressing impulses, understanding the consequences of decisions

2. parietal lobe: major features (see below for details)
   a) either side: cortical sensory syndrome, sensory extinction, contralateral homonymous hemianopia, contralateral neglect
   b) dominant parietal lobe lesion (left in most): language disorders (aphasias), Gerstmann's syndrome (p.98), bilateral astereognosis
   c) non-dominant parietal lobe lesions: topographic memory loss, anosognosia and dressing apraxia
3. occipital lobe: homonymous hemianopsia
4. cerebellum
   a) lesions of the cerebellar hemisphere cause ataxia in the *ipsilateral* limbs
   b) lesions of the cerebellar vermis cause truncal ataxia
5. brainstem: usually produces a mixture of cranial nerve deficits and long tract findings (see below for some specific brainstem syndromes)
6. pineal region
   a) Parinaud's syndrome (p.99)

3.2.2 Parietal lobe syndromes

See reference.[12 (p 308–12)]

Parietal lobe anatomy

The parietal lobe is located behind the central sulcus, above the Sylvian fissure, merging posteriorly into the occipital lobe (the border on the medial surface of brain is defined by a line connecting the parieto-occipital sulcus to the pre-occipital notch).

Parietal lobe neurophysiology

- either side: anterior parietal cortex organizes tactile precepts (probably contralateral) and integrates with visual and auditory sensation to build awareness of body and its spatial relations
- dominant side (on left in 97% of adults): understanding language, includes "cross-modal matching" (auditory-visual, visual-tactile, etc.). Dysphasia present with dominant lobe lesions often impedes assessment
- non-dominant side (right in most): integrates visual and proprioceptive sensation to allow manipulation of body and objects, and for certain constructional activities

Clinical syndromes of parietal lobe disease

Overview

1. *unilateral* parietal lobe disease (dominant or non-dominant):
   a) cortical sensory syndrome (see below) and sensory extinction (neglecting 1 of 2 simultaneously presented stimuli). Large lesion → hemianesthesia
   b) congenital injury → mild hemiparesis & contralateral muscle atrophy
   c) homonymous hemianopia or visual inattentiveness
   d) occasionally: anosognosia
   e) neglect of contralateral half of body and visual space (more common with right side lesions)
   f) abolition of *optokinetic nystagmus* to one side
2. additional effects of dominant parietal lobe lesion (left in most):
   a) language disorders (aphasias)
   b) speech-related or verbally mediated functions, e.g. cross-modal matching (e.g. patient understands spoken words and can read, but cannot understand sentences with elements of relationships)

   c) Gerstmann's syndrome, classically:
      - agraphia without alexia (patients can read but cannot write)
      - left-right confusion
      - digit agnosia: inability to identify finger by name
      - acalculia
   d) tactile agnosia (bilateral astereognosis)
   e) bilateral ideomotor apraxia (inability to carry out verbal commands for activities that can otherwise be performed spontaneously with ease)
3. additional effects of non-dominant parietal lobe lesions (usually right):
   a) topographic memory loss
   b) anosognosia and dressing apraxia

Cortical sensory syndrome

Lesion of postcentral gyrus, especially area that maps to hand.
- sensory deficits:
  a) loss of position sense and of passive movement sense
  b) inability to localize tactile, thermal, and noxious stimuli
  c) astereognosis (inability to judge object size, shape, and identity by feel)
  d) agraphesthesia (cannot interpret numbers written on hand)
  e) loss of two point discrimination
- preserved sensations: pain, touch, pressure, vibration, temperature
- other features
  a) easy fatigability of sensory perceptions
  b) difficulty distinguishing simultaneous stimulations
  c) prolongation of superficial pain with hyperpathia
  d) touch hallucinations

Anton-Babinski syndrome

A unilateral asomatagnosia. May seem more common with non-dominant (usually right) parietal lesions because it may be obscured by the aphasia that occurs with dominant (left) sided lesions.
1. anosognosia (indifference or unawareness of deficits, patient may deny that paralyzed extremity is theirs)
2. apathy (indifference to failure)
3. allocheiria (one-sided stimuli perceived contralaterally)
4. dressing apraxia: neglect of one side of body in dressing and grooming
5. extinction: patient is unaware of contralateral stimulus when presented with double-sided simultaneous stimulation
6. inattention to an entire visual field (with or without homonymous hemianopia), with deviation of head, eyes, and torsion of body to unaffected side

Parietal lobe aphasias

1. Wernicke's aphasia: lesion of auditory association areas or their separation from angular gyrus and primary auditory cortex. A *fluent* aphasia (normal sentence length & intonation, devoid of meaning). May include paraphasias. Lesion in region of Wernicke's area (Brodmann areas 40 & 39, ▶ Fig. 1.1)
2. Broca's (motor) aphasia: in reality, "apraxia" of motor sequencing for speech (speech and phonation muscles aren't paralyzed, and function for other activities), producing faltering, dysarthric speech. Lesion in region of Broca's area (Brodmann area 44, ▶ Fig. 1.1)
3. global aphasia: usually due to lesion that destroys large portion of language center; all aspects of speech and language affected
   a) unable to speak except for some clichés, habitual phrases, or expletives
   b) anomia (inability to name objects or parts of objects)
   c) verbal and motor perseveration
   d) unable to understand all except for a few words
   e) inability to read or write
4. conduction aphasia: due to disruption of connections between frontal and temporal speech areas, usually involving supramarginal gyrus. Similar to Wernicke's (fluent spontaneous speech and paraphasias), but patients understand spoken or written words, and are aware of their deficit. Repetition is severely affected

5. pure word blindness: AKA alexia without agraphia (rare) due to lesion in parieto-occipital lobe that interrupts connections between left angular gyrus and both occipital lobes. Patients can write, but are unable to read what they've written, and frequently seem unconcerned about this. Often accompanied by loss of ability to name colors. Reading and naming numbers usually preserved

3.2.3 Foster Kennedy syndrome

Named after neurologist Robert Foster Kennedy. Usually from olfactory groove or medial third sphenoid wing tumor (usually meningioma). Now rare due to early detection by CT or MRI. Classic triad:
1. ipsilateral anosmia
2. *ipsilateral* central scotoma (with optic *atrophy* due pressure on optic nerve)
3. *contralateral* papilledema (from elevated ICP)

Occasionally ipsilateral proptosis will also occur due to orbital invasion by tumor.

3.2.4 Brain stem and related syndromes

Weber's syndrome

Cr. N. III palsy with contralateral hemiparesis; also see Lacunar strokes (p. 1267). Third nerve palsies from parenchymal lesions may be relatively pupil sparing.

Benedikt's syndrome

Similar to Weber's, plus red nucleus lesion. Cr. N. III palsy with contralateral hemiparesis except arm which has hyperkinesia, ataxia, and a coarse intention tremor. Lesion: midbrain tegmentum involving red nucleus, brachium conjunctivum, and fascicles of III.

Millard-Gubler syndrome

Facial (VII) & abducens (VI) palsy + contralateral hemiplegia (corticospinal tract) from lesion in base of pons (usually ischemic infarct, occasionally tumor).

3.2.5 Parinaud's syndrome

Definition

AKA dorsal midbrain syndrome, AKA pretectal syndrome. As originally described, a supranuclear paralysis of vertical gaze resulting from damage to the mesencephalon.[13]

There are a number of somewhat varying descriptions, however most include:
- supranuclear upward gaze palsy (i.e. upgaze palsy affecting both voluntary saccadic and pursuit movements, with preservation of vestibulo-ocular or oculocephalic (doll's eyes) reflexes in most cases). Horizontal eye movements are spared
- lid retraction (Collier's sign): NB: upgaze palsy + lid retraction produces the "setting sun sign"
- convergence palsy
- accommodation palsy
- less common associations: pseudoabducens palsy (AKA thalamic esotropia), see-saw nystagmus, fixed pupils, dissociated light-near response (pseudo-Argyll Robertson), convergence spasm, nystagmus retractorius, internuclear ophthalmoplegia (INO)

Skew deviation may be a unilateral variant of Parinaud's syndrome.

Syndrome of the Sylvian aqueduct: Parinaud's syndrome (PS) combined with downgaze palsy.

Differential diagnosis

Etiologies
1. masses pressing directly on quadrigeminal plate (e.g. pineal region tumors)
2. elevated ICP: secondary to compression of mesencephalic tectum by dilated suprapineal recess, e.g. in hydrocephalus

3. stroke or hemorrhage in upper brainstem
4. multiple sclerosis (MS)
5. occasionally seen with toxoplasmosis

Conditions affecting ocular motility that could mimic the upgaze palsy of PS:
1. Guillain-Barré syndrome
2. myasthenia gravis
3. botulism
4. hypothyroidism
5. there may be a gradual benign loss of upgaze with senescence

3.3 Jugular foramen syndromes

3.3.1 Applied anatomy

The jugular foramen (JF) is one of a pair of openings between the lateral part of the occipital bone and the petrous part of the temporal bone. The foramen is usually divided in 2 by a bony spine from the petrous temporal bone that attaches via a fibrous bridge (which is bony in 26%) to the jugular process of the occipital bone.[14] The right JF is usually larger than the left.[14,15] The carotid ridge separates the JF from the nearby carotid canal. Contents of jugular foramen (JF): Cr. N. IX, X, XI, petrosal sinus, sigmoid sinus, some meningeal branches from the ascending pharyngeal and occipital arteries.[16]

Nearby: Cr. N. XII passes through the hypoglossal canal just above the occipital condyle. The carotid artery with the sympathetic plexus enters the carotid canal.

Compartmentalization of the jugular foramen remains controversial. As many as 4 foramina have been described over the years. Although it had been recognized previously, an early 2-compartment description was published in 1967 by Hovelacque.[17] In this, the bony spine (± its fibrous septum) divide the foramen into:
- pars vascularis: the larger posterolateral compartment containing the vagal nerve (and branching Arnold's nerve), spinal accessory nerve and the internal jugular vein
- pars nervosa: the smaller anteromedial compartment containing the glossopharyngeal nerve (and branching Jacobson's nerve), inferior petrosal sinus and meningeal branch of the ascending pharyngeal artery

A publication in 1997 described these 3 compartments[18]:
- Sigmoid: large posterolateral compartment containing sigmoid sinus
- Petrosal: smaller anteromedial compartment containing petrosal sinus
- Intrajugular or neural: CN 9, 10 and 11

3.3.2 Clinical syndromes

General information

A number of eponymous syndromes with some conflicting findings in the literature have been described. See ▶ Table 3.2 for a summary and ▶ Fig. 3.2 for a schematic diagram of deficits in various JF syndromes.

Vernet's syndrome: CN IX, X & XI palsy

AKA syndrome of the jugular foramen. Usually due to intracranial lesion.

Etiologies include: jugular foramen tumors, ICA dissections, mycotic aneurysms of the external carotid, thrombosis of the jugular vein, following carotid endarterectomy.

Symptoms: unilateral paralysis of the palate, vocal cords, sternocleidomastoid, trapezius, with loss of taste in the posterior 1/3 tongue, anesthesia of the soft palate, larynx and pharynx.

Collet-Sicard syndrome

Palsies of CN IX, X, XI & XII without sympathetic involvement. More likely with lesion outside skull. If caused by an intracranial lesion, it would have to be of such a large size that it would usually produce brain stem compression → long tract findings.

Table 3.2 Cranial nerve dysfunction in jugular foramen syndromes

Nerve	Result of lesion	Syndrome					
		Vernet	Collet Sicard	Villaret	Tapia	Jackson	Schmidt
IX	loss of taste and sensation in posterior third of tongue	X	X	X			
X	paralysis of vocal cords & palate, anesthesia of pharynx & larynx	X	X	X	X	X	X
XI	weak trapezius & SCM	X	X	X	±	X	X
XII	tongue paralysis & atrophy		X	X	X	X	
sympathetics	Horner's syndrome			X	±		

Key: X indicates dysfunction / deficit (lesion) of that nerve; ± indicates involvement may or may not occur

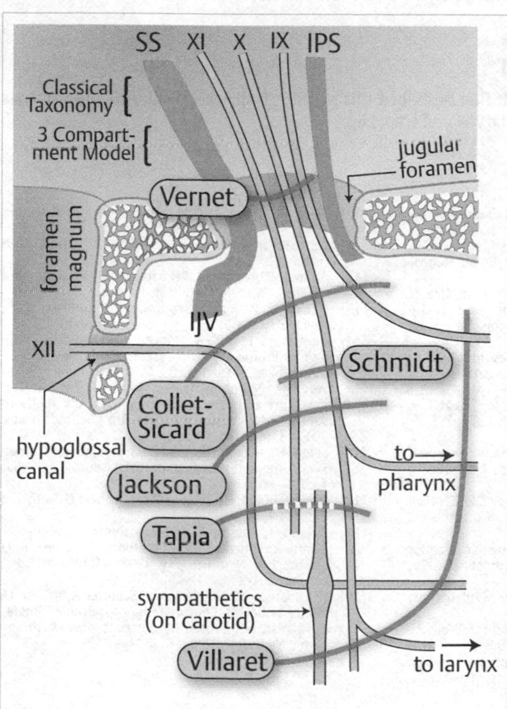

Fig. 3.2 Schematic diagram of the jugular foramen (coronal section through left jugular foramen viewed from the front). Includes the classic 2 compartment model and the 3 compartment classification of Katsuta et al.[18] Jugular foramen syndromes are illustrated: a solid line through a nerve indicates a deficit, dashed line indicates ± involvement.

Etiologies include: condylar and Jefferson's fractures, internal carotid dissection, primary and metastatic tumors, Lyme disease and fibromuscular dysplasia.

Symptoms: unilateral paralysis of the palate, vocal cords, sternocleidomastoid, trapezius, tongue, loss of taste in posterior 1/3 tongue, anesthesia of soft palate, larynx and pharynx.

3

Villaret's syndrome: CN IX, X, XI & XII palsy + sympathetic dysfunction

AKA posterior retropharyngeal syndrome, AKA the nervous syndrome of the posterior retroparotid space). Collet-Sicard syndrome with sympathetic involvement. Usually due to retropharyngeal leasions.

Etiologies include: parotid tumors, metastases, external carotid aneurysm and osteomyelitis of the skull base.

Symptoms: as with Collet-Sicard + Horner's syndrome.

Tapia syndrome: CN X & XII palsy (± XI)

AKA Matador's disease (first described in a bullfighter by Antonio Garcia Tapia). Some authors describe an intracranial and extracranial form.[19]

Etiologies include: oral intubation (majority of cases prior to 2013), metastases, rarely associated with carotid or vertebral artery dissections.

Symptoms: hoarseness of voice, dysphagia secondary to incoordination of tongue and food bolus propulsion, unilateral atrophy and paralysis of the tongue, ± paralysis of sternocleidomastoid & trapezius, sparing the soft palate.

(Hughlings) Jackson's syndrome: CN X, XI & XII palsy

First described in 1864 with unilateral paralysis of the soft palate, larynx, sternocleidomastoid, trapezius and tongue.

Schmidt syndrome: CN X & XI

AKA vago-spinal syndrome. Schmidt first described this in 1892. Unilateral vocal cord and paralysis of sternocleidomastoid, soft palate, larynx and trapezius.

References

[1] Neuwelt EA, Barnett PA, McCormick CI, Frenkel EP, et al. Osmotic Blood-Brain Barrier Modification: Monoclonal Antibody, Albumin, and Methotrexate Delivery to Cerebrospinal Fluid and Brain. Neurosurgery. 1985; 17:419–423

[2] Neuwelt EA, Maravilla KR, Frenkel EP, et al. Use of Enhanced Computerized Tomography to Evaluate Osmotic Blood-Brain Barrier Disruption. Neurosurgery. 1980; 6:49–56

[3] Marcus JC. Flexor Plantar Responses in Children With Upper Motor Neuron Lesions. Arch Neurol. 1992; 49:1198–1199

[4] Dohrmann GJ, Nowack WJ. The Upgoing Great Toe: Optimal Method of Elicitation. Lancet. 1973; 1:339–341

[5] Houten JK, Noce LA. Clinical correlations of cervical myelopathy and the Hoffmann sign. J Neurosurg Spine. 2008; 9:237–242

[6] Glaser JA, Cure JK, Bailey KL, Morrow DL. Cervical spinal cord compression and the Hoffmann sign. Iowa Orthop J. 2001; 21:49–52

[7] MacDiarmid SA. The ABCs of Neurogenic Bladder for the Neurosurgeon. Contemp Neurosurg. 1999; 21:1–8

[8] Youmans JR. Neurological Surgery. Philadelphia 1982

[9] Wein AJ, Walsh PC, Retik AB, Vaughan ED, Wein AJ. In: Neuromuscular Dysfunction of the Lower Urinary Tract and Its Treatment. Campbell's Urology. 7th ed. Philadelphia: W.B. Saunders; 1998:953–1006

[10] Tolterodine for Overactive Bladder. Med Letter. 1998; 40:101–102

[11] Tamsulosin for Benign Prostatic Hyperplasia. Med Letter. 1997; 39

[12] Adams RD, Victor M. Principles of Neurology. 2nd ed. New York: McGraw-Hill; 1981

[13] Pearce JM. Parinaud's syndrome. J Neurol Neurosurg Psychiatry. 2005; 76

[14] Rhoton AL, Jr, Buza R. Microsurgical anatomy of the jugular foramen. J Neurosurg. 1975; 42:541–550

[15] Osunwoke EA, Oladipo GS, Gwuinereama IU, Ngaokere JO. Morphometric analysis of the foramen magnum and jugular foramen in adult skulls in southern Nigerian population. Am J Sci Indust Res. 2012; 3:446–448

[16] Svien HJ, Baker HL, Rivers MH. Jugular Foramen Syndrome and Allied Syndromes. Neurology. 1963; 13:797–809

[17] Hovelacque A. Osteologie. Paris, France: G. Doin and Cie; 1967; 2

[18] Katsuta T, Rhoton AL, Jr, Matsushima T. The jugular foramen: microsurgical anatomy and operative approaches. Neurosurgery. 1997; 41:149–201; discussion 201-2

[19] Krasnianski M, Neudecker S, Schluter A, Krause U, Winterholler M. Central Tapia's syndrome ("matador's disease") caused by metastatic hemangiosarcoma. Neurology. 2003; 61:868–869

Part II

General and Neurology

4

4 Neuroanesthesia

4.1 General information

▶ Table 4.1 shows the American Society of Anesthesiologists (ASA) grading system to estimate anesthetic risk for various conditions.

For issues related to intracranial pressure (ICP), cerebral perfusion pressure (CPP), intracranial constituents, etc., see ICP principles (p. 856). For cerebral blood flow (CBF) and cerebral metabolic rate of oxygen consumption ($CMRO_2$), see CBF and oxygen utilization (p. 1264).

Parameters of primary relevance to neurological surgery that can be modulated by the anesthesiologist:

1. blood pressure: one of the factors that determines CPP as well as spinal cord perfusion. May need to be manipulated (e.g. reduced when working on an aneurysm, or increased to enhance collateral circulation during cross clamping). Measurement by arterial line is most accurate and depending on the patient's presentation and the planned procedure, often should be placed prior to induction of anesthesia. For intracranial procedures, the arterial line should be calibrated at the external auditory meatus to most closely reflect intracranial blood pressure
2. jugular venous pressure: one of the factors that influences ICP
3. arterial CO_2 tension ($PaCO_2$): CO_2 is the most potent cerebral vasodilator. Hyperventilation reduces $PaCO_2$ (hypocapnea) which decreases CBV but also CBF. Goal is generally end tidal CO_2 ($ETCO_2$) of 25–30 mm Hg with a correlating $PaCO_2$ of 30–35. Use with care for stereotactic procedures to minimize shift of intracranial contents when using this method to control ICP[4]
4. arterial O_2 tension
5. hematocrit: in neurosurgery it is critical to balance oxygen carrying capacity (decreased by anemia) against improved blood rheology (impaired by elevated Hct)
6. patient temperature: mild hypothermia provides some protection against ischemia by reducing the cerebral metabolic rate of oxygen ($CMRO_2$) by ≈ 7% for each 1° C drop
7. blood glucose level: hyperglycemia exacerbates ischemic deficits[5]
8. $CMRO_2$: reduced with certain neuro-protective agents and by hypothermia which helps protect against ischemic injury
9. in cases where a lumbar drain or a ventricular drain has been placed: CSF output
10. elevation of the head of the patient: lowering the head increases arterial blood flow, but also increases ICP by impairing venous outflow
11. intravascular volume: hypovolemia can impair blood flow in neurovascular cases. In surgery in the prone position, excessive fluids may contribute to facial edema which is one of the risk factors for PION (p. 1056)
12. positioning injuries: during the procedure, the patient's position may change and be unnoticed due to draping. Careful and frequent examination of the patient's position may prevent injuries associated with prolonged malpositioning
13. post operative nausea and vomiting (PONV): may adversely affect ICP and may negatively impact recent cervical surgical procedures. Avoidance of anesthetic agents known to cause PONV or pretreatment to prevent PONV may be prudent

4.2 Drugs used in neuroanesthesia

4.2.1 Inhalational agents

General information

Most reduce cerebral metabolism (except nitrous oxide) by suppressing neuronal activity. These agents disturb cerebral autoregulation and cause cerebral vasodilatation which increases cerebral blood volume (CBV) and can increase ICP. With administration > 2 hrs they increase CSF volume which can also potentially contribute to increased ICP. Most agents increase the CO_2 reactivity of cerebral blood vessels. These agents affect intra-operative EP monitoring (p. 107).

Drug info: Nitrous oxide

A potent vasodilator that markedly increases CBF and minimally increases cerebral metabolism. Contributes to post-op N/V.

Nitrous oxide, pneumocephalus and air embolism: The solubility of nitrous oxide (N_2O) is ≈ 34 times that of nitrogen.[6] When N_2O comes out of solution in an airtight space it can increase the pressure which may convert pneumocephalus to "tension pneumocephalus." It may also aggravate air embolism. Thus caution must be used especially in the sitting position where significant post-op pneumocephalus and air embolism are common. The risk of tension pneumocephalus may be reduced by filling the cavity with fluid in conjunction with turning off N_2O about 10 minutes prior to completion of dural closure. See Pneumocephalus (p. 887).

Halogenated agents

Agents in primary usage today are shown below. All suppress EEG activity and may provide some degree of cerebral protection.

Drug info: Isoflurane (Forane®)

Can produce isoelectric EEG without metabolic toxicity. Improves neurologic outcome in cases of incomplete global ischemia (although in experimental studies on rats, the amount of tissue injury was greater than with thiopental[7]).

Drug info: Desflurane (Suprane®)

A cerebral vasodilator, increases CBF and ICP. Decreases $CMRO_2$ which tends to cause a compensatory vasoconstriction.

Drug info: Sevoflurane (Ultane®)

Mildly increases CBP and ICP, and reduces $CMRO_2$. Mild negative inotrope, cardiac output not as well maintained as with isoflurane or desflurane.

4.2.2 Intravenous anesthetic agents

Agents generally used for induction

1. propofol: exact mechanism of action unknown. Short half-life with no active metabolites. May be used for induction and as a continuous infusion during total intravenous anesthesia (TIVA). Causes dose dependent decrease in mean arterial blood pressure (MAP) and ICP. See also information other than use in induction (p. 106). Is more rapidly cleared than, and has largely replaced, thiopental
2. barbiturates: produce significant reduction in $CMRO_2$ and scavenge free radicals among other effects (p. 1202). Produce dose-dependent EEG suppression which can be taken all the way to isoelectric. Minimally affect EPs. Most are anticonvulsant, but methohexital (Brevital®) (p. 132) can lower the seizure threshold. Myocardial suppression and peripheral vasodilatation from barbiturates may cause hypotension and compromise CPP, especially in hypovolemic patients
   * sodium thiopental (Pentothal®): the most common agent. Rapid onset, short acting. Minimal effect on ICP, CBF and $CMRO_2$
3. etomidate (Amidate®): a carboxylated imidazole derivative. Anesthetic and amnestic, but no analgesic properties. Sometimes produces myoclonic activity which may be confused with seizures. Impairs renal function and should be avoided in patients with known renal disease. May

produce adrenal insufficiency. See Miscellaneous drugs in neuroanesthesia (p. 106) for information other than use in induction.
4. ketamine: NMDA receptor antagonist. Produces a dissociative anesthesia. Maintains cardiac output. May slightly increase both heart rate and blood pressure. ICP increases in parallel with increased cardiac output.

Narcotics in anesthesia

Nonsynthetic narcotics

Narcotics increase CSF absorption and minimally reduce cerebral metabolism. They slow the EEG but will *not* produce an isoelectric tracing. ✖ All narcotics cause dose-dependent respiratory depression which can result in hypercarbia and concomitant increased ICP in non-ventilated patients. Often also contribute to post-op N/V

Morphine: does not significantly cross the BBB.

✖ Disadvantages in neuro patients:

1. causes histamine release which
   a) may produce hypotension
   b) may cause cerebrovascular vasodilation → increased ICP[8 (p 1593)]
   c) the above together may compromise CPP
2. in renal or hepatic insufficiency, the metabolite morphine-6-glucuronide can accumulate which may cause confusion

Synthetic narcotics

These do *not* cause histamine release, unlike morphine and meperidine.

✱ Remifentanil (Ultiva®); see also detailed information (p. 133): reduces $CMRO_2$, CBV and ICP. Large doses may be neurotoxic to limbic system and associated areas. May be used for awake craniotomy (p. 1432).

Fentanyl: crosses the BBB. Reduces $CMRO_2$, CBV and ICP. May be given as bolus and/or as a continuous infusion.

Sufentanil: more potent then fentanyl. Does not increase CBF. ✖ Raises ICP (may be due to hypoventilation – which can occur with any narcotic) and is thus often not appropriate for neurosurgical cases. Expensive.

4.2.3 Miscellaneous drugs in neuroanesthesia

► **Benzodiazepines.** These drugs are GABA agonists and decrease $CMRO_2$. They also provide anticonvulsant action and produce amnesia. See also agents and reversal (p. 205).

► **Etomidate** (p. 105). Used primarily for induction (p. 105).

- a cerebrovasoconstrictor which therefore: reduces CBF and ICP; reduces $CMRO_2$ but no longer promoted as a cerebral protectant based on experimental studies[9] and a drop in $pBtO_2$ with temporary MCA clipping[10]
- does not suppress brainstem activity
- suppresses adrenocortical function cortisol production. This usually occurs with prolonged administration, but can occur even after single dose for induction and may persist up to 8 hrs (no adverse outcomes from short-term suppression have been reported)
- increases activity of seizure foci which may be used for mapping foci during seizure surgery but may also induce seizures

► **Propofol.** A sedative hypnotic. Useful for induction (p. 105). Reduces cerebral metabolism, CBF and ICP. Has been described for cerebral protection (p. 1203) and for sedation (p. 133). Short half-life permits rapid awakening which may be useful for awake craniotomy (p. 1434). Not analgesic.

► **Lidocaine.** Given IV, suppresses laryngeal reflexes which may help blunt ICP elevations that normally follow endotracheal intubation or suctioning. Anticonvulsant at low doses, may provoke seizures at high concentrations.

► **Esmolol.** Selective beta-1 adrenergic antagonist, blunts the sympathetic response to laryngoscopy and intubation. Less sedating than equipotent doses of lidocaine or fentanyl used for the same purpose. Half life: 9 minutes. See also dosing, etc. (p. 127)

► **Dexmedetomidine (Precedex®).** Alpha 2 adrenergic receptor agonist, used for control of hypertension post operatively, as well as for its sedating qualities during awake craniotomy either alone or in conjunction with propofol (p. 105). Also used to help patients tolerate endotracheal tube without sedatives/narcotics to facilitate extubation.

4.2.4 Paralytics for intubation

Paralytics (neuromuscular blocking agents (NMBA)): administered to facilitate tracheal intubation and to improve surgical conditions when indicated. Administration of paralytics ideally should always be guided by neuromuscular twitch monitoring. Also see Sedatives & paralytics (p. 132). In addition to paralytics, all conscious patients should also receive a sedative to blunt awareness.

Paralytics should not be given until it has been determined that patient can be ventilated manually, unless treating laryngospasm (may be tested with thiopental). Use with caution in non-fixated patients with unstable C-spine.

Due to long action, pancuronium (Pavulon®) is not indicated as the primary paralytic for intubation, but may be useful once patient is intubated or in *low* dose as an adjunct to succinylcholine.

Drug info: Succinylcholine (Anectine®)

The only depolarizing agent. May be used to secure airway for emergency intubation, but due to possible side effects (p. 135), should not be used acutely following injury or in adolescents or children (a short acting nondepolarizing blocker is preferred). May transiently increase ICP. Prior dosing with 10% of the ED95 dose of a non-depolarizing muscle relaxant reduces muscle fasciculations.

℞ Intubating dose: 1–1.5 mg/kg (supplied as 20 mg/ml → 3.5–5 cc for a 70 kg patient), onset 60–90 sec, duration 3–10 min, may repeat same dose × 1.

Drug info: Rocuronium (Zemuron®)

Intermediate acting, aminosteroid, non-depolarizing muscle relaxant. The only nondepolarizing neuromuscular blocking agent approved for rapid sequence intubation. Duration of action and onset are dose dependent. ℞ (p. 135).

Drug info: Vecuronium (Norcuron®)

See details (p. 136).

Aminosteroid with activity similar to that of rocuronium, however, does not cause histamine release and is not approved for rapid sequence intubation. ℞.

Drug info: Cisatracurium (Nimbex®)

See details (p. 136).

Metabolized by Hoffman degradation (temperature dependent), intermediate acting, no significant increases in histamine. ℞

4.3 Anesthetic requirements for intra-operative evoked potential monitoring

For details of intra-operative evoked potential (EP) monitoring itself, see **Intra-operative evoked potentials** (p. 239).

All volatile anesthetics produce dose-dependent reduction in SSEP peak amplitude and an increase in peak latency. Adding nitrous oxide increases this sensitivity to anesthetic agents.

Anesthesia issues related to intra-operative evoked potential (EPs) monitoring:

1. induction: minimize pentothal dose (produces ≈ 30 minutes of suppression of EPs), or use etomidate (which increases both SSEP amplitude and latency[11])
2. total intravenous anesthesia (TIVA) is ideal (i.e. no inhalational agents)
3. nitrous/narcotic technique is a distant second choice
4. if inhalational anesthetic agents are required:
   a) use < 1 MAC (maximal alveolar concentration), ideally < 0.5 MAC
   b) avoid older agents such as Halothane
5. nondepolarizing muscle relaxants have little effect on EP (in monkeys[12])
6. propofol has a mild effect on EP: total anesthesia with propofol causes less EP depression than inhalational agents at the same depth of anesthesia[13]
7. benzodiazepines have a mild-to-moderate depressant effect on EPs
8. continuous infusion of anesthetic drugs is preferred over intermittent boluses
9. SSEPs can be affected by hyper- or hypo-thermia, and changes in BP
10. hypocapnia (down to end tidal CO_2 = 21) causes minimal reduction in peak latencies[14]
11. antiepileptic drugs: phenytoin, carbamazipine and phenobarbital do not affect SSEP[15]

4.4 Malignant hyperthermia

4.4.1 General information

Malignant hyperthermia (MH) is a hypermetabolic state of skeletal muscle due to idiopathic block of Ca^{++} re-entry into sarcoplasmic reticulum. Transmitted by a multifactorial genetic predisposition. Total body O_2 consumption increases × 2–3.

Incidence: 1 in 15,000 anesthetic administrations in peds. 1 in 40,000 adults. 50% had previous anesthesia without MH. Frequently associated with administration of halogenated inhalational agents and the use of succinylcholine (fulminant form: muscle rigidity almost immediately after succinylcholine, may involve masseters → difficulty intubating). Initial attack and recrudescence may also occur post-op. 30% mortality.[16]

4.4.2 Presentation

1. earliest possible sign: *increase* in end-tidal pCO_2
2. tachycardia (early) and other arrhythmias
3. with progression:
   a) coagulation disorder (DIC) (bleeding from surgical wound and body orifices)
   b) ABG: increasing metabolic acidosis & decreasing pO_2
   c) pulmonary edema
   d) elevated body temperature (may reach ≥ 44° C (113° F) at rate of 1° C/5-min) (normal patients become hypothermic with general anesthesia)
   e) limb muscle rigidity (common, but late)
   f) rhabdomyolysis → elevated CPK & myoglobin (late)
4. terminal:
   a) hypotension
   b) bradycardia
   c) cardiac arrest

4.4.3 Treatment

1. eliminate offending agents (stop the operation, D/C inhalation anesthesia and change tubing on anesthesia machine)
2. dantrolene sodium (Dantrium®) 2.5 mg/kg IV usually effective, infuse until symptoms subside, up to 10 mg/kg
3. hyperventilation with 100% O_2
4. surface and cavity cooling: IV, in wound, per NG, PR
5. bicarbonate 1–2 mEq/kg for acidosis
6. IV insulin and glucose (lowers K^+, glucose acts as energy substrate)
7. procainamide for arrhythmias
8. diuresis: volume loading + osmotic diuretics

4.4.4 Prevention

1. identification of patients at risk:
   a) only reliable test: 4 cm viable muscle biopsy for in-vitro tests at a few regional test centers (abnormal contracture to caffeine or halothane)
   b) family history: any relative with syndrome puts patient at risk
   c) related traits: 50% of MH patients have heavy musculature, Duchenne type muscular dystrophy, or scoliosis
   d) patients who exhibit masseter spasm in response to succinylcholine
2. in patients at risk: avoid succinylcholine (nondepolarizing blockers preferred if paralysis essential), may safely have non-halogenated anesthetics (narcotics, barbiturates, benzodiazepines, droperidol, nitrous…)
3. prophylactic oral dantrolene: 4–8 mg/kg/day for 1–2 days (last dose given 2 hrs before anesthesia) is usually effective

References

[1] Schneider AJ. Assessment of Risk Factors and Surgical Outcome. Surg Clin N Am. 1983; 63:1113–1126

[2] Vacanti CJ, VanHouten RJ, Hill RC. A Statistical Analysis of the Relationship of Physical Status to Post-operative Mortality in 68,388 Cases. Anesth Analg Curr Res. 1970; 49:564–566

[3] Marx GF, Mateo CV, Orkin LR. Computer Analysis of Postanesthetic Deaths. Anesthesiology. 1973; 39:54–58

[4] Benveniste R, Germano IM. Evaluation of factors predicting accurate resection of high-grade gliomas by using frameless image-guided stereotactic guidance. Neurosurg Focus. 2003; 14

[5] Martin A, Rojas S, Chamorro A, Falcon C, Bargallo N, Planas AM. Why does acute hyperglycemia worsen the outcome of transient focal cerebral ischemia? Role of corticosteroids, inflammation, and protein O-glycosylation. Stroke. 2006; 37:1288–1295

[6] Raggio JF, Fleischer AS, Sung YF, et al. Expanding Pneumocephalus due to Nitrous Oxide Anesthesia: Case Report. Neurosurgery. 1979; 4:261–263

[7] Drummond JC, Cole DJ, Patel PM, Reynolds LW. Focal Cerebral Ischemia during Anesthesia with Etomidate, Isofluorane, or Thiopental: A Comparison of the Extent of Cerebral Injury. Neurosurgery. 1995; 37:742–749

[8] Shapiro HM, Miller RD. In: Neurosurgical Anesthesia and Intracranial Hypertension. Anesthesia. 2nd ed. New York: Churchill Livingstone; 1986:1563–1620

[9] Drummond JC, McKay LD, Cole DJ, Patel PM. The role of nitric oxide synthase inhibition in the adverse effects of etomidate in the setting of focal cerebral ischemia in rats. Anesth Analg. 2005; 100:841–6, table of contents

[10] Hoffman WE, Charbel FT, Edelman G, Misra M, Ausman JI. Comparison of the effect of etomidate and desflurane on brain tissue gases and pH during prolonged middle cerebral artery occlusion. Anesthesiology. 1998; 88:1188–1194

[11] Koht A, Schutz W, Schmidt G, Schramm J, Watanabe E. Effects of etomidate, midazolam, and thiopental on median nerve somatosensory evoked potentials and the additive effects of fentanyl and nitrous oxide. Anesth Analg. 1988; 67:435–441

[12] Sloan TB. Nondepolarizing neuromuscular blockade does not alter sensory evoked potentials. J Clin Monit. 1994; 10:4–10

[13] Liu EH, Wong HK, Chia CP, Lim HJ, Chen ZY, Lee TL. Effects of isoflurane and propofol on cortical somatosensory evoked potentials during comparable depth of anaesthesia as guided by bispectral index. Br J Anaesth. 2005; 94:193–197

[14] Schubert A, Drummond JC. The effect of acute hypocapnia on human median nerve somatosensory evoked responses. Anesth Analg. 1986; 65:240–244

[15] Borah NC, Matheshwari MC. Effect of antiepileptic drugs on short-latency somatosensory evoked potentials. Acta Neurol Scand. 1985; 71:331–333

[16] Nelson TE, Flewellen EH. The Malignant Hyperthermia Syndrome. N Engl J Med. 1983; 309:416–418

5

5 Sodium Homeostasis and Osmolality

5.1 Serum osmolality and sodium concentration

Clinical significance of various serum osmolarity values is shown in ▶ Table 5.1.

▶ **Serum osmolality.** May be estimated using Eq (5.1).

$$\text{Osmolarity (mOsm/L)} = 2 \times \{[\text{Na}^+] + [\text{K}^+]\} + \frac{[\text{BUN}]}{2.8} + \frac{[\text{glucose}]}{18} \tag{5.1}$$

(with [Na^+] in mEq/L or mmol/L, and glucose and BUN in mg/dl).

NB: terms in square brackets [] represent the serum concentrations (in mEq/L for electrolytes).

▶ **Sodium content.** In the diet: usually expressed in grams Na^+ (not NaCl), a low sodium diet is considered 2 gm of Na^+ per day or less.

1 teaspoon of table salt (NaCl) has 2.3 gm of Na^+.

1 mg NaCl has 17 mEq Na^+. 1 mg Na^+ has 43 mEq Na^+.

Normal saline has 0.9 gm of NaCl/100 ml. 3% NaCl has 3 gm NaCl/100 ml.

5.2 Hyponatremia

5.2.1 General information

Key concepts

- definition: serum [Na^+] < 135 mEq/L. Common etiologies:
  - SIADH: hypotonic hyponatremia (effective serum osmol < 275 mOsm/L) with inappropriately high urinary conentration (urine osmol > 100 mOsm/L) and euvolemia or hypervolemia
  - cerebral salt wasting **(CSW)**: similar to SIADH but with extracellular fluid volume *depletion* due to renal sodium loss (urinary [Na] > 20 mEq/L)
- minimum W/U: ✓ serum [Na^+], ✓ serum osmolality, ✓urine osmolality, ✓ clinical assessment of volume status. If volume status is high or low: ✓ urinary [Na^+] ✓TSH (to R/O hypothyroidism)
- treatment: based on acuity, severity, symptoms & etiology; see SIADH (p. 115) or CSW (p. 118) as appropriate
- risk of overly rapid correction: osmotic demyelination (including central pontine myelinolysis)

▶ **Classification.** [Na^+] < 135 mEq/L = mild, < 130 = moderate, < 125 = severe hyponatremia.

▶ **Hyponatremia in neurosurgical patients.** Chiefly seen in:

- syndrome of inappropriate antidiuretic hormone secretion (p. 114), SIADH (p. 114): dilutional hyponatremia with normal or *elevated intravascular volume.* The most common type of

Table 5.1 Clinical correlates of serum osmolality

Value (mOsm/L)	Comment
282–295	normal
< 240 or > 321	panic values
> 320	risk of renal failure
> 384	produces stupor
> 400	risk of generalized seizures
> 420	usually fatal

hyponatremia.[1] Usually treated with *fluid restriction*. May be associated with numerous intracranial abnormalities (▶ Table 5.2) and following transsphenoidal surgery

- cerebral salt wasting (CSW): inappropriate natriuresis with *volume depletion*. Treated with *volume replacement* (opposite to SIADH) and *sodium*; symptoms from derangements due to CSW may be exacerbated by fluid restriction (p. 118).[2] Etiology of 6% of cases of hyponatremia following aneurysmal SAH[3]

Table 5.2 Etiologies of SIAD[a]

Malignant tumors
1. especially bronchogenic small-cell Ca 2. tumors of GI or GU tract 3. lymphomas 4. Ewing's sarcoma
CNS disorders
1. infection: a) encephalitis b) meningitis: especially in peds c) TB meningitis d) AIDS e) brain abscess 2. head trauma: 4.6% prevalence 3. increased ICP: hydrocephalus, SDH... 4. SAH 5. brain tumors 6. cavernous sinus thrombosis 7. ✱ post craniotomy, especially following surgery for pituitary tumors, craniopharyngiomas, hypothalamic tumors 8. MS 9. Guillain-Barré 10. Shy-Drager 11. delirium tremens (DTs)
Pulmonary disorders
1. infection: pneumonia (bacterial & viral), abscess, TB, aspergillosis 2. asthma 3. respiratory failure associated with positive pressure respiration
Drugs
1. drugs that release ADH or potentiate it a) chlorpropramide (Diabinese®): increases renal sensitivity to ADH b) carbamazepine (Tegretol®), even more common with oxcarbazepine c) HCTZ d) SSRIs, TCAs e) clofibrate f) vincristine g) antipsychotics h) NSAIDs i) MDMA ("ecstasy") 2. ADH analogues a) DDAVP b) oxytocin: ADH cross activity, may also be contaminated with ADH
Endocrine disturbances
1. adrenal insufficiency 2. hypothyroidism
Miscellaneous
1. anemia 2. stress, severe pain, nausea or hypotension (all can stimulate ADH release), postoperative state 3. acute intermittent porphyria (AIP)
[a]excerpted and modified[9,1]

▸ **Other etiologies of hyponatremia:**
- renal failure
- volume overload (e.g. as in congestive heart failure)
- pseudohyponatremia: osmotically active solutes (e.g. glucose, mannitol, marked hyperlipidemia, or hyperproteinemia (which can occur in multiple myeloma)[4]) draw water from cells and also reduce the water fraction of plasma and produce artifactually low sodium values (an artifact of *indirect* lab techniques). For every 100 mg/dl increase of glucose, serum [Na] decreases by 1.6–2.4 mEq/L. It is necessary to measure serum osmolality to rule-out pseudohyponatremia
- postoperative hyponatremia: a rare condition usually described in young, otherwise healthy women undergoing elective surgery[5] and may be related to administration of even only mildly hypotonic fluids (sometimes in modest amounts)[6] and the actions of ADH (which may be increased due to stress, pain or medications)

5

5.2.2 Evaluation of hyponatremia

▸ Fig. 5.1 shows an algorithm for evaluating the etiology of hyponatremia[7] which drives treatment decisions. Work-up requires assessment of:
1. serum sodium: must be < 135 mEq/L to qualify as hyponatremia
2. the *effective* serum osmolality(AKA tonicity) is shown in Eq (5.2)

$$\text{effective serum osmolality} = \text{measured osmolality} - \frac{[\text{BUN}](\text{mg/dl})}{2.8} \tag{5.2}$$

and should be used when the blood urea nitrogen (BUN) level is elevated (for a normal [BUN] of 7–18 mg/dl, just subtract 5 from the measured osmolality). Values < 275 mOsm/kg indicate hypotonic hyponatremia
1. urine osmolality: values > 100 mOsm/kg are inappropriately high if serum tonicity is < 275 mOsm/kg
2. volume status: differentiates SIADH from CSW
   a) clinical assessment: better for hypervolemia (edema, upward trend in patient weights) but is insensitive in identifying extracellular fluid depletion as an etiology of hyponatremia[8] (look for dry mucous membranes, loss of skin turgor, orthostatic hypotension)
   b) normal saline infusion test used in uncertain cases. If baseline urine osmolality is < 500 mOsm/kg, it is usually safe to infuse 2 L of 0.9% saline over 24–48 hours. Correction of the hyponatremia suggests extracellular fluid volume depletion was the cause
   c) central venous pressure (CVP) may be used: CVP < 5–6 cm H_2O suggests hypovolemia in patients with normal cardiac function[3,7]
3. check urinary [Na^+] if volume status is high or low
4. determine duration of hyponatremia:
   a) duration documented as < 48 hours is considered acute
   b) hyponatremia of > 48 hours duration or of unknown duration is chronic
   c) hyponatremia that occurs outside the hospital is usually chronic and asymptomatic except in marathoners and MDMA ("ecstasy") drug users

5.2.3 Symptoms

Due to slow compensatory mechanisms in the brain, a gradual decline in serum sodium is better tolerated than a rapid drop. Symptoms of mild ([Na] < 130 mEq/L) or gradual hyponatremia include: anorexia, headache, difficulty concentrating, irritability, dysgeusia and muscle weakness. Severe hyponatremia (< 125 mEq/L) or a rapid drop (> 0.5 mEq/hr) can cause neuromuscular excitability, cerebral edema, muscle twitching and cramps, nausea/vomiting, confusion, seizures, respiratory arrest and possibly permanent neurologic injury, coma or death.

5.2.4 Syndrome of inappropriate antidiuresis (SIAD)

This term covers excess water retention in the face of hyponatremia, including cases due to inappropriate ADH secretion (SIADH) as well as others without increased circulating levels of ADH (e.g.

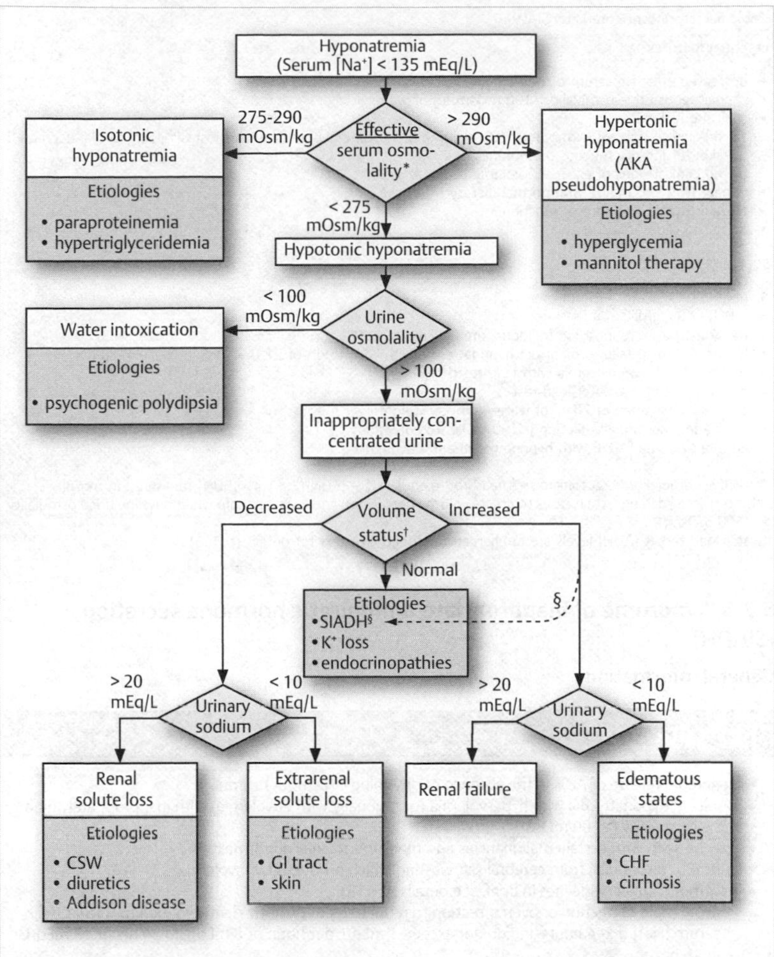

Fig. 5.1 Evaluation of the etiology of hyponatremia (adapted[7])
* effective serum osmolality = measured osmolality – [BUN]/2.8 (Eq (5.2))
† volume status is usually assessed clinically, but this may be insensitive to volume depletion
§ SIADH may be associated with euvolemia or hypervolemia

heightened response to ADH, certain drugs…). A partial list of etiologies is shown in ▶ Table 5.2 (see references[1,9] for details).

The diagnostic criteria of SIAD is shown in ▶ Table 5.3. It is critical to *measure serum osmolality* to rule-out pseudohyponatremia (p. 112), an artifact of indirect lab techniques.

Table 5.3 Diagnostic criteria for SIAD[1]

Essential features
• decreased effective serum osmolality[a] (<275 mOsm/kg of water) • simulatneous urine osmolality>100 mOsm/kg of water • clinical euvolemia a) no clinical signs of extracellular (EC) volume orthostatic hypotension (orthostasis, tachycardia, decreased skin turgor, dry mucous membranes...) b) no clinical signs of excess EC volume (edema, ascites...) • urinary [Na]>40 mEq/L with normal dietary Na intake • normal thyroid and adrenal function • no recent diuretic use
Supplemental features
• plasma [uric acid]<4 mg/dl • [BUN]<10 mg/dl • fractional Na excretion>1%; fractional urea excretion>55% • NS infusion test: failure to correct hyponatremia with IV infusion of 2 L 0.9% saline over 24–48 hrs • [b]correction of hyponatremia with fluid restriction • abnormal result on water load test[c]: a) <80% excretion of 20 ml of water/kg body weight over 5 hours, or b) inadequate urinary dilution (<100 mOsm/kg of water) • elevated plasma [ADH] with hyponatremia and euvolemia
[a]effective osmolality (AKA tonicity) = (measured osmolality) – [BUN]/2.8 with [BUN] measured in mg/dl [b]this test is used in uncertain cases (corrects volume depletion), and is usually safe when baseline urine osmolality is<500 mOsm/L [c]water load test & [ADH] levels are rarely recommended; see text for details (p. 115)

5.2.5 Syndrome of inappropriate antidiuretic hormone secretion (SIADH)

General information

Key concepts

- definition: release of ADH in the absence of physiologic (osmotic) stimuli
- results in hyponatremia with hypervolemia (occasionally with euvolemia) with inappropriately high urine osmolality (>100 mOsm/L)
- may be seen with certain malignancies and many intracranial abnormalities
- critical to distinguish from cerebral salt wasting which produces hypovolemia
- treatment: initial guidelines in brief, see details (p. 115)
  - avoid rapid correction or overcorrection to reduce risk of osmotic demyelination (p. 115). Check serum [Na⁺] q 2–4 hours and do not exceed 1 mEq/L per hour, or 8 mEq/L in 24 hrs or 18 mEq/L in 48 hrs
  - severe ([Na⁺] < 125 mEq/L of < 48 hrs duration or with severe symptoms (coma, Sz): start 3% saline at 1–2 ml/kg body weight/hr + furosemide 20 mg IV qd
  - severe ([Na⁺] < 125 mEq/L of duration > 48 hours or unknown without severe symptoms: normal saline infusion @ 100 ml/hr + furosemide 20 mg IV qd
  - chronic or unknown duration and asymptomatic: fluid restriction (▶ Table 5.4) with dietary salt and protein, and, if necessary, adjuvant drugs (demeclocycline, conivaptan...)

SIADH, AKA Schwartz-Bartter syndrome, was first described with bronchogenic cancer which is one cause of SIAD. SIADH is the release of antidiuretic hormone (ADH), AKA arginine vasopressin (AVP) (p. 151), in the absence of physiologic (osmotic) stimuli. Result: elevated urine osmolality, and expansion of the extracellular fluid volume leading to a dilutional hyponatremia which can produce fluid overload (hypervolemia), but SIADH may also occur with euvolemia. For unclear reasons, edema does not occur.

The hyponatremia of SIADH must be differentiated from that due to cerebral salt wasting (CSW) due to differences in treatment recommendations (p. 118).

Etiologies: ▶ Table 5.2.

Table 5.4 Fluid restriction recommendations[1]

Solute ratio[a]	Recommended fluid intake
> 1	< 500 ml/d
1	500–700 ml/d
< 1	< 1 L/d

[a]solute ratio defined as: $\frac{\text{urinary [Na]+urinary [K]}}{\text{plasma [Na]}}$

Diagnosis of SIADH

In general, 3 diagnostic criteria are: hyponatremia, inappropriately concentrated urine, and no evidence of renal or adrenal dysfunction. In more detail:

1. low serum sodium (hyponatremia): usually < 134 mEq/L
2. low effective serum osmolality: < 275 mOsm/L
3. high urinary sodium (salt wasting): at least > 18 mEq/L, often 50–150. Note: there has not been an adequate explanation of the high urinary sodium in SIADH
4. high ratio of urine:serum osmolality: often 1.5–2.5:1, but may be 1:1
5. normal renal function (check BUN & creatinine): BUN commonly < 10
6. normal adrenal function (no hypotension, no hyperkalemia)
7. no hypothyroidism
8. no signs of dehydration or overhydration (in many patients with acute brain disease, there is significant hypovolemia often due to CSW (p. 118) and as this is a stimulus for ADH secretion, the ADH release may be "appropriate"[10]). In uncertain cases, the normal saline infusion test (p. 112) may be used.

If further testing is required, the following are options, but are rarely recommended:

1. measure serum or urinary levels of ADH. Rarely indicated since urine osmolality > 100 mOsm/kg is usually sufficient to indicate excessive ADH.[1] ADH is normally undetectable in etiologies of hyponatremia other than SIADH
2. water-load test: considered to be the definitive test.[11] The patient is asked to consume a water load of 20 ml/kg up to 1500 ml. In the absence of adrenal or renal insufficiency, the failure to excrete 65% of the water load in 4 hrs or 80% in 5 hrs indicates SIAD.
   ✖ CONTRAINDICATIONS: this test is dangerous if the starting serum [Na⁺] is ≤ 124 mEq/L or if the patient has symptoms of hyponatremia

Symptoms of SIADH

Symptoms of SIADH are those of hyponatremia (p. 112) and possibly fluid overload. If mild, or if descent of [Na⁺] is gradual, it may be tolerated. [Na⁺] < 120–125 mEq/L is almost always symptomatic. These patients often have a paradoxical (inappropriate) thirst.

Treatment of hyponatremia with SIADH

Management is based on the severity and duration of hyponatremia, and the presence of symptoms. Two caveats:

1. ✖ be sure that hyponatremia is not due to CSW (p. 118) before restricting fluids
2. avoid too rapid correction and avoid correcting to normal or supranormal (overcorrection) sodium to reduce the risk of osmotic demyelination syndrome

Osmotic demyelination syndrome

A complication associated with some cases of treatment for hyponatremia. While excessively slow correction of acute hyponatremia is associated with increased morbidity and mortality,[12] some cases of inordinately rapid treatment have been associated with osmotic demyelination syndrome (which includes central pontine myelinolysis (CPM) a rare disorder of pontine white matter[13] (▶ Fig. 5.2) and extrapontine myelinolysis (▶ Fig. 5.3), as well as other areas of cerebral white matter). First described in alcoholics,[14] producing insidious flaccid quadriplegia, mental status changes, and cranial nerve abnormalities with a pseudobulbar palsy appearance. In one review,[15] no patient developed CPM when treated slowly as

5

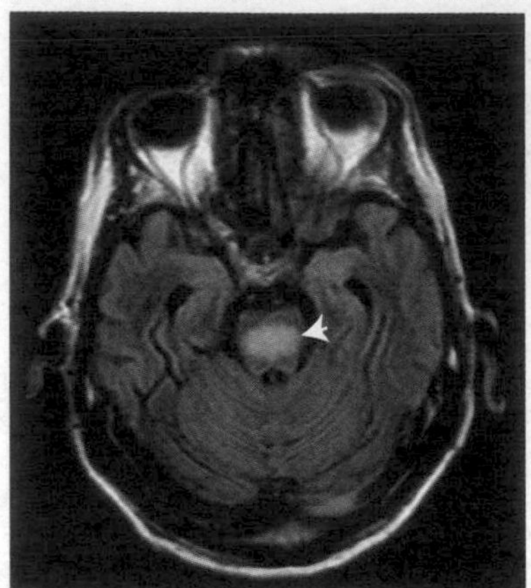

Fig. 5.2 Central pontine myelinolysis (arrowhead). Axial FLAIR MRI

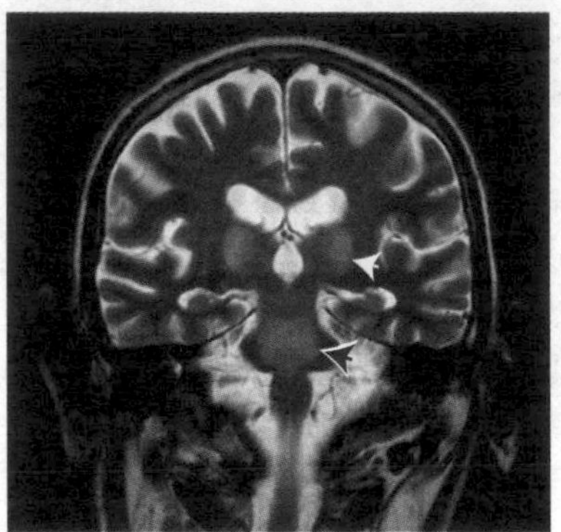

Fig. 5.3 Osmotic demyelination of pons (black arrowhead) & thalamus (white arrowhead). Coronal T2WI MRI

outlined below. And yet, the rate of correction correlates poorly with CPM; it may be that the magnitude is another critical variable.[16] Features common to patients who develop CPM are[15]:

- delay in the diagnosis of hyponatremia with resultant respiratory arrest or seizure with probable hypoxemic event
- rapid correction to normo- or hyper-natremia (> 135 mEq/L) within 48 hours of initiating therapy
- increase of serum sodium by > 25 mEq/L within 48 hours of initiation of therapy
- over-correcting serum sodium in patients with hepatic encephalopathy
- NB: many patients developing CPM were victims of chronic debilitating disease, malnourishment, or alcoholism and never had hyponatremia. Many had an episode of hypoxia/anoxia[17]
- presence of hyponatremia > 24 hrs prior to treatment[16]

The only definitive treatment is treatment of the underlying cause

- if caused by anemia: usually responds to transfusion
- if caused by malignancy, may respond to antineoplastic therapy
- most drug related cases respond rapidly to discontinuation of the offending drug

Treatment algorithms

▶ Fig. 5.4 depicts an algorithm for selecting the correct SIADH treatment protocol.

▶ **Aggressive treatment protocol.** Indications (also refer to ▶ Fig. 5.4):

1. severe hyponatremia (serum [Na^+] < 125 mEq/L)

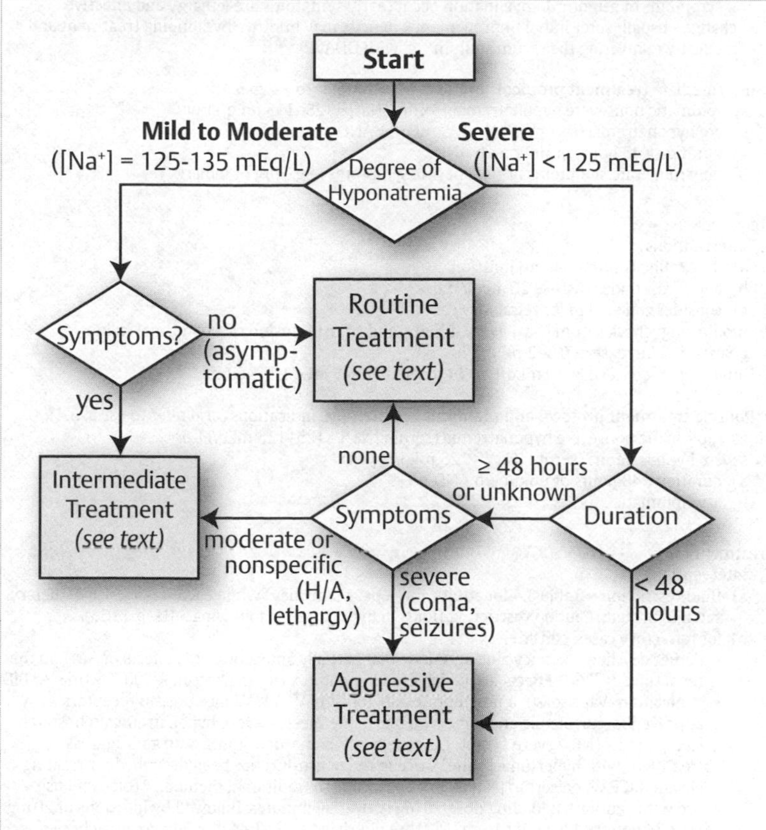

Fig. 5.4 Treatment protocol selection for hyponatremia in SIADH

2. AND either
   a) duration known to be < 48 hours
   b) or severe symptoms (coma, seizures)

Treatment
- transfer patient to ICU
- interventions
  - 3% saline: start infusion 1–2 ml/kg body weight per hour (infusion rate may be doubled to 2–4 ml/kg/hr for limited periods in patients with coma or seizures[1])
  - and furosemide (Lasix®) 20 mg IV q d (furosemide accelerates the increase in $[Na^+]$ and prevents volume overload with subsequent increase in atrial natriuretic factor and resultant urinary dumping of the extra Na^+ being administered)
- monitoring and adjustments
  - check serum $[Na^+]$ every 2–3 hours and adjust infusion rate of 3% saline
    - goal: raise serum sodium by 1–2 mEq/L/hr[18] (use lower end of range for hyponatremia > 48 hours duration or unknown duration)
    - limits: do not exceed 8–10 mEq/L in 24 hrs and 18–25 mEq/L in 48 hrs[1] (use lower end of these ranges for hyponatremia > 48 hours duration or unknown duration)
  - measure K^+ lost in urine and replace accordingly

- if symptoms of osmotic demyelination occur (early symptoms are lethargy and affective changes, usually after initial improvement): deficits may improve by stopping treatment and modestly relowering the serum sodium e.g. with DDAVP[19,20]

► **Intermediate treatment protocol.** Indications (also refer to ► Fig. 5.4):
1. symptomatic nonsevere hyponatremia (serum [Na⁺] = 125–135 mEq/L), or
2. severe hyponatremia (serum [Na⁺] < 125 mEq/L), AND
   a) duration > 48 hours or unknown AND
   b) only moderate symptoms or nonspecific symptoms (e.g. H/A, or lethargy)

Treatment
1. interventions
   a) 0.9% saline (normal saline) infusion
   b) and furosemide (Lasix®) 20 mg IV q d
   c) consider conivaptan for refractory cases
2. monitoring: check serum [Na⁺] every 4 hours and adjust infusion rate of normal saline
3. goals: [Na⁺] increase of 0.5–2 mEq/L/hr
4. limits: do not exceed 8–10 mEq/L in 24 hrs and 18–25 mEq/L in 48 hrs[1]

► **Routine treatment protocol and maintenance therapy.** Indications (also refer to ► Fig. 5.4):
1. asymptomatic nonsevere hyponatremia (serum [Na⁺] = 125–135 mEq/L), or
2. severe hyponatremia (serum [Na⁺] < 125 mEq/L) AND
   a) duration > 48 hours or unknown AND
   b) asymptomatic

Treatment
1. interventions
   a) fluid restriction ► Table 5.4 for adults, for peds: 1 L/m²/day) while encouraging use of dietary salt and protein. Caution restricting fluids in hyponatremia following SAH (p. 1166).
   b) for refractory cases, consider
      - demeclocycline: a tetracycline antibiotic that partially antagonizes the effects of ADH on the renal tubules.[21,22,23] Effects are variable, and nephrotoxicity may occur. ℞ 300–600 mg PO BID
      - conivaptan (Vaprisol®): a nonpeptide antagonist of V1A & V2 vasopressin receptors. FDA approved for euvolemic and hypervolemic moderate-to-severe hyponatremia in hospitalized patients (NB: severe symptoms of seizures, coma, delirium… warrants aggressive treatment with hypertonic saline[1]). Use in the neuro-ICU has been described for treating elevated ICP when serum [Na] is not responding to traditional methods[24] (off-label use – use with caution). ℞ loading dose 20 mg IV over 30 minutes, followed by infusions of 20 mg over 24 hours × 3 days. If serum [Na⁺] are not rising as desired, the infusion may be increased to the maximal dose of 40 mg over 24 hours. Use is approved for up to 4 days total. Caution re drug interactions
      - lithium: not very effective and many side effects. Not recommended

5.2.6 Cerebral salt wasting

Cerebral salt wasting (CSW): renal loss of sodium as a result of intracranial disease, producing hyponatremia and a decrease in extracellular fluid volume.[11] CAUTION: patients with aneurysmal SAH may have CSW with hyponatremia which mimics SIADH, however there is usually also hypovolemia in CSW. In this setting, fluid restriction may exacerbate vasospasm induced ischemia.[11,25,26,27]

The mechanism whereby the kidneys fail to conserve sodium in CSW is not known, and may be either a result of an as yet unidentified natriuretic factor or direct neural control mechanisms (see Hyponatremia following SAH (p. 1166)).

Laboratory tests (serum and urinary electrolytes and osmolalities) may be identical with SIADH and CSW.[28] Furthermore, hypovolemia in CSW may stimulate ADH release. To differentiate: CVP, PCWP, and plasma volume (a nuclear medicine study) are low in hypovolemia (i.e. CSW). ► Table 5.5 compares some features of CSW and SIADH, the two most important differences being extracellular volume and salt balance. An elevated serum [K⁺] with hyponatremia is incompatible with the diagnosis of SIADH.

Treatment of CSW
- Goals:
  - volume replacement
  - positive salt balance

Table 5.5 Comparison of CSW and SIADH[11]

Parameter	CSW	SIADH
* Plasma volume	↓ (<35 ml/kg)	↑ or WNL
* Salt balance	negative	variable
Signs & symptoms of dehydration	present	absent
Weight	↓	↑ or no Δ
PCWP	↓ (<8 mm Hg)	↑ or WNL
CVP	↓ (<6 mm Hg)	↑ or WNL
Orthostatic hypotension	+	±
Hematocrit	↑	↓ or no Δ
Serum osmolality	↑ or WNL[a]	↓
Ratio of serum [BUN]:[creatinine]	↑	WNL
Serum [protein]	↑	WNL
Urinary [Na+]	↑↑	↑
Serum [K+]	↑ or no Δ	↓ or no Δ
Serum [uric acid]	WNL	↓

Abbreviations: ↓ = decreased, ↑ = increased, ↑↑ = significantly increased, WNL = within normal limits, no Δ = no change, [] = concentration, + = present, ± = may or may not be present
[a]In reality, serum osmolality is usually ↓ in CSW

- avoid excessively rapid correction of hyponatremia or overcorrection which may be associated with osmotic demyelination (p. 115) as with SIADH (p. 115).
- Interventions
  - Hydrate patient with 0.9% NS at 100–125 ml/hr. For severe cases, 3% saline at 25–50 cc/hr is occasionally required.
  - Do not give furosemide.
  - Salt may also be simultaneously replaced orally.
  - Blood products may be needed if anemia is present.
  - Medications
    a) Fludrocortisone acetate acts directly on the renal tubule to increase sodium absorption. Benefits of giving 0.2 mg IV or PO q d in CSW have been reported,[29] but significant complications of pulmonary edema, hypokalemia and HTN may occur.
    b) Urea: an alternative treatment using urea may be applicable to the hyponatremia of either SIADH or CSW, and therefore may be used before the cause has been ascertained: urea (Ureaphil®) 0.5 grams/kg (dissolve 40 gm in 100–150 ml NS) IV over 30–60 mins q 8 hrs.[30] Use NS + 20 mEq KCl/L at 2 ml/kg/hr as the main IV until the hyponatremia is corrected (unlike mannitol, urea does not increase ADH secretion). They supplemented with colloids (viz. 250 ml of 5% albumin IV q 8–12 hrs x 72 hrs).

5.3 Hypernatremia

5.3.1 General information

Definition: serum sodium > 150 mEq/L. In neurosurgical patients, this is most often seen in the setting of diabetes insipidus (DI).

Since normal total body water (TBW) is ≈ 60% of the patient's normal body weight, the patient's current TBW may be estimated by Eq (5.3).

$$TBW_{current} = \frac{[Na^+]_{normal} \times TBW_{normal}}{[Na^+]_{current}} = \frac{140mEq/L \times 0.6 \times \text{usual body wt(kg)}}{[Na^+]_{current}} \quad (5.3)$$

The free water deficit to be replaced is given by Eq (5.4). Correction must be made slowly to avoid exacerbating cerebral edema. *One half* the water deficit is replaced over 24 hours, and the remainder is given over 1–2 additional days. Judicious replacement of deficient ADH in cases of true DI must also be made.

$$\begin{aligned}\text{free water deficit} &= 0.6 \times \text{usual body wt (kg)} - TBW_{current} \\ &= \frac{[Na^+]_{current} - 140mEq/L}{[Na^+]_{current}} \times 0.6 \times \text{usual body wt (kg)}\end{aligned} \quad (5.4)$$

5.3.2 Diabetes insipidus

General information

Key concepts

- due to low levels of ADH (or, rarely, renal insensitivity to ADH)
- high output of dilute urine (< 200 mOsmol/L or SG < 1.003) with normal or high serum osmolality and high serum sodium
- often accompanied by craving for water, especially ice-water
- danger of severe dehydration if not managed carefully

Diabetes insipidus (DI) is due to insufficient ADH activity at the kidneys, and results in the excessive renal loss of water and electrolytes. DI may be produced by two different etiologies:
- central or neurogenic DI: subnormal levels of ADH caused by hypothalamic-pituitary axis dysfunction. This is the type most often seen by neurosurgeons
- "nephrogenic DI": due to relative resistance of the kidney to normal or supra-normal levels of ADH. Seen with some drugs (drugs: l)

Etiologies of DI[31]:
1. (neurogenic AKA central) diabetes insipidus
   a) familial (autosomal dominant)
   b) idiopathic
   c) posttraumatic (brain injury, including surgery)
   d) tumor: craniopharyngioma, metastasis, lymphoma…
   e) granuloma: neurosarcoidosis, histiocytosis
   f) infectious: meningitis, encephalitis
   g) autoimmune
   h) vascular: aneurysm, Sheehan's syndrome (rarely causes DI)
2. nephrogenic diabetes insipidus
   a) familial (X-linked recessive)
   b) hypokalemia
   c) hypercalcemia
   d) Sjögren's syndrome
   e) drugs: lithium, demeclocycline, colchicine…
   f) chronic renal disease: pyelonephritis, amyloidosis, sickle cell disease, polycystic kidney disease, sarcoidosis

Central DI

85% of ADH secretory capacity must be lost before clinical DI ensues. Characteristic features: high urine output (polyuria) with low urine osmolality, and (in the conscious patient) craving for water (polydipsia), especially ice-water.

Differential diagnosis of DI:

1. (neurogenic) diabetes insipidus (true DI)
2. nephrogenic diabetes insipidus
3. psychogenic
   a) idiopathic: from resetting of the osmostat
   b) psychogenic polydipsia (excess free water intake)
4. osmotic diuresis: e.g. following mannitol, or with renal glucose spilling
5. diuretic use: furosemide, hydrochlorothiazide…

Central DI may be seen in the following situations:

1. following transsphenoidal surgery or removal of craniopharyngioma: (usually transient, therefore avoid long-acting agents until it can be determined if long-term replacement is required). Injury to the posterior pituitary or stalk usually causes one of three patterns of DI[32]:
   a) transient DI: supra-normal urine output (UO) and polydipsia which typically normalizes ≈ 12–36 hrs post-op
   b) "prolonged" DI: UO stays supra-normal for prolonged period (may be months) or even permanently: only about one–third of these patients will not return to near-normal at one year post-op
   c) "triphasic response": least common
      - phase 1: injury to pituitary reduces ADH levels for 4–5 days → DI (polyuria/polydipsia)
      - phase 2: cell death liberates ADH for the next 4–5 days → transient normalization or even SIADH-like water retention (✖ *NB*: there is a danger of inadvertently continuing vasopressin therapy beyond the initial DI phase into this phase causing significant hemodilution)
      - phase 3: reduced or absent ADH secretion → either transient DI (as in "A" above) or a "prolonged" DI (as in "B" above)
2. central herniation (p. 303): shearing of pituitary stalk may occur
3. brain death: hypothalamic production of ADH ceases
4. with certain tumors:
   a) pituitary adenomas: DI is rare even with very large macroadenomas. DI may occur with pituitary apoplexy (p. 720)
   b) craniopharyngioma: DI usually only occurs postoperatively since damage to pituitary or lower stalk does not prevent production and release of ADH by hypothalamic nuclei
   c) suprasellar germ cell tumors
   d) rarely with a colloid cyst
   e) hypothalamic tumors: Langerhans cell histiocytosis
5. mass lesions pressing on hypothalamus: e.g. a-comm aneurysm
6. following head injury: primarily with basal (clival) skull fractures (p. 884)
7. with encephalitis or meningitis
8. drug induced:
   a) ethanol and phenytoin can inhibit ADH release
   b) exogenous steroids may seem to "bring out" DI because they may correct adrenal insufficiency (below) and they inhibit ADH release
9. granulomatous diseases
   a) Wegener's granulomatosis (p. 199): a vasculitis
   b) neurosarcoidosis involving the hypothalamus (p. 189)
10. inflammatory: autoimmune hypophysitis (p. 1373) [33] or lymphocytic infundibuloneurohypophysitis[34] (distinct conditions)

Diagnosis

The following are usually adequate to make the diagnosis of DI, especially in the appropriate clinical setting:

1. dilute urine:
   a) urine osmolality < 200 mOsm/L (usually 50–150) or specific gravity (SG) < 1.003 (may be 1.001 to 1.005). (Note that normally, urine osmolality averages between 500–800 mOsm/L; extreme range: 50–1400.)
   b) or the inability to concentrate urine to > 300 mOsm/L in the presence of clinical dehydration
   c) NB: large doses of mannitol as may be used in head trauma can mask this by producing a more concentrated urine
2. urine output (UO) > 250 cc/hr (peds: > 3 cc/kg/hr)
3. normal or above-normal serum sodium

5

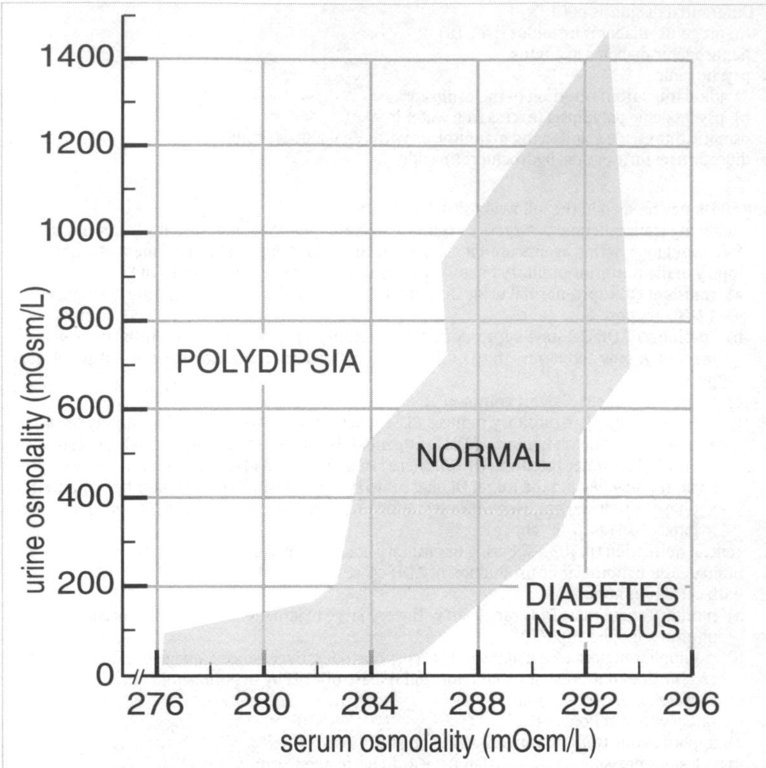

Fig. 5.5 Interpretation of simultaneous serum vs. urine osmolality (Provided by Arnold M. Moses, M.D., used with permission)

4. normal adrenal function: DI cannot occur in primary adrenal insufficiency because a minimum of mineralocorticoid activity is needed for the kidney to make free water, thus steroids may "bring out" underlying DI by correcting adrenal insufficiency

In uncertain cases, plot urine and simultaneous serum osmolality on the graph in ► Fig. 5.5.
1. low serum osmolality: usually indicates psychogenic polydipsia (pathological drinking of water)
2. if the point falls in the "normal" range, a *supervised* water deprivation test is needed to determine if the patient can concentrate their urine with dehydration (caution: see below)
3. high serum osmolality:
   - diagnosis of DI is established and no further testing to establish the diagnosis is required
   - further testing is only needed to differentiate central from nephrogenic DI, if desired to differentiate central from nephrogenic DI, give aqueous Pitressin® 5 U SQ
   - in central DI the urine osmolality should double within 1–2 hours
4. plotting more than one data point may help as some patients tend to "vacillate" around the border zones

Water deprivation test

If still unclear, the diagnosis of DI is confirmed by a water deprivation test (✖ CAUTION: perform only under close supervision as rapid and potentially fatal dehydration may ensue in DI). This test is rarely necessary if serum osmolality > 298 mOsm/L. (Note that in compensated DI, serum osmolality is more likely to be lower and to overlap with normal.[35])

Δ in urinary Osm	Interpretation
< 5% increase	normal
6–67% increase	partial ADH deficiency
> 67% increase	severe ADH deficiency

Table 5.6 Highest urinary osmolality after Pitressin in water deprivation test

- Stop IVs and make the patient NPO
- Monitoring:
  - check urine osmolality q hr
  - check patient weight q 1 hr
- continue the test until one of the following occurs:
  - normal response occurs: urine output decreases, and urine osmolality rises to 600–850 mOsm/L
  - 6–8 hours lapse
  - urine osmolality plateaus (i.e. changes < 30 mOsm in 3 consecutive hours)
  - patient loses 3% of body weight
- if the patient fails to demonstrate the normal response, then:
  - give exogenous ADH (5 U aqueous Pitressin® SQ), which normally increases urine osmolality to > 300 mOsm/L
  - check urine osmolality 30 and 60 minutes later
  - compare highest urine osmolality after Pitressin® to the osmolality just before Pitressin® according to ▶ Table 5.6

Treatment of DI

In *conscious* ambulatory patient

If DI is mild, and the patient's natural thirst mechanism is intact, instruct patient to drink *only* when thirsty and they usually "keep up" with losses and will not become overhydrated.

If severe, the patient may not be able to maintain adequate intake of fluid or tolerate the frequent trips to bathroom. In these cases, treatment typically involves a vasopressin analogue. See below for a synopsis of vasopressin analogues. Typically start with either:

1. desmopressin (DDAVP®)
   a) PO: 0.1 mg PO BID, adjust up or down PRN urine output (typical dosage range: 0.1–0.8 mg/d in divided doses)
   b) nasal spray: 2.5 mcg (0.025 ml) by nasal insufflation BID, titrate up to 20 mcg BID as needed (the nasal spray may be used for doses that are multiples of 10 mcg)

   OR
2. ADH enhancing medications (works primarily in chronic partial ADH deficiency. Will not work in total absence of ADH)
   - clofibrate (Atromid S®) 500 mg PO QID
   - chlorpropramide: increases renal sensitivity to ADH
   - hydrochlorothiazide: thiazide diuretics may act by depleting Na^+ which increases reabsorption in proximal tubules and shifting fluid away from distal tubules which is where ADH works. ℞: e.g. Dyazide® 1 PO q d (may increase up to 2 per day PRN)

In *conscious* ambulatory patient with impaired thirst mechanisms

If thirst mechanisms are *not* intact in conscious ambulatory patient, they run the risk of dehydration or fluid overload. For these patients:

1. have patient follow UO and daily weights, balance fluid intake and output using antidiuretic medication as needed to keep UO reasonable
2. check serial labs (approximately q weekly) including serum sodium, BUN

In non-ambulatory, comatose/stuporous, or brain-dead patient; see also Medical Management of the Potential Organ Donor (p. 313)

1. follow I's & O's q 1 hr, with urine specific gravity (**SG**) q 4 hrs and whenever urine output (**UO**) > 250 ml/hr
2. labs: serum electrolytes with osmolality q 6 hrs

5

Table 5.7 Available preparations of vasopressin analogues

Generic name	Trade name	Route	Concentration	Availability	Manufacturer
desmopressin	DDAVP®	SQ, IM, IV	4 mcg/ml	1 & 10 ml	Aventis
desmopressin	DDAVP® Nasal Spray	nasal spray	100 mcg/ml, each spray delivers 10 mcg	50 doses per bottle	Aventis
desmopressin	DDAVP® Tablets	PO		0.1 & 0.2 mg	Aventis
arginine vasopressin	aqueous Pitressin®	SQ, IM	20 U/ml (50 mcg/ml)	0.5 and 1 ml	Parke-Davis

Table 5.8 Mean time of hypertonic urine[a] (relative to plasma)[b]

Generic name	Route	Dose	Mean duration of action[c]
desmopressin	SQ, IM, IV	0.5 mcg	8 hrs
desmopressin[d]	SQ, IM, IV	1.0 mcg	12 hrs
desmopressin	SQ, IM, IV	2.0 mcg	16 hrs
desmopressin	SQ, IM, IV	4.0 mcg	20 hrs
desmopressin	intranasal	10 mcg (0.1 ml)	12 hrs
desmopressin	intranasal	15 mcg (0.15 ml)	16 hrs
desmopressin	intranasal	20 mcg (0.2 ml)	20 hrs
arginine vasopressin	SQ, IM	5 U (12.5 mcg)	4 hrs (range: 4–8)

[a]provided by Arnold M. Moses, M.D., used with permission
[b]onset of antidiuretic action of these preparations is 30–45 minutes following administration (except pituitary powder in oil which takes 2–4 hrs to start working)
[c]times may vary from patient to patient, but are usually consistent in any individual
[d]Note: 1 mcg BID of desmopressin is as effective as 4 mcg q d, but would obviously be less expensive

3. IV fluid management:
   BASE IV: D5 1/2 NS + 20 mEq KCl/L at appropriate rate (75–100 ml/hr)
   PLUS: replace UO above base IV rate ml for ml with 1/2 NS
   NB: for post-op patients, if the patient received significant intraoperative fluids, then they may have an ***appropriate*** post-op diuresis, in this case use 1/2 NS to replace only ≈ 2/3 of UO that exceeds the basal IV rate
4. if unable to keep up with fluid loss with IV (or NG) replacement (usually with UO > 300 ml/hr), then EITHER
   - 5 U arginine vasopressin (aqueous Pitressin®) IVP/IM/SQ q 4–6 hrs (avoid tannate oil suspension due to erratic absorption and variable duration)
     OR
   - vasopressin IV drip: start at 0.2 U/min & titrate (max: 0.9 U/min)
     OR
   - desmopressin injection SQ/IV titrated to UO, usual adult dose: 0.5–1 ml (2–4 mcg) daily in 2 divided doses

Vasopressin analogues

▶ Table 5.6, ▶ Table 5.7 and ▶ Table 5.8 shows dosing forms and duration of action of vasopressin analogues.

Pitressin® is aqueous solution of 8-arginine vasopressin and should be used with caution in patients with vascular disease (especially coronary arteries). ✖ Caution – soundalikes: sometimes pitocin is confused with pitressin because of similarities of the name.

DDAVP (1-deamino-8-D-arginine vasopressin) AKA desmopressin. More potent and longer acting than vasopressin.

References

[1] Ellison DH, Berl T. Clinical practice. The syndrome of inappropriate antidiuresis. N Engl J Med. 2007; 356:2064–2072

[2] Diringer M, Ladenson PW, Borel C, et al. Sodium and Water Regulation in a Patient With Cerebral Salt Wasting. Arch Neurol. 1989; 46:928–930

[3] Sherlock M, O'Sullivan E, Agha A, Behan LA, Rawluk D, Brennan P, Tormey W, Thompson CJ. The incidence and pathophysiology of hyponatraemia after subarachnoid haemorrhage. Clin Endocrinol (Oxf). 2006; 64:250–254

[4] Weisberg LS. Pseudohyponatremia: a reappraisal. Am J Med. 1989; 86:315–318

[5] Arieff AI. Hyponatremia, Convulsions, Respiratory Arrest and Permanent Brain Damage After Elective Surgery in Healthy Women. N Engl J Med. 1986; 314:1529–1535

[6] Steele A, Gowrishankar M, Abrahamson S, et al. Postoperative Hyponatremia despite Near-Isotonic Saline Infusion: A Phenomenon of Desalination. Ann Intern Med. 1997; 126:20–25

[7] Powers CJ, Friedman AH. Diagnosis and management of hyponatremia in neurosurgical patients. Contemp Neurosurg. 2007; 29:1–5

[8] Chung HM, Kluge R, Schrier RW, Anderson RJ. Clinical assessment of extracellular fluid volume in hyponatremia. Am J Med. 1987; 83:905–908

[9] Lester MC, Nelson PB. Neurological Aspects of Vasopressin Release and the Syndrome of Inappropriate Secretion of Antidiuretic Hormone. Neurosurgery. 1981; 8:725–740

[10] Kröll M, Juhler M, Lindholm J. Hyponatremia in Acute Brain Disease. J Int Med. 1992; 232:291–297

[11] Harrigan MR. Cerebral Salt Wasting Syndrome: A Review. Neurosurgery. 1996; 38:152–160

[12] Ayus JC, Krothapalli RK, Arieff AI. Changing Concepts on Treatment of Severe Symptomatic Hyponatremia: Rapid Correction and Possible Relation to Central Pontine Myelinolysis. Am J Med. 1985; 78:879–902

[13] Fraser CL, Arieff AI. Symptomatic Hyponatremia: Management and Relation to Central Pontine Myelinolysis. Sem Neurol. 1984; 4:445–452

[14] Adams RD, Victor M, Mancall EL. Central Pontine Myelinolysis: A Hitherto Undescribed Disease Occurring in Alcoholic and Malnourished Patients. Arch Neurol Psychiatr. 1959; 81:154–172

[15] Ayus JC, Krothapalli RK, Arieff AI. Treatment of Symptomatic Hyponatremia and Its Relation to Brain Damage. N Engl J Med. 1987; 317:1190–1195

[16] Berl T. Treating Hyponatremia: What is All the Controversy About? Ann Intern Med. 1990; 113:417–419

[17] Arieff AI. Hyponatremia Associated with Permanent Brain Damage. Adv Intern Med. 1987; 32:325–344

[18] Adrogue HJ, Madias NE. Hyponatremia. N Engl J Med. 2000; 342:1581–1589

[19] Soupart A, Ngassa M, Decaux G. Therapeutic relowering of the serum sodium in a patient after excessive correction of hyponatremia. Clin Nephrol. 1999; 51:383–386

[20] Oya S, Tsutsumi K, Ueki K, Kirino T. Reinduction of hyponatremia to treat central pontine myelinolysis. Neurology. 2001; 57:1931–1932

[21] De Troyer A, Demanet JC. Correction of Antidiuresis by Demeclocycline. N Engl J Med. 1975; 293:915–918

[22] Perks WH, Mohr P, Liversedge LA. Demeclocycline in Inappropriate ADH Syndrome. Lancet. 1976; 2

[23] Forrest JN, Cox M, Hong C, et al. Superiority of Demeclocycline over Lithium in the Treatment of Chronic Syndrome of Inappropriate Secretion of Antidiuretic Hormone. N Engl J Med. 1978; 298:173–177

[24] Wright WL, Asbury WH, Gilmore JL, Samuels OB. Conivaptan for hyponatremia in the neurocritical care unit. Neurocrit Care. 2009; 11:6–13

[25] Maroon JC, Nelson PB. Hypovolemia in Patients with Subarachnoid Hemorrhage: Therapeutic Implications. Neurosurgery. 1979; 4:223–226

[26] Wijdicks EFM, Vermeulen M, Hijdra A, et al. Hyponatremia and Cerebral Infarction in Patients with Ruptured Intracranial Aneurysms: Is Fluid Restriction Harmful? Ann Neurol. 1985; 17:137–140

[27] Wijdicks EFM, Vermeulen M, ten Haaf JA, et al. Volume Depletion and Natriuresis in Patients with a Ruptured Intracranial Aneurysm. Ann Neurol. 1985; 18:211–216

[28] Nelson PB, Seif SM, Maroon JC, et al. Hyponatremia in Intracranial Disease. Perhaps Not the Syndrome of Inappropriate Secretion of Antidiuretic Hormone (SIADH). J Neurosurg. 1981; 55:938–941

[29] Hasan D, Lindsay KW, Wijdicks EFM, et al. Effect of Fludrocortisone Acetate in Patients with Subarachnoid Hemorrhage. Stroke. 1989; 20:1156–1161

[30] Reeder RF, Harbaugh RE. Administration of Intravenous Urea and Normal Saline for the Treatment of Hyponatremia in Neurosurgical Patients. J Neurosurg. 1989; 70:201–206

[31] Thibonnier M, Barrow DL, Selman W. In: Antidiuretic Hormone: Regulation, Disorders, and Clinical Evaluation. Neuroendocrinology. Baltimore: Williams and Wilkins; 1992:19–30

[32] Verbalis JG, Robinson AG, Moses AM. Postoperative and Post-Traumatic Diabetes Insipidus. Front Horm Res. 1985; 13:247–265

[33] Abe T, Matsumoto K, Sanno N, Osamura Y. Lymphocytic Hypophysitis: Case Report. Neurosurgery. 1995; 36:1016–1019

[34] Imura H, Nakao K, Shimatsu A, et al. Lymphocytic Infundibuloneurohypophysitis as a Cause of Central Diabetes Insipidus. N Engl J Med. 1993; 329:683–689

[35] Miller M, Dalakos T, Moses AM, et al. Recognition of partial defects in antidiuretic hormone secretion. Ann Intern Med. 1970; 73:721–729

6 General Neurocritical Care

6.1 Parenteral agents for hypertension

Drug info: ✱ Nicardipine (Cardene®)

Calcium channel blocker (CCB) that may be given IV. Does not require arterial line, *does not raise ICP*. Does not reduce heart rate, but may be used in conjunction with e.g. labetalol or esmolol if that is desired. **Side effects:** H/A 15%, nausea 5%, hypotension 5%, reflex tachycardia 3.5%.

℞ start at 5 mg/hr IV (off label: 10 mg/hr may be used in situations where urgent reduction is needed). Increase by 2.5 mg/hr every 5–15 minutes up to a maximum of 15 mg/hr. Decrease to 3 mg/hr once control is achieved. ✖ Ampules contain 25 mg and *must be diluted* before administration.

6

Drug info: Nitroglycerin (NTG)

Raises ICP (less than with nitroprusside due to preferential venous action[1]). Vasodilator, venous > arterial (large coronaries > small). Result: decreases LV filling pressure (pre-load). Does not cause "coronary steal" (cf nitroprusside).

℞ 10–20 mcg/min IV drip (increase by 5–10 mcg/min q 5–10 min). For angina pectoris: 0.4 mg SL q 5 min × 3 doses, check BP before each dose.

Drug info: Labetalol (Normodyne®, Trandate®)

Blocks α_1 selective, β non-selective (potency < propranolol). ICP reduces or no change.[2] Pulse rate: decreases or no change. Cardiac output does not change. Does not exacerbate coronary ischemia. May be used in controlled CHF, but not in overt CHF. Contraindicated in asthma. Renal failure: same dose. **Side effects:** fatigue, dizziness, orthostatic hypotension.

Intravenous (IV)

Onset 5 mins, peak 10 mins, duration 3–6 hrs.

℞ IV: patient supine; check BP q 5 min; give each dose slow IVP (over 2 min) q 10 minutes until desired BP achieved; dose sequence: 20, 40, 80, 80, then 80 mg (300 mg total). Once controlled, use ≈ same total dose IVP q 8 hrs.

℞ *IV drip* (alternative): add 40 ml (200 mg) to 160 ml of IVF (result: 1 mg/ml); run at 2 ml/min (2 mg/min) until desired BP (usual effective dose = 50–200 mg) or until 300 mg given; then titrate rate (bradycardia limits dose, increase slowly since effect takes 10–20 minutes).

Oral (PO)

Undergoes first pass liver degradation, therefore requires higher doses PO. PO onset: 2 hrs, peak: 4 hrs.

℞ *PO*: to convert IV → PO, start with 200 mg PO BID. To start with PO, give 100 mg BID, and increase 100 mg/dose q 2 day; max. = 2400 mg/day.

Drug info: Enalaprilat (Vasotec®)

An angiotensin-converting enzyme (ACE) inhibitor. The active metabolite of the orally administered drug enalapril (see below). Acts within ≈ 15 mins of administration.

Side effects: hyperkalemia occurs in ≈ 1%. Do not use during pregnancy.

℞ IV: start with 1.25 mg slow IV over 5 mins, may increase up to 5 mg q 6 hrs PRN.

Drug info: Esmolol (Brevibloc®)

Cardioselective short-acting beta blocker.[3] Being investigated for hypertensive emergencies. Metabolized by RBC esterase. Elimination half-life: 9 mins. Therapeutic response (> 20% decrease in heart rate, HR < 100, or conversion to sinus rhythm) in 72%. **Side effects:** dose related hypotension (in 20–50%), generally resolves within 30 mins of D/C. Bronchospasm less likely than other beta blockers. Avoid in CHF.

℞ 500 mcg/kg loading dose over 1 min, follow with 4 min infusion starting with 50 mcg/kg/min. Repeat loading dose and increment infusion rate by 50 mcg/kg/min q 5 mins. Rarely > 100 mcg/kg/min required. Doses > 200 mcg/kg/min add little.

Drug info: Fenoldopam (Corlopam®)

Vasodilator. Onset of action < 5 minutes, duration 30 mins.

℞ IV infusion (no bolus doses): start with 0.1–0.3 mcg/kg/min, titrate by 0.1 mcg/kg/min q 15 min up to a maximum of 1.6 mcg/kg/min.

Drug info: Propranolol (Inderal®)

Main use IV is to counteract tachycardia with vasodilators (usually doesn't lower BP acutely when used alone), but esmolol and labetalol are more commonly used for this.

℞ IV: load with 1 10 mg slow IVP, follow with 3 mg/hr. PO: 80–640 mg q d in divided doses.

6.2 Hypotension (shock)

6.2.1 Classification

1. hypovolemic: first sign usually tachycardia. > 20–40% of blood volume loss must occur before perfusion of vital organs is impaired. Includes:
   a) hemorrhage (external or internal)
   b) bowel obstruction (with third spacing)
2. septic: most often due to gram negative sepsis
3. cardiogenic: includes MI, cardiomyopathy, dysrhythmias (including A-fib)
4. neurogenic: e.g. paralysis due to spinal cord injury. Blood pools in venous capacitance vessels
5. miscellaneous
   a) anaphylaxis
   b) insulin reaction

6.2.2 Cardiovascular agents for shock

Plasma expanders. Includes:

1. crystalloids: normal saline has less tendency to promote cerebral edema than others; see IV fluids (p. 870), under control of elevated ICP
2. colloids: e.g. hetastarch (Hespan®). ✖ CAUTION: repeated administration over a period of days may prolong PT/PTT and clotting times and may increase the risk of rebleeding in aneurysmal SAH (p. 1167).[4]
3. blood products: expensive. Risk of transmissible diseases or transfusion reaction

Drug info: Dopamine

See ▶ Table 6.1 for a summary of the effects of dopamine (DA) at various dosages. DA is primarily a vasoconstrictor (β_1 effects usually overridden by α-activity). 25% of dopamine given is rapidly converted to norepinephrine (NE). At doses > 10 mcg/kg/min one is essentially giving NE. May cause significant hyperglycemia at high doses.

℞ Start with 2–5 mcg/kg/min and titrate.

Table 6.1 Dopamine dosage

Dose (mcg/kg/min)	Effect	Result
0.5–2.0 (sometimes up to 5)	dopaminergic	renal, mesenteric, coronary, & cerebral vasodilatation, (+) inotrope
2–10	β_1	positive inotrope
> 10	α, β & dopaminergic	releases nor-epi (vasoconstrictor)

Drug info: Dobutamine (Dobutrex®)

Vasodilates by β_1 (primary) and by increased CO from (+) inotropy (β_2); result: little or no fall in BP, less tachycardia than DA. No alpha release nor vasoconstriction. May be used synergistically with nitroprusside. Tachyphylaxis after ≈ 72 hrs. Pulse increases > 10% may exacerbate myocardial ischemia, more common at doses > 20 mcg/kg/min. Optimal use requires hemodynamic monitoring. Possible platelet function inhibition.

℞ usual range 2.5–10 mcg/kg/min; rarely doses up to 40 used (to prepare: put 50 mg in 250 ml D5 W to yield 200 mcg/ml).

Drug info: Amrinone (Inocor®)

Nonadrenergic cardiotonic. Phosphodiesterase inhibitor, effects similar to dobutamine (including exacerbation of myocardial ischemia). 2% incidence of thrombocytopenia.

℞ 0.75 mg/kg initially over 2–3 min, then drip 5–10 mcg/kg/min.

Drug info: Phenylephrine (Neo-Synephrine®)

Pure alpha sympathomimetic. Useful in hypotension associated with tachycardia (atrial tachyarrhythmias). Elevates BP by increasing SVR via vasoconstriction, causes reflex increase in parasympathetic tone (with resultant slowing of pulse). Lack of β action means non-inotropic, no cardiac acceleration, and no relaxation of bronchial smooth muscle. Cardiac output and renal blood flow may decrease. Avoid in spinal cord injuries (p. 950).

℞ pressor range: 100–180 mcg/min; maintenance: 40–60 mcg/min. To prepare: put 40 mg (4 amps) in 500 ml D5 W to yield 80 mcg/ml; a rate of 8 ml/hr = 10 mcg/min.

Drug info: Norepinephrine

Primarily vasoconstrictor (? counterproductive in cerebral vasospasm, ? decreases CBF). β-agonist at low doses. Increases pulmonary vascular resistance.

Drug info: Epinephrine (adrenalin globally)

℞ 0.5–1.0 mg of 1:10,000 solution IVP; may repeat q 5 minutes (may bolus per ET tube). Drip: start at 1.0 mcg/min, titrate up to 8 mcg/min (to prepare: put 1 mg in 100 ml NS or D5W).

Drug info: Isoproterenol (Isuprel®)

Positive chronotropic and inotropic, → increased cardiac O_2 consumption, arrhythmias, vasodilatation (by β_1 action) skeletal muscle > cerebral vessels.

Drug info: Levophed

Direct β stimulation (positive inotropic and chronotropic).

℞ start drip at 8–12 mcg/min; maintenance 2–4 mcg/min (0.5–1.0 ml/min) (to prepare: put 2 mg in 500 ml NS or D5 W to yield 4 mcg/cc).

6.3 Acid inhibitors

6.3.1 Stress ulcers in neurosurgery

See reference.[5]

The risk of developing stress ulcers (SU) AKA Cushing's ulcers is high in critically ill patients with CNS pathology. These lesions are AKA Cushing's ulcers due to Cushing's classic treatise.[6] 17% of SUs produce clinically significant hemorrhage. CNS risk factors include intracranial pathology: brain injury (especially Glasgow Coma scale score < 9), brain tumors, intracerebral hemorrhage, SIADH, CNS infection, ischemic stroke, as well as spinal cord injury. The odds are increased with the coexistence of extra-CNS risk factors including: long-term use of steroids (usually > 3 weeks), burns > 25% of body surface area, hypotension, respiratory failure, coagulopathies, renal or hepatic failure and sepsis.

The pathogenesis of SUs is incompletely understood, but probably results from an imbalance of destructive factors (acid, pepsin & bile) relative to protective factors (mucosal blood flow, mucus-bicarbonate layer, endothelial cell replenishment & protaglandins).[5] CNS pathology, especially that involving the diencephalon or brain stem, can lead to reduction of vagal output which leads to hypersecretion of gastric acid and pepsin. There is a peak in acid and pepsin production 3–5 days after CNS injury.

6.3.2 Prophylaxis for stress ulcers

There is strong evidence that reduction of gastric acid (whether by antacids or agents that inhibit acid secretion) reduces the incidence of GI bleeding from stress ulcers in critically ill patients. Elevating gastric pH > 4.5 also inactivates pepsin.

Other therapies that don't involve alterations of pH that may be effective include sucralfate (see below) and enteral nutrition (controversial).[5] Titrated antacids or sucralfate appear to be superior to H2 antagonists in reducing the incidence of SUs.

Routine prophylaxis when steroids are used is not warranted unless one of the following risk factors are present: prior PUD, concurrent use of NSAIDs, hepatic or renal failure, malnourishment, or prolonged steroid therapy > 3 weeks.

6.3.3 Possible increased pneumonia and mortality from altering gastric pH

Whereas bringing gastric pH to a more neutral level reduces the risk of SUs, pH > 4 permits bacterial colonization of the normally sterile stomach. This may increase the risk of pneumonia from aspiration, and there is a suggestion that mortality may also be increased.[7] Sucralfate may be as effective in reducing bleeding, but may be associated with lower rates of pneumonia and mortality. There is insufficient data to determine the net result of sucralfate compared to no treatment.[7]

6.3.4 Histamine2 (H2) antagonists

Drug info: Ranitidine (Zantac®)

℞ Adult age ≤ 65 yrs: 150 mg PO BID, or 50 mg IVPB q 8 hrs. For age > 65 with normal renal function: 50 mg IV q 12 hrs.

IV drip (provides a more consistently higher pH without peaks and troughs; some controversy that this may increase gastric bacterial concentration with increased risk of aspiration pneumonia has not been borne out): 6.25 mg/hr (e.g. inject 150 mg into 42 ml of IVF yielding 3.125 mg/ml, run at 2 ml/hr).

Drug info: Famotidine (Pepcid®)

℞ Adult: 20 mg PO q hs for maintenance; 40 mg PO q hs for active ulcer therapy; IV: 20 mg q 12 hrs (for hypersecretory conditions, 20 mg IVPB q 6 hrs).[8] **Supplied:** 20 & 40 mg tablets, 40 mg/5 ml suspension, and 20 & 40 mg orally disintegrating tablets as Pepcid RPD. Available OTC in 10 mg tablets as Pepcid AC. Available IV.

Drug info: Nizatidine (Axid®)

℞ 300 mg PO q d or 150 mg PO BID. **Supplied:** 150 & 300 mg pulvules. Available OTC in 75 mg tablets as Axid AR.

6.3.5 Gastric acid secretion inhibitors (proton pump inhibitors)

These agents reduce gastric acid by specific inhibition of the final step in acid secretion by gastric parietal cells (by inhibiting the (H^+, K^+)-ATPase enzyme system on the cell surface, the so-called "acid pump"). They block acid secretion regardless of the stimulus (Zollinger-Ellison syndrome, hypergastrinemia…). Full recovery of acid secretion upon discontinuation may not occur for weeks. ✖ Not indicated for long-term treatment as the trophic effects of the resultant elevated levels of gastrin may lead to gastric carcinoid tumors.

Drug info: Omeprazole (Prilosec®)

Inhibition of some hepatic P-450 enzymes results in reduced clearance of warfarin and phenytoin. Decreases the effectiveness of prednisone.

℞ *Adult*: for peptic ulcers and gastro-esophageal reflux disease (GERD) 20–40 mg PO daily. For Zollinger-Ellison syndrome: 20 mg PO q d to 120 mg PO TID (dose adjusted to keep basal acid output < 60 mEq/hr). **Side effects:** N/V, H/A, diarrhea, abdominal pain or rash in 1–5% of patients. **Supplied:** 10, 20 & 40 mg delayed-release capsules. Available OTC in 20.6 mg tablets as Prilosec OTC.

Drug info: *Lansoprazole (Prevacid®)

Found *not* to have an affect on a number of other drugs metabolized by cytochrome P-450 including: phenytoin, warfarin and prednisone.

℞ *Adult*: 15 mg (for duodenal ulcer, GERD, or maintenance therapy) or 30 mg (for gastric ulcer or erosive esophagitis) PO q d, short-term treatment × 4 wks. **Supplied:** 15 & 30 mg delayed-release capsules.

Drug info: Pantoprazole (Protonix®)

℞ PO: 40 mg PO q d for up to 8 wks. IV: 40 mg IV q d × 7–10 d. **Supplied:** PO: 40 mg delayed-release capsules.

6.3.6 Miscellaneous

Drug info: Sucralfate (Carafate®)

Minimally absorbed from GI tract. Acts by coating ulcerated areas of mucosa, does not inhibit acid secretion. This may actually result in a lower incidence of pneumonia and mortality than agents that affect gastric pH (see above).

℞ 1 gm PO QID on an empty stomach. Do not give antacids within one half-hour of sucralfate.

References

[1] Cottrell JE, Patel K, Turndorf H, et al. ICP Changes Induced by Sodium Nitroprusside in Patients with Intracranial Mass Lesions. J Neurosurg. 1978; 48:329–331
[2] Orlowski JP, Shiesley D, Vidt DG, Barnett GH, et al. Labetalol to Control Blood Pressure After Cerebrovascular Surgery. Crit Care Med. 1988; 16:765–768
[3] Esmolol - A Short-Acting IV Beta Blocker. Med Letter. 1987; 29:57–58
[4] Trumble ER, Muizelaar JP, Myseros JS. Coagulopathy with the Use of Hetastarch in the Treatment of Vasospasm. J Neurosurg. 1995; 82:44–47
[5] Lu WY, Rhoney DH, Boling WB, et al. A Review of Stress Ulcer Prophylaxis in the Neurosurgical Intensive Care Unit. Neurosurgery. 1997; 41:416–426
[6] Cushing H. Peptic Ulcers and the Interbrain. Surg Gynecol Obstet. 1932; 55:1–34
[7] Cook DJ, Reeve BK, Guyatt GH, et al. Stress Ulcer Prophylaxis in Critically Ill Patients: Resolving Discordant Meta-Analyses. JAMA. 1996; 275:308–314
[8] Famotidine (Pepcid). Med Letter. 1987; 29:17–18

7 Sedatives, Paralytics, Analgesics

7.1 Sedatives and paralytics

7.1.1 Richmond agitation-sedation scale (RASS)

A validated scale[1,2] that uses positive numbers for agitation and negative numbers for sedation as shown in ▶ Table 7.1. Useful for quantitating the desired level of sedation when titrating sedatives for agitated patients.

Procedure for performing RASS assessment:

1. on observation, patient is alert, restless or agitated: score 0 to + 4
2. if patient is not alert, state patient's name and verbally instruct to open eyes and look at speaker: score –1 to –3
3. if no response to verbal stimulus, physically stimulate by shaking shoulder and/or sternal rub: score –4 or –5

7.1.2 Conscious sedation

Use of these agents requires ability to provide immediate emergency ventilatory support (including intubation). Agents include:

1. midazolam (Versed®) (p. 870) with fentanyl
2. fentanyl
3. pentobarbital (Nembutal®): a barbiturate. ℞ for 70 kg adult: 100 mg slow IVP

Drug info: Methohexital (Brevital®)

More potent and shorter acting than thiopental (useful e.g. for percutaneous rhizotomy where patient needs to be sedated and awakened repeatedly). Lasts 5–7 min. Similar cautions with the added problem that methohexital may *induce* seizures. May no longer be available in the U.S.

℞ Adult: 1 gm% solution (add 50 ml diluent to 500 mg to yield 10 mg/ml), 2 ml test dose, then 5–12 ml IVP at rate of 1 ml/5 secs, then 2 to 4 ml q 4–7 min PRN.

Table 7.1 Richmond agitation-sedation scale

	Score	Term	Description	
Agitation	+ 4	combative	overly combative, violent, immediate danger to staff	
	+ 3	very agitated	pulls or removes tubes or catheters; aggressive	
	+ 2	agitated	frequent non-purposeful movements, fights ventilator	
	+ 1	restless	anxious, but movements not aggressive /vigorous	
	0	alert & calm		
Sedation	–1	drowsy	not fully alert, but has sustained awakening (eye-opening/contact) to voice (≥ 10 seconds)	verbal stimulation
	–2	light sedation	briefly awakens with eye contact to voice (< 10 seconds)	
	–3	moderate sedation	movement or eye opening to voice (no eye contact)	
	–4	deep sedation	no response to voice, but movement or eye-opening to physical stimulation	physical stimulation
	–5	unarousable	no response to voice or pjysical stimulation	

7.1.3 Sedation

Generally requires intubation and mechanical ventilatory support in the ICU. Doses are generally lower than those used by anesthesiologists for general anesthesia.

Drug info: Thiopental (Pentothal®)

A short acting barbiturate. 1st dose causes unconsciousness in 20–30 secs (circulation time), depth increases up to 40 secs, duration = 5 mins (terminated by redistribution), consciousness returns over 20–30 mins.

Side effects: dose related respiratory depression, irritation if extravasated, intra-arterial injection → necrosis, agitation if injected slowly, an *antianalgesic*, myocardial depressant, hypotension in hypovolemic patients.

℞ Adult: initial concentration should not exceed 2.5%,
give 50 mg test dose moderately rapid IVP, then if tolerated give 100–200 mg IVP over 20–30 secs (500 mg may be required in large patient).

7

Drug info: ✱ Remifentanil (Ultiva®)

Ultrashort acting micro-opioid receptor agonist. Potency similar to fentanyl. Rapidly crosses BBB. Onset: < 1 min. Offset: 3–10 mins. *Lowers ICP.* Metabolism: non-hepatic hydrolysis by nonspecific blood and tissue esterases, ∴ no accumulation. Synergy with thiopental, propofol, isoflurane, midazolam requires reducing doses of these agents by up to 75%. **Side effects:** bradycardia, hypotension (these side effects may be blunted by pretreatment with anticholinergics), N/V, muscle rigidity, pruritis (aspecially facial) dose dependent respiratory depression at doses > 0.05 mcg/kg/min.

℞ Adult: avoid bolus doses. Start with drip of 0.05 mcg/kg/min. Titrate in 0.025 mcg/kg/min increments tp a maximum of 0.1–0.2 mcg/kg/min. Add a sedative if adequate sedation not achieved at maximum dose. Wean infusion in 25% decrements over 10 minues after extubation. **Supplied:** vials of 1, 2 or 5 mg powder to be reconstituted to 1 mg/ml solution.

Drug info: Fentanyl (Sublimaze®)

Narcotic, potency ≈ 100 × morphine. High lipid solubility → rapid onset. Offset (small doses): 20–30 mins. Unlike morphine and meperidine, does not cause histamine release. *Lowers ICP.* **Side effects:** dose dependent respiratory depression, large doses given rapidly may cause chest wall rigidity. Repeated dosing may cause accumulation. Diminished sensitivity to CO_2 stimulation, may persist longer than the depression of respiratory rate (up to 4 hours).

℞ Adult: 25–100 mcg (0.5–2 ml) IVP, repeat PRN. **Supplied:** 50 mcg/ml; requires refrigeration.

Drug info: ✱ Propofol (Diprivan®)

A sedative hypnotic. Also useful in high doses during aneurysm surgery as a neuroprotectant (p. 1203). Protection seems to be less than with barbiturates. Offset time increases after ≈ 12 hours of use.

℞ for sedation: start at 5–10 mcg/kg/min. Increase by 5–10 mcg/kg/min q 5–10 minutes PRN desired sedation (up to a max of 50 mcg/kg/min).

Side effects: include Propofol Infusion Syndrome: hyperkalemia, hepatomegaly, lipemia, metabolic acidosis, myocardial failure, rhabdomyolosis, renal failure and sometimes death.[3] First identified in children, but may occur at any age. NB: *metabolic acidosis* of unknown etiology in a patient on propofol is propofol infusion syndrome until proven otherwise. Use with caution at doses > 50 mcg/kg/min or at any dose for > 48 hrs. Also note that the lipid carrier provides 1.1 kCal/ml and hypertriglyceridemia may occur.

Supplied: 500 mg suspended in a 50 ml bottle of fat emulsion. The bottle and tubing must be changed every 12 hours since it contains no bacteriostatic agent.

Drug info: ✻ Precedex® (Dexmedetomidine)

An alpha-2 adrenoceptor agonist. Acts in locus ceruleur and dorsal root ganglia. Has both sedative and analgesic properties and dramatically reduce the risk of respiratory depression and the amount of narcotic analgesics required. Reduces shivering.

℞: usual loading dose is 1 mcg/kg IV over 10 minutes (loading dose not needed if patient already sedated with other agents), followed by continuous IV infusion of 0.2–1.0 mcg/kg/hr titrated to desired effect, not to exceed 24 hours (for short sedation or use as a "transition" drug). **Side effects:** clinically significant bradycardia and sinus arrest have occurred in young, healthy volunteers with increased vagal tone (anticholinergics such as atropine 0.2 mg IV or glycopyrrolate 0.2 mg IV may help). Use with caution in patients with advanced heart block, baseline bradycardia, using other drugs that lower heartrate, and hypovolemia. **Supplied:** 2 ml vials of 100 mcg/ml to be diluted in 48 ml NS for a final concentration of 4 mcg/ml for IV use.

7

7.2 Paralytics (neuromuscular blocking agents)

7.2.1 General information

CAUTION: requires ventilation (intubation or Ambu-bag/mask). Reminder: paralyzed patients may still be conscious and therefore able to feel pain, the simultaneous use of sedation is thus required for conscious patients.

Early routine use in head-injured patients lowers ICP (e.g. from suctioning[4]) and mortality, but does not improve overall outcome.[5]

Neuromuscular blocking agents (NMBAs) are classified clinically by time to onset and duration of paralysis as shown in ▶ Table 7.2. Additional information for some agents follows the table along with some considerations for neurosurgical patients.

Table 7.2 Onset and duration of muscle relaxants

Clinical class	Agent	Trade name (®)	Onset (min)	Duration (min)	Spontaneous recovery (min)	Comment
Ultra-short	succinylcholine	Anectine	1	5–10	20	shortest onset and duration; plasma cholinesterase dependent; many side effects
Short	rocuronium	Zemuron	1–1.5	20–35	40–60	close to succinylcholine in onset in large doses; some vagolytic action in children
Intermediate	vecuronium	Norcuron	3–5	20–35	40–60	minimal cardiovascular side effects (bradycardia reported); no histamine release
	cisatracurium	Nimbex	1.5–2	40–60	60–80	no histamine release at recommended doses

7.2.2 Ultra-short acting paralytics

Drug info: Succinylcholine (Anectine®)

The only depolarizing ganglionic blocker (the rest are competitive blockers). Rapidly inactivated by plasma pseudocholinesterases. A single dose produces fasciculations then paralysis. Onset: 1 min. Duration of action: 5–10 min.

Indications

Due to significant side effects (see below), use is now limited primarily to the following indications. Adults: generally recommended only for emergency intubations where the airway is not controlled. In children: only when intubation is needed with a full stomach, or if laryngospasm occurs during attempted intubation using other agents.

Side effects

✖ CAUTIONS: usually increases serum K^+ by 0.5 mEq/L (on rare occasion causes severe *hyperkalemia* ($[K^+]$ up to 12 mEq/L) in patients with neuronal or muscular pathology, causing cardiac complications which cannot be blocked), therefore contraindicated in acute phase of injury following major burns, multiple trauma or extensive denervation of skeletal muscle or upper motor neuron injury. Do not use for routine intubations in adolescents and children (may cause cardiac arrest even in apparently healthy youngsters, many of whom have undiagnosed myopathies). Linked to malignant hyperthermia (p. 108).

May cause dysrhythmias, especially sinus bradycardia (treat with atropine). May get autonomic stimulation from ACh-like action → HTN, and brady- or tachycardia (especially in peds with repeated doses). The fasciculations may increase ICP, intragastric pressure, and intraocular pressure (contraindicated in penetrating eye injury, especially to anterior chamber; OK in glaucoma).

Precurarization with a "priming dose" of a nondepolarizing blocker (usually ≈ 10% of the intubating dose, e.g. *pancuronium* 0.5–1 mg IV 3–5 minutes prior to succinylcholine) in patients with elevated ICP or increased intraocular pressure (to ameliorate further pressure increases during fasciculation phase) and in patients who have eaten recently (controversial[6]). Phase II block (similar to nondepolarizing blocker) may develop with excessive doses or in patients with abnormal pseudocholinesterase.

Dosing

℞ Adult: 0.6–1.1 mg/kg (2–3 ml/70 kg) IVP (err on high side to allow time for procedure & to avoid multi-dosing complications), may repeat this dose × 1.

℞ Peds (CAUTION: *Not* recommended for routine use, see above) *Children*: 1.1 mg/kg. *Infants* (< 1 mos): 2 mg/kg.

Supplied: 20 mg/ml concentration.

7.2.3 Short acting paralytics

Drug info: Rocuronium (Zemuron®)

In large doses, has speed of onset that approaches succinylcholine. However, in these doses, paralysis usually lasts ≈ 1–2 hrs. Expensive.

℞ Adult: initial dose 0.6–1 mg/kg. May be used as infusion of 10–12 mcg/kg/min.

7

7.2.4 Intermediate acting paralytics

Drug info: ✻ Vecuronium (Norcuron®)

Nondepolarizing (competitive) NMBA. Adequate paralysis for intubation within 2.5–3 minutes of administration. About one-third more potent than pancuronium, shorter duration of action (lasts ≈ 30 minutes after initial dose). Unlike pancuronium, very little vagal (i.e. cardiovascular) effects. No CNS active metabolites. Does not affect ICP or CPP. Hepatically metabolized. Due to active metabolites, paralysis has been reported to take 6 hrs to 7 days to recede following discontinuation of the drug after ≥ 2 days use in patients with renal failure.[7] Must be mixed to use.

Dosing

Supplied: 10 mg freeze-dried cakes requiring reconstitution. Use within 24 hrs of mixing.

℞ Adult and children > 10 years age: 0.1 mg/kg (for most adults use 8–10 mg as initial dose). May repeat q 1 hr PRN. Infusion: 1–2 mcg/kg/min.

℞ Pediatric: *children* (1–10 yrs) require slightly higher dose and more frequent dosing than adult. *Infants* (7 weeks - 1 yr): slightly more sensitive on a mg/kg basis than adults, takes ≈ 1.5 × longer to recover. Use in neonates and continuous infusion in children is insufficiently studied.

7

Drug info: ✻ Cisatracurium (Nimbex®)

Nondepolarizing (competitive) blocker. This isomer of atracurium does not release histamine unlike its parent compound (see below). Provides about 1 hour of paralysis. Also undergoes Hofmann degradation, with laudanosine as one of its metabolites.

℞ Adult and children > 12 years age: 0.15 or 0.2 mg/kg as part of propofol/nitrous oxide/oxygen induction-intubation technique produces muscle paralysis adequate for intubation within 2 or 1.5 minutes, respectively. Infusion: 1–3 mcg/kg/min.

℞ Pediatric: *children* (2–12 yrs): 0.1 mg/kg given over 5–10 seconds during inhalational or opioid anesthesia.

7.2.5 Reversal of competitive muscle blockade

Reversal is usually not attempted until patient has at least 1 twitch to a train of 4 stimulus, otherwise reversal may be incomplete if patient is profoundly blocked and blockade may reoccur as the reversal wears off (a response of 1/4 indicates 90% muscle blockade)

- neostigmine (Prostigmin®): 2.5 mg (minimum) to 5 mg (maximum) IV
  (start low, no efficacy from > 5 mg and can produce severe weakness especially if the maximum dose is exceeded in the absence of neuromuscular blockade)
- *PLUS* (to prevent bradycardia…),
  - EITHER
    0.5 mg atropine for each mg of neostigmine
  - OR
    0.2 mg glycopyrrolate (Robinul®) for each mg of neostigmine

7.3 Analgesics

7.3.1 General information

For a discussion of types of pain and pain procedures (p. 476).

Three types of pain medication

1. non-opioid pain medication (see below)
   a) nonsteroidal anti-inflammatory drugs: aspirin, ibuprofen…
   b) acetaminophen
2. opioids (p. 138)
   a) agonists
   b) partial agonists
   c) mixed agonist/antagonists

3. drugs that are not strictly analgesics, but which act as adjuvants (p. 143) when added to any of the above: tricyclic antidepressants, anticonvulsants, caffeine, hydroxyzine, corticosteroids (p. 143)

7.3.2 Guiding principles

The key to good pain control is the early use of adequate levels of effective analgesics. For cancer pain, scheduled dosing is superior to PRN dosing, and "rescue" medication should be available.[8] Non-opioid analgesics should be continued as more potent medications and invasive techniques are utilized.

7.3.3 Analgesics for some specific types of pain

Visceral or deafferentation pain

May sometimes be effectively treated with tricyclic antidepressants (p. 477).

Tryptophan may be effective (p. 143).

Carbamazepine (Tegretol®) may be useful for paroxysmal, lancinating pain.

7

Pain from metastatic bone disease

Steroids, aspirin, or NSAIDs are especially helpful, probably by reducing prostaglandin mediated sensitization of A-delta and C fibers, and therefore may be preferred to APAP.

7.3.4 Nonopioid analgesics

Acetaminophen

Table 7.3 Acetaminophen dosing

Medication	Dosage
acetaminophen (APAP) (Tylenol®)	adult dose: 650 or 1000 mg PO/PR q 4–6 hrs, not to exceed 4000 mg/day[a] pediatric dose: infants: 10–15 mg/kg PO/PR q 4–6 hrs children: 1 grain/yr age (= 65 mg/yr up to 650 mg) PO/PR q 4–6 hrs not to exceed 15 mg/kg q 4 hrs

[a]hepatic toxicity from APAP: usually with doses ≥ 10 gm/day, rare at doses < 4000 mg. However, may occur at lower doses (even at high therapeutic doses) in alcoholics, fasting patients, and those taking cytochrome P-450 enzyme-inducing drugs

Nonsteroidal anti-inflammatory drugs (NSAIDs)

The anti-inflammatory properties of NSAIDs is primarily due to inhibition of the enzyme cyclooxygenase (COX) which participates in the synthesis of prostaglandins and thromboxanes.[9]

Characteristics of nonselective nonsteroidal anti-inflammatory drugs:

1. all are given orally except ketorolac tromethamine (Toradol®) (see below)
2. no dependence develops
3. additive effect improves the pain relief with opioid analgesics
4. NSAIDs (and APAP) demonstrate a ceiling effect: a maximum dose above which no further analgesia is obtained. For aspirin and APAP, this is usually between 650–1300 mg, and is often higher for other NSAIDs which may also have a longer duration of action
5. risk of GI upset is common, more serious risks of hepatotoxicity,[10] or GI ulceration, hemorrhage, or perforation are less common
6. taking medication with meals or antacids has not been proven effective in reducing GI side effects. Misoprostol (Cytotec®), a prostaglandin, may be effective in mitigating NSAID-induced gastric erosion or peptic ulcer. Contraindicated in pregnancy. ℞ 200 mcg PO QID with food as long as patient is on NSAIDs. If not tolerated, use 100 mcg. ✖ CAUTION: an abortifacient. Should not be given to pregnant women or women of childbearing potential
7. most reversibly inhibit platelet function and prolong bleeding time (nonacetlyated salicylates have less antiplatelet action, e.g. salsalate, trisalicylate, nabumetome). Aspirin, unlike all other

NSAIDS, *irreversibly* binds to cyclooxygenase and thus inhibits platelet function for the 8–10 day life of the platelet

8. all cause sodium and water retention and carry the risk of NSAID-induced nephrotoxicity[11] (by reducing synthesis of renal vasodilator prostaglandins → reduced renal blood flow which can → renal insufficiency, interstitial nephritis, nephrotic syndrome, hyperkalemia)
9. non-aspirin NSAIDs increase the risk of heart attack or stroke[12]

Drug info: Ketorolac tromethamine (Toradol®)

The only parenteral NSAID approved for use in pain control in the U.S. Analgesic effect is more potent than anti-inflammatory effect. Half-life ≈ 6 hrs. May be useful to control pain in the following situations:

1. where the avoidance of sedation or respiratory depression is critical
2. when constipation cannot be tolerated
3. for patients who are nauseated by narcotics
4. where narcotic dependency is a serious concern
5. when epidural morphine has been used and further analgesia is needed without risk of respiratory depression (agonist type narcotics are contraindicated)
6. cautions:
   a) not indicated for use > 72 hrs (complications have been reported primarily with prolonged use of the oral form)
   b) use with caution in postoperative patients since (as with most NSAIDs) bleeding time is prolonged by platelet function inhibition (risk of GI or op-site hemorrhage is small, but is increased in patients > 75 yrs old, when used > 5 days, and when used in higher doses[13])
   c) even though IM dosing circumvents the GI system, gastric mucosal irritation and erosions may occur as with all NSAIDs (avoid use with PUD)
   d) as with all NSAIDs, use with caution in patients at risk for renal side effects

℞ Parenteral:For single dose administration: 30 mg IV or 60 mg IM in healthy adult. For multiple dosing: 30 mg IV or IM q 6 hrs PRN. Maximum dosage: 120 mg/day. Parenteral use should not exceed 5 days (3 days may be a better guideline).

For patient weight < 50 kg, age > 65 yrs, or reduced renal function (creatinine clearance < 50 ml/min), all of the above dosages are halved (max daily dose: 60 mg). Creatinine clearance can be estimated using the Cockcroft-Gault equation[14] shown in Eq (7.1), with normal values ≥ 60 ml/min.

$$\text{Creatinine clearance(ml/min)} = \frac{[140 - \text{age(years)}] \times \text{ideal wt(kg)}}{72 \times \text{serum creatinine (mg/dl)}} \times (0.85 \text{ for females}) \qquad (7.1)$$

℞ PO: Indicated only as a continuation of IV or IM therapy, not for routine use as an NSAID. Switching from IM to PO: start with 10 mg PO q 4–6 hrs (combined PO and IM dose should be ≤ 120 mg on the day of transition). **Supplied:** 10 mg tablets.

7.3.5 Opioid analgesics

General information

Narcotics are most commonly used for moderate to severe acute pain or cancer pain (some experts characterize cancer pain as recurrent acute pain and not chronic pain).

Characteristics of narcotics:

1. no ceiling effect (p. 137): i.e. increasing dosage increases the effectiveness (although with weak opioids for moderate pain, side effects may limit dosages to relatively low levels[8])
2. with chronic use, tolerance develops (physical and psychological)
3. overdose possible (p. 207), with the potential for respiratory depression with all, and seizures with some

Table 7.4 Nonsteroidal anti-inflammatory drugs (NSAIDs)[a]

Generic name	Proprietary (®)	Typical adult oral dose[b]	Tabs/caps availability (mg)[c]	Daily maximum dose (mg)
aspirin[d]	(many)	500–1000 mg PO q 4–6 hrs (ceiling dose ≈ 1 gm)	325, 500	4000
diclofenac	Voltaren, Cataflam	start at 25 mg QID; additional dose q hs PRN; increase up to 50 mg TID or QID, or 75 mg BID	25, 50, 75	200
etodolac		for acute pain: 200–400 mg q 6–8 hrs	200, 300 caps, 400 tabs	1200
fenoprofen	Nalfon	200 mg q 4–6 hrs; for rheumatoid arthritis 300–600 mg TID-QID	200, 300, 600	3200
flurbiprofen		50 mg TID-QID or 100 mg TID	50, 100	300
ketoprofen	immediate release	start at 75 mg TID or 50 mg QID, ↑ to 150–300 mg daily DIV TID-QID	25, 50, 75	300
	extended release	150 mg q d	ER[c] 150	
ketorolac		see below	see below	
ibuprofen[e]	Motrin	400–800 mg QID (ceiling dose: 800 mg)	300, 400, 600, 800	3200
indomethacin		25 mg TID, ↑ by 25 mg total per day PRN	25, 50, SR 75	150–200
meclofenamate		50 mg q 4–6 hrs; ↑ to 100 mg QID if needed	50, 100	400
mefenamic	Ponstel	500 mg initial; then 250 mg q 6 hrs	250	
nabumetome[f]	Relafen	1000–2000 mg/d given in 1 or 2 doses	500, 750	2000
naproxen	Naprosyn	500 mg, then 250 mg q 6–8 hrs	250, 375, 500	< 1250
naproxen sodium	Anaprox	550 mg, followed by 275 mg q 6–8 hrs	275, DS = 550	1375
oxaprozin	Daypro	1200 mg q d (1st day may take 1800)	600	1800
piroxicam	Feldene	10–20 mg q d (steady state takes 7–12 d)	10, 20	
sulindac		200 mg BID; ↓ to 150 BID when pain controlled	150, 200	400
salsalate		3000 mg divided BID-TID (e.g. 500 mg 2-tabs TID)	500, 750	
tolmetin		400 mg TID (bioavailability is reduced by food)	200, DS = 400, 600	1800

[a]NSAIDs increase the risk of cardiovascular thrombotic events (heart attack or stroke)[12]
[b]when dosage ranges are given, use the smallest effective dose
[c]abbreviations: DS = double strength; SR = slow release; ER = extended release; DOC = drug of choice
[d]aspirin: has unique effectiveness in pain from bone metastases
[e]ibuprofen: is available as a suspension (PediaProfen®) 100 mg/ml; dose for children 6 mos to 12 yrs age is 5–10 mg/kg with a maximum of 40 mg/kg/day (not FDA approved for children because of possible Reye's syndrome)
[f]unlike most NSAIDs, nabumetome does not interfere with platelet function

7

Mild to moderate pain

Table 7.5 Weak opioids for mild to moderate pain

Medication	Dosage	
codeine	usual adult dose: 30–60 mg IM/PO q 3 hrs PRN; use with caution in nursing mothers[a] and children (30 mg PO is equivalent to 300 mg aspirin) pediatric dose: 0.5–1 mg/kg/dose q 4–6 hrs PO or IV PRN	
pentazocine	pentazocine is a mixed agonist-antagonist	
	Talwin®	→ 12.5 mg pentazocine, 325 mg ASA. ℞: 2 PO TID-QID PRN
	with naloxone	→ 50 mg pentazocine, 0.5 mg naloxone. ℞: 1–2 PO q 3–4 hrs PRN up to 12 tabs/day
tramadol (Ultram®)	(see below)	

[a]1–28% of women are ultrafast metabolizers of codeine and the resultant morphine may be passed on to the infant via the breast milk

7

Some useful medications are shown in ▶ Table 7.5.

Codeine and congener pentazocine, are usually no more effective that ASA or APAP and are usually combined with these drugs.

Drug info: Tramadol (Ultram®)

An oral opioid agonist that binds to μ-opioid receptors, and is also a centrally acting analgesic that inhibits reuptake of norepinephrine and serotonin. For acute pain, 100 mg is comparable to codeine 60 mg with ASA or APAP.[15,16] There has been no report of respiratory depression when oral dosing recommendations are followed. Seizures and opioid-like dependence have been reported.[16]

℞ 50 to 100 mg PO q 4–6 hrs PRN pain up to a maximum of 400 mg/day (or 300 mg/d for older patients). For moderately severe acute pain, an initial dose of 100 mg followed by 50 mg doses may suffice. **Supplied:** 50 mg tabs.

Moderate to severe pain

Table 7.6 Opioids for moderate to severe pain

Medication	Dosage
hydrocodone	(Vicodin®, Lorcet®, Lortab®...): 5 mg hydrocodone + 500 mg acetaminophen; (Vicodin ES®, Lortab 7.5/500®): 7.5 mg hydrocodone + 500 mg APAP; ℞ 1 tab PO q 6 hrs PRN (may increase up to 2 tabs PO q 3–4 hrs not to exceed 8 pills/24 hrs).
	(Lorcet® Plus, Lorcet® 10/650): 7.5 or 10 mg hydrocodone (respectively) + 650 mg APAP; ℞ 1 tab PO q 6 hrs PRN (not to exceed 6 tabs in 24 hrs).
	(Lortab® 10/500: 10 mg. hydrocodone + 500 mg APAP); ℞: 1–2 PO q 4 hrs PRN up to 6 tabs/day.
	(Norco®): 10 mg hydrocodone + 325 mg APAP scored tabs; ℞: 1 PO q 4 hrs PRN up to 6 tabs/day.
oxycodone	**Supplied** : usually available in combination as: aspirin 325 mg with oxycodone 5 mg (Percodan®) or acetaminophen (APAP) (Tylox® = APAP 500 mg + oxycodone 5 mg) (Percocet® = oxycodone/APAP in 2.5/325, 5/325, 7.5/500, 10/650) dose: 1 PO q 3–4 hrs PRN (may increase up to 2 PO q 3 hrs[a])

Table 7.6 continued

Medication	Dosage		
	Supplied :also available alone as OxyIR® 5 mg, OxyFast® oral solution of 20 mg/ml, or in controlled-release tablets as OxyContin® 10, 20, 40, 80[b] & 160[b] mg (which last 12 hours, achieving steady state in 24–36 hours). ℞ Adult: OxyContin® tablets are taken whole and are not to be divided, chewed or crushed. It is intended for management of moderate to severe pain when continuous around-the-clock analgesic is needed for an extended period of time and is not intended for use as a PRN analgesic. For opiate naive patients, start with 10 mg PO q 12 hrs. For patients on narcotic medications, a conversion table is provided below for some medications. Titrate dose every 1–2 days, increasing dose by 25–50% q 12 hrs.		
	Conversion table for starting OxyContin®		
	Preparation currently being used	Dose	Suggested starting dose of OxyContin®
	oxycodone combination pills (Tylox, Percodan...) or Lortab, Vicodin or Tylenol #3	1–5 pills/day	10–20 mg PO q 12 hrs
		6–9 pills/day	20–30 mg PO q 12 hrs
		10–12 pills/day	30–40 mg PO q 12 hrs
	IV PCA morphine	determine total MSO4 dose used per 24 hrs	multiply total MSO4 dose in 24 hrs × 1.3 for total OxyContin dose in 24 hrs
hydromorphone	Dilaudid®: (see ► Table 7.7)		
morphine	used in low doses (see ► Table 7.7)		

[a]not to exceed 4000 mg of acetaminophen/24 hrs (see footnote to ► Table 7.3)
[b]for use only in opioid-tolerant patients

Severe pain

Table 7.7 *Equianalgesic* doses for SEVERE pain, AGONIST opioids (parenteral route is referenced to 10 mg IM morphine)

Drug name: generic (proprietary®)	Route	Dose (mg)	Peak (hrs)	Duration (hrs)	Comments
morphine	IM	10	0.5–1	4–6	respiratory depression long acting PO forms: MS Contin®, Avinza® (see below)
	PO	20–60[a]	1.5–2	4–7	
codeine (not recommended at these doses)	IM	130		3–5	these high doses cause unacceptable side effects
	PO	200			
methadone[b] (Dolophine®)	IM	10	0.5–1	4–6	long half-life[b]
	PO	20	1.5–2	4–7	
oxycodone (e.g. Tylox®[c]) (OxyContin®)	IM	15			
	PO	30	1	3–4	combination (Tylox®) or liquid
	PO	30–40		12	*OxyContin*, see ► Table 7.6
oxymorphone	IM	1		3–5	available as suppository
	PR	10			
hydromorphone (Dilaudid®)	IM	1.5	0.5–1	3–4	

Table 7.7 continued

Drug name: generic (proprietary®)	Route	Dose (mg)	Peak (hrs)	Duration (hrs)	Comments
	PO	7.5	1.5–2	3–4	supplied: 1, 2, 3, & 4 mg tabs
fentanyl (Sublimaze®)	IV	0.1		1–2	not recommended for acute pain control, esp. in narcotic naive pts.
transdermal fentanyl patch (Duragesic®)[d]	transdermal	[e]	12–24	72	patches of 25, 50, 75, 100 or 125 mcg/hr (use lowest effective)

[a]IM:PO potency ratio for morphine is 1:6 for single doses, but changes to 1:2–3 with chronic dosing
[b]due to long half-life, repeated dosing can lead to accumulation and CNS depression (must reduce dose after ≈ 3 days, even though the analgesic half-life does not change), especially in the elderly or debilitated patient. Use should be limited to physicians with experience using these drugs
[c]may not be practical for use in severe pain since 1 Tylox® contains only 5 mg oxycodone (the acetaminophen limits the dosage), may use OxyContin® for higher doses of oxycodone
[d] ✖ should not be used as routine post-op analgesic (risk of respiratory depression). Apply 1 patch to upper torso, replace q 72 hrs PRN.
[e]conversion from total daily parenteral morphine as follows:
8–27 mg MSO4/day → Duragesic 25 mcg/hr
28–37 mg MSO4/day → Duragesic 50 mcg/hr
38–52 mg MSO4/day → Duragesic 75 mcg/hr
53–67 mg MSO4/day → Duragesic 100 mcg/hr
68–82 mg MSO4/day → Duragesic 125 mcg/hr

7

Table 7.8 *Equianalgesic* doses for SEVERE pain, AGONIST/ANTAGONIST opioids (referenced to 10 mg IM morphine)

Drug name: generic (proprietary®)	Route	Dose (mg)	Peak (hrs)	Duration (hrs)	Comments
buprenorphine (Buprenex®)	IM	0.4			partial agonist
	SL	0.3			
Mixed agonist/antagonist[a]					
butorphanol	IM	2	0.5–1	4–6	
nalbuphine	IM	10	1	3–6	no sigma receptor occupation[b]
	IV	140 mcg/kg	0.5	2–5	
pentazocine (Talwin®[c])	IM[b]	20–40	0.5–1	4–6	
	PO[b]	180 (start @ 50)	1.5–2	4–7	

[a]all can precipitate withdrawal symptoms in patients physically dependent on agonists
[b]most agonist/antagonist drugs occupy sigma receptors (Stadol > Nubain), which may cause hallucinations
[c]Talwin Injectable (for IM use) contains only pentazocine. Talwin® Compound tablets contain ASA, therefore for high PO doses, use Talwin Nx which contains no ASA (▶ Table 7.5)

Drug info: Avinza® (extended release morphine)

Once daily oral morphine formulation using a spherical oral drug absorption system (SODAS) (numerous ammonio-methacrylate copolymer beads, ≈ 1 mm dia.). Potential for overdosage and/or abuse.

℞: Dosage is titrated based on patient's opioid tolerance and degree of pain. Taken as 1 capsule p. o. q d. Not to be taken "PRN." Not for post-op pain. ✖ CAUTION: To prevent potentially fatal doses of morphine, capsules are to be swallowed whole, and are not to be chewed, crushed or dissolved. However, the contents of the capsule (the beads) may be sprinkled on apple-sauce for those unable to swallow the capsules, but the beads are not to be chewed or crushed. **Side effects**:Due to the potentially nephrotoxic effect of fumaric acid used in SODAS, the maximum dose of Avinza is 1600 mg/d. Doses ≥ 60 mg are for opioid tolerant patients only. **Supplied**:30, 60, 90 & 120 mg capsules.

7.3.6 Adjuvant pain medications

The following may have efficacy in enhancing the effectiveness of opioid analgesics (and thereby may reduce the required dose).

Tricyclic antidepressants:

Tryptophan: an amino acid and a precursor of serotonin, may work by increasing serotonin levels. Requires high doses and has hypnotic effects, therefore 1.5–2 gm given usually q hs. Must give daily MVI as chronic tryptophan therapy depletes vitamin B6.

Antihistamines: histamines play a role in nociception. Antihistamines, which are also anxiolytic, antiemetic, and mildly hypnotic, are effective as analgesics or as adjuvants. Hydroxyzine (Atarax®, Vistaril®): ℞ start with 50 mg PO q AM and 100 mg PO q hs. May increase up to ≈ 200 mg daily.

Anticonvulsant-class drugs: carbamazepine, clonazepam, phenytoin, gabapentin or pregabalin tend to be more effective in neuropathic pain, e.g. from diabetic neuropathy, trigeminal neuralgia, post-herpetic neuralgia, glossopharyngeal neuralgia, and neuralgias due to nerve injury or infiltration with cancer.[16] See index for entries.

Phenothiazines: some cause mild reduction in nociception. Most are tranquilizing and antiemetic. Best known for this use is fluphenazine (Prolixin®), usually given with a tricyclic antidepressant for neuropathic pain, **Diabetic neuropathy, Treatment** (p.545). Phenothiazines may reduce the seizure threshold.

Corticosteroids: in addition to the reduction of toxic effects of radiation or chemotherapy, they may potentiate narcotic analgesics. There are also a number of nonspecific beneficial effects: increased appetite, sense of well being, antiemetic. Side effects may limit usefulness (p.146).

Caffeine: although it possesses no intrinsic analgesic properties, doses of 65–200 mg enhance the analgesic effect of APAP, ASA or ibuprofen in for pain including: H/A, oral surgery pain and post-partum pain.

References

[1] Sessler CN, Gosnell MS, Grap MJ, Brophy GM, O'Neal PV, Keane KA, Tesoro EP, Elswick RK. The Richmond Agitation-Sedation Scale: validity and reliability in adult intensive care unit patients. Am J Respir Crit Care Med. 2002; 166:1338–1344

[2] Ely EW, Truman B, Shintani A, Thomason JW, Wheeler AP, Gordon S, Francis J, Speroff T, Gautam S, Margolin R, Sessler CN, Dittus RS, Bernard GR. Monitoring sedation status over time in ICU patients: reliability and validity of the Richmond Agitation-Sedation Scale (RASS). JAMA. 2003; 289:2983–2991

[3] Kang TM. Propofol infusion syndrome in critically ill patients. Ann Pharmacother. 2002; 36:1453–1456

[4] Werba A, Weinstabi C, Petricek W, et al. Vecuronium Prevents Increases in Intracranial Pressure During Routine Tracheobronchial Suctioning in Neurosurgical Patients. Anaesthetist. 1991; 40:328–331

[5] Hsiang JK, Chesnut RM, Crisp CD, et al. Early, Routine Paralysis for Intracranial Pressure Control in Severe Head Injury: Is It Necessary? Crit Care Med. 1994; 22:1471–1476

[6] Ohlinger MJ, Rhoney DH. Neuromuscular Blocking Agents in the Neurosurgical Intensive Care Unit. Surg Neurol. 1998; 49:217–221

[7] Segredo V, Caldwell JE, Matthay MA, et al. Persistent Paralysis in Critically Ill Patients After Long-Term Administration of Vecuronium. N Engl J Med. 1992; 327:524–528

[8] Marshall KA. Managing Cancer Pain: Basic Principles and Invasive Treatment. Mayo Clin Proc. 1996; 71:472–477

[9] Celecoxib for Arthritis. Med Letter. 1999; 41:11–12

[10] Helfgott SM, Sandberg-Cook J, Zakim D, Nestler J. Diclofenac-Associated Hepatotoxicity. JAMA. 1990; 264:2660–2662

[11] Henrich WL. Analgesic Nephropathy. Am J Med Sci. 1988; 295:561–568

[12] U.S. Food and Drug Administration (FDA). FDA Drug Safety Communication: FDA strengthens warning that non-aspirin nonsteroidal anti-inflammatory drugs (NSAIDs) can cause heart attacks or strokes. 2015

[13] Strom BL, Berlin JA, Kinman JL, et al. Parenteral Ketorolac and Risk of Gastrointestinal and Operative Site Bleeding. JAMA. 1996; 275:376–382

[14] Cockcroft DW, Gault MH. Prediction of creatinine clearance from serum creatinine. Nephron. 1976; 16:31–41

[15] Tramadol - A new oral analgesic. Med Letter. 1995; 37:59–60

[16] Drugs for Pain. Med Letter. 1998; 40:79–84

8 Endocrinology

8.1 Corticosteroids

8.1.1 General information

Under normal, basal conditions, the zona fasciculata of the adrenal cortex secretes 15–25 mg/day of cortisol (hydrocortisone is the name for the identical pharmaceutical compound for administration), and 1.5–4 mg/day of corticosterone. Cortisol has a half-life of ≈ 90 minutes. The release of cortisol by the adrenal glands is stimulated by adrenocorticotrophic hormone (ACTH) from the pituitary which in turn is stimulated by corticotropin releasing hormone (CRH) from the hypothalamus.

8.1.2 Replacement therapy

In primary adrenocortical insufficiency (Addison's disease), both glucocorticoids and mineralocorticoids must be replaced. In secondary adrenal insufficiency caused by deficient corticotropin (ACTH) release by the pituitary, mineralocorticoid secretion is usually normal and only glucocorticoids need to be replaced.

► Table 8.1 shows equivalent daily corticosteroid doses for replacement therapy.

Physiologic replacement (in the absence of stress) can be accomplished with either:

1. hydrocortisone: 20 mg PO q AM and 10 mg PO q PM
2. or prednisone: 5 mg PO q AM and 2.5 mg PO q PM

Cortisol and cortisone are useful for chronic primary adrenocortical insufficiency or for Addisonian crisis. Because of mineralocorticoid activity, use for chronic therapy of other conditions (e.g. hypopituitarism) may result in salt and fluid retention, hypertension and hypokalemia.

8.1.3 Hypothalamic-pituitary-adrenal axis suppression

General information

Chronic steroid administration suppresses the hypothalamic-pituitary-adrenal (HPA) axis, and eventually causes adrenal atrophy. When the HPA is suppressed, if exogenous steroids are abruptly

Table 8.1 Equivalent corticosteroid doses[a]

Steroid: generic (proprietary)	Equiv dose (mg)	Route	Dosing	Mineralocorticoid potency	Oral dosing forms
cortisone acetate	25	PO, IM	2/3 in AM, 1/3 in PM	2+	tabs: 5, 10 & 25 mg
hydrocortisone AKA cortisol (Cortef®)	20	PO	2/3 in AM, 1/3 in PM	2+	tabs: 5, 10 & 20 mg
(Solu-Cortef®)		IV, IM[b]			
prednisone	5	PO only	divided BID-TID	1+	tabs: 1, 2.5, 5, 10, 20, 50 mg[c]
methylprednisolone	4	PO, IV, IM		0	Tabs[d]: 2, 4, 8, 16, 24, 32 mg
dexamethasone	0.75	PO, IV	divided BID-QID	0	scored tabs: 0.25, 0.5, 0.75, 1.5, 4, 6 mg

[a]doses given are daily doses. Steroids listed are used primarily as glucocorticoids: equivalent glucocorticoid PO or IV dose is given; IM may differ
[b]IM route recommended only for emergencies where IV access cannot be rapidly obtained
[c]Sterapred Uni-Pak® contains 21 tabs of 5 mgs prednisone and tapers dosage from 30 to 5 mgs over 6 days; "DS" contains 10 mg tabs and tapers from 60 mg to 10 mg over 6 days; "DS 12-Day" contains 48 10 mg tabs and tapers from 60 mg to 20 mg over 12 days
[d]Medrol Dosepak® contains 21 tabs of 4 mgs methylprednisolone and tapers dosage from 24 mg/d to 4 mg/d over 6 days

stopped or if acute illness develops (which increases the steroid requirements), symptoms of adrenocortical insufficiency (AI) may ensue ▶ Table 8.2. Severe cases of AI may progress to Addisonian crisis (p. 147). Recovery of adrenal cortex lags behind the pituitary, so basal ACTH levels increase before cortisol levels do.

HPA suppression depends on the specific glucocorticoid used, the route, frequency, time, and duration of treatment. Suppression is unlikely with < 40 mg prednisone (or equivalent) given in the morning for less than ≈ 7 days, or with every-other-day therapy of < 40 mg for ≈ 5 weeks.[1] Some adrenal atrophy may occur after 3–4 days of high dose steroids, and some axis suppression will almost certainly occur after 2 weeks of 40–60 mg hydrocortisone (or equivalent) daily. After a month or more of steroids, the HPA axis may be depressed for as long as one year.

Measuring morning plasma hydrocortisone can evaluate the degree of recovery of basal adrenocortical function, but does *not* assess adequacy of stress response.

Steroid withdrawal

See reference.[1]

In addition to the above dangers of hypocortisolism in the presence of HPA suppression, too rapid a taper may cause a flare-up of the underlying condition for which steroids were prescribed.

When the risk of HPA suppression is low (as is the case with short courses of steroids for less than ≈ 5–7 days[2] generally prescribed for most neurosurgical indications) abrupt discontinuation usually carries a low risk of AI. For up to ≈ 2 weeks of use, steroids are usually safely withdrawn by tapering over 1–2 weeks. For longer treatment, or when withdrawal problems develop, use the following *conservative taper*:

1. make small decrements (equivalent to 2.5–5 mg prednisone) every 3–7 d. Patient may experience mild withdrawal symptoms of[3]:
   a) fatigue
   b) anorexia
   c) nausea
   d) orthostatic dizziness
2. “backtrack” (i.e. increase the dose and resume a more gradual taper) if any of the following occur:
   a) exacerbation of the underlying condition for which steroids were used
   b) evidence of steroid withdrawal symptoms (▶ Table 8.2)
   c) intercurrent infection or need for surgery; see Stress doses (p. 146)
3. once “physiologic” doses of glucocorticoid have been reached (about 20 mg hydrocortisone/day or equivalent (▶ Table 8.1):
   a) the patient is switched to 20 mg hydrocortisone PO q AM (do not use long acting preparations)
   b) after ≈ 2–4 weeks, a morning cortisol level is checked (prior to the AM hydrocortisone dose), and the hydrocortisone is tapered by 2.5 mg weekly until 10 mg/d is reached (lower limits of physiologic)
   c) then, every 2–4 weeks, the AM cortisol level is drawn (prior to AM dose) until the 8 AM cortisol is > 10 mcg/100 ml, indicating return of baseline adrenal function
   d) when this return of baseline adrenal function occurs:
      - daily steroids are stopped, but stress doses must still be given when needed (see below)
      - monthly cosyntropin stimulation (p. 735) tests are performed until normal. The need for stress doses of steroids ceases when a positive test is obtained. The risk for adrenal insufficiency persist ≈ 2 years after cessation of chronic steroids (especially the first year)

Table 8.2 Symptoms of adrenal insufficiency (AI)

- fatigue
- weakness
- arthralgia
- anorexia
- nausea
- hypotension
- orthostatic dizziness
- hypoglycemia
- dyspnea
- Addisonian crisis (p. 147) (if severe; with risk of death)

Steroid stress doses

During physiologic "stress" the normal adrenal gland produces ≈ 250–300 mg hydrocortisone/day. With chronic glucocorticoid therapy (either at present, or within last 1–2 yrs), suppression of the normal "stress-response" necessitates supplemental doses.

In patients with a suppressed HPA axis:

- for mild illness (e.g. UTI, common cold), single dental extraction: double the daily dose (if off steroids, give 40 mg hydrocortisone BID)
- for moderate stress (e.g. flu), minor surgery under local anesthesia (endoscopy, multiple dental extractions…): give 50 mg hydrocortisone BID
- for major illness (pneumonia, systemic infections, high fever), severe trauma, or emergency surgery under general anesthesia: give 100 mg hydrocortisone IV q 6–8 hrs for 3–4 days until the stress is resolved
- for elective surgery, see ▶ Table 8.3 for guidelines

8.1.4 Steroid side effects

8

Although deleterious side effects of steroids are more common with prolonged administration,[4] some can occur even with short treatment courses. Some evidence suggests that low-dose glucocorticoids (≤ 10 mg/d of prednisolone or prednisone equivalent) for rheumatoid arthritis does not increase osteoporotic fractures, blood pressure, cardiovascular disease, or peptic ulcers,[5] but weight gain and skin changes are common. Possible side effects include[3,6]:

- cardiovascular and renal
  - hypertension
  - sodium and water retention
  - hypokalemic alkalosis
- CNS
  - progressive multifocal leukoencephalopathy (PML) (p. 331)
  - mental agitation or "steroid psychosis"
  - spinal cord compression from spinal epidural lipomatosis (p. 1408): rare
  - pseudotumor cerebri, Idiopathic intracranial hypertension (IIH) (p. 766)
- endocrine
  - caution: because of growth suppressant effect in children, daily glucocorticoid dosing over prolonged periods should be reserved for the most urgent indications
  - secondary amenorrhea
  - suppression of hypothalamic-pituitary-adrenal axis: reduces endogenous steroid production → risk of adrenal insufficiency with steroid withdrawal (see above)
  - Cushingoid features with prolonged usage (iatrogenic Cushing's syndrome): obesity, hypertension, hirsutism…
- GI: risk increased only with steroid therapy > 3 weeks duration and regimens of prednisone > 400–1000 mg/d or dexamethasone > 40 mg/d[7]
  - gastritis and steroid ulcers: incidence lowered with the use of antacids and/or H2 antagonists (e.g. cimetidine, ranitidine…)
  - pancreatitis

Table 8.3 Steroid stress doses for elective surgery

On day of surgery, 50 mg cortisone acetate IM, followed by 200 mg hydrocortisone IV infused over 24 hrs			
Post-op day	Hydrocortisone (mg)		
	8 AM	4 PM	10 PM
1	50	50	50
2	50	25	25
3	40	20	20
4	30	20	10
5	25	20	5
6	25	15	–
7	20	10	–

- intestinal or sigmoid diverticular perforation[8]: incidence ≈ 0.7%. Since steroids may mask signs of peritonitis, this should be considered in patients on steroids with abdominal discomfort, especially in the elderly and those with a history of diverticular disease. Abdominal x-ray usually shows free intraperitoneal air
- inhibition of fibroblasts
  - impaired wound healing or wound breakdown
  - subcutaneous tissue atrophy
- metabolic
  - glucose intolerance (diabetes) and disturbance of nitrogen metabolism
  - hyperosmolar nonketotic coma
  - hyperlipidemia
  - tend to increase BUN as a result of protein catabolism
- ophthalmologic
  - posterior subcapsular cataracts
  - glaucoma
- musculoskeletal
  - avascular necrosis (AVN) of the hip or other bones: usually with prolonged administration →cushingoid habitus and increased marrow fat within the bone[9] (prednisone 60 mg/d for several months is probably the minimum necessary dose, whereas 20 mg/d for several months will probably *not* produce AVN[10]). Many cases blamed on steroids may instead be due to alcohol use, cigarette smoking,[11] liver disease, underlying vascular inflammation…
  - osteoporosis: may predispose to vertebral compression fractures which occur in 30–50% of patients on prolonged glucocorticoids. Steroid induced bone loss may be reversed with cyclical administration of etidronate[12] in 4 cycles of 400 mg/d ✖ 14 days followed by 76 days of oral calcium supplements of 500 mg/d (not proven to reduced rate of VB fractures)
  - muscle weakness (steroid myopathy): often worse in proximal muscles
- infectious
  - immunosuppression: with possible superinfection, especially fungal, parasitic
  - possible reactivation of TB, chickenpox
- hematologic
  - hypercoagulopathy from inhibition of tissue plasminogen activator
  - steroids cause demargination of white blood cells, which may artifactually elevate the WBC count even in the absence of infection
- miscellaneous
  - hiccups: may respond to chlorpromazine (Thorazine®) 25–50 mg PO TID-QID ✖ 2–3 days (if symptoms persist, give 25–50 mg IM)
  - steroids readily cross the placenta, and fetal adrenal hypoplasia may occur with the administration of large doses during pregnancy

8.1.5 Hypocortisolism

General information

AKA adrenal insufficiency.

Assessment: 8 A.M. serum cortisol level is the best way to test for hypocortisolism. Each lab should provide a lower limit of normal for their lab, which may be broken down further by age and gender.

Addisonian crisis

General information

AKA adrenal crisis. An adrenal insufficiency emergency.

Symptoms: mental status changes (confusion, lethargy, or agitation), muscle weakness.

Signs: postural hypotension or shock, hyperthermia (as high as 105° F, 45.6 C)

Labs

Hyponatremia, hyperkalemia, hypoglycemia.

Treatment of Addisonian crisis

If possible, draw serum for cortisol determination (do not wait for these results to institute therapy). Give fluids sufficient for dehydration and shock.

For "glucocorticoid emergency"
- hydrocortisone sodium succinate (Solu-Cortef®): 100 mg IV STAT and then 50 mg IV q 6 hrs AND
- cortisone acetate 75–100 mg IM STAT, and then 50–75 mg IM q 6 hrs

For "mineralocorticoid emergency"
Usually not necessary in secondary adrenal insufficiency (e.g. panhypopituitarism)
- desoxycorticosterone acetate (Doca®): 5 mg IM BID
OR
- fludrocortisone (Florinef®): 0.05- 0.2 mg PO q d

✖ methylprednisolone is NOT recommended for emergency treatment.

8.2 Hypothyroidism

8.2.1 General information

8

Chronic primary hypothyroidism may result in (non-pathologic) enlargement of the pituitary gland. Plasma TSH determination will distinguish primary hypothyroidism (high TSH) from secondary hypothyroidism (low TSH). Wound healing and cardiac function may be compromised, and surgery under general anesthesia should be postponed if possible until thyroid levels are normalized. Effects of anesthesia may be markedly prolonged, and dosages should be adjusted accordingly.

8.2.2 Thyroid replacement

Caution in patients with adrenal insufficiency

Primary hypothyroidism may be associated with immunologic destruction of adrenal cortex (Schmidt syndrome). Secondary hypothyroidism may be associated with and may mask reduced adrenal function. ✖ Thyroid replacement without adrenal replacement in patients with adrenal insufficiency (as may occur in panhypopituitarism) may precipitate adrenal crisis (thus give ≈ 300–400 mg hydrocortisone IV over 24 hrs in addition to thyroid replacement).

8.2.3 Routine thyroid replacement dosing

Drug info: Levothyroxine (Synthroid®)

Almost pure T4 (contains no T3 as most T3 is produced peripherally from T4).
Dose required to prevent myxedema coma (not to achieve euthyroidism):
- Maintenance: ℞ 0.05 mg po q d
- when patient has been hypothyroid: ℞ start at 0.05 mg po q d and increase by 0.025 mg every 2–3 weeks

For euthyroidism (approximate dose, follow levels and clinical evaluation):
- for most adults < 60 years age: ℞ 0.18 mg/day
- for elderly patients: ℞ 0.12 mg/day

Drug info: Desiccated thyroid (e.g. Armour thyroid®)

Typical dose: ℞ 60 mg (1 grain) to 300 mg daily.

Thyroid replacement in myxedema coma

Myxedema coma is an emergency of hypothyroidism and carries 50% mortality.
Symptoms: altered mental status or unresponsiveness.

Signs: hypotension, bradycardia, hyponatremia, hypoglycemia, hypothermia, hypoventilation, occasionally seizures.

Treatment

Drugs may need to be given IV due to reduced gastric motility.

1. general supportive care:
   a) hypotension: treat with IV fluids (responds poorly to pressors until thyroid replacement accomplished)
   b) hyponatremia: will correct with thyroid replacement; avoid hypertonic saline
   c) hypoglycemia: IV glucose
   d) symptoms of hypocortisolism: thyroid replacement may precipitate adrenal crisis (*see caution above*); give 300–400 mg hydrocortisone IV over 24 hrs
   e) hypothermia: avoid active warming since this increases metabolic demand, use blankets to warm gradually
   f) hypoventilation: check ABG, intubate if necessary
2. thyroid replacement (for average -sized adult):
   a) IV replacement: ℞ 0.5 mg of levothyroxine IV, followed by 0.05–0.2 mg/d IV until patient able to tolerate PO or NG meds
   b) nasogastric replacement: liothyronine (Cytomel®) is primarily T_3, has a rapid onset of action, much shorter half-life than T4, and should be reserved for emergencies.
      ℞: liothyronine 0.05–0.1 mg per NG initially, followed by 0.025 mg BID per NG

8

8.3 Pituitary embryology and neuroendocrinology

8.3.1 Embryology and derivation of the pituitary gland

The posterior pituitary (neurohypophysis) derives from downward evagination of neural crest cells (brain neuroectoderm) from the floor of the third ventricle. The residual recess in the floor of the third ventricle is called the median eminence. The anterior pituitary gland (adenohypophysis) develops from an evagination of epithelial ectoderm of the oropharynx, the evagination is known as Rathke's pouch and is eventually separated from the oropharynx by the sphenoid bone. Cleft-like remnants of Rathke's pouch separates the adenohypophysis and neurohypophysis. The adenohypophysis is comprised of the pars distalis (anterior lobe), the pars intermedia (intermediate lobe) and the pars tuberalis (extension of adenohypophyseal cells on the anterior aspect of the pituitary stalk). The pituitary gland is functionally *outside* the blood-brain barrier.

8.3.2 Pituitary hormones, their targets and their controls

General Information

The pituitary gland releases 8 hormones, 6 from the anterior pituitary, 2 from the posterior pituitary (▶ Fig. 8.1). The anterior pituitary is one of only two sites in the body having a portal circulation (the other being the liver). 6 hypothalamic hormones released in a pulsatile fashion are conveyed in blood from hypothalamic capillaries through this portal circulation via the pituitary stalk to a second capillary bed in the anterior pituitary where they control release of hormones by adenohypophyseal gland cells.

Hormones released from the posterior pituitary (ADH & oxytocin) are synthesized in *neurons* in the hypothalamus (*not* gland cells) and are conveyed along their *axons* also in the pituitary stalk to the posterior pituitary gland where they are released.

The complete homeostatic loop (including negative feedback of the hypothalamic hormones) will not be covered here, and the reader is referred to physiology texts.

Propiomelanocortin (POMC), AKA proopiomelanocortin

241 amino acid polypeptide hormone precursor synthesized primarily in corticotroph cell of the anterior pituitary (but also found in the hypothalamus). Contains amino acid sequences for ACTH, alpha-melanocyte-stimulating hormone (**α-MSH**), β-lipotropin, γ-lipotropin, β-endorphin and met-enkephalin.

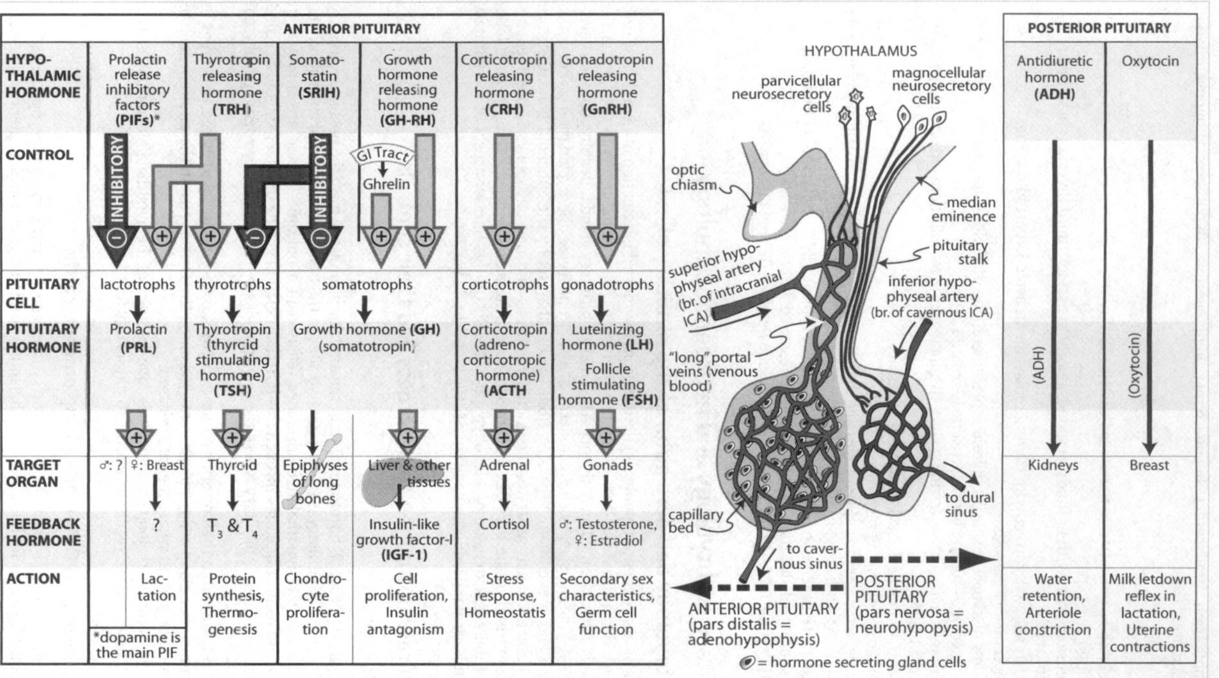

Fig. 8.1 Pituitary neuroendocrinology

Corticotropin AKA adrenocorticotrophic hormone (ACTH)

A 39 amino acid trophic hormone synthesized from POMC. The first 13 amino acids at the amino terminal of ACTH are identical to **α-MSH.** Active half-life is ≈ 10 minutes. Produces a diurnal peak in cortisol (the highest peak occurs in the early morning, with a second, lesser peak in the late afternoon) and also increases in response to stress.

Control: CRH from the hypothalamus stimulates the release of ACTH.

Prolactin (PRL)

AKA somatomammotropin. 199 amino-acid protein weighing 23,000 daltons. Levels are higher in females than males, and are higher still in pregnancy (see ▶ Table 46.3). Secreted in pulsatile fashion with a frequency and amplitude that varies during menstrual cycle (range: 5–27 ng/ml) (≈ 9 pulses/24 hours in the late luteal phase, ≈ 14 pulses/24 hours in the late follicular phase, the pulse amplitude increases from early to late follicular and luteal phases). There is also diurnal variation: levels begin to rise 1 hour after the onset of sleep, peak ≈ 5:00–7:00 AM, and nadir in midmorning after awakening. Heterogeneity of the molecule may produce different results between bioassays and immunoassays.

Control: PRL is the only pituitary hormone predominantly under *inhibitory* control from the hypothalamus by prolactin inhibitory factors (PRIFs), with dopamine being the primary PRIF. Prolactin releasing factors (PRFs) include: thyrotropin-releasing hormone (TRH) and vasoactive intestinal peptide (VIP). The physiologic role of PRFs is not established. For DDx of hyperprolactinemia see ▶ Table 46.4.

8

Growth hormone (GH)

A 191 amino-acid polypeptide trophic hormone. GH normally has pulsatile secretion (≈ 5–10 pulses/24 hours, primarily at night, up to 30 mcg/L), levels may be undetectable (< 0.2 mcg/L) by standard assays between pulses.[13] Insulin-like growth factor-1 (IGF-1) (formerly AKA somatomedin-C) is the protein secreted primarily by the liver in response to GH that is responsible for most of GH's systemic effects (see levels (p. 736)). GH also acts directly on epiphyseal end-plates of long bone to stimulate chondrocyte proliferation.

Control: GH is under dual hypothalamic control via the hypophysial portal system. GH-releasing hormone (GHRH) from the arcuate nucleus stimulates pituitary *secretion* and *synthesis* of GH and induces GH gene transcription. Somatostatin from the periventricular nucleus suppresses GH *release* only, and has no effect on synthesis. GH *release* is also stimulated by ghrelin,[14] a peptide synthesized primarily in the GI tract in response to certain nutrients (may act partially or totally via hypothalamic GHRH).

Thyrotropin AKA thyroid stimulating hormone (TSH)

Glycoprotein trophic hormone secreted by thyrotroph cells of the anterior pituitary.

Control: TSH is also under dual hypothalamic control. TRH stimulates production and release of TSH. Somatostatin inhibits the release of TSH.

Gonadotropins

Follicle stimulating hormone (FSH) and luteinizing hormone (LH) (AKA lutropin) are released from the pituitary in response to gonadotropin releasing hormone 1 (GnRH, formerly luteinizing hormone releasing hormone LH-RH) synthesized primarily in the preoptic area of the hypothalamus.

Antidiuretic hormone (ADH)

AKA arginine vasopressin (AVP). The major source of this nanopeptide hormone is the magnocellular portion of the supraoptic nucleus of the hypothalamus. It is conveyed along *axons* in the supraoptic-hypophyseal tract to the posterior pituitary gland where it is released into the systemic circulation. All actions of ADH result from binding of the hormone to specific membrane bound receptors on the surface of target cells.[15] One of the major effects of ADH is to increase the permeability of the distal renal tubules resulting in increased reabsorption of water, diluting the circulating blood and producing a concentrated urine. The most powerful physiologic stimulus for ADH release is an increase in serum osmolality, a less potent stimulus is a reduction of intravascular volume. ADH is also released in glucocorticoid deficiency, and is inhibited by exogenous glucocorticoids and adrenergic drugs. ADH is also a potent vasoconstrictor.

Oxytocin

A nonapeptide. Oxytocin is a neurotransmitter as well as a hormone. The hypothalamus is the main source of pituitary oxytocin which is stored in nerve endings in the neurohypophysis and is involved in the milk letdown reflex for breastfeeding as well as in uterine contraction during labor.

References

[1] Byyny RL. Withdrawal from Glucocorticoid Therapy. N Engl J Med. 1976; 295:30–32

[2] Szabo GC, Winkler SR. Withdrawal of Glucocorticoid Therapy in Neurosurgical Patients. Surg Neurol. 1995; 44

[3] Kountz DS. An Algorithm for Corticosteroid Withdrawal. Am Fam Physician. 1989; 39:250–254

[4] Marshall LF, King J, Langfitt TW. The Complication of High-Dose Corticosteroid Therapy in Neurosurgical Patients: A Prospective Study. Ann Neurol. 1977; 1:201–203

[5] Da Silva JA, Jacobs JW, Kirwan JR, Boers M, Saag KG, Ines LB, de Koning EJ, Buttgereit F, Cutolo M, Capell H, Rau R, Bijlsma JW. Safety of low dose glucocorticoid treatment in rheumatoid arthritis: published evidence and prospective trial data. Ann Rheum Dis. 2006; 65:285–293

[6] Braughler JM, Hall ED. Current Application of "High-Dose" Steroid Therapy for CNS Injury: A Pharmacological Perspective. J Neurosurg. 1985; 62:806–810

[7] Lu WY, Rhoney DH, Boling WB, et al. A Review of Stress Ulcer Prophylaxis in the Neurosurgical Intensive Care Unit. Neurosurgery. 1997; 41:416–426

[8] Weiner HL, Rezai AR, Cooper PR. Sigmoid Diverticular Perforation in Neurosurgical Patients Receiving High-Dose Corticosteroids. Neurosurgery. 1993; 33:40–43

[9] Zizic TM, Marcoux C, Hungerfold DS, et al. Corticosteroid Therapy Associated with Ischemic Necrosis of Bone in Systemic Lupus Erythematosus. Am J Med. 1985; 79:597–603

[10] Zizic TM. Avascular Necrosis of Bone. Current Opinions in Rheumatology. 1990; 2:26–37

[11] Matsuo K, Hirohata T, Sugioka T, et al. Influence of Alcohol Intake, Cigarette Smoking and Occupational Status on Idiopathic Necrosis of the Femoral Head. Clin Orthop. 1988; 234:115–123

[12] Struys A, Snelder AA, Mulder H. Cyclical Etidronate Reverses Bone Loss of the Spine and Proximal Femur in Patients With Established Corticosteroid-Induced Osteoporosis. Am J Med. 1995; 99:235–242

[13] Peacey SR, Toogood AA, Veldhuis JD, Thorner MO, Shalet SM. The relationship between 24-hour growth hormone secretion and insulin-like growth factor I in patients with successfully treated acromegaly: impact of surgery or radiotherapy. J Clin Endocrinol Metab. 2001; 86:259–266

[14] Tannenbaum GS, Epelbaum J, Bowers CY. Interrelationship between the novel peptide ghrelin and somatostatin/growth hormone-releasing hormone in regulation of pulsatile growth hormone secretion. Endocrinology. 2003; 144:967–974

[15] Thibonnier M, Barrow DL, Selman W. In: Antidiuretic Hormone: Regulation, Disorders, and Clinical Evaluation. Neuroendocrinology. Baltimore: Williams and Wilkins; 1992:19–30

9 Hematology

9.1 General information

Circulating blood volumes for adults and peds are shown in ▶ Table 9.1.

9.2 Blood component therapy

9.2.1 Massive transfusions

Definition: replacement of > 1 blood volume (in average adult ≈ 20 U) in < 24 hrs for adult, or > 2 × circulating blood volume in peds, may cause dilution of effective platelets and coagulation factors. When operating on a pediatric patient, you can usually safely replace up to 1.5 × the circulating blood volume before problems with coagulopathy ensue.

Blood component therapy required for massive transfusions:

1. PRBCs
2. platelets (4 U in adult)
3. FFP

9.2.2 Cellular component

Red blood cell therapy

General information

Major histocompatibilities of blood are shown in ▶ Table 9.2.

Whole blood

1 U (≈ 510 cc) = 450 cc blood + 63 cc preservative.

Recommended transfusion criteria:

- exchange transfusions in neonates
- acute burn debridement and grafting in children

Packed red blood cells (PRBCs)

Recommended transfusion criteria:

1. acute blood loss ≥ 15% of patient's blood volume
2. in asymptomatic patient: hemoglobin (Hb) ≤ 8 gm or Hct ≤ 24%

Table 9.1 Circulating blood volume

Age	Vol (cc/kg[a])
premature infant	85–100
term infant < 1 month	85
infant > 1 mos (& adult)	75

[a]cc per kg of body weight

Table 9.2 Blood compatibility (ABO)

Blood type	Antibody present	Compatible blood (PRBC)	Compatible plasma	Compatible platelets or cryoprecipitate
A	B	A, 0	A, AB	0
B	A	B, 0	B, AB	
AB	none	AB, A, B, 0	AB	
0	A, B	0	AB, A, B, 0	

3. symptoms of anemia at rest
4. preoperative Hb ≤ 15 gm or Hct < 45% in the neonate

Amount to transfuse:
Adult: 1 U (250–300 cc) raises Hct by 3–4%.
For peds, use Eq (9.1).

$$\text{ml of PRBC to transfuse} = \frac{(\text{estimated blood volume [ml]}) \times (\text{Hct increment desired [\%]})}{70\%} \tag{9.1}$$

(where the Hct of PRBCs ranges 70–80%)

Give no faster than 2–3 cc/kg/hr.

Autologous blood transfusion

Predonated whole blood may be stored 35 days. PRBCs may be stored 42 days.

Patients may donate every 3 days to 1 week as long as they maintain Hct ≥ 34% (supplement with ferrous sulfate). The following patients require physician release before donating: patients with coronary artery disease, angina, cerebrovascular disease, seizure disorder, pregnancy (because of possible vasovagal episode) or patients with malignancy.

Try to time last donation > 72 hrs prior to surgery to allow patient to replenish some of the depleted RBCs before surgery.

9

9.2.3 Platelets

General information

Normal platelet count (PC) is 150K-400K (abbreviation used here: 150K = 150,000/mm^3 = 150 × 109/l). Thrombocytopenia is defined as PC < 150K. Bleeding (spontaneously or with invasive procedures) is rarely a problem with PC > 50K. Spontaneous hemorrhage is very likely with PC < 5K. Spontaneous intracranial hemorrhage is uncommon with PC > 30K, and is more common in adults than children. Based on patients with ITP, the risk of fatal hemorrhage in patients with PC < 30K is 0.0162–0.0389 cases per patient-year[1] (risk of death from infection is higher). Intracranial bleeding is usually subarachnoid or intraparenchymal, with petechial hemorrhages common.

1 unit of platelets contains 5.5 × 1010 (minimum) to 10 × 1010 platelets. The volume of 6 units is 250–300 ml. Platelets may be stored up to 5 days.

Recommended platelet transfusion criteria

Indications for platelet transfusion[2]:

1. thrombocytopenia due to ↓ production (with or without increased destruction) (the most common causes are aplastic anemia and leukemia)
   a) PC < 10K even if no bleeding (prophylactic transfusion to prevent bleeding)
   b) PC < 20K and bleeding
   c) PC < 30K and patient at risk for bleeding: complaints of H/A, presence of confluent (c.f. scattered) petechiae, continuous bleeding from a wound, increasing retinal hemorrhage
   d) PC < 50K AND
      - major surgery planned within 12 hours
      - PC rapidly falling
      - patient < 48 hours post-op
      - patient requires lumbar puncture
      - acute blood loss of > 1 blood volume in < 24 hours
2. platelet transfusions have limited usefulness when thrombocytopenia is due to platelet destruction (e.g. by antibodies as in ITTP) or consumption (if production is adequate or increased, platelet transfusion usually will not be useful)
3. documented platelet dysfunction in a patient scheduled for surgery or in a patient with advanced hepatic and/or renal insufficiency (consider pharmacologic enhancement of platelet function, e.g. desmopressin[3])

Other indications for platelet transfusion:

1. patients who have been on Plavix® or aspirin who need urgent surgery that cannot be postponed for ≈ 5 days to allow new platelets to be synthesized

Dosage

Approximately 25% of platelets are lost just with transfusion.

Peds: 1 U/m^2 raises PC by ≈ 10K, usually give 4 U/m^2.

Adult: 1 U raises platelet count by ≈ 5–10K. Typical dose for thrombocytopenic bleeding adult: 6–10 U (usual order: "8-pack"). Alternatively, 1 U of pheresed platelets may be given (obtained from a single donor by apheresis, equivalent to 8–10 U of pooled donor platelets).

Check PC 1–2 hrs after transfusion. The increase in PC will be less in DIC, sepsis, splenomegaly, with platelet antibodies, or if the patient is on chemotherapy. In the absence of increased consumption, platelets will be needed q 3–5 days.

9.2.4 Plasma proteins

FFP (fresh frozen plasma)

General information

1 bag = 200–250 ml (usually referred to as a "unit", not to be confused with 1 unit of factor activity which is defined as 1 ml). FFP is plasma separated from RBCs and platelets, and contains all coagulation factors and natural inhibitors. FFP has an out-date period of 12 months. The risk of AIDS and hepatitis for each unit of FFP is equal to that of a whole unit of blood.

Recommended transfusion criteria

Recommendations (modified[2]):

1. history or clinical course suggestive of coagulopathy due to congenital or acquired coagulation factor deficiency with active bleeding or pre-op, with PT > 18 sec or APTT > 1.5 × upper limit of normal (usually > 55 sec), fibrinogen functioning normally and level > 1 g/l, and coagulation factor assay < 25% activity
2. proven coagulation factor deficiency with active bleeding or scheduled for surgery or other invasive procedure
   a) congenital deficiency of factor II, V, VII, X, XI or XII
   b) deficiency of factor VIII or IX if safe replacement factors unavailable
   c) von Willebrand's disease unresponsive to DDAVP
   d) multiple coagulation factor deficiency as in hepatic dysfunction, vitamin K depletion or DIC
3. reversal of warfarin (Coumadin®) (p. 166) effect (PT > 18 sec, or INR > 1.6) in patient actively bleeding or requiring emergency surgery or procedure with insufficient time for vitamin K to correct (which usually requires > 6–12 hrs)
4. deficiency of antithrombin III, heparin cofactor II, or protein C or S
5. massive blood transfusion: replacement of > 1 blood volume (≈ 5 L in 70 kg adult) within several hours with evidence of coagulation deficiency as in (1) and with continued bleeding
6. treatment of thrombotic thrombocytopenic purpura, hemolytic uremic syndrome
7. ✖ because of associated hazards and suitable alternatives, the use of FFP as a volume expander is relatively contraindicated

Dosage

Usual starting dose is 2 bags of FFP (400–600 ml). If PT is 18–22 secs or APTT is 55–70 secs, 1 bag may suffice. Doses as high as 10–15 ml/kg may be needed for some patients. Monitor PT/PTT (or specific factor assay) and clinical bleeding. Since factor VII has a shorter half-life (≈ 6 hrs) than the other factors, PT may become prolonged before APTT.

Remember: if patient is also receiving platelets, that for every 5–6 units of platelets the patient is also receiving coagulation factors equivalent to ≈ 1 bag of FFP.

Albumin and plasma protein fraction (PPF, AKA Plasmanate®)

Usually from outdated blood, treated to inactivate hepatitis B virus. Ratio of albumin:globulin percentage in "albumin" is 96%:4%, in PPF it is 83%:17%. Available in 5% (oncotically and osmotically equivalent to plasma) and 25% (contraindicated in dehydrated patients). 25% albumin may be diluted to 5% by mixing 1 volume of 25% albumin to 4 volumes of D5 W or 0.9% NS (✖ caution: mixing with sterile water will result in a hypotonic solution that can cause hemolysis and possible renal failure).

Expensive for use simply as a volume expander (≈ $60–80 per unit). Indicated only when total protein < 5.2 gm% (otherwise, use crystalloid which is equally effective). Rapid infusion (> 10 cc/min) has been reported to cause hypotension (due to Na-acetate and Hageman factor fragments). Use in ARDS is controversial. In neurosurgical patients, may be considered as an adjunct for volume

9

expansion (along with crystalloids) for hyperdynamic therapy (p. 1186) when the hematocrit is < 40% following SAH where there is concern about increasing the risk of rebleeding e.g. with the use of hetastarch (p. 1165).

Cryoprecipitate

Recommended transfusion criteria:
1. hemophilia A
2. von Willebrand disease
3. documented fibrinogen/factor VIII deficiency
4. documented disseminated intravascular coagulation (DIC): along with other modes of therapy

Prothrombin complex concentrate (PCC) (Kcentra® and others)

Derived from fresh-frozen human plasma, contains clotting factors II, VII, IX and X, with protein C & S to prevent thrombosis. Primary indication is to be given IV to reverse warfarin in emergency situations. However it is also used in other settings. Requires much lower volume than FFP to work. Also, when the INR gets down to about 1.4, PCC will continue to reduce the INR whereas FFP will have little or no benefit.

Optimal dosing is not known. Doses of 15-50 IU/kg have been given to hemophiliacs but the clotting deficit differs in vitamin-K depletion than in clotting factor absence. A reasonable dose that is often used is 25 IU/kg.

9

9.2.5 Anticoagulation considerations in neurosurgery

General information

Most of these issues have not been studied in a rigorous, prospective fashion. Yet, these questions frequently arise. The following is to be considered a framework of guidelines, and is not to be construed as a standard of care. ▶ Table 9.3 acts as an index to the topics discussed below.

Contraindications to heparin

Contraindications to heparin therapy are constantly being reevaluated. Massive PE producing hemodynamic compromise should be treated with anticoagulation in most cases despite intracranial risks. Contraindications to full anticoagulation with heparin include:
- recent severe head injury
- recent craniotomy: see below
- patients with coagulopathies
- hemorrhagic infarction
- bleeding ulcer or other inaccessible bleeding site

Table 9.3 Anticoagulation issues in neurosurgery

General neurosurgical contraindications to full anticoagulation with heparin (p. 156)
Starting/continuing anticoagulation in the presence of the following neurosurgical conditions

• incidental aneurysm (p. 157)
• subarachnoid hemorrhage (p. 157)
• brain tumor (p. 157)
• following craniotomy (p. 157)
• acute epidural/subdural hematoma
• chronic subdural hematoma
• ischemic stroke
  ◦ after tPA (p. 1287)
  ◦ for prevention of (p. 1270)
• intracerebral hemorrhage (p. 1341)

Managing patients who are already anticoagulated who need a neurosurgical procedure
• warfarin (Coumadin®) (p. 157) • heparin (p. 160) • LMW-heparin (p. 160) • antiplatelet drugs (aspirin, Plavix, NSAIDs) (p. 160)
Recommendations for DVT prophylaxis in neurosurgical patients (p. 168)

- uncontrollable hypertension
- severe hepatic or renal disease
- <4–6 hours before an invasive procedure (see below)
- brain tumor: see below

Patients with unruptured (incidental) cerebral aneurysms

Anticoagulation may not increase the risk of hemorrhage (i.e. rupture), however, should rupture occur, anticoagulation would most likely increase volume of hemorrhage and thus increase morbidity and mortality.

The decision to start/continue anticoagulant depends on the indication for the drugs, the size of the aneurysm (a small aneurysm < 4 mm is not as worrisome). Patients needing Plavix® for drug-eluting cardiac stents should probably be left on their drugs.

Patients on anticoagulation/antiplatelet drugs who develop SAH

Coumadin and antiplatelet drugs are usually reversed.

In patients with brain tumor

Some authors are reluctant to administer full-dose heparin to a patient with a brain tumor,[4] although a number of studies found no higher risk in these patients when treated with heparin or oral anticoagulation[5,6,7] (PT should be followed very closely, one study recommended maintaining PT ≈ 1.25 × control[7]).

9

Post-operatively following craniotomy

Requires individualization based on the reason for the craniotomy. Surgery for parenchymal lesions where the surgery disrupts small vessels (e.g. brain tumor) is probably higher risk for hemorrhage than e.g. aneurysm surgery (expert opinion). Options:

Full anticoagulation: most neurosurgeons would probably not fully anticoagulate patients < 3–5 days following craniotomy,[8] and some recommend at least 2 weeks. However, one study found no increased incidence of bleeding when anticoagulation was resumed 3 days post craniotomy.[9]

Low-dose (prophylactic) anticoagulation: either with mini-dose heparin (5000 U SQ 2 hrs prior to craniotomy and continuing q 12 hrs post-op × 7 d) or enoxaparin (Lovenox) (30 mg SQ BID or as a single dose of 40 MG SQ q d). – RPDB study[10]: assessed *safety* (not efficacy), 55 patients undergoing craniotomy for tumor received mini-dose heparin as indicated had no increased bleeding tendency by any of the parameters measured. RPNB study[11]: incidence of post-op hemorrhage increased to 11% with enoxaparin.

Management of anticoagulants prior to neurosurgical procedures

Pre-operative laboratory assessment of the coagulation pathway and platelet function is routinely used even though these studies rarely contribute critical information in the patient with a negative history for bleeding tendencies. There are no randomized studies to assess the value of coagulation laboratory measurements to patient care. This section encompasses the use of antiplatelet and anticoagulation medicines, their monitoring, and their reversal.

▶ Table 9.4 summarizes this information.

Warfarin

Management guidelines

Patients on warfarin who must be anticoagulated as long as possible (e.g. mechanical heart valves) may be "bridged" to LMW heparin injections, e.g. Lovenox (p. 165), as follows: stop warfarin at least 3 days prior to the procedure, and begin self-administered LMW heparin injections which are discontinued as outlined in ▶ Table 9.4.

Patients with less critical anticoagulation needs (e.g. chronic a-fib) can usually stop the warfarin at least 4–5 days before the procedure, and a PT/INR is then checked on admission to the hospital. Patients must be advised that during the time that they are not anticoagulated, they are at risk of possible complications from the condition for which they are receiving the agents (*annual* risk for mechanical valve: ≈ 6%; for a-fib: depends on several factors including age & history of prior stroke, an average for patients > 65 years age is ≈ 5–6%; see details (p. 1304).

9

Table 9.4 Anticoagulants

Drug Name (Brand)	Administration	Mechanism	Monitoring	Metabolism	Reversal strategy	Hold time[a]	Comments
Unfractionated Heparin	IV for therapeutic anticoagulation; SQ for prophylaxis	Binds artithrombin III. Inhibits conversion of prothrombin → thrombin and fibrinogen → fibrin	aPTT, ACT, or antifactor Xa	Liver; excreted in urine; $T_{1/2}$ 60–90 min	1 mg protamine sulfate/ 100 u heparin administered	Full anticoagulation 4–6 hrs, consider repeat aPTT; SQ "mini-dose" 12 hrs	Heparin produced since 2009 is 10% less potent; incidence of HIT is variable and reportedly 1–2%; "heparin rebound" may occur 8–9 hrs after protamine infusion[31,32]
Enoxaparin (Lovenox, Sanofi Aventis) (a LMWH)	SQ for DVT prophylaxis and therapeutic anticoagulation	Binds antithrombin III and accelerates activity; inhibits thrombin and factor Xa	Antifactor Xa (therapeutic level 0.4–0.8 units/ml)	Liver; renal clearance, caution in patients with CrCl < 30 ml/min	protamine sulfate (1 mg/ 1 mg enoxaparin given in last 8 hrs); will only partially reverse effects (60%)	12 hrs after prophylactic dose; 24 hrs after therapeutic dose	more selective inhibitor of factor Xa than thrombin[33,31,32]
Fondaparinux (Arixtra, GlaskoSmithKline)	SQ for DVT prophylaxis and therapeutic anticoagulation	Inhibits factor Xa	Antifactor Xa; Prophylactic dose (0.4–0.5 mg/l); Therapeutic dose (1.2–1.26 mg/l)	Unknown; Excreted in urine; $T_{1/2}$ 17–21 hrs	No approved antidote; consider rVIIa, but no studies examining the role of rVIIa in reversing fondaparinaux in the setting of bleeding, hemodialysis reduces ≈ 20%	2–4 days in patients with normal renal function	Does not cause HIT, useful in patients with HIT; recommend 50% dose reduction if CrCl 30–50, contraindicated if CrCl < 30[33,31,32]
Warfarin (Coumadin, Bristol-Myers Squibb)	PO	Vitamin K antagonist. Vitamin K dependent factors: II, VII, IX, X, protein C & S.	PT; INR (goal varies with indication)	Liver; excreted in urine ≈ 92%, bile; $T_{1/2}$ 20–60 hrs (highly variable)	Vitamin K10 mg IV x 3 days and/or PCC (25–100 UI/kg) or FFP (15 ml/kg)[b] [31]	5 days	Consider decreasing dose with hepatic impairment
Argatroban (GlaskoSmithKline)	IV for prophylaxis and treatment of thrombosis in patients with HIT	Direct thrombin inhibitor	aPTT (goal 1.5–3x normal); ACT	Liver; excreted in feces ≈ 65% and urine ≈ 22%; $T_{1/2}$ 39–51 min	No reversal agent; supportive care; Hemodialysis can remove some drug from bloodstream, but unknown effect on bleeding, consider FFP or cryoprecipitate	2–4 hrs	Liver disease consider decreasing start dose and titrate slowly[32,28]
Dabigatran (Pradaxa®, Boehringer Ingelheim)	PO, BID dosing	Direct thrombin inhibitor, reversible	No routine monitoring; normal aPTT implies no effect	Liver; renal clearance in urine; $T_{1/2}$ 12–17 hrs	Praxbind (see text below)	1–2 days, longer if renal CrCl < 50 ml/min (see ▶ Table 9.5)	For prevention of stroke with atrial fibrillation (afib); PCC shown to be most effective but unproven in human studies[34,31,32]

Drug Name (Brand)	Administration	Mechanism	Monitoring	Metabolism	Reversal strategy	Hold time[a]	Comments
Rivaroxaban (Xarelto®, Bayer HealthCare)	PO daily dosing	Factor Xa inhibitor	No routine monitoring; normal antifactor Xa indicates no effect	Liver; renal clearance≈66%, feces≈28%; $T_{1/2}$ 5–9h	No specific antagonist; rVIIa has been shown to partially reverse in animal models	24 hrs (see ▶ Table 9.5)	For prevention of stroke in afib and DVT treatment; Caution use with CrCl 15–50; CrCl < 30 avoid use[35,34]
Apixaban (Eliquis®, Bristol-Myers Squibb)	PO, BID dosing	Factor Xa inhibitor	No routine monitoring; normal antifactor Xa indicates no effect	Liver≈75% renal clearance≈25%; $T_{1/2}$ 12h	Consider PCC, or rVIIa. rVIIa decreases bleeding time in animal model but does not reverse anticoagulant effect.	48 hrs (see ▶ Table 9.5)	For prevention of stroke in afib and DVT prophylaxis after orthopedic surgery. Decrease dose if Cr > 1.5; do not use with severe hepatic impairment[34,31]
Antithrombin, recombinant (ATryn, Lundbeck)	IV	Inhibits thrombin and factor Xa	AT levels	$T_{1/2}$ 11.6–17.7h			For thromboembolism prophylaxis in hereditary antithrombin deficiency
Antithrombin III (Thrombate III, Grifols)	IV	Forms bond with thrombin	AT levels	$T_{1/2}$ 2–3 days			For thromboembolism prophylaxis in hereditary antithrombin deficiency
Dalteparin (Fragmin, Eisai)	SQ for DVT prophylaxis and therapeutic anticoagulation	Accelerates activity of antithrombin III (inhibits thrombin and factor Xa)		Liver, urine; $T_{1/2}$ 3–5h (longer with renal impairment)			Caution when use with CrCl < 30; caution with hepatic impairment
Bivalirudin (Angiomax®, The Medicines Company)	IV	Direct thrombin inhibitor (reversible)	ACT	Plasma; excreted in urine; $T_{1/2}$ 25 min (longer with renal impairment)	None		Caution when use with CrCl < 30
Desirudin (Iprivask®, Canyon)	SC	Direct thrombin inhibitor (selectively inhibits free and clot-bound thrombin	aPTT	Kidney; excreted in urine; $T_{1/2}$ 2h (longer with renal impairment)	None		CrCl < 60 use caution, decrease initial dose[31]

Abbreviations: PCC = prothrombin complex concentrate, IV = intravenous, SQ = subcutaneous, aPTT = partial thromboplastin time, DVT = deep venous thrombosis, HIT = heparin induced thrombocytopenia, ACT = activated clotting time, AT = anti-thrombin, CrCl = creatinine clearance

[a] Hold time is the recommended time to wait after discontinuing the drug before doing an elective operation in order to eliminate the effects of the drug

[b] Intravenous vitamin K has a more rapid onset than subcutaneous vitamin K and current formulations, made with micelles of lecithin and glycol, seem to have a lower complication profile than older formulations containing polyethylated castor oil.[36]

Table 9.5 Recommendations for holding new oral anticoagulants prior to invasive procedures related to renal function.[31]

	Dabigatran	Apixaban	Rivoraxaban
CrCl > 80 ml/min	≥ 72 hr	≥ 48 hr	≥ 48 hr
CrCl 50–80 ml/min	≥ 72 hr	≥ 48 hr	≥ 48 hr
CrCl 30–49 ml/min	≥ 96 hr	≥ 72 hr	≥ 72 hr
CrCl < 30 ml/min	≥ 120 hr	≥ 96 hr	≥ 96 hr

The recommended minimum interval between last dose and procedure is based on renal function and procedure risk. Generally, neurosurgical procedures including minor procedures such as LPs are considered interventions with a high bleeding risk

For non-emergent neurosurgical procedures

For procedures where post-op mass effect from bleeding would pose serious risk (which includes most neurosurgical operations), it is recommended that the PT should be ≈ ≤ 13.5 sec (i.e. ≤ upper limits of normal) or the INR should be ≈ ≤ 1.4 (e.g. for reference, this INR is considered safe for performing a percutaneous needle liver biopsy). See also reversal of anticoagulation (p. 166).

For emergent neurosurgical procedures

9

Give FFP (start with 2 units) and vitamin K (10–20 mg IV at ≤ 1 mg/min) as soon as possible; see also reversal of anticoagulation (p. 166). The timing of surgery is then based on the urgency of the situation and the nature of the procedure (e.g. the decision might be to evacuate a spinal epidural hematoma in an acutely paralyzed patient before anticoagulation is fully reversed).

Heparin

For emergencies: if it would be deleterious to wait 4–6 hours after discontinuing heparin and then repeating the PTT to verify that anticoagulation has been corrected, then heparin can be reversed with protamine (p. 166).

For non-emergencies

IV heparin: stop the drip ≈ 4–6 hours prior to the planned procedure. Option: recheck PTT just prior to starting the procedure.

"Mini-dose" SQ heparin: not mandatory to stop for craniotomy, but if desired to discontinue, then give last dose ≥ 12 hours prior to surgery.

Low-molecular weight heparins (LMWH)

For emergencies: can be reversed with protamine (p. 166).

Non-emergencies: See ▶ Table 9.4. Longer times are needed in renal failure. A factor Xa level can be used to check anticoagulation status, but this usually must be sent out, making it unsuitable for acute management.

Antiplatelet drugs and neurosurgical procedures

Platelet mechanistics and platelet function tests

Platelets are important for maintaining vascular endothelial integrity and are constantly involved with hemostasis in conjunction with coagulation factors. Severe thrombocytopenia can result in petechial hemorrhages or spontaneous intracerebral hemorrhage (ICH). Vascular wall disturbance is the initial stimulus for platelet deposition and activation. Platelets adhere to collagen via surface receptors GPIb-V-IX and von Willebrand factor. This adhesion sets off a cascade of reactions, which result in platelet aggregation forming a hemostatic plug. Historically, bleeding time (BT) was used as the screening test for abnormalities of platelet function. Due to unreliability, many institutions have replaced the BT with the platelet function assay (PFA) using the PFA-100 (platelet function analyzer). There are limited studies confirming its use according to the International Society of Thrombosis and Hemostasis.[12,13]

In the PFA-100, primary hemostasis is simulated under "high-shear" flow by movement of citrated blood through a membrane-impregnated capillary in two collagen-coated cartridges; one stimulates platelets with adenosine diphosphate (ADP) and the other with epinephrine.[14] This interaction with the collagen induces a platelet plug, which closes an aperture. Results are reported as closure time in seconds. This method is eligible as a screening test for primary hemostatic disease such as von Willebrand disease as well as for monitoring the effect of antiplatelet therapy. The PFA-100 works for testing with aspirin but not with thienopyridine drug class (e.g. clopidogrel). Newly available PFA cartridges detect P2Y12 receptor blockade in patients on theinopyridine drugs.[15] VerifyNow® measures agonist-induced aggregation as an increase in light transmittance. The system contains a preparation of human fibrinogen-coated beads, which cause a change in light transmittance by ADP-induced platelet aggregation.[15] There is little correlation between PFA-100 results and VerifyNow Assay.

Agents

► **Plavix® (clopidogrel)** (p. 1275) **and aspirin.** Cause permanent inhibition of platelet function that persists ≈ 5 days after discontinuation of the drug and can increase the risk of bleeding. For elective cases, 5–7 days off these drugs is recommended (surveys of German neurosurgeons[16,17]: an average of 7 days was used for low-dose ASA, with a few who do *spine* surgery even while the patient is on ASA).

Cardiac stents: dual antiplatelet therapy (e.g. ASA + Plavix®) are mandatory for 4 weeks (90 days is preferable[18]) after placement of a bare metal cardiac stent, and for at least 1 year with drug-eluting stents (DES) (the risk declines from ≈ 6% to ≈ 3%).[19] Even short gaps in drug therapy (e.g. to perform neurosurgical procedures) is associated with significant risk of acute stent occlusion (and therefore elective surgery during this time is discouraged[20]). DES are so effective in suppressing endothelialization that lifetime dual antiplatelet therapy may be required. Bridging DES patients with antithrombin, anticoagulants, or glycoprotein IIb/IIIa agents has not been proven effective.[20]

Reversal of antiplatelet drugs: While heparin and warfarin can be reliably and measurably reversed, the situation is less clear with antiplatelet agents.[21] Agents used pre-op to reverse these drugs include: Desmopressin (p. 166) (DDAVP®)[16,17] and FFP.[16]

Reversal of Plavix for emergency surgery (p. 154): platelets may be given, however, Plavix effects persists for up to a couple of days after the last dose, and can actually inhibit platelets given after the drug is discontinued (the half-life of aspirin is lower and should not be an issue after 1 day). In cases with continued oozing in the first day or so after discontinuing Plavix, the following regimen is an option:

1. recombinant activated coagulation factor VII (rFVIIa): even though the defect is in the platelets, rFVIIa works, via a mechanism not mediated by protein clotting factors. Very expensive (≈ $10,000 per dose), but this must be balanced against the cost of repeat craniotomy, increased ICU stay and additional morbidity
   a) initial dose[22]: 90–120 mcg/kg
   b) same dose 2 hrs later
   c) 3rd dose 6 hrs after initial dose
2. platelets every 8 hours for 24 hours, *either*
   a) 6 U of regular platelets
   b) if patient is on fluid or volume restriction: 1 unit of pheresed platelets

► **Herbal products and supplements.** Herbal products and supplements often affect platelet aggregation and the coagulation cascade by means that cannot be detected by laboratory tests. The increasing popularity of these unregulated products requires screening patients for their use. There are limited studies regarding the use of herbal supplements in neurosurgery and for an elective operation waiting 7–14 days after cessation of their use is warranted.

Fish Oil (Omega-3 Fatty Acids) is widely used among the cardiac and general population for treatment of dyslipidemia and hypertriglyceridemia. Fish oil may affect platelet aggregation by a reduction in arachnadonic acid and thomboxane and adenosine diphosphate receptor blockade. Fish oil may also potentially lengthen bleeding times.[23,24,25]

Garlic (Allium sativum) has increased in popularity as a supplement. Purported benefits include: lowering blood pressure, preventing infection and myocardial infarction, and treating hypercholesterolemia. Garlic has an antiplatelet affect through ADP receptor blockade, and reducing calcium and thromboxane.[26] There is particular concern with garlic as it may potentiate the antiplatelet or anticoagulant affect of aspirin or warfarin.[27]

Ginkgo (Ginkgo biloba)has also become a popular supplement found in many formulations from capsules to energy drinks. Ginkgo has been used to treat a number of ailments including memory loss, depression, anxiety, dizziness, claudication, erectile dysfunction, tinnitus and headache. Ginkgo affects bleeding via an antiplatelet effect and antagonism of platelet-activating factor.[28,29] See Ginkgo biloba under Spontaneous subdural hematoma (p. 901).

Ginseng (Panax ginseng)has also been found to have antiplatelet activity through thromboxane inhibition and platelet-activating factor.[30]

Some authors also advocate cautious use of **ginger** and **vitamin E** when planning surgery, but the exact antiplatelet mechanism is unclear.[25]

Table 9.6 Platelet function inhibitors

Drug Name (Brand)	Class/Target	Mechanism	Administration	Monitoring	Metabolism	Reversal strategy	Hold time[a]	Comments
Aspirin (Acetylsalicylic acid)	COX-1	Direct action, irreversible	PO	PFA, Arachidonic acid-based tests (VerifyNow)	Gut, plasma, and liver; renal clearance; $T_{1/2}$ 15–20 min	Platelet transfusion; Desmopressin[b]	7–10 days	Prevalence of aspirin resistance is 5–60%; therapeutic effect for lifetime of platelets (9 days), 10% of circulating platelets are replaced in 24-hr period[37,31,32]
Clopidogrel (Plavix®, Sanofi Aventis)	Thienopyridines/$P2Y_{12}$	Prodrug, irreversible	PO	PFA, VerifyNow P2Y12 (PRU Test)	Liver; renal clearance $T_{1/2}$ 8 hrs	Platelet transfusion (10 concentrate units every 12 hrs for 48 hrs); Desmopressin[b]	7–10 day	Prevalence of clopidogrel resistance is 8–35%[37,31,32]
Ticlodipine (Ticlid, Roche)	Thienopyridines/$P2Y_{12}$	Prodrug, irreversible	PO	Bleeding time	Liver; renal clearance; $T_{1/2}$ 4–5 days	NA		Effective in ≈96% of patients with clopidogrel resistance
Prasugrel (Effient®, Eli Lilly)	Thienopyridines/$P2Y_{12}$	Prodrug, irreversible	PO	PFA, VerifyNow P2Y12 (PRU Test)	Liver; renal clearance ≈68%, feces≈27%; $T_{1/2}$ 3.7 hrs	Platelet transfusion; active metabolite not removed by dialysis		Used for coronary artery disease[31]
Ticagrelor (Brilinta, AstraZeneca)	Cyclopentyltriaxolopyrimidine/$P2Y_{12}$	Direct-acting, reversible	PO	NA	Liver; excreted in bile primarily; $T_{1/2}$ 9 hrs (active metabolite)	NA, not removed by dialysis		
Dipyridamole (Persantine, Boehringer Ingelheim)	cGMP V	Prodrug, reversible	PO	NA	Liver; excretion in bile; $T_{1/2}$ 10–12 hrs	Dialysis is no benefit		
Abciximab (ReoPro, Eli Lilly)	GPIIb/IIIa	Reversible	IV	aPTT, ACT, VerifyNow IIb/IIIa test	Proteolytic cleavage; $T_{1/2}$ 30 min	Platelet transfusion, no antagonist		Platelet function returns to ≈50% of baseline 24hrs after infusion; low-level inhibition may continue for up to 7 weeks[32]
Eptifibatide	GPIIb/IIIa	Reversible	IV	aPTT, ACT,	Renal clearance 75%;	May be removed by		CrCl < 50 adjust infusion

Table 9.6 continued

Drug Name (Brand)	Class/Target	Mechanism	Adminis-tration	Monitoring	Metabolism	Reversal strategy	Hold time[a]	Comments
(Integrilin, Millennium/ Merck)				VerifyNow IIb/IIIa test	$T_{1/2}$ 2.5 hrs	dialysis		rate; platelet function returns to ≈50% 4hrs after infusion D/C'd[32]
Triofiban (Aggrastat, Medicure)	GPIIb/IIIa	Reversible	IV		Renal clearance 65%, feces 25%; $T_{1/2}$ 2–3 hrs	May be removed by dialysis		CrCl < 30 adjust infusion rate; platelet coagulation is inhibited within 5 min, and remains inhibited for 3–8h[32]

Abbreviations: PCC = prothrombin complex concentrate, IV = intravenous. SQ = subcutaneous, aPTT = partial thromboplastin time, ACT = activated clotting time, CrCl = creatinine clearance, D/C = discontinue

[a] Hold time is the recommended time to wait after discontinuing the drug before doing an elective operation in order to eliminate the effects of the drug

[b] Desmopressin enhances platelet adhesion to vessel wall by increased concentrations of factor VIII and von Willebrand factor. Desmopressin increased platelet adhesion in randomized trial in both aspirin group and control group.[38]

9

Table 9.7 Recommended INRs[39]

Indication	INR
• mechanical prosthetic heart valve • prevention of recurrent MI	2.5–3.5
antiphospholipid antibody syndrome (p. 1270) [40]	≥ 3
all other indications (*DVT prophylaxis* and treatment, PE, atrial fibrillation, recurrent systemic embolism, tissue heart valves)	2–3

Anticoagulants

See also platelet function inhibitors (p. 164).

Warfarin

Drug info: Warfarin (Coumadin®)

An oral vitamin K antagonist. To anticoagulate average weight patient, give 10 mg PO q d × 2–4 days, then ≈ 5 mg q d. Follow coagulation studies, titrate to PT = 1.2–1.5 × control (or INR ≈ 2–3) for most conditions (e.g. DVT, single TIA). Higher PT ratios of 1.5–2 × control (INR ≈ 3–4) may be needed for recurrent systemic embolism, mechanical heart valves... (the recommended ranges for the International Normalized Ratio (INR) are shown in ▶ Table 9.7).

Starting warfarin: During the first ≈ 3 days of warfarin therapy, patients may actually be hypercoagulable (secondary to reduction of vitamin-K dependent anticoagulation factors protein C and protein S), putting them at risk of "Coumadin necrosis." Therefore patients should be "bridged" by starting either Lovenox (p. 165) which can be self-administered as an outpatient, or heparain (with a therapeutic PTT).

Supplied: scored tabs of 1, 2, 2.5, 5, 7.5 and 10 mg. IV form: 5 mg/vial.

Heparin

Drug info: Heparin

℞ Full anticoagulation in an average weight patient, give 5000 U bolus IV, follow with 1000 U/hr IV drip. Titrate to therapeutic anticoagulation of APTT = 2–2.5 × control (for DVT, some recommend 1.5–2 × control[41]).

℞ prophylactic AKA low-dose ("mini-dose") heparin: 5000 IU SQ q 8 or 12 hrs. Routine monitoring of APTT is usually not done, although occasionally patients may become fully anticoagulated on this regimen.

Side effects: (see Anticoagulant considerations in neurosurgery above): hemorrhage, thrombosis[42] (heparin activates anti-thrombin III and can cause platelet aggregation) which can result in MIs, DVTs, PEs, strokes, etc. Heparin induced thrombocytopenia (HIT): transient mild thrombocytopenia is fairly common in the first few days after initiating heparin therapy, however severe thrombocytopenia occurs in 1–2% of patients receiving heparin > 4 days (usually has a delayed onset of 6–12 days, and is due to consumption in heparin-induced thrombosis or to antibodies formed against a heparin-platelet protein complex). The incidence of HIT in SAH is 5–6% and was similar with enoxaparin.[43] Consider use of fondaparinux in thrombocytopenic patients. Chronic therapy may cause osteoporosis.

Low molecular weight heparins

See references.[44,45]

Low molecular weight heparins (LMWH) (average molecular weight = 3000–8000 daltons) are derived from unfractionated heparin (average MW = 12,000–15,000 daltons). LMWHs differ from unfractionated heparin because they have a higher ratio of anti-factor Xa to anti-factor IIa (antithrombin) activity which theoretically should produce antithrombic effects with fewer hemorrhagic complications. Realization of this benefit has been very minor in clinical trials. LMWH have greater bioavailability after sub-Q injection leading to more predictable plasma levels which eliminates the need to monitor biologic activity (such as APTT). LMWH have a longer half-life and therefore require fewer doses per day. LMWH have a lower incidence of thrombocytopenia. More effective in DVT prophylaxis than warfarin in orthopedic surgery.[46]

Spinal epidural hematomas: There have been a number of case reports of spinal epidural hematomas occurring in patients on LMWH (primarily enoxaparin) who also underwent spinal/epidural anesthesia or lumbar puncture, primarily in elderly women undergoing orthopedic surgery. Some have had significant neurologic sequelae, including permanent paralysis.[47] The risk is further increased by the use of NSAIDs, platelet inhibitors, or other anticoagulants, and with traumatic or repeated epidural or spinal puncture.

► **Available low molecular weight heparins.** Drugs include:
- enoxaparin (Lovenox®): see below
- dalteparin (Fragmin®): ℞ 2500 anti-Xa U SQ q d
- ardeparin (Normiflo®): half-life = 3.3 hrs. ℞ 50 anti-Xa U/kg SQ q 12 hrs
- danaparoid (Orgaran®): a heparinoid. Even higher anti-Xa:anti-IIa ratio than LMWHs. Does not require laboratory monitoring. ℞ 750 anti-Xa U SQ BID
- tinzaparin (Logiparin®, Innohep®): not available in U.S. ℞ 175 anti-Xa U per kg SQ once daily

Drug info: Enoxaparin (Lovenox®)

℞ dosage established following hip replacement is 30 mg SQ BID × 7–14 days (alternative: 40 mg SQ q d). **Pharmacokinetics:** After SQ injection, peak serum concentration occurs in 3–5 hrs. Half-life: 4.5 hrs.

9

Direct thrombin inhibitors

Drug info: Dabigatran (Pradaxa®, Rendix®)

An oral anticoagulant in the class of direct thrombin inhibitors. Administered as the prodrug dabigatran etexilate. Must be stopped 24 hrs prior to surgery.

Reversal of anticoagulation: Praxbind (idarucizumab) IV for emergencies. Reverses pradaxa within 4 hrs, lasts 24 hrs.[48]

Drug info: Bivalirudin (Angiomax® or Angiox®)

A reversible direct thrombin inhibitor (DTI) that increases the rapidity of plasminogen activator-mediated recanalization. No effective reversal.

℞: IV loading dose of 0.5 mg/kg IV, followed by continuous infusion of 1.75 mg/kg/hr. Intraarterial: inject 15 mg in 10 ml of heparinized saline via a microcatheter.

Factor Xa inhibitors

Drug info: Fondaparinux (Arixtra®)

A synthetic analog of the pentasaccharide binding sequence of heparin. Increases factor Xa inhibition without affecting factor IIa (thrombin).[49] Unlike heparin, fondaparinux does not bind to other plasma proteins or platelet factor-4 and does not cause heparin-induced thrombocytopenia (HIT) and can therefore be used in patients with HIT. May be more effective than enoxaparin (Lovenox®) for preventing post-op DVTs. **Side effects:** Bleeding is the most common side effect (may be increased by concurrent NSAID use). ✖ Contraindicated with severe renal impairment (CrCl < 30 ml/min).[50]

℞: 2.5 mg SQ injection q d. **Supplied:** 2.5 mg single-dose syringes. **Pharmacokinetics:** Peak activity occurs in 2–3 hrs. Half-life: 17-21 hrs. Anticoagulation effect lasts 3-5 half-lives. Elimination: in urine (in renal insufficiency reduce dose by 50% for CrCl 30-50 ml/min). STOP: 2-4 days pre-op (longer with kidney dysfunction)

Coagulopathies

Correction of coagulopathies or reversal of anticoagulants

Also refer to recommended normal values for coagulation studies in neurosurgery (p. 157).

Platelets

See indications and administration guidelines (p. 154).

Fresh frozen plasma

To reverse warfarin anticoagulation, use the following as a starting point and recheck PT/PTT afterwards:

- when patient is "therapeutically anticoagulated" start with 2–3 units FFP (approximately 15 ml/kg is usually needed)
- for severely prolonged PT/PTT, start with 6 units FFP

Prothrombin complex concentrate (PCC)

Warfarin induced anticoagulation may be reversed up to 4 or 5 times more quickly with PCC (Kcentra) (contains coag factors II, IX, and X) than with FFP.[51] Patient may become hyperthrombotic with this.

Drug info: Vitamin K (Mephyton®)

To reverse elevated PT from *warfarin* , give aqueous colloidal solution of vitamin K1 (phytonadione, Mephyton®). Doses > 10 mg may produce warfarin resistance for up to 1 week. FFP may be administered concurrently for more rapid correction (see above). See recommended levels of PT (p. 157).

℞ adult: start with 10–15 mg IM; the effect takes 6–12 hrs (in absence of liver disease). Repeat dose if needed. The average total dose needed to reverse therapeutic anticoagulation is 25–35 mg.

IV administration has been associated with severe reactions (possibly anaphylactic), including hypotension and even fatalities (even with proper precautions to dilute and administer slowly), therefore IV route is reserved only for situations where other routes are not feasible and the serious risk is justified. ℞ IV (when IM route not feasible): 10–20 mg IV at a rate of injection not to exceed 1 mg/min (e.g. put 10 mg in 50 ml of D5 W and give over 30 minutes).

Drug info: Protamine sulfate

For heparin: 1 mg protamine reverses ≈ 100 U *heparin* (give slowly, not to exceed 50 mg in any 10 min period). Therapy should be guided by coagulation studies.

Reversal of low molecular weight heparins (LMWH): slow IV injection of a 1% solution of protamine can also be used to reverse LMWHs as follows:

Enoxaparin (Lovenox®): ≈ 60% of Lovenox can be reversed with 1 mg of protamine for every mg of Lovenox given (maximum dose = 50 mg) within the last 8 hrs, and 0.5 mg of protamine for every mg of Lovenox given from 8–12 hrs prior. Protamine is probably not needed for Lovenox given > 12 hrs earlier.

Dalteparin (Fragmin®) or ardeparin (Normiflo®): 1 mg of protamine for every 100 anti-Xa IU of the LMWH (maximum dose = 50 mg) with a second infusion of 0.5 mg protamine for every 100 anti-Xa IU of LMWH if the APTT remains elevated 2–4 hours after the first dose is completed.

Danaparoid and Hirudin: no known reversing agent.

Drug info: Desmopressin (DDAVP®)

Causes an increase in factor III coagulant activity and von Willebrand factor which helps coagulation and platelet activity in hemophilia A and in von Willebrand's disease Type I (where the factors are normal in makeup but low in concentration, ✖ but may cause thrombocytopenia in von Willebrand's disease Type IIB where factors may be abnormal or missing).

℞ 0.3 mcg/kg (use 50 ml of diluent for doses ≤ 3 mcg, use 10 ml for doses > 3 mcg) given over 15–30 minutes 30 minutes prior to a surgical procedure.

Elevated pre-op PTT

In a patient with no history of coagulopathy, a significantly elevated pre-op PTT is commonly due to either a factor deficiency or to lupus anticoagulant. Work-up:

1. mixing study
2. lupus coagulant

If the mixing study corrects the elevated PTT, then there is probably a factor deficiency. Consult a hematologist.

Lupus anticoagulant: If the test for lupus anticoagulant is positive, then the major risk to the patient with surgery is *not* bleeding, rather it is thromboembolism. Management recommendations:

1. as soon as feasible post-op, start patient on heparin (p.164) or LMW heparin (p.164), e.g. Lovenox
2. at the same time start warfarin, and maintain therapeutic anticoagulation for 3–4 weeks (the risk of DVT/PE is actually highest in the first few weeks post-op)
3. mobilize as soon as possible post-op
4. consider vena-cava interruption filter in patients for whom anticoagulation is contraindicated

Disseminated intravascular coagulation (DIC)

Abnormal intravascular coagulation which consumes clotting factors and platelets, coupled with abnormal activation of fibrinolytic system. Head trauma is an independent risk factor for DIC, possibly because the brain is rich in thromboplastin which may be released into systemic circulation with trauma.[52] Other risk factors: shock, sepsis.

Presentation

Diffuse bleeding, cutaneous petechia, shock.

Labs

1. fibrinogen degradation products (FDP) > 16 mcg/ml (1–8 = normal; 8–16 = borderline; 32 = definitely abnormal; some labs require > 40 for diagnosis of DIC) (the most common abnormality)
2. fibrinogen < 100 mcg/dl (some use 130)
3. PT > 16; PTT > 50
4. platelets < 50,000 (relatively uncommon)

Chronic DIC

PT & PTT may be normal; platelet & fibrinogen low, fibrin split products elevated.

Treatment

1. remove inciting stimulus if possible (treat infections, debride injured tissue, stop transfusions if suspected)
2. vigorous fluid resuscitation
3. anticoagulants, if not contraindicated (p.156)
4. FFP if PT or PTT elevated, or fibrinogen < 130
5. platelet transfusion if platelet count < 100 K

Pseudo-DIC

Increased fibrin split products, normal fibrinogen.
Seen in conditions such as liver failure.

Thromboembolism in neurosurgery

Deep-vein thrombosis (DVT)

DVT is of concern primarily because of the potential for material (clot, platelet clumps…) to dislodge and form emboli (including pulmonary emboli, (PE)) which may cause pulmonary infarction, sudden death (from cardiac arrest), or cerebral infarction (from a paradoxical embolus, which may occur in the presence of a patent foramen ovale, see Cardiogenic brain embolism (p.1304)). The reported mortality from DVT in the LEs ranges from 9–50%.[53] DVT limited to the calf has a low threat (< 1%) of embolization, however, these clots later extend into the proximal deep veins in 30–50% of cases,[53] from where embolization may occur (in 40–50%), or they may produce postphlebitic syndrome.

Neurosurgical patients are particularly prone to developing DVTs (estimated risk: 19–50%) due at least in part to the relatively high frequency of the following:

1. long operating times of some procedures
2. prolonged bed rest pre- and/or post-op

3. alterations in coagulation status
   a) in patients with brain tumors (see below) or head injury[54]
      - related to the condition itself
      - due to release of brain thromboplastins during brain surgery
   b) increased blood viscosity with concomitant "sludging"
      - from dehydration therapy sometimes used to reduce cerebral edema
      - from volume loss following SAH (cerebral salt wasting)
   c) use of high-dose glucocorticoids

Specific "neurological" risk factors for DVT and PE include[53]:
1. spinal cord injury (p.952)
2. brain tumor: autopsy prevalence of DVT = 28%, of PE = 8.4%. Incidence using 125I-fibrinogen[55]: meningioma 72%, malignant glioma 60%, metastasis 20%. Risk may be reduced by pre-op use of aspirin[56]
3. subarachnoid hemorrhage
4. head trauma: especially severe TBI (p.918)
5. stroke: incidence of PE = 1–19.8%, with mortality of 25–100%
6. neurosurgical operation: risk is higher following craniotomy for supratentorial tumors (7% of 492 patients) than p-fossa tumors (0 out of 141)[57]

Prophylaxis against DVT

Options include:
1. general measures
   a) passive range of motion
   b) ambulate appropriate patients as early as possible
2. mechanical techniques (minimal risk of complications):
   a) pneumatic compression boots[58] (PCBs) or sequential compression devices (SCDs): reduces the incidence of DVTs and probably PEs. Do not use if DVTs already present. Continue use until patient able to walk 3–4 hrs per day
   b) TED Stockings®: (TEDS) applies graduated pressure, higher distally. As effective as PCB. No evidence that the benefit is additive.[53] Care should be taken to avoid a tourniquet effect at the proximal end (note: TEDS® is a registered trademark. "TED" stands for thromboembolic disease)
   c) electrical stimulation of calf muscles
   d) rotating beds
3. anticoagulation; see also contraindications and considerations of anticoagulation in neurosurgery (p.156)
   a) full anticoagulation is associated with perioperative complications[59]
   b) "low-dose" anticoagulation[60] (low-dose heparin): 5000 IU SQ q 8 or 12 hrs, starting 2 hrs pre-op or on admission to hospital. Potential for hazardous hemorrhage within brain or spinal canal has limited its use
   c) low molecular weight heparins and heparinoids (p.164): not a homogeneous group. Efficacy in neurosurgical prophylaxis has not been determined
   d) aspirin: role in DVT prophylaxis is limited because ASA inhibits platelet aggregation, and platelets play only a minor role in DVT
4. combination of PCBs and "mini-dose" heparin starting on the morning of post-op day 1 (with no evidence of significant complications)[61]

Recommendations

Recommended prophylaxis varies with the risk of developing DVT, as illustrated in ▶ Table 9.8.[53] See also details of prophylaxis in cervical spinal cord injuries (p.952).

Diagnosis of DVT

(For PE, see below). The clinical diagnosis of DVT is very unreliable. A patient with the "classic signs" of a hot, swollen, and tender calf, or a positive Homans' sign (calf pain on dorsiflexion of the ankle) will have a DVT only 20–50% of the time.[53] 50–60% of patients with DVT will not have these findings.

Laboratory tests

- contrast venography: the "gold standard", however it is invasive and carries risk of iodine reaction, occasionally produces phlebitis, not readily repeated

Table 9.8 Risk & prophylaxis of DVT in neurosurgical patients[a]

Risk group	Estimated risk of calf DVT	Typical neurosurgical patients	Treatment recommendation
low risk	< 10%	age < 40 yrs, minimal general risk factors, surgery with < 30 minutes general anesthesia	no prophylaxis, or PCB/TEDS
moderate risk	10–40%	age ≥ 40 yrs, malignancy, prolonged bed rest, extensive surgery, varicose veins, obesity, surgery > 30 minutes duration (except simple lumbar discectomy), SAH, head injury	PCB/TEDs; or for patients without ICH or SAH, mini-dose heparin
high risk	40–80%	history of DVT or PE, paralysis[b] (para- or quadriplegia or hemiparesis), brain tumor (especially meningioma or malignant glioma)	PCB/TEDS + (in patients without ICH or SAH) mini-dose heparin

[a]abbreviations: DVT = deep venous thrombosis, PCB = pneumatic compression device, TEDS = TED (thromboembolic disease) Stockings®, ICH = intracerebral hemorrhage, SAH = subarachnoid hemorrhage
[b]see specifics regarding DVT prophylaxis in cervical SCI (p. 952)

- Doppler ultrasound with high-resolution real-time B-mode imaging: 95% sensitive and 99% specific for proximal DVT. Less effective for calf DVT.[62] As a result, it is recommended that patients with initially negative studies undergo repeat studies over the next 7–10 days to R/O proximal extension. Requires more skill on the part of the tester than IPG. May be used in immobilized or casted LE (unlike IPG). Widely accepted as the non-invasive test of choice for DVT[63]
- impedance plethysmography (IPG): looks for reduced electrical impedance produced by blood flow from the calf following relaxation of a pneumatic tourniquet. Good in detecting proximal DVT, not sensitive for calf DVT. A positive study indicates DVT that should be treated, a negative study can occur with non-occlusive DVT or with good collaterals, and should be repeated over a 2 week period
- 125I-fibrinogen: radiolabeled fibrinogen is incorporated into the developing thrombus. Better for calf DVT than proximal DVT. Expensive, and many false positives. Risk of HIV transmission has resulted in withdrawal of use
- D-dimer (a specific fibrin degradation product): high levels are associated with DVT and PE[64]

Treatment of DVT

1. bed rest, with elevation of involved leg(s)
2. unless anticoagulation is contraindicated (p. 156): start heparin as outlined in Anticoagulation (p. 156), aim for APTT = 1.5–2 × control; or fixed dose of LMW heparinoids, e.g. tinzaparin (Logiparin®,[65] or in the U.S. enoxaparin (Lovenox®) (p. 165). *Simultaneously* initiate warfarin therapy. Heparin can be stopped after ≈ 5 days[66]
3. in patients where anticoagulation is contraindicated, consider inferior vena cava interruption or placement of a filter (e.g. Greenfield filter)
4. in non-paralyzed patients, cautiously begin to ambulate after ≈ 7–10 days
5. wear anti-embolic stocking on affected LE indefinitely (limb is always at risk of recurrent DVT)

Pulmonary embolism (PE)

See reference.[67]

Prevention of PE

Prevention of PE is best accomplished by prevention of DVT (p. 168).[68]

Presentation of PE

Post-op PE generally occurs 10–14 days following surgery.[68] The reported incidence[68] ranges from 0.4–5%. A series (on a service with routine use of elastic stockings and, in high risk patients, "minidose" heparin) found a post-op incidence of ≈ 0.4%, with a doubling of this number if only patients with major pathology (brain tumor, head trauma, or cerebrovascular or spinal pathology) were considered[68] (another series dealing only with brain tumors found a 4% incidence[57]).

Clinical diagnosis is nonspecific (differential diagnosis of symptoms is large, and ranges from atelectasis to MI or cardiac tamponade).

9

Common findings: sudden dyspnea (the most frequent finding), tachypnea, tachycardia, fever, hypotension, 3rd or 4th heart sound. *Triad* (rare): hemoptysis, pleuritic chest pain, dyspnea. Auscultation: pleuritic friction rub or rales (rare). Shock and CHF (mimics MI) indicates massive life-threatening PE. Mortality reported ranges from 9–60%,[68] with a significant number of deaths within the first hour.

Diagnosis of PE

A negative D-dimer test (see above) reliably excludes PE in patients with a low clinical probability of PE[69] or in those with nondiagnostic VQ scan.[64]

Alternatively, one can check for DVT utilizing IPG, Doppler, or venography (see above). If positive, this indicates a possible source of PE, and since the treatment is similar for both, no further search for PE need be made and treatment is started. If negative, further testing may be needed (e.g.VQ scan, see below).

Laboratory tests

D-dimer: see above.

General diagnostic tests

None are very sensitive or specific.

- EKG: "classic" S1Q3T3 is rare. Usually just nonspecific-ST & T changes occur. Tachycardia may be the only finding
- CXR: normal in 25–30%. When abnormal, usually shows infiltrate and elevated hemidiaphragm
- ABG: not very sensitive. $pO_2 > 90$ on room air virtually excludes *massive* PE

9

Specific radiographic evaluation

- **Test of choice: contrast enhanced chest CT. Occasionally chest CTA may be employed. Can provide insight into alternate diagnoses**
- pulmonary angiogram: historically, the "gold standard." Invasive, expensive, and labor intensive. 3–4% risk of significant complications. Not indicated in most cases
- ventilation-perfusion scan (VQ scan): CXR is also needed. A perfusion defect with no ventilation defect in a patient with no previous history of PE strongly suggests acute PE. Equivocal studies occur when an area of malperfusion corresponds to an area of reduced ventilation (on ventilation scan) or infiltrate (on CXR). Probabilities of PE based on VQ scan are shown in ▶ Table 9.9.[70] A technically adequate normal VQ scan virtually rules out PE. Patients with low or intermediate probability scans should have a test for DVT or quantitative D-dimer (see above). If test for DVT is positive, treat; if it is negative, the choice is to follow serial IPG or Doppler studies for 2 weeks, or (rarely) to do a pulmonary angiogram
- thin-section contrast-enhanced chest CT: more accurate in patients with COPD who often have an indeterminate VQ scan

Treatment

If diagnosis is seriously entertained, start *heparin* – unless contraindicated (p.156) – without waiting for results of diagnostic studies. For an average 70 kg patient, begin with 5000–7500 unit IV bolus, followed by 1000 U/hr drip (less for smaller patient). Follow PTT and titrate drip rate for PTT 1.5 to 2 × control.

The use of heparin shortly after surgery and in patients with brain tumors is controversial, and vena caval interruption may be an alternate consideration (e.g. Greenfield filter).

Patients with massive PEs may be hemodynamically unstable. They usually require ICU care, often with PA catheter and pressors.

Table 9.9 Probability of PE based on VQ scan

Scan results	Incidence of PE
high probability	90–95%
intermediate probability or indeterminate	30–40%
low probability	10–15%
normal	0–5%

9.3 Extramedullary hematopoiesis

9.3.1 General information

In chronic anemias (especially thalassemia major, AKA Cooley's anemia), low hematocrit results in chronic over-stimulation of bone marrow to produce RBCs. This results in systemic bony abnormalities, cardiomyopathy (due to hemochromatosis caused by increased breakdown of defective RBCs).

Pertinent to the CNS, there are three sites where extramedullary hematopoiesis (EMH) can cause findings:

- skull: produces "hair-on-end" appearance on skull x-ray
- vertebral bodies: may result in epidural cord compression[71] (see below)
- choroid plexus

9.3.2 Epidural cord compression from EMH

The exuberant tissue is very radiosensitive, however, the patient may be somewhat dependent on the hematopoietic capacity of the tissue.

9.3.3 Treatment

Surgical excision followed by radiation therapy has been the recommended treatment. Repeated blood transfusions may help reduce EMH and may be useful post-op instead of RTX except for refractory cases.[71]

Surgery on these patients is difficult because of:

1. low platelet count
2. poor condition of bone
3. cardiomyopathy: increased anesthetic risk
4. anemia, coupled with the fact that most of these patients are "iron-toxic" from multiple previous transfusions
5. total removal of the mass is not always possible

9

References

[1] Cohen YC, Djulbegovic B, Shamai-Lubovitz O, Mozes B. The bleeding risk and natural history of idiopathic thrombocytopenic purpura in patients with persistent low platelet counts. Arch Intern Med. 2000; 160:1630–1638

[2] Fresh-Frozen Plasma Cryoprecipitate and Platelets Administration Practice Guidelines Development Task Force of the College of American Pathologists. Practice Parameter for the Use of Fresh-Frozen Plasma, Cryoprecipitate, and Platelets. JAMA. 1994; 271:777–781

[3] Mannucci PM. Desmopressin: A nontransfusion form of treatment for congenital and acquired bleeding disorders. Blood. 1988; 72:1449–1455

[4] So W, Hugenholtz H, Richard MT. Complications of Anticoagulant Therapy in Patients with Known Central Nervous System Lesions. Can J Surg. 1983; 26:181–183

[5] Ruff R, Posner J. Incidence and Treatment of Peripheral Thrombosis in Patients with Glioma. Ann Neurol. 1983; 13:334–336

[6] Olin JW, Young JR, Graor RA, et al. Treatment of Deep Vein Thrombosis and Pulmonary Emboli in Patients with Primary and Metastatic Brain Tumors: Anticoagulants or Inferior Vena Cava Filter? Arch Intern Med. 1987; 147:2177–2179

[7] Altschuler E, Moosa H, Selker RG, Vertosick FT. The Risk and Efficacy of Anticoagulant Therapy in the Treatment of Thromboembolic Complications in Patients with Primary Malignant Brain Tumors. Neurosurgery. 1990; 27:74–77

[8] Stern WE, Youmans J. In: Preoperative Evaluation: Complications, Their Prevention and Treatment. Neurological Surgery. 2nd ed. Philadelphia: W. B. Saunders; 1982:1051–1116

[9] Kawamata T, Takeshita M, Kubo O, et al. Management of Intracranial Hemorrhage Associated with Anticoagulant Therapy. Surg Neurol. 1995; 44:438–443

[10] Constantini S, Kanner A, Friedman A, Shoshan Y, Israel Z, Ashkenazi E, Gertel M, Even A, Shevach Y, Shalit M, Umansky F, Rappaport ZH. Safety of perioperative minidose heparin in patients undergoing brain tumor surgery: a prospective, randomized, double-blind study. J Neurosurg. 2001; 94:918–921

[11] Dickinson LD, Miller LD, Patel CP, Gupta SK. Enoxaparin increases the incidence of postoperative intracranial hemorrhage when initiated preoperatively for deep venous thrombosis prophylaxis in patients with brain tumors. Neurosurgery. 1998; 43:1074–1081

[12] Posan E, McBane RD, Grill DE, Motsko CL, Nichols WL. Comparison of PFA-100 testing and bleeding time for detecting platelet hypofunction and von Willebrand disease in clinical practice. Thromb Haemost. 2003; 90:483–490

[13] Hayward CP, Harrison P, Cattaneo M, Ortel TL, Rao AK. Platelet function analyzer (PFA)-100 closure time in the evaluation of platelet disorders and platelet function. J Thromb Haemost. 2006; 4:312–319

[14] Beshay JE, Morgan H, Madden C, Yu W, Sarode R. Emergency reversal of anticoagulation and antiplatelet therapies in neurosurgical patients. J Neurosurg. 2010; 112:307–318

[15] Seidel H, Rahman MM, Scharf RE. Monitoring of antiplatelet therapy. Current limitations, challenges, and perspectives. Hamostaseologie. 2011; 31:41–51

[16] Korinth MC. Low-dose aspirin before intracranial surgery–results of a survey among neurosurgeons in Germany. Acta Neurochir (Wien). 2006; 148:1189–96; discussion 1196

[17] Korinth MC, Gilsbach JM, Weinzierl MR. Low-dose aspirin before spinal surgery: results of a survey among neurosurgeons in Germany. Eur Spine J. 2007; 16:365–372

[18] Nuttall GA, Brown MJ, Stombaugh JW, Michon PB, Hathaway MF, Lindeen KC, Hanson AC, Schroeder DR, Oliver WC, Holmes DR, Rihal CS. Time and

cardiac risk of surgery after bare-metal stent percutaneous coronary intervention. Anesthesiology. 2008; 109:588–595
[19] Rabbitts JA, Nuttall GA, Brown MJ, Hanson AC, Oliver WC, Holmes DR, Rihal CS. Cardiac risk of noncardiac surgery after percutaneous coronary intervention with drug-eluting stents. Anesthesiology. 2008; 109:596–604
[20] Landesberg G, Beattie WS, Mosseri M, Jaffe AS, Alpert JS. Perioperative myocardial infarction. Circulation. 2009; 119:2936–2944
[21] Ross IB, Dhillon GS. Ventriculostomy-related cerebral hemorrhages after endovascular aneurysm treatment. AJNR Am J Neuroradiol. 2003; 24:1528–1531
[22] NovoSeven for non-hemophilia hemostasis. Med Letter. 2004; 46:33–34
[23] Goodnight SH, Jr, Harris WS, Connor WE. The effects of dietary omega 3 fatty acids on platelet composition and function in man: a prospective, controlled study. Blood. 1981; 58:880–885
[24] Ang-Lee MK, Moss J, Yuan CS. Herbal medicines and perioperative care. JAMA. 2001; 286:208–216
[25] Stanger MJ, Thompson LA, Young AJ, Lieberman HR. Anticoagulant activity of select dietary supplements. Nutr Rev. 2012; 70:107–117
[26] Allison GL, Lowe GM, Rahman K. Aged garlic extract and its constituents inhibit platelet aggregation through multiple mechanisms. J Nutr. 2006; 136:782S–788S
[27] Saw JT, Bahari MB, Ang HH, Lim YH. Potential drug-herb interaction with antiplatelet/anticoagulant drugs. Complement Ther Clin Pract. 2006; 12:236–241
[28] Lee CJ, Ansell JE. Direct thrombin inhibitors. Br J Clin Pharmacol. 2011; 72:581–592
[29] Birks J, Grimley Evans J. Ginkgo biloba for cognitive impairment and dementia. Cochrane Database Syst Rev. 2009. DOI: 10.1002/14651858.CD003120.pub3
[30] Teng CM, Kuo SC, Ko FN, Lee JC, Lee LG, Chen SC, Huang TF. Antiplatelet actions of panaxynol and ginsenosides isolated from ginseng. Biochim Biophys Acta. 1989; 990:315–320
[31] Baron TH, Kamath PS, McBane RD. Management of antithrombotic therapy in patients undergoing invasive procedures. N Engl J Med. 2013; 368:2113–2124
[32] Ryan J, Bolster F, Crosbie I, Kavanagh E. Antiplatelet medications and evolving antithrombotic medication. Skeletal Radiol. 2013; 42:753–764
[33] Hirsh J, Bauer KA, Donati MB, Gould M, Samama MM, Weitz JI. Parenteral anticoagulants: American College of Chest Physicians Evidence-Based Clinical Practice Guidelines (8th Edition). Chest. 2008; 133:141S–159S
[34] Kaatz S, Kouides PA, Garcia DA, Spyropolous AC, Crowther M, Douketis JD, Chan AK, James A, Moll S, Ortel TL, Van Cott EM, Ansell J. Guidance on the emergent reversal of oral thrombin and factor Xa inhibitors. Am J Hematol. 2012; 87 Suppl 1:S141–S145
[35] Rivaroxaban-once daily, oral, direct factor Xa inhibition compared with vitamin K antagonism for prevention of stroke and Embolism Trial in Atrial Fibrillation: rationale and design of the ROCKET AF study. Am Heart J. 2010; 159:340–347 e1
[36] Tran HA, Chunilal SD, Harper PL, Tran H, Wood EM, Gallus AS. An update of consensus guidelines for warfarin reversal. Med J Aust. 2013; 198:198–199
[37] James RF, Palys V, Lomboy JR, Lamm JR, Jr, Simon SD. The role of anticoagulants, antiplatelet agents, and their reversal strategies in the management of intracerebral hemorrhage. Neurosurg Focus. 2013; 34. DOI: 10.3171/2013.2.FOCUS1328
[38] Lethagen S, Olofsson L, Frick K, Berntorp E, Bjorkman S. Effect kinetics of desmopressin-induced platelet retention in healthy volunteers treated with aspirin or placebo. Haemophilia. 2000; 6:15–20
[39] Hirsh J, Dalen JE, Deykin D, Poller L. Oral Anticoagulants: Mechanism of Action, Clinical Effectiveness, and Optimal Therapeutic Range. Chest. 1992; 102:312–326
[40] Khamashta MA, Cuadrado MJ, Mujic F, et al. The Management of Thrombosis in the Antiphospholipid-Antibody Syndrome. N Engl J Med. 1995; 332:993–997
[41] Hyers TM, Hull RD, Weg JG. Antithrombotic Therapy for Venous Thromboembolic Disease. Chest. 1989; 95:37S–51S
[42] Atkinson JLD, Sundt TM, Kazmier FJ, Bowie EJW, et al. Heparin-induced thrombocytopenia and thrombosis in ischemic stroke. Mayo Clin Proc. 1988; 63:353–361
[43] Kim GH, Hahn DK, Kellner CP, Komotar RJ, Starke R, Garrett MC, Yao J, Cleveland J, Mayer SA, Connolly ES. The incidence of heparin-induced thrombocytopenia Type II in patients with subarachnoid hemorrhage treated with heparin versus enoxaparin. J Neurosurg. 2009; 110:50–57
[44] Dalteparin - Another Low-Molecular-Weight Heparin. Med Letter. 1995; 37:115–116
[45] Ardeparin and Danaparoid for Prevention of Deep Vein Thrombosis. Med Letter. 1997; 39:94–95
[46] Geerts WH, Bergqvist D, Pineo GF, Heit JA, Samama CM, Lassen MR, Colwell CW. Prevention of venous thromboembolism: American College of Chest Physicians Evidence-Based Clinical Practice Guidelines (8th Edition). Chest. 2008; 133:381S–453S
[47] FDA Public Health Advisory. Rockville, MD 1997
[48] U.S. Food and Drug Administration (FDA). FDA approves Praxbind, the first reversal agent for the anticoagulant Pradaxa. 2015
[49] Fondaparinux (Arixtra), a new anticoagulant. Med Letter. 2002; 44:43–44
[50] Garcia DA, Baglin TP, Weitz JI, Samama MM, American College of Chest Physicians. Parenteral anticoagulants: Antithrombotic Therapy and Prevention of Thrombosis, 9th ed: American College of Chest Physicians Evidence-Based Clinical Practice Guidelines. Chest. 2012; 141:e24S–e43S
[51] Fredriksson K, Norrving B, Stromblad LG. Emergency Reversal of Anticoagulation After Intracerebral Hemorrhage. Stroke. 1992; 23:972–977
[52] Kaufman HH, Hui K-S, Mattson JC, et al. Clinicopathological Correlations of Disseminated Intravascular Coagulation in Patients with Head Injury. Neurosurgery. 1984; 15:34–42
[53] Hamilton MG, Hull RD, Pineo GF. Venous Thromboembolism in Neurosurgery and Neurology Patients: A Review. Neurosurgery. 1994; 34:280–296
[54] Olson JD, Kaufman HH, Moake J, et al. The Incidence and Significance of Hemostatic Abnormalities in Patients with Head Injuries. Neurosurgery. 1989; 24:825–832
[55] Sawaya R, Zuccarello M, El-Kalliny M. Brain Tumors and Thromboembolism: Clinical, Hemostatic, and Biochemical Correlations. J Neurosurg. 1989; 70
[56] Quevedo JF, Buckner JC, Schmidt JL, Dinapoli RP, O'Fallon JR. Thromboembolism in Patients With High-Grade Glioma. Mayo Clin Proc. 1994; 69:329–332
[57] Constantini S, Karnowski R, Pomeranz S, Rappaport ZH. Thromboembolic Phenomena in Neurosurgical Patients Operated Upon for Primary and Metastatic Brain Tumors. Acta Neurochir. 1991; 109:93–97
[58] Black PM, Baker MF, Snook CP. Experience with External Pneumatic Calf Compression in Neurology and Neurosurgery. Neurosurgery. 1986; 18:440–444
[59] Snyder M, Renaudin J. Intracranial Hemorrhage Associated with Anticoagulation Therapy. Surg Neurol. 1977; 7:31–34
[60] Cerrato D, Ariano C, Fiacchino F. Deep Vein Thrombosis and Low-Dose Heparin Prophylaxis in Neurosurgical Patients. J Neurosurg. 1978; 49:378–381
[61] Frim DM, Barker FG, Poletti CE, Hamilton AJ. Postoperative Low-Dose Heparin Decreases Thromboembolic Complications in Neurosurgical Patients. Neurosurgery. 1992; 30:830–833
[62] Rose SC, Zwiebel WJ, Murdock LE, et al. Insensitivity of Color Doppler Flow Imaging for Detection of Acute Calf Deep Venous Thrombosis in Asymptomatic Postoperative Patients. J Vasc Interv Radiol. 1993; 4:111–117

[63] Wells PS, Anderson DR, Bormanis J, et al. Value of Assessment of Pretest Probability of Deep-Vein Thrombosis in Clinical Management. Lancet. 1997; 350:1795–1798

[64] Ginsberg JS, Wells PS, Kearon C, Anderson D, et al. Sensitivity and Specificity of a Rapid Whole-Blood Assay for D-dimer in the Diagnosis of Pulmonary Embolism. Ann Intern Med. 1998; 129:1006–1011

[65] Hull RD, Raskob GE, Pineo GF, et al. Subcutaneous Low-Molecular-Weight Heparin Compared with Continuous Intravenous Heparin in the Treatment of Proximal-Vein Thrombosis. N Engl J Med. 1992; 326:975–982

[66] Hull RD, Raskob GE, Rosenbloom D, et al. Heparin for Five Days as Compared with Ten Days in the Initial Treatment of Proximal Venous Thrombosis. N Engl J Med. 1990; 322:1260–1264

[67] Wenger NK, Schwartz GR. In: Principles and Practice of Emergency Medicine. Philadelphia: W.B. Saunders; 1978:949–952

[68] Inci S, Erbengi A, Berker M. Pulmonary Embolism in Neurosurgical Patients. Surg Neurol. 1995; 43:123–129

[69] Wells PS, Ginsberg JS, Anderson DR, et al. Use of a Clinical Model for Safe Management of Patients with Suspected Pulmonary Embolism. Ann Intern Med. 1998; 129:997–1005

[70] The PIOPED Investigators. Value of the Ventilation/Perfusion Scan in Acute Pulmonary Embolism. Results of the Prospective Investigation of Pulmonary Embolism Diagnosis (PIOPED). JAMA. 1990; 263:2753–2759

[71] Mann KS, Yue CP, Chan KH, et al. Paraplegia due to Extramedullary Hematopoiesis in Thalassemia: Case Report. J Neurosurg. 1987; 66:938–940

10 Neurology for Neurosurgeons

10.1 Dementia

▶ **Definition.** Loss of intellectual abilities previously attained (memory, judgement, abstract thought, and other higher cortical functions) severe enough to interfere with social and/or occupational functioning.[1] Memory deficit is the cardinal feature, however, the DSM-IV definition requires impairment in at least one other domain (language, perception, visuospatial function, calculation, judgement, abstraction, problem-solving skills). Affects 3–11% of community-dwelling adults > 65 yrs of age, with a greater presence among institutionalized residents.[2]

Risk factors: advanced age, family history of dementia, and apolipoprotein E-4 allele.

▶ **Delirium vs. dementia (critical distinction).** Delirium AKA acute confusional state. Distinct from dementia, however, patients with dementia are at increased risk of developing delirium.[3,4] A primary disorder of attention that subsequently affects all other aspects of cognition.[5] Often represents life-threatening illness, e.g. hypoxia, sepsis, uremic encephalopathy, electrolyte abnormality, drug intoxication, MI. 50% of patients die within 2 yrs of this diagnosis.

Unlike dementia, delirium has acute onset, motor signs (tremor, myoclonus, asterixis), slurred speech, altered consciousness (hyperalert/agitated or lethargic, or fluctuations), hallucinations may be florid. EEG shows pronounced diffuse slowing.

▶ **Brain biopsy for dementia.** Clinical criteria are usually sufficient for the diagnosis of most dementias. Biopsy should be reserved for cases of a chronic progressive cerebral disorder with an unusual clinical course where all other possible diagnostic methods have been exhausted and have failed to provide adequate diagnostic certainty.[6] Biopsy may disclose CJD, low grade astrocytoma, and AD among others. The high incidence of CJD among patients selected for biopsy under these criteria necessitates appropriate precautions; see Creutzfeldt-Jakob disease (p. 367).In a report of 50 brain biopsies performed to assess progressive neurodegenerative disease of unclear etiology,[7] the diagnostic yield was only 20% (6% were only suggestive of a diagnosis, 66% were abnormal but nonspecific, 8% were normal). The yield was highest in those with focal MRI abnormalities. Among the 10 patients with diagnostic biopsies, the biopsy result led to a meaningful therapeutic intervention in only 4.

▶ **Recommendations.** Based on the above, the following recommendations are made for patients with an otherwise unexplained neurodegenerative disease:

1. those with a focal abnormality on MRI: stereotactic biopsy
2. those without focal abnormality (possibly including SPECT or PET scan): brain biopsy should only be performed within an investigative protocol

▶ **Recommendations for specimen.** Ideally the biopsy specimen should[8]:

1. be large enough (usually 1 cm^3)
2. be taken from an affected area
3. include grey and white matter, pia and dura
4. be handled carefully to minimize artifact (electrocautery should not be used on the specimen side of the incision)

10.2 Headache

10.2.1 General information

Headache (H/A) may be broadly categorized as follows:

1. chronic recurring headaches
   a) vascular type (migraine): see below
   b) muscle contraction (tension) headaches
2. headache due to pathology
   a) systemic pathology
   b) intracranial pathology: a wide variety of etiologies including:
      - subarachnoid hemorrhage: *sudden* onset, severe, usually with vomiting, apoplexy, focal deficits possible;see differential diagnosis of paroxysmal H/A (p. 1158)

   - increased intracranial pressure from any cause (tumor, communicating hydrocephalus, inflammation, pseudotumor cerebri…)
   - irritation or inflammation of meninges: meningitis
   - tumor (p. 590): with or without elevated ICP

c) local pathology of the eye, nasopharynx, or extracranial tissues (including giant cell arteritis (p. 195)
d) following head trauma: postconcussive syndrome (p. 923)
e) following craniotomy: "syndrome of the trephined" (p. 1431)

A severe new H/A, or a change in the pattern of a longstanding or recurrent H/A (including developing associated N/V, or an abnormal neurologic exam) warrants further investigation with CT or MRI.[9]

Unilateral H/A that never changes side over a period ≥ 1 year warrants an MRI; this would be atypical in migraine and may be a presentation of an occipital AVM (p. 1239).

10.2.2 Migraine

General information

Migraine attacks usually occur in individuals predisposed to the condition, and may be activated by factors such as bright light, stress, diet changes, trauma, administration of radiologic contrast media (especially angiography) and vasodilators.

Classification

Based on the 1962 ad hoc committee on headache (H/A). See also index under Headache, e.g. for: crash migraine (thunderclap headache) (p. 1158), post-myelogram headache (p. 1508)...

Common migraine

Episodic H/A with N/V and photophobia, without aura or neurologic deficit.

Classic migraine

Common migraine + aura. May have H/A with occasional focal neurologic deficit(s) that resolve completely in ≤ 24 hrs.

Over half of the transient neurologic disturbances are visual, and usually consist of positive phenomena (spark photopsia, stars, complex geometric patterns, fortification spectra) which may leave negative phenomena (scotoma, hemianopia, monocular or binocular visual loss…) in their wake. The second most common symptoms are somatosensory involving the hand and lower face. Less frequently, deficits may consist of aphasia, hemiparesis, or unilateral clumsiness. A *slow march-like progression* of deficit is characteristic. The risk of stroke is probably increased in patients with migraine.[10]

Complicated migraine

Occasional attacks of classic migraine with minimal or no associated H/A, and complete resolution of neurologic deficit in ≤ 30 days.

Migraine equivalent

Neurologic symptoms (N/V, visual aura, etc.) without H/A (acephalgic migraine). Seen mostly in children. Usually develops into typical migraine with age. Aura may be shortened by opening and swallowing contents of a 10 mg nifedipine capsule.[11]

Hemiplegic migraine

H/A typically precedes hemiplegia which may persist even after H/A resolves.

Cluster headache

AKA histaminic migraine. Actually a neurovascular event, distinct from true migraine. Recurrent unilateral attacks of severe pain. Usually oculofrontal or oculotemporal with occasional radiation into the jaw, usually recurring on the same side of the head. Ipsilateral autonomic symptoms (conjunctival injection, nasal congestion, rhinorrhea, lacrimation, facial flushing) are common. Partial Horner's syndrome (ptosis and miosis) sometimes occurs. Male:female ratio is ≈ 5:1. 25% of patients have a personal or family history of migraine.

Headaches characteristically have no prodrome, last 30–90 minutes, and recur one or more times daily usually for 4–12 weeks, often at a similar time of day, following which there is typically a remission for an average of 12 months.[12]

Prophylaxis for cluster H/A is only minimally effective:

1. β-adrenergic blockers are less effective
2. lithium: becoming drug of choice (response rate 60–80%). 300 mg PO TID and follow levels (desired: 0.7–1.2 mEq/L)
3. occasionally ergotamines are used
4. naproxen (Naprosyn®)
5. methysergide (Sansert®) 2–4 mg PO TID is effective in 20–40% of cases, must cycle patient off the drug to prevent retroperitoneal fibrosis, etc. (also see below)

Treatment for cluster H/A (prophylaxis is only minimally effective):

Treatment is difficult because there is no prodrome and the H/A often stop after 1–2 hrs. Treatment of acute attacks includes:

- 100% O_2 by face mask with patient sitting for ≤ 15 min or until attack aborted
- ergotamine: see below
- SQ sumatriptan: usually aborts attack within 15 minutes (see below)
- steroids: see below
- refractory cases may be considered for:
  - percutaneous radiofrequency sphenopalatine ganglion blockade[13]
  - occipital nerve stimulation[14]
  - hypothalamic deep brain stimulation

10

Basilar artery migraine

Essentially restricted to adolescence. Recurrent episodes lasting minutes to hours of transient neurologic deficits in distribution of vertebrobasilar system. Deficits include: vertigo (most common), gait ataxia, visual disturbance (scotomata, bilateral blindness), dysarthria, followed by severe H/A and occasionally nausea and vomiting.[15] Family history of migraine is present in 86%.

10.3 Parkinsonism

10.3.1 General information

Parkinsonism may be primary or secondary to other conditions. All result from a relative loss of dopamine mediated inhibition of the effects of acetylcholine in the basal ganglia.

10.3.2 Idiopathic paralysis agitans (IPA)

Clinical

Classical Parkinson's disease AKA shaking palsy. Affects ≈ 1% of Americans > age 50 yrs,[16] it is frequently underdiagnosed.[17] Male:female ratio is 3:2. Not clearly environmentally or genetically induced, but may be influenced by these factors.

The classic triad is shown in ▶ Table 10.1. Other signs may include: postural instability, micrographia, mask-like facies. Gait consists of small, shuffling steps (marche á petits pas) or festinating gait.

Clinically distinguishing IPA from secondary parkinsonism (see below)

May be difficult early. IPA generally exhibits gradual onset of bradykinesia with tremor that is often asymmetrical, and initially responds well to levodopa. Other disorders are suggested with rapid progression of symptoms, when the initial response to levodopa is equivocal, or when there is early midline symptoms (ataxia or impairment of gait and balance, sphincter disturbance…) or the

Table 10.1 Classic triad of Parkinson's disease

- tremor (resting, 4–7/second)
- rigidity (cogwheel)
- bradykinesia

presence of other features such as early dementia, sensory findings, profound orthostatic hypotension, or abnormalities of extraocular movements.[18,19]

Pathophysiology

Degeneration primarily of pigmented (neuromelanin-laden) dopaminergic neurons of the pars compacta of the substantia nigra, resulting in reduced levels of dopamine in the neostriatum (caudate nucleus, putamen, globus pallidus). This decreases the activity of inhibitory neurons with predominantly D2 class of dopamine receptors which project directly to the internal segment of the globus pallidus (GPi), and also increases (by loss of inhibition) activity of neurons with predominantly D1 receptors which project indirectly to the globus pallidus externa (GPe) and subthalamic nucleus.[20] The net result is increased activity in GPi which has inhibitory projections to the thalamus which then suppresses activity in the supplemental motor cortex among other locations.

Histologically: Lewy bodies (eosinophilic intraneuronal hyaline inclusions) are the hallmark of IPA.

10.3.3 Secondary parkinsonism

General information

The differential diagnosis of Parkinson's disease includes the following etiologies of secondary parkinsonism or Parkinson-like conditions (sometimes of these are occasionally referred to as "Parkinson plus" syndromes or parkinsonian disorders) (see above for distinguishing features):

1. olivopontocerebellar degeneration (OPC)
2. striato-nigral degeneration (SND): more aggressive than parkinsonism
3. postencephalitic parkinsonism: followed an epidemic of encephalitis lethargica (von Economo disease) in the 1920s, victims are no longer living. Distinguishing features: oculogyric crisis, tremor involves not only extremities but also trunk and head, asymmetrical, no Lewy bodies
4. progressive supranuclear palsy (PSNP): impaired vertical gaze (see below)
5. multiple system atrophy (Shy-Drager syndrome): see below
6. drug induced: includes:
   a) prescription drugs (elderly females seem more susceptible)
      - antipsychotics (AKA neuroleptics): haloperidol (Haldol®) which works by blocking post-synaptic dopamine receptors
      - phenothiazine antiemetics: prochlorperazine (Compazine®)
      - metoclopramide (Reglan®)
      - reserpine
   b) MPTP (1-methyl-4-phenyl-1,2,3,6-tetrahydropyridine): a commercially available chemical intermediate which is also a by-product of the synthesis of MPPP (a meperidine analog) that was synthesized and self-injected by a graduate student,[21] and later produced by illicit drug manufacturers to be sold as "synthetic heroin" and unwittingly injected by some IV drug abusers in northern California in 1983[22] (there is also a case report of a chemist who worked with MPTP who developed parkinsonism).[23] MPTP was subsequently discovered to be a potent neurotoxin for dopaminergic neurons (with continued toxic effects that persisted for years[24]). As a rule, the response to levodopa is dramatic, but short-lived with frequent side effects. In contrast to classic IPA, the locus coeruleus and dorsal motor vagus nucleus were essentially normal, and the symptoms differ slightly
   c) there is an as yet unproven assertion that methylenedioxymethamphetamine (MDMA) AKA "ecstasy" (on the street), may hasten the onset of Parkinsonism (a study demonstrating a link had to be withdrawn because of a mislabeling of drugs)
7. toxic: poisoning with
   a) carbon monoxide: symmetric low densities in the globus pallidus on CT
   b) manganese: may be seen in miners, welders, and pyrotechnics workers. Manganese is excreted by the liver, ∴ people with hepatic insufficiency are more susceptible. Imaging: symmetrical high signal abnormalities on T1WI primarily in the globus pallidus with essentially no findings on T2WI or GRASS (almost pathognomonic)
8. ischemic (lacunes in basal ganglia): produces so-called arteriosclerotic parkinsonism AKA vascular parkinsonism: "lower-half" parkinsonism (gait disturbance predominates[17]). Also causes pseudobulbar deficits, emotional lability. Tremor is rare
9. posttraumatic: parkinsonian symptoms may occur in chronic traumatic encephalopathy, see dementia pugilistica (p. 924). There are usually other features not normally present in IPA (e.g. cerebellar findings)

10. normal pressure hydrocephalus (NPH): urinary incontinence (p. 404)...
11. neoplasm in the region of the substantia nigra
12. Riley-Day (familial dysautonomia)
13. parkinson-dementia complex of Guam: classic IPA + amyotrophic lateral sclerosis (ALS). Pathologically has features of parkinsonism and Alzheimer's disease but no Lewy bodies nor senile plaques
14. Huntington's disease (HD): whereas adults typically show chorea, when HD manifests in a young person it may resemble IPA
15. (spontaneous) intracranial hypotension (p. 389) may present with findings mimicking IPA

Multiple system atrophy (MSA)

AKA Shy-Drager syndrome. Parkinsonism (indistinguishable from IPA), PLUS idiopathic orthostatic hypotension, PLUS other signs of autonomic nervous system (ANS) dysfunction (ANS findings may precede parkinsonism and may include urinary sphincter disturbance and hypersensitivity to noradrenaline or tyramine infusions). Degeneration of preganglionic lateral horn neurons of thoracic spinal cord. Unlike IPA, most do not respond to dopa therapy. NB: classic IPA may eventually produce orthostatic hypotension from inactivity or as a result of progressive autonomic failure.

Progressive supranuclear palsy (PSNP)

AKA Steele-Richardson-Olszewski syndrome.[25]

Triad:

1. progressive supranuclear ophthalmoplegia (chiefly vertical gaze): paresis of voluntary vertical eye movement, but still moves to vertical doll's eyes maneuver
2. pseudobulbar palsy (mask-like facies with marked dysarthria and dysphagia, hyperactive jaw jerk, emotional incontinence usually mild)
3. axial dystonia (especially of neck and upper trunk)

Associated findings: subcortical dementia (inconstant), motor findings of pyramidal, extrapyramidal and cerebellar systems. Average age of onset: 60 yrs. Males comprise 60%. Response to anti-parkinson drugs is usually very short lived. Average survival after diagnosis: 5.7 yrs.

Differentiating from Parkinson's disease (IPA):

Patients with PSNP have a pseudo-parkinsonism. They have mask facies, but do not walk bent forward (they walk erect), and they do not have a tremor. They tend to fall backwards.

Course

1. early:
   a) many falls: due to dysequilibrium + downgaze palsy (can't see floor)
   b) eye findings may be normal initially, subsequently may develop difficulty looking down (especially to command, less to following), calorics have normal tonic component but absent nystagmus (cortical component)
   c) slurred speech
   d) personality changes
   e) difficulty eating: due to pseudobulbar palsy + inability to look down at food on plate
2. late:
   a) eyes fixed centrally (no response to oculocephalics or oculovestibulars): ocular immotility is due to frontal lobe lesions
   b) neck stiffens in extension (retrocollis)

Treatment for Parkinson's disease

Medical treatment for Parkinson's disease is beyond the scope of this book.

Surgical treatment

Before the introduction of L-dopa in the late 1960's, stereotactic thalamotomy was widely used for Parkinson's disease. The location ultimately targeted for lesioning was the ventrolateral nucleus. The procedure worked better for relieving the tremor than for the bradykinesia, however it was the latter symptom that was most disabling. This procedure cannot be done bilaterally without significant risk to speech function. The procedure fell out of favor when more effective drugs became available.[26]

See Surgical treatment of Parkinson's disease (p. 1524) for further information.

10.4 Multiple sclerosis

Key concepts

- an idiopathic demyelinating disease of the CNS producing exacerbating and remitting symptoms disseminated in space and time
- classic clinical findings: optic neuritis, paresthesias, INO and bladder symptoms
- diagnostic criteria (McDonald criteria) use clinical and/or lab results (MRI, CSF...) to stratify patients as: MS, probable MS, or not MS
- MRI: multiple usually enhancing lesions involving optic nerves & white matter of brain (especially periventricular white matter), cerebellum and spinal cord

10.4.1 General information

An idiopathic demyelinating disease (thus affecting only white matter) of the cerebrum, optic nerves, and spinal cord (especially the corticospinal tracts and the posterior columns). Does *not* affect peripheral myelin. Pathologically produces multiple plaques of various age in diffuse locations in the CNS, especially in the periventricular white matter. Lesions initially evoke an inflammatory response with monocytes and lymphocytic perivascular cuffing, but with age settle down to glial scars.

10.4.2 Epidemiology

Usual age of onset: 10–59 years, with the greatest peak between ages 20–40 years. The female:male incidence is approximately 2:1.[27]

Prevalence varies with latitude, and is < 1 per 100,000 near the equator, and is ≈ 30–80 per 100,000 in the northern U.S. and Canada.

10.4.3 Classification

Typically causes exacerbations and remissions in various locations in the CNS (*dissemination in space and time*). Common symptoms: visual disturbances (diplopia, blurring, field cuts or scotoma), spastic paraparesis, and bladder disturbances. Nomenclature for the time course of MS is shown in ▶ Table 10.2.[28] Relapsing-remitting MS is the most common pattern (≥ 70%) at onset, and has the best response to therapy, but > 50% of cases eventually become secondary progressive MS. Only 10% have primary progressive MS, and these patients tend to be older at onset (40–60 years) and frequently develop progressive myelopathy.[29] Progressive relapsing MS is very uncommon. Deficits present > 6 months usually persist.

Table 10.2 Clinical categories of MS

Category	Definition
relapsing-remitting	episodes of acute worsening with recovery and a stable course between relapses
secondary progressive	gradual neurologic deterioration ± superimposed acute relapses in a patient who previously had relapsing-remitting MS
primary progressive	gradual, nearly continuous neurologic deterioration from the onset of symptoms
progressive relapsing	gradual neurologic deterioration from the onset of symptoms, but with subsequent superimposed relapses

10.4.4 Clinical signs and symptoms

Visual disturbances

Disturbances of visual acuity may be caused by optic or retrobulbar neuritis which is the presenting symptom of MS in 15% of cases, and which occurs at some time in 50% of MS patients. The percentage of patients with an attack of optic neuritis and no prior attack that will go on to develop MS ranges from 17–87% depending on the series.[30] Symptoms: acute visual loss in one or both eyes with mild pain (often on eye movement).

Diplopia may be due to internuclear ophthalmoplegia (INO) (p. 565) from a plaque in the MLF. INO is an important sign because it rarely occurs in other conditions besides MS or brainstem stroke.

Motor findings

Extremity weakness (mono, para, or quadriparesis) and gait ataxia are among the most common symptoms of MS. Spasticity of the LEs is often due to pyramidal tract involvement. Scanning speech results from cerebellar lesions.

Sensory findings

Posterior column involvement often causes loss of proprioception. Paresthesias of extremities, trunk, or face occur. Lhermitte's sign (electric shock-like pain radiating down the spine on neck flexion) is common, but is not pathognomonic. Trigeminal neuralgia occurs in ≈ 2%, and is more often bilateral and occurs at a younger age than the population in general.[31]

Mental disturbances

Euphoria (la belle indifference) and depression occur in ≈ 50% of patients.

Reflex changes

Hyperreflexia and Babinski signs are common. *Abdominal cutaneous reflexes* disappear in 70–80%.

GU symptoms

Urinary frequency, urgency, and incontinence are common. Impotence in males and reduced libido in either sex is often seen.

10.4.5 Differential diagnosis

The plethora of possible signs and symptoms in MS causes the differential diagnosis to extend to almost all conditions causing focal or diffuse dysfunction of the CNS. Conditions that may closely mimic MS clinically and on diagnostic testing include:

1. acute disseminated encephalomyelitis (ADEM) (p. 182): generally monophasic. May also have CSF-OCB (p. 182). Corpus callosum involvement is uncommon
2. CNS lymphoma (p. 710)
3. other closely related demyelinating diseases: e.g. Devic syndrome (p. 1409)
4. vasculitis
5. encephalitis: patients are usually very ill
6. chronic white matter changes: seen in older patients

10.4.6 Diagnostic criteria

No single clinical feature or diagnostic test is adequate for the accurate diagnosis of MS. Therefore, clinical information is integrated with paraclinical studies. Diagnosing MS after a single, acute remitting clinically isolated syndrome (CIS) is very risky. 50–70% of patients with a CIS suggestive of MS will have multifocal MRI abnormalities characteristic of MS. The presence of these MRI abnormalities increases the risk of developing MS in 1–3 years (with greater prognostic significance than CSF-OCB). The more MRI lesions, the higher the risk.[32] Criteria for the diagnosis of MS[33] follows.

Definitions

See references.[33,34]

The following definitions are used in the classification system that follows:

1. attack (exacerbation, relapse): neurologic disturbance lasting > 24 hrs[35] typical of MS when clinicopathological studies determine that the cause is demyelinating or inflammatory lesions
2. remission: ≥ 30 days should separate the onset of the first attack from the onset of a second
3. historical information: reporting of symptoms by the patient (confirmation by observer desirable), adequate to locate a lesion of MS, and has no other explanation (i.e. manifestations must not be attributable to another condition)
4. clinical evidence (signs): neuro dysfunction recorded by competent examiner
5. paraclinical evidence: tests or procedures demonstrating CNS lesion which has not produced signs; e.g. Uhthoff phenomenon or sign (worsening of symptoms with hot bath or shower), BAER, imaging procedures (CT, MRI), expert urological assessment
6. typical of MS: signs & symptoms (S/S) known to occur frequently in MS. Thus excludes gray matter lesions, peripheral nervous system lesions, and non-specific complaints such as H/A, depression, convulsive seizures, etc.
7. separate lesions: S/S cannot be explained on basis of single lesion (optic neuritis of both eyes simultaneously or within 15 days represents single lesion)
8. laboratory support: in this study, the only considerations were CSF oligoclonal bands (CSF-OCB) (see below) (OCB must not be present in serum) or increased CSF IgG production (CSF-IgG) (serum IgG must be normal). This assumes that syphilis, SSPE, sarcoidosis, etc. have been ruled out

Diagnosis of MS

The 2010"McDonald MS Diagnostic criteria"[36] are shown in ▶ Table 10.3.

MRI

MRI is the preferred imaging study in evaluating MS[39] and can demonstrate dissemination of lesions in time and space. Recommended[33] brain MRI criteria for diagnosing MS are shown in ▶ Table 10.3.[40,41] Lesions are normally > 3 mm diameter.[33] MRI shows multiple white matter abnormalities in 80% of patients with MS (compared to 29% for CT).[42,43] Lesions are high signal on T2, and acute lesions tend to enhance with gadolinium more than old lesions do. Periventricular lesions may blend in with the signal from CSF in the ventricles on T2, these lesions are shown to better advantage on FLAIR (fluid attenuation) MRI (p.229). These lesions are ovoid and are oriented perpendicular to the ependymal surface and are sometimes called Dawson's fingers (after neuropathologist James Dawson).

Spinal cord lesions normally show little or no swelling, should be ≥ 3 mm but < 2 vertebral segments, occupy only a portion of the cross-section of the cord, and must be hyperintense on T2.[44]

Specificity of MRI is ≈ 94%,[45] however, encephalitis as well as UBOs seen in aging may mimic MS lesions. DWI should be normal, however plaques can sometimes exhibit "shine through" (p.232) so the ADC map must be checked to rule-out infarct.

Focal tumefactive demyelinating lesions (TDL) may occur in isolation or, more commonly, in patients with established MS (concentric sclerosis of Balo). TDL may represent an intermediate position between MS and ADEM (p.182).[46] TDLs tend to be symmetric. TDLs may enhance, and show perilesional edema (but less than MS) and thus be mistaken for neoplasms. Biopsy results may be confusing. MRS may not be able to differentiate from neoplasm.[47]

CSF

CSF analysis can support the diagnosis in some cases, but cannot document dissemination of lesions in time or space. The CSF in MS is clear and colorless. The OP is normal. Total CSF protein is < 55 mg/dl in ≈ 75% of patients, and < 108 mg/dl in 99.7% (values near 100 should prompt a search for an alternative diagnosis). The WBC count is ≤ 5 cells/mcl in 70% of patients, and only 1% have a count > 20 cells/mcl (high values may be seen in the acute myelitis).

In ≈ 90% of patients with MS, CSF-IgG is increased relative to other CSF proteins, and a characteristic pattern occurs. Agarose gel electrophoresis shows a few IgG bands in the gamma region (oligoclonal bands) that are not present in the serum (higher resolution isoelectric focusing can demonstrate 10–15 bands). CSF-OCB are not specific for MS, and can occur in CNS infections and less commonly with strokes or tumors. The predictive value of the absence of IgG in a patient with suspected MS has not been satisfactorily elucidated.

Table 10.3 2010 McDonald MS Diagnostic Criteria[36]

The diagnosis of MS requires elimination of more likely diagnoses and demonstration of lesions disseminated in space (DIS) and time (DIT)		
Clinical (attacks)	**Lesions**	**Additional criteria to make the diagnosis**
≥ 2	Objective clinical evidence of ≥ 2 lesions or objective clinical evidence of 1 lesion with reasonable historical evidence of a prior attack	None. If additional tests are done, results must still be consistent with MS
≥ 2	Objective clinical evidence of 1 lesion	DIS; or wait for further clinical attack implicating a different CNS location
1	Objective clinical evidence of ≥ 2 lesions	DIT; or wait for a second clinical attack
1	Objective clinical evidence of 1 lesion	DIS or wait for further clinical attack implicating a different CNS location and DIT; or wait for a second clinical attack
0 (progression from onset)		One year of disease progression (retrospective or prospective) and at least 2 of: • DIS in the brain based on ≥ 1 T2 MRI lesion in periventricular, juxtacortical or infratentorial regions • DIS in the spinal cord based on ≥ 2 T2 MRI lesions • or positive CSF
Paraclinical evidence in diagnosis of MS		
Evidence for DIS[37]	≥ 1 T2 MRI lesion in at least 2 out of 4 areas of the CNS: periventricular, juxtacortical, infratentorial or spinal cord • Gadolinium enhancement of lesions is not required • If the patient has a brainstem or spinal cord syndrome, the symptomatic lesions are excluded and do not contribute to lesion count	
Evidence for DIT[38]	• New T2 and/or gadolinium-enhancing MRI lesion(s) on follow-up MRI, with reference to a baseline study, irrespective of the timing of the baseline MRI or • Simultaneous presence of asymptomatic gadolinium-enhancing and non-enhancing lesions at any time	
Evidence for positive CSF	Oligoclonal bands in CSF (and not serum) or elevated IgG index	

Recommended criteria have been published,[48] most of which pertain to specifics of laboratory analysis, pertinent clinical excerpts are shown in ▶ Table 10.4.

10.5 Acute disseminated encephalomyelitis

AKA ADEM. Acute demyelinating condition, has been associated with relatively recent history of vaccination. Like MS, may also demonstrate oligoclonal bands in CSF. ADEM is generally monophasic, and lesions occur within a couple of weeks. There is usuallly a good response to high-dose IV corticosteroids.

10.6 Motor neuron diseases

10.6.1 General information

Degenerative diseases of motor neurons. See also comparison of upper motor neuron (UMN) with lower motor neuron (LMN) (p. 504) and the paralysis they produce. Five subtypes of which ALS is the most common (see below).

Table 10.4 CSF criteria for MS

1. qualitative assessment of IgG is the most informative analysis and is best performed using IEF with some form of immunodetection (blotting or fixation)
2. analysis should be performed on unconcentrated CSF and must be compared to simultaneously run serum sample in the same assay
3. runs should use the same amount of IgG from serum and CSF
4. each run should contain positive and negative controls
5. quantitative analysis should be made in terms of one of the 5 recognized staining patterns for OCB
6. an individual experienced in the techniques should report the results
7. all other tests performed on the CSF (including WBC, protein & glucose, lactate) should be taken into consideration
8. evaluation using light chains for immunodetection may be helpful in certain cases to resolve equivocal oligoclonal IgG patterns
9. if clinical suspicion is high but CSF results are equivocal, negative or show only a single band, consider repeating the LP
10. to measure IgG levels, nonlinear formulas that consider integrity of the blood-CSF barrier should be used (e. g. the ratio of CSF to serum albumin (AKA Qalb) is a measure of leakiness)
11. labs analyzing CSF should have internal as well as external quality assessment controls
12. quantitative IgG is a complementary test, but is not a substitute for qualitative IgG testing which has the highest sensitivity and specificity

Three patterns of involvement:

1. mixed UMN & LMN degeneration: amyotrophic lateral sclerosis (ALS) (see below). The most common of the motor neuron diseases
2. UMN degeneration: primary lateral sclerosis. Rare, onset after age 50. No LMN signs. Slower progression than ALS (yrs to decades). Pseudobulbar palsy is common.[49] Usually does not shorten longevity. May present with falling due to balance problems or low back and neck pain due to axial muscle weakness
3. LMN degeneration: progressive muscular atrophy (PMA) and spinal muscular atrophy (SMA)

10

10.6.2 Amyotrophic lateral sclerosis

Key concepts

- degeneration of anterior horn cells and corticospinal tracts in the cervical spine and medulla (bulb) of unknown etiology
- a mixed upper and lower motor neuron disease (UMN → mild spasticity in LEs; LMN → atrophy and fasciculations in UEs)
- clinically: progressive muscle wasting, weakness, and fasciculations
- no cognitive, sensory, nor autonomic dysfunction

In the U.S. amyotrophic lateral sclerosis (ALS) is AKA Lou Gehrig's disease named after the New York Yankee first baseman who announced that he had the disease in 1939. AKA motor neuron disease (singular).

Epidemiology

See reference.[30]

Prevalence: 4–6/100,000. Incidence: 0.8–1.2/100,000.

Familial in 8–10% of cases. Familial cases usually follow autosomal dominant inheritance, but occasionally demonstrate a recessive pattern.

Onset usually after 40 years of age.

Pathology

Etiology is not known with certainty. Histology: degeneration of anterior horn alpha-motoneurons (in the spinal cord *and* in brain stem motor nuclei) (LMNs) and corticospinal tracts (UMNs). Produces mixed UMN & LMN findings, with a great deal of variability depending on which predominates at any given time.

Clinical

Characterized by progressive muscle wasting, weakness, and fasciculations.

Involvement is of voluntary muscles, sparing the voluntary eye muscles and urinary sphincter.

Classically, presents initially with weakness and atrophy of the hands (lower motor neuron) with spasticity and hyperreflexia of the lower extremities (upper motor neuron). However, LEs may be hyporeflexic if the lower motor neuron deficits predominate.

Dysarthria and dysphagia are caused by a combination of upper and lower motor neuron pathology. Tongue atrophy and fasciculations may also occur.

Although cognitive deficits are generally considered to be absent in ALS, in actuality 1–2% of cases are associated with dementia, and cognitive changes may occasionally predate the usual features of ALS.[50]

Differential diagnosis

At times, it may be very difficult to distinguish ALS from cervical spondylotic myelopathy; see discussion of differentiating features (p. 1086).

Diagnostic studies

EMG

Not absolutely necessary to make diagnosis in most cases. Fibrillations and positive sharp waves are found in advanced cases (may be absent early, especially if upper motor neuron pathology predominates). LMN findings in the LE in the absence of lumbar spine disease, or fibrillation potentials in the tongue are suggestive of ALS.

LP (CSF)

May have slightly elevated protein.

10

Treatment

Much of care is directed towards minimizing disability:

1. risk of aspiration may be reduced with
   a) tracheostomy
   b) gastrostomy tube to allow continued feeding
   c) vocal cord injection with Teflon
2. noninvasive ventilation: e.g. BiPAP spasticity that occurs when upper motor neuron deficits predominate may be treated (usually with short-lived response) with:
   a) baclofen (p. 1530): also may relieve the commonly occurring cramps
   b) diazepam
3. riluzole (Rilutek®): inhibits presynaptic release of glutamate. Doses of 50-200 mg/d increases tracheostomy-free survival at 9 & 12 months, but the improvement is more modest or may be nonexistent by ≈ 18 months [51,52]

Prognosis

Most patients die within 5 years of onset (median survival: 3–4 yrs). Those with prominent oropharyngeal symptoms may have a shorter life-span usually due to complications of aspiration.

10.7 Guillain-Barré syndrome

10.7.1 General

Key concepts

- acute onset of peripheral neuropathy with progressive muscle weakness (more severe *proximally*) with areflexia, reaches maximum over 3 days to 3 weeks
- cranial neuropathy: also common, may include facial diplegia, ophthalmoplegia
- little or no sensory involvement (paresthesias are not uncommon)
- onset often 3 days-5 weeks following viral URI, immunization, *Campylobacter jejuni enteritis*, or surgery
- pathology: focal segmental demyelination with endoneurial monocytic infiltrate
- elevated CSF protein without pleocytosis (albuminocytologic dissociation)

Guillain-Barré syndrome (GBS) AKA acute polyradiculoneuritis, among others, is actually a collection of syndromes having inflammatory polyradiculoneuropathy in common. Its most frequent form is acute inflammatory demyelinating polyradiculoneuropathy (AIDP). First described as an ascending paralysis, most forms are characterized by *symmetric* weakness and areflexia. Mild cases may present only with ataxia, whereas fulminant cases may ascend to complete tetraplegia with paralysis of respiratory muscles and cranial nerves. There are also a number of variants (p. 186).

GBS is the most common acquired demyelinating neuropathy. Incidence is ≈ 1–3/100,000. The lifetime risk for any one individual getting GBS is ≈ 1/1,000.

GBS is triggered by both humoral and cell mediated autoimmune response to an immune sensitizing event. Frequent (but not essential) antecedents: viral infection, surgery, immunization, mycoplasma infection, enteral infection with Campylobacter jejuni (≈ 4 days of intense diarrhea). Higher frequency in the following conditions than in general population: Hodgkin's disease, lymphoma, lupus.

Most cases involve antibodies to gangliosides and glycolipids in peripheral myelin (axon antibodies occur in some forms). For unknown reasons serum creatine kinase can be mildly elevated, and may correlate with muscle type pain.[53]

10.7.2 Diagnostic criteria

See reference.[54]

features required for diagnosis:

- progressive motor weakness of more than 1 limb (from minimal weakness ± ataxia to paralysis, may include bulbar or facial or EOM palsy). Unlike most neuropathies, proximal muscles are affected more than distal
- areflexia (usually universal, but distal areflexia with definite hyporeflexia of biceps and knee jerks suffices if other features consistent)

features strongly supportive of diagnosis:

- clinical features (in order of importance)
  - progression: motor weakness peaks at 2 wks in 50%, by 3 wks in 80%, and by 4 wks in > 90%
  - relative symmetry
  - mild sensory symptoms/signs (e.g. mild paresthesias in hands or feet)
  - *cranial nerve* involvement: *facial weakness* in 50%, usually *bilateral*. GBS presents initially in EOMs or other Cr. N. in < 5% of cases. Oropharyngeal muscles may be affected
  - recovery usually by 2–4 wks after progression stops, may be delayed by months (most patients recover functionally)
  - autonomic dysfunction (may fluctuate): tachycardia and other arrhythmias, postural hypotension, HTN, vasomotor symptoms
  - afebrile at onset of neuritic symptoms
  - variants (not ranked):
    - fever at onset of neuritic symptoms
    - severe sensory loss with pain
    - progression > 4 wks
    - cessation of progression without recovery
    - sphincter dysfunction (usually spared): e.g. bladder paralysis
    - CNS involvement (controversial): e.g. ataxia, dysarthria, Babinski signs
- CSF: albuminocytologic dissociation (↑ protein without pleocytosis)
  - protein: elevated after 1 wk of symptoms, > 55 mg/dl
  - cells: 10 or fewer mononuclear leukocytes/ml
  - variants
    - no CSF protein rise 1–10 wks after onset (rare)
    - 11–50 monocytes/ml
    - electrodiagnostics: 80% have NCV slowing or block at some time (may take several weeks in some). NCV usually < 60% of normal, but not in all nerves

features casting doubt on diagnosis:

- marked, persistent, asymmetry of weakness
- persistent bowel or bladder dysfunction
- > 50 monocytes/ml CSF
- PMNs in CSF
- sharp sensory level

features of conditions in the differential diagnosis (see below)

10.7.3 Guillain-Barré variants

General information

A number of variants have been described (some may simply be incomplete forms of typical Guillain-Berré). Autonomic dysfunction may occur in some.

Miller-Fisher variant of GBS

Ataxia, areflexia and ophthalmoplegia. May also have ptosis. 5% of cases of GBS. Serum marker: anti-GQ1b antibodies.

Acute motor axonal neuropathy (AMAN)

This variant and AIDP are the most common to follow Campylobacter jejuni enteritis.

Pharyngeal-cervical-brachial variant

Facial, oropharyngeal, cervical, and UE weakness, sparing the LEs.

Pure sensory variant

Sensory loss accompanied by areflexia.

Atypical GBS

May be accompanied by rhabdomyolysis.[55]

10.7.4 Differential diagnosis

Also see conditions in the differential diagnosis under Myelopathy (p. 1407)

1. Guillain-Barré syndrome (including one of its variants)
2. critical illness polyneuropathy (p. 542): EMG: ↓ CMAP & SNAP
3. current hexacarbon abuse: volatile solvents (n-hexane, methyl n-butyl ketone), glue sniffing
4. acute intermittent porphyria (AIP): a disorder of porphyrin metabolism. CSF protein is not elevated in AIP. Recurrent painful abdominal crises are common. Check urine delta-aminolevulinic acid or porphobilinogen
5. recent diphtheritic infection: diphtheritic polyneuropathy has a longer latency and a slower crescendo of symptoms
6. lead neuropathy: UE weakness with wrist drop. May be asymmetrical
7. poliomyelitis: usually *asymmetric*, has meningeal irritation
8. hypophosphatemia (may occur in chronic IV hyperalimentation)
9. botulism: difficult to distinguish clinically from GBS. Normal NCV and a facilitating response to repetitive nerve stimulation on electrodiagnostics
10. toxic neuropathy (e.g. from nitrofurantoin, dapsone, thallium or arsenic)
11. tick paralysis: may cause an ascending motor neuropathy without sensory impairment. Careful examination of the scalp for tick(s)
12. chronic immune demyelinating polyradiculoneuropathy (CIDP) AKA chronic relapsing GBS, chronic relapsing polyneuritis.[56] ICD9: 357.81 chronic inflammatory demyelinating polyneuritis. Similar to GBS, but long time course (symptoms must be present > 2 mos). CIDP produces progressive, symmetrical, proximal & distal weakness, depression of muscle stretch reflexes, and variable sensory loss. Cranial nerves are usually spared (facial muscles may be involved). Balance difficulties are common. Need for respiratory support is rare. Peak incidence: age 40–60 yrs. Electrodiagnostics and nerve biopsy findings are indicative of demyelination. CSF findings are similar to GBS (see above). Most respond to immunosuppressive therapy (especially prednisolone & plasmapheresis) but relapses are common. Refractory cases may be treated with IV gamma-globulin, cyclosporin-A,[57] total body lymphoid irradiation or interferon-α[58]
13. critical illness myopathy: ICD9: 359.81 chronic illness myopathy. Muscles not excitable with direct stimulation. EMG: low or normal CMAP with normal SNAP. Muscle biopsy: abnormalities may range from Type II fiber atrophy to necrosis (severe necrosis may not recover)
14. motor neuron disease (p. 182): AKA ALS. Hyperreflexia in LEs
15. myasthenia gravis: weakness worsens towards the end of the day and with repeat efforts. Positive assay for circulating anti-acetylcholine receptor antibodies
16. spinal cord injury

10.7.5 Imaging

No characteristic finding, however, diffuse enhancement of cauda equina and nerve roots occurs in up to 95% of cases.[59] Thought to be due to disruption of the blood-nerve barrier from inflammation. Conspicuous nerve root enhancement correlates with pain, GBS disability grade, and duration of recovery.[59]

10.7.6 Treatment

Immunoglobulins may be helpful. In *severe* cases, early plasmapheresis hastens the recovery and reduces the residual deficit. Its role in mild cases is uncertain. Steroids are not helpful.[60] Mechanical ventilation and measures to prevent aspiration are used as appropriate. In cases of facial diplegia, the eyes must be protected from exposure (neuroparalytic) keratitis.

10.7.7 Outcome

Recovery may not be complete for several months. 35% of untreated patients have residual weakness and atrophy. Recurrence of GBS after achieving maximal recovery occurs in ≈ 2%.

10.8 Myelitis

10.8.1 General information

AKA acute transverse myelitis (ATM). The terminology is confusing: myelitis overlaps with "myelopathy." Both are pathologic conditions of the spinal cord. Myelitis indicates inflammation, and etiologies include: infectious/post-infectious, autoimmune, and idiopathic. Myelopathy is generally reserved for compressive, toxic, or metabolic etiologies[61]; see also differential diagnosis (p. 1407).

10

10.8.2 Etiology

Many so-called "causes" remain unproven. Immunologic response against the CNS (most likely via cell mediated component) is the probable common mechanism. Animal model: experimental allergic encephalomyelitis (requires myelin basic protein of CNS, not peripheral).

Generally accepted etiologies include (items with an asterisk * may be more properly associated with myelopathy rather than myelitis):

1. infectious and post-infectious
   a) primary infectious myelitis
      - viral: poliomyelitis, myelitis with viral encephalomyelitis, herpes zoster, rabies
      - bacterial: including tuberculoma of spinal cord
      - spirochetal: AKA syphilitic myelitis. Causes syphilitic endarteritis
      - fungal (aspergillosis, blastomycosis, cryptococcosis)
      - parasitic (Echinococcus, cysticercosis, paragonimiasis, schistosomiasis)
   b) post-infectious: including post-exanthematous, influenza
2. post-traumatic
3. physical agents
   a) decompression sickness (dysbarism)
   b) electrical injury*
   c) post-irradiation
4. paraneoplastic syndrome (remote effect of cancer): most common primary is lung, but prostate, ovary and rectum have also been described[62]
5. metabolic
   a) diabetes mellitus*
   b) pernicious anemia*
   c) chronic liver disease*
6. toxins
   a) cresyl phosphates*
   b) intra-arterial contrast agents*
   c) spinal anesthetics
   d) myelographic contrast agents
   e) following chemonucleolysis[63]
7. arachnoiditis
8. autoimmune
   a) multiple sclerosis (MS), especially Devic syndrome (p. 1409)
   b) following vaccination (smallpox, rabies)

9. collagen vascular disease
   a) systemic lupus erythematosus
   b) mixed connective tissue disease

10.8.3 Clinical

Presentation

34 patients with ATM[64]: age of onset ranged 15–55 yrs, with 66% occurring in 3rd and 4th decade. 12 patients (35%) had a viral-like prodrome. Presenting symptoms are shown in ▶ Table 10.5, with other presenting symptoms of unspecified frequency including[65]: fever and rash.

Presenting level

The levels at presentation in 62 patients with ATM are shown in ▶ Table 10.6.[65] The thoracic level is the most common sensory level. Infrequently, ATM is the presenting symptom of MS (≈ 3–6% of patients with ATM develop MS).

Progression

Progression is usually rapid, with 66% reaching maximal deficit by 24 hrs, however the interval between first symptom and maximal deficit varies from 2 hrs-14 days.[65] Findings at the time of maximal deficit are shown in ▶ Table 10.7.

10.8.4 Evaluation

Imaging should be done to rule-out a compressive lesion. Myelogram, CT & MRI: no characteristic finding. One paper reports 2 patients with fusiform cord enlargement.[67] MRI may be able to demonstrate the area of involvement within the cord. MRI may show the "central dot sign",[68] an area of high signal on axial T2WI usually centrally located with a small dot of isointense signal in the core of the hyperintensity.

CSF: normal during acute phase in 38% of LPs. Remainder (62%) had elevated protein (usually > 40 mg%) or pleocytosis (lymphocytes, PMNs, or both) or both.

Table 10.5 Presenting symptoms in myelitis

Symptom	Series A[a]	Series B[b]
pain (back or radicular)	35%	35%
muscle weakness	32%	13%
sensory deficit or paresthesias	26%	46%
sphincter disturbance	12%	6%

[a]series A: 34 patients with ATM[64]
[b]series B: 52 patients with acute or subacute transverse myelitis[66]

Table 10.6 Level of sensory deficit

Level	%
cervical	8%
high thoracic	36%
low thoracic	32%
lumbar	8%
unknown	16%

Table 10.7 Symptoms at time of *maximal* deficit (62 patients with ATM[65])

Symptom	%
sensory deficit or paresthesias	100%
muscle weakness	97%
sphincter disturbance (hesitancy, retention, overflow incontinence)	94%
pain in back, abdomen, or limbs	34%
fever	27%
nuchal rigidity	13%

Evaluation scheme

In a patient developing acute myelopathy/paraplegia, especially when ATM is considered likely, the first test of choice is an emergency MRI. If not readily available, a myelogram (with CT to follow) directed at the region of the sensory level is performed (CSF may be sent in this circumstance once block is ruled out).

10.8.5 Treatment

No treatment has been studied in a randomized controlled trial.

1. steroids: not beneficial for all causes of myelitis,[69] especially with ASIA A (complete loss of spinal cord function).[70] Rx: high-dose IV methylprednisolone 3-5 days (doses quoted include 500 mg/d, and 1000 mg/d[71]). The decision to introduce additional treatment measures is based on the response to steroids and the MRI appearance after ≈ 5 days of steroids
2. plasma exchange (PLEX) for patients that do not respond to steroids within 3-5 days
3. other forms of immune suppression may be attempted for failure of above therapies, including: cyclophosphamide (usually under the direction of an oncologist)
4. in cases of focal spinal cord enlargement, surgical decompression may be considered in cases that fail to respond to the above

10.8.6 Prognosis

In a series of 34 ATM patients with ≥ 5 yrs follow-up (F/U)[64]: 9 patients (26%) had good recovery (ambulate well, mild urinary symptoms, minimal sensory and UMN signs); 9 (26%) had fair recovery (functional gait with some degree of spasticity, urinary urgency, obvious sensory signs, paraparesis); 11 (32%) poor (paraplegic, absent sphincter control); 5 (15%) died within 4 mos of illness. 18 patients (62% of survivors) became ambulatory (in these cases, all could walk with support by 3–6 mos).

In a series of 59 patients[65] (F/U period unspecified): 22 (37%) had good recovery; 14 (24%) poor; 3 died in acute stage (respiratory insufficiency in 2, sepsis in 1). Recovery occurred between 4 weeks and 3 mos after onset (no improvement occurred after 3 mos).

10.9 Neurosarcoidosis

10.9.1 General

Key concepts

- neurologic involvement of sarcoidosis (a systemic granulomatous disease)
- may produce multiple cranial nerve palsies
- the most common neurologic manifestation is diabetes insipidus
- corticosteroids are beneficial for systemic as well as neurologic involvement

Sarcoidosis is a granulomatous disease that is usually systemic, and may include the CNS (so-called neurosarcoidosis AKA neurosarcoid). Only 1–3% of cases have CNS findings without systemic manifestations.[72] The cause of the disease is unknown. An exaggerated cellular immune response for unknown reasons is the currently favored hypothesis. Organs commonly involved include lungs, skin, lymph nodes, bones, eyes, muscles, and parotid glands.[30]

10.9.2 Pathology

CNS sarcoidosis primarily involves the leptomeninges, however parenchymal invasion often occurs. Adhesive arachnoiditis with nodule formation may also occur (nodules have a predilection for the posterior fossa). Diffuse meningitis or meningoencephalitis may occur, and may be most pronounced at the base of the brain (basal meningitis) and in the subependymal region of the third ventricle (including the hypothalamus).

Constant microscopic features of neurosarcoidosis include noncaseating granulomas with lymphocytic infiltrates. Langhans giant cells may or may not be present.

10.9.3 Epidemiology

Incidence of sarcoidosis is ≈ 3–50 cases/100,000 population; neurosarcoidosis occurs in ≈ 5% of cases (reported range: 1–27%). In one series, the median age of onset of neurologic symptoms was 44 years.

10.9.4 Clinical findings

Clinical findings include multiple cranial nerve palsies in 50–70% (particularly facial n., including diplegia), peripheral neuropathy, and myopathy.[73] Occasionally the lesions may produce mass effect,[74] and hydrocephalus may result from adhesive basal arachnoiditis. Patients may have low grade fever. Intracranial hypertension is common and may be dangerous. Hypothalamic involvement may produce disorders of ADH (diabetes insipidus, disordered thirst). Rare involvement of the pituitary may produce pituitary insufficiency. Seizures occur in 15%.

10

0.4% of patients with sarcoidosis develop spinal cord involvement,[75] and in 16% of these, the spinal cord was the only identifiable site of involvement.

10.9.5 Laboratory

CBC: mild leukocytosis and eosinophilia may occur.

Serum angiotensin-converting enzyme (ACE): abnormally elevated in 83% of patients with active pulmonary sarcoidosis, but in only 11% with inactive disease.[76] False positive rate: 2–3%; may also be elevated in primary biliary cirrhosis.

CSF: similar to any subacute meningitis: elevated pressure, mild pleocytosis (10–200 cells/mm^3) mostly lymphocytes, elevated protein (up to 2,000 mg/dl), mild hypoglycorrhachia (15–40 mg/dl). CSF ACE is elevated in ≈ 55% of cases with neurosarcoidosis (normal in patients with sarcoidosis not involving the CNS).[77] No organisms are recovered on culture or gram stain.

10.9.6 Imaging

CXR

Usually demonstrates characteristic findings of sarcoidosis (hilar adenopathy, mediastinal lymph nodes…).

MRI

Gadolinium enhancement of the leptomeninges and/or optic nerve may be the only abnormal finding(s). Meningeal enhancement was seen in 38% of neurosarcoidosis patients.[78] Lesons may be solitary or multiple, and may be located intra- or extraparenchymal, periventricular, and/or in basal cisterns. Lesions may be seen on FLAIR that would otherwise have been missed. Hydrocephalus may occur.

Gallium scan

Nuclear medicine scan with 67Ga citrate (p. 236). Described findings include:

1. Panda sign[79]: uptake in lacrimal glands, parotid glands & nasopharynx (normal). Not specific for sarcoidosis
2. lambda distribution[80]: uptake in hilar lymph nodes
3. leopard man sign[81]: diffuse dappled pattern due to uptake in soft tissues, skin, muscles, mediastinum, and lacrimal glands

Table 10.8 Differential diagnosis of neurosarcoidosis

1. Hodgkin's disease
2. chronic granulomatous meningitis:
   a) Hansen's disease (leprosy)
   b) syphilis
   c) cryptococcosis
   d) tuberculosis
3. multiple sclerosis
4. CNS lymphoma
5. pseudotumor cerebri
6. granulomatous angiitis

10.9.7 Differential diagnosis

Differentiating granulomatous angiitis (**GA**) from neurosarcoidosis that involves only the CNS can be done on histologic criteria: the inflammatory reaction in sarcoidosis is not limited to the region immediately surrounding blood vessels as it is in GA, where extensive disruption of the vessel wall may occur.

10.9.8 Diagnosis

Making the diagnosis is relatively easy when systemic involvement occurs: characteristic findings on CXR, biopsy of skin or liver nodules, muscle biopsy, serum ACE assay.

Isolated neurosarcoidosis may be more difficult to diagnose, and may require biopsy (see below).

10.9.9 Biopsy

In uncertain cases, biopsy may be indicated. Whenever possible, MRI should be used to localize a supratentorial region of involvement. If a mass lesion cannot be biopsied, a meningeal biopsy may be done and should include all layers of meninges and cerebral cortex. Cultures and stains for fungus and acid-fast bacteria (TB) should be performed in addition to microscopic examination.

10.9.10 Treatment

Antibiotics have not been proven to be of benefit. Immunosuppression primarily with corticosteroids are beneficial for systemic as well as neurologic involvement. Therapy may be initiated with prednisone 60 mg PO qd in adults, and tapered based on response. Therapy with cyclosporine may allow a reduction in steroid dosage in refractory cases.[82] Treatment for unresponsive cases include: methotrexate, cytoxan, cyclophosphamide, azathioprine, low dose XRT. CSF shunting is indicated if hydrocephalus develops.

10.9.11 Prognosis

Usually a benign disease. Peripheral and cranial nerve palsies recover slowly.

References

[1] Consensus Conference. Differential Diagnosis of Dementing Diseases. JAMA. 1987; 258:3411–3416
[2] Fleming KC, Adams AC, Petersen RC. Dementia: Diagnosis and Evaluation. Mayo Clin Proc. 1995; 70:1093–1107
[3] Lipowski ZJ. Delerium (Acute Confusional States). JAMA. 1987; 258:1789–1792
[4] Pompei P, Foreman M, Rudberg MA, et al. Delerium in Hospitalized Older Persons: Outcomes and Predictors. J Am Geriatr Soc. 1994; 42:809–815
[5] Petersen RC. Acute Confusional State: Don't Mistake it for Dementia. Postgrad Med. 1992; 92:141–148
[6] Hulette CM, Earl NL, Crain BJ. Evaluation of Cerebral Biopsies for the Diagnosis of Dementia. Arch Neurol. 1992; 49:28–31
[7] Javedan SP, Tamargo RJ. Diagnostic Yield of Brain Biopsy in Neurodegenerative Disorders. Neurosurgery. 1997; 41:823–830
[8] Groves R, Moller J. The Value of the Cerebral Cortical Biopsy. Acta Neurol Scand. 1966; 42:477–482
[9] Forsyth PA, Posner JB. Headaches in Patients with Brain Tumors: A Study of 111 Patients. Neurology. 1993; 43:1678–1683
[10] Welch KMA, Levine SR. Migraine-related stroke in the context of the International Headache Society Classification of head pain. Arch Neurol. 1990; 47:458–462
[11] Lance JW. Treatment of Migraine. Lancet. 1992; 339:1207–1209
[12] Kittrelle JP, Grouse DS, Seybold ME. Cluster Headache: Local Anesthetic Abortive Agents. Arch Neurol. 1985; 42:496–498
[13] Sanders M, Zuurmond WWA. Efficacy of Sphenopalatine Ganglion Blockade in 66 Patients Suffering from Cluster Headache: A 12- to 70-Month Follow-Up Evaluation. J Neurosurg. 1997; 87:876–880

10

[14] Burns B, Watkins L, Goadsby PJ. Treatment of medically intractable cluster headache by occipital nerve stimulation: long-term follow-up of 8 patients. Lancet. 2007; 369:1099–1106
[15] Lapkin ML, Golden GS. Basilar Artery Migraine: A Review of 30 Cases. Am J Dis Child. 1978; 132:278–281
[16] Mitchell SL, Kiely DK, Kiel DP, Lipsitz LA. The Epidemiology, Clinical Characteristics, and Natural History of Older Nursing Home Residents with a Diagnosis of Parkinson's Disease. J Am Geriatr Soc. 1996; 44:394–399
[17] Lang AE, Lozano AM. Parkinson's Disease. First of Two Parts. N Engl J Med. 1998; 339:1044–1053
[18] Koller WC, Silver DE, Lieberman A. An Algorithm for the Management of Parkinson's Disease. Neurology. 1994; 44:S5–52
[19] Young R. Update on Parkinson's Disease. Am Fam Physician. 1999; 59:2155–2167
[20] Kondziolka D, Bonaroti EA, Lunsford LD. Pallidotomy for Parkinson's Disease. Contemp Neurosurg. 1996; 18:1–6
[21] Davis GC, Williams AC, Markey SP, et al. Chronic Parkinsonism Secondary to Intravenous Injection of Meperidine Analogues. Psychiatry Res. 1979; 1:249–254
[22] Langston JW, Ballard P, Tetrud JW, Irwin I. Chronic Parkinsonism in Humans Due to a Product of Meperidine-Analog Synthesis. Science. 1983; 219:979–980
[23] Langston JW, Ballard PA, Jr. Parkinson's Disease in a Chemist Working with 1-Methyl-4-phenyl-1,2,5,6-tetrahydropyridine. N Engl J Med. 1983; 309
[24] Langston JW, Forno LS, Tetrud J, Reeves AG, Kaplan JA, Karluk D. Evidence of Active Nerve Cell Degeneration in the Substantia Nigra of Humans Years After 1-Methyl-4-phenyl-1,2,3,6-tetrahydropyridine Exposure. Ann Neurol. 1999; 46:598–605
[25] Kristensen MO. Progressive Supranuclear Palsy - 10 Years Later. Acta Neurol Scand. 1985; 71:177–189
[26] Gildenberg PL. Whatever Happened to Stereotactic Surgery? Neurosurgery. 1987; 20:983–987
[27] Pugliatti M, Rosati G, Raine CS, McFarland HF, Hohlfeld R. In: Epidemiology of multiple sclerosis. Multiple sclerosis: a comprehensive text. Philadelphia: Saunders Elsevier; 2008
[28] Lublin FD, Reingold SC. Defining the Clinical Course of Multiple Sclerosis: Results of an International Survey. Neurology. 1996; 46:907–911
[29] Rudick RA, Cohen JA, Weinstock-Guttman B, et al. Management of Multiple Sclerosis. N Engl J Med. 1997; 22:1604–1611
[30] Rowland LP. Merritt's Textbook of Neurology. Philadelphia 1989
[31] Jensen TS, Rasmussen P, Reske-Nielsen E. Association of Trigeminal Neuralgia with Multiple Sclerosis. Arch Neurol. 1982; 65:182–189
[32] Filippi M, Horsfield MA, Morrissey SP, et al. Quantitative Brain MRI Lesion Load Predicts the Course of Clinically Isolated Syndromes Suggestive of Multiple Sclerosis. Neurology. 1994; 44:635–641
[33] McDonald WI, Compston A, Edan G, et al. Recommended diagnostic criteria for multiple sclerosis: Guidelines from the international panel on the diagnosis of multiple sclerosis. Ann Neurol. 2001; 50:121–127
[34] Polman CH, Reingold SC, Edan G, Filippi M, Hartung HP, Kappos L, Lublin FD, Metz LM, McFarland HF, O'Connor PW, Sandberg-Wollheim M, Thompson AJ, Weinshenker BG, Wolinsky JS. Diagnostic criteria for multiple sclerosis: 2005 revisions to the "McDonald Criteria". Ann Neurol. 2005; 58:840–846
[35] Poser CM, Paty DW, Scheinberg L, et al. New Diagnostic Criteria for Multiple Sclerosis: Guidelines for Research Protocols. Ann Neurol. 1983; 13:227–231
[36] Polman CH, Reingold SC, Banwell B, Clanet M, Cohen JA, Filippi M, Fujihara K, Havrdova E, Hutchinson M, Kappos L, Lublin FD, Montalban X, O'Connor P, Sandberg-Wollheim M, Thompson AJ, Waubant E, Weinshenker B, Wolinsky JS. Diagnostic criteria for multiple sclerosis: 2010 revisions to the McDonald criteria. Ann Neurol. 2011; 69:292–302
[37] Swanton JK, Rovira A, Tintore M, Altmann DR, Barkhof F, Filippi M, Huerga E, Miszkiel KA, Plant GT, Polman C, Rovaris M, Thompson AJ, Montalban X, Miller DH. MRI criteria for multiple sclerosis in patients presenting with clinically isolated syndromes: a multicentre retrospective study. Lancet Neurol. 2007; 6:677–686
[38] Montalban X, Tintore M, Swanton J, Barkhof F, Fazekas F, Filippi M, Frederiksen J, Kappos L, Palace J, Polman C, Rovaris M, de Stefano N, Thompson A, Yousry T, Rovira A, Miller DH. MRI criteria for MS in patients with clinically isolated syndromes. Neurology. 2010; 74:427–434
[39] Swanson JW. Multiple Sclerosis: Update in Diagnosis and Review of Prognostic Factors. Mayo Clin Proc. 1989; 64:577–586
[40] Barkhof F, Filippi M, Miller DH, et al. Comparison of MR imaging criteria at first presentation to predict conversion to clinically definite multiple sclerosis. Brain. 1997; 120:2059–2069
[41] Tintore M, Rovira A, Martinez M, et al. Isolated demyelinating syndromes: comparison of different MR imaging criteria to predict conversion to clinically definite multiple sclerosis. AJNR. 2000; 21:702–706
[42] Stewart JM, Houser OW, Baker HL, O'Brien PC, et al. Magnetic Resonance Imaging and Clinical Relationships in Multiple Sclerosis. Mayo Clin Proc. 1987; 62:174–184
[43] Mushlin AI, Detsky AS, Phelps CE, et al. The Accuracy of Magnetic Resonance Imaging in Patients With Suspected Multiple Sclerosis. JAMA. 1993; 269:3146–3151
[44] Kidd C, Thorpe JW, Thompson AJ, et al. Spinal cord imaging MRI using multi-array coils and fast spin echo. II. Findings in multiple sclerosis. Neurology. 1993; 43:2632–2637
[45] Kent DL, Larson EB. Magnetic Resonance Imaging of the Brain and Spine. Ann Intern Med. 1988; 108:402–424
[46] Kepes JJ. Large focal tumor-like demyelinating lesions of the brain: intermediate entity between multiple sclerosis and acute disseminated encephalomyelitis? A study of 31 patients. Ann Neurol. 1993; 33:18–27
[47] Law M, Meltzer DE, Cha S. Spectroscopic magnetic resonance imaging of a tumefactive demyelinating lesion. Neuroradiology. 2002; 44:986–989
[48] Freedman MS, Thompson EJ, Deisenhammer D, et al. Recommended standard of cerebrospinal fluid analysis in the diagnosis of multiple sclerosis: A consensus statement. Arch Neurol. 2005; 62:865–870
[49] Rowland LP. Diagnosis of amyotrophic lateral sclerosis. J Neurol Sci. 1998; 160:S6–24
[50] Peavy GM, Herzog AG, Rubin NP, Mesulam M-M. Neuropsychological Aspects of Dementia of Motor Neuron Disease: A Report of Two Cases. Neurology. 1992; 42:1004–1008
[51] Bensimon G, Lacomblez L, Meininger V, et al. A Controlled Trial of Riluzole in Amyotrophic Lateral Sclerosis. N Engl J Med. 1994; 24:585–591
[52] Lacomblez L, Bensimon G, Guillet P, et al. Riluzole: A Double-Blind Randomized Placebo-Controlled Dose-Range Study in Amyotrophic Lateral Sclerosis (ALS). Electroenceph Clin Neurophysiol. 1995; 97
[53] Ropper AH, Shahani BT. Pain in Guillain-Barre syndrome. Arch Neurol. 1984; 41:511–514
[54] Asbury AK, Arnaso BGW, Karp HR, et al. Criteria for Diagnosis of Guillain-Barre Syndrome. Ann Neurol. 1978; 3:565–566
[55] Scott AJ, Duncan R, Henderson L, Jamal GA, Kennedy PG. Acute rhabdomyolysis associated with atypical Guillain-Barre syndrome. Postgrad Med J. 1991; 67:73–74
[56] Mendell JR. Chronic Inflammatory Demyelinating Polyradiculoneuropathy. Annu Rev Med. 1993; 44:211–219
[57] Mahattanakul W, Crawford TO, Griffin JW, et al. Treatment of Chronic Inflammatory Demyelinating Polyneuropathy with Cyclosporin-A. J Neurol Neurosurg Psychiatry. 1996; 60:185–187

[58] Gorson KC, Ropper AH, Clark BD, et al. Treatment of Chronic Inflammatory Demyelinating Polyneuropathy with Interferon-a 2a. Neurology. 1998; 50:84–87
[59] Gorson KC, Ropper AH, Muriello MA, Blair R. Prospective evaluation of MRI lumbosacral nerve root enhancement in acute Guillain-Barre syndrome. Neurology. 1996; 47:813–817
[60] Guillain-Barré Syndrome Steroid Trial Group. Double-Blind Trial of Intravenous Methylprednisolone in Guillain-Barré Syndrome. Lancet. 1993; 341:586–590
[61] Kincaid JC, Dyken ML, Baker AB, Joynt RJ. In: Myelitis and Myelopathy. Clinical Neurology. Hagerstown: Harper and Row; 1984:1–32
[62] Altrocchi PH. Acute Transverse Myelopathy. Arch Neurol. 1963; 9:111–119
[63] Eguro H. Transverse Myelitis following Chemonucleolysis: Report of a Case. J Bone Joint Surg. 1983; 65A:1328–1329
[64] Lipton HL, Teasdall RD. Acute Transverse Myelopathy in Adults: A Follow-Up Study. Arch Neurol. 1973; 28:252–257
[65] Berman M, Feldman S, Alter M, et al. Acute Transverse Myelitis: Incidence and Etiologic Considerations. Neurology. 1981; 31:966–971
[66] Ropper AH, Poskanzer DC. The Prognosis of Acute and Subacute Transverse Myelopathy Based on Early Signs and Symptoms. Ann Neurol. 1978; 4:51–59
[67] Merine D, Wang H, Kumar AJ, et al. CT Myelography and MRI of Acute Transverse Myelitis. J Comput Assist Tomogr. 1987; 11:606–608
[68] Berg B, Franklin G, Cuneo R, et al. Nonsurgical Cure of Brain Abscesses. Ann Neurol. 1978; 3:474–478
[69] Kalita J, Misra UK. Is methyl prednisolone useful in acute transverse myelitis? Spinal Cord. 2001; 39:471–476
[70] Greenberg BM, Thomas KP, Krishnan C, Kaplin AI, Calabresi PA, Kerr DA. Idiopathic transverse myelitis: corticosteroids, plasma exchange, or cyclophosphamide. Neurology. 2007; 68:1614–1617
[71] Britt RH, Enzmann DR, Yeager AS. Neuropathological and CT Findings in Experimental Brain Abscess. J Neurosurg. 1981; 55:590–603
[72] Stern BJ, Krumholz A, Johns C, Scott P, et al. Sarcoidosis and its Neurological Manifestations. Arch Neurol. 1985; 42:909–917
[73] Oksanen V. Neurosarcoidosis: Clinical Presentation and Course in 50 Patients. Acta Neurol Scand. 1986; 73:283–290
[74] de Tribolet N, Zander E. Intracranial Sarcoidosis Presenting Angiographically as a Subdural Hematoma. Surg Neurol. 1978; 9:169–171
[75] Saleh S, Saw C, Marzouk K, Sharma O. Sarcoidosis of the spinal cord: literature review and report of eight cases. J Natl Med Assoc. 2006; 98:965–976
[76] Rohrbach MS, DeRemee RA. Pulmonary Sarcoidosis and Serum Angiotensin-Converting Enzyme. Mayo Clin Proc. 1982; 57:64–66
[77] Oksanen V. New Cerebrospinal Fluid, Neurophysiological and Neuroradiological Examinations in the Diagnosis and Follow-Up of Neurosarcoidosis. Sarcoidosis. 1987; 4:105–110
[78] Zajicek JP, Scolding NJ, Foster O, Rovaris M, Evanson J, Moseley IF, Scadding JW, Thompson EJ, Chamoun V, Miller DH, McDonald WI, Mitchell D. Central nervous system sarcoidosis–diagnosis and management. QJM. 1999; 92:103–117
[79] Kurdziel KA. The Panda Sign. Radiology. 2000; 215:884–885
[80] Sulavik SB, Spencer RP, Weed DA, Shapiro HR, Shiue ST, Castriotta RJ. Recognition of distinctive patterns of gallium-67 distribution in sarcoidosis. J Nucl Med. 1990; 31:1909–1914
[81] Fayad F, Duet M, Orcel P, Liote F. Systemic sarcoidosis: the "leopard-man" sign. Joint Bone Spine. 2006; 73:109–112
[82] Stern BJ, Schonfeld SA, Sewell C, et al. The Treatment of Neurosarcoidosis With Cyclosporine. Arch Neurol. 1992; 49:1065–1072

11 Neurovascular Disorders and Neurotoxicology

11.1 Posterior reversible encephalopathy syndrome (PRES)

11.1.1 General information

AKA reversible posterior leukoencephalopathy syndrome (RPLS). A group of encephalopathies with characteristic pattern of widespread vasogenic brain edema seen on CT or MRI with some predominance in the parietal and occipital regions.[1] The most common PRES pattern involves watershed zones with involvement of the cortex, subcortical and deep white matter to a variable extent.[1] A small number of patients with PRES will go on to infarction.

Patients may present with headache, seizures, mental status changes and focal neurologic deficit. Intracerebral hemorrhage (ICH) and SAH may occur in up to 15%.[1]

11.1.2 Associated findings and conditions

Includes:

1. hypertensive encephalopathy: commonly seen in the setting of subacute blood pressure elevations (as may occur with malignant hypertension). Imaging studies show symmetric confluent lesions with mild mass effect and patchy enhancement primarily in the subcortical white matter of the *occipital lobes*[2] which may produce cortical blindness
   a) moderate to severe hypertension is seen in ≈ 75% of patients with PRES[1] although the upper limits of autoregulation are often not reached
   b) in addition to hemispheric patterns of edema isolated brain stem and cerebellar edema have been described. Posterior fossa edema has been reported to cause obstructive hydrocephalus in a severe case[3]
2. preeclampsia/eclampsia associated with cerebral edema.[4] The condition is often temporary, but (permanent) infarctions also occur. Restricted diffusion on MR imaging is seen in 11–26% of cases. Abnormal DWI areas on MRI may be associated with a worse prognosis[5]
   a) may present (e.g. with blindness) during pregnancy complicated by preeclampsia or eclampsia[6]
   b) may develop 4–9 days post-partum and may be associated with vasospasm[7] even in patients not meeting clinical criteria for the diagnosis of eclampsia
   c) toxemia is attributed to the placenta. Delivery and removal of the placenta is felt to be curative[8]
3. infection, sepsis and shock: blood pressure was normal in 40% (edema was greater in the normotensive patients). Gram positive organisms predominate[9]
4. autoimmune disease: PRES has been described in patients with lupus, scleroderma, Wegener's granulomatosis and polyarteritis nodosa.[1] These patients often receive regimens of immunosuppressive medications (tacrolimus, cyclosporine), which have also been linked to cases of PRES
5. cancer chemotherapy: PRES occurs in patients receiving multi-drug high dose chemotherapy most commonly for hematopoietic malignancies
6. transplantation: PRES has been reported both with bone marrow and solid organ transplantation
   a) incidence: 3–16% with bone marrow transplantation depending on the preconditioning regimen and whether or not it is myeloablative[1]
   b) highest incidence in the first month following allogeneic bone marrow transplant[1]
   c) lower incidence following solid organ transplants. Occurs earlier following liver transplantation, usually within 2 months. Occurs later in renal transplants[1]
7. cyclosporine post-transplant neurotoxicity[9]

11.1.3 Treatment

Disordered autoregulation mandates tight control of blood pressure to reduce the risk of ICH. The underlying cause needs to be addressed (i.e. control HTN, hold immunosuppressives or chemotherapeutics, delivery of the placenta, etc.).

11.2 Crossed cerebellar diaschisis

Hypometabolism of cerebellar cortex contralateral to a cerebral hemispheric lesion (lesions include: stroke, brain tumor…). Lesions in the motor cortex, anterior corona radiata, and thalamus produce the most marked suppression of metabolism. Theory: hypometabolism is due to disconnection of cerebro-ponto-cerebellar pathways → decreased oxygen and glucose consumption → decreased CO_2 production → local arterial constriction (down-regulation of cerebellar blood flow).

11.3 Vasculitis and vasculopathy

11.3.1 General information

The vasculitides are a group of disorders characterized by inflammation and necrosis of blood vessels. Vasculitis may be primary or secondary. Those that may affect the CNS are listed in ▶ Table 11.1, all of these cause tissue ischemia (even after the inflammation is quiescent) that may range in effect from neuropraxia to infarction.

11.3.2 Giant cell arteritis (GCA)

Key concepts

- formerly often referred to as temporal arteritis
- a chronic vasculitis of large and medium caliber vessels, primarily involving cranial branches of the arteries arising from the aortic arch
- age > 50 years; affects women twice as often as men
- important possible late complications: blindness, stroke, thoracic aortic aneurysms and aortic dissections
- temporal artery biopsy is recommended for all patients suspected of GCA
- corticosteroids are the drug of choice for treatment

AKA temporal arteritis (TA), AKA cranial arteritis. A chronic granulomatous arteritis of unknown etiology involving primarily the cranial branches of the aortic arch (especially the external carotid artery (ECA)),[11] which if untreated, may lead to blindness. Takayasu's arteritis is similar to GCA, but tends to affect large arteries in young women; it has 2 phases: inflammatory (treated with corticosteroids) and stenotic (treated with arterial bypasses).

Epidemiology

Seen almost exclusively in Caucasians > 50 yrs age (mean age of onset is 70). Incidence: 17.8 per 100,000 people ≥ 50 years old[12] (range: 0.49–23). Prevalence: ≈ 223 (autopsy incidence may be much

Table 11.1 Vasculitides that may affect the CNS[10]

Vasculitis	Frequency of neuro involvement	Type of CNS involvement[a]				
		Acute encephalopathy	Seizure	Cranial nerve	Spinal cord	ICH or SAH
periarteritis nodosa[b] (PAN)[c]	20–40%	++	++	+	+	+
hypersensitivity vasculitis[b]	10%	+	+	0	0	+
giant cell (temporal) arteritis[b]	10%	+	0	++	0	0
Takayasu's arteritis	10–36%	+	++	++	+	+
Wegener's granulomatosis[b]	23–50%	+	++	++	+	+
lymphomatoid granulomatosis[b]	20–30%	++	+	++	+	0
isolated angiitis of the CNS[b]	100%	++	+	++	++	+
Behçet's disease[b]	10–29%	++	+	++	+	+

[a]KEY: 0 = uncommon or unreported; + = not uncommon; ++ = common; ICH = intracerebral hemorrhage; SAH = subarachnoid hemorrhage
[b]see section that follows for these topics
[c]PAN: a group of disorders, frequencies may vary by subgroup

higher).[13] More common in northern latitudes and among individuals of Scandinavian descent suggesting a genetic and environmental causes.[11] Female:male ratio is ≈ 2:1 (reported range: 1.05–7.4:1). 50% of GCA patients also have polymyalgia rheumatica (PMR) (p. 198).

Pathology

Discontinuous (so-called "skip lesions") inflammatory reaction of lymphocytes, plasma cells, macrophages, ± giant cells (if absent, intimal proliferation may be prominent); predominantly in media of involved arteries. Arteries preferentially involved include the ophthalmic and posterior ciliary branches and the entire distribution of the external carotid system (of which the STA is a terminal branch). Other arteries in the body may be involved (reported involvement of abdominal aorta, femoral, brachial and mesenteric arteries are rarely symptomatic). Unlike PAN, GCA generally spares the renal arteries.

Clinical

Various combinations of symptoms of giant cell arteritis are listed in ▶ Table 11.2. Onset is usually insidious, although occasionally it may be abrupt.[14]

Details of some findings:

1. H/A: the most common presenting symptom. May be nonspecific or located in one or both temporal areas, forehead, or occiput. May be superficial or burning with paroxysmal lancinating pain
2. symptoms relating to ECA blood supply (strongly suggestive of GCA, but not pathognomonic[16]): jaw claudication, tongue, or pharyngeal muscles
3. ophthalmologic symptoms: due to arteritis and occlusion of branches of ophthalmic artery or posterior ciliary arteries
   a) symptoms include: amaurosis fugax (precedes permanent visual loss in 44%), blindness, visual field cuts, diplopia, ptosis, ocular pain, corneal edema, chemosis
   b) blindness: incidence is ≈ 7%, and once it occurs, recovery of sight is unlikely
4. systemic symptoms
   a) nonspecific constitutional symptoms: fever (may present as FUO in 15% of cases), anorexia, weight loss, fatigue, malaise
   b) 30% have neurologic manifestations. 14% are neuropathies including mononeuropathies and peripheral polyneuropathies of the arms or legs[17]
   c) musculoskeletal symptoms
      - PMR (p. 198) is the most common (occurs in 40% of patients):
      - peripheral arthritis, swelling & pitting edema of hands & feet in 25%
      - arm claudication from stenosis of subclavian and axillary arteries
   d) thoracic aortic aneurysms: 17 times as likely in GCA. Annual CXRs are adequate for screening
5. temporal arteries on physical examination may exhibit tenderness, swelling, erythema, reduced pulsations, or nodularity. Normal in 33%
6. the presence of systemic symptoms correlates with a *lower* incidence of blindness or stroke

Differential diagnosis

1. periarteritis nodosa (PAN) (p. 199)
2. hypersensitivity vasculitis
3. atherosclerotic occlusive disease
4. malignancy: shares systemic also has symptoms of low grade fever, malaise and weight loss
5. infection
6. trigeminal neuralgia (p. 479)
7. ophthalmoplegic migraine
8. dental problems

Table 11.2 Signs and symptoms of GCA[15,11]

Frequent (>50% of cases)	Occasional (10–50% of cases)	Rare (<10% of cases)
H/A: 66% temporal artery tenderness	visual symptoms weight loss fever (low grade) proximal myalgias jaw claudication facial pain scalp tenderness	blindness extremity claudication tongue claudication ear pain synovitis stroke angina

Evaluation

Laboratory studies

1. ESR > 40 mm/hr (usually > 50) by Westergren method (if > 80 mm/hr with above clinical syndromes, highly suggestive of GCA). ESR is normal in up to 22.5%[18]
2. C-reactive protein: another acute phase reactant that is more sensitive than ESR. Has the advantage that it can be performed on frozen sera
3. CBC: may show mild normochromic anemia[19]
4. rheumatoid factor, ANA, and serum complement usually normal
5. LFTs abnormal in 30% (usually elevated alkaline phosphatase)
6. tests for rheumatoid factor and ANA are usually negative
7. temporal artery angiography not helpful (angiography elsewhere indicated if suspicion of large artery involvement exists)
8. CT: usually not helpful, one report described calcified areas corresponding to the temporal arteries[20]
9. temporal artery biopsy: see below

Temporal artery biopsy

Sensitivity and specificity are shown in ▶ Table 11.3.

Indications and timing

Current recommendations: temporal artery biopsy in all patients suspected of having GCA.[11] May be controversial. Arguments for: toxicity of a long course of steroids in an elderly patient, and a high rate of false initial responses of other illnesses to steroids. Arguments against: since a negative biopsy cannot exclude the diagnosis, cases with a negative biopsy but a strong clinical suspicion are often treated as though they have GCA.[22] In general, however, biopsy is considered prudent before embarking on a long course of high-dose steroid therapy.[16] Complications of biopsy are rare and include bleeding, infection, and only in the setting of active vasculitis has scalp necrosis been reported (not linked to biopsy).

In general, perform biopsy before starting steroids if biopsy can be done immediately.[11] Otherwise, start steroids to preserve vision and perform biopsy usually within 1 week (pathologic changes can be seen after more than 2 weeks of therapy,[23] therefore do not withhold steroids to await biopsy).

Technique of temporal artery biopsy

Biopsy side of involvement if laterality exists. The yield is increased by removing a portion of artery that is involved clinically (a tender or inflamed segment).[24] Mark the frontal branch of the STA with a skin marker (spare the main trunk and parietal branch if possible). Infiltrate local anesthetic. The incision is made parallel to the artery and if possible behind the hairline. The incision is taken down to the fascia of the temporalis muscle, to which the STA is superficial.[25] Optimal length of STA biopsy: 4–6 cm (if an abnormal segment of STA can be palpated, some say that a smaller biopsy to include this area may be sufficient, but this is probably unreliable as the muscle may be tender, etc.). Step-sectioning by pathologist through the entire length of the biopsy specimen also increases the yield.

Frozen sections can be performed. Biopsy of the contralateral side if the first side is negative in cases where clinical suspicion is high increases the yield only by 5–10%.

Treatment

No known cure. Steroids can produce symptomatic relief and usually prevent blindness (progression of ocular problems 24–48 hrs after institution of adequate steroids is rare). Totally blind patients or those with longstanding partial visual loss are unlikely to respond to any treatment.

1. for most cases:
   a) start with *prednisone* , 40–60 mg/d PO divided BID-QID (qod dosing is usually not effective in initial management)
   b) if no response after 72 hrs, and diagnosis certain, ↑ to 10–25 mg QID

Table 11.3 Temporal artery biopsy

sensitivity	≈ 90% (reported range[15,21] is 9–97%)
specificity	near 100%
predictive value	≈ 94%

11

c) once response occurs (usually within 3–7 days), give entire dose as q AM dose for 3–6 weeks until symptoms resolved and ESR normalizes (occurs in 87% of patients within ≈ 4 weeks) or stabilizes at < 40–50 mm/hr
d) once quiescent, a gradual taper is performed to prevent exacerbations: reduce by 10 mg/d q 2–4 weeks to 40 mg/d, then by 5 mg/d q 2–4 wks to 20 mg/d, then by 2.5 mg/d q 2–4 wks to 5–7.5 mg/d which is maintained for several months, followed by 1 mg/d decrements q 1–3 mos (usual length of treatment is 6–24 mos; do *not* D/C steroids when ESR normalizes)
e) if symptoms recur during treatment, prednisone dose is temporarily increased until symptoms resolve (isolated rise in ESR is not sufficient reason to increase steroids[11])
f) patients should be followed closely for ≈ 2 years
2. in severely ill patients: methylprednisolone, 15–20 mg IV QID
3. anticoagulant therapy: controversial
4. acute blindness (onset within 24–36 hrs) in a patient with giant cell arteritis:
a) consider up to 500 mg methylprednisolone IV over 30–60 mins (no controlled studies show reversal of blindness)
b) some have used intermittent inhalation of 5% carbon dioxide and oxygen

Outcome

Complications of steroid therapy occur in ≈ 50% of patients. Most are not life threatening, and include vertebral compression fractures in ≈ 36%, peptic ulcer disease in ≈ 12%, proximal myopathy, cataracts, exacerbation of diabetes; also see Possible deleterious side effects of steroids (p. 146).

30–50% of patients will have spontaneous exacerbations of GCA (especially during the first 2 years) regardless of the corticosteroid regimen.[11]

Survival parallels that of the general population. Onset of blindness after initiation of steroid therapy is rare.

11.3.3 Polymyalgia rheumatica (PMR)

11

General information

PMR and giant cell arteritis (GCA) (p. 195) may be different points on a continuum of the same disease. Both have in increased frequency of HLA-DR4 and systemic monocyte activation. 15% of patients with PMR eventually develop GCA.

Epidemiology

See reference.[11]

Both GCA & PMR occur in people ≥ 50 years old. The incidence increases with age and peaks between 70–80 years and is higher at higher latitudes.[11]

PMR is more common than GCA. Prevalence: 500/100,000).[26] Incidence: 52.5 per 100,000 people ≥ age 50, higher in females (61.7) than males (39.9).[27]

Features

See reference.[11]

- an inflammatory condition of unknown etiology
- clinical characteristics
  a) aching and morning stiffness in the cervical region and shoulder & pelvic girdles lasting > 1 month. The pain usually increases with movement
    ◦ shoulder pain: present in 70–95% of patients. Radiates toward elbow
    ◦ hip & neck pain: 50–70%. Hip pain radiates towards knees
  b) age ≥ 50 years
  c) ESR ≥ 40 mm/hr (7–20% have normal ESR[28])
  d) usually responds rapidly to low dose corticosteroids (≤ 20 mg prednisone/day) see below
  e) systemic symptoms (present in ≈ 33%): fever, malaise or fatigue, anorexia and weight loss
- favorable prognosis: usually remits in 1–3 years

Treatment

PMR responds to either to low doses of steroids[26] (10–20 mg prednisone/day) or sometimes to NSAIDs (response to steroids is much more rapid). The initial dose of steroids is maintained for 2–4 weeks, and then by ≤ 10% of the daily dose every 1–2 weeks[11] while observing for signs of GCA.

11.3.4 Other vasculitides

Periarteritis nodosa

AKA polyarteritis nodosa. Actually a group of necrotizing vasculitides, including:

- classic periarteritis nodosa (PAN): a multisystem disease with inflammatory necrosis, thrombosis (occlusion), and hemorrhage of arteries and arterioles in every organ except lung & spleen. Nodules may be palpated along medium sized muscular arteries. Commonly produces mononeuritis multiplex, weight loss, fever, and tachycardia. Peripheral nerve manifestations are attributed to arteritic occlusion of vasa nervorum. CNS manifestations are uncommon and include H/A, seizures, SAH, retinal hemorrhages, and stroke in ≈ 13%
- allergic angiitis and granulomatosis (Churg-Strauss syndrome)
- systemic necrotizing vasculitis

These patients do better when treated with cyclophosphamide rather than steroids.

Wegener's granulomatosis

General information

A systemic necrotizing granulomatous vasculitis involving the respiratory tract (lung → cough/hemoptysis, and/or nasal airways → serosanguinous nasal drainage ± septal perforation→ characteristic "saddle nose deformity") and frequently the kidneys (no reported cases of kidney involvement without respiratory).[29]

Nasal obstruction and crusting are the usual initial findings. Arthralgia (not true arthritis) is present in > 50%.

Neurologic involvement usually consists of cranial nerve dysfunction (usually II, III, IV, & VI; less often V, VII, & VIII; and least commonly IX, X, XI, & XII) and peripheral neuropathies, with diabetes insipidus (occasionally preceding other symptoms by up to 9 months). Focal lesions of the brain and spinal cord occur less frequently.

Differential diagnosis

Differential diagnosis includes:

- "lethal midline granuloma" (may be similar or identical to polymorphic reticulosis) may evolve into lymphoma. May cause fulminant local destruction of the nasal tissue. Differentiation is crucial as this condition is treated by radiation; one should avoid immune suppression (e.g. cyclophosphamide). Probably does not involve true granulomas. Renal and tracheal involvement do not occur
- fungal disease: Sporothrix schenckii & Coccidioides may cause identical syndrome
- other vasculitides: especially Churg-Strauss syndrome (asthma and peripheral eosinophilia usually seen), and PAN (granulomas usually lacking)

Evaluation

Biopsy of upper airways consists of removing all crusts, and obtaining as much friable mucosa as possible. This tissue should be fixed in formaldehyde and examined pathologically within 24 hrs (do not freeze). A sample should also be cultured (including fungal and acid-fast cultures). Renal biopsy should not be done when more specific tissue is available from the upper airway.

Treatment

Untreated, Wegener's granulomatosis is rapidly fatal, with a median survival of 5 months, and more than 90% of patients are dead within 2 years of diagnosis.[30] For fulminating disease: prednisone 60–80 mg/d until disease is controlled (documented by decreasing ESR and improvement of serum creatinine).

When disease is stable: cyclophosphamide (Cytoxan®) ≈ 2 mg/kg daily (takes 2–3 weeks to have an effect). Continue 1 year beyond last evidence of active disease. Low-dose weekly methotrexate may be an acceptable alternative to cyclophosphamide in selected patients.[30]

11.3.5 Lymphomatoid granulomatosis

Rare; affects mainly the lungs, skin (erythematous macules or indurated plaques in 40%) and nervous system (CNS in 20%, peripheral neuropathies in 15%). Sinuses, lymph nodes, and spleen are usually spared.

11.3.6 Behçet's syndrome

Relapsing ocular lesions and recurrent oral and genital ulcers, with occasional skin lesions, thrombophlebitis, and arthritis.[10] H/A occur in > 50%. Neurologic involvement includes pseudotumor, cerebellar ataxia, paraplegia, seizures, and dural sinus thrombosis. Only 5% have neurologic symptoms as the presenting complaint.

86% have CSF pleocytosis and protein elevation. Cerebral angiography is usually normal. CT may show focal areas of enhancing low density.

Steroids usually ameliorate ocular and cerebral symptoms, but usually have no effect on skin and genital lesions. Uncontrolled trials of cytotoxic agents → some benefit. Thalidomide may be effective (uncontrolled studies), but carries risk of serious adverse effects (teratogenicity, peripheral neuropathy…).[31]

Although painful, the disease is usually benign. Neurologic involvement portends a worse prognosis.

11.3.7 Isolated CNS vasculitis

General information

AKA isolated angiitis of the CNS. Rare (≈ 20 cases reported[32] as of 1983); limited to vessels of CNS. Small vessel vasculitis is ≈ always present → segmental inflammation and necrosis of small leptomeningeal and parenchymal blood vessels with surrounding tissue ischemia or hemorrhage.[10]

Presentation

Combinations of H/A, confusion, dementia, and lethargy. Occasionally seizures. Focal and multifocal brain disturbance occurs in > 80%. Visual symptoms are frequent (secondary either to involvement of choroidal and retinal arteries, or to involvement of visual cortex → visual hallucinations).

Evaluation

11

ESR & WBC count are usually normal. CSF may be normal or have pleocytosis and/or elevated protein. CT may show enhancing areas of low density.

Angiography (required for diagnosis): characteristically shows multiple areas of symmetrical narrowing ("string of pearls" configuration). If normal, it does not exclude diagnosis.

Histological diagnosis (recommended): all biopsy material should be cultured. Brain parenchyma biopsy infrequently shows vasculitis. Leptomeningeal biopsy invariably shows involvement.

Treatment and outcome

Reportedly fatal if untreated, but may smolder for years.

Rarity of this condition makes treatment uncertain. Recommended: cyclophosphamide (Cytoxan®) 2 mg/kg/d and prednisone 1 mg/kg/d qod therapy.

NB: this condition is thought to be T-cell mediated, but prednisone causes more B-cell suppression, therefore breakthrough during prednisone therapy is not uncommon.

11.3.8 Hypersensitivity vasculitis

Neurologic involvement is not a prominent feature of this group of vasculitides, which include:

- drug induced allergic vasculitis: A number of drugs are associated with the development of cerebral vasculitis. These include methamphetamines ("speed"), cocaine (frank vasculitis occurs[33] but is rare), heroin and ephedrine
- cutaneous vasculitis
- serum sickness: may → encephalopathy, seizures, coma, peripheral neuropathy and brachial plexopathy
- Henoch-Schönlein purpura

11.3.9 Fibromuscular dysplasia

General information

A vasculopathy (angiopathy) affecting primarily branches of the aorta, with renal artery involvement in 85% of cases (the most common site) and commonly associated with hypertension. The disease has an incidence of ≈ 1%, and results in multifocal arterial constrictions and intervening regions of aneurysmal dilatation.

The second most commonly involved site is the cervical internal carotid (primarily near C1–2), with fibromuscular dysplasia (FMD) appearing on 1% of carotid angiograms, making FMD the second most common cause of extracranial carotid stenosis.[34] Bilateral cervical ICA involvement occurs in ≈ 80% of cases. 50% of patients with carotid FMD have renal FMD. Patients with FMD have an increased risk of intracranial aneurysms and neoplasms, and are probably at higher risk of carotid dissection.

Aneurysms and fibromuscular dysplasia: The reported incidence of aneurysms with FMD[35] ranges from 20–50%.

Etiology

The actual etiology remains unknown, although congenital defects of the media (muscular layer) and internal elastic layer of the arteries has been identified which may predispose the arteries to injury from otherwise well-tolerated trauma. A high familial rate of strokes, HTN, and migraine have supported the suggestion that FMD is an autosomal dominant trait with reduced penetrance in males.[36]

Presentation

Most patients have recurrent, multiple symptoms shown in ▶ Table 11.4.

Up to 50% of patients present with episodes of transient cerebral ischemia or infarction. However, FMD may also be an incidental finding and some cases have been followed for 5 years without recurrence of ischemic symptoms suggesting that FMD may be a relatively benign condition.

Headaches are commonly unilateral and may be mistaken for typical migraine. Syncope may be caused by involvement of the carotid sinus.

Horner's syndrome occurs in ≈ 8% of cases. T-wave changes on EKG may be seen in up to one-third of cases, and may be due to involvement of the coronary arteries.

Diagnosis

The "gold-standard" for the diagnosis of FMD is the angiogram. The three angiographic types of FMD[37] are shown in ▶ Table 11.5.

Treatment

Medical therapy including antiplatelet medication (e.g. aspirin) has been recommended.

Direct surgical treatment is problem ridden due to the difficult location (high carotid artery, near the base of the skull), and the friable nature of the vessels making anastamosis or arteriotomy closure difficult.

Transluminal angioplasty has achieved some degree of success. Carotid cavernous fistulas and arterial rupture have been reported as complications.

Table 11.4 Previous symptoms in 37 cases of aortocranial FMD[36]

Symptom	%
H/A	78%
mental distress	48%
tinnitus	38%
vertigo	34%
cardiac arrhythmia	31%
TIA	31%
syncope	31%
carotidynia	21%
epilepsy	15%
hearing impairment	12%
abdominal angina	8%
angina/MI	8%

Table 11.5 Angiographic classification of FMD

Type	Findings
1	most common (80–100% of reported cases). Multiple, irregularly spaced, concentric narrowings with normal or dilated intervening segments giving rise to the so-called "string of pearls" appearance. Corresponds with arterial medial fibroplasia
2	focal tubular stenosis, seen in ≈ 7% of cases. Less characteristic for FMD than Type 1, and may also be seen in Takayasu's arteritis and other conditions
3	"atypical FMD." Rare. May take on various appearances, most commonly consisting of diverticular outpouchings of one wall of the artery

11.3.10 Miscellaneous vasculopathies

CADASIL

Key concepts

- clinical: migraines, dementia, TIAs, psychiatric disturbances
- MRI: white matter abnormalities
- autosomal dominant inheritance
- anticoagulants controversial, generally discouraged

An acronym for Cerebral Autosomal Dominant Arteriopathy with Subcortical Infarcts and Leukoencephalopathy.[38] A familial disease with onset in early adulthood (mean age at onset: 45 ± 11 yrs), mapped to chromosome 19. Clinical and neuroradiologic features are similar to those seen with multiple subcortical infarcts from HTN, except there is no evidence of HTN. The vasculopathy is distinct from that seen in lipohyalinosis, arteriosclerosis and amyloid angiopathy, and causes thickening of the media (by eosinophilic, granular material) of leptomeningeal and perforating arteries measuring 100–400 mcm in diameter.

Clinical involvement

Recurrent subcortical infarcts (84%), progressive or stepwise dementia (31%), migraine with aura (22%), and depression (20%). All symptomatic and 18% of asymptomatic patients had prominent subcortical white-matter and basal ganglia hyperintensities on T2WI MRI.

Treatment

Warfarin (Coumadin®) is used by some.

11.3.11 Paraneoplastic syndromes affecting the nervous system

General information

Paraneoplastic syndromes (PNS), AKA "remote effects of cancer." Develop acutely or subacutely. May mimic or be mimicked by metastatic disease. The neurologic disability is usually severe, and may precede other manifestations of the cancer by 6–12 mos. Often one particular neural cell type is predominantly affected. The presence of a PNS may portend a more benign course of the cancer.

16% of patients with lung Ca, and 4% with breast Ca will develop a PNS.

Pathogenesis unknown. Theories: ? toxin; ? competition for essential substrate; ? opportunistic infection; ? auto-immune process.

Types of syndromes

1. affecting cerebrum or cerebellum
   a) encephalitis
      - diffuse
      - limbic and brainstem: usually due to small-cell lung Ca or testicular Ca[39] as a result of serum antineuronal antibodies

   b) “limbic encephalitis” (mesial): dementia (decreased memory, psychiatric symptoms, hallucinations)
   c) pan-cerebellar degeneration (PCD) AKA subacute cerebellar degeneration*: (see below)
   d) opsoclonus-myoclonus syndrome*: in peds, usually indicates neuroblastoma
2. affecting spinal cord
   a) poliomyelitis (anterior horn syndrome): mimics ALS (weakness, hyporeflexia, fasciculations)
   b) subacute necrotizing (transverse) myelitis: rapid necrosis of spinal cord
   c) ganglionitis* (dorsal root ganglion): chronic or subacute. Pure sensory neuronopathy (not neuropathy)
3. affecting peripheral nervous system
   a) chronic sensory-motor: typical neuropathy (as in DM or EtOH abuse)
   b) pure sensory (p. 1268) [40]
   c) pure motor: rare. Almost always due to lymphoma (mostly Hodgkin's)
   d) acute inflammatory demyelinating polyradiculopathy, AKA Guillain-Barré (p. 184)
   e) Eaton-Lambert (EL) myasthenic syndrome*: rare. 66% of patients with this syndrome will have cancer, most common primary is oat cell Ca of lung. Pre-synaptic neuromuscular junction (PSNMJ) blockade due to antibodies against the PSNMJ; NB: true myasthenia gravis (MG) is a post-synaptic block. Worse in AM, improves during day with recruitment (opposite of MG, which is worse at night or with exercise due to depletion). Mostly motor, but often accompanied by paresthesias. MG is affects mostly nicotinic receptors, but EL also affects muscarinic receptors, and therefore autonomic symptoms may occur: dry mouth, males may have impotence. Repetitive nerve stimulation on EMG: for MG use 2–5 Hz stimulation, for EL use > 10 Hz, MG: decremental response with low frequency, with EL there is incremental response (more response with repeat stimulation).
   f) myasthenia gravis
   g) polymyositis: in age > 60 yrs, 25% of patients with this have a malignancy*, most often linked to bronchogenic Ca
   h) type IIb muscle fiber atrophy: the most common paraneoplastic syndrome; mainly proximal muscle weakness (same as in other endocrine myopathies, e.g. hypothyroid, steroid)

* “classic” neurologic PNS. In a patient without previous cancer history presenting with one of these syndromes with an asterisk, work-up for occult malignancy has high yield.

Pan-cerebellar degeneration

Severe Purkinje cell loss (due to anti-Purkinje cell antibody) → severe pan-cerebellar dysfunction. Presents with vertigo, gait and upper and lower extremity ataxia, dysarthria, N/V, diplopia, oscillopsia, nystagmus, oculomotor dysmetria. Usually not treatable nor remitting even with immune suppression. 20% of patients improve with treatment of the primary cancer. CT is WNL early, late → cerebellar atrophy. In 70% of cases, cerebellar findings precede diagnosis of cancer.

The most common primary malignancies in pan-cerebellar degeneration are shown in ▶ Table 11.6.

Evaluation

- LP: CSF for cell count, cytology and IgG. Typically WBCs and IgG are elevated
- Evaluation for primary
  - CT of chest/abdomen/pelvis
  - lymph node exam
  - pelvic exam and mammogram in women

Table 11.6 Common primaries with pan-cerebellar degeneration

Women	Men
ovarian Ca breast uterus Hodgkin's lymphoma	lung Ca Hodgkin's lymphoma

11

11.4 Neurotoxicology

11.4.1 Ethanol

General information

The acute and chronic effects of ethyl alcohol (ethanol, EtOH) abuse on the nervous system (not to mention the effects of EtOH on other organ systems) are protean,[41] and are beyond the scope of this text). Neuromuscular effects include:

1. acute intoxication: see below
2. effects of chronic alcohol abuse
   a) **Wernicke's encephalopathy** (p.206)
   b) cerebellar degeneration: due to degeneration of Purkinje cells in the cerebellar cortex, predominantly in the anterior superior vermis
   c) central pontine myelinolysis (p.115)
   d) stroke: increased risk of
      - intracerebral hemorrhage (p.1330)
      - ischemic stroke[42]
      - possibly aneurysmal SAH
   e) peripheral neuropathy (p.541)
   f) skeletal myopathy
3. effects of alcohol withdrawal: usually seen in habituated drinkers with cessation or reduction of ethanol intake
   a) alcohol withdrawal syndromes: see below
   b) seizures: up to 33% of patients have a generalized tonic-clonic seizure 7–30 hrs after cessation of drinking – Alcohol withdrawal seizures (p.464)
   c) delirium tremens (**DTs**): see below

Acute intoxication

11

The primary effect of EtOH on the CNS is depression of neuronal excitability, impulse conduction, and neurotransmitter release due to direct effects on the cell membranes. ▶ Table 11.7 shows the clinical effects associated with specific EtOH concentrations. Mellanby effect: the severity of intoxication is greater at any given level when blood alcohol levels are rising than when falling.

In most jurisdictions, individuals with blood ethanol levels ≥ 21.7 mmol/l (100 mg/dl) are defined as legally intoxicated, and a number of states have changed this to 80 mg/dl. However, even levels of 10.2 mmol/l (47 mg/dl) are associated with increased risk of involvement in motor vehicle accidents. Chronic alcoholism leads to increased tolerance; in habituated individuals survival with levels exceeding 1000 mg/dl has been reported.

Alcohol withdrawal syndrome

General information

Compensation for the CNS depressant effects of EtOH occurs in chronic alcoholism. Consequently, rebound CNS hyperactivity may result from falling EtOH levels. Clinical signs of EtOH withdrawal are classified as major or minor (the degree of autonomic hyperactivity and the presence/absence of DTs differentiates these), as well as early (24–48 hrs) or late (> 48 hrs).

Signs/symptoms include: tremulousness, hyperreflexia, insomnia, N/V, autonomic hyperactivity (tachycardia, systolic HTN), agitation, myalgias, mild confusion. If EtOH withdrawal seizures (p.464) occur, they tend to be early. Perceptual disturbances or frank hallucinosis may also occur early.

Table 11.7 Blood ethanol concentrations

[blood EtOH]		Clinical effect
mmol/liter	mg/dl	
5.4	25	mild intoxication: altered mood, impaired cognition, incoordination
> 21.7	100	vestibular and cerebellar dysfunction: increased nystagmus, diplopia, dysarthria, ataxia
> 108.5	500	usually fatal from respiratory depression

Hallucinosis consists of visual and/or auditory hallucinations with an otherwise clear sensorium (which distinguishes this from the hallucinations of DTs). DTs can occur 3–4 days after cessation of drinking (see below).

Suppressed by benzodiazepines, resumption of drinking, β-adrenergic antagonists, or α2-agonists.

Prevention of and treatment for alcohol withdrawal syndrome

See reference.[43]

Mild EtOH withdrawal is managed with a quiet, supportive environment, reorientation and one-to-one contact. If symptoms progress, institute pharmacologic treatment.

Benzodiazepines

Benzodiazepines (BDZs) are the mainstay of treatment. They reduce autonomic hyperactivity, and may prevent seizures and/or DTs. All BDZs are effective. Initial doses are shown in ▶ Table 11.8 and are higher than those used for treating anxiety. Symptom triggered dosing with repeated evaluation utilizing a standardized protocol (e.g. CIWA-Ar[44]) may be more efficacious than fixed-dose schedules.[45] Avoid IM administration (erratic absorption).

Adjunctive medications

Associated conditions commonly seen in patients experiencing alcohol withdrawal syndrome include dehydration, fluid and electrolyte disturbances, infection, pancreatitis, and alcoholic ketoacidosis, and should be treated accordingly.

Other medications used for EtOH withdrawal itself include:

1. drugs useful for controlling HTN (caution: these agents should not be used alone because they do not prevent progression to more severe levels of withdrawal, and they may mask symptoms of withdrawal)
   a) β-blockers: also treat most associated *tachyarrhythmias*
      - *atenolol* (Tenormin®): reduces length of withdrawal and BDZ requirement
      - ✖ avoid propranolol (psychotoxic reactions)
   b) α-agonists: do not use together with β-blockers
2. phenobarbital: an alternative to BDZs. Long acting, and helps prophylax against seizures
3. baclofen: a small study[47] found 10 mg PO q d X 30 days resulted in rapid reduction of symptoms after the initial dose and continued abstinence
4. "supportive" medications
   a) *thiamine* : 100 mg IM q d × 3 d (can be given IV if needed, but there is risk of adverse reaction). Rationale: high-concentration glucose may precipitate acute Wernicke's encephalopathy in patients with thiamine deficiency
   b) folate 1 mg IM, IV or PO q d × 3 d
   c) MgSO4 1 gm × 1 on admission: helpful only if magnesium levels are low, reduces seizure risk. Be sure renal function is normal before administering
   d) vitamin B12 for macrocytic anemia: 100 mcg IM (do not give before folate)
   e) multivitamins: of benefit only if patient is malnourished

11

Table 11.8 Guidelines for BDZ doses for EtOH withdrawal[a]

Drug	Dose	
	Oral	IV
chlordiazepoxide (Librium®)	100 mg initially, then 25–50 mg PO TID-QID, gradually taper over ≈ 4 days). Additional doses may be needed for continuing agitation, up to 50 mg PO hourly[46]	–
lorazepam (Ativan®)	4 mg initially, then 1–2 mg PO q 4 hrs	1–2 mg q 1–2 hrs
diazepam (Valium®)	20 mg PO initially, then 10 mg PO BID-QID	5–10 mg initially
midazolam (Versed®)		titrate drip to desired effect

[a]modify as appropriate based on patient response

5. seizures: see indications for treatment (p.464)
   a) **phenytoin** (Dilantin®) (p.446): load with 18 mg/kg = 1200 mg/70 kg
   b) continued seizures may sometimes be effectively treated with *paraldehyde* if available
6. ethanol drip: not widely used. 5% EtOH in D5 W, start at 20 cc/hr, and titrate to a blood level of 100–150 mg/dl

Delirium tremens (DTs)

When DTs occur, they usually begin within 4 days of the onset of EtOH withdrawal, and typically persist for 1–3 days.

Signs and symptoms include: profound disorientation, agitation, tremor, insomnia, hallucinations, severe autonomic instability (tachycardia, HTN, diaphoresis, hyperthermia).[48] Mortality is 5–10% (higher in elderly), but can be reduced with treatment (including treating associated medical problems and treatment for seizures).

Haloperidol and phenothiazines may control hallucinations, but can lower the seizure threshold. HTN and tachyarrhythmias should be treated as outline above under alcohol withdrawal syndrome.

Wernicke's encephalopathy (WE)

General information

AKA Wernicke-Korsakoff encephalopathy (not to be confused with Korsakoff's syndrome or Korsakoff's psychosis). Classic triad: encephalopathy (consisting of global confusion), ophthalmoplegia, and ataxia (NB: all 3 are present in only 10–33% of cases).

Due to thiamine deficiency. Body stores of thiamine are adequate only for up to ≈ 18 days. May be seen in:

1. a certain susceptible subset of thiamine deficient alcoholics. Thiamine deficiency here is due to a combination of inadequate intake, reduced absorption, decreased hepatic storage, and impaired utilization
2. hyperemesis (as in some pregnancies)
3. starvation: including anorexia nervosa, rapid weight loss
4. gastroplication (bariatric surgery)
5. hemodialysis
6. cancers
7. AIDS
8. prolonged IV hyperalimentation

Clinical

Oculomotor abnormalities occur in 96% and include: nystagmus (horizontal > vertical), lateral rectus palsy, conjugate-gaze palsies.

Gait ataxia is seen in 87%, and results from a combination of polyneuropathy, cerebellar dysfunction, and vestibular impairment.

Systemic symptoms may include: vomiting, fever.

Diagnostic testing

MRI: May show high signal in T2WI and FLAIR images in the paraventricular (medial) thalamus, the floor of the 4th ventricle, and periaqueductal gray of the midbrain. These changes may resolve with treatment.[49] Atrophy of the mammillary bodies may also be seen. Normal MRI does not R/O the diagnosis.

Treatment

Wernicke's encephalopathy (WE) is a medical emergency. When WE is suspected, 100 mg thiamine should be given IM or IV (oral route is unreliable, see above) daily for 5 days. ✖ IV glucose can precipitate acute WE in thiamine deficient patients, ∴ give thiamine before glucose.

Thiamine administration improves eye findings within hours to days; ataxia and confusion improve in days to weeks. Many patients that survive are left with horizontal nystagmus, ataxia, and 80% have Korsakoff's syndrome (AKA Korsakoff's psychosis), a disabling memory disturbance involving retrograde and anterograde amnesia.

11.4.2 Opioids

Includes heroin (which is usually injected IV, but the powder can be snorted or smoked) as well as prescription drugs. Opioids produce small pupils (miosis).

Overdose may produce:
1. respiratory depression
2. pulmonary edema
3. coma
4. hypotension and bradycardia
5. seizures
6. fatal overdose may occur with any agent, but is more likely with synthetic opioids such as fentanyl (Sublimaze®) among users unfamiliar with their high potency

Reversal of intoxication[50]

A test dose of naloxone (Narcan®) 0.2 mg IV avoids sudden complete reversal of all opioid effects. If no significant reaction occurs, an additional 1.8 mg (for a total dose of 2 mg) will reverse the toxicity of most opioids. If needed, the dose may be repeated q 2–3 minutes up to a total of 10 mg, although even larger doses may be needed with pentazocine or buprenorphine (Buprenex®). Naloxone may precipitate narcotic withdrawal symptoms in opioid dependent patients, with anxiety or agitation, piloerection, yawning, sneezing, rhinorrhea, nausea, vomiting, diarrhea, abdominal cramps, muscle spasms... which are uncomfortable but not life threatening. Clonidine (Catapres®) may be helpful for some narcotic withdrawal symptoms.

With longer acting opioids, especially methadone (Dolophine®), repeat doses of naloxone may be obviated by the use of nalmefene (Revex®), a long-acting narcotic antagonist which is not appropriate for the initial treatment of opioid overdosage.

11.4.3 Cocaine

Cocaine is extracted from Erythroxylon coca leaves (and other Erythroxylon species) and is thus unrelated to opioids. It blocks the re-uptake of nor-epinephrine by presynaptic adrenergic nerve terminals. It is available in 2 forms: cocaine hydrochloride (heat labile and water soluble, it is usually taken PO, IV or by nasal insufflation) and as the highly purified cocaine alkaloid (free base or crack cocaine, which is heat stable but insoluble in water and is usually smoked).

Peak toxicity occurs 60–90 minutes after ingestion (except for "body packers"), 30–60 minutes after snorting, and minutes after IV injection or smoking (freebase or crack).[50]

11

Acute pharmacologic effects of cocaine

Effects on body systems outside the nervous system include: tachycardia, acute myocardial infarction, arrhythmias, rupture of ascending aorta (aortic dissection), abruptio placenta, hyperthermia, intestinal ischemia, and sudden death.

Acute pharmacologic effects pertinent to the nervous system include:
1. mental status: initial CNS stimulation that first manifests as a sense of well-being and euphoria. Sometimes dysphoric agitation results, occasionally with delirium. Stimulation is followed by depression. Paranoia and toxic psychosis may occur with overdosage or chronic use. Addiction may occur
2. pupillary dilatation (mydriasis)
3. hypertension: from adrenergic stimulation

Non-pharmacologic effects related to the nervous system
1. pituitary degeneration: from chronic intranasal use
2. cerebral vasculitis: less common than with amphetamines
3. seizures: possibly related to the local anesthetic properties of cocaine
4. stroke[51]
   a) intracerebral hemorrhage: see Intracerebral hemorrhage, Etiologies (p. 1332)
   b) subarachnoid hemorrhage[52,53]: possibly as a result of HTN in the presence of aneurysms or AVMs, however, sometimes no lesion is demonstrated on angiography.[54] May possibly be due to cerebral vasculitis
   c) ischemic stroke[55]: may result from vasoconstriction
   d) thrombotic stroke[50]
   e) TIA[56]
5. anterior spinal artery syndrome[56]
6. effects of maternal cocaine use on the fetal nervous system include[57]: microcephaly, disorders of neuronal migration, neuronal differentiation and myelination, cerebral infarction, subarachnoid and intracerebral hemorrhage, and sudden infant death syndrome (SIDS) in the postnatal period

Treatment of toxicity

Most cocaine toxicity is too short-lived to be treated. Anxiety, agitation or seizures may be treated with IV benzodiazepines, e.g. lorazepam (p.471). Refractory HTN may be treated with nicardipine (p.126) or phentolamine (Regitine®) (p.655). IV lidocaine used to treat cardiac arrhythmias may cause seizures.[50]

11.4.4 Amphetamines

Toxicity is similar to that of cocaine (see above), but longer in duration (may last up to several hours). Cerebral vasculitis may occur with prolonged abuse which may lead to cerebral infarction.

Elimination of amphetamines requires adequate urine output. Antipsychotic drugs such as haloperidol (Haldol®) should not be used because of risk of seizures.

11.4.5 Carbon monoxide

General information

Carbon monoxide (CO) is the largest source of death from poisoning in the U.S.A.

Normal cellular function requires ≈ 5 ml O_2/100 ml blood. Blood normally contains ≈ 20 ml O_2/100 ml.

CO binds to hemoglobin (Hb) with an affinity ≈ 250 times that of O_2, and it causes a left shift of the Hb/O_2 dissociation curve. It also binds to intracellular myoglobin.

Only ≈ 6% of patients show the classic "cherry-red" color of blood.

Clinical findings

Clinical findings related to CO-Hb levels are shown in ▶ Table 11.9.

Diagnostic studies

11

EKG changes are common, usually non-specific ST-T wave changes.

In cases of severe intoxication, CT may show symmetrical low attenuation in the globus pallidus; see differential diagnosis (p.1386).

Outcome

Prognosticators
1. outcome is more closely correlated with hypotension than with actual CO-Hb level
2. coma
3. metabolic acidosis
4. EEG
5. CT/MRI changes: in one study, the presence of MRI lesions after 1 month did not accurately predict subsequent outcome
6. CO-Hb level
7. other factors probably have an effect, including: age, severity of exposure

Approximately 40% of patients exposed to significant levels of CO die. 30–40% have transient symptoms but make a full recovery. 10–30% have persistent neurological sequelae including CO-encephalopathy (may be delayed in onset) – impaired memory, irritability, parietal lobe symptoms including various agnosias.

Brain lesions:
1. white matter lesions:
   a) multifocal small necrotic lesions in deep hemispheres
   b) extensive necrotic zones along lateral ventricles
   c) Grinker's myelinopathy (not necrosis)
2. grey matter lesions:
   a) bilateral necrosis of globus pallidus
   b) lesions of hippocampal formation and focal cortical necrosis

Table 11.9 Levels of CO-Hb

CO-Hb level (%)	Signs/symptoms[a]
0–10	none
10–20	mild H/A, mild DOE
20–30	throbbing H/A
30–40	severe H/A, dizziness, dimming of vision, impaired judgement
40–50	confusion, tachypnea, tachycardia, possible syncope
50–60	syncope, seizures, coma
60–70	coma, hypotension, respiratory failure, death
>70	rapidly fatal

[a]NB: smokers may have CO-Hb levels of 15% without signs or symptoms

References

[1] Bartynski WS. Posterior reversible encephalopathy syndrome, part 1: fundamental imaging and clinical features. AJNR Am J Neuroradiol. 2008; 29:1036–1042

[2] Port JD, Beauchamp NJ. Reversible Intracerebral Pathologic Entities Mediated by Vascular Autoregulatory Dysfunction. Radiographics. 1998; 18:353–367

[3] Lin KL, Hsu WC, Wang HS, Lui TN. Hypertension-induced cerebellar encephalopathy and hydrocephalus in a male. Pediatr Neurol. 2006; 34:72–75

[4] Schaefer PW, Buonanno FS, Gonzalez RG, Schwamm LH. Diffusion-Weighted Imaging Discriminates Between Cytotoxic and Vasogenic Edema in a Patient with Eclampsia. Stroke. 1997; 28:1082–1085

[5] Covarrubias DJ, Luetmer PH, Campeau NG. Posterior reversible encephalopathy syndrome: prognostic utility of quantitative diffusion-weighted MR images. AJNR Am J Neuroradiol. 2002; 23:1038–1048

[6] Beeson JH, Duda EE. Computed Axial Tomography Scan Demonstration of Cerebral Edema in Eclampsia Preceded by Blindness. Obstet Gynecol. 1982; 60:529–532

[7] Raps EC, Galetta SL, Broderick M, Atlas SW. Delayed Peripartum Vasculopathy: Cerebral Eclampsia Revisited. Ann Neurol. 1993; 33:222–225

[8] Dekker GA, Sibai BM. Etiology and pathogenesis of preeclampsia: current concepts. Am J Obstet Gynecol. 1998; 179:1359–1375

[9] Bartynski WS, Boardman JF, Zeigler ZR, Shadduck RK, Lister J. Posterior reversible encephalopathy syndrome in infection, sepsis, and shock. AJNR Am J Neuroradiol. 2006; 27:2179–2190

[10] Moore PM, Cupps TR. Neurologic Complications of Vasculitis. Ann Neurol. 1983; 14:155–167

[11] Salvarani C, Cantini F, Boiardi L, Hunder GG. Polymyalgia rheumatica and giant-cell arteritis. N Engl J Med. 2002; 347:261–271

[12] Salvarani C, Gabriel SE, O'Fallon WM, Hunder GG. The incidence of giant cell arteritis in Olmstead County, Minnesota: apparent fluctuations in a cyclic pattern. Ann Intern Med. 1995; 123:192–194

[13] Machado EB, Michet CJ, Ballard DJ, et al. Trends in Incidence and Clinical Presentation of Temporal Arteritis in Olmstead County, Minnesota, 1950-1985. Arthritis Rheum. 1988; 31:745–749

[14] Hunder GG. Giant Cell (Temporal) Arteritis. Rheum Dis Clin N Amer. 1990; 16:399–409

[15] Allen NB, Studenski SA. Polymyalgia Rheumatica and Temporal Arteritis. Med Clin N Amer. 1986; 70:369–384

[16] Hall S, Hunder GG. Is Temporal Artery Biopsy Prudent? Mayo Clin Proc. 1984; 59:793–796

[17] Caselli RJ, Danube JR, Hunder GG, Whisnant JP. Peripheral neuropathic syndromes in giant cell (temporal) arteritis. Neurology. 1988; 38:685–689

[18] Salvarani C, Hunder GG. Giant cell arteritis with low erythrocyte sedimentation rate: frequency of occurrence in a population-based study. Arthritis Rheum. 2001; 45:140–145

[19] Baumel B, Elsner LS. Diagnosis and Treatment of Headache in the Elderly. Med Clin N Amer. 1991; 75:661–675

[20] Karacostas D, Taskos N, Nikolaides T. CT Findings in Temporal Arteritis: A Report of Two Cases. Neurorad. 1986; 28

[21] McDonnell PJ, Moore GW, Miller NR, et al. Temporal Arteritis: A Clinicopathologic Study. Ophthalmology. 1986; 93:518–530

[22] Hall S, Lie JT, Kurland LT, et al. The Therapeutic Impact of Temporal Artery Biopsy. Lancet. 1983; 2:1217–1220

[23] Achkar AA, Lie JT, Hunder GG, O'Fallon WM, Gabriel SE. How does previous corticosteroid treatment affect the biopsy findings in giant cell (temporal) arteritis? Ann Intern Med. 1994; 120:987–992

[24] Hunder GG, Kelley WN, Harris ED, Ruddy S, Sledge CB. In: Giant Cell Arteritis and Polymyalgia Rheumatica. Textbook of Rheumatology. 4th ed. Philadelphia: W. B. Saunders; 1993:1103–1112

[25] Kent RB, Thomas L. Temporal Artery Biopsy. Am Surg. 1989; 56:16–21

[26] Chuang TY, Hunder GG, Ilstrup DM, et al. Polymyalgia Rheumatica: A 10-Year Epidemiologic and Clinical Study. Ann Intern Med. 1982; 97:672–680

[27] Salvarani C, Gabriel SE, O'Fallon WM, Hunder GG. Epidemiology of polymyalgia rheumatica in Olmstead County, Minnesota, 1970-1991. Arthritis Rheum. 1995; 38:369–373

[28] Cantini F, Salvarani C, Olivieri I, et al. Erythrocyte sedimentation rate and C-reactive protein in the evaluation of disease activity and severity in

polymyalgia rheumatica: a prospective follow-up study. Semin Arthritis Rheum. 2000; 30:17–24
[29] McDonald TJ, DeRemee RA. Wegener's Granulomatosis. Laryngoscope. 1983; 93:220–231
[30] Sneller MC. Wegener's Granulomatosis. JAMA. 1995; 273:1288–1291
[31] New Uses of Thalidomide. Med Letter. 1996; 38:15–16
[32] Cupps TR, Moore PM, Fauci AS. Isolated Angitis of the Central Nervous System: Prospective Diagnostic and Therapeutic Experience. Am J Med. 1983; 74:97–105
[33] Kaye BR, Fainstat M. Cerebral Vasculitis Associated with Cocaine Abuse. JAMA. 1987; 258:2104–2106
[34] Hasso AN, Bird CR, Zinke DE, et al. Fibromuscular Dysplasia of the Internal Carotid Artery: Percutaneous Transluminal Angioplasty. AJR. 1981; 136:955–960
[35] Mettinger KL. Fibromuscular Dysplasia and the Brain II: Current Concept of the Disease. Stroke. 1982; 13:53–58
[36] Mettinger KL, Ericson K. Fibromuscular Dysplasia and the Brain: Observations on Angiographic, Clinical, and Genetic Characteristics. Stroke. 1982; 13:46–52
[37] Osborn AG, Anderson RE. Angiographic Spectrum of Cervical and Intracranial Fibromuscular Dysplasia. Stroke. 1977; 8:617–626
[38] Chabriat H, Vahedi K, Iba-Zizen MT, et al. Clinical Spectrum of CADASIL: A Study of Seven Families. Lancet. 1995; 346:934–939
[39] Voltz R, Gultekin SH, Rosenfeld MR, et al. A Serologic Marker of Paraneoplastic Limbic and Brain-Stem Encepahlitis in Patients with Testicular Cancer. N Engl J Med. 1999; 340:1788–1795
[40] Denny-Brown D. Primary Sensory Neuropathy with Muscular Changes Associated with Carcinoma. J Neurol Neurosurg Psychiatry. 1948; 11:73–87
[41] Charness ME, Simon RP, Greenberg DA. Ethanol and the Nervous System. N Engl J Med. 1989; 321:442–454
[42] Gorelick PB. Alcohol and stroke. Stroke. 1987; 18:268–271
[43] Lohr RH. Treatment of Alcohol Withdrawal in Hospitalized Patients. Mayo Clin Proc. 1995; 70:777–782
[44] Sullivan JT, Sykora K, Schneiderman J, et al. Assessment of Alcohol Withdrawal: The Revised Clinical Institute Withdrawal Assessment for Alcohol Scale (CIWA-Ar). Br J Addict. 1989; 84:1353–1357
[45] Saitz R, Mayo-Smith MF, Roberts MS, et al. Individualized Treatment for Alcohol Withdrawal: A Randomized Double-Blind Controlled Trial. JAMA. 1994; 272:519–523
[46] Lechtenberg R, Worner TM. Seizure Risk With Recurrent Alcohol Detoxification. Arch Neurol. 1990; 47:535–538
[47] Addolorato G, Caputo F, Capristo E, Janiri L, Bernardi M, Agabio R, Colombo G, Gessa GL, Gasbarrini G. Rapid suppression of alcohol withdrawal syndrome by baclofen. Am J Med. 2002; 112:226–229
[48] Treatment of Alcohol Withdrawal. Med Letter. 1986; 28:75–76
[49] Watson WD, Verma A, Lenart MJ, Quast TM, Gauerke SJ, McKenna GJ. MRI in acute Wernicke's encephalopathy. Neurology. 2003; 61
[50] Acute Reactions to Drugs of Abuse. Med Letter. 1996; 38:43–46
[51] Fessler RD, Esshaki CM, Stankewitz RC, et al. The Neurovascular Complications of Cocaine. Surg Neurol. 1997; 47:339–345
[52] Lichtenfeld PJ, Rubin DB, Feldman RS. Subarachnoid Hemorrhage Precipitated by Cocaine Snorting. Arch Neurol. 1984; 41:223–224
[53] Oyesiku NM, Collohan ART, Barrow DL, Reisner A. Cocaine-Induced Aneurysmal Rupture: An Emergent Negative Factor in the Natural History of Intracranial Aneurysms? Neurosurgery. 1993; 32:518–526
[54] Schwartz KA, Cohen JA. Subarachnoid Hemorrhage Precipitated by Cocaine Snorting. Arch Neurol. 1984; 41
[55] Levine SR, Brust JCM, Futrell N, Ho KL, et al. Cerebrovascular Complications of the Use of the 'Crack' Form of Alkaloidal Cocaine. N Engl J Med. 1990; 323:699–704
[56] Mody CK, Miller BL, McIntyre HB, et al. Neurologic Complications of Cocaine Abuse. Neurology. 1988; 38:1189–1193
[57] Volpe JJ. Effect of Cocaine Use on the Fetus. N Engl J Med. 1992; 327:399–407

Part III

Imaging and Diagnostics

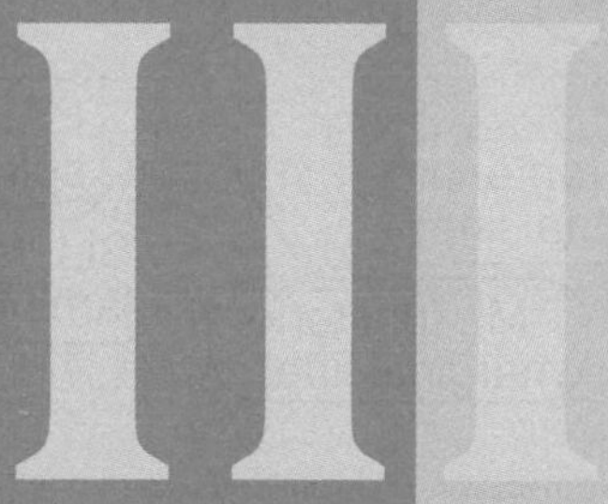

12

12 Plain Radiology and Contrast Agents

12.1 C-Spine x-rays

12.1.1 Normal findings

For radiographic signs of cervical spine trauma, see ▶ Table 63.2, and for guidelines for diagnosing clinical instability, see ▶ Table 65.4.

Contour lines

On a lateral C-spine x-ray, there are 4 contour lines (AKA arcuate lines). Normally each should form a smooth, gentle curve (▶ Fig. 12.1):

1. posterior marginal line (PML): along posterior cortical surfaces of vertebral bodies (VB). Marks the anterior margin of spinal canal
2. anterior marginal line (AML): along anterior cortical surfaces of VBs

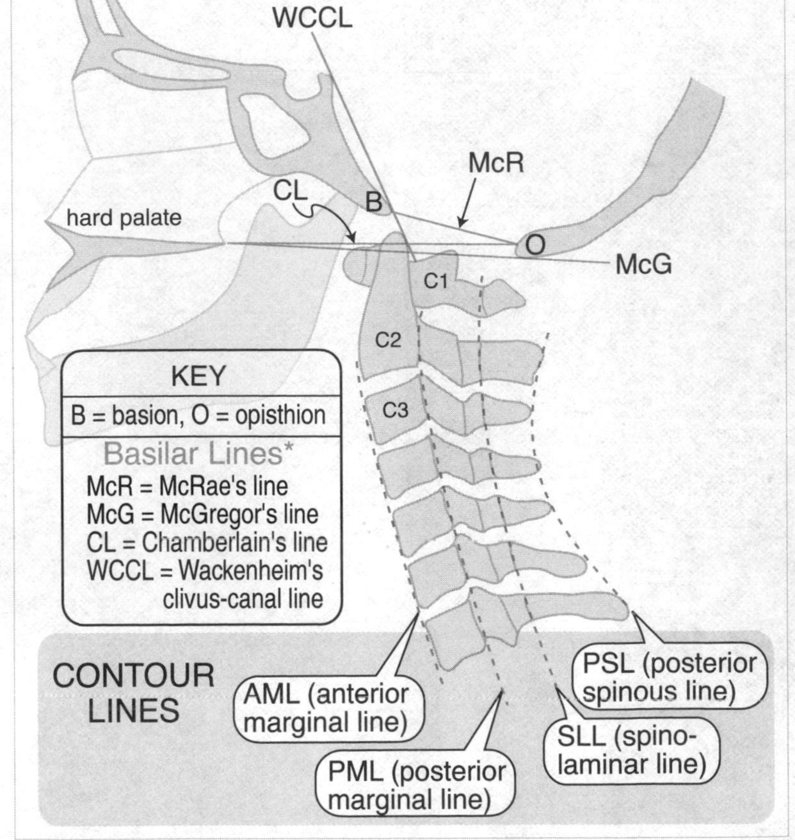

Fig. 12.1 Spinal contour lines and lines used to diagnose basilar invagination
Lateral view through craniocervical junction.
* See discussion of the basilar lines (p. 218)

Table 12.1 Normal ADI

Patient		ADI
adults	males	≤ 3 mm
	females	≤ 2.5 mm
pediatrics[7] (≤ 15 yrs)		≤ 4 mm

3. spinolaminar line (SLL): along base of spinous processes. The posterior margin of the spinal canal
4. posterior spinous line (PSL): along tips of spinous processes

Relation of atlas to occiput

See also criteria for atlantooccipital dislocation (AOD) (p. 965).

Relation of atlas to axis

These measurements are useful for atlantoaxial subluxation/dislocation (p. 968) e.g. in trauma, rheumatoid arthritis (p. 1134) or Down syndrome (p. 1138).

12.1.2 Rule of Spence

On AP or open-mouth odontoid x ray, if the sum total overhang of both C1 lateral masses on C2 is ≥ 7 mm (x + y in ▶ Fig. 12.7), the transverse atlantal ligament (TAL) is probably disrupted[1,2] (when corrected for an 18% magnification factor, it has been suggested that the criteria be increased to ≥ 8.2 mm[3])

12.1.3 (Anterior) atlantodental interval (ADI)

Note: the term ADI usually refers to the anterior atlantodental Interval (there is also a posterior ADI (p. 213) and a lateral ADI which can be seen on AP radiographs).

AKA predental space. The distance between the anterior margin of the dens and the closest point of the anterior arch of C1 ("C1 button") on a lateral C-spine x-ray (▶ Fig. 12.2). The normal maximal ADI is variously given in the range of 2 to 4 mm.[4,5] Commonly accepted upper limits are shown in ▶ Table 12.1. An abnormally increased ADI is a surrogate marker for TAL disruption[6]

12.1.4 Posterior atlantodental interval (PADI)

AKA the neural canal width (NCW).[8] The PADI is the AP diameter of the *bony* canal at C1 and is measured from the back of the odontoid to the anterior aspect of the posterior C1 ring (▶ Fig. 12.2). It is more useful than the ADI for some conditions, e.g. AAS in rheumatoid arthritis (p. 1134) or Down syndrome (p. 1138).

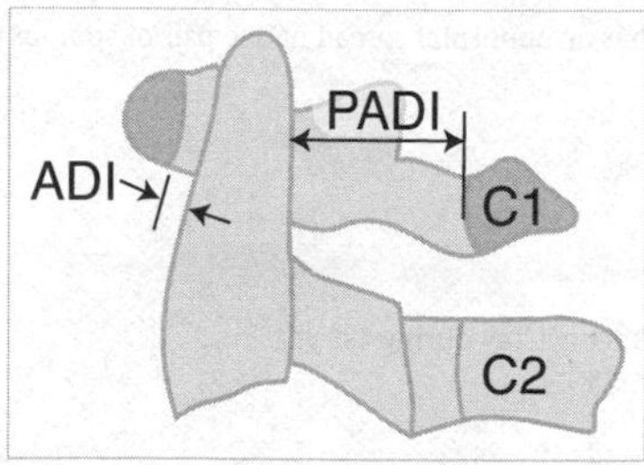

Fig. 12.2 The atlantodental interval (ADI) (p. 213) and posterior atlantodental interval (PADI) on a lateral C-spine x-ray

12

Table 12.2 Normal prevertebral soft tissue

Space	Level	Maximum normal width (mm)		
		Adults		Peds
		MDCT	Lateral X-Ray	
retropharyngeal	C1	8.5	10	unreliable
	C2–4	6–7[a]	5–7	
retrotracheal	C5–7	18	22	14

[a]CT data was deemed unreliable at C4[11]

Canal diameter

Normal canal diameter on lateral C-spine x-ray (from spinolaminar line (SLL) to posterior vertebral body with 6 foot tube to film distance)[9]: 17 ± 5 mm. In the presence of osteophytic spurs, measure from the back of the spur to the SLL.

Cervical spinal stenosis: various cutoffs for the normal minimum AP diameter have been suggested.[10] On a plain lateral C-spine x-ray this is usually measured from the posterior vertebral body (or the posterior aspect of an osteophyte) to the spinolaminar line. Some use 15 mm. Most agree that stenosis is present when the AP diameter is < 12 mm in an adult. This measurement is less critical than it once was, it is a surrogate marker for stenosis severe enough to compress the spinal cord, which now may be demonstrated directly with MRI (or myelography).

Prevertebral soft tissue

Abnormally increased prevertebral soft tissue (PVST) may indicate the presence of a vertebral fracture, dislocation, or ligamentous disruption.[12] Normal values for lateral C-spine x-ray and CT scan are shown in ▶ Table 12.2. Plain films are subjcet to errors due to magnification and rotation. Multidetector CT (MDCT) eliminates these shortcomings.[11]

Increased PVST is more likely with anterior than posterior injuries.[13] NB: the sensitivity of these measurements is only ≈ 60% at C3 and 5% at C6.[12] False positives may occur with basal skull/facial fractures, especially with fracture of the pterygoid plates. An ET-tube may allow fluid to accumulate in the posterior oropharynx which can obscure this measurement. In this setting, one can look for a thin fat layer between the prevertebral muscles and the posterior pharynx on cervical CT; the prevertebral tissue (posterior to this line) will be thickened (no measurements available at this time). MRI can also demonstrate abnormal signal within the prevertebral tissue.

Interspinous distances

C-spine AP: a fracture/dislocation or ligament disruption may be diagnosed if the interspinous distance is 1.5 times that at both adjacent levels (measured from center of spinous processes).[14] Also look for a malalignment of spinous processes below a certain level which may be evidence of rotation due to a unilaterally locked facet.

C-spine lateral: look for **"fanning"** or **"flaring"** which is an abnormal spread of one pair of spinous processes that may also indicate ligament disruption.

12.1.5 Pediatric C-spine

C1 (atlas)

Ossification centers[15]: usually 3 (▶ Fig. 12.3)
- 1 (sometimes 2) for body (not ossified at birth; appears on x-ray during 1st yr)
- 1 for each neural arch (appear bilaterally ≈ 7th fetal week)

Synchondroses[15]:
- synchondrosis of the spinous process: fuses by ≈ 3 yrs age
- 2 neurocentral synchondroses: fuse by ≈ age 7 yrs

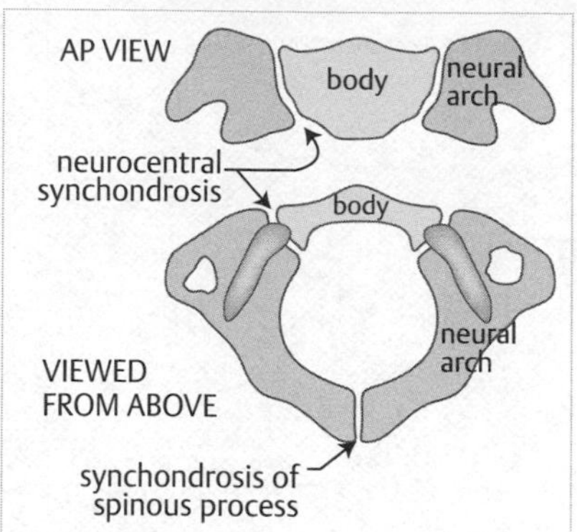

Fig. 12.3 Pediatric C1 (atlas)

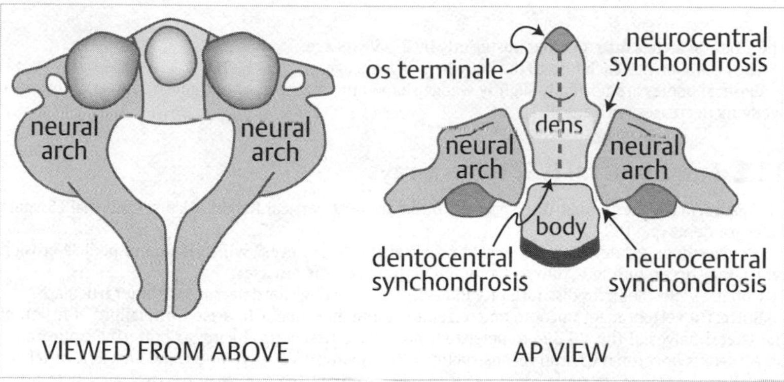

Fig. 12.4 Pediatric C2 (axis)

The ossification centers of C1 fail to completely close in 5% of adults (usually posteriorly). When present, the rare anterior defect is usually associated with a posterior defect.

C2 (axis)

Developmentally there are 5 ossification centers. The two halves of the odontoid fuse together in the midline (dashed line in ▶ Fig. 12.4) at 7 months development, so that at birth there are 4 primary ossification centers (▶ Fig. 12.4):

- odontoid process
- vertebral body
- 2 neural arches

The posterior arches fuse together by 2-3 years of age. The anterior synchondroses normally fuse between 3-6 years of age. However, the dentocentral synchondrosis (AKA subdental synchondrosis) may be visible on x-ray until ≈ 11 years of age. A secondary ossification center (os terminale) appears at the summit of the dens between 3–6 years of age, and fuses with the dens by age 12 years.[15]

C3–7

3 ossification centers at birth[16] (see ▶ Fig. 12.5).

- vertebral body
- 2 neural arches

12

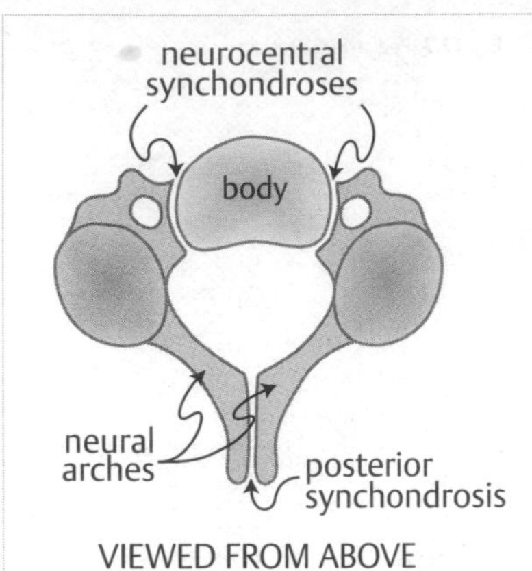

Fig. 12.5 Pediatric C3-7

The 2 neural arches fuse together posteriorly by 2-3 years age.

The neural arches each fuse to the body by 3 6 years age.

Cervical bodies are normally slightly wedge shaped in pediatric population (narrower anteriorly). Wedging decreases with age.

12.2 Lumbosacral (LS) spine x-rays

12

L4–5 is normally the lumbar disc space with the greatest vertical height. Also see Normal LS spine measurements (p. 1102).

AP view: look for defect or non visualization of the "owl's eyes" which is due to pedicle erosion which may occur with lytic tumors (common with metastatic disease).

Oblique views: look for discontinuity in neck of "Scotty dog" for defect in pars interarticularis.

Butterfly vertebra: An uncommon congenital anomaly thought to arise from failure of fusion of the lateral halves of the VB due to persistent notochord tissue, producing a "butterfly" appearance on AP x-rays or coronal CT scan reconstructions. The involved VB is widened, and adjacent vertebrae may show a compensatory deformity as if to fill in some of the gap. May be associated with other spinal and rib malformations.[17] On lateral views may simulate compression fracture. In severe cases, there may be significant kyphosis and/or scoliosis. Often asymptomatic, requiring no treatment. May be associated with lipomyelomeningocele (p. 269).

12.3 Skull x-rays

Water's view: AKA submental vertex view. X-ray tube angled up 45° (perpendicular to clivus). Towne's view: x-ray tube angled down 45°, to view occiput.

12.3.1 Sella turcica

Normal adult dimensions on skull x-ray

Technique: true lateral, 91 cm target to film distance, central ray 2.5 cm anterior and 1.9 cm superior to EAM. ▶ Table 12.3 shows normal values (▶ Fig. 12.6 shows how measurements are made).

Depth (D): defined as the greatest measurement from floor to diaphragma sellae.

Length (L): defined as the greatest AP diameter.

Abnormal findings

Pituitary adenomas tend to enlarge the sella, in contrast to craniopharyngiomas which erode the posterior clinoids. Empty sella syndrome tends to balloon the sella symmetrically, and also does not erode the clinoids. Tuberculum meningiomas usually do not enlarge the sella, and may be associated with enlargement of the sphenoid sinus; see sphenoid pneumosinus dilatans (p. 1372).

Table 12.3 Normal sella turcica dimensions (▸ Fig. 12.6)

Dimension	Max	Min	Avg
D (depth) (mm)	12	4	8.1
L (length) (mm)	16	5	10.6

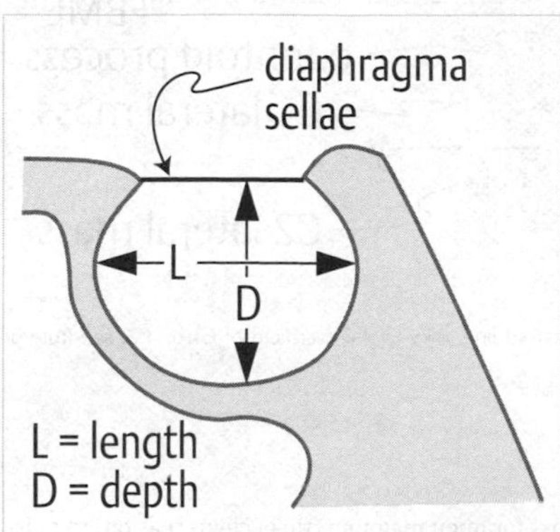

Fig. 12.6 Measurements of the sella turcica (lateral view)

"J" shaped sella suggests optic nerve glioma. It can also occur congenitally in Hurler syndrome (a mucopolysaccharidosis).

12

12.3.2 Basilar invagination and basilar impression (BI)

Terminology

The terms basilar impression and basilar invagination are often used interchangeably in the literature: historically, basilar invagination (AKA cranial settling) denoted upward indentation of skull base usually due to acquired softening of bone (see below), often associated with atlanto-occipital fusion, while basilar impression implied normal bone. Making a distinction seems pointless (the abbreviation (BI) will be used for either). Common feature: upward displacement of the upper cervical spine (including odontoid process, AKA cranial migration of the odontoid) through the foramen magnum into the p-fossa.

Platybasia: flattening of the skull base. Originally assessed on plain x-rays (which are subject to error due to skull rotation or difficulty identifying landmarks), now more commonly evaluated on CT or MRI. May or may not be associated with BI, and may occur in association with craniofacial abnormalities, Chiari malformation, Paget's disease…

Quantitated by measuring the basal angle, which on plain x-rays, measured the angle between lines drawn from the nasion to center of sella and then to the anterior foramen magnum,[18] but on MRI was felt to be better represented by the angle between a line drawn along the floor of the anterior fossa to the dorsum sellae and a second line drawn along the posterior clivus.[19] Normal mean basal angle: 130°. Platybasia: > 145° (abnormally obtuse basal angle).

Two subtypes of BI

See reference.[20]

Type I: BI without Chiari malformation. Tip of odontoid tends to be above CL, McR, and WCCL in ▸ Fig. 12.7. Brainstem compression is due to odontoid process invagination. 85% can be reduced with traction. Treatment: transoral surgery is recommended, usually accompanied by posterior fusion

Type II: BI + Chiari malformation. Odontoid tip tends to be above CL, but not McR or WCCL. Brainstem compression is due to reduced p-fossa volume. Only 15% can be reduced with traction. Foramen magnum decompression is appropriate

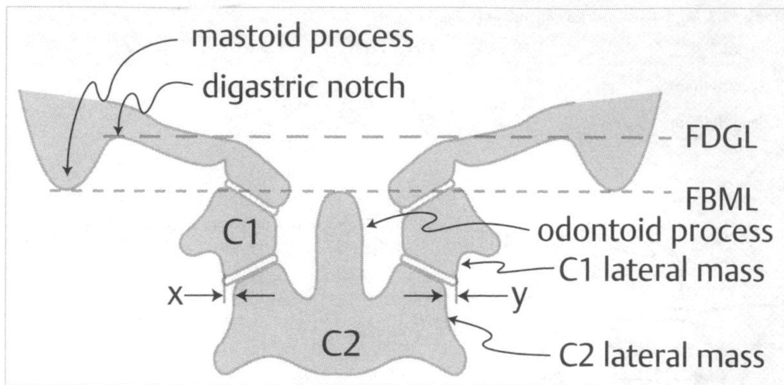

Fig. 12.7 AP view through craniocervical junction
FDGL = Fischgold's digastric line, FBML = Fischgold's bimastoid line, x + y = total overhang of C1 on C2; see Rule of Spence (p. 970)

Measurements used in BI

(► Fig. 12.1 and ► Fig. 12.7):

1. McRae's line ("McR" in ► Fig. 12.1): drawn across foramen magnum (tip of clivus (basion) to opisthion).[21] The mean position of the odontoid tip below the line is 5 mm (± 1.8 mm SD) on CT and 4.6 mm (± 2.6 mm SD) on MRI.[22] No part of odontoid should be above this line (the most accurate measure for BI).
2. Chamberlain's line ("CL" in ► Fig. 12.1)[23]: posterior hard palate to posterior margin of foramen magnum (opisthion). Less than 3 mm or half of dens should be above this line, with 6 mm being definitely pathologic. Seldom used because the opisthion is often hard to see on plain film and may also be invaginated. On CT[24] and MRI[22] the normal odontoid tip is 1.4 mm (± 2.4) below the line
3. McGregor's baseline ("McG" in ► Fig. 12.1)[25]: posterior margin of hard palate to most caudal point of occiput. No more than 4.5 mm of dens should be above this. On CT[24] and MRI[22] the normal odontoid tip is 0.8 mm (± 2.4) above the line
4. Wackenheim's clivus-canal line ("WCCL" in ► Fig. 12.1): the odontoid should be tangential to or below the line that extends the course of the clivus (the clivus baseline). If the clivus is concave or convex, this baseline is drawn to connect the basion to the base of the posterior clinoids on the clivus[26]
5. (Fischgold's) digastric line ("FDGL" in ► Fig. 12.7): joins the digastric notches. The normal distance from this line to the middle of the atlanto-occipital joint is 10 mm (decreased in BI).[27] No part of odontoid should be above this line. More accurate than the bimastoid line (FBML)
6. Fischgold's bimastoid line ("FBML" in ► Fig. 12.7): joins tips of mastoid processes. The odontoid tip averages 2 mm above this line (range: 3 mm below to 10 mm above) and this line should cross the atlanto-occipital joint

Conditions associated with BI

1. congenital conditions (BI is the most common congenital anomaly of the craniocervical junction, it is often accompanied by other anomalies[28(p 148–9)])
   a) Down syndrome
   b) Klippel-Feil syndrome (p. 271)
   c) Chiari malformation (p. 277): in a series of 100 patients, 92 had BI[29]
   d) syringomyelia
2. acquired conditions
   a) rheumatoid arthritis (in part due to incompetence of transverse ligament, see Basilar impression in rheumatoid arthritis (p. 1137)
   b) post-traumatic
3. conditions with BI associated with softening of bone include[30]:
   a) Paget's disease

b) osteogenesis imperfecta: patients have blue discolored sclera and early hearing loss and due to a genetic defect that causes defective Type 1 collagen. Bones are weak ("brittle-bone disease"). Autosomal dominant inheritance. There are 4 common types of OI and some uncommon ones
c) osteomalacia
d) rickets
e) hyperparathyroidism

12.4 Contrast agents in neuroradiology

Also see Intraoperative dyes (p. 1426) for visible dyes useful in the operating room.

12.4.1 Iodinated contrast agents

General precautions

Water-soluble contrast agents have superseded non-water-soluble ones such as Pantopaque® (ethyl iodophenylundecylate or iophendylate meglumine).

✖ Caution: iodinated contrast (IV or intra-arterial) may delay excretion of metformin (Glucophage®, Avandamet®), an oral hypoglycemic agent used in diabetes type II, and can be associated with lactic acidosis and renal failure (particularly in patients with CHF or those consuming alcohol). The manufacturer recommends withholding metformin 48 hrs prior to and following contrast administration (or longer if there is evidence of declining renal function following use of contrast). Metformin should also be held ≈ 48 hours before any surgery, and should not be restarted post-op until the patient has fully recovered and is eating and drinking normally.

Maximum dose of iodine with normal renal function is ≈ 86 gm in a 24 hour period.

Intrathecal contrast agents

Inadvertent intrathecal injection of unapproved contrast agents

✖ Caution: serious reactions can occur with inadvertent intrathecal injection (e.g. for myelography, cisternography, ventriculography…) of iodinated contrast media that are not specifically indicated for intrathecal use (including ionic contrast agents as well as some non-ionic agents (e.g. Optiray®, Reno-60…)). This can cause uncontrollable seizures, intracerebral hemorrhage, cerebral edema, coma, paralysis, arachnoiditis, myoclonus (tonic-clonic muscle spasms), rhabdomyolysis with subsequent renal failure, hyperthermia, and respiratory compromise, with a significant fatality rate.[31]

Management suggestions for inadvertent intrathecal injection include:

1. immediately remove CSF + contrast if the error is recognized when the opportunity is available (e.g. withdraw fluid through myelography needle)
2. elevate head of bed ≈ 45° (to keep contrast out of head)
3. if there is a question about what may have occurred (i.e. it is not certain if an inappropriate contrast agent was used) send blood and CSF with contrast for high-performance liquid chromatography for identification of agent[32]
4. antihistamines: e.g. diphenhydramine (Benadryl®) 50 mg deep IM
5. respiration: supplemental oxygen, and if needed, intubation
6. control HTN
7. IV hydration
8. IV steroids
9. sedation if patient is agitated
10. treat fever with acetaminophen and if needed with a cooling blanket
11. pharmacologic paralysis if necessary to manage muscle activity
12. anticonvulsant medication: more than one agent may be required (e.g. phenytoin + phenobarbital + a benzodiazepine)
13. consider unenhanced brain CT scan: may help assess if contrast has diffused intracranially, but this requires placing patient flat and may not be advisable
14. insert lumbar subarachnoid drain with CSF drainage (e.g. 10 cc q hr)
15. monitor: electrolytes, anticonvulsant levels, creatine kinase (CK)
16. repeat EEGs to assess seizure activity while sedated/paralyzed

Iohexol (Omnipaque®)

The primary approved agent employed for intrathecal use today is iohexol (Omnipaque®).

A non-ionic triiodinated compound. Concentration is expressed as follows: e.g. Omnipaque 300 contains the equivalent of 300 mg of organic iodine per ml of media (300 mgI/ml).

Used for myelography, cisternography as well as IV contrasted CT. Uses and concentrations are shown in ▶ Table 12.4.

Intrathecal use

NB: only Omnipaque 180, 210, 240 and 300 are labeled for intrathecal use. 140 and 350 are *not* FDA approved for intrathecal use, however, some neuroradiologists will use Omnipaque 140 or diluted 180 e.g. for CT ventriculography (off-label usage).

Consider discontinuing neuroleptic drugs (including: phenothiazines, e.g. chlorpromazine, prochlorperazine, and promethazine) at least 48 hours prior to procedure. Elevate HOB ≥ 30° for the first few hours after the procedure. Hydrate orally or IV.

Use with caution in patients with seizure history, severe cardiovascular disease, chronic alcoholism or multiple sclerosis.

Iohexol undergoes slow diffusion from the intrathecal space to the systemic circulation and is eliminated by renal excretion with no significant metabolism or deiodination.

Maximum dosage: a total dose of 3060 mg iodine should not be exceeded in an adult during a single myelogram (some say up to 4500 mg is OK) (e.g. 15 cc of Omnipaque 300 = 15 ml × 300 mgI/ml= 4500 mg of iodine).

Iopamidol (e.g. Isovue 300, Isovue 370®)

Triiodinated, non-ionic, water-soluble. Used for intravascular and intrathecal radiographic contrast. Isovue 300 and 370 contains 300 and 270 mg iodine/ml, respectively.

Table 12.4 Iohexol concentrations for adults

Procedure	Concentration (mgI/ml)	Volume (ml)
lumbar myelography via LP	180 240	10–17 7–12.5
thoracic myelography via LP or cervical injection	240 300	6–12.5 6–10
cervical myelography via LP	240 300	6–12.5 6–10
cervical myelography via C1–2 puncture	180 240 300	7–10 6–12.5 4–10
complete myelography via LP	240 300	6–12.5 6–10
cerebral arteriography[a]	300	≈ 6–12 ml/vessel
IV contrast enhanced CT scan of the brain	240 350	120–250 ml IV drip 70–150 ml bolus[b]
CT cisternography via LP or C1–2 puncture	300 350	12 12
CT ventriculography via ventricular catheter	180[c]	2–3
plain film ventriculography via ventricular catheter	180	2–3
plain film "shunt-o-gram" injected via shunt into ventricles	180	2–3
plain film "shunt-o-gram" injected via shunt distal to valve so as not to enter into ventricles (to check distal shunt function)	300 350	10–12 10–12

[a]most centers use Optiray®, see text
[b]follow with 250 ml bolus of 0.45% NS to rehydrate patient
[c]180 will be very dense on CT, and some use 1–3 ml of 140 or diluted 180%(dilute approximately 2 parts contrast to 1 part preservative-free normal saline)

Non-intrathecal contrast agents

For inadvertent intrathecal injection of contrast agents *not* intended for intrathecal use, see above.

Ioversol (Optiray®)

✖ Not for intrathecal use (see above).
Uses and concentrations include:

- arteriography: Optiray 300 (ioversol 64%) or Optiray 320 (ioversol 68%). Total procedural dose should not usually exceed 200 ml
- IV contrast enhanced CT scan of brain:
  a) adult: 50–150 ml of Optiray 300, 320, or 100–250 ml of Optiray 240. Typically: 100 ml of Optiray 320
  b) pediatrics: 1–3 ml/kg of Optiray 320

Iopromide (Ultravist®)

✖ Not for intrathecal use (see above). Available in 150, 240, 300 & 370 mg iodine/ml. Osmolality of Ultravist 300 is 607.

Cerebral angiography (300 mg/ml): maximum dose is 150 ml per procedure.

Contrast enhanced CT (CECT) (300 mg/ml). ℞ *Pediatrics* (> 2 years age): typical dose in is 1–2 ml/kg IV, maximum dose is 3 ml/kg per procedure. *Adult*:typical dose is 50–200 ml, maximum dose is 200 ml.

Iodixanol (Visipaque®)

✖ Not for intrathecal use (see above). Triiodinated, non-ionic, *isosmolar* to blood. For intravascular use. FDA approved for CECT, some angiographers use Visipaque 270 for cerebral angiography (slightly lower opacification, but also slightly lower iodine dose). Available in 270 and 320 mg iodine/ml.

Iodinated contrast with allergies or renally insufficiency

Allergy prep

Indicated for patients with previous history of reaction to IV iodinated contrast material. Minor previous reactions such as hives and itching merit preparation with this regimen whenever possible. Patients with anaphylactic shock or severe edema causing compromise of the airway should probably not receive IV iodine even with this prep, unless absolutely necessary. ✖ Caution: in spite of this regimen, the patient may still have serious reaction (modified[33]). This prep has also been used for the rare gadolinium allergy.

1. utilize non-ionic contrast medium (e.g. iohexol) whenever possible
2. have emergency equipment available during study
3. medications:
   a) steroid (▶ Table 8.1 for further details of steroid dosing)
      - prednisone 50 mg PO: 20–24 hrs, 8–12 hrs & 2 hrs before study
      - equivalent dose of IV Solumedrol® (methylprednisolone): ≈ 25 mg
   b) diphenhydramine (Benadryl®) 50 mg, *EITHER* IM 1 hr before, *OR* IV 5 min before study
   c) optional: H2 antagonist, e.g. cimetidine 300 mg PO or IV 1 hr before study

Medications for an *emergency* scan when 24 hour prep is not possible:

- hydrocortisone 100 mg IV then scan within 2 hours

Prep for renal insufficiency or patients with DM

For patients with DM or mild renal insufficiency (e.g. slight serum creatinine elevation, > 1.2 mg/dl (U.S.) which is > 100 mcmol/L) 1 mg/dl of creatinine (used in the U.S.) = 88.4 mcmol/L, to mitigate against iodine contrast-induced nephropathy:

- N-acetyl cysteine (Mucomyst; the actual efficacy of NAC has not been proven, and may be no better than hydration alone): regimens all accompany hydration and include:
  a) 800 mg PO q 8 hrs for 24 hours before the study,[34] followed by 600 mg PO BID for 24 hours after the study
  b) 600 mg PO BID X 2 days before the study, 600 mg PO BID for 24 hours after
  c) 600-mg IV bolus before the study, and 600 mg PO BID for 48 hours after[35]

12

- hydration: 1 L of sterile water with 3 amps of sodium bicarbonate IV at 100 ml/hr, start 1 hour prior to the study, and continue until entire L given

12.4.2 Reactions to intravascular contrast media

General information

See also treatment of inadvertent intrathecal injection of ionic contrast agents (p. 219)

✖ Beta blockers

Beta blockers can increase the risk of contrast media reactions, and may mask some manifestations of an anaphylactoid reaction. They also make use of epinephrine inadvisable since the alpha effects of epinephrine will predominate (bronchospasm, vasoconstriction, increased vagal tone). If treatment is required for hypotension after beta-blocker administration, may try glucagon 2–3 mg IV bolus, followed by 5 mg IV drip over 1 hour (glucagon has positive inotropic and chronotropic effect that is not mediated through adrenergic pathways).

Idiosyncratic reactions and treatment

Hypotension with tachycardia (anaphylactoid reaction)

1. mild: Trendelenburg position. IV fluids
2. if no response but remains mild:
   epinephrine (use with caution in patients with coronary artery disease, limited cardiac reserve, hypertension, or unclipped cerebral aneurysm)
   a) 0.3–0.5 ml of 1:1000 SQ (0.3–0.5 mg) q 15–20 mins (peds: 0.01 mg/kg)
   b) or, ASEP recommendations (especially for elderly or patients in shock): 10 ml of 1:100,000 IV over 5 to 10 min (put 0.1 ml of 1:1000 in 10 ml of NS, or dilute 1 amp of 1:10,000 to 10 ml with NS)
3. moderate to severe or worsening (anaphylaxis): add:
   a) IV colloidal fluids, e.g. hetastarch (Hespan®) 6% (colloids are required since there is extravascular shift of fluids due to see page, these agents also carry a small risk of allergic reaction)
   b) epinephrine (see above). May repeat × 1
   c) O_2 2–6 L/min per NC. Intubate if necessary
   d) EKG to R/O ischemic changes
4. if shock develops: add dopamine (p. 128), start at 5 mcg/kg/min

Hypotension with bradycardia (vasovagal reaction)

1. mild:
   a) Trendelenburg position
   b) IV fluids
2. if no response, add:
   a) atropine 0.75 mg IV, may repeat up to 2–3 mg over 15 mins PRN. Use with caution in patients with underlying heart disease
   b) EKG and/or cardiac monitor: especially if atropine or dopamine are used
3. if no response: add dopamine (p. 128), start at 5 mcg/kg/min

Urticaria

1. mild: self limited. No treatment necessary
2. moderate:
   a) diphenhydramine (Benadryl®) 50 mg PO or deep IM (avoid IV, can cause anaphylaxis itself)
   b) cimetidine (Tagamet®) 300 mg PO or IV diluted to 20 ml and given over 20 mins. H2 receptors contribute to wheal and flare of reaction
3. severe: treat as above for moderate reaction, and add:
   a) epinephrine (see above)
   b) maintain IV line

Facial or laryngeal angioedema

1. epinephrine: see above. May repeat up to 1 mg
2. if respiratory distress: O_2 2–6 L/min. Intubate if necessary (orotracheal may be very difficult due to swelling of tongue, nasotracheal intubation or emergency cricothyrotomy may be required)

3. diphenhydramine: see above
4. cimetidine: see above
5. if angioedema is accessible, add ice pack
6. maintain IV line
7. steroids are usually effective only for *chronic* angioedema

Bronchospasm
1. mild to moderate:
   a) epinephrine: see above. May repeat up to 1 ml
   b) if respiratory distress: O_2 2–6 L/min. Intubate if necessary
   c) maintain IV line
   d) inhalational therapy with a β-adrenergic agonist, e.g. albuterol (Proventil®) if respiratory therapy is available, otherwise, metered dose inhaler e.g. pirbuterol (Maxair®) or metaproterenol (Metaprel®), 2 puffs
2. severe: treat as above for moderate reaction, and add:
   a) aminophylline 250–500 mg in 10–20 cc NS slow IV over 15–30 mins. Monitor for hypotension and arrhythmias
   b) intubate
3. prolonged: add the following (will not have immediate effect):
   a) hydrocortisone 250 mg IV
   b) diphenhydramine: see above
   c) cimetidine: see above

Pulmonary edema
1. O_2 2–6 L/min per NC. Intubate if necessary
2. raise head and body
3. furosemide (Lasix®) 40 mg IV
4. EKG
5. if hypoxia develops (may manifest as agitation or combativeness), add:
   a) morphine 8–15 mg IV. May cause respiratory depression, be prepared to intubate
   b) epinephrine: see above. ✖ CAUTION: use only if MI can be R/O as cause of the pulmonary edema. Patients with acute intracranial pathology may be at risk of neurogenic pulmonary edema (p. 1178)

Seizures
If seizure is not self limited, start with lorazepam (Ativan®) 2–4 mg IV for an adult. Take precautions for status epilepticus (p. 470) and proceed to other drugs as indicated (p. 471).

12.5 Radiation safety for neurosurgeons

12.5.1 General information

Radiation exposure has both a deterministic component (exposure over a certain threshold will cause a specific injury) as well as a stochastic component (any dose increases the *chances* of an adverse event, and the higher the cumulative dose, the higher the chances).

12.5.2 Units

See reference.[36]

Absorbed dose: the amount of energy absorbed per unit mass. Expressed in Gray or rads.

Gray (Gy): the SI unit. 1 Gy = 100 cGy = 100 rads = an absorbed dose of 1 Joule/kg.

Rad: 1 rad = an absorbed dose of 100 ergs/gram = 0.01 joule/kg = 0.01 Gy = 1 cGy.

The biological effect (dose equivalent) of radiation: can be expressed in rem or Sieverts.

Sievert (Sv): the SI unit. The dose equivalent in sieverts is equal to the absorbed dose in grays multiplied by a "quality factor" (Q) which differs for different sources of radiation, e.g. high-energy protons have a Q of 10, x-rays have a Q of 1. 1 Sv=100 rems.

Roentgen-equivalent man (rem): the absorbed dose in rads multiplied by Q. 1 rem is estimated to cause ≈ 300 additional cases of cancer per million persons (one third of which are fatal). 1 rem = 0.01 sievert.

12.5.3 Typical radiation exposure

The average annual exposure to radiation is 360 mrem (about 30 mrem are due to background cosmic radiation, ≈ 20% of the total dose is due to radioactive potassium-40 which is in every cell). Exposure from a transcontinental airline flight is ≈ 5 mrem.

CXR: causes about 0.01–0.04 rem of exposure to the chest.

Spine x-ray with obliques: 5 rem.

CAT scan (brain, noncontrast): median effective dose to the head = 0.2 rem, but the range varied 13 fold within and across institutions.[37]

Spine CT: 5 rem.

Cerebral arteriogram: ≈ 10–20 rem (including fluoroscopy).[38]

Cerebral embolization: 34 rem.

Bone scan: 4 rem.

C-arm fluoroscopy[39]: exposure is shown in ▶ Table 12.5.

Doses during a minimally invasive TLIF[40]:

Patient exposure: mean 60 mGy to the skin in the AP plane (range: 8–250 mGy), 79 mGy in the lateral plane.

Surgeon exposure: 76 mrem to dominant hand, 27 mrem at the waist under a lead apron, and 32 mrem to an unprotected thyroid level detector.

12.5.4 Occupational exposure

The U.S. Nuclear Regulatory Commission (NRC) maximal recommended annual occupational dose limits for radiation are shown in ▶ Table 12.6.[41] The 1990 recommendations of the International Commission on Radiological Protection (ICRP) was to keep exposure ≤ 2 rem/year averaged over 5 years.[42]

ALARA: an acronym for "As Low As Reasonably Achievable" by which the NRC means making every reasonable effort to keep radiation dose as far below the limits as possible consistent with the purpose for which the licensed activity is undertaken.[43]

Steps to reduce occupational radiation dose (to staff) during surgery:

1. increase the distance from the radiation source: radiation exposure is proportional to the inverse *square* of the distance. Conventional wisdom is to try to keep 6 feet away. In a AANS publication, 3 m (10 ft) was recommended[44]
   Lead aprons/shields may or may not work. Distance ALWAYS works[45] (inverse square law – double the distance and get 1/4 the radiation).
2. shielding: shielding is less effective at higher kV (used with larger patients). Portable lead "doors" are more effective than aprons. Wrap-around 2-piece aprons are better than front side aprons. With front aprons the wearer must always face the x-ray source, otherwise the apron can actually reflect some radiation back onto the wearer. Non-lead aprons may not provide the rated protection at levels > 100 keV[46]
3. don't overuse magnification: most fluoro systems increase the radiation emitted × ≈ 4 to compensate for the associated reduction in image brightness
4. "boost" mode can double the radiation output. Use should be kept to a minimum
5. use live fluoro only when absolutely necessary
6. for lateral imaging, when possible stand on the "downstream" (image intensifier (ImI)) side of the C-arm: scatter is the most significant cause of exposure here and is higher on the *source side*[47] (this asymmetry is not as significant for C-spine[48])
7. keep the ImI as close to the patient as possible (reduces patient & staff exposure and improves image quality)
8. on AP images (with the patient prone or supine): position the x-ray tube *under* the table with the ImI over the patient (lowers scatter exposure to staff)[49]
9. *collimate* the beam as much as possible: reduces radiation to patient and to staff, and results in less image degradation
10. keep hands, arms, etc. out of the primary beam at all times (consider using leaded gloves if hands need to be within the beam or nearby for an extended time)
11. minimize number of images: plan your shot, avoid frequent "checks" or peeks
12. use image guided navigation when possible and practical
13. leaded glasses are recommended only for personnel with very high fluoro times: cataracts can be induced by single doses of 200 rads (very high), cumulative doses of 750 rads have not been associated with cataracts

Table 12.5 Radiation exposure with fluoroscopy[39a]

Distance from beam		Typical team member	Deep exposure	Superficial exposure
feet	meters		(mrem/min)	
Direct beam		patient	4000	
1	0.3	surgeon	20	29
2	0.6	assistant	6	10
3	0.9	scrub tech	0	≤2
5	1.5	anesthesiologist	0[b]	0[b]

[a]in a mock OR set up for maximal scatter
[b]after 10 minutes of exposure

Table 12.6 Annual occupational radiation dose limits

Target organ	Recommended MAXIMAL dose (rem/yr)
whole body	5
lens of eye	15
skin, hands, feet	50
other organs (including thyroid)	15

References

[1] Spence KF, Decker S, Sell KW. Bursting Atlantal Fracture Associated with Rupture of the Transverse Ligament. J Bone Joint Surg. 1970; 52A:543–549

[2] Fielding JW, Cochran GB, Lawsing JF, III, Hohl M. Tears of the transverse ligament of the atlas. A clinical and biomechanical study. J Bone Joint Surg Am. 1974; 56:1683–1691

[3] Heller JG, Viroslav S, Hudson T. Jefferson fractures: the role of magnification artifact in assessing transverse ligament integrity. J Spinal Disord. 1993; 6:392–396

[4] Hinck VC, Hopkins CE. Measurement of the Atlanto-Dental Interval in the Adult. Am J Roentgenol Radium Ther Nucl Med. 1960; 84:945–951

[5] Meijers KAE, van Beusekom GT, Luyendijk W, et al. Dislocation of the Cervical Spine with Cord Compression in Rheumatoid Arthritis. J Bone Joint Surg. 1974; 56B:668–680

[6] Panjabi MM, Oda T, Crisco JJ, III, Oxland TR, Katz L, Nolte LP. Experimental study of atlas injuries. I. Biomechanical analysis of their mechanisms and fracture patterns. Spine. 1991; 16:S460–S465

[7] Powers B, Miller MD, Kramer RS, et al. Traumatic Anterior Atlanto-Occipital Dislocation. Neurosurgery. 1979; 4:12–17

[8] Brockmeyer D. Down syndrome and craniovertebral instability. Topic review and treatment recommendations. Pediatr Neurosurg. 1999; 31:71–77

[9] Schmidek HH, Sweet WH. Operative Neurosurgical Techniques. New York 1982

[10] Epstein N, Epstein JA, Benjamin V, Ransohoff J. Traumatic Myelopathy in Patients With Cervical Spinal Stenosis Without Fracture or Dislocation: Methods of Diagnosis, Management, and Prognosis. Spine. 1980; 5:489–496

[11] Rojas CA, Vermess D, Bertozzi JC, Whitlow J, Guidi C, Martinez CR. Normal thickness and appearance of the prevertebral soft tissues on multidetector CT. AJNR Am J Neuroradiol. 2009; 30:136–141

[12] DeBenhe K, Havel C. Utility of Prevertebral Soft Tissue Measurements in Identifying Patients with Cervical Spine Injury. Ann Emerg Med. 1994; 24:1119–1124

[13] Miles KA, Finlay D. Is Prevertebral Soft Tissue Swelling a Useful Sign in Injury of the Cervical Spine? Injury. 1988; 19:177–179

[14] Naidich JB, Naidich TP, Garfein C, et al. The Widened Interspinous Distance: A Useful Sign of Anterior Cervical Dislocation. Radiology. 1977; 123:113–116

[15] Bailey DK. The Normal Cervical Spine in Infants and Children. Radiology. 1952; 59:712–719

[16] Yoganandan N, Pintar FA, Lew SM, Rao RD, Rangarajan N. Quantitative Analyses of Pediatric Cervical Spine Ossification Patterns Using Computed Tomography. Ann Adv Automot Med. 2011; 55:159–168

[17] Fischer FJ, Vandemark RE. Sagittal cleft (butterfly) vertebra. J Bone Joint Surg. 1945; 27:695–698

[18] Poppel MH, Jacobson HG, Duff BK, Gottlieb C. Basilar impression and platybasia in Paget's disease. Br J Radiol. 1953; 21:171–181

[19] Koenigsberg RA, Vakil N, Hong TA, Htaik T, Faerber E, Maiorano T, Dua M, Faro S, Gonzales C. Evaluation of platybasia with MR imaging. AJNR Am J Neuroradiol. 2005; 26:89–92

[20] Goel A, Bhatjiwale M, Desai K. Basilar invagination: a study based on 190 surgically treated patients. J Neurosurg. 1998; 88:962–968

[21] McRae DL. The Significance of Abnormalities of the Cervical Spine. AJR. 1960; 70:23–46

[22] Cronin CG, Lohan DG, Mhuircheartigh JN, Meehan CP, Murphy JM, Roche C. MRI evaluation and measurement of the normal odontoid peg position. Clin Radiol. 2007; 62:897–903

12

[23] Chamberlain WE. Basilar Impression (Platybasia); Bizarre Developmental Anomaly of Occipital Bone and Upper Cervical Spine with Striking and Misleading Neurologic Manifestations. Yale J Biol Med. 1939; 11:487–496
[24] Cronin CG, Lohan DG, Mhuircheartigh JN, Meehan CP, Murphy J, Roche C. CT evaluation of Chamberlain's, McGregor's, and McRae's skull-base lines. Clin Radiol. 2009; 64:64–69
[25] McGregor J. The Significance of Certain Measurements of the Skull in the Diagnosis of Basilar Impression. Br J Radiol. 1948; 21:171–181
[26] VanGilder JC, Menezes AH, Dolan KD. In: Radiology of the Normal Craniovertebral Junction. The Craniovertebral Junction and Its Abnormalities. NY: Futura Publishing; 1987:29–68
[27] Hinck VC, Hopkins CE, Savara BS. Diagnostic Criteria of Basilar Impression. Radiology. 1961; 76
[28] The Cervical Spine Research Society. The Cervical Spine. Philadelphia 1983
[29] Menezes AH. Primary craniovertebral anomalies and the hindbrain herniation syndrome (Chiari I): data base analysis. Pediatr Neurosurg. 1995; 23:260–269
[30] Jacobson G, Bleeker HH. Pseudosubluxation of the Axis in Children. Am J Roentgenol. 1959; 82:472–481
[31] Rivera E, Hardjasudarma M, Willis BK, Pippins DN. Inadvertent Use of Ionic Contrast Material in Myelography: Case Report and Management Guidelines. Neurosurgery. 1995; 36:413–415
[32] Bohn HP, Reich L, Suljaga-Petchel K. Inadvertent Intrathecal Use of Ionic Contrast Media for Myelography. AJNR. 1992; 13:1515–1519
[33] Lasser EC, Berry CC, Talner LB, Santini LC, et al. Pretreatment with Corticosteroids to Alleviate Reactions to Intravenous Contrast Material. N Engl J Med. 1987; 317:825–829
[34] Allaqaband S, Tumuluri R, Malik AM, Gupta A, Volkert P, Shalev Y, Bajwa TK. Prospective randomized study of N-acetylcysteine, fenoldopam, and saline for prevention of radiocontrast-induced nephropathy. Catheter Cardiovasc Interv. 2002; 57:279–283
[35] Marenzi G, Assanelli E, Marana I, Lauri G, Campodonico J, Grazi M, De Metrio M, Galli S, Fabbiocchi F, Montorsi P, Veglia F, Bartorelli AL. N-acetylcysteine and contrast-induced nephropathy in primary angioplasty. N Engl J Med. 2006; 354:2773–2782
[36] Units of radiation dose. 1991
[37] Smith-Bindman R, Lipson J, Marcus R, Kim KP, Mahesh M, Gould R, Berrington de Gonzalez A, Miglioretti DL. Radiation dose associated with common computed tomography examinations and the associated lifetime attributable risk of cancer. Arch Intern Med. 2009; 169:2078–2086
[38] Thompson TP, Maitz AH, Kondziolka D, Lunsford LD. Radiation, Radiobiology, and Neurosurgery. Contemp Neurosurg. 1999; 21:1–5
[39] Mehlman CT, DiPasquale TG. Radiation exposure to the orthopaedic surgical team during fluoroscopy: "how far away is far enough?". J Orthop Trauma. 1997; 11:392–398
[40] Bindal RK, Glaze S, Ognoskie M, Tunner V, Malone R, Ghosh S. Surgeon and patient radiation exposure in minimally invasive transforaminal lumbar interbody fusion. J Neurosurg Spine. 2008; 9:570–573
[41] Occupational dose limits for adults. 1991
[42] 1990 Recommendations of the International Commission on Radiological Protection. Ann ICRP. 1991; 21
[43] Definitions. 1991
[44] McCormick PW. Fluoroscopy: Reducing radiation exposure in the OR. Rolling Meadows, IL 2008
[45] Rechtine GR. Radiation satety for the orthopaedic surgeon: Or, C-arm friend or foe. Tampa, FL 2009
[46] Scuderi GJ, Brusovanik GV, Campbell DR, Henry RP, Kwon B, Vaccaro AR. Evaluation of non-lead-based protective radiological material in spinal surgery. Spine J. 2006; 6:577–582
[47] Boone JM, Pfeiffer DE, Strauss KJ, Rossi RP, Lin PJ, Shepard JS, Conway BJ. A survey of fluoroscopic exposure rates: AAPM Task Group No. 11 Report. Med Phys. 1993; 20:789–794
[48] Giordano BD, Baumhauer JF, Morgan TL, Rechtine GR. Cervical spine imaging using standard C-arm fluoroscopy: patient and surgeon exposure to ionizing radiation. Spine. 2008; 33:1970–1976
[49] Faulkner K, Moores BM. An assessment of the radiation dose received by staff using fluoroscopic equipment. Br J Radiol. 1982; 55:272–276

13 Imaging and Angiography

13.1 CAT scan (AKA CT scan)

13.1.1 General information

CAT scans employ ionizing radiation (x-rays) with the attendant risks; see Radiation safety for neurosurgeons (p.223).

Attenuation of the x-ray beam on a CT scan is defined in Hounsfield units. These units are not absolute, and vary between CT scanner models. Some sample values are shown in ▶ Table 13.1.

13.1.2 Noncontrast vs. IV contrast enhanced CT scan (CECT)

Noncontrast CT scans are often employed in emergency situations (to quickly rule-out most acute abnormalities), to evaluate bone in great detail, or as a screening test. It excels in demonstrating acute blood (EDH, SDH, IPH, SAH), fractures, foreign bodies, pneumocephalus and hydrocephalus. It is weak in demonstrating acute stroke (DWI MRI is preferred), and often has poor signal quality in the posterior fossa (due to bone artifact).

IV enhanced CT scans are used primarily for imaging neoplasms or vascular malformations, especially in patients with contraindications to MRI. All CT contrast agents contain iodine.

Typical IV dose of contrast: 60–65 ml of e.g. Isovue 300® (p.220) which delivers 18–19.5 grams of iodine.

13.1.3 CT angiography (CTA)

Employs rapid injection of iodinated contrast at 3–4 cc/sec, typically 65–75 ml of e.g. Isovue 300®. Optimal results in patients who can hold their breath for 30–40 seconds (for spiral CT).

Table 13.1 Hounsfield units for a sample CT scanner

Definitions	Hounsfield units	Comment
no attenuation (air)	−1000	definition
water	0	definition
dense bone	+ 1000	definition
Cranial CT		
brain (grey matter)	30 to 40	
brain (white matter)	20 to 35	
cerebral edema	10 to 14	
CSF	+ 5	
bone	+ 600	
blood clot[a]	75 to 80	acute SDH or EDH, fresh SAH
fat	−35 to −40	
calcium	100 to 300	
enhanced vessels	90–100	
Spine CT		
disc material	55–70	disc density is ≈ 2 × thecal sac
thecal sac	20–30	

[a]Hct < 23% will cause an acute SDH to be isodense with brain

Various methods may be used to determine timing of CT after injection: may be based on time to peak in aorta after a small test injection, or can be based empirically on time, or give injection and look for peak in the region of interest.

Accuracy is diminished for vessels that are perpendicular to the axial CT plane. Also in the vicinity of dense clot, CTA has trouble resolving the adjacent vessels.

13.1.4 CT perfusion (CTP)

Requires use of iodinated contrast. Areas of interest are selected from an unenhanced CT scan in the 3 supratentorial vascular territories. Contrast is given at a standard rate (e.g. 40 ml IV at 5 ml/sec). Scans through the regions of interest are repeated at intervals, e.g. every 2 seconds for 1 minute.

Acetazolamide (ACZ) (Diamox®) challenge: after the above, a bolus of 1000 mg of IV ACZ is given, and scans are repeated at intervals for approximately 10 minutes, with a final scan usually at 15 minutes.

Parameters then calculated from the images: cerebral blood volume (CBV), CBF, meant transit times (MTT), and time to peak (TTP). In ischemic stroke, MTT is almost always increased and CBF is decreased.

Abnormalities that can be demonstrated:

1. flow significant stenosis: decreased CBV & CBF, increased MTT and TTP
2. steal: after ACZ challenge (see above), CBV & CBF decrease, often with increases in the corresponding contralateral territory; MTT increases

In comparison to perfusion weighted MRI (PWI) (p. 232):

1. PWI acquires multiple slices of the whole brain over and over. CTP is limited to a given slice or several slices (usually 10–20 mm thick), and one has to choose where to place that slice
2. PWI has more artifact than CTP

13.2 Magnetic resonance imaging (MRI)

13.2.1 General information

Definitions[1]

Abbreviations:

- TR: time to repetition
- TE: time to echo
- T_I: time to inversion
- T_1: spin-lattice relaxation time ("time to magnetize") (regrowth)
- T_2: spin-spin relaxation time ("time to demagnetize") (decay)

13.2.2 T_1 weighted image (T1WI)

Short T_1 → high signal (bright). "Anatomic image", somewhat resembles CT. Shorter acquisition time than T2WI. Proton rich tissue (e.g. H_2O) has long T1.

Table 13.2 Range of acquisition data

	short TE (te < 50)	long TE (te > 80)
short TR (TR < 1000)	T1WI	
long TR (TR > 2000)	proton density or spin density	T2WI

Table 13.3 T1WI, MRI intensity change

fat (including bone marrow), blood > 48 hrs old, melanin	white matter	grey matter	calcium	CSF, bone
(note: grey-bar illustrates direction of intensity change and does not show actual grey on MRI)				

Clues to recognizing T1WI: CSF is black, subcutaneous fat is white, TR and TE are short (hundreds and double digits, respectively).

✱ The only objects that appear white on T1WI are: fat, melanin, Onyx® (p.1589), and subacute blood (> 48 hrs old). White matter is higher signal than grey matter (myelin has a high fat content). Most pathology is low signal on T1WI.

13.2.3 T_2 weighted image (T2WI)

Long $T_2 \rightarrow$ high signal (bright). "Pathological image." Most pathology shows up as high signal, including surrounding edema.

Clues to recognizing T2WI: CSF is white, TR & TE are long (thousands and hundreds, respectively).

13.2.4 Spin density image

AKA balanced image, AKA proton density image. Partway between T1WI and T2WI. CSF = grey, approximately isodense with brain. Becoming less commonly used.

13.2.5 FLAIR

Acronym: FLuid-Attenuated Inversion Recovery. Long TR and TE. Resembles a T2WI except the CSF is nulled out (appears dark). The grey/white intensity pattern is reversed from T1WI and is more prominent. Most abnormalities including MS plaques, other white matter lesions, tumors, edema, encephalomalacia, gliosis and acute infarcts appear bright. Periventricular lesions such as MS plaques become more conspicuous. Also good for demonstrating abnormalities in CSF.

Differential diagnosis of increased signal in subarachnoid spaces on FLAIR:

1. subarachnoid hemorrhage (SAH): ✱ the best sequence for detecting acute SAH on MRI
2. meningitis: occurs in some cases
3. meningeal carcinomatosis
4. superior sagittal sinus thrombosis
5. stroke
6. adjacent tumor: ? if related to higher protein
7. previous administration of gadolinium
8. high levels of FIO_2 especially at levels nearing 100% as may be used in patients getting MRI under general anesthesia.[2] Shows up in basal cisterns and in sulci over the convexity, but not in ventricles

13

13.2.6 Echo train (AKA fast spin echo (FSE))

tr is held constant, te is progressively increased utilizing multiple echoes (8–16) rather than one. Image approaches T2WI but with substantially reduced acquisition time (fat is brighter on FSE, which may be rectified by fat suppression techniques).

13.2.7 Gradient echo

AKA T2* (called T2-star), and some manufacturers have trademarked names for this, e.g. "GRASS" (a GE trademarked acronym for Gradient Recalled Acquisition in a Steady State) or FISP. A "fast" T2WI utilizing a partial flip angle. CSF and flowing vessels appear white. Bone, calcium and heavy metals are *dark*. Typical acquisition data: TR = 22, TE = 11, angle 8°. Used e.g. in cervical spine to produce a "myelographic" image, improves MRI's ability to delineate bony spurs. Also shows small old cerebral hemorrhages (seen in 60% of patients presenting with hemorrhagic infarction, and in 18% with ischemic infarcts[3]); these patients may be at increased risk of hemorrhage from anticoagulation. ✱*Gradient-echo T2WI* MRI is the 3–4 × more sensitive test than FLAIR for demonstrating intraparenchymal blood (which appears *dark*) due to high sensitivity to paramagnetic artifact. It is not as sensitive as the more recently introduced SWI.

Table 13.4 T1WI, MRI intensity change

brain edema/water	CSF	grey matter	white matter	bone, fat

(note: grey-bar illustrates direction of intensity change and does not show actual grey level on MRI)

13.2.8 "STIR" image

Acronym for "Short Tau Inversion Recovery." Summates T1 & T2 signals. Causes fat to drop out – sometimes also called fat suppression or "fat sat" (for fat saturation), allows gadolinium enhancement to show up better in areas of fat. Useful primarily in spine and orbit. Very good for showing bone edema (can help in dating spine fractures). The dorsal root ganglion may enhance on fat suppression images.

13.2.9 Contraindications to MRI

General information

An extensive reference[4] details safety issues. Web sites for MRI safety include: *www.MRIsafety.com* and *www.IMRSER.org* . Some issues that come up frequently in neurosurgical patients follows.

Pregnancy and MRI

During the first trimester, MRI can cause reabsorption of products of conception (miscarriage). There are no studies to determine the long term effects of MRI on a fetus after the first trimester (the low risk of MRI in this situation is probably preferable to the known dangers of ionizing radiation of x-rays (including CT)[5]). Gadolinium contrast is contraindicated during all of pregnancy, and is not approved for use in age < 2 years. Breast-feeding must be interrupted for 2 days after administration of gadolinium to the mother.

Common contraindications to MRI

13

1. cardiac pacemakers/defibrillator, implanted neurostimulators, cochlear implants, infusion pumps: may cause temporary or permanent malfunction
2. ferromagnetic aneurysm clips (see below): some centers exclude all patients with any type of aneurysm clip
3. metallic implants or foreign bodies with large component of iron or cobalt (may move in field, or may heat up)
4. Swann-Ganz catheter (pulmonary artery catheter)
5. metallic fragments within the eye
6. placement of a vascular stent, coil or filter within the past 6 weeks
7. shrapnel: BB's (some bullets are OK)
8. *relative* contraindications:
   a) claustrophobic patients: may be able to sedate adequately to perform study
   b) critically ill patients: ability to monitor and access to patient are impaired. Specially designed non-magnetic ventilator may be required. Cannot use most brands of electronic IV pumps/regulators
   c) obese patients: may not physically fit into many closed bore MRI scanners. Open bore scanners may circumvent this but many utilize lower field strength magnets and generally produce inferior quality images in large patients
   d) non-MRI compatible metal implants in the region of interest (or previous surgery with high speed drills which may leave metal filings): may produce susceptibility artifact which can distort the image in that area
   e) programmable shunt valve (p. 418): most will tolerate up to a 3 T MRI without permanent damage, however, the pressure setting may be altered and therefore should be rechecked after having an MRI for any reason

Aneurysm clips and MRI

MRI concerns in patients with a cerebral aneurysm clip:
1. the danger of the MRI magnetic field causing the aneurysm clip to be pulled or torqued off of the aneurysm or to tear the neck
2. the artifact produced by the metal of the clip in the magnetic field
3. heat generated in the region of the clip: not clinically significant

The more ferromagnetic the clip, the larger the force exerted on it by the magnetic field and the greater the image distortion near the clip.

Stainless steel (SS) is classified as martensitic (ferromagnetic) or austenitic (non-ferromagnetic). Cobalt-based superalloys are non-ferromagnetic and include Elgiloy (Sugita clips), Phynox (Yasargil),

Table 13.5 Magnetic remanence of aneurysm clips[6]

Clip	Type of steel	Magnetic remanence (no units)
MRI compatible: no		
Drake DR 12	martensitic SS	100
Heifetz	17–7PH	44
Mayfield	martensitic SS	74
Scoville	EN-58J	64
MRI compatible: yes		
Olivecrona		0
Sugita	Elgiloy	0
Sugita with loop	gold plated	1
McFadden	Vari-Angle	0
Yasargil	316	0
Yasargil	Phynox	0
Yasargil (old)		1
silver clip		0

and Vari-Angle (McFadden). Essentially all modern aneurysm clips are MRI compatible, but patients clipped before the 1990s may have ferromagnetic clips.

▸ Table 13.5 shows the magnetic remanence of various clips which is related to their ferromagnetic properties. If in doubt at the time of aneurysm surgery, apply the following simple test: non-ferromagnetic clips cannot be lifted or dragged with a small magnet.

13

13.2.10 Hemorrhage on MRI

Because its signal characteristics change with time (and location), blood is one of the most complex entities to interpret on MRI. A mnemonic for the changes in appearance of blood on MRI with time is shown in ▸ Table 13.6. See also intracerebral hemorrhage (p. 1330). Blood, hemosiderin and calcium are dark on GRASS images. FLAIR (p. 229) is the best sequence for detecting SAH on MRI (p. 229).

13.2.11 MRI contrast

Current agents are mostly based on gadolinium (a rare earth metal which is paramagnetic in solutions) include: gadopentatate dimeglumine (Magnevist®), gadodiamide (Omniscan®), gadoversetamide (OptiMARK®), gadobenate dimeglumine (MultiHance®) and gadoteridol (ProHance®).

Adverse reactions:

1. anaphylactic reactions: rare (prevalence: 0.03–0.1%)
2. nephrotoxicity: incidence is lower than with iodinated agents used with angiograms or CT and x-ray contrast
3. nephrogenic systemic fibrosis (NSF): a rare, but serious illness characterized by fibrosis of skin, joints and other organs, which is associated with certain gadolinium containing agents given to patients with severe renal failure (most were on dialysis). ✖ Gadolinium is now relatively contraindicated with a GFR of 30–60 ml/min, and is contraindicated with GFR < 30.[7] Safest agents: Dotarem, Gadovist and ProHance.[8] Contrast agents with a linear structure appear to be associated with a higher risk of NSF and include: Omniscan, Multihance, Magnevist and OptiMARK. In patients with end-stage renal disease, the risk is ≈ 2.4% per gadolinium study[9]
4. gadolinium allergy: use the same allergy prep as for iodine allergy (p. 221)
5. as of the time of publication of this book, the FDA is investigating the risk of accumulation of gadolinium in brain tissue after repeated MRI scans using gadolinium based contrast agents (GBCAs).[10] In the meantime, the FDA is recommending that health-care professionals consider

Table 13.6 Variation of brain MRI signal characteristics of intraparenchymal blood over time

Phase	Approximate time after onset	T1 MRI	T2 MRI	Mnemonic[a]
Hyperacute	0-6 hrs[b]	I	B	I be
Acute	6-72 hrs	I	D	iddy
Early subacute	3-7 d	B	D	biddy
Late subacute	7-14 d	B	B	baby
Chronic	> 2 weeks	D	D	doodoo

[a] Mnemonic: B (bright or hyperintense compared to brain), D (dark or hypointense), I (isointense)
[b] Some authors consider up to about 24 hrs as hyperacute

limiting the use of GBCAs to situations where the additional information provided by the contrast is absolutely necessary

6. see also issues related to pregnancy (p. 230)

13.2.12 Magnetic resonance angiography (MRA)

There are 2 ways to obtain an MRA

- Gadolinium enhanced: usually for extracranial vessels (e.g. carotids)
- Noncontrast images using flow related enhancement techniques (most common: 2D time of flight (2D TOF)). Usually for intracranial vessels. Anything that appears bright on T1WI will also show up on MRA, but doesn't necessarily represent blood flow. This includes fat and fat-laden macrophages in an area of old stroke. Using fat-sat T1WI can mitigate this. Has some utility in screening for aneurysms (p. 1161), and for angiographically occult vascular malformations (p. 1246). High-flow AVMs are hard to resolve because arterialized veins can appear similar to arteries.

13.2.13 Diffusion-weighted imaging (DWI) and perfusion-imaging (PWI)

13

Diffusion-weighted imaging

Primary uses: early detection of ischemia (stroke) and differentiating active MS plaques from old ones. DWI is sensitive to random Brownian motion of water molecules.

Two images are generated, an apparent diffusion coefficient (ADC) map (based on a number of variables (time, slice orientation...)), and a trace image (the actual DWI).[11] Freely diffusing water (e.g. in CSF) appears dark on DWI.

The DWI is based on a T2WI, and anything that is bright on T2WI can also be bright on DWI (so-called "shine-through"). Since bright areas on DWI can represent either restricted dffusion or T2 "shine-through." ∴ check the ADC map: if the area is black on the ADC map, then this likely represents true restricted diffusion (recent infarct is the most common etiology).

✱ Intraparenchymal areas of bright signal on DWI that are not bright on the ADC map are abnormal and represent regions of restricted diffusion such as acute stroke.

Differential diagnosis of areas of increased signal (bright) on DWI:

1. ischemic brain: *acute* stroke and areas with hypoperfusion (penumbra). While restricted diffusion usually indicates irreversible cell injury (death), it can sometimes indicate tissue that is just near cell death (penumbra). Acute brain ischemia can light up within minutes.[12,11] The DWI abnormality will persist for ≈ 1 month. The ADC map usually normalizes after ≈ 1 week
2. cerebral abscess (p. 323): DWI = bright, ADC = dark
3. *active* MS plaque (old plaques will not be bright)
4. some tumors: most tumors are dark on DWI, but highly cellular tumors may have decreased diffusion (bright on DWI) (e.g. epidermoids, some meningiomas...)

Other possible uses of DWI:

TIAs: some, but not all,[13] are associated with DWI abnormalities. However, factors other than focal ischemia (e.g. global ischemia, hypoglycemia, status epilepticus...) can produce ADC decline and the DWI images must therefore be interpreted in relation to the clinical setting.[11]

DWI may also be able to distinguish cytotoxic from vasogenic edema (p. 90).[14,15]

Perfusion-weighted MRI

Provides information related to the perfusion status of the microcirculation. PWI is the most sensitvie study for ischemia of the brain (more sensitive than DWI and FLAIR which primarily show *infarcted* tissue). There are several methods currently in use; the bolus-contrast approach is the most widely employed.[11] Ultrafast gradient imaging is used to follow the gradual reduction to normal following administration of contrast (usually gadolinium). A signal wash-out curve is derived and is compared to contrast in an artery. In practical terms, PWI is not widely used because of technical challenges. Time-to-peak and mean-transit-time are 2 common parameters that are displayed (higher signal = longer times beyond normal).

DWI and PWI mismatch

DWI and PWI may be combined to locate areas of diffusion-perfusion mismatch (deficit on PWI that exceeds the zone of diffusion deficit on DWI), thus identifying salvageable brain tissue at risk of infarction – "penumbra" (p.1202) – e.g. to screen for potential candidates for thrombolytic therapy.[16]

13.2.14 Magnetic resonance spectroscopy (MRS)

General information

This section specifically covers proton (H+) MRS which can be performed on almost any MRI scanner (especially units ≥ 1.5 T) with the appropriate software. Spectroscopy of other nuclei (e.g. phosphorous) can be evaluated only with specialized equipment.

Single voxel MRS

General information

A small area is selected on the "scout" MRI and the spectroscopic peaks for that region are displayed in resonance as a function of parts-per-million (ppm). Since only small regions are selected, may be subject to "sampling" error.

Clinically important characteristic peaks are delineated in ▶ Table 13.7.

Table 13.7 Important peaks on proton MRS

Moiety	Resonance (ppm)	Description
lipid	0.5–1.5	slightly overlaps lactate peak at TE ≈ 35
lactate	1.3	a couplet peak. Not present in normal brain. End product of anaerobic glycolysis, ∴ a marker of hypoxia. Present in: ischemia, infection, demyelinating disease, inborn errors of metabolism… At higher TE (e.g. TE = 144), the peak inverts which can help distinguish it from the lipid peak
N-acetyl aspartate (NAA)	2	a neuronal marker. Normally the tallest peak (higher than Cr or Cho). ↓ in ≈ all focal and regional brain abnormalities (tumor, MS, epilepsy, Alzheimer's disease, abscess, brain injury…)
creatine (Cr)	3[a]	useful primarily as a reference for choline. Higher in grey matter than white matter
choline (Cho)	3.2	marker of membrane synthesis. ↑ in neoplasms and some rare conditions of increased cell growth & in the developing brain. ✱ Stroke is low in choline

[a]Cr has another less important peak

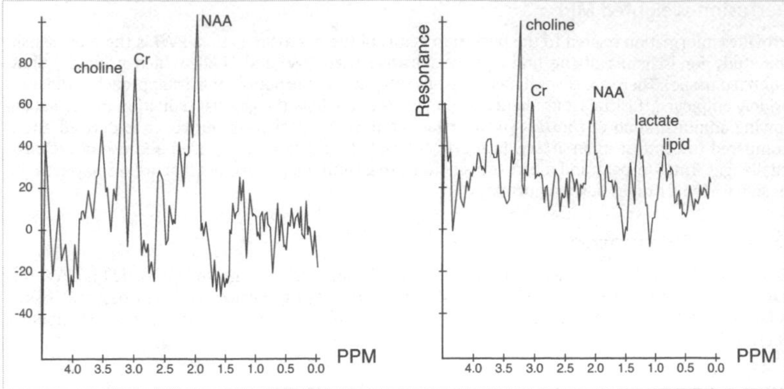

Fig. 13.1 Proton MRS of (A) normal brain, and (B) high grade glioma

Illustrative patterns

Normal brain: See ▶ Fig. 13.1.

Tumor: See ▶ Fig. 13.1. ↓ NAA, ↑ lactate, ↑ lipid, ↑ choline (rule of thumb: with gliomas, the higher the choline, the higher the grade up to grade 3, thereafter necrosis reduces relative choline levels and the lipid peak may be utilized).

Stroke: ↑ lactate peak predominates. Choline is characteristically low.

Abscess[17]: Reduced NAA, Cr & choline peaks, and "atypical peaks" (succinate, acetate…) from bacterial synthesis is pathognomonic for abscess (not always present). Lactate may be elevated.

Multiple sclerosis: Bland pattern. NAA slightly reduced. Lactate and lipid slightly elevated. Choline not elevated.

Possible uses of MRS

13

1. differentiating abscess from neoplasm
2. post-op enhancement vs. recurrence of tumor
3. distinguishing tumor from MS plaques: occasionally cannot be differentiated
4. in AIDS: may be able to help differentiate toxo from lymphoma from PML (PML: ↓ NAA, no significant increase in choline, lactate or lipid)
5. the promise of differentiating tumor infiltration from edema has not materialized
6. some utility in distinguishing tumor from radiation necrosis (p. 1560)
7. large inositol peak may distinguish hemangiopericytoma from meningioma[18])

Multi-voxel MRS

Color coded scan with selected overlay for NAA, choline… one at a time. May reduce risk of sampling error.

13.2.15 Diffusion tensor imaging (DTI) MRI and white matter tracts

AKA diffusion tensor tractography (DTT) MRI. An MRI technique that demonstrates *white matter tracts* by exploiting the difference in diffusion parallel to the nerve axons that comprise white matter tracts from diffusion perpendicular to their course.

Available only with specialized software for specific MRI scanners.

Contraindications are same as for MRI in general (p. 230).

Probably most useful to permit planning surgical approaches that minimize disruption of critical white matter tracts during intraparenchymal brain surgery for deep lesions, especially when a lesion (e.g. tumor, AVM, cerebral hemorrhage…) may displace these tracts from their expected position.

The major divisions of white matter tracts demonstrable by DTT MRI are (▶ Fig. 13.2):

- Projection fibers: tend to be oriented rostro-caudally
  - Corticospinal tract coalesces as corona radiata funnels into internal capsule and forms pyramidal tract

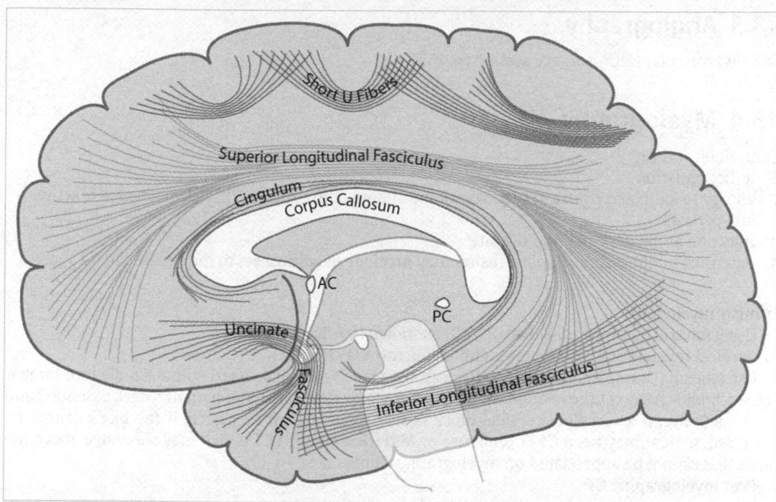

Fig. 13.2 White matter tracts (color conventions for DTI are not used in this anatomic diagram)

- Commisural fibers: medio-laterally oriented, connecting the cerebral hemispheres
  - Corpus callosum
  - Anterior commisure
  - Posterior commisure
- Association fibers: connect regions within the same hemisphere
  - U-fibers: connect adjacent gyri
  - Long association fibers: connect more distant areas
    - Optic radiations: connect lateral geniculate bodies to visual cortex. Pass lateral to the body of the lateral ventricles.
    - Uncinate fasciculus: connects the anterior temporal lobe to the inferior frontal gyrus. Damage can cause language deficits.
    - Superior longitudinal fasciculus (SLF): connects regions of frontal lobe to temporal and occipital lobes. Injury can cause language deficits.
    - Arcuate fasciculus: part of SLF. Classic neuroanatomy teaching: connects the superior and middle frontal gyri (Broca's area (motor speech)) to the superior temporal gyrus (Wernicke's area (language comprehension)). DTI has suggested broader connections, including premotor cortex. Injury causes conduction aphasia
    - Inferior longitudinal fasciculus (ILF): connects temporal and occipital lobes at the level of the optic radiation. Injury can cause deficits in object recognition, visual agnosias, prosopagnosia (face blindness)
    - Cingulum: project from cingulate gyrus to the entorhinal cortex as part of the limbic system

The convention for color coding tracts on DTI images[19]:

- Blue: superior-inferior tracts
- Red: mediolateral (horizontal) tracts
- Green: anterior-posterior tracts

Owing to a number of technical considerations, DTI is somewhat more operator- dependent than conventional MRI.

For surgical planning, the goal is to keep the surgical trajectory roughly parallel (at < 30°angle) to the long axis of the white matter tract that one is trying to preserve (unproven hypothesis[20]).

Surgical "corridors" have been described taking into consideration preservation of white matter tracts:

- Anterior corridor: parallel to association fibers, between the SLF and the cingulum
- Posterior corridor: enters at the parieto-occipital sulcus, passes adjacent to the optic radiations
- Lateral corridor

13

13.3 Angiography

See Endovascular Neurosurgery section (p. 1575).

13.4 Myelography

Contraindications:
1. anticoagulation
2. allergy to iodinated contrast: requires iodine allergy prep (p. 221). NB: risk of adverse reaction still persists
3. infection at the desired puncture site
4. extensive midline lumbar spinal fusion may preclude needle access to the subarachnoid space

Lumbar myelogram

Using iohexol (Omnipaque® 140 or 180) as shown in ▶ Table 12.4.

Cervical myelogram with water soluble contrast via LP

Use iohexol (Omnipaque® 300 or 240) as shown in ▶ Table 12.4. Insert spinal needle into lumbar subarachnoid space, tilt the head of the myelogram table down with the patient's neck extended and then inject dye. If a complete cervical block is seen, have patient flex neck. If the block cannot be traversed, patient may need C1–2 puncture or MRI (first obtain a CT which may show dye above the block that cannot be appreciated on myelography alone).

Post myelographic CT

Increases sensitivity and specificity of myelography (p. 1031). In cases of complete block on myelogram, CT will often show dye distal to the apparent site of the block.

13.5 Radionuclide scanning

13.5.1 Three phase bone scan

Technetium-99 (99mTc) pertechnetate is a radioisotope that may be attached to various substrates for use in bone scanning. It may be used to label polyphosphate (rarely used today), diphosphonate[21] (MDP), or phosphorous (HDP) (the most widely agent used currently). Accumulates in areas of osteoblastic activity.

13

With technetium 99m-HDP, images are obtained immediately after injection (flow phase), at 15 min (blood pooling) and in 4 hours (bone imaging). Cellulitis shows up as increased activity in the first 2 phases, and there is little or diffuse increased activity in the 3rd. Osteomyelitis causes increased uptake in all 3 phases.

Used in evaluation of acute osteomyelitis with sensitivity and specificity of ≈ 95% each, and is usually positive within 2–3 days. False positives can occur in conditions involving increased bone turnover, e.g. fracture, septic arthritis, tumors. False negative can occur in cases with associated bone infarction.

Applications for bone scans include:
1. infection
   a) osteomyelitis of the spine – vertebral osteomyelitis (p. 355) – or skull
   b) discitis (p. 356)
2. tumor
   a) spine metastases (p. 818)
   b) primary bone tumors of the spine (p. 792)
   c) skull tumors (p. 775)
3. diseases involving abnormal bone metabolism
   a) Paget's disease: of the skull or spine (p. 1120)
   b) hyperostosis frontalis interna (p. 780)
4. craniosynostosis (p. 252)
5. fractures: spine or skull
6. "low back problems" (p. 1032): to help identify some of the above conditions

13.5.2 Gallium scan

Nuclear medicine scan with 67Ga citrate which accumulates in areas of inflammation and some malignancies. Utility in neurosurgery for: sarcoidosis (p. 189), chronic vertebral osteomyelitis; see alsocomparison to bone scan (p. 355).

References

[1] Jackson EF, Ginsberg LE, Schomer DF, et al. A Review of MRI Pulse Sequences and Techniques in Neuroimaging. Surg Neurol. 1997; 47:185–199

[2] Anzai Y, Ishikawa M, Shaw DW, Artru A, Yarnykh V, Maravilla KR. Paramagnetic effect of supplemental oxygen on CSF hyperintensity on fluid-attenuated inversion recovery MR images. AJNR Am J Neuroradiol. 2004; 25:274–279

[3] Alemany M, Stenborg A, Terent A, Sonninen P, Raininko R. Coexistence of microhemorrhages and acute spontaneous brain hemorrhage: Correlation with signs of microangiopathy and clinical data. Radiology. 2006; 238:240–247

[4] Shellock FG. Reference Manual for Magnetic Resonance Safety. Salt Lake City, Utah: Amirsys, Inc.; 2003

[5] Edelman RR, Warach S. Magnetic Resonance Imaging (First of Two Parts). N Engl J Med. 1993; 328:708–716

[6] Romner B, Olsson M, Ljunggren B, et al. Magnetic Resonance Imaging and Aneurysm Clips: Magnetic Properties and Image Artifacts. J Neurosurg. 1989; 70:426–431

[7] Kanal E, Barkovich AJ, Bell C, et al. ACR guidance document for safe MR practices: 2007. Am J Roentgenol. 2007; 188:1447–1474

[8] Medicines and Healthcare Products Regulatory Agency. 2007

[9] Deo A, Fogel M, Cowper SE. Nephrogenic systemic fibrosis: a population study examining the relationship of disease development to gadolinium exposure. Clin J Am Soc Nephrol. 2007; 2:264–267

[10] U.S. Food and Drug Administration (FDA). FDA Drug Safety Communication: FDA evaluating the risk of brain deposits with repeated use of gadolinium-based contrast agents for magnetic resonance imaging (MRI). 2015

[11] Fisher M, Albers GW. Applications of diffusion-perfusion magnetic resonance imaging in acute ischemic stroke. Neurology. 1999; 52:1750–1756

[12] Prichard JW, Grossman RI. New reasons for early use of MRI in stroke. Neurology. 1999; 52:1733–1736

[13] Ay H, Buonanno FS, Rordorf G, et al. Normal diffusion-weighted MRI during stroke-like deficits. Neurology. 1999; 52:1784–1792

[14] Ay H, Buonanno FS, Schaefer PW, et al. Posterior Leukoencephalopathy Without Severe Hypertension: Utility of Diffusion-Weighted MRI. Neurology. 1998; 51:1369–1376

[15] Schaefer PW, Buonanno FS, Gonzalez RG, Schwamm LH. Diffusion-Weighted Imaging Discriminates Between Cytotoxic and Vasogenic Edema in a Patient with Eclampsia. Stroke. 1997; 28:1082–1085

[16] Marks MP, Tong DC, Beaulieu C, et al. Evaluation of Early Reperfusion and IV tPA Therapy Using Diffusion- and Perfusion-Weighted MRI. Neurology. 1999; 52:1792–1798

[17] Martinez-Perez I, Moreno A, Alonso J, Aguas J, Conesa G, Capdevila A, Arus C. Diagnosis of brain abscess by magnetic resonance spectroscopy. Report of two cases. J Neurosurg. 1997; 86:708–713

[18] Barba I, Moreno A, Martinez-Perez I, et al. Magnetic resonance spectroscipy of brain hemangiopericytomas: high myoinositol concentrations and discrimination from meningiomas. J Neurosurg. 2001; 94:55–60

[19] Douek P, Turner R, Pekar J, Patronas N, Le Bihan D. MR color mapping of myelin fiber orientation. J Comput Assist Tomogr. 1991; 15:923–929

[20] Kassam AB, Labib MA, Bafaquh M, et. al. Part I: The challenge of functional preservation: an integrated systems approach using diffusion-weighted, image guided, exoscopic-assisted, transsulcal radial corridors. Innovative Neurosurgery. 2015

[21] Handa J, Yamamoto I, Morita R, et al. 99mTc-Polyphosphate and 99mTc-Diphosphonate Bone Scintigraphy in Neurosurgical Practice. Surg Neurol. 1974; 2:307–310

14 Electrodiagnostics

14.1 Electroencephalogram (EEG)

14.1.1 General information

The primary use of EEG is in the diagnosis and management of seizure disorders. Non-convulsive use of EEG is essentially limited to monitoring for burst suppression (see below) (e.g. induced barbiturate coma) or for differential diagnosis of diffuse encephalopathy, including:

1. differentiating psychogenic unresponsiveness from organic: a normal EEG indicates either psychiatric unresponsiveness or locked-in syndrome
2. non-convulsive status epilepticus (seizures): absence or complex partial status
3. subclinical focal abnormalities: e.g. PLEDs (see below), focal slowing…
4. specific patterns diagnostic for certain pathologies: e.g.:
   a) periodic lateralizing epileptiform discharges (PLEDs): may occur with any acute focal cerebral insult (e.g. herpes simplex encephalitis (HSE), abscess, tumor, embolic infarct): seen in 85% of cases of HSE (onset 2–5 d after presentation), if bilateral is ≈ diagnostic of HSE
   b) subacute sclerosing panencephalitis (SSPE) (pathognomonic pattern): periodic high voltage with 4–15 secs separation with accompanying body jerks, no change with painful stimulation (differential diagnosis includes PCP overdose)
   c) Creutzfeldt-Jakob disease (p.367): myoclonic jerks. EEG → bilateral sharp wave 1.5–2 per second (early → slowing; later→ triphasic). May resemble PLEDs, but are reactive to painful stimulation (most PLEDs are not)
   d) triphasic waves: not really specific. May be seen in hepatic encephalopathy, post-anoxia, and hyponatremia
5. objective measure of severity of encephalopathy: usually used for anoxic encephalopathy (e.g. periodic spikes with seizures indicates < 5% chance of normal neurologic outcome, with high mortality). Alpha coma, burst suppression, and electrocerebral silence are all poor prognosticators
6. differentiating hydranencephaly (p.288) from severe hydrocephalus
7. as a clinical confirmatory test in the determination of brain death (p.310)

14.1.2 Common EEG rhythms.

Common EEG rhythms are shown in ▶ Table 14.1.

14.1.3 Burst suppression

Isoelectric intervals interrupted by bursts of 8–12 Hz electrical activity that diminish to 1–4 Hz prior to electrical silence.[1] Often used as an endpoint for titrating neuroprotective drugs such as barbiturates, propofol…

14.2 Evoked potentials

14.2.1 General information

Evoked potentials are averaged EEG waveforms recorded following repetitive stimulation. The process of averaging nulls-out EEG activity that is not time -locked to the stimulus. Resultant waveforms contain peaks that are named N (negative – upward deflection) or P (positive – downward deflection) followed by the latency in milliseconds to the onset of the peak.

Table 14.1 Common EEG rhythms

Rhythm	Symbol	Frequency
delta	Δ	0–3 Hz
theta	θ	4–7 Hz
alpha	α	8–13 Hz
beta	β	> 13 Hz

14.2.2 Sensory evoked potentials (SEP)

General information

May use electrical stimulation of peripheral nerves (somatosensory or (SSEP)), auditory clicks through earphones (auditory or AEP, AKA BAER (brainstem auditory evoked response)) or flashing lights through goggles (visual EP or VEP).

Evoked potentials are most commonly used by neurosurgeons for intraoperative monitoring purposes. SSEP (especially from median nerve stimulation) also has prognostic significance in cervical spondylotic myelopathy[2] although use for this purpose is limited.

Typical waveforms

Abbreviations

Abbreviations used below: BAER = brain stem auditory evoked response; UE/LE SSEP = upper/lower extremity somatosensory evoked potential; PR VER = pattern reversal visual evoked response which requires patient cooperation and visual attention as opposed to flash VER which may even be done through closed eyelids. See also references.[3,4]

14.2.3 Intra-operative evoked potentials

General information

EPs may be used for intra-operative monitoring (e.g. monitoring hearing during resection of vestibular schwannomas, or monitoring SSEPs during some spine surgery), however, their delayed nature often makes them of limited usefulness in avoiding acute intra-operative injury. A 10% increased latency of

Table 14.2 Typical stimulus values for intra-op evoked potentials

Test	Stimulus			Comment
	Freq (Hz)	Duration (mcS)	Magnitude	
BAER	23.5	150	85–100 dB	rarefaction usually better than compression
UE SSEP (median nerve at wrist)	4.7	300–700	up to 50 mA	supramaximal stimulus (sensory threshold + motor threshold)
LE SSEP (posterior tibial at ankle)	4.7	300–700	up to 100 mA	supramaximal stimulus
PR VER	1.97			16 × 16 checks, 1.6 cm each, at 1 meter (subtends 55" arc visual angle)

Table 14.3 Input characteristics for acquiring evoked potentials

Test	Analysis				Electrode derivations
	Input filter (Hz)	Sensitive (mcV)	Duration (mS)	Reps	
BAER	150–3000	25	15	1500	$M_1{}^a$-C_ZZ, $M_2{}^*$-C_Z, ground = FZ
UE SSEP	30–3000	50	55–60	600	F_Z-Erb's point, C_{V7}-F_{PZ}, C_3-F_{PZ}, C_3'-NC (non-cephalic, e.g. shoulder)
LE SSEP	30–3000	50	60	600	popliteal fossa (front to back), C_Z-F_{PZ}, back (L_5-T_{12}) (difficult in obese or elderly), C_I-C_C (optional: somatosensory ipsilateral to contralateral)
PR VER	5–100	50	500	100	O_1-A_1, O_Z-A_1, O_2-A_1, O_Z-C_Z

[a]M= mastoid ("i" is ipsilateral to stimulus, and "c" is contralateral)

a major EP peak, or a drop in amplitude of ≥ 50% is significant and should cause the surgeon to assess all variables (retractors, instruments, blood pressure...). Intra-operative SSEPs may also be used to localize primary sensory cortex in anesthetized patients (as opposed to using brain mapping techniques in awake patients) by looking for phase reversal potentialsacross the central sulcus.[5,6]

Brainstem auditory evoked responses (BAER)

AKA auditory brainstem response (ABR), AKA auditory evoked potential (AEP). Auditory clicks are delivered to the patient by earphones. Peaks ▶ Table 14.4). Once used for assistance in diagnosing vestibular schwannomas, their use for intraoperative monitoring is limited and has been largely replaced by direct eighth cranial nerve monitoring which provides more rapid information for the surgeon.

SSEP monitoring during spine surgery

Paralytics actually improve SSEP recordings by reducing muscle artifact, but will abolish the visible twitch that confirms that the stimulus is being received.

Typical stimulus sites: median, ulnar, and tibial nerves. Impulses ascend in the *ipsilateral* posterior column. UE SSEPs travel primarily in the dorsal columns, but LE SSEPs are carried mostly in the dorsolateral fasciculus (p. 72) which is supplied by the *anterior* spinal artery. Thus, UE and LE SSEPs are more sensitive to direct mechanical effects primarily on the posterior spinal cord (sensory) and may remain unchanged with some injuries to the anterior cord (motor), however, LE SSEPs can detect ischemic effects on the anterior cord by virtue of involvement of the anterior spinal artery.

In a personal series of 809 patients,[7] 17 had SSEP degradation, 14 of these (82%) responded to intra-op interventions (see below), and in 13 of these 14 (93%) there were no new deficits. In the 3 that did not respond, 2 had significant new neurologic deficits.

Table 14.4 Evoked potential waveforms (note: values may differ from lab to lab)

Test	Figure	Possible generators
BAER	CM, P1, P2, P3, P4, P5, P6, P7, Mi-CZ, 0.25 uV, 10 mS	CM cochlear microphonic $P_1$1distal VIII nerve, P_2 $_2$proximal VIII or cochlear nucleus, P_3 $_3$lower pons (? superior olivary complex), $P_4$4mid-upper pons, $P_5$5upper pons or inferior colliculus
UE SSEP	C3'-FPZ, P22, P22 early, N19, Cv7-FPZ, N13/P13, N11, EP, Fz-Ep, 2 uV, 10 mS	$N_9$9(on F_Z-E_PP where E_P is Erb's point) AKA EP: entry of volley into distal brachial plexus, N_{11}11(on C_{V7}-F_{PZ}): root entry zone (cervical region), N_{13}13cervicomedullary junction (recorded from C2), N_{19}19primary sensory cortex, P_{22}22(early) motor cortex, P_{22}22(late) IPSP "reaction" to N_{18}18
LE SSEP	Cv7-FPz, N25, N27, 0.25 uV, Cz-FPz, P40, N30, P22, L5-T12, N50, 50 mS	P_{22}2(on L_5-T_{12}): lumbo-sacral plexus, P_{40}4(on C_Z-F_{PZ}): sensory cortex (analogous to N18 in UE SSEP, reversed in polarity for ? reason), N_{27}2(on C_{V7}-F_{PZ}): ? dorsal column nucleus N_{30}30
PR VER	P100, Oz-Cz, 5 uV, 500 mS	P_{100} striate & pre-striate occipital cortex, with contributions from thalamocortical volleys

Table 14.5 Normal values for evoked potentials[a] (note: values may differ from lab to lab)

Test	Parameters measured	-- Normal values --		Comment
		Mean	+ 2.5 std dev	
BAER	I-V peak latency	4.01 mS	4.63 mS	
	I-III peak latency	2.15 mS	2.66 mS	prolongation suggests lesion between pons & colliculus, often **vestibular schwannoma**
	V absolute latency	5.7 mS	6.27 mS	
	III-V peak latency			prolongation suggests lesion between lower pons & midbrain, may be seen in M.S.
UE SSEP	$N_9$9-N_{18}18 peak latency	9.38 mS	11.35 mS	
LE SSEP	P_{22}22-P_{40}40 peak latency	15.62 mS	20.82 mS	
	P_{40}40 absolute latency	37.20 mS	44.16 mS	
PR VER	P_{100}10 absolute latency		+ 3 S.D.	
	P_{100} inter-eye difference	8–10 mS		Inter-eye difference is more sensitive with full field stimulation. Monocular defect suggests conduction defect in that optic nerve anterior to chiasm (e.g. M.S., glaucoma, compression retinal degeneration). Bilateral defect does not localize.

[a]normal values in boldface are critical values used as cutoff for abnormal results

Transcranial motor evoked potentials (TCMEPs)

Anesthetic requirements: In addition to EP anesthetic requirements, neuromuscular blockade must be minimized to permit ≥ 2 out of 4 twitches.

AKA motor evoked potentials (MEP): transcranial electrical or magnetic stimulation of motor cortex and descending motor axons with recording of motor potentials from distal spinal cord or muscle groups. Using direct electrical stimulation is limited in awake patients by local pain. Due to the large potentials, the acquisition time is shorter and feedback to the surgeon is almost immediate. However, due to patient movement from the muscle contractions, continuous recording is usually not possible (except with monitoring the response over the spinal cord). Useful for surgery involving the spinal cord (cervical or thoracic), no utility for lumbar spine surgery.Seizures occur rarely, usually in patients with increased seizure risk and with high-rate stimulation frequency.

Contraindications to MEP:
1. history of epilepsy/seizures
2. past surgical skull defects
3. metal in head or neck
4. use special care with implanted electronic devices

Descending evoked potentials (DEP)

(Formerly referred to by the misleading term "neurogenic motor evoked potentials"). Rostral stimulation of the spinal cord with recording of a caudal neurogenic response from the spinal cord or peripheral nerve, or a myogenic response from a distal muscle. DEPs can be mediated primarily by sensory nerves and therefore do not represent true motor potentials. However, shown to be sensitive to spinal cord changes and may be useful when TCMEPs cannot be obtained.

14.2.4 Electrophysiologic monitoring criteria to trigger notification of surgeon

Any of the following:
1. SSEP:
   a) 50% decrease in peak signal amplitude from baseline
   b) increase in peak latency > 10%
   c) complete loss of a waveform
2. TCMEP: sustained 50% decrease in signal amplitude
3. DEP: decrease in signal of > 60%

Interventions for loss or degradation of monitoring signal during spine surgery

When compression is the culprit, the prognosis may be good. Vascular injuries generally do not fare as well.

Options/suggestions include (adapted/excerpted from the "Vitale cheklist"[8]):
1. verify that the change is real (check connections, equipment...)
2. place OR on alert status
   a) announce intraoperative pause and stop the case
   b) eliminate possible distractions (music, unnecessary conversations...)
   c) "muster the troops": the attending anesthesiologist, senior neurologist or neurophysiologist and experienced nurse are called to the room. Consult a surgical colleague if necessary
3. anesthetic/metabolic considerations
   a) optimize mean arterial pressure (MAP usually > 85 mm Hg preferred)
   b) check hematocrit for anemia (could contribute to cord ischemia)
   c) optimize blood pH (rule out acidemia) and pCO_2
   d) normalize patient body temperature
   e) check anesthetic technical factors: assess extent of paralytics
   f) discuss possibility of "Stagnara wake up test" (see below) with attending anesthesiologist and scrub nurse
4. technical/neurophysiologic considerations
   a) rule-out 60 Hz. interference from other equipment (OR table, C-arm, microscope... anything with a plug)
   b) verify that stimulating electrodes recording leads are making good contact

14.3 NCS/EMG

14

14.3.1 General information

Electrodiagnostic studies of peripheral nerves consist of two parts:
1. conduction measurements: typically referred to as "NCV" (nerve conduction velocity) but technically should be called NCS (nerve conduction studies) since amplitude, latency and duration of motor & sensory nerves are also evaluated
2. electromyogram (EMG) AKA "needle exam" (see below)

14.3.2 Electromyography

General information

There are 3 phases of an EMG exam:

Phase 1 – insertional activity: the electric response of the muscle to mechanical irritation caused by small movements of the needle

Phase 2 – spontaneous activity: in muscle at rest
1. normal: silent with stationary needle once insertional activity has subsided
2. spontaneous activity: independently produced electrical activity. Usually abnormal (although sometimes seen in normal volunteers).
   a) after denervation (secondary to a nerve injury) or muscle injury:
      - positive sharp waves (PSW)
      - fibrillation potentials (AKA fibrillations or fibs): action potentials arising from *single* muscle fibers. Detectable on EMG; not visible to the naked eye, c.f. fasciculations (p. 505). Earliest onset 7–10 days after denervation, sometimes not for 3–4 weeks. If the nerve recovers, it

may reinnervate the muscle, but with larger motor units resulting in longer duration and decreased numbers
   b) myotonic discharges ("dive bomber" sound on speaker monitor)
   c) complex repetitive discharge (CRD): ephaptic conduction of groups of adjacent muscle fibers. Occurs in neuropathic or myopathic disorders
   d) fasciculation potentials: nonspecific, but typically associated with motor neuron disease (ALS) (p. 183)
   e) other less common spontaneous activity includes: myokymic, neuromytonic and cramp discharges

Phase 3 – volitional activity: evaluated with minimal volitional effort and maximal effort
1. motor unit action potential (MUAP) analysis: includes evaluation of motor unit amplitude, duration, polyphasia and stability. Generally increase amplitude and duration suggest a disorder of the LMN, and reduction of amplitude and duration suggests a primary myopathic disorder
2. with minimal volitional effort. Two possible abnormal findings
   a) reduced recruitment (or fast firing) is always indicative of a neuropathic process
   b) early or increased recruitment: indicative of a myopathic process
3. with maximal effort

Definitions

SNAP: sensory nerve action potential. Key concept: since the ganglion of the sensory nerves lies within the neural foramen, preganglionic lesions (injury to the nerve root *proximal* to the neural foramen, e.g. root compression by herniated disc or root avulsion) does not affect the cell body, and therefore the distal SNAP is unaffected.[9] Postganglionic lesions (distal to the neural foramen, e.g. peripheral nerve injury) reduces SNAP amplitudes and/or slows the sensory conduction velocity.

F-wave: stimulation of a nerve causes orthodromic and antidromic conduction. Some anterior horn cells that are stimulated antidromically will fire orthodromically producing the F-wave. F-wave latency may be prolonged in multilevel radiculopathy (not sensitive). Most helpful in evaluating proximal root slowing, e.g. GBS (p. 184).

H-reflex: practical ≈ only in S1 nerve root, similar information to the ankle jerk. Stimulation of Ia afferent fibers passes through a monosynaptic connection causing an orthodromic alpha-motor action potential that can be measured in the triceps surae.

Volitional activity: the motor unit action potential (MUAP) can be assessed only with voluntary muscle contraction by the patient. Components of the MUAP measured include: amplitude, rise time, duration, and number of phases (crossings of the baseline).

Polyphasic potentials: MUAPs with > 4 phases. Normally comprise < 15% of MUAPs. Following a nerve injury, abnormally increased polyphasic potentials can be seen 6–8 weeks after reinnervation begins, gradually increase over several months, and then begin to wane (as firing becomes more synchronous).

Myotonia: there are a number of myotonic conditions, including myotonic dystrophy in which there is sustained contraction of the muscle. Classic EMG finding: "dive bomber" sound due to myotonic discharges.

EMG for radiculopathy

EMG pearls for the neurosurgeon

General principles:
- EMG – if a reliable motor exam can be done, the EMG will not likely add any information. A normal motor exam will usually be associated with a normal EMG
- EMG is not extremely sensitive for radiculopathy (e.g. irritative radiculopathy might not be picked up), this is more likely in the cervical region than lumbar. However, when abnormal, EMG is very specific
- EMG is best reserved for cases with documented weakness where additional localizing/prognostic information is needed, or when the patient's strength cannot be reliably assessed (inability to cooperate, functional overlay…)
- Timing
  - It takes about 3 weeks after onset of radiculopathy for the EMG to reliably show any findings
  - "Acute changes" begin at about 3 weeks and can last up to about 6 months
  - Chronic changes can be seen starting at about 6 months, and may persist indefinitely

Cervical EMG:
- EMG is most helpful for nerve roots C5-T1. There are no good muscles to reliably test C3-4, and compression here may cause findings in lower nerve roots

Lumbar EMG:
- If lumbar MRI is normal in a patient with evidence of motor weakness (e.g. foot drop), do an EMG to look for peripheral neuropathy (again, a good motor exam can give the same info). If the EMG is negative for peripheral neuropathy (e.g. peroneal nerve palsy) then do an MRI (or CT) of abdomen and pelvis to look for pelvic floor tumor

Findings

Include spontaneous activity (fibs & PSWs, see above).

The earliest possible finding (within 2–3 d) is reduced recruitment with volitional activity, but this occurs only with significant compression of motor fibers.

EMG is useful if there is a concern about possible overlapping peripheral neuropathy (e.g. carpal tunnel syndrome vs. C6 radiculopathy).

EMG criteria for radiculopathy

1. fibrillations and/or positive sharp waves in at least 2 muscles innervated by a single nerve root in question, but by 2 different *peripheral* nerves
2. abnormal paraspinals: this supports the diagnosis, but is not required since paraspinals will be normal in ≈ 50%

Lumbar radiculopathy from herniated disc

With radiculopathy, SNAP is usually normal (see above). Paraspinal muscle fibrillations may occur. Accuracy in predicting level of involvement[10] is ≈ 84%.

Foot drop: the short head of the biceps femoris in the LE is the first muscle innervated by the peroneal division of the sciatic nerve at or just above the popliteal fossa just after the nerve splits off from the sciatic nerve. In cases e.g. of foot drop it is a good muscle to test to determine if there is a peroneal neuropathy vs. a more proximal lesion (i.e. above the popliteal fossa).

Findings with healing radiculopathy (e.g. following discectomy or spontaneous healing):
- motor potentials return first (if nerve injury were "complete", it would take a month to return)
- if lost, sensory potentials return last or may not return
- following laminectomy, paraspinal potentials may no longer be useful for EMG because cutting the muscles during surgery alters their electrical signals resulting in effective denervation due to muscle injury. Fibs and PSWs decrease in amplitude over time but may remain present indefinitely

EMG in plexopathy

Reduction of SNAP with *no paraspinal* muscle fibrillations (the dorsal rami exit proximally to innervate the paraspinals, and are involved ≈ *only* with root lesions).

EMG in nerve root avulsion

Produces muscles weakness and sensory loss with normal SNAP since the lesion is proximal to the dorsal root ganglion (where the cell bodies for the sensory nerves are located).

References

[1] Donnegan JH, Blitt CD. In: The Electroencephalogram. Monitoring in Anesthesia and Critical Care Medicine. New York: Churchill Livingstone; 1985:323–343

[2] Holly LT, Matz PG, Anderson PA, Groff MW, Heary RF, Kaiser MG, Mummaneni PV, Ryken TC, Choudhri TF, Vresilovic EJ, Resnick DK. Clinical prognostic indicators of surgical outcome in cervical spondylotic myelopathy. J Neurosurg: Spine. 2009; 11:112–118

[3] Chiappa KH. Evoked Potentials in Clinical Medicine (First of Two Parts). N Engl J Med. 1982; 306:1140–1150

[4] Chiappa KH. Evoked Potentials in Clinical Medicine (Second of Two Parts). N Engl J Med. 1982; 306:1205–1211

[5] Gregori EM, Goldring S. Localization of Function in the Excision of Lesions from the Sensorimotor Region. J Neurosurg. 1984; 61:1047–1054

[6] Woolsey CN, Erickson TC, Gibson WE. Localization in Somatic Sensory and Motor Areas of Human Cerebral Cortex as Determined by Direct Recording of Evoked Potentials and Electrical Stimulation. J Neurosurg. 1979; 51:476–506

[7] Roh M, Wilson-Holden T, Padberg A. The utility of SSEP monitoring during cervical spine surgery: How often does it prompt intervention and affect outcome. 2002

[8] Vitale MG, Skaggs DL, Pace GI, Wright ML, Matsumoto H, Anderson RCE, Brockmeyer DL, Dormans JP, Emans JB, Erickson MA, Flynn JM, Glotzbecker MP, Ibrahim KN, Lewis SJ, Luhmann SJ, Mendiratta A, Richards BS, III, Sanders JO, Shah SA, Smith JT, Song KM, Sponseller PD, Sucato DJ, Roye DP, Lenke LG. Best Practices in Intraoperative Neuromonitoring in Spine Deformity Surgery: Development of an Intraoperative Checklist to Optimize Response. Spine Deformity. 2014; 2:333–339

[9] Benecke R, Conrad B. The distal sensory nerve action potential as a diagnostic tool for the differentiation of lesions in dorsal roots and peripheral nerves. J Neurol. 1980; 223:231–239

[10] Young A, Getty J, Jackson A, et al. Variations in the Pattern of Muscle Innervation by the L5 and S1 Nerve Roots. Spine. 1983; 8:616–624

Part IV

Developmental Anomalies

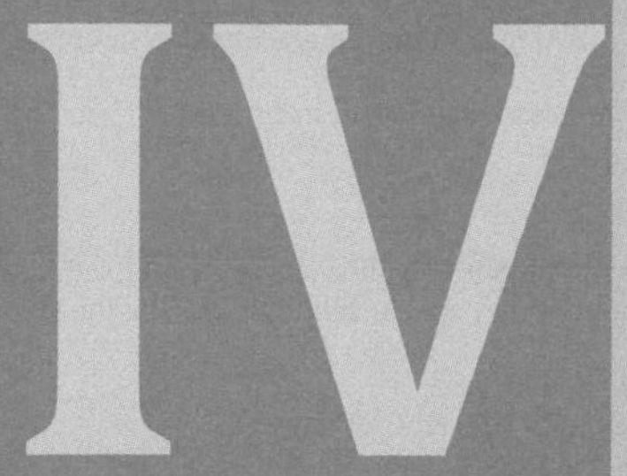

15 Primary Intracranial Anomalies

15.1 Arachnoid cysts, intracranial

15.1.1 General information

Key concepts

- a congenital abnormality, most common in middle fossa, cerebellopontine angle (CPA), suprasellar region, and posterior fossa
- most are asymptomatic (i.e. an incidental finding) except in the suprasellar region
- imaging often shows remodeling of bone; imaging characteristics exactly mimic CSF on CT or MRI in most cases
- recommendation for incidentally discovered arachnoid cyst in adults: a single follow-up imaging study in 6–8 months is usually adequate to rule-out any increase in size. Subsequent studies only if concerning symptoms develop

AKA leptomeningeal cysts, distinct from posttraumatic leptomeningeal cysts (AKA growing skull fractures) (p.915), and unrelated to infection. Arachnoid cysts (AC) are congenital lesions that arise during development from splitting of arachnoid membrane (thus they are technically intra-arachnoid cysts) and contain fluid that is usually identical to CSF. They do not communicate with the ventricles or subarachnoid space. May be unloculated or may have septations. Typically lined with meningothelial cells positive for epithelial membrane antigen (EMA) and negative for carcinoembryonic antigen (CEA). AC may also occur in the spinal canal.

"Temporal lobe agenesis syndrome" is a label that had been used to describe the findings with middle cranial fossa ACs. This term is now obsolete since brain volumes on each side are actually the same,[1] bone expansion and shift of brain matter account for the parenchyma that appears to be replaced by the AC.

Two types of histological findings[2]:

1. "simple arachnoid cysts": arachnoid lining with cells that appear to be capable of active CSF secretion. Middle fossa cysts seem to be exclusively of this type
2. cysts with more complex lining which may also contain neuroglia, ependyma, and other tissue types

15.1.2 Epidemiology of intracranial arachnoid cysts

15

Incidence: 5 per 1000 in autopsy series. Comprise ≈ 1% of intracranial masses.

Male:female ratio is 4:1. More common on the left side.

Bilateral arachnoid cysts may occur in Hurler syndrome (a mucopolysaccharidosis).

15.1.3 Distribution

Almost all occur in relation to an arachnoid cistern (exception: intrasellar, the only one that is extradural, ▶ Table 15.1).

Epidermoid cysts in the cerebellopontine angle (CPA) may mimic an arachnoid cyst, but are high signal on DWI MRI.

See also differential diagnosis of midline posterior fossa arachnoid cysts (p.256).

15.1.4 Presentation

Most ACs are asymptomatic. Those that become symptomatic usually do so in early childhood.[4] The presentation varies with location of the cyst, and oftentimes appear mild considering the large size of some.

Typical presentations are shown in ▶ Table 15.2 [4] and include:

1. symptoms of intracranial hypertension (elevated ICP): H/A, N/V, lethargy
2. seizures
3. sudden deterioration:

Table 15.1 Distribution of arachnoid cysts[3]

Location	%
sylvian fissure	49%
CPA	11%
supracollicular	10%
vermian	9%
sellar & suprasellar	9%
interhemispheric	5%
cerebral convexity	4%
clival	3%

Table 15.2 Typical presentations of arachnoid cysts

Middle fossa cysts	Suprasellar cysts with hydrocephalus	Diffuse supra- or infratentorial cysts with hydrocephalus
seizures headache hemiparesis	intracranial hypertension craniomegaly developmental delay visual loss precocious puberty bobble-head doll syndrome	intracranial hypertension craniomegaly developmental delay

a) due to hemorrhage (into cyst or subdural compartment): middle fossa cysts are notorious for hemorrhage due to tearing of bridging veins. Some sports organizations do not allow participation in contact sports for these patients
b) due to rupture of the cyst
4. as a focal protrusion of the skull
5. with focal signs/symptoms of a space occupying lesion
6. incidental finding discovered during evaluation for unrelated condition
7. suprasellar cysts may additionally present with[5]:
   a) hydrocephalus (probably due to compression of the third ventricle)
   b) endocrine symptoms: occurs in up to 60%. Includes precocious puberty
   c) head bobbing (the so-called "bobble-head doll syndrome"[6]): considered suggestive of suprasellar cysts, but occurs in as few as 10%
   d) visual impairment

15

15.1.5 Evaluation

General information

Routine evaluation with CT or MRI is usually satisfactory. Further evaluation with CSF contrast or flow studies (cisternograms, ventriculograms...) are only occasionally necessary for the diagnosis of midline suprasellar and posterior fossa lesions[4]; for Differential diagnosis, see Intracranial cysts (p. 1374); see ▶ Fig. 15.1 for the classification scheme of Galassi et al for middle fossa cysts.

CT scan

Smooth bordered non-calcified extraparenchymal cystic mass with density similar to CSF and no enhancement with IV contrast. Expansion of nearby bone by remodelling is usually seen, confirming their chronic nature. Often associated with ventriculomegaly (in 64% of supratentorial and 80% of infratentorial cysts).

Convexity or middle fossa cysts exert mass effect on adjacent brain and may compress ipsilateral lateral ventricle and cause midline shift. Suprasellar, quadrigeminal plate, and midline posterior-fossa cysts may compress the third and fourth ventricle and cause hydrocephalus by obstructing the foramina of Monro or the Sylvian aqueduct.

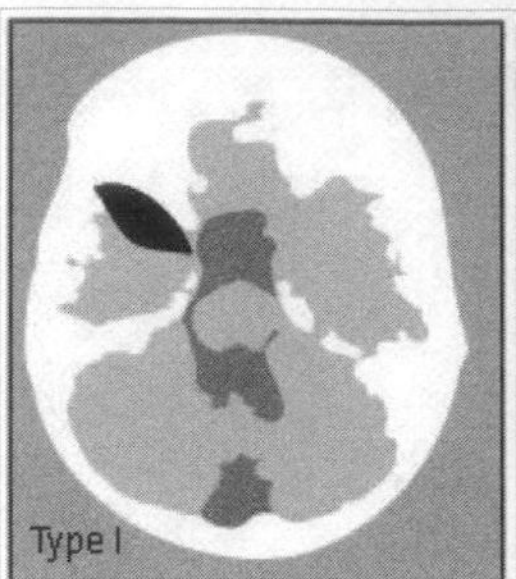

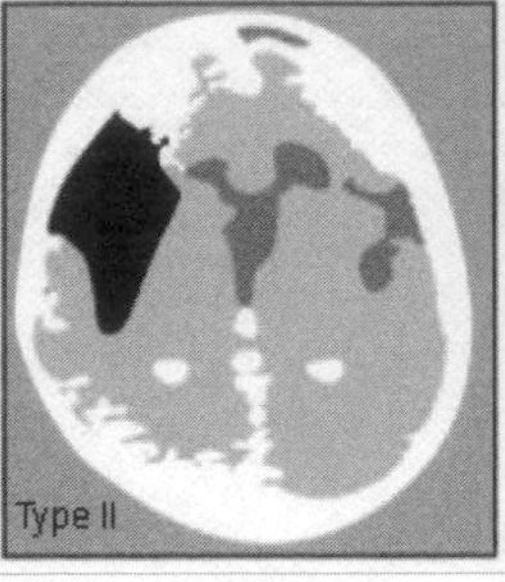

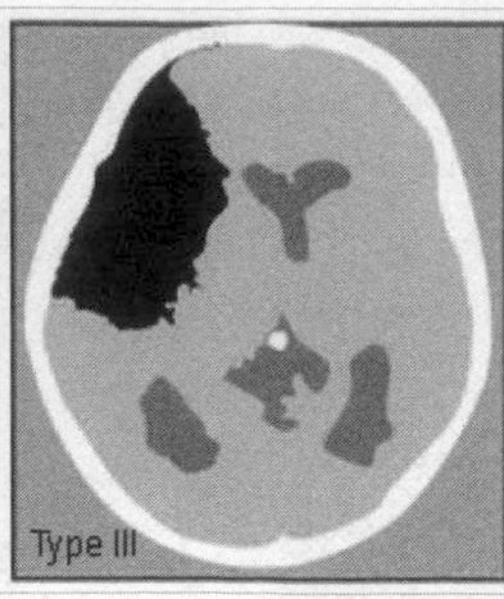

Fig. 15.1 CT Classification of Sylvian fissure arachnoid cysts.[7]
Type I: small, biconvex, located in anterior temporal tip. No mass effect. Communicates with subarachnoid space on water-soluble contrast CT cisternogram (WS-CTC).
Type II: involves proximal and intermediate segments of Sylvian fissure. Completely open insula gives rectangular shape. Partial communication on WS-CTC.
Type III: involves entire Sylvian fissure. Marked midline shift. Bony expansion of middle fossa (elevation of lesser wing of sphenoid, outward expansion of squamous temporal bone). Minimal communication on WS-CTC. Surgical treatment usually does not result in total reexpansion of brain (may approach type II lesion).

MRI

Better than CT in differentiating the CSF contained in arachnoid cysts from the fluid of neoplastic cysts. May also show cyst walls.

Cisternograms and/or ventriculograms

Using either iodinated contrast or radionuclide tracers. Variable rate of opacification has resulted in difficulty correlating results with operative findings. Some cysts are actually diverticula, and may fill with radiotracer or contrast.

15.1.6 Treatment

General information

15

Many (but not all) authors recommend not treating arachnoid cysts that do not cause mass effect or symptoms, regardless of their size and location. For incidentally discovered arachnoid cyst in an adult not considered for surgery: a single follow-up imaging study in 6–8 months is usually adequate to rule-out any changes (since they may grow in size). Subsequent studies may be done if concerning symptoms develop. Pediatric patients may need to be followed until adulthood.

Treatment considerations for cysts (excluding suprasellar cysts)

Surgical treatment options are summarized in ▶ Table 15.3.

Cyst shunting

Probably the best overall treatment. For shunting into peritoneum, use a *low pressure* valve. If there is concurrent ventriculomegaly, one may simultaneously place a ventricular shunt (e.g. through a "Y" connector). Ultrasound, ventriculoscope, or image guidance may assist in locating suprasellar cysts. Shunting of middle fossa ACs may also be accomplished through the lateral ventricle, thus shunting both compartments.[9]

✖ NB: in running the distal shunt tubing from the middle fossa, it should be routed behind the ear (do not tunnel in front of ear to avoid injury to facial nerve – if this anterior route is unavoidable, it may help to solicit the services of a plastic surgeon to help avoid the facial nerve).

Treatment of Suprasellar cysts

These cysts present with some unique treatments options which include:
- transcallosal cystectomy[10]

Table 15.3 Surgical treatment options for arachnoid cysts

Procedure	Advantages	Disadvantages
drainage by needle aspiration or burr hole evacuation	• simple • quick	• high rate of recurrence of cyst and neurologic deficit
craniotomy, excising cyst wall and fenestrating it into basal cisterns	• permits direct inspection of cyst (may help with diagnosis) • loculated cysts (rare) treated more effectively • avoids permanent shunt (in some cases) • allows visualization of bridging vessels (small advantage)	• subsequent scarring may block fenestration allowing reaccumulation of cyst • flow through subarachnoid space may be deficient; many patients develop shunt dependency post-op • significant morbidity and mortality (may be due to abrupt decompression)
endoscopic cyst fenestration through a burr hole[8]	• as above	• as above
shunting of cyst into peritoneum or into vascular system	• definitive treatment • low morbidity/mortality • low rate of recurrence	• patient becomes "shunt dependent" • risk of infection of foreign body (shunt)

- percutaneous ventriculo-cystostomy: procedure of choice of Pierre-Kahn et al.[5] Performed via a paramedian coronal burr hole through the lateral ventricle and foramen of Monro (may be facilitated by using a ventriculoscope[8])
- subfrontal approach (for fenestration or removal): dangerous and ineffective[5]

✖ ventricular drainage is ineffective (actually promotes cyst enlargement) and should not be routinely considered

15.1.7 Outcome

Even following successful treatment a portion of the cyst may remain due to the remodeling of the bone and chronic shift of brain contents. Hydrocephalus may develop following treatment. Endocrinopathies tend to persist even after successful treatment of suprasellar cysts.

15.2 Craniofacial development

15.2.1 Normal development

Fontanelles

Anterior fontanelle: the largest fontanelle. Diamond shaped, 4 cm (AP) × 2.5 cm (transverse) at birth. Normally closes by age 2.5 yrs.

Posterior fontanelle :triangular. Normally closes by age 2–3 mos.

Sphenoid and *mastoid fontanelles*: small, irregular. Normally, former closes by age 2–3 mos, latter by age 1 yr.

Cranial vault

Growth: largely determined by growth of brain. 90% of adult head size is achieved by age 1 yr; 95% by age 6 yrs. Growth essentially ceases at age 7 yrs. By end of 2nd yr, bones have interlocked at sutures and further growth occurs by accretion and absorption.

Skull is unilaminar at birth. Diplöe appear by 4th yr and reach a maximum by age 35 yrs (when diploic veins form).

Mastoid process: formation commences by age 2 yrs, air cell formation occurs during 6th yr.

15.2.2 Craniosynostosis

General

Originally called craniostenosis. Incidence: ≈ 0.6/1000 live births.

Primarily a prenatal deformity, postnatal craniosynostosis (CSO) occurs uncommonly (postnatal causes consist primarily of positional alterations which may not represent true synostosis). CSO is rarely associated with hydrocephalus (HCP).[11] The assertion that CSO may follow CSF shunting for HCP is unproven. Other causes for failure of normal skull growth include lack of brain growth due to any of the causes of arrested development of the cerebral hemispheres (lissencephaly, micropolygyria, some cases of hydranencephaly…).

Treatment is usually surgical. In most instances, the indication for surgery is for cosmesis and to prevent the severe psychological effects of having a disfiguring deformity. However, with multiple CSO, brain growth may be impeded by the unyielding skull. Also, ICP may be pathologically elevated, and although this is more common in multiple CSO,[12] elevated ICP occurs in ≈ 11% of cases with a single stenotic suture. Coronal synostosis can cause amblyopia. Most cases of single suture involvement can be treated with linear excision of the suture. Involvement of multiple sutures or the skull base usually requires the combined efforts of a neurosurgeon and craniofacial surgeon, and may need to be staged in some cases. Risks of surgery include: blood loss, seizures, stroke.

Diagnosis

Many cases of "synostosis" are really due to positional flattening (e.g. "lazy lambdoid", see below). If this is suspected, instruct parents to keep head off of flattened area and recheck patient in 6–8 weeks: if it was positional, it should be improved, if it was CSO then it usually declares itself. The diagnosis of CSO may be aided by:

1. palpation of a bony prominence over the suspected synostotic suture (exception: lambdoidal synostosis, see below)
2. gentle firm pressure with the thumbs fails to cause relative movement of the bones on either side of the suture
3. plain skull x-rays:
   a) lack of normal lucency in center of suture. Some cases with normal x-ray appearance of the suture (even on CT) may be due to focal bony spicule formation[13]
   b) beaten copper calvaria (p. 254), sutural diastasis and erosion of the sella may be seen in cases of increased ICP[14]
4. CT scan:
   a) helps demonstrate cranial contour
   b) may show thickening and/or ridging at the site of synostosis
   c) will demonstrate hydrocephalus if present
   d) may show expansion of the frontal subarachnoid space[15]
   e) three-dimensional CT may help better visualize abnormalities
5. in questionable cases, a technetium bone scan can be performed[16]:
   a) there is little isotope uptake by any of the cranial sutures in the first weeks of life
   b) in prematurely closing sutures, increased activity compared to the other (normal) sutures will be demonstrated
   c) in completely closed sutures, no uptake will be demonstrated
6. MRI: usually reserved for cases with associated intracranial abnormalities. Often not as helpful as CT
7. measurements, such as occipito-frontal-circumference may not be abnormal even in the face of a deformed skull shape

Increased ICP

Evidence of increased ICP in the newborn with craniosynostosis include:

1. radiographic signs (on plain skull x-ray or CT, see above)
2. failure of calvarial growth (unlike the non-synostotic skull where increased ICP causes macrocrania in the newborn, here it is the synostosis that causes the increased ICP and lack of skull growth)
3. papilledema
4. developmental delay

Types of craniosynostosis

Sagittal synostosis

General information

The most common CSO affecting a single suture; 80% male. Results in dolichocephaly or scaphocephaly (boat shaped skull) with frontal bossing, prominent occiput, palpable keel-like sagittal ridge. OFC remains close to normal, but the biparietal diameter is markedly reduced. As many as 44% of patients with nonsyndromic sagittal synostosis have elevated ICP.[17]

Surgical treatment

Skin incision may be longitudinal or transverse. A linear "strip" craniectomy is performed, excising the sagittal suture from the coronal to the lambdoid suture, preferably within the first 3–6 months of life. The width of the strip should be at least 3 cm, no proof exists that interposing artificial substances (e.g. silastic sheeting over the exposed edges of the parietal bone) retards the recurrence of synostosis. Great care is taken to avoid dural laceration with potential injury to the underlying superior sagittal sinus. The child is followed and reoperated if fusion recurs before 6 months age. After ≈ 1 yr age, more extensive cranial remodelling is usually required.

Coronal synostosis

General information

Accounts for 18% of CSO, more common in females. In Crouzon's syndrome this is accompanied by abnormalities of sphenoid, orbital and facial bones (hypoplasia of midface), and in Apert's syndrome is accompanied by syndactyly.[18] Unilateral coronal CSO → plagiocephaly with forehead on affected side flattened or concave above eye (normal side falsely appears to bulge abnormally), supra-orbital margin higher than normal side (on skull x-ray → harlequin eye sign). The orbit rotates out on the abnormal side, and can produce amblyopia. Without treatment, flattened cheeks develop and the nose deviates to the normal side (root of nose tends to rotate towards deformity).

Bilateral coronal CSO (usually in craniofacial dysmorphism with multiple suture CSO, e.g. Apert's) → brachycephaly with broad, flattened forehead (acrocephaly). When combined with premature closure of frontosphenoidal and frontoethmoidal sutures, results in foreshortened anterior fossa with maxillary hypoplasia, shallow orbits, progressive proptosis.

Surgical treatment

Simple strip craniectomy of the involved suture has been used, often with excellent cosmetic result. However, some argument that this may not be adequate has been presented. Therefore, a more current recommendation is to do frontal craniotomy (uni- or bi-lateral) with lateral canthal advancement by taking off orbital bar.

Metopic synostosis

At birth, the frontal bone consists of two halves separated by the frontal or metopic suture. Abnormal closure results in a pointed forehead with a midline ridge (trigonocephaly). Many of these have a 19p chromosome abnormality and are retarded.

15

Lambdoid synostosis

Epidemiology

Long considered a clinical rarity with a reported incidence range 1–9% of CSO,[19] recent reports suggest a higher incidence of 10–20%[20] which may be due to an actual increased incidence, or simply to increased awareness or changing diagnostic criteria. More common in males (male:female = 4:1), and the right side is involved in 70% of cases. Usually presents between 3–18 months of age, but may be seen as early as 1–2 months of age.

Controversy exists regarding the actual criteria for this condition, and some authors differentiate between those cases which appear to have a primary abnormality of the lambdoid suture from those which may be due to positional flattening, the so-called "lazy lambdoid." Others do not make this distinction, and sometimes refer to the condition as occipital plagiocephaly to avoid the need to implicate abnormalities of the lambdoid suture.

Positional flattening (or molding) may be produced by:

1. decreased mobility: patients who constantly lie supine with the head to the same side, e.g. cerebral palsy, mental retardation, prematurity, chronic illness
2. abnormal postures: *congenital torticollis*,[21] congenital disorders of the cervical spine

3. intentional positioning: trend since 1992 to place newborns in a supine sleeping position to reduce the risk of sudden infant death syndrome (SIDS),[22] sometimes with a foam wedge to tilt the child to one side to reduce the risk of aspiration
4. intrauterine etiologies[23]: intrauterine crowding (e.g. from multiparous births or large fetal size), uterine anomalies

Clinical findings

Flattening of the occiput. May be unilateral or bilateral. If unilateral, it is sometimes termed lambdoid plagiocephaly which when severe also produces bulging of the ipsilateral forehead resulting in a "rhomboid" skull with the ipsilateral ear located anterior and inferior to the contralateral ear. The contralateral orbit and forehead may also be flattened. This may be confused with hemifacial microsomia or with plagiocephaly seen in unilateral coronal craniosynostosis. Bilateral lambdoid synostosis produces brachycephaly with both ears displaced anteriorly and inferiorly.[19] Unlike the palpable ridge of sagittal or coronal synostosis, an *indentation* may be palpated along the synostotic lambdoid suture (although a perisutural ridge may be found in some).

Diagnostic evaluation

The physical exam is the most important aspect of diagnosis. Skull x-ray may help differentiate (see below). If the skull x-ray is equivocal, prevent the infant from laying on the affected side for several weeks. A bone scan should be obtained if no improvement occurs (see below). In definite cases of synostosis, and for some cases of refractory positional flattening (which usually corrects with time, but may take up to 2 years) surgical treatment may be indicated.

Skull x-ray: Shows a sclerotic margin along one edge of the lambdoid suture in 70% of cases. Local "beaten copper cranium" (BCC) occasionally may be seen due to indentations in the bone from underlying gyri which may be due to locally increased ICP. BCC produces a characteristic mottled appearance of the bone with lucencies of varying depth having round and poorly marginated edges. BCC correlates with generalized ↑ ICP only when it is seen with sellar erosion and sutural diastasis.[14]

CT scan: Bone windows may show eroded or thinned inner table in the occipital region in 15–20% of cases,[20] > 95% are on the side of the involvement. The suture may appear closed. Brain windows show parenchymal brain abnormalities in < 2%: heterotopias, hydrocephalus, agenesis of the corpus callosum; but ≈ 70% will have significant expansion of the frontal subarachnoid space (may be seen in synostosis of other sutures, see above).

Bone scan: Isotope uptake in the lambdoid suture increases during the first year, with a peak at 3 months of age[24] (following the usual inactivity of the first weeks of life). The findings with synostosis are those typical for CSO (p. 252).

Treatment

Early surgical treatment is indicated in cases with severe craniofacial disfigurement or those with evidence of increased ICP. Otherwise, children may be managed nonsurgically for 3–6 months. The majority of cases will remain static or will improve with time and simple nonsurgical intervention. Approximately 15% will continue to develop a significant cosmetic deformity.

Nonsurgical management[25]:

Although improvement can usually be attained, some degree of permanent disfigurement is frequent.

Repositioning will be effective in ≈ 85% of cases. Patients are placed on the unaffected side or on the abdomen. Infants with occipital flattening from torticollis should have aggressive physical therapy and resolution should be observed within 3–6 months.

More severe involvement may be treated with a trial of molding helmets[26] (however, no controlled study has proven the efficacy).

Surgical treatment:

Required in only ≈ 20% of cases. The ideal age for surgery is between 6 and 18 months. The patient is positioned prone on a well-padded cerebellar headrest (the face should be lifted and gently massaged every ~ 30 minutes by the anesthesiologist to prevent pressure injuries).

Surgical options range from simple unilateral craniectomy of the suture to elaborate reconstruction by a craniofacial team.

Linear craniectomy extends from the sagittal suture to the asterion is often adequate for patients ≤ 12 weeks of age without severe disfigurement. Great care is taken to avoid dural laceration near the asterion which is in the region of the transverse sinus. The excised suture demonstrates an *internal* ridge. Better results are obtained with earlier surgery, more radical surgery may be necessary after the age of 6 months.

Average blood loss for uncomplicated cases is 100–200 ml and therefore transfusion is often required.

Multiple synostoses

Fusion of many or all cranial sutures → oxycephaly (tower skull with undeveloped sinuses and shallow orbits). These patients have elevated ICP.

Craniofacial dysmorphic syndromes

Over 50 syndromes have been described, ▶ Table 15.4, shows a few selected ones.

A number of craniosynostosis syndromes are due to mutations in the FGFR (fibroblast growth factor receptor) genes. FGFR gene-related craniosynostosis syndromes include some classic syndromes (Apert, Crouzon, Pfeiffer…) as well as several newer entities (Beare-Stevenson, Muenke, Jackson-Weiss syndromes). All exhibit autosomal dominant inheritance.

15.2.3 Encephalocele

General information

Cranium bifidum is a defect in the fusion of the cranial bone, it occurs in the midline, and is most common in the occipital region. If meninges and CSF herniate through the defect, it is called a meningocele. If meninges and cerebral tissue protrude, it is called an encephalocele.

Encephalocele AKA cephalocele is an extension of intracranial structures outside of the normal confines of the skull. One case was seen for every five cases of spinal myelomeningoceles.[28] A nasal polypoid mass in a *newborn* should be considered an encephalocele until proven otherwise. See also Differential diagnosis (p. 1388).

Classification

System based on Suwanwela and Suwanwela[29]:

1. occipital: often involves vascular structures
2. cranial vault: comprises ≈ 80% of encephaloceles in Western hemisphere
   a) interfrontal
   b) anterior fontanelle
   c) interparietal: often involves vascular structures
   d) temporal
   e) posterior fontanelle
3. fronto-ethmoidal: AKA sincipital; 15% of encephaloceles; external opening into face in one of the following 3 regions:
   a) nasofrontal: external defect in the nasion
   b) naso-ethmoidal: defect between nasal bone and nasal cartilage
   c) naso-orbital: defect in the antero-inferior portion of medial orbital wall
4. basal: 1.5% of encephaloceles; (see below)
   a) transethmoidal: protrudes into nasal cavity through defect in cribriform plate
   b) spheno-ethmoidal: protrudes into posterior nasal cavity

15

Table 15.4 Selected craniofacial dysmorphic syndromes (modified[27] (p 123–4))

Syndrome	Genetics		Craniofacial findings	Associated findings
	Sporadic	Inherited		
Crouzon (craniofacial dysostosis)	yes (25%)	FGFR AD	CSO of coronal & basal skull sutures, maxillary hypoplasia, shallow orbits, proptosis	HCP rare
Apert (acrocephalosyndactyly)	yes (95%)	FGFR AD	same as Crouzon	syndactyly of digits 2,3,4; shortened UE, HCP common
Kleeblattschadel	yes	AD	CSO with trilobular skull	isolated, or with Apert's or thanatophoric dwarfism

[a]Abbreviations: AD = autosomal dominant; FGFR = fibroblast growth factor receptor gene-related; CSO = craniosynostosis; HCP = hydrocephalus; UE = upper extremities

c) transsphenoidal: protrudes into sphenoid sinus or nasopharynx through patent craniopharyngeal canal (foramen cecum)
d) fronto-sphenoidal or spheno-orbital: protrudes into orbit through superior orbital fissure
5. posterior fossa: usually contains cerebellar tissue and ventricular component

Basal encephalocele
The only group that does not produce a visible soft tissue mass. May present as CSF leak or recurrent meningitis. May be associated with other craniofacial deformities, including: cleft lip, bifid nose, optic-nerve dysplasia, coloboma and microphthalmia, hypothalamic-pituitary dysfunction.

Iniencephaly is characterized by defects around the foramen magnum, rachischisis and retrocollis. Most are stillborn, some survive up to age 17.

Etiology

Two main theories:
1. arrested closure of normal confining tissue allows herniation through persistent defect
2. early outgrowth of neural tissue prevents normal closure of cranial coverings

Treatment

Occipital encephalocele
Surgical excision of the sac and its contents with water-tight dural closure. It must be kept in mind that vascular structures are often included in the sac. Hydrocephalus is often present and may need to be treated separately.

Basal encephalocele
Caution: a transnasal approach to a basal encephalocele (even for biopsy alone) may be fraught with intracranial hemorrhage, meningitis, or persistent CSF leak. Usually a combined intracranial approach (with amputation of the extracranial mass) and transnasal approach is used.

Outcome

Occipital encephalocele
The prognosis is better in occipital meningocele than in encephalocele. The prognosis is worse if a significant amount cerebral tissue is present in the sac, if the ventricles extend into the sac, or if there is hydrocephalus. Less than ≈ 5% of infants with encephalocele develop normally.

15.3 Dandy Walker malformation

15.3.1 General information

Definition: an enlarged posterior fossa with complete or partial agenesis of the cerebellar vermis and cystic dilatation of the fourth ventricle which is distorted and encased in a membrane. The anomaly was first described by Dandy & Blackfan in 1914, and was named Dandy Walker malformation forty years later by Benda to acknowledge Taggart and Walker's contributions in 1942.[30]

15.3.2 Differential diagnosis

Disorders with posterior fossa CSF collections include[31]:
1. Dandy Walker malformation (DWM)
2. Dandy Walker variant (DWV): vermian hypoplasia and cystic dilatation of the fourth ventricle, without enlargement of the posterior fossa
3. persistent Blake's pouch cyst (BPC): tetraventricular hydrocephalus, communicating 4th ventricle and posterior fossa cyst, with or without hypoplasia of both the cerebellar vermis and the medial aspects of the cerebellar hemispheres
4. retrocerebellar arachnoid cyst: anteriorly displaces the 4th ventricle and cerebellum, which can produce significant mass effect
5. Joubert's syndrome: absence or underdevelopment of the cerebellar vermis
6. mega cisterna magna: enlarged posterior fossa secondary to an enlarged cisterna magna with a normal vermis and fourth ventricle)

Differentiating features: DWM and DWV are difficult to distinguish, and may represent a continuum of developmental anomalies that are grouped together as Dandy Walker complex.[32]

Retrocerebellar arachnoid cysts and BPCs may mimic DWM, but these do *not* have vermian agenesis and the cyst does not open into the 4th ventricle. The position of the choroid plexus of the fourth ventricle is normal in arachnoid cysts, absent in Dandy Walker malformations, and displaced into the superior cyst wall in BPC. An intrathecal enhanced CT scan (performed after instilling iodinated contrast into a ventricular catheter) would identify a mega cisterna magna which communicates with the ventricles, while DWM and most but not all arachnoid cysts do not.

15.3.3 Pathophysiology

The etiology of DWM is unknown. Multiple unsatisfactory theories have been abandoned. DWM is likely due to dysembryogenesis, secondary to insults of varying severity to the cerebellum and 4th ventricle. This results in agenesis of the cerebellar vermis with a large posterior fossa cyst communicating with an enlarged 4th ventricle.[32,30]

Hydrocephalus occurs in 70–90% of cases, and Dandy Walker malformation is present in 2–4% of all cases of hydrocephalus.

15.3.4 Risk factors and epidemiology

Gestational exposure to rubella, CMV, toxoplasmosis, warfarin, alcohol, and isotretinoin are thought to be predisposing factors. Autosomal recessive inheritance has been identified in a few cases, but a genetic basis is lacking in most. Incidence: 1 per 25,000–35,000 live births.[30] Male:female=1:3.

15.3.5 Associated abnormalities

CNS abnormalities include agenesis of the corpus callosum in 17%,[33] and occipital encephalocele in 7%. Other findings include heterotopias, spina bifida, syringomyelia, microcephaly, dermoid cysts, porencephaly, and Klippel-Feil deformity. Most have an enlarged posterior fossa with elevation of the torcular herophili. Atresia of the foramina of Magendie and Luschka may occur.[34]

Systemic abnormalities include[33]: facial abnormalities (e.g. angiomas, cleft palates, macroglossia, facial dysmorphia), ocular abnormalities (e.g. coloboma, retinal dysgenesis, microphthalmia), and cardiovascular anomalies (e.g. septal defects, patent ductus arteriosus, aortic coarctation, dextrocardia). Note: be aware of the possibility of a cardiac abnormality when considering surgery on these patients.

15.3.6 Treatment

Early decompression of ventriculomegaly is recommended to achieve maximum cognitive development. In the absence of hydrocephalus, DWM may be followed. When treatment is necessary, the posterior fossa cyst must be shunted. Shunting the lateral ventricles alone is contraindicated because of the risk of upward herniation.[35] However, it is important to confirm patency of the cerebral aqueduct, otherwise the supratentorial ventricles need to be shunted concomitantly. Varying reports exist regarding rates of associated aqueductal stenosis, although it is widely believed to be rare.

Another option once used commonly is excision of the obstructing membrane. This has fallen out of favor due to its associated risks of morbidity and mortality. However, it remains an option for patients with frequent shunt malfunctions.

Newer treatments include endoscopic third ventriculostomy in cases where the aqueduct is patent, however further study is necessary.[36,37]

15.3.7 Prognosis

Prognosis ranges widely as there are various levels of severity of the malformation. Some pediatric neurosurgical literature quotes 12–50% mortality rates, although this is improving with modern shunting techniques. Only 50% have normal IQ. Ataxia, spasticity, and poor fine motor control are common. Seizures occur in 15%.

15.4 Aqueductal stenosis

15.4.1 General information

Aqueductal stenosis (AqS) produces what is sometimes called triventricular hydrocephalus, characterized by a normal sized 4th ventricle and enlarged third and lateral ventricles on MRI or CT. Most cases occur in children, however some present for the first time in adulthood.

15.4.2 Etiologies

1. a congenital malformation: may be associated with Chiari malformation or neurofibromatosis
2. acquired
   a) due to inflammation (following hemorrhage or infection, e.g. syphilis, T.B.)
   b) neoplasm: especially brainstem astrocytomas – including tectal gliomas (p. 634), lipomas
   c) quadrigeminal plate arachnoid cysts

15.4.3 Aqueductal stenosis in infancy

AqS is a frequent cause of congenital hydrocephalus (HCP) (up to 70% of cases[27]), but occasionally may be the *result* of HCP. Patients with congenital AqS usually have HCP at birth or develop it within ≈ 2–3 mos. Congenital AqS may be due to an X-linked recessive gene.[28] Four types of congenital AqS described by Russell (summarized[38]):

1. forking: multiple channels (often narrowed) with normal epithelial lining that do not meet, separated by normal nervous tissue. Usually associated with other congenital abnormalities (spina bifida, myelomeningocele)
2. periaqueductal gliosis: luminal narrowing due to subependymal astrocytic proliferation
3. true stenosis: aqueduct histologically normal
4. septum

15.4.4 Aqueductal stenosis in adulthood

General information

AqS may be an overlooked cause of "normal pressure hydrocephalus" in the adult.[39] It is unknown why some cases of AqS would remain occult, and manifest only in adulthood. In one series of 55 cases,[40] 35% had duration of symptoms < 1 year, 47% for 1–5 years; the longest was 40 yrs. Although most follow this longstanding benign course, there are reports of elevated ICP and sudden death.

Symptoms

15

See ▸ Table 15.5. Headache was the most common symptom, and had characteristics of H/A associated with elevated ICP. Visual changes were next, and usually consisted of blurring or loss of acuity. Endocrine changes included menstrual irregularities, hypothyroidism, and hirsutism.

Signs

Papilledema was the most common finding (53%). Visual fields were normal in 78%, the remainder having reduced peripheral vision, increased blind spots, quadrantic or hemianopic field cuts, or scotomata. Intellectual impairment was present in at least 36%. Other signs included: ataxia (29%), "pyramidal tract signs" in 44% (mild hemi- or para-paresis (22%), spasticity (22%), or Babinski's (20%)), anosmia (9%).

Evaluation

MRI is the test of choice. MRI will show the absence of the normal flow void in the Sylvian aqueduct. Contrast should be given to rule-out tumor.

Treatment (of non-tumoral AqS)

Although treatments of the primary lesion have been attempted (e.g. lysis of aqueductal septum), this has fallen into disfavor with the improved efficacy of CSF shunting and endoscopic third ventriculostomy (ETV).

Table 15.5 Symptoms of aqueductal stenosis presenting in adulthood (55 patients > 16 years age[40])

Symptom	No.	%
H/A	32	58%
visual disturbances	22	40%
mental deterioration	17	31%
gait disturbance	16	29%
frequent falling	13	24%
endocrine disturbance	10	18%
nausea/vomiting	9	16%
seizures	8	15%
incontinence	7	13%
vertigo	6	11%
LE weakness	4	7%
hemiparesis or hemianesthesia	4	7%
diplopia	3	5%
dysarthria	1	
deafness	1	

1. shunting: CSF is usually shunted to the peritoneum or the vascular system, however shunting to subarachnoid space is also feasible (once obstruction at the level of the arachnoid granulations has been ruled out)
2. a Torkildsen shunt (shunting a lateral ventricle to the cisterna magna[41]) may work in adult cases,[38] however pediatric patients with obstructive hydrocephalus may not have an adequately developed subarachnoid space for this to function properly
3. endoscopic third ventriculostomy (p. 415)

Follow-up of at least two years to rule out tumor is recommended.

15.5 Agenesis of the corpus callosum

15.5.1 General information

A failure of commissuration occurring ≈ 2 weeks after conception. Results in expansion of the third ventricle and separation of the lateral ventricles (which develop dilated occipital horns and atria, and concave medial borders).

The corpus callosum (CC) forms from rostrum (genu) to splenium,[42] ∴ in agenesis there may be an anterior portion with absence of the posterior segment (the converse occurs infrequently). Absence of the anterior CC with presence of some posterior CC is indicative of some form of holoprosencephaly.

15.5.2 Incidence

1 in 2,000–3,000 neuroradiological examinations.

15.5.3 Associated neuropathologic findings

See reference.[43]

- porencephaly

- microgyria
- interhemispheric *lipomas* and lipomas of the corpus callosum (p. 260)
- arhinencephaly
- optic atrophy
- colobomas
- hypoplasia of the limbic system
- bundles of Probst: aborted beginnings of corpus callosum, bulge into lateral ventricles
- loss of horizontal orientation of cingulate gyrus
- schizencephaly (p. 288)
- anterior and hippocampal commissures may be totally or partially absent[44]
- hydrocephalus
- cysts in the region of the corpus callosum
- spina bifida with or without myelomeningocele
- absence of the septum pellucidum (p. 260)

15.5.4 Possible presentation

- hydrocephalus
- microcephaly
- seizures (rare)
- precocious puberty
- disconnection syndrome: more likely with *acquired* CC defect than in congenital

May be an incidental finding, and by itself may have no clinical significance. However, may be occur as part of a more complex clinical syndrome or chromosomal abnormality (e.g. Aicardi syndrome: agenesis of CC, seizures, retardation, patches of retinal pigmentation).

15.6 Absence of the septum pellucidum

Etiologies[45 (p 178)]

1. holoprosencephaly (p. 289)
2. schizencephaly (p. 288)
3. agenesis of the corpus callosum (p. 259)
4. Chiari type 2 malformation (p. 284)
5. basal encephalocele
6. porencephaly/hydranencephaly
7. may occur in severe hydrocephalus: thought to be due to necrosis with resorption of the septum
8. septo-optic dysplasia: see below

15

Septo-optic dysplasia[46,45 (p 175–8)]

AKA de Morsier syndrome. Incomplete early morphogenesis of anterior midline structures produces hypoplasia of the optic nerves and possibly optic chiasm (affected patients are blind) and pituitary infundibulum. The septum pellucidum is absent in about half the cases. About half the cases also have schizencephaly (p. 288).

Presentation may be due to secondary hypopituitarism manifesting as dwarfism, isolated growth hormone deficiency, or panhypopituitarism. Occasionally hypersecretion of growth hormone, corticotropin or prolactin may occur, and precocious puberty may occur. Most patients are of normal intelligence although retardation may occur. Septo-optic dysplasia may be a less severe form of holoprosencephaly (p. 289), and occasionally may occur as part of this anomaly (with its attendant poorer prognosis for function or survival). The ventricles may be normal or dilated. May be seen by the neurosurgeon because of concerns of possible hydrocephalus.

15.7 Intracranial lipomas

15.7.1 General information

Intracranial and intraspinal lipomas are felt to be of maldevelopmental origin[47 (p 706)] and may arise from failure of involution of the primitive meninges.[48]

15.7.2 Epidemiology of intracranial lipomas

Incidence: 8 in 10,000 autopsies. Usually found in or near the midsagittal plane, particularly over the corpus callosum; lipomas in this region are frequently associated with agenesis of the corpus callosum (p.259). The tuber cinereum and quadrigeminal plate are less frequently affected.[43] Rarely, the CP angle or cerebellar vermis may be involved. May occur in isolation, but also has been described in association with a number of congenital anomalies, including: trisomy 21, Pai's syndrome, frontal encephalocele, facial anomalies.... Other midline abnormalities may also be found: agenesis of the corpus callosum, myelomeningocele, and spina bifida.[48]

15.7.3 Evaluation

May be diagnosed by CT, MRI (study of choice), and by ultrasound in infants.

CT: Low density, may have peripheral calcification (difficult to appreciate on MRI).[48] Differential diagnosis on CT: primarily between dermoid cyst, teratoma[49] and germinoma.[48]

MRI: characteristic finding is a midline lesion with signal characteristics of fat (high intensity on T1WI, low intensity on T2WI).

15.7.4 Presentation

Often discovered incidentally. Large lipomas may be associated with seizures, hypothalamic dysfunction, or hydrocephalus (possibly from compression of the aqueduct). Associated findings that may or may not be directly related: mental retardation, behavioral disorders and headache.

15.7.5 Treatment

Direct surgical approach is seldom necessary for intracranial lipomas.[49] Shunting may be required for cases where hydrocephalus results from obstruction of CSF circulation.[49]

15.8 Hypothalamic hamartomas

15.8.1 General information

Key concepts

- rare, non-neoplastic congenital malformation, usually occurs in tuber cinereum
- may be parahypothalamic (pedunculated) or intrahypothalamic (sessile)
- presentation: precocious puberty, seizures (usually starting with gelastic seizures (brief unprovoked laughter)), developmental delay
- treatment: GnRH analogs for precocious puberty. Latero-basal craniotomy for pedunculated lesions, transcallosal interforniceal approach for intrahypothalamic lesions, option of endoscopic approach for lesions ≤ 1.5 cm dia, stereotactic radiosurgery may be an alternative

Hypothalamic hamartomas (**HH**; hamartoma: an abnormal conglomeration of cells normally found in the same area) AKA diencephalic hamartomas or hamartomas of the tuber cinereum. Rare, non-neoplastic congenital malformations arising from inferior hypothalamus or tuber cinereum (floor of the third ventricle between the infundibular stalk and the mammillary bodies). May occur as part of Pallister-Hall syndrome (genetics: AD inherited defect in GL13 gene resulting in abnormally short GL13 protein which participates in normal shaping of many organs).

15.8.2 Clinical findings

1. specific types of seizures:
   a) gelastic seizures (brief episodes of unprovoked laughter[50]) are the most characteristic type and are the earliest seizure manifestation. Present in up to 92% of patients.[51] They are resistant to medical management and can lead to cognitive and behavioral deficits.[52] Not pathognomonic. A neocortical origin has been described[53]

b) epileptic encephalopathy: gelastic fits gradually increase in frequency and other seizure types accrue: complex partial seizures, drop attacks, tonic seizures, tonic-clonic seizures, and secondarily generalized seizures. This phase is associated with marked deterioration of cognitive and behavioral abilities. Develops in 52% by a mean age of 7 years[51]

2. precocious puberty: believed to be due to release of gonadotropin-releasing hormone (GnRH) found within hamartoma cells.[54] HH are the most common CNS tumor to cause precocious puberty, other causes include: other CNS tumors – astrocytoma, ependymoma, pineal tumors (p. 658), optic/hypothalamic gliomas (especially in NFT patients) -, CNS XRT, hydrocephalus, CNS inflammation, septo-optic dysplasia (p. 260), and chronic hypothyroidism
3. developmental delay: primarily in patients with seizure disorder (severity correlates with duration of seizures). 46% of patients have borderline intellectual function (mental retardation)
4. behavioral disturbances[55]: aggressive behavior, rage attacks…

15.8.3 Imaging

MRI: nonenhancing, isointense on T1WI, slightly hyperintense or isointense on T2WI.[56]

15.8.4 Pathology

Two subtypes of hypothalamic hamartomas[56,51]:

1. pedunculated or parahypothalamic: narrower base attached to the floor of the hypothalamus (not arising within hypothalamus). No distortion of 3rd ventricle. Generally associated with precocious puberty more than seizures
2. intrathalamic or sessile: within hypothalamus (distorting the 3rd ventricle) or broad attachment to hypothalamus. More often associated with seizures. 66% have developmental delay, 50% have precocious puberty

Microscopic pathology: Clusters of disorganized small neurons surrounded by large pyramidal like neurons in an astrocyte-rich neuropil[57] (in contrast to the usual ganglion cells surrounded by oligodendrocytes found in the hypothalamus).

15.8.5 Treatment

Precocious puberty usually responds well to GnRH analogs.[58]

► **Indications for surgery:**

1. precocious puberty that fails to respond to medical therapy (GnRH analogs)
2. seizures that cannot be adequately controlled medically. Post-op seizure control is related to completeness of resection
3. neurologic deficit from mass effect of the tumor

15

► **Options:**

1. surgical resection
   a) pedunculated lesions: approaches include[59] subtemporal, subfrontal, pterional, orbitozygomatic (most commonly recommended). Risks: cranial neuropathy, stroke[59]
   b) sessile lesions with intraventricular component: transcallosal anterior interforniceal approach.[60,61,62] Risks: memory impairment (forniceal injury), endocrine disturbances, weight gain[60,62]
   c) neuroendoscopic approach: considered for HH ≤ 1.5 cm diameter.[63] Risks: 25% incidence of thalamic cerebrovascular injury
2. stereotactic radiosurgery: especially for small sessile lesions, subtotal resection, or patients refusing or not candidates for surgery. In small series, 3-year outcome showed improvement similar to surgical resection with less neurologic and endocrinologic morbidity[64,65]

References

[1] Van Der Meche F, Braakman R. Arachnoid Cysts in the Middle Cranial Fossa: Cause and Treatment of Progressive and Non-Progressive Symptoms. J Neurol Neurosurg Psychiatry. 1983; 46:1102–1107

[2] Mayr U, Aichner F, Bauer G, et al. Supratentorial Extracerebral Cysts of the Middle Cranial Fossa: A Report of 23 Consecutive Cases of the So-called Temporal Lobe Agenesis Syndrome. Neurochirugia. 1982; 25:51–56

[3] Rengachary SS, Watanabe I. Ultrastructure and Pathogenesis of Intracranial Arachnoid Cysts. J Neuropathol Exp Neurol. 1981; 40:61–83

[4] Harsh GR, Edwards MSB, Wilson CB. Intracranial Arachnoid Cysts in Children. J Neurosurg. 1986; 64:835–842
[5] Pierre-Kahn A, Capelle L, Brauner R, Sainte-Rose C, et al. Presentation and Management of Suprasellar Arachnoid Cysts: Review of 20 Cases. J Neurosurg. 1990; 73:355–359
[6] Altschuler EM, Jungreis CA, Sekhar LN, Jannetta PJ, et al. Operative Treatment of Intracranial Epidermoid Cysts and Cholesterol Granulomas: Report of 21 Cases. Neurosurgery. 1990; 26:606–614
[7] Galassi E, Tognetti F, Gaist G, et al. CT scan and Metrizamide CT Cisternography in Arachnoid Cysts of the Middle Cranial Fossa. Surg Neurol. 1982; 17:363–369
[8] Hopf NJ, Perneczky A. Endoscopic Neurosurgery and Endoscope-Assisted Microneurosurgery for the Treatment of Intracranial Cysts. Neurosurgery. 1998; 43:1330–1337
[9] Page LK. Comment on Albright L: Treatment of Bobble-Head Doll Syndrome by Transcallosal Cystectomy. Neurosurgery. 1981; 8
[10] Albright L. Treatment of Bobble-Head Doll Syndrome by Transcallosal Cystectomy. Neurosurgery. 1981; 8:593–595
[11] Golabi M, Edwards MSB, Ousterhout DK. Craniosynostosis and Hydrocephalus. Neurosurgery. 1987; 21:63–67
[12] Renier D, Sainte-Rose C, Marchac D, Hirsch J-F. Intracranial Pressure in Craniostenosis. J Neurosurg. 1982; 57:370–377
[13] Burke MJ, Winston KR, Williams S. Normal Sutural Fusion and the Etiology of Single Suture Craniosynostosis: The Microspicule Hypothesis. Pediatr Neurosurg. 1995; 22:241–246
[14] Tuite GF, Evanson J, Chong WK, et al. The Beaten Copper Cranium: A Correlation between Intracranial Pressure, Cranial Radiographs, and Computed Tomographic Scans in Children with Craniosynostosis. Neurosurgery. 1996; 39:691–699
[15] Chadduck WM, Chadduck JB, Boop FA. The Subarachnoid Spaces in Craniosynostosis. Neurosurgery. 1992; 30:867–871
[16] Gates GF, Dore EK. Detection of Craniosynostosis by Bone Scanning. Radiology. 1975; 115:665–671
[17] Wall SA, Thomas GP, Johnson D, Byren JC, Jayamohan J, Magdum SA, McAuley DJ, Richards PG. The preoperative incidence of raised intracranial pressure in nonsyndromic sagittal craniosynostosis is underestimated in the literature. J Neurosurg Pediatr. 2014; 14:674–681
[18] Renier D, Arnaud E, Cinalli G, et al. Prognosis for Mental Function in Apert's Sydrome. J Neurosurg. 1996; 85:66–72
[19] Muakkassa KF, Hoffman HJ, Hinton DR, Hendrick EB, et al. Lambdoid Synostosis: Part 2. Review of Cases Managed at The Hospital for Sick Children, 1972-1982. J Neurosurg. 1984; 61:340–347
[20] Keating RF, Goodrich JT. Lambdoid Plagiocephaly. Contemp Neurosurg. 1996; 18:1–7
[21] Morrison DL, MacEwen GD. Congenital Muscular Torticollis: Observations Regarding Clinical Findings, Associated Conditions, and Results of Treatment. J Pediatr Orthop. 1982; 2:500–505
[22] American Academy of Pediatrics Task Force on Infant Positioning and SIDS. Positioning and SIDS. Pediatrics. 1992; 89:1120–1126
[23] Higginbottom MC, Jones KL, James HE. Intrauterine Constraint and Craniosynostosis. Neurosurgery. 1980; 6
[24] Hinton DR, Becker LE, Muakkassa KF, Hoffman HJ, et al. Lambdoid Synostosis: Part 1: The Lambdoid Suture: Normal Development and Pathology of 'Synostosis'. J Neurosurg. 1984; 61:333–339
[25] McComb JG. Treatment of Functional Lambdoid Synostosis. Neurosurg Clin North Am. 1991; 2
[26] Clarren SK. Plagiocephaly and Torticollis: Etiology, Natural History, and Helmet Treatment. J Pediatr. 1981; 98
[27] Section of Pediatric Neurosurgery of the American Association of Neurological Surgeons. Pediatric Neurosurgery. New York 1982
[28] Matson DD. Neurosurgery of Infancy and Childhood. 2nd ed. Springfield: Charles C Thomas; 1969
[29] Suwanwela C, Suwanwela N. A Morphological Classification of Sincipital Encephalomeningoceles. J Neurosurg. 1972; 36:201–211
[30] Incesu L, Khosia A. Dandy-Walker malformation. 2008
[31] Calabro F, Arcuri T, Jinkins JR. Blake's pouch cyst: an entity within the Dandy-Walker continuum. Neuroradiology. 2000; 42:290–295
[32] Forzano F, Mansour S, Ierullo A, Homfray T, Thilaganathan B. Posterior fossa malformation in fetuses: a report of 56 further cases and a review of the literature. Prenat Diagn. 2007; 27:495–501
[33] Hirsch JF, Pierre-Kahn A, Renier D, et al. The Dandy-Walker Malformation: A Review of 40 Cases. J Neurosurg. 1984; 61:515–522
[34] Raimondi AJ, Samuelson G, Yarzagaray L, et al. Atresia of the Foramina of Luschka and Magendie: The Dandy-Walker Cyst. J Neurosurg. 1969; 31:202–216
[35] Mohanty A, Biswas A, Satish S, Praharaj SS, Sastry KV. Treatment options for Dandy-Walker malformation. J Neurosurg. 2006; 105:348–356
[36] Garg A, Suri A, Chandra PS, Kumar R, Sharma BS, Mahapatra AK. Endoscopic third ventriculostomy: 5 years' experience at the All India Institute of Medical Sciences. Pediatr Neurosurg. 2009; 45:1–5
[37] Sikorski CW, Curry DJ. Endoscopic, single-catheter treatment of Dandy-Walker syndrome hydrocephalus: technical case report and review of treatment options. Pediatr Neurosurg. 2005; 41:264–268
[38] Nag TK, Falconer MA. Non-Tumoral Stenosis of the Aqueduct in Adults. Brit Med J. 1966; 2:1168–1170
[39] Vanneste J, Hyman R. Non-Tumoral Aqueduct Stenosis and Normal Pressure Hydrocephalus in the Elderly. J Neurol Neurosurg Psychiatry. 1986; 49:529–535
[40] Harrison MJG, Robert CM, Uttley D. Benign Aqueduct Stenosis in Adults. J Neurol Neurosurg Psychiatry. 1974; 37:1322–1328
[41] Alp MS. What is a Torkildsen shunt? Surg Neurol. 1995; 43:405–406
[42] Davidson HD, Abraham R, Steiner RE. Agenesis of the Corpus Callosum: Magnetic Resonance Imaging. Radiology. 1985; 155:371–373
[43] Atlas SW, Zimmerman RA, Bilaniuk LT, et al. Corpus Callosum and Limbic System: Neuroanatomic MR Evaluation of Developmental Anomalies. Radiology. 1986; 160:355–362
[44] Loeser JD, Alvord EC. Agenesis of the Corpus Callosum. Brain. 1968; 91:553–570
[45] Taveras JM, Pile-Spellman J. Neuroradiology. 3rd ed. Baltimore: Williams and Wilkins; 1996
[46] Jones KL. Smith's Recognizable Patterns of Human Malformation. 4th ed. Philadelphia: W.B. Saunders; 1988
[47] Russell DS, Rubenstein LJ. Pathology of Tumours of the Nervous System. 5th ed. Baltimore: Williams and Wilkins; 1989
[48] Rubio G, Garcci Guijo C, Mallada JJ, MR and CT Diagnosis of Intracranial Lipoma. AJR. 1991; 157:887–888
[49] Kazner E, Stochdorph O, Wende S, Grumme T. Intracranial Lipoma. Diagnostic and Therapeutic Considerations. J Neurosurg. 1980; 52:234–245
[50] Daly D, Mulder D. Gelastic epilepsy. Neurology. 1957; 7:189–192
[51] Nguyen D, Singh S, Zaatreh M, Novotny E, Levy S, Testa F, Spencer SS. Hypothalamic hamartomas: seven cases and review of the literature. Epilepsy Behav. 2003; 4:246–258
[52] Striano S, Meo R, Bilo L, Cirillo S, Nocerino C, Ruosi P, Striano P, Estraneo A. Gelastic epilepsy: symptomatic and cryptogenic cases. Epilepsia. 1999; 40:294–302
[53] Kurle PJ, Sheth RD. Gelastic seizures of neocortical origin confirmed by resective surgery. J Child Neurol. 2000; 15:835–838
[54] Culler FL, James HE, Simon ML, Jones KL. Identification of gonadotropin-releasing hormone in neurons of a hypothalamic hamartoma in a boy with precocious puberty. Neurosurgery. 1985; 17:408–412

[55] Prigatano GP. Cognitive and behavioral dysfunction in children with hypothalamic hamartoma and epilepsy. Semin Pediatr Neurol. 2007; 14:65–72
[56] Arita K, Ikawa F, Kurisu K, Sumida M, Harada K, Uozumi T, Monden S, Yoshida J, Nishi Y. The relationship between magnetic resonance imaging findings and clinical manifestations of hypothalamic hamartoma. J Neurosurg. 1999; 91:212–220
[57] Coons SW, Rekate HL, Prenger EC, Wang N, Drees C, Ng YT, Chung SS, Kerrigan JF. The histopathology of hypothalamic hamartomas: study of 57 cases. J Neuropathol Exp Neurol. 2007; 66:131–141
[58] Chamouilli JM, Razafimahefa B, Pierron H. [Precocious puberty and hypothalamic hamartoma: treatment with triptorelin during eight years]. Arch Pediatr. 1995; 2:438–441
[59] Feiz-Erfan I, Horn EM, Rekate HL, Spetzler RF, Ng YT, Rosenfeld JV, Kerrigan JF,3rd. Surgical strategies for approaching hypothalamic hamartomas causing gelastic seizures in the pediatric population: transventricular compared with skull base approaches. J Neurosurg. 2005; 103:325–332
[60] Rosenfeld JV, Harvey AS, Wrennall J, Zacharin M, Berkovic SF. Transcallosal resection of hypothalamic hamartomas, with control of seizures, in children with gelastic epilepsy. Neurosurgery. 2001; 48:108–118
[61] Ng Y, Rekate HL, Kerrigan JF, et al. Transcallosal resection of a hypothalamic hamartoma: Case report. BNI Quarterly. 2004; 20:13–17
[62] Ng YT, Rekate HL, Prenger EC, Chung SS, Feiz-Erfan I, Wang NC, Varland MR, Kerrigan JF. Transcallosal resection of hypothalamic hamartoma for intractable epilepsy. Epilepsia. 2006; 47:1192–1202
[63] Rekate HL, Feiz-Erfan I, Ng YT, Gonzalez LF, Kerrigan JF. Endoscopic surgery for hypothalamic hamartomas causing medically refractory gelastic epilepsy. Childs Nerv Syst. 2006; 22:874–880
[64] Regis J, Scavarda D, Tamura M, Villeneuve N, Bartolomei F, Brue T, Morange I, Dafonseca D, Chauvel P. Gamma knife surgery for epilepsy related to hypothalamic hamartomas. Semin Pediatr Neurol. 2007; 14:73–79
[65] Mathieu D, Kondziolka D, Niranjan A, Flickinger J, Lunsford LD. Gamma knife radiosurgery for refractory epilepsy caused by hypothalamic hamartomas. Stereotact Funct Neurosurg. 2006; 84:82–87

16 Primary Spinal Anomalies

16.1 Spinal arachnoid cysts

16.1.1 General information

Almost always dorsal, most common in thoracic spine. With a ventral cyst, consider a neurenteric cyst (see below). Most are actually extradural and these are sometimes referred to as arachnoid diverticula – these may be associated with kyphoscoliosis in juveniles or with spinal dysraphism. Intradural arachnoid cysts may be congenital or may follow infection or trauma.

Usually asymptomatic, even if large.

16.1.2 Treatment

When indicated, treatment options include:

1. percutaneous procedures: may be done under MRI[1] or CT guidance. CT guidance usually requires use of intrathecal contrast to delineate the cyst
   a) needle aspiration
   b) needle fenestration[1]
2. open surgical resection or fenestration

16.2 Spinal dysraphism (spina bifida)

16.2.1 Definitions

See reference.[2]

▸ **Spina bifida occulta.** Congenital absence of a spinous process and variable amounts of lamina. No visible exposure of meninges or neural tissue.

The following two entities are grouped together under the term spina bifida aperta (aperta from the Latin for "open") or spina bifida cystica.

▸ **Meningocele.** Congenital defect in vertebral arches with cystic distension of meninges, but no abnormality of neural tissue. One third have some neurologic deficit.

▸ **Myelomeningocele.** Congenital defect in vertebral arches with cystic dilatation of meninges and structural or functional abnormality of spinal cord or cauda equina.

16.2.2 Spina bifida occulta (SBO)

Reported prevalence range of SBO: 5–30% of North Americans (5–10% is probably more realistic). The defect may be palpable, and there may be overlying cutaneous manifestations (in ▸ Table 16.3.

Often an incidental finding, usually of no clinical importance *when it occurs alone*. Numerous reviews have shown no statistical association of SBO with nonspecific LBP.[3,4] An increased incidence of disc herniation was shown in one study.[5]

SBO may occasionally be associated with diastematomyelia, tethered cord, lipoma, or dermoid tumor. When symptomatic from one of these associated conditions, the presentation is usually that of tethered cord; gait disturbance, leg weakness and atrophy, urinary disturbance, foot deformities..., see Tethered cord syndrome (p. 272).

16.2.3 Myelomeningocele

Embryology

The anterior neuropore closes at gestation day 25. The caudal neuropore closes at day 28.

Epidemiology/genetics

Incidence of spina bifida with meningocele or myelomeningocele (MM) is 1–2/1000 live births (0.1–0.2%). Risk increases to 2–3% if there is one previous birth with MM, and 6–8% after two affected children. The risk is also increased in families where close relatives (e.g. siblings) have given birth to

MM children, especially when on the mother's side of the family. Incidence may increase in times of war, famine or economic disasters, but it may be gradually declining overall.[6] Transmission follows non-Mendelian genetics, and is probably multifactorial. Prenatal folate (in the form of folic acid) lowers the incidence of MM (p.290).

Hydrocephalus in myelomeningocele

Hydrocephalus (HCP) develops in 65–85% of patients with MM, and 5–10% of MM patients have clinically overt HCP at birth.[7] Over 80% of MM patients who will develop HCP do so before age 6 mos. Most MM patients will have an associated Chiari type 2 malformation (p.284). Closure of the MM defect may convert a latent HCP to active HCP by eliminating a route of egress of CSF.

Latex allergy in myelomeningocele

Up to 73% of MM patients are allergic to proteins present in latex (the milky sap from the rubber tree Hevea brasiliensis), found only in naturally occurring rubber products (and which are not present in synthetics such as: silicone, vinyl, plastic, neoprene, nitrile...). The allergy is thought to arise from early and frequent exposure to latex products during medical care for these patients, and there is a suggestion that latex-free surgery on these infants may reduce the risk of the development of latex allergy.[8]

Prenatal diagnosis

See Prenatal detection of neural tube defects (p.290).

Intrauterine closure of MM defect

Controversial. Does reduce incidence of Chiari II defect, but it has not been determined if this is clinically significant. Argued whether this reduces incidence of hydrocephalus. Does not improve distal neurologic function.

General management

Assessment and management of lesion

- measure size of defect
- assess whether lesion is ruptured or unruptured
  - ruptured: start antibiotics (e.g. nafcillin and gentamicin; D/C 6 hrs after MM closure, or continue if shunt anticipated in next 5 or 6 days)
  - unruptured: no antibiotics necessary
- cover lesion with telfa, then sponges soaked in lactated ringers or normal saline (form a sterile gauze ring around the lesion if it is cystic and protruding) to prevent desiccation
- Trendelenburg position, patient on stomach (keeps pressure off lesion)
- perform surgical closure within 36 hrs unless there is a contraindication to surgery (simultaneous shunt is not usually done except if overt hydrocephalus (HCP) at birth): see below

16

Neurological assessment and management

- items related to spinal lesion
  - watch for spontaneous movement of the LEs (good spontaneous movement correlates with better later functional outcome[9])
  - assess lowest level of neurologic function ▶ Table 16.1) by checking response of LEs to painful stimulus: although some infants will have a clear demarcation between normal and abnormal levels, at least 50% show some mixture of normal, reflex, and autonomous activity (arising from uninhibited anterior horn motor neurons)[9]
    - differentiating reflex movement from voluntary may be difficult. In general, voluntary movement is not stereotyped with repetitive stimulus and reflex movement usually only persists as long as the noxious stimulus is applied
- items related to the commonly associated Chiari type 2 malformation:
  - measure OFC: risk of developing hydrocephalus (see above). Use OFC graphs (p.395), and also look for abnormal rate of growth (e.g. > 1 cm/day)
  - head U/S within ≈ 24 hrs
  - check for inspiratory stridor, apneic episodes

Table 16.1 Findings in various levels of MM lesion[10]

Paralysis below	Findings
T12	complete paralysis of all muscles in LEs
L1	weak to moderate hip flexion, palpable contraction in sartorius
L2	strong hip flexion and moderate hip adduction
L3	normal hip adduction & almost normal knee extension
L4	normal hip adduction, knee extension & dorsiflexion/inversion of foot; some hip abduction in flexion
L5	normal adduction, flexion & lateral rotation of hip; moderate abduction; normal knee extension, moderate flexion; normal foot dorsiflexion; hip extension absent; • produces dorsiflexed foot and flexed thigh
S1	normal hip flexion & abduction/adduction, moderate extension and lateral rotation; strong knee flexion & inversion/eversion of foot; moderate plantarflexion of foot; extension of all toes, but flexion only of terminal phalanx of great toe; normal medial & lateral hip rotation; complete paralysis of foot intrinsic (except abductor and flexor hallicus brevis); • produces clawing of toes and flattening of sole of foot
S2	difficult to detect abnormality clinically; • with growth this produces clawing of the toes due to weakness of intrinsic muscles of sole of foot (innervated by S3)

Ancillary assessment and management

- evaluation by neonatologist to assess for other abnormalities, especially those that may preclude surgery (e.g. pulmonary immaturity). There is an average incidence of 2–2.5 additional anomalies in MM patients
- bladder: start patient on regular urinary catheterizations, obtain urological consultation (non-emergent)
- AP & lat spine films: assess scoliosis (baseline)
- orthopedic consultation for severe kyphotic or scoliotic spine deformities and for hip or knee deformities

Surgical management

Timing of MM closure

Early closure of MM defect is *not* associated with improvement of neurologic function, but evidence supports lower infection rate with early closure. MM should be closed within 24 hrs whether or not membrane is intact (after ≈ 36 hrs the back lesion is colonized and there is increased risk of postoperative infection).

Simultaneous MM defect closure and VP shunting

In patients without hydrocephalus, most surgeons wait at least ≈ 3 days after MM repair before shunting. In MM patients with clinically overt HCP at birth (ventriculomegaly with enlarged OFC and/or symptoms), MM repair and shunting may be performed in the same sitting without increased incidence of infection, and with shorter hospitalization.[11,12] It may also reduce the risk of MM repair breakdown previously seen during the interval before shunting. Patient is positioned prone, head turned to *right* (to expose the right occiput), right knee and thigh flexed to expose right flank (consider using left flank to prevent confusion with appendectomy scar later in life).

Surgical technique of myelomeningocele repair

Key concepts

- critical goals: 1) free placode from dura (to avoid tethering), 2) water-tight dural closure, 3) skin closure (can be accomplished in essentially all cases). Closure does not restore any neurologic function
- timing goal: surgical closure with latex-free setup ideally ≤ 36 hours after birth
- helpful tips: start at normal dura, open as wide as the defect, trim placode if necessary to close dura, undermine skin to achieve closure (avoid trapping skin → dermoid tumor)
- post-op CSF leak usually means a shunt is required

16

General principles[13]: prevent desiccation – keep the exposed neural tissue moist. Use latex-free environment (reduces development of latex allergy, as well as attack by maternal antibodies that may have crossed through the placenta). Do not allow scrub solutions or chemical antimicrobials to contact neural placode. Do not use monopolar cautery. At every point during the closure, avoid placing tension on the neural placode.

Multiple layer closure is advocated, 5 layers should be attempted, although occasionally only 2 or so layers may be closed. There is no evidence that multiple layer closure either improves neurologic function or prevents later tethering, but there is a suggestion that when tethering does occur, it may be easier to release when a previous multilayered closure was performed. Silastic does not prevent adherence in series with long follow-up (> 6 yrs), and may even render untethering procedures more difficult.

Begin by dividing the abnormal epithelial covering from the normal skin. The pia-arachnoid may be separated from the neural tissue. The placode is folded into a tube and the pia-arachnoid is then approximated around it with 7–0 suture (absorbable suture, e.g. PDS, may make future re-operation easier). It often helps to start with normal dura above, and then work down. The dura can then be isolated around the periphery and followed deep to the spinal canal superiorly. The dura is then also formed into a tube and approximated in a water-tight closure. If the dura cannot be closed, the placode may be judiciously trimmed. The filum terminale should be divided if it can be located. The skin is then mobilized and closed. Dermoid tumors may result from retained skin during the closure, but alternatively dermoids may also be present congenitally.[14]

If there is a kyphotic deformity, it is repaired at the same sitting as the MM defect closure. The kyphotic bone is rongeured, and 2–0 Vicryl is used to suture the adjacent bones. Some surgeons use a brace post-op, some do not.

Post-op management of MM repair

1. keep patient off all incisions
2. bladder catheterization regimen
3. daily OFC measurements
4. *avoid narcotics* (midbrain malformation renders these patient more sensitive to respiratory depression from narcotics)
5. if not shunted
   a) regular head U/S (twice weekly to weekly)
   b) keep patient flat to ↓ CSF pressure on incision
6. if a kyphectomy was done, use of a brace is optional (surgeon preference)

Late problems/issues

Include:

1. hydrocephalus: may mimic ≈ anything listed below. *ALWAYS RULE OUT SHUNT MALFUNCTION* when a MM patient deteriorates
2. syringomyelia (and/or syringobulbia) (p. 1144):
3. Tethered cord syndrome (p. 272) as many as 70% of MM patients have a tethered cord radiographically (some quote 10–20%), but only a minority are symptomatic. Unfortunately there is no good test to check for symptomatic retethering (SSEPs may deteriorate,[15] myelography may help)
   a) scoliosis: early untethering of cord may improve scoliosis; seeScoliosis in tethered cord (p. 272)
   b) symptomatic tethering may manifest as delayed neurological deterioration[16]
4. dermoid tumor at the MM site (p. 784)[17]: incidence ≈ 16%
5. medullary compression at foramen magnum, see symptomatic Chiari II malformation (p. 284)
6. use of growth hormone to increase stature is controversial

16

Outcome

Without any treatment, only 14–30% of MM infants survive infancy; these usually represent the least severely involved; 70% will have normal IQ's. 50% are ambulatory.

With modern treatment, ≈ 85% of MM infants survive. The most common cause of early mortality are complications from the Chiari malformation (respiratory arrest, aspiration...), where late mortality is usually due to shunt malfunction. 80% will have normal IQ. Mental retardation is most closely linked to shunt infection. 40–85% are ambulatory with bracing, however, most choose to use wheelchairs for ease. 3–10% have normal urinary continence, but most may be able to remain dry with intermittent catheterization.

16.2.4 Lipomyeloschisis

General information

Dorsal spinal dysraphism with lipoma. Six forms are described,[18] the following 3 are clinically important as possible causes of progressive neurologic dysfunction via tethering (p.272) and/or compression:

1. (intra)dural lipoma
2. lipomyelomeningocele (see below)
3. fibrolipoma of the filum terminale

Lipomyelomeningocele

General information

A subcutaneous lipoma that passes through a midline defect in the lumbodorsal fascia, vertebral neural arch, and dura, and merges with an abnormally low tethered cord.[18] These may be terminal, dorsal, or transitional (between the two).

The intradural fatty tumor may also be known as lipoma of the cauda equina. In addition to being abnormally low, the conus medullaris is split in the midline dorsally usually at the same level as the bifid spine, and this dorsal myeloschisis may extend superiorly under intact spinal arches.[19] There is a thick fibrovascular band that joins the lamina of the most cephalic vertebrae with the bifid lamina. This band constricts the meningocele sac and neural tissue, causing a kink in the superior surface of the meningocele. Asymptomatic lipomas of the filum terminale occur in 0.2–4%[20,21] of MRIs.

The dura is dehiscent at the level of the dorsal myeloschisis, and reflects onto the placode. The lipoma passes through this dehiscence to become attached to the dorsal surface of the placode, and may continue cephalad under intact arches with the possibility of extension into the central canal superiorly to levels without dorsal myeloschisis. The lipoma is distinct from the normal epidural fat which is looser and more areolar. The subarachnoid space typically bulges to the side contralateral to the lipoma. These lipomas account for 20% of covered lumbosacral masses.

Presentation

In a pediatric series, 56% presented with a back mass, 32% with bladder problems, and 10% because of foot deformities, paralysis or leg pain.[22]

Physical examination

Almost all patients have cutaneous stigmata of the associated spina bifida: fatty subcutaneous pads (located over the midline and usually extends asymmetrically to one side) with or without dimples, port-wine stains, abnormal hair, dermal sinus opening, or skin appendages.[23] Clubbing of the feet (talipes equinovarus) may occur.

The neurologic exam may be normal in up to 50% of patients (most presenting with skin lesion only). The most common neurologic abnormality was sensory loss in the sacral dermatomes.

Evaluation

Plain LS spine x-rays will show spina bifida in most cases. Present in almost all by definition, but some may have segmentation anomalies instead such as butterfly vertebra (p.216). Abnormalities of fusion and sacral defects may also be seen.

The abnormally low conus can be demonstrated on myelogram/CT or on MRI. MRI also demonstrates the lipomatous mass (high signal on T1WI, low signal on T2WI).

All patients should have pre-op urological evaluation to document any deficit.

Treatment

Since symptoms are due to (1) tethering of the spinal cord, especially during growth spurts, and (2) compression due to progressive deposition of fat, especially during periods of rapid weight gain; the goals of surgery are to release the tethering and reduce the bulk of fatty tumor. Simple cosmetic treatment of the subcutaneous fat pad does not prevent neurologic deficit, and may make later definitive repair more difficult or impossible.

Surgical treatment is indicated when the patient reaches 2 months of age, or at the time of diagnosis if the patient presents later in life. Adjuncts to surgical treatment include evoked potential monitoring and laser. Overall, with surgery, 19% will improve, 75% will be unchanged, and 6% will worsen. Foot deformities often progress regardless.

Surgical technique (modified)

See reference.[19]

1. mobilize the subcutaneous mass, it funnels down through the deep fascia
2. open last intact vertebral arch (work from normal dura)
3. identify the fibrovascular band that crosses the most cephalic widely bifid lamina
4. sectioning the fibrovascular band frees the dural tube and releases the sharp kink in the superior surface of the meningocele
5. taking care to preserve dorsal nerve roots, the dura is incised anterior to the dura-lipoma junction
6. similar procedure is carried out with arachnoid membrane
7. dural/arachnoid incisions are continued around entire extent of tethered conus
8. cord and placode are untethered; monitoring techniques described in Tethered cord syndrome (p. 272) are an option
9. ✱ subtotal removal of lipoma: lipoma is then trimmed as completely as possible, intentionally leaving some fat behind to avoid injury to dorsal surface of placode. Superior extension along dorsal surface of cord or into central canal is debulked as much as is safely possible
10. the placode is reformed into a closed neural tube
11. close the pial margins
12. the dura is closed (primarily if possible, or using fascia lata graft if too much tension is placed on folded placode)

16.2.5 Dermal sinus

General information

A tract beginning at the skin surface, lined with epithelium. Usually located at either end of neural tube: cephalic or caudal. Most common location is lumbosacral. Probably results from failure of the cutaneous ectoderm to separate from the neuro-ectoderm at the time of closure of the neural groove.[2]

Spinal dermal sinus

General information

May appear as a dimple or as a sinus, with or without hairs, usually very close to midline, with an opening of only 1–2 mm. Surrounding skin may be normal, pigmented ("port wine" discoloration), or distorted by an underlying mass.

The sinus may terminate superficially, may connect with the coccyx, or may traverse between normal vertebrae or through bifid spines to the dural tube. It may widen at any point along its path to form a cyst; called an epidermoid cyst if lined with stratified squamous epithelium and containing only keratin from desquamated epithelium, or called a dermoid cyst if also lined with dermis (containing skin appendages, such as hair follicles and sebaceous glands) and also containing sebum and hair.

Although innocuous in appearance, they are a potential pathway for intradural infection which may result in meningitis (sometimes recurrent) and/or intrathecal abscess. Less serious, a local infection may occur. The lining dermis contains normal skin appendages which may result in hair, sebum, desquamated epithelium and cholesterol, within the tract. As a result, the contents of the sinus tract are irritating and can cause a sterile (chemical) meningitis with possible delayed *arachnoiditis* if it enters the dural space.

16

Incidence of a presumed sacral sinus (a dimple whose bottom could not be seen on skin retraction): 1.2% of neonates.[24]

Dermal sinuses are similar but distinct from **pilonidal cysts** which may also be congenital (although some authors say they are acquired), contain hair, are located superficial to the postsacral fascia, and may become infected.

If the tract expands intrathecally to form a cyst, the mass may present as a tethered cord or as an intradural tumor. Bladder dysfunction is usually the first manifestation.

The tract from a spinal dermal sinus always courses cephalad as it dives inward from the surface. An occipital sinus may penetrate the skull and can communicate with dermoid cysts as deep as the cerebellum or fourth ventricle.

Evaluation

These tracts are NOT to be probed or injected with contrast as this can precipitate infection or sterile meningitis.

Exam is directed towards detecting abnormalities in sphincter function (anal and urinary), lumbosacral reflexes, and lower extremity sensation and function.

Radiologic evaluation

When seen at birth, *ultrasound* is the best means to evaluate for spina bifida and a possible mass inside the canal.

If seen initially following birth, an MRI should be obtained. Sagittal images may demonstrate the tract and its point of attachment. MRI also optimally demonstrates masses (lipomas, epidermoids…) within the canal.

Plain x-rays and CT are unable to demonstrate the fine tract which may exist between the skin and the dura.

Plain x-rays must be done when embarking on surgery as part of operative planning, as preparation for the possibility of a complete laminectomy.

Treatment

Sinuses above the lumbosacral region should be surgically removed. More caudally located sinuses are slightly controversial. Although ≈ 25% of presumed sacral sinuses seen at birth will regress to a deep dimple on follow-up (time not specified), it is recommended that all dermal sinuses should be surgically explored and fully excised *prior* to the development of neurologic deficit or signs of infection. The results following intradural infection are never as good as when undertaken prior to infection. Surgery within the week of diagnosis is appropriate. Sinuses that terminate on the tip of the coccyx rarely penetrate the dura, and may not need to be treated unless local infection occurs.

Surgical technique

An ellipse is cut around the opening, and the sinus is followed deep until the termination of the tract is encountered. Careful insertion of a lacrimal duct probe under direct vision may facilitate excision without violating the tract. If the tracts penetrates the spine, laminectomy must be performed and the tract followed to its full extent (even if necessary to extend the laminectomy to T12). An extradural cyst may be present. If the tract enters the dura, it usually does so in the midline, and in these cases the dura should be opened and inspected. Extreme care is taken to prevent spilling the contents into the subdural space.

Cranial dermal sinus

General information

Stalk begins with a dimple in the occipital or nasal region. Cutaneous stigmata of hemangioma, subcutaneous dermoid cyst, or abnormal hair formation may occur. Occipital sinuses extend caudally, and if they enter the skull, they do so caudal to the torcular herophili. Presentation may include recurrent bacterial (usually S. aureus) or aseptic meningitis. Evaluation should include MRI to look for intracranial extension and associated anomalies, including an intracranial dermoid cyst.

Treatment

When operating on a cranial dermal sinus, use a sagittally based incision to permit deep exploration. The tract must be followed completely. Be prepared to enter the posterior fossa.

16

16.3 Klippel-Feil syndrome

16.3.1 General information

Congenital fusion of two or more cervical vertebrae. Ranges from fusion of only the bodies (congenital block vertebrae) to fusion of the entire vertebrae (including posterior elements). Results from failure of normal segmentation of cervical somites between 3–8 weeks gestation. Involved vertebral bodies are often flattened and associated disc spaces are absent or hypoplastic. Hemivertebrae may also occur. Neural foramina are smaller than normal and oval. Cervical stenosis is rare. Complete absence of the posterior elements with an enlarged foramen magnum and fixed hyperextension posture is called iniencephaly and is rare. Incidence of Klippel-Feil is unknown due to its rarity and the fact that it is frequently asymptomatic.

May occur in conjunction with other congenital cervical spine anomalies such as basilar impression and atlanto-occipital fusion.

16.3.2 Presentation

Classic clinical triad (all 3 are present in < 50%):
1. low posterior hairline
2. shortened neck (brevicollis)
3. limitation of neck motion (may not be evident if < 3 vertebrae are fused, if fusion is limited only to the lower cervical levels,[25] or if hypermobility of nonfused segments compensates). Limitation of movement is more common in rotation than flexion-extension or lateral bending

Other clinical associations include scoliosis in 60%, facial asymmetry, torticollis, webbing of the neck (called pterygium colli when severe), Sprengel's deformity in 25–35% (raised scapula due to failure of the scapula to properly descend from its region of formation high in the neck to its normal position about the same time as the Klippel-Feil lesion occurs), synkinesis (mirror motions, primarily of hands but occasionally arms also) and less commonly facial nerve palsy, ptosis, cleft or high arched palate. Systemic congenital abnormalities may also occur including: genitourinary (the most frequent being unilateral absence of a kidney), cardiopulmonary, CNS, and in ≈ 30% deafness[26] (due to defective development of the osseous inner ear).

No neurologic symptoms have ever been directly attributed to the fused vertebrae, however symptoms may occur from nonfused segments (less common in short-segment fusions) which may be hypermobile possibly leading to instability or degenerative arthritic changes.

16.3.3 Treatment

Usually directed at detecting and managing the associated systemic anomalies. Patients should have cardiac evaluation (EKG), CXR, and a renal ultrasound. Serial examinations with lateral flexion-extension lateral C-spine x-rays to monitor for instability. Occasionally, judicious fusion of an unstable nonfused segment may be needed at the risk of further loss of mobility. See also recommendations regarding athletic competition (p. 937).

16.4 Tethered cord syndrome

16.4.1 General information

Abnormally low conus medullaris. Usually associated with a short, thickened filum terminale, or with an intradural lipoma (other lesions, e.g. lipoma extending through dura, or diastematomyelia are considered as separate entities). Most common in myelomeningocele (MM). Diagnosis must be made clinically in MM, as almost all of these patients will have tethering radiographically.

16.4.2 Presentation

Presenting signs and symptoms in patients with tethered cord are shown in ▶ Table 16.2.

16

16.4.3 Myelomeningocele patients

If a MM patient has increasing scoliosis, increasing spasticity, worsening gait (in those previously ambulatory), or deteriorating urodynamics[28]:
- always make sure that there is a working shunt with normal ICP
- if painful, should be considered tethered cord until proven otherwise
- if painless, should be considered syringomyelia until proven otherwise
- may be due to brainstem compression – see symptomatic Chiari II malformation (p. 284) – requiring posterior fossa decompression

16.4.4 Scoliosis in tethered cord

Progressive scoliosis may be seen in conjunction with tethered cord. Early untethering of the cord may result in improvement of scoliosis, however, untethering must be done when the scoliosis is mild. When cases of ≤ 10° scoliosis were untethered, 68% had neurologic improvement and the remaining 32% were stabilized, whereas when scoliosis is severe (≥ 50°) ≈ 16% deteriorated.

Table 16.2 Presenting signs and symptoms[27 (p 1331–2)]

Finding	%
cutaneous findings • hypertrichosis • sub-Q lipoma (no intraspinal extension) • miscellaneous (hemangiomatous discoloration, dermal sinus, multiple manifestations)	54% • 22% • 15% • 17%
gait difficulty with LE weakness	93%
visible muscle atrophy, short limb, or ankle deformity	63%
sensory deficit	70%
bladder dysfunction	40%
bladder dysfunction as only deficit	4%
pain in back, leg, or foot arches	37%
scoliosis or kyphosis[a]	29%
posterior spina bifida (lumbar or sacral)	98%
[a]high incidence of scoliosis and kyphosis due to inclusion of series by Hoffman	

16.4.5 Tethered cord in adults

General information

Although most cases of tethered cord present in childhood, cases of adult tethered cord also occur (≈ 50 published cases as of 1982). For comparison of adult and childhood forms, ▶ Table 16.3

Evaluation

Radiographically: low conus medullaris (below L2) and thickened filum terminale (definition of thickened filum: normal diameter < 1 mm; diameters > 2 mm are pathological). NB: apparent filum diameter on CT-myelogram may vary with concentration of contrast material.

It is difficult to differentiate a tethered cord from a congenitally low lying conus (filum diameter is generally normal in the latter).

16.4.6 Pre-op evaluation

Pre-operative *cystometrogram* is strongly recommended, especially if the patient seems continent (postoperative changes in bladder function are not uncommon, possibly due to stretching of the lower fibers of the cauda equina).

Surgical treatment

If the only abnormality is a thickened, shortened filum, then a limited lumbosacral laminectomy may suffice, with division of the filum once identified.

If a lipoma is found, it may be removed with the filum if it separates easily from neural tissues.

Distinguishing features of the filum terminale intraoperatively

The filum is differentiated from nerve roots by presence of characteristic squiggly vessel on surface of filum. Also, under the microscope, the filum has a distinctively whiter appearance than the nerve roots, and ligamentous-like strands can be seen running through it. NB: intra-op electrical stimulation and recording of anal sphincter EMG are more definitive.

Table 16.3 Comparison of childhood and adult tethered cord syndrome[29]

Finding	Childhood tethered cord	Adult tethered cord
pain	uncommon; usually in back and legs, not peri-anal nor perineal	present in 86%, often peri-anal & perineal; diffuse & bilateral; occasionally shock-like
foot deformities	common early; usually progressive cavovarus deformity (club foot)	not seen
progressive spinal deformity	common; usually progressive scoliosis	uncommon (<5%)
motor deficits	common; usually gait abnormalities & regression of gait training	usually presents as leg weakness
urological symptoms	common; usually continuous urinary dribbling, delayed toilet training, recurrent UTIs, enuresis	common; usually urinary frequency, urgency, sensation of incomplete emptying, stress incontinence, overflow incontinence
trophic ulcerations	relatively common in LEs	rare
cutaneous stigmata of dysraphism	present in 80–100% (tuft of hair, dimple, capillary angioma (naevus flammeus)	present in < 50%
aggravating factors	growth spurts	trauma, maneuvers associated with stretching conus, lumbar spondylosis, disc herniation, spinal stenosis

From J Neurosurg, D. Pang and J.E. Wilberger, Vol. 57, pp. 40, 1982, with permission.

Outcome

In MM, it is usually impossible to permanently untether a cord, however, in a growing MM child, it may be that after 2–4 untetherings that the child will be finished growing and tethering may cease to be a problem. Cases that are untethered early in childhood may recur later, especially during the adolescent growth-spurt. Incidence of post-op CSF leak: 15%.

Adult form: surgical release is usually good for pain relief. However, it is poor for return of bladder function.

16.5 Split cord malformation

16.5.1 General information

16

There is no uniformly accepted nomenclature for malformations characterized by duplicate or split spinal cords. Pang et al.[30] have proposed the following.

The term split cord malformation (SCM) should be used for all double spinal cords, all of which appear to have a common embryologic etiology.

16.5.2 Type I SCM

Defined as two hemicords, each with its own central canal and surrounding pia, each within a separate dural tube separated by a dural-sheathed rigid osseocartilaginous (bony) median septum. This has often (but not consistently) been referred to as diastematomyelia. There are abnormalities of the spine at the level of the split (absent disc, dorsal hypertrophic bone where the median "spike" attaches).[31] Two-thirds have overlying skin abnormalities including: nevi, hypertrichosis (tuft of hair), lipomas, dimples or hemangiomas. These patients often have and an orthopedic foot deformity (neurogenic high arches).

Treatment: symptoms are most commonly due to tethering of the cord; and are usually improved by untethering. In addition to untethering, the bony septum must be removed and the dura reconstituted as a single tube (these spines are often very distorted and rotated, therefore start at normal anatomy and work towards defect). ✖ DO NOT cut the tethered filum until *after* the median septum is removed to avoid having the cord retract up against septum.

16.5.3 Type II SCM

Consists of two hemicords within a single dural tube, separated by a nonrigid fibrous median septum. This has sometimes been referred to as diplomyelia. Each hemicord has nerve roots arising from it. There is usually no spine abnormality at the level of the split, but there is usually spina bifida occulta in the lumbosacral region.

Treatment: consists of untethering the cord at the level of the spina bifida occulta, and occasionally at the level of the split.[31]

16.6 Lumbosacral nerve root anomalies

Congenital anomalies of nerve roots are rare. This possibility should be considered in cases of failed back surgery for herniated disc.

Classification system of Cannon et al.[32]

1. Type 1 anomalies: include conjoined nerve root (2 nerve roots arise from a common dural sheath). They separate at various distances from the thecal sac, and exit through the same or separate neural foramina. Neurosurgeons need to be aware of this anomaly to avoid inadvertent injury e.g. during surgery for herniated disc
2. Type 2 anomalies: 2 nerve roots exit through one foramen. Variants[33]:
   a) leaves an unoccupied neural foramen
   b) all foramina occupied, but one foramen has 2 nerve roots
3. Type 3 anomalies: adjacent nerve roots are connected by an anastomosis

References

[1] Takahashi S, Morikawa S, Egawa M, Saruhashi Y, Matsusue Y. Magnetic resonance imaging-guided percutaneous fenestration of a cervical intradural cyst. Case report. J Neurosurg. 2003; 99:313–315
[2] Matson DD. Neurosurgery of Infancy and Childhood. 2nd ed. Springfield: Charles C Thomas; 1969
[3] van Tulder MW, Assendelft WJ, Koes BW, Bouter LM. Spinal radiographic findings and nonspecific low back pain. A systematic review of observational studies. Spine. 1997; 22:427–434
[4] Steinberg EL, Luger E, Arbel R, Menachem A, Dekel S. A comparative roentgenographic analysis of the lumbar spine in male army recruits with and without lower back pain. Clin Radiol. 2003; 58:985–989
[5] Avrahami E, Frishman E, Fridman Z, Azor M. Spina bifida occulta of S1 is not an innocent finding. Spine. 1994; 19:12–15
[6] Lorber J, Ward AM. Spina Bifida - A Vanishing Nightmare? Arch Dis Child. 1985; 60:1086–1091
[7] Stein SC, Schut L. Hydrocephalus in Myelomeningocele. Childs Brain. 1979; 5:413–419
[8] Cremer R, Kleine-Diepenbruck U, Hoppe A, Blaker F. Latex allergy in spina bifida patients–prevention by primary prophylaxis. Allergy. 1998; 53:709–711
[9] Sharrard WJW, McLaurin RL. In: Assessment of the Myelomeningocele Child. Myelomeningocele. New York: Grune and Stratton; 1977:389–410
[10] Sharrard WJW. The Segmental Innervation of the Lower Limb Muscles in Man. Ann R Coll Surgeons (Engl). 1964; 34:106–122
[11] Epstein NE, Rosenthal RD, Zito J, et al. Shunt Placement and Myelomeningocele Repair: Simultaneous versus Sequential Shunting. Childs Nerv Syst. 1985; 1:145–147
[12] Hubballah MY, Hoffman HJ. Early Repair of Myelomeningocele and Simultaneous Insertion of VP Shunt: Technique and Results. Neurosurgery. 1987; 20:21–23
[13] McLone DG. Technique for Closure of Myelomeningocele. Childs Brain. 1980; 6:65–73
[14] Ramos E, Marlin AE, Gaskill SJ. Congenital dermoid tumor in a child at initial myelomeningocele closure: an etiological discussion. J Neurosurg Pediatrics. 2008; 2:414–415
[15] Larson SJ, Sances A, Christenson PC. Evoked Somatosensory Potentials in Man. Arch Neurol. 1966; 15:88–93
[16] Heinz ER, Rosenbaum AE, Scarff TB, Reigel DH, et al. Tethered Spinal Cord Following Meningomyelocele Repair. Radiology. 1979; 131:153–160
[17] Scott RM, Wolpert SM, Bartoshesky LE, Zimbler S, Klauber GT. Dermoid tumors occurring at the site of previous myelomeningocele repair. J Neurosurg. 1986; 65:779–783
[18] Emery JL, Lendon RG. Lipomas of the Cauda Equina and Other Fatty Tumors Related to Neurospinal Dysraphism. Dev Med Child Neurol. 1969; 11:62–70
[19] Naidich TP, McLone DG, Mutluer S. A new understanding of dorsal dysraphism with lipoma (lipomyeloschisis): radiologic evaluation and surgical correction. AJNR. 1983; 4:103–116
[20] Uchino A, Mori T, Ohno M. Thickened fatty filum terminale: MR imaging. Neuroradiology. 1991; 33:331–333
[21] Brown E, Matthes JC, Bazan C, III, Jinkins JR. Prevalence of incidental intraspinal lipoma of the lumbosacral spine as determined by MRI. Spine. 1994; 19:833–836
[22] Bruce DA, Schut L. Spinal Lipomas in Infancy and Childhood. Childs Brain. 1979; 5:192–203
[23] Sato K, Shimoji T, Sumie H, et al. Surgically Confirmed Myelographic Classification of Congenital Intraspinal Lipoma in the Lumbosacral Region. Childs Nerv Syst. 1985; 1:2–11
[24] Powell KR, Cherry JD, Horigan TJ, et al. A Prospective Search for Congenital Dermal Abnormalities of Craniospinal Axis. J Pediatr. 1975; 87:744–750
[25] Gray SW, Romaine CB, Skandalakis JE. Congenital Fusion of the Cervical Vertebrae. Surg Gynecol Obstet. 1964; 118
[26] Hensinger RN, Lang JR, MacEwen GD. Klippel-Feil Syndrome: A Constellation of Associated Anomalies. J Bone Joint Surg. 1974; 56A
[27] Youmans JR. Neurological Surgery. Philadelphia 1982
[28] Park TS, Cail WS, Maggio WM, Mitchell DC. Progressive Spasticity and Scoliosis in Children with Myelomeningocele: Radiological Investigation and Surgical Treatment. J Neurosurg. 1985; 62:367–375

[29] Pang D, Wilberger JE. Tethered Cord Syndrome in Adults. J Neurosurg. 1982; 57:32–47

[30] Pang D, Dias MS, Ahab-Barmada M. Split Cord Malformation: Part I: A Unified Theory of Embryogenesis for Double Spinal Cord Malformations. Neurosurgery. 1992; 31:451–480

[31] Hoffman HJ. Comment on Pang D, et al.: Split Cord Malformation: Part I: A Unified Theory of Embryogenesis for Double Spinal Cord Malformations. Neurosurgery. 1992; 31

[32] Cannon BW, Hunter SE, Picaza JA. Nerve-root anomalies in lumbar-disc surgery. J Neurosurg. 1962; 19:208–214

[33] Neidre A, MacNab I. Anomalies of the lumbosacral nerve roots. Review of 16 cases and classification. Spine. 1983; 8:294–299

17 Primary Craniospinal Anomalies

17.1 Chiari malformations

17.1.1 General information

The term "Chiari malformation" (after pathologist, Hans Chiari) is preferred for type 1 malformations, with the commonly used term "Arnold-Chiari malformation" reserved for type 2 malformation.

The Chiari malformations consists of four types of hindbrain abnormalities, probably unrelated to each other. The majority of Chiari malformations are types 1 or 2 ▶ Table 17.1), a very limited number of cases comprise the remaining types. Chiari zero is a novel condition (p.286).

17.1.2 Type 1 Chiari malformation

General information

Key concepts

- a heterogeneous entity with the common feature of impaired CSF circulation through the foramen magnum
- may be congenital or acquired
- evaluation: MRI of brain and cervical spine (to R/O syringomyelia). Cine MRI to evaluate CSF flow through foramen magnum in uncertain cases
- cerebellar tonsillar herniation on MRI: criteria vary, > 5 mm below the foramen magnum is often cited, but is neither essential nor diagnostic of the condition
- treatment, when indicated, is surgical, but aspects of what that surgery should entail are controversial (enlargement of foramen magnum is usually involved)
- associated with syringomyelia in 30–70% which almost always improves with treatment of the Chiari malformation

AKA primary cerebellar ectopia,[2] AKA adult Chiari malformation (since it tends to be diagnosed in the 2nd or 3rd decade of life). A heterogeneous group of conditions, with the underlying commonality of disruption of normal CSF flow through the foramen magnum (FM). Some cases are congenital, but others are acquired (this section is kept here under developmental for historical and organizational reasons).

Table 17.1 Comparisons of Chiari type 1 and 2 anomalies (adapted[1])

Finding	Chiari type 1 (see below)	Chiari type 2 (p.284)
caudal dislocation of medulla	unusual	yes
caudal dislocation into cervical canal	tonsils	inferior vermis, medulla, 4th ventricle
spina bifida (myelomeningocele)	may be present	rarely absent
hydrocephalus	may be absent	rarely absent
medullary "kink"	absent	present in 55%
course of upper cervical nerves	usually normal	usually cephalad
usual age of presentation	young adult	infancy
usual presentation	cervical pain, suboccipital H/A	progressive hydrocephalus, respiratory distress

17

Classically described as a rare abnormality restricted to caudal displacement of cerebellum with tonsillar herniation below the foramen magnum (below for criteria) and "peg-like elongation of tonsils." Unlike Chiari type 2, the medulla is *not* caudally displaced (some authors disagree on this point[3]), the brainstem is not involved, lower cranial nerves are not elongated, and upper cervical nerves do not course cephalad. Syringomyelia of the spinal cord is present in 30–70%.[4] True hydromyelia probably doesn't occur; CSF flow has not been documented in man, and it is generally not possible to find communication between the syrinx and the central canal in Chiari 1 patients. Hydrocephalus occurs in 7–9% of patients with Chiari type 1 malformation and syringomyelia.[4]

Cerebellar tonsil descent below FM with impaction, while common, is no longer a sine qua non of diagnosis.

Associations

May be associated with

1. a small posterior fossa
   a) underdevelopment of the occipital bone due to a defect in the occipital somites originating from the para-axial mesoderm
   b) low lying tentorium (the roof of the p-fossa)
   c) thickened or elevated occipital bone (the floor of the p-fossa)
   d) space occupying lesion in p-fossa: arachnoid cyst (retrocerebellar or supracerebellar[5]), tumor (e.g. FM meningioma or cerebellar astrocytoma), hypervascular dura
2. has been described with just about anything that takes up intracranial space
   a) chronic subdural hematomas
   b) hydrocephalus
3. following lumboperitoneal shunt (p. 418) or multiple (traumatic) LPs[6]: acquired Chiari 1 malformation (may be asymptomatic)
4. arachnoid web or scar or fibrosis around brainstem and tonsils near FM
5. abnormalities of the upper cervical spine
   a) hypermobility of the craniovertebral junction
   b) Klippel-Feil syndrome
   c) occipitalization of the atlas
   d) anterior indentation at foramen magnum: e.g. basilar invagination or retroversion of the odontoid process
6. Ehlers-Danlos syndrome
7. craniosynostosis: especially cases involving all sutures
8. retained rhomboid roof: rare

Epidemiology

Average age at presentation is 41 years (range: 12–73 yrs). Slight female preponderance (female: male = 1.3:1). Average duration of symptoms clearly related to Chiari malformation is 3.1 yrs (range: 1 month-20 yrs); if nonspecific complaints, e.g. H/A, are included, this becomes 7.3 years.[7] This latency is probably lower in the MRI era.

Clinical

Clinical correlates

Patients with Chiari type 1 malformation may present due to any or all of the following:

1. compression of brain stem at the level of the foramen magnum
2. hydrocephalus
3. syringomyelia
4. isolation of the intracranial pressure compartment from the spinal compartment causing transient elevations of ICP intracranial pressure
5. 15–30% of patients with adult Chiari malformation are asymptomatic[8]

Symptoms

The most common symptom is pain (69%), especially headache which is usually felt in the suboccipital region ▶ Table 17.2). H/A are often brought on by neck extension or valsalva maneuver. Weakness is also prominent, especially unilateral grasp. Lhermitte's sign may also occur. Lower extremity involvement usually consists of bilateral spasticity.

Table 17.2 Presenting *symptoms* in Chiari 1 malformation (71 cases[3])

Symptom	%
pain	69%
H/A	34%
neck (suboccipital, cervical)	13%
girdle	11%
arm	8%
leg	3%
weakness (1 or more limbs)	56%
numbness (1 or more limbs)	52%
loss of temperature sensation	40%
painless burns	15%
unsteadiness	40%
diplopia	13%
dysphasia	8%
tinnitus	7%
vomiting	5%
dysarthria	4%
miscellaneous	
dizziness	3%
deafness	3%
fainting	3%
facial numbness	3%
hiccough	1%
facial hyperhidrosis	1%

Signs

Downbeat nystagmus is considered a characteristic of this condition. 10% will have a normal neurologic exam with occipital H/A as their only complaint. Some patients may present primarily with spasticity.

See ▶ Table 17.3. Three main patterns of clustering of signs[3]:

1. *foramen magnum compression syndrome* (22%): ataxia, corticospinal and sensory deficits, cerebellar signs, lower cranial nerve palsies. 37% have severe H/A
2. *central cord syndrome* (65%): dissociated sensory loss (loss of pain & temperature sensation with preserved touch & JPS), occasional segmental weakness, and long tract signs (syringomyelic syndrome[9]). 11% have lower cranial nerve palsies
3. *cerebellar syndrome* (11%): truncal and limb ataxia, nystagmus, dysarthria

Natural history

The natural history is not known with certainty (only 2 reports on “natural history”). A patient may remain stable for years, with intermittent periods of deterioration. Rarely, spontaneous improvement may occur (debated).

Table 17.3 Presenting *signs* in Chiari I malformation (127 patients[7])

Sign	%
hyperactive lower extremity reflexes	52%
nystagmus[a]	47%
gait disturbance	43%
hand atrophy	35%
upper extremity weakness	33%
"cape" sensory loss	31%
cerebellar signs	27%
hyperactive upper extremity reflexes	26%
lower cranial nerve dysfunction	26%
Babinski sign	24%
lower extremity weakness	17%
dysesthesia	17%
fasciculation	11%
Horner's sign	6%

[a]classically: downbeat nystagmus on vertical movement, and rotatory nystagmus on horizontal movement; also includes oscillopsia[10]

Evaluation

Plain x-rays

Of 70 skull x-rays, only 36% were abnormal (26% showed basilar impression, 7% platybasia, and 1 patient each with Paget's and concave clivus); in 60 C-spine x-rays, 35% were abnormal (including assimilation of atlas, widened canal, cervical fusions, agenesis of posterior arch of atlas).

MRI

MRI of brain and C-spine is the diagnostic test of choice. Easily shows many of the classic abnormalities described earlier, including tonsillar herniation, as well as hydrosyringomyelia which occurs in 20–30% of cases. Also demonstrates ventral brain stem compression when present. Other findings include: hydrocephalus, empty sella.

Tonsillar herniation: Criteria for the descent of the tonsillar tips below the foramen magnum (FM) to diagnose Chiari type 1 malformation have gone through a number of reconsiderations.

17

Σ

Tonsillar herniation identified radiographically is of limited prognostic value in diagnosing Chiari I malformation, and requires clinical correlation.

Initially, > 5 mm was defined as clearly pathologic[11] (with 3–5 mm being borderline). Barkovich[12] found tonsillar positions as shown in ▶ Table 17.4, and ▶ Table 17.5 shows the effect of utilizing 2 vs. 3 mm as the lowest normal position.

The tonsils normally ascend with age[13] as shown in ▶ Table 17.6

Table 17.4 Location of cerebellar tonsils below foramen magnum[12]		
Group	**Mean[a]**	**Range**
normal	1 mm above	8 mm above to 5 mm below
Chiari I	13 mm below	3–29 mm below
[a]based on measurements in 200 normals and 25 Chiari I patients taken in relation to the lower part of the foramen magnum		

Table 17.5 Criteria for Chiari I[12]		
Criteria for lowest extent of tonsils accepted as normal	**Sensitivity for Chiari I**	**Specificity for Chiari I**
2 mm below FM	100%	98.5%
3 mm below FM	96%	99.5%

Table 17.6 Tonsillar position relative to FM at various ages[13]		
Age (years)	**Normal (mm)[a]**	**2 S.D.[b] (mm)**
0–9	−1.5	−6
10–19	−0.4	−5
20–29	−1.1	
30–39	0.0	−4
40–49	0.1	
50–59	0.2	
60–69	0.2	
70–79	0.6	
80–89	1.3	−3
[a]negative number indicates distance below FM [b]S.D. = standard deviation. Descent > 2 S.D. beyond normal is suggested as a criteria for tonsillar ectopia		

Patients with syringohydromyelia without hindbrain herniation that responded to p-fossa decompression have been described[14] (so-called "Chiari zero malformation"). Conversely, 14% of patients with tonsillar herniation > 5 mm are asymptomatic[15] (average extent of ectopia in this group was 11.4 ± 4.86 mm).

Potentially more significant than the absolute tonsillar descent is the amount of compression of the brainstem at the FM, best appreciated on axial T2WI MRI through the FM. Complete obliteration of CSF signal and compression of the brainstem at the FM by impacted tonsils is a common significant finding.

Cine MRI

AKA CSF flow study. May demonstrate blockage of CSF flow at FM. Not widely available. Accuracy is not high, therefore usually does not alter management.

Myelography

Generally used only when MRI cannot be obtained. Only 6% false negative. It is critical to run the intrathecal contrast (dye) all the way up to the foramen magnum. Usually combined with CT scan.

CT

Unenhanced CT is poor for evaluating the foramen magnum region due to bony artifact. It is very good at demonstrating hydrocephalus (as is MRI). When combined with intrathecal iodinated contrast (myelogram), reliability improves. Findings: tonsillar descent with possible complete blockage of dye at foramen magnum.

Treatment

Indications for surgery

Since patients respond best when operated on within 2 years of the onset of symptoms (below), early surgery is recommended for symptomatic patients. Asymptomatic patients may be followed and operated upon if and when they become symptomatic. Patients who have been symptomatic and stable for years may be considered for observation, with surgery indicated for signs of deterioration.

Surgical techniques

The most frequently performed operation is posterior fossa decompression (suboccipital craniectomy), with or without other procedures (usually combined with dural patch grafting and cervical laminectomy of C1, sometimes to C2 or C3). Options for grafts: same incision (pericranium), separate incision (e.g. or fascia lata), and allograft (avoided by many authors because of dissatisfaction with ability to provide water-tight closure and because of infectious risks).

Goals of surgery: decompress the brain stem and reestablish normal flow of CSF at the craniocervical junction.

The patient is positioned prone on chest rolls with the head in a Mayfield head-holder or in a horseshoe headrest. Flex the neck to open the interspace between the occiput and posterior arch of C1. The shoulders are retracted inferiorly with adhesive tape. If a fascia lata graft is to be taken, elevate one thigh on a sandbag. A midline incision from inion to ≈ C2 spinous process is made. The removal of bone above the foramen magnum should be ≈ 3 cm high by ≈ 3 cm wide (keep the posterior-fossa part of these operations *small*, the main thrust is to open the foramen magnum to decompress the tonsils and an upper cervical laminectomy; the compression is *not* in the p-fossa). Excessive removal of occipital bone may allow the cerebellar hemispheres to herniate through the opening ("cerebellar ptosis"), and create additional problems. If a pericranial graft is to be taken, it should be harvested at this time to reduce the amount of blood entering the subsequent dural opening.[16] Pericranial graft can be procured without extending the incision about the inion using the technique of Dr. Robert Ojemann[16] with subgaleal dissection and using a monopolar cautery with a bent tip to incise the periosteum and then a Penfield #1 dissector to free it from the bone surface.

Open the dura in a "Y" shaped incision, and excise the triangular top flap. CAUTION: the transverse sinuses are usually abnormally *low* in Chiari malformations. Suture the patch graft to provide more room for the contents (tonsils + medulla).

An option that is sometimes used in pediatrics is to not initially open the dura but to lyse constricting bands over the dura at the foramen magnum and then and use intraoperative ultrasound to determine if there is adequate room for CSF flow, the dura is then opened only if there is not.

Historical procedures that have been appended to the above: plugging the obex (with muscle or teflon), drainage of syrinx if present (fenestration, usually through dorsal root entry zone, with or without stent or shunt), 4th ventricular shunting, terminal ventriculostomy, and opening foramen of Magendie if obstructed (see reference for illustrations[9]). Current recommendations are that these or other additional procedures beyond dural patch grafting are usually not warranted.

Some authors repeatedly admonish *not* to attempt to remove adhesions binding the tonsils together (to avoid injuring vital structures, including PICAs). Others recommend cautiously separating the tonsils and even shrinking them down with bipolar cautery.

In cases with ventral brain-stem compression, some authors advocate performing a transoral clivus-odontoid resection as they feel these patients may potentially deteriorate with posterior fossa decompression alone.[17] Since this deterioration was reversible with odontoidectomy, it may be reasonable to perform this procedure on patients who show signs of deterioration or progression of basilar impression on serial MRIs after posterior fossa decompression.

Booking the case: Chiari malformation

Also see defaults & disclaimers (p. 27).
1. position: prone
2. equipment:
   a) optional microscope
   b) intra-op Doppler, if used
3. consent:
   a) procedure: surgery through the back of the neck to open the bone at the base of the skull and to insert a "patch" to make more room for the brainstem
   b) alternatives: non-surgical management is usually not effective
   c) complications: CSF leak, brainstem injury/stroke, apnea, failure to improve syrinx (if present)

Operative findings

See ▶ Table 17.7.

Tonsillar herniation is present in all cases (by definition); the most common position being at C1 (62%). Fibrous adhesions between dura, arachnoid and tonsils with occlusion of foramina of Luschka and Magendie in 41%. The tonsils separated easily in 40%.

Surgical complications

After suboccipital craniectomy plus C1–3 laminectomy in 71 patients, with dural patch grafting in 69, one death due to sleep apnea occurred 36 hrs post-op. Respiratory depression was the most common post-op complication (in 10 patients), usually within 5 days, mostly at night. Close respiratory

Table 17.7 Operative findings in Chiari I (71 patients[3])

Finding	%
tonsillar descent	100%
below foramen magnum	4%
C1	62%
C2	25%
C3	3%
unspecified level	6%
adhesions	41%
syringomyelia	32%
dural band (at foramen magnum or C1 arch)	30%
vascular abnormalities[a]	20%
skeletal abnormalities	
inverted foramen magnum	10%
keel of bone	3%
C1 arch atresia	3%
occipitalization of C1 arch	1%
cervicomedullary "hump"	12%

[a]vascular abnormalities: PICA dilated or abnormal course in 8 patients (PICA often descends to lower margin of tonsils[9]); large dural venous lakes in 3

Table 17.8 Long-term follow-up after surgery for Chiari I malformation (69 patients, 4 years mean F/U[3])

early improvement of pre-op symptoms	82%
percent of above that relapsed[a]	21%
early improvement of pre-op signs	70%
no change from pre-op status	16%
worse than pre-op	0

[a]these patients deteriorated to pre-op status (none deteriorated further) within 2–3 years of surgery; relapse occurred in 30% with foramen magnum compression syndrome, and in 21% with central cord syndrome

monitoring is therefore recommended.[3] Other risks of the procedure include: CSF leak, herniation of cerebellar hemispheres, vascular injuries (to PICA…).

Operative results

See ▶ Table 17.8.

Patients with pre-op complaints of pain generally respond well to surgery. Weakness is less responsive to surgery, especially when muscle atrophy is present.[17] Sensation may improve when the posterior columns are unaffected and the deficit is due to spinothalamic involvement alone.

Rhoton feels that the main benefit of operation is to arrest progression.

The most favorable results occurred in patients with cerebellar syndrome (87% showing improvement, no late deterioration). Factors that correlate with a worse outcome are the presence of atrophy, ataxia, scoliosis, and symptoms lasting longer than 2 years.[17]

17.1.3 Type 2 (Arnold)-Chiari malformation

General information

Key concepts

- usually associated with myelomeningocele, often accompanied by hydrocephalus pathology includes: caudally displaced cervicomedullary junction, small posterior fossa, tectal beaking. Is probably not due to tethering
- major clinical findings: swallowing difficulties, apnea, stridor, opisthotonos, downbeat nystagmus
- when symptomatic: always check the shunt first! Then, consider surgical decompression (which cannot correct intrinsic brainstem abnormalities)
- cranial and cervical MRI is the diagnostic test of choice.

17

Usually associated with myelomeningocele (MM), or rarely spina bifida occulta.

Pathophysiology

Probably does *not* result from tethering of the cord by the associated MM. More likely due to primary dysgenesis of the brainstem with multiple other developmental anomalies.[18]

Major findings

Caudally dislocated cervicomedullary junction, pons, 4th ventricle and medulla. Cerebellar tonsils located at or below the foramen magnum. Replacement of normal cervicomedullary junction flexure with a "kink-like deformity."

Other possible associated findings:

1. beaking of tectum
2. absence of the septum pellucidum with enlarged interthalamic adhesion: absence of the septum pellucidum is thought to be due to necrosis with resorption secondary to hydrocephalus, and not a congenital absence[19(p 178)]

3. poorly myelinated cerebellar folia
4. hydrocephalus: present in most
5. heterotopias
6. hypoplasia of falx
7. microgyria
8. degeneration of lower cranial nerve nuclei
9. bony abnormalities:
   a) of cervicomedullary junction
   b) assimilation of atlas
   c) platybasia
   d) basilar impression
   e) Klippel-Feil deformity (p.271)
10. hydromyelia
11. craniolacunia of the skull (see below)

Presentation

Findings are due to brain stem and lower cranial nerve dysfunction. Onset is rare in adulthood. The presentation of neonates differs substantially from older children, and neonates were more likely to develop rapid neurological deterioration with profound brain stem dysfunction over a period of several days than were older children in whom symptoms were more insidious and rarely as severe.[20]

Findings include[21,20]:

1. swallowing difficulties (neurogenic dysphagia) (69%).[22] Manifests as poor feeding, cyanosis during feeding, nasal regurgitation, prolonged feeding time, or pooling of oral secretions. Gag reflex often decreased. More severe in neonates
2. apneic spells (58%): due to impaired ventilatory drive. More common in neonates
3. stridor (56%): more common in neonates, usually worse on inspiration (abductor and occasionally adductor vocal cord paralysis seen on laryngoscopy) due to 10th nerve paresis; usually transient, but may progress to respiratory arrest
4. aspiration (40%)
5. arm weakness (27%) that may progress to quadriparesis[23]
6. opisthotonos (18%)
7. nystagmus: especially downbeat nystagmus
8. weak or absent cry
9. facial weakness

Diagnostic evaluation

Skull films

May demonstrate cephalofacial disproportion from congenital HCP. Craniolacunia (AKA lückenschädel) in 85% (round defects in the skull with sharp borders, separated by irregularly branching bands of bone; *not* due to increased ICP). Low lying internal occipital protuberance (foreshortened posterior fossa). Enlarged foramen magnum in 70%; elongation of upper cervical lamina.[1]

CT and/or MRI findings

Cranial and cervical MRI is the diagnostic test of choice.

- primary findings
  a) "Z" bend deformity of medulla*
  b) cerebellar peg
  c) tectal fusion ("tectal beaking")
  d) enlarged massa intermedia (interthalamic adhesion)*
  e) elongation/cervicallization of medulla
  f) low attachment of tentorium
- associated findings
  a) hydrocephalus
  b) syringomyelia in the area of the cervicomedullary junction (reported incidence in pre MRI era[17] ranges from 48–88%)
  c) trapped fourth ventricle
  d) cerebellomedullary compression
  e) agenesis/dysgenesis of corpus callosum*

* items with an asterisk are best appreciated on MRI

17

Laryngoscopy

Performed in patients with stridor to rule out croup or other upper respiratory tract infection.

Treatment

General information

- insert CSF shunt for hydrocephalus (or check function of existing shunt)
- if neurogenic dysphagia, stridor, or apneic spells occur, expeditious posterior fossa decompression is recommended (see below) (required in 18.7% of MM patients[21]); before recommending decompression, always make sure the patient has a functioning shunt!

Surgical decompression

NB: it has been argued that part of the explanation for the poor operative results in infants is that many of the neurological findings may be due in part to intrinsic (uncorrectable) abnormalities which surgical decompression cannot improve.[24,25] A dissenting view is that the histologic lesions are due to chronic brain stem compression and concomitant ischemia, and that expeditious brain stem decompression should be carried out when any of the following critical warning signs develop: *neurogenic dysphagia, stridor, apneic spells.*[20]

Surgical technique

Decompression of cerebellar tonsils, usually with dural graft to decompress dura. Patients is placed prone, with the neck flexed. A suboccipital craniectomy is combined with a cervical laminectomy which must be carried down to the bottom of the tonsillar tip.[23] A thick constricting dural band is usually found between the C1 arch and foramen magnum. The dura is opened in a "Y" shaped incision. Caution when opening the dura above the level of the foramen magnum in infants as they have a well-developed occipital sinus and may have large dural lakes.[21] DO NOT attempt to dissect tonsils from underlying medulla. In cases with a significant syringomyelic cavity, a syringo-subarachnoid shunt is placed.[20]

Tracheostomy (usually temporary) is recommended if stridor and abductor laryngeal palsy were present pre-op. Close post-op respiratory monitoring is needed for obstruction *and* reduced ventilatory drive (mechanical ventilation is indicated for hypoxia or hypercarbia).

Outcome

68% had complete or near complete resolution of symptoms, 12% had mild to moderate residual deficits, and 20% had no improvement (in general, neonates fared worse than older children).[20]

Respiratory arrest is the most common cause of mortality (8 of 17 patients who died), with the rest due to meningitis/ventriculitis (6 patients), aspiration (2 patients), and biliary atresia (1 patient).[21]

In follow-up ranging 7 mos-6 yrs, 37.8% mortality in operated patients.

Pre-op status and the rapidity of neurologic deterioration were the most important prognosticators. Mortality rate is 71% in infants having cardiopulmonary arrest, vocal cord paralysis or arm weakness within 2 weeks of presentation; compared to 23% mortality in patients with a more gradual deterioration. Bilateral vocal cord paralysis was a particularly poor prognosticator for response to surgery.[20]

17.1.4 Other Chiari malformations

Chiari type 0

Patients with syringohydromyelia without hindbrain herniation that respond to p-fossa decompression have been described[14] (so-called "Chiari zero malformation").

Chiari type 1.5

Obex situated below foramen magnum, does not respond to suboccipital decompression with or without duroplasty.

Chiari type 3

Rare. Both the definition and even the existence are controversial. Most descriptions are based on 1 or 2 cases. Original description cited dislocation of the cerebellum below the foramen magnum into an occipital encephalocele.[26] Some have added herniation of the medulla, fourth ventricle and all of the cerebellum into an occipital and high cervical encephalocele. Some have sided with Raimondi who included occipital encephaloceles associated with caudal displacement of the cerebellum and medulla.[27,28]

Prognosis is poor for most, as it is usually incompatible with life.

Chiari type 4

Originally described as cerebellar hypoplasia without cerebellar herniation.[29] Existence as a distinct clinical entity is debated.[26]

17.2 Neural tube defects

17.2.1 Classification

General information

There is no universally accepted classification system. Two are presented below.

Lemire classification

A system adapted from Lemire.[30]

1. neurulation defects: non-closure of the neural tube results in open lesions
   a) craniorachischisis: total dysraphism. Many die as spontaneous abortion
   b) anencephaly: AKA exencephaly. Due to failure of fusion of the anterior neuropore. Neither cranial vault nor scalp covers the partially destroyed brain. Uniformly fatal. Risk of recurrence in future pregnancies: 3%
   c) meningomyelocele: most common in lumbar region
      - myelomeningocele (MM) (p.265)
      - myelocele
2. postneurulation defects: produces skin-covered (AKA closed) lesions (some may also be considered "migration abnormalities", see below)
   a) cranial
      - microcephaly: see below
      - hydranencephaly: loss of most of cerebral hemispheres, replaced by CSF (see below). Must R/O maximal hydrocephalus (see below)
      - holoprosencephaly: see below
      - lissencephaly: see below
      - porencephaly: see below to distinguish from schizencephaly
      - agenesis of corpus callosum: see below
      - cerebellar hypoplasia/Dandy Walker syndrome (p.256)
      - macroencephaly AKA megalencephaly: see below
   b) spinal
      - diastematomyelia, diplomyelia: see Split cord malformation (p.274)
      - hydromyelia/syringomyelia (p.1144)

Migration abnormalities

A slightly different classification scheme defines the following as abnormalities of neuronal migration (some are considered postneurulation defects, see above):

1. lissencephaly: The most severe neuronal migration abnormality. Maldevelopment of cerebral convolutions (probably an arrest of cortical development at an early fetal age). Infants are severely retarded and usually don't survive > 2 yrs
   a) agyria: completely smooth surface
   b) pachygyria: few broad & flat gyri with shallow sulci
   c) polymicrogyria: small gyri with shallow sulci. May be difficult to diagnose by CT/MRI, and may be confused with pachygyria
2. heterotopia: abnormal foci of (nonenhancing) gray matter which may be located anywhere from the subcortical white matter to (most commonly) the subependymal lining of the ventricles. May manifest as nodules or as a band of cortex. An early migration defect that results from arrest of radial migration. Almost always presents with seizures
3. cortical dysplasia: a cleft that does not communicate with the ventricle. Heterotopias are common. A migration abnormality not quite as severe as schizencephaly

17

4. **schizencephaly**:
   a) sine qua non: cleft that communicates with the ventricle (communication may be confirmed with CT cisternogram if necessary)
   b) cleft lined with cortical grey matter (often abnormal, may have polymicrogyria). This distinguishes it from **porencephaly**, a cystic lesion lined with connective or glial tissue that may communicate with the ventricular system, often caused by vascular infarcts or following intracerebral hemorrhage or penetrating trauma (including repeated ventricular punctures)
   c) two forms:
      - open lipped: large cleft to ventricle. Very severe forms may mimic hydranencephaly (see below)
      - close lipped (walls fused): ✱ look for a dimple in the lateral wall of the lateral ventricle immediately under the cortical cleft (the appearance of which may mimic an enlarged sulcus)
   d) may be unilateral or bilateral
   e) pia and arachnoid fuse
   f) there may be an "abnormal" vein that represents a cortical vein that now looks medullary because it follows the cortex into the cleft)
   g) absence of septum pellucidum in 80–90%
   h) presentation may range from seizures to hemiparesis depending on size and location

17.2.2 Examples of neural tube defects

Hydranencephaly

General information

A post-neurulation defect. Total or near-total absence of the cerebrum (small bands of cerebrum may be consistent with the diagnosis[31]), with intact cranial vault and meninges, the intracranial cavity being filled with CSF. There is usually progressive macrocrania, but head size may be normal (especially at birth), and, occasionally, microcephaly may occur. Facial dysmorphism is rare.

May be due to a variety of causes, the most commonly cited is bilateral ICA infarcts (which results in absence of brain tissue supplied by the anterior and middle cerebral arteries with preservation in the distribution of the PCA). May also be due to infection (congenital or neonatal herpes, toxoplasmosis, equine virus).

Less affected infants may appear normal at birth, but are often hyperirritable and retain primitive reflexes (Moro, grasp, and stepping reflex) beyond 6 mo. They rarely progress beyond spontaneous vowel production and social smiling. Seizures are common.

Differentiation from hydrocephalus

Progressive enlargement of CSF spaces may occur which can mimic severe ("maximal") hydrocephalus (HCP). It is critical to differentiate the two since true HCP may be treated by shunting which may produce some re-expansion of the cortical mantle. Many means to distinguish hydranencephaly and HCP have been described, including:

1. EEG: shows no cortical activity in hydranencephaly (maximal HCP typically produces an abnormal EEG, but background activity will be present throughout the brain[31]) and is one of the best ways to differentiate the two
2. CT,[32,31] MRI or ultrasound: majority of intracranial space is occupied by CSF. Usually do not see frontal lobes or frontal horns of lateral ventricles (there may be remnants of temporal, occipital or subfrontal cortex). A structure consisting of brainstem nodule (rounded thalamic masses, hypothalamus) and medial occipital lobes sitting on the tentorium occupies a midline position surrounded by CSF. Posterior fossa structures are grossly intact. The falx is usually intact (unlike alobar holoprosencephaly), and is not thickened, but may be displaced laterally. In HCP, some cortical mantle is usually identifiable
3. transillumination of the skull: in a darkened room, a bright light is placed against the surface of the skull. To transilluminate, the patient must be < 9 mos old and the cortical mantle under the light source must be < 1 cm thick,[33(p 215)] can also occur if fluid displaces the cortex inward (e.g. subdural effusions). Too insensitive to be very helpful
4. angiography: in "classic" cases resulting from bilateral ICA occlusion, no flow through supraclinoid carotids and a normal posterior circulation is expected

Treatment

Shunting may be performed to control head size, but unlike the case with maximal hydrocephalus, there is no restitution of the cerebral mantle.

Holoprosencephaly

AKA arhinencephaly. Failure of the telencephalic vesicle to cleave into two cerebral hemispheres. The degree of cleavage failure ranges from the severe alobar (single ventricle, no interhemispheric fissure) to semilobar and lobar (less severe malformations). The olfactory bulbs are usually small and the cingulate gyrus remains fused. Median faciocerebral dysplasia is common, and the degree of severity parallels the extent of the cleavage failure ▶ Table 17.9). 80% are associated with trisomy (primarily trisomy 13, and to a lesser extent trisomy 18). Survival beyond infancy is uncommon, most survivors are severely retarded, a minority are able to function in society. Some develop shunt dependent hydrocephalus. The risk of holoprosencephaly is increased in subsequent pregnancies of the same couple.

Microcephaly

Definition: head circumference more than 2 standard deviations below the mean for sex and gestational age. Terms that are sometimes used synonymously: microcrania, microcephalus. Not a single entity, many of the conditions in ▶ Table 17.9 may be associated with microcephaly. It may also result from maternal cocaine abuse.[35] It is important to differentiate microcephaly from a small skull resulting from craniosynostosis in which surgical treatment may provide opportunity for improved cerebral development.

Macroencephaly

Adapted.[36(p 109)] AKA macrencephaly, AKA megalencephaly. Not to be confused with macrocephaly (p. 1403), which is enlargement of the skull. Not a single pathologic entity. An enlarged brain which may be due to: hypertrophy of gray matter alone, gray and white matter, presence of additional structures (glial overgrowth, diffuse gliomas, heterotopias, metabolic storage diseases…).

Conditions in which macrocephaly may be seen include:

- neurocutaneous syndromes (especially neurofibromatosis)
- megalencephaly-capillary malformation syndrome (MCAP): an overgrowth syndrome with megalencephaly (often with hydrocephalus, Chiari malformation, polymicrogyria and seizures), and capillary malformations in the skin (usually on the face)

Brains may weigh up to 1600–2850 grams. IQ may be normal, but developmental delay, retardation, spasticity and hypotonia may occur. Head circumference is 4–7 cm above mean. The usual signs of hydrocephalus (frontal bossing, bulging fontanelle, "setting sun" sign, scalp vein engorgement) are absent. Imaging studies (CT or MRI) show normal sized ventricles and can be used to rule out extra-axial fluid collections.

Table 17.9 The five facies of severe holoprosencephaly[34]

Type of face	Facial features	Cranium and brain findings
cyclopia	single eye or partially divided eye in single orbit; arhinia with proboscis	microcephaly; alobar holoprosencephaly
ethmocephaly	extreme orbital hypotelorism; separate orbits; arhinia with proboscis	microcephaly; alobar holoprosencephaly
cebocephaly	orbital hypotelorism; proboscis-like nose; no median cleft lip	microcephaly; usually has alobar holoprosencephaly
with median cleft lip	orbital hypotelorism; flat nose	microcephaly; sometimes has trigonocephaly; usually has alobar holoprosencephaly
with median philtrum-premaxilla anlage	orbital hypotelorism; bilateral lateral cleft lip with median process representing philtrum-premaxillary anlage; flat nose	microcephaly; sometimes has trigonocephaly; semilobar or lobar holoprosencephaly

17.2.3 Risk factors

1. lack of prenatal folic acid: early administration of folic acid[37,38,39] (0.4 mg/d if no history of neural tube defects; 4 mg/d in a carrier or with previous child with NTD was associated with a 71% reduction in recurrence of NTD[40]) (confirm that vitamin B12 levels are normal)
2. folate antagonists (e.g. carbamazepine) doubles the incidence of MM
3. mothers with 5, 10-methylenetetrahydrofolate reductase (MTHFR) gene polymorphism. The common variant, C677T, substitutes an alanine residue for valine at position 222 in the folate dependent MTHFR enzyme → decreased enzyme activity → reduced levels of tissue folate, and increased levels of homocysteine in the plasma. This polymorphism may be homozygous (TT genotype) or heterozygous (CT genotype); present in ≈10% and 38% of the population, respectively. The effects with the TT genotype are more pronounced than with the heterozygous CT form, and there is an increased risk of neural tube defects, as well as a lesser increased risk of cardiovascular disease[41]
4. use of valproic acid (Depakene®) during pregnancy is associated with a 1–2% risk of NTD[42]
5. maternal heat exposure in the form of hot-tubs, saunas or fever (but not electric blankets) in the first trimester was associated with an increased risk of NTDs[43]
6. obesity (before and during pregnancy) increases the risk of NTD[44,45]
7. maternal cocaine abuse may increase the risk of microcephaly, disorders of neuronal migration, neuronal differentiation and myelination[35]

17.2.4 Prenatal detection of neural tube defects

Serum alpha-fetoprotein (AFP)

See Alpha-fetoprotein (p.600) for background. A high maternal serum AFP (≥ 2 multiples of the median for the appropriate week of gestation) between 15–20 weeks gestation carries a relative risk of 224 for neural tube defects, and an abnormal value (high or low) was associated with 34% of all major congenital defects.[46] The sensitivity of maternal serum AFP for spina bifida was 91% (10 of 11 cases), it was 100% for 9 cases of anencephaly. However, other series show a lower sensitivity. Closed lumbosacral spine defects, accounting for ≈ 20% of spina bifida patients,[47] will probably be missed by serum AFP screening, and may also be missed on ultrasound. Since maternal serum AFP rises during normal pregnancy, an overestimate of gestational age may cause an elevated AFP to be interpreted as normal, and an underestimate may cause a normal level to be interpreted as elevated.[48]

Ultrasound

Prenatal ultrasound will detect 90–95% of cases of spina bifida, and thus in cases of elevated AFP, it can help differentiate NTDs from non-neurologic causes of elevated AFP (e.g. omphalocele), and can help to more accurately estimate gestational age.

Amniocentesis

For pregnancies subsequent to a MM, if prenatal ultrasound does not show spinal dysraphism, then amniocentesis is recommended (even if abortion is not considered, it may allow for optimal postpartum care if MM is diagnosed). *Amniotic* fluid AFP levels are elevated with open neural tube defects, with a peak between weeks 13–15 of pregnancy. Amniocentesis also carries a ≈ 6% risk of fetal loss in this population.

17.3 Neurenteric cysts

17.3.1 General information

No uniformly accepted nomenclature. Working definition: CNS cyst lined by endothelium primarily resembling that of the GI tract, or less often, respiratory tract. Congenital. Not true neoplasms. Most common alternate term: enterogenous cyst. Less common terms include: teratomatous cyst, intestinoma, archenteric cyst,[49] enterogene cyst, and endodermal cyst. Usually affect the upper thoracic and lower cervical spine.[50] Associated developmental vertebral anomalies (e.g. diastematomyelia) are common.[51] Rarely intracranial (see below). Spinal neurenteric cysts (NEC) may have a fistulous or fibrous connection to the GI tract (through a spinal dysraphism) and some call these endodermal sinus cysts. Occurs as a result of persistence of the neurenteric canal (temporary duct between the notochord and the primitive gut (amniotic and yolk sacs) formed during week 3 of embryogenesis by breakdown of the floor of the notochordal canal).

17.3.2 Intracranial neurenteric cysts

General information

Rare, most common in p-fossa. Initially, may be difficult to rule-out metastasis from an extremely well-differentiated primary adenocarcinoma of unknown origin (absence of progressive disease suggests NEC). Locations:

1. posterior fossa
   a) cerebellopontine angle (CPA)[49]: usually intradural, extraaxial (case report of extradural lesion with bone destruction[52])
   b) in midline anterior to brainstem[50]
   c) cisterna magna[53]
2. supratentorial: only 15 case reports as of 2004.[54] Locations: suprasellar[55] (possible confusion with Rathke's cleft cyst), frontal lobe intraparenchymal,[54] quadrigeminal plate region, dural-based extra-axial. Source of endoderm is controversial since the primitive foregut extends cranially only to the midbrain.[56] Theory: colloid cysts, Rathke cleft cysts, and supratentorial NECs may all arise from remnants of Seesel's pouch, a transient endodermally derived diverticulum of the cranial end of the embryonic foregut[57]

Clinical

Most commonly present during the first decade of life.[51] Pain or myelopathy from the intraspinal mass are the most common presentations in older children and adults. Neonates and young children may present with cardiorespiratory compromise from an intrathoracic mass, or with cervical spinal cord compression.[51] Meningitis may occur from the fistulous tract, especially in newborns and infants.

Imaging

Intracranial NEC:
- CT: usually low density, nonenhancing[58]
- T1WI MRI: isointense or sl hyperintense to CSF (may be hyperintense if there are blood products). T2WI isointense to CSF.[58] Nonenhancing

Histology

Most are simple cysts lined by cuboidal-columnar epithelium and mucin secreting goblet cells. Less common types of epithelium described include: stratified squamous and pseudostratified columnar, and ciliated epithelial cells. Mesodermal components may be present, including smooth muscle and adipose tissue, and some have called these teratomatous cysts[59,60] which is not to be confused with teratomas which are true germinal cell neoplasms. May be histologically identical to colloid cysts.

Treatment

Spinal NEC

Surgical removal usually reverses the symptoms. Recurrence is uncommon with complete removal of cyst wall.

Intracranial NEC

Capsule adherent to brainstem may prevent complete resection, which predisposes to delayed recurrence. Apparently successful treatment by evacuation of contents and marsupialization has been reported (5 cases, mean follow-up: 5 yrs[61]). Incomplete removal requires long-term follow-up. Hydrocephalus is shunted if indicated.

References

[1] Carmel PW. Management of the Chiari Malformations in Childhood. Clinical Neurosurg. 1983; 30:385–406

[2] Spillane JD, Pallis C, Jones AM. Developmental Abnormalities in the Region of the Foramen Magnum. Brain. 1957; 80:11–52

[3] Paul KS, Lye RH, Strang FA, et al. Arnold-Chiari Malformation: Review of 71 Cases. J Neurosurg. 1983; 58:183–187

[4] Guinto G, Zamorano C, Dominguez F, Sandoval B, Villasana O, Ortiz A. Chiari I malformation: Part I. Contemp Neurosurg. 2004; 26:1–7

[5] Bahuleyan B, Rao A, Chacko AG, Daniel RT. Supracerebellar arachnoid cyst - a rare cause of acquired Chiari I malformation. Journal of Clinical Neuroscience. 2006; 14:895–898

[6] Sathi S, Stieg PE. "Acquired" Chiari I Malformation After Multiple Lumbar Punctures: Case Report. Neurosurgery. 1993; 32:306–309

[7] Levy WJ, Mason L, Hahn JF. Chiari Malformation Presenting in Adults: A Surgical Experience in 127 Cases. Neurosurgery. 1983; 12:377–390

[8] Bejjani GK, Cockerham KP. Adult Chiari malformation. Contemp Neurosurg. 2001; 23:1–7

[9] Rhoton AL. Microsurgery of Arnold-Chiari Malformation in Adults with and without Hydromyelia. J Neurosurg. 1976; 45:473–483

[10] Gingold SI, Winfield JA. Oscillopsia and Primary Cerebellar Ectopie: Case Report and Review of the Literature. Neurosurgery. 1991; 29:932–936

[11] Aboulezz AO, Sartor K, Geyer CA, Gado MH. Position of cerebellar tonsils in the normal population and in patients with Chiari malformation: a quantitative approach with MR imaging. J Comput Assist Tomogr. 1985; 9:1033–1036

[12] Barkovich AJ, Wippold FJ, Sherman JL, Citrin CM. Significance of Cerebellar Tonsillar Position on MR. AJNR. 1986; 7:795–799

[13] Mikulis DJ, Diaz O, Egglin TK, Sanchez R. Variance of the position of the cerebellar tonsils with age: preliminary report. Radiology. 1992; 183:725–728

[14] Iskandar BJ, Hedlund GL, Grabb PA, Oakes WJ. The resolution of syringohydromyelia without hindbrain herniation after posterior fossa decompression. J Neurosurg. 1998; 89:212–216

[15] Meadows J, Kraut M, Guarnieri M, Haroun RI, Carson BS. Asymptomatic Chiari Type I malformations identified on magnetic resonance imaging. J Neurosurg. 2000; 92:920–926

[16] Stevens EA, Powers AK, Sweasey TA, Tatter SB, Ojemann RG. Simplified harvest of autologous pericranium for duraplasty in Chiari malformation Type I. Technical note. J Neurosurg Spine. 2009; 11:80–83

[17] Dyste GN, Menezes AH, VanGilder JC. Symptomatic Chiari Malformations: An Analysis of Presentation, Management, and Long-Term Outcome. J Neurosurg. 1989; 71:159–168

[18] Peach B. The Arnold-Chiari Malformation. Morphogenesis. Arch Neurol. 1965; 12:527–535

[19] Taveras JM, Pile-Spellman J. Neuroradiology. 3rd ed. Baltimore: Williams and Wilkins; 1996

[20] Pollack IF, Pang D, Albright AL, Krieger D. Outcome Following Hindbrain Decompression of Symptomatic Chiari Malformations in Children Previously Treated with Myelomeningocele Closure and Shunts. J Neurosurg. 1992; 77:881–888

[21] Park TS, Hoffman HJ, Hendrick EB, et al. Experience with Surgical Decompression of the Arnold-Chiari Malformation in Young Infants with Myelomeningocele. Neurosurgery. 1983; 13:147–152

[22] Pollack IF, Pang D, Kocoshis S, Putnam P. Neurogenic Dysphagia Resulting from Chiari Malformations. Neurosurgery. 1992; 30:709–719

[23] Hoffman HJ, Hendrick EB, Humphreys RP. Manifestations and Management of Arnold-Chiari Malformation in Patients with Myelomeningocele. Childs Brain. 1975; 1:255–259

[24] Gilbert JN, Jones KL, Rorke LB, et al. Central Nervous System Anomalies Associated with Myelomeningocele, Hydrocephalus, and the Arnold-Chiari Malformation: Reappraisal of Theories Regarding the Pathogenesis of Posterior Neural Tube Closure Defects. Neurosurgery. 1986; 18:559–564

[25] Bell WO, Charney EB, Bruce DA, et al. Symptomatic Arnold-Chiari Malformation: Review of Experience with 22 Cases. J Neurosurg. 1987; 66:812–816

[26] Brownlee R, Myles T, Hamilton MG, Anson JA, Benzel EC, Awad IA. In: The Chiari III and IV malformations. Syringomyelia and the Chiari Malformations. Park Ridge, IL: American Association of Neurological Surgeons; 1997:83–90

[27] Raimondi AJ. Pediatric neuroradiology. Philadelphia: W. B. Saunders; 1972

[28] Castillo M, Quencer RM, Dominguez R. Chiari III malformation: imaging features. AJNR Am J Neuroradiol. 1992; 13:107–113

[29] Chiari H. Über veränderungen des kleinhirns des pons und der medulla oblongata in folge von congenitaler hydrocephalie des grosshirns. Denkschr Akad Wiss Wien. 1895; 63:71–116

[30] Lemire RJ. Neural Tube Defects. JAMA. 1988; 259:558–562

[31] Sutton LN, Bruce DA, Schut L. Hydranencephaly versus Maximal Hydrocephalus: An Important Clinical Distinction. Neurosurgery. 1980; 6:35–38

[32] Dublin AB, French BN. Diagnostic Image Evaluation of Hydranencephaly and Pictorially Similar Entities with Emphasis on Computed Tomography. Radiology. 1980; 137:81–91

[33] Matson DD. Neurosurgery of Infancy and Childhood. 2nd ed. Springfield: Charles C Thomas; 1969

[34] DeMyer W, Zeman W, Palmer CG. The Face Predicts the Brain: Diagnostic Significance of Median Facial Anomalies for Holoprosencephaly (Arhinencephaly). Pediatrics. 1964; 34:256–263

[35] Volpe JJ. Effect of Cocaine Use on the Fetus. N Engl J Med. 1992; 327:399–407

[36] Section of Pediatric Neurosurgery of the American Association of Neurological Surgeons. Pediatric Neurosurgery. New York 1982

[37] Werler MM, Shapiro S, Mitchell AA. Periconceptual Folic Acid Exposure and Risk of Occurent Neural Tube Defects. JAMA. 1993; 269:1257–1261

[38] Centers for Disease Control. Recommendations for Use of Folic Acid to Reduce Number of Spina Bifida Cases and Other Neural Tube Defects. MMWR. 1992; 41:RR–14

[39] Daly LE, Kirke PN, Molloy A, et al. Folate Levels and Neural Tube Defects. JAMA. 1995; 274:1698–1702

[40] Wald N, Sneddon J. Prevention of neural tube defects: Results of the Medical Research Council Vitamin Study. Lancet. 1991; 338:131–137

[41] Kirke PN, Mills JL, Molloy AM, Brody LC, O'Leary VB, Daly L, Murray S, Conley M, Mayne PD, Smith O, Scott JM. Impact of the MTHFR C677T polymorphism on risk of neural tube defects: case-control study. BMJ. 2004; 328:1535–1536

[42] Oakeshott P, Hunt GM. Valproate and Spina Bifida. Br Med J. 1989; 298:1300–1301

[43] Milunsky A, Ulcickas M, Rothman J, et al. Maternal Heat Exposure and Neural Tube Defects. JAMA. 1992; 268:882–885

[44] Werler MM, Louik C, Shapiro S, Mitchell AA. Prepregnant Weight in Relation to Risk of Neural Tube Defects. JAMA. 1996; 275:1089–1092

[45] Shaw GM, Velie EM, Schaffer D. Risk of Neural Tube Defect-Affected Pregnancies Among Obese Women. JAMA. 1996; 275:1093–1096

[46] Milunsky A, Jick SS, Bruell CL, MacLaughlin DS, Tsung YK, Jick H, Rothman KJ, Willett W. Predictive Values, Relative Risks, and Overall Benefits of High and Low Maternal Serum Alpha-Fetoprotein Screening in Singleton Pregnancies: New epidemiologic data. Am J Obstet Gynecol. 1989; 161:291–297

[47] Burton BK. Alpha-Fetoprotein Screening. Adv Pediatr. 1986; 33:181–196

[48] Bennett MJ, Blau K, Johnson RD, Chamberlain GVP. Some Problems of Alpha-Fetoprotein Screening. Lancet. 1978; 2:1296–1297

[49] Enyon-Lewis NJ, Kitchen N, Scaravilli F, Brookes GB. Neurenteric Cyst of the Cerebellopontine Angle. Neurosurgery. 1998; 42:655–658

[50] Lin J, Feng H, Li F, Chen Z, Wu G. Ventral brainstem enterogenous cyst: an unusual location. Acta Neurochir (Wien). 2004; 146:419–20; discussion 420
[51] LeDoux MS, Faye-Petersen OM, Aronin PA. Lumbosacral Neurenteric Cyst in an Infant. J Neurosurg. 1993; 78:821–825
[52] Inoue T, Kawahara N, Shibahara J, Masumoto T, Usami K, Kirino T. Extradural neurenteric cyst of the cerebellopontine angle. Case report. J Neurosurg. 2004; 100:1091–1093
[53] Boto GR, Lobato RD, Ramos A, Ricoy JR, Alen JF, Benito A. Enterogenous cyst of the cisterna magna. Acta Neurochir (Wien). 2000; 142:715–716
[54] Christov C, Chretien F, Brugieres P, Djindjian M. Giant supratentorial enterogenous cyst: report of a case, literature review, and discussion of pathogenesis. Neurosurgery. 2004; 54:759–63; discussion 763
[55] Fandino J, Garcia-Abeledo M. [Giant intraventricular arachnoid cyst: report of 2 cases]. Rev Neurol. 1998; 26:763–765
[56] Harris CP, Dias MS, Brockmeyer DL, Townsend JJ, Willis BK, Apfelbaum RI. Neurenteric cysts of the posterior fossa: recognition, management, and embryogenesis. Neurosurgery. 1991; 29:893–7; discussion 897-8
[57] Graziani N, Dufour H, Figarella-Branger D, Donnet A, Bouillot P, Grisoli F. Do the suprasellar neurenteric cyst, the Rathke cleft cyst and the colloid cyst constitute a same entity? Acta Neurochir (Wien). 1995; 133:174–180
[58] Shin JH, Byun BJ, Kim DW, Choi DL. Neurenteric cyst in the cerebellopontine angle with xanthogranulomatous changes: serial MR findings with pathologic correlation. AJNR Am J Neuroradiol. 2002; 23:663–665
[59] Morita Y. Neurenteric Cyst or Teratomatous Cyst. J Neurosurg. 1994; 80
[60] Hes R. Neurenteric Cyst or Teratomatous Cyst. J Neurosurg. 1994; 80:179–180
[61] Goel A. Comment on Lin J, et al.: Ventral brainstem enterogenous cyst: an unusual location. Acta Neurochir (Wien). 2004; 146

Part V

Coma and Brain Death

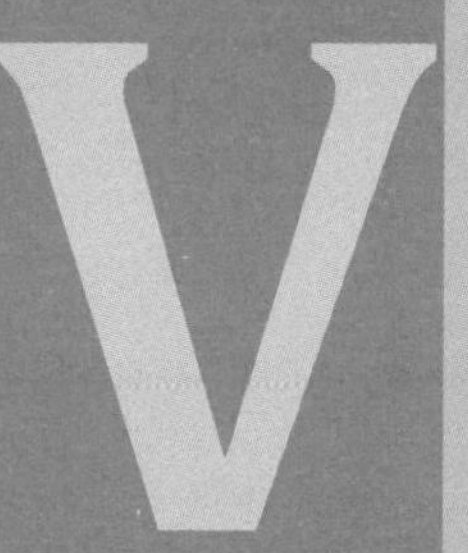

18 Coma

18.1 General information

Consciousness has two components: arousal and content. Impairment of arousal can vary from mild (drowsiness or somnolence), to obtundation, to stupor to coma. Coma is the severest impairment of arousal, and is defined as the inability to obey commands, speak, or open the eyes to pain.

The Glasgow Coma Scale (GCS) is a widely used scoring system with good repeatability and is shown in ▶ Table 18.1 (note: the scale is used to assess level of consciousness and is not designed for following neurologic deficits). General practice is to record a "T" (for "intubated") next to the verbal score and the total score for patients whose verbal axis cannot be assessed because of intubation.[2] No single GCS score defines a cutoff for coma, however, 90% of patients with GCS ≤ 8 and none with GCS ≥ 9 meet the above definition of coma. Thus, GCS ≤ 8 is a generally accepted operational definition of coma.

A number of scales for use in children have been proposed. One is shown in ▶ Table 18.2.[3]

Coma results from one or more of the following:

- dysfunction of high brainstem (central upper pons) or midbrain
- bilateral diencephalic dysfunction
- diffuse lesions in both cerebral hemispheres (cortical or subcortical white matter)

Table 18.1 Glasgow coma[a] scale[1] (recommended for age ≥ 4 yrs)

Points[b]	Best eye opening	Best verbal	Best motor
6	–	–	obeys
5	–	oriented	localizes pain
4	spontaneous	confused	withdraws to pain
3	to speech	inappropriate	flexion (decorticate)
2	to pain[c]	incomprehensible	extensor (decerebrate)
1	none	none	none[d]

[a]technically, this is a scale of impaired consciousness, whereas "coma" implies unresponsiveness
[b]range of total points: 3 (worst) to 15 (normal)
[c]when testing eye opening to pain, use peripheral stimulus (the grimace associated with central pain may cause eye closure)
[d]if no motor response, important to exclude spinal cord transection

Table 18.2 Children's coma scale[a] (for age < 4 yrs)

Points[b]	Best eye	Best verbal		Best motor
6	–	–		obeys
5	–	smiles, oriented to sound, follows objects, interacts		localizes pain
		Crying	**Interaction**	
4	spontaneous	consolable	inappropriate	withdraws to pain
3	to speech	inconsistently consolable	moaning	flexion (decorticate)
2	to pain	inconsolable	restless	extensor (decerebrate)
1	none	none	none	none

[a]same as adult Glasgow coma scale except for verbal response[3]
[b]range of total points: 3 (worst) to 15 (normal)

18.2 Posturing

18.2.1 General information

The following terms do not accurately localize the site of the lesion. Decorticate posturing implies a more rostral lesion than extensor posturing, and prognosis may be slightly better.

18.2.2 Decorticate posturing

Classically attributed to disinhibition by removal of corticospinal pathways above the midbrain.

Overview: abnormal flexion in UE and extension in LE.

Detail:

- UE: slow flexion of arm, wrist and fingers with adduction
- LE: extension, internal rotation, plantarflexion

18.2.3 Decerebrate posturing

Classically attributed to disinhibition of vestibulospinal tract (more caudal) and pontine reticular formation (RF) by removing inhibition of medullary RF (transection at intercollicular level, between vestibular and red nuclei).

Overview: abnormal extension in UE and LE.

Detail:

- Head & trunk: opisthotonos (head and trunk extended), teeth clenched
- UE: arms extended, adducted and hyperpronated (internally rotated), wrists flexed, fingers flexed
- LE: extended and internally rotated, feet plantarflexed and inverted, toes plantarflexed.

18.3 Etiologies of coma

18.3.1 Toxic/metabolic causes of coma

1. electrolyte imbalance: especially hypo- or hypernatremia, hypercalcemia, renal failure with elevated BUN & creatinine, liver failure with elevated ammonia
2. endocrine: hypoglycemia, nonketotic hyperosmolar state, DKA (diabetic ketoacidosis, AKA diabetic coma), myxedema coma, Addisonian crisis (hypoadrenalism)
3. vascular: vasculitis, DIC, hypertensive encephalopathy (p. 194)
4. toxic: EtOH, drug overdose (including narcotics, iatrogenic polypharmacy, barbiturates), lead intoxication, carbon monoxide (CO) poisoning, cyclosporine (causes an encephalopathy that shows white-matter changes on MRI that is often reversible with discontinuation of the drug)
5. infectious/inflammatory: meningitis, encephalitis, sepsis, lupus cerebritis, neurosarcoidosis (p. 189), toxic-shock syndrome
6. neoplastic: leptomeningeal carcinomatosis, rupture of neoplastic cyst
7. nutritional: Wernicke's encephalopathy, vitamin B_{12} deficiency
8. inherited metabolic disorders: porphyria, lactic acidosis
9. organ failure: uremia, hypoxemia, hepatic encephalopathy, Reye's syndrome, anoxic encephalopathy (e.g. post-resuscitation from cardiac arrest), CO_2 narcosis
10. epileptic: status epilepticus (including non-convulsive status), post-ictal state (especially with unobserved seizure)

18.3.2 Structural causes of coma

1. vascular:
   a) bilateral cortical or subcortical infarcts (e.g. with cardioembolism due to SBE, mitral stenosis, A-fib, mural thrombus…)
   b) occlusion of vessel supplying both cerebral hemispheres (e.g. severe bilateral carotid stenosis)
   c) bilateral diencephalic infarcts: well described syndrome. May be due to occlusion of a thalamo-perforator supplying both medial thalamic areas or with "top-of-the-basilar" occlusion. Initially resembles metabolic coma (including diffuse slowing on EEG), patient eventually arouses with apathy, memory loss, vertical gaze paresis
2. infectious: abscess with significant mass effect, subdural empyema, herpes simplex encephalitis
3. trauma: hemorrhagic contusions, edema, hematoma (see below)
4. neoplastic: primary or metastatic

18

5. herniation from mass effect: presumably brainstem compression causes dysfunction of reticular activating system or mass in one hemisphere causing compression of the other results in bilateral hemisphere dysfunction
6. increased intracranial pressure: reduces CBF
7. acute lateral shift (midline shift) of the brain: e.g. due hematoma (subdural or epidural) ▶ Table 18.3)

18.3.3 Pseudocoma

Differential diagnosis:
1. locked-in syndrome: ventral pontine infarction
2. psychiatric: catatonia, conversion reaction
3. neuromuscular weakness: myasthenia gravis, Guillain-Barré

18.3.4 Approach to the comatose patient

General information

This section addresses nontraumatic coma. See Head trauma (p. 824) for that topic.

Initial evaluation: includes measures to protect brain (by providing CBF, O_2, and glucose), assesses upper brainstem (Cr. N. VIII), and rapidly identifies surgical emergencies. Keep "pseudocoma" as a possible etiology in back of mind.

Outline of approach to comatose patient

1. cardiovascular stabilization: establish airway, check circulation (heartbeat, BP, carotid pulse), CPR if necessary
2. obtain blood for tests
   a) STAT: electrolytes (especially Na, glucose, BUN), CBC + diff, ABG
   b) others as appropriate: toxicology screen (serum & urine), calcium, ammonia, antiepileptic drug (AED) levels (if patient is taking AEDs)
3. administer emergency supportive medications
   a) glucose: at least 25 ml of D50 IVP. Due to potentially harmful effect of glucose in global ischemia, if possible check fingerstick glucose first, otherwise glucose is given without exception, unless it is known with certainty that serum glucose is normal
   b) naloxone (Narcan®): in case of narcotic overdose. 1 amp (0.4 mg) IVP
   c) flumazenil (Romazicon®): in case of benzodiazepine overdose. Start with 0.2 mg IV over 30 seconds, wait 30 secs, then give 0.3 mg over 30 secs at 1 minute intervals up to 3 mg or until patient arouses
   d) thiamine: 50–100 mg IVP (3% of Wernicke's present with coma)
4. core neuro exam (assesses midbrain/upper pons, allows emergency measures to be instituted rapidly, more thorough evaluation possible once stabilized): see Core neuro exam below
5. if herniation syndrome or signs of expanding p-fossa lesion with brainstem compression ▶ Table 18.4): initiate measures to lower ICP – see Treatment measures for elevated ICP (p. 866) –, then get a CT scan if patient begins improving, otherwise emergency surgery. ✖ Do *NOT* do LP
6. if meningitis suspected (altered mental status + fever, meningeal signs…)
   a) if no indication of herniation, p-fossa mass (▶ Table 18.4), focal deficit indicating mass effect or papilledema: perform LP, start antibiotics immediately (do not wait for CSF results); see Meningitis (p. 318)
   b) if evidence of possible mass effect, coagulopathy or herniation, CT to R/O mass. If significant delay anticipated, consider empiric antibiotics or careful LP with small gauge needle (≤ 22

18

Table 18.3 Effect of lateral shift on level of consciousness[4]

Amount of midline shift	Level of consciousness
0–3 mm	alert
3–4 mm	drowsy
6–8.5 mm	stuporous
8–13 mm	comatose

Table 18.4 Signs of herniation syndrome or posterior fossa lesion	
Herniation syndromes	**Signs of P-fossa lesion**
also see Herniation syndromes (p. 302)	also see Posterior fossa (infratentorial) tumors (p. 592)
• unilateral sensory or motor deficit • progressive obtundation → coma • unilateral 3rd nerve palsy • decorticate or decerebrate posturing (especially if unilateral)	• initial symptoms of diplopia, vertigo, bilateral limb weakness, ataxia, occipital H/A • rapid onset of deterioration/coma • bilateral motor signs at onset • miosis • absent calorics to horizontal movement, possibly with preserved vertical movements • ocular bobbing • ophthalmoplegia • multiple cranial nerve abnormalities with long tract signs • apneustic, cluster or ataxic respirations

Ga.), measure opening pressure (OP), remove only a small amount of CSF if OP high, replace CSF if patient deteriorates; LP in this setting may be risky, see Lumbar puncture (p. 1504).

7. treat generalized seizures if present. If status epilepticus is suspected, treat as indicated (p. 470); obtain emergency EEG if available
8. treat metabolic abnormalities
   a) restore acid-base balance
   b) restore electrolyte imbalance
   c) maintain body temperature
9. obtain as complete history as possible once stabilized
10. administer specific therapies

Core neuro exam for coma

Respiratory rate and pattern

The most common disorder in impaired consciousness (this information is often lacking in patients that are intubated early in their course):

- Cheyne-Stokes (▶ Fig. 18.1 **a**): breathing gradually crescendos in amplitude and then trails off, followed by an expiratory pause, and then the pattern repeats. Hyperpneic phase is usually longer than apneic. Usually seen with diencephalic lesions or bilateral cerebral hemisphere dysfunction (non-specific), e.g. early increased ICP or metabolic abnormality. Results from an increased ventilatory response to CO_2
- hyperventilation: usually in response to hypoxemia, metabolic acidosis, aspiration, or pulmonary edema. True central neurogenic hyperventilation is rare, and usually results from dysfunction within the pons. If no other brainstem signs are present, may suggest psychiatric disorder
- cluster breathing (▶ Fig. 18.1 **b**): periods of rapid irregular breathing separated by apneic spells, may appear similar to Cheyne-Stokes, may merge with various patterns of gasping respirations. High medulla or lower pons lesion. Often an ominous sign
- apneustic (rare; ▶ Fig. 18.1 **c**): a pause at full inspiration. Indicates pontine lesion, e.g. with basilar artery occlusion
- ataxic (Biot's breathing; (▶ Fig. 18.1 **d**): no pattern in rate or depth of respirations. Seen with medullary lesion. Usually preterminal

Pupil

18

Record size (in mm) in ambient light, and in reaction to direct/consensual light

1. ✱ equal and reactive pupils indicates toxic/metabolic cause with few exceptions (see below) (may have hippus). The light reflex is the most useful sign in distinguishing metabolic from structural coma
   a) the *only* metabolic causes of fixed/dilated pupil: glutethimide toxicity, anoxic encephalopathy, anticholinergics (including topically applied atropine), occasionally with botulism toxin poisoning
   b) narcotics cause small pupils (*miosis*) with a small range of constriction and sluggish reaction to light (in severe overdose, the pupils may be so small that a magnifying glass may be needed to see reaction)

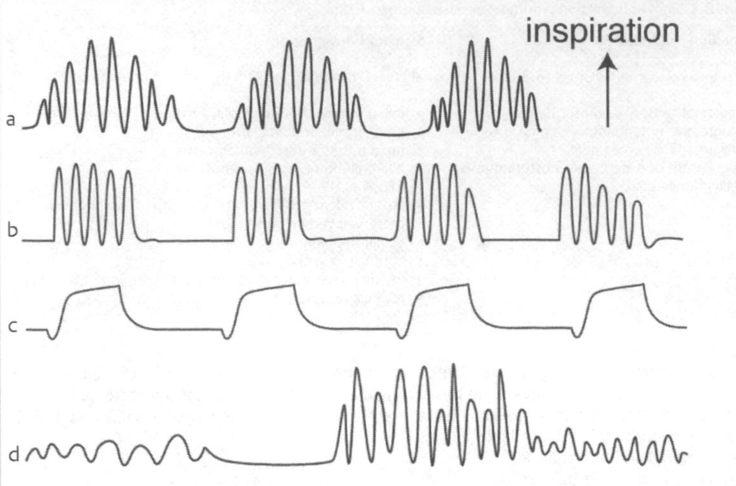

Fig. 18.1 Respiratory rate and pattern.
a) Cheyne-Stokes respiratory pattern
b) Cluster breathing
c) Apneustic respiratory pattern
d) Ataxic respirations

2. unequal; note: an afferent pupillary defect does *not* produce anisocoria, see Alterations in pupillary diameter (p. 561)
   a) fixed and dilated pupil: usually due to oculomotor palsy. Possible herniation, especially if larger pupil associated with ipsilateral 3rd nerve EOM palsy (eye deviated "down and out")
   b) possible Horner's syndrome: consider carotid occlusion/dissection (NB: in Horner's syndrome, the miotic (smaller) pupil is the abnormal one)
3. bilateral pupil abnormalities
   a) pinpoint with minute reaction that can be detected with magnifying glass[5]: pontine lesion (sympathetic input is lost; parasympathetics emerge at Edinger-Westphal nucleus and are unopposed)
   b) bilateral fixed and dilated (7–10 mm): subtotal damage to medulla or immediate post-anoxia or hypothermia (core temperature < 90° F (32.2° C))
   c) midposition (4–6 mm) and fixed: more extensive midbrain lesion, presumably due to interruption of sympathetics and parasympathetics

Extraocular muscle function

18

1. deviations of ocular axes at rest
   a) bilateral conjugate deviation:
      - frontal lobe lesion (frontal center for contralateral gaze): looks toward side of destructive lesion (away from hemiparesis). Looks away from side of seizure focus (looks at jerking side), may be status epilepticus. Reflex eye movements (see below) are normal
      - pontine lesion: eyes look *away* from lesion and towards hemiparesis; calorics impaired on side of lesion
      - "wrong way gaze": medial thalamic hemorrhage. Eyes look away from lesion and towards hemiparesis (an exception to the axiom that the eyes look *towards* a destructive supratentorial lesion)[5]
      - downward deviation: may be associated with unreactive pupils, Parinaud's syndrome (p. 99). Etiologies: thalamic or midbrain pretectal lesions, metabolic coma (especially barbiturates), may follow a seizure
   b) unilateral outward deviation on side of larger pupil (III palsy): uncal herniation
   c) unilateral inward deviation: VI (abducens) nerve

d) skew deviation
   - III or IV nerve/nucleus lesion
   - infratentorial lesion (frequently dorsal midbrain)
2. spontaneous eye movements
   a) "windshield wiper eyes": random roving conjugate eye movements. Non-localizing. Indicates an intact III nucleus and medial longitudinal fasciculus
   b) periodic alternating gaze, AKA "ping-pong gaze": eyes deviate side to side with frequency of ≈ 3–5 per second (pausing 2–3 secs in each direction). Usually indicates bilateral cerebral dysfunction
   c) **ocular bobbing** (p.570): repetitive rapid vertical deviation downward with slow return to neutral position.
3. internuclear ophthalmoplegia (INO) (p.565): due to lesion in medial longitudinal fasciculus (MLF) (fibers crossing to contralateral III nucleus are interrupted). Eye ipsilateral to MLF lesion does not adduct on spontaneous eye movement or in response to reflex maneuvers (e.g. calorics)
4. reflex eye movements (maneuvers to test brainstem)
   a) oculovestibular reflex[a], AKA ice water calorics: first rule-out TM perforation and occlusion of the EAC by cerumen. Elevate the HOB 30°, irrigate one ear with 60–100 ml of ice water[b]. NB: response is inhibited by neuromuscular blocking agents (NMBA)
      - a comatose patient with an *intact* brainstem will have tonic conjugate eye deviation to side of cold stimulus which may be delayed up to one minute or more. There will be no fast component (nystagmus) (the cortical component) even if the brainstem is intact. (NB: oculocephalic reflex[c] (doll's eyes) provides similar information as oculovestibular reflex[d], but poses a greater risk to the spinal cord if C-spine not cleared)
      - no response: symmetrical, could be specific toxin (e.g. neuromuscular block or barbiturates), metabolic cause, brain death or possibly massive infratentorial lesion
      - asymmetric: infratentorial lesion, especially if response inconsistent with 3rd nerve palsy (herniation). Usually maintained in toxic/metabolic coma
      - nystagmus without tonic deviation (i.e. eyes remain in primary position) virtually diagnostic of psychogenic coma
      - contralateral eye fails to adduct: INO (MLF lesion)
   b) optokinetic nystagmus presence strongly suggests psychogeniccoma

Notes:

[a] **Oculovestibular reflexes** (calorics): the anticipated response is commonly misunderstood. In a normal **awake** patient **there is slow deviation towards the side of the cold stimulus with nystagmus** (which is named for the rapid, cortical phase) in the opposite direction (hence the mnemonic "COWS" (cold-opposite, warm-same)). Nystagmus will be **absent** in the comatose patient.

[b] HOB at 30° places the horizontal semicircular canal (SCC) vertically for maximal response.[6(p 56)] – Cold water → downward endolymphatic currents, **away** from the ampulla of the horizontal SCC.[6(p 57)]

[c] **Oculocephalic reflex** ("doll's eyes" or "doll's head"): do not perform if there is any uncertainty about cervical-spine stability. In an **awake** patient, the eyes will either move with the head, or, if the movement is slow enough and the patient is fixating on an object, there will be contraversive conjugate eye movement[7] (c.f. oculovestibular reflex which does not depend on patient's level of cooperation). In a comatose patient with an intact brainstem & cranial nerves, there will also be contraversive conjugate eye movement (a positive doll's eyes response).

[d] Oculovestibular reflexes are absent but oculocephalic are maintained only when vestibular inputs are interrupted, e.g. streptomycin toxicity of labyrinths or bilateral vestibular schwannomas.

Motor

Record muscle tone and reflexes, response to pain, plantar reflex (Babinski). Note asymmetries

1. appropriate: implies corticospinal tracts and cortex intact
2. asymmetric: supratentorial lesion (tone usually increased), unlikely in metabolic
3. inconsistent/variable: seizures, psychiatric
4. symmetric: metabolic (usually decreased). Asterixis, tremor, myoclonus may be present in metabolic coma
5. hyporeflexia: consider myxedema coma, especially in patient presenting weeks after transsphenoidal surgery
6. patterns
   a) decorticate posturing: arms flex, legs extend: large cortical or subcortical lesion
   b) decerebrate posturing: arms and legs extend: brainstem injury at or below lower midbrain

c) arms flexed, legs flaccid: pontine tegmentum
d) arms flaccid, legs appropriate ("man-in-the-barrel syndrome"): anoxic injury (poor prognosis)

Ciliospinal reflex

Pupillary dilatation to noxious cutaneous stimuli: tests integrity of sympathetic pathways
1. bilaterally present: metabolic
2. unilaterally present: possible 3rd nerve lesion (herniation) if on side of larger pupil. Possible pre-existing Horner's syndrome if on side of smaller pupil
3. bilaterally absent: usually not helpful

18.4 Herniation syndromes

18.4.1 General information

Classic teaching has been that shifts in brain tissue (e.g. caused by masses or increased intracranial pressure) through rigid openings in the skull (herniation) compress other structures of the CNS producing the observed symptoms. In actuality it may be that herniation is an epiphenomenon that occurs late in the process and is not actually the cause of the observations.[8] However, herniation models still serve as useful models.

The five most common herniation syndromes are:
- Supratentorial herniation
  - central (transtentorial) herniation (p. 303)
  - uncal herniation (p. 304)
- cingulate herniation: cingulate gyrus herniates under falx (AKA subfalcine herniation). Usually asymptomatic unless ACA kinks and occludes causing bifrontal infarction. Usually warns of impending transtentorial herniation
- Infratentorial herniation
  - upward cerebellar (see below)
  - tonsillar herniation (see below)

18.4.2 Coma from supratentorial mass

See reference.[6]

General information

Central and uncal herniation each causes a different form of rostral-caudal deterioration. Central herniation results in sequential failure of: diencephalon, midbrain, pons, medulla (p. 303). See also uncal herniation (p. 304). "Classic" signs of increased ICP (HTN, bradycardia, altered respiratory pattern) usually seen with p-fossa lesions may be absent in slowly developing supratentorial masses.

Distinction between central and uncal herniation is difficult when dysfunction reaches the midbrain level or below. Predicting the location of the lesion based on the herniation syndrome is unreliable.

Clinical characteristics differentiating uncal from central herniation

- decreased consciousness occurs early in central herniation, late in uncal
- uncal herniation syndrome *rarely* gives rise to decorticate posturing

Differential diagnosis of supratentorial etiologies

1. vascular: stroke, intracerebral hemorrhage, SAH
2. inflammatory: cerebral abscess, subdural empyema, herpes simplex encephalitis
3. neoplastic: primary or metastatic
4. traumatic: epidural or subdural hematoma, depressed skull fracture

18.4.3 Coma from infratentorial mass

General information

NB: it is essential to identify patients with primary posterior fossa lesions (► Table 18.4) as they may require emergent surgical intervention.

Etiologies of infratentorial masses:

1. vascular: brainstem infarction (including basilar artery occlusion), cerebellar infarction or hematoma
2. inflammatory: cerebellar abscess, central pontine myelinolysis, brainstem encephalitis
3. neoplasms: primary or metastatic
4. traumatic: epidural or subdural hematoma

Hydrocephalus

Infratentorial masses can produce obstructive hydrocephalus by compressing the Sylvian aqueduct and/or 4th ventricle.

Upward cerebellar herniation

Occasionally seen with p-fossa masses, may be exacerbated by ventriculostomy. Cerebellar vermis ascends above tentorium, compressing the midbrain, and possibly occluding SCAs → cerebellar infarction. May compress sylvian aqueduct → hydrocephalus.

Tonsillar herniation

Cerebellar tonsils "cone" through foramen magnum, compressing medulla → respiratory arrest. Usually rapidly fatal.

Occurs with either supra- or infra-tentorial masses or with elevated ICP. May be precipitated by LP. In many cases, there may simply be pressure on the brainstem without actual herniation.[9] There are also cases with significant cerebellar herniation through the foramen magnum with the patient remaining alert.[8]

18.4.4 Central herniation

General information

AKA transtentorial herniation AKA tentorial herniation. Usually more chronic than uncal herniation, e.g. due to tumor, especially of frontal, parietal or occipital lobes.

The diencephalon is gradually forced through the tentorial incisura. The pituitary stalk may be sheared, resulting in diabetes insipidus. PCAs may be trapped along the open edge of the incisura, and may occlude producing cortical blindness; see Blindness from hydrocephalus (p. 396). The brainstem suffers ischemia from compression and shearing of perforating arteries from basilar artery → hemorrhages within the brainstem (Duret hemorrhages).

Imaging

MRI or CT: the perimesencephalic cisterns may be compressed.

Skull x-rays: downward displacement of the pineal gland may be identified.[10]

Stages of central herniation

Diencephalic stage

Early. May be due to diffuse bilateral hemisphere dysfunction (e.g. from decreased blood flow from increased ICP) or (more likely) from bilateral diencephalic dysfunction due to downward displacement. This stage warns of impending (irreversible) midbrain damage but is frequently reversible if the cause is treated.

Consciousness: Altered alertness is first sign; usually lethargy, agitation in some. Later: stupor → coma.

Respiration: Sighs, yawns, occasional pauses. Later: Cheyne-Stokes.

Pupils: Small (1 – 3 mm), small range of contraction.

Oculomotor: Conjugate or slightly divergent roving eyes; if conjugate then brainstem intact. Usually positive DOLL'S EYES and conjugate ipsilateral response to cold water calorics (CWC). Impaired upgaze due to compression of superior colliculi and diencephalic pretectum: Parinaud's syndrome (p. 99)

Motor: Early: appropriate response to noxious stimuli, bilateral Babinski, gegenhalten (paratonic resistance). If previously hemiparetic contralateral to lesion: may worsen. Later: motionlessness & grasp reflexes, then DECORTICATE (initially contralateral to lesion in most cases).

18

Midbrain – upper pons stage

When midbrain signs fully developed (in adults), prognosis is very poor (extreme ischemia of midbrain). Fewer than 5% of cases will have a good recovery if treatment is successfully undertaken at this stage.

Respiration: Cheyne-Stokes → sustained tachypnea.

Pupils: Moderately dilated midposition (3–5 mm), fixed. Note: in pontine hemorrhage pinpoint pupils appear because the loss of sympathetics leaves the parasympathetics unopposed, whereas in herniation, the parasympathetics are usually lost, too (3rd nerve injury).

Oculomotor: Doll's eyes & CWC impaired, may be dysconjugate. MLF lesion → internuclear ophthalmoplegia (when doll's or CWC elicited and dysconjugate, medially moving eye moves less than laterally moving eye).

Motor: Decorticate → bilaterally DECEREBRATE (occasionally spontaneously).

Lower pons – upper medullary stage

Respiration: Regular, shallow and rapid (20–40/min).

Pupils: Midposition (3–5 mm), fixed.

Oculomotor: Doll's eyes and CWC unelicitable.

Motor: Flaccid. Bilateral Babinski. Occasionally LE flexion to pain.

Medullary stage (terminal stage)

Respiration: Slow, irregular rate and depth, sighs/gasps. Occasionally hyperpnea alternating with apnea

Pupils: Dilate widely with hypoxia.

Outcome after central herniation

In a series of 153 patients with signs of central herniation (altered level of consciousness, anisocoria or fixed pupils, abnormal motor findings) 9% had good recovery, 18% had functional outcome, 10% were severely disabled, and 60% died.[11]

Factors associated with a better result were young age (especially age ≤ 17 yrs), anisocoria with deteriorating Glasgow Coma Score and nonflaccid motor function. Factors associated with poor outcome were bilaterally fixed pupils, with only 3.5% of these patients having a functional recovery.

18.4.5 Uncal herniation

General information

Usually occurs in rapidly expanding traumatic hematomas, frequently in the lateral middle-fossa or temporal lobe pushing medial uncus and hippocampal gyrus over edge of tentorium, entrapping third nerve and directly compressing midbrain. PCA may be occluded (as with central herniation). For CT criteria see below.

Impaired consciousness is NOT a reliable early sign. Earliest consistent sign: unilaterally dilating pupil. However, it is unlikely that a patient undergoing early uncal herniation would be completely neurologically intact except for anisocoria (do not dismiss confusion, agitation, etc.). Once brainstem findings appear, deterioration may be rapid (deep coma may occur within hours).

CT and/or MRI criteria

See reference.[12]

The tentorial incisura surrounds the interpeduncular and pre-pontine cisterns and brainstem. There is great interpersonal variability in the amount of space in the incisura.

Impending uncal or hippocampal herniation may be indicated by encroachment on lateral aspect of suprasellar cistern → flattening of normal pentagonal shape. Once herniation occurs CT may show: brainstem displacement and flattening, compression of contralateral cerebral peduncle, midbrain rotation with slight increase of ipsilateral subarachnoid space. Also, contralateral hydrocephalus may occur.[13]

Obliteration of parasellar and interpeduncular cisterns occurs as uncus and/or hippocampus are forced through hiatus. Brainstem is elongated in AP direction due to lateral compression. Since dural structures enhance with IV contrast, this may be used to help delineate tentorial margins when necessary.

Stages of uncal herniation

Early third nerve stage

This is *not* a brainstem finding, it is due to 3rd nerve compression.

Pupils: Approach to the comatose patient

Oculomotor: Doll's eyes (oculocephalic reflex) = normal or dysconjugate. CWC (oculovestibular reflex) = slow ipsilateral deviation, impaired nystagmus, may be dysconjugate if external oculomotor ophthalmoplegia (**EOO**).

Respirations: Normal.

Motor: Appropriate response to nociceptive stimulus. Contralateral Babinski.

Late third nerve stage

Midbrain dysfunction occurs almost immediately after symptoms extend beyond those due to focal cerebral lesion (i.e. may skip diencephalic stage, due to lateral pressure on midbrain). Treatment delays may result in irreversible damage.

Pupils: Pupil fully dilates.

Oculomotor: Once pupil blown, then external oculomotor ophthalmoplegia (EOO).

Consciousness: Once EOO occurs: stupor→coma

Respirations: Sustained hyperventilation, rarely Cheyne-Stokes.

Motor: Usually produces contralateral weakness. However, the contralateral cerebral peduncle may be compressed against the tentorial edge causing ipsilateral hemiplegia (*Kernohan's phenomenon*, a false localizing sign). Then bilateral decerebration (decortication unusual).

Midbrain – upper pons stage

Contralateral pupil fixes in midposition or full dilation. Eventually, both midposition (5–6 mm) and fixed.

Oculomotor: Impaired or absent.

Respirations: Sustained hyperpnea.

Motor: Bilateral decerebrate rigidity.

Following the midbrain – upper pons stage

From this point onward, the uncal syndrome is indistinguishable from central herniation (see above).

18.5 Hypoxic coma

Anoxic encephalopathy may be due to anoxemic anoxia (drop in pO_2) or anemic anoxia (following exsanguination or cardiac arrest). Myoclonus is common.

Vulnerable cells:

1. cerebral grey matter: lesions predominate in 3rd cortical layer (white matter is usually better preserved due to lower O_2 requirements)
2. Ammon's horn is also vulnerable, especially the Sommer section
3. in the basal ganglia (BG):
   a) anoxemic anoxia severely affects globus pallidus
   b) anemic anoxia affects the caudate nucleus and putamen
4. in the cerebellum: Purkinje cells, dentate nuclei, and inferior olives are affected

Multivariate analysis yields outcome prognosticators shown in ▶ Table 18.5 and ▶ Table 18.6. NB: this analysis applies *only* to hypoxic-ischemic coma; and is based retrospectively on 210 patients, most S/P cardiac arrest with many medical complications.[14] More recent studies confirm the poor prognosis of unreactive pupils and lack of motor response to pain[15]; if either of these findings are seen within a few hours after cardiac arrest there is an 80% risk of death or permanent vegetative state, and if present at 3 days these this rate rose to 100%.

Glucocorticoids (steroids) have been shown to have no beneficial effect on survival rate or neurological recovery rate after cardiac arrest.[16]

Table 18.5 Patients with BEST chance of regaining independence[a]

Time of exam	Finding
<6 hrs from onset	(pupillary light reflex present) *AND* (GCS-motor > 1) *AND* (spontaneous EOM WNL, i.e. orienting or conjugate roving)
1 day	(GCS-motor > 3) *AND* (GCS-eye improved ≥ 2 from initial)
3 days	(GCS-motor > 3) *AND* (spontaneous EOM WNL)
1 week	GCS-motor = 6
2 weeks	oculocephalic WNL

[a] abbreviations: WNL = within normal limits, GCS = Glasgow Coma Scale ("GCS-motor" refers to the motor score...); EOM = extraocular muscle;

Table 18.6 Patients with virtually NO chance of regaining independence[a]

Time of exam	Finding
<6 hrs	no pupillary light reflex
1 day	(GCS-motor < 4) *AND* (spontaneous eye movements not orienting nor conjugate roving)
3 days	GCS-motor < 4
1 week	(GCS-motor < 6) *AND* (at < 6 hrs spontaneous EOM not orienting nor conjugate roving) *AND* (at 3 d GCS-eye < 4)
2 week	(oculocephalic not WNL) *AND* (at 3 d GCS-motor < 6) *AND* (at 3 d GCS-eye < 4) *AND* (at 2 wk GCS-eye not improved at least 2 points from initial)

[a]abbreviations: WNL = within normal limits, GCS = Glasgow Coma Scale ("GCS-motor" refers to the motor score...); EOM = extraocular muscle;

References

[1] Teasdale G, Jennett B. Assessment of Coma and Impaired Consciousness: a Practical Scale. Lancet. 1974; 2:81–84

[2] Valadka AB, Narayan RK, Narayan RK, Wilberger JE, Povlishock JT. In: Emergency Room Management of the Head-Injured Patient. Neurotrauma. New York: McGraw-Hill; 1996:119–135

[3] Hahn YS, Chyung C, Barthel MJ, Bailes J, Flannery AM, McLone DG. Head Injuries in Children Under 36 Months of Age: Demography and Outcome. Childs Nerv Syst. 1988; 4:34–40

[4] Ropper AH. Lateral Displacement of the Brain and Level of Consciousness in Patients with an Acute Hemispheral Mass. N Engl J Med. 1986; 314:953–958

[5] Fisher CM. Some Neuro-Ophthalmological Observations. J Neurol Neurosurg Psychiatry. 1967; 30:383–392

[6] Plum F, Posner JB. The Diagnosis of Stupor and Coma. 3rd ed. Philadelphia: F A Davis; 1980:87–130

[7] Buettner UW, Zee DS. Vestibular Testing in Comatose Patients. Arch Neurol. 1989; 46:561–563

[8] Fisher CM. Acute Brain Herniation: A Revised Concept. Sem Neurology. 1984; 4:417–421

[9] Fisher CM, Picard EH, Polak A, Ojemann RG, et al. Acute Hypertensive Cerebellar Hemorrhage: Diagnosis and Surgical Treatment. J Nerv Ment Dis. 1965; 140:38–57

[10] Hahn F, Gurney J. CT Signs of Central Descending Transtentorial Herniation. Am J Neuroradiol. 1985; 6:844–845

[11] Andrews BT, Pitts LH. Functional Recovery After Traumatic Transtentorial Herniation. Neurosurgery. 1991; 29:227–231

[12] Osborn AG. Diagnosis of Descending Transtentorial Herniation by Cranial CT. Radiology. 1977; 123:93–96

[13] Stovring J. Descending Tentorial Herniation: Findings on Computerized Tomography. Neuroradiology. 1977; 14:101–105

[14] Levy DE, Caronna JJ, Singer BH, et al. Predicting Outcome from Hypoxic-Ischemic Coma. JAMA. 1985; 253:1420–1426

[15] Zandbergen EGJ, de Haan RJ, Stoutenbeek CP, et al. Systematic Review of Early Prediction of Poor Outcome in Anoxic-Ischemic Coma. Lancet. 1998; 352:1808–1812

[16] Jastremski M, Sutton-Tyrell K, Vaagenes P, et al. Glucocorticoid Treatment Does Not Improve Neurological Recovery Following Cardiac Arrest. JAMA. 1989; 262:3427–3430

19 Brain Death and Organ Donation

19.1 Brain death in adults

The President's Commission for the Study of Ethical Problems in Medicine first published guidelines for the determination of death in 1981[1] which contributed to the approval of the Uniform Determination of Death Act (UDDA; policy statement, see box).[2]

Uniform determination of death act, 1980 (verbatim quote)

"An individual who has sustained either
1. irreversible cessation of circulatory and respiratory functions, or
2. irreversible cessation of all functions of the entire brain, including the brain stem,
is dead.
A determination of death must be made with accepted medical standards."

Most states have adopted the UDDA, although some have enacted amendments stipulating qualifications of the determining clinician(s). Individual hospitals may also mandate that certain protocols be followed.

As reaffirmed in 2010,[3] when the clinical determination of brain death is made in accordance with the original published guidelines,[4] there has been no report of recovery of neurologic function in adults.

19.2 Brain death criteria

19.2.1 General information

This section deals with brain death in adults. For individuals < 5 years age, see Brain death in children (p.312).

When the cause of death is other than natural causes the Medical Examiner or Coroner (depending on the authority in your jurisdiction) will be contacted per hospital policy.

Key point: Criteria shown below may be used to determine the clinical absence of brain and brainstem function. Then to ensure that the total cessation of brain function is irreversible, the clinician must take into consideration the cause of the absence, and exclude conditions that can mimic the clinical appearance of brain death. This may require ancillary confirmatory tests and observation for a period of time.

Waiting periods: There is insufficient evidence to support a specific observation period to ensure that the cessation of neurologic function is irreversible.[3] This requires that the determination of brain death take into consideration all of the available information and circumstances.

19.2.2 Establishing the cause of cessation of brain activity

The cause of the cessation of brain activity (CBA) can usually be determined by a combination of history, physical examination, laboratory tests and imaging studies.

19.2.3 Clinical criteria

See ▶ Table 19.1 for a summary of basic requirements and clinical findings that may be used in determining brain death. Details follow below.

Recommendations[1,5,3]:

1. Absence of **brainstem reflexes**:
   a) ocular examination:
      - *fixed* pupils: no response to bright light (caution after resuscitation: see below). The size of the pupils is unimportant (they are usually midposition (4–6 mm) but may vary to dilated range (9 mm): dilated pupils can be compatible with brain death because cervical sympathetic pathways may remain intact)
      - absent corneal reflexes (corneal reflex: eye closing to corneal, not scleral, stimulation)

Table 19.1 Summary of findings in brain death (see text for details)[3]

Vital signs & general criteria	
• Core temp > 36° C (96.8° F)	
• SBP ≥ 100 mm Hg	
• No drugs that could simulate brain death. Blood alcohol content (BAC) should be < 0.08%	
Absence of brainstem reflexes	
• Fixed pupils	No pupillary reaction to light
• Absent corneal reflexes	Touching cornea with a gauze does not cause eye closure
• Absent oculovestibular reflex (calorics)	No eye movement of any sort to ice water in ear with HOB elevated to 30°
• Absent oculocephalic reflex: "Doll's eyes" (p. 301)	Turning the head does not cause contralateral eye deviation (clear C-spine first)
• Absent gag reflex	No gagging reaction to movement of ET tube
• Absent cough reflex	No coughing in response to bronchial suctioning
No response to deep central pain	**Stimulate areas like supraorbital ridge. No limb movement, no eye movement, no facial movement**
Failed apnea challenge	**No respirations with $pCO_2 > 60$ mm Hg**

- absent oculocephalic "doll's eyes" reflex (p. 301), contraindicated if C-spine not cleared
- absent oculovestibular reflex (cold water calorics): instill 60–100 ml ice water into one ear (✖ do not do if TM perforated) with HOB at 30°. Brain death is excluded if *any* eye movement. Wait at least 1 minute for response, and ≥ 5 min before testing the opposite side (to prevent cancellation of opposing response)

b) absent oropharyngeal reflex (gag) to stimulation of posterior pharynx

c) no cough response to bronchial suctioning

2. apnea test AKA apnea challenge: no spontaneous respirations after disconnection from ventilator (assesses function of medulla). Respirations are defined as abdominal or chest excursions that produce adequate tidal volumes; if there is any question, a spirometer may be connected to the patient.[4] Since elevating $PaCO_2$ increases ICP which could precipitate herniation and vasomotor instability, this test should be reserved for last and only used when the diagnosis of brain death is reasonably certain. Guidelines[6,7]:

   a) Apnea for > 2 minutes with $PaCO_2 > 60$ mm Hg or $PaCO_2 > 20$ mm Hg over baseline or pH < 7.3 (CO_2 is the most potent stimulus for respirations). If patient does not breathe by this point, they won't breathe at a higher $PaCO_2$. Not as valid with severe COPD

   b) to prevent hypoxemia during the test (with the danger of cardiac arrhythmia or myocardial infarction):
   - preoxygenate for ≥ 10 minutes before the test with 100% FIO_2 to $PaO_2 > 200$ mm Hg
   - prior to the test, reduce the ventilator rate to bring the $PaCO_2$ to 35-40 mm Hg (to shorten the test time and thus reduce the risk of hypoxemia)
   - during the test, have passive O_2 flow administered at 6 L/min through either a pediatric oxygen cannula or a No. 14 French tracheal suction catheter (with the side port covered with adhesive tape) passed to the estimated level of the carina

   c) starting from normocapnea, the average time to reach $PaCO_2 = 60$ mm Hg is **6 minutes** (classic teaching is that $PaCO_2$ rises 3 mm Hg/min, but in actuality this the rate at which $PaCO_2$ rises varies widely, with an average 3.7 ± 2.3[6]; or 5.1 mm Hg/min if starting at normocarbia[7]). Sometimes as long as 12 minutes may be necessary

   d) the test is aborted if:
   - the patient breathes (chest or abdominal movement, gasps): incompatible with brain death
   - SBP < 90 mm Hg (hypotension)
   - if O_2 saturation drops < 80% for > 30 seconds (on pulse oximeter)
   - significant cardiac arrhythmias occur

e) if patient does not breathe, send ABG at regular intervals and at the completion of test regardless of reason for termination. If the patient does not breathe for at least 2 minutes *after* a $PaCO_2 > 60$ mm Hg is documented, then the test is valid and is compatible with brain death (if the patient is stable and ABGs results are available within a few minutes, the apnea challenge may be continued while waiting for results in case the $PaCO_2$ is < 60)
f) if $PaCO_2$ stabilizes below 60 mm Hg and the pO_2 remains adequate, try reducing the passive O_2 flow rate slightly (O_2 flow may be washing out CO_2 from lungs)
g) the test is positive (i.e. compatible with brain death) if there are no respirations and $PaCO_2$ is ≥ 60 mm Hg (or there is a 20 mm Hg rise in $PaCO_2$ above baseline)

3. no motor function
   a) no response to deep *central* pain: there should be no movement of limbs, no eye opening or eye movement, no facial movement
   b) true decerebrate or decorticate posturing or seizures are incompatible with the diagnosis of brain death
   c) spinal cord mediated reflex movements (including flexor plantar reflexes, flexor withdrawal, muscle stretch reflexes,[8] and even abdominal and cremasteric reflexes) can be compatible with brain death, and may occasionally consist of complex movements,[9] including bringing one or both arms up to the face,[10] or sitting up (the "Lazarus" sign[11]) especially with hypoxemia (thought to be due to spinal cord ischemia stimulating surviving motor neurons in the upper cervical cord). If complex integrated motor movements occur, it is recommended that confirmatory testing be performed prior to pronouncement of brain death[12]
4. absence of *complicating conditions* (that could simulate brain death on exam):
   a) hypothermia: core temp should be > 36° C (96.8° F). Below this temp, pupils may be fixed and dilated,[13] respirations may be difficult to detect, and recovery is possible[14]
   b) no evidence of remediable exogenous or endogenous intoxication, including drug or metabolic (blood alcohol level should be < 0.08%, barbiturates, benzodiazepines, meprobamate, methaqualone, trichloroethylene, paralytics, hepatic encephalopathy, hyperosmolar coma...). If there is doubt, depending on circumstances, lab tests including drug levels (serum and urine) may be sent. Pseudocholinesterase deficiency is present in 1/3000 patients which can cause succinycholine to last up to 8 hours (instead of 5 mins). A twitch monitor can rule-out NMB (place the electrodes immediately behind the eye or across the zygomatic arch)
   c) shock (neuro exam should be reliable if SBP ≥ 100 mm Hg) and anoxia. Loss of > 45% of circulating blood volume can produce lethargy
   d) immediately post-resuscitation: shock or anoxia may cause fixed and dilated pupils. Atropine (p. 311) may cause slight dilatation but *not* unreactivity. Neuromuscular blockage (e.g. for intubation) does not affect pupils because the iris lacks nicotinic receptors
   e) patients coming out of pentobarbital coma (wait until level ≈ ≤ 10 mcg/ml)
5. confirmation of brain death by use of Ancillary confirmatory tests (preferred tests[3]: EEG, CRAG or angiography, see below) is not required. May be used at the discretion of the physician, generally if there is uncertainty about the reliability of other parts of the exam
6. recommended observation periods: there is insufficient evidence to determine a minimal observation period to ensure that neurologic function has irreversibly ceased[3]:
   a) in situation where overwhelming brain damage from an irreversible condition is well established (e.g. massive intracerebral hemorrhage, gunshot wound traversing the brain...), and no uncertainty in the clinical exam, an ancillary confirmatory tests would usually not be necessary
   b) in clear-cut situations as outlined above, if several hours have passed since the onset of the brain insult, a single neurologic examination consistent with brain death should suffice although many states require two examinations by statute[3] (see state and local laws below)
   c) in less clear-cut situations (e.g. anoxic brain injury, hypothermia...) longer observation periods are appropriate and ancillary confirmatory tests may be considered (see below)

19.2.4 State and local laws

Most states have adopted the Uniform Determination of Death Act (UDDA) regarding brain death. State amendments and local regulations or hospital policies may dictate that more than 1 practitioner must concur on the diagnosis. It is incumbent that the practitioner know the applicable regulations before making the diagnosis.

19.2.5 Ancillary confirmatory tests

General information

There is insufficient evidence that any ancillary test can accurately determine brain death.[3] Preferred tests[3]: EEG, CRAG or angiography.

Cerebral angiography

Requires absence of cerebral blood flow, which is incompatible with brain survival. Pros: highly sensitive for determining death of cerebral hemispheres. Cons: costly, time-consuming, requires transport of the patient to x-ray department, invasive, potentially damaging to organs that may be used for donation, and is not optimal for detecting small amount of blood blow to brainstem. Requires a radiologist and technician. Criteria: absence of intracranial flow at the level of the carotid bifurcation or circle of Willis[5]). Filling of the superior sagittal sinus may occur in a delayed fashion and is not incompatible with brain death. Interobserver validity has not been studied. Not routinely used in the diagnosis of brain death, but may be employed in difficult situations.

EEG

Can be done at bedside. Requires experienced interpreter. Does not detect brainstem activity, and electrocerebral silence (ECS) (i.e. isoelectric EEG) does not exclude the possibility of reversible coma. ∴ Use ECS as a clinical confirmatory test only in patients without drug intoxication, hypothermia, or shock, and not in patients where brainstem activity might be preserved (i.e. situations where the clinical brainstem exam cannot be performed). Note: a practical problem with EEG for brain-death determination is that it is often difficult to get a tracing that is totally free of electrical signal even in patients who are brain dead by other criteria.

Definition of electrocerebral silence on EEG: no electrical activity > 2 mcV with the following requirements:

1. recording from scalp or referential electrode pairs ≥ 10 cm apart
2. 8 scalp electrodes and ear lobe reference electrodes
3. inter-electrode resistance < 10,000 Ω (or impedance < 6,000 Ω) but over 100 Ω
4. sensitivity of 2 mcV/mm
5. time constants 0.3–0.4 sec for part of recording
6. no response to stimuli (pain, noise, light)
7. record > 30 mins
8. repeat EEG in doubtful cases
9. qualified technologist and electroencephalographer with ICU EEG experience
10. telephone transmission not permissible

Cerebral radionuclide angiogram (CRAG)

General information

Can be done using a gamma camera, or more contemporary HMPAO SPECT (for 99mTechnetium hexamethylpropyleneamine oxime single-photon emission CT). May not detect minimal blood flow to the brain, especially brainstem. Necessitates transport to the radiology/nuclear medicine department and requires an experienced interpreter.

May be useful to confirm clinical brain death in the following settings:

1. where complicating conditions are present, e.g. hypothermia, hypotension (shock), drug intoxication… (e.g. patients emerging from barbiturate coma), metabolic abnormalities
2. in patients with severe facial trauma where evaluation of ocular findings may be difficult or confusing
3. in patients with severe COPD or CHF where apnea testing may not be valid
4. to shorten the observation period

19

Technique

Using gallium camera

1. scintillation camera is positioned for an AP head and neck view
2. inject 20–30 mCi of 99mTc-labeled serum albumin or pertechnetate in a volume of 0.5–1.5 ml into a proximal IV port, or a central line, followed by a 30 ml NS flush
3. perform serial dynamic images at 2 second intervals for ≈ 60 seconds
4. then, obtain static images with 400,000 counts in AP and then lateral views at 5, 15 & 30 minutes after injection

5. if a study needs to be repeated because of a previous non-diagnostic study or a previous exam incompatible with brain death, a period of 12 hours should lapse to allow the isotope to clear from the circulation

Findings

No uptake in brain parenchyma = "hollow skull phenomenon" (▶ Fig. 19.1). Termination of carotid circulation at the skull base, and lack of uptake in the ACA and MCA distributions (absent "candelabra effect"). There may be delayed or faint visualization of dural venous sinuses even with brain death[15] due to connections between the extracranial circulation and the venous system.

MRI and MR angiography (MRA)

MRA is very sensitive for detecting loss of blood flow in cavernous ICA, however the specificity has not been accurately evaluated[3] (i.e. might give false positives for brain death in comatose patients) and is not considered a valid confirmatory test.

CT angiography (CTA)

Blood flow on CTA (i.e. not consistent with brain death) was seen in patients with isoelectric EEG. False positive rate had not been determined in comatose non-brain dead patients. CTA is not considered to be a valid confirmatory test for brain death.[3]

Transcranial doppler

See reference.[4]

Not widely used.

1. small peaks in early systolc without diastolic flow or reverberating flow (indicative of significantly increased ICP)
2. initial absence of doppler signals cannot be used as criteria for brain death since 10% of patients do not have temporal insonation windows

SSEPs

One protocol requires bilateral absence of N20-P22 response with median nerve stimulation. An alternative criteria is disappearance of the P14 peak[16] (substrate: medial lemniscus and nucleus cuneatus) on nasopharyngeal electrode recordings. Studies were judged as Class III data and that P14 recordings could be a valuable confirmatory test but that this test has not been used routinely and that interobserver variability needed to be studied.[3]

Atropine

In brain death, 1 amp of atropine (1 mg) IV should not affect the heart rate due to the absence of vagal tone (the normal response to atropine of increased heart rate rules out brain death, but

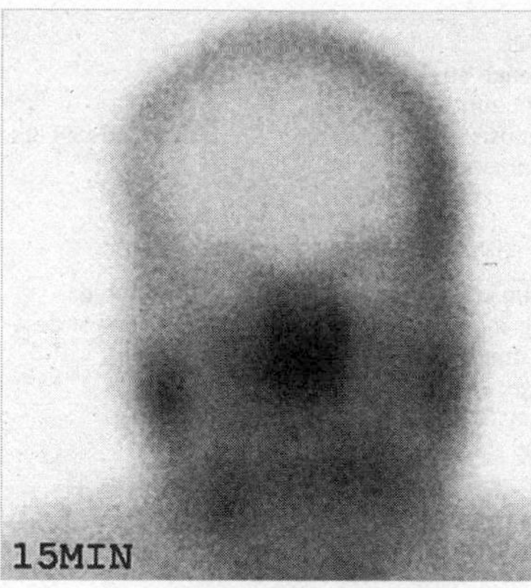

Fig. 19.1 "Hollow-skull" sign on CRAG radionuclide CBF study (static AP view taken15 minutes after injection)

19

absence of the response is not helpful since some conditions such as Guillain-Barre may blunt the response).

Systemic atropine in usual doses causes slight pupillary dilatation,[17,18] but does not eliminate reaction to light (therefore, to eliminate uncertainty, it is prudent to examine the pupils before giving the atropine).

19.2.6 Pitfalls in brain death determination

The following pitfalls may complicate the determination of brain death:

- Movement of body parts after brain death. Movements are sometimes complex in nature, and may occur as long as 32 hours after brain death. Many are mediated by spinal cord discharges as it undergoes cell death. Documented observations include: facial movements, finger tremor, repetitive leg movements, and even sitting up. These movements are often repetitive, usually stereotypical, and do not change with changing stimuli.
- The appearance of breathing. This typically occurs with a ventilator that is set to trigger on detecting respiratory effort. Ventilators may be sensing air movement created by transmission of arterial pulses of the great vessels to the lung or actions of a chest tube.

19.3 Brain death in children

19.3.1 General information

The following is based on 2011 guidelines[19] that are endorsed by the Society of Critical Care Medicine, The Section for Critical Care and Section of Neurology of the American Academy of Pediatrics and the American College of Critical Care Medicine.

Key points[19]:

- The diagnosis of brain death in term newborns, infants and children is a clinical diagnosis requiring absence of neurologic function and a known irreversible cause of loss of function.
- These guidelines are not supported for infants < 37 weeks gestational age because of insufficient data
- Ancillary tests are not required and are not a substitute for a correctly performed neurologic exam
- Two examinations that include apnea testing separated by an observation period is recommended
- Treat and correct conditions that can interfere with the neurologic exam including: hypothermia, hypotension, interfering drugs (high levels of sedatives, analgesics, paralytics, high doses of anticonvulsant drugs) and metabolic disturbances

19.3.2 Clinical examination

Two examinations each including apnea testing, each consistent with brain death, performed by different attending physicians separated by an observation period are required. Apnea testing may be performed by the same physician.

Apnea testing requires documentation of arterial $PaCO_2$ that is 20 mm Hg above the baseline and ≥ 60 mm Hg with no respiratory effort. If apnea testing cannot be safely completed, an ancillary study should be done.

Recommended observation periods between exams:

- For term newborns (37 weeks gestational age) through 30 days of age: 24 hours
- For infants and children (> 30 days to 18 years): 12 hours
- Following cardiopulmonary resuscitation, the diagnosis of brain death should be deferred ≥ 24 hrs if there are concerns or inconsistencies in the examination

19

19.3.3 Ancillary studies

These tests are not required to make the determination of brain death. Use may be considered:

- When apnea testing cannot be safely completed e.g. due to underlying medical conditions or desaturation to < 85% or inability to achieve $paCO_2 \geq 60$ mm Hg
- If there is uncertainty about results of the neurologic examination
- If drugs that interfere with the neurologic exam may be present
- To reduce the inter-examination observation period

When ancillary tests are employed, a second neurologic examination and apnea test should be performed to the extent possible, and there should not be any finding inconsistent with brain death.

19.4 Organ and tissue donation

19.4.1 General considerations

The Center for Medicare Services (CMS) conditions of participation require all hospitals that receive Medicare funds to refer all imminent deaths to the local Organ Procurement Organization (OPO).[20] The OPO is responsible for the determination of suitability and for discussion of donation with the legal next of kin. The discussion must be by trained personnel. The OPO is also responsible for organ donor management, allocation and facilitating recovery of organs in the OR.[20]

19.4.2 Referral of the potential organ donor

Most OPO's have developed a process for referral of the potential organ donor by educating the critical care nurses to referral by a set of "triggers." The triggers usually include patients with a neurologic injury (anoxia, hemorrhage, trauma etc.), on a ventilator and either losing brain stem reflexes, GCS < 5 or for discussion of withdrawal of support. This set of triggers results in the referral of many patients not suitable for donation but allows for the early notification of the OPO and reduces the risk of missed referrals.

19.4.3 Medical management of the potential organ donor

Brain death results in several predictable physiologic aberrations. Many hospitals have developed "Catastrophic Brain Injury" order sets to address these predictable consequences.

Hypotension

With hypovolemia due to diabetes insipidus and destruction of the pontine and medullary vasomotor centers most brain dead patients are hypotensive. Treatment requires restoration of a euvolemic state and support with vasopressors. Usually norepinephrine to supply inotropic support and neosynephrine to increase peripheral vascular resistance is sufficient to support the blood pressure.

Diabetes insipidus

With loss of hypothalamic function brain dead individuals frequently have posterior pituitary dysfunction and diabetes insipidus. This is manifest by large volume dilute urinary output, hypernatremia and hyperosmolar serum. Management options include DDAVP injection (1-2 mcg SC/IV q 12 hours) or a vasopressin drip (0.01 – 0.04 units/min IV). The vasopressin drip may be preferable because the shorter duration of action can help avoid oliguria due to overdosing.

Hypothermia

Loss of temperature regulation frequently causes hypothermia which can worsen coagulopathy and invalidate brain death testing. Application of a warming blanket to support temperature will help restore normal physiology.

19.4.4 Organ Procurement Organization (OPO) process

Authorization

OPO staff will respond to referrals and after discussion with medical staff and nursing staff engage the family in a discussion involving authorization for organ donation. United Network for Organ Sharing (UNOS) data has demonstrated that OPO trained staff have higher authorization rates than medical staff. This is thought to be due to the position of the OPO staff only advocating for donation and if the treating staff advocates for donation there may be a sense of abandonment.

Donor evaluation

The OPO staff will evaluate donor suitability. Donors will be ruled out if there is thought to be a high potential for transmission of malignancy. The OPO will screen for blood-borne pathogens (HIV, HCV, HBV). Each organ will be evaluated for suitability.

- Heart: EF > 50%, no LVH, no CAD
- Lungs: P/F Ratio > 300, normal bronchoscopy
- Liver: ALT, AST, GGTP and bilirubin WNL or returning to normal and no known liver disease

- Kidneys: BUN and Creatinine WNL
- Pancreas: normal lipase, amylase and HgbA1c

Allocation and recovery

Once brain death occurs in a patient authorized or organ donation, the OPO will allocate organs according to UNOS allocation policy and UNOS generated allocation lists. When the transplant centers have accepted organs an OR time will be set and the teams will come to the donor hospital for organ recovery. The time frame from authorization until organ recovery frequently takes 24 to 36 hours or longer.

19.4.5 Organ donation after cardiac death

General information

Key concepts

- candidates: ventilator dependent patients (typically with brain or spinal cord injury) where the family has decided to withdraw support and the medical team expects the patient would progress to asystole less than 60 minutes after withdrawal
- consent from legal next of kin for: organ donation, heparin, and femoral lines
- clearance from medical examiner when applicable (usually, cases of unnatural death)
- counsel the family that the procedure cannot be done in ≈ 20% of cases. They are to be notified immediately if this happens and end-of-life care continues
- the transplant team cannot participate in end-of-life care or declaration of death, and should not be in O.R. until after cardiac death is declared

Candidates for organ donation after cardiac death are typically ventilator dependent patients with brain or spinal cord injuries who are so near death that further treatment is futile, but who do not meet brain death criteria. Organs typically recovered in this manner: kidneys, liver, pancreas, lungs, and rarely the heart.[21]

Ethical concerns related to DCD organ recovery have been raised.[22] The Institute of Medicine has reviewed DCD twice (1997 and 2000) and determined DCD to be ethically sound and OPO's have been encouraged to pursue DCD donation.[23]

Consent

Prior to any discussion of donation, the family should have made their decision to withdraw support and allow the patient to progress to death. After the family has had this discussion with the treating physician, the OPO can discuss DCD with the legal next of kin. Consent must also be obtained for any donation-related procedures prior to death (which typically includes heparin infusion to prolong organ viability[24] and the possibility of femoral catheters). The discussion should also include process to return to ICU if the patient does not progress to asystole.

Clearance from the medical examiner must be obtained in applicable cases (including deaths due to accident, homicide, suicide…).

Procedure

Life sustaining measures are discontinued (typically consisting of extubation) usually in the operating room. Death is pronounced typically ≈ 2 to 5 minutes after cardiac activity becomes insufficient to generate a pulse, because limited data indicates that circulation will not spontaneously return[25] (NB: EKG activity does not need to cease). After declaration of death, cold perfusion of organs is performed and they are procured.

To avoid potential conflicts of interest, no member of the transplant team can participate in end-of-life care nor the declaration of death.[21] About 20% of the time, the progression to cardiac death does not occur in a timeframe that permits organ retrieval. In these cases, organ donation is cancelled, the family must be immediately notified, and end-of-life care continues.

References

[1] Guidelines for the determination of death. Report of the medical consultants on the diagnosis of death to the President's Commission for the Study of Ethical Problems in Medicine and Biomedical and Behavioral Research. JAMA. 1981; 246:2184–2186

[2] National Conference of Commissioners on Uniform State Laws. Uniform Determination of Death Act. 645 N. Michigan Ave., Suite 510, Chicago, IL 60611 1980

[3] Wijdicks EF, Varelas PN, Gronseth GS, Greer DM. Evidence-based guideline update: determining brain death in adults: report of the Quality Standards Subcommittee of the American Academy of Neurology. Neurology. 2010; 74:1911–1918

[4] Wijdicks EF. Determining Brain Death in Adults. Neurology. 1995; 45:1003–1011

[5] Quality Standards Subcommittee of the American Academy of Neurology. Practice Parameters for Determining Brain Death in Adults (Summary Statement). Neurology. 1995; 45:1012–1014

[6] Benzel EC, Gross CD, Hadden TA, et al. The Apnea Test for the Determination of Brain Death. J Neurosurg. 1989; 71:191–194

[7] Benzel EC, Mashburn JP, Conrad S, Modling D. Apnea Testing for the Determination of Brain Death: A Modified Protocol. J Neurosurg. 1992; 76:1029–1031

[8] Ivan LP. Spinal Reflexes in Cerebral Death. Neurology. 1973; 23:650–652

[9] Turmel A, Roux A, Bojanowski MW. Spinal Man After Declaration of Brain Death. Neurosurgery. 1991; 28:298–302

[10] Heytens L, Verlooy J, Gheuens J, et al. Lazarus Sign and Extensor Posturing in a Brain-Dead Patient. J Neurosurg. 1989; 71:449–451

[11] Ropper AH. Unusual Spontaneous Movements in Brain-Dead Patients. Neurology. 1984; 34:1089–1092

[12] Jastremski MS, Powner D, Snyder J, Smith J, Grenvik A. Spontaneous Decerebrate Movement After Declaration of Brain Death. Neurosurgery. 1991; 29:479–480

[13] Treatment of Hypothermia. Med Letter. 1994; 36:116–117

[14] Antretter H, Dapunt OE, Mueller LC. Survival After Prolonged Hypothermia. N Engl J Med. 1994; 330

[15] Goodman JM, Heck LL, Moore BD. Confirmation of Brain Death with Portable Isotope Angiography: A Review of 204 Consecutive Cases. Neurosurgery. 1985; 16:492–497

[16] Wagner W. Scalp, earlobe and nasopharyngeal recordings of the median nerve somatosensory evoked P14 potential in coma and brain death. Detailed latency and amplitude analysis in 181 patients. Brain. 1996; 119 (Pt 5):1507–1521

[17] Greenan J, Prasad J. Comparison of the Ocular Effects of Atropine and Glycopyrrolate with Two IV Induction Agents. Br J Anaesth. 1985; 57:180–183

[18] Goetting MG, Contreras E. Systemic Atropine Administration During Cardiac Arrest Does Not Cause Fixed and Dilated Pupils. Ann Emerg Med. 1991; 20:55–57

[19] Nakagawa TA, Ashwal S, Mathur M, Mysore MR, Bruce D, Conway EE,Jr, Duthie SE, Hamrick S, Harrison R, Kline AM, Lebovitz DJ, Madden MA, Montgomery VL, Perlman JM, Rollins N, Shemie SD, Vohra A, Williams-Phillips JA. Guidelines for the determination of brain death in infants and children: an update of the 1987 Task Force recommendations. Crit Care Med. 2011; 39:2139–2155

[20] U.S. Electronic Code of Federal Regulations. Condition of Participation for Hospitals. 1998

[21] Steinbrook R. Organ donation after cardiac death. N Engl J Med. 2007; 357:209–213

[22] DuBois JM, DeVita M. Donation after cardiac death in the United States: how to move forward. Crit Care Med. 2006; 34:3045–3047

[23] Committee on Non-Heart-Beating Transplantation II, Division of Health Care Services - Institute of Medicine. Non-Heart-Beating Organ Transplantation: Practice and Protocols. Washington, D.C.: National Academy Press; 2000

[24] Bernat JL, D'Alessandro AM, Port FK, Bleck TP, Heard SO, Medina J, Rosenbaum SH, Devita MA, Gaston RS, Merion RM, Barr ML, Marks WH, Nathan H, O'Connor K, Rudow DL, Leichtman AB, Schwab P, Ascher NL, Metzger RA, Mc Bride V, Graham W, Wagner D, Warren J, Delmonico FL. Report of a National Conference on Donation after cardiac death. Am J Transplant. 2006; 6:281–291

[25] DeVita MA. The death watch: certifying death using cardiac criteria. Prog Transplant. 2001; 11:58–66

Part VI

Infection

VI

20 Bacterial Infections of the Parenchyma and Meninges and Complex Infections

20.1 Meningitis

20.1.1 General information

Community acquired meningitis (CAM) is generally more fulminant than meningitis following neurosurgical procedures or trauma (CAM tends to occur with more virulent organisms or in individuals with impaired host defenses). Waterhouse-Friderichspageen syndrome: occurs in 10–20% of children with meningococcal infection (usually disseminated infection in age < 10 yrs), produces large petechial hemorrhages in the skin and mucous membranes, fever, septic shock, adrenal failure (due to hemorrhage into adrenal glands) and DIC. Focal neurologic signs are rare in acute purulent meningitis. Community acquired meningitis is a medical emergency, and should be treated immediately. See Lumbar puncture (p. 323) for a discussion about when to perform an LP.

The remainder of this chapter discusses meningitis that is not community acquired.

20.1.2 Post-neurosurgical procedure meningitis

1. usual organisms: coagulase-negative staphylococci, S. aureus, Enterobacteriaceae, Pseudomonas sp., pneumococci usually with basilar skull fractures and otorhinologic surgery
2. empiric antibiotics: vancomycin (to cover MRSA), adult ℞ 15 mg/kg q 8-12 hours to achieve trough 15-20 mg/dl + cefipime 2 gm IV q 8 hrs
3. if severe PCN allergy, use aztreonam 2gm IV q6-8 H or ciprofloxacin 400 mg IV q8h
4. if severe infection, consider intrathecal therapy delivered daily (use only preservative free drug)
   - vancomycin
   - tobramycin/gentamicin
   - amikacin
   - colistin
5. streamline ABX based on sensitivities, e.g. if organism turns out to be MSSA, change vancomycin oxacillin or nafcillin

For suspected CSF fistula
1. usual organisms: streptococci; see CSF fistula (cranial) (p. 384)
2. treatment/work-up; see CSF fistula (cranial) (p. 384)
3. immunocompromised host (e.g. AIDS)
   a) usual organisms: as above PLUS Cryptococcus neoformans, M. tuberculosis, HIV aseptic meningitis, L. monocytogenes
   b) empiric antifungal agents for cryptococcal meningitis: Induction therapy: Liposomal amphotericin B 3-4 mg/kg IV daily + flucytosine25 mg/kg PO QID for at least 2 weeks followed by
   c) Consolidation therapy: fluconazole 400 mg PO daily for at least 8 weeks followed by
   d) Chronic maintenance therapy: fluconazole 200 mg PO daily

20.1.3 Post craniospinal trauma meningitis (post-traumatic meningitis)

Epidemiology

Occurs in 1–20% of patients with moderate to severe head injuries.[1] Most cases occur within 2 weeks of trauma, although delayed cases have been described.[2] 75% of cases have demonstrable basal skull fracture (p. 884), and 58% had obvious CSF rhinorrhea.

20

Pathogens

As expected from above, there is a high rate of infection with organisms indigenous to the nasal cavity. The most common organisms in a series from Greece were Gram-positive cocci (Staph. hemoliticus, S. warneri, S. cohnii, S. epidermidis, and Strep. pneumonia) and Gram-negative bacilli (E. coli, Klebsiella pneumonia, Acinetobacter anitratus).[1]

Treatment

1. See also CSF Fistula, Treatment (p. 388)
2. antibiotics: appropriate antibiotics are selected based on CSF penetration and organism sensitivities (adapted to the pathogens common in the patient's locale; in the above series, all Gram-negative strains appeared resistant to ampicillin and third-generation cephalosporins, but were sensitive to imipenem and ciprofloxacin; Gram-positive strains were all sensitive to vancomycin). For empiric antibiotics: Vancomycin 15 mg/kg IV q8-12 hours to achieve trough 15-20 mg/dl + meropenem 2gm IV q8h
3. surgical treatment vs. "conservative treatment": controversial. Some feel that any case of post-traumatic CSF rhinorrhea should be explored,[3,4] and that cases of spontaneous cessation often represent obscuration by incarcerated brain, so-called "sham healing" with the potential for later CSF leak and/or meningitis.[2] Others support the notion that cessation (possibly with the assistance of lumbar spinal drainage) is acceptable
4. continue antibiotics for 1 week after CSF is sterilized. If rhinorrhea persists at this time, surgical repair is recommended

20.1.4 Recurrent meningitis

Patients with recurrent meningitis must be evaluated for the presence of abnormal communication with the intraspinal/intracranial compartment. Etiologies include dermal sinus (p. 270) (either spinal or cranial), CSF fistula (p. 384), or neurenteric cyst (p. 290).

20.1.5 Chronic meningitis

Usually due to one of the following etiologies:
1. tuberculosis
2. fungal infections
3. cysticercosis, neurocysticercosis (p. 371)

Differential diagnosis includes:
1. sarcoidosis
2. meningeal carcinomatosis

20.1.6 Antibiotics for specific organisms in meningitis

Specific antibiotics

See reference.[5]

Route is IV unless specified otherwise.
1. S. pneumoniae: PCN G (2nd choice: chloramphenicol)
   a) if MIC ≤ 0.06: PCN G or ampicillin, alternative: third generation cephalosporin (ceftriaxone)
   b) if MIC ≥ 0.12: third generation cephalosporin (ceftriaxone)
   c) if cephalosporin resistance: vancomycin
   d) alternative: moxifloxacin
2. N. meningitidis: PCN G (2nd choice: chloramphenicol)
   a) if MIC ≤ 0.1 PCN G or ampicillin
   b) if MIC ≥ 0.1: third generation cephalosporin (ceftriaxone)
   c) alternative: moxifloxacin, meropenem
3. H. influenza:
   a) beta lactamase negative: ampicillin
   b) beta lactamase positive
      - third generation cephalosporin (ceftriaxone)
      - alternative: aztreonam, ciprofloxacin
4. Group B strep
   a) ampicillin
   b) alternative: vancomycin
5. L. monocytogenes
   a) ampicillin ± IV gentamicin
   b) alternative: IV sulfamethoxazole/trimethoprim
6. S. aureus
   a) if methicillin susceptible
      - oxacillin or nafcillin
      - PCN allergy: vancomycin

   b) if methicillin resistant
      - vancomycin ± rifampin
      - alternative: linezolid ± rifampin
7. aerobic Gram negative bacilli (GNB)
   a) ceftriaxone, or cefotaxime, or moxifloxacin (in order of preference, make alterations based on sensitivities)
   b) if aminoglycoside required, intraventricular therapy may be indicated after the newborn period
8. P. aeruginosa
   a) ceftazidime or cefepime
   b) alternative meropenem or aztreonam
   c) if ventriculitis: consider IT gentamicin or tobramycin
9. Candida spp: Liposomal amphotericin B 3-4 mg/kg IV daily + flucytosine25 mg/kg PO QID

Length of treatment for meningitis

Generally continue antibiotics for 10 – 14 days total. Duration is dependent on organism and clinical response. Treatment should be 21 days for listeria, group B strep and some GN bacilli.

20.2 Cerebral abscess

20.2.1 General information

Key concepts

- may arise from hematogenous spread, contiguous spread, or direct trauma
- risk factors: pulmonary abscess or AV fistulas, congenital cyanotic heart disease, immune compromise, chronic sinusitis/otitis, dental procedures
- symptoms are similar to any other mass lesions but tend to progress rapidly
- peripheral WBC may be normal or slightly ↑, CRP usually ↑
- organisms: Streptococcus is most common, up to 60% are polymicrobial
- imaging: usually round with thin enhancing ring on CT or MRI. T2WI → high signal lesion with thin rim of low intensity surrounded by hi signal (edema). Unlike with tumor, DWI often shows core of restricted diffusion (not reliable)
- treatment: IV antibiotics, needle drainage for some, excision infrequently (for fungal or resistant abscess)

20.2.2 Epidemiology

Approximately 1500–2500 cases per year in the U.S. Incidence is higher in developing countries. Male:female ratio is 1.5–3:1.

20.2.3 Risk factors

Risk factors include: pulmonary abnormalities (infection, AV-fistulas…, see below), congenital cyanotic heart disease (see below), bacterial endocarditis, penetrating head trauma (see below), chronic sinusitis or otitis media, and immunocompromised host (transplant recipients on immunosuppressants, HIV/AIDS).

20.2.4 Vectors

General information

Prior to 1980, the most common source of cerebral abscess was from contiguous spread. Now, hematogenous dissemination is the most common vector. In 10–60% no source can be identified.[6]

Hematogenous spread

Abscesses arising by this means are multiple in 10–50% of cases.[7] No source can be found in up to 25% of cases. The chest is the most common origin:

1. in adults: lung abscess (the most common), bronchiectasis and empyema
2. in children: congenital cyanotic heart disease (CCHD) (estimated risk of abscess is 4–7%, which is ≈ 10-fold increase over general population), especially tetralogy of Fallot (which accounts for ≈ 50% of cases). The increased Hct and low PO_2 in these patients provides an hypoxic environment suitable for abscess proliferation. Those with right-to-left (veno-atrial) shunts additionally lose the filtering effects of the lungs (the brain seems to be a preferential target for these infections over other organs). Streptococcal oral flora is frequent, and may follow dental procedures. Coexisting coagulation defects often further complicate management[8]
3. pulmonary arteriovenous fistulas: ≈ 50% of these patients have Osler-Weber-Rendu syndrome (AKA hereditary hemorrhagic telangectasia), and in up to 5% of these patients a cerebral abscess will eventually develop
4. bacterial endocarditis: only rarely gives rise to brain abscess.[9] More likely to be associated with acute endocarditis than with subacute form
5. dental abscess
6. GI infections: pelvic infections may gain access to the brain via Batson's plexus

In patients with septic embolization, the risk of cerebral abscess formation is elevated in areas of previous infarction or ischemia.[10]

Contiguous spread

1. from purulent sinusitis: spreads by local osteomyelitis or by phlebitis of emissary veins. Virtually always singular. Rare in infants because they lack aerated paranasal and mastoid air cells. This route has become a less common source of cerebral abscess due to improved treatment of sinus disease (with antibiotics and, especially with surgery for chronic otitis media and mastoiditis)
   a) middle-ear and mastoid air sinus infections → temporal lobe and cerebellar abscess. The risk of developing a cerebral abscess in an adult with active chronic otitis media is ≈ 1/10,000 per year[11] (this risk appears low, but in a 30 year-old with active chronic otitis media the lifetime risk becomes ≈ 1 in 200)
   b) ethmoidal and frontal sinusitis → frontal lobe abscess
   c) sphenoid sinusitis: the least common location for sinusitis, but with a high incidence of intracranial complications due to venous extension to the adjacent cavernous sinus → temporal lobe
2. odontogenic → frontal lobe. Rare. Associated with a dental procedure in the past 4 weeks in most cases.[12] May also spread hematogenously

Following penetrating cranial trauma or neurosurgical procedure

Following penetrating trauma: The risk of abscess formation following civilian gunshot wounds to the brain is probably very low with the use of prophylactic antibiotics, except in cases with CSF leak not repaired surgically following traversal of an air sinus. An abscess following penetrating trauma cannot be treated by simple aspiration as with other abscesses, open surgical debridement to remove foreign matter and devitalized tissue is required.

Post-neurosurgical: especially with traversal of an air sinus. Abscess has been reported following use of intracranial pressure monitors and halo traction.[13]

20.2.5 Pathogens

1. cultures from cerebral abscesses are sterile in up to 25% of cases
2. organisms recovered varies with the primary source of infection
3. in general: Streptococcus is the most frequent organism, 33–50% are anaerobic or microaerophilic. Multiple organisms may be cultured to varying degrees (depends on care of technique), usually in only 10–30% of cases, but can approach 60%,[6] and usually includes anaerobes (Bacteroides sp. common)
4. when secondary to fronto-ethmoidal sinusitis: Strep. milleri and Strep. anginosus may be seen
5. from otitis media, mastoiditis, or lung abscess: usually multiple organisms, including anaerobic strep., Bacteroides, Enterobacteriaceae (Proteus)
6. post traumatic: usually due to S. aureus or Enterobacteriaceae
7. odontogenic (dental) source: may be associated with Actinomyces

8. following neurosurgical procedures: Staph. epidermidis and aureus may be seen
9. immunocompromised hosts including transplant patients (both bone marrow and solid organ) and AIDS: fungal infections are more common than otherwise would be seen. Organisms include:
   a) Toxoplasma gondii (p. 334); see also treatment (p. 333)
   b) Nocardia asteroides (p. 336)
   c) Candida albicans
   d) Listeria monocytogenes
   e) mycobacterium
   f) Aspergillus fumigatus often from a primary pulmonary infection
10. infants: Gram negatives are common because IgM fraction of antibodies don't cross the placenta

20.2.6 Presentation

Adults: no findings are specific for abscess, and many are due to edema surrounding the lesion. Most symptoms are due to increased ICP (H/A, N/V, lethargy). Hemiparesis and seizures develop in 30–50% of cases. Symptoms tend to progress more rapidly than with neoplasms.

Newborns: patent sutures and poor ability of infant brain to ward off infection → cranial enlargement. Papilledema is rare before 2 yrs of age. Common findings: seizures, meningitis, irritability, increasing OFC, and failure to thrive. Most newborns with abscess are afebrile. Prognosis is poor.

20.2.7 Stages of cerebral abscess

▶ Table 20.1 shows the four well recognized histologic stages of cerebral abscess, and correlates this with the resistance to insertion of an aspirating needle at the time of surgery. It takes at least 2 weeks to progress through this maturation process, and steroids tend to prolong it.

20.2.8 Evaluation

Bloodwork

Peripheral WBC: may be normal or only mildly elevated in 60–70% of cases (usually > 10,000).

Blood cultures: should be obtained when abscess is suspected, usually negative.

ESR: may be normal (especially in congenital cyanotic heart disease CCHD where polycythemia lowers the ESR).

C-reactive protein (CRP): hepatic synthesis increases with inflammatory conditions, however, infection anywhere in body (including brain abscess and dental abscess) can raise the CRP level. May also be elevated in noninfectious inflammatory conditions and brain tumor. Sensitivity for abscess is ≈ 90%, specificity is ≈ 77%.[14] See also normal values (p. 347).

Table 20.1 Histologic staging of cerebral abscess

Stage	Histologic characteristics (days shown are general estimates)	Resistance to aspirating needle
1	early cerebritis: (days 1–3) early infection & inflammation, poorly demarcated from surrounding brain, toxic changes in neurons, perivascular infiltrates	intermediate resistance
2	late cerebritis: (days 4–9) reticular matrix (collagen precursor) & developing necrotic center	no resistance
3	early capsule: (days 10–13) neovascularity, necrotic center, reticular network surrounds (less well developed along side facing ventricles)	no resistance
4	late capsule: (> day 14) *collagen* capsule[a], necrotic center, gliosis around capsule	firm resistance, "pop" on entering

[a]abscess is ≈ the only process in the brain that leaves a collagen scar, all other scars are glial scars

20

Lumbar puncture (LP)

The role of LP is *very* dubious in abscess. Although LP is abnormal in > 90%, there is no characteristic finding diagnostic of abscess. The OP is usually increased, and the WBC count and protein may be elevated. The offending organism can rarely be identified from CSF obtained by LP (unless abscess ruptures into ventricles) with positive cultures in ≈ 6–22%.[15] There is a risk of transtentorial herniation, especially with large lesions.

Σ

✖ Due to the risk involved and the low yield of useful information, avoid the use of LP in evaluating patients with suspected cerebral abscess if not already done.

Brain imaging

CT

Ring enhancing. Sensitivity ≈ 100%. For CT staging of abscess see below.

MRI

See ▶ Table 20.2 for findings. Enhanced T1WI → thin-walled ring enhancement surrounding low intensity central region (▶ Fig. 89.1). Fluid-fluid levels may be seen. Occasionally gas producing organisms may cause pneumocephalus.

Diffusion MRI: DWI → bright, ADC → dark (restricted diffusion suggesting viscous fluid)[16] (▶ Fig. 89.1). Unlike most tumors which are *dark* on DWI (▶ Fig. 89.2). More reliable with pyogenic abscess, less reliable e.g. with fungal[17] or TB abscess).

MR-spectroscopy: presence of amino acids and either acetate or lactate are diagnostic for abscess.

Infrequently used imaging

Leukocyte scan with 99mTc-HMPAO: patient's own WBCs are tagged and reinjected. Close to 100% sensitivity and specificity (sensitivity will be reduced if patient is treated with steroids within 48 hrs prior to the scan).[14]

Staging cerebral abscess on imaging

CT staging

Late cerebritis (stage 2) has similar features to early capsule (stage 3) on routine contrast and non-contrast CT. There is some therapeutic importance in differentiating these two stages; the following aids in distinguishing[18]:

1. cerebritis: tends to be more ill-defined
   a) ring-enhancement: usually appears by late cerebritis stage, usually *thick*
   b) further diffusion of contrast into central lumen, and/or lack of decay of enhancement on delayed scan 30–60 min after contrast infusion
2. capsule:
   a) faint rim present on pre-contrast CT (necrotic center with edematous surrounding brain cause collagen capsule to be seen)
   b) *thin* ring enhancement *AND* (more importantly) delayed scans → decay of enhancement

NB: Thin ring enhancement but lack of delayed decay correlates better with cerebritis

NB: Steroids reduce degree of contrast enhancement (especially in cerebritis)

Table 20.2 MRI findings with cerebral abscess

Stage	T_1WI	T_2WI
cerebritis	hypointense	hi signal
capsular	lesion center → low signal, capsule → mildly hyperintense, perilesional edema → low signal	center → iso- or hyperintense, capsule → dark (collagen), perilesional edema → hi signal

MRI staging

▶ Table 20.2 shows MRI findings in cerebral abscess. In the cerebritis stage, the margins are ill defined.

Additional evaluation

CXR and chest CT (if indicated) to look for pulmonary source.

Cardiac echo (including TEE, Doppler and/or echo with agitated saline injection (bubble study)): for suspected hematogenous spread, to look for patent foramen ovale or cardiac vegetations.

20.2.9 Treatment

General information

There is no single best method for treating a brain abscess. Treatment usually involves:

- Surgical treatment: needle drainage or excision
- correction of the primary source
- long-term use of antibiotics: often IV x 6-8 weeks and possibly followed by oral route x 4-8 weeks. Duration should be guided by clinical and radiographic response

Surgical vs. pure medical management

General information

In a patient with suspected cerebral abscess, tissue should be obtained in almost every case to confirm diagnosis and to isolate pathogens (preferably before initiation of antibiotics).

Medical treatment

In general, surgical drainage or excision is employed in the treatment. Purely medical treatment of *early* abscess (cerebritis stage)[19] is controversial. NB: pathogens were cultured from well encapsulated abscesses despite adequate levels of appropriate antibiotics in 6 patients who failed medical therapy.[20] Failure may be due to poor blood supply and acidic conditions within the abscess (which may inactivate antibiotics in spite of concentrations exceeding the MIC).

Medical therapy alone is more successful if:

1. treatment is begun in cerebritis stage (before complete encapsulation), even though many of these lesions subsequently go on to become encapsulated
2. small lesions: diameter of abscesses successfully treated with antibiotics alone were 0.8–2.5 cm (1.7 mean). Those that failed were 2–6 cm (4.2 mean).
   * 3 cm is suggested as a cutoff,[21] above this diameter surgery should be included
3. duration of symptoms ≤ 2 wks (correlates with higher incidence of cerebritis stage)
4. patients show definite clinical improvement within the first week

Medical management alone considered if:

1. poor surgical candidate (NB: with local anesthesia, stereotactic biopsy can be done in almost any patient with normal blood clotting)
2. multiple abscesses, especially if small
3. abscess in poorly accessible location: e.g. brain stem[22]
4. concomitant meningitis/ependymitis

Indications for surgical treatment

Indications for initial *surgical* treatment include:

1. significant mass effect exerted by lesion (on CT or MRI)
2. difficulty in diagnosis (especially in adults)
3. proximity to ventricle: indicates likelihood of intraventricular rupture which is associated with poor outcome[23,8]
4. evidence of significantly increased intracranial pressure
5. poor neurologic condition (patients responds only to pain, or does not even response to pain)
6. traumatic abscess associated with foreign material
7. fungal abscess
8. multiloculated abscess
9. follow-up CT/MRI scans cannot be obtained every 1–2 weeks
10. failure of medical management: neurological deterioration, progression of abscess towards ventricles, or after 2 wks if the abscess is enlarged. Also considered if no decrease in size by 4 wks.

Management

General outline

- obtain blood cultures
- initiate antibiotic therapy (preferably after biopsy specimen obtained), regardless of which mode of treatment (medical vs. surgical) is chosen (see below)
- LP (p. 323): avoid in most cases of cerebral abscess
- anticonvulsants: indicated for seizures, prophylactic use is optional
- steroids: controversial. Reduces edema, but may impede therapy (see below)

Antibiotic selection

1. initial antibiotics of choice when pathogen unknown, and especially if S. aureus suspected (if there is no history of trauma or neurosurgical procedure, then the risk of MRSA is low):
   - **vancomycin**: covers MRSA. 15 mg/kg IV q8-12 hours to achieve trough 15-20 mg/dl PLUS
   - a 3rd generation cephalosporin (ceftriaxone); utilize cefepime if post surgical PLUS
   - **metronidazole** (Flagyl®). Adult: 500 mg q6-8 hours
   - alternative to cefepime + metronidazole: meropenem 2gm IV q8h
   - make appropriate changes as sensitivities become available
2. if culture shows only strep, may use PCN G (high dose) alone or with ceftriaxone
3. if cultures show methicillin sensitive staph aureus and the patient does not have a beta lactam allergy, can change vancomycin to nafcillin (adult: 2 gm IV q 4 hrs. peds: 25 mg/kg IV q 6 hrs)
4. Cryptococcus neoformans, Aspergillus sp., Candida sp.: Liposomal amphotericin B 3-4 mg/kg IV daily + flucytosine25 mg/kg PO QID.
5. in AIDS patients: Toxoplasma gondii is a common pathogen, and initial empiric treatment with sulfadiazine + pyrimethamine + leucovorin is often used (p. 332)
6. for suspected or confirmed nocardia asteroides, see details (p. 336)

Antibiotic duration

IV antibiotics for 6–8 wks (most commonly 6), may then D/C *even if the CT abnormalities persist* (neovascularity remains). NB: CT improvement may lag behind clinical improvement. Duration of treatment may be reduced if abscess and capsule entirely excised surgically. Oral antibiotics may be used following IV course.

Glucocorticoids (steroids)

Reduces edema and decreases likelihood of fibrous encapsulation of abscess. May reduce penetration of antibiotics into abscess.[21] Immune suppression may also be deleterious.

✱ Reserved for patients with clinical and imaging evidence of deterioration from marked mass effect, and duration of therapy should be minimized.

Follow-up imaging

If therapy is successful, imaging should show decrease in:

1. degree of ring enhancement
2. edema
3. mass effect
4. size of lesion: takes 1 to 4 wks (2.5 mean). 95% of lesions that will resolve with antibiotics alone decrease in size by 1 month

Surgical treatment

Options

See reference.[24]

1. needle aspiration: the mainstay of surgical treatment. Especially well-suited for multiple or deep lesions (see below) may also be used with thin walled or immature lesions
2. surgical excision: Shortens length of time on antibiotics and reduces risk of recrudescence. Recommended in traumatic abscess to debride foreign material (especially bone), and in fungal abscess because of relative antibiotic resistance (see below)
3. external drainage: controversial. Not frequently used
4. instillation of antibiotics directly into the abscess: has not been extremely efficacious, although it may be used as for refractory Aspergillus abscesses

Needle aspiration

Most often implemented with stereotactic localization especially for deep lesions.[25] May be performed under local anesthesia if necessary (e.g. in patients who are poor surgical candidates for general anesthesia). May be combined with irrigation with antibiotics or normal saline. Repeated aspirations are required in up to 70% of cases. May be the only surgical intervention required (in addition to antibiotics), but sometimes must be followed with excision (especially with multiloculated abscess).

Performed through a trajectory chosen to:

1. minimize the path length through the brain
2. avoid traversing the ventricles or vital neural or vascular structures
3. avoid traversing infected structures outside the intracranial compartment (infected bone, paranasal sinuses, and scalp wounds)
4. in cases of multiples abscesses, target[7]:
   a) when the diagnosis is unknown: the largest lesion or the one causing the most symptoms
   b) once the diagnosis of abscess is confirmed
      - any lesion ≥ 2.5 cm diameter
      - lesions causing significant mass effect
      - enlarging lesions

Cultures

Send aspirated material for the following:

1. stains
   a) Gram stain
   b) acid-fast stain for Mycobacterium (AFB stain, acid-fast resist decolorization with an acid-alcohol mixture and retain the initial dye carbolfuchsin and appear red. The genus Mycobacterium and the genus Nocardia are acid-fast, all other bacteria will be decolorized and stain blue, the color of the counterstain methylene blue)
   c) modified acid-fast stain (for Nocardia, see below) looking for branching acid fast bacillus
   d) special fungal stains (e.g., methenamine silver, mucicarmine)
2. culture
   a) routine cultures: aerobic and anaerobic
   b) fungal culture: this is not only helpful for identifying fungal infections, but since these cultures are kept for longer period and any growth that occurs will be further characterized, fastidious or indolent bacterial organisms may sometimes be identified
   c) TB culture
   d) molecular testing: PCR (mycobacteria, EBV, JC virus)

Excision

Can only be performed during the "chronic" phase (late capsule stage). Abscess is removed as any well encapsulated tumor. The length of time on antibiotics can be shortened to ≈ 3 days in some cases following total excision of an accessible, mature abscess (e.g. located in pole of brain). Recommended for abscesses associated with foreign body and most Nocardia abscesses (see below). May also be needed necessary for: fungal abscess, multiloculated or resistant lesions.

20.2.10 Outcome

In the pre-CT era, mortality ranged from 40–60%. With advances in antibiotics, surgery, and the improved ability to diagnose and follow response with CT and/or MRI, mortality rate has been reduced to ≈ 10%, but morbidity remains high with permanent neurologic deficit or seizures in up to 50% of cases. Current outcomes are shown in ▶ Table 20.3. A worse prognosis is associated with poor neurologic function, intraventricular rupture of abscess, and almost 100% mortality with fungal abscesses in transplant recipients.

Table 20.3 Outcomes with cerebral abscess

mortality (CT era data)[26,7]	0–10%
neurologic disability	45%
late focal or generalized seizures	27%
hemiparesis	29%

20.3 Subdural empyema

20.3.1 General information

Referred to as subdural abscess prior to 1943.[27] Subdural empyema (**SDE**) is a suppurative infection that forms in the subdural space, which has no anatomic barrier to spread over the convexity and into the interhemispheric fissure[28] (and occasionally to the opposite hemisphere and posterior fossa). Antibiotic penetration into this space is poor. Distinguished from abscess which forms within brain substance, surrounded by tissue reaction with fibrin and collagen capsule formation. Hence, SDE tends to be more emergent.

SDE may be complicated by cerebral abscess (seen in 20–25% of imaging studies in patients with SDE), cortical venous thrombosis with risk of venous infarction, or localized cerebritis.

20.3.2 Epidemiology

Less common than cerebral abscess (ratio of abscess:empyema is ≈ 5:1). Found in 32 cases in 10,000 autopsies. Male:female ratio is 3:1.

Location: 70–80% are over the convexity, 10–20% are parafalcine.

20.3.3 Etiologies

See ▶ Table 20.4 for etiologies. Most often occurs as a result of direct extension of local infection (rarely following septicemia). Spread of the infection to the intracranial compartment may occur through the valveless diploic veins, often with associated thrombophlebitis.[29]

Chronic otitis media was the leading cause of SDE in the preantibiotic era, but in the U.S. this has now been surpassed by paranasal sinus disease especially with frontal sinus involvement[30] (may also follow mastoid sinusitis). SDE is a rare but sometimes fatal complication of cranial traction devices.[31,30] Infection of preexisting subdural hematomas (both treated and untreated, in infants and adults) have been reported[30] (bacteremic seeding of an unoperated SDH is very rare).

Trauma includes compound skull fractures and penetrating injuries. Other etiologies include: osteomyelitis, pneumonia, unrelated infection (e.g. foot cellulitis) in diabetics.

20.3.4 Organisms

The causative organism varies with the specific source of the infection. SDE associated with sinusitis is often caused by aerobic and anaerobic streptococci ▶ Table 20.5). Following trauma or neurosurgical procedures, staphylococci and Gram-negative species predominate (whereas S. aureus was not a common pathogen in sinusitis related SDE). Sterile cultures occur in up to 40% (some of which may be due to fastidious anaerobes and/or previous exposure to antibiotics).

Table 20.4 Etiologies of SDE

Location	%
paranasal sinusitis (especially frontal)[a]	67–75
otitis (usually chronic otitis media)[b]	14
post surgical (neuro or ENT)	4
trauma	3
meningitis (more common in peds[32])	2
congenital heart disease	2
misc. (including pulmonary suppuration)	4
undetermined	3

[a]more common in adults
[b]no cases from otitis in a recent series[30]

Table 20.5 Organisms in SDE associated with sinusitis

Organisms	%
Adult cases	
aerobic streptococcus	30–50%
staphylococci	15–20%
microaerophilic and anaerobic strep	15–25%
aerobic Gram-negative rods	5–10%
other anaerobes	5–10%
Childhood	
Organisms are similar to meningitis for the same age group. Antibiotics choice is the same as for meningitis	

Table 20.6 Findings on presentation with SDE[a]

Finding	%
fever	95
H/A	86
meningismus (nuchal rigidity...)	83
hemiparesis	80
altered mental status	76
seizures	44
sinus tenderness, swelling or inflammation	42
nausea and/or vomiting	27
homonymous hemianopsia	18
speech difficulty	17
papilledema	9

[a]from a review of multiple articles[30]

20.3.5 Presentation

Neurologic findings are shown in ▶ Table 20.6. Symptoms are due to mass effect, inflammatory involvement of the brain and meninges, and thrombophlebitis of cerebral veins and/or venous sinuses. SDE should be suspected in the presence of meningismus + unilateral hemisphere dysfunction. Marked tenderness to percussion or pressure over affected air sinuses is common.[28] Forehead or eye swelling (from emissary vein thrombosis) may occur.

Focal neurologic deficit and/or seizures usually occur late.

20.3.6 Evaluation

20

- CT: IV contrast is usually helpful. CT may miss some cases (related to early generation scanners, failure to give IV contrast, poor scan quality…). If normal, repeat the CT at a later time or do an MRI if clinical suspicion persists. Findings: hypodense (but denser than CSF) crescentic or lenticular extracerebral lesion with dense enhancement of medial membrane; inward displacement of gray-white interface; ventricular distortion and effacement of basal cisterns are common findings[33]
- MRI: low signal on T1WI, high signal on T2WI. Pial ependymal line: a non-specific MRI finding in CNS infection

- LP: ✖ potentially hazardous (risk of herniation). Organisms are usually present only in cases originating from meningitis. If no meningitis, usually see findings consistent with a parameningeal inflammatory process: moderate sterile pleocytosis (150–600 WBC/mm³) with PMNs predominating; glucose normal; opening pressure is usually high[28]; protein is usually elevated (range: 75–150 mg/dl)

20.3.7 Treatment

1. surgical drainage: indicated in most cases (nonsurgical management has been reported,[34] but should only be considered with minimal neurologic involvement, limited extension and mass effect of SDE, and early favorable response to antibiotics) usually done relatively emergently
2. early in the course, the pus tends to be more fluid and may be more amenable to burr hole drainage; later, loculations develop which may necessitate craniotomy
3. there has been controversy over the optimal surgical treatment. Early studies indicated a better outcome with craniotomy than with burr holes. Recent studies show less difference
   a) critically ill patients with localized SDE may be candidates for burr-hole drainage (usually inadequate if loculations are present). Repeat procedures may be needed, and up to 20% will later require a craniotomy
   b) craniotomy: to debride and, if possible, drain. A wide craniotomy is often required because of septations. The dura appears white because of pus underneath. Open and wash out subdural space. Do not try to remove material adherent to cortex (may cause infarction)
4. antibiotics: similar to treatment for cerebral abscess
5. anticonvulsants: usually used prophylactically, mandatory if seizures occur

20.3.8 Outcome

See ▸ Table 20.7. Mortality has dropped from near 100% in the per-antibiotic era to ≈ 10%. Neurologic deficits tend to improve following treatment, but were present in 55% of patients at the time of discharge from the hospital.[30] Age ≥ 60 years, obtundation or coma at presentation, and SDE related to surgery or trauma (rather than sinusitis) carry a worse prognosis.[30] Burr-hole drainage may be associated with a worse outcome than with craniotomy, but this may have been influenced by the poorer condition of these patients. Fatal cases may have associated venous infarction of the brain.

20.4 Neurologic involvement in HIV/AIDS

20.4.1 Types of neurologic involvement

General information

40–60% of all patients with acquired immunodeficiency syndrome (AIDS) will develop neurologic symptoms, with one-third of these presenting initially with their neurologic complaint.[35,36] Only ≈ 5% of patients that die with AIDS have a normal brain on autopsy. One study found the CNS complications of AIDS shown in ▸ Table 20.8.

The most common conditions producing *focal* CNS lesions in AIDS[38]:

1. toxoplasmosis
2. primary CNS lymphoma
3. progressive multifocal leukoencephalopathy (PML)
4. cryptococcal abscess
5. TB (tuberculoma)

Table 20.7 Outcome with SDE

Outcome	%
persistent seizures	34%
residual hemiparesis	17%
mortality	10–20%

Table 20.8 CNS complications of AIDS (320 patients[35])

Complication	%
viral syndromes	
subacute encephalitis[a]	17
atypical aseptic meningitis	6.5
herpes simplex encephalitis	2.8
✱ progressive multifocal leukoencephalopathy (PML)	1.9[b]
viral myelitis	0.93
varicella zoster encephalitis	0.31
non-viral infections	
✱ Toxoplasma gondii	>32
Cryptococcus neoformans	13
Candida albicans	1.9
coccidiomycosis	0.31
Treponema pallidum (neurosyphilis)	0.62
atypical Mycobacteria	1.9
Mycobacterium tuberculosis	0.31
Aspergillus fumigatus	0.31
bacteria (E. coli)	0.31
neoplasms	
✱ primary CNS lymphoma	4.7
systemic lymphoma with CNS involvement	3.8
Kaposi's sarcoma (including brain mets)	0.93
stroke (stroke)	
infarct	1.6
intracerebral hemorrhage	1.2
miscellaneous/unknown	7.8

[a]CMV encephalitis occasionally occurs
[b]more recent estimate[37] of the incidence of PML in AIDS: 4%

Primary effects of HIV infection

Aside from opportunistic infection and tumors caused by the immunodeficient state, infection with the Human Immunodeficiency Virus (HIV) itself can cause direct neurologic involvement including:

1. AIDS encephalopathy: the most common neurologic involvement, occurs in ≈ 66% of patients with AIDS involving the CNS
2. AIDS dementia AKA HIV dementia complex
3. aseptic meningitis
4. cranial neuropathies: including "Bell's palsy" (occasionally bilateral)
5. AIDS related myelopathy: vacuolization of spinal cord; see Myelopathy (p. 1407)
6. peripheral neuropathies

20

CNS toxoplasmosis in AIDS

May present as:
1. mass lesion (toxoplasmosis abscess): the most common lesion causing mass effect in AIDS patients (70–80% of cerebral mass lesions in AIDS[39]) (see below for CT/MRI findings)
2. meningoencephalitis
3. encephalopathy

CNS toxoplasmosis occurs late in the course of HIV infection, usually when CD4 counts are < 200 cells/mm^3.

PML in HIV/AIDS

Progressive multifocal leukoecnephalopathy (PML):
1. Is caused by a ubiquitous polyomavirus (a subgroup of papova virus, small nonenveloped viruses with a closed circular double DNA-stranded genome) called "JC virus" (JCV, named after the initials of the patient in whom it was first discovered, not to be confused with Jakob-Creutzfeldt – a prion disease – nor with Jamestown Canyon virus, also confusingly called JC virus, a single-stranded RNA virus that occasionally causes encephalitis in humans). 60–80% of adults have antibodies to JCV[40]
2. frequently manifests in patients with suppressed immune systems, including
   a) AIDS: currently the most common underlying disease associated with PML
   b) prior to AIDS, the most common associated diseases were chronic lymphocytic leukemia & lymphoma
   c) allograft recipients: due to immunosuppression[41]
   d) chronic steroid therapy
   e) PML also occurs with other malignancies, and with autoimmune disorders (e.g. SLE)
3. pathologic findings: focal myelin loss (demyelination, ∴ effects white matter) with sparing of axon cylinders, surrounded by enlarged astrocytes and bizarre oligodendroglial cells with eosinophilic intranuclear inclusion bodies. EM can detect the virus. Sometimes occurs in brainstem and cerebellum
4. clinical findings: mental status changes, blindness, aphasia, progressive cranial nerve, motor, or sensory deficits and ultimately coma. Seizures are rare
5. imaging findings: see below
6. clinical course: usually rapidly progressive to death within a few months, occasionally longer survival occurs inexplicably.[42] There is no effective treatment. Some promise initially with anti-retroviral therapy[43]
7. definitive diagnosis requires brain biopsy (sensitivity: 40–96%) although it is infrequently employed. JCV has been isolated from brain and urine. Polymerase chain reaction (PCR) of JCV DNA from CSF has been reported, and is specific but not sensitive for PML

Primary CNS lymphoma (PCNSL) in AIDS

Occurs in ≈ 10% of patients with AIDS.[44] PCNSL is associated with the Epstein-Barr virus (p.711).

Neurosyphilis

1. AIDS patients can develop neurosyphilis in as little as 4 mos from infection[45] (unlike the 15–20 yrs usually required in non-immunocompromised patients)
2. neurosyphilis can develop in spite of what would otherwise be adequate treatment for early syphilis with benzathine PCN[45,46]
3. CDC recommendations[47]: treat patients having symptomatic or asymptomatic neurosyphilis with:
   - penicillin G 3-4-million units IV q 4 hrs (total of 24-million units/d) for 10-14 days or
   - penicillin G procaine 2.4 million units IM daily + probenecid 500 mg QID orally, both for 10-14 days
   - alternative: Rocephin 2gm IV once daily for 10-14 days for patients with a mild beta-lactam allergy
   - for severe beta-lactam allergy: PCN desensitization

20.4.2 Neuroradiologic findings in AIDS

Overview

MR with gadolinium is recommended as the initial screening procedure of choice for AIDS patients with CNS symptoms (lower false negative rate than CT[38]).

See ▶ Table 20.9 for a comparison of neuroradiologic findings in toxoplasmosis, PCNSL and PML.

Table 20.9 Comparison of neuroradiologic lesions in AIDS[a]

Feature	Toxo	PCNSL	PML
Multiplicity	usually > 5 lesions	multiple but < 5 lesions	may be multiple
Enhancement	ring	homogeneous	none
Location	basal ganglia and grey-white junction	subependymal	usually limited to white matter
Mass effect	mild-moderate	mild	none-minimal
Miscellaneous	lesions surrounded by edema	may extend across corpus callosum	high signal on T2WI, low on T1WI

[a]abbreviations: Toxo = toxoplasmosis, PCNSL = primary CNS lymphoma, PML = progressive multifocal leukoencephalopathy

CT/MRI findings in toxoplasma abscess

See ▶ Table 20.9.

1. most common findings: large area (low density on CT) with mild to moderate edema, ring enhancement with IV contrast in 68% compatible with abscess (of those that did not ring enhance, many showed hypodense areas with less mass effect with slight enhancement adjacent to lesion), well circumscribed margins[48]
2. most commonly located in *basal ganglia* , are also often subcortical
3. often multiple (typically > 5 lesions[49]) and bilateral
4. usually with little to moderate mass effect[38] (in BG, may compress third ventricle and sylvian aqueduct causing obstructive hydrocephalus)
5. most patients with toxoplasmosis had evidence of cerebral atrophy

CT/MRI findings in PML

See ▶ Table 20.9. Note: the appearance of PML may differ in AIDS patients from its appearance in non-AIDS patients.

1. CT: diffuse areas of low density. MRI: high intensity on T2WI
2. normally involves only white matter (spares cortex), however in AIDS patients gray matter involvement has been reported
3. no enhancement (on either CT or MRI), unlike most toxoplasmosis lesions
4. no mass effect
5. no edema
6. lesions may be solitary on 36% of CTs and on 13% of MRIs
7. borders are usually more ill-defined than in toxoplasmosis[48]

CT/MRI findings in primary CNS lymphoma (PCNSL)

See ▶ Table 20.9. NB: the appearance of PCNSL may differ in AIDS patients from non-AIDS patients.

1. multiple lesions with mild mass effect and edema that tend to ring-enhance on CT, or appear as areas of hypointensity surrounding central area of high intensity (target lesions) on T2WI MRI (unlike non-AIDS cases which tend to enhance homogeneously[50])
2. there is a greater tendency to multicentricity in AIDS patients than in the nonimmunosuppressed population[51]

20.4.3 Management of intracerebral lesions

20

Neurosurgical consultation is often requested for biopsy in an AIDS patient with questionable lesion (s). The diagnostic dilemma is usually for low density lesions on CT, and in the United States is primarily between the following:

- toxoplasmosis: treated with pyrimethamine and sulfadiazine + leucovorin (see below)
- PML: no proven effective treatment (initiate or optimize antiretroviral therapy may help[43])
- CNS lymphoma: usually treated with RTX; see CNS lymphoma (p. 710)

- note: cryptococcus is more common than PML or lymphoma, but usually manifests as cryptococcal meningitis (p. 376), and *not* as a *ring enhancing* lesion

Recommendations

PML can usually be identified radiographically. However, radiographic imaging alone cannot reliably differentiate toxoplasmosis from lymphoma or from some other concurrent conditions (patients with toxoplasmosis may have other simultaneous diseases). Therefore, the following recommendations are made:

1. obtain baseline toxoplasmosis serology (IgG) on all known AIDS patients (NB: 50% of the general population have been infected by toxo and have positive titer by age 6 years, 80–90% will be positive by middle adulthood).
2. multiple enhancing lesions with basal ganglion involvement in a patient whose toxo titer is positive have a high probability of being toxo
3. primary CNS lymphoma (PCNSL): with a *single* lesions, lymphoma is more likely than toxo. If the possibility of PCNSL is strong
   a) consider LP (contraindicated in presence of mass effect)
      - high volume LP for cytology: PCNSL can be diagnosed in ≈ 10–25% of cases using ≈ 10 ml of CSF
      - or send CSF for polymerase chain reaction (PCR) amplification of viral DNA of Epstein-Barr virus or JC-virus[52] (the agents responsible for AIDS-related PCNSL and PML, respectively)
   b) some centers recommend early biopsy to identify PCNSL cases to avoid delaying RTX for 3 weeks while assessing response to antibiotics[38]; instead of biopsy, a few centers advocate empiric radiation treatment (for possible lymphoma)
4. in patient with possible toxoplasmosis (i.e. positive toxo serology and imaging findings typical for toxo) even if other conditions have not been excluded:
   a) initial therapy: sulfadiazine 1000 mg four times daily for patients < 60 kg or 1500 mg four time daily for patients ≥ 60 kg + pyrimethamine 200 mg loading dose, then 50 mg daily for patients < 60 kg or 75 mg daily for patients ≥ 60 kg + folinic acid 10-25 mg daily to prevent pyrimethamine induced hematologic toxicity
   b) for patients who cannot take sulfadiazine (including those who develop sulfa allergy), change sulfadiazine to clindamicin 600 mg IV or PO q 6 hrs
   c) alternative regimens:
      - atovaquone 1500 mg PO BID + pyrimethamine 200 mg loading dose, then 50 mg daily for patients < 60 kg or 75 mg daily for patients ≥ 60 kg + folinic acid 10-25 mg daily
      - atovaquone 1500 mg PO BID + sulfadiazine 1000 mg four times daily for patients < 60 kg or 1500 mg four time daily for patients ≥ 60 kg
   d) there should be a clinical and radiographic response within 2-3 weeks[53]
   e) if no response to therapy after 3 weeks (some recommend 7-10 days[54]), then consider alternative diagnosis (brain biopsy should be considered)
   f) if response is good, reduce dosage of sulfadiazine after 6to 50% of the above dose for chronic maintenance therapy: sulfadiazine 1000 mg twice daily for patients < 60 kg or 1500 mg four twice daily for patients ≥ 60 kg + pyrimethamine 25-50 mg daily + folinic acid 10-25 mg daily
   g) chronic maintenance therapy can be discontinued in asymptomatic patients who have completed initial therapy if they are receiving antiretroviral therapy (ART), have a suppressed HIV viral load, and have maintained a CD4 count > 200 cells/mcl for at least six months
5. perform biopsy in the following settings:
   a) in patient with a negative toxo titer (note: patients occasionally have negative titer because of anergy)
   b) accessible lesion(s) atypical for toxo (i.e. non-enhancing, sparing basal ganglia, periventricular location)
   c) in the presence of extraneural infections or malignancies that may involve the CNS
   d) lesion that could be either lymphoma or toxo (e.g. single lesion, see 3. A.)
   e) in patients who have lesions not inconsistent with toxo but fail to respond to appropriate anti-toxo medications in the recommended time (see above)
   f) the role of biopsy for *non-enhancing* lesions is less well defined as the diagnosis does not influence therapy (most are PML or biopsies are non-diagnostic), it may be useful only for prognostic purposes[54]
   g) note: the risk of open biopsy in AIDS patients may be higher than nonimmunocompromised patients. Stereotactic biopsy may be especially well suited, with up to 96% efficacy, fairly low morbidity (major risk: significant hemorrhage, ≈ 8% incidence) and low mortality[55,56]
6. stereotactic biopsy guidelines:
   a) if multiple lesions are present, choose the most accessible lesion in the least eloquent brain area, or the lesion not responding to treatment

b) biopsy the center of non-enhancing lesions, or the enhancing portion of ring-enhancing lesions
c) recommended studies on biopsy: histology; immunoperoxidase stain for Toxoplasma gondii; stains for TB and fungus; culture for TB, fungi, pyogens

20.4.4 Prognosis

Patients with CNS toxo have a median survival of 446 days, which is similar to that with PML but longer than AIDS-related PCNSL.[49]

Patients with CNS lymphoma in AIDS survive on average a shorter time than similarly treated CNS lymphoma in nonimmunosuppressed patients (3 months vs. 13.5 mos). Median survival is < 1 month with no treatment. CNS lymphoma in AIDS tends to occur late in the disease, and patients often die of unrelated causes (e.g. Pneumocystis carinii pneumonia).[54]

20.5 Lyme disease – neurologic manifestations

20.5.1 General information

Lyme disease (LD) is a complex multisystem disease caused by various species of Borrelia spirochetes (in North America: Borrelia burgdorferi) transmitted to humans by the Ixodes scapularis or pacificus ticks (the American dog tick is not involved). It was first recognized in Lyme, Connecticut in 1975, and is now the most common arthropod-borne infection in the U.S.[57]

20.5.2 Clinical findings

There are 3 clinical stages which can overlap or occur separately.

► **Stage 1 (early localized disease, erythema migrans and flu-like illness).** Systemic signs of infection usually begin with a flu-like illness within days to weeks of infection, symptoms include: fever, chills, malaise, fatigue or lethargy, backache, headache, arthralgia, and myalgia. Regional or generalized lymphadenopathy may occur.

The hallmark of LD is erythema chronicum migrans (ECM) (classically a "bulls-eye rash") which begins 3–30 days after the tick bite, and occurs in 60–75% of patients. ECM usually begins in the thigh, inguinal region, or axilla, and consists of an expanding macular rash with bright red borders and central clearing and induration that usually fades without scarring in 3–4 weeks. In addition to ECM, other dermatologic findings include: malar rash (13%), diffuse erythema, and urticaria. Within 30 days of the tick bite, spirochetes may be demonstrated in acellular spinal fluid.

► **Stage 2 (early disseminated disease).** Several weeks to months after infection, untreated patients develop signs of more serious organ involvement. Cardiac and neurologic involvement may occur. Manifestations include:

1. cardiac: occurs in 8%. Conduction defects (usually A-V block, generally brief and mild) and myopericarditis
2. ocular: panophthalmitis, ischemic optic atrophy, and interstitial keratitis occur rarely
3. neurologic: occurs in 10–15% of patients with stage 2 disease
   a) the clinical triad of neurologic manifestations of Lyme disease is[58]:
      - cranial neuritis (especially that mimicking Bell's palsy: Lyme disease is the most common cause of bilateral "Bell's palsy" (facial diplegia) in endemic areas)
      - meningitis
      - radiculopathy
   b) other possible neurologic involvement includes: encephalitis, myelitis, peripheral neuritis

Neurologic findings are frequently migratory, and ≈ 60% of patients have multiple neurologic findings simultaneously. In Europe, Bannwarth's syndrome (chronic lymphocytic meningitis, peripheral neuropathy, and radiculopathy) is the most common manifestation, and primarily affects the peripheral nervous system.[59] Neurologic symptoms usually resolve gradually.

► **Stage 3 (late disease).** Arthritis and chronic neurologic syndromes may occur in this stage. Arthralgias are common in stage 1, but true arthritis usually does not begin for months to years after infection, and is seen in ≈ 60% of cases.[60] When arthritis occurs, it may affect the knee (89%), hip (9%), shoulder (9%), ankle (7%) and/or elbow (2%).[61] Neurologic involvement includes[62]:

1. encephalopathy (chronic, manifestation may be subtle)
2. encephalomyelitis (chronic, manifestation may be subtle)
3. peripheral neuropathy (chronic, manifestation may be subtle)
4. ataxia
5. dementia
6. sleep disorder
7. neuropsychiatric disease and fatigue syndromes

20.5.3 Diagnosis

Diagnostic criteria

There is no test indicative of active infection. The spirochete is difficult to culture from infected humans. Diagnosis is easy if a history of travel to endemic areas, tick bite, and ECM are identified. ▶ Table 20.10 shows the CDC criteria for diagnosis.

Serology

It takes 7–10 days from initial infection to develop antibodies to B. burgdorferi, but it takes ≈ 2–3 wks before antibodies can reliably be detected in untreated patients (antibiotics can reduce the immune response).[64] If the first serum test is negative, it should be repeated in 4–6 weeks if the clinical suspicion of LD is strong (seroconversion from negative to positive is supportive of B. burgdorferi infection). False positives can occur with other borrelial and treponemal infections (e.g. syphilis, however, VDRL test will differentiate the two).

Enzyme-linked immunosorbent assay (ELISA) detects IgM or IgG. Antibodies to B. burgdorferi is the usual test method. IgM is elevated acutely, and IgG gradually rises and is elevated in almost all patients at 4–6 weeks and is usually highest in patients with arthritis.[57] Western blot may help identify false-positive ELISA results (more sensitive and specific than ELISA, however, results may vary between labs). Amplification of B. burgdorferi DNA by polymerase chain reaction (PCR) yields a more very sensitive test that may have significant false positives, and can be positive even if the DNA is from dead organisms.

CSF

Elevated CSF IgG antibody titer to B. burgdorferi may occur with neurologic involvement.[65] CSF findings in late disease are usually compatible with aseptic meningitis. Oligoclonal bands and increased ratio of IgG to albumin may occur.[66]

20.5.4 Treatment

See references.[67,68,62]

Antibiotic therapy is more effective early in the illness.

20.6 Nocardia brain abscess

20.6.1 General information

Nocardia infections may involve the CNS in multiple ways.

Table 20.10 CDC criteria for diagnosis of Lyme disease[63]

Area	Criteria
In endemic area	• erythema chronicum migrans (ECM) • antibody titer ≥ 1:256 by IFA[a] and involvement of ≥ 1 organ system[b]
In non-endemic area	• ECM with antibody titer ≥ 1:256 • ECM with involvement of ≥ 2 organ systems[b] • antibody titer ≥ 1:256 by IFA[a] and involvement of ≥ 1 organ system[b]

[a]IFA = immunofluorescence antibody
[b]either musculoskeletal, neurologic or cardiac

Nocardiosis is caused primarily by Nocardia asteroides (other Nocardia species such as N. brasiliensis are less common), a soil-born aerobic actinomycete (a bacteria, not a fungus) that is usually inoculated through the respiratory tract and produces a localized or disseminated infection. Hematogenous spread frequently results in cutaneous lesions and CNS involvement. Nocardia is responsible for 2% of all brain abscesses, the majority of these are N. asteroides.

Nocardiosis occurs primarily in patients with chronic debilitating illnesses including:

1. neoplasms: leukemia, lymphoma…
2. conditions requiring long-term corticosteroid treatment
3. Cushing's disease
4. Paget's disease of bone
5. AIDS
6. renal or cardiac organ transplant recipients

The diagnosis is suspected in high-risk patients presenting with soft-tissue abscesses and CNS lesions. CNS involvement occurs in about one-third and includes:

1. cerebral abscess: often multiloculated
2. meningitis
3. ventriculitis in patients with CSF shunt[69]
4. epidural spinal cord compression from vertebral osteomyelitis[70]

20.6.2 Diagnosis

Brain biopsy may not be needed in high-risk patients with confirmed nocardia infection in other sites,[69] except possibly in AIDS patients where the risk of multiple organism infections or infection plus tumor (particularly lymphoma) is considerable.

20.6.3 Treatment

General information

Surgical indications (p. 324) are the same as for other abscesses.

Antibiotics

See references.[71,72]

- Primary choice: trimethoprim-sulfamethoxazole (TMP-SMZ 15 mg/kg IV of trimethoprim component per day in two to four divided doses PLUS imipenem 500 mg IV q6h ± amikacin 7.5 mg/kg IV q12h (if CNS disease with multiorgan involvement)
- Alternative if sulfa allergy: imipenem 500 mg IV q6h PLUS amikacin 7.5 mg/kg IV q12h

Antimicrobial susceptibility testing should be conducted on all isolates.

Duration: because of risks of relapse or hematogenous spread, treatment is recommended forat least one year with CNS involvement, possibly indefinitely in for immunocompromised hosts.

References

[1] Baltas I, Tsoulfa S, Sakellariou P, et al. Posttraumatic Meningitis: Bacteriology, Hydrocephalus, and Outcome. Neurosurgery. 1994; 35:422–427

[2] Eljamel MSM, Foy PM. Post-Traumatic CSF Fistulae, the Case for Surgical Repair. Br J Neurosurg. 1990; 4:479–483

[3] Lewin W. Cerebrospinal Fluid Rhinorrhea in Closed Head Injuries. Clin Neurosurg. 1966; 12:237–252

[4] Horwitz NH, Levy CS. Comment on Baltas I, et al.: Posttraumatic Meningitis: Bacteriology, Hydrocephalus, and Outcome. Neurosurgery. 1994; 35

[5] van de Beek D, Brouwer MC, Thwaites GE, Tunkel AR. Advances in treatment of bacterial meningitis. Lancet. 2012; 380:1693–1702

[6] Calfee DP, Wispelwey B. Brain abscess. Semin Neurol. 2000; 20:353–360

[7] Mamelak AN, Mampalam TJ, Obana WG, Rosenblum ML. Improved Management of Multiple Brain Abscesses: A Combined Surgical and Medical Approach. Neurosurgery. 1995; 36:76–86

[8] Takeshita M, Kagawa M, Yato S, et al. Current treatment of brain abscess in patients with congenital cyanotic heart disease. Neurosurgery. 1997; 41:1270–1279

[9] Kanter MC, Hart RG. Neurologic Complications of Infective Endocarditis. Neurology. 1991; 41:1015–1020

[10] Garvey G. Current Concepts of Bacterial Infections of the Central Nervous System: Bacterial Meningitis and Bacterial Brain Abscess. J Neurosurg. 1983; 59:735–744

[11] Nunez DA, Browning GG. Risks of Developing an Otogenic Intracranial Abscess. J Laryngol Otol. 1990; 104:468–472

[12] Hollin SA, Hayashi H, Gross SW. Intracranial Abscesses of Odontogenic Origin. Oral Surg. 1967; 23:277–293

[13] Williams FH, Nelms DK, McGaharan KM. Brain Abscess: A Rare Complication of Halo Usage. Arch Phys Med Rehabil. 1992; 73:490–492

[14] Grimstad IA, Hirschberg H, Rootwelt K. 99mTc-hexamethylpropyleneamine oxime leukocyte scintigraphy and C-reactive protein levels in the differential diagnosis of brain abscesses. J Neurosurg. 1992; 77:732–736
[15] Fritz DP, Nelson PB, Roos KL. In: Brain Abscess. Central Nervous System Infectious Diseases and Therapy. New York: Marcel Dekker; 1997:481–498
[16] Desprechins B, Stadnik T, Koerts G, Shabana W, Breucq C, Osteaux M. Use of diffusion-weighted MR imaging in differential diagnosis between intracerebral necrotic tumors and cerebral abscesses. AJNR Am J Neuroradiol. 1999; 20:1252–1257
[17] Mueller-Mang C, Castillo M, Mang TG, Cartes-Zumelzu F, Weber M, Thurnher MM. Fungal versus bacterial brain abscesses: is diffusion-weighted MR imaging a useful tool in the differential diagnosis? Neuroradiology. 2007; 49:651–657
[18] Britt RH, Enzmann DR. Clinical Stages of Human Brain Abscesses on Serial CT Scans After Contrast Infusion. J Neurosurg. 1983; 59:972–989
[19] Heineman HS, Braude AI, Osterholm JL. Intracranial Suppurative Disease. JAMA. 1971; 218:1542–1547
[20] Black P, Graybill JR, Charache P. Penetration of Brain Abscess by Systemically Administered Antibiotics. J Neurosurg. 1973; 38:705–709
[21] Rosenblum ML, Hoff JT, Norman D, et al. Nonoperative Treatment of Brain Abscesses in Selected High-risk Patients. J Neurosurg. 1980; 52:217–225
[22] Ruelle A, Zerbi D, Zuccarello M, Andrioli G. Brain Stem Abscess Treated Successfully by Medical Therapy. Neurosurgery. 1991; 28:742–746
[23] Zeidman SM, Geisler FH, Olivi A. Intraventricular Rupture of a Purulent Brain Abscess: Case Report. Neurosurgery. 1995; 36:189–193
[24] Stephanov S. Surgical Treatment of Brain Abscess. Neurosurgery. 1988; 22:724–730
[25] Hollander D, Villemure J-G, Leblanc R. Thalamic Abscess: A Stereotactically Treatable Lesion. Appl Neurophysiol. 1987; 50:168–171
[26] Rosenblum ML, Hoff JT, Norman D, et al. Decreased Mortality from Brain Abscesses Since Advent of CT. J Neurosurg. 1978; 49:658–668
[27] Stephanov S, Sidani AH. Intracranial subdural empyema and its management. A review of the literature with comment. Swiss Surg. 2002; 8:159–163
[28] Kubik CS, Adams RD. Subdural Empyema. Brain. 1943; 66:18–42
[29] Maniglia AJ, Goodwin WJ, Arnold JE, Ganz E. Intracranial Abscess Secondary to Nasal, Sinus, and Orbital Infections in Adults and Children. Arch Otolaryngol Head Neck Surg. 1989; 115:1424–1429
[30] Dill SR, Cobbs CG, McDonald CK. Subdural Empyema: Analysis of 32 Cases and Review. Clin Inf Dis. 1995; 20:372–386
[31] Garfin SR, Botte MJ, Triggs KJ, Nickel VL. Subdural Abscess Associated with Halo-Pin Traction. J Bone Joint Surg. 1988; 70A:1338–1340
[32] Jacobson PL, Farmer TW. Subdural Empyema Complicating Meningitis in Infants: Improved Prognosis. Neurology. 1981; 31:190–193
[33] Weisberg L. Subdural Empyema: Clinical and Computed Tomographic Correlations. Arch Neurol. 1986; 43:497–500
[34] Mauser HW, Ravijst RAP, Elderson A, van Gijn J, Tulleken CAF. Nonsurgical Treatment of Subdural Empyema: Case Report. J Neurosurg. 1985; 63:128–130
[35] Levy RM, Bredesen DE, Rosenblum ML. Neurological manifestations of the acquired immunodeficiency syndrome (AIDS): Experience at UCSF and review of the literature. J Neurosurg. 1985; 62:475–495
[36] Simpson DM, Tagliati M. Neurologic Manifestations of HIV Infection. Ann Intern Med. 1994; 121:769–785
[37] Berger JR, Kaszovitz B, Post JD, et al. Progressive Multifocal Leukoencephalopathy Associated with Human Immunodeficiency Virus Infection: A Review of the Literature with a Report of Sixteen Cases. Ann Intern Med. 1987; 107:78–87
[38] Ciricillo SF, Rosenblum ML. Use of CT and MR Imaging to Distinguish Intracranial Lesions and to Define the Need for Biopsy in AIDS Patients. J Neurosurg. 1990; 73:720–724
[39] Chaisson RE, Griffin DE. Progressive Multifocal Leukoencephalopathy in AIDS. JAMA. 1990; 364:79–82
[40] Demeter LM, Mandell GL, Bennett JE. In: JC, BK, and other polyomaviruses; progressive multifocal leukoencephalopathy. Mandell, Douglas and Bennett Principles and Practice of Infectious Diseases. 4th edition ed. New York: Churchill Livingstone; 1995:1400–1406
[41] Krupp LB, Lipton RB, Swerdlow ML, Leeds NE, Llena J. Progressive Multifocal Leukoencephalopathy: Clinical and Radiographic Features. Ann Neurol. 1985; 17:344–349
[42] Berger JR, Mucke L. Prolonged Survival and Partial Recovery in AIDS-Associated Progressive Multifocal Leukoencephalopathy. Neurology. 1988; 38:1060–1065
[43] Elliot B, Aromin I, Gold R, Flanigan T, Mileno M. 2.5 year remission of AIDS-associated progressive multifocal leukoencephalopathy with combined antiretroviral therapy. Lancet. 1997; 349
[44] Jean WC, Hall WA. Management of Cranial and Spinal Infections. Contemp Neurosurg. 1998; 20:1–10
[45] Johns DR, Tierney M, Felenstein D. Alterations in the Natural History of Neurosyphilis by Concurrent Infection with the Human Immunodeficiency Virus. N Engl J Med. 1987; 316:1569–1592
[46] Lukehart SA, Hook EW, Baker-Zander SA, Collier AC, et al. Invasion of the Central Nervous System by Treponema pallidum: Implications for Diagnosis and Treatment. Ann Int Med. 1988; 109:855–862
[47] Workowski KA, Bolan GA. Sexually transmitted diseases treatment guidelines, 2015. MMWR Recomm Rep. 2015; 64:1–137
[48] Jarvik JG, Hesselink JR, Kennedy C, et al. Acquired Immunodeficiency Syndrome: Magnetic Resonance Patterns of Brain Involvement with Pathologic Correlation. Arch Neurol. 1988; 45:731–736
[49] Sadler M, Brink NS, Gazzard BG. Management of Intracerebral Lesions in Patients with HIV: A Retrospective Study with Discussion of Diagnostic Problems. Q J Med. 1998; 91:205–217
[50] Schwaighofer BW, Hesselink JR, Press GA, et al. Primary Intracranial CNS Lymphoma: MR Manifestations. AJNR. 1989; 10:725–729
[51] So YT, Beckstead JH, Davis RL. Primary central nervous system lymphoma in acquired immune deficiency syndrome: A clinical and pathological study. Ann Neurol. 1986; 20:566–572
[52] Cinque P, Brytting M, Vago L, et al. Epstein-Barr Virus DNA in Cerebrospinal Fluid from Patients with AIDS-Related Primary Lymphoma of the Central Nervous System. Lancet. 1991; 342:398–401
[53] Cohn JA, Meeking MC, Cohen W, et al. Evaluation of the policy of empiric treatment of suspected toxoplasma encephalitis in patients with the acquired immunodeficiency syndrome. Am J Med. 1989; 86:521–527
[54] Chappell ET, Guthrie BL, Orenstein J. The Role of Stereotactic Biopsy in the Management of HIV-Related Focal Brain Lesions. Neurosurgery. 1992; 30:825–829
[55] Levy RM, Russell E, Yungbluth M, et al. The efficacy of image-guided stereotactis brain biopsy in neurologically symptomatic acquired immunodeficiency syndrome patients. Neurosurgery. 1992; 30:186–190
[56] Nicolato A, Gerosa M, Piovan E, et al. Computerized Tomography and Magnetic Resonance Guided Stereotactic Brain Biopsy in Nonimmunocompromised and AIDS Patients. Surg Neurol. 1997; 48:267–277
[57] Nocton JJ, Steere AC. Lyme Disease. Adv Int Med. 1995; 40:69–117
[58] Pachner AR, Steere AC. The Triad of Neurologic Manifestations of Lyme Disease: Meningitis, Cranial Neuritis, and Radiculoneuritis. Neurology. 1985; 35:47–53

[59] Pachner AR, Duray P, Steere. Central Nervous System Manifestations of Lyme Disease. Arch Neurol. 1990; 46:790–795
[60] Steere AC, Schoen RT, Taylor E. The Clinical Evolution of Lyme Arthritis. Ann Intern Med. 1987; 107:735–731
[61] Centers for Disease Control. Lyme Disease - Connecticut. MMWR. 1988; 37:1–3
[62] Sigal LH. Lyme Disease Overdiagnosis: Cause and Cure. Hosp Pract. 1996; 31:13–15
[63] Weinstein A, Bujak DI. Lyme Disease: A Review of its Clinical Features. NY State J Med. 1989; 89:566–571
[64] Magnarelli LA. Current Status of Laboratory Diagnosis for Lyme Disease. Am J Med. 1995; 98 (S4A):10–2S
[65] Wilkse B, Scheirz G, Preac-Mursic V, et al. Intrathecal Production of Specific Antibodies Against Borrelia burgdorferi in Patients with Lymphocytic Meningoradiculitis (Bannwarth's Syndrome). J Infect Dis. 1986; 153:304–314
[66] Henriksson A, Link H, Cruz M, et al. Immunoglobulin Abnormalities in Cerebrospinal Fluid and Blood Over the Course of Lymphocytic Meningoradiculitis (Bannwarth's Syndrome). Ann Neurol. 1986; 20:337–345
[67] Treatment of Lyme Disease. Med Letter. 1988; 30:65–66
[68] Steere AC. Lyme Disease. N Engl J Med. 1989; 321:586–596
[69] Byrne E, Brophy BP, Pettett LV. Nocardia Cerebral Abscess: New Concepts in Diagnosis, Management, and Prognosis. J Neurol Neurosurg Psychiatry. 1979; 42:1038–1045
[70] Awad I, Bay JW, Petersen JM. Nocardial Osteomyelitis of the Spine with Epidural Spinal Cord Compression - A Case Report. Neurosurgery. 1984; 15:254–256
[71] Sorrell TC, Iredell JR, Mandell GL, Bennett JE, Dolin R. Principles and Practice of Infectious Diseases. 6th ed. Philadelphia: Elsevier; 2005
[72] Lerner PI. Nocardiosis. Clin Infect Dis. 1996; 22:891–903; quiz 904-5

21 Skull, Spine, and Post-Surgical Infections

21.1 Shunt infection

21.1.1 Epidemiology

Acceptable shunt infection rate[1]: < 5–7% (although many published series have a rate near 20%,[2] possibly due to different patient population).

Risk of early infection after shunt surgery: reported range is 3–20% per procedure (typically ≈ 7%).

Over 50% of staph infections occur within 2 weeks post-shunt, 70% within 2 mos. Source is often the patient's own skin.[1] It is estimated that in ≈ 3% of operations for shunt insertion the CSF is already infected (therefore CSF during shunt insertion is recommended).

21.1.2 Morbidity of shunt infections in children

Children with shunt infections have an increased mortality rate and risk of seizure than those without shunt infection. Those with myelomeningocele who develop ventriculitis after shunting have a lower IQ compared to those without infection.[3] Mortality ranges from 10–15%.

21.1.3 Risk factors for shunt infection

Many factors have been blamed. Some that seem to be better documented include:
- young age of patient[2]: in myelomeningocele (MM) patients, waiting until the child is 2 weeks old may significantly lower the infection rate
- length of procedure
- open neural tube defect

21.1.4 Pathogens

Early infection

Most commonly:
- Staph. epidermidis (coagulase-negative staph): 60–75% of infections (most common)
- S. aureus
- Gram-negative bacilli (GNB): 6–20% (may come from intestinal perforation)

In neonates E. coli and Strep. hemoliticus dominate.

Late infection (> 6 months after procedure)

Risk: 2.7–31% per patient (typically 6%). Almost all are S. epidermidis. 3.5% of patients account for 27% of infections.[4]

"Late" shunt infections may be due to:
- an indolent infection due to Staph. epidermidis
- seeding of a vascular shunt during episode of septicemia (probably very rare)
- colonization from an episode of meningitis

Fungal infections

Candida spp. infections

Candida spp. are responsible for the majority of fungal ventricular shunt infections. Usually occurs in children < 1 year age. Incidence: 1–7%.[5] The 4th leading pathogen causing meningitis in neurosurgical patients in 1 study,[6] possibly related to the use of prophylactic antibiotics used for ICP monitoring and CSF drainage. Higher incidence in VP shunt patients with abdominal infections and shunts placed in patients with previous bacterial meningitis.[7] CSF typically shows: elevated WBCs and protein, normal glucose. Management recommendations:
1. completely remove the contaminated shunt (may be more important than with bacterial infections)
2. place a fresh external ventricular drain (if patient is shunt dependent)
3. treat with antifungal therapy

21

4. place a fresh shunt after ≥ 5–7 days of therapy and clinical response is apparent
5. continue antifungal agents for 6–8 weeks

21.1.5 Presentation

Signs and symptoms

Non-specific syndrome: fever, N/V, H/A, lethargy, anorexia, irritability. May also present as shunt malfunction; 29% of patients presenting with shunt malfunction had positive cultures.

Erythema and tenderness along shunt tubing may occur.

Distal infection of ventriculoperitoneal shunts may mimic acute abdomen.

In neonates may manifest as apneic episodes, anemia, hepatosplenomegaly, and stiff neck.[8] S. epidermidis infections tend to be indolent (smoldering). GNB infections usually cause more severe illness; abdominal findings are more common; main clinical manifestation is fever, usually intermittent and low grade.

Shunt nephritis[9]: may occur with chronic low level infection of a ventriculovascular shunt causing immune complex deposition in renal glomeruli, characterized by proteinuria and hematuria.

Blood tests

WBC: < 10K in one fourth of shunt infections. It is > 20K in one-third.

ESR: rarely normal in shunt infections.

Blood cultures: positive in less than one-third of cases.

CSF: WBC is usually not > 100 cells/mm^3. Gram stains may be positive ≈ 50% (yield with S. epidermidis is much lower). Protein is often elevated, glucose may be low or normal. Rapid antigen tests used for community acquired meningitis are usually not helpful for the organisms that tend to cause shunt infections. CSF cultures are negative in 40% of cases (higher culture yield if CSF WBC count is > 20K).

Evaluation of shunt for infection

1. history and physical directed at determining presence of above signs and symptoms with emphasis on
   a) history suggestive of infection at another site
      - exposure to others with viral syndromes, including sick siblings
      - GI source (e.g. acute gastroenteritis). Often associated with diarrhea.
      - otitis media (check tympanic membranes)
      - tonsillitis/pharyngitis
      - appendicitis (peritoneal inflammation may impede VP shunt outflow)
      - URI
      - UTI
      - pneumonia
   b) physical exam to R/O meningismus (stiff neck, photophobia…)
2. bloodwork
   a) serum WBC count with differential
   b) acute phase reactants: ESR & CRP
   c) blood cultures
3. shunt tap: should be done in cases of suspected shunt infection. Clip hair (do nto shave) and prep carefully to avoid introducing infection. GNB requires different therapy and has higher morbidity than staph, thus it is desirable to identify these rare patients: > 90% of these had positive Gram-stained CSF smear (only a few Gram-positive infections have positive results). GNB have higher protein and lower glucose, and neutrophils predominate in differential (unpublished data[1])
4. imaging
   a) CT: usually not helpful for diagnosing infection. Ependymal enhancement when it occurs is diagnostic of ventriculitis. CT may demonstrate shunt malfunction
   b) abdominal U/S or CT: the presence of an abdominal pseudocyst is suggestive of infection
5. LP: usually NOT recommended. ✖ May be hazardous in obstructive hydrocephalus (HCP) with a nonfunctioning shunt. Often does not yield the pathogen even in communicating HCP, especially if the infection is limited to a ventriculitis. If positive, may obviate a shunt tap

21.1.6 Treatment

Antibiotics alone (without removal of shunt hardware)

Although eradication of shunt infections without removal of hardware has been reported,[10(p 595–7),11] this has a lower success rate than with shunt removal,[12] may require protracted treatment (up to 45 days in some), risks problems associated with draining infected CSF into the peritoneum (reduced CSF absorption, abdominal signs/symptoms including tenderness to full-blown peritonitis[10(p 235)]) or vascular system – shunt nephritis (p. 340), sepsis... – and often requires at least partial shunt revision at some point in most cases. Treatment with antibiotics without shunt removal is therefore recommended only in cases where the patient: is terminally ill, is a poor anesthetic risk, or has slit ventricles that might be difficult to catheterize.

Removal of shunt hardware

In most instances, during the initial treatment with antibiotics the shunt is either externalized (i.e. tubing is diverted at some point distal to the ventricular catheter and connected to a closed drainage system), or sometimes the entire shunt may be removed. In the latter case, some means of CSF drainage must be provided in shunt dependent cases; either by insertion of an external ventricular drain (EVD), or by intermittent ventricular taps (rarely employed) or LPs (with communicating HCP). EVD allows easy monitoring of CSF flow, control of ICP, and repeated sampling for signs of resolution of infection (normalization of WBC count and surveillance cultures). In addition, EVD allows for possible administration of intrathecal antibiotics. In symptomatic patients or those with a positive CSF culture,[13] any hardware removed should be cultured as only ≈ 8% are sterile in shunt infections. Skin organisms are fastidious and may take several days to grow.

If there is an abdominal pseudocyst, the fluid should be drained through the peritoneal catheter before removing it.

Antibiotics

Empiric antibiotics

See reference.[14]

1. Vancomycin (adult) 15 mg/kg IV q8-12 hours to achieve trough 15-20 mg/dl for MRSA coverage + cefepime 2gm IV q8h or meropenem 2gm q8h to cover gram negative pathogens. Streamline therapy based on culture and sensitivity results
2. intraventricular injection of preservative-free antibiotics may be used in addition to IV therapy. Clamp EVD for one hour after injection

Treatment for specific organisms

Positive cultures from shunt hardware removed at the time of shunt revision in the absence of clinical symptoms or a positive CSF culture may be due to contamination and do not always require treatment.[13]

1. S. aureus and S. epidermidis
   a) if methicillin sensitive: nafcillin or oxacillin ± IT vancomycin
   b) if methicillin resistant: continue IV vancomycin + PO rifampin ± IT vancomycin
2. Enterococcus: IV ampicillin ± IT gent
3. other streptococci: either antistreptococcal or above enterococcal regimen
4. aerobic GNR: base on susceptibilities. Both IV beta-lactam & IT aminoglycoside indicated
5. Serratia marcescens: a rare cause of VP shunt infection[15] but the high morbidity may warrant aggressive antibiotic therapy (IV ceftriaxone + IT aminoglycoside) and surgical therapy
6. Corynebacterium spp. & Proprionibacterium spp. (diphtheroids)
   a) if PCN sensitive: use enterococcal regimen above
   b) if PCN resistant: IV + IT vancomycin
7. Candida spp.: see protocol and drugs (p. 320). Systemic antifungal therapy and removal of shunt is warranted. Avoid echinocandins (antifungal drugs that inhibit synthesis of glucan in the fungal cell wall) as they have poor CNS penetration

Subsequent management

Once the CSF is sterile × 3 days, convert the EVD to a shunt (if an EVD was not used, it is still recommended that the shunt be replace with new hardware). Continue antibiotics an additional 10–14 days.

Managing ventriculoperitoneal shunts in patients with peritonitis

Peritonitis may occur as a result of:
1. perforation of a viscus (sometimes as a result of penetration by the peritoneal catheter tip,[16] more common with obsolete Raimondi wire-reinforced tubing)
2. spontaneous bacterial peritonitis (SBP): absence of an identifiable intra-abdominal source. Most commonly diagnosed in patients with cirrhotic ascites[17]
3. or as a result of seeding through a VP shunt in a patient with a shunt infection: predominantly gram-positive, cutaneous organisms[18]

Concerns following an episode of peritonitis in a patient with VP shunt:
1. ascending infection into the CNS: uncommon, especially in the acute setting while on appropriate antibiotics with shunts containing a 1-way valve (as most do). CSF grows predominantly mixed, gram-negative intestinal flora[18]
2. contamination of the distal shunt: prevents permanent eradication of infection (appendicitis in the absence of peritonitis does not produce shunt infection[18])
3. shunt malfunction due to distal shunt obstruction: often as a result of walling off of the catheter tip, usually by omentum in reaction to the infection

Management recommendations following an episode of peritonitis (many viable options):
1. immediate appropriate treatment of peritonitis, usually managed by general surgeon (e.g. for ruptured appendix: appendectomy and appropriate antibiotics), with initial attempt to address shunt not being mandatory
2. anecdotally, cases have been managed successfully by cleaning off the peritoneal catheter with bacitracin solution, and then wrapping the catheter in a bacitracin soaked lap sponge until the time to close the abdomen
3. if the peritonitis was diffuse or if the shunt catheter is believed to have been contaminated, an option is to externalize the distal catheter, preferably once the patient has stabilized from the peritonitis (afebrile, stable vital signs, normal WBC)
   a) externalization is done in a manner to avoid pulling contaminated catheter up towards hopefully sterile portions of the shunt. This can be accomplished by reopening the skin incision used for inserting the peritoneal catheter, and making a second incision over the shunt tubing, well above this entry point. The catheter is then divided at the upper incision. The catheter is grasped at the lower incision and is pulled, extracting both ends (the peritoneal end and the end just cut). The remaining catheter coming from above is connected to an external drainage system
   b) CSF cultures are monitored daily
   c) if 3 consecutive cultures are negative, a new distal catheter may be implanted
   d) if cultures continuously grow organisms, then the shunt may be contaminated and should then be replaced with an entirely new shunt system
   e) when it is time to replace the shunt, some authors[19,20] recommend using an alternative site other than the peritoneum, but this is not mandatory[18]

21.2 External ventricular drain (EVD)-related infection

21.2.1 General information

Key concepts

- Common organisms: S. epidermidis and S. aureus followed by gram negative bacilli and proprionibacterium acne.
- Diagnosis: Hypoglycorrhea (CSF glucose/Blood glucose < 0.2), rising cell index, and CSF pleocytosis > 1000 in the presence of positive CSF culture suggests EVD-related infection

- In CSF drain-related ventriculitis the diagnostic utility of CSF leucocyte count, glucose and protein is limited as noninfectious entities like intracranial hemorrhage and neurosurgical procedures can also cause abnormalities in these parameters.
- Management: remove EVD when clinically acceptable. Empiric coverage with IV vancomycin (for gram positives) + IV ceftazidime or cefepime (for gram negatives). Consider intraventricular/intrathecal antimicrobial for resistant organisms or non-responsiveness to IV antimicrobials.
- Prevention: antibiotic-coated catheters and catheter tunneling decrease infection rate.

21.2.2 Definitions

Suggested classification system and approach to a patient with suspected external ventricular drain (EVD) AKA ventriculostomy infection (modification of Lozier's definitions).[21]
- **Cell index**, see Eq (21.1) [22,23]
- **Contamination:** isolated positive CSF culture and/or Gram stain, with expected CSF cell count and glucose with NO attributable symptoms or signs.
- **Ventriculostomy colonization:** Multiple positive CSF cultures and/or Gram stain, with expected CSF cell count and glucose levels with NO attributable symptoms or signs.
- **Possible ventriculostomy-related infection:** Progresive rise in cell index or progressive decrease in CSF: blood glucose ratio or an extreme value for CSF WBC count (> 1000/micro L) or CSF:blood glucose ratio (< 0.2), with attributable symptoms and signs, but NEGATIVE Gram stain & cultures
- **Probable ventriculostomy-related infection:** CSF WBC count or CSF: blood glucose ratio MORE abnormal than expected, but NOT an extreme value (CSF WBC count 1000/micro L or CSF:blood glucose ratio < 0.2) and stable (not progressively worsening) attributable symptoms and signs and POSITVE Gram stain & cultures
- **Definitive meningitis:** Progressive rise in cell index or progressive decrease in CSF: blood glucose ratio or an extreme value for CSF WBC count (> 1000/micro L) or CSF:blood glucose ratio (< 0.2), with attributable symptoms or signs and a POSITIVE Gram stain & cultures

$$\text{Cell index} = \frac{Leucocytes\ (CSF)\ /\ Erythroctyes\ (CSF)}{Leucocytes\ (Blood)\ /\ Erythrocytes\ (Blood)} \tag{21.1}$$

21.2.3 Epidemiology

▶ **Incidence.** The incidence of EVD infection is approximately 9.5%.[24]

▶ **Risk factors.** Factors associated with EVD infections[21]:
- Duration of EVD[21,25,26]
- Site leakage
- Blood in CSF (IVH and SAH)[27]
- Irrigation and flushing[25,26]

21.2.4 Microbiology

- Unlike organisms that cause acute community-acquired meningitis those causing neurosurgical procedure-related meningitis are slow to grow on cultures and may require anaerobic media.
- The usual organisms that cause EVD-related infections are either:
  - Organisms that usually colonize the skin, especially the scalp (coagulase negative Staphylococcus, Staphylococcus aureus, and Propionibacterium acnes).
  - Organisms that can be present in the healthcare environment: S. aureus, both methicillin sensitive and resistant, gram-negative bacteria like E. coli, Klebsiella, pseudomonas, and Acinitobacter species, some of which can be multi-drug resistance.
- Infectious organisms can form a polysaccharide layer (biofilm) on the surface of catheters which increases the resistant to antimicrobials.

21.2.5 Clinical presentation

Clinical signs and symptoms may include the following; however, these symptoms are nonspecific as they are commonplace in the neuro-ICU as a result of the underlying pathology (e.g. intracranial hemorrhage or hydrocephalus)[28]

- change in mental status
- fever: alternative sources of fever may include intracranial hemorrhage, central fever, thrombotic episodes, drug fevers, in addition to non-CNS infection like blood- borne infections, hospital-acquired pneumonias and urinary tract infections
- meningisumus: stiff neck, Brudzinski or Kernig's sign.

21.2.6 Diagnosis

► **Blood parameters.** These parameters can suggest the diagnosis but should not be relied upon exclusively.

- A prospective study showed likely EVD infections in the presence of these parameters[29]: peripheral WBC count > 15 in EVD infections (vs. < 11 in non-infected)
- Serum inflammatory markers: there is very limited literature on the diagnostic utility of ESR and CRP. Procalcitonin alone was found not to be helpful.[30]

► **CSF parameters.** There are limited studies on the diagnostic accuracy of CSF parameters in post craniotomy meningitis and ventriculitis. Often the surgery itself can cause "chemical meningitis" or postoperative meningitis, particularly posterior fossa surgeries or in the presence of intraventricular hemorrhage. The CSF leucocyte and CSF glucose values can look very similar to infectious meningitis making it hard to distinguish these entities based on these parameters. The following could help in confirming underlying EVD infection.

- Hypoglycorrhachia (low CSF glucose): ratio of [CSF glucose]/[blood glucose] < 0.2
- CSF pleocytosis > 1000 or rising Cell index (p. 343)
- CSF protein was not a reliable predictor for incipient ventricular catheter infection[31]

Routine CSF sampling: CSF sampling should be performed only when symptoms appear. There is no evidence of benefit to obtaining CSF cultures or cell count at the time of EVD insertion (false positive cultures may occur from contamination).[32]

21.2.7 Principles of management

- It is difficult to achieve high CSF antimicrobial levels due to blood-CSF barrier.
- Some hospital-acquired organisms have higher MICs (minimal inhibitory concentration) for antimicrobials than community-acquired organisms.
- Organisms often form biofilms on the catheters which resist antimicrobial penetration. For this reason, catheter should be removed if it is safe to do so.
- Empiric antibiotics: initiate if ventriculitis is suspected once the appropriate sampling has been obtained
  - If no penicillin allergy:
    - vancomycin as a continuous infusion or divided doses (2–3) of 60 mg per kg of body weight per day after a loading dose of 15 mg per kg of body weight, aiming for trough (15 – 25 mcg/ml) PLUS
    - ceftazidime 2 g IV Q 8 hrs or cefepime 2 g IV Q 8hrs
  - For penicillin allergy:
    - vancomycin as a continuous infusion or divided doses (2–3) of 60 mg per kg of body weight per day after a loading dose of 15 mg per kg of body weight PLUS
    - meropenem 2 g IV q8 or aztreonam 2 g IV Q 6 hrs
- Switch to more selective agents as appropriate based on culture and susceptibility when they become available (see ► Table 21.1)
- Duration of treatment should be individualized to the patient but as a rule of thumb: treat for 2 weeks if the infection was with S. aureus and S. epidermidis, and 3 weeks if it was gram negatives.[33]
- Failing to respond to systemic treatment or infection with a resistant organism might require Intrathecal/Intraventricular antibiotic administration. Choose the antimicrobial based on susceptibility. Dosages for intraventricular antibiotics:
  - Vancomycin: for slit ventricles 5 mg, 10 mg with normal-sized ventricles, 15–20 mg for patients with enlarged ventricles.

Table 21.1 Selective antibacterial agents (based on culture and susceptibility)

Bacteria	Specific antimicrobial regimen
MRSA and MRSE (with an MIC ≤ 1 mcg/ml)	Vancomycin continuous infusion or divided doses (2–3/d) of 60 mg per kg of body weight per day after a loading dose of 15 mg per kg of body weight. If the catheter is retained can add rifampin 300 mg IV q 12 hrs
MRSA and MRSE (with MIC > 1 mcg/ml) or patient with vancomycin allergy	Linezolid 600 mg IV or PO q 12 hrs
MSSA and MSSE	Nafcillin 2 g IV q4
Propionobacter acne	Penicillin G 2 MU IV q4
Pseudomonas	Ceftazidime 2 g IV Q8, Cefepime 2 g IV Q8, or Meropenem 2 g q 8 hrs
E. coli or other enterobacteriaceae	Ceftriaxone 2 g IV Q 12 hrs or meropenem 2 g IV q 8 hrs
Enterobacter or Citrobacter	Cefepime 2 g IV Q 8 hrs or meropenem 2 g IV q 8 hrs

  - Aminoglycoside: Dosing can also be tailored to ventricular size. Frequency can be adjusted based on drain output as well: once daily for drain output > 100 ml/day, every other day if drain output = 50–100 ml/day, every third day if drainage < 50 ml/day
    - Gentamicin: 4–8 mg
    - Tobramycin: 5–20 mg
    - Amikacin: 5–30 mg
  - Colistimethate sodium: 10 mg CMS, which is 125,000 IU or 3.75 mg CBA (Colistin Base units)
  - Daptomycin: 2–5 mg
- After IT administration of an antimicrobial, clamp the drain for 15–60 minutes to allow the antimicrobial concentration to equilibrate in the CSF before opening the drain[34]
- Expert opinion: wait at least 7–10 days after the CSF cultures become sterile to implant a shunt if needed.

21.2.8 Prevention

- Tunneling > 5 cm away from the burr hole.[35]
- Antibiotic coated catheters (e.g., Rifampin + minocycline) significantly reduce the risk of EVD infection.[36,37,38,39,40]
- Routine catheter exchange at day 5 *did not* show reduction in the rate of infection.[41,42,43] Therefore a single catheter may be employed as long as clinically required.[44]
- Prolonged antibiotic prophylaxis while the EVD is in place does not decrease the risk of infection and may select for resistant organisms. *However one dose pre-procedure antimicrobial may be administered.*

21.3 Wound infections

21.3.1 Laminectomy wound infection

General information

Occurs in 0.9–5% of cases.[45] May range from superficial to severe dehiscent wound infection to deeper infection (discitis/osteomyelitis ± epidural abscess). The risk is increased with age, long term steroid use, obesity, and possibly DM. Intraoperative mild hypothermia (as commonly occurs in the operating room) may also increase the risk of wound infection (as demonstrated with colorectal resection[46]). Most are caused by S. aureus.

Superficial wound infection

Management

1. culture the wound and/or any purulent drainage

2. start the patient empirically on vancomycin plus cefepime or meropenem
3. modify antibiotics appropriately when culture and sensitivity results available
4. debride wound of all necrotic and devascularized tissue and any visible suture material (foreign bodies). Superficial wound infections may be debrided in the office or treatment room, deep infections must be done in OR
5. shallow defects may be allowed to heal by secondary intention, and the following is one possible regimen
   a) pack the wound defect with 1/4" Iodophor® gauze
   b) dressing changes at least BID (for hospitalized patients, change q 8 hrs), remove and trim ≈ 0.5–1" of packing with each dressing change
      - while wound is purulent, utilize 1/2 strength Betadine® wet to dry dressings
      - when purulence subsides, switch to normal saline wet to dry
   c) antibiotics, may be useful as an adjunct to wound treatment initially, switch to oral antibiotics as early as possible, a duration of 10–14 days total is probably adequate if local wound care is being done
6. some prefer to close wound by primary intention,[47] it is critical that there be no tension on the wound for healing to occur. Some close over an irrigation system or antibiotic beads. Retention sutures may be helpful[48]
7. with large defects or when bone and/or dura becomes exposed, the use of a muscle flap (often performed by a plastic surgeon) is probably required[45]
8. CSF leakage requires exploration in the OR with watertight dural closure to prevent meningitis

Postoperative discitis

Epidemiology

Incidence after lumbar discectomy[49]: 0.2–4% (realistic estimate is probably at the lower end of this range). May also occur after LP, myelogram, cervical laminectomy, lumbar sympathectomy, discography, fusions (with or without instrumentation) and other procedures. Very rare after ACDF. Risk factors include: advanced age, obesity, immunosuppression, systemic infection at the time of surgery.

Pathophysiology

There is some controversy as to whether some cases of post-op discitis are not infectious,[50] an autoimmune process has been implicated in some of these so-called "avascular" or "chemical" or "aseptic" discitis cases. These cases are less common than infectious ones. ESR and CRP abnormalities may be less pronounced in these patients, and biopsy of the disc space fails to grow organisms or show signs of infection (infiltrates of lymphocytes or PMNS) on microscopy.[50]

In septic cases, various mechanisms for infection have been proposed: direct inoculation at the time of surgery, infection following aseptic necrosis of disc material...

Pathogens

See ▶ Table 21.2. Most studies report S. aureus as the most commonly identified organism, accounting for ≈ 60% of positive cultures,[49] followed by other staph species. Also reported: Gram-negative organisms (including E. coli), Strep viridans, Streptococcus species anaerobes, TB and fungi. Enteric flora in post-op discitis may due to unrecognized breach of the anterior longitudinal ligament with bowel perforation.

Blood cultures were positive in 2 of 6 patients (both S. aureus) in one series.[51]

For culture techniques, see surgical management section below.

Clinical

1. interval from operation to onset of symptoms: 3 days to 8 mos (most commonly 1–4 wks post-op, usually after an initial period of pain relief and recovery from surgery). 80% present by 3 wks

Table 21.2 Culture results (14 patients, Craig needle biopsy)

Organism	No. of patients
Staphylococcus epidermidis	4
S. aureus	3
No growth	7

2. symptoms:
   a) moderate to (usually) severe back pain at the site of operation was the most common symptom, exacerbated by virtually any motion of the spine, often accompanied by paraspinal muscle spasms. Back pain is usually out of proportion to the findings
   b) fever (> 38° C in 9 patients; literature reports only 30–50% are febrile) and chills
   c) pain radiating to hip, leg, scrotum, groin, abdomen or perineum (true sciatica is uncommon)
3. signs: in 27 patients,[51] all had paravertebral muscle spasm and limited range of motion of the spine. 13 (48%) were virtually immobilized by pain. Point tenderness over the infected level occurred in 9, expressible pus in 2 (literature reports 0–8%). No new neurologic deficits were noted. Only 10–12% have associated wound infection[52]
4. lab findings:
   a) ESR: in a series of 27 patients,[51] 96% had ESR > 20 mm/hr (60 = ave.; > 40 in 17 patients; > 100 in 5 patients; the single patient < 20 was on steroids). ESR increases after uncomplicated discectomy, peaking at 2–5 days, and can fluctuate for 3–6 weeks before normalizing.[53] An elevated ESR that never decreases after surgery is a strong indicator of discitis. NB: ESR in anemic patients is unreliable and no reference range can be established (use CRP in these cases)
   b) *C-reactive protein* (CRP)[53]: an acute phase protein synthesized by hepatocytes that because of rapid decomposition may be a more specific indicator of post-op infection than ESR. Values vary from lab to lab, but CRP is normally not detectable in the blood (i.e. < 0.6 mg/dl = 6 mg/L). After uncomplicated discectomy (i.e. in the absence of discitis), CRP peaks ≈ 2–3 days post-op (to 4.6 ± 2.1 mg/dl after lumbar microdiscectomy, 9.2 ± 4.7 after conventional lumbar discectomy, 7.0 ± 2.3 after anterior lumbar fusion, and 17.3 ± 3.9 after PLIF), and returns to normal between 5–14 days post-op
   c) *WBC*: > 10,000 in only 8/27 patients[51] (prevalence in literature: 18–30%)

Radiographic evaluation

In postoperative discitis (POD), the average time from surgery to changes on plain x-ray is 3 mos (range: 1–8 mos). Average time from first change to spontaneous spinal fusion: 2 yrs.

MRI: The triad of gadolinium enhancement shown in ▶ Table 21.3 is strongly suggestive of discitis (some asymptomatic patients may have some of these findings, but they rarely have all).[54]

MRI also rules-out other causes of post-op pain (epidural abscess, recurrent/residual disc herniation…).

Management

1. initial labs (in addition to routine): ESR, C-reactive protein, CBC, blood cultures
2. analgesics + muscle relaxants (e.g. diazepam (Valium®) 10 mg PO TID)
3. antibiotics:
   a) IV antibiotics for 1-6 wks then PO for 1-6 mos
   b) most start with anti-staphylococcal antibiotics (initial empiric therapy: vancomycin ± PO rifampin) and cefepime or meropenem. Modify based on sensitivities if positive cultures are obtained
   c) duration of therapy depends on depth of infection and presence of hardware
      - superficial infection: 1-2 weeks
      - deep infection 4-8 weeks, possibly up to 12 weeks in complex cases
      - consider chronic PO therapy if hardware not removed
4. activity restriction (one of the following used, usually until significant pain relief):
   a) spinal immobilization with brace
   b) strict bed rest
   c) advance activity with brace as tolerated
5. some authors recommend steroid therapy initially to assist pain relief

Table 21.3 Gadolinium enhancement in discitis

Location of gadolinium enhancement	Number (out of 15 post-op patients without discitis)	Number (out of 7 patients with discitis)
1. vertebral bone marrow	1	7
2. disc space	3	5
3. posterior annulus fibrosus	13	7

6. cultures: performed if radiographs suspicious, usually performed utilizing percutaneous CT-guided technique
   a) sites
      - disc aspiration if evidence of disc space involvement
      - needling of paraspinal mass if present
   b) send culture for the following
      - Stains: (**a**) Gram stain (**b**) fungal stain (**c**) AFB stain
      - Cultures: (**a**) routine cultures: aerobic and anaerobic (**b**) fungal culture: this is not only helpful for fungus, but since these cultures are kept for longer period and any growth that occurs will be further characterized, fastidious or indolent bacterial organisms may sometimes be identified (**c**) AFB (TB) culture
7. 3 out of 27 patients underwent anterior discectomy and fusion after unsuccessful medical therapy[51]

Outcome

9 patients developed bony bridging in 12–18 mos; 10 developed bony fusion in 18–24 mos.[51]

All patients eventually become pain free (or significantly improve). This is not the case in all series, where some report 60% were pain free at F/U, others found slight back pain in most patients, and yet others report severe chronic LBP in 75%.[49] 67–88% return to their previous work, and 12–25% received disability pension; these numbers are similar to the outcome from disc surgery in general.

No difference in outcome was found for the various activity restrictions specified, except for earlier pain relief with first two types listed above.

21.3.2 Craniotomy wound infection

Also; see under meningitis, post-neurosurgical procedure (p. 318).

C-reactive protein

Following uncomplicated craniotomy for microsurgery for brain tumors, C-reactive protein (CRP) peaked on post-op day (POD) 2 with a mean value of 32 ± 38 mg/l.[55] Values declined from POD 3 through 5, reaching a mean of 6.7 ± 11 on POD 5. These values may be lower than with most post-op infections.

21.4 Osteomyelitis of the skull

21.4.1 General information

The skull is normally very resistant to osteomyelitis, and hematogenous infection is rare. Most infections are due to contiguous spread (usually from an infected air sinus, occasionally from scalp abscess) or to penetrating trauma (including surgery and fetal scalp monitors[56]). With longstanding infection, edema and swelling in the area may become visible (usually over the forehead, but also may occur over the mastoids), and is called "Pott puffy tumor" (after Percival Pott).

21.4.2 Pathogens

Staphylococcus is the most common organism, with S. aureus predominating, followed by S. epidermidis. In neonates, E. coli may be the infecting organism.

21.4.3 Imaging

Imaging findings may include: bony resorption, periosteal reaction, contrast enhancement.

21.4.4 Treatment

Antibiotics alone are rarely curative. Treatment usually involves surgical debridement of infected skull, biting off infected bone with rongeurs until a normal snapping sound replaces the more muted sound made by rongeuring infected bone. In the case of an infected craniotomy bone flap, the flap usually must be removed and discarded, and the edges of the skull rongeured back to healthy bone. Bone suspected of infection should be sent for cultures.

Closure of the scalp is then performed either leaving an bone defect (for later cranioplasty) or cranioplasty can be performed using titanium mesh.

Debridement surgery is followed by at least 6–12 weeks of antibiotics.[57] Until MRSA is ruled out: vancomycin + cefepime or meropenem. Culture results guide choice of antibiotic. Once MRSA is ruled out, vancomycin may be changed to a penicillinase resistant synthetic penicillin (e.g. nafcillin). Most treatment failures occurred in patients treated with < 4 weeks of antibiotics following surgery.

Cranioplasty may be performed ≈ 6 months post-op if there are no signs of residual infection.

21.5 Spine infections

Spine infections may be divided into the following major categories:

1. vertebral osteomyelitis (p. 353) (spondylitis):
   a) pyogenic
   b) nonpyogenic, granulomatous
      - tuberculous spondylitis
      - brucellosis
      - aspergillosis
      - blastomycosis
      - coccidiomycosis
      - infection with Candida tropicalis
2. discitis (p. 356): usually associated with vertebral osteomyelitis (spondylodiscitis) (p. 353)
   a) spontaneous
   b) post-operative/post-procedure
3. spinal epidural abscess (see below)
4. spinal subdural empyema
5. meningitis
6. spinal cord abscess

MRI experience suggests that patients with infectious spondylitis will develop an associated epidural abscess if untreated, and that epidural empyema is unusual in the absence of vertebral osteomyelitis.[58] Thus, the discovery of one of these conditions should prompt a search for the other.

21.5.1 Spinal epidural abscess

General information

Key concepts

- should be considered in a patient with back pain, fever, and spine tenderness
- major risk factors: diabetes, IV drug abuse, chronic renal failure, alcoholism
- may produce progressive myelopathy, sometimes with precipitous deterioration, therefore early surgery has been advocated by some even if no neuro deficit
- fever, sweats or rigors are common, but normal WBC and temperature can occur
- classical presentation of a skin boil (furuncle) occurs in only ≈ 15% somewhere on the body
- treatment: controversial. Many patients improve with antibiotics alone, but some may deteriorate precipitously

Epidemiology

Incidence: 0.2–1.2 per 10,000 hospital admissions annually,[59] possibly on the rise.[60] Average age: 57.5 ± 16.6 years.[61]

Thoracic level is the most common site (≈ 50%), followed by lumbar (35%) then cervical (15%).[61] 82% were posterior to the cord, and 18% anterior in one series.[59] SEA may span from 1 to 13 levels.[62]

Spinal epidural abscess (SEA) is often associated with vertebral osteomyelitis (in one series of 40 cases, osteomyelitis occurred in all cases of anterior SEA, in 85% of circumferential SEA, and no cases of posterior SEA) and intervertebral discitis.

Co-morbid conditions

Chronic diseases associated with compromised immunity were identified in 65% of 40 cases.[63] Associated conditions included diabetes mellitus (32%), IV drug abuse (18%), chronic renal failure (12%), alcoholism (10%), and the following in only 1 or 2 patients: cancer, recurrent UTI, Pott's disease, and positivity for HIV. Chronic steroid use and recent spinal procedure or trauma (e.g. GSW) are also risk factors.[62] Skin infection (e.g. furuncle).

Clinical features

Usually presents with excruciating pain localized over spine with tenderness to percussion. Radicular symptoms follow with subsequent distal cord findings, often beginning with bowel/bladder disturbance, abdominal distension, weakness progressing to para- and quadriplegia. Average time is 3 days from back pain to root symptoms; 4.5 days from root pain to weakness; 24 hrs from weakness to paraplegia.

Fever, sweats or rigors are common, but are not always present.[62]

A furuncle (skin boil) somewhere on the body may be identified in 15%.

Patients may be encephalopathic. This may range from mild to severe and may further delay diagnosis. Meningismus with a positive Kernig's sign may occur.

Patients with post-operative SEA may demonstrate surprisingly few signs or symptoms (including lack of leukocytosis, lack of fever) aside from local pain.[64]

Pathophysiology of spinal cord dysfunction

Although some cord symptoms may be due to mechanical compression (including that due to vertebral body collapse), this is not always found.[65] A vascular mechanism has also been postulated, and various combinations of arterial and venous pathology have been described[59] (one autopsy series showed little arterial compromise, but did show venous compression and thrombosis, thrombophlebitis of epidural veins, and venous infarction and edema of the spinal cord[66]). Occasionally, there may be infection of the spinal cord itself, possibly by extension through the meninges.

Differential diagnosis

SEA should be considered in any patient with backache, fever, and spine tenderness,[67] especially diabetics, IV drug abusers or immunocompromised patients. Also see Differential diagnosis, Myelopathy (p. 1407).

Differential diagnosis:

1. meningitis
2. acute transverse myelitis (paralysis is usually more rapid, radiographic studies are normal)
3. intervertebral disc herniation
4. spinal cord tumors
5. post-op SEA may appear similar to pseudomeningocele[64]

Source site of infection

1. hematogenous spread is the most common source (26–50% of cases) either to the epidural space or to the vertebra with extension to epidural space. Reported foci include:
   a) skin infections (most common): furuncle may be found in 15% of cases
   b) parenteral injections, especially with *IV drug abuse*[68]
   c) bacterial endocarditis
   d) UTI
   e) respiratory infection (including otitis media, sinusitis, or pneumonia)
   f) pharyngeal or dental abscess
2. direct extension from:
   a) decubitus ulcer
   b) psoas abscess: see below
   c) penetrating trauma, including: abdominal wounds, neck wounds, GSW
   d) pharyngeal infections
   e) mediastinitis
   f) pyelonephritis with perinephric abscess
   g) dermal sinus

3. following spinal procedures (3 of 8 of these patients had readily identified perioperative infections of periodonta, UTI, or AV-fistula[63])
   a) open procedures: especially lumbar discectomy (incidence[64] ≈ 0.67%)
   b) closed procedures: e.g. epidural catheter insertion for spinal epidural anesthesia,[69,70,71] lumbar puncture[72]...
4. a history of recent back trauma is common (in up to 30%)
5. no source can be identified in up to 50% of patients in some series[73]

Organisms

Operative cultures are most useful in identifying the responsible organism, these cultures may be negative (possibly more common in patients previously on antibiotics) and in these cases blood cultures may be positive. No organism may be identified in 29–50% of cases.

1. *Staph. aureus*: the most common organism (cultured in > 50%) possibly due to its propensity to form abscesses, its ubiquity, and its ability to infect normal and immunocompromised hosts (these facts help explain why many SEA arise from skin foci)
2. aerobic & anaerobic streptococcus: second most common
3. E.coli
4. Pseudomonas aeruginosa
5. Diplococcus pneumoniae
6. Serratia marcescens
7. Enterobacter
8. chronic infections:
   a) TB is the most common of these, and although it has become less widespread in the U.S. it is still responsible for 25% of cases of SEA,[74] it is usually associated with vertebral osteomyelitis, see Pott's disease (p.354)
   b) fungal: cryptococcosis, aspergillosis, brucellosis
   c) parasitic: Echinococcus
9. multiple organisms in ≈ 10%
10. anaerobes cultured in ≈ 8%

Laboratory tests

CBC: leukocytosis common in acute group (average WBC = 16,700/mm^3), but usually normal in chronic (ave. WBC = 9,800/mm^3).[59]

ESR elevated in most,[75] usually > 30,[63] CRP.

LP: performed cautiously in suspected cases at a level distant to the clinically suspected site (C1–2 puncture may be needed to do myelogram) with constant aspiration while approaching thecal sac to detect pus (danger of transmitting infection to subarachnoid space); if pus is encountered, stop advancing, send the fluid for culture, and abort the procedure. CSF protein & WBC usually elevated; glucose normal (indicative of parameningeal infection). 5 of 19 cases grew organisms identical to abscess.

Blood cultures: may be helpful in identifying organism in some cases.

Anergy battery: (e.g. mumps and Candida) to assess immune system.

Radiographic studies

Plain films

Usually normal unless there is osteomyelitis of adjacent vertebral bodies (more common in infections anterior to dura). Look for lytic lesions, demineralization, and scalloping of endplates (may take 4–6 weeks after onset of infection).

MRI

Imaging study of choice. Differentiates other conditions (especially transverse myelitis or spinal cord infarction) better than myelo/CT, and doesn't require LP.

Typical findings: T1WI → hypo- or iso-intense epidural mass, vertebral osteomyelitis shows up as reduced signal in bone. T2WI → high intensity epidural mass that often enhances with gadolinium (3 patterns of enhancement: 1) dense homogeneous, 2) inhomogeneous with scattered areas of sparse or no uptake, and 3) thin peripheral enhancement[76]) but may show minimal enhancement in the acute stage when comprised primarily of pus with little granulation tissue. Vertebral osteomyelitis shows up as increased signal in bone, associated discitis produces increased signal in disc and loss of intranuclear cleft. Unenhanced MRI may miss some SEA,[77] gadopentetate dimeglumine enhancement may slightly increase sensitivity.[78]

Myelogram-CT

Usually shows findings of extradural compression (e.g. "paintbrush appearance" when complete block is present). In the event of complete block, C1–2 puncture may be needed to delineate upper extent (unless post-myelographic CT shows dye above the lesion). See cautions above regarding LP.

CT scan

Intraspinal gas has been described on plain CT.[79] Post-myelographic CT is more sensitive.

Treatment

General information

Controversial. In most cases, treatment consists of early surgical evacuation combined with antibiotics as the treatment of choice. Argument: although there are reports of management with antibiotics alone[80,81,82] ± immobilization,[58] rapid and irreversible deterioration has occurred even in patients treated with appropriate antibiotics who were initially neurologically intact.[63,61] 86% of those who deteriorated were initially treated it with antibiotics alone.[62] Therefore it has been recommended that nonsurgical management be reserved for the following patients (reference[80] modified[62]):

1. those with prohibitive operative risk factors
2. involvement of an extensive length of the spinal canal
3. complete paralysis for > 3 days

To add fuel to the argument, in many cases, at the time of surgery, instead of a true abscess, inflammatory tissue that is not easily or effectively debrided is encountered.

Surgery

Goals are establishing diagnosis and causative organism, drainage of pus and debridement of granulation tissue, and bony stabilization if necessary. Most SEA are posterior to the dura and are approached with extensive laminectomy. For posteriorly located SEA and no evidence of vertebral osteomyelitis, instability will usually not follow simple laminectomy and appropriate postoperative antibiotics.[73] Thorough antibiotic irrigation is employed intra-operatively. Primary closure is often employed. Post-op drainage is not necessary in cases with only granulation tissue and no pus. For recurrent infections, reoperation and post-op suction-irrigation may be needed.[83]

Patients with associated osteomyelitis of the vertebral body may develop instability after laminectomy alone[84] especially if significant bony destruction is present. Thus for anterior SEA, usually with osteomyelitis (especially Pott's disease), a posterolateral extracavitary approach is utilized whenever possible (to avoid transabdominal or transthoracic approach in these debilitated patients) with removal of devitalized bone usually followed by posterior instrumentation and fusion. Strut grafting with autologous bone (rib or fibula) can be done acutely in Pott's disease with little risk of graft infection. With purulent osteomyelitis, metal hardware is not contraindicated (titanium is more resistant to harboring bacteria than stainless steel for several reasons, including the fact that titanium does not permit bacteria to form a glycocalyx on its surface), but bone grafting may run the risk of perpetuating the infection. In this situation, some surgeons use beads of calcium sulfate bone void filler impregnated with antibiotic (e.g. Stimulan® Rapid Cure™ antibiotic beads).

Specific antibiotics

If organism and source unknown, S. aureus most likely. Empiric antibiotics:

- Ceftriaxone or cefepime (use when pseudomonas is a concern)
  PLUS
- metronidazole
  PLUS
- vancomycin:
  - until methicillin resistant S. aureus (MRSA) can be ruled out
  - once MRSA is ruled out switch to synthetic penicillin (e.g. nafcillin or oxacillin)
- ± rifampin PO

Modify antibiotics based on culture results or knowledge of source (e.g. IV drug abusers have a higher incidence of Gram-negative organisms).

Modify antibiotics based on culture results or knowledge of source (e.g. IV drug abusers have a higher incidence of Gram-negative organisms).

Duration of treatment

For spinal epidural abscess (SEA), treatment should continue for a minimum of 6 weeks. Longer therapy may be warranted in complicated infections and for patients who have spinal implants or hardware. Immobilization for at least 6 weeks during antibiotic therapy is recommended.

Outcome

Fatal in 4–31%[85](the higher end of the range tends to be in older patients and in those paralyzed before surgery[63]). Patients with severe neurologic deficit rarely improve, even with surgical intervention within 6–12 hrs of onset of paralysis, although a few series have shown a chance for some recovery with treatment within 36 hrs of paralysis.[67,86] Reversal of paralysis of caudal spinal cord segments if present for more than a few hours is rare (exception: Pott's disease has 50% return). Mortality is usually due to original focus of infection or as a complication of residual paraplegia (e.g. pulmonary embolism).

21.5.2 Vertebral osteomyelitis

General information

Key concepts

- presentation and risk factors similar to spinal epidural abscess (p. 349)
- percutaneous needle biopsy for C&S and to rule-out tumor can usually be done by neurosurgeon or interventional radiologist
- treatment: most cases can be managed nonsurgically with long-term antibiotics
- surgery is considered for instability, and infrequently for severe resistance to Abx

For differential diagnosis, see Destructive lesions of the spine (p. 1392). Often associated with discitis, which may be grouped together under the term spondylodiscitis. VO has features similar to spinal epidural abscess (SEA) (p. 349).

Vertebral body collapse and kyphotic deformity may occur with possible retropulsion of necrotic bone and disc fragments, compressing the spinal cord or cauda equina.

Complications that may accrue

1. spinal epidural abscess
2. subdural abscess
3. meningitis
4. bony instability
5. progressive neurologic impairment
6. unique to cervical spine involvement: pharyngeal abscess
7. unique to thoracic spine involvement: mediastinitis

Epidemiology

Vertebral osteomyelitis (VO) comprises 2–4% of all cases of osteomyelitis.[87] Incidence is 1:250,000 in general population. Incidence appears to be rising. Male:female ratio is 2:1. Incidence increases with age, most patients are > 50 years old. The lumbar spine is the most common site, followed by thoracic, cervical and sacrum.[88] Thoracic VO may → empyema.

Risk factors

1. IV drug abuse[89]
2. diabetes mellitus: susceptible to unusual bacterial infections and even fungal osteomyelitis
3. hemodialysis: a diagnostic challenge since radiographic changes of osteomyelitis can occur even in the absence of infection, see Destructive lesions of the spine (p. 1392)
4. immunosuppression
   a) AIDS
   b) chronic corticosteroid use
   c) ethanol abuse
5. infectious endocarditis
6. following spinal surgery or invasive diagnostic or therapeutic procedures
7. may occur in elderly patients with no other identifiable risk factors[90]

Clinical

Signs/symptoms: localized pain (90%), fever (52%, with fever spikes and chills being rare), weight loss, paraspinal muscle spasm, radicular symptoms (50–93%) or myelopathy. VO sometimes produces few systemic effects (e.g. WBC and/or ESR may be normal). ≈ 17% of patients with VO have neurologic symptoms. The risk of paralysis may be higher in the older patient, in cervical VO (vs. thoracic or lumbar), in those with DM or rheumatoid arthritis, and in those with VO due to S. aureus.[84] Neurologic findings are uncommon initially, which may delay the diagnosis.[91] Sensory involvement is less common than motor and long-tract signs because compression is primarily anterior.

Pathogenesis

Source of infection

Sources of spontaneous VO: UTI (the most common), respiratory tract, soft-tissues (e.g. skin boils, IV drug abuse...), dental flora. In 37% of cases a source is never identified.[92]

Potential routes of spread

Three main routes: arterial, venous, and direct extension:

1. hematogenous: hematogenously disseminated spondylodiscitis in adults usually involves bone initially, and once infection is established in the subchondral space, spread is to the adjacent disc and thence to the next VB[93]
   a) arterial
   b) via spinal epidural venous plexus (Batson's plexus[94])
2. direct extension (e.g. following surgery/LP, trauma, or local infection)

Organisms

1. Staphylococcus aureus is the most common pathogen (> 50%) as in SEA
2. E. coli is a distant second
3. organisms associated with some primary infection sites[95]:
   a) IV drug abusers: Pseudomonas aeruginosa and *S. aureus* are common
   b) urinary tract infections: E. coli & Proteus spp. are common
   c) respiratory tract infections: Streptococcus pneumoniae
   d) alcohol abuse: Klebsiella pneumoniae
   e) endocarditis:
      - acute endocarditis: Staph. aureus
      - subacute endocarditis: Streptococcus spp.
4. tuberculous VO: Mycobacterium tuberculosis (see below)
5. unusual organisms include: nocardia (p.335)
6. Mycobacterium avium complex (M. Avium and M. intracellulare) (MAC) can cause pulmonary disease in nonimmunocompromised patients (usually elderly or on chronic steroids), but can also cause VO similar to TB[96] as part of disseminated disease which usually occurs in HIV patients
7. polymicrobial infections: *rare* (< 2.5% of pyogenic VO infections)

Tuberculous vertebral osteomyelitis: AKA tuberculous spondylitis, AKA Pott's disease. More common in third world countries. Typically symptomatic for many months. Usually affects more than one level. The most common levels involved are the lower thoracic and upper lumbar levels. Has a predilection for the vertebral body, sparing the posterior elements. Psoas abscess is common (the psoas major muscle attaches to the bodies and intervertebral discs from T12-L5). Sclerosis of the involved vertebral body may occur. Definitive diagnosis requires the identification of acid fast bacilli on culture or Gram stain of biopsy material (may be done percutaneously).

Neurologic deficit develops in 10–47% of patients,[97] and may be due to medullary and radicular artery inflammation in most cases. The infection itself rarely extends into the spinal canal,[98] however, epidural granulation tissue or fibrosis or a kyphotic bony deformity may cause cord compression.[97]

The role of surgical debridement and fusion with TB is controversial, and good results may be obtained with either medical treatment or surgery. Surgery may be more appropriate when definite cord compression is documented or for complications such as abscess or sinus formation[99] or spinal instability.

Diagnostic tests

Laboratories

WBC: elevated in only ≈ 35% (rarely > 12,000), associated with poor prognosis.

ESR: elevated in almost all. Usually > 40 mm/hr. Mean: 85.

CRP: may be more sensitive than ESR, and may tend to normalize more quickly with appropriate treatment.[100] See also normal values (p. 347).

Cultures/biopsy

Culture: blood (positive in ≈ 50%), urine and any focal suppurative process.

Needle biopsy with cultures: can usually be done percutaneously via transpedicular approach with CT or fluoroscopic guidance. May be helpful even if blood cultures are positive (different organisms retrieved in 15%[101]) ∴ an attempt at direct culture from the involved site should be made. Ideally, cultures should be done before antibiotics are started. The yield of needle biopsy cultures ranges from 60–90%. Open biopsy is more sensitive, but morbidity is higher.

Imaging

A comparison of sensitivities and specificities of various imaging modalities is shown in ▶ Table 21.4. NB: CT may be negative if done too early in the course.

MRI: T1WI → confluent low signal in vertebral bodies and intervertebral disc space. T2WI → increased intensity of involved VBs and disc space.[102] Contrast: enhancement of VB and disc, also look for paraspinal and epidural mass.

CT scan: helpful for demonstrating bony involvement as well as detailed bony anatomy in case instrumentation is required during treatment.

Plain x-ray: changes take from 2–8 weeks from the onset of infection to develop. Earliest changes are loss of cortical endplate margins and loss of disc space height.

Bone scan: three phase bone scan (p. 236) has reasonably good sensitivity and specificity. Gallium scan (p. 236) has better accuracy, findings include increased uptake in the 2 adjacent VBs with loss of intervening disc.[103] Indium-111 labeled WBC scan: low sensitivity for vertebral osteomyelitis.

Work-up

In patients with suspected vertebral osteomyelitis (VO) (see text above for details):

1. clinical: history of IV drug abuse, DM, immunocompromise, skin boil
2. physical exam: R/O radiculopathy & myelopathy, point tenderness over spine
3. diagnostic tests:
   a) bloodwork: WBC, ESR & CRP (a normal ESR is almost incompatible with VO), blood cultures
   b) imaging:
      - MRI without and with contrast
      - If MRI is contraindicated: CT-myelogram assesses bony anatomy and can demonstrate spinal canal compromise. Bone scan may occasionally be helpful if the diagnosis is still uncertain when suspicion is high
   c) percutaneous needle biopsy with cultures: usually by radiologist. Cultures should include: fungal, aerobic and anaerobic bacterial, and TB

Treatment

Also see more details (p. 352). 90% of cases can be managed non-surgically with antibiotics and immobilization. Characteristics of potential candidates for non-surgical treatment are listed in ▶ Table 21.5. Must also take into account level(s) involved and patient's condition.

Table 21.4 Accuracy of various imaging modalities for vertebral osteomyelitis[102]

Modality	Sensitivity	Specificity	Accuracy
plain x-rays	82%	57%	73%
bone scan	90%	78%	86%
gallium scan	92%	100%	93%
bone scan + gallium scan	90%	100%	94%
MRI	96%	92%	94%

Table 21.5 Candidates for non-surgical treatment in pyogenic spontaneous spondylodiscitis[95]

- organism identified
- antibiotic sensitivity
- single disc space involvement with little VB involvement
- minimal or no neurologic deficit
- minimal or no spinal instability

In cases with high suspicion for VO, antibiotics may be started as soon as biopsy has been performed (some treat even earlier). For details of antimicrobials, see Treatment (p. 352) under spinal epidural abscess.

Improvement on imaging can lag behind clinical response and ESR/CRP.

Indications for neurosurgical intervention (note: intervention by a general surgeon may be indicated for empyema, psoas abscess…):

1. progression of disease despite adequate best-case antibiotic therapy
2. spinal instability
3. spinal epidural abscess (p. 349)
4. chronic infection refractory to medical management

For patients not being treated surgically:

1. percutaneous biopsy to obtain ID & sensitivity of organism
2. antibiotics:
   a) IV antibiotics for at least 6 weeks (the rate of treatment failure is increased when IV antibiotics are given for < 4 weeks[95]; longer, e.g. 12 weeks, if ESR not normalizing or if extensive bone involvement and paravertebral infection)
   b) followed by 6–8 weeks of oral agents[95]
3. pain medication as appropriate for pain
4. TLSO brace: to reduce pain (due to movement at involved site) and to reduce stress on weakened bone until healing
5. check upright films in the TLSO to verify stability in the brace
6. follow-up at approximately 8 and 12 weeks with x-rays in brace, then consider discontinuing brace if infection and pain are under control

Surgical treatment

Decompression of neural elements, removal of inflammatory tissue and infected bone to decrease bioburden. Use of instrumented fusion is not contraindicated even for pyogenic infections. Although not routinely used, bone morphogenic protein (rhBMP-2) in 14 patients undergoing circumferential fusion for refractory infections did not produce complications.[104]

21.5.3 Discitis

General information

Infection of the nucleus pulposus. May start in the cartilaginous endplate and spread to the disc and vertebral body (VB). Similar to vertebral osteomyelitis, except osteomyelitis primarily involves the VB and spreads secondarily to the disc space.

Setting: may be "post-op" or "spontaneous"

- Spontaneous discitis: Occurs in the absence of any procedure. Discussed below
- Post-op discitis: Can occur following a number of procedures; see Postoperative discitis (p. 346). This is covered under post-op infections

Many radiographic features of spondylodiscitis and tumor (metastatic and primary) are similar, but tumors rarely involve the disc space, whereas most infections begin in, or before too long, involve the disc space; for more details, see Differentiating factors (p. 1392).

Two distinct types:

1. juvenile: age usually < 20 yrs (see below)
2. adult: usually occurs in susceptible patients (diabetics, IV drug abusers)

Juvenile discitis

Age usually < 20 yrs, with a peak between 2–3 years. Probably due to the presence of primordial feeding arteries that nourish the nucleus pulposus and which involute at ≈ 20–30 yrs age. Lumbar spine is more commonly involved than thoracic or cervical.

Common presentation in young children: refusal to walk or stand progressing to refusal to sit. Back pain is most common in children > 9 yrs age. Low grade fever may be present. ESR is usually 2–3 × normal. WBC is sometimes elevated. *H. flu* is a more commonly seen pathogen in this group.

In most cases, there is complete resolution in 9–22 weeks without recurrence in long-term follow-up studies.[97 (p 365–71)] Surgery is reserved for the rare case that progresses in spite of antibiotics, for spinal instability, or for recurrent cases.

Most authors reserve antibiotics for patients with[97 (p 365–71)]:

1. positive cultures (blood cultures or biopsy cultures)
2. elevated WBC count, constitutional symptoms, or high fever
3. poor response to rest or immobilization
4. neurologic sequelae (very rare)

Antibiotics should be given for a total of 4–6 weeks. Start with IV antibiotics, and when clinical symptoms improve convert to PO for the remainder of therapy.

Clinical

1. symptoms:
   a) pain (the primary symptom)
      - local pain, moderate to severe, exacerbated by virtually any motion of the spine, usually well localized to the level of involvement
      - radiating to abdomen,[105] hip, leg, scrotum, groin, or perineum
      - radicular symptoms: occurs in 50%[52] to 93%[106] depending on the series

   b) fever and chills: up to 70% are afebrile
2. signs:
   a) localized tenderness
   b) paravertebral muscle spasm
   c) limitation of movement

Work-up

Overview

See following sections for details.

- blood tests
  - WBC
  - ESR & CRP
  - blood cultures
- imaging
  - MRI of the region of concern without and with contrast: the diagnostic test of choice.
  - If MRI is contraindicated: CT-myelogram, bone scan
- percutaneous needle biopsy: usually performed by interventional radiologist
- a source of the infection should be sought
  - thorough history for possible risk factors: skin lesions, IV drug abuse, immunocompromise
  - echocardiogram TEE: rule-out endocarditis or valvular vegetations

Radiographic evaluation

General information

A characteristic radiographic finding that helps distinguish infection from metastatic disease is that destruction of the disc space is highly suggestive of infection, whereas in general, *tumor* does *not* cross the disc space; see Differentiating factors (p. 1392).

Plain x-rays

Usually not helpful for early diagnosis. Sequence of changes on plain films:

- earliest changes: interspace narrowing with some demineralization of the VB. Not seen < 2–4 wks following onset of clinical symptoms, nor later than 8 wks

- sclerosis (eburnation) of adjacent cortical margins with increased density of adjacent areas of VB representing new bone formation, starting 4–12 weeks following onset of clinical symptoms
- irregularity of the adjacent vertebral endplates, with sparing of the pedicles (except for tuberculosis, which may involve the pedicles)
- in 50% of cases, the infection remains confined to the disc space, in the other 50% it spreads to adjacent VB
- a late finding is widening (ballooning) of the disc space with erosion of the VB
- circumferential bone formation may lead to exuberant spur formation between VBs 6–8 months into course of illness
- spontaneous fusion of the VB may occur

MRI

Without and with gadolinium contrast. Demonstrates involvement of disc space and of VBs. MRI can R/O paravertebral or epidural spinal abscess but is poor in assessing bony fusion and bone integrity. As sensitive as radionuclide bone scan. Characteristic finding: decreased signal from the disc and adjacent portion of VBs on T1WI, and increased signal from these structures on T2WI. Enhancement is common. Characteristic findings may occur 3–5 days after onset of *symptoms.*

CT and myelo-CT

Like MRI, may also R/O paravertebral or epidural spinal abscess, and while it is better for assessing bony fusion and integrity, by itself it is poor for demonstrating canal compromise. With the addition of water soluble intrathecal contrast (myelo-CT), also assesses the spinal canal for compromise.

Diagnostic criteria

Three basic changes on CT[107] (if all 3 are present, pathognomonic for discitis; if only the 1st 2 are present, then only 87% specific for discitis):

1. endplate fragmentation
2. paravertebral soft-tissue swelling with obliteration of fat planes
3. paravertebral abscess

Nuclear medicine

Very sensitive for discitis and vertebral osteomyelitis (85% sensitivity), but may be negative in up to 85% of patients with Pott's disease. Uses either technetium-99 (abnormal as early as 7 days following onset of clinical symptoms) or gallium-67 (abnormal within 14 days). A positive scan shows focal increased uptake in adjacent endplates, and may be differentiated from osteomyelitis which will involve only one endplate. A positive scan is not specific for infection, and may also occur with neoplasms, fractures, and degenerative changes.

Laboratory studies

ESR: In non-immunocompromised patients, ESR will be elevated in almost all cases with an average value of 60 mm/hr (although discitis with a normal ESR occurs rarely, it should call the diagnosis into question. ESR may be useful to follow as an indicator of response to treatment.

C-reactive protein (CRP): Often used in conjunction with ESR

WBC: Peripheral WBC is often normal, and rarely is elevated above 12,000.

PPD (Purified Protein Derivative, AKA Mantoux screening test): May be helpful to R/O Pott's disease in cases of spontaneous discitis (p. 354), may be negative in 14% of cases.[108]

Cultures: An attempt should be made to obtain direct cultures from the involved disc space. These may be obtained percutaneously (e.g. Craig needle biopsy) with CT or other radiographic guidance (reported up to 60% positive culture rate), or from intra-operative specimen (NB: surgery for open biopsy alone is usually not indicated). Staining for acid fast bacilli (AFB) to identify *Mycobacterium tuberculosis* (TB) should be done in all cases.

Blood cultures may be positive in ≈ 50% of cases, and can be helpful in guiding choice of antimicrobial agent when positive.

Pathogens

Staphylococcus aureus is the most common organism when direct cultures are obtained, followed by S. albus and S. epidermidis. Gram negative organisms may also be found, including E. coli and Proteus species.

Pseudomonas aeruginosa may be more common in IV drug abusers.

H. flu is common in juvenile discitis (see below).

Mycobacterium tuberculosis: Tuberculous spondylitis (Pott's disease) may also occur.

Treatment

General information

Outcome is generally good, and antibiotics together with spinal bracing (immobilization) are adequate treatment in ≈ 75% of cases. Occasionally surgery is required. See also under postoperative discitis for other aspects of management (p.347).

Most patients are started on strict bed rest, and are then mobilized with or without a brace as tolerated

Spinal bracing

Probably does not affect final outcome. Affords earlier pain relief for some, and may allow return to activity at an earlier time. For thoracic or upper lumbar discitis, the patient is fitted with a clamshell-type body jacket which is used for 6–8 weeks on the average. As a practical matter, most patients find that the discomfort from the brace is worse than that without the brace. Alternative forms of immobilization include spica cast (provides better immobilization for lower lumbar discitis) or a corset-type brace (less immobilization but better tolerated).

Antibiotics

Choice of antibiotics is guided by the results of direct cultures when positive. In the 40–50% of cases where no organism is isolated, broad spectrum antibiotics should be used. Positive blood culture results may also help guide choice of antibiotics.

Two alternative treatment plans suggested:

1. treat with IV antibiotics for an arbitrary period of time, usually ≈ 4–6 weeks, followed with oral antibiotics for an additional 4–6 weeks
2. treat with IV antibiotics until the ESR normalizes, then change to PO

Surgery

Required in only ≈ 25% of cases.

Indications for surgery:

1. situations where the diagnosis is uncertain, especially when neoplasm is a strong consideration (CT guided needle biopsy usually helps here)
2. decompression of neural structures, especially with associated spinal epidural abscess or compression by reactive granulation tissue. Ascending numbness, weakness, or onset of neurogenic bladder herald cauda equina syndrome
3. drainage of associated abscess, especially septated abscesses that might be recalcitrant to CT guided percutaneous needling
4. rarely, to fuse an unstable spine. Most cases go on to spontaneous fusion

Approaches

- anterior approaches: generally used in the cervical or thoracic regions. Removes some or most of the offending infected tissue
  - cervical spine: anterior discectomy and fusion for limited involvement; corpectomy with strut graft and plating with posterior instrumentation (360° fusion) for more extensive involvement
  - thoracic spine: a posterolateral approach (e.g. transpedicular or costotransversectomy approach) or lateral approach (e.g. trans-thoracic or retro-coelomic) may be used
- posterior laminectomy
  - may be used in the lumbar region (below the conus medullaris)
  - ✖ laminectomy alone is not appropriate in the thoracic or cervical spine when there is anterior compression of the spinal cord.

21.5.4 Psoas abscess

General information

1. Applied anatomy of psoas muscle:
   a) one of 2 heads of the iliopsoas muscle (the other head is iliacus)
   b) origin: inner surface of ilium, base of sacrum, and transverse processes, vertebral bodies (VB) and intervertebral discs of spinal column starting from the inferior margin of T12 VB, extending to the upper part of L5 VB. Insertion: lesser trochanter of the femur. Psoas is the primary hip flexor
   c) 30% of people also have a psoas minor which lies anterior to the psoas major

21

Table 21.6 Conditions associated with secondary psoas abscess[111]

Organ system	Condition
gastrointestinal	diverticulitis, appendicitis, Crohn's disease, colorectal cancer
genitourinary	UTI, cancer
musculoskeletal infections	vertebral osteomyelitis, infectious sacroiliitis, septic arthritis
other	endocarditis, femoral artery catheterization, infected abdominal aortic aneurysm graft, hepatocellular Ca, intrauterine contraceptive device, trauma, sepsis, dialysis (peritoneal or long-term hemodialysis)

   d) innervation: branches of L2–4 nerve roots proximal to the formation of the femoral nerve
   e) susceptibility to infection
      - rich vascular supply makes it vulnerable to hematogenous spread
      - proximity to structures that may be a source of infection: sigmoid colon, jejunum, vermiform appendix, ureters, aorta, renal pelvis, pancreas, iliac lymph nodes and spine
2. may be primary (no identifiable underlying disease) or secondary in which it may be associated with one of the conditions shown in ▶ Table 21.6
3. risk factors: IV drug abuse, HIV/AIDS, age > 65 years, DM, immunosuppression, renal failure

Clinical findings

Physical findings: signs of iliopsoas inflammation include:
1. active: pain on flexing the hip against resistance
2. passive: with the patient lying on the unaffected side, hyperextension of the affected hip stretches the psoas muscle and produces pain.

Diagnostic tests

1. routine infection work-up: WBC (often elevated), blood cultures, U/A + C&S (pyuria may be seen)
2. AP abdominal x-ray: psoas shadow may be obliterated
3. CT: sensitivity is 80–100% (MRI is not better).[109] Enlargement of psoas muscle on affected side best seen inside iliac wing.

Treatment often includes drainage of the psoas abscess either surgically or percutaneously with CT-guidance.

Mortality rates associated with psoas abscess: 2.4% with primary, 19% with secondary, with sepsis being the usual cause of death.[110]

References

[1] Yogev R. Cerebrospinal Fluid Shunt Infections: A Personal View. Pediatr Infect Dis. 1985; 4:113–118

[2] Ammirati M, Raimondi A. Cerebrospinal Fluid Shunt Infections in Children: A Study of the Relationship between the Etiology of the Hydrocephalus, Age at the Time of Shunt Placement, and Infection. Childs Nerv Syst. 1987; 3:106–109

[3] McLone D, Czyzewski D, Raimondi A, Sommers R. Central Nervous System Infection as a Limiting Factor in the Intelligence of Children with Myelomeningocele. Pediatrics. 1982; 70:338–342

[4] Amacher AL, Wellington J. Infantile Hydrocephalus: Long-Term Results of Surgical Therapy. Childs Brain. 1984; 11:217–229

[5] Sanchez-Portocarrero J, Martin-Rabadan P, Saldana CJ, Perez-Cecilia E. Candida cerebrospinal fluid shunt infection. Report of two new cases and review of the literature. Diagn Microbiol Infect Dis. 1994; 20:33–40

[6] Nguyen MH, Yu VL. Meningitis caused by Candida species: an emerging problem in neurosurgical patients. Clin Infect Dis. 1995; 21:323–327

[7] Geers TA, Gordon SM. Clinical significance of Candida species isolated from cerebrospinal fluid following neurosurgery. Clin Infect Dis. 1999; 28:1139–1147

[8] O'Brien M, Parent A, Davis B. Management of Ventricular Shunt Infections. Childs Brain. 1979; 5:304–309

[9] Wald SL, McLaurin RL. Shunt-Associated Glomerulonephritis. Neurosurgery. 1978; 3:146–150

[10] Section of Pediatric Neurosurgery of the American Association of Neurological Surgeons. Pediatric Neurosurgery. New York 1982

[11] Frame PT, McLaurin RL. Treatment of CSF Shunt Infections with Intrashunt Plus Oral Antibiotic Therapy. J Neurosurg. 1984; 60:354–360

[12] James HE, Walsh JW, Wilson HD, et al. Prospective Randomized Study of Therapy in Cerebrospinal Fluid Shunt Infection. Neurosurgery. 1980; 7:459–463

[13] Steinbok P, Cochrane DD, Kestle JRW. The Significance of Bacteriologically Positive Ventriculoperitoneal Shunt Components in the Absence of Other Signs of Shunt Infection. J Neurosurg. 1996; 84:617–623

[14] van de Beek D, Drake JM, Tunkel AR. Nosocomial bacterial meningitis. N Engl J Med. 2010; 362:146–154

[15] Tumialan LM, Lin F, Gupta SK. Spontaneous bacterial peritonitis causing Serratia marcescens and Proteus mirabilis ventriculoperitoneal shunt infection. Case report. J Neurosurg. 2006; 105:320–324

[16] Vinchon M, Baroncini M, Laurent T, Patrick D. Bowel perforation caused by peritoneal shunt catheters: diagnosis and treatment. Neurosurgery. 2006; 58:ONS76–82; discussion ONS76–82

[17] Gaskill SJ, Marlin AE. Spontaneous bacterial peritonitis in patients with ventriculoperitoneal shunts. Pediatr Neurosurg. 1997; 26:115–119

[18] Rush DS, Walsh JW, Belin RP, Pulito AR. Ventricular Sepsis and Abdominally Related Complications in Children with Cerebrospinal Fluid Shunts. Surgery. 1985; 97:420–427

[19] Bayston R. Epidemiology, diagnosis, treatment, and prevention of cerebrospinal fluid shunt infections. Neurosurg Clin N Am. 2001; 12:703–8, viii

[20] Salomao JF, Leibinger RD. Abdominal pseudocysts complicating CSF shunting in infants and children. Report of 18 cases. Pediatr Neurosurg. 1999; 31:274–278

[21] Lozier AP, Sciacca RR, Romanoli M, et al. Ventriculostomy-related infection: a critical review of the literature. Neurosurgery. 2002; 51:170–182

[22] Pfausler B, Beer R, Engelhardt K, Kemmler G, Mohsenipour I, Schmutzhard E. Cell index–a new parameter for the early diagnosis of ventriculostomy (external ventricular drainage)-related ventriculitis in patients with intraventricular hemorrhage? Acta Neurochir (Wien). 2004; 146:477–481

[23] Beer R, Lackner P, Pfausler B, Schmutzhard E. Nosocomial ventriculitis and meningitis in neurocritical care patients. J Neurol. 2008; 255:1617–1624

[24] Kim JH, Desai NS, Ricci J, Stieg PE, Rosengart AJ, Hartl R, Fraser JF. Factors contributing to ventriculostomy infection. World Neurosurg. 2012; 77:135–140

[25] Aucoin PJ, Kotilainen HR, Gantz NM, Davidson R, Kellogg P, Stone B. Intracranial pressure monitors. Epidemiologic study of risk factors and infections. Am J Med. 1986; 80:369–376

[26] Mayhall CG, Archer NH, Lamb VA, Spadora AC, Baggett JW, Ward JD, Narayan RK. Ventriculostomy-related infections. A prospective epidemiologic study. N Engl J Med. 1984; 310:553–559

[27] Mayhall CG, Archer NH, Lamb VA, Spadora AC, Baggett JW, Ward JD, Narayan RK. Ventriculostomy-related infections. A prospective epidemiologic study. N Engl J Med. 1984; 310:553–559

[28] Schade RP, Schinkel J, Roelandse FW, Geskus RB, Visser LG, van Dijk JM, Voormolen JH, Van Pelt H, Kuijper EJ. Lack of value of routine analysis of cerebrospinal fluid for prediction and diagnosis of external drainage-related bacterial meningitis. J Neurosurg. 2006; 104:101–108

[29] Schuhmann MU, Ostrowski KR, Draper EJ, Chu JW, Ham SD, Sood S, McAllister JP. The value of C-reactive protein in the management of shunt infections. J Neurosurg. 2005; 103:223–230

[30] Martinez R, Gaul C, Buchfelder M, Erbguth F, Tschaikowsky K. Serum procalcitonin monitoring for differential diagnosis of ventriculitis in adult intensive care patients. Intensive Care Med. 2002; 28:208–210

[31] Pfisterer W, Muhlbauer M, Czech T, Reinprecht A. Early diagnosis of external ventricular drainage infection: results of a prospective study. J Neurol Neurosurg Psychiatry. 2003; 74:929–932

[32] Hader WJ, Steinbok P. The value of routine cultures of the cerebrospinal fluid in patients with external ventricular drains. Neurosurgery. 2000; 46:1149–53; discussion 1153-5

[33] The management of neurosurgical patients with postoperative bacterial or aseptic meningitis or external ventricular drain-associated ventriculitis. Infection in Neurosurgery Working Party of the British Society for Antimicrobial Chemotherapy. Br J Neurosurg. 2000; 14:7–12

[34] Cook AM, Mieure KD, Owen RD, Pesaturo AB, Hatton J. Intracerebroventricular administration of drugs. Pharmacotherapy. 2009; 29:832–845

[35] Friedman WA, Vries JK. Percutaneous tunnel ventriculostomy. Summary of 100 procedures. J Neurosurg. 1980; 53:662–665

[36] Harrop JS, Sharan AD, Ratliff J, Prasad S, Jabbour P, Evans JJ, Veznedaroglu E, Andrews DW, Maltenfort M, Liebman K, Flomenberg P, Sell B, Baranoski AS, Fonshell C, Reiter D, Rosenwasser RH. Impact of a standardized protocol and antibiotic-impregnated catheters on ventriculostomy infection rates in cerebrovascular patients. Neurosurgery. 2010; 67:187–91; discussion 191

[37] Zabramski JM, Spetzler RF, Sonntag VK. Impact of a standardized protocol and antibiotic-impregnated catheters on ventriculostomy infection rates in cerebrovascular patients. Neurosurgery. 2011; 69. DOI: 10.1227/NEU.0b013e31821756ca

[38] Sonabend AM, Korenfeld Y, Crisman C, Badjatia N, Mayer SA, Connolly ES, Jr. Prevention of ventriculostomy-related infections with prophylactic antibiotics and antibiotic-coated external ventricular drains: a systematic review. Neurosurgery. 2011; 68:996–1005

[39] Zabramski JM, Whiting D, Darouiche RO, Horner TG, Olson J, Robertson C, Hamilton AJ. Efficacy of antimicrobial-impregnated external ventricular drain catheters: a prospective, randomized, controlled trial. J Neurosurg. 2003; 98:725–730

[40] Poon WS, Ng S, Wai S. CSF antibiotic prophylaxis for neurosurgical patients with ventriculostomy: a randomised study. Acta Neurochir Suppl. 1998; 71:146–148

[41] Holloway KL, Barnes T, Choi S, et al. Ventriculostomy Infections: The Effect of Monitoring Duration and Catheter Exchange in 584 Patients. J Neurosurg. 1996; 85:419–424

[42] Wong GK, Poon WS, Wai S, Yu LM, Lyon D, Lam JM. Failure of regular external ventricular drain exchange to reduce cerebrospinal fluid infection: result of a randomised controlled trial. J Neurol Neurosurg Psychiatry. 2002; 73:759–761

[43] Lo CH, Spelman D, Bailey M, Cooper DJ, Rosenfeld JV, Brecknell JE. External ventricular drain infections are independent of drain duration: an argument against elective revision. J Neurosurg. 2007; 106:378–383

[44] Khalil BA, Sarsam Z, Buxton N. External ventricular drains: is there a time limit in children? Childs Nerv Syst. 2005; 21:355–357

[45] Shektman A, Granick MS, Solomon MP, et al. Management of Infected Laminectomy Wounds. Neurosurgery. 1994; 35:307–309

[46] Kurz A, Sessler DI, Lenhardt R. Perioperative Normothermia to Reduce the Incidence of Surgical-Wound Infection and Shorten Hospitalization. N Engl J Med. 1996; 334:1209–1215

[47] Dernbach PD, Gomez H, Hahn J. Primary Closure of Infected Spinal Wounds. Neurosurgery. 1990; 26:707–709

[48] Ebersold MJ. Comment on Shektman A, et al.: Primary Closure of Infected Spinal Wounds. Neurosurgery. 1994; 35

[49] Iversen E, Nielsen VAH, Hansen LG. Prognosis in Postoperative Discitis. A Retrospective Study of 111 Cases. Acta Orthop Scand. 1992; 63:305–309

[50] Fouquet B, Goupille P, Jattiot F, et al. Discitis After Lumbar Disc Surgery. Features of "Aseptic" and "Septic" Forms.. Spine. 1992; 17:356–358

[51] Rawlings CE, Wilkins RH, Gallis HA, et al. Postoperative Intervertebral Disc Space Infection. Neurosurgery. 1983; 13:371–376

[52] Malik GM, McCormick P. Management of Spine and Intervertebral Disc Space Infection. Contemp Neurosurg. 1988; 10:1–6

[53] Thelander U, Larsson S. Quantitation of C-Reactive Protein Levels and Erythrocyte Sedimentation Rate After Spinal Surgery. Spine. 1992; 17:400–404

[54] Boden SD, Davis DO, Dina TS, et al. Postoperative Diskitis: Distinguishing Early MR Imaging Findings from Normal Postoperative Disk Space Changes. Radiology. 1992; 184:765–771

[55] Mirzayan MJ, Gharabaghi A, Samii M, Tatagiba M, Krauss JK, Rosahl SK. Response of C-reactive protein after craniotomy for microsurgery of intracranial tumors. Neurosurgery. 2007; 60:621–5; discussion 625

[56] Listinsky JL, Wood BP, Ekholm SE. Parietal Osteomyelitis and Epidural Abscess: A Delayed Complication of Fetal Monitoring. Pediatr Radiol. 1986; 16:150–151

[57] Bernard L, Dinh A, Ghout I, Simo D, Zeller V, Issartel B, Le Moing V, Belmatoug N, Lesprit P, Bru JP, Therby A, Bouhour D, Denes E, Debard A, Chirouze C, Fevre K, Dupon M, Aegerter P, Mulleman D. Antibiotic treatment for 6 weeks versus 12 weeks in patients with pyogenic vertebral osteomyelitis: an open-label, non-inferiority, randomised, controlled trial. Lancet. 2015; 385:875–882

[58] Cahill DW. Infections of the Spine. Contemp Neurosurg. 1993; 15:1–8

[59] Baker AS, Ojemann RG, Swartz MN, et al. Spinal Epidural Abscess. N Engl J Med. 1975; 293:463–468

[60] Nussbaum ES, Rigamonti D, Standiford H, et al. Spinal Epidural Abscess: A Report of 40 Cases and Review. Surg Neurol. 1992; 38:225–231

[61] Danner RL, Hartman BJ. Update of Spinal Epidural Abscess: 35 Cases and Review of the Literature. Rev Infect Dis. 1987; 9:265–274

[62] Curry WT, Jr, Hoh BL, Amin-Hanjani S, Eskandar EN. Spinal epidural abscess: clinical presentation, management, and outcome. Surg Neurol. 2005; 63:364–71; discussion 371

[63] Hlavin ML, Kaminski HJ, Ross JS, Ganz E. Spinal Epidural Abscess: A Ten-Year Perspective. Neurosurgery. 1990; 27:177–184

[64] Spiegelmann R, Findler G, Faibel M, et al. Postoperative Spinal Epidural Empyema: Clinical and Computed Tomography Features. Spine. 1991; 16:1146–1149

[65] Browder J, Meyers R. Pyogenic Infections of the Spinal Epidural Space. Surgery. 1941; 10:296–308

[66] Russell NA, Vaughan R, Morley TP. Spinal Epidural Infection. Can J Neurol Sci. 1979; 6:325–328

[67] Heusner AP. Nontuberculous Spinal Epidural Infections. N Engl J Med. 1948; 239:845–854

[68] Koppel BS, Tuchman AJ, Mangiardi JR, et al. Epidural Spinal Infection in Intravenous Drug Abusers. Arch Neurol. 1988; 45:1331–1337

[69] Abdel-Magid RA, Kotb HIM. Spinal Epidural Abscess After Spinal Anesthesia: A Favorable Outcome. Neurosurgery. 1990; 27:310–311

[70] Loarie DJ, Fairley HB. Epidural Abscess Following Spinal Anesthesia. Anesth Analg. 1978; 57:351–353

[71] Strong WE. Epidural Abscess Associated with Epidural Catheterization: A Rare Event? Report of Two Cases with Markedly Delayed Presentation. Anesthesiology. 1991; 74:943–946

[72] Bergman I, Wald ER, Meyer JD, Painter MJ. Epidural Abscess and Vertebral Osteomyelitis following Serial Lumbar Punctures. Pediatrics. 1983; 72:476–480

[73] Rea GL, McGregor JM, Miller CA, Miner ME. Surgical Treatment of the Spontaneous Spinal Epidural Abscess. Surg Neurol. 1992; 37:274–279

[74] Kaufman DM, Kaplan JG, Litman N. Infectious Agents in Spinal Epidural Abscesses. Neurology. 1980; 30:844–850

[75] Wilkins RH, Rengachary SS. Neurosurgery. New York 1985

[76] Post MJD, Sze G, Quencer RM, et al. Gadolinium-Enhanced MR in Spinal Infection. J Comput Assist Tomogr. 1990; 14:721–729

[77] Post MJD, Quencer RM, Montalvo BM, et al. Spinal infection: evaluation with MR imaging and intraoperative ultrasound. Radiology. 1988; 169:765–771

[78] Sandhu FS, Dillon WP. Spinal Epidural Abscess: Evaluation with Contrast-Enhanced MR Imaging. AJNR. 1991; 158:1087–1093

[79] Kirzner H, Oh YK, Lee SH. Intraspinal Air: A CT Finding of Epidural Abscess. AJR. 1988; 151:1217–1218

[80] Leys D, Lesoin F, Viaud C, et al. Decreased Morbidity from Acute Bacterial Spinal Epidural Abscess using Computed Tomography and Nonsurgical Treatment in Selected Patients. Ann Neurol. 1985; 17:350–355

[81] Mampalam TJ, Rosegay H, Andrews BT, Rosenblum ML, Pitts LH. Nonoperative Treatment of Spinal Epidural Infections. J Neurosurg. 1989; 71:208–210

[82] Hanigan WC, Asner NG, Elwood PW. Magnetic Resonance Imaging and the Nonoperative Treatment of Spinal Epidural Abscess. Surg Neurol. 1990; 34:408–413

[83] Garrido E, Rosenwasser RH. Experience with the Suction-Irrigation Technique in the Management of Spinal Epidural Infection. Neurosurgery. 1983; 12:678–679

[84] Eismont FJ, Bohlman HH, Soni PL, Goldberg VM, et al. Pyogenic and Fungal Vertebral Osteomyelitis with Paralysis. J Bone Joint Surg. 1983; 65A:19–29

[85] Pereira CE, Lynch JC. Spinal epidural abscess: an analysis of 24 cases. Surg Neurol. 2005; 63:S26–S29

[86] Curling OD, Gower DJ, McWhorter JM. Changing Concepts in Spinal Epidural Abscess: A Report of 29 Cases. Neurosurgery. 1990; 27:185–192

[87] Schmorl G, Junghanns H. The Human Spine in Health and Disease. New York: Grune & Stratton; 1971

[88] Waldvogel FA, Vasey H. Osteomyelitis: The Past Decade. N Engl J Med. 1980; 303:360–370

[89] Holzman RS, Bishko R. Osteomyelitis in Heroin Addicts. Ann Intern Med. 1971; 75:693–696

[90] Cahill DW, Love LC, Rechtine GR. Pyogenic Osteomyelitis of the Spine in the Elderly. J Neurosurg. 1991; 74:878–886

[91] Burke DR, Brant-Zawadzki MB. CT of Pyogenic Spine Infection. Neuroradiology. 1985; 27:131–137

[92] Sapico FL, Montgomerie JZ. Pyogenic Vertebral Osteomyelitis: Report of Nine Cases and Review of the Literature. Rev Infect Dis. 1979; 1:754–776

[93] Skaf GS, Fehlings MG, Bouclaous CH. Medical and surgical management of pyogenic and nonpyogenic spondylodiscitis: Part I. Contemp Neurosurg. 2004; 26:1–5

[94] Batson OV. The Function of the Vertebral Veins and Their Role in the Spread of Metastases. Ann Surg. 1940; 112

[95] Skaf GS, Fehlings MG, Bouclaous CH. Medical and surgical management of pyogenic and nonpyogenic spondylodiscitis: Part II. Contemp Neurosurg. 2004; 26:1–5

[96] Weiner BK, Love TW, Fraser RD. Mycobacterium avium intracellulare: vertebral osteomyelitis. J Spinal Disord. 1998; 11:89–91

[97] Rothman RH, Simeone FA. The Spine. Philadelphia 1992

[98] Kinnier WSA. In: Tuberculosis of the Skull and Spine. Neurology. London: Edward Arnold; 1940:575–583

[99] Medical Research Council Working Party on Tuberculosis of the Spine. Controlled Trial of Short-Course Regimens of Chemotherapy in the Ambulatory Treatment of Spinal Tuberculosis: Results at Three Years of a Study in Korea. J Bone Joint Surg. 1993; 75B:240–248

[100] Rath SA, Nelf U, Schneider O, et al. Neurosurgical management of thoracic and lumbar vertebral osteomyelitis and discitis in adults: a review of 43 consecutive surgically treated patients. Neurosurgery. 1996; 38:926–933

[101] Patzakis MJ, Rao S, Wilkins J, Moore TM, Harvey PJ. Analysis of 61 cases of vertebral osteomyelitis. Clin Orthop. 1991; 264:178–183

[102] Modic MT, Feiglin DH, Piraino DW, et al. Vertebral Osteomyelitis: Assessment Using MR. Radiology. 1985; 157:157–166

[103] Hadjipavlou AG, Cesani-Vazquez F, Villaneuva-Meyer J, et al. The effectiveness of gallium citrate Ga 67 radionuclide imaging in vertebral osteomyelitis revisited. Am J Orthop. 1998; 27:179–183

[104] Allen RT, Lee YP, Stimson E, Garfin SR. Bone morphogenetic protein-2 (BMP-2) in the treatment of pyogenic vertebral osteomyelitis. Spine. 2007; 32:2996–3006
[105] Sullivan CR, Symmonds RE. Disk Infections and Abdominal Pain. JAMA. 1964; 188:655–658
[106] Kemp HBS, Jackson JW, Jeremiah JD, et al. Pyogenic Infections Occurring Primarily in Intervertebral Discs. J Bone Joint Surg. 1973; 55B:698–714
[107] Kopecky KK, Gilmor RL, Scott JA, et al. Pitfalls of CT in Diagnosis of Discitis. Neuroradiology. 1985; 27:57–66
[108] Lifeso RM, Weaver P, Harder EH. Tuberculous Spondylitis in Adults. J Bone Joint Surg. 1985; 67A:1405–1413
[109] Taiwo B. Psoas abscess: a primer for the internist. South Med J. 2001; 94:2–5
[110] Gruenwald I, Abrahamson J, Cohen O. Psoas abscess: case report and review of the literature. J Urol. 1992; 147:1624–1626
[111] Riyad NYM, Sallam A, Nur A. Pyogenic psoas abscess: Discussion of its Epidemiology, Etiology, Bacteriology, Diagnosis, Treatment and Prognosis - Case Report. Kuwait Medical Journal. 2003; 35:44–47

22 Other Nonbacterial Infections

22.1 Viral encephalitis

Encephalitides that come to the attention of the neurosurgeon usually cause imaging findings that may mimic mass lesions, for cases where biopsy may be helpful, and shunting for hydrocephalus is needed. Those covered in this book:

1. herpes simplex encephalitis: see below
2. multifocal herpes varicella-zoster virus leukoencephalitis (p.366)
3. progressive multifocal leukoencephalopathy (PML) (p.331)

22.1.1 Herpes simplex encephalitis

General information

Key concepts

- a hemorrhagic viral encephalitis with a predilection for temporal lobes
- definitive diagnosis requires brain biopsy
- optimal treatment: early administration of IV acyclovir

Herpes simplex encephalitis (HSE) AKA multifocal necrotizing encephalomyelitis, is caused by the herpes simplex virus (HSV) type I. It produces an acute, often (but not always) hemorrhagic, necrotizing encephalitis with edema. There is a predilection for the temporal and orbitofrontal lobes and limbic system.

Epidemiology

Estimated incidence of HSE: 1 in 750,000 to 1 million persons/yr. Equally distributed between male and females, in all races, in all ages (over 33% of cases occur in children 6 mos to 18 yrs), throughout the year.[1]

Presentation

Patients are often confused and disoriented at onset, and progress to coma within days. Adult presentations are shown in ▶ Table 22.1, and for pediatrics in ▶ Table 22.2. Other symptoms include headache.

Diagnostic studies

Diagnosis can often be made on the basis of history, CSF, and MRI. Treatment should be instituted rapidly without waiting for biopsy, before the onset of coma.

1. CSF: leukocytosis (mostly monos), RBCs 500–1000/mm^3, (NB: 3% have no pleocytosis), protein rises markedly as disease progresses. HSV antibodies may appear in the CSF but takes at least ≈ 14 days and is thus not useful for early diagnosis

Table 22.1 Herpes simplex encephalitis – adult presentation

Symptom	%
altered consciousness	97%
fever	90%
seizures (usually focal onset)	67%
personality changes	71%
hemiparesis	33%

Table 22.2 Herpes simplex encephalitis – presentation in age < 10 yrs
irritability
altered mentation
malaise
seizure
disorientation
dysphasia
hemiparesis
fever
papilledema (except in age ≤ 2 yrs)

2. EEG: periodic lateralizing epileptiform discharges (PLEDs) (triphasic high-voltage discharges every few seconds) usually from the temporal lobe. EEG may vary rapidly over few days (unusual in conditions mimicking HSE)
3. CT: edema predominantly localized in temporal lobes (poorer prognosis once hemorrhagic lesions visible). In one review, 38% of initial CTs were normal[2] (many were on early generation CT scanners or were done within 3 days of onset). Hemorrhages were apparent in only 12% of the initially abnormal CTs
4. MRI: more sensitive than CT,[3] demonstrates edema as high signal on T2WI, primarily within the temporal lobe, with some extension across sylvian fissure ("transsylvian sign"),[2] especially suggestive of HSE if bilateral. Differentiate from MCA infarct (which may also span sylvian fissure) by typical arterial distribution of the latter. Enhancement doesn't occur until the 2nd week
5. technetium brain scan: process localized to temporal lobes
6. brain biopsy: false negatives may occur[4]; see details below

Brain biopsy

Indications: reserved for questionable cases. May not be necessary in patients with fever, encephalopathy, compatible CSF findings, focal neuro findings (focal seizure, hemiparesis, or cranial nerve palsy), and supporting evidence of at least one of the following: focal EEG, CT, MRI or technetium brain scan abnormality.

Should be performed within ≤ 48 hrs of starting acyclovir (otherwise false negatives may occur).

Biopsy results: of 432 brain biopsies performed using the technique below, 45% had HSE, 22% had identifiable but non HSE pathology (e.g. vascular disease, other viral infection, adrenal leukodystrophy, bacterial infection…), and 33% remained without a diagnosis.[5]

Technique

1. anterior inferior temporal lobe is preferred site
   a) the side chosen for biopsy is the one showing maximal involvement based on clinical information (e.g. localizing seizures), EEG and/or imaging studies[6]
   b) 10 × 10 × 5 mm deep specimen obtained from anterior portion of the inferior temporal gyrus with NO COAGULATION on specimen side (cut surface with #11 blade, then cauterize pial surface on *non*-specimen side)
   c) 2nd specimen obtained from beneath surface specimen with fenestrated pituitary biopsy forceps
2. virus isolation is the most specific (100%) and sensitive (96–97%) test for HSE. Other findings (less accurate): perivascular cuffing, lymphocytic infiltration, hemorrhagic necrosis, neuronophagia, intranuclear inclusions (present in 50%)
3. if electron microscopy (EM) or immunohistofluorescence is available, 70% may be diagnosed within ≈ 3 hrs of biopsy
4. biopsy tissue handling
   a) avoid macerating specimens for histology
   b) tissue for EM: placed in glutaraldehyde
   c) tissue for permanent histology: placed in formalin
   d) tissue for culture:

22

- handling: specimen is placed in sterile specimen container and sent directly to virology lab. If lab is closed, tissue may be placed in regular refrigerator for up to 24 hrs or placed in –70° C freezer for indefinite time (virus remains viable for up to 5 yrs). ✖ DO NOT place specimen in regular *freezer* (destroys virus)
- cultures generally take at least 1 week to become positive
- cultures checked for 3 weeks before being declared negative

Treatment

General treatment measures

General supportive measures: to control elevated ICP from edema, includes: elevate HOB, mannitol, hyperventilation (dexamethasone unproven efficacy); also see Treatment measures for elevated ICP (p. 866). Anticonvulsants are used for seizure prophylaxis.

Antiviral medications

Acyclovir is the drug of choice for HSE.

Drug info: Acyclovir (Zovirax®)

℞ Adult: 30 mg/kg/day, in divided q 8 hr doses in minimum volume of 100 ml IV fluid over 1 hr (caution: this fluid load may be hazardous, especially since cerebral edema is already usually problematic) for 14–21 days (some relapses have been reported after only 10 days of treatment).

℞ Children > 6 mos age: 500 mg/m² IV q 8 hrs × 10 days.

℞ Neonatal: 10 mg/kg IV q 8 hrs for 10 days.

Drug info: Vidarabine (Vira-A®)

Six month mortality following treatment with acyclovir was influenced by:

- age (6% under age 30, 36% over age 30)
- Glasgow coma score (GCS) at time of treatment initiation (25% for GCS ≤ 10, 0% for GCS > 10)
- duration of disease before therapy (0% for initiating therapy within 4 days of onset of symptoms, 35% if after 4 days)

22.1.2 Multifocal varicella-zoster leukoencephalitis

Caused by the herpes varicella-zoster virus (VZV) which is responsible for varicella (chickenpox), herpes zoster (HZ) (shingles), and post-herpetic neuralgia (p. 493). VZV is a herpesvirus that is distinct from the herpes simplex virus.

Symptomatic zoster-related encephalitis occurs in < 5% of immunocompromised patients (including AIDS patients) with cutaneous zoster.[7] It typically follows cutaneous HZ by a short time (average time: 9 days) although cases have been reported where many months have lapsed.[8]

Manifestations include:, altered level of consciousness, headache, photophobia, meningismus. Although focal neurologic deficits may occur, these are uncommon.

Recently, vasculopathy following VZV reactivation has been increasingly recognized.[9]

MRI may show multiple, discrete, round and oval lesions with minimal edema (best seen on T2WI) and minimal enhancement.

Unlike herpes simplex virus, VZV is difficult to isolate in culture. On brain biopsy, look for multiple discrete lesions within grey and white matter, with Cowdry type A intranuclear inclusion bodies in oligodendrocytes, astrocytes, and neurons, and a positive direct fluorescent antibody test directed against VZV.

There is a case report of VZV encephalitis treated with IV acyclovir.[7]

22.2 Creutzfeldt-Jakob disease

22.2.1 General information

Key concepts

- an invariably fatal encephalopathy characterized by rapidly progressive dementia, ataxia and myoclonus
- death usually occurs within 1 yr of onset of symptoms
- 3 forms: 1) transmissible (possibly via prions), 2) autosomal dominant inherited, 3) sporadic
- characteristic EEG finding: bilateral sharp wave (0.5–2 per second)
- pathology: status spongiosus without inflammatory response

Creutzfeldt-Jakob disease (CJD) is one of 4 known rare human diseases associated with transmissible spongiform encephalopathy agents, also called prions (proteinaceous infectious particles). Although sometimes also referred to as a "slow virus", these agents contain no nucleic acids and are also resistant to processes that inactivate conventional viruses (▶ Table 22.4). Prions do not provoke an immune response. The other human prion diseases are kuru, Gerstmann-Sträussler-Scheinker disease, and fatal familial insomnia (described in 2 families[10,11,12]). The protease-resistant protein associated with disease is designated PrPres or PrPSc, and is an isoform of a naturally occurring protease-sensitive protein designated PrPsen or PrPC. In the abnormal state, PrPsen which is a predominantly alpha-helical structure, undergoes a post-translational conformation change to PrPres which has large beta-sheets, and which accumulates in neural cells, disrupting function and leading to cell death and vacuolization.[13] The famous choreographer George Balanchine died of CJD in 1983.

CJD occurs in 3 forms: transmissible, inherited and sporadic.

22.2.2 Epidemiology

Annual incidence of CJD: 0.5–1.5 per million population[13] with little change over time and no geographic clustering (except in locations with large numbers of familial cases). Over 200 people die of CJD in the U.S. each year.

22.2.3 Acquired prion diseases

Natural route of infection is unknown and virulence appears low, with lack of significant dissemination by respiratory, enteric, or sexual contact. There is no increased incidence in spouses (only a single conjugal pair of cases has been verified), physicians or laboratory workers. There is no evidence of transplacental transmission. The only known cases of horizontal transmission of CJD have occurred iatrogenically (see below). Kuru has been transmitted via handling and ingestion of infected brains in ritualistic funereal cannibalism practiced among the Fore (pronounced: "fore-ay") linguistic group in the eastern highlands of Papua, New Guinea,[14] a practice which was generally abandoned in the 1950s. Kuru is a subacute, uniformly fatal disease involving cerebellar degeneration (the word "kuru" means "to tremble" in the local language[15 (p 6)]).

Most noniatrogenically transmitted cases of CJD occur in patients > 50 yrs old, and is rare in age < 30. The incubation period can range from months to decades. The onset of symptoms following direct inoculation is usually faster (common range: 16–28 mos), but still may be much longer (up to 30 years with corneal transplant,[16] and 4–21 yrs with hGH transmission). In experimental models of CJD, higher inoculation doses produce shorter incubation periods.[17]

22.2.4 Inherited CJD

5–15% of cases of CJD occur in an autosomal dominant inheritance pattern with abnormalities in the amyloid gene[18] on chromosome 20 with a penetrance of 0.56.[19] Since familial CJD is dominantly inherited, analysis for the PrP gene is not indicated unless there is a history of dementia in a first degree relative.

22.2.5 Sporadic CJD

In ≈ 90% of cases of CJD, no infectious or familial source can be identified,[18] and these cases are considered sporadic. 80% occur in persons 50–70 yrs old.[13] Sporadic cases show no abnormality in the PrP gene.

There appears to be a genetic susceptibility in the sporadic and iatrogenically transmitted CJD cases, with the majority of these showing specific changes in the human prion protein.

22.2.6 New variant CJD

Cases of atypical CJD are well-recognized. A new variant of CJD (vCJD) was identified in 10 cases of unusually young individuals (median age at death: 29 yrs) during 1994–95 in the United Kingdom,[20] and has been strongly linked to the 1980s epidemic of bovine spongiform encephalopathy (BSE), dubbed ("mad cow" disease) by the lay press. The BSE epidemic may have been exacerbated by the practice of feeding discarded sheep organs (called offals) to the cows (a practice banned since 1989). This raises the question of possible transmission and mutation of the sheep slow-virus disease, scrapie (which resembles kuru in man) to cows. None of the vCJD patients had periodic spikes on EEG characteristic of classic CJD, the clinical course was atypical (having prominent psychiatric symptoms and early cerebellar ataxia, somewhat similar to kuru), and brain plaques showed unusual features also reminiscent of amyloid plaques seen in kuru. A comparison of vCJD to sporadic CJD is shown in ▶ Table 22.3.

22.2.7 Iatrogenic transmission of CJD

Described only in cases of direct contact with infected organs, tissues or surgical instruments. Has been reported with: corneal transplants,[21,16] intracerebral EEG electrodes sterilized with 70% alcohol and formaldehyde vapor after use on a CJD patient,[22] operations in neurosurgical O.R.s after procedures on CJD patients, in recipients of pituitary-derived human growth hormone (hGH)[23] (most cases have occurred in France[17]; there is no longer a risk of CJD with growth hormone in the U.S. since distribution of pituitary derived hGH was halted in 1985 and current hGH is obtained from recombinant DNA technology), and dural graft with cadaveric dura mater (Lyodura®) (most cases have occurred in Japan[17]). Ethylene oxide, autoclaving, formalin and ionizing radiation do not inactivate the CJD agent[24,25,26] (see ▶ Table 22.4 for other ineffective procedures). Recommended sterilization procedures for suspected CJD tissues and contaminated materials also appear in ▶ Table 22.4.

22.2.8 Pathology

The typical form of CJD produces the classic histologic triad of neuronal loss, astrocytic proliferation, and cytoplasmic vacuoles in neurons and astrocytes (status spongiosus), all in the absence of an inflammatory response. There is a predilection for cerebral cortex and basal ganglia, but all parts of the CNS may be involved. In 5–10% of cases, these changes are accompanied by the deposition of amyloid plaques (plaques are common in kuru, vCJD and some familial spongiform encephalopathies). Immunostaining for PrPres is definitive.

Table 22.3 Comparison of vCJD to sporadic CJD[13]

Characteristic	vCJD	sporadic
mean age at onset (yr)	29	60
mean duration of disease (mo)	14	5
most consistent and prominent early signs	psychiatric abnormalities, sensory symptoms	dementia, myoclonus
cerebellar signs (%)	100	40
periodic complexes on EEG (%)	0	94
pathological changes	diffuse amyloid plaques	sparse plaques in 5–10%

Cysticercosis is the most common parasitic infection involving the CNS[40] and in some low-income countries it is the most common cause of acquired epilepsy.[41] It is caused by Cysticercus cellulosae, the larval stage of the pork tapeworm Taenia solium, which has a marked predilection for neural tissue. Cysticercosis is endemic in areas of Mexico, Eastern Europe, Asia, Central and South America, and Africa. The incidence of neurocysticercosis (encystment of larva in the brain) may reach 4% in some areas.[42] The incubation period varies from months to decades, but 83% of cases show symptoms within 7 years of exposure.

Life cycle of T. Solium

Stages

There are 3 stages to the life cycle: larva, embryo (or oncosphere) and adult. T. solium can infect man in two different ways: as the adult worm or as the larva.

Infection with the adult worm (taeniasis – a parasitic infection)

Human intestinal tapeworm infection (taeniasis) results from eating undercooked infested (measly) pork. The encysted larvae are released in the small bowel and can then mature within the intestine into an adult over about 2 months. The scolex (head) of the segmented adult worm attaches by means of four suckers and two rows of hooklets to the wall of the small intestine where the worm absorbs food directly through its cuticle. Man is the only known definitive host for the adult tapeworm, for which the GI tract is the sole habitat. Proglottids (mature segments, each containing reproductive organs) produce eggs which are liberally excreted along with gravid proglottid segments in the feces.

Infection with the larva

The disease *cysticercosis* occurs when animals or humans become an intermediate host for the larval stage by ingesting viable *eggs* produced by the proglottid. The most common routes of ingestion of viable eggs are:

1. food (usually vegetables) or water contaminated with human feces containing eggs or gravid proglottids (this is the means whereby pigs acquire the disease)
2. fecal-oral autoinoculation in an individual harboring the adult form of the tapeworm due to lack of good sanitary habits or facilities
3. autoinfection by reverse peristalsis of gravid proglottids from the intestine into the stomach (unproven theoretical possibility)

In the duodenum of man and pig, the shell of the ova dissolves and the thusly hatched embryos (oncospheres) burrow through the small bowel wall to enter the lymphatics or systemic circulation and gain access to the following commonly involved sites:

- brain: involved in 60–92% of cases of cysticercosis. Latency from ingestion of eggs to symptomatic neurocysticercosis: 2–5 years[43]
- skeletal muscle
- eye: immunologically privileged, like brain
- subcutaneous tissue
- heart

Once in the tissue of the intermediary host, embryos develop a cyst wall in ≈ 2 months (immature cyst) which matures in ≈ 4 months to a larva. Larval cysts are usually rapidly eliminated by the immune system. Many larvae die naturally within 5–7 yrs or with cysticidal therapy producing an inflammatory reaction with collapse of the cyst (granular nodular stage), these sometimes calcify (nodular calcified stage). In pigs, the larva lie dormant in the muscle, "waiting" to be eaten after which the cycle repeats.

Types of neurologic involvement

Spinal cord and peripheral nerves involvement is rare.

Giant cysts: definition: cyst with diameter > 50 mm.[44]

Two types of cysts tend to develop in the brain[45]:

1. cysticercus cellulosae: regular, round or oval thin-walled cyst, ranging in size from ≈ 3 to 20 mm tending to form in the *parenchyma* or narrow *subarachnoid* spaces. This cyst contains a scolex (head), is usually static, and produces only mild inflammation during the active phase

Table 22.4 Operating room sterilization procedures for CJD[27]

Fully effective (recommended) procedures • steam autoclaving for 1 hr at 132°C, or • immersion in 1N sodium hydroxide (NaOH) for 1 hr at room temperature
Partially effective procedures • steam autoclaving at either 121° C or 132° C for 15–30 mins, or • immersion in 1N NaOH for 15 mins, or lower concentrations (< 0.5N) for 1 hr at room temp, or • immersion in sodium hypochlorite (household bleach) undiluted or up to 1:10 dilution (0.5%) for 1 hr[28]
✖ *Ineffective* procedures: • boiling, UV or ionizing radiation, ethylene oxide, ethanol, formalin, beta-propiolactone, detergents, quaternary ammonium compounds, Lysol®, alcoholic iodine, acetone, potassium permanganate, routine autoclaving

Table 22.5 Major clinical signs in sporadic CJD[13]

Sign	Freq (%)
cognitive deficits[a]	100
myoclonus	> 80
pyramidal tract signs	> 50
cerebellar signs	> 50
extrapyramidal signs	> 50
cortical visual deficits	> 20
abnormal extraocular movements	> 20
lower motor-neuron signs	< 20
vestibular dysfunction	< 20
seizures	< 20
sensory deficits	< 20
autonomic abnormalities	< 20

[a]dementia, psychiatric and behavioral abnormalities

22.2.9 Presentation

One-third initially express vague feelings of fatigue, sleep disorders, or reduced appetite. Another third have neurologic symptoms including memory loss, confusion, or uncharacteristic behavior. The last third have focal signs including cerebellar ataxia, aphasia, visual deficits (including cortical blindness), or hemiparesis.

The typical course is inexorable, progression of dementia, often noticeably worse week by week, with subsequent rapid development of pyramidal tract findings (limb weakness and stiffness, pathologic reflexes), and late extrapyramidal findings (tremor, rigidity, dysarthria, bradykinesia) and myoclonus (often stimulus triggered). Clinical signs of sporadic CJD are shown in ▶ Table 22.5.

Supranuclear gaze palsy is an occasional finding, also usually late.[19] In early stages, CJD may resemble Alzheimer's disease (SDAT). 10% of cases present as ataxia without dementia or myoclonus. Cases with predominant spinal cord findings may be initially mistaken for ALS.

Myoclonus subsides in the terminal phases, and akinetic mutism ensues.

22.2.10 Diagnosis

Diagnostic criteria

The complete "diagnostic triad" (dementia, myoclonus and periodic EEG activity) may be absent in up to 25% of cases. Diagnostic criteria have been published[29] as shown in ▶ Table 22.6. No patients in

Table 22.6 Diagnostic criteria[a] of CJD[29]

Pathologically confirmed (with unequivocal spongiform changes)
- clinically: requires brain biopsy (see text)
- found at autopsy

Clinical criteria	Mental deterioration	Myoclonus	1–2 Hz periodic EEG complexes	Any movement disorder or periodic EEG activity	Duration of illness (months)
clinically definite	+	+	+		<12
clinically probable	+	+ OR +			<18
clinically possible	+			+	<24

[a]in patients with normal metabolic status and spinal fluid. If there are early cerebellar or visual symptoms and then muscular rigidity, or if another family member has died of pathologically verified CJD, then upgrade the degree of certainty to the next higher category

their series with a diagnosis other than CJD fulfilled the criteria for clinically definite CJD. The most common condition other than CJD fulfilling the criteria for clinically probable CJD was SDAT (especially difficult to distinguish in the early stages). There is a CSF immunoassay for the 14–3-3 brain protein (see below).

Differential diagnosis

CSF examination to exclude infections such as tertiary syphilis or SSPE is recommended. Toxicity from bismuth, bromides and lithium must be ruled-out. Myoclonus is usually more prominent early in toxic/metabolic disorders than in CJD, and seizures in CJD are usually late.[13]

Diagnostic tests

1. imaging: no characteristic CT or MR finding. These studies are frequently normal, but are essential to rule-out other conditions (e.g. herpes-simplex encephalitis, recent stroke…). Diffuse atrophy may be present, especially late. MRI may show increased intensity on T2WI in areas typically involved (basal ganglion, striatum) in up to 79% of cases (retrospectively).[30] This is nonspecific but may help differentiate CJD from SDAT[31]
2. blood tests: serum assays for S-100 protein are so insensitive and nonspecific[32] that it can only be used as an diagnostic adjunct
3. CSF:
   a) routine labs: usually normal, although protein may occasionally be elevated
   b) abnormal proteins:
      - abnormal proteins (designated 130 & 131) have been identified in the CSF of patients with CJD,[33] but the assay is technically difficult and is therefore not practical for routine clinical use
      - proteins 130/131 were identified as the *normal* neuronal protein 14–3-3, and a relatively simple immunoassay for this was developed for use on as little as 50 mcl of CSF.[34] Detection of the 14–3-3 protein in the CSF has 96% sensitivity and specificity for CJD among patients with dementia. False positives may occur in other conditions involving extensive neuronal destruction including: acute stroke, herpes encephalitis, multi-infarct dementia, primary CNS lymphoma and rarely SDAT (most cases of SDAT test negative). Requires CSF (cannot be done on blood)
4. EEG: characteristic finding of bilateral, symmetrical, periodic bi- or triphasic synchronous sharp-wave complexes, AKA periodic spikes, AKA pseudoperiodic sharp-wave complexes (0.5–2 per second) have ≈ 70% sensitivity and 86% specificity.[35] They resemble PLEDs (p.238), but are responsive to noxious stimulus (may be absent in familial CJD[19] and in the recent UK variant (see above))
5. SPECT scan: may be abnormal in vCJD even when EEG is normal,[36] however the findings are not specific for vCJD
6. brain biopsy: see below
7. tonsillar biopsy: patients with variant CJD (vCJD) may have detectable levels of variant type 4 of the abnormal prion protein (PrPSc) in their lymphoreticular system, which may be accessed by a 1 cm wedge-biopsy of one palatine tonsil (using careful aseptic precautions)[37]

Brain biopsy

Due to lack of an effective treatment and the potential for iatrogenic infection in surgery, biopsy is reserved for cases where establishing the diagnosis is deemed important, or as part of a research study,[6] or when diagnostic tests are equivocal and other potentially treatable etiologies are suspected.

Technique: to prevent aerosolization of the infectious agent, a manual saw is recommended over a power craniotome, and every effort should be made to avoid cutting the dura with the saw. Recommended decontamination procedures should be followed (▶ Table 22.4 and references). Specimens should be clearly labeled as being from suspected CJD patients to alert laboratory personnel to the hazard. Tissue should be fixed in a saturated 15% phenolized formalin (15 g of phenol per dl of 10% neutral buffered formalin with the undissolved phenol layering at the bottom of the solution).[38]

Analysis for classic histologic findings (see above) and/or immunostaining for PrPres are the gold standards of diagnosis.

22.2.11 Treatment and prognosis

Given the lack of demonstrated infectivity (with tissues other than brain or CSF), isolation precautions such as gowns or masks are felt to be unnecessary.[13]

There is no known treatment. The disease is rapidly progressive. Median survival is 5 months, and 80% of patients with sporadic CJD die within 1 year of diagnosis.[13]

22.3 Parasitic infections of the CNS

22.3.1 General information

A number of parasitic infections may involve the central nervous system. Immunosuppression (including HIV) increases the susceptibility.[39] CNS parasitic infections include (those that potentially involve neurosurgical intervention have a dagger (†):

1. cysticercosis†: see Neurocysticercosis below
2. toxoplasmosis†: may occur as a congenital TORCH infection, or in the adult usually with AIDS; see Neurologic manifestations of AIDS (p.329). Toxoplasma gondii is an obligate intracellular protozoan that is ubiquitous but does not cause clinical infection except in immunocompromised hosts. Histologic features: necrosis containing 2–3 nm tachyzoites (cysts)
3. echinococcus† (p.375)
4. amebiasis†: ≈ exclusively Naegleria fowleri (p.377)
5. schistosomiasis
6. malaria
7. African trypanosomiasis.

† parasitic infections with a dagger are those that are more likely to come to neurosurgical attention.

22.3.2 Neurocysticercosis

General information

Key concepts

- intracranial encystment of larva of Taenia solium (pork tapeworm)
- the most common parasitic infection of the CNS
- neurological symptoms: seizures or progressive intracranial hypertension
- occurs from ingesting the parasite's eggs, not from eating infested meat
- characteristic imaging finding: low density cysts with eccentric punctate high density (the scolex = tapeworm head). Hydrocephalus is common
- medical treatment: all patients get steroids. Start antihelmintic drugs (praziquantel or albendazole) when no signs of intracranial hypertension
- biopsy sometimes needed for diagnosis. Surgery: may be required for spinal, intraventricular or subarachnoid cysts (more refractory to medical therapy) or for giant cysts (> 50 mm) when intracranial hypertension persists despite steroids

2. cysticercus racemosus: larger (4–12 cm), grows actively producing grape-like clusters in the basal subarachnoid spaces and produces intense inflammation. There are *no larvae* in these cysts. These cysts usually degenerate in 2–5 years, in which the capsule thickens and the clear cyst contents are replace by a whitish gel which undergoes calcium deposition with concomitant shrinkage of the cyst

Location of the cysts tends to fall into 1 of 4 groups:
1. meningeal: found in 27–56% of cases with neural involvement. Cysts are adherent or free-floating and are located either in:
   a) dorsolateral subarachnoid space: usually *C. cellulosae* type, causing minimal symptoms
   b) basal subarachnoid space: usually the expanding *C. racemosus* form producing arachnoiditis and fibrosis comprising a chronic meningitis with hypoglycorrhachia. Can obstruct foramina of Luschka and Magendie producing hydrocephalus, or can cause entrapment of basal cisterns → cranial neuropathies (including visual disturbance). Extremely high mortality with this form
2. parenchymal: found in 30–63%; focal or generalized seizures occurs in ≈ 50% of cases (up to 92% in some series)
3. ventricular: found in 12–18%, possibly gaining access via the choroid plexus. Pedunculated or free floating cysts occur, can block CSF flow and cause hydrocephalus with intermittent intracranial hypertension (Brun syndrome). There may be adjacent ependymal enhancement (ependymitis)
4. mixed lesions: found in ≈ 23%

Clinical

Presentation: seizures, signs of elevated ICP (36% of patients with CNS cysticercosis present with increased ICP[46]), focal deficits related to the location of the cyst, and altered mental status are the most common findings. Increased ICP may be due to hydrocephalus or to giant cysts. Symptoms may also be produced by the immunologic reaction to the infestation (cysticercotic encephalitis). Cranial nerve palsies can occur with basal arachnoiditis. Subcutaneous nodules may sometimes be felt.

Diagnosis

General information

Diagnosis is usually made by imaging studies and confirmatory serologic tests.

Laboratory evaluation

Mild peripheral eosinophilia can occur, but is inconsistent and thus unreliable.

CSF may be normal. Eosinophils are seen in 12–60% of cases and suggests parasitic infection. Protein may be elevated.

Stool: less than 33% of cases have T. solium ova in the stool.

Serology

Most centers use enzyme-linked immunoelectrotransfer blot (EIBT) against glycoprotein antigens (western blot) which is ≈ 100% specific and 98% sensitive,[47] although sensitivity is less (70%) in cases with a solitary cyst.[48] May be used on serum or CSF. EIBT has effectively superseded ELISA where titer is considered significant at 1:64 in serum, and 1:8 in the CSF; checking for titer exceeding these thresholds in the serum produces a test that is more sensitive and in the CSF is more specific for cysticercosis. False negative rates are higher in cases without meningitis.

Radiographic evaluation

Soft-tissue x-rays may show calcifications in subcutaneous nodules, and in thigh and shoulder muscles.

Skull x-rays show calcifications in 13–15% of cases with neurocysticercosis. May be single or multiple. Usually circular or oval in shape.

CT

The following findings on brain CT have been described (modified[45,49]):
1. ring enhancing cysts of various sizes representing living cysticerci. Little inflammatory response (edema) occurs as long as larva is alive. Characteristic finding: small (< 2.5 cm) low density cysts with eccentric punctate high density that may represent the scolex

2. low density with ring enhancement seen as an intermediate stage between living cyst and calcified remnant representing intermediate stage in granuloma formation. Resultant inflammatory reaction can cause edema, and basal arachnoiditis in cysts located in basal subarachnoid space. Often ring enhancing
3. intraparenchymal punctate calcifications (granuloma) sometimes with, but usually without surrounding enhancement, seen with dead parasites
4. hydrocephalus. Sometimes with intraventricular cysts which may be isointense with CSF on plain CT[50] and may require contrast CT ventriculography[51] or MRI to be demonstrated

MRI

Early findings: nonenhancing cystic structure(s) with eccentric T1WI hyperintensity (scolex) with no inflammatory response. Lesions may be seen in parenchyma, ventricle, and subarachnoid space. The cyst collapses in later stages of parasitic evolution, with initial edema that gradually resolves with time.

Treatment

Overview

Combination of:
1. antihelmintic medication: antiparasitic and/or cysticidal regimens
2. antiepileptics: to treat seizures, which may sometimes be medically refractory
3. steroids (see below)
4. surgery:
   a) surgical resection of lesions when appropriate
   b) ventricular CSF diversionary procedures

Steroids

Corticosteroids should be used in all patients. May temporarily relieve symptoms, and may help decrease edema that tends to occur initially during treatment with antihelmintic drugs. If possible, start 2–3 d before antihelmintics (e.g. dexamethasone 8 mg q 8 hours[44]), on day 3 decrease to 4 mg q 8 hours, on day 6 change to prednisone 0.4 mg/kg per day divided TID. Taper steroids after antihelmintics are discontinued. In patients with symptoms of intracranial hypertension: antihelmintic treatment is started after symptoms subside (usually after 3 doses). ✖ Any cysticercocidal drug may cause irreversible damage when used to treat ocular or spinal cysts, even with corticosteroid use.

Antiepileptics

Seizures usually respond to a single AED. However, the risk of seizures may be lifelong. Risk factors for recurrent seizures: calcified brain lesions, multiple seizures, multiple brain cysts.[52]

Antihelmintic drugs

Since many lesions resolve on their own, and there are significant side effects to these drugs, their use is controversial.[53]

Praziquantel (Biltricide®) is an antihelmintic with activity against all known species of schistosomas. Several regimens have been published:
- 50 mg/kg/d divided in 3 doses (same dose for pediatrics) for 15 days (doses of 100 mg/kg/d have been recommended[44] because steroids reduce serum concentration by 50%[54]). Produces a significant reduction in symptoms and in number of cysts seen on CT[40]
- 10–100 mg/kg/d × 3–21 days
- high dose single day regimen: 25–30 mg/kg q 2 hrs × 3 doses
- for intestinal infestation: single oral dose of 5–10 mg/kg

Albendazole (Zentel®) 15 mg/kg per day divided in 2–3 doses, taken with a fatty meal to enhance absorption (same dose for pediatrics), may be given for 3 months,[55,56] can be stopped sooner if imaging shows resolution.[44] More parasiticidal than praziquantel and may have fewer side effects.

Niclosamide (Niclocide® and others) may be given orally to treat adult tapeworms in the *GI tract*. ℞ 1 gm (2 tablets) chewed PO, repeated in 1 hour (total = 2 gm).

Intraventricular disease: There is no consensus on the efficacy of medical treatment for intraventricular cysts.[46,44,57]

Surgery

Surgery may sometimes be necessary to establish the diagnosis. Stereotactic biopsy may be well suited for some cases, especially with deep lesions.

CSF diversion is necessary for patients with symptomatic hydrocephalus, although tubing may become obstructed by granulomatous inflammatory debris.[58]

Surgery may be indicated for spinal cysts[42] and for intraventricular cysts which may be less responsive to medical therapy. The latter may sometimes be dealt with using stereotactic techniques and/or endoscopic instrumentation,[51] however, shunting and antihelmintics may suffice.[57] Surgery may also be needed for giant cysts when intracranial hypertension does not respond to steroids.[44] Antihelmintics may be required even after complete surgical removal because of possibility of relapse.[44]

Follow-up

CT or MRI scan every 6 months until lesions disappear or calcify.[44]

Contacts

Both patients with cysticercosis and their personal contacts should be screened for tapeworm infection since a single dose of niclosamide or praziquantel will eliminate the tapeworm.[59] Close contacts of persons with tapeworms should have screening by medical history and serologic testing for cysticercosis; if suggestive of cysticercosis a neurologic exam and CT or MRI should be done.

22.3.3 Echinococcosis

General information

AKA hydatid (cyst) disease. Caused by encysted larvae of the dog tapeworm Echinococcus granulosa in endemic areas (Uruguay, Australia, New Zealand…). The dog is the primary definitive host of the adult worm. Intermediate hosts for the larval stage include sheep and man. Ova are excreted in dog feces and contaminate herbage eaten by sheep. After ingestion, the embryos hatch and the parasite burrows through the duodenal wall to gain hematogenous access to multiple organs (liver, lungs, heart, bone, brain). Dogs eat these infested organs and the parasite enters the intestine where it remains.

Man is infected either by eating food contaminated with ova, or by direct contact with infected dogs. CNS involvement occurs in only ≈ 3%. Produces cerebral cysts that are confined to the white matter. Primary cysts are usually solitary, secondary cysts (e.g. from embolization from cardiac cysts that rupture or from iatrogenic rupture of cerebral cysts) are usually multiple. The CT density of the cyst is similar to CSF, it does not enhance (although rim enhancement may occur if there is an inflammatory reaction), and there is little surrounding edema. It contains germinating parasitic particles called "hydatid sand" containing ≈ 400,000 scoleces/ml. The cyst enlarges slowly (rates of ≈ 1 cm per year are quoted, but this is variable and may be higher in children), and usually does not present until quite large with findings of increased ICP, seizures, or focal deficit. Patients often have eosinophilia and may have positive serologic tests for hydatid disease.

Treatment

Treatment is surgical removal of the intact cyst. Every effort must be made to avoid rupturing these cysts during removal, or else the scoleces may contaminate the adjacent tissues with possible recurrence of multiple cysts or allergic reaction. May use adjunctive medical treatment with albendazole (Zentel®) 400 mg PO BID (pediatric dose: 15 mg/kg/d) × 28 days, taken with a fatty meal, repeated as necessary.[56]

The Dowling technique is recommended[60]:

1. the head is positioned so that the cyst points straight up towards the ceiling when the OR table is 30° head up
2. drilling burr holes and performing craniotomy must be done very carefully to avoid rupturing the cyst or tearing the dura which is thin and under tension
3. do not coagulate with anything but low-power bipolar (to avoid cyst rupture)
4. open the dura circumferentially away from the dome of the cyst as it may be adherent to the dura
5. keep the surface of the cyst moist to prevent desiccation and rupture
6. open the thinned overlying cortex gently, separating it from the cyst with irrigation and cottonoids. The cortical opening need only be ≈ 3/4 the cyst diameter but no less

7. insert a soft rubber catheter between the cyst and the brain, and gently irrigate with saline as the head of the OR table is slowly lowered 45° while the surgeon supports the adjacent cortex with his/her fingers
8. continue irrigating more saline and float the cyst out and into a saline filled receptacle
9. if the cyst is ruptured during the procedure, immediately place a sucker in the cyst to aspirate the contents, remove the capsule, and wash the cavity with saline for 5 minutes. Change instruments and gloves. Placing 10% formalin soaked cottonoids on the cavity for a few minutes is controversial[61 (p 3750)]

22.4 Fungal infections of the CNS

22.4.1 General information

Most are medically treated conditions that do not require neurosurgical intervention. They tend to present either with chronic meningitis or brain abscess. Some of the more common ones or those of particular relevance to neurosurgery include:

1. cryptococcosis: see below
   a) cryptococcal meningitis
   b) cryptococcoma (mucinous pseudocyst): rare
2. candidiasis: the most common fungal infection of the CNS, but rarely diagnosed before autopsy. Very rare in healthy individuals. Most are C. albicans
   a) candidal meningitis (p. 320): the most common CNS infection; see ℞ (p. 320)
   b) parenchymal infection: candida brain abscesses are rare
   c) following ventricular shunt placement: almost all fungal VP shunt infections are due to Candida spp. (p. 339) [62]
3. aspergillosis (p. 322): may be associated with cerebral abscess in organ transplant patients
4. coccidiomycosis: caused by the dimorphic fungus Coccidioides immitis. Endemic in southwestern U.S. (including San Joaquin Valley in southern California), Mexico, and Central America. Usually presents as meningitis, with rare reports of parenchymal lesions[63]
5. mucormycosis (phycomycosis) (p. 568): usually occurs in diabetics

22.4.2 Cryptococcal involvement of the CNS

General information

Cryptococcal CNS involvement with cryptococcus is diagnosed more frequently in living patients than any other fungal disease. Occurs in healthy or immunocompromised patients. In HIV, Cryptococcus neoformans is the typical agent.

1. cryptococcoma (mucinous pseudocyst): a parenchymal collection which occurs almost exclusively in AIDS patients. Much less common than cryptococcal meningitis. No enhancement of the lesion or the meninges. Usually 3–10 mm in diameter and are frequently located in the basal ganglia (due to spread by small perforating vessels)
2. cryptococcal meningitis (p. 376)
   a) occurs in 4–6% of patients with AIDS.[64] Typical symptoms: fever, malaise and H/A.[65] Meningeal signs (nuchal rigidity, photophobia...) occur in only ≈ 25%. Encephalopathic symptoms (lethargy, altered mentation...) usually from increased ICP occur in a minority
   b) can also occur without AIDS: gatti variety can infect the brain of immunocompetent hosts[66]
   c) may be associated with increased ICP (with or without hydrocephalus on CT/MRI), decreased visual acuity, and/or cranial nerve deficits. Dilation of Virchow-Robbins spaces may be seen on imaging; on MRI the signal is similar to CSF on T1WI & T2WI but will be higher signal on FLAIR
   d) late deterioration in the absence of documented infection may respond to decadron 4 mg q 6 hrs transitioned to prednisone 25 mg p.o. q d[67]

Diagnosis

LP

Opening pressure (OP) should be measured in the lateral decubitus position.[68] OP is usually elevated, and is > 20 cm H_2O in up to 75%.

CSF: cryptococcal antigen titer is invariably high with cryptococcal meningitis or meningoencepahlitis.

Serum cryptococcal antigen: almost always elevated with CNS involvement.[68]

Management

2009 CDC guidelines for CNS cryptoccal infection in *HIV*-infected adolescents/adults[68]:

1. antifungal agents: the recommended initial standard treatment[68] is amphotericin B deoxycholate (Amphocin®) 0.7 mg/kg IV q d, plus fluconazole (an oral triazole) 100 mg/kg po q d in 4 divided doses
2. patients with clinical signs of increased ICP (confusion, blurred vision, papilledema, LE clonus…) should have LP to measure ICP
3. management of intracranial hypertension (ICHT) (OP ≥ 25 cm H_2O) with or without hydrocephalus; corticosteroids, acetazolamide and mannitol have not been shown to be effective[69]:
   a) daily LPs: drain enough CSF to reduce ICP by 50% (typically 20–30 ml)[70]
   b) daily LPs may be suspended when pressures are normal for several consecutive days
   c) lumbar drain: occasionally needed for extremely high OPs (> 40 cm H_2O) when frequent LPs are required to or fail to control symptoms[69]
   d) CSF shunt: considered when daily LPs are no longer tolerated or when signs and symptoms of ICHT are not being relieved (neither dissemination of infection through the distal shunt nor creation of a nidus of infection refractory to medical therapy has been described[71]). Options:
      - lumboperitoneal shunt
      - VP or VA shunt[72,73]
4. antifungal treatment is continued for ≥ 2 weeks if renal function is normal (most immunocompetent patients will be successfully treated with 6 weeks of therapy[69])
5. after 2 weeks of treatment, repeat the LP to look for clearance of the organism from the CSF. Positive CSF cultures after 2 weeks of treatment are predictive of future relapse and are associated with worse outcome
6. treatment failures: defined as lack of clinical improvement after 2 weeks of appropriate therapy including management of ICHT, or relapse after an initial response, defined as either a positive CSF culture and/or rising CSF cryptococcal Ag titer with a compatible clinical picture. Management:
   a) optimal management has not been defined
   b) trials with alternative antifungals (e.g. flucytosine) or higher doses of fluconazole
7. maintenance therapy (secondary prophylaxis): HIV patients who have completed 10 weeks of treatment should be maintained on fluconazole 200 mg q d until immune reconstitution occurs, otherwise lifetime treatment is indicated[68]
8. the risk of recurrence is low for patient who remain asymptomatic after a complete course of therapy and have sustained increase (> 6 months) of CD4 + counts to ≥ 200 cells/mcl. Some experts perform an LP to document negative CSF culture and antigen before stopping maintenance therapy

22.5 Amebic infections of the CNS

22.5.1 General information

Naegleria fowleri: the only ameba (alternative spelling: amoeba) known to cause CNS infection in humans → primary amebic meningoencephalitis (PAM): diffuse encephalitis with hemorrhagic necrosis and prurulent meningitis involving brain and spinal cord. Rare (only 95 cases in the U.S. as of 2002, and ≈ 200 cases worldwide as of 2004). The ameba lives in fresh water and soil and typically gains entry to the CNS by invading nasal olfactory mucosa. PAM usually occurs within 5 days of exposure, usually from diving in warm freshwater.

Associated cerebral edema may cause increased ICP and, ultimately, herniation. Fatal in ≈ 95% of cases, usually within 1 week.

CSF: cloudy and often hemorrhagic, ↑ leukocytes, ↑ protein, normal or ↓ glucose, Gram stain negative (no bacteria or fungi), wet prep → motile trophozoites (may be confused with WBCs).

22.5.2 Treatment

Drug of choice: amphotericin B (lipid preparations (Abelcet®) achieve higher MICs (minimal inhibitory concentrations) than other amphotericin preparations). Miconazole may be synergistic with amphotericin B.

Surgical intervention: ventriculostomy with CSF drainage may be indicated when findings are suggestive of increased ICP. In one survivor, surgical drainage of a brain abscess was performed in addition to treatment with a 6-week course of amphotericin B, rifampicin, and chloramphenicol.

22

References

[1] Wilkins RH, Rengachary SS. Neurosurgery. New York 1985

[2] Neils EW, Lukin R, Tomsick TA, Tew JM. Magnetic Resonance Imaging and Computerized Tomography Scanning of Herpes Simplex Encephalitis. J Neurosurg. 1987; 67:592–594

[3] Schroth G, Gawehn J, Thron A, et al. The Early Diagnosis of Herpes Simplex Encephalitis by MRI. Neurology. 1987; 37:179–183

[4] Whitley RJ, Soong S-J, Dolin R, et al. Adenosine Arabinoside Therapy of Biopsy-Proved Herpes Simplex Encephalitis: National Institute of Allergy and Infectious Diseases Collaborative Antiviral Study. N Engl J Med. 1977; 297:289–294

[5] Whitley RJ, Cobbs CG, Alford CA, et al. Diseases that Mimic Herpes Simplex Encephalitis: Diagnosis, Presentation, and Outcome. JAMA. 1989; 262:234–239

[6] Schlitt MJ, Morawetz RB, Bonnin JM, Zeiger HE, Whitley RJ. Brain Biopsy for Encephalitis. Clin Neurosurg. 1986; 33:591–602

[7] Carmack MA, Twiss J, Enzmann DR, et al. Multifocal Leukoencephalitis Caused by Varicella-Zoster Virus in a Child with Leukemia: Successful Treatment with Acyclovir. Pediatr Infect Dis J. 1993; 12:402–406

[8] Horten B, Price RW, Jiminez D. Multifocal Varicella-Zoster Virus Leukoencephalitis Temporally Remote from Herpes Zoster. Ann Neurol. 1981; 9:251–266

[9] Gilden D, Cohrs RJ, Mahalingam R, Nagel MA. Varicella zoster virus vasculopathies: diverse clinical manifestations, laboratory features, pathogenesis, and treatment. Lancet neurology. 2009; 8. DOI: 10.1016/s1474-4422(09)70134-6

[10] Medori R, Montagna P, Tritschler HJ, et al. Fatal Familial Insomnia: A Second Kindred with Mutation of Prion Protein Gene at Codon 178. Neurology. 1992; 42:669–670

[11] Medori R, Tritschler HJ, LeBlanc A, et al. Fatal Familial Insomnia, a Prion Disease with a Mutation at Codon 178 of the Prion Protein Gene. N Engl J Med. 1992; 326:444–449

[12] Manetto V, Medori R, Cortelli P, et al. Fatal familial insomnia: Clinical and pathologic study of five new cases. Neurology. 1992; 42:312–319

[13] Johnson RT, Gibbs CJ. Creutzfeldt-Jakob Disease and Related Transmissible Spongiform Encephalopathies. N Engl J Med. 1998; 339:1994–2004

[14] Gajdusek DC. Unconventional Viruses and the Origin and Disappearance of Kuru. Science. 1977; 197:943–960

[15] Klitzman R. The Trembling Mountain. A Personal Account of Kuru, Cannibals, and Mad Cow Disease. New York: Plenum Trade; 1998

[16] Heckmann JG, Lang CJG, Petruch F, et al. Transmission of Creutzfeldt-Jakob Disease via a Corneal Transplant. J Neurol Neurosurg Psychiatry. 1997; 63:388–390

[17] Brown P, Preece M, Brandel J-P, et al. Iatrogenic Creutzfeldt-Jakob Disease at the Millennium. Neurology. 2000; 55:1075–1081

[18] Hsiao K, Prusiner SB. Inherited Human Prion Diseases. Neurology. 1990; 40:1820–1827

[19] Bertoni JM, Brown P, Goldfarb LG, Rubenstein R, Gajdusek C. Familial Creutzfeldt-Jakob Disease (Codon 200 Mutation) With Supranuclear Palsy. JAMA. 1992; 268:2413–2415

[20] Will RG, Zeidler JW, Cousens SN, et al. A new variant of Creutzfeldt-Jakob disease in the UK. Lancet. 1996; 347:921–925

[21] Duffy P, Wolf J, Collins G, et al. Possible Person to Person Transmission of Creutzfeldt-Jakob Disease. N Engl J Med. 1974; 290:692–693

[22] Bernoulli C, Siegfried J, Baumgartner G, et al. Danger of Accidental Person-To-Person Transmission of Creutzfeldt-Jakob Disease by Surgery. Lancet. 1977; 1:478–479

[23] Fradkin JE, Schonberger LB, Mills JL, et al. Creutzfeldt-Jakob Disease in Pituitary Growth Hormone Recipients in the United States. JAMA. 1991; 265:880–884

[24] Centers for Disease Control (Morbidity and Mortality Weekly Report). Rapidly Progressive Dementia in a Patient Who Received a Cadaveric Dura Mater Graft. JAMA. 1987; 257:1036–1037

[25] Thadani V, Penar PL, Partington J, et al. Creutzfeldt-Jakob disease probably acquired from a cadaveric dura mater graft. J Neurosurg. 1988; 69:766–769

[26] Centers for Disease Control. Creutzfeldt-Jakob Disease in a Second Patient Who Received a Cadaveric Dura Mater Graft. MMWR. 1989; 39:37–43

[27] Rosenberg RN, White CL, Brown P, et al. Precautions in Handling Tissues, Fluids and Other Contaminated Materials from Patients with Documented or Suspected Creutzfeldt-Jakob Disease. Ann Neurol. 1986; 12:75–77

[28] Brown P, Gibbs CJ, Amyx JL, et al. Chemical disinfection of Creutzfeldt-Jakob virus. N Engl J Med. 1982; 306:1279–1282

[29] Brown P, Cathala F, Castaigne P, Gajdusek DC. Creutzfeldt-Jakob Disease: Clinical Analysis of a Consecutive Series of 230 Neuropathologically Verified Cases. Ann Neurol. 1986; 20:597–602

[30] Finkenstaedt M, Szudra A, Zerr I, et al. MR Imaging of Creutzfeldt-Jakob Disease. Radiology. 1996; 199:793–798

[31] Gertz H-J, Henkes H, Cervos-Navarro J. Creutzfeldt-Jakob Disease: Correlation of MRI and Neuropathologic Findings. Neurology. 1988; 38:1481–1482

[32] Otto M, Wiltfang J, Schutz E, et al. Diagnosis of Creutzfeldt-Jakob Disease by Measurement of S100 Protein in Serum: Prospective Case-Control Study. Br Med J. 1998; 316:577–582

[33] Harrington MG, Merril CR, Asher DM, Gajdusek DC. Abnormal Proteins in the Cerebrospinal Fluid of Patients with Creutzfeldt-Jakob Disease. N Engl J Med. 1986; 315:279–283

[34] Hsich G, Kenney K, Gibbs CJ, et al. The 14-3-3 Brain Protein in Cerebrospinal Fluid as a Marker for Transmissible Spongiform Encephaloptahies. N Engl J Med. 1996; 335:924–930

[35] Steinhoff BJ, Räcker S, Herrendorf G, et al. Accuracy and Reliability of Periodic Sharp Wave Complexes in Creutzfeldt-Jakob Disease. Arch Neurol. 1996; 53:162–166

[36] de Silva R, Patterson J, Hadley D, et al. Single photon emission computed tomography in the identification of new variant Creutzfeldt-Jakob disease: Case reports. Br Med J. 1998; 316:593–594

[37] Hill AF, Butterworth RJ, Joiner S, et al. Investigation of Variant Creutzfeldt-Jakob Disease and Other Human Prion Diseases with Tonsil Biopsy Samples. Lancet. 1999; 353:183–189

[38] Brumbach RA. Routine Use of Phenolized Formalin in Fixation of Autopsy Brain Tissue to Reduce Risk of Inadvertent Transmission of Creutzfeldt-Jakob Disease. N Engl J Med. 1988; 319

[39] Walker M, Kublin JG, Zunt JR. Parasitic central nervous system infections in immunocompromised hosts: malaria, microsporidiosis, leishmaniasis, and African trypanosomiasis. Clin Infect Dis. 2006; 42:115–125

[40] Sotelo J, Escobedo F, , et al. Therapy of parenchymal brain cysticercosis with praziquantel. N Engl J Med. 1984; 310:1001–1007

[41] Garcia HH, Gonzales AE, Evans CAW, Gilman RH, The Cysticercosis Working Group in Peru. Taenia solium cysticersosis. Lancet. 2003; 362:547–556

[42] Sotelo J, Guerrero V, Rubio F. Neurocysticercosis: A new classification based on active and inactive forms. Arch Intern Med. 1985; 145:442–445

[43] Garcia HH, Del Brutto OH, for The Cysticercosis Working Group in Peru. Neurocysticercosis: updated concepts about an old disease. Lancet Neurology. 2005; 4:653–661

[44] Proano JV, Madrazo I, Avelar F, Lopez-Felix B, Diaz G, Grijalva I. Medical treatment for neurocysticercosis characterized by giant subarachnoid cysts. N Engl J Med. 2001; 345:879–885

[45] Leblanc R, Knowles KF, Melanson D, MacLean JD, et al. Neurocysticercosis: Surgical and Medical

Management with Praziquantel. Neurosurgery. 1986; 18:419–427
[46] Colli BO, Carlotti CG, Machado HR, Assirati JA. Treatment of Patients with Intraventricular Cysticercosis. Contemp Neurosurg. 1999; 21:1–7
[47] Wilson M, Bryan RT, Fried JA, et al. Clinical Evaluation of the Cysticercosis Enzyme-Linked Immunoelectrotransfer Blot in Patients with Neurocysticercosis. J Infect Dis. 1991; 164:1007–1009
[48] Prabhakaran V, Rajshekhar V, Murrell KD, Oommen A. Taenia solium metacestode glycoproteins as diagnostic antigens for solitary cysticercus granuloma in Indian patients. Trans R Soc Trop Med Hyg. 2004; 98:478–484
[49] Enzman DR. In: Cysticercosis. Imaging of Infections and Inflammations of the Central Nervous System: Computed Tomography, Ultrasound, and Nuclear Magnetic Resonance. New York: Raven Press; 1984:103–122
[50] Madrazo I, Renteria JAG, Paredes G, Olhagaray B. Diagnosis of Intraventricular and Cisternal Cysticercosis by Computerized Tomography with Positive Intraventricular Contract Medium. J Neurosurg. 1981; 55:947–951
[51] Apuzzo MLJ, Dobkin WR, Zee C-S, Chan JC, et al. Surgical Considerations in Treatment of Intraventricular Cysticercosis: An Analysis of 45 Cases. J Neurosurg. 1984; 60:400–407
[52] Del Brutto OH. Prognostic factors for seizure recurrence after withdrawal of entiepileptic drugs in patients with neurocysticercosis. Neurology. 1994; 44:1706–1709
[53] Abba K, Ramaratnam S, Ranganathan LN. Anthelmintics for people with neurocysticercosis. Cochrane Database Syst Rev. 2010. DOI: 10.1002/14651858.CD000215.pub3
[54] Jung H, Hurtado M, Sanchez M, Medina MT, Sotelo J. Plasma and CSF levels of albendazole and praziquantel in patients with neurocysticercosis. Clin Neuropharmacol. 1990; 13:559–564
[55] Sotelo J, Penagos P, Escobedo F, Del Brutto OH. Short Course of Albendazole Therapy for Neurocysticercosis. Arch Neurol. 1988; 45:1130–1133
[56] Drugs for Parasitic Infections. Med Letter. 1995; 37:99–108
[57] Bandres JC, White AC, Jr, Samo T, Murphy EC, Harris RL. Extraparenchymal neurocysticercosis: report of five cases and review of management. Clin Infect Dis. 1992; 15:799–811
[58] McCormick GF, Zee C-S, Heiden J. Cysticercosis Cerebri. Arch Neurol. 1982; 39:534–539
[59] Centers for Disease Control. Locally acquired neurocysticercosis. MMWR. 1992; 41:1–4
[60] Carrea R, Dowling E, Guevara JA. Surgical Treatment of Hydatid Cysts of the Central Nervous System in the Pediatric Age (Dowling's Technique). Childs Brain. 1975; 1:4–21
[61] Youmans JR. Neurological Surgery. Philadelphia 1990
[62] Sanchez-Portocarrero J, Martin-Rabadan P, Saldana CJ, Perez-Cecilia E. Candida cerebrospinal fluid shunt infection. Report of two new cases and review of the literature. Diagn Microbiol Infect Dis. 1994; 20:33–40
[63] Mendel E, Milefchik EN, Ahmadi J, Gruen P. Coccidioidomycotic Brain Abscess: Case Report. J Neurosurg. 1994; 80:140–142
[64] Chuck SL, Sande MA. Infections with cryptococcus neoformans in the acquired immunodeficiency syndrome. N Engl J Med. 1989; 321:794–799
[65] Aberg JA, Powderly WG, Dolin R, Masur H, Saag MS. In: Cryptococcosis. AIDS Therapy. New York: Churcill Livingstone; 2002:498–510
[66] Lan S, Chang W, Lu C, Lui C, Chang H. Cerebral infarction in chronic meningitis: a comparison of tuberculous meningitis and cryptococcal meningitis. Q J Med. 2001; 94:247–253
[67] Lane M, McBride J, Archer J. Steroid responsive late deterioration in Cryptococcus neoformans variety gattii meningitis. Neurology. 2004; 63:713–714
[68] Kaplan JE, Benson C, Holmes KH, Brooks JT, Pau A, Masur H, Centers for Disease Control, Prevention, National Institutes of Health. Guidelines for prevention and treatment of opportunistic infections in HIV-infected adults and adolescents. MMWR Recomm Rep. 2009; 58:1–207; quiz CE1-4
[69] Saag MS, Graybill RJ, Larsen RA, Pappas PG, Perfect JR, et al. Practice guidelines for the management of crytpococcal disease. Clin Infect Dis. 2000; 30:710–718
[70] Fessler RD, Sobel J, Guyot L, Crane L, Vazquez J, Szuba MJ, Diaz FG. Management of elevated intracranial pressure in patients with Cryptococcal meningitis. J Acquir Immune Defic Syndr Hum Retrovirol. 1998; 17:137–142
[71] Park MK, Hospenthal DR, Bennett JE. Treatment of hydrocephalus secondary to cryptococcal meningitis by use of shunting. Clin Infect Dis. 1999; 28:629–633
[72] Bach MC, Tally PW, Godofsky EW. Use of cerebrospinal fluid shunts in patients having acquired immunodeficiency syndrome with cryptococcal meningitis and uncontrollable intracranial hypertension. J Neurosurg. 1997; 41:1280–1283
[73] Liliang PC, Liang CL, Chang WN, Lu K, Lu CH. Use of ventriculoperitoneal shunts to treat uncontrollable intracranial hypertension in patients who have cryptococcal meningitis without hydrocephalus. Clin Infect Dis. 2002; 34:E64–E68

Part VII

Hydrocephalus and Cerebrospinal Fluid (CSF)

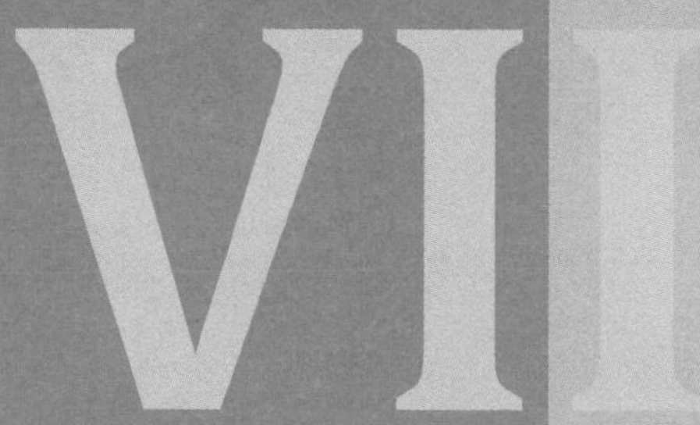

23 Cerebrospinal Fluid

23.1 General information

Cerebrospinal fluid (CSF) surrounds the brain and spinal cord, and may function as a shock absorber for the CNS. It may also serve an immunological function analogous to the lymphatic system.[1] It circulates within the subarachnoid space, between the arachnoid and the pial membranes.

CSF is normally a clear colorless fluid with a specific gravity of 1.007 and a pH of ≈ 7.33–7.35.

23.2 Production

23.2.1 Location

80% of CSF is produced by the choroid plexuses, located in both lateral ventricles (accounts for ≈ 95% of CSF produced in the choroid plexuses) and in the 4th ventricle. Most of the rest of intracranial production occurs in the interstitial space.[2] A small amount may also be produced by the ependymal lining of the ventricles. In the spine, it is produced primarily in the dura of the nerve root sleeves. ▶ Table 23.1 shows properties of CSF production, volumes and pressures.

23.2.2 Production rate

In the adult, CSF is produced at a rate of about 0.3 ml/min ▶ Table 23.1). In terms that are clinically relevant, this approximates 450 ml/24hrs, which means that in an adult (where the average total CSF volume in the body is 150 ml), the CSF is "turned over" ≈ 3 times every day. The rate of formation is independent of the intracranial pressure[3] (except in the limiting case when ICP becomes so high that cerebral blood flow is reduced[4]).

23.3 Absorption

CSF is absorbed primarily by arachnoid villi (granulations) that extend into the dural venous sinuses. Other sites of absorption include the choroid plexuses and lymphatics. The rate of absorption is pressure dependent.[5]

23.4 CSF constituents

23.4.1 Cellular components of CSF

In normal adult CSF, there are 0–5 lymphocytes or mononuclear cells per mm³, and no polys (PMNs) or RBCs. In the absence of RBCs, 5–10 WBCs per mm³ is suspicious, and > 10 WBCs per mm³ is definitely abnormal.

Table 23.1 Normal CSF production, volumes, and pressure

Property	Peds		Adult
	Newborn	1–10 yrs	
total volume (ml)	5		150 (50% intracranial, 50% spinal)
formation rate	25 ml/d		≈ 0.3–0.35 ml/min (≈ 450–750 ml/d)
pressure[a] (cm of fluid)	9–12	mean: 10 normal: < 15	adult: 7–15 (> 18 usually abnormal) young adult: < 18–20

[a]as measured in the lumbar subarachnoid space, with the patient relaxed in the lateral decubitus position

23.4.2 Noncellular components of CSF

Table 23.2 CSF solutes.[6(p 169),7] For CEA, AFP, & hCG, see Tumor markers (p. 598)

Constituent	Units	CSF	Plasma	CSF:plasma ratio
osmolarity	mOsm/L	295	295	1.0
H_2O content		99%	93%	
sodium	mEq/L	138	138	1.0
potassium	mEq/L	2.8	4.5	0.6
chloride	mEq/L	119	102	1.2
calcium	mEq/L	2.1	4.8	0.4
pCO_2	mm Hg	47	41[a]	1.1
pH		7.33	7.41	
pO_2	mm Hg	43	104[a]	0.4
glucose	mg/dl	60	90	0.67
lactate	mEq/L	1.6	1.0[a]	1.6
pyruvate	mEq/L	0.08	0.11[a]	0.73
lactate:pyruvate		26	17.6[a]	
total protein[b]	mg/dl	35	7000	0.005
albumin	mg/L	155	36600	0.004
IgG	mg/L	12.3	9870	0.001

[a]arterial plasma
[b]Note: CSF protein is lower in ventricular fluid than in lumbar subarachnoid space
Data from Table 6–1 of "Cerebrospinal Fluid in Diseases of the Nervous System" by Robert A. Fishman, M.D., © 1980, W. B. Saunders Co., Philadelphia, PA, used with permission

23.4.3 Variation with site

The composition of CSF differs slightly in the ventricles where the majority of it is produced compared to the lumbar subarachnoid space.

23.4.4 CSF variations with age

Table 23.3 Variations with age

Age group	WBC /mm³	RBC /mm³	Protein (mg/dl)	Glucose (mg/dl)	Glucose ratio (CSF:plasma)
newborn					
preemie	10	many	150	20–65	0.5–1.6
term	7–8	mod	80	30–120	0.4–2.5
infants					
1–12 mos	5–6	0	15–80		
1–2 yrs	2–3	0	15		

Table 23.3 continued

Age group	WBC /mm³	RBC /mm³	Protein (mg/dl)	Glucose (mg/dl)	Glucose ratio (CSF:plasma)
young child	2–3	0	20		
child 5–15 yrs	2–3	0	25		
adolescent & adult	3	0	30	40–80	0.5
senile	5	0	40[a]		

[a]normal CSF protein rises ≈ 1 mg/dl per year of age in the adult

23.5 Cranial CSF fistula

Key concepts

- suspect in posttraumatic otorrhea/rhinorrhea or recurrent meningitis
- management strategy: 1) confirm the fluid is CSF, 2) identify the site of origin of the leak, 3) determine etiology/mechanism
- most bedside tests are unreliable and include: "reservoir sign", target/halo sign, qualitative glucose
- most accurate confirmatory test is β2-transferrin
- CT cisternography is the test of choice for localizing site of fistula

23.5.1 General information

AKA CSF leak. CSF fistula should be suspected in patients with otorrhea or rhinorrhea after head trauma, or in patients with recurrent meningitis.

23.5.2 Possible routes of egress of CSF

1. mastoid air cells (especially after p-fossa surgery, e.g. for vestibular schwannoma (VS))
2. sphenoid air cells (especially post-transsphenoidal surgery)
3. cribriform plate/ethmoidal roof (floor of frontal fossa)
4. frontal sinus air cells
5. herniation into empty sella and then into sphenoid air sinus
6. along path of internal carotid artery
7. Rosenmüller's fossa: located just inferior to cavernous sinus, may be exposed by drilling off anterior clinoids to allow access to ophthalmic artery aneurysms
8. site of the opening of the transient lateral craniopharyngeal canal
9. percutaneously through a surgical or traumatic wound
10. petrous ridge or internal auditory canal: following temporal bone fracture or vestibular schwannoma surgery. Then either:
    a) rhinorrhea: through middle ear → eustachian tube → nasopharynx
    b) otorrhea: via perforated tympanic membrane → external auditory canal

23.5.3 Traumatic vs. nontraumatic etiology

Description

Two major subgroups of CSF fistula (omitting the ambiguous category of "spontaneous")[8]:

1. traumatic (or posttraumatic): may occur acutely or may be delayed
   a) post-procedure (iatrogenic). Including: post-transsphenoidal surgery and post skull base surgery
   b) posttraumatic (more common): 67–77% of cases
2. nontraumatic
   a) high pressure
      - hydrocephalus
      - tumor

Table 23.4 CSF findings in various pathologic conditions (adult values)[a]

Condition	OP (cm H_2O)	Appearance	Cells (per mm^3)	Protein (mg%)	Glucose (% serum)	Miscellaneous
normal	7–18	clear colorless	0 PMN, 0 RBC 0–5 monos	15–45	50	
acute purulent meningitis	Freq ↑	turbid	few-20K (WBCs mostly PMNs)	100–1000	< 20	few cells early or if treated
viral meningitis & encephalitis	nl	nl	few-350 WBCs (mostly monos)	40–100	nl	PMNs early
Guillain-Barré	nl	nl	nl	50–1000	nl	protein ↑ freq. IgG
polio	nl	nl	50–250 (monos)	40–100	nl	
TB meningitis[b]	freq ↑	opalescent, yellow, fibrin clot on standing	50–500 (lympho-cytes and monocytes)	60–700	20–40	PMN early, (+) AFB culture, (+) Ziel-Neelson stain
fungal meningitis	Freq ↑	opalescent	30–300 (monos)	100–700	< 30	(+) India ink prep with cryptococcus
amebic meningoencephalitis (Naegleria)	freq ↑	cloudy, may be hemorrhagic	↑ WBCs (400–26K), ↑ RBCs	↑	nl or ↓	negative Gram stain; wet mount → motile trophozoites (p.377)
parameningeal infection	↑ if block	nl	WBCs nl or ↑(0–800)	↑	nl	e.g. spinal epidural abscess
traumatic[c] (bloody) tap	nl	bloody; supernatant colorless	RBC:WBC ratio ≈ as in peripheral	slight ↑	nl	RBCs ↓ in successive tubes; no xanthochromia
SAH[c]	↑	bloody; supernatant xanthochromic	early: ↑RBCs	50–400	nl or ↓	RBCs disappear In 2 wks, xanthochromia may persist for weeks
			late: ↑WBCs	100–800		
multiple sclerosis (MS)[d]	nl	nl	5–50 monos	nl-800	nl	usually ↑ gamma globulins (oligoclonal)

[a]abbreviations: OP = opening pressure; nl = normal; ↑ = increased; ↓ = decreased; freq = frequently
[b]the CSF findings in TB meningitis are almost pathognomonic when they occur in combination; 20–30% have acid-fast bacilli in their CSF sediment smears
[c]to differentiate traumatic tap from SAH, see Differentiating SAH from traumatic tap (p.1506)
[d]see more information on the CSF in MS (p.181)

b) normal pressure
- congenital defects
- bony erosion from infection or necrosis
- focal atrophy (olfactory or sellar)

Traumatic fistula

Occur in 2–3% of all patients with head injury, 60% occur within days of trauma, 95% within 3 months.[9] 70% of cases of CSF rhinorrhea stop within 1 wk, and usually within 6 mos in the rest. Non-traumatic cases cease spontaneously in only 33%. Adult:child ratio is 10:1, rare before age 2 yrs. In children the incidence of CSF leaks is less than 1% of closed head injuries.[10] Anosmia is common in traumatic leaks (78%), rare in spontaneous.[11] Most (80–85%) CSF otorrhea ceases in 5–10 days.

CSF fistula occurred in 8.9% of 101 cases of penetrating trauma, and increases the infection rate over those penetrating injuries without fistula (50% vs. 4.6%).[12] It is reported to occur post-op in up to 30% of cases of skull-base surgery.[13]

Nontraumatic CSF fistula

General information

Nontraumatic leaks primarily occur in adults > 30 yrs. Often insidious. May be mistaken for allergic rhinitis. Unlike traumatic leaks, these tend to be intermittent, the sense of smell is usually preserved, and pneumocephalus is uncommon.[14]

Sometimes associated with the following[15]

1. agenesis of the floor of the anterior fossa (cribriform plate) or middle fossa
2. empty sella syndrome (p. 773): primary or post transsphenoidal surgery
3. increased ICP and/or hydrocephalus
4. infection of the paranasal sinuses
5. tumor: including pituitary adenomas (p. 718), meningiomas
6. a persistent remnant of the craniopharyngeal canal[16]
7. AVM[14]
8. congenital anomalies: most involve dehiscence of bone
   a) dehiscence of the footplate of the stapes (a congenital abnormality) which can produce CSF rhinorrhea via the eustachian tube[14]
   b) dehiscence below foramen rotundum

Spontaneous posterior fossa CSF fistula

1. pediatric: usually presents with either meningitis or hearing loss
   a) preserved labyrinthine function (hearing and balance): these usually present with meningitis. 3 usual routes of fistula:
      - facial canal: can fistulize into middle ear
      - petromastoid canal: along path of arterial supply to mucosa of mastoid air sinuses
      - Hyrtl's fissure (AKA tympanomeningeal fissure): links p-fossa to hypotympanum
   b) anomalies of labyrinth (hearing lost): one of several types of Mundini dysplasias, usually presenting with rounded labyrinth/cochlea that permits CSF to erode through oval or round window into auditory canal
2. adult: usually presents with conductive hearing loss with serous effusion, meningitis (often following an episode of otitis media), or cerebral abscess. Occurs most commonly through middle fossa. May be due to arachnoid granulations eroding into air sinus compartment

23.6 Spinal CSF fistula

Often presents with postural headache associated with neck stiffness and tenderness.[17]

23.7 Meningitis in CSF fistula

Incidence with posttraumatic CSF leak: 5–10%, increases as leak persists > 7 days. Meningitis is more common with spontaneous fistula. Risk may be higher in fistula following a neurosurgical procedure than in post-traumatic fistula possibly due to elevated ICP common in latter (forces CSF outward).

Meningitis may promote inflammatory changes at the site of the leak, with a resultant cessation of the leak. However, this often proves to be a temporary resolution, providing a false sense of security.

Pneumococcal meningitis is the most common pathogen (83% of cases[18]), mortality is lower than in pneumococcal meningitis without underlying fistula (< 10% vs. 50%), possibly because the latter is frequently seen in elderly debilitated patients. Prognosis in children is worse.[9]

23.8 Evaluation of the patient with CSF fistula

23.8.1 Determining if rhinorrhea or otorrhea is due to a CSF fistula

1. characteristics of the fluid suggesting the presence of CSF
   a) fluid is as clear as water (unless infected or admixed with blood)
   b) fluid does not cause excoriation within or outside the nose
   c) patients with CSF rhinorrhea describe the taste as salty
2. confirmatory tests
   a) β_2-transferrin: present in CSF, but absent in tears, saliva, nasal exudates and serum (except for newborns and patients with liver disease).[19,20] The only other source is the vitreous fluid of the eye. It may be detected by protein electrophoresis. A minimum of ≈ 0.5 ml needs to be collected, placed in a sterile urine container, packed in dry ice, and shipped to a lab that can perform this study. Very sensitive & specific
   b) collect fluid and obtain *quantitative* glucose (urine glucose detection strips are too sensitive, and may be positive even with excess mucus). Test the fluid shortly after collection to minimize fermentation. Normal CSF glucose is > 30 mg% (usually lower with meningitis) whereas lacrimal secretions and mucus are usually < 5 mg%. A negative test is more helpful since it rules out CSF (except in hypoglycorrhachia (low glucose in the CSF)), but there is a 45–75% chance of false positive[21 (p 1638)]
   c) "ring sign": when a CSF leak is suspected but the fluid is blood tinged, allow the fluid to drip onto linen (sheet or pillowcase). A ring of blood with a larger concentric ring of clear fluid (so called "double ring" or halo sign) suggests the presence of CSF. An old, but unreliable, sign
   d) reservoir sign: a gush of fluid that occurs with a certain head position. Most commonly when first sitting up after a period of recumbency. Thought to indicate drainage of CSF pooled in the sphenoid sinus. Not reliable[22]
3. radiographic signs: pneumocephalus on CT or skull x-ray. Pneumocephalus occurs in ≈ 20% of patients with CSF leaks[23 (p 280)]
4. cisternogram: intrathecal injection of radionuclide tracer followed by scintigram or injection of radiopaque contrast followed by CT scan (see below)
5. anosmia is present in ≈ 5% of CSF leaks
6. following skull-base surgery (especially involving greater superficial petrosal nerve) there may be a pseudo-CSF rhinorrhea possibly due to nasal hypersecretion from imbalanced autonomic regulation of the nasal mucosa[13] ipsilateral to the surgery. Often accompanied by nasal stuffiness and absent ipsilateral lacrimation, and occasionally by facial flushing

Localizing the site of CSF fistula

90% of the time, localization does not require water-soluble contrast CT cisternography (WS-CTC) (see below).

1. CT: to detect pneumocephalus, fractures, skull base defects, hydrocephalus and obstructive neoplasms. Include thin *coronal* cuts or reconstructions through anterior fossa all the way back to the sella turcica
   a) non-contrast (optional): to demonstrate bony anatomy
   b) with IV contrast: leak site is usually associated with abnormal enhancement of adjacent brain parenchyma (possibly from inflammation)
2. water-soluble contrast CT cisternography (procedure of choice): see below
3. plain skull x-ray (helpful in only 21%)
4. MRI: may provide additional information for localization and can R/O p-fossa mass, tumor, and empty sella better than CT. Both CT and MRI can R/O hydrocephalus. T2WI fast spin-echo sequences with fat suppression and video image reversal have been used to visualize CSF flow (sensitivity and specificity are 0.87 and 0.57 respectively)[24]
5. older tests (abandoned in favor of above):
   a) radionuclide cisternography (RNC): not a contemporary test. Poor localization. Some of the studied radiopharmaceuticals are no longer available
   b) intrathecal (visible) dye studies: some success with indigo carmine or fluorescein (p. 1426) with little or no complications.
      ✖ methylene blue (p. 1426) is neurotoxic and should not be used

Water-soluble contrast CT cisternography

Procedure of choice. This test is performed if:

1. no site identified on plain CT (with coronals)

2. when patient is leaking clinically (the site is only sometimes identified in the absence of an active leak)
3. when multiple bony defects are identified, and it is essential to determine which site is actively leaking
4. if a bony defect seen on plain CT does not have associated changes of abnormal enhancement of adjacent brain parenchyma

Technique[25]: Use iohexol (p.219) 6–7 ml of 190–220 mg/ml injected into lumbar subarachnoid space via 22 gauge spinal needle (or 5 ml via C1–2 puncture). Patient positioned in -70° Trendelenburg × 3 min prone with neck gently flexed, in CT they are kept prone with head hyperextended with 5 mm coronal cuts with 3 mm overlap (use 1.5 mm cuts if necessary). May need provocative maneuvers (coronal scans prone (brow up) or in position of leak, intrathecal saline infusion (requires Harvard pump)[26]…).

Look for accumulation of contrast in air sinuses. Apparent discontinuity of bone on CT without extravasation of contrast is probably not the site of leakage (bone discontinuities may be mimicked by partial volume averaging on CT).

23.9 Treatment for CSF fistula

23.9.1 Initial treatment

Acutely after trauma, observation is justified as most cases cease spontaneously.

Prophylactic antibiotics: Controversial. There was no difference in the incidence or morbidity of meningitis between treated and untreated patients.[27] Furthermore, the risk of selecting resistant strains appears real[9] and is therefore usually avoided.

23.9.2 For persistent posttraumatic or post-op leaks

Non-surgical treatment

1. measures to lower ICP:
   a) bed rest: although recumbency may ameliorate symptoms, there is no other benefit from bed rest[28]
   b) avoid straining (stool softeners) and avoid blowing nose
   c) acetazolamide (250 mg PO QID) to reduce CSF production
   d) modest fluid restriction; caution post-transsphenoidal because of possible DI (p.120): 1500 ml/day in adults, 75% of maintenance/day in peds
2. if leak persists (caution: first R/O obstructive hydrocephalus with CT or MRI)
   a) LP: q d to BID (lower pressure to near atmospheric or until H/A)
   OR
   b) continuous lumbar drainage (CLD): via percutaneous catheter. Two (of many) management options:
      - keep HOB elevated 10–15° and place drip chamber at shoulder level (lower the chamber if leak persists) and leave open to drain (uses pressure to regulate drainage – may be dangerous e.g. if drainage bag falls to floor)
      - allow 15–20 cc to drain, then clamp tubing. Repeat q 1 hour
   c) CLD may require ICU monitoring. If patient deteriorates with drain in place: immediately stop drainage, place patient flat in bed (or slight Trendelenburg), start 100% O_2, get CT or bedside cross-table skull x-ray (to R/O tension pneumocephalus due to drawing in of air)
3. surgical treatment in persistent cases (see below)

Surgical treatment

General information

If the site of leakage is not identified prior to attempted surgical treatment, 30% develop a recurrent leak post-op, with 5–15% of these developing meningitis before leak is stopped.[26]

Indications for surgical intervention

1. **traumatic** CSF leak that persists > 2 weeks in spite of non-surgical measures
2. **spontaneous** leaks and those of **delayed onset following trauma** or surgery: usually require surgery because of a high incidence of recurrence
3. leaks complicated by recurrent **meningitis**

Leaks through cribriform plate/ethmoidal roof

Extradural approach: Generally preferred by ENT surgeons.[29] If a frontal craniotomy is being performed, an intradural approach should be used since problems may arise in dissecting the dura off of the floor of the frontal fossa, wherein the dura almost always tears and then it is difficult to know if an identified tear is the cause of the leak or if it is iatrogenic. Fluorescein dye mixed with CSF injected intrathecally may help demonstrate the leak intraoperatively. *CAUTION*: must be diluted with CSF to reduce risk of seizures (p.1426).

Intradural approach

Generally the procedure of choice.[30] If the fistula site is unidentified preoperatively, use a bifrontal bone flap.

General techniques of *intradural* approach:

Close bone defects with fat, muscle, cartilage, or bone.

Close dural defect with fascia lata, temporalis muscle fascia, or pericranium. Fibrin glue may be used to help hold tissue in place.

If the leak is unidentified pre-op and intra-op, then pack both cribriform plates and sphenoid sinus (incise dura over tuberculum sellae, drill through bone to reach sphenoid sinus, remove mucosa or pack it inferiorly, pack with fat).

Post op: lumbar drain after craniotomy is controversial. Some feel CSF pressure may help enhance the seal.[31] If used, place the drip chamber at the level of shoulder for 3–5 days (for precautions, see above).

Consider shunt (LP or VP) if elevated ICP or hydrocephalus is demonstrated.

Leaks into sphenoid sinus (including post-transsphenoidal surgery leak)

1. LP BID or CLD: as long as pressure > 150 mm H_2O or CSF xanthochromic
   a) if leak persists > 3 days: repack sphenoid sinus and pterygoid recesses with fat, muscle, cartilage and/or fascia lata (must reconstruct floor of sella, packing alone is inadequate). Some recommend against muscle since it putrefies and shrinks. Continue LP or CLD as above for 3–5 days post-op
   b) if leak persists > 5 days: lumboperitoneal shunt (first R/O obstructive hydrocephalus)
2. more difficult surgical approach: intracranial (intradural) approach to medial aspect of middle cranial fossa
3. consider transnasal sellar injection of fibrin glue under local anesthesia[32]

Petrous bone

May present as otorrhea or as rhinorrhea (via the eustachian tube).

1. following posterior fossa surgery: see also treatment following vestibular schwannoma surgery (p.685)
2. following mastoid bone fractures: may be approached via extensive mastoidectomy[14]
3. due to dehiscence of the footplate of the stapes: may require obliteration of the middle ear and eustachian tube through a tympanomeatal flap[14]

23.10 Intracranial hypotension (spontaneous)

23.10.1 General information

Intracranial hypotension may be spontaneous or post-traumatic (including iatrogenic, e.g. post-LP). This chapter addresses spontaneous intracranial hypotension (SIH).

Key concepts

- orthostatic headache (headache that is improved in recumbency)
- diagnosed clinically with assistance of LP
- characteristic findings on imaging not required for dx : "SEEPS" (sagging brain, pachymeningeal enhancement, engorged veins, pituitary hyperemia, subdural fluid)
- excludes patients with history of dural puncture, penetrating spinal trauma, spinal surgery or procedures
- epidural blood patch provides relief in the majority of patients

Epidemiology

Incidence 5:100,000, prevalence 1:50,000.[33,34] More common in females[33,34,35,36] with mean age of presentation in the 40's.[34,35]

Clinical

The syndrome of spontaneous intracranial hypotension is characterized by the following in the absence of antecedent trauma or dural puncture:
1. orthostatic headache: dramatically worse when upright, improved in recumbency
2. low CSF pressure
3. diffuse pachymeningeal enhancement (cerebral and/or spinal) on MRI

Most patients have orthostatic headache with sudden onset, but other headaches have been described such as thunderclap, non-positional, exertional headaches, headaches at the end of the day, and even paradoxical headaches with worsening upon lying.[36,37] Atypical patients have been described without headache, without pachymeningeal enhancement on MRI,[38] with clinical signs of encephalopathy, cervical myelopathy or parkinsonism.[39] Since some patients may have normal intracranial pressure, the term "CSF hypovolemia" has been suggested.[40]

Diagnosis

Diagnostic criteria per IHS Classification (ICHD-III)[41]:
1. any headache fulfilling criterion C (see below)
2. low CSF pressure (< 6 cm of water) and/or evidence of CSF leakage on imaging
3. headache has developed in temporal relation to the low CSF pressure or CSF leakage, or has led to its discovery
4. not better accounted for by another ICHD-III

Compared to older criteria,[36,42] current diagnostic criteria exclude the need for the headache to worsen within 15 minutes from sitting or standing, eliminate the need for specific associated symptoms used previously to aid in diagnosis although some of these symptoms are often seen (neck stiffness, tinnitus, hypacusia, photophobia, nausea), exclude the need for MRI as there is no change seen in 20-25% of patients,[33,36,37,43] and exclude the effectiveness of epidural blood patch within 72hrs, as it has no effect in approximately 25% of patients.[33,36,44]

Median delay from presentation to diagnosis of SIH is 4 months.[34,35] This delay may be detrimental to patient outcomes. Therefore, brain MRI without and with contrast is recommended in patients with new onset orthostatic headaches.[35]

Pathophysiology

The underlying cause of SIH is a spontaneous CSF leak.[34] Evidence supports an underlying weakness of the meninges as a contributing factor, for instance connective tissue disorders like Marfan syndrome, and Ehlers-Danlos syndrome.[17,33,34,45] Spinal diverticula, at the cervicothoracic junction or thoracic spine, thoracic being more common,[34,36,37] and excluding lumbosacral perineural cysts, are thought to be the source of CSF leak in most patients. No relationship has been found between cranial leaks and SIH.[33,46] Other causes of dural injury are degenerative disc disease, osteophytes and bony spurs.[34] The orthostatic headache is believed to be caused by the descent of the brain, causing strain on intracranial structures sensitive to pain.[33,37,47]

Evaluation

1. radiographic studies
   a) MRI Brain: findings (mnemonic **SEEPS**)
      - Sagging of the brain caused by the loss of buoyancy from low CSF volume.[33,37] Associated with low lying cerebellar tonsils occurred, seen in 36% of patients,[39] effacement of peri-chiasmatic and prepontine cisterns, bowing of the optic chiasm, flattening of pons, and ventricular collapse[33,36,37,48]
      - Enhancement of the pachymeninges, sparing the leptomeninges, is common from dilation of subdural blood vessels[33,46,48]
      - Engorgement of veins. Can also see venous distension sign as transverse sinus becomes dilated and convex[49]
      - Pituitary hyperemia
      - Subdural fluid collections seen in 50% of patients.[34,50] Can be hygromas versus hematomas, with hygromas being twice as frequent as hematomas. Occasionally may require intervention
   b) CT Brain is not as conclusive but can help identify these changes. 11% of SIH patients also have pseudo-SAH finding on CT caused by effacement of basal cisterns due to sagging of the brain[51,52]
   c) CT Myelogram with iodinated contrast: Study of choice for diagnosis and localization of CSF leak. Timed images immediately after contrast injection or at delayed intervals after injections can help localize intermittent leaks[34,37]
   d) MRI with intrathecal gadolinium: Alternative to CT myelogram. Injection of 0.5 ml of gadolinium followed by full spine T1 with fat suppression imaging an hour after injection. Contrast remains for 24 hours, hence it can aide in detection of intermittent leaks. Prospective cohort study localized leak in 67% of patients with SIH. In another study, MRI 15 minutes after gadolinium injection identified CSF leak in 21% of SIH patients with a negative CT myelogram. No side effects were reported, but intrathecal gadolinium is not FDA approved (off-label use)[44,53,54]
   e) spinal MRI: May show evidence of CSF leak, but is more likely to help localize extrathecal fluid collections for patients with local symptoms.[33] If there is focal spine pain, the leak will often be near this location. Other findings include: dural enhancement, dilated veins, deformed dural sac, meningeal diverticula, syringomyelia, and retrospinal fluid collections at C1-C2.[34,55,56,57,58,59,60,61,62]
   f) radioisotope cisternography: Poor resolution, may leave as many as one third of leaks unidentified.[34,37] Can be used especially if CT myelogram fails
2. lumbar puncture: CSF pressure < 6 cm of water is part of the diagnostic criteria. Patients have been identified with normal CSF pressure.[34,43,63] Associated CSF findings that have been identified include: lymphocytic pleocytosis, high protein level and xanthochromia[37,34,51]
3. positive response to EBP can also be used to support the diagnosis.

Treatment

None of these treatments have been evaluated by randomized clinical trials.

- conservative medical management: bed rest, hydration, analgesics, caffeine, and abdominal binder. Limited effect has been reported with intravenous caffeine, steroids and theophylline[33,34,36,37]
- epidural blood patch (EBP): see technique (p. 1509). Injection of autologous blood (10-20 ml) into epidural space. Evidence shows patients respond well and usually immediately.[34,52] However, some patients require more than one EBP and relief in headache may not be permanent.[41] If unsuccessful, can repeat blood patch with same or larger amount of blood. Positioning the patient in Trendelenberg position after injection aides in movement of blood to cover more segments for increased effectiveness.[37,34] May not be effective in up to 25-33%[33,34,36,44,64]
- directed epidural blood patch to site of leak if the above fails
- percutaneous placement of fibrin sealant at site of leak: can provide relief in patients that fail to improve with conservative measures and epidural blood patch[37,34,64,65]
- surgical intervention: last resource for patients without relief with conservative measures, EBP or fibrin sealant in which the exact site of leak has been identified. Meningeal diverticula can be ligated with suture, aneurysm clips or muscle pledget with gel foam and fibrin sealant, technique that may also be effective if a dural defect is identified[37,34]

Outcome

After appropriate treatment, clinical improvement is seen and precedes radiographic improvement. MRI usually takes days to weeks to normalize. Complete resolution of HA was achieved in 70% of patients (usually in days to weeks). Resolution was more likely if receiving EBP and less likely if they had multiple sites of CSF leak.[39] Patients with MRI changes characteristic of SIH and an identifiable focal CSF leak have better outcomes when compared to patients with multilevel CSF leaks.[37,34,66] CSF leak can recur in approximately 10% of patients. An association between longer interval from symptom onset to diagnosis and poorer outcome has been reported.[35]

References

[1] Binhammer RT. CSF anatomy with emphasis on relations to nasal cavity and labyrinthine fluids. Ear Nose Throat J. 1992; 71:292–299

[2] Sato O, Bering EA. Extraventricular Formation of Cerebrospinal Fluid. Brain Nerv. 1967; 19:883–885

[3] Lorenzo AV, Page LK, Wlaters GV. Relationship Between Cerebrospinal Fluid Formation, Absorption, and Pressure in Human Hydrocephalus. Brain. 1970; 93:679–692

[4] Bering EA, Sato O. Hydrocephalus: Changes in Formation and Absorption of Cerebrospinal fluid within the Cerebral Ventricles. J Neurosurg. 1963; 20:1050–1063

[5] Griffith HB, Jamjoom AB. The Treatment of Childhood Hydrocephalus by Choroid Plexus Coagulation and Artificial Cerebrospinal Fluid Perfusion. Br J Neurosurg. 1990; 4:95–100

[6] Fishman RA. Cerebrospinal Fluid in Diseases of the Nervous System. Philadelphia: W. B. Saunders; 1980

[7] Felgenhauer K. Protein Size and Cerebrospinal Fluid Composition. Klin Wochenschr. 1974; 52:1158–1164

[8] Ommaya AK. Spinal fluid fistulae. Clin Neurosurg. 1975; 23:363–392

[9] Spetzler RF, Zabramski JM. Cerebrospinal Fluid Fistula. Contemp Neurosurg. 1986; 8:1–7

[10] Shulman K. Later complications of head injuries in children. Clin Neurosurg. 1971; 19:371–380

[11] Manelfe C, Cellerier P, Sobel D, et al. CSF Rhinorrhea: Evaluation with Metrizamide Cisternography. AJNR. 1982; 3:25–30

[12] Meirowsky AM, Ceveness WF, Dillon JD, et al. CSF Fistulas Complicating Missile Wounds of the Brain. J Neurosurg. 1981; 54:44–48

[13] Cusimano MD, Sekhar LN. Pseudo-Cerebrospinal Fluid Rhinorrhea. J Neurosurg. 1994; 80:26–30

[14] Calcaterra TC, English GM. In: Cerebrospinal Rhinorrhea. Otolaryngology. Philadelphia: Lippincott-Raven; 1992:1–7

[15] Nutkiewicz A, DeFeo DR, Kohout RI, et al. Cerebrospinal Fluid Rhinorrhea as a Presentation of Pituitary Adenoma. Neurosurgery. 1980; 6:195–197

[16] Jonhston WH. Cerebrospinal Rhinorrhea: The Study of One Case and Reports of Twenty Others Collected from the Literature Published Since Nineteen Hundred. Ann Otolaryngol. 1926; 35

[17] Schievink WI, Meyer FB, Atkinson JLD, Mokri B. Spontaneous Spinal Cerebrospinal Fluid Leaks and Intracranial Hypotension. J Neurosurg. 1996; 84:598–605

[18] Hand WL, Sanford JP. Posttraumatic Bacterial Meningitis. Ann Int Medicine. 1970; 72:869–874

[19] Ryall RG, Peacock MK, Simpson DA. Usefulness of ß2-Transferrin Assay in the Detection of Cerebrospinal Fluid Leaks Following Head Injury. J Neurosurg. 1992; 77:737–739

[20] Fransen P, Sindic CJM, Thauvoy C, Laterre C, Stroobandt G. Highly Sensitive Detection of Beta-2 Transferrin in Rhinorrhea and Otorrhea as a Marker for Cerebrospinal Fluid (CSF) Leakage. Acta Neurochir. 1991; 109:98–101

[21] Wilkins RH, Rengachary SS. Neurosurgery. New York 1985

[22] Kaufman B, Nulsen FE, Weiss MH, Brodkey JS, White RJ, Sykora GF. Acquired spontaneous, nontraumatic normal-pressure cerebrospinal fluid fistulas originating from the middle fossa. Radiology. 1977; 122:379–387

[23] Bakay L. Head Injury. Boston: Little Brown; 1980

[24] El Gammal T, Sobol W, Wadlington VR, Sillers MJ, Crews C, Fisher WS,3rd, Lee JY. Cerebrospinal fluid fistula: detection with MR cisternography. AJNR Am J Neuroradiol. 1998; 19:627–631

[25] Ahmadi J, Weiss MH, Segall HD, et al. Evaluation of CSF Rhinorrhea by Metrizamide CT Cisternography. Neurosurgery. 1985; 16:54–60

[26] Naidich TP, Moran CJ. Precise Anatomic Localization of Atraumatic Sphenoethmoidal CSF Rhinorrhea by Metrizamide CT Cisternography. J Neurosurg. 1980; 53:222–228

[27] Klastersky J, Sadeghi M, Brihaye J. Antimicrobial Prophylaxis in Patients with Rhinorrhea or Otorrhea: A Double Blind Study. Surg Neurol. 1976; 6:111–114

[28] Allen C, Glasziou P, Del Mar C. Bed Rest: A Potentially Harmful Treatment Needing More Careful Evaluation. Lancet. 1999; 354:1229–1233

[29] Calcaterra TC. Extracranial Repair of Cerebrospinal Rhinorrhea. Ann Otol Rhinol Laryngol. 1980; 89:108–116

[30] Lewin W. Cerebrospinal Fluid Rhinorrhea in Closed Head Injuries. Br J Surgery. 1954; 17:1–18

[31] Dagi TF, George ED, Schmidek HH, Sweet WH. In: Surgical Management of Cranial Cerebrospinal Fluid Fistulas. Operative Neurosurgical Techniques. 3rd ed. Philadelphia: W.B. Saunders; 1995:117–131

[32] Fujii T, Misumi S, Onoda K, et al. Simple Management of CSF Rhinorrhea After Pituitary Surgery. Surg Neurol. 1986; 26:345–348

[33] Hoffmann J, Goadsby PJ. Update on intracranial hypertension and hypotension. Curr Opin Neurol. 2013; 26:240–247

[34] Schievink WI. Spontaneous spinal cerebrospinal fluid leaks. Cephalalgia. 2008; 28:1345–1356

[35] Mea E, Chiapparini L, Savoiardo M, Franzini A, Bussone G, Leone M. Clinical features and outcomes in spontaneous intracranial hypotension: a survey of 90 consecutive patients. Neurol Sci. 2009; 30 Suppl 1:S11–S13

[36] Schievink WI, Maya MM, Louy C, Moser FG, Tourje J. Diagnostic criteria for spontaneous spinal CSF leaks and intracranial hypotension. AJNR Am J Neuroradiol. 2008; 29:853–856

[37] Schievink WI. Spontaneous spinal cerebrospinal fluid leaks and intracranial hypotension. JAMA. 2006; 295:2286–2296

[38] Schievink WI, Tourje J. Intracranial hypotension without meningeal enhancement on magnetic resonance imaging. J Neurosurg. 2000; 92:475–477

[39] Chung SJ, Kim JS, Lee MC. Syndrome of cerebral spinal fluid hypovolemia: clinical and imaging features and outcome. Neurology. 2000; 55:1321–1327

[40] Mokri B. Spontaneous cerebrospinal fluid leaks, from intracranial hypotension to cerebrospinal fluid hypovolemia: evolution of a concept. Mayo Clin Proc. 1999; 74:1113–1123

[41] The International Classification of Headache Disorders, 3rd edition (beta version). Cephalalgia. 2013; 33:629–808

[42] Headache Classification Subcommittee of the International Headache Society. The International Classification of Headache Disorders: 2nd edition. Cephalalgia. 2004; 24 Suppl 1:9–160

[43] Schoffer KL, Benstead TJ, Grant I. Spontaneous intracranial hypotension in the absence of magnetic resonance imaging abnormalities. Can J Neurol Sci. 2002; 29:253–257

[44] Vanopdenbosch LJ, Dedeken P, Casselman JW, Vlaminck SA. MRI with intrathecal gadolinium to detect a CSF leak: a prospective open-label cohort study. J Neurol Neurosurg Psychiatry. 2011; 82:456–458

[45] Schievink WI, Gordon OK, Tourje J. Connective tissue disorders with spontaneous spinal cerebrospinal fluid leaks and intracranial hypotension: a prospective study. Neurosurgery. 2004; 54:65–70; discussion 70-1

[46] Schievink WI, Schwartz MS, Maya MM, Moser FG, Rozen TD. Lack of causal association between spontaneous intracranial hypotension and cranial cerebrospinal fluid leaks. J Neurosurg. 2012; 116:749–754

[47] Mea E, Franzini A, D'Amico D, Leone M, Cecchini AP, Tullo V, Chiapparini L, Bussone G. Treatment of alterations in CSF dynamics. Neurol Sci. 2011; 32 Suppl 1:S117–S120

[48] Fishman RA, Dillon WP. Dural enhancement and cerebral displacement secondary to intracranial hypotension. Neurology. 1993; 43:609–611

[49] Farb RI, Forghani R, Lee SK, Mikulis DJ, Agid R. The venous distension sign: a diagnostic sign of intracranial hypotension at MR imaging of the brain. AJNR Am J Neuroradiol. 2007; 28:1489–1493

[50] Schievink WI, Maya MM, Moser FG, Tourje J. Spectrum of subdural fluid collections in spontaneous intracranial hypotension. J Neurosurg. 2005; 103:608–613

[51] Ferrante E, Regna-Gladin C, Arpino I, Rubino F, Porrinis L, Ferrante MM, Citterio A. Pseudo-subarachnoid hemorrhage: a potential imaging pitfall associated with spontaneous intracranial hypotension. Clin Neurol Neurosurg. 2013; 115:2324–2328

[52] Zada G, Pezeshkian P, Giannotta S. Spontaneous intracranial hypotension and immediate improvement following epidural blood patch placement demonstrated by intracranial pressure monitoring. Case report. J Neurosurg. 2007; 106:1089–1090

[53] Akbar JJ, Luetmer PH, Schwartz KM, Hunt CH, Diehn FE, Eckel LJ. The role of MR myelography with intrathecal gadolinium in localization of spinal CSF leaks in patients with spontaneous intracranial hypotension. AJNR Am J Neuroradiol. 2012; 33:535–540

[54] Albayram S, Kilic F, Ozer H, Baghaki S, Kocer N, Islak C. Gadolinium-enhanced MR cisternography to evaluate dural leaks in intracranial hypotension syndrome. AJNR Am J Neuroradiol. 2008; 29:116–121

[55] Moayeri NN, Henson JW, Schaefer PW, Zervas NT. Spinal dural enhancement on magnetic resonance imaging associated with spontaneous intracranial hypotension. Report of three cases and review of the literature. J Neurosurg. 1998; 88:912–918

[56] Rabin BM, Roychowdhury S, Meyer JR, Cohen BA, LaPat KD, Russell EJ. Spontaneous intracranial hypotension: spinal MR findings. AJNR Am J Neuroradiol. 1998; 19:1034–1039

[57] Dillon WP. Spinal manifestations of intracranial hypotension. AJNR Am J Neuroradiol. 2001; 22:1233–1234

[58] Yousry I, Forderreuther S, Moriggl B, Holtmannspotter M, Naidich TP, Straube A, Yousry TA. Cervical MR imaging in postural headache: MR signs and pathophysiological implications. AJNR Am J Neuroradiol. 2001; 22:1239–1250

[59] Sharma P, Sharma A, Chacko AG. Syringomyelia in spontaneous intracranial hypotension. Case report. J Neurosurg. 2001; 95:905–908

[60] Chiapparini L, Farina L, D'Incerti L, Erbetta A, Pareyson D, Carriero MR, Savoiardo M. Spinal radiological findings in nine patients with spontaneous intracranial hypotension. Neuroradiology. 2002; 44:143–50; discussion 151-2

[61] Burtis MT, Ulmer JL, Miller GA, Barboli AC, Koss SA, Brown WD. Intradural spinal vein enlargement in craniospinal hypotension. AJNR Am J Neuroradiol. 2005; 26:34–38

[62] Watanabe A, Horikoshi T, Uchida M, Koizumi H, Yagishita T, Kinouchi H. Diagnostic value of spinal MR imaging in spontaneous intracranial hypotension syndrome. AJNR Am J Neuroradiol. 2009; 30:147–151

[63] Mokri B, Piepgras DG, Miller GM. Syndrome of orthostatic headaches and diffuse pachymeningeal gadolinium enhancement. Mayo Clin Proc. 1997; 72:400–413

[64] Schievink WI, Maya MM, Moser FM. Treatment of spontaneous intracranial hypotension with percutaneous placement of a fibrin sealant. Report of four cases. J Neurosurg. 2004; 100:1098–1100

[65] Gladstone JP, Nelson K, Patel N, Dodick DW. Spontaneous CSF leak treated with percutaneous CT-guided fibrin glue. Neurology. 2005; 64:1818–1819

[66] Schievink WI, Maya MM, Louy C. Cranial MRI predicts outcome of spontaneous intracranial hypotension. Neurology. 2005; 64:1282–1284

23

24 Hydrocephalus – General Aspects

24.1 Basic definition

An abnormal accumulation of cerebrospinal fluid within the ventricles of the brain.

24.2 Epidemiology

Estimated prevalence: 1–1.5%.

Incidence of congenital hydrocephalus is ≈ 0.9–1.8/1000 births (reported range from 0.2 to 3.5/1000 births[1]).

24.3 Etiologies of hydrocephalus

24.3.1 General information

Hydrocephalus (HCP) is either due to subnormal CSF reabsorption or, rarely, CSF overproduction.

- subnormal CSF reabsorption. Two main functional subdivisions:
  1. obstructive hydrocephalus (AKA non-communicating): block proximal to the arachnoid granulations (AG) On CT or MRI: enlargement of ventricles proximal to block (e.g. obstruction of aqueduct of Sylvius → lateral and 3rd ventricular enlargement out of proportion to the 4th ventricle, sometimes referred to as triventricular hydrocephalus)
  2. communicating hydrocephalus (AKA non-obstructive): defect in CSF reabsorption by the AG
- CSF overproduction: rare. As with some choroid plexus papillomas; even here, reabsorption is probably defective in some as normal individuals could probably tolerate the slightly elevated CSF production rate of these tumors.

24.3.2 Specific etiologies of hydrocephalus

The etiologies in one series of pediatric patients is shown in ▶ Table 24.1.

1. congenital
   a) Chiari Type 2 malformation and/or myelomeningocele (MM) (usually occur together)
   b) Chiari Type 1 malformation: HCP may occur with 4th ventricle outlet obstruction
   c) primary aqueductal stenosis (usually presents in infancy, rarely in adulthood)
   d) secondary aqueductal gliosis: due to intrauterine infection or germinal matrix hemorrhage[3]
   e) Dandy Walker malformation (p. 256): atresia of foramina of Luschka & Magendie. The incidence of this in patients with HCP is 2.4%
   f) X-linked inherited disorder (p. 401): rare
2. acquired
   a) infectious (the most common cause of communicating HCP)
      - post-meningitis; especially purulent and basal, including TB, cryptococcus (p. 376)
      - cysticercosis
   b) post-hemorrhagic (2nd most common cause of communicating HCP)
      - post-SAH
      - post-intraventricular hemorrhage (IVH): many will develop *transient* HCP. 20–50% of patients with large IVH develop permanent HCP requiring a shunt

Table 24.1 Etiologies of HCP in 170 pediatric patients with HCP[2]	
congenital (without myelomeningocele)	38%
congenital (with MM)	29%
perinatal hemorrhage	11%
trauma/subarachnoid hemorrhage	4.7%
Tumor	11%
previous infection	7.6%

c) secondary to masses
   - non neoplastic: e.g. vascular malformation
   - neoplastic: most produce obstructive HCP by blocking CSF pathways, especially tumors around aqueduct, e.g. medulloblastoma. A colloid cyst can block CSF flow at the foramen of Monro. Pituitary tumor: suprasellar extension of tumor or expansion from pituitary apoplexy

d) post-op: 20% of pediatric patients develop permanent hydrocephalus (requiring shunt) following p-fossa tumor removal. May be delayed up to 1 yr
e) neurosarcoidosis (p. 189)
f) "constitutional ventriculomegaly": asymptomatic. Needs no treatment
g) associated with spinal tumors[4]: ? due to ↑ protein?, ↑ venous pressure?, previous hemorrhage in some?

24.3.3 Special forms of hydrocephalus

These are covered in subsequent sections
- normal pressure hydrocephalus (NPH) (p. 403)
- entrapped fourth ventricle (p. 402)
- arrested hydrocephalus (p. 402)

24.4 Signs and symptoms of HCP

24.4.1 In older children (with rigid cranial vault) and adults

Symptoms are those of increased ICP, including: papilledema, H/A, N/V, gait changes, upgaze and/or abducens palsy. Slowly enlarging ventricles may initially be asymptomatic.

24.4.2 In young children

Overview

- abnormalities in head circumference (OFC) (see below)
- cranium enlarges at a rate > facial growth
- irritability, poor head control, N/V
- fontanelle full and bulging
- enlargement and engorgement of scalp veins: due to reversal of flow from intracerebral sinuses due to increased intracranial pressure[5]
- Macewen's sign: cracked pot sound on percussing over dilated ventricles
- 6th nerve (abducens) palsy: the long intracranial course is postulated to render this nerve very sensitive to pressure
- **"setting sun sign" (upward gaze palsy)** (p. 99): Parinaud's syndrome (p. 99) from pressure on region of suprapineal recess
- hyperactive reflexes
- irregular respirations with apneic spells
- splaying of cranial sutures (may be seen on plain skull x-ray)

Occipital-frontal circumference

The occipital-frontal circumference (OFC) should be followed in every growing child (as part of a "well-baby" check-up, and especially in infants with documented or suspected hydrocephalus (HCP)). As a rule of thumb, the OFC of a normal infant should equal the distance from crown to rump.[6 (rule No. 335)] for the differential diagnosis of macrocephaly (p. 1403).

Measurement technique[7]: use a non-stretchable tape, measure the circumference of the head just above the supraorbital ridge anteriorly and around the most prominent part of the occiput posteriorly (keeping above the ears). Pull the tape snug to compress hair (exclude any braids or hairclips). Take 2 separate measurements (reposition the tape each time), if the measurements are within 2 mm, record the largest value. If the measurements disagree by > 2 mm, take a third measurement and record the average of the 2 closest measures.

Normal head growth: parallels normal curves as seen on the graphs on the inside front cover of this book, or in ▸ Fig. 24.1 and ▸ Fig. 24.2 for preemies. Any of the following may signify treatable conditions such as active HCP, subdural hematoma, or subdural effusions, and should prompt an evaluation of the intracranial contents (e.g. CT, head U/S …):

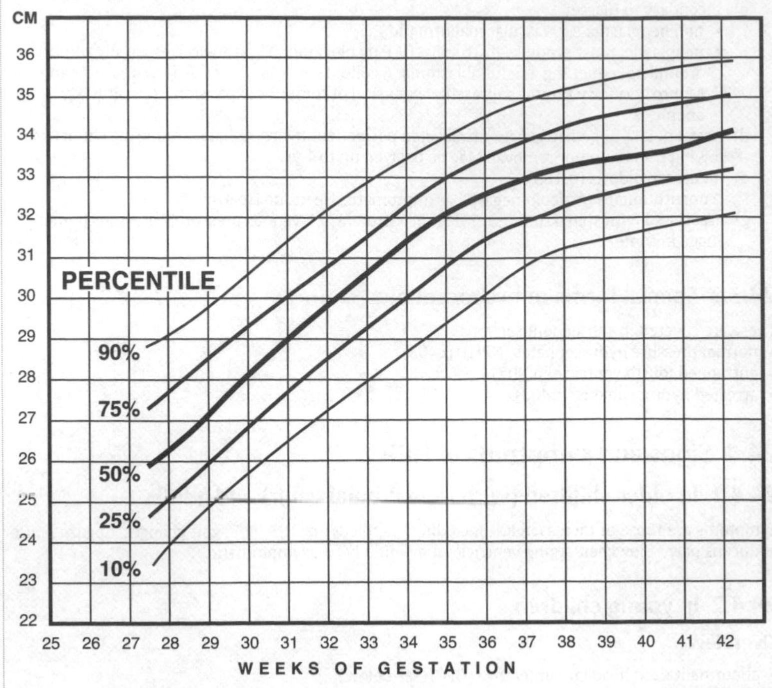

Fig. 24.1 OFC for premature infants as a function of gestational age

1. Progressive upward deviations from the normal curve (crossing curves)
2. continued head growth of more than 1.25 cm/wk
3. OFC approaching 2 standard deviations (SD) above normal
4. head circumference out of proportion to body length or weight, even if within normal limits for age (▸ Fig. 24.2)[8]

These conditions may also be seen in the "catch-up phase" of brain growth in premature infants after they recover from their acute medical illnesses, see **Catch-up phase of brain growth** (p. 1351). Deviations below the curves or head growth in the premature infant in the neonatal period of less than 0.5 cm/wk (excluding the first few weeks of life) may indicate microcephaly (p. 289).

Technique: measure circumference around forehead and occiput (excluding ears) three consecutive times, and use the *largest* value. OFC is then plotted on a graph of average values as a function of age[9] and followed for each individual patient. Use the graphs on the inside front cover for most children and adolescents. The graph in ▸ Fig. 24.1 shows the OFC for premature infants as a function of gestational age up to term.

The graph in ▸ Fig. 24.2 shows the relationship of head circumference, weight and length for various gestational ages.

24.4.3 Blindness from hydrocephalus

General information

Blindness is a rare complication of hydrocephalus and/or shunt malfunction. Possible causes include:

1. occlusion of posterior cerebral arteries (**PCA** caused by downward transtentorial herniation
2. chronic papilledema causing injury to optic nerve at the optic disc
3. dilatation of the 3rd ventricle with compression of optic chiasm

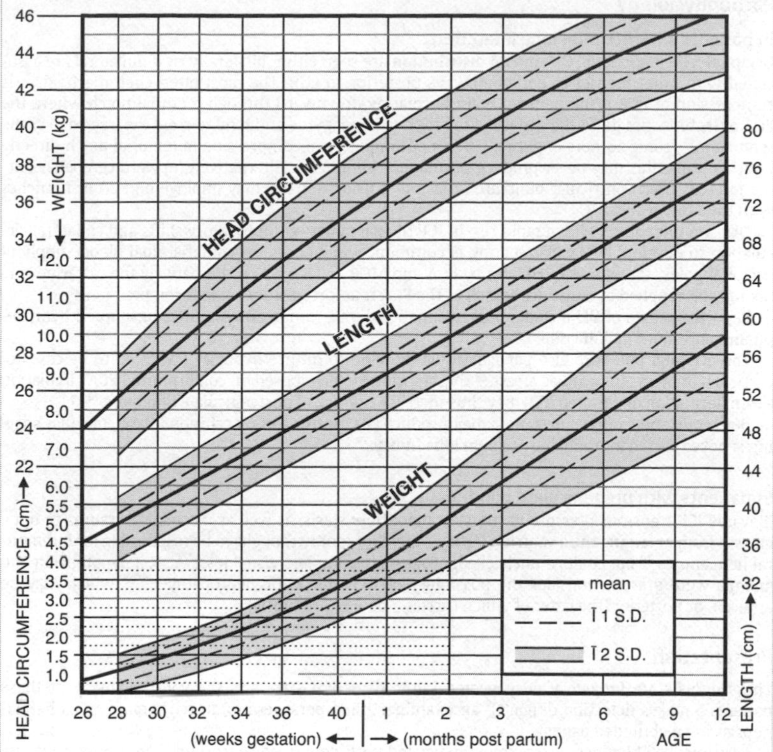

Fig. 24.2 Head circumference, weight and length
(Redrawn from Journal of Pediatrics, "Growth Graphs for the Clinical Assessment of Infants of Varying Gestational Age", Babson S G, Benda G I, vol 89, pp 815, with permission)

Ocular motility or visual field defects are more common with shunt malfunction than is blindness.[10,11,12,13] One series found 34 reported cases of permanent blindness in children attributed to shunt malfunction with concomitant increased ICP[14] (these authors were based in a referral center for visually impaired children, thus incidence not estimated). Another series of 100 patients with tentorial herniation (most from acute EDH and/or SDH) proven by CT; 48 patients operated; only 19 of 100 survived > 1 month (all were in operated group); 9 of 100 developed occipital lobe infarct (2 died, 3 vegetative state, remaining 4 moderate to severe disability).[15]

Types of visual disturbance

9 of 14 had pregeniculate (anterior visual pathway) blindness with marked optic nerve atrophy (early), and reduced pupillary light reflexes. 5 of 14 had postgeniculate (cortical) blindness with normal light responses and minimal or no optic nerve atrophy (or atrophy late). A few patients had evidence of damage in both sites.

Cortical blindness: due to lesions posterior to lateral geniculate bodies (LGB), may also be seen with hypoxic injuries or trauma.[16] Occasionally associated with Anton's syndrome (denial of visual deficit) and with Ridoch's phenomenon (appreciation of moving objects without perception of stationary stimuli).

24

Pathophysiology

In patients with occipital lobe infarction

Occipital lobe infarctions (OLI) in PCA distribution are seen either bilaterally, or if unilateral are associated with other injuries to optic pathways posterior to LGB. The most often cited mechanism is compression of PCA resulting from brain herniating downward through tentorial notch where the PCA or its branches lie on the surface of the hippocampal gyrus and tend to cross the free edge of the tentorium[17] (some authors implicate parahippocampal gyral compression in tentorial notch directly injuring LGBs; this may never produce permanent blindness). Alternatively, upward cerebellar herniation (e.g. from ventricular puncture in face of a p-fossa mass) may impinge on PCA or branches with the same results.[18]

OLIs are more likely with a rapid rise in ICP (doesn't allow compensatory shifts and collateral circulation to develop).[19] Macular sparing is common, possibly due to potential dual blood supply of occipital poles (sometimes filled both by PCA and MCA collaterals[20]), alternatively the calcarine cortex may be supplied by a distinct branch of the PCA that fortuitously escapes compression.[21]

Reported causes of OLI include: post traumatic edema, tumor, abscess, SDH, unshunted hydrocephalus, and shunt malfunction.[17,22,23]

The occipital poles are also particularly vulnerable to diffuse hypoxia[24]; attested to by cases of cortical blindness after cardiac arrest.[25] Hypotension superimposed on compromised PCA circulation (from herniation or elevated ICP) may thus increase the risk of postgeniculate blindness.[14,19]

Both coup and contrecoup trauma may produce OLI. Unlike a PCA occlusion infarct, macular sparing is not expected in traumatic occipital lobe injury.[17]

In patients with pregeniculate blindness

Elevated ICP transmits pressure to retina → bloodflow stasis, as well as mechanical trauma to optic chiasm from enlarging third ventricle (latter more commonly thought to be responsible for bitemporal hemianopia,[10] but could, if unchecked, progress to complete visual loss). Also, if hypotension and anemia were present, consider the possibility of ischemic optic neuropathy[26,27,28] which may be anterior, or posterior (the latter of which carries a poorer prognosis).

Presentation

These deficits are frequency unsuspected (altered mental state and the youth of many of these patients[14] makes detection difficult); an examiner must persevere to detect homonymous hemianopsias in an obtunded patient.[17]

Pregeniculate blindness is less often associated with depressed sensorium than is postgeniculate (where direct compression and vascular compromise of midbrain are more likely[14]).

Prognosis

Cortical blindness after diffuse anoxia frequently improves (occasionally to normal); usually slowly (weeks to years quoted; several mos usually adequate).[25] Many reports of blindness after shunt malfunction are pre-CT era, thus the presence or extent of occipital lobe infarction not ascertained. Some optimistic outcomes reported,[29] however, permanent blindness or severe visual handicap are also described[17,23]; no reliable predictor has been identified. As with infarcts elsewhere, younger patients fare better,[24] but extensive calcarine infarcts are probably incompatible with significant visual recovery.

24.5 CT/MRI criteria for hydrocephalus

24.5.1 General information

In general, hydrocephalus is best demonstrated on CT or MRI (▶ Fig. 24.3). Occasionally, other means of determining the presence of hydrocephalus must be employed. Most experienced clinicians can recognize HCP by its appearance on CT or MRI. Numerous methods have been devised to attempt to quantitatively define radiographic criteria for hydrocephalus (HCP) (most date back to the early CT experience, and some are used definitionally for research purposes). Some are presented here for completeness. See also radiologic features of chronic HCP (p. 400).

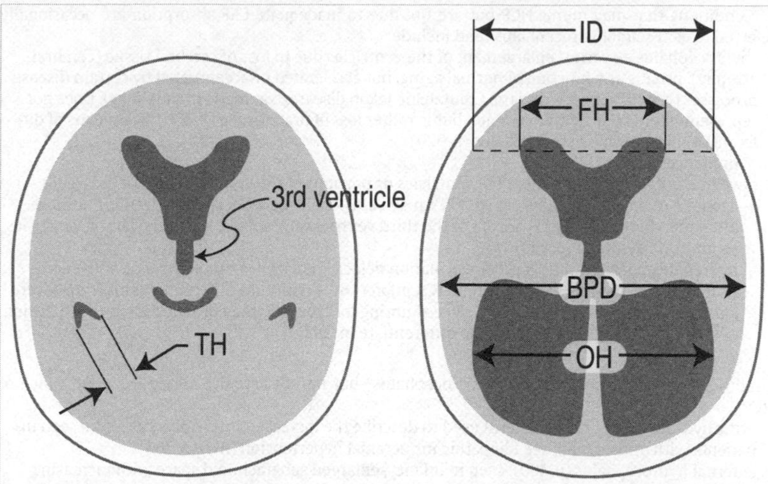

Fig. 24.3 Linear ventricular measurement for CT, MRI or U/S
Abbreviations: TH = temporal horns, FH = frontal horns, ID = internal diameter, BPD = biparietal diameter, OH = occipital horns

24.5.2 Specific imaging criteria for hydrocephalus

HCP is suggested when either[30]:

1. the size of both temporal horns (TH) is ≥ 2 mm in width (▶ Fig. 24.3; in the absence of HCP, the temporal horns should be barely visible), and the sylvian & interhemispheric fissures and cerebral sulci are not visible
   OR
2. both TH are ≥ 2 mm, *and* the ratio $\frac{FH}{ID} > 0.5$ (where FH is the largest width of the frontal horns, and ID is the internal diameter from inner-table to inner-table at this level, ▶ Fig. 24.3)

Other features suggestive of hydrocephalus (see ▶ Fig. 24.3 for measurements):

1. ballooning of frontal horns of lateral ventricles ("Mickey Mouse" ventricles) and/or 3rd ventricle (the 3rd ventricle should normally be slit-like)
2. periventricular low density on CT, or periventricular high intensity signal on T2WI on MRI suggesting transependymal absorption of CSF (note: a misnomer: CSF does not actually penetrate the ependymal lining, proven with CSF labeling studies; probably represents stasis of fluid in brain adjacent to ventricles)
3. used alone, the ratio

$$\frac{FH}{ID}\begin{cases} < 40\% & \text{normal} \\ 40-50\% & \text{borderline} \\ > 50\% & \text{suggests hydrocephalus} \end{cases}$$

4. Evans ratio (originally described for ventriculography[31], or index; note: measurements that rely on the frontal horn diameter tend to underestimate hydrocephalus in pediatrics possibly because of disproportionate dilatation of the occipital horns in peds[32]): ratio of FH to *maximal* biparietal diameter (BPD) measured in the same CT slice: > 0.3 suggests hydrocephalus
5. sagittal MRI may show thinning of the corpus callosum (generally present with chronic HCP) and/or upward bowing of the corpus callosum

24.6 Differential diagnosis of hydrocephalus

For etiologies of HCP, see above.

Conditions that may mimic HCP but are not due to inadequate CSF absorption are occasionally referred to as "Pseudohydrocephalus" and include:

- "hydrocephalus ex vacuo" enlargement of the ventricles due to loss of cerebral tissue (cerebral atrophy), usually as a function of normal aging, but accelerated or accentuated by certain disease processes (e.g. Alzheimer's disease, Creutzfeldt-Jakob disease, traumatic brain injury). Does not represent altered CSF hydrodynamics, but is rather loss of brain tissue (p. 400). See means of differentiating from true hydrocephalus (p. 920)
- hydranencephaly (p. 288)
- developmental anomalies where the ventricles or portions of the ventricles appear enlarged:
  - agenesis of the corpus callosum (p. 259): may occasionally be associated with HCP, but more often merely represents expansion of the third ventricle and separation of the lateral ventricles
  - septo-optic dysplasia (p. 260)
  - hydranencephaly (p. 288): a post-neurulation defect. Total or near-total absence of the cerebrum most commonly due to bilateral ICA infarcts. It is critical to differentiate this from severe ("maximal") hydrocephalus (HCP) since shunting for true HCP may produce some re-expansion of the cortical mantle; see means to differentiate (p. 288)

Conditions that have been dubbed "hydrocephalus" but do not actually mimic the appearance of HCP

- otitic hydrocephalus: obsolete term used to describe the increased intracranial pressure seen in patients with otitis media; see Idiopathic intracranial hypertension (IIH) (p. 766)
- external hydrocephalus (p. 400): seen in infancy, enlarged subarachnoid space with increasing OFCs and normal or mildly dilated ventricles

24.7 Chronic HCP

Features indicative of chronic hydrocephalus (as opposed to acute hydrocephalus):

1. beaten copper cranium (some refer to beaten silver appearance) on plain skull x-ray.[33] By itself, does not correlate with increased ICP, however when associated with #3 and #4 below, does suggest ↑ ICP. May be seen in craniosynostosis; see description (p. 252)
2. 3rd ventricle herniating into sella (seen on CT or MRI)
3. erosion of sella turcica (may be due to #2 above) which sometimes produces an empty sella, and erosion of the dorsum sella
4. the temporal horns may be less prominent on imaging than in acute HCP
5. macrocrania: by convention, OFC greater than 98th percentile[34(p 203)]
6. atrophy of corpus callosum: best appreciated on sagittal MRI
7. in infants
   a) sutural diastasis
   b) delayed closure of fontanelles
   c) failure to thrive or developmental delay

24.8 External hydrocephalus (AKA benign external hydrocephalus)

24.8.1 General information

Key concepts

- enlarged subarachnoid spaces over the frontal poles in the first year of life
- ventricles are normal or minimally enlarged
- may be distinguished from subdural hematoma by the "cortical vein sign"
- usually resolves spontaneously by 2 years of age

Enlarged subarachnoid space (usually over the cortical sulci of the frontal poles) seen in infancy (primarily in the first year of life) usually accompanied by abnormally increasing head circumference with normal or mildly dilated ventricles.[35] There are often enlarged basal cisterns and widening of the anterior interhemispheric fissure. No other symptoms or signs should be present (although there may be slight delay only in motor milestones due to the large head). Etiology is unclear, but a defect in CSF resorption is postulated. External hydrocephalus (EH) may be a variant of communicating hydrocephalus.[36] No predisposing factor may be found in some cases, although EH may be associated with some craniosynostoses[37] (especially plagiocephaly) or it may follow intraventricular hemorrhage or superior vena cava obstruction.

24.8.2 Differential diagnosis

EH is probably distinct from **benign subdural collections (or extra-axial fluid) of infancy** (p.903). ✱ EH must be distinguished from **symptomatic chronic extra-axial fluid collections** (p.904) (or chronic subdural hematoma), which may be accompanied by seizures, vomiting, headache… and may be the result of child abuse. With EH, MRI or CT may demonstrate cortical veins extending from the surface of the brain to the inner table of the skull coursing through the fluid collection ("cortical vein sign"), whereas the collections in subdural hematomas compress the subarachnoid space which apposes the veins to the surface to the brain.[38,39]

24.8.3 Treatment

EH usually compensates by 12–18 mos age without shunting.[40] Recommend: follow serial ultrasound and/or CT to rule out abnormal ventricular enlargement. Emphasize to parents that this does not represent cortical atrophy. Due to increased risk for positional molding, parents may need to periodically reposition the head while the child is sleeping.[41]

A shunt may rarely be indicated when the collections are bloody (consider the possibility of child abuse) or for cosmetic reasons for severe macrocrania or frontal bossing.

24.9 X-linked hydrocephalus

24.9.1 General information

Inherited hydrocephalus (HCP) with phenotypic expression in males passed on through carrier mothers who are phenotypically normal. Classical phenotypic expression will skip single generations.

Incidence: 1/25,000 to 1/60,000. Prevalence: ≈ 2 cases per 100 cases of hydrocephalus.

Gene located on Xq28.[42,43,44]

24.9.2 Pathophysiology

L1CAM membrane bound receptor plays a significant role in CNS development for axonal migration to appropriate target locations through Integrin cell adhesion molecules and MAP Kinase signal cascade.[42,43,44]

Abnormal gene expression results in poor differentiation and maturation of cortical neurons macroscopic anatomical abnormalities (bilateral absence of pyramidal tracts, see below).

Cytoplasmic domain loss of function mutations result in severe L1 syndrome, whereas mutations retaining expression of some functional protein (component imbedded in cell membrane) leads to mild L1 syndrome.

24.9.3 L1 syndromes

Classical syndromes include CRASH (corpus callosum hypoplasia, retardation, adducted thumbs (clasp thumbs), spastic paralysis, HCP), MSAS (mental handicap, aphasia, shuffling gate, adducted thumbs), HSAS (HCP with stenosis of the aqueduct of sylvius). Spectrum of disease also includes x-linked agenesis of the corpus callosum (ACC), and spastic paraparesis type 1.[42,43]

Recent deliniations[44]:

- mild L1 syndrome: adducted thumbs, spastic paralysis, hypoplasia of CC
- severe L1 syndrome: as in mild L1 syndrome plus anterior cerebellar vermis hypoplasia, large massa intermedia, enlarged quadrigeminal plate, rippled ventricular wall following VP shunt placement (pathognomonic for X-linked HCP). Profound mental retardation in virtually all cases

Radiographic findings likely present if severe L1[45]:

1. severe symmetric HCP with predominant posterior horn dilation
2. hypoplastic CC/ACC
3. hypoplastic anterior cerebellar vermis

4. large massa intermedia
5. large quadrigeminal plate
6. rippled ventricular wall following VP shunt placement (pathognomonic)

Treatment: no intervention demonstrates improvement in retardation status in observational papers.

1. VP shunt: main purpose is management of head size for improved care by caregiver. Does not improve neurologic outcome
2. there are no current genetic therapies for L1CAM protein abnormalities
3. prenatal U/S: early (≈ 20–24 weeks gestational age) with frequent repeat scan in known carrier mothers. May allow for medically indicated termination early on
4. male infants with HCP and ≥ 2 clinical/radiographic signs should undergo genetic testing for L1CAM mutation detection for future pregnancy counseling[42]

24.10 "Arrested hydrocephalus"

24.10.1 General information

The exact definition of this term is not generally agreed upon, and some use the term compensated hydrocephalus interchangeably. Most clinicians use these terms to refer to a situation where there is no progression or deleterious sequelae due to hydrocephalus that would require the presence of a CSF shunt. Patients and families should be advised to seek medical attention if they develop symptoms of intracranial hypertension (decompensation) which may include: headaches, vomiting, ataxia or visual symptoms.[41]

Arrested hydrocephalus satisfies the following criteria in the absence of a CSF shunt:

1. near normal ventricular size
2. normal head growth curve
3. continued psychomotor development

24.10.2 Shunt independence

The concept of becoming independent of a shunt is not universally accepted.[46] Some feel that shunt independence occurs more commonly when the HCP is due to a block at the level of the arachnoid granulations (communicating hydrocephalus),[47] but others have shown that it can occur regardless of the etiology.[48] These patients must be followed closely as there are reports of death as late as 5 years after apparent shunt independence, sometimes without warning.[47]

24.10.3 When to remove a disconnected or non-functioning shunt?

Note: a disconnected shunt may continue to function by CSF flow through an endothelialized subcutaneous tract. Recommendations on whether or not to repair vs. remove a disconnected or non-functioning shunt:

1. when in doubt, shunt
2. indications for shunt repair (vs. removal)
   a) marginally functioning shunts
   b) the presence of any signs or symptoms of increased ICP (vomiting, upgaze palsy, sometimes H/A alone[49]...)
   c) changes in cognitive function, ↓ attention span, or emotional changes
   d) patients with aqueductal stenosis or spina bifida: most are shunt dependent
3. because of risks associated with shunt removal, surgery for this purpose alone should be performed only in the situation of a shunt infection[50]
4. patients with a nonfunctioning shunt should be followed closely with serial CTs, and possibly with serial neuropsychological evaluations

24.11 Entrapped fourth ventricle

24.11.1 General information

AKA isolated fourth ventricle: 4th ventricle that neither communicates with the 3rd ventricle (through sylvian aqueduct) nor with the basal cisterns (through foramina of Luschka or Magendie). Usually seen with chronic shunting of the lateral ventricles, especially with post-infectious hydrocephalus (fungal, in particular) or in those with repeated shunt infections. Possibly as a result of adhesions forming from prolonged apposition of the ependymal lining of the aqueduct due to the diversion of CSF through the shunt. Occurs in 2–3% of shunted patients.[51] May also occur in Dandy Walker malformation (p. 256) if the aqueduct is also obstructed. The choroid plexus of the 4th ventricle continues to produce CSF which enlarges the ventricle when there is 4th ventricular outlet obstruction or obstruction at the level of the arachnoid granulations.

24.11.2 Presentation

Presentation may include:
1. headache
2. lower cranial nerve palsies: swallowing difficulties
3. pressure on the floor of the 4th ventricle may compress the facial colliculus (p. 576) → facial diplegia and bilateral abducens palsy
4. ataxia
5. reduced level of consciousness
6. nausea/vomiting
7. may also be an incidental finding (NB: some "atypical" findings, such as reduced attention span, may be related)

24.11.3 Treatment

Treatment of the entrapped 4th ventricle may alleviate associated slit ventricles.[52] Most surgeons advocate shunting the ventricle either with a separate VP shunt, or linking into an existing shunt. Options:
1. usual first choice: insertion from below the tonsils under direct vision. The catheter may be brought out at the dural suture line, and may be anchored here by use of an angle adapter sutured to the dura
2. passage through a cerebellar hemisphere: potential complications include delayed injury to the brainstem by the catheter tip as the brainstem moves into its normal position with drainage of the 4th ventricle. This may be avoided by bringing the catheter into the 4th ventricle at a slight angle through the cerebellar hemisphere
3. Torkildsen shunt (ventriculocisternal shunt) is an option for obstructive hydrocephalus if it is certain that the arachnoid granulations are functional (usually not the case with hydrocephalus of infantile onset)
4. an LP shunt may be considered when the 4th ventricle outlets are patent

Cranial nerve palsies may occur with shunting of the 4th ventricle usually as a result of penetration of the brainstem by the catheter either at the time of catheter insertion, or in a delayed fashion as the 4th ventricle decreases in size,[53] but also possibly as a result of overshunting causing traction on the lower cranial nerves as the brainstem shifts posteriorly.[51]

24.12 Normal pressure hydrocephalus (NPH)

24.12.1 General information

Key concepts

- triad (not pathognomonic): dementia, gait disturbance, urinary incontinence
- communicating hydrocephalus on CT or MRI
- normal pressure on random LP
- symptoms may be remediable with CSF shunting

Normal pressure hydrocephalus (NPH), AKA Hakim-Adams syndrome, first described in 1965,[54] is clinically important because it may cause treatable symptoms, including one of the few forms of remediable dementia.

As originally described, the hydrocephalus of NPH was considered to be *idiopathic* (*iNPH*). However, in some cases of hydrocephalus with normal pressure, a predisposing condition may be identified, suggesting that the ICP may have been elevated at some point in time. These patients may also respond to shunting.

Possible etiologies of "secondary NPH" include:

1. post-SAH
2. post-traumatic
3. post-meningitis
4. following posterior fossa surgery
5. tumors, including carcinomatous meningitis
6. also seen in ≈ 15% of patients with Alzheimer's disease (AD)
7. deficiency of the arachnoid granulations
8. aqueductal stenosis may be an overlooked cause

To further complicate things, some patients considered to have NPH may actually have episodic elevations in ICP.

Throughout this text, discussion focuses on *idiopathic* NPH unless stated otherwise.

It is becoming increasingly acknowledged that the ventricular enlargement is likely not the primary underlying pathologic entity. Research continues in an effort to improve the understanding of this complicated condition.

24.12.2 Epidemiology

Incidence for idiopathic NPH (iNPH) may be as high as 5.5 per 100,000 per year.[55]

The mean age for iNPH is older than that for secondary NPH.

24.12.3 Clinical

Clinical triad

See reference.[56]

The triad is not pathognomonic, and similar features may also be seen e.g. in vascular dementia,[57] Alzheimer's dementia and Parkinson's disease.

1. gait disturbance: usually precedes other symptoms. Wide based with short, shuffling steps and unsteadiness on turning. Patients often feel like they are "glued to the floor" (so-called "magnetic gait") and may have difficulty initiating steps or turns. Absence of appendicular ataxia
2. dementia: primarily memory impairment with bradyphrenia (slowness of thought) and bradykinesia ► Table 24.2 shows some differentiating features with Alzheimer's disease)
3. urinary incontinence: usually unwitting (NB: a patient demented for any reason or with mobility impairment may have incontinence)

Table 24.2 Comparison of cognitive deficits in Alzheimer's disease (AD) and NPH[a,b]

Feature	AD	NPH
memory	↓	± auditory memory
executive function[c]	↓	±
attention concentration	↓	±
orientation	↓	
writing	↓	
learning	↓	
fine motor speed and accuracy	±	↓
psychomotor skills	±	slowed
language and reading	±	
behavioral or personality changes		±

[a]modified[58]
[b]Key: ↓ = impaired; ± = borderline impaired
[c]see ► Table 24.3 for definition of executive function

Table 24.3 Diagnostic guidelines for NPH[58]

Probable NPH
History[a]: must include:
1. insidious onset (vs. acute) 2. onset age ≥ 40 years 3. duration ≥ 3–6 months 4. no antecedent head trauma, ICH, meningitis or other known cause of secondary hydrocephalus 5. progression over time 6. no other neurological, psychiatric or general medical conditions that are sufficient to explain the presenting symptoms
Brain imaging: CT or MRI *after* onset of symptoms must show:
1. ventricular enlargement not attributable to cerebral atrophy or congenital enlargement ((Evan's index[b] > 0.3 or comparable measure) 2. no macroscopic obstruction to CSF flow 3. ≥ 1 of the following supportive features a) enlarged temporal horns not entirely attributable to hippocampal atrophy b) callosal angle ≥ 40° c) evidence of altered brain water content, including periventricular changes not attributable to microvascular ischemic changes or demyelination d) aqueductal or 4th ventricle flow void on MRI Other imaging findings that may support *Probable* designation but are not required: 1. pre-morbid study showing smaller or nonhydrocephalic ventricles 2. radionuclide cisternogram showing delayed clearance of radiotracer over the convexities after 48–72 hours 3. cine-MRI or other technique showing increased ventricular flow rate 4. SPECT showing decreased periventricular perfusion that is not altered by acetazolamide challenge
Physiological
CSF opening pressure (OP) on lateral decubitus LP: 5–18 mm Hg (70–245 mm H_2O)
Clinical: must show gait/balance disturbance, plus impairment in cognition and/or urinary function
1. **gait/imbalance:** ≥ 2 of the following (not entirely attributable to other conditions a) decreased step height b) decreased step length c) decreased cadence (speed of walking) d) increased trunk sway while walking e) widened standing base f) toes turn outward while walking g) retropulsion (spontaneous or provoked) h) en bloc turning (≥ 3 steps to turn 180°) i) impaired walking balance: ≥ 2 corrections out of 8 tandem steps 2. **cognition:** documented impairment (adjusted for age & education) and/or decrease in performance on cognitive screening instrument (e.g. Monumental State examination), or evidence of ≥ 2 of the following not fully attributable to other conditions: a) psychomotor slowing (increased response latency) b) decreased fine motor speed c) decreased fine motor accuracy d) difficulty dividing or maintaining attention e) impaired recall, especially for recent events f) executive dysfunction: e.g. impairment in multistep procedures, working memory, formulation of abstractions/similarities, insight g) behavioral or personality changes 3. **urinary dysfunction:** a) any one of the following • episodic or persistent incontinence not attributable to primary urological disorder • persistent urinary incontinence • urinary and fecal incontinence b) or, any 2 of the following: • urinary urgency: frequent perception of a pressing need to void • urinary frequency (pollakiuria): voiding > 6 times in 12 hours with normal fluid intake • nocturia: needing to void > 2 times in an average night
Possible NPH
History: reported symptoms may:
1. have subacute or indeterminate mode of onset 2. onset at any age after childhood

Table 24.3 continued

3. duration: < 3 months or indeterminate 4. may follow events such as mild head trauma, remote history of ICH, or childhood or adult meningitis or other conditions judged not likely to be causally related 5. coexist with other neurological, psychiatric, or general medical disorders but judged not to be entirely attributable to these conditions 6. be nonprogressive or not clearly progressive
Clinical: symptoms of either:
1. incontinence and/or cognitive impairment in the absence of observable gait/balance disturbance 2. gait disturbance or dementia alone
Brain imaging: ventricular enlargement consistent with hydrocephalus but associated with any of the following:
1. cerebral atrophy of sufficient severity to potentially explain ventricular enlargement 2. structural lesions that may influence ventricular size
Physiological
OP not available or outside of the range delineated for *Probable NPH*
Unlikely NPH
1. no ventriculomegaly 2. signs of increased ICP (e.g. papilledema) 3. no component of the clinical triad of NPH 4. symptoms explained by other causes (e.g. spinal stenosis)
[a]history should be verified by individual familiar with premorbid and current condition [b]See definition and illustration of Evan's index (p. 399)

Other clinical features

Age usually > 60 yrs. Slight male preponderance. Also below for other clinical information.

True aphasia is unusual, but speech output may be disturbed by impaired motivation or executive dysfunction.[58] As NPH progresses, cognitive impairment may become more generalized and less responsive to treatment.[58] Symptoms identical to those of idiopathic parkinsonism may occur in 11%.[59]

Case reports of a variety of psychiatric disturbances associated with NPH include: depression,[60] bipolar disorder,[61] aggressiveness,[62] paranoia.[63]

Symptoms not expected with NPH

Although a variety of clinical features have been demonstrated to occur infrequently (e.g. SIADH,[64] syncope…), clinical features *not* expected solely as a result of NPH include: papilledema, seizures (prior to shunting), headaches.[58]

24.12.4 Imaging in NPH

CT and MRI

Features on CT[65] and MRI[66]

1. prerequisite: ventricular enlargement without block (i.e. communicating hydrocephalus)
2. features that correlate with favorable response to shunt. These features suggest that the hydrocephalus is *not* due to atrophy alone. (Note: atrophy / hydrocephalus ex vacuo, as in conditions such as Alzheimer's disease, lessens the chance of, but does not preclude, responding to a shunt (cortical atrophy is a common finding in healthy individuals of advanced age[67])
   a) periventricular low density on CT or high intensity on T2WI MRI: may represent transependymal absorption of CSF. May resolve with shunting
   b) compression of convexity sulci (note: focal sulcal dilation may sometimes be seen and may represent atypical reservoirs of CSF which may diminish after shunting and should not be considered as atrophy[68])
   c) rounding of the frontal horns

Although some patients improve with no change in ventricles,[69] clinical improvement most often accompanies reduction of ventricular size.

Radionuclide cisternography

Usefulness remains controversial. One study found that the cisternogram does not increase the diagnostic accuracy of clinical and CT criteria.[70] Use has been abandoned by most researchers.[71]

24.12.5 Ancillary tests for NPH

Lumbar puncture (LP)

Opening pressure

Normal LP opening pressure (OP) in the left lateral decubitus position averages 12.2 ± 3.4 cm H_2O (8.8 ± 0.9 mm Hg)[72] and should be < 180 mm H_2O (OP > 24 cm H_2O suggests noncommunicating hydrocephalus rather than NPH[58,73]). In NPH the average OP is 15 ± 4.5 cm H_2O (11 ± 3.3 mm Hg), slightly higher than, but overlapping with, normal. Based on expert opinion, an upper limit of 24 cm H_2O (17.6 mm Hg) is suggested for the definition of NPH. Patients with an initial OP > 10 cm H_2O have a higher response rate to shunting.

CSF labs

Send CSF for routine labs (p. 1506) to R/O infection, elevated protein (e.g. with tumor), SAH.

"Tap Test"

Consists of lumbar puncture with removal of a specific quantity of CSF and assessment of response.

The tap test has not undergone rigorous prospective evaluation. A *positive* response to withdrawal of 40–50 ml of CSF has a PPV in the range of 73–100%,[74,75,76] but sensitivity is low (26–61%). (Note: what constitutes a ***significant*** "response" has not been standardized, most experts prefer demonstrating objective improvement in gait, taking into account the fact that NPH patients can have day-to-day fluctuations in symptoms.)

Resistance testing

CSF Ro is considered to be the impedance of CSF absorptive mechanisms. 1/Ro is the conductance. Techniques and thresholds are center-specific. No clinical study has adequately addressed the fact that Ro normally increases with age.[77]

Determination of CSF Ro *may* have a higher sensitivity (57–100%) but a similar PPV (75–92%) to the tap test.

Methodology

Numerous methods have been devised to measure Ro. Two illustrative methods:

1. bolus method[78]: a known volume (usually ≈ 4 ml) is injected via LP at a rate of 1 ml/sec
2. Katzman test[79]: infuse saline through LP at a known rate, Ro is given by Eq (24.1) (up to 19% of patients experience H/A after infusion studies[80])

$$Ro = \frac{\text{(final steady state pressure)} - \text{(initial pressure)}}{\text{infusion rate}} \tag{24.1}$$

Ambulatory lumbar drainage (ALD)

See reference.[74]

A lumbar subarachnoid drain is placed with Tuohy needle, connected through a drip chamber to a closed drainage system. The drip chamber is placed at the level of the patient's ear when they are recumbent, or at the level of the shoulder when sitting or ambulating.

A properly functioning drain should put out ≈ 300 ml of CSF per day.

If symptoms of nerve root irritation develop during the drainage, the catheter should be withdrawn several millimeters. Daily surveillance CSF cell counts and cultures should be performed (NB: a pleocytosis of ≈ 100 cells/mm^3 can be seen normally just as a result of the presence of a drain).

A 5 day trial is recommended (mean time to improvement: 3 days).

Continuous CSF pressure monitoring

Some patients with a normal OP on LP demonstrate pressure peaks > 270 mm H_2O or recurrent B-waves.[81] These patients also, and may have a higher response rate to shunting than those without these findings.

Miscellaneous

Cerebral blood flow (CBF) measurements: Although some studies indicate otherwise, CBF measurements show no specific findings in NPH, and are not helpful in predicting who will respond to shunting. However, increased CBF after shunting correlates with clinical improvement.[82]

EEG: There are no specific EEG findings in NPH.

24.12.6 Diagnostic criteria

Practice guideline: Diagnosis of NPH

Level II[58]: Since strict diagnostic criteria cannot be formulated for NPH because of a lack of knowledge of the underlying pathophysiology at this time, it is recommended that the diagnosis be made in terms of Probable, Possible, and Unlikely NPH as described in ▶ Table 24.3.

Guidelines for diagnosis of NPH are shown in ▶ Table 24.3.

24.12.7 Differential diagnosis of NPH

▶ Table 24.4 shows conditions with presentations similar to findings in NPH in the differential diagnosis.[58,83] ▶ Table 24.5 compares some features of NPH, Alzheimer's disease, and Parkinson's disease.

24.12.8 Treatment

Management algorithm

1. based on history, physical exam, and imaging studies, categorize the patient as probable, possible, or unlikely NPH based on ▶ Table 24.3. For probable and possible NPH, without further testing, the degree of certainty of the diagnosis of NPH is ≈ 50–61%.[70,84,85] In an otherwise healthy patient in whom the diagnosis of NPH seems highly probable, it is not unreasonable to proceed to shunting[73]
2. otherwise, to increase the certainty of response to shunting, one or more of the following tests is recommended[73]
   a) "tap test": withdrawal of 40–50 ml of CSF via LP
      - positive response (p. 407) increases likelihood of responding to a shunt (PPV) to the range of 73–100%
      - due to low sensitivity (26–61%), a negative response does not rule out the possibility of responding, and a subsequent supplemental test should be performed[73]
      - if OP > 17.6 mm Hg (24 cm H_2O), consider further search for cause of secondary hydrocephalus (does not rule-out shunting as a treatment)
   b) resistance testing: sensitivity (57–100%) > tap test, similar PPV (75–92%)
   c) external lumbar drainage

CSF diversionary procedures

VP shunt is the procedure of choice. Lumbar-peritoneal shunts have been used, but disadvantages include: tendency to overshunt, difficult to tap, tendency to migrate. For most, use a *medium pressure* valve[86] (closing pressure 65–90 mm H_2O) to minimize the risk of subdural hematomas (see below), although response rate may be higher with a low-pressure valve.[87] Gradually sit patient up over a period of several days; proceed more slowly in patients who develop low-pressure headaches. Alternatively, the risk of developing SDH may be decreased with use of a programmable shunt valve, set initially at a high pressure (to reduce risk of subdural hematoma) and gradually decreasing the pressure setting over a number of weeks.

Follow patients clinically and with CT for ≈ 6–12 months.

Patients who do not improve and whose ventricles do not change on imaging should be evaluated for shunt malfunction. If not obstructed, and if no subdural fluid collections have developed, a lower pressure valve may be tried (or a lower pressure selected on a programmable shunt).

Potential complications of shunting for NPH

Complication rates may be as high as ≈ 35% (due in part to the frailty of the elderly brain).[88,89]

Table 24.4 Conditions with similar presentation to NPH

Conditions with similar presentation to NPH
Neurodegenerative disorders • Alzheimer's disease • Parkinson's disease • Lewy body disease • Huntington's disease • frontotemporal dementia • corticobasal degeneration • progressive supranuclear palsy • amyotrophic lateral stenosis • multisystem atrophy • spongiform encephalopathy
Vascular dementia • cerebrovascular disease • multi-infarct dementia • Binswanger's disease • CADASIL • vertebrobasilar insufficiency (VBI)
Other hydrocephalic disorders • aqueductal stenosis • arrested hydrocephalus • long-standing overt ventriculomegaly syndrome • noncommunicating hydrocephalus
Infectious disease • Lyme disease • HIV • syphilis
Urological disorders • urinary tract infection • bladder or prostate cancer • benign prostatic hypertrophy (BPH)
Miscellaneous • vitamin B12 deficiency • collagen vascular diseases • epilepsy • depression • traumatic brain injury • spinal stenosis • Chiari malformation • Wernicke's encephalopathy • carcinomatous meningitis • spinal cord tumor

Potential complications include[90]:

1. subdural hematomas or hygroma (p. 426): higher risk with low pressure valve and older patients who tend to have cerebral atrophy. Usually accompanied by headache, most resolve spontaneously or remain stable. Approximately one–third require evacuation and tying off of shunt (temporarily or permanently). Risk may be reduced by gradual mobilization post-op
2. shunt infection
3. intracerebral hemorrhage
4. seizures (p. 417)
5. delayed complications include: above, plus shunt obstruction or disconnection

Endoscopic third ventriculostomy (ETV)

Initially reported for NPH in 1999.[91] Mechanistically, it is difficult to explain why ETV would work for NPH, but it has been advocated by some[92] in highly selected patients, using nonvalidated outcome measures, quoting post-op improvement in 69% of patients. At this time, ETV should not be considered a first line treatment for most cases of NPH.

Table 24.5 Comparison of NPH, Alzheimer's & Parkinson's disease[a]

Feature	NPH	AD	IPA
gait disturbance[b]	+	±	±
postural instability	±		+
urinary disturbance	±	±	±
memory or cognitive impairment	±	+	±
difficulty performing familiar tasks	±	+	±
behavioral changes	±	+	±
limb rigidity			+
limb tremor			+
bradykinesia			+

[a]abbreviations: AD + Alzheimer's disease; IPA = idiopathic paralysis agitans (Parkinson's disease); + = feature present; ± = feature partial or late
[b]in NPH, the gait is often wide based, in IPA often narrow stance

24.12.9 Outcome

The most likely symptom to improve with shunting is *incontinence*, then gait disturbance, and lastly dementia. Black et al.[86] give the following markers for good candidates for improvement with shunting:

- clinical: presence of the classic triad (p. 404).[88] Also 77% of patients with gait disturbance as the primary symptom improved with shunting. Patients with dementia and *no* gait disturbance rarely respond to shunting
- LP: OP > 100 mm H_2O
- isotope cisternogram: typical NPH pattern. The mixed or normal pattern has no correlation with response to shunting
- continuous CSF pressure recording: pressure > 180 mm H_2O or frequent Lundberg B waves (p. 864)
- CT or MRI: large ventricles with flattened sulci (little atrophy)

Response is better when symptoms have been present for a shorter time.

NB: NPH patients with co-existing Alzheimer's disease (AD) may still improve with VP shunts, thus AD should not exclude these patients from shunting.[93] However, patients with AD *alone* (without NPH) did not respond to shunting in a RPDB placebo-controlled trial.[94]

In general, most responders eventually relapse, often after ≈ 5–7 years of good response. Shunt malfunction and subdural collections must be ruled out before ascribing this to the natural course of the underlying condition.

24.13 Hydrocephalus and pregnancy

24.13.1 General information

Patients with CSF shunts may become pregnant, and there are case reports of patients developing hydrocephalus during pregnancy requiring shunting.[95]

Any of the shunt problems discussed in the following sections may occur in a pregnant patient with a shunt. With VP shunts, distal shunt problems may be higher in pregnancy. The following are management suggestions modified from Wisoff et al.[95]

24.13.2 Preconception management of patients with shunts

1. evaluation, including:
   a) evaluation of shunt function: preconception baseline MRI or CT. Further evaluation of shunt patency if any suspicion of malfunction. Patients with slit ventricles may have reduced compliance and may become symptomatic with very small changes in volume
   b) assessment of medications, especially anticonvulsants

2. counselling, including:
   a) genetic counselling: if the HCP is due to a neural tube defect (NTD), then there is a 2–3% chance that the baby will have a NTD
   b) other recommendations include early administration of prenatal vitamins, and avoiding teratogenic drugs and excessive heat (e.g. hot-tubs): Neural tube defects, Risk factors (p.290).

24.13.3 Gravid management

1. close observation for signs of increased ICP: headache, N/V, lethargy, ataxia, seizures… Caution: these signs may mimic pre-eclampsia (which must also be ruled out). 58% of patients exhibit signs of increased ICP, which may be due to:
   a) decompensation of partial shunt malfunction
   b) shunt malfunction
   c) some show signs of increased ICP in spite of adequate shunt function, may be due to increased cerebral hydration and venous engorgement
   d) enlargement of tumor during pregnancy
   e) cerebral venous thrombosis: including dural sinus thrombosis & cortical venous thrombosis
   f) encephalopathy related to disordered autoregulation
2. patients developing symptoms of increased ICP should have CT or MRI to compare ventricle size to preconception baseline study
   a) if no change from preconception study, puncture shunt to measure ICP and culture CSF. Consider radioisotope shunt-o-gram
   b) if all studies are negative, then physiologic changes may be responsible. Treatment is bed rest, fluid restriction, and in severe cases steroids and/or diuretics. If symptoms do not abate, then early delivery is recommended as soon as fetal lung maturity can be documented (give prophylactic antibiotics for 48 hrs before delivery)
   c) if ventricles have enlarged and/or shunt malfunction is demonstrated on testing, shunt revision is performed
      - in first two trimesters: VP shunt is preferred (do not use peritoneal trocar method after first trimester) and is tolerated well
      - in third trimester: VA or ventriculopleural shunt is used to avoid uterine trauma or induction of labor

24.13.4 Intrapartum management

1. prophylactic antibiotics are recommended during labor and delivery to reduce the incidence of shunt infection. Since coliforms are the most common pathogen in L&D, Wisoff et al. recommend ampicillin 2 gm IV q 6 hrs, and gentamicin 1.5 mg/kg IV q 8 hrs in labor and × 48 hrs post partum[95]
2. in patients without symptoms: a vaginal delivery is performed if obstetrically feasible (lower risk of forming adhesions or infection of distal shunt). A shortened second stage is preferred since the increase in CSF pressure in this stage is probably greater than during other valsalva maneuvers[96]
3. in the patient who becomes symptomatic near term or during labor, after stabilizing the patient a C-section under general anesthesia (epidurals are contraindicated with elevated ICP) is performed with careful fluid monitoring and, in severe cases, steroids and diuretics

References

[1] Lemire RJ. Neural Tube Defects. JAMA. 1988; 259:558–562

[2] Amacher AL, Wellington J. Infantile Hydrocephalus: Long-Term Results of Surgical Therapy. Childs Brain. 1984; 11:217–229

[3] Hill A, Rozdilsky B. Congenital Hydrocephalus Secondary to Intra-Uterine Germinal Matrix/Intraventricular Hemorrhage. Dev Med Child Neurol. 1984; 26:509–527

[4] Kudo H, Tamaki N, Kim S, et al. Intraspinal Tumors Associated with Hydrocephalus. Neurosurgery. 1987; 21:726–731

[5] Schmidek HH, Auer LM, Kapp JP. The Cerebral Venous System. Neurosurgery. 1985; 17:663–678

[6] Parker T. Never Trust a Calm Dog: And Other Rules of Thumb. New York: Harper Perennial; 1990

[7] U.S. Department of Health and Human Services - Health Resources and Services Administration. Accurately Weighing and Measuring: Technique.

[8] Babson SG, Benda GI. Growth Graphs for the Clinical Assessment of Infants of Varying Gestational Age. J Pediatr. 1976; 89:814–820

[9] Nelhaus G. Head Circumference from Birth to Eighteen Years. Pediatrics. 1968; 41:106–114

[10] Humphrey PRD, Moseley IF, Russell RWR. Visual Field Defects in Obstructive Hydrocephalus. J Neurol Neurosurg Psychiatry. 1982; 45:591–597

[11] Calogero JA, Alexander E. Unilateral Amaurosis in a Hydrocephalic Child with an Obstructed Shunt. J Neurosurg. 1971; 34:236–240

[12] Kojima N, Kuwamura K, Tamaki N, et al. Reversible Congruous Homonymous Hemianopia as a Symptom of Shunt Malfunction. Surg Neurol. 1984; 22:253–256

[13] Black PM, Chapman PH. Transient Abducens Paresis After Shunting for Hydrocephalus. J Neurosurg. 1981; 55:467–469

[14] Arroyo HA, Jan JE, McCormick AQ, et al. Permanent Visual Loss After Shunt Malfunction. Neurology. 1985; 35:25–29

[15] Sato M, Tanaka S, Kohama A, et al. Occipital Lobe Infarction Caused by Tentorial Herniation. Neurosurgery. 1986; 18:300–305

[16] Joynt RJ, Honch GW, Rubin AJ, Trudell RG, Frederiks JAM. In: Occipital Lobe Syndromes. Handbook of Clinical Neurology. Holland: Elsevier Science Publishers; 1985:49–62

[17] Hoyt WF. Vascular Lesions of the Visual Cortex with Brain Herniation Through the Tentorial Incisura. Arch Ophthalm. 1960; 64:44–57

[18] Rinaldi I, Botton JE, Troland CE. Cortical Visual Disturbances Following Ventriculography and/or Ventricular Decompression. J Neurosurg. 1962; 19:568–576

[19] Lindenberg R, Walsh FB. Vascular Compressions Involving Intracranial Visual Pathways. Tr Am Acad Ophth Otol. 1964; 68:677–694

[20] Glaser JS, Duane TD, Jaeger EA. In: Topical Diagnosis: Retrochiasmal Visual Pathways and Higher Cortical Function. Clinical Ophthalmology. 2nd ed. Philadelphia: Harper and Row; 1983:4–10

[21] Lindenberg R. Compression of Brain Arteries as Pathogenetic Factor for Tissue Necrosis and their Areas of Predilection. J Neuropath Exp Neurol. 1955; 14:223–243

[22] Barnet AB, Manson JI, Wilner E. Acute Cerebral Blindness in Childhood. Neurology. 1970; 20:1147–1156

[23] Keane JR. Blindness Following Tentorial Herniation. Ann Neurol. 1980; 8:186–190

[24] Hoyt WF, Walsh FB. Cortical Blindness with Partial Recovery Following Cerebral Anoxia from Cardiac Arrest. Arch Ophthalm. 1958; 60:1061–1069

[25] Weinberger HA, van der Woude R, Maier HC. Prognosis of Cortical Blindness Following Cardiac Arrest in Children. JAMA. 1962; 179:126–129

[26] Slavin ML. Ischemic Optic Neuropathy After Cardiac Arrest. Am J Ophthalmol. 1987; 104:435–436

[27] Sweeney PJ, Breuer AC, Selhorst JB, et al. Ischemic Optic Neuropathy: A Complication of Cardiopulmonary Bypass Surgery. Neurology. 1982; 32:560–562

[28] Drance SM, Morgan RW, Sweeney VP. Shock-Induced Optic Neuropathy. A Cause of Nonprogressive Glaucoma. N Engl J Med. 1973; 288:392–395

[29] Lorber J. Recovery of Vision Following Prolonged Blindness in Children with Hydrocephalus or Following Pyogenic Meningitis. Clin Pediatr. 1967; 6:699–703

[30] LeMay M, Hochberg FH. Ventricular Differences Between Hydrostatic Hydrocephalus and Hydrocephalus Ex Vacuo by CT. Neuroradiology. 1979; 17:191–195

[31] Evans WA. An encepahlographic ratio for estimating ventricular and cerebral atrophy. Arch Neurol Psychiatry. 1942; 47:931–937

[32] O'Hayon BB, Drake JM, Ossip MG, Tuli S, Clarke M. Frontal and Occipital Horn Ratio: A Linear Estimate of Ventricular Size for Multiple Imaging Modalities in Pediatric Hydrocephalus. Pediatric Neurosurgery. 1998; 29:245–249

[33] Tuite GF, Evanson J, Chong WK, et al. The Beaten Copper Cranium: A Correlation between Intracranial Pressure, Cranial Radiographs, and Computed Tomographic Scans in Children with Craniosynostosis. Neurosurgery. 1996; 39:691–699

[34] Section of Pediatric Neurosurgery of the American Association of Neurological Surgeons. Pediatric Neurosurgery. New York 1982

[35] Alvarez LA, Maytal J, Shinnar S. Idiopathic External Hydrocephalus: Natural History and Relationship to Benign Familial Macrocephaly. Pediatrics. 1986; 77:901–907

[36] Barlow CF. CSF Dynamics in Hydrocephalus - With Special Attention to External Hydrocephalus. Brain Dev. 1984; 6:119–127

[37] Chadduck WM, Chadduck JB, Boop FA. The Subarachnoid Spaces in Craniosynostosis. Neurosurgery. 1992; 30:867–871

[38] McCluney KW, Yeakley JW, Fenstermacher JW. Subdural Hygroma Versus Atrophy on MR Brain Scans: "The Cortical Vein Sign". AJNR. 1992; 13:1335–1339

[39] Kuzma BB, Goodman JM. Differentiating External Hydrocephalus from Chronic Subdural Hematoma. Surg Neurol. 1998; 50:86–88

[40] Ment LR, Duncan CC, Geehr R. Benign Enlargement of the Subarachnoid Spaces in the Infant. J Neurosurg. 1981; 54:504–508

[41] Sutton LN. Current Management of Hydrocephalus in Children. Contemp Neurosurg. 1997; 19:1–7

[42] Weller S, Gartner J. Genetic and clinical aspects of X-linked hydrocephalus (L1 disease): Mutations in the L1CAM gene. Hum Mutat. 2001; 18:1–12

[43] Grupe A, Hultgren B, Ryan A, Ma YH, Bauer M, Stewart TA. Transgenic knockouts reveal a critical requirement for pancreatic beta cell glucokinase in maintaining glucose homeostasis. Cell. 1995; 83:69–78

[44] Yamasaki M, Arita N, Hiraga S, Izumoto S, Morimoto K, Nakatani S, Fujitani K, Sato N, Hayakawa T. A clinical and neuroradiological study of X-linked hydrocephalus in Japan. J Neurosurg. 1995; 83:50–55

[45] Kanemura Y, Okamoto N, Sakamoto H, Shofuda T, Kamiguchi H, Yamasaki M. Molecular mechanisms and neuroimaging criteria for severe L1 syndrome with X-linked hydrocephalus. J Neurosurg. 2006; 105:403–412

[46] Foltz EL, Shurtleff DB. Five-Year Comparative Study of Hydrocephalus in Children with and without Operation (113 Cases). J Neurosurg. 1963; 20:1064–1079

[47] Rekate HL, Nulsen FE, Mack HL, et al. Establishing the Diagnosis of Shunt Independence. Monogr Neural Sci. 1982; 8:223–226

[48] Holtzer GJ, De Lange SA. Shunt-Independent Arrest of Hydrocephalus. J Neurosurg. 1973; 39:698–701

[49] Hemmer R. Can a Shunt Be Removed? Monogr Neural Sci. 1982; 8:227–228

[50] Epstein F. Diagnosis and Management of Arrested Hydrocephalus. Monogr Neural Sci. 1982; 8:105–107

[51] Pang D, Zwienenberg-Lee M, Smith M, Zovickian J. Progressive cranial nerve palsy following shunt placement in an isolated fourth ventricle: case report. J Neurosurg. 2005; 102:326–331

[52] Oi S, Matsumoto S. Slit ventricles as a cause of isolated ventricles after shunting. Childs Nerv Syst. 1985; 1:189–193

[53] Eder HG, Leber KA, Gruber W. Complications after shunting isolated IV ventricles. Childs Nerv Syst. 1997; 13:13–16

[54] Hakim S, Adams RD. The Special Clinical Problem of Symptomatic Hydrocephalus with Normal CSF Pressure. J Neurol Sci. 1965; 2:307–327

[55] Brean A, Eide PK. Prevalence of probable idiopathic normal pressure hydrocephalus in a Norwegian population. Acta Neurol Scand. 2008; 118:48–53

[56] Adams RD, Fisher CM, Hakim S, Ojemann RG, et al. Symptomatic Occult Hydrocephalus with 'Normal' Cerebrospinal Fluid Pressure. N Engl J Med. 1965; 273:117–126

[57] Thal LJ, Grundman M, Klauber MR. Dementia: Characteristics of a Referral Population and Factors Associated with Progression. Neurology. 1988; 38:1083–1090

[58] Relkin N, Marmarou A, Klinge P, Bergsneider M, Black PMcL. INPH Guidelines, Part II: Diagnosing idiopathic normal-pressure hydrocephalus. Neurosurgery. 2005; 57:S2–4 to 16

[59] Knutsson E, Lying-Tunell U. Gait apraxia in normal-pressure hydrocephalus. Neurology. 1985; 35:155–160

[60] Rosen H, Swigar ME. Depression and normal pressure hydrocephalus. A dilemma in neuropsychiatric differential diagnosis. J Nerv Ment Dis. 1976; 163:35–40

[61] Schneider U, Malmadier A, Dengler R, Sollmann WP, Emrich HM. Mood cycles associated with normal

pressure hydrocephalus. Am J Psychiatry. 1996; 153:1366–1367
[62] Crowell RM, Tew JM,Jr, Mark VH. Aggressive dementia associated with normal pressure hydrocephalus. Report of two unusual cases. Neurology. 1973; 23:461–464
[63] Bloom KK, Kraft WA. Paranoia–an unusual presentation of hydrocephalus. Am J Phys Med Rehabil. 1998; 77:157–159
[64] Yoshino M, Yoshino Y, Taniguchi M, Nakamura S, Ikeda T. Syndrome of inappropriate secretion of antidiuretic hormone associated with idiopathic normal pressure hydrocephalus. Intern Med. 1999; 38:290–292
[65] Vassilouthis J. The Syndrome of Normal-Pressure Hydrocephalus. J Neurosurg. 1984; 61:501–509
[66] Jack CR, Mokri B, Laws ER, Houser OW, et al. MR Findings in Normal Pressure Hydrocephalus: Significance and Comparison with Other Forms of Dementia. J Comput Assist Tomogr. 1987; 11:923–931
[67] Schwartz M, Creasey H, Grady CL, et al. Computed Tomographic Analysis of Brain Morphometrics in 30 Healthy Men, Aged 21 to 81 Years. Ann Neurol. 1985; 17:146–157
[68] Holodny AI, George AE, de Leon MJ, et al. Focal Dilation and Paradoxical Collapse of Cortical Fissures and Sulci in Patients with Normal-Pressure Hydrocephalus. J Neurosurg. 1998; 89:742–747
[69] Shenkin HA, Greenberg JO, Grossman CB. Ventricular Size After Shunting For Idiopathic Normal Pressure Hydrocephalus. J Neurol Neurosurg Psychiatry. 1975; 38:833–837
[70] Vanneste J, Augustijn P, Davies GAG, Dirven C, et al. Normal-Pressure Hydrocephalus: Is Cisternography Still Useful in Selecting Patients for a Shunt? Arch Neurol. 1992; 49:366–370
[71] Relkin Norm. Neuroradiology Assessment of iNPH. Banff, Alberta, Canada 2015
[72] Bono F, Lupo MR, Serra P, Cantafio C, et al. Obesity does not induce abnormal CSF pressure in subjects with normal cerebral MR venography. Neurology. 2002; 59:1641–1643
[73] Marmarou A, Bergsneider M, Klinge P, Relkin N, Black PMcL. INPH Guidelines, Part III: The value of supplemental prognostic tests for the preoperative assessment of idiopathic normal-pressure hydrocephalus. Neurosurgery. 2005; 57:S2–17 to 28
[74] Haan J, Thomeer RTWM. Predictive Value of Temporary External Lumbar Drainage in Normal Pressure Hydrocephalus. Neurosurgery. 1988; 22:388–391
[75] Malm J, Kristensen B, Karlsson T, Fagerlund M, Elfverson J, Ekstedt J. The predictive value of cerebrospinal fluid dynamic tests in patients with the idiopathic adult hydrocephalus syndrome. Arch Neurol. 1995; 52:783–789
[76] Walchenbach R, Geiger E, Thomeer RT, Vanneste JA. The value of temporary external lumbar CSF drainage in predicting the outcome of shunting on normal pressure hydrocephalus. J Neurol Neurosurg Psychiatry. 2002; 72:503–506
[77] Czosnyka M, Czosnyka ZH, Whitfield PC, Donovan T, Pickard JD. Age dependence of cerebrospinal pressure-volume compensation in patients with hydrocephalus. J Neurosurg. 2001; 94:482–486
[78] Marmarou A, Shulman K, Rosende RM. A nonlinear analysis of the cerebrospinal fluid system and intracranial pressure dynamics. J Neurosurg. 1978; 48:332–344
[79] Katzman R, Hussey F. A simple constant-infusion manometric test for measurement of CSF absorption. I. Rationale and method. Neurology. 1970; 20:534–544
[80] Meier U, Bartels P. The importance of the intrathecal infusion test in the diagnostic of normal-pressure hydrocephalus. Eur Neurol. 2001; 46:178–186
[81] Symon L, Dorsch NWC, Stephens RJ. Pressure Waves in So-Called Low-Pressure Hydrocephalus. Lancet. 1972; 2:1291–1292
[82] Tamaki N, Kusunoki T, Wakabayashi T, et al. Cerebral Hemodynamics in Normal-Pressure Hydrocephalus: Evaluation by 133Xe Inhalation Method and Dynamic CT Study. J Neurosurg. 1984; 61:510–514
[83] Bech-Azeddine R, Waldemar G, Knudsen GM, Hogh P, Brahn P, Wildschiotz G, Gjerris F, Paulson OB, Juhler M. Idiopathic nromal pressure hydrocephalus: Evaluation and findings in a multidisciplinary memory clinic. Eur J Neurol. 2001; 8:601–611
[84] Vanneste J, Augustijn P, Tan WF, Dirven C. Shunting normal pressure hydrocephalus: The predictive value of combined clinical and CT data. J Neurol Neurosurg Psychiatry. 1993; 56:251–256
[85] Takeuchi T, Kasahara E, Iwasaki M, Mima T, Mori K. Indications for shunting in patients with idiopathic normal pressure hydrocephalus presenting with dementia and brain atrophy (atypical idiopathic normal pressure hydrocephalus). Neurol Med Chir (Tokyo). 2000; 40:38–47
[86] Black PM, Ojemann RG, Tzouras A. CSF Shunts for Dementia, Incontinence and Gait Disturbance. Clin Neurosurg. 1985; 32:632–651
[87] McQuarrie IG, Saint-Louis L, Scherer PB. Treatment of Normal-Pressure Hydrocephalus with Low versus Medium Pressure Cerebrospinal Fluid Shunts. Neurosurgery. 1984; 15:484–488
[88] Black PM. Idiopathic Normal-Pressure Hydrocephalus: Results of Shunting in 62 Patients. J Neurosurg. 1980; 52:371–377
[89] Peterson RC, Mokri B, Laws ER. Surgical Treatment of Idiopathic Hydrocephalus in Elderly Patients. Neurology. 1985; 35:307–311
[90] Udvarhelyi GB, Wood JH, James AE. Results and Complications in 55 Shunted Patients with Normal Pressure Hydrocephalus. Surg Neurol. 1975; 3:271–275
[91] Mitchell P, Mathew B. Third ventriculostomy in normal pressure hydrocephalus. Br J Neurosurg. 1999; 13:382–385
[92] Gangemi M, Maiuri F, Naddeo M, Godano U, Mascari C, Broggi G, Ferroli P. Endoscopic third ventriculostomy in idiopathic normal pressure hydrocephalus: an Italian multicenter study. Neurosurgery. 2008; 63:62–7; discussion 67-9
[93] Golomb J, et al. Alzheimer's Disease Comorbidity in Normal Pressure Hydrocephalus: Prevalence and Shunt Response. J Neurol Neurosurg Psychiatry. 2000; 68:778–781
[94] Silverberg GD, Mayo M, Saul T, Fellmann J, Carvalho J, McGuire D. Continuous CSF drainage in AD: results of a double-blind, randomized, placebo-controlled study. Neurology. 2008; 71:202–209
[95] Wisoff JH, Kratzert KJ, Handwerker SM, Young BK, Epstein F. Pregnancy in Patients with Cerebrospinal Fluid Shunts: Report of a Series and Review of the Literature. Neurosurgery. 1991; 29:827–831
[96] Marx GF, Zemaitis MT, Orkin LR. CSF Pressures During Labor and Obstetrical Anesthesia. Anesthesiology. 1981; 22:348–354

25 Treatment of Hydrocephalus

25.1 Medical treatment of hydrocephalus

HCP remains a surgically treated condition. Acetazolamide may be helpful for temporizing (see below).

25.1.1 Diuretic therapy

25

May be tried in premature infants with bloody CSF (as long as there is no evidence of active hydrocephalus) while waiting to see if there will be resumption of normal CSF absorption. However, at best this should only be considered as an adjunct to definitive treatment or as a temporizing measure.

Satisfactory control of HCP was reported in ≈ 50% of patients of age < 1 year who had stable vital signs, normal renal function and no symptoms of elevated ICP (apnea, lethargy, vomiting) using the following[1] with the following regimen:

1. acetazolamide (a carbonic anhydrase inhibitor): 25 mg/kg/day PO divided TID × 1 day, increase 25 mg/kg/day each day until 100 mg/kg/day is reached
2. simultaneously start furosemide: 1 mg/kg/day PO divided TID
3. to counteract acidosis, use tricitrate (Polycitra®):
   a) start 4 ml/kg/day divided QID (each ml is equivalent to 2 mEq of bicarbonate, and contains 1 mEq K^+ and 1 mEq Na^+)
   b) measure serial electrolytes, and adjust dosage to maintain serum HCO_3 > 18 mEq/L
   c) change to Polycitra-K® (2 mEq K^+ per ml, no Na^+) if serum potassium becomes low, or to sodium bicarbonate if serum sodium becomes low
4. watch for electrolyte imbalance and acetazolamide side effects: lethargy, tachypnea, diarrhea, paresthesias (e.g. tingling in the fingertips)
5. perform weekly U/S or CT scan and insert ventricular shunt if progressive ventriculomegaly occurs. Otherwise, maintain therapy for a 6 month trial, then taper dosage over 2–4 weeks. Resume 3–4 mos of treatment if progressive HCP occurs

25.2 Spinal taps

HCP after intraventricular hemorrhage may be only transient. Serial taps (ventricular or LP[2]) may temporize until resorption resumes but LPs can only be performed for *communicating* HCP. If reabsorption does not resume when the protein content of the CSF is < 100 mg/dl, then it is unlikely that spontaneous resorption will occur in the near future (i.e. a shunt will usually be necessary).

25.3 Surgical

25.3.1 Goals of therapy

Normal sized ventricles is not the goal of therapy (some children have a paucity of brain tissue). Goals are optimum neurologic function (which usually requires normal intracranial pressure) and a good cosmetic result.

25.3.2 Surgical options

Options include

- third ventriculostomy: currently, endoscopic method is preferred (see below)
- shunting: various shunts are described below. The techniques of shunt placement are covered for VP shunts (p. 1515), for VA shunt (p. 1516), for ventriculopleural shunts (p. 1515), and for LP shunt (p. 1517)
- eliminating the obstruction: e.g. opening a stenosed sylvian aqueduct. Often higher morbidity and lower success rate than simple CSF diversion with shunts, except perhaps in the case of tumor
- choroid plexectomy: described by Dandy in 1918 for communicating hydrocephalus.[3] May reduce the rate but does not totally halt CSF production (only a portion of CSF is secreted by the choroid plexus, other sources include the ependymal lining of the ventricles and the dural sleeves of spinal nerve roots). Open surgery was associated with a high mortality rate (possibly due to replacement

of CSF by air). Endoscopic choroid plexus coagulation was originally described in 1910 and was recently resurrected[4]

25.4 Endoscopic third ventriculostomy

25.4.1 Indications

Endoscopic third ventriculostomy (ETV) may be used in patients with obstructive HCP. May also be an option in managing shunt infection (as a means to remove all hardware without subjecting the patient to increased ICP). ETV has also been proposed as an option for patients who developed subdural hematomas after shunting (the shunt is removed before the ETV is performed). ETV may also be indicated for slit ventricle syndrome (p. 424).

25.4.2 Contraindications

Communicating hydrocephalus has traditionally been considered a contraindication to ETV. However, it has been occasionally used for NPH.[5] Relative contraindications to ETV would be the presence of any of the conditions associated with a low success rate (see below).

25.4.3 Complications

- hypothalamic injury: may result in hyperphagia
- injury to pituitary stalk or gland: may result in hormonal abnormalities including diabetes insipidus, amenorrhea
- transient 3rd and 6th nerve palsies
- injury to basilar artery, p-comm, or PCA: a fixed endoscope sheath seated just distal to the foramen of Monro within the third ventricle may allow for safe egress of blood extacranially)
- uncontrollable bleeding
- cardiac arrest[6]
- traumatic basilar artery aneurysm[7]: possibly related to thermal injury from use of laser in performing ETV

25.4.4 Technique

See dedicated section on technique (p. 1517).

25.4.5 Success rate

Overall success rate is ≈ 56% (range of 60–94% for nontumoral aqueductal stenosis[7] (AqS)). Highest maintained patency rate is with previously untreated acquired AqS. Success rate in infants may be poor because they may not have a normally developed subarachnoid space. There is a low success rate (only ≈ 20% of TVs will remain patent) if there is pre-existing pathology including:

1. tumor
2. previous shunt
3. previous SAH
4. previous whole brain radiation (success with focal stereotactic radiosurgery is not known)
5. significant adhesions visible when perforating through the floor of the third ventricle at the time of performance of ETV

The ETV Success Score (see ▶ Table 25.1)[8,9] is a validated[10,11] means of predicting the likelihood of success of ETV and therefore may assist in selecting appropriate patients for the procedure.

Total of the 3 scores (1 from each category: age, etiology and shunt history) expressed as a percent is the approximate chance of an ETV lasting 6 months without failure. Scores < 40% correlated with a very low chance of success. Scores > 80% correlated with a better chance of success compared to shunting from the outset.

Intermediate scores (50-70%) ETV had a higher initial failure rate compared to shunting, but after 3-6 months the balance shifted in favor of ETV.[9]

In one series, clinical improvement after ETV was achieved in 76% (72 of 95 patients), including 6 patients requiring second ETVs (three of which had partially functioning shunts that were left in place at the time of ETV).

Table 25.1 ETV Success Score

Category	Description	Value	Score
Age	<1 month	0%	___%
	1 to<6 months	10%	
	6 months to<1 year	30%	
	1 to>10 years	40%	
	≥10 years	50%	
Etiology	• post infectious	0%	___%
	• myelomeningocele • post IVH • non-tectal brain tumor	20%	
	• aqueductal stenosis • tectal tumor • other	30%	
Shunt history	• previous shunt	0%	___%
	• no previous shunt	10%	
		Total (range 0-90%)	___%

25.5 Shunts

25.5.1 Types of shunts

1. ventriculoperitoneal (**VP**) shunt:
   a) most commonly used shunt in modern era
   b) lateral ventricle is the usual proximal location
   c) intraperitoneal pressure: normal is near atmospheric
2. ventriculo-atrial (**VA**) shunt ("vascular shunt"):
   a) shunts ventricles through jugular vein to superior vena cava, so-called "ventriculo-atrial" shunt because it shunts the cerebral ventricles to the vascular system with the catheter tip in the region of the right cardiac atrium)
   b) treatment of choice when abdominal abnormalities are present (extensive abdominal surgery, peritonitis, morbid obesity, in preemies who have had NEC and may not tolerate VP shunt…)
   c) shorter length of tubing results in lower distal pressure and less siphon effect than VP shunt, however pulsatile pressures may alter CSF hydrodynamics
3. Torkildsen shunt:
   a) shunts ventricle to cisternal space
   b) rarely used
   c) effective only in acquired obstructive HCP, as patients with congenital HCP frequently do not develop normal subarachnoid CSF pathways
4. miscellaneous: various distal projections used historically or in patients who have had significant problems with traditional shunt locations (e.g. peritonitis with VP shunt, SBE with vascular shunts):
   a) pleural space (ventriculopleural shunt): not a first choice, but a viable alternative if the peritoneum is not available.[12] To avoid symptomatic hydrothorax necessitating relocating distal end, it is recommended only for patients > 7 yrs age (although some feel that these may be placed as young as 2 yrs age, and that hydrothorax is primarily a sign of infection regardless of age). Pressure in pleural space is less than atmospheric
   b) gall bladder
   c) ureter or bladder: causes electrolyte imbalances due to losses through urine
5. lumboperitoneal (LP) shunt; see insertion technique (p. 1517)
   a) only for communicating HCP: primarily pseudotumor cerebri or CSF fistula.[13] Useful in situations with small ventricles
   b) over age 2 yrs, percutaneous insertion with Tuohy needle is preferred

6. cyst or subdural shunt: from arachnoid cyst or subdural hygroma cavity, usually to peritoneum

25.5.2 Disadvantages/complications of various shunts

Complications that may occur with any shunt

1. obstruction: the most common cause of shunt malfunction
   a) proximal: ventricular catheter (the most common site)
   b) valve mechanism
   c) distal: reported incidence of 12–34%.[14] Occurs in peritoneal catheter in VP shunt (see below), in atrial catheter in VA shunt
2. disconnection at a junction, or break at any point
3. infection: may produce obstruction
4. hardware erosion through skin, usually only in debilitated patients (especially preemies with enlarged heads and thin scalp from chronic HCP, who lay on one side of head due to elongated cranium). May also indicate silicone allergy (see below)
5. *seizures* (ventricular shunts only): there is ≈ 5.5% risk of seizures in the first year after placement of a shunt which drops to ≈ 1.1% after the 3rd year[15] (NB: this does not mean that the shunt was the cause of all of these seizures). Seizure risk is questionably higher with frontal catheters than with parieto-occipital
6. act as a conduit for extraneural metastases of certain tumors (e.g. medulloblastoma). This is probably a relatively low risk[16]
7. silicone allergy[17]: rare (if it occurs at all). May resemble shunt infection with skin breakdown and fungating granulomas. CSF is initially sterile but later infections may occur. May require fabrication of a custom silicone-free device (e.g. polyurethane)

Disadvantages/complications with VP shunt

1. inguinal hernia: incidence = 17% (many shunts are inserted while processus vaginalis is patent)[18]
2. need to lengthen catheter with growth: may be obviated by using long peritoneal catheter (p.1515)
3. obstruction of peritoneal catheter:
   a) may be more likely with distal slit openings ("slit valves") due to occlusion by omentum or by trapping debris from the shunt system[14]
   b) by peritoneal cyst (or pseudocyst)[19]: usually associated with infection, may also be due to reaction to talc from surgical gloves (the omentum tends to "wall off" a nidus of irritation). It may rarely be necessary to differentiate a CSF collection from a urine collection in patients with overdistended bladders that have ruptured (e.g. secondary to neurogenic bladder). Fluid can be aspirated percutaneously and analyzed for BUN and creatinine (which should be absent in CSF)
   c) severe peritoneal adhesions: reduce surface area for CSF resorption
   d) malposition of catheter tip:
      - at time of surgery: e.g. in preperitoneal fat
      - tubing may pull out of peritoneal cavity with growth
4. peritonitis from shunt infection
5. hydrocele
6. CSF ascites
7. tip migration
   a) into scrotum[20]
   b) perforation of a viscus[21]: stomach,[22] bladder… More common with older spring-reinforced (Raimondi) shunt tubing
   c) through the diaphragm[23]
8. intestinal obstruction (as opposed to perforation): rare
9. volvulus[24]
10. intestinal strangulation: occurred only in patients in whom attempt was made to remove peritoneal tubing using traction on the catheter applied at the cephalad incision with subsequent breakage of the tubing leaving a residual intraabdominal segment (immediate peritoneal exploration is recommended under these circumstances)[25]
11. overshunting (p.424): more likely than with VA shunt. Some recommend LP shunt for communicating hydrocephalus

Disadvantages/complications with VA shunt

1. requires repeated lengthening in growing child
2. higher risk of infection, septicemia
3. possible retrograde flow of blood into ventricles if valve malfunctions (rare)
4. shunt embolus
5. vascular complications: perforation, thrombophlebitis, pulmonary micro-emboli may cause pulmonary hypertension[26] (incidence ≈ 0.3%)

Disadvantages/complications with LP shunt

1. if at all possible, should not be used in growing child unless ventricular access is unavailable (e.g. due to slit ventricles) because of:
   a) laminectomy in children causes scoliosis in 14%[27]
   b) risk of progressive cerebellar tonsillar herniation (Chiari I malformation)[28] in up to 70% of cases[29,30]
2. overshunting harder to control when it occurs (a special horizontal-vertical (H-V) valve increases resistance when upright, see below)
3. difficult access to proximal end for revision or assessment of patency; see Lumboperitoneal (LP) shunt evaluation (p. 1518).
4. lumbar nerve root irritation (radiculopathy)
5. leakage of CSF around catheter
6. pressure regulation is difficult
7. bilateral 6th and even 7th cranial nerve dysfunction from overshunting
8. high incidence of arachnoiditis and adhesions

Programmable shunt valves

A number of externally programmable shunts available in the U.S., including:
- Strata by Medtronic (p. 429)
- Polaris by Sophysa (p. 431)
- Codman Hakim (p. 429)
- Certas Plus by Codman
- proGav by Aesculap

All are programmed externally with a magnet, and can potentially be inadvertently reprogrammed by external magnetic fields including those encountered during an MRI (the Polaris valve and the Certas Plus valve are promoted as being less susceptible to inadvertent reprogramming. ✱ Therefore, valve settings should be rechecked after an MRI scan performed for any reason, or if there is ever a concern about shunt function. The pressure setting on all of these valves can be checked on a plain x-ray taken perpendicular to the shunt valve (see ► Fig. 25.1 to identify the programmable valve type, then see the corresponding section for that valve to determine the shunt pressure setting). Some can also be checked using a special hand-held compass-like device provided by the manufacturer to most hospitals and clinics that deal with their valves.

In all systems on the market, increasing the programmed number results in higher valve opening pressures and therefore *less* CSF drainage at any given CSF pressure.

X-ray appearance of some shunt valves

► Fig. 25.1 depicts *idealized* x-ray appearances of some common shunts. It is intended to help differentiate shunt systems on x-ray, and is not to scale. Appearance may vary with orientation relative to the x-ray beam. Manufacturer's diagrams of these shunts appears in section 25.7.

Miscellaneous shunt hardware

1. tumor filter: used to prevent peritoneal or vascular seeding in tumors that may metastasize through CSF (e.g. medulloblastoma,[31] PNETs, ependymoma); may eventually become occluded by tumor cells and need replacement; may be able to radiate tumor filter to "sterilize" it. Not often used despite the fact that the risk of "shunt mets" appears to be low[16]
2. devices to avoid overdrainage when the patient is upright
   a) antisiphon devices (ASD): prevents siphoning effect when patient is erect. Some valves have ASDs integrated into the valve. ASDs always increase the resistance of the shunt
   b) "horizontal-vertical valve" (H-V valve) (p. 433) used primarily with LP shunts

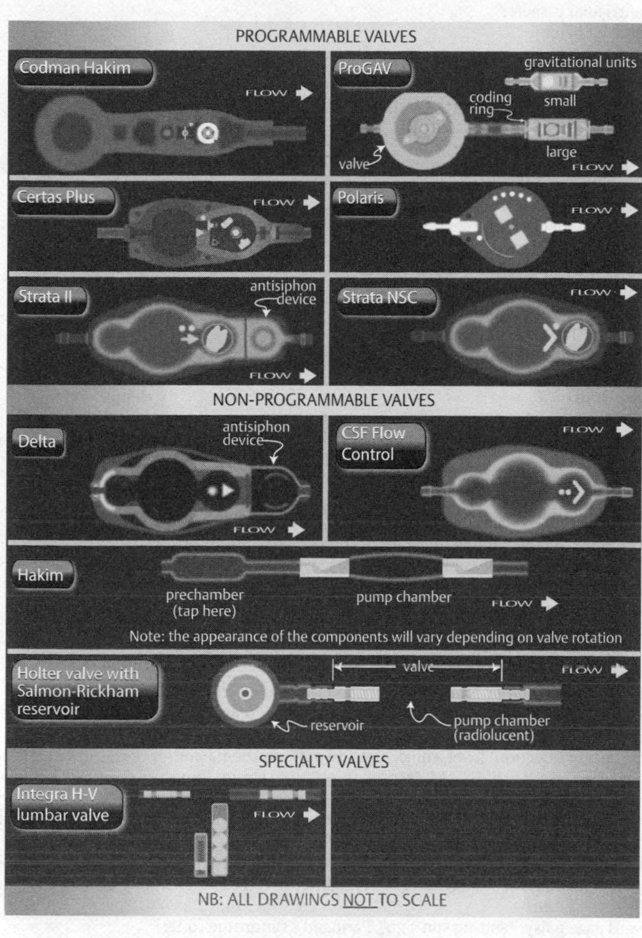

Fig. 25.1 X-ray appearance of common shunts
For x-ray appearance of programmable valves and the corresponding pressures, see the individual valve.

3. with a standard 90 cm long 1.2 mm inner diameter distal catheter, the hydrodynamic resistance of most shunts increases by 2–2.5 mm Hg/(ml/min)[32]

25.6 Shunt problems

25.6.1 Risks associated with shunt insertion

1. intraparenchymal or intraventricular hemorrhage: risk ≈ 4% (in the absence of coagulopathy[33])
2. seizures

3. malposition
   a) of ventricular catheter
   b) of distal catheter
4. infection

25.6.2 Problems in patients with established CSF shunt

Shunt "problems" usually involve one or more of the following (**undershunting and infection account for most common shunt problems**):
1. undershunting (see below): obstruction (rate: ≈ 10% per year), breakage...
2. infection (p.339): range 1–40%. A serious complication. Often associated with obstruction.
3. Having a shunt infection decrease IQ
4. overshunting:
   a) slit ventricle syndrome
   b) subdural hematomas... (p.424)
   c) "spinal headache"
5. seizures (p.417)
6. problems related to the distal catheter
   a) peritoneal (p.417)
   b) atrial (p.418)
7. skin breakdown over hardware (p.417): may indicate infection or silicone allergy

25.6.3 Evaluation of the patient with a shunt

History and physical

1. history directed at determining presence of shunt-related symptoms
   a) acute symptoms of increased ICP
      - H/A: effect of posture, position, activity, migraine-like symptoms (visual aura...)
      - N/V
      - diplopia
      - lethargy
      - ataxia
      - infants: apnea and/or bradycardia; irritability; poor feeding
      - seizures: either new onset, or if pre-existing, an increase in frequency, or difficulty in control
   b) symptoms of infection: fever, chills, night-sweats, erythema and/or tenderness over shunt tubing. Diarrhea may indicate infection unrelated to shunt. Exposure to other sick individuals
2. physical exam: the following includes signs of increased intracranial pressure
   a) for children: OFC (p.395). Plot on graph of normal curves (use existing chart for that patient if available) loof for OFC crossing curves
   b) fontanelle tension (if open): a soft pulsating fontanelle varying with respirations is normal, a tense bulging fontanelle suggests obstruction, a sunken fontanelle may be normal or may represent overshunting
   c) upward gaze palsy: "setting sun sign", Parinaud's syndrome (p.99)
   d) abducens palsy (p.567): false localizing sign
   e) field cut, or blindness; see Blindness from hydrocephalus (p.396)
   f) swelling around shunt tubing: caused by CSF dissecting along tract of an obstructed shunt
3. shunt history
   a) type of shunt: VP, VA, pleural, LP
   b) initial insertion of shunt: reason (MM, post-meningitis, etc.) and patient age
   c) date of last revision and reason for revision
   d) presence of accessory hardware in system (e.g. antisiphon device, etc.)
4. ability of shunt to pump and refill
   a) ✖ caution: may exacerbate obstruction, especially if shunt is occluded by ependyma due to overshunting: controversial
   b) difficult to depress: suggests distal occlusion
   c) slow to refill (generally, any valve should refill in 15–30 secs): suggests proximal (ventricular) occlusion or slit ventricles
5. evidence of CSF dissecting along tract outside of shunt tubing
6. in children presenting only with vomiting, especially those with cerebral palsy and feeding gastrostomy tubes, rule-out gastroesophageal reflux

Radiographic evaluation

1. "shunt series" (plain x-rays to visualize entire shunt)
   a) Purpose: R/O disconnection/breakage or migration of tip (NB: a disconnected shunt may continue to function by CSF flow through a subcutaneous fibrous tract)
   b) For a VP shunt: AP & lateral skull, CXR and abdominal x-ray
   c) the following hardware may be radiolucent and can mimic disconnection:
      - the central silastic part of older Holter style valves
      - connectors ("Y" & "T" as well as straight)
      - antisiphon devices
      - tumor filters
   d) obtain most recent x-rays available to compare for breaks (essential for "complicated" shunts involving multiple ventricular or cyst ends or accessory hardware)
2. in infants with open fontanelles, ultrasound is optimal method of evaluation (especially if previous U/S available)
3. *CT* required if fontanelles closed, may be desirable in complicated shunt systems (e.g. cyst shunts). Minimize the number of CTs in pediatric patients
4. *MRI*: shunt hardware is difficult to see. May show transependymal absorption of CSF, loculations… Programmable valves must be evaluated and reprogrammed after MRI
5. "shunt-o-gram" if it is still unclear if shunt is functioning
   a) radionuclide: see below
   b) x-ray: using iodinated contrast: see below

25

"Shunt-o-gram"

Indications

When shunt function cannot be reliably ascertained using other methods.

Procedure

Shave hair over reservoir & prep (e.g. with Betadine). With patient supine tap the shunt by inserting a 25 gauge butterfly needle into the reservoir. Measure the pressure with a manometer. Patients with multiple ventricular catheters need to have each injected to verify its patency.

Radionuclide "shunt-o-gram" AKA radionuclide shuntography[34]: after tapping the shunt, drain 2–3 ml of CSF and send 1 ml of CSF for C&S. Inject radio-isotope (e.g. for VP shunt in an adult, use 1 mCi of 99m-Tc (technetium) pertechnetate (usable range: 0.5 to 3 mCi) in 1 cc of fluid) while occluding distal flow (by compressing valve or occluding ports). Flush in isotope with remaining CSF.

Immediately image the abdomen with the gamma camera to rule out direct injection into distal tubing. Image the cranium to verify flow into ventricles (proximal patency). for diffusion of the isotope within the abdomen to rule out pseudocyst formation around catheter.

Interpretation: If spontaneous flow into abdomen occurs within 20 minutes, the shunt is patent. If there is no flow on delayed imaging, it is occluded. The valve can be pumped to look for diffusion of isotope within the abdomen to rule out pseudocyst formation around the catheter tip. If it takes > 20 minutes, or if the patient has to be stood up to get flow, this is indeterminate and you should use other information to decide whether or not to revise the shunt.

X-ray "shunt-o-gram": after tapping the shunt, drain ≈ 1 ml of CSF and send for C&S. Inject e.g. iohexol (Omnipaque 180) (p.219) while occluding distal flow (by compressing valve or occluding ports).

Pseudocyst (peritoneal) with VP shunt

An abdominal pseudocyst is usually an indication of infection.

Treatment algorithm

One of many viable surgical protocols to deal with this:

1. open abdominal incision over tubing, and divide tubing at this site
2. verify which cut end is the peritoneal end and which is the distal shunt (with a working shunt, pumping the valve should cause CSF to come out the distal shunt)
3. attempt to drain the cyst through the remaining peritoneal end
   a) when you can't draw any more fluid, or if you don't get any to begin with, withdraw the catheter a little at a time and aspirate at each step
   b) send any fluid obtained for culture
   c) if tubing does not pull out smoothly, the abdomen may need to be opened (consider consulting general surgeon)

4. verify function of remaining shunt
   a) if the remaining shunt is functioning
      - connect it to sterile collection system
      - monitor output volumes & send surveillance cultures of CSF qod
      - after 3 consecutive cultures are negative, internalize distal end of shunt (using fresh distal catheter). The choice of target for distal end (peritoneum, pleura, vein) depends on whether abdominal cyst fluid is infected and if the peritoneal cavity still seems suitable)
   b) if the shunt is not functioning, a new external ventricular catheter should be inserted and connected to a collection system
      - monitor output volumes & send surveillance cultures of CSF qod
      - after 3 consecutive cultures are negative, remove the old shunt and place a totally new shunt. The choice of target for distal end (peritoneum, pleura, vein) depends on whether abdominal cyst fluid is infected and if the peritoneal cavity still seems suitable)
5. shunt tap: indications vary, generally performed if occlusion suspected or if surgical exploration is considered or if infection is strongly suspected; see Tapping a shunt (p. 422)
6. shunt exploration: sometimes even after thorough evaluation the only means to definitively prove or disprove the functioning of various shunt components is to operate and isolate and test each part of the system independently. Even when infection is not suspected, CSF and any removed hardware should be cultured.

Tapping a shunt

Indications

Indications to tap a shunt or ventricular access device (e.g. Ommaya reservoir) include:

1. to obtain CSF specimen
   a) to evaluate for shunt infection
   b) for cytology: e.g. in PNET to look for malignant cells in CSF
   c) to remove blood: e.g. in intraventricular hemorrhage
2. to evaluate shunt function
   a) measuring pressures
   b) contrast studies:
      - proximal injection of contrast (iodinated or radio-labeled)
      - distal injection of contrast
3. as a temporizing measure to allow function of a distally occluded shunt[35,36]
4. to inject medication
   a) antibiotics: for shunt infection or ventriculitis
   b) chemotherapeutic (antineoplastic) agents
5. for catheters placed within tumor cyst (not a true shunt):
   a) periodic withdrawal of accumulated fluid
   b) for injection of radioactive liquid (usually phosphorous) for ablation

Technique

For LP shunt, see Lumboperitoneal (LP) shunt evaluation (p. 1518).

There is a risk of introducing infection with every entry into the shunt system. With care, this may be kept to a minimum.

1. shave area
2. prep: e.g. povidone iodine solution × 5 minutes
3. use 25 gauge butterfly needle or smaller (ideally a noncoring needle should be used): for routine taps, the needle should only be introduced into shunt components specifically designed to be tapped

To measure pressures

A 25 Ga butterfly needle and an LP tray (with manometer, specimen tubes, 3-way stopcock valve...) are helpful. Steps are outlined in ▶ Table 25.2.

25.6.4 Undershunting

General information

The shunt malfunction rate is ≈ 17% during the first year of placement in the pediatric population.

Table 25.2 Steps in tapping a shunt

Step	Information provided
• After shave and prep, insert 25 Ga butterfly needle into the reservoir and look for spontaneous flow into butterfly tubing • measure pressure in manometer	• spontaneous flow indicates proximal end not completely occluded • pressure is that of ventricular system (normal is < 15 cm of CSF in relaxed recumbent patient)
• then measure the pressure with distal occluder compressed (if present)	• rise in pressure indicates some function of valve and distal shunt
• if no spontaneous flow, try to aspirate CSF with syringe	• if CSF is easily aspirated, it may be that pressure seen by ventricular system is very low. There should be spontaneous flow after that when the end of the tubing is lowered • if no CSF obtained or if difficult to aspirate, indicates proximal occlusion
• if still no flow, carefully inject 1–2 ml of preservative free saline into ventricular catheter and see if spontaneous flow of more than the amount injected occurs	• may dislodge clot or debris from catheter • if only the 1–2 ml that were injected returns, indicates there is not a patent catheter in an open CSF space (possibilities include: occluded catheter, tip lodged in brain, slit ventricles)
• send any CSF for: C&S, protein/glucose, cell count	• checks for infection
• fill manometer with sterile saline with the valve turned off to the shunt • compress *proximal* (inlet) occluder if present • Open valve to shunt and measure runoff pressure after ≈ 60 seconds	• measures forward transmission pressure (through valve and peritoneal catheter in valves with a proximal occluder); forward pressure should be less than ventricular pressure (and absolute pressure should be < 8 cm H_2O)
• if no distal flow, keep inlet occluder compressed and inject 3–5 ml of saline into distal shunt and recheck distal runoff pressure • ✖ do not inject more than ≈ 1–2 ml into ventricles to avoid increasing ICP	• if peritoneal catheter is in a loculated compartment the pressure will be considerably higher after injection

Etiologies

May be due to one or a number of the following:

1. blockage (occlusion)
   a) possible causes of occlusion:
      • proximal obstruction by choroid plexus
      • buildup of proteinaceous accretions
      • blood
      • cells (inflammatory or tumor)
      • secondary to infection
   b) site of blockage
      • blockage of ventricular end (most common): usually by choroid plexus, may also be due to glial adhesions, intraventricular blood
      • blockage of intermediate hardware (valves, connectors, etc., tumor filters may become obstructed by tumor cells, antisiphon devices may close due to variable overlying subcutaneous tissue pressures[37])
      • blocked distal end, also see VP shunt (p. 417)
   c) disconnection, kinking or breakage of system at any point: with age, silicone elastomers used in catheters calcify and break down, and become more rigid and fragile which may promote subcutaneous attachment.[38] Barium impregnation may accelerate this process. Tube fractures often occur near the clavicle, presumably due to the increased motion there

Signs and symptoms of undershunting

Signs and symptoms are those of active hydrocephalus. See "Evaluation of patient with shunt" (p. 420).

25.6.5 Shunt infection

See Shunt infection (p. 339) for evaluation and treatment.

25.6.6 "Overshunting"

General information

Possible complications of overshunting include[39]:
1. slit ventricles: including slit ventricle syndrome (see below)
2. intracranial hypotension: see below
3. subdural hematomas (p. 426)
4. craniosynostosis and microcephaly (p. 427): controversial
5. stenosis or occlusion of sylvian aqueduct

25

10–12% of long-term ventricular shunt patients will develop one of the above problems within 6.5 yrs of initial shunting.[39] Some experts feel that problems related to overshunting could be reduced by utilizing LP shunts for communicating hydrocephalus, and reserving ventricular shunts for obstructive HCP.[39] VP shunts may also be more likely to overdrain than VA shunts because of the longer tubing → greater siphoning effect.

Intracranial hypotension

AKA low ICP syndrome. Very rare. Symptoms similar to those of spinal H/A (postural in nature, *relieved by recumbency*). Although usually not associated with the following symptoms,[40] they may occur[39]: N/V, lethargy, or neurologic signs (e.g. diplopia, upgaze palsy). Sometimes the symptoms resemble those of high ICP except that they are relieved when prostrate. Acute effects that may occur include[39]: tachycardia, loss of consciousness, other brain stem deficits due to a rostral shift of the intracranial contents or to low ICP.

Etiology is a siphoning effect due to the column of CSF in the shunt tube when the patient is erect.[41] Ventricles may be slit-like (as in slit ventricle syndrome (SVS)) or may be normal in appearance. Sometimes it is necessary to document a drop in ICP when going from supine to erect to diagnose this condition. These patients may also develop shunt occlusion and then the distinction from SVS blurs (see below).

With short-term symptoms, an antisiphon device (ASD) is the treatment of choice. However, patients with long-standing overshunting may not tolerate efforts to return intraventricular pressures to normal levels.[39,42]

Slit ventricles

"Slit ventricles" refers to complete collapse of the ventricles. In a survey, a frontal-occipital horn ratio[43] < 0.2 was most often interpreted as representing SVS. May be seen in:
1. overshunting
2. with entrapped (isolated) fourth ventricle (p. 402)
3. some patients with idiopathic intracranial hypertension (AKA pseudotumor cerebri) (p. 766) have slit-like ventricles with consistently elevated ICP

Slit ventricles may be:
1. asymptomatic:
   a) slit ventricles (totally collapsed lateral ventricles) may be seen on CT in 3 -80% of patients after shunting,[40,44] most are asymptomatic
   b) these patients may occasionally present with symptoms unrelated to the shunt, e.g. true migraine
2. slit ventricle syndrome (SVS): seen in < 12% of all shunted patients. Subtypes:
   a) intermittent shunt occlusion: overshunting leads to ventricular collapse (slit ventricles) which causes the ependymal lining to occlude the inlet ports of the ventricular catheter (by coaptation) producing shunt obstruction. With time, many of these patients develop low ventricular compliance,[45] where even minimal dilatation results in high pressure which produces symptoms. Expansion then eventually reopens the inlet ports allowing resumption of drainage (hence the intermittent symptoms). Symptoms may resemble shunt malfunction: intermittent headaches unrelated to posture, often with N/V, drowsiness, irritability and impaired

mentation. Signs may include 6th cranial nerve palsy. Incidence in shunted patients: 2–5%.[40, 46] CT or MRI scans may also show evidence of transependymal absorption of CSF
   b) total shunt malfunction (AKA normal volume hydrocephalus[45]): may occur and yet ventricles remain slit-like if the ventricles cannot expand because of subependymal gliosis, or due to the law of Laplace (which states that the pressure required to expand a large container is lower than the pressure required to expand a small container)
   c) venous hypertension with normal shunt function: may result from partial venous occlusion that occurs in some conditions (e.g. at the level of the jugular foramen in Crouzon's syndrome). Usually subsides by adulthood
3. intracranial hypotension: symptoms often relieved by recumbency (see above)

Evaluation of slit ventricles

The shunt valve fills slowly if pumped when the ventricles are collapsed.

Monitoring CSF pressure: either via lumbar drain, or with a butterfly inserted into the shunt reservoir (with this method, pressure can be followed during postural changes to look for negative pressure when upright; possibly higher risk of infection with this). These patients are also monitored for pressure spikes, especially during sleep.

Alternatively, these patients may be evaluated by "shunt-o-gram" (see above).

Treatment

In treating a patient with slit ventricles in imaging studies, it is important to ascertain into which of the categories (see above) the patient falls. If the patient can be categorized, then the specific treatment listed below should be employed. Otherwise, it is probably most common to initially treat the patient empirically as intracranial hypotension, and then to move on to other methods for treatment failures.

Treatment of asymptomatic slit ventricles

Prophylactic upgrading to a higher pressure valve or insertion of an antisiphon device as initially advocated has largely been abandoned. However, this may be appropriate at the time of shunt revision when done for other reasons.[44]

Treatment of intracranial hypotension

Postural H/A due to intracranial hypotension (true overshunting) is usually self limited, however, if symptoms persist after ≈ 3 days of bed-rest and analgesics and a trial with a tight abdominal binder, the valve should be checked for proper closing pressure. If it is low, replace with a higher pressure valve. If it is not low, an ASD (which, by itself, also increases the resistance of the system) alone or together with a higher pressure valve may be needed.[47]

Treatment of slit ventricle syndrome

Patients with symptoms of SVS are actually suffering from intermittent high pressure. If total shunt malfunction is the cause, then shunt revision is indicated. For intermittent occlusion, treatment options include:

1. if symptoms occur early after shunt insertion or revision, initial expectant management may be indicated since symptoms will spontaneously resolve in many patients as they equilibrate to the new intracranial pressure
2. revision of the proximal shunt. This may be difficult due to the small size of the ventricles. One can attempt to follow the existing tract and insert a longer or shorter length of tubing based on the pre-op imaging studies. Some advocate the placement of a second ventricular catheter, leaving the first one in place
3. patients may "respond" (fortuitously) to either of the following interventions because the slight ventricular enlargement elevates the ependyma off of the inlet ports (this may *not* always be the therapy of choice):
   a) valve upgrade[48] or
   b) ASD insertion[40,47]: the procedure of choice in some opinions.[39] First described in 1973[49]
4. subtemporal decompression[50,51,52] sometimes with dural incision.[50] This results in dilatation of the temporal horns (evidence for elevated pressure) in most, but not all[52] cases
5. third ventriculostomy (p.415) [53]

25.6.7 Problems unrelated to shunting

For H/A consistent with migraine that are not postural, a trial with migraine-specific medications is warranted (Fiorinal®). See treatment of idiopathic intracranial hypertension (pseudotumor cerebri) (p.771).

25.6.8 Subdural hematomas

General information

May be due to collapse of brain with tearing of bridging veins. Incidence: 4–23% in adults, 2.8–5.4% in children, and is higher with normal pressure hydrocephalus (20–46%) than with "hypertensive hydrocephalus" (0.4–5%).[54,55] The risk of SDH is higher in the setting of longstanding hydrocephalus with a large head and little brain parenchyma (craniocerebral disproportion) with a thin cerebral mantle, as usually occurs in children with macrocephaly and large ventricles on initial evaluation. These patients have an "extremely delicate balance between subdural and intraventricular pressure".[54] By the same token, SDH can also follow shunting in elderly patients who have severe brain atrophy. The development of SDH may also be facilitated by negative pressures in the ventricles as a result of a siphoning effect when the patient is upright.[55,56] There is also a low risk of epidural hematoma following CSF shunting.[55]

Characteristics of the fluid

The collections may be on the same side as the shunt in 32%, on the opposite side in 21%, and bilateral in 47%.[55]

At the time of discovery, the SDHs are usually subacute to chronic, and the previously large ventricles are usually collapsed. Only 1 of 19 cases showed colorless fluid.[55] In all cases tested (even the 1 with clear fluid), the protein was elevated compared to CSF.

Treatment

Indications for treatment

Small (< 1–2 cm thick) asymptomatic collections in patients with closed cranial sutures may be followed with serial imaging studies. SDH were symptomatic in ≈ 40% of cases (symptoms often resemble those of shunt malfunction), and these require treatment. Treatment of SDH in children with open sutures has been advocated[55] to prevent later symptoms and/or development of macrocrania. The controversy arises with large asymptomatic SDH in older children or adults. Many authors recommend not treating asymptomatic lesions regardless of appearance,[54,57] whereas others vary their recommendations based on diverse criteria including size, appearance (chronic, acute, mixed…), etc.

Treatment techniques

A number of techniques have been described. Most involve evacuation of the SDHs by any of the usual methods (e.g. burr holes for chronic collections, craniotomy for acute collections) together with:

1. reducing the degree of shunting (i.e. to establish a lower pressure in the subdural space than in the intraventricular space, to cause the ventricles to re-expand and to prevent reaccumulation of the SDH)
   a) in shunt dependent cases
      - replacing the valve with a higher pressure unit (upgrading the valve)
      - increasing the pressure on a programmable pressure valve[58,59]
      - using a Portnoy device that can be turned off and on externally. Be sure that care providers can reliably open the device in an emergency
   b) in non-shunt dependent cases
      - any of the methods outlined above for shunt dependent cases, or
      - temporarily tying off the shunt[60]
   c) insertion of an anti-siphon device[49]
2. drainage of the subdural space to
   a) the cisterna magna[61]
   b) to the peritoneum (subdural peritoneal shunt) with a low pressure valve (or no valve[55]). Some authors have the care-giver frequently pump the subdural valve

The goal is to achieve a delicate balance between undershunting (producing symptoms of active hydrocephalus) and overshunting (promoting the return of the SDH). Following surgery the patient should be mobilized slowly to prevent recurrence of the SDH.

25.6.9 Miscellaneous shunt issues

Craniosynostosis, microcephaly and skull deformities

See also Craniosynostosis (p.252). A number of skull changes have been described in infants after shunting, including[62]: thickening and inward growth of the bone of the skull base and cranial vault, decrease in size of the sella turcica, reduction in size of the cranial foramina, and craniosynostosis. The most common skull deformity was dolichocephaly from sagittal synostosis.[63] Microcephaly accounted for ≈ 6% of skull deformities after shunting (about half of these had sagittal synostosis). Some of these changes were reversible (except when complete synostosis was present) if intracranial hypertension recurred.

Laparoscopic surgery in patients with VP shunts

Issues regarding safety of laparoscopic surgery in patients with VP shunts:
1. laparoscopic surgery: abdominal insufflation with CO_2 is used to create a pneumoperitoneum permitting the general surgeon to work. Typical insufflation pressure: 15 mm Hg (see conversion factors between mm Hg and cm of water (p.861)). In thin patients, 10 mm Hg may suffice. Transient additional increases in pressure may occur, e.g. when the surgeon leans on the patient's abdomen
2. concerns for patients with VP shunts:
   a) in some cases insufflation → ↑ ICP[64] which may be due to:
      - compression of vena cava → reduced venous return from head, as in valsalva maneuver (independent of presence of a shunt)
      - absorption of CO_2 from the peritoneum → ↑ in arterial CO_2 causing cerebral arterial dilatation thereby increasing ICP
      - ↓ CSF drainage due to ↑ pressure against which CSF must flow
      - retrograde passage of air/debris into intracranial compartment through an incompetent shunt valve (this also has potential for infection in the presence of peritonitis). This risk is minimal even with in vitro back-pressures up to 80 mm Hg.[65] Retrograde flow may also occur with a valveless shunt (rarely used)
      - in one case report monitoring TCDs,[66] there was no change during laparoscopic surgery in a patient with a VP shunt (except during periods of very high pressure)
   b) occlusion of the distal catheter by air, debris[67] or soft tissue
   c) extremely high intraabdominal pressures (> 80 mm Hg in vitro) may damage the valve,[65] which could cause malfunction after the laparoscopy

Prophylactic management options:
1. very controversial, special precautions may not be necessary[68]
2. one can temporarily occlude the peritoneal catheter (e.g. by a hemoclip applied by the general surgeon through the laparoscope under minimal initial insufflation pressure; the clip is removed at the end of the procedure), or, temporary externalization of the shunt by the neurosurgeon, with internalization at the end of the procedure (this engenders an increased risk of infection)
3. ICP monitoring during laparoscopy
4. using low insufflation pressures (e.g. < 10 mm Hg)

25.7 Specific shunt systems

The following describes the salient features of some commonly used shunt systems. Diagrams are for general information only, and are not to scale.

25.7.1 Comparison of nonprogrammable shunt valves

▶ Fig. 25.2 compares opening pressures for some common nonprogrammable shunt valves. Symbols superimposed on the pressure bars show the x-ray markings on the valves.

25.7.2 Comparison of programmable shunt valves

▶ Fig. 25.3 shows a comparison of operating pressures of some common programmable shunt valves.

25.7.3 PS Medical/Medtronic CSF flow controlled valve

Manufactured by Medtronic Inc.

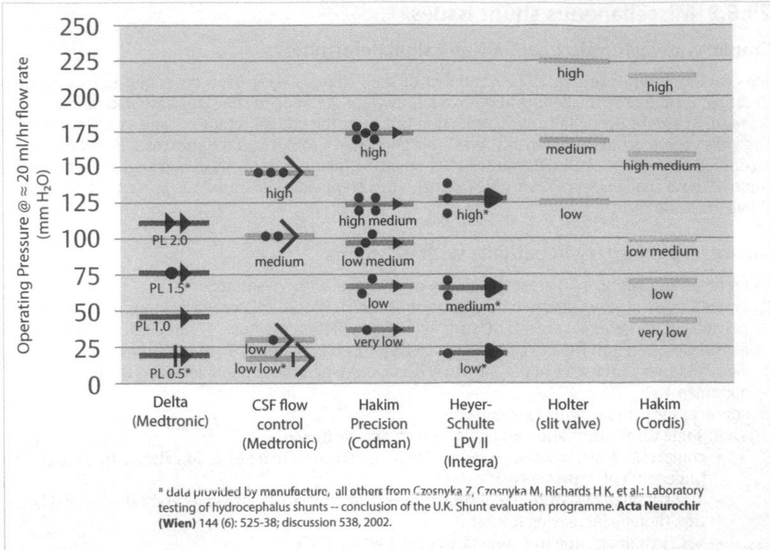

Fig. 25.2 Opening pressures of nonprogrammable shunt valves.

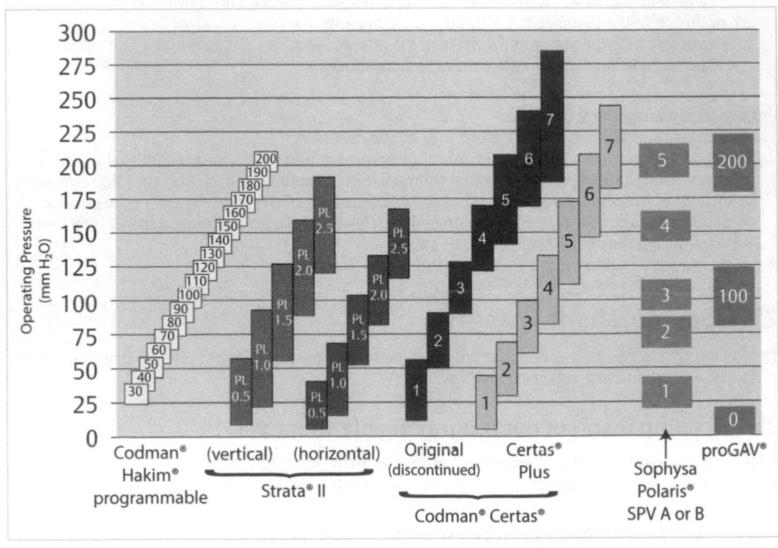

Fig. 25.3 Operating pressures of programmable shunt valves. Modified from figure courtesy of Codman Neuro, used with permission.

A single one-way membrane valve design. The radio-opaque arrowhead points in the direction of flow (▶ Fig. 25.4).

Pumping the valve

To pump the shunt in the "forward" direction, first occlude the inlet port (▶ Fig. 25.5) with pressure from one finger on the "inlet occluder" (prevents back-flow into the ventricle during the next step). Then while maintaining this pressure, depress the reservoir dome with a second finger. Release both fingers, and repeat. The one-way valve regulates shunt pressure and prevents reflux of CSF during normal use and during the release phase of shunt pumping.

X-ray characteristics

The three available valve pressures are indicated by radio-opaque dots on the valve (allows x-ray identification of valve pressure): one dot = low pressure, two dots = medium, three dots = high.

25.7.4 Strata® programmable valve

The Medtronic Strata valve is an externally adjustable valve that is programmed (using a magnet) to one of five performance level ("P/L") settings (▶ Fig. 25.6).

Also, see general information regarding programmable valves (p. 418).

25.7.5 Codman Hakim programmable valve

Manufactured by Codman Inc.

18 pressure settings. Programmed by an AC powered programming unit that requires confirmatory x-ray after re-programming. Newer programming units with acoustic monitoring may obviate

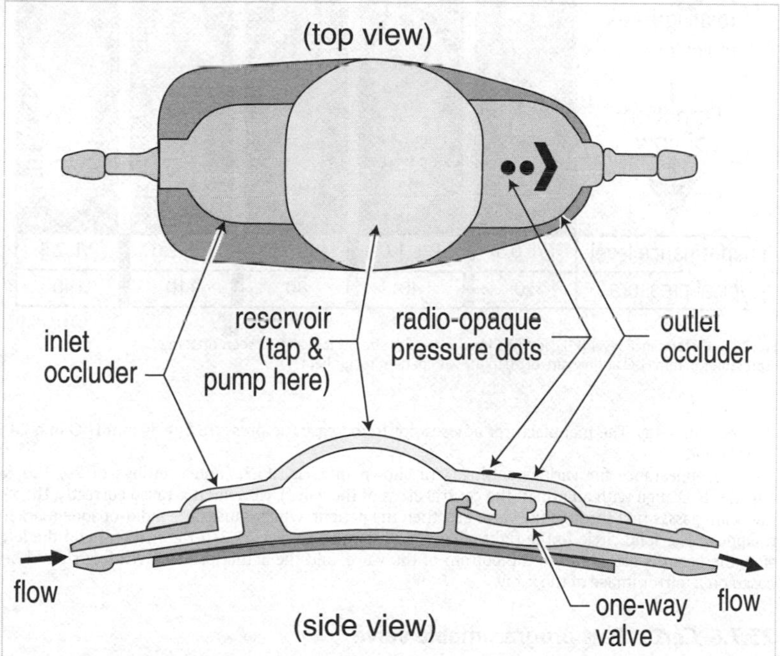

Fig. 25.4 PS Medical standard contoured valve

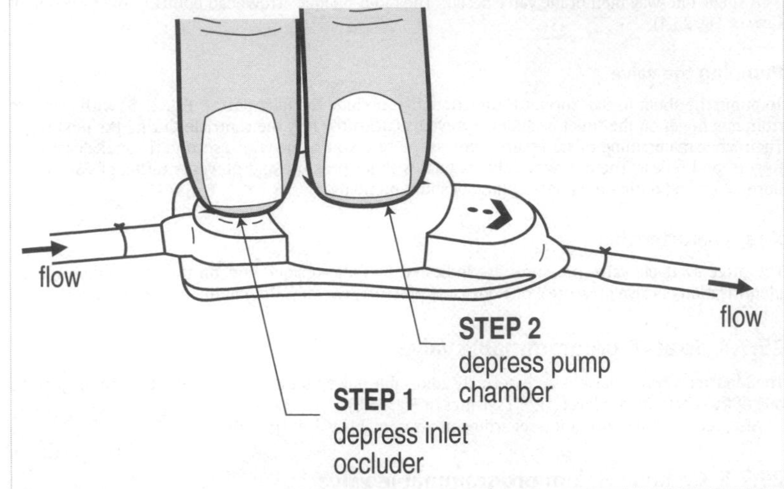

Fig. 25.5 Pumping the PS Medical valve

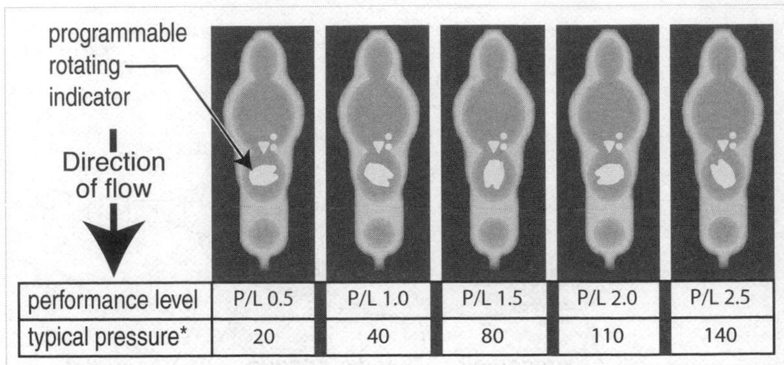

performance level	P/L 0.5	P/L 1.0	P/L 1.5	P/L 2.0	P/L 2.5
typical pressure*	20	40	80	110	140

Fig. 25.6 Performance level (P/L) settings for the regular size Strata valve as seen on x-ray
* pressures in mm H_2O at flow rate of 20 ml/hr with patient recumbent

the need for x-ray. The manufacturer advises not to increase the pressure by > 40 mm H_2O in a 24-hour period.

X-ray appearance for various settings are shown in ▶ Fig. 25.7. (note: settings of 70, 120 & 170 mm H_2O align with an arm of the central cross of the valve). NB: when x-rayed correctly, the x-ray beam passes first through the valve and then the patient, which causes the radio-opaque marker to appear as a solid circle to the right of center as shown in ▶ Fig. 25.7. If the marker is on the left side, the beam is passing from the bottom of the valve, and the actual pressure reading should be based on a mirror image of the x-ray.

25.7.6 Certas Plus programmable valve

Manufactured by Codman Inc.

The x-ray appearance is shown in ▶ Fig. 25.8, and the pressure settings appear in ▶ Table 25.2.

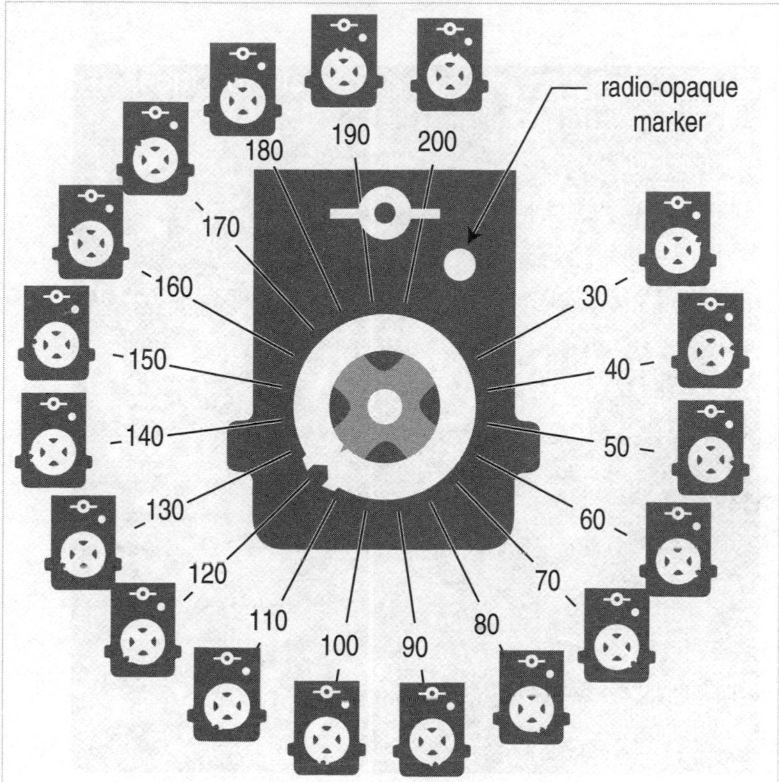

Fig. 25.7 X-ray appearance of Codman Hakim programmable valve at its various settings in mm Hg (e.g. the large central image shows a setting of 120 mm H_2O)

25.7.7 Polaris programmable valve

Manufactured by Sophysa.

The Polaris valve is an externally programmable valve that uses two attracting Samarium-Cobalt magnets to lock the pressure setting and to resist inadvertent reprogramming by environmentally encountered magnets such as MRI scanners, cell phones, headphones...

Available in 4 models (different pressure ranges, each identified by a unique number of radio-opaque dots), each with 5 externally adjustable positions. The x-ray appearance and corresponding pressures are shown in ▶ Fig. 25.9.

25.7.8 Heyer-Schulte

Distributed by Integra Neurosciences.

The LPV® II valve is shown in ▶ Fig. 25.10. To pump the shunt, occlude inlet port with one finger, then depress reservoir with another finger (as for the PS Medical valve, see above). This valve may be injected in either direction by depressing the appropriate occluder while injecting into the reservoir.

25.7.9 Hakim (Cordis) shunt

Distributed by Integra Neurosciences.

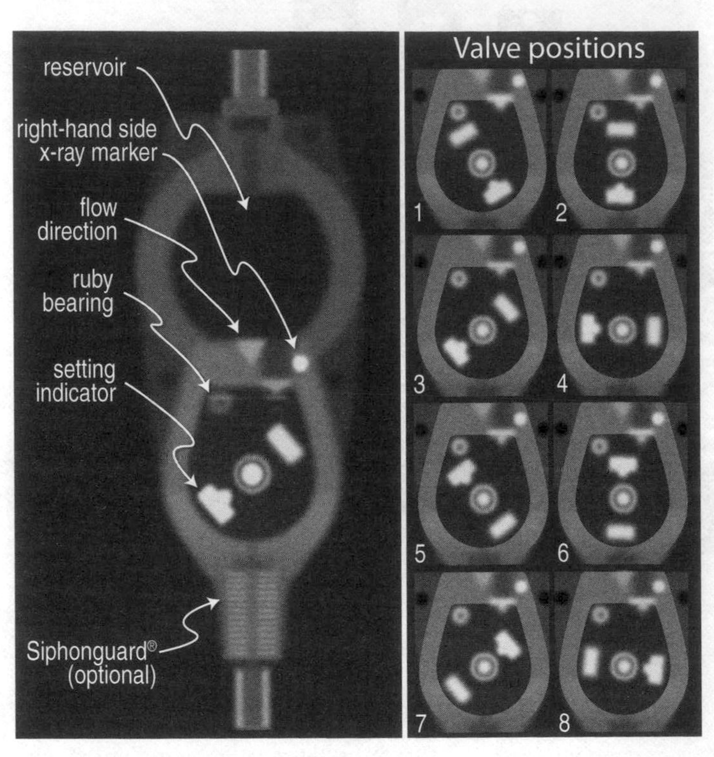

Fig. 25.8 Certas Plus Valve, x-ray appearance

Table 25.3 Certas pressure settings

Setting number	Mean pressure (mm H_2O) measured at 20 ml/hr flow rate	
	Certas (discontinued)	Certas Plus
1	36	25
2	71	50
3	109	80
4	146	110
5	178	145
6	206	180
7	238	215
8	> 400	(virtual off)

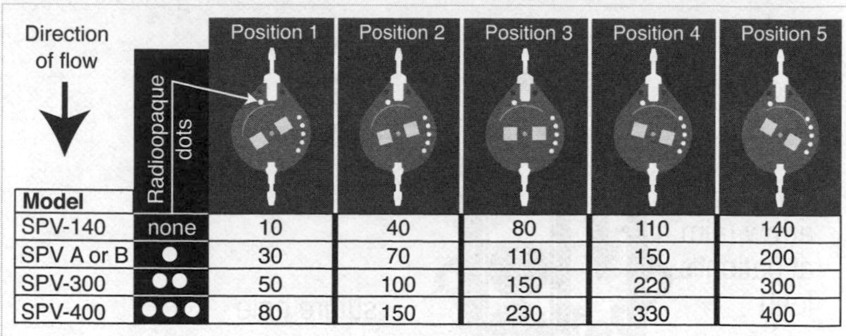

Model	Radiopaque dots	Position 1	Position 2	Position 3	Position 4	Position 5
SPV-140	none	10	40	80	110	140
SPV A or B	●	30	70	110	150	200
SPV-300	●●	50	100	150	220	300
SPV-400	●●●	80	150	230	330	400

Fig. 25.9 Programmable settings for Polaris valve models as seen on x-ray (pressures in mm H_2O)

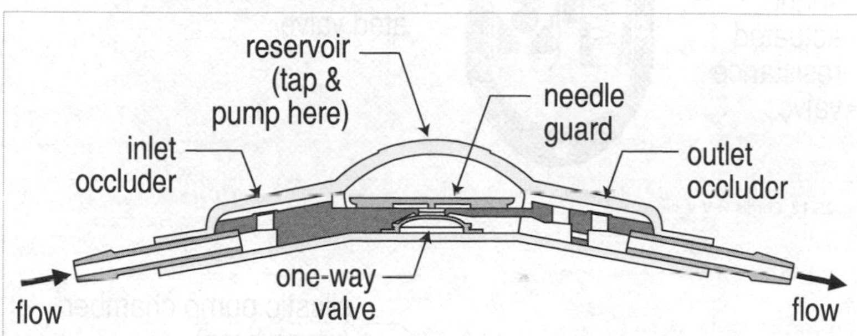

Fig. 25.10 Heyer-Schulte LPV® II(low-profile) valve (side view)

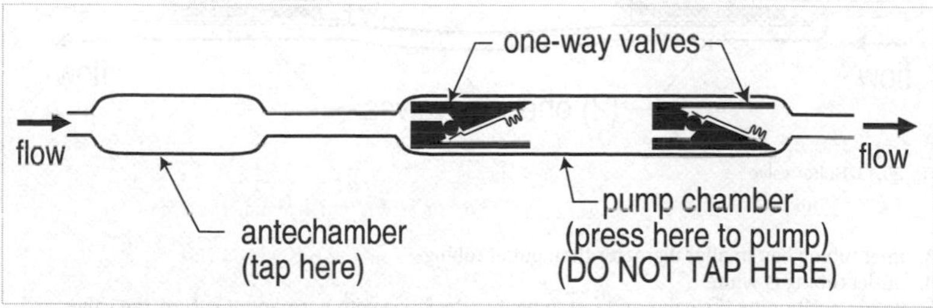

Fig. 25.11 Hakim Standard Mechanism

A dual ball-valve mechanism (▸ Fig. 25.11). To pump shunt, depress the indicated portion of the valve. NB: *do not* tap here, as the silicone elastomer housing is not self-sealing. The antechamber is provided for this type of access.

25.7.10 Integra (Cordis) horizontal-vertical lumbar valve

▸ Fig. 25.12. May be used in lumboperitoneal shunt to increase the transmission pressure when the patient is upright to prevent overshunting. Markings used to orient the device during implantation:

1. an arrow on the inlet side of the unit indicates direction of flow
2. inlet tubing is clear

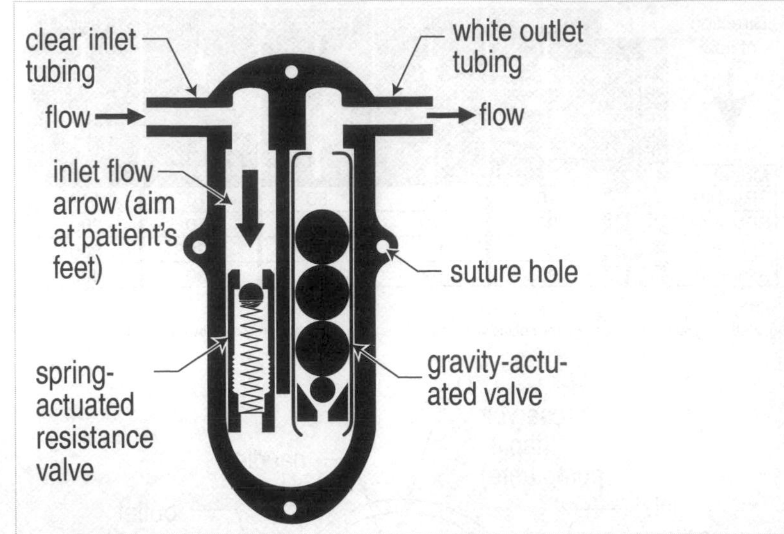

Fig. 25.12 Cordis H-V valve

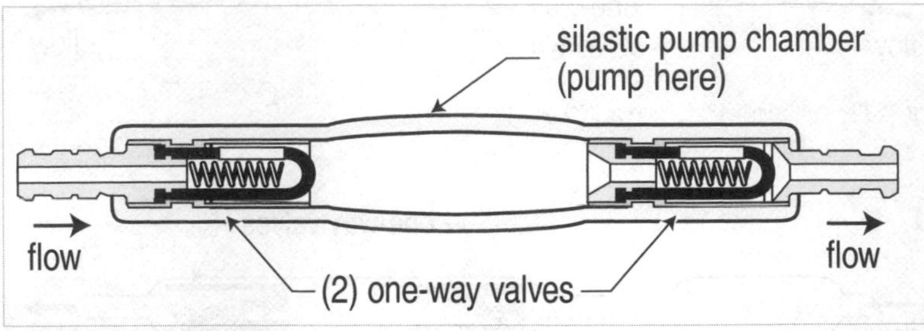

Fig. 25.13 Holter valve

3. inlet tubing has smaller diameter than outlet tubing
4. outlet tubing is white
5. before positioning the valve and fastening it to the fascia with permanent suture, the valve should be connected to both the subarachnoid catheter (inlet) and the peritoneal catheter (outlet). The arrow on the inlet valve should point towards the patient's feet

25.7.11 Holter valve

A dual slit valve mechanism (▶ Fig. 25.13). Usually used in combination with a Rickham or Salmon-Rickham reservoir (▶ Fig. 25.14).

To pump the shunt, simply depress the indicated portion of the valve.

X-ray characteristics

The silastic tube between the two one-way valves is radiolucent (▶ Fig. 25.1).

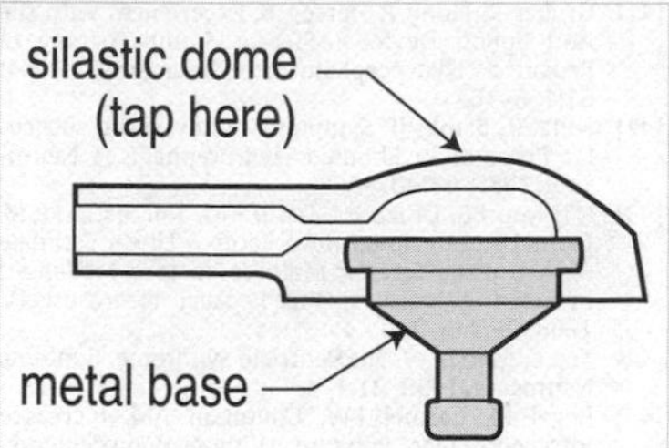

Fig. 25.14 Salmon-Rickham Reservoir

25.7.12 Salmon-Rickham reservoir

Similar to standard Rickham reservoir except for lower profile (▶ Fig. 25.14).

25.8 Surgical insertion techniques

For surgical techniques, refer to the section on insertion of Ventricular shunts (p. 1514).

25.9 Instructions to patients

All patients and families of patients with hydrocephalus should be instructed regarding the following:

1. signs and symptoms of shunt malfunction or infection
2. not to pump the shunt unless instructed to do so for a specific purpose
3. prophylactic antibiotics: for the following situations (mandatory in vascular shunts, sometimes recommended in other shunts)
   a) dental procedures other than routine cleaning
   b) instrumentation of the bladder: not practical for patients who catheterize to void. Important for cystoscopy, CMG, etc. where septicemia may occur
4. in a growing child: the need for periodic evaluation, including assessment of distal shunt length

References

[1] Shinnar S, Gammon K, Bergman EW, et al. Management of Hydrocephalus in Infancy: Use of Acetazolamide and Furosemide to Avoid Cerebrospinal Fluid Shunts. J Pediatr. 1985; 107:31–37

[2] Kreusser KL, Tarby TJ, Kovnar E, et al. Serial LPs for at Least Temporary Amelioration of Neonatal Posthemorrhagic Hydrocephalus. Pediatrics. 1985; 75:719–724

[3] Dandy WE. Extirpation of the Choroid Plexus of the Lateral Ventricle in Communicating Hydrocephalus. Ann Surg. 1918; 68:569–579

[4] Griffith HB, Jamjoom AB. The Treatment of Childhood Hydrocephalus by Choroid Plexus Coagulation and Artificial Cerebrospinal Fluid Perfusion. Br J Neurosurg. 1990; 4:95–100

[5] Gangemi M, Maiuri F, Naddeo M, Godano U, Mascari C, Broggi G, Ferroli P. Endoscopic third ventriculostomy in idiopathic normal pressure hydrocephalus: an Italian multicenter study. Neurosurgery. 2008; 63:62–7; discussion 67-9

[6] Handler MH, Abbott R, Lee M. A Near-Fatal Complication of Endoscopic Third Ventriculostomy: Case Report. Neurosurgery. 1994; 35:525–528

[7] McLaughlin MR, Wahlig JB, Kaufmann AM, Albright AL. Traumatic Basilar Aneurysm After Endoscopic Third Ventriculostomy: Case Report. Neurosurgery. 1997; 41:1400–1404

[8] Kulkarni AV, Drake JM, Mallucci CL, Sgouros S, Roth J, Constantini S. Endoscopic third ventriculostomy in the treatment of childhood hydrocephalus. J Pediatr. 2009; 155:254–9 e1

[9] Kulkarni AV, Drake JM, Kestle JR, Mallucci CL, Sgouros S, Constantini S. Predicting who will benefit from endoscopic third ventriculostomy compared with shunt insertion in childhood hydrocephalus using the ETV Success Score. J Neurosurg Pediatr. 2010; 6:310–315

[10] Naftel RP, Reed GT, Kulkarni AV, Wellons JC. Evaluating the Children's Hospital of Alabama endoscopic third ventriculostomy experience using the Endoscopic Third Ventriculostomy Success Score: an external validation study. J Neurosurg Pediatr. 2011; 8:494–501

[11] Durnford AJ, Kirkham FJ, Mathad N, Sparrow OC. Endoscopic third ventriculostomy in the treatment of childhood hydrocephalus: validation of a success score that predicts long-term outcome. J Neurosurg Pediatr. 2011; 8:489–493

[12] Jones RFC, Currie BG, Kwok BCT. Ventriculopleural Shunts for Hydrocephalus: A Useful Alernative. Neurosurgery. 1988; 23:753–755

[13] James HE, Tibbs PA. Diverse Clinical Application of Percutaneous Lumboperitoneal Shunts. Neurosurgery. 1981; 8:39–42

[14] Cozzens JW, Chandler JP. Increased Risk of Distal Ventriculoperitoneal Shunt Obstruction Associated With Slit Valves or Distal Slits in the Peritoneal Catheter. J Neurosurg. 1997; 87:682–686

[15] Dan NG, Wade MJ. The Incidence of Epilepsy After Ventricular Shunting Procedures. J Neurosurg. 1986; 65:19–21

[16] Berger MS, Baumeister B, Geyer JR, Milstein J, et al. The Risks of Metastases from Shunting in Children with Primary Central Nervous System Tumors. J Neurosurg. 1991; 74:872–877

[17] Jimenez DF, Keating R, Goodrich JT. Silicone Allergy in Ventriculoperitoneal Shunts. Childs Nerv Syst. 1994; 10:59–63
[18] Moazam F, Glenn JD, Kaplan BJ, et al. Inguinal Hernias After Ventriculoperitoneal Shunt Procedures in Pediatric Patients. Surg Gynecol Obstet. 1984; 159:570–572
[19] Bryant MS, Bremer AM, Tepas JJ, et al. Abdominal Complications of Ventriculoperitoneal Shunts. Am Surg. 1988; 54:50–55
[20] Ram Z, Findler G, Guttman I, et al. Ventriculoperitoneal Shunt Malfunction due to Migration of the Abdominal Catheter into the Scrotum. J Pediatr Surg. 1987; 22:1045–1046
[21] Rush DS, Walsh JW. Abdominal Complications of CSF-Peritoneal Shunts. Monogr Neural Sci. 1982; 8:52–54
[22] Alonso-Vanegas M, Alvarez JL, Delgado L, et al. Gastric Perforation due to Ventriculo-Peritoneal Shunt. Pediatr Neurosurg. 1994; 21:192–194
[23] Lourie H, Bajwa S. Transdiaphragmatic Migration of a Ventriculoperitoneal Catheter. Neurosurgery. 1985; 17:324–326
[24] Sakoda TH, Maxwell JA, Brackett CE. Intestinal Volvulus Secondary to a Ventriculoperitoneal Shunt. Case Report. J Neurosurg. 1971; 35:95–96
[25] Couldwell WT, LeMay DR, McComb JG. Experience with Use of Extended Length Peritoneal Shunt Catheters. J Neurosurg. 1996; 85:425–427
[26] Pascual JMS, Prakash UBS. Development of Pulmonary Hypertension After Placement of a Ventriculoatrial Shunt. Mayo Clin Proc. 1993; 68:1177–1182
[27] Chumas PD, Kulkarni AV, Drake JM, Hoffman HJ, Humphreys RP, Rutka JT. Lumboperitoneal Shunting: A Retrospective Study in the Pediatric Population. Neurosurgery. 1993; 32:376–383
[28] Welch K, Shillito J, Strand R, Fischer EG, Winston KR. Chiari I "malformation": An acquired disorder? J Neurosurg. 1982; 55:604–609
[29] Chumas PD, Armstrong DC, Drake JM, et al. Tonsillar Herniation: The Rule Rather than the Exception After Lumboperitoneal Shunting in the Pediatric Population. J Neurosurg. 1993; 78:568–573
[30] Payner TD, Prenger E, Berger TS, Crone KR. Acquired Chiari Malformations: Incidence, Diagnosis, and Management. Neurosurgery. 1994; 34:429–434
[31] Kessler LA, Dugan P, Concannon JP. Systemic Metastases of Medulloblastoma Promoted by Shunting. Surg Neurol. 1975; 3:147–152
[32] Czosnyka Z, Czosnyka M, Richards HK, Pickard JD. Laboratory testing of hydrocephalus shunts – conclusion of the U.K. Shunt evaluation programme. Acta Neurochir (Wien). 2002; 144:525–38; discussion 538
[33] Savitz MH, Bobroff LM. Low incidence of delayed intracerebral hemorrhage secondary to ventriculoperitoneal shunt insertion. J Neurosurg. 1999; 91:32–34
[34] French BN, Swanson M. Radionuclide Imaging Shuntography for the Evaluation of Shunt Patency. Monogr Neural Sci. 1982; 8:39–42
[35] Chan KH, Mann KS. Prolonged Therapeutic External Ventricular Drainage: A Prospective Study. Neurosurgery. 1988; 23:436–438
[36] Mann KS, Yue CP, Ong GB. Percutaneous Sump Drainage: A Palliation for Oft-Recurring Intracranial Cystic Lesions. Surg Neurol. 1983; 19:86–90
[37] Hassan M, Higashi S, Yamashita J. Risks in Using Siphon-Reducing Devices in Adult Patients with Normal-Pressure Hydrocephalus: Bench Test Investigations with Delta valves. J Neurosurg. 1996; 84:634–641
[38] Boch A-L, Hermelin É, Sainte-Rose C, Sgouros S. Mechanical Dysfunction of Ventriculoperitoneal Shunts Caused by Calcification of the Silicone Rubber Catheter. J Neurosurg. 1998; 88:975–982
[39] Pudenz RH, Foltz EL. Hydrocephalus: Overdrainage by Ventricular Shunts. A Review and Recommendations. Surg Neurol. 1991; 35:200–212
[40] McLaurin RL, Olivi A. Slit-Ventricle Syndrome: Review of 15 Cases. Pediat Neurosci. 1987; 13:118–124
[41] Gruber R, Jenny P, Herzog B. Experiences with the Anti-Siphon Device (ASD) in Shunt Therapy of Pediatric Hydrpcephalus. J Neurosurg. 1984; 61:156–162
[42] Foltz EL, Blanks JP. Symptomatic Low Intraventricular Pressure in Shunted Hydrocephalus. J Neurosurg. 1988; 68:401–408
[43] O'Hayon BB, Drake JM, Ossip MG, Tuli S, Clarke M. Frontal and Occipital Horn Ratio: A Linear Estimate of Ventricular Size for Multiple Imaging Modalities in Pediatric Hydrocephalus. Pediatric Neurosurgery. 1998; 29:245–249
[44] Teo C, Morris W. Slit Ventricle Syndrome. Contemp Neurosurg. 1999; 21:1–4
[45] Engel M, Carmel PW, Chutorian AM. Increased Intraventricular Pressure Without Ventriculomegaly in Children with Shunts: "Normal Volume" Hydrocephalus. Neurosurgery. 1979; 5:549–552
[46] Kiekens R, Mortier W, Pothmann R. The Slit-Ventricle Syndrome After Shunting in Hydrocephalic Children. Neuropediatrics. 1982; 13:190–194
[47] Hyde-Rowan MD, Rekate HL, Nulsen FE. Reexpansion of Previously Collapsed Ventricles: The Slit Ventricle Syndrome. J Neurosurg. 1982; 56:536–539
[48] Salmon JH. The Collapsed Ventricle: Management and Prevention. Surg Neurol. 1978; 9:349–352
[49] Portnoy HD, Schult RR, Fox JL, et al. Anti-Siphon and Reversible Occlusion Valves for Shunting in Hydrocephalus and Preventing Postshunt Subdural Hematoma. J Neurosurg. 1973; 38:729–738
[50] Epstein FJ, Fleischer AS, Hochwald GM, et al. Subtemporal Craniectomy for Recurrent Shunt Obstruction Secondary to Small Ventricles. J Neurosurg. 1974; 41:29–31
[51] Holness RO, Hoffman HJ, Hendrick EB. Subtemporal Decompression for the Slit-Ventricle Syndrome After Shunting in Hydrocephalic Children. Childs Brain. 1979; 5:137–144
[52] Linder M, Diehl J, Sklar FH. Subtemporal Decompressions for Shunt-Dependent Ventricles: Mechanism of Action. Surg Neurol. 1983; 19:520–523
[53] Reddy K, Fewer HD, West M, Hill NC. Slit Ventricle Syndrome with Aqueduct Stenosis: Third Ventriculostomy as Definitive Treatment. Neurosurgery. 1988; 23:756–759
[54] Puca A, Fernandez E, Colosimo C, et al. Hydrocephalus and Macrocrania: Surgical or Non-Surgical Treatment of Postshunting Subdural Hematoma. Surg Neurol. 1996; 45:76–82
[55] Hoppe-Hirsch E, Sainte Rose C, Renier D, Hirsch J-F. Pericerebral Collections After Shunting. Childs Nerv Syst. 1987; 3:97–102
[56] McCullogh DC, Fox JL. Negative Intracranial Pressure Hydrocephalus in Adults with Shunts and its Relationship to the Production of Subdural Hematoma. J Neurosurg. 1974; 40:372–375
[57] Schut L. Comment on Puca A, et al.: Hydrocephalus and Macrocrania: Surgical or Non-Surgical Treatment of Postshunting Subdural Hematoma. Surg Neurol. 1996; 45
[58] Dietrich U, Lumenta C, Sprick C, et al. Subdural Hematoma in a Case of Hydrocephalus and Macrocrania: Experience with a Pressure-Adjustable Valve. Childs Nerv Syst. 1987; 3:242–244
[59] Kamano S, Nakano Y, Imanishi T, Hattori M. Management with a Programmable Pressure Valve of Subdural Hematomas Caused by a Ventriculoperitoneal Shunt: Case Report. Surg Neurol. 1991; 35:381–383
[60] Illingworth RD. Subdural Hematoma After the Treatment of Chronic Hydrocephalus by Ventriculocaval Shunts. J Neurol Neurosurg Psychiatry. 1970; 33:95–99
[61] Davidoff LM, Feiring EH. Subdural Hematoma Occurring in Surgically Treated Hydrocephalic Children with a Note on a Method of Handling Persistent Accumulations. J Neurosurg. 1963; 10:557–563
[62] Kaufman B, Weiss MH, Young HF, Nulsen FE. Effects of Prolonged Cerebrospinal Fluid Shunting on the Skull and Brain. J Neurosurg. 1973; 38:288–297

[63] Faulhauer K, Schmitz P. Overdrainage Phenomena in Shunt Treated Hydrocephalus. Acta Neurochir. 1978; 45:89–101
[64] Al-Mufarrej F, Nolan C, Sookhai S, Broe P. Laparoscopic procedures in adults with ventriculoperitoneal shunts. Surg Laparosc Endosc Percutan Tech. 2005; 15:28–29
[65] Neale ML, Falk GL. In vitro assessment of back pressure on ventriculoperitoneal shunt valves. Is laparoscopy safe? Surg Endosc. 1999; 13:512–515
[66] Ravaoherisoa J, Meyer P, Afriat R, Meyer Y, Sauvanet E, Tricot A, Carli P. Laparoscopic surgery in a patient with ventriculoperitoneal shunt: monitoring of shunt function with transcranial Doppler. Br J Anaesth. 2004; 92:434–437
[67] Baskin JJ, Vishteh AG, Wesche DE, Rekate HL, Carrion CA. Ventriculoperitoneal shunt failure as a complication of laparoscopic surgery. J Soc Laparoendosc Surg. 1998; 2:177–180
[68] Collure DW, Bumpers HL, Luchette FA, Weaver WL, Hoover EL. Laparoscopic cholecystectomy in patients with ventriculoperitoneal (VP) shunts. Surg Endosc. 1995; 9:409–410

Part VIII

Seizures

VIII

26 Seizure Classification and Anti-Convulsant Pharmacology

26.1 Seizure classification

Definition of a seizure: an abnormal paroxysmal cerebral neuronal discharge that results in alteration of sensation, motor function, behavior or consciousness. Seizures may be classified by type, etiology, and by epileptic syndromes.

26.1.1 Classification of major seizure types

Generalized seizures

1. Tonic–clonic (in any combination)
2. Absence
   - Typical
   - Atypical
   - Absence with special features: Myoclonic absence, Eyelid myoclonia
3. Myoclonic
   - Myoclonic
   - Myoclonic atonic
   - Myoclonic tonic
4. Clonic
5. Tonic
6. Atonic
7. Focal seizures
8. Unknown
   - Epileptic spasms

Primary generalized seizures

Primary generalized: bilaterally symmetrical and synchronous involving both cerebral hemispheres at the onset, no local onset, consciousness lost from the start. Represents ≈ 40% of all seizures

1. generalized tonic-clonic (GTC) (née: grand-mal seizure): generalized seizure that evolves from tonic to clonic motor activity. This is a specific type and does *NOT* include partial seizures that generalize secondarily
2. clonic seizures: fairly symmetric, bilateral synchronous semirhythmic jerking of the UE & LE, usually with elbow flexion and knee extension
3. tonic seizures: sudden sustained increased tone with a characteristic guttural cry or grunt as air is forced through adducted vocal cords
4. absence (née: petit-mal seizure): impaired consciousness with mild or no motor involvement (see below)
   a) typical absences
   b) atypical absences: more heterogeneous with more variable EEG pattern then typical absence. Seizures may last longer
5. myoclonic seizures: shocklike body jerks (1 or more in succession) with generalized EEG discharges
6. atonic seizures (AKA astatic seizures or "drop attacks"): sudden brief loss of tone that may cause falls

Partial seizures

Partial (née focal seizure): implies one hemisphere involved at onset. About 57% of all seizures. A new onset of partial seizure represents a structural lesion until proven otherwise

1. simple partial seizure (no impairment of consciousness)
   a) with motor signs (including Jacksonian)
   b) with sensory symptoms (special sensory or somatosensory)
   c) with autonomic signs or symptoms
   d) with psychic symptoms (disturbance of higher cerebral function)

2. complex partial seizure (many used to be classified as psychomotor seizure, often attributed to temporal lobe but they can arise from any cortical area): any alteration of consciousness, usually LOC or automatisms (including lip smacking, chewing, or picking with the fingers) with autonomic aura (usually an epigastric rising sensation)
   a) simple partial onset followed by impairment of consciousness (may have premonitory aura)
      - without automatisms
      - with automatisms
   b) with impairment of consciousness at onset
      - without automatisms (impairment of consciousness only)
      - with automatisms
   c) partial seizure with secondary generalization
      - simple partial evolving to generalized
      - complex partial evolving to generalized
      - simple partial evolving to complex partial evolving to generalized

Unclassified epileptic seizures

≈ 3% of all seizures

26.1.2 Epileptic syndromes

General information

This list is not all inclusive (see reference[1,2]).

1. symptomatic (AKA "secondary"): seizures of known etiology (e.g. stroke, tumor…)
   a) temporal lobe epilepsies:
      - mesial temporal sclerosis: see below
2. idiopathic (AKA "primary"): no underlying cause. Includes:
   a) juvenile myoclonic epilepsy: see below
3. cryptogenic: seizures presumed to be symptomatic but with unknown etiology
   a) West syndrome (infantile spasms, Blitz-Nick-Salaam Krämpfe): see below
   b) Lennox-Gastaut syndrome: see below
4. special syndromes: situation-related seizures
   a) febrile seizures (p. 467)
   b) seizures occurring only with acute metabolic or toxic event: e.g. alcohol

KEY distinctions (having therapeutic implications)

In generalized tonic-clonic seizures: primary generalized vs. partial with secondary generalization (often, local onset may not be observed).

In staring spells: absence vs. complex partial.

Epilepsy

A disorder, not a single disease. Characterized by recurrent (2 or more), unprovoked seizures.

Absence seizure

Formerly called petit-mal seizure. Impaired consciousness with mild or no motor involvement (automatisms occur more commonly with bursts lasting > 7 secs). *No post-ictal confusion.* Aura rare. May be induced by hyperventilation × 2–3 mins. EEG shows spike and wave at exactly 3 per second.

Uncinate seizures

Obsolete term: "uncal fits." Seizures originating in the inferior medial temporal lobe, usually in the hippocampal region. May produce olfactory hallucinations (kakosmia or cacosmia: the perception of bad odors where none exist).

Mesial temporal sclerosis

See references.[3,4]

The most common cause of intractable temporal lobe epilepsy. Specific pathologic basis: hippocampal sclerosis (cell loss in hippocampus on one side). Characteristics are shown in ▶ Table 26.1. See also differential diagnosis (p. 1386).

Table 26.1 Syndrome of mesial temporal-lobe epilepsy[5]

History

- higher incidence of complicated febrile seizures than in other types of epilepsy
- common family history of epilepsy
- onset in latter half of first decade of life
- auras in isolation are common
- infrequent secondarily generalized seizures
- seizures often remit for several years until adolescence or early adulthood
- seizures often become medically refractory
- common interictal behavioral disturbances (especially depression)

Clinical features of seizures

- most have aura (especially epigastric, emotional, olfactory or gustatory) × several secs
- CPS often begin with arrest & stare; oroalimentary & complex automatisms are common. Posturing of contralateral arm may occur. Seizure usually lasts 1–2 mins
- postictal disorientation, recent-memory deficit, amnesia of ictus and (in dominant hemisphere) aphasia usually lasts several mins

Neurologic and laboratory features

- neuro exam: normal except memory deficit
- MRI: hippocampal atrophy and signal alteration with ipsilateral dilatation of temporal horn of lateral ventricle
- unilateral or bilateral independent anterior temporal EEG spikes with maximal amplitude in basal electrodes
- external ictal EEG activity only with CPS, usually initial or delayed focal rhythmic onset pattern of 5–7 Hz, maximal in 1 basal temporal derivation
- interictal fluorodeoxyglucose PET scan: hypometabolism in temporal lobe and possibly ipsilateral thalamus and basal ganglia
- neuropsychological testing: memory dysfunction specific to involved temporal lobe
- Wada test (p. 1553): amnesia with contralateral amobarbital injection

Adult seizures are initially responsive to medical therapy but become more varied and refractory, and may respond to seizure surgery.

Juvenile myoclonic epilepsy

See reference.[6]

Sometimes called bilateral myoclonus. 5–10% of cases of epilepsy. An idiopathic generalized epilepsy syndrome with age-related onset consisting of 3 seizure types:

1. myoclonic jerks: predominantly after waking
2. generalized tonic-clonic seizures
3. absence

EEG → polyspike discharges. Strong family history (some studies showing linkage to the HLA region on the short arm of chromosome 6).

Most are responsive to depakene.

West syndrome

This term is being used less frequently as it appears not to be a homogeneous group and as specific etiologies for infantile spasms are identified. Classically a seizure disorder that usually appears in first year of life, and consists of recurrent, gross flexion and occasionally extension of the trunk and limbs (massive myoclonus, AKA infantile spasms, AKA salaam seizures, AKA jackknife spasms). Seizures tend to diminish with age, often abating by 5 yrs. Usually associated with mental retardation. 50% may develop complex-partial seizures, some of the rest may develop Lennox-Gastaut syndrome (see below). An associated brain lesion may be found in some.

EEG → the majority show either interictal hypsarrhythmia (huge spike/wave plus slow wave resembling muscle artifact) or modified hypsarrhythmia at some point.

Usually dramatic response of seizures and EEG findings to ACTH or corticosteroids.

Lennox-Gastaut syndrome

Rare condition that begins in childhood as atonic seizures ("drop attacks"). Often develops into tonic seizures with mental retardation. Seizures are often polymorphic, difficult to treat medically, and may occur as often as 50 per day. May also present with status epilepticus. Approximately 50% of patients have reduced seizures with valproic acid. Corpus callosotomy may reduce the number of atonic seizures.

26.1.3 Miscellaneous seizure information

Factors that lower the seizure threshold

Factors that lower the seizure threshold (i.e. make it easier to provoke a seizure) in individuals with or without a prior seizure history include many items listed under Etiologies of New onset seizures (see below) as well as:

1. sleep deprivation
2. hyperventilation
3. photic stimulation (in some)
4. infection: systemic (febrile seizures (p. 467)), CNS (meningitis…)
5. metabolic disturbances: electrolyte imbalance (especially profound hypoglycemia), pH disturbance (especially alkalosis), drugs… (see below)
6. head trauma: closed head injury, penetrating trauma (p. 463)
7. cerebral ischemia: stroke (see below)
8. "kindling": a concept that repeated seizures may facilitate the development of later seizures

Todd's paralysis

A post-ictal phenomena in which there is partial or total paralysis usually in areas involved in a partial seizure. More common in patients with structural lesions as the source of the seizure. The paralysis usually resolves slowly over a period of an hour or so. Thought to be due to depletion of neurons in the wake of the extensive electrical discharges of a seizure. Other similar phenomena include post-ictal aphasia and hemianopsia.

26.2 Antiepileptic drugs

26.2.1 General information

The goal of antiepileptic drugs (AEDs) is seizure control (a contentious term, usually taken as reduction of seizure frequency and severity to the point to permit the patient to live a normal lifestyle without epilepsy-related limitations) with minimal or no drug toxicity. ≈ 75% of epileptics can achieve satisfactory seizure control with medical therapy.[7]

26.2.2 Classification of AEDs

AEDs can be grouped as shown in ▶ Table 26.2.

The following agents are considered "broad spectrum" (treat a variety of seizure types):

1. valproic acid
2. lamotrigine (Lamictal®)
3. levetiracetam (Keppra®)

These agents are not considered broad spectrum:

1. phenytoin (Dilantin® and others)
2. carbamazepine (Tegretol®)

Agents that interfere with platelet function and may increase the risk of bleeding complications:

1. valproic acid
2. phenytoin (Dilantin® and others)

26

Table 26.2 Classification of AEDs

Drug	Indications[a]
Barbiturates	
pentobarbital (Nembutal®)	**status**
phenobarbital	**status, GTC, partial Sz,** febrile Sz, neonatal Sz
primidone (Mysoline®)	
Benzodiazepines	
clonazepam (Klonopin®)	**Lennox-Gastaut, akinetic, myoclonic**
clorazepate (Tranxene-SD®)	**adj – partial Sz**
diazepam (Valium®)	**status**
lorazepam (Ativan®)	**status**
GABA analogues	
gabapentin (Neurontin®)	**adj – partial Sz**
tiagabine (Gabitril®)	**adj – partial Sz**
Hydantoins	
fosphenytoin (Cerebyx®)	**status, Sz during neurosurgery, short-term replacement for oral PHT**
phenytoin (Dilantin®)	**GTC, CP, Sz during or after neurosurgery**
Phenyltriazenes	
lamotrigine (Lamictal®)	**adj – partial Sz, adj – Lennox-Gastaut**
Succinimides	
ethosuximide (Zarontin®)	**ABS**
methsuximide (Celontin®)	**ABS** refractory to other drugs
Miscellaneous	
acetazolamide (Diamox®)	
carbamazepine (Tegretol®, Carbatrol®)	**partial Sz + complex symptomology, GTC, mixed Sz,** ✖ not for absence
felbamate (Felbatol®)	use only with extreme caution – see text
levetiracetam (Keppra®)	**adj – partial Sz**
oxcarbazepine (Trileptal®)	**mono or adj – partial Sz**
topiramate (Topamax®)	**adj – partial Sz** or **primarily GTC**
valproate (Depakene®...)	**CP (alone or with other types), ABS, adj – multiple Sz types**
zonisamide (Zonegran®)	**adj – partial Sz**

[a]Indications for seizure types (does not include other uses, e.g. for chronic pain). FDA approved indications are in bold, off-label indications appear in plain text.
Abbreviations: ABS = absence, adj = adjunctive therapy, CP = complex partial, GTC = generalized tonic-clonic, PHT = phenytoin, Sz = seizure, status = status epilepticus

26.2.3 Choice of antiepileptic drug

Antiepileptic drugs (AED) for various seizure types

Boldface drugs are drug of choice (DOC).

1. primary generalized
   a) GTC (generalized tonic-clonic):
      - **valproic acid (VA)** (p. 451): if no evidence of focality some studies show fewer side effects and better control than PHT
      - carbamazepine (p. 449)
      - **phenytoin (PHT)** (p. 446)
      - phenobarbital (PB) (p. 451)
      - primidone (PRM) (p. 452)
   b) absence:
      - **ethosuximide**
      - **valproic acid (VA)**
      - clonazepam
      - methsuximide (p. 453)
   c) myoclonic → benzodiazepines
   d) tonic or atonic:
      - benzodiazepines
      - felbamate (p. 453)
      - vigabatrin (p. 456)
2. partial (simple or complex, with or without secondary generalization): the well controlled Veterans Administration Cooperative Study[8] ranked the following drugs (based on seizure control and side effects) in this order (VA may compare favorably with CBZ for secondarily GTC, but is less effective for complex partial seizures[9]):
   a) **carbamazepine (CBZ):** most effective, least side effects
   b) **phenytoin (PHT):** ↓
   c) phenobarbital (PB): ↓
   d) primidone (PRM): slightly less effective, more side effects
3. second line drugs for any of the above seizure types:
   a) valproate
   b) lamotrigine (p. 456): effective for many types of generalized seizures, but are not FDA approved for this yet
   c) topiramate (p. 456): effective for many types of generalized seizures, but are not FDA approved for this yet

26.2.4 Anticonvulsant pharmacology

See reference.[10]

General guidelines

Monotherapy versus polytherapy

1. increase a given medication until seizures are controlled or side effects become intolerable (do not rely solely on therapeutic levels, which is only the range in which most patients have seizure control without side effects)
2. try monotherapy with a different drugs before resorting to two drugs together. 80% of epileptics can be controlled on monotherapy, however, failure of monotherapy indicates an 80% chance that the seizures will not be controllable pharmacologically. Only ≈ 10% benefit significantly from the addition of a second drug.[9] When > 2 AEDs are required, consider nonepileptic seizures (p. 464)
3. when first evaluating patients on multiple drugs, withdraw the most sedating ones first (usually barbiturates and clonazepam)

26

Generally, dosing intervals should be less than one half-life. Without loading dose, it takes about 5 *half-lives* to reach steady state.

Many AEDs affect liver function tests (LFTs), however, only rarely do the drugs cause enough hepatic dysfunction to warrant discontinuation. Guideline: discontinue an AED if the GGT exceeds twice normal.

Specific anticonvulsants

Table 26.3 Anticonvulsants: Abbreviations

AED	antiepileptic drug
ABS	absence
EC	enteric coated
DIV	divided
DOC	drug of choice
GTC	generalized tonic-clonic seizure
S/C-P	simple or complex partial
Pharmacokinetics: Unless otherwise specified, numbers are given for *oral* dosing form.	
$t_{1/2}$	half-life
t_{PEAK}	time to peak serum level
t_{SS}	time to steady state (approximately $5 \times t_{1/2}$)
$t_{D/C}$	time to discontinue (recommended withdrawal period over which drug should be tapered)
MDF	minimum dosing frequency. "Therapeutic level" is the average therapeutic range.

Drug info: Phenytoin (PHT) (Dilantin®)

Indications

GTC, S/C-P, occasionally in ABS.

Pharmacokinetics

Pharmacokinetics are complicated: at low concentrations, kinetics are 1st order (elimination proportional to concentration), metabolism saturates near the therapeutic level resulting in zero-order kinetics (elimination at a constant rate). ≈ 90% of total drug is protein bound. Oral bioavailability is ≈ 90% whereas IV bioavailability is ≈ 95%; this small difference may be significant when patients are near limits of therapeutic range (due to zero-order kinetics).

Table 26.4 Pharmacokinetics of phenytoin				
$t_{1/2}$ (half-life)	t_{PEAK} (peak serum levels)	t_{SS} (steady state)	$t_{D/C}$ (discontinue)	Therapeutic level[a]
≈ 24 hrs (range: 9–140 hrs)[b]	oral suspension: 1.5–3 hrs regular capsules: 1.5–3 hrs extended release capsules: 4–12 hrs	7–21 days	4 wks	10–20 mcg/ml

[a]therapeutic level as measured in most labs: 10–20 mcg/ml (NB: it is the free PHT that is the important moiety; this is usually ≈ 1% of total PHT, thus therapeutic free PHT levels are 1–2 mcg/ml; some labs are able to measure free PHT directly).
[b] $t_{1/2}$ for phenytoin

26

Renal failure: dosage adjustment not needed. However, serum protein binding may be altered in uremia which can obfuscate interpretation of serum phenytoin levels. Eq (26.1) may be used to convert serum PHT concentration in a uremic patient C (observed), to the expected PHT level in nonuremic patients C (nonuremic).

$$C(\text{nonuremic}) = \frac{C(\text{observed})}{0.1 \times \text{albumin} + 0.1} \tag{26.1}$$

Oral dose

℞ Adult: usual maintenance dose= 300–600 mg/d divided BID or TID (MDF = q d, for single daily dosing, either the phenytoin-sodium capsules or the extended release form should be used). Oral *loading* dose: 300 mg PO q 4 hrs until 17 mg/kg are given. Peds: oral maintenance: 4–7 mg/kg/d (MDF = BID). **Supplied** : (oral forms): 100 mg tablets of phenytoin-sodium (sodium-salt); 30 & 100 mg Kapseals® (extended release); 50 mg chewable Infatabs® (phenytoin-acid); oral suspension 125 mg/5-ml in 8 oz. (240 ml) bottles or individual 5 ml unit dose packs; pediatric suspension 30 mg/5-ml. Phenytek® 200 & 300 mg capsules.

Dosage changes

Table 26.5 Guidelines for changing phenytoin dosage

Present level (mg/dl)	Change to make
<6	100 mg/day
6–8	50 mg/day
>8	25–30 mg/day

Because of zero-order kinetics, at near-therapeutic levels a small dosage change can cause large level changes. Although computer models are necessary for a high degree of accuracy, the dosing change guidelines in ▶ Table 26.5 or the nomogram in ▶ Fig. 26.1 [11] may be used as a quick approximation.

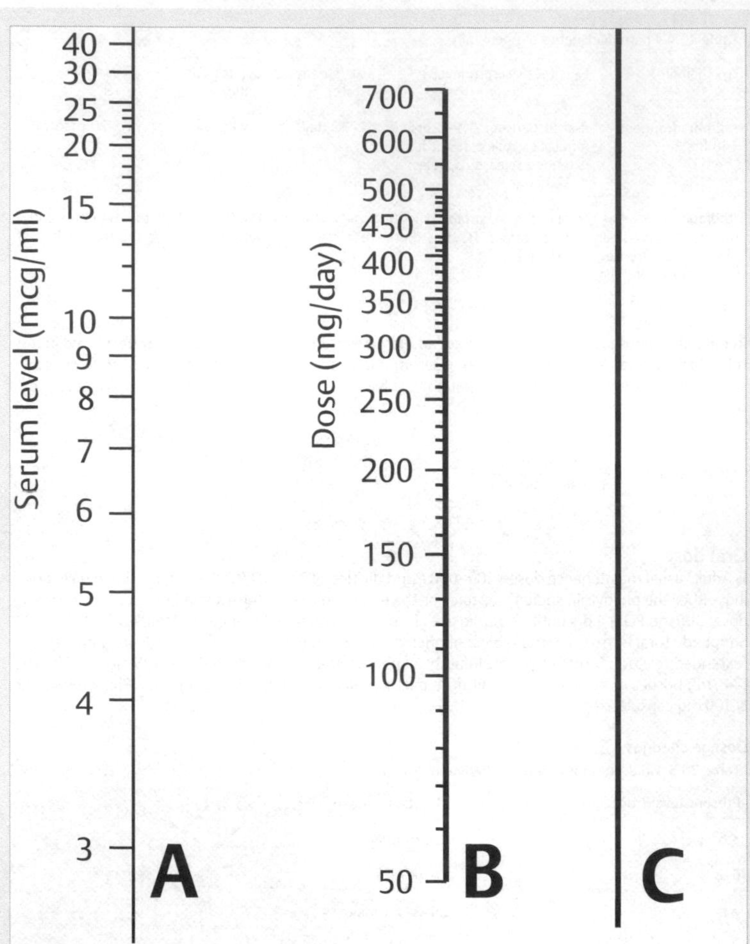

Fig. 26.1 Nomogram for adjusting phenytoin dose.
Directions for using nomogram (assumes steady state)
(a) draw line connecting serum level on line A with current dose on line B
(b) mark point where this line intersects line C
(c) connect point on C to the desired serum level on A
(d) read new dosage on line B (Reproduced from Therapeutic Drug Monitoring, "Predicting Phenytoin Dose - A Revised Nomogram", Rambeck B, et al, Vol. 1, pp. 325-33, 1979, with permission)

GI absorption of phenytoin suspension or capsules may be decreased by up to 70% when given with nasogastric feedings of Osmolyte® or Isocal®,[12,13] and the suspension has been reported to have erratic absorption. Hold NG feeding for 2 hrs before and 1 hour after phenytoin dose.

Parenteral dose

Phenytoin is a negative inotrope and can cause hypotension.

Conventional phenytoin may be given slow IVP or by IV drip (see below). The IM route should NOT be used (unreliable absorption, crystallization and sterile abscesses may develop). IV must be given slowly to reduce risk of arrhythmias and hypotension, viz. Adult: < 50 mg/min, Peds: < 1–3 mg/kg/min. The only compatible solution is NS, inject at site nearest vein to avoid precipitation.

℞ *loading*. Adult: 18 mg/kg slow IV. Peds: 20 mg/kg slow IV.

℞ *maintenance*. Adult: 200–500 mg/d (MDF = q d). Most adults have therapeutic levels on 100 mg PO TID. Peds: 4–7 mg/kg/d (MDF = BID).

Drip loading method:

Requires cardiac monitoring, and BP check q 5 minutes.

℞ Add 500 mg PHT to 50 ml NS to yield 10 mg/ml, run at 2 ml/min (20 mg/min) long enough to give 18 mg/kg (for 70 kg patient: 1200 mg over 60 mins). For more rapid administration, up to 40 mg/min may be used, or use fosphenytoin (see below). Decrease rate if hypotension occurs.

Fosphenytoin sodium injection

Fosphenytoin sodium (FOS) injection (Cerebyx®) is a newer formulation for administering IV phenytoin, and is indicated for short term use (≤ 5 days) when the enteral route is not usable. It is completely converted in vivo to phenytoin by organ and blood phosphatases with a conversion half-life of 10 minutes. Product labeling is given in terms of phenytoin equivalents (PE). Safety in pediatric patients has not been established. **Supplied:** 50 mg PE/ml in 2 & 10 ml vials (100 mg PE and 500 mg PE respectively).

26

Advantages of FOS (over conventional IV phenytoin):

1. less venous irritation (due to lower pH of 8.6–9 compared to 12 for phenytoin) resulting in less pain and IV extravasation
2. FOS is water soluble and therefore may be infused with dextrose or saline
3. tolerated well by IM injection (however, the IM route should not be used for status epilepticus)
4. does not come combined with propylene glycol (which can cause cardiac arrhythmias and/or hypotension itself)
5. the maximum administration rate is 3 × as fast (i.e. 150 mg PE/min)

Side effects of phenytoin

May interfere with cognitive function. May produce SLE-like syndrome, hepatic granulomas, megaloblastic anemia, cerebellar degeneration (chronic doses), hirsutism, gingival hypertrophy, hemorrhage in newborn if mother on PHT, toxic epidermal necrolysis (Stevens-Johnson variant). PHT antagonizes vitamin D → osteomalacia and rickets. Most hypersensitivity reactions occur within 2 months of initiating therapy.[12] In cases of maculopapular erythematous rash, the drug may be stopped and the patient may be rechallenged; often the rash will not recur the second time. *Teratogenic* (fetal hydantoin syndrome[14]).

Signs of phenytoin toxicity may develop at concentrations above 20 mcg/ml (toxicity is more common at levels > 30 mcg/ml) and include nystagmus (may also occur at therapeutic levels), diplopia, ataxia, asterixis, slurred speech, confusion, and CNS depression.

Drug-drug interactions: fluoxetine (Prozac®) results in elevated phenytoin levels (ave: 161% above baseline).[15] Phenytoin may impair the efficacy of: corticosteroids, warfarin, digoxin, doxycycline, estrogens, furosemide, oral contraceptives, quinidine, rifampin, theophylline, vitamin D.

Drug info: Carbamazepine (CBZ) (Tegretol®)

Indications

Partial seizures with or without secondary generalization. Trigeminal neuralgia. An IV form for use in e.g. status epilepticus is in development.

Dose

℞ oral route. Adult range: 600–2000 mg/d. Peds: 20–30 mg/kg/d. MDF = BID.

Before starting, check: CBC & platelet count (consider reticulocyte count) & serum Fe. Package insert says "recheck at frequent intervals, perhaps q week × 3 mos, then q month × 3 yrs."

Do not start CBZ (or discontinue it if patient already on CBZ) if: WBC < 4K, RBC < 3 × 106, Hct < 32%, platelets < 100K, reticulocytes < 0.3%, Fe > 150 mcg%.

Start low and increment slowly: 200 mg PO q d × 1 wk, BID × 1 wk, TID × 1 wk. As an inpatient, dosage changes may be made every 3 days, monitoring for signs of side effects. As an outpatient, changes should be made only ≈ weekly, with levels after each change. Carbatrol® (extended release CBZ) is usually dosed BID.

Supplied : oral form. Scored tabs 200 mg. Chewable scored tabs 100 mg. Suspension 100 mg/5-ml. IV form: not available in the U.S. at the time of this writing. Carbatrol® (extended release CBZ): 200 & 300 mg tablets.

Caveats with oral forms: oral absorption is erratic, and smaller more frequent doses are preferred.[16] Oral suspension is absorbed more readily, and also ✖ should *not* be administered simultaneously with other liquid medicinal agents as it may result in the precipitation of a rubbery, orange mass. ✖ May aggravate hyponatremia by SIADH-like effect.

Pharmacokinetics

Table 26.6 Pharmacokinetics of carbamazepine

$t_{1/2}$ (half-life)	t_{PEAK} (peak levels)	t_{SS} (steady state)	$t_{D/C}$ (discontinue)	Therapeutic level(mcg/ml)[a]
single dose: 20–55 hrs after chronic therapy: 10–30 hrs (adults), 8–20 hrs (peds)	4–24 hrs	up to 10 days[b]	4 wks	6–12

[a]may be misleading since the active metabolite carbamazepine-10,11-epoxide may cause toxicity and must be assayed separately
[b] t_{SS} may subsequently fall due to autoinduction which plateaus at 4–6 wks

CBZ induces hepatic enzymes that result in increased metabolism of itself (autoinduction) as well as other drugs over a period of ≈ 3–4 weeks.

Side effects

✖ Drug-drug interaction: caution, cimetidine, erythromycin and isoniazid may cause dramatic elevation of CBZ levels due to inhibition of hepatic cytochrome oxidase that degrades CBZ.[17] Side effects include:

1. drowsiness and GI upset: minimized by slow dose escalation
2. relative leukopenia in many: usually does not require discontinuing drug
3. transient diplopia
4. ataxia
5. less effect on cognitive function than PHT
6. hematological toxicity: rare. May be serious → agranulocytosis & aplastic anemia
7. Stevens-Johnson syndrome
8. SIADH
9. hepatitis (occasionally fatal) reported

Drug info: Oxcarbazepine (Trileptal®)

Very similar efficacy profile to carbamazepine with the following differences:

1. there is no autoinduction (C-P450 is not involved in metabolism) and therefore minimal drug-drug interactions
2. no blood testing is required since:
   a) there is no liver toxicity
   b) there is no hematologic toxicity
   c) there is no need to check drug levels
3. dosing is BID
4. kinetics are linear
5. more expensive

Dose

℞: starting dose for pain control is 150 mg PO BID, for seizures it is 300 mg PO BID. Maximum dose 2400 mg/day total. **Supplied:** 150, 300 & 600 mg scored tablets. 300 mg/5 ml oral suspension.

Drug info: Valproate

Available as valproic acid (Depakene®) and divalproex sodium (Depakote®).

Indications

Effective in primary GTC. Also useful in ABS with GTC, juvenile myoclonic epilepsy, and partial seizures (not FDA approved for latter). Also FDA approved for migraine prophylaxis. Note: severe GI upset and short half-life make valproic acid much less useful than Depakote® (divalproex sodium).

Dose

Adult range: 600–3000 mg/d. Peds range: 15–60 mg/kg/d. MDF = q d.

℞ Start at 15 mg/kg/d, increment at 1 wk intervals by 5–10 mg/kg/d. Max recommended adult dose: 60 mg/kg/d. If daily dose > 250 mg is required, it should be divided. **Supplied:** Oral: capsules 250 mg. Syrup 250 mg/5-ml. Depakote® (enteric coated) tabs: 125, 250, & 500 mg; sprinkle capsules125 mg. IV: Depacon® for IV injection 500 mg/5 ml vial.

26

Pharmacokinetics

Table 26.7 Pharmacokinetics of valproate

$t_{1/2}$ (half-life)	t_{PEAK} (peak serum levels)	t_{SS} (steady state)	$t_{D/C}$ (discontinue)	Therapeutic level(mcg/ml)
8–20 hrs	(uncoated) 1–4 hrs	2–4 days	4 wks	50–100

Valproic acid (VA) is 90% protein bound. ASA displaces VA from serum proteins.

Side effects

Serious side effects are rare. *Pancreatitis* has been reported, sometimes life-threatening. Fatal liver failure has occurred especially if age < 2 yrs and in combination with other AEDs. *Teratogenic* (below). Drowsiness (temporary), minimal cognitive deficits, N/V (minimized with Depakote), liver dysfunction, hyperammonemia (even without liver dysfunction), weight gain, mild hair loss, tremor (dose related; similar to benign familial tremor; if severe and valproic acid is absolutely necessary, the tremor may be treated with beta blockers). May interfere with platelet function, caution with surgery on these patients.

Contraindications

✖ Pregnancy: causes neural tube defects (NTD) in ≈ 1–2% of patients.[18] Since a correlation between peak VA levels and the risk of NTDs has been found, if VA must be used, some experts recommend changing from BID to TID dosing. ✖ Patients ≤ 2 yrs age (risk of hepatotoxicity).

Drug info: Phenobarbital

Indications

Used as alternative in GTC and partial (not DOC). Had been DOC for febrile seizures, dubious benefit.[19] About as effective as PHT, but very sedating. Also used for status epilepticus (p. 469).

Dose

Same dose PO, IV, or IM. MDF = q d.[20,21] Start slowly to minimize sedation.

℞ Adult *loading*: 20 mg/kg *slow* IV (administer at rate < 100 mg/min). *Maintenance*: 30–250 mg/d (usually divided BID-TID). Peds *loading:* 15–20 mg/kg. *Maintenance:* 2–6 mg/kg/d (usually divided BID). **Supplied:** tabs 15 mg, 30 mg, 60 mg, 100 mg; elixir 20 mg/5-ml.

Pharmacokinetics

Table 26.8 Pharmacokinetics of phenobarbital

$t_{1/2}$ (half-life)	t_{PEAK} (peak levels)	t_{SS} (steady state)	$t_{D/C}$ (discontinue)	Therapeutic level
adult: 5 d (range: 50–160 hrs) peds: 30–70 hrs	PO & IM: 1–6 hrs	16–21 days (may take up to 30 days)	≈ 6–8 wks (reduce ≈ 25% per week)	15–30 mcg/ml

Phenobarbital is a potent inducer of hepatic enzymes that metabolize other AEDs.

Side effects

Cognitive impairment (may be subtle and may outlast administration of the drug by at least several months[19]), thus avoid in peds; sedation; paradoxical hyperactivity (especially in peds); may cause hemorrhage in newborn if mother is on phenobarbital.

Drug info: Primidone (Mysoline®)

Indications

Same as phenobarbital (not DOC). NB: when used in combination therapy, low doses (50–125 mg/day) may add significant seizure control to the primary AED with few side effects.

26

Dose

℞ Adult: 250–1500 mg/d. Peds: 15–30 mg/kg/d; MDF = BID.

Start at 125 mg/d × 1 wk, and inc. slowly to avoid sedation. **Supplied:** (oral only): scored tabs 50 mg, 250 mg; suspension 250 mg/5-ml.

Pharmacokinetics

Metabolites include phenylethylmalonamide (PEMA) and phenobarbital. Therefore always check phenobarbital level at same time as primidone level.

Table 26.9 Pharmacokinetics of primidone

$t_{1/2}$ (half-life)	t_{PEAK} (peak levels)	t_{SS} (steady state)	$t_{D/C}$ (discontinue)	Therapeutic level (mcg/ml)
Primidone: 4–12 hrs derived phenobarbital: 50–160 hrs	2–5 hrs	up to 30 days	same as phenobarbital	primidone: 1–15 derived phenobarbital: 10–30

Side effects

Same as phenobarbital, plus: loss of libido, rare macrocytic anemia.

Drug info: Ethosuximide (Zarontin®)

Indications

DOC in ABS.

Dose

℞ Adult: 500–1500 mg/d. Peds: 10–40 mg/kg/d; MDF = q d. **Supplied:** oral only; capsules 250 mg; syrup 250 mg/5-ml.

Pharmacokinetics

Table 26.10 Pharmacokinetics of ethosuximide

$t_{1/2}$ (half-life)	t_{PEAK} (peak levels)	t_{SS} (steady state)	Therapeutic level (mcg/ml)
adult: 40–70 hrs peds: 20–40 hrs	1–4 hrs	adult: up to 14 days peds: up to 7 days	40–100

Side effects

N/V; lethargy; hiccups; H/A; rarely: eosinophilia, leukopenia, erythema multiforme, Stevens-Johnson syndrome, SLE-like syndrome. Toxic levels→ psychotic behavior.

Drug info: Methsuximide (Celontin®)

Indications

Indicated for absence seizures refractory to other drugs.

Dose

℞ optimum dose must be determined by trial. Start with 300 mg PO q d, increase by 300 mg at weekly intervals PRN to a maximum of 1200 mg/d. **Supplied:** 150 & 300 mg capsules.

Drug info: Felbamate (Felbatol®)

26

✖ CAUTION: Due to an unacceptably high rate of aplastic anemia and hepatic failure, felbamate (FBM) should not be used except in those circumstances where the benefit clearly outweighs the risk; then, hematologic consultation is recommended by the manufacturer. See Side effects below (also for drug-drug interactions).

FBM is efficacious for monotherapy and adjunctive therapy for partial seizures (complex and secondary generalization), and reduces the frequency of atonic and GTC seizures in Lennox-Gastaut syndrome.

Pharmacokinetics

Table 26.11 Pharmacokinetics of felbamate

$t_{1/2}$ (half-life)	t_{PEAK} (peak levels)	t_{SS} (steady state)	Therapeutic level (mcg/ml)
20–23 hrs	1–3 hrs	5–7 days	not established

Dose

Table 26.12 Effect of felbamate on other AED levels

AED	Change in level	Recommended dosing change
phenytoin	↑ 30–50%	↓ 20–33%
carbamazepine	↓ 30% total ↑ 50–60% epoxide	↓ 20–33%
valproic acid	↑ 25–100%	↓ 33%

℞: CAUTION see above. Felbamate is *not* to be used as a first-line drug. Patient or guardian should sign informed consent release. Start with 1200 mg/d divided BID, TID, or QID, and decrease other AEDs by one-third. Increase felbamate biweekly in 600 mg increments to usual dose of 1600–3600 mg/d (max: 45 mg/kg/d). Slow down increments and/or reduce other AEDs further if side effects become severe. Administer at upper end of range when used as monotherapy. **Supplied:** (oral only) 400 & 600 mg scored tablets; suspension 600 mg/5-ml.

Side effects

Felbamate has been associated with aplastic anemia (usually discovered after 5–30 wks of therapy) in ≈ 2–5 cases per million persons per yr, and hepatic failure (some fatal, necessitating baseline and serial LFTs every 1–2 wks). Other side effects: insomnia, anorexia, N/V, H/A. Felbamate is a potent metabolic inhibitor, thus it is necessary to reduce the dose of phenytoin, valproate or carbamazepine when used with felbamate[22] (▶ Table 26.12, general rule: drop dose by one third).

Drug info: Levetiracetam (Keppra®)

No identified drug-drug interactions. Less than 10% protein bound. Linear pharmacokinetics, no level monitoring needed.

Indications

Adjunctive therapy for partial onset Sz with secondary generalization in patients 4 years of age and older. Myoclonic seizures (juvenile myoclonic epilepsy). Generalized tonic-clonic.

Dose

℞ start with 500 mg PO BID. Increment by 1000 mg/d q 2 weeks PRN to a maximum of 3000 mg/d. Keppra XR: the same dose of levetiracetam can be converted to Keppra XR for q d dosing.

IV: 500–1500 mg diluted in 100 ml of diluent (LR, D5 W, normal saline) infused over 15 minutes BID.

26

Supplied: 250, 500, 750 & 1000 mg scored film-coated tabs; 100 mg/ml oral solution. Keppra XR (extended release) 500 mg.

IV: 1 vial (5 ml) contains 500 mg.

Side effects

PO or IV: somnolence and fatigue in 15%. Dizziness in 9%. Asthenia 15% and infection 13% (nasopharyngitis and influenza may or may not have been related).

Keppra XR: somnolence 8%, irritability 6%.

Drug info: Clonazepam (Klonopin®)

A benzodiazepine derivative.

Indications

✖ *Not* a recommended drug for seizures (see below).

Used for myoclonic, atonic, and absence seizures (in absence, less effective than valproate or ethosuximide, and tolerance may develop).

NB: clonazepam usually works very well for several months, and then tends to become less effective, leaving only the sedating effects. Also, many cases have been reported of patients having seizures during withdrawal, including status epilepticus (even in patients with no history of status). Thus, may need to taper this drug over 3–6 months.

Dose

℞ Adult: start at 1.5 mg/d DIV TID, increase by 0.5–1 mg q 3 d, usual dosage range is 1–12 mg/d (max 20 mg/d); MDF = q d. Peds: start at 0.01–0.03 mg/kg/d DIV BID or TID, increase by 0.25–0.5 mg/kg/d q 3 d; usual dosage range is 0.01–0.02 mg/kg/d; MDF = q d. **Supplied:** oral only; scored tabs: 0.5 mg, 1 mg, 2 mg.

Pharmacokinetics

Table 26.13 Pharmacokinetics of clonazepam

$t_{1/2}$ (half-life)	t_{PEAK} (peak levels)	t_{SS} (steady state)	$t_{D/C}$ (discontinue)	Therapeutic level (mcg/ml)
20–60 hrs	1–3 hrs	up to 14 days	≈ 3–6 months[a]	0.013–0.072

[a]CAUTION: withdrawal seizures are common, see text above

Side effects

Ataxia; drowsiness; behavior changes.

Drug info: Zonisamide (Zonegran®)

Indications
 Adjunctive therapy for partial Sz in adults.

Drug info: Acetazolamide (Diamox®)

The anti-epileptic effect may be either due to direct inhibition of CNS carbonic anhydrase (which also reduces CSF production rate) or due to the slight CNS acidosis that results.

Indications

Centricephalic epilepsies (absence, nonfocal seizures). Best results are in absence seizures; however benefit has also been observed in GTC, myoclonic jerk.

Side effects

Do not use in first trimester of pregnancy (may be teratogenic). The diuretic effect causes renal loss of HCO3 which may lead to an acidotic state with long-term therapy. A sulfonamide, therefore any typical reaction to this class may occur (anaphylaxis, fever, rash, Stevens-Johnson syndrome, toxic epidermal necrolysis...). Paresthesias: medication should be discontinued.

Dose

℞ Adult: 8–30 mg/kg/d in divided doses (max 1 gm/d, higher doses do not improve control). When given with another AED, the suggested starting dose is 250 mg once daily, and this is gradually increased. **Supplied:** tablets 125, 250 mg. Diamox sequels® are sustained release 500 mg capsules. Sterile cryodessicated powder is also available in 500 mg vials for parenteral (IV) use.

Drug info: Gabapentin (Neurontin®)

Although developed to be a GABA agonist, it does not interact at any known GABA receptor. Efficacious for primary generalized seizures and partial seizures (with or without secondary generalization). Ineffective for absence seizures. Very low incidence of known side-effects. No known drug interactions (probably because it is renally excreted). Also used for central pain

Dose

℞ Adult: 300 mg PO × 1 day 1; 300 mg BID day 2; 300 mg TID day 3; then increase rapidly up to usual doses of ≈ 800–1800 mg per day. Doses of 1800–3600 may be needed in intractable patients. ✖ Dosage must be reduced in patients with renal insufficiency or on dialysis, see Eq (7.1) to estimate. **Supplied:** 100, 300, 400, 600, 800 mg capsules. 50 mg/ml suspension.

Pharmacokinetics

Gabapentin is not metabolized, and 93% is excreted unchanged renally with plasma clearance directly proportional to creatinine clearance.[23] Does not affect hepatic microsomal enzymes, and does not affect metabolism of other AEDs. Antacids decrease bioavailablilty by ≈ 20%, therefore give gabapentin > 2 hrs after the antacid.[24]

Table 26.14 Pharmacokinetics of gabapentin

$t_{1/2}$ (half-life)	t_{PEAK} (peak levels)	t_{SS} (steady state)	Therapeutic level (mcg/ml)
5–7 hrs[a]	2–3 hrs	1–2 days	not established

[a]with normal renal function

Side effects

Somnolence, dizziness, ataxia, fatigue, nystagmus; all reduce after 2–3 weeks of drug therapy. Increased appetite. Not known to be teratogenic.

26

Drug info: Lamotrigine (Lamictal®)

Anticonvulsant effect may be due to presynaptic inhibition of glutamate release.[23]

Efficacious as *adjunctive* therapy for partial seizures (with or without secondary generalization) and Lennox-Gastaut syndrome. Preliminary data suggest it may also be useful as an adjunct for refractory generalized seizures, or as monotherapy for newly diagnosed partial or generalized seizures.[25] Also FDA approved for bipolar disorder.

Side effects

Somnolence, dizziness, diplopia. ✖ Serious rashes requiring hospitalization and discontinuation of therapy have been reported (rash usually begins 2 weeks after initiating therapy and may be severe and potentially life-threatening, including Stevens-Johnson syndrome (more of a concern with simultaneous use of valproate), and rarely, toxic epidermal necrolysis (TEN)). Incidence of significant epidermal reaction may be decreased by a slow ramping-up of dosage. May increase seizure frequency in some patients with severe myoclonic epilepsy of infancy.[26] Metabolism of lamotrigine is affected by concurrent use of other AEDs.

26

Dose

℞ Adult: In adults receiving enzyme-inducing AEDs (PHT, CBZ, or phenobarbital), start with 50 mg PO q d x 2 wks, then 50 mg BID × 2 wks, then ↑ by 100 mg/d q week until the usual maintenance dose of 200–700 mg/d (divided into 2 doses) is reached. For patients on valproic acid (VA) alone, the maintenance dose was 100–200 mg/d (divided into 2 doses), and VA levels drop by ≈ 25% within a few weeks of starting lamotrigine. For patients on both enzyme-inducing AEDs *and* VA, the starting dose is 25 mg PO qod × 2 wks, then 25 mg qd × 2 wks, then ↑ by 25–50 mg/d q 1–2 wks up to a maintenance of 100–150 mg/d (divided into 2 doses). Instruct patients that rash, fever or lymphadenopathy may herald a serious reaction and that a physician should be contacted immediately. Peds: not indicated for use in patients < 16 yrs old due to higher incidence of potentially life-threatening rash in the pediatric population.[23] **Supplied:** 25, 100, 150 & 200 mg tablets. 2, 5 & 25 mg chewable dispersible tablets.

Pharmacokinetics[25]

Table 26.15 Pharmacokinetics of lamotrigine

$t_{1/2}$ (half-life)	t_{PEAK} (peak levels)	t_{SS} (steady state)	Therapeutic level (mcg/ml)
24 hrs[a]	1.5–5 hrs	4–7 days	controversial[27]

[a]half-life is shortened to ≈ 15 hrs by PHT and CBZ, whereas valproic acid increases it to 59 hrs

Drug info: Vigabatrin

Indications

Effective in treating partial seizures. Less so for generalized seizures.

Dose

℞ Adult: 1500–3000 mg/d.

Drug info: Topiramate (Topamax®)

May block voltage-sensitive sodium channels and enhance GABA activity at GABAA receptors and attenuate some glutamate receptors.[23]

Indications[28]

As an oral adjunct to other drugs in treating refractory partial onset seizures.

Dose

℞ Adult: start with 50 mg/d and increase slowly up to 200–400 mg/d,[29] with no significant benefit noted at dosages > 600 mg/d.[30] **Supplied:** 25, 100, & 200 mg tabs.

Pharmacokinetics

30% is metabolized in the liver, the rest is excreted unchanged in the urine.

Table 26.16 Pharmacokinetics of topiramate

$t_{1/2}$ (half-life)	t_{ss} (steady state)	Therapeutic level
19–25 hrs	5–7 days	not established

Side effects

May increase phenytoin concentration by up to 25%. Levels of topiramate are reduced by other AEDs (phenytoin, carbamazepine, valproic acid and possibly others).

Cognitive impairment (word finding difficulty, problems with concentration…), weight loss, dizziness, ataxia, diplopia, paresthesias, nervousness and confusion have been troublesome. ≈ 1.5% incidence of renal stones which usually pass spontaneously[23]

Oligohidrosis (reduced sweating) and hyperthermia, primarily in children in association with elevated environmental temperatures and/or vigorous physical activity.

Drug info: Tiagabine (Gabitril®)

A GABA uptake inhibitor, with cognitive problems of a similar frequency to that with topiramate.[31]

℞ Adult: start with 4 mg/d, increase weekly by 4–8 mg to a maximum of 32–56 mg (divided BID to QID). **Supplied:** 4, 12, 16 & 20 mg tablets.

Drug info: Lacosamide (Vimpat®)

Enhances slow inactivation of voltage gated sodium channels, affecting only neurons that are depolarized of active over a prolonged period (as in a seizure).

Indications

Partial onset seizures. Painful diabetic neuropathy.

Dose

℞ Adult: 200–400 mg. **Supplied:** mg tabs.

26.2.5 Withdrawal of antiepileptic drugs

General information

Most seizure recurrences develop during the first 6 months after AED withdrawal.[32]

Indications for AED withdrawal

There is no agreement on how long a patient should be seizure-free before withdrawal of anticonvulsants, nor is there agreement on the prognostic value of EEGs and on the best time period over which to withdraw AEDs.

The following is based on a study of 92 patients with *idiopathic* epilepsy, who had been free of seizures for two years.[33] Generalization, e.g. to posttraumatic seizures, may not be appropriate. Taper was by 1 "unit" q 2 weeks (where a unit is defined as 200 mg for CBZ or valproic acid, or 100 mg for PHT). Follow-up: mean = 26 mos (range: 6–62).

26

31 patients (34%) relapsed, with the average time to relapse being 8 mos (range: 1–36). Using actuarial methods, the risk for recurrence is 5.9%/month for 3 months, then 2.7%/month for 3 months, then 0.5%/month for 3 months. Factors found to affect the likelihood of relapse include:
1. seizure type: 37% relapse rate for generalized seizures; 16% for complex or simple partial; 54% for complex partial with secondary generalization
2. number of seizures before control attained: those with ≥ 100 seizures before control had statistically significant higher relapse rate than those with < 100
3. the number of drugs that had to be tried before single drug therapy successfully controlled seizures: 29% if 1st drug worked, 40% if a change to a 2nd drug was needed, and 80% if a change to a 3rd drug was required
4. EEG class (▶ Table 26.17): class 4 had worst prognosis for relapse. Epileptiform discharges on EEG serves to discourage AED withdrawal[34]

26

In a larger randomized study,[35] the most important factors identified to predict freedom from recurrent seizures were:
1. longer seizure-free period
2. use of only one AED (vs. multiple AEDs)
3. seizures other than tonic-clonic seizures

Withdrawal times

The recommended withdrawal times in ▶ Table 26.18 should be used only as guidelines.

26.2.6 Pregnancy and antiepileptic drugs

General information

Women of childbearing potential with epilepsy should undergo counseling regarding pregnancy.[36]

Birth control

AEDs that induce liver microsomal cytochrome P450 enzymes (▶ Table 26.19) increase the failure rate of oral contraceptives up to fourfold.[37] Patients desiring to use BCPs should employ barrier contraceptive measures until ovulation is consistently suppressed, and they should watch for breakthrough bleeding which may indicate a need for a change in the hormone dosage.[32] Non-oral hormonal contraceptives (e.g. levonorgestrel implant (Norplant®)) circumvents first pass liver degradation but should combined with a barrier method because of declining effectiveness with time.

Table 26.17 EEG class and seizure relapse rate

Class	EEG description		Relapse rate	No. of relapses/ patients at risk
	Before treatment	Before withdrawal		
1	normal	normal	34%	11/31
2	abnormal	normal	11%	4/35
3	abnormal	improved	50%	2/4
4	abnormal	unchanged	74%	14/19

Table 26.18 Recommended AED withdrawal times

AED	Recommended withdrawal period
phenytoin, valproic acid, carbamazepine	2–4 weeks
phenobarbital	6–8 weeks (25% per week)
clonazepam	3–6 months; see CAUTION (p. 454)

Table 26.19 Effect of AEDs on liver cytochrome P_{450}[a]

Inducers	Noninducers
carbamazepine phenobarbital phenytoin felbamate primidone	valproic acid benzodiazepines gabapentin lamotrigine

[a]references[32,38]

Table 26.20 Changes in free AED levels during pregnancy[39]

Drug	Change
carbamazepine	↓ 11%
phenobarbital	↓ 50%
phenytoin	↓ 31%
valproic acid	↑ 25%

Complications during pregnancy

Women with epilepsy have more complications with pregnancy than mothers without epilepsy, but > 90% of pregnancies have a favorable outcome.[32]

There is an increase in the number of gravid seizures in ≈ 17% (reported range: 17–30%) of epileptic women, which may be due to noncompliance or to changes of free drug levels of AEDs during pregnancy (▸ Table 26.20). Isolated seizures can occasionally be deleterious, but usually cause no problem. Status epilepticus poses serious risk to mother and fetus during pregnancy and should be treated aggressively.

There is also a slightly increased risk of toxemia (HTN of pregnancy) and fetal loss.

Birth defects

The incidence of fetal malformations in offspring of patients with a known seizure disorder is ≈ 4–5%, or approximately double that of the general population.[40] The degree to which this is due to the use of AEDs vs. genetic and environmental factors is unknown. All AEDs have the potential to cause deleterious effects on the infant. Polytherapy is associated with an increased risk over monotherapy in a more than additive manner.

Generally, the risk of seizures (with possible concomitant maternal and fetal hypoxia and acidosis) is felt to outweigh the teratogenic risk of most AEDs, but this must be evaluated on a case-by-case basis. Occasionally patients may be weaned off AEDs.

Specific drugs

Carbamazepine (CBZ) produced an increased incidence of "minor" malformations (but not of "major" malformations) in one study[41] (this study may have had methodologic problems), and may increase the incidence of neural tube defects (NTD).[42] In utero exposure to phenytoin may lead to the fetal hydantoin syndrome[14,43] and a child with an IQ lower by ≈ 10 points.[44] Phenobarbital produced the highest incidence of major malformations (9.1%) in one prospective study[45] and was also associated with most of the increase in fetal death or anomalies in another study.[46] Valproate (VA) causes the highest incidence of NTD (1-2%[18]), which can be detected with amniocentesis and allow an abortion if desired. TID dosing may reduce the risk of NTD (p. 451). Benzodiazepines given shortly before delivery can produce the "floppy infant syndrome".[47] Similar effects may occur with other sedating AEDs such as phenobarbital.

Drug recommendations

A general consensus is that for most women of childbearing potential who require AEDs, that monotherapy with the lowest dose of CBZ that is effective is the method of choice if the seizure disorder is responsive to it.[48] If ineffective, then monotherapy with valproic acid (with TID dosing) is currently the recommended second choice. Folate supplementation (after confirming normal B12 levels) should be used in all.

26

References

[1] Commission on Classification and Terminology of the International League Against Epilepsy. Guidelines for Epidemiologic Studies on Epilepsy. Epilepsia. 1989; 30:389–399

[2] Mosewich RK, So EL. A Clinical Approach to the Classification of Seizures and Epileptic Syndromes. Mayo Clin Proc. 1996; 71:405–414

[3] French JA, Williamson PD, Thadani VM, et al. Characteristics of Medial Temporal Lobe Epilepsy. I. Results of History and Physical Examination. Ann Neurol. 1993; 34:774–780

[4] Williamson PD, French JA, Thadani VM, et al. Characteristics of Medial Temporal Lobe Epilepsy. II. Interictal and Ictal Scalp Electroencephalography, Neuropsychological Testing, Neuroimaging, Surgical Results, and Pathology. Ann Neurol. 1993; 34:781–787

[5] Engel JJ. Surgery for Seizures. N Engl J Med. 1996; 334:647–652

[6] Grunewald RA, Panayiotopoulos CP. Juvenile Myoclonic Epilepsy: A Review. Arch Neurol. 1993; 50:594–598

[7] Brodie MJ, Dichter MA. Antiepileptic Drugs. N Engl J Med. 1996; 334:168–175

[8] Mattson RH, Cramer JA, Collins JF, et al. Comparison of Carbamezepine, Phenobarbital, Phenytoin, and Primidone in Partial and Secondarily Generalized Tonic-Clonic Seizures. N Engl J Med. 1985; 313:145–151

[9] Mattson RH, Cramer JA, Collins JF, et al. A Comparison of Valproate with Carbamezepine for the Treatment of Complex Partial Seizures and Secondarily Generalized Tonic-Clonic Seizures in Adults. N Engl J Med. 1992; 327:765–771

[10] Drugs for Epilepsy. Med Letter. 1986; 28:91–93

[11] Rambeck B, Boenigk HE, Dunlop A, et al. Predicting Phenytoin Dose - A Revised Nomogram. Ther Drug Monit. 1979; 1:325–333

[12] Saklad JJ, Graves RH, Sharp WP. Interaction of Oral Phenytoin with Enteral Feedings. J Parent Ent Nutr. 1986; 10:322–323

[13] Worden JP, Wood CA, Workman CH. Phenytoin and Nasogastric Feedings. Neurology. 1984; 34

[14] Buehler BA, Delimont D, van Waes M, et al. Prenatal Prediction of Risk of the Fetal Hydantoin Syndrome. N Engl J Med. 1990; 322:1567–1572

[15] Public Health Service. Fluoxetine-Phenytoin Interaction. FDA Medical Bulletin. 1994; 24:3–4

[16] Winkler SR, Luer MS. Antiepileptic Drug Review: Part 1. Surg Neurol. 1998; 49:449–452

[17] Oles KS, Waqar M, Penry JK. Catastrophic Neurologic Signs due to Drug Interaction: Tegretol and Darvon. Surg Neurol. 1989; 32:144–151

[18] Oakeshott P, Hunt GM. Valproate and Spina Bifida. Br Med J. 1989; 298:1300–1301

[19] Farwell JR, Lee YJ, Hirtz DG, Sulzbacher SI, et al. Phenobarbital for Febrile Seizures - Effects on Intelligence and on Seizure Recurrence. N Engl J Med. 1990; 322:364–369

[20] Wroblewski BA, Garvin WH. Once-Daily Administration of Phenobarbital in Adults: Clinical Efficacy and Benefit. Arch Neurol. 1985; 42:699–700

[21] Davis AG, Mutchie KD, Thompson JA, Myers GG. Once-Daily Dosing with Phenobarbital in Children with Seizure Disorders. Pediatrics. 1981; 68:824–827

[22] Felbamate. Med Letter. 1993; 35:107 109

[23] Winkler SR, Luer MS. Antiepileptic Drug Review: Part 2. Surg Neurol. 1998; 49:566–568

[24] Gabapentin - A new anticonvulsant. Med Letter. 1994; 36:39–40

[25] Lamotrigine for Epilepsy. Med Letter. 1995; 37:21–23

[26] Guerrini R, Dravet C, Genton P, et al. Lamotrigine and Seizure Aggravation in Severe Myoclonic Epilepsy. Epilepsia. 1998; 39:508–512

[27] Sondergaard Khinchi M, Nielsen KA, Dahl M, Wolf P. Lamotrigine therapeutic thresholds. Seizure. 2008; 17:391–395

[28] Topiramate for Epilepsy. Med Letter. 1997; 39:51–52

[29] Faught E, Wilder BJ, Ramsay RE, et al. Topiramate Placebo-Controlled Dose-Ranging Trial in Refractory Partial Epilepsy using 200-, 400-, and 600-mg Daily Dosages. Neurology. 1996; 46:1684–1690

[30] Privitera M, Fincham R, Penry J, et al. Topiramate Placebo-Controlled Dose-Ranging Trial in Refractory Partial Epilepsy using 600-, 800-, and 1,000-mg Daily Dosages. Neurology. 1996; 46:1678–1683

[31] Tiagabine for Epilepsy. Med Letter. 1998; 40:45–46

[32] Shuster EA. Epilepsy in Women. Mayo Clin Proc. 1996; 71:991–999

[33] Callaghan N, Garrett A, Goggin T. Withdrawal of Anticonvulsant Drugs in Patients Free of Seizures for Two Years. N Engl J Med. 1988; 318:942–946

[34] Anderson T, Braathen G, Persson A, et al. A Comparison Between One and Three Years of Treatment in Uncomplicated Childhood Epilepsy: A Prospective Study. II. The EEG as Predictor of Outcome After Withdrawal of Treatment. Epilepsia. 1997; 38:225–232

[35] Medical Research Council Antiepileptic Drug Withdrawal Study Group. Randomized study of antiepileptic drug withdrawal in patients in remission. Lancet. 1991; 337:1175–1180

[36] Delgado-Escueta A, Janz D. Consensus Guidelines: Preconception Counseling, Management, and Care of the Pregnant Woman with Epilepsy. Neurology. 1992; 42:149–160

[37] Mattson RH, Cramer JA, Darney PD, Naftolin F. Use of Oral Contraceptives by Women with Epilepsy. JAMA. 1986; 256:238–240

[38] Perucca E, Hedges A, Makki KA, et al. A Comparative Study of the Relative Enzyme Inducing Properties of Anticonvulsant Drugs in Epileptic Patients. Br J Clin Pharmacol. 1984; 18:401–410

[39] Yerby MS, Freil PN, McCormick K. Antiepileptic Drug Disposition During Pregnancy. Neurology. 1992; 42:12–16

[40] Dias MS, Sekhar LN. Intracranial Hemorrhage from Aneurysms and Arteriovenous Malformations during Pregnancy and the Puerperium. Neurosurgery. 1990; 27:855–866

[41] Jones KL, Lacro RV, Johnson KA, Adams J. Patterns of Malformations in the Children of Women Treated With Carbamazepine During Pregnancy. N Engl J Med. 1989; 310:1661–1666

[42] Rosa FW. Spina Bifida in Infants of Women Treated with Carbamazepine During Pregnancy. N Engl J Med. 1991; 324:674–677

[43] Hanson JW, Smith DW. The Fetal Hydantoin Syndrome. J Pediatr. 1975; 87:285–290

[44] Scolnik D, Nulman I, Rovet J, et al. Neurodevelopment of Children Exposed In Utero to Phenytoin and Carbamazepine Monotherapy. JAMA. 1994; 271:767–770

[45] Nakane Y, Okuma T, Takahashi R, et al. Multi-Institutional Study of the Teratogenicity and Fetal Toxicity of Antiepileptic Drugs: A Report of a Collaberative Study Group in Japan. Epilepsia. 1980; 21:663–680

[46] Waters CH, Belai Y, Gott PS, et al. Outcomes of Pregnancy Associated with Antiepileptic Drugs. Arch Neurol. 1994; 51:250–253

[47] Kanto JH. Use of Benzodiazepines During Pregnancy, Labor, and Lactation, with Particular Reference to Pharmacokinetic Considerations. Drugs. 1982; 23:354–380

[48] Saunders M. Epilepsy in Women of Childbearing Age: If Anticonvulsants Cannot be Avoided, Use Carbamazepine. Br Med J. 1989; 199

27 Special Types of Seizures

27.1 New onset seizures

27.1.1 General information

The age adjusted *incidence* of new onset seizures in Rochester, Minnesota was 44 per 100,000 person years.[1]

27.1.2 Etiologies

In patients presenting with a first-time seizure, etiologies include (modified[2]):
1. following neurologic insult: either acutely (i.e. < 1 week) or remotely (> 1 week, and usually < 3 mos from insult)
   a) stroke: 4.2% had a seizure within 14 days of a stroke. Risk increased with severity of stroke[3]
   b) head trauma: closed head injury, penetrating trauma (p. 463)
   c) CNS infection: meningitis, cerebral abscess, subdural empyema
   d) febrile seizures (p. 467)
   e) birth asphyxia
2. underlying CNS abnormality
   a) congenital CNS abnormalities
   b) degenerative CNS disease
   c) CNS tumor: metastatic or primary
   d) hydrocephalus
   e) AVM
3. acute systemic metabolic disturbance
   a) electrolyte disorders: uremia, hyponatremia, hypoglycemia (especially profound hypoglycemia), hypercalcemia
   b) drug related, including:
      - alcohol-withdrawal (p. 464)
      - cocaine toxicity (p. 207)
      - opioids (narcotics)
      - phenothiazine antiemetics (p. 143)
      - with administration of flumazenil (Romazicon®) to treat benzodiazepine (BDZ) overdose (especially when BDZs are taken with other seizure lowering drugs such as tricyclic antidepressants or cocaine
      - phencyclidine (PCP): originally used as an animal tranquilizer
      - cyclosporine: can affect Mg^{++} levels
   c) eclampsia
4. idiopathic

In 166 *pediatric* patients presenting to an emergency department with either a chief complaint of, or a discharge diagnosis of a first-time seizure[4]:
1. 110 were found to actually have either a recurrent seizure or a non-ictal event
2. of the 56 patients actually thought to have had a first-time seizure
   a) 71% were febrile seizures
   b) 21% were idiopathic
   c) 7% were "symptomatic" (hyponatremia, meningitis, drug intoxication...)

In a prospective study of 244 patients with a new-onset unprovoked seizure, only 27% had further seizures during follow-up.[2,5] Recurrent seizures were more common in patients with a family seizure history, spike-and-waves on EEG, or a history of a CNS insult (stroke, head injury...). No patient seizure-free for 3 years had a recurrence. Following a second seizure, the risk of further seizures was high.

27.1.3 Evaluation

Adults

A new-onset seizure in an *adult* in the absence of obvious cause (e.g. alcohol withdrawal) should prompt a search for an underlying basis (the onset of idiopathic seizures, i.e. epilepsy, is most common before or during adolescence). A CT or MRI (without and with enhancement) should be performed. A systemic work-up should be done to identify the presence of any factors listed previously (see above). If all this is negative, then an MRI should be performed if not already done. If this is negative also, a repeat study (CT or MRI) should be done in ≈ 6 months and at 1 and possibly 2 years to rule-out a tumor which might not be evident on the initial study.

Pediatrics

Among pediatric patients with first-time seizures, laboratory and radiologic evaluations were often costly and not helpful.[4] A detailed history and physical exam were more helpful.

Management

Management of an adult with the new onset of idiopathic seizures (i.e. no abnormality found on CT or MRI, no evidence of drug withdrawal) is controversial. In one study, an EEG was performed, which if normal was followed by a sleep deprived EEG with the following observations[6]:

1. there is substantial interobserver variation in interpreting such EEGs
2. if both EEGs were normal, the 2-yr recurrence rate of seizures was 12%
3. if one or both EEGs showed epileptic discharges, the 2-yr recurrence rate was 83%
4. the presence of nonepileptic abnormalities in one or both EEGs had a 41% 2-yr recurrence rate
5. the recurrence rate with focal epileptic discharges (87%) was slightly higher than for generalized epileptic discharges (78%)

The conclusion is that EEGs thus obtained have moderate predictive value, and may be factored into the decision of whether or not to treat such seizures with AEDs.

27.2 Posttraumatic seizures

27.2.1 General information

Key concepts

- 2 categories: early (≤ 7 days) and late (> 7 days) after head trauma
- anticonvulsants (AEDs) may be used to prevent early posttraumatic seizures (PTS) in patients at high risk for seizures
- prophylactic AEDs do NOT reduce the frequency of late PTS
- discontinue AEDs after 1 week except for cases meeting specific criteria (see text)

Posttraumatic seizures (PTS) are often divided (arbitrarily) into: early (occurring within 1 week of injury) and late (thereafter).[7] There may be justification for a third category: "immediate", i.e. within minutes to an hour or so.

27.2.2 Early PTS (≤ 7 days after head trauma)

30% incidence in severe head injury ("severe" defined as: LOC > 24 hrs, amnesia > 24 hrs, focal neuro deficit, documented contusion, or intracranial hematoma) and ≈ 1% in mild to moderate injuries. Occurs in 2.6% of children < 15 yrs age with head injury causing at least brief LOC or amnesia.[8]

Early PTS may precipitate adverse events as a result of elevation of ICP, alterations in BP, changes in oxygenation, and excess neurotransmitter release.[9]

27.2.3 7 days after head trauma)",3,7,2,0,0mm,0mm,0mm,0mm>Late onset PTS (> 7 days after head trauma)

Estimated incidence 10–13% within 2 yrs after "significant" head trauma (includes LOC > 2 mins, GCS < 8 on admission, epidural hematoma...) for all age groups.[10,11] Relative risk: 3.6 times control population. Incidence in severe head injury > > moderate > mild.[8]

The incidence of early PTS is higher in children than adults, but late seizures are much less frequent in children (in children who have PTS, 94.5% develop them within 24 hrs of the injury[12]). Most patients who have not had a seizure within 3 yrs of penetrating head injury will not develop seizures.[13] Risk of late PTS in children does not appear related to the occurrence of early PTS (in adults: only true for mild injuries). Risk of developing late PTS may be higher after repeated head injuries.

27.2.4 Penetrating trauma

The incidence of PTS is higher with penetrating head injuries than with closed head injuries (occurs in 50% of penetrating trauma cases followed 15 yrs[14]).

27.2.5 Treatment

General information

Some early retrospective studies suggested that early administration of PHT prevents early PTS, and reduces the risk of late PTS even after discontinuation of the drug. Later prospective studies disputed this but were criticized for not maintaining satisfactory levels and for lacking statistical power.[7,11] A prospective double blind study of patients at high risk of PTS (excluding penetrating trauma) showed a 73% reduction of risk of *early* PTS by administering 20 mg/kg loading dose of PHT within 24 hrs of injury and maintaining high therapeutic levels; but after 1 week there was no benefit in continuing the drug (based on intention to treat).[15] Carbamazepine (Tegretol®) has also been shown to be effective in reducing the risk of early PTS.

Phenytoin has adverse cognitive effects when given long-term as prophylaxis against PTS.[16]

27

Treatment guidelines

Based on available information (see above) it appears that:

1. no treatment studied effectively impedes epileptogenesis (i.e. neuronal changes that ultimately lead to late PTS)
2. in high-risk patients (► Table 27.1), AEDS reduces the incidence of *early* PTS
3. however, no study has shown that reducing early PTS improves outcome[17]
4. once epilepsy has developed, continued AEDs reduces the recurrence of further seizures

The following are therefore offered as guidelines.

Initiation of AEDs

AEDs may be considered for short term use especially if a seizure could be detrimental. Early post-traumatic seizures were effectively reduced when phenytoin was used for 2 weeks following head injury with no significant increased risk of adverse effects.[18]

Acutely, seizures may elevate ICP, and may adversely affect blood pressure and oxygen delivery, and may worsen other injuries (e.g. spinal cord injury in the setting of an unstable cervical spine). There may also be negative psychological effects on the family, loss of driving privileges, and possibly deleterious effects of excess neurotransmitters.[9]

Option: begin AEDs (usually levetiracetam, phenytoin or carbamazepine) within 24 hrs of injury in the presence of any of the high risk criteria shown in ► Table 27.1 (modified[9,12,13,19]). When using PHT, load with 20 mg/kg and maintain high therapeutic levels. Switch to phenobarbital if PHT not tolerated.

Discontinuation of AEDs

1. taper AEDs after 1 week of therapy except in the following:
   a) penetrating brain injury
   b) development of late PTS (i.e. a seizure > 7 days following head trauma)

Table 27.1 High risk criteria for PTS

1. acute subdural, epidural, or intracerebral hematoma SDH, EDH or ICH
2. open-depressed skull fracture with parenchymal injury
3. seizure within the first 24 hrs after injury
4. Glasgow Coma Scale score < 10
5. penetrating brain injury
6. history of significant alcohol abuse
7. ± cortical (hemorrhagic) contusion on CT

   c) prior seizure history
   d) patients undergoing craniotomy[20]
2. for patients *not* meeting the criteria to discontinue AEDs after 1 week (see above):
   a) maintain ≈ 6–12 mos of therapeutic AED levels
   b) recommend EEG to rule-out presence of a seizure focus before discontinuing AEDs (shown to have poor predictive value is poor, however probably advisable for legal purposes) for the following:
      • repeated seizures
      • presence of high risk criteria shown in ▶ Table 27.1.

27.3 Alcohol withdrawal seizures

27.3.1 General information

Also, see Alcohol withdrawal syndrome (p.204). The withdrawal syndrome may begin hours after the EtOH peak; see also prevention and treatment (p.205). Ethanol withdrawal seizures are classically seen in up to 33% (some say 75%) of habituated drinkers within 7–30 hours of cessation or reduction of ethanol intake. They typically consist of 1–6 tonic-clonic generalized seizures without focality within a 6 hour period.[21] Seizures usually occur before delirium develops. They may also occur during intoxication (without withdrawal).

The seizure risk persists for 48 hrs (risk of delirium tremens (DTs) continues beyond that), thus a single loading dose of PHT is frequently adequate for prophylaxis. However, since most EtOH withdrawal seizures are single, brief, and self-limited, PHT has *not* been shown to be of benefit in uncomplicated cases and is thus *usually not indicated*. Chlordiazepoxide (Librium®) or other benzodiazepines (p.205) administered during detoxification reduces the risk withdrawal seizures.[22]

27.3.2 Evaluation

The following patients should have a CT scan of the brain, and should be admitted for further evaluation as well as for observation for additional seizures or for DTs:
1. those with their first EtOH withdrawal seizure
2. those with focal findings
3. those having more than 6 seizures in 6 hrs
4. those with evidence of trauma

Other causes of seizure should also be considered, e.g. a febrile patient may require an LP to rule-out meningitis.

27.3.3 Treatment

A brief single seizure may not warrant treatment, except as outlined below. A seizure that continues beyond 3–4 minutes may be treated with diazepam or lorazepam, with further measures used as in status epilepticus (p.468) if seizures persist. Loading with phenytoin (18 mg/kg = 1200 mg/70 kg) and long-term treatment is indicated for:
1. a history of previous alcohol withdrawal seizures
2. recurrent seizures after admission
3. history of a prior seizure disorder unrelated to alcohol
4. presence of other risk factors for seizure (e.g. subdural hematoma)

27.4 Nonepileptic seizures

27.4.1 General information

AKA pseudoseizures (some prefer not to use this term since it may connote voluntary feigning of seizures), with the term psychogenic seizures being preferred for nonepileptic seizures (NES) with a psychologic etiology (psychogenic seizures are real events and may not be under voluntary control).[23]

One of the hazards of NES is that patients may end up needlessly taking AEDs, which in some cases may worsen NES. Possible etiologies of NES are given in ▶ Table 27.2. Most NES are psychogenic.

Table 27.2 Differential diagnosis of nonepileptic seizures[23]

psychologic disorders (psychogenic seizure) a) somatoform disorders: especially conversion disorder b) anxiety disorders: especially panic attack and posttraumatic stress disorder c) dissociative disorders d) psychotic disorders e) impulse control disorders f) attention-deficit disorders[a] g) factitious disorders: including Munchausen's syndrome
cardiovascular disorders a) syncope b) cardiac arrhythmias c) transient ischemic attacks d) breath-holding spells[a]
migraine syndromes a) complicated migraines[a] b) basilar migraines
movement disorders a) tremors b) dyskinesias c) tics[a], spasms d) other (including shivering)
parasomnias & sleep-related disorders a) night terrors[a], nightmares[a], somnambulism[a] b) narcolepsy, cataplexy c) rapid eye movement behavior disorder d) nocturnal paroxysmal dystonia
gastrointestinal disorders a) episodic nausea or colic[a] b) cyclic vomiting syndrome[a]
other a) malingering b) cognitive disorders with episodic behavioral or speech symptoms c) medication effects or toxicity d) daydreams[a]
[a]usually encountered in children

27

DDx for seizures:

1. psychogenic: 20–90% of patients with intractable seizures referred to epilepsy centers. These patients carry the diagnosis of seizures from 5–7 years. Up to 50% of these may have legitimate seizures at some time as well.[24]
2. tic: can be suppressed, is not repetitive (if repetitive, may be hemifacial spasm)
3. movement disorder: myoclonus (can be epileptic or non-epileptic)
   a) cataplexy: e.g. with narcolepsy often provoked by laughter or other emotional stimulus (can rarely be caught on EEG, when it is it shows REM intrusion into wakefulness)
   b) parasomnia: a sleep movement disorder (occurs during sleep). Includes: night terrors (occurs in slow wave sleep, vs. nightmare which occurs in REM), sleep walking, REM behavior disorders (usually occurs in older men, and there is a high probability they will go on to have degenerative brain disease (used to be called paroxysmal nocturnal PNT). Head banging is a benign parasomnia
4. syncope: 90% of the time people who faint have myoclonic jerks or shaking[25]
5. TIA

27.4.2 Differentiating NES from epileptic seizures

General information

Distinguishing between epileptic seizures (ES) and NES is a common clinical dilemma. There are unusual seizures that may fool experts.[26] Some frontal lobe and temporal lobe complex partial seizures may produce bizarre behaviors that do not correspond to classic ES findings and may not produce discernible abnormalities with scalp-electrode EEG (and therefore may be misdiagnosed even with video-EEG monitoring, although this is more likely with partial seizures than with generalized). A multidisciplinary team approach may be required.

▶ Table 27.3 contrasts some features of true seizures vs. NES, and ▶ Table 27.4 lists some features often associated with NES, however, no characteristics are definitively diagnostic of NES since a number of them may also occur with ES.

Features common to both true seizures and NES: verbal unresponsiveness, rarity of automatisms and whole-body flaccidity, rarity of urinary incontinence. Reminder: some seizures can be bizarre and can resemble NES (sometimes called pseudo-pseudoseizures). 10% of patients with psychogenic seizures actually have epilepsy.

Table 27.3 Features of ES vs. NES[24]

Feature	Epileptic seizure	NES
% males	72%	20%
Clonic UE movement		
in-phase	96%	20%
out-of-phase	0	56%
Clonic LE movement		
in-phase	88%	16%
out-of-phase	0	56%
Vocalizations		
none	16%	56%
start of seizure	24%	44%
middle	60% "epileptic cry"	0
types	only sounds of tonic or clonic respiratory muscle contraction	moans, screams, grunts, snorts, gagging, retching, understandable statements, gasps
Head turning		
unilateral	64%	16%
side-to-side	8% (slow, low amplitude)	36% (violent, high amplitude)

Table 27.4 Features often associated with NES[23]

- frequent seizures despite therapeutic AEDs
- multiple different-physician visits
- lingering prodrome or gradual ictal onset (over minutes)
- prolonged duration (> 5 mins)
- manifestations altered by distraction
- suggestible or inducible seizures
- intermittent arrhythmic and out-of-phase convulsive activity
- fluctuating intensity and severity during Sz
- side-to-side rolling, pelvic thrusting, wild movements
- bilateral motor activity with preserved consciousness
- nonphysiologic spread of neurologic signs
- absence of labored breathing or drooling after generalized convulsion
- expression of relief or indifference
- crying or whimpering
- no postictal confusion or lethargy
- disproportionate postictal mental status changes
- absence of stereotypy

Features suggestive of non-epileptic seizures:
1. arching of the back: 90% specific for NES
2. asynchronous movement
3. stop & go: seizures usually build and then gradually subside
4. forced eye closing during entire seizure
5. provoked with stimuli that would not cause a seizure (e.g. tuning fork to the head, alcohol pad to the neck, IV saline…)
6. bilateral shaking with preserved awareness. Exception: supplementary motor area seizures (mesial frontal area) these seizures are usually tonic (not clonic)
7. weeping (whining): highly specific
8. multiple or variable seizure types (ES is usually stereotypical), fluctuating level of consciousness, denial of correlation of Sz with stress

If any two of the following are demonstrated, 96% of time this will be NES:
1. out-of-phase clonic UE movement
2. out-of-phase clonic LE movement
3. no vocalization or vocalization at start of event

Lateral tongue laceration is very specific for seizures.

History

Attempt to document: prodromal symptoms, precipitating factors, time and environment of Sz, mode and duration of progression, ictal and postictal events, frequency and stereotypy of manifestations. Determine if patient has history of psychiatric conditions, and if they are acquainted with individuals who have ES.

Psychological testing

May help. Differences occur in ES and NES on the Minnesota Multiphasic Personality Inventory (MMPI) scales in hypochondriasis, depression hysteria, and schizophrenia.[27]

Prolactin levels after seizures

Transient elevations in human serum prolactin (HSP) levels occur following 80% of generalized motor, 45% of complex partial, and only 15% of simple partial seizures.[28] Peak levels are reached in 15–20 minutes, and gradually return to baseline over the subsequent hour.[29,30,31] It has been suggested that drawing a serum prolactin level shortly after a questionable seizure may be helpful in differentiating NES (which may have elevated cortisol levels but normal HSP levels[32]).

Repetitive seizures are associated with progressively smaller HSP elevations,[33] and no rise follows absence seizures or status epilepticus (whether convulsive or absence).[34] Greater than twofold HSP elevations consistently follow seizures that produce intense widespread high frequency mesial temporal lobe discharges; whereas such elevations do not occur in seizures not involving these limbic structures.[35]Furthermore, there may be higher baseline HSP levels in cases with right-sided interictal EEG discharges compared to those with left-sided,[36] and the presence of psychopathology may affect postictal HSP elevations.[37]

Therefore, the presence of HSP peaks may be strongly indicative of true seizures, but the absence may be due to a variety of complex phenomena.[38] The overall classification accuracy is ≈ 72%.[31]

27.5 Febrile seizures

27.5.1 Definitions

See reference.[39]

▶ **Febrile seizure.** A seizure in infants or children associated with fever with no defined cause and unaccompanied by acute neurologic illness (includes seizures during vaccination fevers)

▶ **Complex febrile seizure.** A convulsion that lasts longer than 15 minutes, is focal, or multiple (more than one convulsion per episode of fever)

▶ **Simple febrile seizure.** Not complex

▶ **Recurrent febrile seizure.** More than one episode of fever associated with seizures

27.5.2 Epidemiology

See reference.[39]

Febrile convulsions are the most common type of seizure. Excluding children with pre-existing neurologic or developmental abnormalities, the prevalence of febrile seizures is ≈ 2.7% (range: 2–5% in U.S. children aged 6 mos-6 yrs). The risk for developing epilepsy after a simple febrile seizure is ≈ 1%, and for a complex febrile seizure is 6% (9% for prolonged seizure, 29% for focal seizure). An underlying neurological or developmental abnormality or a family history of epilepsy increases the risk of developing epilepsy. The notion that the younger the child with a febrile seizure the greater the risk of epilepsy is unproven.

27.5.3 Treatment

27

In one study, the IQ in the group treated with phenobarbital was 8.4 points lower (95% confidence interval) than the placebo group, and there remained a significant difference several months after discontinuing the drug.[40] Furthermore, there was no significant reduction in seizures in the phenobarbital group. And yet, no other drug really appears well suited to treating this entity: carbamazepine and phenytoin appear ineffective, valproate may be effective but has serious risks in the < 2 yrs age group. Given the low incidence (1%) of having afebrile seizures (i.e. epilepsy) after a *simple* febrile seizure and the fact that AEDs probably do not prevent this development, there is little support for prescribing anticonvulsants in these cases. The recurrence rate of febrile seizures in children with a history of one or more febrile seizure can be reduced by administering diazepam 0.33 mg/kg PO q 8 hrs during a febrile episode (temp > 38.1° C) and continuing until 24 hrs after the fever subsides.[41]

27.6 Status epilepticus

27.6.1 General information

Key concepts

- definition: Sz > 5 mins, or persistent Sz after 1st & 2nd line AEDs
- morbidity and mortality are high in untreated status epilepticus (SE)
- most common etiology: patient with known Sz disorder with low AED levels
- de novo SE in acute illness is considered a manifestation of the illness which should be treated at the same time as the SE
- see ► Table 27.5 for treatment measures

► **Definition.** A seizure lasting > 5 minutes or persistent seizure activity after sequential administration of appropriate first and second-line AEDs.[42]

► **Features important to management:**
- 61% of seizures that persist > 5 mins will continue > 1 hour[43]
- in patients with no prior Sz history, status epilepticus (SE) is usually a manifestation of illness-related cortical irritation or injury[42] and treatment of the underlying disorder (in addition to treating the SE) is critical
- a relapse of Sz. in a patient with a known Sz. disorder and subtherapeutic AED levels usually responds to a bolus of the maintenance AEDs. However, SE should be treated by the standard protocol[42]
- most cases of convulsive status in adults start as partial seizures that generalize secondarily
- the choice of 1st and 2nd-line AEDs is arbitrary, *dose*[42] and starting treatment in < 30 minutes[44] are more important determinants of success in aborting SE

27.6.2 Types of status epilepticus

See reference.[45]
- generalized status
  1. convulsive (tonic-clonic, tonic-clonic-tonic, or clonic): generalized convulsive tonic-clonic status epilepticus (SE) is the most frequent type.[46] A medical emergency
  2. absence (note: in status, this may present in twilight state)

Table 27.5 Summary of initial steps for status epilepticus (adults and children > 13 kg; see text for details)[50]

ABC's. Start O_2. Turn patient on their side. Check VS. Do a neuro exam
Monitor/labs: Pulse oximetry. EKG/telemetry. ✓ Fingerstick glucose. Blood tests (do not wait for results to begin ℞):✓ electrolytes, ✓ CBC, ✓ ABG, ✓ AED levels, ✓ LFTs, ✓ Mg^{++}, ✓ Ca^{++}, ✓ head CT
Large bore IV X 2. Start IV fluids
• thiamine 100 mg IV and/or 50 ml of 50% dextrose (if needed based on fingerstick glucose)
First-line AED: • lorazepam (Ativan®) 4 mg IV for adults, 2 mg IV for children > 13 kg @ < 2 mg/min OR • midazolam (Versed®) 10 mg IM for adults, 5 mg IM for children > 13 kg OR (if no IV access or midazolam injections not available) • diazepam can be given rectally in Diastat® gel formulation (0.2-0.5 mg/kg) Repeat loading dose of benzodiazepine if necessary
Second-line AED: given with failure of (or simultaneously with administration of) repeat dose of benzodiazepine • fosphenytoin: 15-20 mg PE/kg IV @ < 150 mg PE/min (preferred drug: faster infusion rate, less irritation) OR • phenytoin: 15-20 mg/kg IV @ < 50 mg/min (less expensive) If no response to loading dose, an additional 10 mg/kg IV may be given after 20 min. NB: following infusion rate guidelines is imperative. Significant cardiovascular risk is associated with rapid infusion of phenytoin/fosphenytoin.
✓ phenytoin level ≈ 10 min after PHT loading dose; repeat 10 min later additional dose if required
Alternative second-line AEDs: • sodium valproate: 20-30 mg/kg IV bolus (max rate: 100 mg/min) – has been shown to be equal or superior to phenytoin in a few small studies OR • phenobarbital: 20 mg/kg IV (start infusing @ 50-100 mg/min) – commonly used 2nd or 3rd line AED. A repeat dose of 25-30 mg/kg can be given 10 min after first dose. OR • Levetiracetam (Keppra®): 20 mg/kg IV bolus of over 15 minutes – evidence for Keppra as a first or second line drug is less clear
If seizures continue > 30 mins and are refractory to 1st and 2nd line AEDs: intubate in ICU and begin continuous infusion therapy (CIT) of: • Midazolam: 0.2 mg/kg IV loading dose followed by 0.2-0.6 mg/kg/hr OR • Propofol: 2 mg/kg IV loading dose followed by 2-5 mg/kg/hr
If Sz persist, ensure that correctable conditions have been ruled-out and/or treated
novel therapeutic options (not systematically studied): shock therapy...

3. secondarily generalized: accounts for ≈ 75% of generalized SE
4. myoclonic
5. atonic (drop attack): especially in Lennox-Gastaut syndrome (p. 443)

- partial status (usually related to an anatomic abnormality)
  1. simple (AKA epilepsy partialis continua)
  2. complex (note: in status, this may present in twilight state) most often from frontal lobe focus. Urgent treatment is required (several case reports of permanent deficits following this)
  3. secondarily generalized
- non-convulsive SE
  1. benign variants (typical absence SE, complex partial SE)
  2. electrical SE during sleep
  3. atypical absence SE
  4. tonic SE (associated with learning disability in children) SE in coma

Alternatively, SE can be broken down as follows:
- with prominent motor effects
- without prominent motor effects

27

- boundary syndromes (syndromes which combine encephalopathy, behavioral disturbances, delirium, or psychosis with SE-like EEG findings)

27.6.3 Epidemiology

Incidence is ≈ 150,000 new cases/year in the U.S. in the outpatient setting.[42] Most cases occur in young children (among children, 73% were < 5 yrs old[47]), the next most affected group is patients > 60 yrs age. In > 50% of cases, SE is the patient's first seizure.[46] One out of six patients presenting with a first time seizure will present in SE

27.6.4 Etiologies

Most common causes: low level of AED (34%), remote symptomatic cause (24%), cerebrovascular accident (22%), metabolic disturbances (15%), and hypoxia (13%).

A more comprehensive list:

1. a patient with a known seizure disorder having low AED levels for any reason (non-compliance, intercurrent infection preventing PO intake of meds, drug-drug interactions → lowering effectiveness of AEDs…)
2. febrile seizures: a common precipitator in young patients. 5–6% of patients presenting with SE have a history of prior febrile seizures
3. stroke: the most commonly identified cause in the elderly
4. CNS infection: in children, most are bacterial, the most common organisms were H. influenza and S. pneumoniae
5. idiopathic: accounts for ≈ one-third (in children, usually associated with fever)
6. epilepsy: is present or is subsequently diagnosed in ≈ 50% of patients presenting with SE. About 10% of adults ultimately diagnosed as having epilepsy will present in SE
7. electrolyte imbalance: hyponatremia (most common in children, usually due to water intoxication[47]), hypoglycemia, hypocalcemia, uremia, hypomagnesemia…
8. illicit drug intoxication: especially cocaine, amphetamines
9. precipitous drug withdrawal: barbiturates, benzodiazepines, alcohol or narcotics
10. proconvulsant drugs, including: β-lactam antibiotics (penicillins, cephalosporins), certain antidepressants (bupropion), clonazapine, bronchodilators, immunosuppressants
11. traumatic brain injury: acute as well as old
12. hypoxia/ischemia
13. tumor

In children < 1 yr age, 75% had an acute cause: 28% were secondary to CNS infection, 30% due to electrolyte disorders, 19% associated with fever.[47] In adults, a structural lesion is more likely. In an adult, the most common cause of SE is subtherapeutic AED levels in a patient with a known seizure disorder.

27.6.5 Morbidity and mortality from SE

Outcomes are related to underlying cause and duration of SE. Mean duration of SE in patients without neurologic sequelae is 1.5 hrs (therefore, proceed to pentobarbital anesthesia before ≈ 1 hour of SE). Recent mortality: < 10–12% (only ≈ 2% of deaths are directly attributable to SE or its complications; the rest are due to the underlying process producing the SE). Mortality in lowest amongst children (≈ 6%[47]), patients with SE related to subtherapeutic AEDs, and patients with unprovoked SE.[48] The highest mortality occurs in elderly patients and those with SE resulting from anoxia or stroke.[48] 1% of patients die during the episode itself.

Morbidity and mortality is due to[49]:

1. CNS injury from repetitive electric discharges: irreversible changes begin to appear in neurons after as little as 20 minutes of convulsive activity. Cell death is very common after 60 mins
2. systemic stress from the seizure (cardiac, respiratory, renal, metabolic)
3. CNS damage by the acute insult that provoked the SE

27.6.6 Treatment

General treatment measures for status epilepticus

Treatment success, like morbidity/mortality, may be time dependent. One review showed that first-line AED therapy aborted SE in 60% of patients if initiated within the first 30 minutes, and efficacy decreased as seizure duration increased [Lowenstein 1993]. As such, treatment should be initiated as soon as possible and should be directed at stabilizing the patient, stopping the seizure, and identifying the cause (determining if there is an acute insult to the brain) and if possible also treating the underlying process. Treatment often must be initiated prior to the availability of test results to confirm the diagnosis and may even be initiated in the pre-hospital setting.

1. "ABC's"
   a) Airway: oral airway if feasible. Turn patient on their side to avoid aspiration
   b) Breathing: O_2 by nasal cannula or bag-valve-mask. Consider intubation if respirations compromised or if seizure persists > 30 min
   c) Circulation: CPR if needed. Large bore proximal IV access (2 if possible: 1 for phenytoin (PHT) (Dilantin®), not necessary if fosphenytoin is available): start with NS KVO
2. Simultaneous with ABCs, AEDs should be prepared and/or given if SE suspected
3. neurologic exam
4. monitor: EKG & baseline vital signs. Pulse oximeter. Frequent blood pressure checks
5. bloodwork: STAT capillary blood (fingerstick) glucose (to R/O hypoglycemia), electrolytes (including glucose), CBC, LFTs, Mg^{++}, Ca^{++}, AED levels, ABG
6. head CT (usually without contrast)
7. correct any electrolyte imbalance (SE due to electrolyte imbalance responds more readily to correction than to AEDs[47])
8. if CNS infection is a major consideration, perform LP for CSF analysis (especially in febrile children) unless contraindicated (p. 1504). WBC pleocytosis up to $80 \times 106/L$ can occur following SE (benign postictal pleocytosis), and these patients should be treated with antibiotics until infection can be ruled out by negative cultures
9. *general* meds for unknown patient:
   a) glucose:
      - in patients with poor nutrition (e.g. alcoholics): giving glucose in thiamine deficiency can precipitate Wernicke's encephalopathy (p. 206) ∴ prior to glucose bolus give thiamine 50–100 mg IV
      - if fingerstick glucose can be obtained immediately and it shows hypoglycemia, or if no fingerstick glucose can be done: give 25–50 ml of D50 IV push for adults (2 ml/kg of 25% glucose for peds). If at all possible, draw blood for definitive serum glucose first
   b) naloxone (Narcan®) 0.4 mg IVP (in case of narcotics)
   c) ± bicarbonate to counter acidosis (1–2 amps depending on length of seizure)
   d) for neonate < 2 years: consider pyridoxine 100 mg IV push (pyridoxine-dependent seizures constitute a rare autosomal recessive condition that generally presents in the early neonatal period[43])
10. administer specific anticonvulsants for seizures lasting > 5- 10 mins (see below)
11. EEG monitor if possible
12. if paralytics are used (e.g. to intubate), use short acting agents and be aware that muscle paralysis alone may stop visible seizure manifestations, but does not stop the electrical seizure activity in the brain, which can lead to permanent neurologic damage if prolonged (see above).

Medications for generalized convulsive status epilepticus

General information

There are no randomized trials for refractory status epilepticus, although there is published data regarding specific treatment options. Numerous protocols exist. ▶ Table 27.5 shows a summary of medications for a status epilepticus protocol that is outlined in further detail below (adapted[42,45,50,51]). "Peds dosing" refers to patients < 40 kg or approximately 12 yrs of age. Rapid treatment is indicated as delays are associated with neuronal injury and reduced response to medications.

Prehospital phase

1. impending SE: may be heralded by a crescendo in Sz. A 1–3 d course of lorazepam may preempt the development of SE
2. SE treatment may be initiated in the home setting with buccal midazolam or rectal diazepam

Hospital phase

Start IV drugs at half the maximal rate, and titrate up to maximal rate if VS stable.

1. First line drugs
   a) benzodiazepine[52] (main side effect: respiratory depression in ≈ 12%; be prepared to intubate). Onset of action is rapid (1–2 mins):
      - lorazepam (Ativan®) 4 mg IV for adults, 2 mg IV for children @ < 2 mg/min

27

- *OR* midazolam (Versed®) 10 mg IM for adults, 5 mg IM for children > 13 kg–Repeat dose of benzodiazepine if necessary after 10 min.
- If no IV access or if midazolam injections not available, diazepam can be given rectally in Diastat® gel formulation (0.2-0.5 mg/kg)

2. If seizures persist after first dose of benzodiazepine, initiate second line agent in a different IV.
   a) load with fosphenytoin (Cerebyx®) or phenytoin (Dilantin®) as listed below. Do not worry about acutely overdosing, but do follow dosing rates, monitor BP for hypotension and EKG for arrhythmias. After giving the following loading dose, start on maintenance. Fosphenytoin has the advantage of being less irritating and able to infuse at a faster rate, but phenytoin is less expensive and does not need to be metabolized.
      - fosphenytoin: 15-20 mg PE/kg IV @ 150 mg PE/min
      - *OR* phenytoin: 15-20 mg/kg IV @ 50 mg/min
        - if no response to loading dose, an additional 10 mg/kg IV may be given after 20 min.
        - if pt is on PHT and a recent level is known: a rule of thumb is giving 0.74 mg/kg to an adult raises the level by ≈1 mcg/ml
        - if on PHT and level not known: adult: give 500 mg @ < 50 mg/min
   b) There are several good alternatives to fosphenytoin/phenytoin as second-line AEDs:
      - Sodium valproate: 20-30 mg/kg IV bolus (max rate: 100 mg/min) – has been shown to be equal or superior to phenytoin in a few small studies
      - Phenobarbital: 20 mg/kg IV (start infusing @ 50-100 mg/min) – commonly used 2nd or 3rd line AED. A repeat dose of 25-30 mg/kg can be given 10 min after first dose.
      - Levetiracetam (Keppra®): 20 mg/kg IV bolus of over 15 minutes – evidence for Keppra as a first or second line drug is less clear
3. Traditionally, a third line agent was given prior to continuous infusion therapy (CIT), however was successful in only 7%.[52] As such, most new protocols proceed directly to anesthetic administration. If seizures are continuing after above therapies have been administered (15-30 min after initial presentation), begin CIT as follows:
   - Midazolam: 0.2 mg/kg IV loading dose followed by 0.2-0.6 mg/kg/hr
   - *OR* Propofol: 2 mg/kg IV loading dose followed by 2-10 mg/kg/hr
4. At this time, lab results and tests should be available. Ensure that all reversible etiologies have been addressed and that a CT head has been performed.
5. Pentobarbital is often reserved for SE that is refractory to all of the above interventions. If necessary, Pentobarbital is administered as follows:
   - Pentobarbital: 5 mg/kg IV followed by 1-5 mg/kg/hr
6. While some practitioners will try additional drugs (carbamazepine, oxcarbazepine, topiramate, levetiracetam, lamotrigine, gabapentin), these are likely to be of limited utility.
7. Experimental interventions include: lidocaine infusion, inhalational anesthesia, direct brain stimulation, transcranial magnetic stimulation, electroconvulsive therapy (shock therapy), surgical intervention if a seizure focus is identified

Remember: Paralytics stop the visible manifestations of the seizure and they may be useful for intubation and/or in order to obtain head imaging; however, they do not stop the abnormal electrical brain activity or the neurological damage that results.

Efficacy of drug therapy

Studies vary widely, but it appears that approximately 2/3 of patients will respond to initial therapy with the other 1/3 progressing to refractory SE.[50]

Medications to avoid in status epilepticus

1. narcotics
2. phenothiazines: including promethazine (Phenergan®)
3. neuromuscular blocking agents in the absence of AED therapy: seizures may continue and cause neurologic injury but would not be clinically evident

27.6.7 Medications for non-convulsive status epilepticus

In non-convulsive status epilepticus, the first and second line AEDs listed in ▶ Table 27.5 should be utilized. However, many practitioners avoid escalating to the anesthetic options (CIT, pentobarbital) instead opting for trials of additional AEDs first (carbamazepine, oxcarbazepine, topiramate, lamotrigine, etc).

27.6.8 Miscellaneous status epilepticus

Myoclonic status

Treatment: valproic acid (drug of choice). Place NG, give 20 mg/kg per NG loading dose. Maintenance: 40 mg/kg/d divided.

Can add lorazepam (Ativan®) or clonazepam (Klonopin®) to help with acute control.

Absence status epilepticus

Almost always responds to diazepam.

References

[1] Hauser WA, Annegers JF, Kurland LT. Incidence of Epilepsy and Unprovoked Seizures in Rochester, Minnesota, 1935-1984. Epilepsia. 1993; 34:453–468

[2] Hauser WA, Anderson VE, Loewenson RB, McRoberts SM. Seizure Recurrence After a First Unprovoked Seizure. New Engl J Med. 1982; 307:522–528

[3] Reith J, Jorgensen HS, Nakayama H, et al. Seizures in acute stroke: Predictors and prognostic significance. The Copenhagen stroke study. Stroke. 1997; 28:1585–1589

[4] Landfish N, Gieron-Korthals M, Weibley RE, Panzarino V. New Onset Childhood Seizures: Emergency Department Experience. J Fla Med Assoc. 1992; 79:697–700

[5] Hauser WA, Rich SS, Jacobs MP, Anderson VE. Patterns of Seizure Occurrence and Recurrence Risks in Patients with Newly Diagnosed Epilepsy. Epilepsia. 1983; 24:516–517

[6] van Donselaar C, Schimsheimer R-J, Geerts AT, Declerck AC. Value of the Electroencephalogram in Adult Patients With Untreated Idiopathic First Seizures. Arch Neurol. 1992; 49:231–237

[7] Young B, Rapp RP, Norton JA, et al. Failure of Prophylactically Administered Phenytoin to Prevent Late Posttraumatic Seizures. J Neurosurg. 1983; 58:236–241

[8] Annegers JF, Grabow JD, Groover RV, et al. Seizures After Head Trauma: A Population Study. Neurology. 1980; 30:683–689

[9] Bullock R, Chesnut RM, Clifton G, et al. Guidelines for the Management of Severe Head Injury. 1995

[10] McQueen JK, Blackwood DHR, Harris P, et al. Low Risk of Late Posttraumatic Seizures Following Severe Head Injury. J Neurol Neurosurg Psychiatry. 1983; 46:899–904

[11] Young B, Rapp RP, Norton JA, et al. Failure of Prophylactically Administered Phenytoin to Prevent Early Posttraumatic Seizures. J Neurosurg. 1983; 58:231–235

[12] Hahn YS, Fuchs S, Flannery AM, Barthel MJ, McLone DG. Factors Influencing Posttraumatic Seizures in Children. Neurosurgery. 1988; 22:864–867

[13] Weiss GH, Salazar AM, Vance SC, et al. Predicting Posttraumatic Epilepsy in Penetrating Head Injury. Arch Neurol. 1986; 43:771–773

[14] Temkin NR, Dikmen SS, Winn HR. Posttraumatic Seizures. Neurosurg Clin North Amer. 1991; 2:425–435

[15] Temkin NR, Dikmen SS, Wilensky AJ, Keihm J, et al. A Randomized, Double-Blind Study of Phenytoin for the Prevention of Post-Traumatic Seizures. N Engl J Med. 1990; 323:497–502

[16] Dikmen SS, Temkin NR, Miller B, Machamer J, et al. Neurobehavioral Effects of Phenytoin Prophylaxis of Posttraumatic Seizures. JAMA. 1991; 265:1271–1277

[17] Brain Trauma Foundation, Povlishock JT, Bullock MR. Antiseizure prophylaxis. J Neurotrauma. 2007; 24:S83–S86

[18] Haltiner AM, Newell DW, Temkin NR, et al. Side Effects and Mortality Associated with Use of Phenytoin for Early Posttraumatic Seizure Prophylaxis. J Neurosurg. 1999; 91:588–592

[19] Yablon SA. Posttraumatic Seizures. Arch Phys Med Rehabil. 1993; 74:983–1001

[20] North JB, Penhall RK, Hanieh A, Frewin DB, et al. Phenytoin and Postoperative Epilepsy: A Double-Blind Study. J Neurosurg. 1983; 58:672–677

[21] Charness ME, Simon RP, Greenberg DA. Ethanol and the Nervous System. N Engl J Med. 1989; 321:442–454

[22] Lechtenberg R, Worner TM. Seizure Risk With Recurrent Alcohol Detoxification. Arch Neurol. 1990; 47:535–538

[23] Chabolla DR, Krahn LE, So EL, Rummans TA. Psychogenic Nonepileptic Seizures. Mayo Clin Proc. 1996; 71:493–500

[24] Gates JR, Ramani V, Whalen S, et al. Ictal Characteristics of Pseudoseizures. Arch Neurol. 1985; 42:1183–1187

[25] Lempert T, Bauer M, Schmidt D. Syncope: a videometric analysis of 56 episodes of transient cerebral hypoxia. Ann Neurol. 1994; 36:233–237

[26] King DW, Gallagher BB, Marvin AJ, et al. Pseudoseizures: Diagnostic Evaluation. Neurology. 1982; 32:18–23

[27] Henrichs TF, Tucker DM, Farha J, Novelly RA. MMPI Indices in the Identification of Patients Evidencing Pseudoseizures. Epilepsia. 1988; 29:184–187

[28] Wyllie E, Luders H, MacMillan JP, et al. Serum Prolactin Levels After Epileptic Seizures. Neurology. 1984; 34:1601–1604

[29] Dana-Haeri J, Trimble MR, Oxley J. Prolactin and Gonadotropin Changes Following Generalized and Partial Seizures. J Neurol Neurosurg Psychiatry. 1983; 46:331–335

[30] Prichard PB, Wannamaker BB, Sagel J, et al. Serum Prolactin and Cortisol Levels in Evaluation of Pseudoepileptic Seizures. Ann Neurol. 1985; 18:87–89

[31] Laxer KD, Mullooly JP, Howell B. Prolactin Changes After Seizures Classified by EEG Monitoring. Neurology. 1985; 35:31–35

[32] Abbott RJ, Browning MCK, Davidson DLW. Serum Prolactin and Cortisol Concentrations After Grand Mal Seizures. J Neurol Neurosurg Psychiatry. 1980; 43:163–167

[33] Jackel RA, Malkowicz D, Trivedi R, Sussman NM, et al. Reduction of Prolactin Response with Repetitive Seizures. Epilepsia. 1987; 28

[34] Tomson T, Lindbom U, Nilsson BY, Svanborg E, et al. Serum Prolactin During Status Epilepticus. J Neurol Neurosurg Psychiatry. 1989; 52:1435–1437

[35] Sperling MR, Pritchard PB, Engel J, et al. Prolactin in Partial Epilepsy: An Indicator of Limbic Seizures. Ann Neurol. 1986; 20:716–722

[36] Meierkord H, Shorvon S, Lightman S, Trimble M. Comparison of the Effects of Frontal and Temporal Lobe Partial Seizures on Prolactin Levels. Arch Neurol. 1992; 49:225–230

[37] Dana-Haeri J, Trimble MR. Prolactin and Gonadotropin Changes Following Partial Seizures in Epileptic Patients With and Without Psychopathology. Biol Psychiatry. 1984; 19:329–336

[38] Herzog AG. Prolactin: Quo Vadis? Arch Neurol. 1992; 49:223–224

[39] Verity CM, Golding J. Risk of Epilepsy After Febrile Convulsions: A National Cohort Study. BMJ. 1991; 303:1373–1376

[40] Farwell JR, Lee YJ, Hirtz DG, Sulzbacher SI, et al. Phenobarbital for Febrile Seizures - Effects on Intelligence and on Seizure Recurrence. N Engl J Med. 1990; 322:364–369
[41] Rosman NP, Colton T, Labazzo J, et al. A Controlled Trial of Diazepam Administered During Febrile Ilnesses to Prevent Recurrence of Febrile Seizures. N Engl J Med. 1993; 329:79–84
[42] Costello DJ, Cole AJ. Treatment of acute seizures and status epilepticus. J Intensive Care Med. 2007; 22:319–347
[43] Abend NS, Dlugos DJ. Treatment of refractory status epilepticus: literature review and a proposed protocol. Pediatr Neurol. 2008; 38:377–390
[44] Eriksson K, Metsaranta P, Huhtala H, Auvinen A, Kuusela AL, Koivikko M. Treatment delay and the risk of prolonged status epilepticus. Neurology. 2005; 65:1316–1318
[45] Varelas PN, Spanaki MV, Mirski MA. Status epilepticus: an update. Curr Neurol Neurosci Rep. 2013; 13. DOI: 10.1007/s11910-013-0357-0
[46] Hauser WA. Status Epilepticus: Epidemiologic Considerations. Neurology. 1990; 40:9–13
[47] Phillips SA, Shanahan RJ. Etiology and Mortality of Status Epilepticus in Children. Arch Neurol. 1989; 46:74–76
[48] Delorenzo RJ, Pellock JM, Towne AR, Boggs JG. Epidemiology of Status Epilepticus. J Clin Neurophysiol. 1995; 12:312–325
[49] Fountain NB, Lothman EW. Pathophysiology of Status Epilepticus. J Clin Neurophysiol. 1995; 12:326–342
[50] Betjemann JP, Lowenstein DH. Status epilepticus in adults. Lancet Neurol. 2015; 14:615–624
[51] Kinney M, Craig J. Grand Rounds: An Update on Convulsive Status Epilepticus. Ulster Med J. 2015; 84:88–93
[52] Treiman DM, Meyers PD, Walton NY, Collins JF, Colling C, Rowan AJ, Handforth A, Faught E, Calabrese VP, Uthman BM, Ramsay RE, Mamdani MB. A comparison of four treatments for generalized convulsive status epilepticus. Veterans Affairs Status Epilepticus Cooperative Study Group. N Engl J Med. 1998; 339:792–798

Part IX

Pain

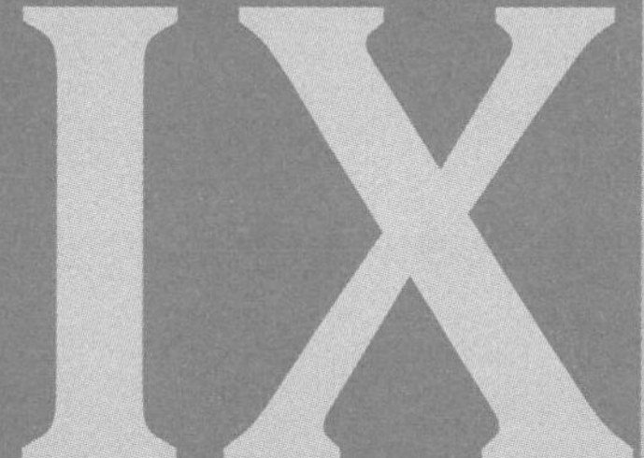

28 Pain

28.1 General information

For pain medication, see Analgesics (p. 136).

Major types of pain:

1. nociceptive
   a) somatic: well localized. Described as sharp, stabbing, aching or cramping. Results from tissue injury or inflammation, or from nerve or plexus compression. Responds to treating the underlying pathology or by interrupting the nociceptive pathway
   b) visceral: poorly localized. Poor response to primary pain medications
2. deafferentation: poorly localized. Described as crushing, tearing, tingling or numbness. Also causes burning dysesthesia numbness often with lancinating pain, and hyperpathia. Unaffected by ablative procedures
3. "sympathetically maintained" pain and the likes, e.g. causalgia (p. 497)

28.2 Neuropathic pain syndromes

28

28.2.1 General information

Definition: Neuropathic pain: pain caused by a lesion of the peripheral and/or central nervous system manifesting with sensory symptoms and signs (Backonja[1] modified from the International Association for the Study of Pain[2]).

Neuropathic pain syndromes (NPS) are typified by painful diabetic neuropathy (PDN) and postherpetic neuralgia (PHN). Common chronic NPSs are shown in ▶ Table 28.1,[3] divided into central or peripheral nervous system origin of the pain. The pain of PDN and PHN is typically burning and aching, and is continuous. and is characteristically refractory to medical and surgical treatment.

Table 28.1 Common neuropathic pain syndromes

Peripheral neuropathic pain
acute & chronic inflammatory demyelinating polyradiculoneuropathy (CIDP) alcoholic polyneuropathy chemotherapy induced polyneuropathy complex regional pain syndrome (CRPS) entrapment neuropathies HIV sensory neuropathy iatrogenic neuralgias (e.g. postthoracotomy pain) idiopathic sensory neuropathy neoplastic nerve compression or infiltration nutritional-deficiency neuropathies painful diabetic neuropathy (PDN) phantom limb pain postherpetic neuralgia (PHN) postradiation plexopathy radiculopathy toxic exposure-related neuropathies trigeminal neuralgia posttraumatic neuralgias
Central neuropathic pain
cervical spondylotic myelopathy HIV myelopathy multiple sclerosis-related pain Parkinson disease-related pain postischemic myelopathy postradiation myelopathy poststroke pain posttraumatic spinal cord injury pain syringomyelia

28.2.2 Medical treatment of neuropathic pain

General information

Treatment traditionally includes narcotic analgesics,[4] and tricyclic antidepressants (see below). For further details and other treatment measures, see PHN (p.494).

Tricyclic antidepressants

Use is often limited by anticholinergic and central effects and by limited pain relief.[5,6] Possibly because serotonin potentiates the analgesic effect of endorphins and elevates pain thresholds, serotonin re-uptake blockers are more effective than norepinephrine re-uptake blockers, e.g. trazodone (Desyrel®) blocks only serotonin. Also useful: amitriptyline (Elavil®) 75 mg daily; desipramine (Norpramin®) 10–25 mg/d; doxepin (Sinequan®) 75–150 mg/d. Some benefit may also derive from the fact that many patients with chronic pain are depressed. **Side effects:** anticholinergic effects and orthostatic hypotension, especially in the elderly. ✖ Not recommended for use in patients with ischemic heart disease.

Gabapentin

Effective in postherpetic neuralgia (PHN) (p.495) and painful diabetic neuropathy. Benefit also reported in pain associated with: trigeminal neuralgia, cancer,[7] multiples sclerosis, HIV-related sensory neuropathy, CRPS, spinal cord injury, post-operative state,[8] migraine[9] (a number of these studies may have been sponsored by the manufacturer[10]). See also side effects, dosing & availability... (p.455)

Lidocaine patch (Lidoderm®)

May be effective.[3] ℞: apply patch for up to 12 hrs/day up to a maximum of 3 patches at a time to the intact skin over the most painful area (may trim patch to appropriate size). **Supplied:** 5% lidocaine (p.496).

Tramadol (Ultram®)

A centrally acting analgesic (p.140).[3]

28.3 Craniofacial pain syndromes

28.3.1 General information

Possible pathways for *facial* pain include: trigeminal nerve (portio major as well as portio minor (motor root)), facial nerve (usually deep facial pain), and eighth nerve.[11] Etiologies (adapted[12 (p 2328),13]).

1. cephalic neuralgias
   a) trigeminal neuralgia (see below)
      - vascular compression of Cr. N. V at root entry zone: the most common cause
      - MS: plaque within Cr. N. V nucleus
   b) glossopharyngeal neuralgia (p.492): pain usually in base of tongue and adjacent pharynx
   c) geniculate neuralgia (p.493): otalgia and deep prosopalgia
   d) tic convulsif (p.493): geniculate neuralgia with hemifacial spasm
   e) occipital neuralgia (p.515)
   f) superior laryngeal neuralgia: a branch of the vagus, results primarily in laryngeal pain and occasionally pain on the auricle
   g) sphenopalatine neuralgia
   h) herpes zoster: pain is continuous (not paroxysmal). Characteristic vesicles and crusting usually follow pain, most often in distribution of V1 (isolated V1 TGN is rare). In rare cases without vesicles, diagnosis may be difficult
   i) postherpetic neuralgia (Ramsay-Hunt syndrome) (p.493)
   j) supraorbital neuralgia (SON) (p.491)
   k) trigeminal neuropathic pain (AKA trigeminal deafferentation pain)[13]: may follow injuries from sinus or dental surgery, head trauma
   l) trigeminal deafferentation pain: follows trigeminal denervation including therapeutic measures to treat trigeminal neuralgia[13]

28

m) short-lasting unilateral neuralgiform headache with conjunctival injection and tearing (SUNCT)[14]: rare. Usually affects males 23–77 years old. Brief (< 2 minutes) pain (burning, stabbing or shock-like) usually near the eye, occurring multiple times per day. Associated autonomic findings (the "hallmark of SUNCT"): ptosis, conjunctival injection, lacrimation, rhinorrhea, hyperemia. May be due to CPA AVM. Microvascular decompression or trigeminal rhizotomy may be effective in some cases refractory to medical treatment with AEDs or corticosteroids. Note: lacrimation (the most common) or other autonomic signs may occur in V1 trigeminal neuralgia but are usually mild, and appear only in the later stages of the condition and with long lasting attacks.[15] Dramatic lacrimation and conjunctival injection from the onset of symptoms with SUNCT are the best characteristics to distinguish this from trigeminal neuralgia.[16] May also occur in cluster headache (p. 175).

2. ophthalmic pain
   a) Tolosa-Hunt syndrome (p. 569): painful ophthalmoplegia
   b) (Raeder's) paratrigeminal neuralgia (p. 569): unilateral Horner's syndrome + trigeminal neuralgia
   c) orbital pseudotumor (p. 569): proptosis, pain, and EOM dysfunction
   d) diabetic (oculomotor) neuritis
   e) optic neuritis
   f) iritis
   g) glaucoma
   h) anterior uveitis

3. otalgia (see below)
4. masticatory disorders
   a) dental or periodontal disease
   b) nerve injury (inferior and/or superior alveolar nerves)
   c) temporo-mandibular joint (TMJ) dysfunction
   d) elongated styloid process
   e) temporal & masseter myositis
5. vascular pain syndromes
   a) migraine headaches: see Migraine (p. 175)
      - simple migraine: includes classic migraine, common migraine
      - complicated migraine: includes hemiplegic migraine, ophthalmoplegic migraine
   b) cluster H/A (p. 175); subtypes: episodic, chronic, chronic paroxysmal hemicrania
   c) giant cell arteritis (p. 195) (temporal arteritis). Tenderness over STA
   d) toxic or metabolic vascular H/A (fever, hypercapnia, EtOH, nitrites, hypoxia, hypoglycemia, caffeine withdrawal)
   e) hypertensive H/A
   f) aneurysm or AVM (due either to mass effect or hemorrhage)
   g) carotidynia: e.g. with carotid dissection (p. 1324)
   h) basilar dolichoectasia with fifth n. compression or indentation of the pons
6. sinusitis (maximally, frontal, ethmoidal, sphenoidal)
7. dental disease
8. neoplasm: may cause referred pain or fifth nerve compression
   a) extracranial
   b) intracranial tumor: primarily posterior fossa lesions, neoplastic compression of trigeminal nerve usually causes sensory deficit (p. 481)
9. atypical facial pain (AFP) (prosopalgia): traditionally a "wastebasket" category used for many things. It has been proposed[13] to reserve this term for a psychogenic disorder. May be suspected by
10. primary (nonvascular) H/A: including
    a) tension (muscle contraction) H/A
    b) post-traumatic H/A

28.3.2 Otalgia

General information

Because of redundant innervation of the region of the ear, *primary* otalgia may have its source in the 5th, 7th, 9th, or 10th cranial nerves or the occipital nerves.[17] As a result, sectioning of the 5th, 9th or 10th nerve or a component of the 7th (nervus intermedius, chorda tympani, geniculate ganglion) has been performed with varying results.[18] Also, microvascular decompression (MVD) of the corresponding nerve may also be done.[19]

Work-up includes: neurotologic evaluation to rule out causes of secondary otalgia (otitis media or externa, temporal bone neoplasms…). CT or MRI should be done in any case where no cause is found.

Primary otalgia

Primary otalgia is unilateral in most (≈ 80%). Trigger mechanisms are identified in slightly more than half, with cold air or water being the most common.[18] About 75% have associated aural symptoms: hearing loss, tinnitus, vertigo. Pain relief upon cocainization or nerve block of the pharyngeal tonsils suggests glossopharyngeal neuralgia (p.492), however, the overlap of innervation limits the certainty.

An initial trial with medications used in trigeminal neuralgia (carbamazepine, phenytoin, baclofen…) (p.481) is the first line of defense. In intractable cases not responding to pharyngeal anesthesia, suboccipital exploration of the 7th (nervus intermedius) and lower cranial nerves may be indicated. If significant vascular compression is found, one may consider MVD alone. If MVD fails, or if no significant vessels are found, Rupa et al. recommend sectioning the nervus intermedius, the 9th and upper 2 fibers of 10th nerve, and a geniculate ganglionectomy (or, if glossopharyngeal neuralgia is strongly suspected, just 9th and upper 2 fibers of 10th).[18]

28.3.3 Trigeminal neuralgia

28

General information

Key concepts

- sharp, electric shock-like paroxysmal lancinating pain in the distribution of one or more branches of the trigeminal nerve on one side
- characterized by periods of remission and initial response to carbamazepine
- neurologic exam must be intact (only exception: mild sensory loss)
- 80–90% of cases are caused by compression of the trigeminal nerve at the root entry zone by the superior cerebellar artery. In MS patients, may be due to MS plaque (MS patients are usually less responsive to procedures)
- 75% will ultimately fail medical therapy and require a procedure (main options: microvascular decompression, percutaneous rhizotomy or radiosurgery). Choice of modality depends on patient age, location of symptoms, prior treatment and the side effect profile of the treatment modality

Trigeminal neuralgia (TGN) (AKA tic douloureux): paroxysmal lancinating electric-like pain lasting a few seconds, often triggered by sensory stimuli, confined to the distribution of one or more branches of the trigeminal nerve (▶ Fig. 28.1) on one side of the face, with no neurologic deficit. The term "atypical facial pain" (AFP) is sometimes used to describe any other type of facial pain.

Rarely, TGN manifests as status trigeminus, a rapid succession of tic-like spasms triggered by seemingly any stimulus. IV carbamazepine (where available) or phenytoin may be effective for this.

Epidemiology

See ▶ Table 28.2. Annual incidence 4/100,000. There is no correlation with herpes simplex infection.[20] There is a tendency for spontaneous remission with pain free intervals of weeks or months being characteristic, regardless of treatment. 2% of patients with MS have TGN,[21] whereas ≈ 18% of patients with bilateral trigeminal neuralgia have MS.[22]

Pathophysiology

Probably due to ephaptic transmission in trigeminal nerve from large-diameter partially demyelinated A fibers to thinly myelinated A-delta and C (nociceptive) fibers. Pathogenesis may be due to:

1. vascular compression of the trigeminal nerve at the root entry zone (NB: compression may be seen in up to 50% of autopsies in patients without TGN[25]):
   a) most commonly (80%) by the SCA; see Neurovascular compression syndromes (p.1534) for more details
   b) persistent primitive trigeminal artery (p.83) [26]
   c) dolichoectatic basilar artery[27(p 1108)]

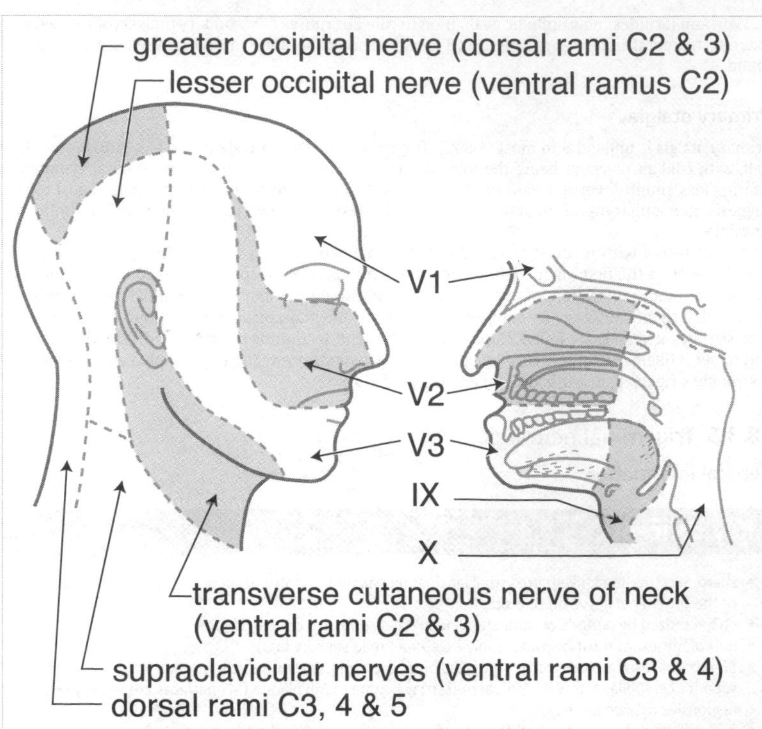

Fig. 28.1 Pain/temperature innervation of the head*
* KEY: V1 = ophthalmic nerve; V2 = maxillary nerve; V3 = mandibular nerve; IX = glossopharyngeal nerve; X = vagus

Table 28.2 Epidemiology of trigeminal neuralgia[23,24]

age (years)	typically > 50 (average 63)
female:male	1.8:1
Laterality	
right	60%
left	39%
both	1%
Division involved	
V1 only	2%
V2 only	20%
V3 only	17%
V1 & V2	14%
V2 & V3	42%
all three	5%

2. posterior fossa tumor (below)
3. in MS, plaque within brainstem may cause TGN that is often poorly responsive to microvascular decompression

In addition to the sensory division of the trigeminal nerve, other possible pain pathways include[11]: the motor branch of the 5th nerve (portio minor), or the 7th or 8th nerve.

Tumors and trigeminal neuralgia

In > 2000 patients with facial pain seen over 10 yrs, only 16 harbored tumor (< 0.8% incidence).[28] 3 tumors outside cranial vault included nasal carcinoma and skull base mets; all had hypalgesia and atypical facial pain (AFP). 6 middle fossa tumors included 2 meningiomas, 2 schwannomas (1 primary tumor of Gasserian ganglion), and 1 pituitary adenoma. Posterior fossa tumors are the most likely to cause symptoms that most closely resemble true TGN; of these, vestibular schwannoma (VS) is most common. 2 of 7 VSs had tumors contralateral to the neuralgia (presumably due to brainstem shift). Patients with true TGN initially responded to carbamazepine, none with AFP did.

When facial pain is caused by tumor, especially with peripheral tumors, the pain is frequently atypical (usually constant), neurologic abnormalities are often present (usually sensory loss, although some are neurologically normal at first), and the age is often younger than typical TGN.

Differential diagnosis

See Craniofacial pain syndromes (p. 477).

Evaluation

History and physical (in addition to routine)
1. history
   a) accurate description of pain localization to determine which divisions of trigeminal nerve need to be treated
   b) determine time of onset of TGN, trigger mechanisms
   c) ascertain presence and length of pain-free intervals (lack of any pain-free interval is atypical for TGN)
   d) determine duration, side-effects, dosages, and responses to medications tried
   e) inquire about symptoms that may indicate the presence of conditions other than TGN: e.g. history of herpetic vesicles, excessive tearing of the eye (may indicate SUNCT (p. 478), facial twitching (tic convulsif), tongue pain (glossopharyngeal neuralgia), sensory loss (tumor…), progressive relentless pain (tumor, herpes…), symptoms that suggest MS
2. physical exam: the exam should be normal in TGN, any neurologic deficit (except very mild sensory loss) in previously unoperated patient should prompt search for structural cause, e.g. tumor (see below). This exam also serves as a baseline for post-op comparison
   a) assess sensation in all 3 divisions of trigeminal nerve bilaterally (include corneal reflexes)
   b) assess masseter function (bite) and pterygoid function (on opening mouth, chin deviates to weak side)
   c) assess EOM function

Imaging

MRI is often used to evaluate these patients for possible intracranial tumors or MS plaques, especially in cases with atypical features. The yield in typical cases is low.

Medical therapy for trigeminal neuralgia

Drug info: Carbamazepine (Tegretol®)

Complete or acceptable relief in 69% (if 600–800 mg/d are tolerated and give no relief, diagnosis of TGN is suspect[21]). **Side effects:** Drowsiness. Rash in 5–10%. Possible Stevens-Johnson syndrome. Relative leukopenia is common (usually does not require discontinuing drug). See precautions under carbamazepine (**CBZ**, Tegretol®) (p. 450).

℞ 100 mg PO BID, increase by 200 mg/d up to maximum of 1200 mg/d divided TID. **Supplied:** See supply information (p. 450).

Drug info: Carbamazepine (Tegretol®)

Rapidly metabolized to carbamazepine, similar efficacy, often tolerated at higher doses than carbamazepine. **Side effects :** symptomatic hyponatremia.

℞ for trigeminal neuralgia: 300 mg PO BID, increase by 600 mg/d q week. Usual dose: 450–1200 mg. Maximum of 2400 mg/d. **Supplied :** 150, 300, 600 mg tablets; 500 mg/5-ml suspension.

Drug info: Baclofen (Lioresal®)

2nd DOC (not as effective as carbamazepine, but fewer side-effects). Caution: teratogenic in rats. Avoid abrupt withdrawal (can cause hallucinations and seizures). May be more effective if used in conjunction with low dose carbamazepine.

℞ Start low, 5 mg PO TID, increase q 3 d by 5 mg/dose; not to exceed 20 mg QID (80 mg/d); use smallest effective dose.

28

Drug info: Gabapentin (Neurontin®)

An anticonvulsant, may act synergistically with carbamazepine and baclofen. **Side effects :** include ataxia, sedation and rash.

℞ start with 100 mg po BID, titrate to 5–7 mg/kg/day (3600 mg/d max).

Miscellaneous drugs

Also possibly effective:

1. phenytoin (Dilantin®): may be useful IV in patients in too much pain to open their mouths to take carbamazepine orally
2. capsaicin (Zostrix®): 1 gm applied TID for several days resulted in remission of symptoms in 10 of 12 patients (4 relapsed in < 4 mos, but remained pain free for 1 yr after 2nd course)[29]
3. clonazepam (Klonopin®) (p. 454): works in 25%
4. lamotrigine (Lamictal®)
5. amitriptyline (Elavil®): more commonly used for atypical facial pain
6. botulinum **toxin** (Botox®): reduces transmission of CGRP producing a direct effect on the sensory nerve fibers

Surgical therapy for trigeminal neuralgia

Indications for surgery

Reserved for cases refractory to medical management, or when side effects of medications exceed risks and drawbacks of surgery.

Surgical options

1. peripheral trigeminal nerve branch procedures to block or ablate the division involved with *pain*, or can be used to block the trigger[30]:
   a) means of blocking
      - local blocks (phenol, alcohol)
      - neurectomy of trigeminal branch involved
   b) nerve branches:
      - V1 (ophthalmic division) at the supraorbital, supratrochlear, or infraorbital nerves
      - V2 (maxillary division) at the foramen rotundum
      - V3 (mandibular division) block at the foramen ovale, or neurectomy of inferior dental nerve

2. blocking the *trigger*: either via percutaneous rhizotomy or alcohol block
3. percutaneous trigeminal rhizotomy (PTR): AKA percutaneous (stereotactic) rhizotomy (PSR) of trigeminal (Gasserian) ganglion (see below) (not truly a stereotactic procedure in the current sense of the word, therefore the term percutaneous trigeminal rhizotomy is preferred). Objective is to selectively destroy A-delta and C fibers (nociceptive) while preserving A-alpha and beta fibers (touch). Ideally, a retrogasserian lesion (not a ganglionic lesion). May also be used to block trigger. Lesioning techniques include (see below for comparison of techniques):
   a) *radiofrequency* rhizotomy (RFR) (originated by Sweet and Wespic[31]). Uses radiofrequency energy to thermocoagulate the pain fibers. Requires the patient to be awake at intervals during the procedure
   b) *glycerol* injection into Meckel's cave[32,33]: possibly lower incidence of sensory loss and anesthesia dolorosa than with radiofrequency lesion.[34] Water soluble contrast cisternography was recommended in original description, may not be essential[35]
   c) mechanotrauma (percutaneous microcompression (PMC) rhizolysis): via inflation of No. 4 Fogarty catheter balloon.[36,37,38] Does not require the patient to be awake
   d) injection of sterile boiling water
4. Spiller-Frazier subtemporal extradural approach with retrogasserian rhizotomy (rarely used today). Original Spiller-Frazier technique involved avulsion of the nerve, which was met with unacceptably high risk of bleeding. The approach may be used to expose the ganglion and then mildly traumatize it
5. intradural retrogasserian trigeminal nerve section (sensory portion ± motor root, see below): may be performed during MVD if no vascular compression is identified
6. cutting descending trigeminal tract in lower medulla (99.5% success): rarely used
7. microvascular decompression (MVD)[39]: (see below) microsurgical exploration of root entry zone, usually via posterior fossa craniectomy, and displacement of vessel impinging on nerve (if such a vessel is found). Usually with the placement of a non-absorbable "insulator" (Ivalon® sponge or shredded Teflon felt; see relative merits of Ivalon® vs. Teflon felt (p. 1536)
8. complete section of the nerve proximal to the ganglion via a p-fossa crani
9. stereotactic radiosurgery: see below
10. motor cortex stimulation[40]: (somewhat analogous to spinal cord stimulation for spinal or extremity pain). Better for neuropathic trigeminal pain (as distinct from trigeminal neuralgia)

Selection of surgical option

Some pearls that influence treatment option choices (expert opinion[41]):

1. V3 neuralgia: RF. Can selectively treat V3 without involving other divisions
2. V1 or V2: balloon compression. Causes numbness in all 3 divisions, but unlike the lesion with RF the corneal numbness is better tolerated and the corneal reflex is often preserved
3. bilateral pain: glycerol. It has the shortest duration of effect, which is an advantage if you think you may need to treat the other side at some point
4. SRS: due to latency until pain relief, suboptimal for patients who need immediate pain relief

Peripheral nerve ablation and neurectomies

Limited to pain or trigger points in territory of supraorbital/supratrochlear, infraorbital, or inferior dental nerves. Neurectomy may be a consideration especially for elderly patients who are not candidates for MVD (neurectomy may be done under local anesthesia) with pain in the forehead (to avoid anesthesia of the eye, as could occur with RFR). Disadvantages include sensory loss in the distribution of the nerve and a high rate of pain recurrence due to nerve regeneration (usually in 18–36 months) which often responds to repeat neurectomy.[42] May also be used following PTR.

Supraorbital and supratrochlear nerve: See also information on supraorbital neuralgia (SON) or supratrochelar neuralgia (STN) (p. 491). SON may be treated with rhizotomy (e.g. with alcohol or radiofrequency) or with neurectomy. Alcohol injection is used with caution for STN because of risk of injury to the superior oblique muscle. For neurectomy, these nerves are exposed through a 2 cm incision parallel to and just above the medial portion of the eyebrow (never through the eyebrow as this can create an unsightly "bi-brow"; shaving the eyebrow is also discouraged since it occasionally does not grow back). The incision is carried down to the bone and the periosteum is elevated caudally towards the supraorbital foramen or notch. The nerves will be visible on the undersurface of the periosteal flap. The supraorbital nerve is freed in its foramen/notch, and is then avulsed by grasping it with a mosquito hemostat and twisting the clamp. The nerve avulses "like pulling a worm out of a hole." The distal portion of the nerve should be located at the site were the periosteum was incised and it, too, should be avulsed. The process can be repeated for the more medially situated supratrochlear nerve.

Other nerves: Not covered here, other nerve branches that may be cut or avulsed include: infratrochlear, lacrimal (the branch of V1 at the lateral edge of the orbit), infraorbital nerve, inferior alveolar, lingual and mental nerves.[43(p 290)]

Percutaneous trigeminal rhizotomy (PTR)

Recommended for patients who: are poor risk for general anesthesia (elderly or those with increased risk for general anesthesia), wish to avoid "major" surgery, have unresectable intracranial tumors, have MS, have impaired hearing on the other side, or have limited life expectancy (<5 yrs).[34] For "atypical facial pain", denervating the painful region of the face benefits <20% of patients, and worsens 20%.[44] Recurrences are easily treated by repeat procedures. May be used to treat failures of peripheral nerve ablation.

▶ **Choice of lesion technique.** Recurrence rates and incidence of dysesthesias are comparable among the various lesioning techniques. Incidence of intraoperative hypertension is less with PMC than with radiofrequency rhizotomy (RFR) lesion[38] (no reports of intracerebral hemorrhage). Bradycardia occurs regularly with PMC which may not be harmful (some prophylax with atropine[45]). RFR requires a patient who is able to cooperate; PMC can be done with the patient asleep. Paralysis of ipsilateral trigeminal motor root (e.g. pterygoids) is more common after PMC (usually temporary) than RFR, and so PMC should not be done if there is already contralateral paralysis from a previous procedure. See also description of technique (p. 486).

28

Complications with percutaneous radiofrequency (note: some "numbness" is actually expected in most successful PTRs and occurs in 98% of cases,[24] and is not considered a complication here)

1. mortality: only 17 deaths in over 22,000 procedures (includes lesser experienced neurosurgeons and patients often considered poor surgical risks)[21]
2. dysesthesias[24] (sometimes called "annoying paresthesias"): higher rate in more complete lesions
   a) minor: 9%
   b) major (requiring medical treatment): 2%
   c) anesthesia dolorosa (severe, constant, burning aching pain that is refractory to all treatment): 0.2–4%
3. meningitis[23]: 0.3%
4. alterations in salivation[46]: 20% (increased in 17%, decreased in 3%)
5. partial masseter weakness (usually not perceived by patient, ▶ Table 28.3)
6. oculomotor paresis (usually temporary, ▶ Table 28.3)
7. reduced hearing (secondary to paresis of tensor tympani, ▶ Table 28.3)
8. **neuroparalytic keratitis** (keratitis due to fifth nerve deficit which impairs sensation, ▶ Table 28.3)
9. intracranial hemorrhage: personal report of 7 cases (6 fatal) in >14,000 procedures, probably due to transient HTN (SBP up to 300 torr)
10. alterations in lacrimation[46]: 20% (increased in 17%, decreased in 3%)
11. herpes simplex eruption: prescribe antiherpetic drug if patient develops symptoms, e.g. Acyclovir® (p. 366).
12. bradycardia and hypotension: 1% with RFR compared to up to 15% with glycerol injection)
13. rare[47,48]:
    a) temporal lobe abscess
    b) aseptic meningitis
    c) intracerebral abscess: 0.1%

Table 28.3 Complications with percutaneous radiofrequency

Complication	850 cases[56]		315 cases[46]
	straight electrode (N = 700)	curved electrode (N = 150)	
partial masseter weakness (usually not perceived by patient)	15–24%	7%	50%
oculomotor paresis (usually temporary)	2%	0	
reduced hearing (secondary to paresis of tensor tympani)	0	0	27%
neuroparalytic keratitis (keratitis due to fifth nerve deficit which impairs sensation)	4%	2%	0

d) trigeminal trophic syndrome (TTS)[49]: triad of unilateral crescentic nasal alar ulceration with anesthesia and paresthesia of the trigeminal dermatome (may present with severe pruritus and self-induced skin lesions from scratching). A result of trigeminal nerve injury. Treatment has included: carbamazepine, diazepam, amitriptyline, chlorpromazine, clonazepam or pimozide[50]
e) complications related to needle placement[51]:
   - carotid cavernous fistula (CCF): may occur with any percutaneous technique[52] (including balloon microcompression[53])
   - blindness: from penetration of inferior orbital fissure[54]
   - injury to other cranial nerves: II, III, IV, VI[55]
f) subarachnoid hemorrhage
g) seizures

Microvascular decompression (MVD)

See also more detailed information (p. 488).

Recommended for patients with inadequate medical control of pain with > 5 years anticipated survival and able to tolerate a small craniotomy[34] (surgical morbidity increases with age). Relief is often long lived, persevering 10 yrs in 70%. Incidence of facial anesthesia is much less than with PTR, and anesthesia dolorosa does not occur. Mortality: < 1%. Incidence of aseptic meningitis (AKA hemogenic meningitis): 20%. 1–10% major neurologic morbidity. Failure rate: 20–25%.

1–2% of patients with MS will have a demyelinating plaque at the root entry zone, this usually does not respond to MVD, and one should attempt a PTR.

Stereotactic radiosurgery (SRS)

The first use of SRS by Leksell was for the treatment of TGN. Initially, this was reserved for refractory cases following multiple operations,[57] now becoming more widely practiced. The least invasive procedure. Generally recommended for patients with co-morbidities, high-risk medical illness, pain refractory to prior surgical procedures, or those on anticoagulants (anticoagulation does not have to be reversed to have SRS).

Treatment plan: 4 -5 mm isocenter in the trigeminal nerve root entry zone identified on MRI. Use 70–80 Gy at the *center*, keeping the 80% isodose curve outside of the brainstem.

Results: Significant pain reduction after initial SRS: 80–96%,[58,59,60,61] but only ≈ 65% become pain free. Median latency to pain relief: 3 months (range: 1 d-13 months).[62] Recurrent pain occurs within three years in 10–25%. Patients with TN and multiple sclerosis are less likely to respond to SRS than those without MS. SRS can be repeated, but only after four months following the original procedure.

Favorable prognosticators: higher radiation doses, previously unoperated patient, absence of atypical pain component, normal pre-treatment sensory function.[63]

Side effects: Hypesthesia occurred in 20% after initial SRS, and in 32% of those requiring repeat treatment[62] (higher rates associated with higher radiation doses[59]).

Management of surgical treatment failures

90% of recurrences are in distribution of previously involved divisions; 10% are in new division and may represent progression of the underlying process. Some treatment failures are not persistent TN, but rather represent trigeminal neuropathic pain (AKA trigeminal deafferentation pain).

PTR may be repeated in patients who have a recurrence with some preservation of facial sensation. Attempted repeat PTR is often productive, and failures can be managed as below.

MVD may be performed in patients failing PTR, but the success rate may be reduced[64] (91% for patients undergoing MVD first, vs. 43% for those having MVD following PTR; note: 91% may be an unrealistically high success rate, and taking patients that fail PTR may select for a more difficult subgroup). Repeat MVD may also be performed, with attention given to possible slippage of the insulating sponge, or the fact that the true offending vessel may be “artificially” moved away from the nerve secondary to the surgical positioning.

SRS can be repeated, using the same dose, with reported significant reduction in pain in 89%, and complete relief in 58%.[62]

Intradural retrogasserian trigeminal nerve section

May be used as a measure of last resort in patients who have recurrent TGN following one or more PTRs in the presence of total facial anesthesia, or in patients undergoing posterior-fossa craniectomy for the purpose of MVD when no impinging vessel can be identified. In the latter case, a partial rhizotomy is performed by sectioning 2/3 of nerve, with resulting partial anesthesia. In the case of patients with facial anesthesia pre-op, consideration should be given to sectioning the motor division (portio minor) as an alternate pain pathway.[11]

Percutaneous trigeminal rhizotomy (PTR)

Due to concerns about hemorrhage, check coagulation profile (PT/PTT, consider bleeding time), and discontinue ASA and NSAIDs, preferably 10 days pre-op. Procedure may be performed in OR with fluoro, or in angiography suite in x-ray department.

Booking the case: Percutaneous trigeminal rhizotomy

(For any of the percutaneous methods: balloon, glycerol, RFR)

Also see defaults & disclaimers (p. 27) and pre-op orders (see below).

1. position: supine
2. anesthesia: MAC with sedation
3. equipment:
   a) lesion generator and needle kit for radiofrequency rhizotomy
   b) C-arm fluoroscopy (2 C-arms for balloon compression)
   c) calibrated inflatable balloons (as in kyphoplasty) for balloon rhizotomy
4. consent (in lay terms for the patient – not all-inclusive):
   a) procedure: put a needle into the cheek to numb the nerve to the face
   b) alternatives: medical treatment, surgery through the back of the skull (microvascular decompression), radiation (stereotactic radiosurgery)
   c) complications: facial numbness is anticipated, rarely: stroke, bleeding, blindness

28

Pre-op orders (RFR)

1. NPO after MN except meds
2. continue Tegretol® & other meds PO with sips of water
3. AM of procedure: IV NS @ KVO in arm contralateral to neuralgia
4. atropine 0.4 mg IM PRN (✖ contraindications include rapid a-fib)
5. non-disposable LP tray to accompany patient

Technique: Percutaneous trigeminal radiofrequency rhizotomy (RFR)

Adapted technique.[65]

NB: needle insertion and/or lesioning may cause HTN, consider monitoring BP. Use either a straight electrode (bare 5 mm for 1 division, 7.5 mm for 2 divisions, or 10 mm for total lesions) or a curved electrode.[56]

Electrode insertion

1. attach ground electrode to patient's upper arm
2. prep the cheek on the involved side with Betadine
3. entry point: under short-acting anesthetic agent – e.g. propofol (Diprivan®) (p. 133) or methohexital (Brevitol®) (p. 132) –, insert electrode-needle 2.5–3 cm lateral to oral commissure
4. trajectory:
   a) palpate the buccal mucosa with a gloved finger inside the mouth (lateral to the teeth) and with the other hand pass the electrode medial to the coronoid process of the mandible (keeping the needle deep to the oral mucosa, i.e. outside the oral cavity) initially aiming towards the plane intersecting a point 3 cm anterior to EAM and the medial aspect of the pupil when the eye is directed forward. Be careful not to contaminate the field with the hand that was in the patient's mouth
   b) as insertion progresses, use fluoroscopy to direct the tip towards the intersection of the top of the petrous bone with the clivus (5–10 mm below floor of sella along clivus)
   c) upon entering foramen ovale the masseter often contracts, causing the jaw to briefly close. Remove the stylet, look for CSF to verify location (may not occur in re-do cases), and insert electrode through needle

In difficult cases, intraoperative fluoroscopy may assist in localizing the needle to Meckel's cave and to R/O e.g. entry into superior orbital fissure (which can cause blindness after lesioning), or entry into foramen spinosum (middle meningeal artery). If necessary to visualize (e.g. when there is difficulty entering), the foramen ovale is optimally seen on a submental x-ray by hyperextending neck 20° and rotating head 15–20° away from side of pain.[66]

Impedance measurements: from the tip of the electrode when available may help indicate location of needle tip. Impedance: CSF (or any fluid) low (≈ 40–120 Ω); connective tissue, muscle, or nerve is usually 200–300 Ω (may be up to 400 Ω); if > 400 Ω this likely indicates electrode is contacting periosteum or bone. After starting the lesion, impedance often goes down by 30 Ω transiently, and then as the lesioning continues it gradually returns to baseline or ≈ 20 Ω above it. If char develops on the electrode tip, the impedance will read higher than where it started.

Stimulation and repositioning

Once the foramen ovale is entered, the needle is positioned with the following guidelines: for V3 division lesion the curved electrode should be just short of the clivus and pointing down, for V2 it is at the clivus and directed up, for V1 it is 5 mm beyond clivus and pointing up. ✖ At no time should the needle tip extend > 8 mm beyond clival line (to avoid Cr. N. III or VI complications).

The patient is allowed to wake up and is stimulated through the electrode with the following settings: frequency = 50–75 Hz, 1 mS duration, start at 0.1 V amplitude and slowly increase (usually 0.2–0.5 V is adequate, higher voltages may indicate that the needle is not near the target and that stimulation is due to far-field currents, however, in previously lesioned patients up to 4 V may sometimes be necessary). If stimulation does not reproduce pain in the distribution of the patient's TGN, then the amplitude is returned to 0, the electrode is repositioned (straight electrode: advance needle < 5 mm at a time, until the tip is in the vicinity of the clival line; curved tip electrode: advance and/or rotate) and then slowly elevate the voltage again from 0 and repeat the repositioning-stimulating process until stimulation reproduces the distribution of tic pain. If previous lesions have produced analgesia and the patient cannot feel the stimulating current, one may stimulate at 2 Hz. and watch for masseter twitch (requires preserved motor root).

Lesioning

When stimulation produces pain in the involved distribution of the TGN, perform the first lesion under short-acting anesthesia at 60–70° C × 90 sec. A facial flush may be noted.[66] After every lesion, perform a post-lesion assessment (see below). The goal is analgesia (but not anesthesia) in the areas of tic pain and hypalgesia in areas of trigger points. An average of three lesions are necessary at the first sitting, each ≈ 5° C higher than the previous for 90 seconds. Anesthetic may not be needed after the first lesion if moderate analgesia has been produced by previous lesions.

Post-lesion assessment

After each lesion and at completion of procedure, assess:

1. sensitivity to pinprick and light touch in all three divisions of trigeminal nerve (grading: normal, hypalgesic, analgesic, anesthetic)
2. corneal reflex bilaterally
3. EOM function
4. masseter muscle strength (patient clenches teeth, palpate cheeks for contraction)
5. pterygoid muscle strength (ask patient to open mouth, chin deviates towards side of pterygoid weakness)

Post-op care (PTR)

Include in post-op orders:

1. ice pack to face on side of procedure for 4 hrs
2. soft diet
3. routine activity when alert
4. avoid narcotics (usually not necessary)
5. if corneal reflex impaired: risk of neuroparalytic keratitis. Natural tears 2 gtt q 2 hrs while awake to eye on affected side. Lacrilube® to eye & tape eye shut q hs

Prior to discharge from hospital, repeat post-lesion assessment (see above). Patients are then weaned off of carbamazepine as tolerated.

Percutaneous microcompression rhizolysis balloon (PMC)

Via inflation of No. 4 Fogarty catheter balloon.

Technique

1. the needle is placed as with RFR (p. 486).
2. aim for balloon placement in the medial foramen ovale (to avoid entering the middle fossa). After placing the balloon, insert the stylet to visualize where the balloon will go. Use Omnipaque 240 to fill the balloon
3. inflate to 1.4 atmospheres of pressure

Table 28.4 Comparison of outcomes of percutaneous techniques to MVD

Parameter	Percutaneous techniques (PTR)			MVD
	RFR[a]	Glycerol	Balloon	
initial success rate[11,24]	91–99%	91%	93%	85–98%
medium-term recurrence rate	19% at 6 yrs[23]	54% at 4 yrs	21% at 2 yrs	15% in 5 yrs
long-term recurrence rate	80% at 12 yrs[46b]			30% at 10 yrs
facial numbness[24]	98%	60%	72%	2%

[a]abbreviations: RFR = radiofrequency rhizotomy; MVD = microvascular decompression; balloon = balloon microcompression
[b]this author included initial failures to PTR requiring repeat procedures during same hospitalization

28

Results

Results of various PTR techniques compared to microvascular decompression (MVD) are shown in ► Table 28.4. Recurrence rate is higher in patients with multiple sclerosis (50% at 3 yrs mean F/U).[67]

Microvascular decompression (MVD) for trigeminal neuralgia

Indications

1. patients unable to achieve adequate medical control of trigeminal neuralgia with ≥ 5 yrs anticipated survival, without significant medical or surgical risk factors[34] (although a small p-fossa exploration is usually well tolerated, surgical morbidity increases with age)
2. may be used in patients who do not fit the above criteria, but have intractable pain and fail PTR
3. patient with tic involving V1 for whom the risk of exposure keratitis due to corneal anesthesia would be unacceptable (e.g. already blind in contralateral eye) or patient wishing to avoid facial anesthesia for any reason
4. ✖ patients with MS are usually not considered candidates for MVD due to low response rate

Booking the case: Microvascular decompression

Also see defaults & disclaimers (p. 27) and pre-op preparation (see below).
1. position: park bench
2. equipment: microscope
3. implants: Ivalon sponge or shredded Teflon
4. intra-op monitoring: (optional) BAER, facial EMG (monitors VII and portio minor (motor) of VII), VIII (CNAP (compound nerve action potential) using Cueva electrode placed directly on VIII nerve referenced to ipsilateral earlobe)
5. consent (in lay terms for the patient – not all-inclusive):
   a) procedure: surgery behind the ear to move a blood vessel from the sensory nerve of the face, if no offending vessel can be identified then possible partial sectioning of the appropriate part of the trigeminal nerve with associated numbness)
   b) alternatives: needle procedures through the cheek (percutaneous rhizotomy), radiation (stereotactic radiosurgery)
   c) complications: (in addition to usual craniotomy complications), CSF leak, hearing loss (≈ 10%), facial numbness, pain near incision (occipital neuralgia or lesser occipital neuralgia), rarely: diplopia, facial paralysis, failure of the procedure

Technique

Also see Paramedian suboccipital craniectomy (p. 1447), for important pointers, including use of armored endotracheal tube.

Preoperative preparation
An MRI is recommended (with FIESTA sequence or equivalent, if available) to rule-out mass lesion or vascular abnormality. Baseline BAER are performed by some[68] (see below for intra-op monitoring).

O.R. setup
Setup for lateral oblique suboccipital (posterior-fossa) craniotomy (p. 1446). Microscope: observer's eyepiece is placed on the side opposite to that of the tic.

Positioning
See reference.[69]

1. lateral oblique position (p. 1446), symptomatic side *up*, axillary roll
2. thorax elevated 10–15° to reduce venous pressure
3. 3-pin skull fixation. Head position:
   a) head rotation: head rotated 10–15° away from the affected side. Do not exceed 30° rotation
   b) lateral head tilt
      - for trigeminal neuralgia or VIII nerve approach: the head is parallel to the floor (if it is lower, nerves VII & VIII will obscure view of V)
      - for VII nerve or lower, the vertex is tilted 15° *down* from the horizontal
   c) flex neck: leave 2 fingerbreadths room between the chin and the sternum
4. upper shoulder retracted caudally with adhesive tape
5. option: lumbar spinal drain. Drain 20–30 cc during craniotomy, then drain off small amounts from time-to-time during the case to keep the field mostly dry, but occasionally letting CSF build up to bathe cranial nerves

Intra-operative monitoring
Option: intra-operative monitoring of facial EMG and BAER (assesses acoustic nerve).[68]

Approach

1. skin incision[69]: vertical incision 3–5 cm in length, 5 mm medial to mastoid notch, a small "5–6-4" incision (p. 1448); in thick or short-necked patients, a slightly longer incision that angles inferomedially is used. 75% of the incision is inferior to the transverse sinus, 25% superior
2. burr hole:
   a) 1 cm inferior and 1 cm medial to the asterion[70(p 60)]
   b) if the asterion is not easily identified or if there are concerns about the reliability of the asterion as a landmark for the junction of the transverse and sigmoid sinuses,[71] place the burr hole directly over the mastoid emissary vein which drains superolaterally into the sigmoid sinus
3. craniotomy: top of bone opening as close as possible to transverse sinus. The position of the transverse sinus can be approximated by a line drawn from the posterior base of the zygomatic process to the inion, or roughly ≈ 2 finger-breadths above the upper end of the mastoid notch. Lateral limit of bone opening is sigmoid sinus. A triangular bony opening with a leg along each sinus works well. Craniectomy diameter needs to be only ≈ 3 cm. Apply bone wax liberally (blocks off any possible opening into the mastoid air cells)
4. dural opening: either a curvilinear with each end at a sinus and the convexity *away* from the junction (Jannetta) or an inverted "T" (with one incision towards each sinus and the third towards junction of sinuses)
5. minimal or no retraction of cerebellum is usually required
6. allow CSF to drain before proceeding: this may require gentle advancement of a cottonoid in the CPA. A lumbar drain should be placed if CSF cannot be drained
7. follow the junction of tentorium with temporal bone deep. Place a retractor that both medially displaces the cerebellum *and* slightly "lifts" the cerebellum towards the surgeon (medial displacement alone is not as effective)
8. petrosal vein: coagulate and divide the petrosal vein complex (usually 2–3 veins connecting to the tentorial dura). If the vein is torn, the dural side is tamponaded (sometimes up to 30 minutes is needed) while the free end is coagulated
9. V is deeper than the VII/VIII complex, which should not even be seen with this approach. If VII/VIII are seen, move the retractor superiorly as even gentle traction may cause hearing loss (▶ Fig. 1.9). There is often a hillock of bone just posterior to Meckel's cave obscuring the site where the fifth nerve enters the cave

Decompression of nerve

1. arachnoid overlying the fifth nerve is sharply divided (caution re Cranial Nerve IV which follows the tentorial opening in the arachnoid rostral to the fifth nerve). Intra-op changes in BAER are often attributed to retraction of arachnoid that is tethered to the VII/VIII complex
2. the fifth nerve may be markedly atrophic if previous PTRs have been done
3. identify the smaller motor root (portio minor) of the fifth nerve
4. arteries and/or veins compressing V should be dissected off the nerve. NB: vessels located proximally are the most likely offenders, however, the dorsal root entry zone (which is the sensitive part of the nerve) may be variable in location and peripheral vessels may be culpable. The nerve should be inspected and freed of vessels from its origin at the brainstem all the way to its entrance into Meckel's cave.[69] Veins may be coagulated and then should be divided (to prevent recanalization)
5. the most common cause of compression is the superior cerebellar artery (SCA)
6. check the nerve at the junction with brainstem for any residual compression prior to the next step
7. insulating material is interposed between nerve and vessel to prevent re-compression. Options include:
   a) e.g. Ivalon®, (polyvinyl formyl alcohol) sponge (Ivalon Surgical Products, 1040 OCL Parkway, Eudora, KS, 66025, U.S.A. distributed by Fabco in the U.S.A. (860) 536–8499, toll free: (888) 813–8214, http://fabco.net/catalog/ivalon-ophthalmic/) cut in a saddle shape. Note: if an Ivalon block is used instead of pre-packaged sterile pads, it must be rinsed thoroughly to remove formalin, then autoclaved. Ivalon should be hydrated in NS for 10 minutes prior to cutting it
   b) shredded Teflon felt; see merits of Ivalon® vs. Teflon or muscle (p. 1536)
8. Wilson recommends performing a partial sensory rhizotomy of the inferior one-half to two-thirds of the portio major for the following: cases where no vascular contact with the nerve or no deformity of the nerve is identified, in most cases of patients undergoing a repeat MVD, or for cases with duration of symptoms > 8–9 yrs as this latter group tends to have a lower success rate with MVD alone[72]
9. if the procedure is for a failed MVD and it is desired to partially divide the nerve, the nerve is organized somatotopically with V1 fibers superiorly, and V3 inferiorly. If the goal is total elimination of pain pathways and there is concern about pain conduction through ancillary pathways, consider also dividing the motor root (portio minor)

Closure

1. bone wax should be applied liberally to the exposed lateral bone edges (to paraphrase Dr. Jannetta[69] and Mr. Miyagi,[73] "Wax in, wax out.")
2. irrigate gently with *warm* saline (avoid "jet" irrigation which can damage the VIII nerve)
3. intra-op BAER decline may occur on dural closure and should prompt re-opening of the dura and checking for tension on the VIII nerve from a vessel or Telfa
4. perform several Valsalva maneuvers to ensure watertight closure of dura
5. the bone defect should be covered e.g. with burr hole cover to reduce chance of pain associated with uncovered craniectomy
6. after fascial closure, Valsalva maneuver is performed again to ensure watertight closure
7. use 4–0 running locked nylon to approximate skin in watertight fashion (avoid excessive tension)

Post-op care following MVD

Include in post-op orders

1. admit to ICU
2. arterial-line for continuous BP monitoring
3. analgesics (e.g. codeine 30–60 mg IM q 3 hrs)
4. anti-emetics (e.g. ondansetron 4 mg IV q 6 hrs)
5. medication to aggressively treat HTN (viz. SBP > 160 mm Hg)

Post-op H/A, nausea and pain

Patients routinely have H/A and nausea for 2–3 days (there tends to be less intracranial air and less "pneumoencephalogram sickness" if the park-bench position is used instead of the sitting position). However, *severe* H/A should prompt a STAT CT to R/O bleeding. If the CT is negative, severe H/A may be due to transient elevation of CSF pressure that occurs in some, and which usually responds to 1, or at most 2, LPs to halve the pressure. Aseptic meningitis usually responds to steroids. Some patients have continued but lessened tic douloureux pain for several days post-op, this usually subsides.[69]

Complications

The short list:

1. cerebellar injury
2. hearing loss
3. CSF leak

The long list:

1. mortality: 0.22–2% in experienced hands (> 900 procedures)[74,75]
2. meningitis
   a) aseptic meningitis (AKA hemogenic meningitis): H/A, meningismus, mild fever, culture negative CSF, pleocytosis. Incidence: ≈ 2% (up to 20% has been reported). Usually occurs 3–7 days post-op. Responds to LP + steroids
   b) bacterial meningitis: 0.9%
3. major neurologic morbidity: 1–10% (higher rates with less experienced surgeons), including:
   a) deafness: 1%
   b) vestibular nerve dysfunction
   c) facial nerve dysfunction
4. mild facial sensory loss: 25%
5. cranial nerve palsies[76]:
   a) fourth nerve (diplopia): 4.3% (only ≈ 0.1% are permanent)
   b) facial nerve: 1.6% (most are transient)
   c) eighth nerve (hearing loss): 3%
6. postoperative hemorrhage[77]: subdural, intracerebral (1%[24]), subarachnoid
7. seizures: including status epilepticus[77]
8. infarction[77]: including posterior cerebral artery distribution, brain stem
9. CSF leak: resolves with lumbar drainage in most cases
10. pneumonia: 0.6%

Outcome

1. success rate: 75–80% (rates may be lower in patients having prior destructive procedure); good but not total relief in an additional ≈ 10%
2. recurrence rate in large series is difficult to ascertain from literature; in a series of 40 patients followed 8.5 yrs mean[75]:
   a) major recurrence (recurrent tic not controlled by medications) rate: 31%
   b) minor recurrence (mild or controlled by medications) rate: 17%
   c) using Kaplan-Meier curve, expect 70% to be either pain free or have minor recurrence by 8.5 years (or ≈ 80% at 5 years)
   the risk for a *major* recurrence after MVD is 3.5% annually
   the risk for a *minor* recurrence after MVD is 1.5% annually
   d) major recurrence rate is lower for patients having major arterial cross-compression of the nerve discovered at the time of surgery (patients with venous compression had much higher rate)
   e) this study found no correlation between previous destructive surgery and major recurrence rate (in 11 patients)

Some feel that the longer one waits before performing a MVD, the lower the success rate.

28.3.4 Supraorbital and supratrochlear neuralgia

Anatomy

The supraorbital and supratrochlear nerves arise from the frontal nerve and are 2 of the 5 branches of V1 (ophthalmic division of the trigeminal nerve). The supraorbital nerve is the largest branch. It exits the orbit through the supraorbital notch or foramen, usually within the medial third of the orbital roof (mean distance from exit to medial angle of orbit: 20 mm (range: 5–47)[78]). The supratrochlear nerve exits the orbit without a foramen or notch 3–38 mm medial to the supraorbital nerve (mean: 15.3 mm)[78]), the most medial branch varies from 8–30 mm lateral to the patient's midline.[78]

Supraorbital neuralgia characteristics

Trigeminal neuralgia (TGN) may present with pain in the distribution of the supraorbital nerve, however, the supraorbital nerve may be involved in supraorbital neuralgia (SON), a distinct syndrome with different clinical characteristics. SON is a rare condition slightly more common in women, with onset typically 40–50 years of age.[79] Characteristics[80]: 1) unilateral pain in the distribution of the supraorbital nerve (▶ Fig. 93.2), 2) tenderness in the region of the supraorbital notch or along the distribution of the nerve, and 3) temporary relief with nerve block.

The pain is usually chronic-continuous or remitting-intermittent.[79]

SON may be:

1. primary (no identifiable etiology): these cases lack any sensory loss
2. secondary (e.g. due to trauma to the area, or resulting from chronic pressure such as with wearing swim goggles): more common than primary SON. Most cases remit within one year[79] with elimination of the offending pressure

Supratrochlear neuralgia

Cases of pain isolated to the supratrochlear nerve appear to exist. Supratrochlear neuralgia (STN) may be differentiated from SON by restriction of pain in the more medial forehead, and with relief on blockade of the supratrochlear nerve alone.

Differential diagnosis

1. migraine: suggested by nausea, vomiting and photophobia
2. associated autonomic activity is rare with SON, and should prompt consideration of cluster H/A (p. 175) or SUNCT (p. 478)
3. TGN: typical TGN features *lacking* in SON include characteristic triggers and pain consisting exclusively of paroxysmal/ultra-brief electric shock-like pain
4. hemicrania continua: continuous unilateral pain that tends to be located more posteriorly and is absolutely responsive to indomethacin[80]
5. trochleitis: inflammation of the trochlea/superior-oblique muscle complex, may mimic supratrochlear neuralgia with pain of the medial upper orbit extending a short distance to the forehead.[81] The pain is typically exacerbated by supraduction of the eye and to palpation of the trochlea, and is relieved with injection of local anesthetic or, by the usually definitive treatment of infiltration of corticosteroids close to the trochlea. Diplopia is rare and minimal
6. nummular (coin-like) H/A[82]: round or oval 2–6 cm diameter area of pressure-like continuous head pain without underlying structural abnormality. In 13 patients, 9 (70%) the area was located at the parieto-occipital junction. 9 (70%) demonstrated hypoesthesia and touch provoked paresthesias in the affected area

Treatment

Gabapentin (800–2400 mg/d) or pregabalin (150 mg/d) is helpful for some.[83]

Topical capsaicin (p. 482) applied to the symptomatic area may help.

Refractory cases may respond to rhizotomy with alcohol (providing an average of 8.5 months relief[84]) or with radiofrequency ablation.

Persistent cases may require exploration and decompression of the nerve by lysing bands overlying the supraorbital notch,[85] or, ultimately, to neurectomy (p. 483) which provides an average of 33.2 months relief.[86]

28.3.5 Glossopharyngeal neuralgia

Epidemiology

Incidence: 1 case for every 70 of trigeminal neuralgia.[87 (p 3604–5)]

Clinical

Severe, lancinating pain in the distribution of the glossopharyngeal and vagus nerves (throat & base of tongue most commonly involved, radiates to ear (otalgia), occasionally to neck), occasionally with salivation and coughing. Rarely: hypotension,[88] syncope,[89] cardiac arrest and convulsions may accompany. May be triggered by swallowing, talking, chewing. Trigger zones are rare.

Treatment

Pain may be reduced by cocainization of tonsillar pillars and fossa. Usually, the persistence and severity of pain requires surgical intervention. One may either perform microvascular decompression, or nerve division via extra- or intra-cranial approach (latter may be required for permanent relief).

Intracranial approach: Section of preganglionic glossopharyngeal nerve (IX) and upper one–third or two fibers (whichever is larger) of vagus (X). IX is readily identified at its dural exit zone where it is separated from X by a dural septum. The upper third of X is usually composed of a single rootlet, or less commonly, multiple small rootlets. Initial post-op dysphagia usually resolves. Cardiovascular complications following vagal section have been reported, warrants close monitoring × 24 hrs.

28.3.6 Geniculate neuralgia

General information

Geniculate neuralgia (GeN) AKA Hunt's neuralgia AKA nervus intermedius neuralgia: a very rare neuralgia affecting the nervus intermedius (the somatic sensory branch of the facial nerve primarily innervating mechanoreceptors of the hair follicles on the inner surface of the pinna and deep mechanoreceptors of nasal and buccal cavities and chemoreceptors in the taste buds on the anterior 2/3 of the tongue).

Symptoms: unilateral paroxysmal otalgia (lancinating pain experienced deep within the ear, often described as an "ice pick in the ear") radiating to the auricle, with occasional burning sensations around the ipsilateral eye and cheek, and prosopalgia (pain referred to deep facial structures, including orbit, posterior nasal and palatal regions). During pain attacks, some patients have: salivation, bitter taste, tinnitus, or vertigo.

28

GeN occasionally has cutaneous trigger points in the anterior EAC and tragus, and pain may also be triggered by cold, noise, or swallowing.

Work-up includes neuro-otologic evaluation with audiometry and ENG. Some patients may require imaging (MRI or high-resolution CT) and angio (to R/O aneurysm).

Variants

Tic convulsif (AKA convulsive tic): GeN combined with hemifacial spasm, usually due to neurovascular compression of both the sensory and motor roots of the facial nerve,[17] most often by AICA. First described by Cushing in 1920.

GeN may be associated with herpetic infections of the geniculate ganglion (AKA herpetic ganglionitis, AKA Ramsay Hunt syndrome (RHS)) in which case herpetic lesions appear on pinna, in EAC, and possibly on TM. May include facial palsy, decreased auditory acuity, tinnitus or vertigo. Unlike idiopathic GeN, RHS is more chronic and less paroxysmal, tends to remit with time, and is usually refractory to carbamazepine. Idiopathic GeN tends to be more painful than RHS, and does not remit spontaneously.

Treatment

1. medical therapy
   a) mild cases may respond to carbamazepine, sometimes in combination with phenytoin
   b) may respond to valproate (Depakote®) 250 mg PO BID
   c) topical antibiotics for secondary infections of herpetic lesions
   d) local anesthetic to EAC
2. surgery: for severe cases where medical treatment fails or is not tolerated
   a) microvascular decompression together with division of the nervus intermedius (nerve of Wrisberg)[90]). To find the nerve, a micro nerve hook is hooked around the VII nerve, the hook is rotated 90°, and the nerve is fished out from in front of VII. Operating under local anesthesia allows verification by stimulating nerve
   b) geniculate ganglion section[91]

28.4 Postherpetic neuralgia

28.4.1 General information

Herpes zoster (HZ) (Greek: zoster – girdle) (shingles in lay terms): painful vesicular cutaneous eruptions caused by the herpes varicella zoster virus (VZV) (the etiologic agent of chickenpox, a herpesvirus that is distinct from herpes simplex virus). It occurs in a dermatomal distribution over one side of the thorax in ≈ 65% of cases (rarely, infections occur without vesicles, called zoster sine herpete). In 20% of cases it involves the trigeminal nerve (with a predilection for the ophthalmic division, called herpes zoster ophthalmicus). Pain usually resolves after 2–4 weeks. When the pain persists > 1 month after the vesicular eruption has healed, this pain syndrome is known as postherpetic neuralgia (PHN). PHN can follow a herpes varicella infection in any site and is difficult to treat by any means (medical or surgical). It can occasionally be seen in a limb, and follows a dermatomal distribution (*not* a peripheral nerve distribution). PHN may remit spontaneously, but if it hasn't done so by 6 mos this is unlikely.

28.4.2 Epidemiology

Incidence of herpes zoster is ≈ 125/100,000/year in the general population, or about 850,000 cases per year in the U.S.[92] Both sexes are equally affected. There is no seasonal variance. HZ is also more common in those with reduced immunity and in those with a coexistent malignancy (especially lympho-proliferative).[93,94] PHN occurs in ≈ 10% of cases of HZ.[92] Both HZ and PHN are more common in older patients (PHN is rare in age < 40 yrs, and usually occurs in age > 60) and in those with diabetes mellitus. PHN is more likely after ophthalmic HZ than after spinal segmental involvement.

28.4.3 Etiology

It is postulated that the VZV lies dormant in the sensory ganglia (dorsal root ganglia of the spine, trigeminal (semilunar) ganglion for facial involvement) until such time that the patient's immune system is weakened and then the virus erupts. Inflammatory changes within the nerve are present early and are later replaced by fibrosis.

28

28.4.4 Clinical

PHN is usually described as a constant burning and aching. There may be superimposed shocks or jabs. It rarely produces throbbing or cramping pain. Pain may be spontaneous, or may be triggered by light cutaneous stimulation (allodynia) (e.g. by clothing), and may be relieved by constant pressure. The pain is present to some degree at all times with no pain-free intervals. Scars and pigmentary changes from the acute vesicular eruption are usually visible. It is not known if PHN can follow zoster sine herpete. The involved area may demonstrate hypesthesia, hypalgesia, paresthesias and dysesthesias.

28.4.5 Medical treatment

For herpes zoster

Varicella vaccination of older individuals can increase immunity to herpes zoster, but it will be several years before it can be determined if this will reduce PHN.[92]

Treatment for the pain of the *acute* attack of herpes zoster may be accomplished with epidural or paravertebral somatic (intercostal) nerve block.[95 (p 4018)]

Oral antiherpetic drugs: Also effective (they shorten the duration of pain) and also reduce the incidence of PHN. They may cause thrombotic thrombocytopenic purpura/hemolytic uremic syndrome (TTP/HUS) when used in severely immunocompromised patients at high doses. These drugs include:

Acyclovir (Zovirax®): poorly absorbed from the GI tract (15–30% bioavailability). ℞ 800 mg PO q 4 hrs 5 times/d × 7 d.

Valacyclovir (Valtrex®)[96] is a prodrug of acyclovir and is more completely absorbed and should be equally as effective with fewer daily doses. ℞ 1,000 mg PO TID starting within 72 hrs of onset of the rash × 7 days.

Famciclovir (Famvir®): ℞ 500 mg PO TID × 7 d.

For post-herpetic neuralgia

General information

Most drugs useful for trigeminal neuralgia (p. 481) are less effective for PHN. Some treatment alternatives for PHN are summarized in ▶ Table 28.5. Details of some drugs follows. It is suggested to initiate therapy with lidocaine skin patches (p. 496) since this modality has the lowest potential for serious side effects.[92]

Table 28.5 Medical treatments for PHN[a]

Treatment	Efficacy
PHN treatments that appear effective	
tricyclic antidepressants	widely used for PHN (see text)
lidocaine patch (Lidoderm®)[97]	effective, few side effects (p. 496)
intrathecal steroids + lidocaine (see text)	appears very effective, larger studies & long-term follow-up needed
Gabapentin	proven efficacy (see text)
oxycodone CR 10 mg PO BID[4]	proven efficacy
Treatments of questionable efficacy	
SSRIs[b]	may be effective
SNRIs	may be effective
Tramadol	may be effective
topical capsaicin	controversial (see text)
Iontophoresis	insufficient evidence
nonsteroidal creams	questionable
aspirin suspended in acetone, ether or chloroform	questionable
EMLA cream	questionable
Treatments that are not useful	
dextromethorphan, benzodiazepines, acyclovir, acupuncture	no benefit[98]
ketamine (NMDA receptor antagonist)	may be beneficial, but hepatotoxic
Preventative treatment	
oral antiherpetic drugs given during HZ infection	shortens length of HZ, may reduce incidence of PHN
varicella vaccination of older patients	trials of this strategy are in progress[92]

[a]modified with permission from Rubin M, Relief for postherpetic neuralgia, **Neurology Alert**, 6: 33–4, 2001
[b]abbreviations: oxycodone CR = controlled release (Oxycontin®); HZ = herpes zoster; PHN = postherpetic neuralgia; SNRIs = serotonin-norepinephrine reuptake inhibitor; SSRIs = selective serotonin reuptake inhibitors (e. g. Prosac®),

Antiepileptic drugs

Drug info: Gabapentin (Neurontin®)

FDA approved only for partial seizures and postherpetic neuralgia (PHN).

Side effects : dizziness and somnolence (usually during titration, often diminish with time). Ataxia, fatigue, peripheral edema, confusion and depression may occur.

Rx For PHN, start with 300 mg on Day 1, 300 mg BID on Day 2, and 300 mg TID on Day 3. Dose may be titrated up to 1800 mg/d divided TID. To limit daytime drowsiness, patients may need to start with 100 mg at hs and increase slowly over 3–8. Although doses up to 3600 mg/day (the antiseizure dose) were studied[99] there was no significant benefit for PHN over 1800 mg/d. Lower doses are required for renal insufficiency. **Supplied:** 100, 300 & 400 mg capsules; 600 & 800 mg scored tabs. 50 mg/ml suspension.

Drug info: Oxcarbazepine (Trileptal®)

℞ 150 mg PO BID.

Drug info: Zonisamide (Zonegran®)

℞ Initiate therapy with 100 mg PO q PM × 2 wks, then increase dose by 100 mg/d q 2 wks up to 400 mg/d. Bioavailability is not affected by food. Steady state is achieved within 14 days of dosage changes. **Supplied :** 100 mg capsules.

Tricyclic antidepressants (TCA)

Drug info: Amitriptyline (Elavil®)

28

Helpful in ≈ 66% of patients at a mean dose of 75 mg/d even without antidepres-sant effect.[5] **Side effects:** see Amitriptyline, side effects (p. 545), minimized by starting low and slowly incrementing dose.

℞ Start with 12.5–25 mg PO q hs, and increase by the same amount q 2–5 days to a maximum of 150 mg/d.

Drug info: Nortriptyline (Pamelor®)

Fewer side effects than amitriptyline.

℞ Start with 10–20 mg PO q hs, and increase gradually.

Topical treatment

Drug info: Capsaicin (Zostrix®)

A vanillyl alkaloid derived from hot peppers, available without prescription for topical treatment of the pain of herpes zoster and diabetic neuropathy. Beneficial in some patients with either of these conditions (response rate at 8 weeks was 90% for PHN, 71% for diabetic neuropathy, vs. 50% with placebo in either group), although the high placebo response rate is disturbing and many authorities are skeptical.[100] Expensive. **Side effects:** include burning and erythema at the application site (usually subsides by 2–4 weeks).

℞ Manufacturer recommends massaging the medication into the affected area of the skin TID-QID (apply a very thin coat). Some authorities recommend q 2 hr application. Avoid contact with eyes or damaged skin. Supplied as Zostrix® (0.25% capsaicin) or Zostrix-HP® (0.75%).

Drug info: Lidocaine patch 5% (Lidoderm®)

Often better tolerated by elderly patients than TCAs (due to pre-existing cognitive impairments, cardiac disease, or systemic illness).

℞ Apply up to 3 patches of 5% lidocaine (to cover a maximum of 420 cm^2) to intact skin q 12 hrs to cover as much of the area of greatest pain as possible.[97]

Intrathecal steroids

Over 90% of patients receiving intrathecal methylprednisolone (60 mg) + 3% lidocaine (3 ml) given once per week for up to 4 weeks, reported good to excellent pain relief for up to 2 years.[101] This technique was not studied for use in PHN involving the trigeminal nerve. Further clinical trials are needed to verify the efficacy and safety[92] (potential long-term side effects include adhesive arachnoiditis).

Surgical treatment

There is no operation that is uniformly successful in treating PHN. Numerous operations have been shown to work occasionally. Procedures that have been tried include:

1. nerve blocks: once PHN is established, nerve blocks provide only temporary relief[102]
2. cordotomy: although percutaneous cordotomy (p. 1542) may work when the level of PHN is at least 3–4 segments below the cordotomy, this procedure is not recommended for pain of benign etiology because of possible complications and the high likelihood of pain recurrence
3. rhizotomy: including retrogasserian for facial involvement
4. neurectomies
5. sympathectomy
6. DREZ (p. 1550) [103]: often offers good early relief, but recurrence rate is high.
7. acupuncture[104]
8. TENS
9. spinal cord stimulation (p. 1547)
10. undermining the skin
11. motor cortex stimulation: for *facial* PHN

28

28.5 Complex regional pain syndrome (CRPS)

28.5.1 General information

The terminology is confusing. Formerly also called causalgia (reflex sympathetic dystrophy). The term causalgia (Greek: kausis – burning, algos – pain) was introduced by Weir Mitchell in 1864. It was used to describe a rare syndrome that followed a minority of *partial* peripheral nerve injuries in the American civil war. *Triad*: burning pain, autonomic dysfunction and trophic changes.

CRPS Type II (AKA major causalgia) follows nerve injury (originally described after high velocity missile injuries). CRPS Type I (AKA reflex sympathetic dystrophy or causalgia minor) denoted less severe forms, and has been described after non-penetrating trauma.[105] Shoulder-hand syndrome and Sudeck's atrophy are other variant designations. In 1916, the autonomic nervous system was implicated by René Leriche, and the term reflex sympathetic dystrophy (RSD) later came into use[106] (but RSD may be distinct from causalgia[107]).

Post-op CRPS has been described following carpal tunnel surgery as well as surgery on the lumbar[108] and cervical spine.

At best, CRPS must be regarded as a symptom complex, and not as a discrete syndrome nor medical entity (for a cogent editorial on the subject, see the essay by Ochoa[109]). Patients exhibiting CRPS phenomenology are not a homogeneous group, and include[110]:

1. actual CRPS (for these, Mailis proposes the term "physiogenic RSD"): a complex set of neuropathic phenomena that may occur with or without nerve injury
2. medical conditions distinct from CRPS but with signs and symptoms that mimic CRPS: vascular, inflammatory, neurologic…
3. the product of mere immobilization: as in severe pain avoidance behavior, or at times psychiatric disorders
4. part of a factitious disorder with either a psychological basis (e.g. Munchausen's syndrome) or for secondary gain (financial, drug seeking…) i.e. malingering

28.5.2 Pathogenesis

Early theories invoked ephaptic transmission between sympathetics and afferent pain fibers. This theory is rarely cited currently. Another more recent postulate involves nor-epinephrine released at sympathetic terminals together with hypersensitivity secondary to denervation or sprouting. Many modern hypotheses do not even embrace involvement of the autonomic nervous system in all cases.[106,107,110]

Thus, many of the alterations seen in CRPS may simply be epiphenomena rather than part of the etiopathogenetic mechanism.

28.5.3 Clinical

CRPS may be described as a phenomenology, i.e. a variable complex of signs and symptoms due to multiple etiologies included in this nonhomogeneous group.[110] No diagnostic criteria for the condition have been established, and various investigators select different factors to include or exclude patients from their studies.

28.5.4 Symptoms

Pain: affecting a limb, usually burning, and prominent in the hand or foot. Onset in the majority is within 24 hrs of injury (unless injury causes anesthesia, then hrs or days may intervene); however, CRPS may take days to weeks to develop. Median, ulnar and sciatic nerves are the most commonly cited involved nerves. However, it is not always possible to identify a specific nerve that has been injured. Almost any sensory stimulus worsens the pain (allodynia is pain induced by a nonnoxious stimulus).

28.5.5 Signs

The physical exam is often difficult due to pain.

Vascular changes: either vasodilator (warm and pink) or vasoconstrictor (cold, mottled blue). Trophic changes (may be partly or wholly due to immobility): dry/scaly skin, stiff joints, tapering fingers, ridged uncut nails, either long/course hair or loss of hair, sweating alterations (varies from anhidrosis to hyperhidrosis).

28.5.6 Diagnostic aids

In the absence of an agreed upon etiology or pathophysiology, there can be no basis for specific tests, and the lack of a "gold-standard" diagnostic criteria makes it impossible to verify the authenticity of any diagnostic marker. Numerous tests have been presented as aids to the diagnosis of CRPS, and essentially all have eventually been refuted. Candidates have included:

1. thermography: discredited in clinical practice
2. three-phase bone scan: typical CRPS changes also occur after sympathectomy,[111] which has traditionally been considered curative of CRPS
3. osteoporosis on x-ray,[112] particularly periarticular demineralization: nonspecific
4. response to sympathetic block (once thought to be the sine qua non for causalgia major and minor, the response sought was relief (complete or significant) with sympathetic block of appropriate trunk (stellate for UE, lumbar for LE)): has failed to hold up once stringent placebo-controlled trials were executed
5. various autonomic tests[113]: resting sweat output, resting skin temperature, quantitative sudomotor axon reflex test

28.5.7 Treatment

In the absence of a delineated pathophysiology, treatment is judged purely by subjective impression of improvement. CRPS treatment studies have had an unusually high placebo response rate.[114] Medical therapy is usually ineffective. Proposed treatments include:

1. tricyclic antidepressants
2. 18–25% have satisfactory long-lasting relief after a series of sympathetic blocks, see Stellate ganglion block (p. 1521) and Lumbar sympathetic block (p. 1521), although one report found no long-lasting benefit in any of 30 patients[115]
3. intravenous regional sympathetic block, particularly for UE CRPS: agents used include *guanethedine*[116] 20 mg, reserpine, bretylium…, injected IV with arterial tourniquet (sphygmomanometer cuff) inflated for 10 min. If no relief, repeat in 3–4 wks. No better than placebo in several trials[117, 118]
4. surgical sympathectomy (p. 1537): some purport that this relieves pain in > 90% of patients (with a few retaining some tenderness or hyperpathia). Others opine that there is no rational reason to consider sympathectomy since sympathetic blocks have been shown to be no more effective than placebo[106]
5. spinal cord stimulation: some success has been reported

References

[1] Backonja MM. Defining neuropathic pain. Anesth Analg. 2003; 97:785–790

[2] Merskey H, Bogduk N. Classification of Chronic Pain: Descriptions of Chronic Pain Syndromes and Definitions of Pain Terms. 2nd ed. Seattle, WA: IASP Press; 1994

[3] Dworkin RH, Backonja M, Rowbotham MC, Allen RR, Argoff CR, Bennett GJ, Bushnell MC, Farrar JT, Galer BS, Haythornthwaite JA, Hewitt DJ, Loeser JD, Max MB, Saltarelli M, Schmader KE, Stein C, Thompson D, Turk DC, Wallace MS, Watkins LR, Weinstein SM. Advances in neuropathic pain: diagnosis, mechanisms, and treatment recommendations. Arch Neurol. 2003; 60:1524–1534

[4] Watson CPN, Babul N. Efficacy of oxycodone in neuropathic pain: a randomized trial in postherpetic neuralgia. Neurology. 1998; 50:1837–1841

[5] Watson CP, Evans RJ, Reed K, Merserkey H, et al. Amitriptyline versus Placebo in Postherpetic Neuralgia. Neurology. 1982; 32:671–673

[6] Max MB, Lynch SA, Muir J, Shoaf SE, et al. Effects of Desipramine, Amitriptyline, and Fluoxetine on Pain in Diabetic Neuropathy. N Engl J Med. 1992; 326:1250–1256

[7] Bennett MI, Simpson KH. Gabapentin in the treatment of neuropathic pain. Palliat Med. 2004; 18:5–11

[8] Dierking G, Duedahl TH, Rasmussen ML, Fomsgaard JS, Moiniche S, Romsing J, Dahl JB. Effects of gabapentin on postoperative morphine consumption and pain after abdominal hysterectomy: a randomized, double-blind trial. Acta Anaesthesiol Scand. 2004; 48:322–327

[9] Mathew NT, Rapoport A, Saper J, Magnus L, Klapper J, Ramadan N, Stacey B, Tepper S. Efficacy of gabapentin in migraine prophylaxis. Headache. 2001; 41:119–128

[10] Gabapentin (Neurontin®) for chronic pain. Med Letter. 2004; 46:29–31

[11] Keller JT, van Loveren H. Pathophysiology of the Pain of Trigeminal Neuralgia and Atypical Facial Pain: A Neuroanatomical Perspective. Clin Neurosurg. 1985; 32:275–293

[12] Wilkins RH, Rengachary SS. Neurosurgery. New York 1985

[13] Burchiel KJ. A new classification for facial pain. Neurosurgery. 2003; 91:1164–1167

[14] Pareja JA, Sjaastad O. SUNCT syndrome. A clinical review. Headache. 1997; 37:195–195

[15] Sjaastad O, Pareja JA, Zukerman E, Jansen J, Kruszewski P. Trigeminal neuralgia. Clinical manifestations of first division involvement. Headache. 1997; 37:346–357

[16] Pareja JA, Baron M, Gili P, Yanguela J, Caminero AB, Dobato JL, Barriga FJ, Vela L, Sanchez-del-Rio M. Objective assessment of autonomic signs during triggered first division trigeminal neuralgia. Cephalalgia. 2002; 22:251–255

[17] Yeh HS, Tew JM. Tic Convulsif, the Combination of Geniculate Neuralgia and Hemifacial Spasm Relieved by Vascular Decompression. Neurology. 1984; 34:682–683

[18] Rupa V, Saunders RL, Weider DJ. Geniculate Neuralgia: The Surgical Management of Primary Otalgia. J Neurosurg. 1991; 75:505–511

[19] Young RF. Geniculate Neuralgia. J Neurosurg. 1992; 76

[20] Wepsic JG. Tic Douloureaux: Etiology, Refined Treatment. N Engl J Med. 1973; 288:680–681

[21] Sweet WH. The Treatment of Trigeminal Neuralgia (Tic Douloureux). N Engl J Med. 1986; 315:174–177

[22] Brisman R. Bilateral Trigeminal Neuralgia. J Neurosurg. 1987; 67:44–48

[23] van Loveren H, Tew JM, Keller JT, et al. A 10-Year Experience in the Treatment of Trigeminal Neuralgia: Comparison of Percutaneous Stereotaxic Rhizotomy and Posterior Fossa Exploration. J Neurosurg. 1982; 57:757–764

[24] Taha JM, Tew JM. Comparison of Surgical Treatments for Trigeminal Neuralgia: Reevaluation of Radiofrequency Rhizotomy. Neurosurgery. 1996; 38:865–871

[25] Hardy DG, Rhoton AL. Microsurgical Relationships of the Superior Cerebellar Artery and the Trigeminal Nerve. J Neurosurg. 1978; 49:669–678

[26] Morita A, Fukushima T, Miyazaki S, et al. Tic Douloureux Caused by Primitive Trigeminal Artery or its Variant. J Neurosurg. 1989; 70:415–419

[27] Apfelbaum RI, Carter LP, Spetzler RF, Hamilton MG. In: Trigeminal Neuralgia: Vascular Decompression. Neurovascular Surgery. New York: McGraw-Hill; 1995:1107–1117

[28] Bullitt E, Tew JM, Boyd J. Intracranial Tumors in Patients with Facial Pain. J Neurosurg. 1986; 64:865–871

[29] Fusco BM, Alessandri M. Analgesic Effect of Capsaicin in Idiopathic Trigeminal Neuralgia. Anesth Analg. 1992; 74:375–377

[30] Poppen JL. An Atlas of Neurosurgical Techniques. Philadelphia: W. B. Saunders; 1960

[31] Sweet WH, Wepsic JG. Controlled Thermocoagulation of Trigeminal Ganglion and Rootlets for Differential Destruction of Pain Fibers. Part I. Trigeminal Neuralgia. J Neurosurg. 1974; 40:143–156

[32] Hakanson S. Trigeminal Neuralgia Treated by the Injection of Glycerol into the Trigeminal Cistern. Neurosurgery. 1981; 9:638–646

[33] Sweet WH, Poletti CE, Macon JB. Treatment of Trigeminal Neuralgia and Other Facial Pains by the Retrogasserian Injection of Glycerol. Neurosurgery. 1981; 9:647–653

[34] Lunsford LD, Apfelbaum RI. Choice of Surgical Therapeutic Modalities for Treatment of Trigeminal Neuralgia. Clin Neurosurg. 1985; 32:319–333

[35] Young RF. Glycerol Rhizolysis for Treatment of Trigeminal Neuralgia. J Neurosurg. 1988; 69:39–45

[36] Mullan S, Lichtor T. Percutaneous Microcompression of the Trigeminal Ganglion for Trigeminal Neuralgia. J Neurosurg. 1983; 59:1007–1012

[37] Belber CJ, Rak RA. Balloon Compression Rhizolysis in the Surgical Management of Trigeminal Neuralgia. Neurosurgery. 1987; 20:908–913

[38] Lichtor T, Mullan JF. A 10-Year Follow-Up Review of Percutaneous Microcompression of the Trigeminal Ganglion. J Neurosurg. 1990; 72:49–54

[39] Taarnhoj P. Decompression of the Posterior Trigeminal Root in Trigeminal Neuralgia. J Neurosurg. 1982; 57:14–17

[40] Henderson JM, Lad SP. Motor cortex stimulation and neuropathic facial pain. Neurosurg Focus. 2006; 21

[41] van Loveren H, Greenberg MS. Tampa 2009

[42] Murali R, Rovit RL. Are peripheral neurectomies of value in the treatment of trigeminal neuralgia? An analysis of new cases and cases involving previous radiofrequency Gasserian thermocoagulation. J Neurosurg. 1996; 85:435–437

[43] Wilkins RH, Burchiel KJ. In: Trigeminal neuralgia: Historical overview, with emphasis on surgical treatment. Surgical Management of Pain. New York: Thieme Medical Publishers, Inc.; 2002:288–301

[44] Tew JM, van Loveren H, Schmidek HH, Sweet WH. In: Percutaneous Rhizotomy in the Treatment of Intractable Facial Pain (Trigeminal, Glossopharyngeal, and Vagal Nerves). Operative Neurosurgical Techniques. 2nd ed. Philadelphia: W B Saunders; 1988:1111–1123

[45] Brown JA, Preul MC. Percutaneous Trigeminal Ganglion Compression for Trigeminal Neuralgia. Experience in 22 Cases and Review of the Literature. J Neurosurg. 1989; 70:900–904

[46] Menzel J, Piotrowski W, Penzholz H. Long-Term Results of Gasserian Ganglion Electrocoagulation. J Neurosurg. 1975; 42:140–143

[47] Wepsic JG. Complications of Percutaneous Surgery for Pain. Clin Neurosurg. 1976; 23:454–464

[48] Tew JM, Keller JT. The Treatment of Trigeminal Neuralgia by Percutaneous Radiofrequency Technique. Clin Neurosurg. 1977; 24:557–578

[49] Luksic I, Sestan-Crnek S, Virag M, Macan D. Trigeminal trophic syndrome of all three nerve branches: an underrecognized complication after brain surgery. J Neurosurg. 2008; 108:170–173
[50] Setyadi HG, Cohen PR, Schulze KE, Mason SH, Martinelli PT, Alford EL, Taffet GE, Nelson BR. Trigeminal trophic syndrome. South Med J. 2007; 100:43–48
[51] Kaplan M, Erol FS, Ozveren MF, Topsakal C, Sam B, Tekdemir I. Review of complications due to foramen ovale puncture. J Clin Neurosci. 2007; 14:563–568
[52] Sekhar L, Heros RC, Kerber CW. Carotid-Cavernous Fistula Following Percutaneous Retrogasserian Procedures. J Neurosurg. 1979; 51:700–706
[53] Kuether TA, O'Neill OR, Nesbit GM, Barnwell SL. Direct Carotid Cavernous Fistula After Trigeminal Balloon Microcompression Gangliolysis: Case Report. Neurosurgery. 1996; 39:853–856
[54] Agazzi S, Chang S, Drucker MD, Youssef AS, Van Loveren HR. Sudden blindness as a complication of percutaneous trigeminal procedures: mechanism analysis and prevention. J Neurosurg. 2009; 110:638–641
[55] Kanpolat Y, Savas A, Bekar A, Berk C. Percutaneous controlled radiofrequency trigeminal rhizotomy for the treatment of idiopathic trigeminal neuralgia: 25-year experience with 1,600 patients. Neurosurgery. 2001; 48:524–32; discussion 532-4
[56] Tobler WD, Tew JM, Cosman E, Keller J, et al. Improved outcome in the treatment of trigeminal neuralgia by percutaneous stereotactic rhizotomy with a new, curved tip electrode. Neurosurgery. 1983; 12:313–317
[57] Lunsford LD. Comment on Taha J M and Tew J M: Comparison of Surgical Treatments for Trigeminal Neuralgia: Reevaluation of Radiofrequency Rhizotomy. Neurosurgery. 1996; 38
[58] Brisman R. Gamma knife surgery with a dose fo 75 to 76.8 Gray for trigeminal neuralgia. J Neurosurg. 2004; 100:848–854
[59] Pollock BE, Phuong LK, Foote RL, Stafford SL, Gorman DA. High-dose trigeminal neuralgia radiosurgery associated with increased risk of trigeminal nerve dysfunction. Neurosurgery. 2001; 49:58–62; discussion 62-4
[60] Kondziolka D, Lunsford LD, Flickinger JC. Stereotactic radiosurgery for the treatment of trigeminal neuralgia. Clin J Pain. 2002; 18:42–47
[61] Massager N, Lorenzoni J, Devriendt D, Desmedt F, Brotchi J, Levivier M. Gamma knife surgery for idiopathic trigeminal neuralgia performed using a far-anterior cisternal target and a high dose of radiation. J Neurosurg. 2004; 100:597–605
[62] Urgosik D, Liscak R, Novotny J, Jr, Vymazal J, Vladyka V. Treatment of essential trigeminal neuralgia with gamma knife surgery. J Neurosurg. 2005; 102 Suppl:29–33
[63] Maesawa S, Salame C, Flickinger JC, Pirris S, Kondziolka D, Lunsford LD. Clinical outcomes after stereotactic radiosurgery for idiopathic trigeminal neuralgia. J Neurosurg. 2001; 94:14–20
[64] Barba D, Alksne JF. Success of Microvascular Decompression with and without Prior Surgical Therapy for Trigeminal Neuralgia. J Neurosurg. 1984; 60:104–107
[65] Schmidek HH, Sweet WH. Operative Neurosurgical Techniques. New York 1982
[66] Onofrio BM. Radiofrequency Percutaneous Gasserian Ganglion Lesions: Results in 140 Patients with Trigeminal Pain. J Neurosurg. 1975; 42:132–139
[67] Kondziolka D, Lunsford LD, Bissonette DJ. Long-Term Results After Glycerol Rhizotomy for Multiple Sclerosis-Related Trigeminal Neuralgia. Can J Neurol Sci. 1994; 21:137–140
[68] Burchiel KJ, Favre J. Current Techniques for Pain Control. Contemp Neurosurg. 1997; 19:1–6
[69] McLaughlin MR, Jannetta PJ, Clyde BL, Subach BR, Comey CH, Resnick DK. Microvascular decompression of cranial nerves: Lessons learned after 4400 operations. J Neurosurg. 1999; 90:1–8
[70] Tew JM, van Loveren HR. Atlas of Operative Microneurosurgery. Philadelphia: W. B. Saunders; 1994; 1: Aneurysms and Arteriovenous Malformations
[71] Day JD, Tschabitscher M. Anatomic position of the asterion. Neurosurgery. 1998; 42:198–199
[72] Bederson JB, Wilson CB. Evaluation of Microvascular Decompression and Partial Sensory Rhizotomty in 252 Cases of Trigeminal Neuralgia. J Neurosurg. 1989; 71:359–367
[73] Avildsen JG. The Karate Kid. 1984
[74] Jannetta PJ. Microsurgical Management of Trigeminal Neuralgia. Arch Neurol. 1985; 42
[75] Burchiel KJ, Clarke H, Haglund M, et al. Long-Term Efficacy of Microvascular Decompression in Trigeminal Neuralgia. J Neurosurg. 1988; 69:35–38
[76] Schmidek HH, Sweet WH. Operative Neurosurgical Techniques. Philadelphia 1988
[77] Hanakita J, Kondo A. Serious Complications of Microvascular Decompression Operations for Trigeminal Neuralgia and Hemifacial Spasm. Neurosurgery. 1988; 22:348–352
[78] Andersen NB, Bovim G, Sjaastad O. The frontotemporal peripheral nerves. Topographic variations of the supraorbital, supratrochlear and auriculotemporal nerves and their possible clinical significance. Surg Radiol Anat. 2001; 23:97–104
[79] Pareja JA, Caminero AB. Supraorbital neuralgia. Curr Pain Headache Rep. 2006; 10:302–305
[80] Headache Classification Committee of the International Headache Society. Classification and diagnostic criteria for headache disorders, cranial neuralgias, and facial pain, 2nd edition. Cephalalgia. 2004; 24:9–160
[81] Pareja JA, Pareja J, Yanguela J. Nummular headache, trochleitis, supraorbital neuralgia, and other epicranial headaches and neuralgias: the epicranias. J Headache Pain. 2003; 4:125–131
[82] Pareja JA, Caminero AB, Serra J, Barriga FJ, Baron M, Dobato JL, Vela L, Sanchez del Rio M. Numular headache: a coin-shaped cephalgia. Neurology. 2002; 58:1678–1679
[83] Caminero AB, Pareja JA. Supraorbital neuralgia: a clinical study. Cephalalgia. 2001; 21:216–223
[84] Stookey B, Ransohoff J. Trigeminal Neuralgia: Its History and Treatment. Springfield, IL: Charles C Thomas; 1959
[85] Sjaastad O, Stolt-Nielsen A, Pareja JA, Vincent M. Supraorbital neuralgia: on the clinical manifestations and a possible therapeutic approach. Headache. 1999; 39:204–212
[86] Grantham EG, Segerberg LH. An evaluation of palliative surgical procedures in trigeminal neuralgia. J Neurosurg. 1952; 9:390–394
[87] Youmans JR. Neurological Surgery. Philadelphia 1982
[88] Weinstein RE, Herec D, Friedman JH. Hypotension due to Glossopharyngeal Neuralgia. Arch Neurol. 1986; 43:90–92
[89] Ferrante L, Artico M, Nardacci B, et al. Glossopharyngeal Neuralgia with Cardiac Syncope. Neurosurgery. 1995; 36:58–63
[90] Lovely TJ, Jannetta PJ. Surgical management of geniculate neuralgia. Am J Otol. 1997; 18:512–517
[91] Pulec JL. Geniculate neuralgia: diagnosis and surgical management. Laryngoscope. 1976; 86:955–964
[92] Watson CPN. A new treatment for postherpetic neuralgia. N Engl J Med. 2000; 343:1563–1565
[93] Loeser JD. Herpes Zoster and Postherpetic Neuralgia. Pain. 1986; 25:149–164
[94] Schimpff S, Serpick A, Stoler B, Rumack B, et al. Varicella-Zoster Infection in Patients with Cancer. Ann Intern Med. 1972; 76:241–254
[95] Youmans JR. Neurological Surgery. Philadelphia 1990
[96] Valacyclovir. Med Letter. 1996; 38:3–4
[97] Rowbotham MC, Davies PS, Verkempinck C, et al. Lidocaine patch: double-blind controlled trial of a new treatment method for postherpetic neuralgia. Pain. 1996; 65:39–44
[98] Alper BS, Lewis PR. Treatment of postherpetic neuralgia: a systematic review of the literature. J Fam Pract. 2002; 51:121–128

[99] Rowbotham MC, Harden N, Stacey B, et al. Gabapentin for the treatment of postherpetic neuralgia: A randomized controlled trial. JAMA. 1998; 280:1837–1842
[100] Capsaicin - A Topical Analgesic. Med Letter. 1992; 34:62–63
[101] Kotani N, Kushikata T, Hashimoto H, et al. Intrathecal methylprednisolone for intractable postherpetic neuralgia. N Engl J Med. 2000; 343:1514–1519
[102] Dan K, Higa K, Noda B, Fields H, Dubner R, Cervero F. In: Nerve block for herpetic pain. Advances in Pain Research and Therapy. New York: Raven Press; 1985:831–838
[103] Friedman AH, Nashold BS. Dorsal Root Entry Zone Lesions for the Treatment of Postherpetic Neuralgia. Neurosurgery. 1984; 15:969–970
[104] Lewith GT, Field J, Machin D. Acupuncture Compared with Placebo in Post-Herpetic Pain. Pain. 1983; 17:361–368
[105] Sternschein MJ, Myers SJ, Frewin DB, et al. Causalgia. Arch Phys Med Rehabil. 1975; 56:58–63
[106] Schott GD. An Unsympathetic View of Pain. Lancet. 1995; 345:634–636
[107] Ochoa JL, Verdugo RJ. Reflex Sympathetic Dystrophy: A Common Clinical Avenue for Somatoform Expression. Neurol Clin. 1995; 13:351–363
[108] Sachs BL, Zindrick MR, Beasley RD. Reflex Sympathetic Dystrophy After Operative Procedures on the Lumbar Spine. J Bone Joint Surg. 1993; 75A:721–725
[109] Ochoa JL. Reflex? Sympathetic? Dystrophy? Triple Questioned Again. Mayo Clin Proc. 1995; 70:1124–1125
[110] Mailis A. Is Diabetic Autonomic Neuropathy Protective Against Reflex Sympathetic Dystrophy? Clin J Pain. 1995; 11:77–81
[111] Mailis A, Meindok H, Papagapiou M, Pham D. Alterations of the Three-Phase Bone Scan After Sympathectomy. Clin J Pain. 1994; 10:146–155
[112] Kozin F, Genant HK, Bekerman C, et al. The Reflex Sympathetic Dystrophy Syndrome. Am J Med. 1976; 60:332–338
[113] Chelimsky TC, Low PA, Naessens JM, et al. Value of Autonomic Testing in Reflex Sympathetic Dystrophy. Mayo Clin Proc. 1995; 70:1029–1040
[114] Ochoa JL. Pain Mechanisms in Neuropathy. Curr Opin Neurol. 1994; 7:407–414
[115] Dotson R, Ochoa JL, Cline M, Yarnitsky D. A Reassessment of Sympathetic Blocks as Long Term Therapeutic Modality for "RSD". Pain. 1990; 5
[116] Hannington-Kiff JG. Relief of Sudek's Atrophy by Regional Intravenous Guanethidine. Lancet. 1977; 1:1132–1133
[117] Blanchard J, Ramamurthy W, Walsh N, et al. Intravenous Regional Sympatholysis: A Double-Blind Comparison of Guanethedine, Reserpine, and Normal Saline. J Pain Symptom Manage. 1990; 5:357–361
[118] Jadad AR, Carroll D, Glynn CJ, McQuay HJ. Intravenous Regional Sympathetic Blockade for Pain Relief in Reflex Sympathetic Dystrophy: A Systematic Review and a Randomized, Double-Blind Crossover Study. J Pain Symptom Manage. 1995; 10:13–20

Part X

Peripheral Nerves

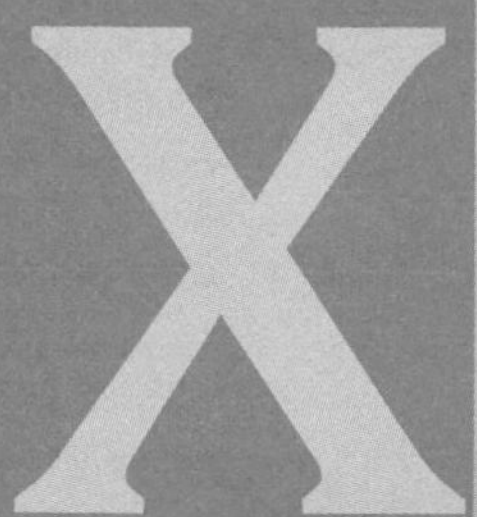

29 Peripheral Nerves

29.1 General information

29.1.1 Peripheral nervous system definition

The peripheral nervous system (PNS) consists of those structures (including cranial nerves III-XII, spinal nerves, nerves of the extremities, and the cervical, brachial and lumbosacral plexi) containing nerve fibers or axons that connect the central nervous system (CNS) with motor and sensory, somatic and visceral, end organs.[1] ▶ Table 29.1 shows classification of motor and sensory nerves.

29.1.2 Grading strength and reflexes

Muscle strength grading most commonly employs the Royal Medical Research Council of Great Britain (MRC) scale,[2] a common modification of which is shown in ▶ Table 29.2. Muscle stretch reflexes may be graded as shown in ▶ Table 29.3.[2]

29.1.3 Upper motor neuron vs. lower motor neuron

29

Lower motor neurons (LMN) (first-order motor neuron): cell bodies (soma) reside in spinal cord (in anterior gray matter) or in brainstem (for cranial nerve motor nuclei). Axons connect directly to neuromuscular junction of muscles.

Upper motor neurons (UMN) (second-order motor neurons): some soma reside in the primary motor cortex (precentral gyrus) of the brain. Axons project to LMNs.

See ▶ Table 29.4 for comparison of weakness due to UMN vs. LMN.

Table 29.1 Motor & sensory classification of nerves

Sensory	Sensory & motor	Greatest fiber diameter (mcm)	Greatest conduction velocity (m/sec)	Motor/ sensory	Comments
Ia	A-alpha	22	120	motor	large alpha motor neurons of lamina IX (extrafusal) sensory-primary afferents (anulospiral of muscle spindles for proprioception)
Ib	A-alpha	22	120	sensory	Golgi tendon organs, touch & pressure receptors
II	A-beta	13	70	sensory	secondary afferents (flower spray) of muscle spindles, crude touch, pressure receptors, Pacinian corpucsles (vibratory) (to posterior columns[a])
	A-gamma	8	40	motor	small γ motor neurons of lamina IX (intrafusal)
III	A-delta	5	15	sensory	small, lightly myelinated, fine touch, pressure, pain & temperature
	B	3	14	motor	small, lightly myelinated preganglionic autonomic fibers
IV	C	1	2	motor	all post-ganglionic autonomic
				sensory	unmyelinated pain & temp (to spinothalamic tract)

[a]these fibers to the posterior columns are more medial in the root entry zone than the C-fibers (important in DREZ lesions where the goal is to lesion C-fibers and spare A-beta)

Table 29.2 Muscle grading (modified Medical Research Council system)

Grade	Strength	
0	no contraction (total paralysis)	
1	flicker or trace contraction (palpable or visible)	
2	active movement with gravity eliminated	
3	active movement through full ROM against gravity	
4	active movement against resistance; subdivisions →	4– Slight resistance 4 Moderate resistance 4 + Slight resistance
5	normal strength (against full resistance)	
NT	not testable	

Table 29.3 Muscle stretch reflex (deep tendon reflex) grading scale

Grade	Definition
0	no contraction (total paralysis)
0.5 +	elicitable only with reinforcement[a]
1 +	low normal
2 +	normal
3 +	more brisk than normal (hyperreflexic)
4 +	hyperreflexic with clonus
5 +	sustained clonus

[a]In the LEs, reinforcement consists of having the patient hook the tips of the fingers of the left hand into the tips of the hooked fingers of the right hand and pulling (Jendrassik maneuver). Reinforcement in the UEs consists of having the patient clench their teeth

Table 29.4 Upper vs. lower motor neuron paralysis

	Upper motor neuron paralysis	Lower motor neuron paralysis
possible etiologies	stroke (motor strip, internal capsule...), spinal cord injury, cervical spondylotic myelopathy	herniated intervertebral disk, nerve entrapment syndrome, polio, progressive muscular atrophy (PMA)
muscle tone	initially flaccid; later spastic with clasp-knife resistance	flaccid
tendon reflexes	hyperactive; clonus may be present	absent
pathologic reflexes (e.g. Babinski, Hoffman)	present (after days to weeks)	absent
muscle manifestations	spontaneous spasms may occur; some *atrophy of disuse* may occur	fibrillations, fasciculations *Atrophy* after days to weeks due to trophic influence

29.1.4 Fasciculations vs. fibrillations

Fasciculations are coarse muscle contractions that are visible to the naked eye, whereas fibrillations are *not* visible and require EMG to detect; AKA fibrillation potentials (p. 242).

29

Fasciculations represent discharge of a group of muscle fibers (all or part of an entire motor unit), and occur most often in diseases involving anterior horn cells, including:

1. amyotrophic lateral sclerosis (ALS) (p. 183)
2. spinal muscular atrophy (p. 1413)
3. polio
4. syringomyelia

29.2 Muscle innervation

29.2.1 Muscles, roots, trunks, cords and nerves of the upper extremities

Table 29.5 Muscle innervation – shoulder & upper extremity[a]

	Muscle	Action to test	Roots[b]	Trunk[c]	Cord[d]	Nerve
	deep neck	flex, ext, rotation of neck	C1–4	–	–	cervical
	trapezius	elevates shoulder, abducts arm > 90°	XI, C3, 4			(spinal acc + roots)
	diaphragm	inspiration	C3–5			phrenic
•	serratus anterior	forward shoulder thrust	C5–7	–	–	long thoracic
	levator scapulae	elevate scapula	C3, 4, **5**			dorsal scapular
	rhomboids	adduct & elevate scapula	C4, 5			
	supraspinatus	abduct arm (15–30°)	C4, **5**, 6	S		suprascapular
•	infraspinatus	exorotation of humerus	**C5**, 6	S	–	
	latissimus dorsi	adduct arm	C5, 6, **7**, 8			thoracodorsal
	teres major, subscapularis		C5–7			subscaspular
•	deltoid	abduct arm (30–90°)	**C5**, 6	S	P	axillary
	teres minor	exorotate & adduct humerus	C4,5			
•	biceps brachii	flex forearm (with hand supinated), & supinate forearm	**C5**, C6	S	L	musculocutaneous
	coracobrachialis	flex humerus at shoulder	C5–7			
	brachialis	flex forearm	C5, 6			
•	flexor carpi ulnaris	ulnar flexion of wrist	C7, **8**, T1	M, I	M	ulnar
•	flexor digitorum profundus III & IV (ulnar part)	flex distal phalanx of Dig 4–5	C7, **8**, T1	M, I	M	
	adductor pollicis	thumb adduction	C8, **T1**		M	
	abductor digiti minimi	abduction Dig 5	C8, T1		M	
	opponens digiti minimi	opposition Dig 5	C7, 8, T1			
	flexor digiti minimi brevis	flexion Dig 5	C7, **8**, **T1**		M	
•	interossei	flex proximal phalanx, extend 2 distal phalanges, abduct or adduct fingers	C8, **T1**	I	M	

Table 29.5 continued

	Muscle	Action to test	Roots[b]	Trunk[c]	Cord[d]	Nerve
	lumbricals 3 & 4	flex proximal phalanges & extend 2 distal phalanges of Dig 4–5	C7, **8**			
•	pronator teres	forearm pronation	C6,7	S,M	L	median
•	flexor carpi radialis	radial flexion of wrist	" "	S,M	L	
	palmaris longus	wrist flexion	C7, 8, T1			
•	flexor digitorum superficialis	flexion middle phalanx Dig 2–5, flex wrist	C7, **8**, T1	M, I	M	
•	abductor pollicis brevis	abduct thumb metacarpal	C8, **T1**	I	M	
	flexor pollicis brevis	flex prox phalanx thumb	C8, **T1**			
•	opponens pollicis	opposes thumb metacarp	C8, **T1**	I	M	
	lumbricals 1 & 2	flex proximal phalanx & extend 2 distal phalanges Dig 2–3	C8, **T1**			
•	flexor digitorum profundus I & II (radial part)	flex distal phalanx of Dig 2–3; flex wrist	C7, **8**, T1	M, I	M	anterior interosseous
•	flexor pollicis longus	flex distal phalanx thumb	C7, **8**, T1			
•	triceps brachii	forearm extension	C6, **7**, 8	all	P	radial
•	brachioradialis	forearm flexion (with thumb pointed up)	C5, **6**	S	P	
•	extensor carpi radialis	radial wrist extension	C5, **6**	S,M	P	
•	supinator	forearm supination	C6, 7	S	P	
•	extensor digitorum	extension of wrist & phalanges of Dig 2–5	**C7**, C8	M, I	P	posterior interosseous (PIN)
	extensor carpi ulnaris	ulnar wrist extension	**C7**, C8			
•	abductor pollicis longus	abduction thumb metacarpal & radial wrist extens.	**C7**, C8	M, I	P	
	extensor pollicis brevis & longus	thumb extension & radial wrist extension	**C7**, C8			
	extensor indicis proprius	extension Dig 2 & wrist extension	**C7**, C8			
	pectoralis major: clavicular head	push arm forward against resistance	**C5**, 6			lateral pectoral
	pectoralis major: sternocostal head	adduct arm	C6, 7, 8			lateral & medial pectoral

[a]NB: items marked with a bullet (•) are clinically important muscle/nerves.
NB: Dig ® U.S. digit numbering convention: 1=thumb, 2=index finger, 3=middle, 4=ring, 5=little.
[b]Major innervation is indicated in boldface. Differing opinions exist, most shown are based on reference.[3]
[c] **Trunk** (trunks of brachial plexus): S = superior, M = middle, I = inferior, all = all three.
[d]**Cord** (cords of brachial plexus): P = posterior, L = lateral, M = medial.

29

29.2.2 Thumb innervation/movement

Table 29.6 The 3 innervations of the thumb

Action	Nerve	Muscle(s)
abduction, flexion, opposition[a]	median	abductor pollicis brevis, flexor pollicis brevis, opponens pollicis
adduction	ulnar	adductor pollicis
extension	radial[b]	extensor pollicis brevis & longus

[a]occasional anomalous innervation by ulnar nerve
[b]via the posterior interosseous nerve

Flexion/extension: occurs in the plane of the palm.

Abduction/adduction: occur in a plane at right angles to palm.

Opposition: bringing the thumb across the hand.

29.2.3 Muscles, roots, trunks, cords and nerves of the lower extremities

Table 29.7 Muscle innervation – hip & lower extremity[a]

	Muscle	Action	Roots[b]	Plexus[c]	Nerves
•	iliopsoas[d]	hip flexion	**L1, 2,** 3	L	femoral & L1, 2, 3
	sartorius	hip flex & thigh evert	L2, 3		femoral
•	quadriceps femoris	leg (knee) extension	**L2, 3, 4**	L	
	pectineus	thigh adduction	L2, 3		obturator
•	adductor longus		**L2, 3, 4**	L	
	adductor brevis		L2–4		
	adductor magnus		L3, 4		
	gracilis		L2–4		
	obturator externus	thigh adduction & lateral rotation	L3, 4		
•	gluteus medius/minimus	thigh abduction & medial rotation	**L4, 5,** S1	S	superior gluteal
	tensor fasciae lata	thigh flexion	L4, 5		
	piriformis	lateral thigh rotation	L5, S1		
•	gluteus maximus	thigh abduction (patient prone)	**L5, S1,** 2	S	inferior gluteal
	obturator internus	lateral thigh rotation	L5, S1	S	muscular branches
	gemelli		L4, 5, S1	S	
	quadratus femoris		L4, 5, S1	S	
•	biceps femoris[e]	leg flexion (& assist thigh extension)	L5, **S1,** 2		sciatic (trunk)
•	semitendinosus[e]		L5, **S1,** 2		
•	semimembranosus[e]		L5, **S1,** 2		
•	tibialis anterior	foot dorsiflexion & supination	**L4, 5**[f]	S	deep peroneal
•	extensor digitorum longus	extension toes 2–5 & foot dorsiflexion	**L5,** S1		

Table 29.7 continued

	Muscle	Action	Roots[b]	Plexus[c]	Nerves
•	extensor hallucis longus (EHL)[g]	great toe extension & foot dorsiflexion	**L5**[f], S1	S	
•	extensor digitorum brevis	extension great toe & toes 2–5	**L5**, S1	S	
•	peroneus longus & brevis	P-flex pronated foot & eversion	L5, S1	L/S	superficial peroneal
•	posterior tibialis	P-flex supinated foot & inversion	L4, 5	S	tibial
	flexor digitorum longus	P-flex sup foot, flex terminal phalanx toes 2–5	L5, **S1, 2**		
	flexor hallucis longus	P-flex sup foot, flex terminal phalanx great toe	L5, **S1, 2**		
	flexor digitorum brevis	flex mid phalanx toes 2–5	S2, 3		
	flexor hallucis brevis	flex proximal phalanx great toe	L5, S1, 2		
•	gastrocnemius	knee flexion, ankle P-flex	**S1, 2**	S	
	plantaris		**S1, 2**		
•	soleus	ankle P-flex	**S1, 2**	S	
•	abductor hallicus[h]	(cannot test[h])	**S1, 2**	S	
	perineal & sphincters	voluntary contract pelvic floor	S2–4		pudendal

NB: items marked with a bullet (•) are clinically important muscle/nerves.
[a]Abbreviations: P-flex = plantarflexion, D-flex = dorsiflexion, phlnx = phalanx.
[b]Major innervation is indicated in boldface type. E.g. when roots are shown as L4, 5, this indicates L5 is the main innervation, but both L4 & L5 contribute.
[c]Plexus: L = lumbar, S = sacral
[d]iliopsoas is the term for the combined iliacus and psoas major muscles
[e] **"hamstrings"**: familiar term for the grouped: semitendinosus and semimembranosus (together, the medial hamstrings) and the biceps femoris (lateral hamstrings)
[f] although many references, including some venerable ones, cite AT as being primarily L4, many clinicians agree that L5 innervation is probably more significant
[g] EHL is the best L5 muscle to test clinically (although S1 radiculopathy can also weaken this muscle)
[h]abductor hallicus cannot be tested clinically, but is important for EMG

29.3 Peripheral nerve injury/surgery

29.3.1 Nerve action potentials

Stimulating a healthy nerve fiber with an electrical stimulus of an amplitude and duration that exceeds its threshold will produce a conducted impulse, or nerve action potential (NAP).[4(p 103)] Medium-sized axons (fibers) have a lower threshold than large ones which have lower threshold than small or fine axons.[4(p 103)]

29.3.2 Use of NAP with lesion in continuity

There is some degree of continuity in ≥ 60% of nerve injuries.[4(p 104)]

For a lesion in continuity (LIC), if surgical repair is needed, it may be too late if one waits until there is failure of anticipated clinical improvement. Presence of a NAP (regardless of amplitude or latency) distal to an LIC in the first few months after an injury usually indicates that operative intervention will not be needed. For recommended timing to obtain NAP recording, ► Table 29.8.[4(p 106)]

Table 29.8 Recommended timing to obtain NAP recording	
Injury	**Timing**
relatively focal contusions	2–4 months
stretch injuries (esp. brachial plexus)	4–5 months
partial injuries & entrapments, compressive lesions and tumors	any time
to identify an area of conduction block (regardless if lesion is from neuropraxia, axonotmesis, or neurotmesis)	acutely

29.3.3 Timing of surgical repair

The longer the distance from the injury site to the functional unit to be reinnervated, the earlier surgical intervention should be considered.[4(p 74)]

24 month rule[4(p 74)]: after 24 months of denervation, most muscles cannot recover useful function even with reinnervation. Exceptions: facial muscles, large bulky muscles such as biceps, brachialis, gastrocs, and some lesions in continuity with some preserved innervation.

29.3.4 Brachial plexus

General information

29

Formed by *ventral* rami (the dorsal rami innervate the paraspinal muscles), most commonly of nerve roots C5-T1 (schematically depicted in ▶ Fig. 29.1.

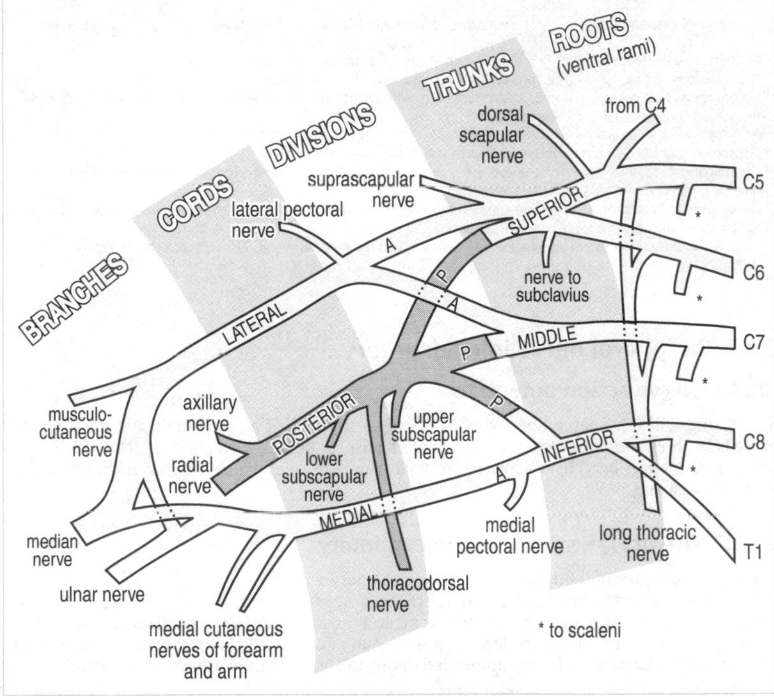

Fig. 29.1 Schematic diagram of the brachial plexus (By Permission: Churchill Livingstone, Edinburgh, 1973, R. Warwick & P. Williams: Gray's Anatomy 35th Edition © Longman Group UK Limited)

► Table 29.5 shows action, etc. of specific muscles. Also see ► Fig. 29.1. ↯ indicates that the nerve supplies the muscles listed; ↳ denotes a branch of the preceding nerve.

Nerves arising from the brachial plexus

Radial nerve (C5-C8)

See ► Fig. 29.2.

Radial nerve (and its branches) innervate the extensors of arm and forearm:

- ↯ triceps (all 3 heads)
- ↯ anconeus
- ↯ brachioradialis
- ↯ extensor carpi radialis longus & brevis (latter originates ≈ at terminal branch)
- ↯ supinator (originates near the terminal branch)
- ↳ continues into forearm as **posterior interosseous nerve** (C7, C8)
  - ↯ extensor carpi ulnaris
  - ↯ extensor digitorum
  - ↯ extensor digiti minimi
  - ↯ extensor pollicis brevis & longus
  - ↯ abductor pollicis longus
  - ↯ extensor indicus

Axillary nerve (C5, C6)

See ► Fig. 29.2.

- ↯ teres minor
- ↯ deltoid

Median nerve (C5-T1)

See ► Fig. 29.3, also see Martin-Gruber anastomosis (p. 514).

- nothing in arm
- all forearm pronators and flexors except the two supplied by ulnar nerve
  - ↯ pronator teres
  - ↯ flexor carpi radialis
  - ↯ palmaris longus
  - ↯ flexor digitorum superficialis
- in the hand ⇒ only the "LOAF muscles"
  - ↯ Lumbricals 1 & 2
  - ↯ Opponens pollicis
  - ↯ Abductor pollicis brevis
  - ↯ Flexor pollicis brevis (C8, T1)
- ↳ branch at or just distal to elbow anterior interosseous nerve (purely *motor*)
- ↯ flexor digitorum profundus I & II
- ↯ flexor pollicis longus
  - ↯ pronator quadratus

Ulnar nerve (C8, T1)

► Fig. 29.3. (Note: This is classic winging of the scapula. A variant of winging can occur with loss of trapezius muscle, e.g. with accessory nerve injury, and typically manifests when the patient pushes forward with the elbow held at the side of the thorax.)

- nothing in arm
- only 2 muscles in forearm:
  - ↯ flexor carpi ulnaris
  - ↯ half of flexor digitorum profundus (parts III & IV)
- all hand muscles excluding "LOAF" muscles (see above), viz.:
  - ↯ adductor pollicis
  - ↯ all interossei (4 dorsal & 3 palmar)
  - ↯ lumbricals 3 & 4
  - ↯ 3 hypothenar muscles: abductor, opponens & flexor digiti minimi
  - ↯ deep part of flexor pollicis brevis (by deep branch of ulnar nerve)
  - ↯ palmaris brevis (by the superficial branch of the ulnar nerve)

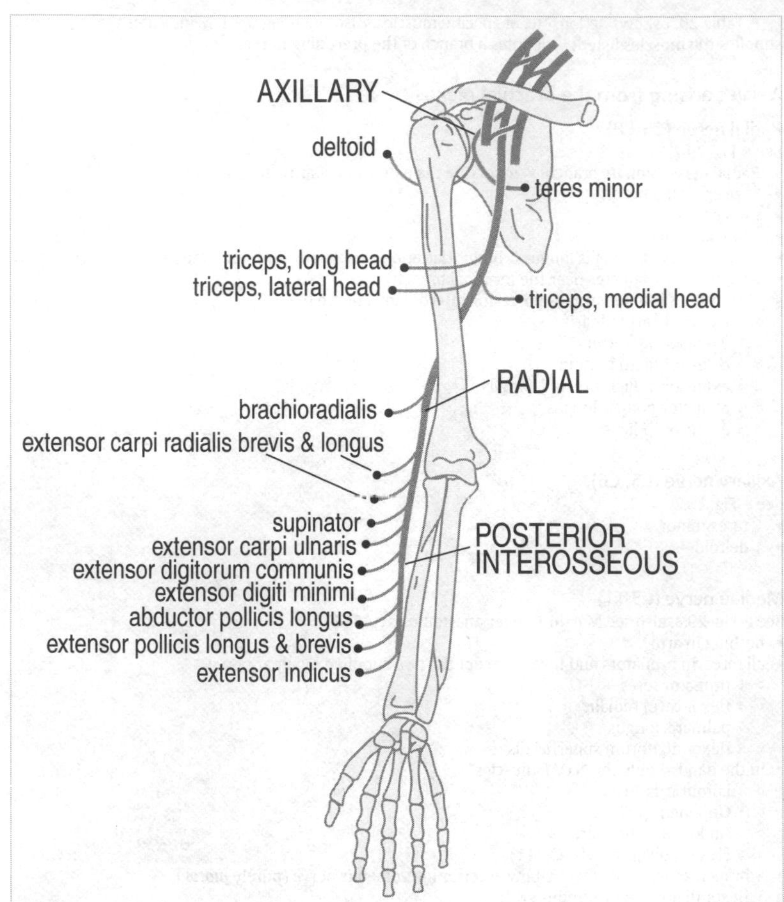

Fig. 29.2 Muscles of the radial and axillary nerves

Musculocutaneous nerve (C5, C6)

Supplies arm flexors

- ↯ Coracobrachialis
- ↯ biceps
- ↯ brachialis

↳ lateral cutaneous nerve of the forearm (terminal branch) supplies cutaneous sensation to radial aspect of forearm

Dorsal scapular nerve (C4, C5)

- ↯ rhomboids (major & minor)
- ↯ levator scapulae

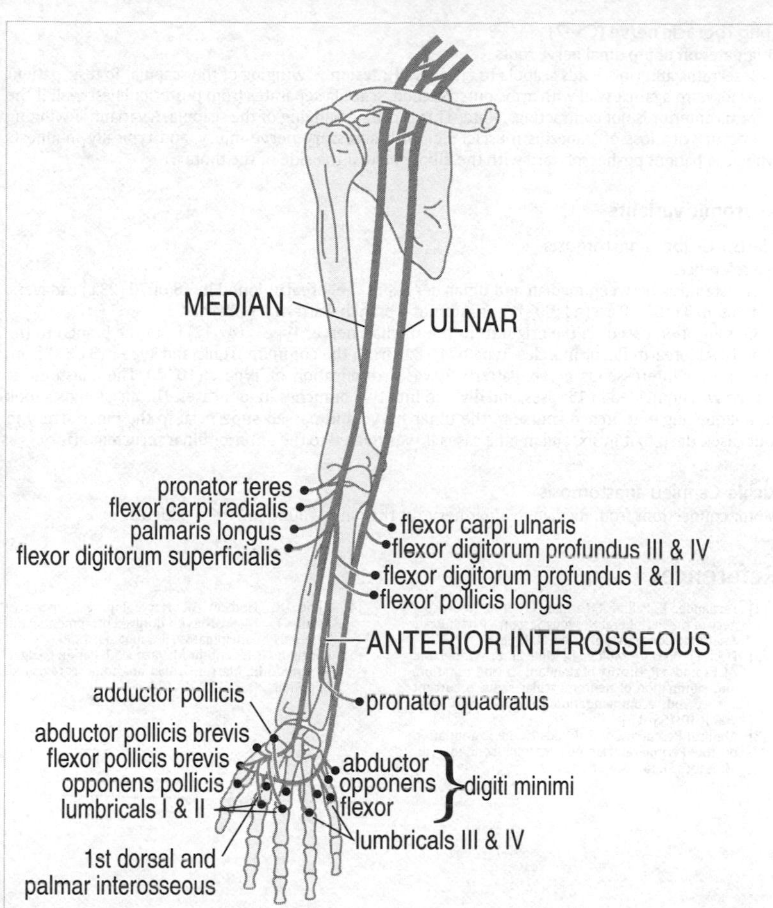

Fig. 29.3 Muscles of the median and ulnar nerves

Suprascapular nerve (C5, C6)

- ♮ Supraspinatus
- ♮ Infraspinatus

Subscapular nerve (C5–7)

- ♮ teres major
- ♮ subscapularis

Thoracodorsal nerve (C6, C7, C8)

- ♮ latissimus dorsi

Long thoracic nerve (C5–7)

Originates off of proximal nerve roots

↯ serratus anterior (holds scapula to chest wall): lesion → winging of the scapula. To test: patient leans forward against wall with arms outstretched, scapula separates from posterior chest wall if the serratus anterior is not contracting. (Note: This is classic winging of the scapula. A variant of winging can occur with loss of trapezius muscle, e.g. with accessory nerve injury, and typically manifests when the patient pushes forward with the elbow held at the side of the thorax.)

Anatomic variants

Martin-Gruber anastomosis

See reference.[5]

Anastamosis between median and ulnar nerves in the forearm found in 16 of 70 (23%) cadavers, bilateral in 3 (19%). Pattern I (90%): 1 anastamotic branch, Pattern II (10%) had 2.

Classification based on the origin from the median nerve: Type a (47.3%) from the branch to the superficial forearm flexor muscles, Type b (10.6%) from the common trunk, and Type c (31.6%) from the anterior interosseous nerve. Pattern II was a duplication of Type c (10.5%). The anastomotic branch was undivided in 15 cases, and divided into two branches in four cases. The anastomosis took an oblique angle or arched course to the ulnar nerve and passed superficial to the ulnar artery in four cases, deep to it in six, and in nine cases it was related to the anterior ulnar recurrent artery.[5]

Richie-Cannieu anastomosis

Motor connections from median to ulnar nerve at the palm. Found in 70% of patients.

References

[1] Fernandez E, Pallini R, La Marca F, et al. Neurosurgery of the Peripheral Nervous System - Part I: Basic Anatomic Concepts. Surg Neurol. 1996; 46:47–48

[2] Dyck PJ, Boes CJ, Mulder D, Millikan C, Windebank AJ, Espinosa R. History of standard scoring, notation, and summation of neuromuscular signs. A current survey and recommendation. J Peripher Nerv Syst. 2005; 10:158–173

[3] Medical Research Council. Aids to the Examination of the Peripheral Nervous System. London: Her Majesty's Stationery Office; 1976

[4] Kline DG, Hudson AR. Nerve Injuries: Operative Results for Major Nerve Injuries, Entrapments, and Tumors. Philadelphia: W. B. Saunders; 1995

[5] Rodriguez-Niedenfuhr M, Vazquez T, Parkin I, Logan B, Sanudo JR. Martin-Gruber anastomosis revisited. Clin Anat. 2002; 15:129–134

30 Entrapment Neuropathies

30.1 General information

Entrapment neuropathy is a peripheral nerve injury resulting from compression either by external forces or from nearby anatomic structures. Mechanism can vary from one or two significant compressive insults to many localized, repetitive mild compressions of a nerve. Certain nerves are particularly vulnerable at specific locations by virtue of being superficial, fixed in position, traversing a confined space, or in proximity to a joint. The most common symptom is pain (frequently at rest, more severe at night, often with retrograde radiation causing more proximal lesion to be suspected) with tenderness at the point of entrapment. Referred pain is so common that Frank Mayfield once said that patients with nerve entrapment don't know where the problem is located. Always consider the possibility of a systemic cause. Entrapment neuropathies may be associated with:

1. diabetes mellitus
2. hypothyroidism: due to glycogen deposition in Schwann cells
3. acromegaly
4. amyloidosis: primary or secondary (as in multiple myeloma)
5. carcinomatosis
6. polymyalgia rheumatica (p. 198)
7. rheumatoid arthritis: 45% incidence of 1 or more entrapment neuropathies
8. gout

30.2 Mechanism of injury

Brief compression primarily affects myelinated fibers, and classically spares unmyelinated fibers (except in cases of severe acute compression). Acute compression compromises axoplasmic flow which can reduce membrane excitability. Chronic compression affects both myelinated and unmyelinated fibers and can produce segmental demyelination in the former, and if the insult persists, axolysis and wallerian degeneration will occur in both types. The issue of ischemia is more controversial.[1] Some contend that simultaneous venous stasis at the site of compression can produce ischemia which can lead to edema outside the axonal sheath which may further exacerbate the ischemia. Eventually, fibrosis, neuroma formation, and progressive neuropathy can occur.

30.3 Occipital nerve entrapment

30.3.1 General information

Greater occipital nerve (nerve of Arnold) is a sensory branch of C2 (▶ Fig. 28.1 for dermatome). Entrapment presents as occipital neuralgia: pain in occiput usually with a trigger point near the superior nuchal line. Pressure here reproduces pain radiating up along back of head towards vertex.

More common in women.

30.3.2 Differential diagnosis

1. headache
   a) may be mimicked by migraine headache
   b) may be part of muscle contraction (tension) headache
2. myofascial pain[2]: the pain may be widely separated from the trigger point
3. vertebrobasilar disease including aneurysm and SAH
4. cervical spondylosis
5. pain from Chiari I malformation (p. 277)

30.3.3 Possible causes of entrapment

1. trauma
   a) direct trauma (including iatrogenic placement of suture through the nerve during surgical procedures, e.g. in closing a posterior fossa craniectomy)
   b) following traumatic cervical extension[3] which may crush the C2 root and ganglion between the C1 arch and C2 lamina
   c) fractures of the upper cervical spine

2. atlanto-axial subluxation (AAS) (e.g. in rheumatoid arthritis) or arthrosis
3. entrapment by hypertrophic C1–2 (epistrophic) ligament[4]
4. neuromas
5. arthritis of the C2–3 zygapophyseal joint

30.3.4 Treatment

General information

> Σ
>
> For idiopathic occipital neuralgia: available evidence is from small, retrospective, case series studies and is insufficient to conclude that either local injection or surgery are effective. Nerve blocks with steroids and local anesthetics provide only temporary relief. Surgical procedures such as nerve root decompression or neurectomy may provide effective pain relief for some patients; however, patient-selection criteria for these procedures have not been defined, and recurrence is common.

In idiopathic cases with no neurologic deficit, the condition is usually self limited.

Non surgical treatment

1. greater occipital nerve block with local anesthetic and steroids (see below)
   a) may provide relief typically lasting ≈ 1 month[5]
   b) is no longer considered diagnostic because it is not sufficiently specific
2. physical therapy: massage and daily stretching exercises
3. TENS unit: provided ≥ 50% relief in 13 patients for up to 5 yrs[6]
4. oral antiinflammatory agents
5. centrally acting pain medications: Neurontin, Paxil, Elavil...
6. botulinum toxin injection[7]: although this study had quite a few placebo responders

If these measures do not provide permanent relief in *disabling* cases, surgical treatment may be considered, although caution is advised by many due to poor results.[2,8] Alcohol neurolysis may be tried. A collar is *not* indicated as it may irritate the condition.

Occipital nerve block

Inject trigger point(s) if one or more can be identified (there is usually a trigger point near the superior nuchal line). The nerve may also be blocked at the point where it emerges from the dorsal neck muscles.

If the pathology is more proximal (e.g. at C2 spinal ganglion), then block of the ganglion may be required. Technique[9] (done under fluoroscopy): shave hair below the mastoid process; prep with iodine; infiltrate with local; insert a 20 gauge spinal needle midway between C1 and C2, halfway between the midline and the lateral margin of the dorsal neck muscles. Aim rostrally, the final target is the midpoint of the C1–2 joint on AP fluoro, and almost but not touching the inferior articular process of C1. Infiltrate 1–3 ml of anesthetic and check for analgesia in the C2 distribution.

Surgical treatment

1. decompression of C2 nerve root if compressed between C1 and C2[4]
2. in cases of AAS, decompression and atlanto-axial fusion (p. 1479) may work

Surgical treatment options for *idiopathic* occipital neuralgia:
1. peripheral occipital nerve procedures: these may not be effective for proximal compression of the C2 root or ganglion:
   a) occipital neurectomy (see below)
      - peripheral avulsion of the nerve
      - avulsion of the greater occipital nerve as it exits between the transverse process of C2 and the inferior oblique muscle
   b) alcohol injection of greater occipital nerve

2. occipital nerve stimulators
3. release of the nerve within the trapezius muscle. Immediate results: relief in 46%, improvement in 36%. Only 56% reported improvement at 14.5 mos[10]
4. intradural division of the C2 dorsal route via a posterior intradural approach
5. ganglionectomy

Occipital neurectomy: The occipital nerve usually pierces the cervical muscles ≈ 2.5 cm lateral to the midline, just below the inion. Palpation or doppler localization of the pulse of the accompanying greater occipital artery sometimes helps to locate the nerve. However, relief only occurs in ≈ 50%, and recurrence, usually within a year, is common.

30.4 Median nerve entrapment

30.4.1 General information

The two most common sites of entrapment of the median nerve:
1. at the wrist by the transverse carpal ligament: carpal tunnel syndrome (see below)
2. in upper forearm by pronator teres muscle: pronator teres syndrome (p. 521)

30.4.2 Anatomy

Contributing nerve roots: C5 through T1. The median nerve arises from the medial and lateral cords of the brachial plexus (▶ Fig. 29.1), and descends the upper arm adjacent to the lateral side of the brachial artery. It crosses to the medial side of the artery at the level of the coracobrachialis. In the cubital fossa, the median nerve passes behind the lacertus fibrosus (bicipital aponeurosis) and enters the upper forearm between the two heads of the pronator teres and supplies this muscle.

Just beyond this point, it branches to form the purely motor anterior interosseous nerve which supplies all but 2 muscles of finger and wrist flexion. It descends adherent to deep surface of flexor digitorum superficialis (FDS), lying on the flexor digitorum profundus. Near the wrist, it emerges from the lateral edge of FDS becoming more superficial, lying medial to the tendon of flexor carpi radialis, just lateral to and partially under the cover of the palmaris longus tendon. It passes under the transverse carpal ligament (TCL) through the carpal tunnel which also contains the tendons of the flexor digitorum profundus and superficialis deep to the nerve (9 tendons total, 2 to each finger, 1 to the thumb[11]). The motor branch arises deep to the TCL, but may anomalously pierce the TCL. It supplies the "LOAF muscles" (Lumbricals 1 & 2, Opponens pollicis, and Abductor and Flexor pollicis brevis).

The TCL attaches medially to pisiform and hook of hamate, laterally to trapezium and tubercles of scaphoid. TCL is continuous proximally with fascia over FDS and antebrachial fascia, distally with the flexor retinaculum of the hand. The TCL extends distally into the palm to ≈ 3 cm beyond the distal wrist crease. The palmaris longus tendon, which is absent in 10% of population, partially attaches to the TCL.

Palmar cutaneous branch (PCB) of median nerve: arises from the radial aspect of the median nerve approximately 5.5 cm proximal to styloid process of the radius, underneath the cover of FDS of the middle finger. It crosses the wrist *above* the TCL to provide sensory innervation to the base of the thenar eminence (and is thus spared in carpal tunnel syndrome).

The sensory distribution of the *average* median nerve is shown in ▶ Fig. 30.1.

30.4.3 Injuries to the main trunk of the median nerve

General information

Above the elbow, the median nerve may rarely be compressed by Struther's ligament (see below). At the elbow and forearm, the median nerve may rarely be trapped at any of three sites: 1) lacertus fibrosus (bicipital aponeurosis),[12] 2) pronator teres, 3) sublimis bridge. Neuropathy may also result from direct or indirect trauma or external pressure ("honeymoon paralysis").[12] Longstanding compression of the main trunk of the median nerve produces a "benediction hand" when trying to make a fist (index finger extended, middle finger partially flexed; due to weakness of flexor digitorum profundus I & II).

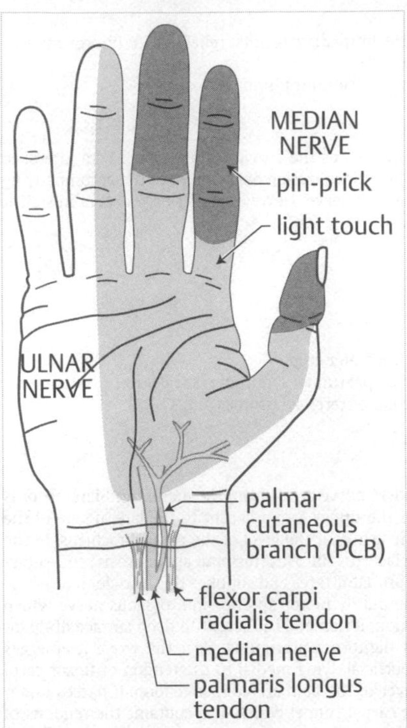

Fig. 30.1 Sensory distribution of the median and ulnar nerves in the hand palmar surface.

30

Struther's ligament

Distinct from struthers arcade (p. 527) which is a normal finding. The supracondylar process (SCP) is an anatomical variant located 5–7 cm above medial epicondyle, present in 0.7–2.7% of population. Struther's ligament bridges the SCP to the medial epicondyle. The median nerve and brachial artery pass underneath, the ulnar nerve may also. Usually asymptomatic, but occasionally may cause typical median nerve syndrome.

Pronator (teres) syndrome

From direct trauma or repeated pronation with tight hand-grip. Trapped where nerve dives between 2 heads of pronator teres. Causes vague aching and easy fatiguing of forearm muscles with weak grip and poorly localized paresthesias in index finger and thumb. Nocturnal exacerbation is *absent*. Pain in palm distinguishes this from carpal tunnel syndrome (CTS) since the median palmar cutaneous branch (PCB) exits before the TCL and is spared in CTS.

Treat with resting forearm. Surgical decompression indicated for cases that progress while on rest or when continued trauma is unavoidable.

Anterior interosseous neuropathy

General information

Key concepts

- weakness of 3 muscles: FDP I & II, FPL, & pronator quadratus. No sensory loss
- loss of flexion of the distal phalanges of the thumb and index finger (pinch sign)

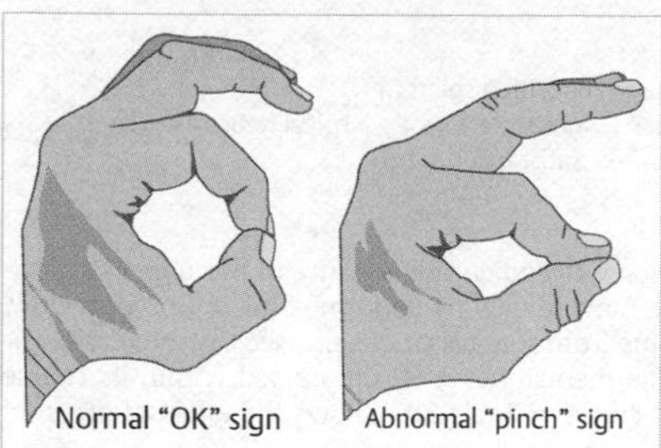

Fig. 30.2 "Pinch sign" seen with AIN

The anterior interosseous nerve is a purely motor branch of the median nerve that arises in the upper forearm. Anterior interosseous neuropathy (AIN) produces no sensory loss and weakness of the 3 muscles supplied by the nerve:

1. flexor digitorum profundus (FDP) I & II: flexion of distal phalanx of digits 2 & 3
2. flexor pollicis longus (FPL): flexion of distal phalanx of thumb
3. pronator quadratus (in the distal forearm): difficult to isolate clinically

Etiologies of AIN

Include: idiopathic, amyotrophy, ulna/radius fractures, penetrating injuries, forearm lacerations.

Clinical

Symptoms: Patients complain of difficulty grasping small objects between the thumb and the index finger. Idiopathic cases may be preceded with forearm aching.

Physical exam: Sensory: *no* sensory loss.

Strength: digits 1, 2 & 3 are examined individually. The proximal interphalangeal joints are stabilized by the examiner and the patient is asked to flex the DIP. With AIN, there is no significant flexion of the DIP.

Pinch sign: the patient attempts to forcefully pinch the *tips* of the index finger and thumb as in making an "OK" sign (▶ Fig. 30.2, left), with AIN the terminal phalanges extend and the pulps touch instead of the tips[13] (▶ Fig. 30.2, right).

Diagnosis

In addition to the physical exam, EMG may be helpful.

EMG: primarily assesses pronator quadratus & flexor pollicis longus (FDP I & II is difficult on EMG because it has dual innervation with the ulnar nerve innervated portion being more superficial than the median nerve innervated portion). Important to evaluate pronator teres (abnormalities suggest involvement more proximal than forearm).

Management

In the absence of an identifiable cause of nerve injury, expectant management is recommended for 8–12 weeks, following which exploration is indicated which may reveal a constricting band near the origin.

30.4.4 Carpal tunnel syndrome

General information

Key concepts

- the most common compression neuropathy. Involves median nerve in the wrist
- symptoms: tingling in the hand, worse at night and with elevation of hands
- physical exam is not very sensitive:
  - sensory: decreased pinprick in digits 1–3 and the radial half of 4
  - sensitivity: Tinels (tapping on wrist) 60%, Phalens (flexion of wrist) 80%
- electrodiagnostics: sensory latency @ wrist > 3.7 ms is the most sensitive test

- treatment:
  - mild cases: nonsurgical treatment (NSAIDs, neutral position splint...)
  - unresponsive or severe cases (neurologic deficits, duration > 1 year): surgical neurolysis (decompression) of the median nerve at the wrist has 70% satisfaction rate

Carpal tunnel syndrome (CTS) is the most common entrapment neuropathy in the upper extremity.[14,15,16] Carpal tunnel release (CTR) is one of the most frequently performed hand procedures.[17,18] The majority of patients have a satisfactory outcome from surgical treatment; see Outcome of surgical treatment (carpal tunnel release) (p. 526). The median nerve is compressed within its course through the carpal tunnel just distal to the wrist crease. ▶ Table 30.1 shows the effect of pressure within the carpal tunnel.

Epidemiology

Usually occurs in middle aged patients. Ratio of female:male = 4:1. It is bilateral in over 50% of cases, but is usually worse in the dominant hand. The prevalence of CTS and UNE is increased in diabetics.

Common etiologies

See reference.[19]

In most cases, no specific etiology can be identified. CTS is very common in the geriatric population without any additional risk factors. The following etiologies tend to be more common in younger patients:

30

1. "classic" CTS: chronic time course, usually over a period of months to years
   a) trauma: often job-related (may also be associated with avocations)
      - repetitive movements of hand or /wrist: e.g. carpenter's
      - repeated forceful grasping or pinching of tools or other objects
      - awkward positions of hand and/or wrist, including wrist extension, ulnar deviation, or especially forced wrist flexion
      - direct pressure over carpal tunnel
      - use of vibrating hand tools
   b) systemic conditions: in addition to systemic causes listed for entrapment neuropathies (p. 515) – especially rheumatoid arthritis, diabetes -, also consider:
      - obesity
      - local trauma
      - pregnancy: 54% remained symptomatic 1 year post-partum, and patients with onset early in pregnancy were less likely to improve[20]
      - mucopolysaccharidosis V
      - tuberculous tenosynovitis
      - multiple myeloma (p. 714) (amyloid deposition in flexor retinaculum)
   c) patients with A-V dialysis shunts in the forearm have an increased incidence of CTS, possibly on an ischemic basis (steal and/or venous stasis) or possibly from the underlying renal disorder
2. "acute" CTS: an uncommon condition where the symptoms of CTS appear suddenly and severely, usually following some type of exertion or trauma. Etiologies:
   a) median artery thrombosis: < 10% of individuals have a persistent median artery
   b) hemorrhage or hematoma in the transverse carpal ligament

Table 30.1 Pressure within carpal tunnel

Pressure (mm Hg)	Description
< 20	normal
20–30	venular flow retarded
30	axonal transport impaired
40	sensory & motor dysfunction
60–80	blood flow ceases

Signs and symptoms

The physical exam for CTS is fairly insensitive. Signs and symptoms may include:

1. dysesthesias:
   a) characteristically patients are awakened at night by a painful numbness in the hand (often described as the "hand falling asleep") that often subjectively feels like a loss of circulation of blood. They often seek relief by: shaking or dangling or swinging the hand, opening and closing or rubbing the fingers, running hot or cold water over the hand, or pacing the floor. It may radiate up the arm, occasionally as far as shoulder
   b) daytime activities that characteristically elicit symptoms usually involve prolonged hand elevation: holding a book or newspaper to read, driving a car, holding a telephone receiver, brushing the hair
   c) distribution of symptoms:
      - on palmar side in radial 3.5 fingers (palmar side of thumb, index finger, middle finger, and radial half of ring finger)
      - dorsal side of these same fingers distal to the PIP joint
      - radial half of palm
      - subjective involvement of little finger occurs not infrequently for reasons that are not clear
2. weakness of hand, especially grip. Characteristically manifests as difficulty opening jars. May be associated with thenar atrophy (late change, severe atrophy is seldom seen with current awareness of CTS by most physicians). An occasional patient may present with severe atrophy and no history of pain
3. clumsiness of the hand and/or difficulty with fine motor skills: probably due mostly to numbness more than a motor deficit. Often presents as difficulties buttoning buttons or zipping zippers, putting on earrings, fastening bra straps...
4. hypesthesia in median nerve sensory distribution: usually best appreciated in finger *tips*, loss of 2-point discrimination may be more sensitive test
5. Phalen's test: 30–60 secs wrist flexion to a 90° angle exaggerates or reproduces pain or tingling. Positive in 80% of cases (80% sensitive)[21]
6. Tinel's sign at the wrist: paresthesias or pain in median nerve distribution produced by gently percussing over the carpal tunnel. Positive in 60% of cases. May also be present in other conditions. Reverse Tinel's sign: produces symptoms radiating up the forearm for variable distance
7. ischemic testing: place blood pressure cuff proximal to wrist, inflation x 30–60 seconds may reproduce CTS pain

30

Differential diagnosis

Differential diagnosis includes (modified[22]):

1. cervical radiculopathy: coexists in 70% of patients with either median or ulnar neuropathy (C6 radiculopathy may mimic CTS). Usually relieved by rest, and exacerbated by neck movement. Sensory impairment has dermatomal distribution. It has been postulated that cervical nerve root compression may interrupt axoplasmic flow and predispose the nerve to compressive injury distally (the term double-crush syndrome was coined to describe this[23]), and although this has been challenged[24] it has not been disproven
2. thoracic outlet syndrome (p. 554): loss of bulk in hand muscles other than thenar. Sensory impairment in ulnar side of hand and forearm
3. pronator teres syndrome (p. 518): more prominent palmar pain than with CTS (median palmar cutaneous branch does not pass through carpal tunnel)
4. de Quervain's syndrome: tenosynovitis of the abductor pollicis longus and extensor pollicis brevis tendons often caused by repetitive hand movements. Results in *pain and tenderness* in the wrist near the thumb. Onset in 25% of cases is during pregnancy, and many in 1st postpartum year. Usually responds to wrist splints and/or steroid injections. NCVs should be normal. Finkelstein's test: the thumb is passively abducted while thumb abductors are palpated, positive if this aggravates the pain[25]
5. reflex sympathetic dystrophy: may respond to sympathetic block (p. 1521)
6. tenosynovitis of any of the flexor ligaments: may occasionally be due to TB or fungus. Usually a long, indolent course. Fluid accumulation may be present

Diagnostic tests

Electrodiagnostics (EDX)

Electromyogram (EMG) and nerve conduction study (NCS) which includes measurement of nerve conduction velocities (NCV): may help confirm the diagnosis of CTS and distinguish it from cervical root abnormalities and from tendonitis.

CTS is predominantly a demyelinating injury although it can progress to axonal loss.[26] Two sensory comparison techniques that clearly agree (either normal or abnormal) are adequate to confirm or refute the diagnosis. For borderline abnormalities additional sensory comparison testing or the combined sensory index (CSI) can clarify the diagnosis. If sensory responses are absent, the median motor latency in comparison to the ulnar latency can help localize a focal abnormality.[27]

Practice guideline: Electrodiagnostic criteria for CTS

The practice guideline for CTS recommends diagnostic examination strategies[28,29,30]:

1. Standard: perform a median sensory nerve conduction study (NCS) across the wrist with conduction distance of 13 to 14 cm. If abnormal, compare to an adjacent sensory nerve in the symptomatic limb
2. Standard: if the initial median sensory NCS across the wrist is normal then additional comparison studies are recommended
3. Guideline: motor NCS of the median nerve recording from the thenar muscle and of 1 other nerve in the symptomatic limb
4. Option: supplementary NCS
5. Option: needle electromyography (EMG) of cervical root screen muscles including a thenar muscle

30

NCV: Electrophysiologic studies support a diagnosis of carpal tunnel syndrome (CTS) using median nerve conduction studies across the transverse carpal ligament. Characteristic abnormalities: prolongation of sensory and motor distal latencies, slowing of the conduction velocity and decreased amplitudes of sensory and motor responses. Guidelines regarding recommended studies are published by the American Association of Neuromuscular and Electrodiagnostic Medicine (AANEM), AAPM&R, and AAN. Adhering to the guidelines, sensitivity is greater than 85% and specificity is greater than 95%.[28] Sensory latencies are more sensitive than motor. (Note: although up to 15% of cases may have normal electrodiagnostic studies, great reservation should be exercised in considering operating on CTS with normal sensory NCV and amplitude.)

Normal findings are shown in ▶ Table 30.2. Abnormal values also listed are a rough guide, but the correlation between severity of EDX findings and symptoms in CTS is not well established.[27] Nevertheless, classification as follows can in part predict the outcome of carpal tunnel release (surgery) with normal and very severe NCS abnormalities having a worse prognosis than patients with moderate NCS abnormalities.[27,31]

EDX interpretation (reports may also include the degree of slowing in the summary of findings or interpretation[27,32,33]):

- mild: Prolonged (relative or absolute) median nerve sensory latencies with normal motor studies. No evidence of axonal loss
- moderate: Prolonged (relative or absolute) median nerve sensory latencies with prolongation of motor distal latency. No evidence of axonal loss.
- severe: Any of the aforementioned NCS abnormalities with evidence of axonal loss on EMG.

Table 30.2 Distal conduction latencies through *carpal tunnel*[a]

Degree of involvement[b]	Sensory		Motor	
	latency[c] (mSec)	amplitude (mcV)	latency[d] (mSec)	amplitude (mV)
normal	<3.7	>25	<4.5	>4
mild[b]	3.7–4.0		4.4–6.9	
moderate[b]	4.1–5.0		7.0–9.9	
severe[b]	>5 or unobtainable		>10	

[a]assumes normal proximal NCV
[b]severity does not reliably correlate with latency (see text)
[c]to index finger. Sensory latency is measured to the peak of the waveform
[d]to abductor pollicis brevis

Additional comparison studies for uncertain cases compare median nerve sensory conduction velocity to that of the ulnar nerve (or radial nerve): normal median nerve should be at least 4 m/sec faster than the ulnar, reversal of this pattern suggests median nerve injury. Alternatively, the sensory latencies for the palmar median and ulnar nerves can be compared; the median nerve latency should not be ≥ 0.3 mS longer than the ulnar.

EMG: normal in up to 31% of cases of CTS. In relatively advanced CTS, it may show increased polyphasicity, positive waves, fibrillation potentials, and decreased motor unit numbers on maximal voluntary thenar muscle contraction. EMG may detect cervical radiculopathy if motor involvement is present.

With severe "end stage" CTS, sensory and motor potentials may not be recordable, and EMG is not helpful in localizing (i.e. differentiating CTS from other etiologies).

Laboratory tests

Recommended in cases where an underlying peripheral neuropathy is suspected (e.g. unclear etiology in a young individual with no risk factors such as repetitive hand use). This same protocol is a useful initial workup for any case of peripheral neuropathy:

1. thyroid hormone levels (T4 (total or free) & TSH): to R/O myxedema
2. CBC: anemia is common in multiple myeloma, also to R/O amyloidosis
3. electrolytes:
   a) to R/O chronic renal failure that could cause uremic neuropathy
   b) blood glucose: R/O diabetes
4. in cases suspicious for multiple myeloma: see full details (p. 714)
   a) 24 hour urine for kappa Bence-Jones protein
   b) bloodwork: serum protein electrophoresis (SPEP) and immune electrophoresis (IEP) (looking for IgG kappa band)
   c) skeletal radiologic survey
   d) anemia is common on the CBC

Imaging studies

Not routinely done unless a mass lesion is suspected.

Wrist MRI: very sensitive. Findings with CTS include: flattening or swelling of the nerve, palmar bowing of the flexor retinaculum, May also demonstrate ganglion cysts, lipomas... Enhancement may occur with hypervascular edema.

Diagnostic ultrasound: faster and less expensive than MRI, and can assess bloodflow and changes with different wrist positions. 18 MHz probes may improve images.

Management of CTS

Practice guideline: Management of CTS

American Association of Orthopedic Surgeons (AAOS) Clinical Practice Guideline endorsed by American Association of Neurological Surgeons, Congress of Neurological Surgeons, American Society of Plastic Surgeons, American Academy of PM&R and AANEM[34]

1. A course of non-operative treatment is an option in patients diagnosed with CTS. Early surgery is an option when there is clinical evidence of median nerve denervation or the patient elects to proceed directly to surgical treatment (Grade C, Level V)
2. another non-operative treatment or surgery is suggested when the current treatment fails to resolve the symptoms within 2- 7 weeks (Grade B, Level I and II)
3. There is not sufficient evidence to provide specific treatment recommendations for CTS when found in association with diabetes, coexisting cervical radiculopathy, hypothyroidism, polyneuropathy, pregnancy, rheumatoid arthritis and CTS in the workplace. (inconclusive)
4. Management specifics
   - local steroid injection or splinting is suggested when treating patients with CTS before considering surgery (Grade B, Level I and II)
   - oral steroids or ultrasound are options for treatment of CTS (Grade C, Level II)
   - carpal tunnel release is recommended for treatment of CTS (Grade A, level I)

Notwithstanding the AAOS recommendations, multiple studies report the results of carpal tunnel release in diabetics are good even when polyneuropathy is present.[35,36]

Non-surgical management

Options include:

1. rest
2. medications: non-steroidal anti-inflammatory drugs (NSAIDs), diuretics, and pyridoxine (vitamin B6) have been studied with no evidence of efficacy[11]
3. treatment of associated conditions (e.g. hypothyroidism or DM) is appropriate, but there is no data as to whether this relieves CTS[11]
4. **neutral position splints**: alleviates symptoms in > 80% of patients[37] (usually within a few days) and reduces prolonged sensory latencies.[38] Relapse is common (works best when patient does not return to heavy manual labor). A trial of at least 2–4 weeks is recommended
5. *steroid injection*: symptoms improve in > 75% of patients.[11] 33% relapse within 15 mos. Repeat injections are possible, but most clinicians limit to 3/year
   a) use 10–25 mg hydrocortisone. *Avoid local anesthetics* (may mask symptoms of intra-neural injection)
   b) inject into carpal tunnel (deep to transverse carpal ligament) to *ulnar side* of palmaris longus to avoid median nerve (in patients without palmaris longus, inject in line with fourth digit)
   c) median nerve injuries have been reported with this technique,[39] primarily due to intra-neural injection (all steroids are neurotoxic upon intrafascicular injection, and so are some of the carrier agents)
   d) risk factors for recurrence: severe electrodiagnostic abnormalities, constant numbness, impaired sensation, & weakness or atrophy of thenar muscles[11]

Surgical treatment

General information

30

The operation is commonly called a carpal tunnel release (CTR), AKA neurolysis or neuroplasty of the median nerve at the wrist.

Indications

Surgical intervention is recommended for: constant numbness, symptoms > 1 year duration, sensory loss, or thenar weakness/atrophy.[11] Surgical treatment of cases due to amyloidosis from multiple myeloma is also effective.

With bilateral CTS, in general one operates on the more *painful* hand first. However if the condition is severe in both hands (on EMG) and if it has progressed beyond the painful stage and is only causing weakness and/or numbness, it may be best to operate on the "better" hand first in order to try and maximize recovery of the median nerve at least on that side. Simultaneous bilateral procedures may also be done.[40] In severe cases, nerve recovery may not occur, it may be necessary to wait up to a year to determine extent of recovery.

Success rate

> 70% of patients report satisfaction with their surgical results,[41] with 70–90% being free of nocturnal pain.[41,42]

Surgical techniques

A number of techniques are popular, including: incision through palm of hand, transverse incision through wrist crease (with or without a retinaculatome[43]), and endoscopic techniques (using single or dual incisions). The efficacies of the various approaches have not been compared in an adequately powered randomized study[11] and there is no consensus on the superiority of any one technique[14,44,45,46] including endoscopic vs. open CTR.

Transpalmar approach (▶ Fig. 30.3): For a right-handed surgeon, sit in patient's "axilla" (facing head of patient) for left sided CTS. Sit above patient's arm (facing feet) for right sided CTS. Usually performed under local or regional anesthesia on outpatient basis. Magnification (operating loupes) are helpful.

Incision along imaginary line extending proximally from space between digits 3 and 4 (usually stay just to the ulnar side of the interthenar crease to avoid the PCB). The location of the median nerve may also be estimated by the palmaris longus tendon (stay slightly to ulnar side of tendon). Incision starts at distal wrist flexion crease, and the length depends on thickness of hand (it may extend as far distally as a line even with the crotch of the thumb). Optionally: curve ulnarward at proximal wrist flexion crease (to facilitate retraction).

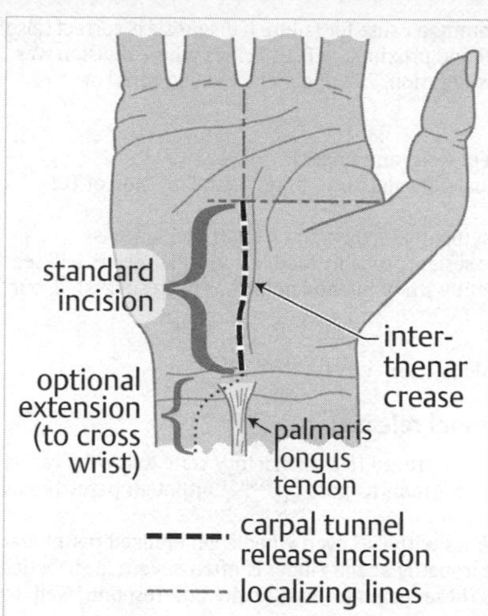

Fig. 30.3 Transpalmar incision for carpal tunnel syndrome

The median nerve is carefully approached through the TCL with progressively deepening incisions made with a 15 blade. All approaches to CTS surgery require complete division of TCL at and distal to the wrist. If tendons of the flexor digitorum superficialis are encountered, you need to look radially (towards the thumb) to find the nerve. In selected cases, the epineurium may be opened; however, internal neurolysis probably does more harm than good and in general should be avoided.

Close with absorbable 4–0 inverted sutures. Approximate skin edges with 4–0 nylon running or interrupted vertical mattress. Pad palm with several fluffs (opened dressing sponge). Cover with Kerlix®.

Post-op: wrap hand with thumb exposed. Wrist elevation and rest is recommended for several days. Analgesics for mild-to-moderate pain (e.g. acetaminophen with codeine) for 3–4 days. Sutures are removed at 7–10 days. No heavy work with hand for 2–3 weeks.

Complications of carpal tunnel surgery

See reference.[47]

1. pain due to neuroma formation following transection of **palmar cutaneous branch** (PCB) of the median nerve
   a) branches of PCB may cross interthenar crease
   b) avoid by: using magnification and making incision slightly to ulnar side of interthenar crease
   c) treated by ligating this branch where it originates from median nerve in forearm (results in small area of numbness at base of thenar eminence)
2. neuroma of dorsal sensory branch of radial nerve
   a) caused by extending incision proximally and radially
   b) may be treated by neurolysis of neuroma
3. injury to recurrent thenar (motor) branch of median nerve
   a) anomaly may cause nerve to lie above or to pierce TCL
   b) avoided by: staying to *ulnar side* of midline
4. direct injury to median nerve
5. volar displacement and entrapment of median nerve in healing edges of TCL
6. hypertrophic scar causing compression of median nerve
   a) usually caused by incision crossing wrist perpendicular to flexion crease
   b) avoid by not crossing flexion crease, or in cases where necessary (e.g. in releasing Guyon's canal entrapment of ulnar nerve, in tenosynovectomy for rheumatoid arthritis, or in dealing with an anomalous superficialis or palmaris muscle) by crossing wrist obliquely at 45° angle directed toward ulnar side[47] (see optional extension line in ▶ Fig. 30.3)
7. failure to improve symptoms
   a) incorrect diagnosis: if EMG or NCV not done pre-op, they should be done after surgical failure (to R/O e.g. cervical root involvement (look for posterior myotome involvement), or generalized peripheral neuropathy)

   b) incomplete transection of TCL: the most common cause for failure if diagnosis is correct (also possibility of accessory ligament or fascial band proximal to TCL in cases where division was complete). When this is identified on re-exploration, 75% of patients will be cured or improved after division is completed
8. joint stiffness
   a) caused by excessively long immobilization of wrist and fingers
9. injury to superficial palmar arch (arterial): usually results from "blind" distal division of TCL
10. bowstringing of flexor tendons
11. complex regional pain syndrome AKA reflex sympathetic dystrophy: exact incidence is unknown, reported in 4 of 132 patients in one series (probably too high, most surgeons will see only one or two cases in their career). Treatment with IV phentolamine has been suggested, but most cases are self limited after ≈ 2 weeks
12. infection: usually causes exquisite tenderness
13. hematoma: also usually quite painful and tender

Outcome of surgical treatment (carpal tunnel release)

75-90% of patients have symptom resolution or are improved to a satisfactory state following carpal tunnel release.[17,44,48] Clinical improvement peaks at 6 months post-op[49,50,51] although paresthesias may take ≥ 9 months to resolve.[44,52,53,54]

The results of decompression are good in diabetics with CTS even when a generalized peripheral neuropathy is present.[55] In comparison, ulnar neuropathy at the elbow is often severe in diabetics and predominantly motor with axonal injury. These patients usually do not respond well to surgery.[35]

Managing surgical treatment failures

30

Less than satisfactory outcomes following CTR should be categorized as:
1. new symptoms: may include neuropathic pain out of proportion to the surgery, new areas of numbness/ paresthesias or marked weakness of the thenar muscles.[56] When present immediately post-op, this suggests iatrogenic injury to branches of the median nerve
2. persistent symptoms (primary failure or failure to improve) defined as symptoms which remain unchanged compared to preop. Etiologies include: incorrect initial diagnosis, incomplete release of the transverse carpal ligament and severe (i.e. irreversible) CTS at initial diagnosis.[14]
3. or recurrent symptoms: requires symptom free interval before return of symptoms (there is no standardization of either the level of recurrent symptoms or length of interval,[44] although 6 months has been used in some studies[56]). Etiologies include: circumferential fibrosis around the median nerve, soft tissue adhesions, synovial proliferation, tenosynovitis, ganglions, amyloid deposits and subtle palmar subluxation.[14,56]

▶ **Electrodiagnostic (EDX) studies.** Following CTR, distal motor latency improves after 3 months and 6 months and may continue to improve for up to 2 years.[50,57,58] Electrophysiologic abnormalities may improve but may not return to normal range after CTR even with clinical improvement.[44,51] Electrophysiologic studies are most helpful when it is possible to compare to pre-op studies.[14,17,56,59,60] There are no guidelines or standard recommendations for when to obtain postoperative studies for surgical failures. It is reasonable to obtain repeat studies at 3 to 6 months following carpal tunnel release for persistent symptoms and at onset for new or recurrent symptoms. If the repeat nerve conduction studies are worse or if the EMG needle exam has findings of denervation (fibrillation potentials and positive sharp waves) not previously present, then repeat surgery is indicated.[17,56] If the preoperative study is not available, repeating the EDX study with comparison at 2 points in time to evaluate for improvement or worsening is advised. Prolonged latencies alone are not an indication for reoperation.[61]

30.5 Ulnar nerve entrapment

30.5.1 General information

Ulnar nerve has components of C7, C8 and T1 nerve roots. Even though this is the second most prevalent entrapment neuropathy after CTS, it is still relatively uncommon. Potential sites of compression:
1. above elbow: possibly by the arcade of Struthers
2. at the elbow: retroepicondylar groove ("ulnar groove"): between the medial epicondyle and the olecranon process. Compression by fascia or by dynamic compression or repetitive trauma

3. cubital: just distal to the ulnar groove, under the aponeurosis between the heads of the flexor carpi ulnaris (FCU)
4. at the point of exit from the FCU
5. wrist: Guyon's canal

Etiologies: structural, mechanical or idiopathic.

Motor findings include:

1. wasting of the interossei may occur, and is most evident in the first dorsal interosseous (in the thumb web space)
2. Wartenberg's sign: one of the earliest findings of ulnar nerve entrapment (abducted little finger due to weakness of the third palmar interosseous muscle–patient may complain that the little finger doesn't make it in when they reach into their pocket)
3. Froment's prehensile thumb sign: grasping a sheet of paper between thumb and the extended index finger results in extension of the proximal phalanx of the thumb and flexion of the distal phalanx as a result of substituting flexor pollicis longus (which is spared since it is innervated by anterior interosseous nerve) for the weak adductor pollicis[62 (p 18)]
4. claw deformity of the hand (main en griffe): in severe ulnar nerve injuries on attempted finger *extension* (some have called this "benediction hand", which differs from that with the same name in median nerve injury where the named sign occurs on trying to make a fist. Fingers 4 and 5 and to a lesser extent 3 are hyperextended at the MCP joints (extensor digitorum is unopposed by interossei and "ulnar" lumbricals III & IV) and flexed at the interphalangeal joints (due to pull of long flexor muscles). NB: C8 radiculopathy can also cause benediction sign[63])

Sensory findings: Disturbance of sensation involving:

1. The little finger and ulnar half of the ring finger
2. Sensory loss over the ulnar side of the dorsum of the hand. This will be spared in ulnar nerve entrapment at the wrist (dorsal ulnar cutaneous nerve branches proximal to the wrist)

30

30.5.2 Injury above elbow

May occur with injury to the medial cord of the brachial plexus.

In the upper arm, the ulnar nerve descends anterior to the medial head of triceps; in 70% of people it passes under arcade of Struthers – distinct from Struther's ligament (p. 518) – a flat, thin, aponeurotic band. This is not normally a point of entrapment, but may cause kinking after ulnar nerve transposition if not adequately divided.[64 (p 1781)]

30.5.3 Ulnar nerve entrapment at elbow (UNE)

General information

Entrapment at or just distal to the elbow produces the cubital tunnel syndrome. (Technically, the cubital tunnel is formed by the fibrous arch between the two heads of the FCU,[65 (p 877)] the proximal entrance to which is just distal to the retrocondylar groove. However, common vernacular usually includes entrapment within the groove itself as being "cubital tunnel syndrome.")

Can also present as so-called tardy ulnar palsy because of delayed onset following bony injury at the elbow, initial case reports occurred ≥ 12 years later, with the majority commencing > 10 years following the original injury The elbow is the most vulnerable point of ulnar nerve: here the nerve is superficial, fixed, and crosses a joint. Most cases are idiopathic, although there may be a history of elbow fracture (especially lateral condyle of the humerus, with associated cubitus valgus deformity), dislocation, arthritis, or repeated minor trauma. The aponeurotic arch extending over the ulnar groove and attaching on the medial epicondyle may become thickened and can compress the nerve, especially with elbow flexion.[65 (p 884)] The ulnar nerve may also be injured during anesthesia (p. 548).[66] In contrast to CTS which is predominantly demyelinating, UNE has more axonal loss even when chronic.[31]

Presentation

Typically presents with discomfort (pain, numbness and/or tingling) in little finger and ulnar half of ring finger, elbow pain, and hand weakness. Early symptoms may be purely motor (see Froment's sign and claw deformity above) – unlike the median nerve where sensory involvement is almost always present. Symptoms may be exacerbated by the cold, and are often somewhat vague and may be described as a loss of finger coordination or clumsiness. Cramping and easy fatiguing of the ulnar

Table 30.3 Stewart classification system for severity of ulnar nerve injury(Stewart[67] after Bartels[68])

Grade	Description
1 (mild)	sensory symptoms ± motor symptoms; ± sensory loss; no muscle atrophy or weakness
2 (moderate)	sensory symptoms with detectable sensory loss. Mild atrophy; 4 or 4 + muscle strength
3 (severe)	usually constant sensory symptoms with detectable sensory loss. Moderate to marked atrophy; 4- or less muscle strength.

innervated muscles of the hand may occur. Pain may *not* be a significant feature, but if present tends to be aching in nature along the ulnar aspect of the elbow or forearm. Atrophy of interossei is common by the time of presentation.

The ulnar nerve is usually tender and may be palpably enlarged in the ulnar groove. Tinel's sign may be positive over the elbow, but this is not very specific.

Grading: the classification system proposed by Stewart[67] is shown in ► Table 30.3.

Evaluation

Electrodiagnostic studies

The literature review from AANEM Practice Parameters for EDX studies in ulnar neuropathy at the elbow (UNE) report sensitivities to range from 37% to 86% with specificities of 95%.[28,29,30]

30

EDX interpretation: Reports should include localization and may comment on whether the lesion is predominantly demyelinating or axonal. Reports may use grading classification.[69]

The following suggest a focal lesion involving the ulnar nerve at the elbow. Multiple internally consistent abnormalities are more convincing than isolated abnormalities. These are listed in order of strength of evidence.

Sensory abnormalities of the distal sensory or mixed nerve action potential (NAP), especially loss of amplitude, are not localizing for ulnar neuropathy (in contradistinction to median nerve/carpal tunnel), the motor component of the exam for the ulnar nerve is more useful for localization of the site of entrapment.

Practice guideline: Electrodiagnostic criteria for ulnar neuropathy at the elbow

Not all criteria need to be present and an EMG needle exam is not required[29,70]:

1. absolute motor nerve conduction velocity (NCV) < 50 m/sec from below elbow (BE) to above elbow (AE)
2. drop of NCV > 10 m/sec comparing BE to wrist segment to the AE to BE segment
3. amplitude of compound motor action potential (CMAP) normally decreases with distance, but a drop > 20% from BE to AE is abnormal (in the absence of anomalous innervation, e.g. Martin-Gruber anastomosis (p. 514))
4. if ulnar motor studies with stimulation at the wrist, above and below the elbow recording from ADQ are inconclusive, the following may be of benefit:
   - NCS recorded from the FDI (first dorsal interosseus muscle, innervated by ulnar nerve)
   - inching study recording latencies and amplitudes at cm increments.
   - with severe UNE and wallerian degeneration -comparison of AE to BE with axilla to AE
   - needle EMG should always include FDI and ulnar innervated forearm muscles (flexor digitorum profundus (FDP) to ring or little finger and/or abductor digiti quinti/minimi (ADQ)). If abnormal then extend to include non-ulnar innervated C8, medial cord, lower trunk muscles and cervical paraspinals to exclude brachial plexopathy/cervical radiculopathy.

The 2 most important parameters that predict a good outcome are preserved compound muscle action potential (CMAP) amplitudes in ulnar hand muscles and conduction block (CB) with slowed conduction velocity across the elbow which is consistent with demyelination and has a better prognosis.[26,71] Poor prognosis correlates with small or absent CMAP and no CB consistent with axonal loss.[26]

Diagnostic ultrasound

Localizing ulnar nerve lesions with electrodiagnostic studies can be difficult. There has been a recent renewed interest in diagnostic ultrasound using high frequency (18 MHz) probes to help with localization, and also for identification of pathology, including nerve swelling, transection,[72] and neuroma, that exceeds MRI in some aspects and at a lower cost and with faster acquisition time.

Management of ulnar neuropathy at the elbow

There are no Clinical Practice Guidelines for treatment of UNE endorsed by AANEM, AAOS, CNS, AANS, AAPM&R, or Am Society of Plastic Surgeons. A fundamental difficulty in treating UNE are the multiple etiologies and locations so that the natural history and responses to treatment vary widely. The primary management decision is conservative versus surgical treatment.

A Cochrane Database Review concluded the available evidence is not sufficient to identify the best treatment for UNE on the basis of clinical, neurophysiologic and imaging characteristics.[73,74]

Nonsurgical treatment (see below) may be considered for the patient with intermittent symptoms, no atrophy and mild EDX findings. Surgical intervention has been advised for patients who fail conservative management, although the best nonsurgical management and duration of treatment are not well defined.[74]

Suggested protocol:

- mild or moderate UNE (grade 1 and 2, table 30.3): treat conservatively as studies report improvement or complete recovery in 30-90%.[31,67] Follow these patients every 2 months to detect deterioration. If worsening occurs image with CT or MRI. Surgical exploration is indicated regardless of imaging results
- severe (grade 3) UNE: initiate conservative treatment, obtain imaging and f/u in 1 month. If there is worsening or if structural abnormality found or both then surgical intervention. If stable or improving and imaging normal then follow at monthly intervals. Surgical intervention for worsening.[67]

There is a probable increased prevalence of UNE in diabetics. The UNE is often more severe with predominant axonal injury and these patients do not respond well to surgery.[35]

Non-surgical treatment

Patient education on positions to avoid (prolonged elbow bending to ≥ 90° flexion). Avoid trauma to the elbow, including resting it on firm surfaces (tables, rigid armrests in motor vehicles…), an elbow pad may help. Results are often better when definite traumatic etiology can be identified and eliminated.

Surgical treatment

General approach

Most operations utilize a "lazy omega" skin incision centered over the medial epicondyle, extending at least ≈ 6 cm proximal and distal to elbow with the central "hump" directed anteriorly. The ulnar nerve is most constant and therefore most easily found immediately at the entrance to the ulnar groove. It may then be followed proximally and distally. Nerve branches that should be preserved include: posterior branches of the medial antebrachial cutaneous nerve (or else numbness or dysesthesias along medial forearm may occur) and branches to the flexor carpi ulnaris (which may branch early). Small articular branches at or proximal to the elbow joint can be preserved with simple decompression but may need to be sacrificed in transposition if they cannot be dissected far enough along the ulnar nerve. Internal neurolysis should be avoided as it may promote intraneural fibrosis.

The choice of one of the options below will determine subsequent steps.

Surgical options primarily consist of:

1. simple nerve decompression without transposition[75] (see below). Includes all of the following:
   a) at the elbow: division of the cubital tunnel retinaculum
   b) distal to the elbow: dividing the aponeurosis connecting the two heads of the flexor carpi ulnaris, some advocate resuturing the aponeurosis underneath the nerve
   c) proximal to the elbow: dividing the medial intermuscular septum (between distal biceps and triceps muscles) and the arcade of Struthers (if present)
   d) preservation of the branch to the flexor carpi ulnaris and the dorsal cutaneous branch to the hand (arises 5 cm proximal to wrist)

2. nerve decompression and transposition (extent of surgery differs because degree of entrapment varies; all forms of transposition require fashioning a sling to retain the nerve in its new location). Transposition may be to:
   a) subcutaneous tissue: this leaves the nerve fairly superficial and vulnerable to further trauma
   b) within the flexor carpi ulnaris muscle (intramuscular transposition): some contend this actually worsens the condition due to intramuscular fibrosis
   c) a submuscular position: below
3. medial epicondylectomy. Usually combined with decompression. Normally reserved for patients with a bony deformity
4. sometimes excision of neuroma and possibly jump graft may be required

Submuscular transposition

Placement under pronator teres, within a groove fashioned in the flexor carpi ulnaris (FCU). Usually requires general anesthesia (endotracheal or laryngeal mask airway).

Some key concepts[76(p 247, 260–5),77]:

1. the skin incision must extend at least ≈ 8 cm distal and proximal to the medial epicondyle to mobilize the nerve (spare the medial antecubital cutaneous nerve in the subcutaneous fatty tissue just distal to the elbow)
2. the nerve is mobilized, sparing branches to flexor carpi ulnaris (FCU) and the ulnar flexor profundi branch(es) (usually arise 2–4 cm distal to olecranon)
3. the medial intermuscular septum (between distal biceps and triceps muscles) must be cut in the distal arm to prevent the nerve from being kinked over it
4. the pronator teres muscle must be sectioned completely through just distal to the medial epicondyle
   a) start by undermining the muscle just distal to the medial epicondyle
   b) a mosquito hemostat may be passed under the muscle to assist
   c) the muscle is cut sharply, cautery is used to treat bleeding areas
5. a trough is cut in the volar aspect of the FCU to accommodate the nerve
6. after the pronator teres is reattached over the nerve, make sure that the nerve can slide back-and-forth easily under the muscle
7. test the elbow through a range of motion after the transposition to look for snapping of the medial portion of the triceps over the medial epicondyle[78]

30

Transposition vs. decompression

Σ

For most cases, simple decompression is recommended over transposition. Possible exceptions include: bony deformity, nerve subluxation

Randomized studies have shown similar success but lower complication rate with simple decompression vs. transposition.[73,79,80] Advantages of simple decompression include[68,81]: shorter operation that can be done more easily under local anesthesia, avoidance of nerve kinking and muscular fibrosis around the transposed nerve, reduced risk of wound infection[73] and scar formation,[67] and preservation of cutaneous branches, ulnar branches, and nourishing blood vessels (vasa nervorum[67]) that are sometimes sacrificed with transposition, rendering portions of the nerve ischemic.

Arguments against simple decompression: Continued dynamic compression with elbow flexion, possible nerve subluxation (if present pre-op, simple decompression may make this worse; to avoid nerve subluxation and loss of vascular supply with simple decompression, avoid a 360° freeing of the nerve) and incomplete release of pressure points.

Results with surgery

Not as good as with CTS, possibly due in part to the fact that patients tend to present much later. Overall, a good to excellent result is obtained in 60%, fair result in 25%, and a poor result (no improvement or worsening) in 15%.[82(p 2530)] These results may be worse in patients with symptoms present > 1 year, with only 30% of these symptomatically improved in one series.[75] Lower success rate is also seen in older patients and those with certain medical conditions (diabetes, alcoholism…). Pain and sensory changes respond better than muscle weakness and atrophy.

30.5.4 Entrapment in the forearm

Very rare. Just distal to the elbow, the ulnar nerve passes from the retroepicondylar groove to pass under the fascial band connecting the two heads of the flexor carpi ulnaris (FCU), superficial to the flexor superficialis and pronator teres. Findings with entrapment in the forearm are similar to tardy ulnar nerve palsy (see above).

Surgical treatment consists of steps outlined for nerve distal to the elbow in ulnar nerve decompression (see above). A technique for locating the course of the ulnar nerve distal to the elbow: the surgeon takes the little finger of his/her own hand (using the hand contralateral to the patient's side that is being decompressed) and places the proximal phalanx in the ulnar groove aiming it toward the ulnar side of the wrist.[76 (p 262)]

30.5.5 Entrapment in the wrist or hand

At the wrist, the terminal ulnar nerve enters Guyon's canal, the roof of which is the palmar fascia and palmaris brevis, the floor is the flexor retinaculum of the palm and the pisohamate ligament.

► **Guyon's canal.** Is *superficial* to the transverse carpal ligament (which overlies the carpal tunnel and compresses the median nerve in carpal tunnel syndrome).

The canal contains no tendons, only the ulnar nerve and artery. At the middle of the canal the nerve divides into a deep and superficial branch. The superficial branch is mostly sensory (except for the branch to palmaris brevis), and supplies hypothenar eminence and ulnar half of ring finger. The deep (muscular) branch innervates hypothenar muscles, lumbricals 3 & 4, and all interossei. Occasionally the abductor digiti minimi branch arises from the main trunk or superficial branch.

Shea and McClain[83] divided lesions of the ulnar nerve in Guyon's canal into 3 types shown in ► Table 30.4. Injury to the distal motor branch can also occur in the palm and produces findings similar to a Type II injury.

Injury is most often due to a ganglion of the wrist,[84] but also may be due to trauma (use of pneumatic drill, pliers, repetitively slamming a stapler, leaning on palm while riding bicycle). Symptoms are similar to those of ulnar nerve involvement at the elbow, except there will never be sensory loss in the *dorsum* of the hand in the ulnar nerve territory because the dorsal cutaneous branch leaves the nerve in the forearm 5–8 cm proximal to the wrist (sparing of flexor carpi ulnaris and flexor digitorum profundus III & IV is not helpful in localizing because these are so rarely involved even in proximal lesions). Electrodiagnostics are usually helpful in localizing the site of the lesion. Pain, when present, may be exacerbated by tapping over pisiform (Tinel's sign). It may also radiate up the forearm.

Surgical decompression may be indicated in refractory cases. To locate: find the ulnar artery, and the nerve is on the ulnar side of the artery. Controversial whether simple decompression vs. subcutaneous transposition is best, the outcome is similar but there may be more complications in the transposition group[79,80] but studies are small.

Table 30.4 Types of ulnar nerve lesions in Guyon's canal

Type	Location of compression	Weakness	Sensory deficit
Type I	just proximal to or within Guyon's canal	all intrinsic hand muscles innervated by ulnar n.	palmar ulnar distribution[a]
Type II	along deep branch	muscles innervated by deep branch[b]	none
Type III	distal end of Guyon's canal	none	palmar ulnar distribution[a]

[a]palmar ulnar distribution: the hypothenar eminence and ulnar half of ring finger, both on the palmar surface only (the dorsum is innervated by the dorsal cutaneous nerve)
[b]depending on the location, may spare hypothenar muscles

30

30.6 Radial nerve injuries

See reference.[85(p 1443–45)]

30.6.1 Applied anatomy

The radial nerve arises from the posterior divisions of the 3 trunks of the brachial plexus. Receives contributions from C5 to C8. The nerve winds laterally along the spiral groove of the humerus where it is vulnerable to compression or injury from fracture.

Distinguish radial nerve injury from injury of posterior cord of brachial plexus by sparing of deltoid (axillary nerve) and latissimus dorsi (thoracodorsal nerve).

30.6.2 Axillary compression

Etiologies: crutch misuse; poor arm position during (drunken) sleep.

30.6.3 Mid-upper arm compression

Etiologies

1. "Saturday night palsy": improper positioning of arm in sleep (especially when drunk and therefore less likely to self-reposition in response to the accompanying discomfort, e.g. due to a bedmate's head resting on the arm)
2. from positioning under general anesthesia
3. from callus due to old humeral fracture

Clinical: weakness of wrist extensors (wrist drop) and finger extensors. ✱ Key: *triceps is normal* because takeoff of nerve to triceps is proximal to spiral groove. Involvement of distal nerve is variable, may include thumb extensor palsy and paresthesias in radial nerve distribution. Differential diagnosis: isolated wrist and finger extensor weakness can also occur in lead poisoning (usually bilateral, more common in adults).

Forearm compression

General information

The radial nerve enters the anterior compartment of the arm just above the elbow. It gives off branches to brachialis, brachioradialis, and extensor carpi radialis (ECR) longus before dividing into the posterior interosseous nerve and the superficial radial nerve. The posterior interosseous nerve dives into the supinator muscle through a fibrous band known as the arcade of Frohse.

Posterior interosseous neuropathy

Posterior interosseous neuropathy (often referred to by its acronym "PIN") may result from: lipomas, ganglia, fibromas, rheumatoid arthritis changes at elbow, entrapment at the arcade of Frohse (rare), and occasionally from strenuous use of the arm.

Treatment: cases that do not respond to 4–8 weeks of expectant management should be explored, and any constrictions lysed (including arcade of Frohse).

Radial tunnel syndrome

AKA supinator syndrome. Controversial. The "radial tunnel" extends from just above the elbow to just distal to it, and is composed of different structures (muscles, fibrous bands…) depending on the level.[86] It contains the radial nerve and its two main branches (posterior interosseous and superficial radial nerves). Repeated forceful supination or pronation or inflammation of supinator muscle attachments (as in tennis elbow) may traumatize the nerve (sometimes by ECR brevis). Characteristic finding: pain in the region of the common extensor origin at the lateral epicondyle on resisted extension of the middle finger which tightens the ECR brevis. May be mistakenly diagnosed as resistant "tennis elbow" (lateral epicondylitis must be excluded). There may also be peristhesias in the distribution of the superficial radial nerve and local tenderness along the radial nerve anterior to the radial head. Even though the site of entrapment is similar to PIN, unlike PIN, there is usually no muscle weakness. Surgery: rarely required, consists of nerve decompression.[86]

Injury in the hand

The distal cutaneous branches of the superficial radial nerve cross the extensor pollicis longus tendon, and can often be palpated at this point with the thumb in extension. Injury to the medial branch of this nerve occurs commonly e.g. with handcuff injuries, and causes a small area of sensory loss in the dorsal web-space of the thumb.

30.7 Axillary nerve injuries

Isolated neuropathy of the axillary nerve may occur in the following situations[87]:
1. shoulder dislocation: the nerve is tethered to the joint capsule[88]
2. sleeping in the prone position with the arms abducted above the head
3. compression from a thoracic harness
4. injection injury in the high posterior aspect of the shoulder
5. entrapment of the nerve in the quadrilateral space (bounded by the teres major and minor muscles, long head of triceps, and neck of humerus) which contains the axillary nerve and the posterior humeral circumflex artery. Arteriogram may show loss of filling of the artery with the arm abducted and externally rotated

30.8 Suprascapular nerve

► **General information.** The suprascapular nerve is a mixed peripheral nerve arising from the superior trunk of the brachial plexus, with contributions from C5 & C6. There is often a history of shoulder trauma or frozen shoulder. Entrapment results in weakness & atrophy of infra- and supraspinatus (IS & SS) and deep, poorly localized (referred) shoulder pain (the sensory part of the nerve innervates the posterior joint capsule but has no cutaneous representation).

30

► **Etiologies**
1. nerve entrapment within the suprascapular notch beneath the transverse scapular (suprascapular) ligament (TSL)[89]
2. repetitive shoulder trauma: may be bilateral when the injury is from activities such as weightlifting
3. ganglion or tumor[90] (MRI is the test of choice for imaging these)
4. paralabral cyst from labral tear (the tendon of the long head of the biceps attaches to the superior glenoid labrum; test of choice for labral tears is MR arthrography)

► **Differential diagnosis**[89]
1. pathology in or around shoulder joint
   a) rotator cuff injuries (distinction may be very difficult)
   b) adhesive capsulitis
   c) bicipital tenosynovitis
   d) arthritis
2. cases of Parsonage-Turner syndrome limited to the suprascapular nerve; see Neuralgic amyotrophy (p. 543)
3. **cervical radiculopathy (≈ C5)**
4. **upper brachial plexus lesion**

NB: cervical radiculopathy and upper brachial plexus lesion will also produce rhomboid and deltoid weakness and, usually, cutaneous sensory loss.

Diagnosis requires temporary relief with nerve block, and EMG abnormalities of SS & IS (in rotator cuff tears, fibrillation potentials will be absent). Transient pain relief with a suprascapular nerve block helps verify the diagnosis.[91]

► **Treatment.** In cases where a mass is not the underlying cause, initial treatment consists of resting the affected UE, PT (including gentle conditioning), NSAIDs, topical capsaicin cream, and sometimes corticosteroid injection.

Surgical treatment is indicated for documented cases that fail to improve with conservative treatment (PT, NSAIDs, steroid/local anesthetic injection...). Position: lateral decubitus. Incision: 2 cm above and parallel to the scapular spine (atrophy of SS facilitates this). Only the trapezius needs to be split along its fibers (caution re spinal accessory nerve). To locate suprascapular notch, follow omohyoid to where it attaches to scapula and palpate just lateral to this. The suprascapular artery and vein pass over the TSL and should be preserved. Elevate the TSL with a dull nerve hook and divide it (exposure of the nerve and/or resection of the bony notch are not necessary).

30.9 Meralgia paresthetica

30.9.1 General information

AKA Originally known as the Bernhardt-Roth syndrome, and sometimes called "swashbuckler's disease", meralgia paresthetica (MP) (Greek: meros – thigh, algos – pain) is a condition often caused by entrapment of the lateral femoral cutaneous nerve (LFCN) of the thigh, (a purely sensory branch with contributions from L2 and L3 nerve roots, see ▶ Fig. 1.14 for distribution) where it enters the thigh though the opening between the inguinal ligament and its attachment to the anterior superior iliac spine (ASIS). Anatomic variation is common, and the nerve may actually pass through the ligament, and as many as four branches may be found. May also be an initial manifestation of diabetes (diabetic neuropathy).

30.9.2 Signs and symptoms

Burning dysesthesias in the lateral aspect of the upper thigh, occasionally just above the knee, usually with increased sensitivity to clothing (hyperpathia). There may be decreased sensation in this distribution. Spontaneous rubbing or massaging the area in order to obtain relief is very characteristic.[92] MP may be bilateral in up to 20% of cases. Sitting or lying prone usually ameliorates the symptoms.

There may be point tenderness at the site of entrapment (where pressure may reproduce the pain), which is often located where the nerve exits the pelvis medial to the ASIS. Hip extension may also cause pain.

30

30.9.3 Occurrence

Usually seen in obese patients, may be exacerbated by wearing tight belts or girdles, and by prolonged standing or walking. Recently found in long distance runners. Higher incidence in diabetics. May also occur post-op in slender patients positioned prone, tends to be *bilateral* (p. 549).

Possible etiologies are too numerous to list, more common ones include: tight clothing or belts, surgical scars post-abdominal surgery, cardiac catheterization (p. 549), pregnancy, iliac crest bone graft harvesting, ascites, obesity, metabolic neuropathies, and abdominal or pelvic mass.

30.9.4 Differential diagnosis

1. femoral neuropathy: sensory changes tend to be more anteromedial than MP
2. L2 or L3 radiculopathy: look for motor weakness (thigh flexion or knee extension)
3. nerve compression by abdominal or pelvic tumor (suspected if concomitant GI or GU symptoms)

The condition can usually be diagnosed on clinical grounds. When it is felt to be necessary, confirmatory tests may help (but frequently are disappointing), including:

1. EMG: may be difficult, the electromyographer cannot always find the nerve)
2. MRI or CT/myelography: when disc disease is suspected
3. pelvic imaging (MRI or CT)
4. somatosensory evoked potentials
5. response to local anesthetic injections
6. recent promise of diagnostic ultrasound using high frequency (18 MHz) probes

30.9.5 Treatment

Nonsurgical management

Tends to regress spontaneously, but recurrence is common. Nonsurgical measures achieve relief in ≈ 91% of cases and should be tried prior to considering surgery[93]:

1. remove offending articles (constricting belts, braces, casts, tight garments…)
2. in obese patients: weight loss and exercises to strengthen the abdominal muscles is usually effective, but is rarely achieved by the patient
3. elimination of activities involving hip extension

4. application of ice to the area of presumed constriction × 30 minutes TID
5. NSAID of choice × 7–10 days
6. capsaicin ointment applied TID (p. 496)
7. lidoderm patches (p. 477) in areas of hyperesthesia may help[94]
8. centrally acting pain medications (e.g. gabapentin, carbamazepine…) are rarely effective
9. if the above measures fail, injection of 5–10 ml of local anesthetic (with or without steroids) at the point of tenderness, or medial to the ASIS may provide temporary or sometimes long lasting relief, and confirms the diagnosis

Surgical treatment

Options include:
1. surgical decompression (neurolysis) of the nerve: higher failure and recurrence rate than neurectomy
2. decompression and transposition
3. selective L2 nerve stimulation
4. division of the nerve (neurectomy) may be more effective, but risks denervation pain, and leaves an anesthetic area (usually a minor nuisance). May be best reserved for treatment failures

Technique

See references.[93,95]

The operation is best performed under general anesthesia. A 4–6 cm oblique incision is centered 2 cm distal to the point of tenderness. Since the course of the nerve is variable, the operation is exploratory in nature, and generous exposure is required. If the nerve can't be located, it is usually because the exposure is too superficial. If the nerve still cannot be found, a small abdominal muscle incision can be made and the nerve may be located in the retroperitoneal area. CAUTION: cases have occurred where the femoral nerve has erroneously been divided.

If neurectomy instead of neurolysis is elected, electrical stimulation should be performed prior to sectioning to rule out a motor component (which would disqualify the nerve as the LFCN). If the nerve is to be divided, it should be placed on stretch and then cut to allow the proximal end to retract back into the pelvis. Any segment of apparent pathology should be resected for microscopic analysis. Neurectomy results in anesthesia in the distribution of the LFCN that is rarely distressing and gradually reduces in size.

A supra-inguinal ligament approach has also been described.[95]

30.10 Obturator nerve entrapment

Controversial if this exists. The obturator nerve is composed of L2–4 roots. It courses along the pelvic wall to provide sensation to the inner thigh, and motor to the thigh adductors (gracilis and adductors longus, brevis, and magnus). It may be compressed by pelvic tumors, also from the pressure of the fetal head or forceps during parturition.

The result is numbness of the medial thigh and weak thigh adduction.

30.11 Femoral nerve entrapment

Composed of roots L2–4. Entrapment is a rare cause of femoral neuropathy. More commonly due to fracture or surgery. See Femoral neuropathy (p. 546).

30.12 Common peroneal nerve palsy

30.12.1 General information and applied anatomy

The peroneal nerve is the most common nerve to develop acute compression palsy.

Functional anatomy: the sciatic nerve (L4-S3) consists of 2 separate nerves within a common sheath that separate at a variable location in the thigh (the peroneal division of the sciatic nerve is more vulnerable to injury than the tibial division); see ▶ Fig. 92.1 for diagram:
1. posterior tibial nerve, or, just tibial nerve (AKA medial popliteal nerve) which provides for foot inversion among other motor functions
2. common peroneal nerve (CPN), or, just peroneal nerve (AKA lateral popliteal nerve): high injuries may involve the lateral hamstring (short head of the biceps femoris) in addition to the following.

30

The CPN passes behind the fibular head where it is superficial and fixed, making it vulnerable to pressure or trauma (e.g. from crossing the legs at the knee). Just distal to this, the CPN divides into:

a) deep peroneal nerve (AKA anterior tibial nerve): primarily motor
   - motor: foot and toe extension (extensor hallicus longus (EHL), anterior tibialis (AT), extensor digitorum longus (EDL))
   - sensory: very small area between great toe and second toe
b) superficial peroneal nerve (AKA musculocutaneous nerve)
   - motor: foot eversion (peroneus longus and brevis)
   - sensory: lateral distal leg and dorsum of foot

30.12.2 Causes of common peroneal nerve injury

The most frequent cause of serious peroneal nerve injury is knee injury ± fracture; see also causes of foot drop other than peroneal nerve palsy (p. 1417).

1. entrapment as it crosses the fibular neck or as it penetrates the peroneus longus
2. diabetes mellitus and other metabolic peripheral neuropathies
3. inflammatory neuropathy: including Hansen's disease (leprosy)
4. traumatic: e.g. clipping injury in football players, stretch injury due to dislocating force applied to the knee, fibular fracture, injury during hip or knee replacement surgery
5. penetrating injury
6. masses in the area of the fibular head/proximal lower leg: popliteal fossa cysts (Baker cyst), anterior tibial artery aneurysm[96] (rare)
7. pressure at fibular head: e.g. from crossing the legs at the knee, casts, obstetrical stirrups…
8. traction injuries: severe inversion sprains of the ankle
9. intraneural tumors: neurofibroma, schwannoma, neurogenic sarcoma, ganglion cysts
10. vascular: venous thrombosis
11. weight loss

30.12.3 Findings in peroneal nerve palsy

General information

1. sensory changes (uncommon): involves lateral aspect of lower half of leg
2. muscle involvement: See ▶ Table 30.5

Common peroneal nerve palsy (most common) produces weak ankle dorsiflexion (foot drop) due to anterior tibialis palsy, weak foot eversion, and sensory impairment in areas innervated by deep and superficial peroneal nerve (lateral calf and dorsum of foot). There may be a Tinel's sign with percussion over the nerve near the fibular neck. Occasionally, only the deep peroneal nerve is involved, resulting in foot drop with minimal sensory loss. Must differentiate from other causes of foot drop (p. 1416).

Examination/clinical correlation

See reference.[76(p 293)]

- buttock level injury: unless the injury is one that permits spontaneous regeneration, prognosis is poor for return of peroneal nerve function even with surgery

Table 30.5 Muscle involvement in peroneal nerve palsy

Muscle	Nerve	Action	Involvement
EHL	deep peroneal	great toe dorsiflexion	Most commonly involved ↓ ↓ ↓ Least commonly involved (often spared)
anterior tibialis		ankle dorsiflexion	
EDL		toe extension	
peroneus longus & brevis	superficial peroneal	foot eversion	

- thigh level injury: also difficult to get improvement with surgical repair. Some peroneus function may occur at ≥ 6 mos, early contraction of AT may take ≥ 1 yr
- knee level injury: with successful regeneration, peroneus contraction may begin by 3–5 months. First signs: quivering of muscle lateral to the proximal fibula on attempted foot eversion, or tightening of tendon posterior and behind the lateral malleolus on attempted ankle dorsiflexion

30.12.4 Evaluation

EMG

EMG takes 2–4 weeks from the onset of symptoms to become positive. Stimulate above and below fibular head for prognostic information: if absent in both sites, the prognosis is poor (indicates retrograde degeneration has occurred). Wallerian degeneration takes ≈ 5 days to cause deterioration.

In addition to the expected findings of denervation – PSWs & fibs (p. 242) – in the anterior tibialis, evaluate:

1. L5 innervated muscles outside the distribution of the common peroneal nerve:
   a) posterior tibialis
   b) flexor digitorum longus
2. L5 muscles whose nerve originates above the knee (these muscles are *spared* in cases of compression of the peroneal nerve at the fibular head due to the fact that the nerve takeoff is proximal to the popliteal fossa):
   a) biceps femoris (short or long head)
   b) tensor fascia lata
3. paraspinal muscles: signs of denervation solidifies the location of the lesion as nerve root; not helpful if negative

MRI

May demonstrate causes such as tumor or a ganglion cyst arising from the superior tibiofibular articulation.

30.12.5 Treatment

General information

When treatment can eliminate a reversible cause, the outcome is usually good. Surgical exploration and decompression may be considered when there is no reversible cause or when improvement does not occur.

Nonsurgical management

Bracing: ankle-foot-orthosis (AFO) compensates for loss of ankle dorsiflexion which inserts unobtrusively into a shoe. If this is inadequate, or to stabilize the ankle, a spring-loaded kick-up foot brace built into a shoe may be used. The patient should be instructed in techniques to avoid contracture of the Achilles tendon (heel cord) which would impair ankle dorsiflexion if nerve function returns.

Surgical management

At the level of the popliteal fossa the skin incision is made just medial to the tendon of the short head of the biceps femoris (lateral hamstring) as the peroneal nerve is best located deep to or slightly medial to this tendon. The incision is carried distally slightly laterally along the surgical neck of the fibula. The biceps femoris is retracted laterally and the nerve is isolated and tagged with a Penrose drain. The sensory sural nerve branches off the peroneal nerve at variable sites ranging from the sciatic portion of the nerve (proximal to the flexor crease) or distal to this.

In cases of compression, the fascia from the lateral gastrocnemius and soleus overlying the nerve distal to the fibular head is lysed and the nerve is exposed in 360°. As the nerve crosses the fibular neck it divides into superficial and deep branches. The superficial branch travels directly distally to supply the peroneus longus and brevis (foot evertors). The deep branches curve anteriorly to the anterior tibialis, EHL, and toe extensors.

If a graft is needed, the contralateral sural nerve is usually used, which may be supplemented with the ipsilateral sural nerve if needed.

30.13 Tarsal tunnel

30.13.1 General information

Entrapment of (posterior) tibial nerve may occur in the tarsal tunnel, posterior and inferior to *medial* malleolus. The tunnel is covered by the flexor retinaculum (laciniate ligament) which extends downward from the medial malleolus to the tubercle of the calcaneus. There is often (but not necessarily) a history of old ankle dislocation or fracture. The nerve may be trapped at the retinacular ligament. This results in pain and paresthesias in the toes and sole of foot (often sparing the heel because the sensory branches often originate proximal to the tunnel), typically worse at night. May cause clawing of toes secondary to weakness of intrinsic foot muscles. Often caused by fracture or dislocation, also rheumatoid arthritis, rarely tumors.

30.13.2 Exam

Percussion of nerve at medial malleolus produces paresthesias that radiate distally (Tinel's sign). Maximal inversion and eversion of the foot tend to exacerbate. Dorsiflexion-eversion test: examiner maximally everts and dorsiflexes the ankle while dorsiflexing the toes at the MTP joints for 5–10 seconds. Positive test reproduces the pain.

30.13.3 Diagnosis

EMG and NCV studies may help.

30.13.4 Nonsurgical management

External ankle support to improve foot mechanics.

30.13.5 Surgical management

Surgical decompression is indicated for confirmed cases that fail to improve. A curvilinear incision is used, ≈ 1.5 cm posterior and inferior to the medial malleolus. The flexor retinaculum is divided, as are any septa underneath, and the distal branches should be followed until they dive into the muscle.

References

[1] Neary D, Ochoa JL, Gilliatt RW. Subclinical Entrapment Neuropathy in Man. J Neurol Sci. 1975; 24:283–298

[2] Graff-Radford SB, Jaeger B, Reeves JL. Myofascial Pain May Present Clinically as Occipital Neuralgia. Neurosurgery. 1986; 19:610–613

[3] Hunter CR, Mayfield FH. Role of the Upper Cervical Roots in the Production of Pain in the Head. Am J Surg. 1949; 48:743–751

[4] Poletti CE, Sweet WH. Entrapment of the C2 Root and Ganglion by the Atlanto-Epistrophic Ligament: Clinical Syndrome and Surgical Anatomy. Neurosurgery. 1990; 27:288–291

[5] Anthony M. Headache and the greater occipital nerve. Clin Neurol Neurosurg. 1992; 94:297–301

[6] Weiner RL, Reed KL. Peripheral neurostimulation for control of intractable occipital neuralgia. Neuromodulation. 1999; 2:217–221

[7] Freund BJ, Schwartz M. Treatment of chronic cervical-associated headache with botulinum toxin A: a pilot study. Headache. 2000; 40:231–236

[8] Weinberger LM. Cervico-Occipital Pain and Its Surgical Treatment. Am J Surg. 1978; 135:243–247

[9] Bogduk N. Local Anesthetic Blocks of the Second Cervical Ganglion. A Technique with Application in Occipital Headache. Cephalalgia. 1981; 1:41–50

[10] Bovim G, Fredriksen TA, Stolt-Nielsen A, Sjaastad O. Neurolysis of the greater occipital nerve in cervicogenic headache. A follow up study. Headache. 1992; 32:175–179

[11] Katz JN, Simmons BP. Clinical practice. Carpal tunnel syndrome. N Engl J Med. 2002; 346:1807–1812

[12] Laha RK, Lunsford LD, Dujovny M. Lacertus Fibrosus Compression of the Median Nerve. J Neurosurg. 1978; 48:838–841

[13] Nakano KK, Lundergan C, Okihiro M. Anterior Interosseous Nerve Syndromes: Diagnostic Methods and Alternative Treatments. Arch Neurol. 1977; 34:477–480

[14] Stewart JD. In: Median Nerve. Focal Peripheral Neuropathies . 4th ed. West Vancouver, Canada: JBJ Publishing; 2010:214–239

[15] Yasargil MG, Antic J, Laciga R, et al. Microsurgical Pterional Approach to Aneurysms of the Basilar Bifurcation. Surg Neurol. 1976; 6

[16] Atroshi I, Gummesson C, Johnsson R, Ornstein E, Ranstam J, Rosen I. Prevalence of carpal tunnel syndrome in a general population. JAMA. 1999; 282:153–158

[17] Mosier BA, Hughes TB. Recurrent carpal tunnel syndrome. Hand Clin. 2013; 29:427–434

[18] Jain NB, Higgins LD, Losina E, Collins J, Blazar PE, Katz JN. Epidemiology of musculoskeletal upper extremity ambulatory surgery in the United States. BMC Musculoskelet Disord. 2014; 15. DOI: 10.1186/1471-2474-15-4

[19] Feldman RG, Goldman R, Keyserling WM. Classical Syndromes in Occupational Medicine: Peripheral Nerve Entrapment Syndromes and Ergonomic Factors. Am J Ind Med. 1983; 4:661–681

[20] Padua L, Aprile I, Caliandro P, et al. Carpal tunnel syndrome in pregnancy: multiperspective follow-up of untreated cases. Neurology. 2002; 59:1643–1646

[21] Phalen GS. The Carpal Tunnel Syndrome. Clinical Evaluation of 598 Hands. Clin Ortho Rel Res. 1972; 83

[22] Sandzen SC. Carpal Tunnel Syndrome. Am Fam Physician. 1981; 24:190–204

[23] Upton RM, McComas AJ. The Double Crush in Nerve Entrapment Syndromes. Lancet. 1973; 11:359–362

[24] Wilbourn AJ, Gilliatt RW. Double-Crush Syndrome: A Critical Analysis. Neurology. 1997; 49:21–29

[25] Rempel DM, Harrison RJ, Barnhart S. Work-Related Cumulative Trauma Disorders of the Upper Extremity. JAMA. 1992; 267:838–842

[26] Robinson LR. How electrodiagnosis predicts clinical outcome of focal peripheral nerve lesions. Muscle Nerve. 2015; 52:321–333

[27] Werner RA, Andary M. Electrodiagnostic evaluation of carpal tunnel syndrome. Muscle Nerve. 2011; 44:597–607

[28] Jablecki CK, Andary MT, Floeter MK, Miller RG, Quartly CA, Vennix MJ, Wilson JR, American Association of Electrodiagnostic Medicine, American Academy of Neurology, American Academy of Physical Medicine, Rehabilitation. Practice parameter: Electrodiagnostic studies in carpal tunnel syndrome. Report of the American Association of Electrodiagnostic Medicine, American Academy of Neurology, and the American Academy of Physical Medicine and Rehabilitation. Neurology. 2002; 58:1589–1592

[29] Campbell WW. Guidelines in electrodiagnostic medicine. Practice parameter for electrodiagnostic studies in ulnar neuropathy at the elbow. Muscle Nerve Suppl. 1999; 8:S171–S205

[30] American Association of Electrodiagnostic Medicine. Chapter 9: Practice parameter for needle electromyographic evaluation of patients with suspected cervical radiculopathy: Summary statement. Muscle Nerve. 1999; 22:S209–S211

[31] Bland JD. A neurophysiological grading scale for carpal tunnel syndrome. Muscle Nerve. 2000; 23:1280–1283

[32] Robinson L, Kliot M. Stop using arbitrary grading schemes in carpal tunnel syndrome. Muscle Nerve. 2008; 37. DOI: 10.1002/mus.21012

[33] Bland JD. Stop using arbitrary grading schemes in carpal tunnel syndrome. Muscle Nerve. 2008; 38:1527; author reply 1527–1527; author reply 1528

[34] Keith MW, Masear V, Chung KC, Amadio PC, Andary M, Barth RW, Maupin K, Graham B, Watters WC,3rd, Turkelson CM, Haralson RH,3rd, Wies JL, McGowan R. American Academy of Orthopaedic Surgeons clinical practice guideline on the treatment of carpal tunnel syndrome. J Bone Joint Surg Am. 2010; 92:218–219

[35] Stewart JD. Mononeuropathies in Diabetics. 2012

[36] Thomsen NO, Cederlund R, Rosen I, Bjork J, Dahlin LB. Clinical outcomes of surgical release among diabetic patients with carpal tunnel syndrome: prospective follow-up with matched controls. J Hand Surg Am. 2009; 34:1177–1187

[37] Burke DT, Burke MM, Stewart GW, Cambre A. Splinting for carpal tunnel syndrome: in search of the optimal angle. Arch Phys Med Rehabil. 1994; 75:1241–1244

[38] Walker WC, Metzler M, Cifu DX, Swartz Z. Neutral wrist splinting in carpal tunnel syndrome: a comparison of night-only versus full-time wear instructions. Arch Phys Med Rehabil. 2000; 81:424–429

[39] Linskey ME, Segal R. Median Nerve Injury from Local Steroid Injection in Carpal Tunnel Syndrome. Neurosurgery. 1990; 26:512–515

[40] Pagnanelli DM, Barrer SJ. Bilateral Carpal Tunel Release at One Operation: Report of 228 Patients. Neurosurgery. 1992; 31:1030–1034

[41] Katz JN, Keller RB, Simmons BP, Rogers WD, Bessette L, Fossel AH, Mooney NA. Maine Carpal Tunnel Study: outcomes of operative and nonoperative therapy for carpal tunnel syndrome in a community-based cohort. J Hand Surg Am. 1998; 23:697–710

[42] Brown RA, Gelberman RH, Seiler JG, III, Abrahamsson SO, Weiland AJ, Urbaniak JR, Schoenfeld DA, Furcolo D. Carpal tunnel release. A prospective, randomized assessment of open and endoscopic methods. J Bone Joint Surg. 1993; 75:1265–1275

[43] Pagnanelli DM, Barrer SJ. Carpal Tunel Syndrome: Surgical Treatment Using the Paine Retinaculatome. J Neurosurg. 1991; 75:77–81

[44] Louie D, Earp B, Blazar P. Long-term outcomes of carpal tunnel release: a critical review of the literature. Hand (N Y). 2012; 7:242–246

[45] Atroshi I, Larsson GU, Ornstein E, Hofer M, Johnsson R, Ranstam J. Outcomes of endoscopic surgery compared with open surgery for carpal tunnel syndrome among employed patients: randomised controlled trial. BMJ. 2006; 332. DOI: 10.1136/bmj.38863.632789.1F

[46] Atroshi I, Hofer M, Larsson GU, Ornstein E, Johnsson R, Ranstam J. Open compared with 2-portal endoscopic carpal tunnel release: a 5-year follow-up of a randomized controlled trial. J Hand Surg Am. 2009; 34:266–272

[47] Louis DS, Greene TL, Noellert RC. Complications of Carpal Tunnel Surgery. J Neurosurg. 1985; 62:352–356

[48] Louie DL, Earp BE, Collins JE, Losina E, Katz JN, Black EM, Simmons BP, Blazar PE. Outcomes of open carpal tunnel release at a minimum of ten years. J Bone Joint Surg Am. 2013; 95:1067–1073

[49] Guyette TM, Wilgis EF. Timing of improvement after carpal tunnel release. J Surg Orthop Adv. 2004; 13:206–209

[50] Zyluk A, Puchalski P. A comparison of the results of carpal tunnel release in patients in different age groups. Neurol Neurochir Pol. 2013; 47:241–246

[51] Padua L, Lo Monaco M, Padua R, Tamburrelli F, Gregori B, Tonali P. Carpal tunnel syndrome: neurophysiological results of surgery based on preoperative electrodiagnostic testing. J Hand Surg Br. 1997; 22:599–601

[52] Nancollas MP, Peimer CA, Wheeler DR, Sherwin FS. Long-term results of carpal tunnel release. J Hand Surg Br. 1995; 20:470–474

[53] Katz JN, Fossel KK, Simmons BP, Swartz RA, Fossel AH, Koris MJ. Symptoms, functional status, and neuromuscular impairment following carpal tunnel release. J Hand Surg Am. 1995; 20:549–555

[54] Pensy RA, Burke FD, Bradley MJ, Dubin NH, Wilgis EF. A 6-year outcome of patients who cancelled carpal tunnel surgery. J Hand Surg Eur Vol. 2011; 36:642–647

[55] Thomsen NO, Rosen I, Dahlin LB. Neurophysiologic recovery after carpal tunnel release in diabetic patients. Clin Neurophysiol. 2010; 121:1569–1573

[56] Jones NF, Ahn HC, Eo S. Revision surgery for persistent and recurrent carpal tunnel syndrome and for failed carpal tunnel release. Plast Reconstr Surg. 2012; 129:683–692

[57] Ginanneschi F, Milani P, Reale F, Rossi A. Short-term electrophysiological conduction change in median nerve fibres after carpal tunnel release. Clin Neurol Neurosurg. 2008; 110:1025–1030

[58] Shurr DG, Blair WF, Bassett G. Electromyographic changes after carpal tunnel release. J Hand Surg Am. 1986; 11:876–880

[59] Schrijver HM, Gerritsen AA, Strijers RL, Uitdehaag BM, Scholten RJ, de Vet HC, Bouter LM. Correlating nerve conduction studies and clinical outcome measures on carpal tunnel syndrome: lessons from a randomized controlled trial. J Clin Neurophysiol. 2005; 22:216–221

[60] Rotman MB, Enkvetchakul BV, Megerian JT, Gozani SN. Time course and predictors of median nerve conduction after carpal tunnel release. J Hand Surg Am. 2004; 29:367–372

[61] Stolp KA. Upper extremity Focal Neuropathies. 2013

[62] Brazis PW, Masdeu JC, Biller J. Localization in Clinical Neurology. 2nd ed. Boston: Little Brown and Company; 1990

[63] Harrop JS, Hanna A, Silva MT, Sharan A, Benzel EC, Stewart TJ. Neurological manifestations of cervical spondylosis: an overview of signs, symptoms, and pathophysiology. Neurosurgery. 2007; 60:S1-14-20

[64] Wilkins RH, Rengachary SS. Neurosurgery. New York 1985

[65] Dumitru D. Elecctrodiagnostic Medicine. Philadelphia: Hanley and Belfus; 1995

[66] Bonney G. Iatrogenic Injuries of Nerves. J Bone Joint Surg. 1986; 68B:9–13

[67] Stewart JD. In: Ulnar Nerve. Focal Peripheral Neuropathies . 4th ed. West Vancouver, Canada: JBJ Publishing; 2010:258–313

[68] Bartels RHMA, Menovsky T, Van Overbeeke JJ, Verhagen WIM. Surgical Management of Ulnar Nerve Compression at the Elbow: An Analysis of the Literature. J Neurosurg. 1988; 89:722–727

[69] Padua L, Aprile I, Mazza O, Padua R, Pietracci E, Caliandro P, Pauri F, D'Amico P, Tonali P. Neurophysiological classification of ulnar entrapment across the elbow. Neurol Sci. 2001; 22:11–16

[70] Practice parameter: electrodiagnostic studies in ulnar neuropathy at the elbow. American Association of Electrodiagnostic Medicine, American Academy of Neurology, and American Academy of Physical Medicine and Rehabilitation. Neurology. 1999; 52:688–690

[71] Beekman R, Wokke JH, Schoemaker MC, Lee ML, Visser LH. Ulnar neuropathy at the elbow: follow-up and prognostic factors determining outcome. Neurology. 2004; 63:1675–1680

[72] Cartwright MS, Chloros GD, Walker FO, Wiesler ER, Campbell WW. Diagnostic ultrasound for nerve transection. Muscle Nerve. 2007; 35:796–799

[73] Caliandro P, La Torre G, Padua R, Giannini F, Padua L. Treatment for ulnar neuropathy at the elbow. Cochrane Database Syst Rev. 2012; 7. DOI: 10.1002/14651858.CD006839.pub3

[74] Elhassan B, Steinmann SP. Entrapment neuropathy of the ulnar nerve. J Am Acad Orthop Surg. 2007; 15:672–681

[75] Le Roux PD, Ensign TD, Burchiel KJ. Surgical Decompression Without Transposition for Ulnar Neuropathy: Factors Determining Outcome. Neurosurgery. 1990; 27:709–714

[76] Kline DG, Hudson AR. Nerve Injuries: Operative Results for Major Nerve Injuries, Entrapments, and Tumors. Philadelphia: W. B. Saunders; 1995

[77] Janjua RM, Fernandez J, Tender G, Kline DG. Submuscular transposition of the ulnar nerve for the treatment of cubital tunnel syndrome. Neurosurgery. 2008; 63:321–4; discussion 324-5

[78] Spinner RJ, O'Driscoll SW, Jupiter JB, Goldner RD. Unrecognized dislocation of the medial portion of the triceps: another cause of failed ulnar nerve transposition. J Neurosurg. 2000; 92:52–57

[79] Bartels RH, Verhagen WI, van der Wilt GJ, Meulstee J, van Rossum LG, Grotenhuis JA. Prospective randomized controlled study comparing simple decompression versus anterior subcutaneous transposition for idiopathic neuropathy of the ulnar nerve at the elbow: Part 1. Neurosurgery. 2005; 56:522–30; discussion 522-30

[80] Biggs M, Curtis JA. Randomized, prospective study comparing ulnar neurolysis in situ with submuscular transposition. Neurosurgery. 2006; 58:296–304; discussion 296-304

[81] Tindall SC. Comment on LeRoux P D, et al.: Surgical Decompression without Transposition for Ulnar Neuropathy: Factors Determining Outcome. Neurosurgery. 1990; 27

[82] Youmans JR. Neurological Surgery. Philadelphia 1990

[83] Shea JD, McClain EJ. Ulnar-Nerve Compression Syndromes at and Below the Wrist. J Bone Joint Surg. 1969; 51A:1095–1103

[84] Cavallo M, Poppi M, Martinelli P, Gaist G. Distal Ulnar Neuropathy from Carpal Ganglia: A Clinical and Electrophysiological Study. Neurosurgery. 1988; 22:902–905

[85] Dyck PJ, Thomas PK. Peripheral Neuropathy. 2nd ed. Philadelphia: W. B. Saunders; 1984

[86] Roles NC, Maudsley RH. Radial Tunnel Syndrome: Resistant Tennis Elbow as a Nerve Entrapment. J Bone Joint Surg. 1972; 54B:499–508

[87] McKowen HC, Voorhies RM. Axillary Nerve Entrapment in the Quadrilateral Space: Case Report. J Neurosurg. 1987; 66:932–934

[88] de Laat EAT, Visser CPJ, Coene LNJEM, Pahlplatz PVM, Tavy DLJ. Nerve Lesions in Primary Shoulder Dislocations and Humeral Neck Fractures. J Bone Joint Surg. 1994; 76B:381–383

[89] Hadley MN, Sonntag VKH, Pittman HW. Suprascapular Nerve Entrapment: A Summary of Seven Cases. J Neurosurg. 1986; 64:843–848

[90] Fritz RC, Helms CA, Steinbach LS, et al. Suprascapular nerve entrapment: Evaluation with MR imaging. Radiology. 1992; 182:437–444

[91] Callahan JD, Scully TB, Shapiro SA, Worth RM. Suprascapular Nerve Entrapment: A Series of 27 Cases. J Neurosurg. 1991; 74:893–896

[92] Stevens HI. Meralgia Paresthetica. Arch Neurol Psychiatry. 1957; 77:557–574

[93] Williams PH, Trzil KP. Management of Meralgia Paresthetica. J Neurosurg. 1991; 74:76–80

[94] Devers A, Galer BS. Topical lidocaine patch relieves a variety of neuropathic pain conditions: an open-label study. Clin J Pain. 2000; 16:205–208

[95] Aldrich EF, Van den Heever C. Suprainguinal Ligament Approach for Surgical Treatment of Meralgia Paresthetica. Technical Note. J Neurosurg. 1989; 70:492–494

[96] Kars HZ, Topaktas S, Dogan K. Aneurysmal Peroneal Nerve Compression. Neurosurgery. 1992; 30:930–931

31 Non-Entrapment Peripheral Neuropathies

31.1 Definitions

► **Peripheral neuropathy.** (The term polyneuropathy is also sometimes used.) Diffuse lesions of peripheral nerves producing weakness, sensory disturbance, and/or reflex changes

► **Mononeuropathy.** A disorder of a single nerve, often due to trauma or entrapment

► **Mononeuropathy multiplex.** Involvement of 2 or more nerves, usually due to a systemic abnormality (e.g. vasculitis, rheumatoid arthritis, DM…). Treatment is directed at the underlying disorder

31.2 Etiologies of peripheral neuropathy

A mnemonic for etiologies of peripheral neuropathies is "GRAND THERAPIST" See ► Table 31.1). Diabetes, alcoholism, and Guillain-Barré (italicized in table) account for 90% of cases. Other etiologies include: arteritis/vasculitis, monoclonal gammopathy (p. 547), hepatitis C virus-associated cryoglobulinemia, acute idiopathic polyneuritis, Sjögren's syndrome (disease).

31.3 Classification

1. inherited neuropathies
   a) Charcot-Marie-Tooth (CMT) (AKA peroneal muscular atrophy, AKA Hereditary Motor and Sensory Neuropathy (HMSN)): Up to 7 types, (the most common form is autosomal dominant, but X-linked recessive forms also exist). CMT Types 1 & 2 together make up the most common inherited disorder of peripheral nerves (up to 40/100,000). The most common forms involve demyelination. Progressive loss of motor (primarily *distal* LE) and, to a lesser degree, sensory function (predominantly proprioception and vibration), with atrophy in UEs & LEs. Earliest findings: pes cavus with hammer toes, foot drop and frequent ankle sprains. Patients are more susceptible to entrapment neuropathies due to underlying compromise of peripheral nerves. Patients with Type 1 usual maintain ability to ambulate, whereas Type 2 usually lose ambulation by their teenage years
   b) hereditary neuropathy with liability to pressure palsies (HNPP): similar to CMT but due to focal areas of irregular thickening of myelin sheaths ("tomaculous" changes), mild trauma or pressure can produce nerve palsies that may last for months
2. acquired neuropathies: see sections below for details
   a) acquired pure *sensory* neuropathies (in the absence of autonomic dysfunction) are rare. May be seen with pyridoxine therapy or paraneoplastic syndromes (see below)
   b) entrapment neuropathies (p. 515)
3. pseudoneuropathy
   a) definition: psychogenic somatoform disorders or malingering, reproducing the pains, paresthesias, hyperalgesia, weakness, and even objective findings such as changes in color and temperature which may mimic neuropathic symptoms[2]

Table 31.1 Mnemonic for etiologies of peripheral neuropathy

G-R-A-N-D	T-H-E-R-A-P-I-S-T
Guillain-Barré (p. 184) Renal; uremic neuropathy (p. 549) *Alcoholism* (see below) Nutritional (B12 deficiency…) *Diabetes*; see below or Drugs (p. 546)	Traumatic Hereditary Endocrine or Entrapment Radiation Amyloid (p. 549) or AIDS (p. 547) Porphyria (should be under hereditary) or Psychiatric or Paraneoplastic (see below) or Pseudoneuropathy (see below) or PMR (p. 198) or Polycythema vera[1] Infectious/post-infectious (e.g. Hansen's disease) Sarcoidosis, see neurosarcoidosis (p. 189), or "Systemic" Toxins, including heavy metals, e.g. lead toxicity (plumbism) (p. 1017)

31

31.4 Clinical

31.4.1 Presentation

Peripheral neuropathies can present as loss of sensation, pain, weakness, incoordination and difficulty ambulating.

31.4.2 Evaluation

Initial (screening) work-up for peripheral neuropathies of unknown etiology:
1. bloodwork: Hgb-A1C, TSH, ESR and vitamin B12
2. EMG

31.5 Syndromes of peripheral neuropathy

31.5.1 Critical illness polyneuropathy (CIP)

AKA neuropathy of critical illness, ICU neuropathy... See DDx under Guillain-Barré syndrome (p. 186).

May occur in up to 70% of septic patients (not all are significantly symptomatic). Affects primarily distal muscles.

Diagnostic criteria:
1. presence of sepsis, multi-organ failure, respiratory failure, or septic inflammatory response syndrome (SIRS)
2. difficulty weaning from ventilator or extremity weakness
3. EMG: ↓ amplitudes of compound muscle action potentials (CMAP) & SNAP
4. widespread muscle denervation potentials
5. normal or only mild increase in serum CPK levels

31

Recovery occurs in weeks to months (faster than Guillain-Barré).

Treatment is supportive. Complete recovery occurs in 50%.

31.5.2 Paraneoplastic syndromes affecting the nervous system

Occurs in < 1% of cancer patients. Peripheral *sensory* neuropathy of unknown etiology has been associated with cancer since its earliest description.[3] Therefore, However, in patients with sensory neuropathy of unknown etiology, occult neoplasms should be ruled out. If the work-up is negative, the patient should be followed since up to 35% of patients will be found to have cancer after a mean interval of 28 months after the onset of neuropathy (range: 3–72 months)[4] (no one particular cancer type predominated, in spite of the fact that historically lung cancer is the most frequent neoplasm associated with sensory neuropathy[5]).

31.5.3 Alcohol neuropathy

Characteristically produces a diffuse sensory neuropathy, with absent achilles reflexes.

31.5.4 Brachial plexus neuropathy

See reference.[6(p 918)]

Evaluation

When the etiology is unclear, check CXR (with apical lordotic view), glucose, ESR and ANA.

If no improvement by ≈ 4 weeks, obtain MRI of the plexus (idiopathic brachial plexitis will usually start to show some improvement by this time, therefore tumor should be ruled out if no improvement).

Differential diagnosis of etiologies of brachial plexopathy

1. Pancoast syndrome or Pancoast tumor AKA superior sulcus tumor. Clinical: various combinations of pain in the shoulder radiating into the upper extremity in the ulnar nerve distribution from

involvement of the lower brachial plexus, atrophy of hand muscles, Horner's syndrome (p.564), UE edema. Etiologies:

a) neoplasms:
   - most common: bronchogenic cancer, usually non-small cell (NSCLC) (squamous cell or adenocarcinoma) arising in the pulmonary apex
   - metastases

b) infections

c) inflammatory: granulomas, amyloid

2. (idiopathic) brachial plexitis AKA neuralgic amyotrophy: most commonly upper plexus or diffuse (see below)
3. cervical rib
4. viral
5. following radiation treatment: often diffuse (see below)
6. diabetes
7. vasculitis
8. inherited: dominant genetics
9. trauma (p.550)

Neuralgic amyotrophy of the upper extremity

General information

AKA idiopathic brachial plexus neuropathy AKA (paralytic) brachial neuritis, AKA brachial plexitis, AKA Parsonage-Turner syndrome,[7] AKA immune-mediated brachial plexus neuropathy, among others. Idiopathic. Not clearly infectious or inflammatory; allergic mechanism possible. Prognosis is generally good. Common patterns: single or multiple mononeuropathy, plexopathy, or some combination. Demographics are shown in ▶ Table 31.2.

In a review of 99 cases[8]: predominant symptom is acute onset of intense *pain*, with weakness developing simultaneously or after a variable period (70% occur within 2 weeks of pain) usually as the pain lessened.[7,9] Weakness never preceded pain, onset of weakness was sudden in 80%. Pain was usually constant, and described as "sharp", "stabbing", "throbbing" or "aching." Arm movement exacerbated pain, and muscle soreness was noted in 15%. Pain lasted hours to several weeks. Paresthesias occurred in 35%. Pain usually lacked radicular features. When bilateral, weakness is usually asymmetric.

Exam

Weakness or paralysis in 96%, confined to shoulder girdle in 50%. In descending order of involvement: deltoid, spinati, serratus anterior, biceps brachii, and triceps. Winging of the scapula occurred in 20%. Sensory loss occurred in 60% of plexus lesions, of mixed variety (superficial cutaneous and proprioceptive). Sensory loss most common in outer surface of upper arm (circumflex nerve distribution) and radial aspect of forearm. Reflexes were variable.

Table 31.2 Neuralgic amyotrophy

incidence	1.64 per 100,000 population
male:female	2.4:1
age range at onset	3 mos – 75 years
prodrome	• ≈ 45% had viral prodrome (URI in 25%) • may follow vaccination
onset	rapid onset of pain or paralysis/paresis
initial symptom	pain in 95%
weakness	• 50% confined to shoulder girdle • 10% confined to a single peripheral nerve
sensory deficit	67%, usually axillary and antebrachial cutaneous
laterality	• 66% unilateral (right side 54%) • 34% bilateral
lab tests	normal

Overall distribution judged to predominantly involve *upper* plexus in 56%, diffuse plexus in 38%, and lower in 6%.

EMG/NCV

May help localize the portion of the plexus involved, and may detect subclinical involvement of the contralateral extremity. Must wait ≥ 3 weeks from onset for findings. Differentiating from cervical radiculopathy: SNAP should be normal in radiculopathy whereas some involvement usually occurs in plexitis. Cervical paraspinals will usually be normal in plexitis (except for very severe cases where there can be some retrograde involvement), and will be abnormal (fibrillations) in radiculopathy (except in cases where there has been enough time that significant recovery has occurred).

Outcome

Functional recovery is better in patients with primarily upper plexus involvement. After 1 year, 60% of upper plexus lesions were functioning normally, whereas none with lower involvement were (latter took 1.5–3 years). Rate of recovery estimated to be 36% within 1 year, 75% within 2, and 89% by 3 years. Recurrence was seen in only 5%. No evidence that steroids altered the course of the disease although it is still often prescribed in the acute phase.

Radiation induced brachial plexus neuropathy

Often follows external beam irradiation in the region of the axilla for breast carcinoma. Produces sensory loss with or without weakness. CT or MRI or biopsy may be needed to rule-out tumor invasion of the brachial plexus.

31.5.5 Lumbosacral plexus neuropathy

See reference.[10]

31

General information

Analogous to idiopathic brachial plexitis (see above). It is controversial whether this actually exists in isolation without diabetes. Often starts with LE pain of abrupt onset, followed in days or a few weeks by weakness with or without muscle atrophy. Sensory symptoms are less prominent, and usually involve paresthesias. Objective sensory loss is only occasionally seen. There may be tenderness over the femoral nerve.

Differential diagnosis

May be confused with femoral neuropathy or L4 radiculopathy when quadriceps weakness and wasting occurs. Similarly, L5 radiculopathy or peroneal neuropathy may be erroneously suspected when foot drop is seen. Straight leg raising may occasionally be positive. Conspicuously absent are: back pain, exacerbation of pain by Valsalva maneuver or back motion, and significant sensory involvement. See differential diagnosis of foot drop (p. 1417) and other causes of sciatica (p. 1410).

Etiologies

Other etiologies are similar to that for brachial plexus neuropathy (see above) except that under tumor, a pelvic mass should also be included (check prostate on rectal exam).

Evaluation

Evaluation is as for brachial plexus neuropathy (see above), except that instead of a brachial plexus MRI, a lumbar MRI and pelvic CT should be done to rule out masses.

EMG is key to diagnosis: evidence of patchy denervation (fibrillation potentials, and motor unit potentials that are either decreased in number or increased in amplitude or duration and polyphasic) involving at least 2 segmental levels with *sparing* of the paraspinal muscles is highly diagnostic (once diabetes, etc. have been ruled-out).

Outcome

Recovery from pain precedes return of strength. Improvement is generally monophasic, slow (years), and incomplete.

31.5.6 Diabetic neuropathy

General information

≈ 50% of patients with DM develop neuropathic symptoms or show slowing of nerve conduction velocities on electrodiagnostic testing. Neuropathy may sometimes be the initial manifestation of diabetes. Diabetic neuropathy is reduced by tight control of blood glucose.[11]

Syndromes

Disagreement exists over the number of distinct clinical syndromes; there is probably a continuum[12] and they likely occur in various combinations. Some of the more readily identified syndromes include:

1. primary sensory polyneuropathy: symmetric, affecting feet and legs more than hands. Chronic, slowly-progressive. Often with accelerated loss of distal vibratory sense (normal loss with aging is ≈ 1% per year after age 40). Presents as pain, paresthesias, and dysesthesias. Soles of feet may be tender to pressure. Meralgia paresthetica (p. 534) may be first manifestation
2. autonomic neuropathy: involving bladder, bowel, and circulatory reflexes (resulting in orthostatic hypotension). May produce impotence, impaired micturition, diarrhea, constipation, impaired pupillary light response
3. diabetic plexus neuropathy[13] or proximal neuropathy: possibly secondary to vascular injury to nerves (similar to a diabetic mononeuritis):
   a) one that occurs in patients > 50 years old with mild diabetes type II that is often confused with femoral neuropathy. Causes severe pain in the hip, anterior thigh, knee, and sometimes medial calf. Weakness of the quadriceps, iliopsoas, and occasionally thigh adductors. Loss of knee jerk. Possible sensory loss over medial thigh and lower leg. Pain usually improves in weeks, the weakness in months
   b) ✱ diabetic amyotrophy: occurs in similar patient population often with recently diagnosed DM. Alternative names include[14]: Bruns-Garland syndrome, ischemic mononeuropathy multiplex....[15] Abrupt onset of asymmetric pain (usually deep aching/burning with superimposed lancinating paroxysms, most severe at night) in back, hip, buttocks, thigh, or leg. Progressive weakness in proximal or proximal and distal muscles, often preceded by weight loss. Patellar reflexes are absent or reduced. Sensory loss is minimal. Proximal muscles (especially thigh) may atrophy. EMG findings consistent with demyelination invariably accompanied by axonal degeneration, with involvement of paraspinals and no evidence of myopathy. Symptoms may progress steadily or stepwise for weeks or even up to 18 months, and then gradually resolve. Opposite extremity may become involved during the course or may occur months or years later. Sural nerve biopsy may suggest demyelination
   c) diabetic proximal neuropathy (DPN): fairly similar findings to diabetic amyotrophy except for subacute onset of symmetric LE involvement that usually start with weakness may be a variant.[16] ▶ Table 31.3 (adapted[16]) compares DPN to diabetic amyotrophy and chronic inflammatory demyelinating polyradiculoneuropathy (CIDP)

Treatment

Treatment of Bruns-Garland syndrome is primarily expectant, although immunotherapy (steroids, immune globulin, or plasma exchange) may be considered in severe or progressive cases (efficacy is unproven).[16]

For sensory polyneuropathy, good control of blood sugar contributes to reduction of symptoms. Adjunctive agents that have been used include:

1. mexiletine (Mexitil®): start at 150 mg q 8 hrs, and titrate to symptoms to a maximum of 10 mg/kg/d
2. amitriptyline (Elavil®) and fluphenazine (Prolixin®): ℞: start with 25 mg amitriptyline PO q hs and 1 mg fluphenazine PO TID; and work up to 75 mg amitriptyline PO q hs[17] (≈ 100 mg qd amitriptyline alone may also be effective[18]). Usefulness has been challenged,[19] but many studies do show benefit.[18,20] **Side effects:** that may limit use include sedation, confusion, fatigue, malaise, hypomania, rash, urinary retention, and orthostatic hypotension
3. desipramine (Norpramin®): more selective blocker of norepinephrine reuptake (which seems more effective for this condition than serotonin reuptake blockers). Effectiveness at mean doses of 110 mg/day ≈ same as amitriptyline and therefore may be useful for patients unable to tolerate amitriptyline.[18] **Side effects:** include insomnia (may be minimized by AM dosing), orthostatic hypotension, rash, bundle branch block, tremor, pyrexia. **Supplied** : 10, 25, 50, 75, 100 & 150 mg tablets
4. capsaicin (Zostrix®) (p. 496): effective in some

Table 31.3 Comparison of diabetic amyotrophy, diabetic proximal neuropathy (DPN), & CIDP

Description	Diabetic amyotrophy	DPN	CIDP
Onset	acute	subacute	gradual
Initial symptoms	asymmetric pain→ weakness	symmetric weakness	symmetric weakness
UE weakness	no	uncommon	yes
Sensory loss	minimal	minimal	moderate
Areflexia	LE	LE	generalized
CSF protein	variable	increased	increased
Axonal pathologic changes	common	typical	uncommon
Conduction slowing	patchy	patchy	diffuse
Prognosis	good	good	poor without treatment
Response to immunotherapy	unknown	possible	yes
Course	monophasic	monophasic	progressive

5. paroxetine (Paxil®): a selective serotonin reuptake inhibitor (SSRI) antidepressant. ℞: 20 mg PO q AM. If necessary, increase by 10 mg/d q week up to a maximum of 50 mg/day (except in elderly, debilitated, or renal or hepatic failure where maximum is 40 mg/day). **Supplied** : 20 mg (scored) & 30 mg tablets
6. gabapentin (Neurontin®) doses of 1800–3600 mg/d produces at least moderate pain relief from painful diabetic neuropathy in 60% of patients[21] and was ≈ as efficacious as amitriptyline.[22] Dosage must be reduced with renal insufficiency. See details (p. 455)
7. pregabalin (Lyrica®) ℞: start with 50 mg TID and increase up to a maximum of 100 mg PO TID within 1 week in patients with creatinine clearance ≥ 60 ml/min, see Eq (7.1) to estimate. Dosage must be reduced with renal insufficiency. **Supplied**: 25, 50, 75, 100, 150, 200, 225, 300 mg capsules

31

31.5.7 Drug-induced neuropathy

Many drugs have been implicated as possible causes of peripheral neuropathy. Those that are better established or more notorious include:

1. thalidomide: neuropathy may occur with chronic use, and may be irreversible[23]
2. metronidazole (Flagyl®)
3. phenytoin (Dilantin®)
4. amitriptyline (Elavil®)
5. dapsone: a rare complication reported with use in nonleprosy patients is a reversible peripheral neuropathy that may be due to axonal degeneration, producing a Guillain-Barré-like syndrome (p. 184).
6. nitrofurantoin (Macrodantin®): may additionally cause optic neuritis
7. cholesterol lowering drugs: e.g. lovastatin (Mevacor®), indapamide (Lozol®), gemfibrozil (Lopid®)
8. thallium: may produce tremors, leg pains, paresthesias in the hands and feet, polyneuritis in the LE, psychosis, delirium, seizures, encephalopathy
9. arsenic: may produce numbness, burning and tingling of the extremities
10. chemotherapy: cisplatin, vincristine…

31.5.8 Femoral neuropathy

Clinical findings

1. motor deficits:
   a) wasting and weakness of the quadriceps femoris (knee extension)
   b) weakness of iliopsoas (hip flexion): if present, indicates very proximal pathology (lumbar root or plexus lesion) as the branches to the iliopsoas arise just distal to the neural foramina

2. diminution of the patellar (knee jerk) reflex
3. sensory findings:
   a) sensory loss over the anterior thigh and medial calf
   b) pain in same distribution may occur
4. mechanical signs: positive femoral stretch test (p. 1048)

Etiologies

1. diabetes: the most frequent cause
2. femoral nerve entrapment: rare
   a) may occur secondary to inguinal hernia or may be injured by deep sutures placed during herniorrhaphy
   b) secondary to prolonged pelvic surgery from retractor compression (usually bilateral)
3. intraabdominal tumor
4. femoral arterial catheterization: see below
5. retroperitoneal hematoma (e.g. in hemophiliac or on anticoagulants)
6. during surgery (p. 549)

Differential diagnosis

1. L4 radiculopathy: L4 radiculopathy should not cause iliopsoas weakness; see L4 involvement (p. 1412).
2. diabetic plexus neuropathy (see above)
3. (idiopathic) lumbosacral plexus neuropathy (see above)

31.5.9 AIDS neuropathy

General information

3.3% of patients with AIDS will develop peripheral nerve disorders[24] (whereas none who were just HIV positive developed neuropathy). The most common disorder is distal symmetric polyneuropathy (DSP), usually consisting of vague numbness and tingling, and sometimes painful feet (although it may also be painless). There may be subtle reduction of light tough and vibratory sense. Other neuropathies include mononeuropathies – usually meralgia paresthetica (p. 534) – mononeuropathy multiplex, or lumbar polyradiculopathy. Drugs used to treat HIV can also cause neuropathies (see below).

The DSP in AIDS patients is often associated with CMV infection, Mycobacterium avium intracellulare infection, or may be due to lymphomatous invasion of the nerve or lymphomatous meningitis. May demonstrate a mixed axonal demyelinating type of neuropathy on electrodiagnostic testing.

Neuropathies associated with drugs used to treat HIV

1. nucleoside reverse transcriptase inhibitors
   a) zidovudine (Retrovir®) (formerly AZT)
   b) didanosine (ddI; Videx®); (formerly dideoxyinosine) can cause a painful dose-related neuropathy[25]
   c) stavudine (d4T; Zerit®): can cause sensory neuropathy which usually improves when d4T is discontinued, and may not recur if restarted at lower dose[25]
   d) zalcitabine (ddC; Hivid®): the least potent of the nucleoside analogs, therefore rarely used; dose-related neuropathy can be severe and persistent. More common in patients with DM or didanosine treatment[25]
2. protease inhibitors
   a) ritonavir (Norvir®): can cause peripheral paresthesias
   b) amprenavir (Agenerase®): can cause perioral paresthesias

31.5.10 Neuropathy associated with monoclonal gammopathy

General information

Monoclonal gammopathies include myeloma (p. 714), Waldenstrom's macroglobulinemia, and non-malignant entities such as monoclonal gammopathy of undetermined significance (MGUS). Much effort has gone into determining which benign gammopathies are or are not likely to progress, and will not be addressed here.

31

≈ 10% of patients with neuropathy with no apparent etiology will be determined to have a monoclonal gammopathy (malignant or otherwise).

Etiologies

1. antibodies directed primarily against oligosaccharides of peripheral nerves, e.g. myelin associated glycoprotein (MAG), producing demyelinating neuropathy
2. cryoglobulins may damage vaso-nervorum (small blood vessels nourishing peripheral nerves)
3. in malignant gammopathies, tumor cells can invade the peripheral nerves (lymphomatosis)
4. amyloidosis (p.549): deposition of amyloid in peripheral nerves
5. thalidomide (p.546) used to treat some myelomas may cause neuropathy

Treatment

1. IgM monoclonal gammopathies: reduce the IgM antibody concentration
2. IgG or IgA monoclonal gammopathies:
   a) treatment for myeloma related neuropathy is directed at treating the myeloma
   b) solitary plasmacytoma: excision or XRT can improve the neuropathy

31.5.11 Perioperative neuropathies

General information

Also, below. Represent ≈ 1/3 of all anesthesia-associated malpractice claims in the U.S.[26] Most often involves ulnar nerve or brachial plexus. In many cases, a nerve that is abnormal but asymptomatic may become symptomatic as a result of any of the following factors: stretch or compression of the nerve, generalized ischemia or metabolic derangement. The injury may be permanent or temporary. Occurs almost exclusively in adults.[27]

Types of perioperative neuropathies

Examples include:

1. ulnar neuropathy: controversial. Often blamed on external nerve compression or stretch as a result of malpositioning. Although this may be true in some cases, in one series this was felt to be a factor in only ≈ 17% of cases.[28] Patient-related characteristics associated with these neuropathies are shown in ▶ Table 31.4.[29] Many of these patients have abnormal contralateral nerve conduction, suggesting a possible predisposing condition.[30] Many patients do not complain of symptoms until > 48 hours post-op[29,30,31] (if it were due to compression, deficit would be maximal immediately post-op). Risk may be reduced by padding the arm at, and especially distal to, the elbow, and avoiding flexion of the elbow (especially avoiding > 110° flexion which tightens the cubital tunnel retinaculum) and by reducing the amount of time spent convalescing in the recumbent position with leaning on the elbows[31]
2. brachial plexus neuropathy: may be mistaken for ulnar neuropathy. May be associated with:
   a) median sternotomy (most common with internal mammary dissection). Posterior sternal retraction displaces the upper ribs and may stretch or compress the C6 through T1 roots (which are major contributors to the ulnar nerve)
   b) head-down (Trendelenburg) positions where the patient is stabilized with a shoulder brace. The brace should be placed over the acromioclavicular joint(s), and non-slip mattresses and flexion of the knees may be used as adjuncts[27]
   c) prone position (rare): especially with shoulder abduction and elbow flexion with contralateral head rotation[27]
3. median neuropathy: perioperative median nerve injury may result from stretch of the nerve. Rare. Seems to occur primarily in middle-aged muscular males with reduced extension of the elbows due to muscle mass. This may result in stretching of the nerve after muscle relaxants are

Table 31.4 Patient-related characteristics in anesthesia-related ulnar neuropathy
male gender
obesity (body mass index ≥ 38)
prolonged post-op bed rest

given. Padding should be placed under the forearms and hands of these patients to maintain mild elbow flexion[27]

4. lower extremity neuropathies: most occur in patients undergoing procedures in the lithotomy position.[27] Frequency of involvement in a large series of patients undergoing procedures in the lithotomy position[32]: common peroneal 81%, sciatic 15%, and femoral 4%. Risk factors other than position: prolonged duration of procedure, extremely thin body habitus, and cigarette smoking in the preoperative period
   a) common peroneal neuropathy: susceptible to injury in the posterior popliteal fossa where it wraps around the fibular head. May be compressed by leg holders, which should be padded in this area
   b) femoral neuropathy: compression of the nerve by self-retaining abdominal wall retractor or rendering the nerve ischemic by occlusion of the external iliac artery.[27] Hemorrhage into the iliopsoas muscle may also compress the nerve. Cutaneous branches of the femoral nerve may be injured during labor and/or delivery[33] (most are transient)
   c) sciatic neuropathy: stretch injuries may occur with hyperflexion of the hip and extension of the knee as may occur in some variants of the lithotomy position
   d) meralgia paresthetica[34]: tends to occur bilaterally in young, slender males positioned prone, with operations lasting 6–10 + hours. Onset: 1–8 days post-op. Spontaneous recovery typically occurs over an average of 5.8 months

Management

Once a neuropathy is detected, determine if it is sensory, motor, or both. Pure sensory neuropathies are more often temporary than motor,[29] and expectant management for ≈ 5 days is suggested (have the patient avoid postures or activities that may further injure the nerve). Neurologic consultation should be requested for all motor neuropathies and for sensory neuropathies persisting > 5 days[27] (EMG evaluation will not usually be helpful earlier than ≈ 3 weeks after onset).

31.5.12 Other neuropathies

Amyloid neuropathy

Amyloid is an insoluble extracellular protein aggregate that can be deposited in peripheral nerves. Amyloidosis occurs in a number of conditions, e.g. in ≈ 15% of patients with **multiple myeloma** (p. 714). The neuropathy predominantly produces a progressive autonomic neuropathy and symmetric dissociated sensory loss (reduced pain and temperature, preserved vibratory sense). There is usually less prominent motor involvement. May predispose to pressure injury of nerves (especially carpal tunnel syndrome, see laboratory tests (p. 523)).

Uremic neuropathy

Occurs in chronic renal failure. Early symptoms include calf cramps ("Charlie horses"), dysesthetic pain in feet (similar to painful diabetic neuropathy) and "restless legs." Achilles reflexes are lost. A stocking sensory loss is followed later by LE weakness that starts distally and ascends. The offending toxin is not known. Dialysis or renal transplantation relieves the symptoms.

Neuropathy after cardiac catheterization

In a series of ≈ 10,000 patients followed after femoral artery catheterization[35] (e.g. for coronary angiography or angioplasty), neuropathy occurred in 0.2% (with an estimated range in the literature up to ≈ 3%). Risk factors identified include: patients developing retroperitoneal hematomas or pseudoaneurysms after the procedure, procedures requiring larger introducer sheaths (e.g. angioplasty & stent placement > diagnostic catheterization), excessive anticoagulation (PTT > 90 for at least 12 hours).

Two groups of patients were identified and are shown in ► Table 31.5.

Excruciating pain after the catheterization procedure often preceded the development or recognition of neuropathy.

Treatment

After considering available information, the recommendation is to repair pseudoaneurysms surgically, but to treat the neuropathy conservatively. A case could *not* be made that surgical drainage of hematoma reduced the risk of neuropathy. Weakness from femoral or obturator neuropathy was treated with inpatient rehabilitation.

Table 31.5 Neuropathy after cardiac catheterization (N = 9585)[35]

Catheterization complication	Neurologic complication
Group I (4 patients)	
groin hematoma or pseudoaneurysm	sensory neuropathy in all 4 cases • in distribution of medial & intermediate femoral cutaneous nerves → isolated sensory neuropathy (dysesthesia & sensory loss) of the anterior and medial thigh • no motor deficit
Group II (16 patients)	
large retroperitoneal hematoma	femoral neuropathy • sensory in all 16 cases: dysesthesia of the anterior/medial thigh & medial calf • motor in 13 cases: iliopsoas & quadriceps weakness
	obturator neuropathy in 4 cases • sensory: upper medial thigh • motor: obturator weakness
	lateral femoral cutaneous nerve → meralgia paresthetica

Outcome

Group I patients all had resolution in < 5 mos. In group II, 50% had complete resolution in 2 mos. 6 patients had persistent symptoms, 5 had mild femoral *sensory* neuropathy (1 of whom felt it was at least somewhat disabling), 1 had mild persistent quadriceps weakness and occasionally walks with a cane.

31

31.6 Peripheral nerve injuries

31.6.1 General information

Anatomy of peripheral nerves

See ▶ Fig. 31.1. Endoneurium surrounds myelinated and unmyelinated axons. These bundles are gathered into fascicles surrounded by perineurium. The epineurium encases the nerve trunk, containing fascicles separated by interfascicular epineurium or mesoneurium.

Nerve regeneration

Peripheral nerves regenerate ≈1 mm/day (about 1 inch/month). Divide this figure into distance that the nerve has to traverse (from knowledge of anatomy) for guide as to how long to wait before considering failure of therapy (either operative or non-operative). However, this rule may not be applicable to long distances (> ≈ 12 inches), and it may take longer to traverse regions of entrapment, scar or nerve injury. There may also be fibrosis of the muscle beyond salvage.

Peripheral nerve injury classification

▶ Table 31.6

There are numerous classification systems. The Seddon classification is an older 3-tiered system, The Sunderland system has 5 tiers, essentially dividing axonotmesis into 3 subgroups. Others have added a 6th category as shown in ▶ Table 31.6.

31.6.2 Brachial plexus injuries

Etiologies

Etiologies include:

1. penetrating trauma
2. traction (stretch injuries): more likely to affect the posterior and lateral cords than the medial cord and median nerve
3. first rib fractures
4. compression by hematoma

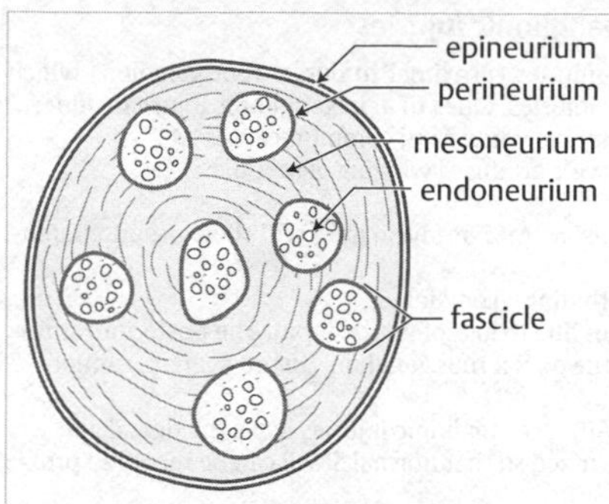

Fig. 31.1 Anatomy of a peripheral nerve

Table 31.6 Classification of peripheral nerve injury[a]

Seddon system	Sunderland system
Neuropraxia	**First-degree**
Features common to both systems Physiologic transection (nerve in continuity). Basement membrane intact. Compression or ischemia → local conduction block (impaired axonal transport). ✱ *No* wallerian degeneration[b]. Motor involvement is typically > sensory. Autonomic function is preserved	
Recovers in hours to months; average is 6–8 weeks	Focal demyelination may occur. Recovery is usually complete in 2–3 weeks (not the "1 mm/day rule")
Axonotmesis	**Second-degree**
Features common to both systems Complete interruption of axons and myelin sheaths. Supporting structures (including endoneurium) intact. ✱ Wallerian degeneration occurs	
	Recovers at 1 mm/day as axon follows "tubule." Sometimes may only be diagnosed retrospectively. Recovery is poor in lesions requiring > 18 months to reach target muscle
	Third-degree
	Endoneurium disrupted, epineurium & perineurium intact. Nerve may not appear seriously damaged on gross inspection. Recovery may range from poor to complete and depends on degree of intrafascicular fibrosis
	Fourth-degree
	Interruption of all neural & supporting elements. Epineurium intact. Grossly: nerve is usually indurated & enlarged
Neurotmesis	**Fifth-degree**
Nerve completely severed or disorganized by scar tissue. Spontaneous regeneration impossible	Complete transection with loss of continuity
	Sixth-degree[c]
	Mixed lesion. Combination of elements of first through fourth degree. There may be some preserved sensory fascicles (may produce a positive Tinel's sign)

[a]comparing and showing approximate equivalence of Seddon and Sunderland systems
[b]wallerian degeneration after British physiologist Augustus Volney Waller (1816–1870), AKA orthograde degeneration, AKA secondary degeneration: degeneration of the axon distal to a focal lesion
[c]not part of original Sunderland system

Differentiating preganglionic from postganglionic injuries

Initial exam seeks to differentiate preganglionic injuries (proximal to dorsal root ganglion) which cannot be repaired surgically, from postganglionic injuries. Clues to a preganglionic injury include:

1. Horner's syndrome: pre-ganglionic injury interrupts white rami communicantes
2. paralysis of serratus anterior (long thoracic nerve): produces winging of scapula
3. paralysis of rhomboids (dorsal scapular nerve)
4. early neuropathic pain suggests nerve root avulsion. MRI or myelogram will show pseudomeningoceles at the avulsed levels
5. EMG: requires ≥ 3 weeks from injury for some findings. Look for:
   a) denervation potentials in paraspinal muscles due to loss of neural input. The posterior ramus of the spinal nerve originates just distal to the dorsal root ganglion. Due to overlap, cannot localize to a specific segment
   b) normal sensory nerve action potential (SNAP): preganglionic injuries leave the dorsal ganglion sensory cell body and the distal axon intact, so that normal SNAP can be recorded proximally even in an anesthetic region
6. pseudomeningocele on myelography or MRI: suggests nerve root avulsion (very proximal), however, 15% of pseudomeningoceles are not associated with avulsions, and 20% of avulsions do not have pseudomeningoceles[36,37]

Types of brachial plexus injuries

(Duchene)-Erb's palsy

Upper brachial plexus injury (C5 & 6, some authors include C7) e.g. from forceful separation of humeral head from shoulder, commonly due to difficult parturition (see below) or motorcycle accident (downward force on shoulder can cause traumatic nerve root avulsion from the spinal cord). Paralysis of deltoid, biceps, rhomboids, brachioradialis, supra- & infra-spinatus, and occasionally supinator. C7 involvement produces weak wrist extension.

Motor: arm hangs at side internally rotated & extended at elbow and flexed at the wrist ("Bellhop's tip position"). Hand motion is unaffected.

Klumpke's palsy

Injury to lower brachial plexus (C8 & T1, some authors include C7), from traction of abducted arm e.g. in catching oneself during a fall from a height, or by Pancoast tumor (lung apex tumor – check CXR with apical lordotic view). Characteristic claw deformity (also seen with ulnar nerve injury) with weakness and wasting of small hand muscles. Possible Horner's syndrome if T1 involved.

Birth brachial plexus injury (BBPI)

Incidence is 0.3–2.0 per 1000 live births (0.1% in infants with birthweight < 4000 gm[38]). Rarely, a congenital case may be mistaken for BBPI.[39] Some contend that the plexus injury may occur when uterine contractions push the shoulder against the mother's pubic bone or with lowering of the shoulder with opposite inclination of the cervical spine.[39]

Classification of BBPI injuries: Upper plexus injuries are most common, with about half having C5 & C6 injuries, and 25% involving C7 also.[40] Combined upper and lower lesions occur in $\approx$ 20%. Pure lower lesions (C7-T1) are rare, constituting only $\approx$ 2% and seen most commonly in breech deliveries. Lesions are bilateral in $\approx$ 4%. A 4-level scale of intensity is shown ▶ Table 31.7.[41]

Risk factors:

1. shoulder dystocia
2. high birth weight
3. primiparous mother
4. forceps[42] or vacuum assisted delivery
5. breech presentation[43]
6. prolonged labor
7. previous birth complicated by BBPI

Management of BBPI: Most surgeons observe all patients until age 3 months. Conservative surgeons may wait up to 9 months. More aggressive surgeons will explore the plexus at age 3 months if not antigravity in deltoid, biceps or triceps. In cases of proven avulsion (pseudomeningocele and EMG indicative of a preganglionic injury), nerve transfers are a valid option at 3 months.[44] EMG may show signs of reinnervation, but the recovery may not be robust enough.

Table 31.7 Birth brachial plexus injury

Group	Lesion	Manifestation	Spontaneous recovery rate
1	C5 or C6 roots or superior trunk	paralysis of shoulder abduction, elbow flexion & forearm supination. Finger flexion is norma	90%
2	above + involvement of C7 or medial trunk	above + paralysis of finger extensors (but not flexors)	65%
3	above + finger flexors	essentially no hand movement. No Horner's syndrome	≈ < 50%
4	complete brachial plexus	flail arm + Horner's syndrome	0%
	"dominant C7" paralysis variant	selective loss of shoulder abduction & elbow extension	

Table 31.8 Indications for neurosurgical intervention in GSW to the brachial plexus[45]

1. complete loss in the distribution of at least one element
   a) no improvement clinically or on EMG in 2–5 months
   b) deficit in distribution that is responsive to surgery (e.g. C5, C6, C7, upper or middle trunk, lateral or posterior cords or their outflows)
   c) injuries with loss only in lower elements are *not* operated
2. incomplete loss with failure to control pain medically
3. pseudoaneurysm, clot or fistula involving plexus
4. true causalgia requiring sympathectomy

Management of brachial plexus injuries

1. most injuries show maximal deficit at onset. Progressive deficit is usually due to vascular injuries (pseudoaneurysm, A-V fistula, or expansile clot), these should be explored immediately
2. clean, sharp, relatively fresh lacerating injuries (usually iatrogenic, scalpel induced) should be explored acutely and repaired with tension-free end-to-end anastamoses within 24–48 hours (after that then ends will more edematous and therefore more difficult to suture)
3. penetrating non-missile injuries with severe or complete deficit should be explored as soon as the primary wound heals
4. gunshot wounds (GSW) to the brachial plexus: deficit is usually due to axonotmesis or neurotmesis (see below). Sometimes nerves may be divided. Nerves showing partial function usually recover spontaneously; those with complete dysfunction rarely do so. Surgery is of little benefit for discrete injuries to the lower trunk, medial cord, or C8/T1 roots. Most are managed conservatively for 2–5 months. Indications for surgery are shown in ▸ Table 31.8
5. traction injuries: incomplete postganglionic injuries tend to improve spontaneously. If recovery is not satisfactory, perform EMG at 4–5 months and explore at 6 months
6. neuromas in continuity: those that do not conduct a SNAP have complete internal disruption and require resection and grafting. Methods of repair:
   a) neurolysis:
      - external neurolysis: most commonly performed in exploration. Value is questionable
      - internal neurolysis: splitting the nerve into fascicles. Not recommended unless a clear neuroma in continuity is found eccentric in the nerve that conducts SNAP
   b) nerve grafting. Sural nerve is the most commonly used interposition graft following resection of neuroma in continuity
   c) nerve transfers. Donor nerve options:
      - spinal accessory nerve
      - intercostal nerves to musculocutaneous nerve
      - fascicles of the ulnar nerve for the median nerve (Oberlin procedure)
      - anterior interosseus nerve to median nerve

31.7 Missile injuries of peripheral nerves

This section deals primarily with gunshot wounds (GSW). Most injuries from a single bullet are due to shock and cavitation from the missile causing axonotmesis or neurotmesis, and are not from direct nerve transection. Approximately 70% will recover with expectant management.

31

However, if there is a lack of improvement on serial examinations including electrodiagnostic studies, intervention should be undertaken by about 5–6 months to avoid further difficulties due to nerve fibrosis and muscle atrophy.

See ▶ Table 31.8 for indications for surgery for missile injuries of the brachial plexus.

31.8 Thoracic outlet syndrome

31.8.1 General information

The thoracic outlet is a confined area at the apex of the lung bordered by the 1st rib below and the clavicle above through which passes the subclavian artery, vein, and brachial plexus.

Thoracic outlet syndrome (TOS) is a term implying compression of one or more of the enclosed structures producing a heterogeneous group of disorders. TOS tends to be diagnosed more often by general and vascular surgeons than by neurologists and neurosurgeons. Four unrelated conditions with different structures involved:

1. noncontroversial", with characteristic symptom complex, reproducible clinical findings, confirmatory laboratory tests. Low incidence[46]
   - arterial vascular: producing arm, hand and finger pallor and ischemia
   - venous vascular: producing arm swelling and edema
   - true neurologic: compressing the lower trunk or median cord of the brachial plexus (see below)
2. disputed neurologic: includes scalenus anticus syndrome (see below)

31.8.2 Differential diagnosis

1. herniated cervical disc
2. cervical arthrosis
3. lung cancer (pancoast tumor)
4. tardy ulnar nerve palsy
5. carpal tunnel syndrome
6. orthopedic shoulder problems
7. complex regional pain syndrome (reflex sympathetic dystrophy)

31

31.8.3 True neurologic TOS

General information

A rare condition primarily affecting adult women, usually unilateral.

Neurologic structures involved

1. most common: compression of the C8/T1 roots
2. or proximal lower trunk of the brachial plexus (BP)
3. less common: compression of the median cord of the BP

Etiologies

1. constricting band extending from the first rib to a rudimentary "cervical rib" or to an elongated C7 transverse process
2. scalenus (anticus) syndrome: controversial (below)
3. compression beneath the pectoralis minor tendon under the coracoid process: may result from repetitive movements of the arms above the head (shoulder elevation and hyperabduction)

Signs and symptoms

1. ✱ sensory changes in distribution of median cord (mainly along medial forearm), *sparing* median nerve sensory fibers (pass through upper and middle trunks)
2. hand clumsiness or weakness and wasting, especially abductor pollicis brevis and ulnar hand intrinsics (C8/T1 denervation/atrophy)
3. there may be tenderness over Erb's point (2 to 3 cm above the clavicle in front of the C6 transverse process)
4. may be painless
5. usually unilateral

Confirmatory tests

1. EMG: unreliable (may be negative). Most common abnormality in neurogenic TOS is loss of medial antebrachial cutaneous SNAP
2. MRI does not show bony abnormalities well, but may occasionally demonstrate a kink in the lower BP. Can also rule-out conditions that may mimic TOS such as herniated cervical disc
3. cervical spine x-rays with obliques and apical lordotic CXR may demonstrate bony abnormalities. However, not every cervical rib produces symptoms (some patients with bilateral cervical ribs may have unilateral TOS).

Treatment

Controversial. Conservative treatment (usually including stretching and physical therapy) is about equally as effective as surgery and avoids attendant risks.

Decompression can be achieved by removing the muscles that surround the nerves (scalenectomy), by transaxillary first rib resection, or both.

31.8.4 Scalenus (anticus) syndrome (disputed neurologic TOS)

Controversial. More commonly diagnosed in the 1940s and 1950s. There is a lack of consensus regarding the pathophysiology (including structures involved), clinical presentation, helpful tests, and optimal treatment. Removal of first thoracic rib is often advocated for treatment, frequently via a transaxillary approach. Unfortunately, injuries, especially to the lower trunk of the brachial plexus, may result from the surgery.

Other variations include an "upper plexus" type for which total anterior scalenectomy is advocated. Again, very controversial.

References

[1] Poza JJ, Cobo AM, Marti-Masso JF. Peripheral neuropathy associated with polycythemia vera. Neurologia. 1996; 11:276–279

[2] Ochoa JL, Verdugo RJ. Reflex Sympathetic Dystrophy: A Common Clinical Avenue for Somatoform Expression. Neurol Clin. 1995; 13:351–363

[3] Denny-Brown D. Primary Sensory Neuropathy with Muscular Changes Associated with Carcinoma. J Neurol Neurosurg Psychiatry. 1948; 11:73–87

[4] Camerlingo M, Nemni R, Ferraro B, et al. Malignancy and Sensory Neuropathy of Unexplained Cause: A Prospective Study of 51 Patients. Arch Neurol. 1998; 55:981–984

[5] McLeod JG, Dyck PJ, Thomas PK. In: Paraneoplastic Neuropathies. Peripheral Neuropathy. Philadelphia: W.B. Saunders; 1993:1583–1590

[6] Adams RD, Victor M. Principles of Neurology. 2nd ed. New York: McGraw-Hill; 1981

[7] Turner JW, Parsonage MJ. Neuralgic amyotrophy (paralytic brachial neuritis); with special reference to prognosis. Lancet. 1957; 273

[8] Tsairis P, Dyck PJ, Mulder DW. Natural History of Brachial Plexus Neuropathy: Report on 99 Patients. Arch Neurol. 1972; 27:109–117

[9] Misamore GW, Lehman DE. Parsonage-Turner syndrome (acute brachial neuritis). J Bone Joint Surg. 1996; 78:1405–1408

[10] Evans BA, Stevens JC, Dyck PJ. Lumbosacral Plexus Neuropathy. Neurology. 1981; 31:1327–1330

[11] The Diabetes Control and Complications Trial Research Group. The Effect of Intensive Treatment of Diabetes on the Development and Progression of Long-Term Complications in Insulin-Dependent Diabetes Mellitus. N Engl J Med. 1993; 329:977–986

[12] Asbury AK. Proximal Diabetic Neuropathy. Ann Neurol. 1977; 2:179–180

[13] Dyck PJ, Thomas PK. Peripheral Neuropathy. 2nd ed. Philadelphia: W. B. Saunders; 1984

[14] Garland H. Diabetic Amyotrophy. BMJ. 1955; 2:1287–1290

[15] Barohn RJ, Sahenk Z, Warmolts JR, Mendell JR. The Bruns-Garland Syndrome (Diabetic Amyotrophy): Revisited 100 Years Later. Arch Neurol. 1991; 48:1130–1135

[16] Pascoe MK, Low PA, Windebank AJ. Subacute Diabetic Proximal Neuropathy. Mayo Clin Proc. 1997; 72:1123–1132

[17] Davis JL, Lewis SB, Gerich JE, et al. Peripheral Diabetic Neuropathy Treated with Amitriptyline and Fluphenazine. JAMA. 1977; 21:2291–2292

[18] Max MB, Lynch SA, Muir J, Shoaf SE, et al. Effects of Desipramine, Amitriptyline, and Fluoxetine on Pain in Diabetic Neuropathy. N Engl J Med. 1992; 326:1250–1256

[19] Mendel CM, Klein RF, Chappell DA, et al. A Trial of Amitriptyline and Fluphenazine in the Treatment of Painful Diabetic Neuropathy. JAMA. 1986; 255:637–639

[20] Mendel CM, Grunfeld C. Amitriptyline and Fluphenazine for Painful Diabetic Neuropathy. JAMA. 1986; 256:712–714

[21] Backonja M, Beydoun A, Edwards KR, Schwartz SL, Fonseca V, Hes M, LaMoreaux L, Garofalo E. Gabapentin for the symptomatic treatment of painful neuropathy in patients with diabetes mellitus: a randomized controlled trial. JAMA. 1998; 280:1831–1836

[22] Morello CM, Leckband SG, Stoner CP, Moorhouse DF, Sahagian GA. Randomized double-blind study comparing the efficacy of gabapentin with amitriptyline on diabetic peripheral neuropathy pain. Arch Intern Med. 1999; 159:1931–1937

[23] New Uses of Thalidomide. Med Letter. 1996; 38:15–16

[24] Fuller GN, Jacobs JM, Guiloff RJ. Nature and Incidence of Peripheral Nerve Syndromes in HIV Infection. J Neurol Neurosurg Psychiatry. 1993; 56:372–381

[25] Drugs for HIV Infection. Med Letter. 2000; 42:1–6

[26] Kroll DA, Caplan RA, Posner K, et al. Nerve Injury Associated with Anesthesia. Anesthesiology. 1990; 73:202–207

[27] Warner MA. Perioperative Neuropathies. Mayo Clin Proc. 1998; 73:567–574

[28] Wadsworth TG, Williams JR. Cubital Tunnel External Compression Syndrome. Br Med J. 1973; 1:662–666

[29] Warner MA, Marner ME, Martin JT. Ulnar Neuropathy: Incidence, Outcome, and Risk Factors in

Sedated or Anesthesthetized Patients. Anesthesiology. 1994; 81:1332–1340

[30] Alvine FG, Schurrer ME. Postoperative Ulnar-Nerve Palsy: Are There Predisposing Factors? J Bone Joint Surg. 1987; 69A:255–259

[31] Stewart JD, Shantz SH. Perioperative ulnar neuropathies: A medicolegal review. Can J Neurol Sci. 2003; 30:15–19

[32] Warner MA, Martin JT, Schroeder DR, et al. Lower-Extremity Motor Neuropathy Associated with Surgery Performed on Patients in a Lithotomy Position. Anesthesiology. 1994; 81:6–12

[33] O'Donnell D, Rottman R, Kotelko D, et al. Incidence of Maternal Postpartum Neurologic Dysfunction. Anesthesiology. 1994; 81

[34] Sanabria EAM, Nagashima T, Yamashita H, Ehara K, Kohmura E. Postoperative bilateral meralgia paresthetica after spine surgery: An overlooked entity? Spinal Surgery. 2003; 17:195–202

[35] Kent CK, Moscucci M, Gallagher SG, et al. Neuropathies After Cardiac Catheterization: Incidence, Clinical Patterns, and Long-Term Outcome. J Vasc Surg. 1994; 19:1008–1014

[36] Carvalho GA, Nikkhah G, Matthies C, Penkert G, Samii M. Diagnosis of root avulsions in traumatic brachial plexus injuries: value of computerized tomography myelography and magnetic resonance imaging. J Neurosurg. 1997; 86:69–76

[37] Hashimoto T, Mitomo M, Hirabuki N, Miura T, Kawai R, Nakamura H, Kawai H, Ono K, Kozuka T. Nerve root avulsion of birth palsy: comparison of myelography with CT myelography and somatosensory evoked potential. Radiology. 1991; 178:841–845

[38] Rouse DJ, Owen J, Goldenberg RL, Cliver SP. The effectiveness and costs of elective cesarean delivery for fetal macrosomia diagnosed by ultrasound. JAMA. 1996; 276:1480–1486

[39] Gilbert A, Brockman R, Carlioz H. Surgical Treatment of Brachial Plexus Birth Palsy. Clin Orthop. 1991; 264:39–47

[40] Boome RS, Kaye JC. Obstetric Traction Injuries of the Brachial Plexus: Natural History, Indications for Surgical Repair and Results. J Bone Joint Surg. 1988; 70B:571–576

[41] van Ouwerkerk WJ, van der Sluijs JA, Nollet F, Barkhof F, Slooff AC. Management of obstetric brachial plexus lesions: state of the art and future developments. Childs Nerv Syst. 2000; 16:638–644

[42] Piatt JH, Hudson AR, Hoffman HJ. Preliminary Experiences with Brachial Plexus Explorations in Children: Birth Injury and Vehicular Trauma. Neurosurgery. 1988; 22:715–723

[43] Hunt D. Surgical Management of Brachial Plexus Birth Injuries. Dev Med Child Neurol. 1988; 30:821–828

[44] Anand P, Birch R. Restoration of sensory function and lack of long-term chronic pain syndromes after brachial plexus injury in human neonates. Brain. 2002; 125:113–122

[45] Kline DG, Hudson AR. Nerve Injuries: Operative Results for Major Nerve Injuries, Entrapments, and Tumors. Philadelphia: W. B. Saunders; 1995

[46] Wilbourn AJ. The Thoracic Outlet Syndrome is Overdiagnosed. Arch Neurol. 1990; 47:328–330

Part XI

Neurophthalmology and Neurotology

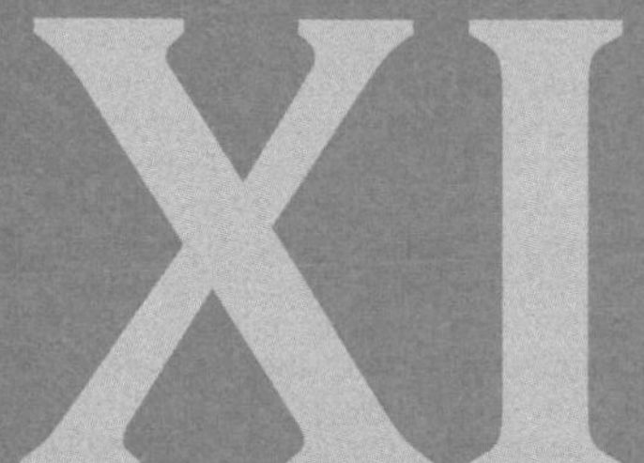

32 Neurophthalmology

32.1 Nystagmus

32.1.1 Definition

Involuntary rhythmic oscillation of the eyes, usually conjugate. Most common form is jerk nystagmus, in which the direction of the nystagmus is defined for the direction of the fast (cortical) component (which is *not* the abnormal component). Horizontal or upward gaze-provoked nystagmus may be due to sedatives or AEDs; otherwise vertical nystagmus is indicative of posterior fossa pathology.

32.1.2 Localizing lesion for various forms of nystagmus

1. seesaw nystagmus: intorting eye moves up, extorting eye moves down, pattern then reverses. Lesion in diencephalon. Also reported with chiasmal compression (occasionally accompanied with bitemporal hemianopia in parasellar masses)
2. convergence nystagmus: slow abduction of eyes followed by adducting (converging) jerks, usually associated with features of Parinaud's syndrome. May be associated with nystagmus retractorius (see below) with similar location of lesion
3. nystagmus retractorius: resulting from co-contraction of all EOM's. May accompany convergence nystagmus. Lesion in upper midbrain tegmentum (usually vascular disease or tumor, especially pinealoma)
4. downbeat nystagmus: nystagmus with the fast phase downward while in primary position. Most patients have a structural lesion in the posterior fossa, especially at the *cervicomedullary junction* (foramen magnum (FM)),[1] including *Chiari I malformation*, basilar impression, p-fossa tumors, syringobulbia.[2] Uncommonly occurs in multiple sclerosis (MS), spinocerebellar degeneration, and in some metabolic conditions (hypomagnesemia, thiamine deficiency, alcohol intoxication or withdrawal, or treatment with phenytoin, carbamazepine or lithium[3])
5. upbeat nystagmus: lesion in medulla
6. abducting nystagmus occurs in INO. Lesion in pons (MLF)
7. Brun's nystagmus: lesion in pontomedullary junction (PMJ)
8. vestibular nystagmus: lesion in PMJ
9. ocular myoclonus: lesion in myoclonic triangle
10. periodic alternating nystagmus (PAN): lesion in FM and cerebellum
11. square wave jerks, macro square wave jerks, macro saccadic oscillations. Lesion in cerebellar pathways
12. "nystagmoid" eye movements (not true nystagmus)
    a) ocular bobbing (p. 570): lesion in pontine tegmentum
    b) ocular dysmetria: overshoot of eye on attempted fixation followed by diminishing oscillations until eye "hones in" on target. Lesion in cerebellum or pathways (may be seen in Friedreich's ataxia)
    c) ping-pong gaze (p. 301)
    d) "windshield wiper eyes" (p. 301)

32.2 Papilledema

32.2.1 General information

AKA choked (optic) disk. Thought to be caused by axoplasmic stasis. One theory: elevated ICP is transmitted through the subarachnoid space of the optic nerve sheath to the region of the optic disc. Elevated ICP will usually obliterate retinal venous pulsation if the pressure is transmitted to the point where the central retinal vein passes through the subarachnoid space (≈ 1 cm posterior to the globe). Papilledema (PPD) may also be dependent on the ratio of retinal arterial to retinal venous pressure, with ratios < 1.5:1 more commonly associated with papilledema than higher ratios.

Elevated ICP generally causes *bilateral* papilledema PPD (see below for unilateral papilledema). Papilledema may appear similar to optic neuritis on funduscopy, but the latter is usually associated with more severe visual loss and tenderness to eye pressure over the eye.

Pseudopapilledema may mimic papilledema in that the optic disc may appear swollen, but, unlike true papilledema, the peripapillary vessels are not obscured. It may be unilateral or bilateral. There are a number of benign conditions that can cause pseudopapilledema (including a small optic cup, buried disc drusen…), and extensive workup is generally not indicated.

Papilledema typically takes 24–48 hours to develop following a sustained rise in ICP. It is rarely seen as early as ≈ 6 hours after onset, but not earlier. Papilledema does not cause visual blurring or reduction of visual fields unless very severe and prolonged.

32.2.2 Differential diagnosis of unilateral papilledema

1. compressive lesions
   a) orbital tumors
   b) tumors of optic nerve sheath (meningiomas)
   c) optic nerve tumors (optic gliomas)
2. local inflammatory disorder
3. Foster Kennedy syndrome (p.99)
4. demyelinating disease (e.g. multiple sclerosis)
5. elevated ICP in the setting of something that prevents manifestation in one eye, including:
   a) blockage which prevents transmission of elevated CSF pressure to that optic disc[4]
   b) prosthetic eye (artificial eye)

32.3 Visual fields

32.3.1 General information

Normal human visual field: extends approximately from 35° nasally in each eye, to 90°temporally, and 50° above and below the horizontal meridian. The normal physiological blind spot (due to absence of light receptors in the optic disc due to penetration of the retina by the optic nerve and vessels) is located to the temporal side of the macular visual area in each eye.

32.3.2 Macular sparing/splitting

Macular splitting can occur both in lesions anterior or posterior to the lateral geniculate body (LGB). However, macular sparing tends to occur with lesions posterior to the LGB. Homonymous hemiaopsia with macular sparing tends to occur with lesions in the optic radiation or infarcts of primary visual cortex. There is more than 1 way for this to occur: input from the macula is spread over a large portion of the optic radiation and primary visual cortex, and the occipital pole (primary visual cortex) receives dual blood supply.

32.4 Visual field deficits

Can be tested by:

1. bedside confrontational testing: detects only gross peripheral field deficits. Stimulus is brought in from non-seeing to seeing field (towards macular vision area) along 8 meridians
2. formal perimetry
   a) using a tangent screen
   b) Goldmann perimetry
   c) automated perimetry exam: Humphrey visual field (HVF)

► **Knee of Wilbrand.** (Named for Hermann Wilbrand (1851–1935) German neurophthalmologist – the name of this physician is variously listed as: Hermann or Herman, and erroneously as von Willebrand, Willebrand, or Wildbrand…). A 1-2 mm anterior "bend" of the decussating fibers of the optic chiasm into the contralateral optic nerve before continuing to the optic tract.[5] Initially identified histologically postmortem in subjects who had monocular enucleation. Optic nerve injury close to the chiasm produces a junctional scotoma involving an ipsilateral nerve fiber bundle defect and contralateral superior temporal quadrantanopia or contralateral temporal hemianopia stemming from injury to the proximal optic nerve and decussating "knee" fibers.[5,6] Controversy as to the existence or significance of Wilbrand's knee initially arose after further cadaveric studies suggested that Wilbrand's knee is an anatomic artifact resulting from buckling of the decussating fibers into the contralateral optic nerve as the optic nerve and chiasm atrophy following enucleation.[5] However, advanced optical imaging techniques have demonstrated a forward bend of the anterior inferior decussating fibers in chiasms with no pre-mortem pathology.[7] However, case series with

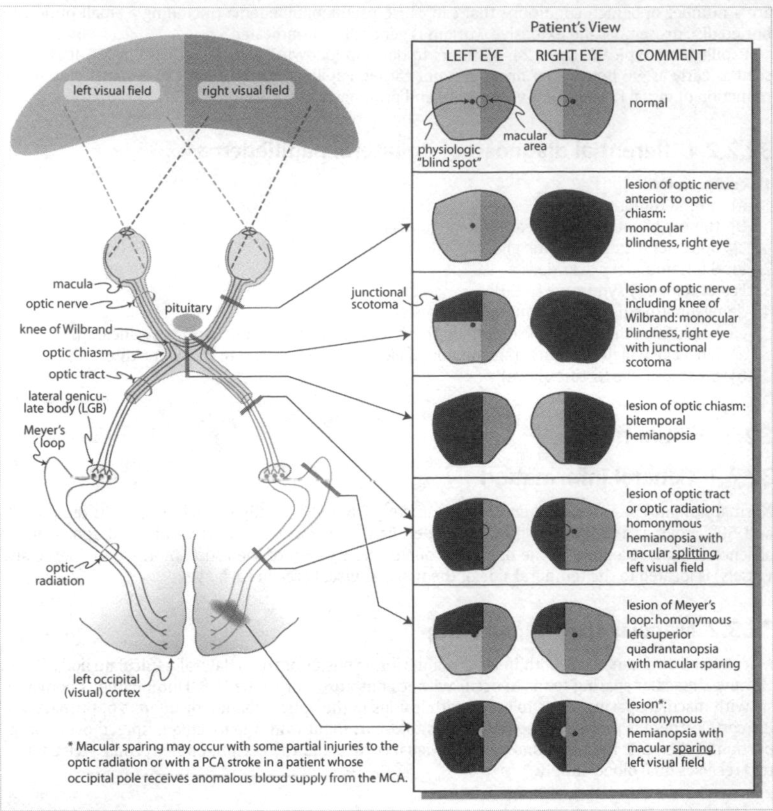

Fig. 32.1 Visual field deficits

intraoperative sectioning of the optic nerve at the level of the chiasm have not been shown to develop contralateral visual field deficits.[8,9]

▸ **Visual field deficit patterns.** ▸ Fig. 32.1.

1. bitemporal hemianopsia
2. posterior cerebral artery occlusion → infarction in the anterior visual cortex → contralateral homonymous hemianopia with macular sparing

32.5 Pupillary diameter

32.5.1 Pupilodilator (sympathetic)

Pupilodilator muscle fibers are sympathetic and are arranged radially in the iris.

First-order sympathetic nerve fibers arise in the posterolateral hypothalamus, and descend uncrossed in the lateral tegmentum of the midbrain, pons, medulla and cervical spinal cord to the intermediolateral cell column of the spinal cord from C8-T2 (ciliospinal center of Budge). Here they synapse with lateral horn cells (neurotransmitter: ACh) and give off 2nd order neurons (preganglionics).

Second-order neurons enter the sympathetic chain and ascend but do not synapse until they reach the superior cervical ganglion, where they give rise to 3rd order neurons.

Third-order neurons (postganglionics) course upward with the common carotid artery, those that mediate sweat in the face split off with the ECA. The rest travel with the ICA passing over the carotid sinus. Some fibers accompany V1 (ophthalmic division of trigeminal nerve), passing through (without synapsing) the ciliary ganglion, reaching the pupilodilator muscle of the eye as 2 long ciliary nerves (neurotransmitter: NE). Other fibers from the ICA travel with the ophthalmic artery to innervate the lacrimal gland and Müller's muscle (AKA the orbital muscle).

32.5.2 Pupilloconstrictor (parasympathetic)

Pupilloconstrictor muscle fibers are arranged as a sphincter in the iris.

Parasympathetic preganglionic fibers arise in the Edinger-Westphal nucleus (in high midbrain, superior colliculus level) and are situated peripherally on the intracranial portion of the oculomotor nerve (p.565).

32.5.3 Pupillary light reflex

Mediated by rods and cones of the retina which are stimulated by light, and transmit via their axons in the optic nerve. As with the visual path, temporal retinal fibers remain ipsilateral, whereas nasal retinal fibers decussate in the optic chiasm. Fibers subserving the light reflex bypass the lateral geniculate body (LGB) (unlike fibers for vision which enter the LGB) to synapse in the pretectal nuclear complex at the level of the superior colliculus. Intercalating neurons connect to both Edinger-Westphal parasympathetic motor nuclei. The preganglionic fibers travel within the third nerve to the ciliary ganglion as described above under Pupilloconstrictor (parasympathetic).

Monocular light normally stimulates bilaterally symmetric (i.e. equal) pupillary constriction (ipsilateral response is called direct, contralateral response is consensual).

32.5.4 Pupillary exam

To perform a complete bedside pupillary exam (see following sections for rationale for various aspects of the pupillary exam):

1. measure pupil size in a darkened room: anisocoria augmented in the dark indicates the smaller pupil is abnormal and suggests a sympathetic lesion
2. measure pupil size in a lighted room: anisocoria intensified in the light suggests the larger pupil is abnormal and that the defect is in the parasympathetics
3. note the reaction to bright light (direct and consensual)
4. near response (it is necessary to check this only if the light reaction is not good): the pupil normally constricts on convergence, and this response should be greater than the light reflex (accommodation is not necessary, and a visually handicapped patient can be instructed to follow their own finger as it is brought in)
   a) light-near dissociation: pupillary constriction on convergence but absent light response (Argyll Robertson pupil). Etiologies:
      - classically described in syphilis
      - Parinaud's syndrome (p.99): dorsal midbrain lesion
      - oculomotor neuropathy (usually causes a tonic pupil as in oculomotor compression, see below): DM, EtOH
      - Adie's pupil: see below
5. swinging flashlight test: alternate the flashlight from one eye to the other with as little delay as possible; watch ≥ 5 seconds for the pupil to redilate (dilation after initial constriction is called pupillary escape and is normal – due to retinal adaptation). Normal: direct and consensual light reflexes are equal. Afferent pupillary defect (see below): consensual reflex is stronger than the direct (i.e. pupil is larger on direct illumination than contralateral illumination)

32.5.5 Alterations in pupillary diameter

Anisocoria

General information

▶ **Definition.** Unequal pupil sizes (usually ≥ 1 mm difference).

▶ **Note.** An afferent pupillary defect (APD) (even with total blindness in one eye) alone does *not* produce anisocoria (i.e. an APD together with anisocoria indicates two separate lesions).

32

Evaluation

1. history is critically important. Check for exposure to drugs that affect pupillary size, trauma. Look at old photos (e.g. driver's license) for physiologic anisocoria
2. exam: see Pupillary exam above
3. a non-contrast CT is usually not helpful and can provide a false sense of security

Differential diagnosis

1. physiologic anisocoria: occurs in ≈ 20% of population (more common in people with a light iris). Familial and nonfamilial varieties exist. The difference in pupils is usually < 0.4 mm. The inequality is the same in a light and dark room (or slightly worse in the dark)
2. pharmacologic pupil (see below): the most common cause of *sudden onset* of anisocoria
   a) mydriatics (pupillary dilators):
      - sympathomimetics (stimulate the dilator pupillae): usually cause only 1–2 mm of dilation, may react slightly to light. Includes: phenylephrine, clonidine, naphazoline (an ingredient in OTC eye drops for allergies), eye contact with cocaine, certain plants (e.g. jimsonweed)
      - parasympatholytics (inhibit the sphincter pupillae): cause maximal dilation (up to 8 mm) that does *not* react to light. Includes: tropicamide, atropine, scopolamine (including patches for motion sickness), certain plants (e.g. deadly nightshade)
   b) miotics (pupillary constrictors): pilocarpine, organophosphates (pesticides), flea powders containing anticholinesterase
3. Horner's syndrome: interruption of sympathetics to pupilodilator. The abnormal pupil is the *smaller* (miotic) pupil. If there is ptosis it will be on the side of the *small* pupil. See etiologies, etc. (p. 564)
4. third nerve palsy (p. 565). If there is ptosis, it will be on the side of the *large* pupil
   a) oculomotor neuropathy ("peripheral" neuropathy of the third nerve): usually spares the pupil. Etiologies: DM (usually resolves in ≈ 8 weeks), EtOH…
   b) third nerve compression: tends *not* to spare pupil (i.e. pupil is dilated). Produces loss of parasympathetic tone. Etiologies include:
      - aneurysm:
        p-comm (the most common aneurysm to cause this)
        basilar bifurcation (occasionally compresses the posterior III nerve)
      - uncal herniation: below
      - tumor
      - cavernous sinus lesions: including cavernous internal carotid aneurysm, carotid-cavernous fistula, cavernous sinus tumors
5. Adie's pupil (AKA tonic pupil): see below
6. local trauma to the eye: traumatic iridoplegia. Injury to the pupillary sphincter muscle may produce mydriasis or less often miosis, shape may be irregular
7. pontine lesions
8. eye prosthesis (artificial eye) AKA pseudoanisocoria
9. occasionally some patients have anisocoria that occurs only during migraine[10]
10. iritis
11. keratitis or corneal abrasion

32

Marcus Gunn pupil

AKA (relative) afferent pupillary defect (APD or RAPD), AKA amaurotic pupil. Finding: consensual pupillary reflex to light is stronger than the direct (normal responses are equal). Contrary to some textbooks, the amaurotic pupil is *not* larger than the other.[11] The presence of the consensual reflex is evidence of a preserved third nerve (with parasympathetics) on the side of the impaired direct reflex. Best detected with the swinging flashlight test (see above).

Etiologies

Lesion *anterior to the chiasm* ipsilateral to the side of the impaired direct reflex:

1. either in the retina (e.g. retinal detachment, retinal infarct e.g. from embolus)
2. or optic nerve, as may occur in:
   a) optic or retrobulbar neuritis: commonly seen in MS, but may also occur after vaccinations or viral infections, and usually improves gradually
   b) trauma to the optic nerve: indirect (p. 836) or direct
   c) compression by tumor anterior to the chiasm

Adie's pupil (tonic pupil)

An iris palsy resulting in a dilated pupil, due to impaired postganglionic parasympathetics. Thought to be due to a viral infection of the ciliary ganglion. When associated with loss of all muscle tendon reflexes it is called Holmes-Adie's (is not limited to knee jerks, as some texts indicate). Typically seen in a woman in her twenties.

Slit-lamp exam shows some parts of iris contract and others don't.

These patients exhibit light-near dissociation (see above): in checking near response it is necessary to wait a few seconds.

Denervation supersensitivity: usually occurs after several weeks (not in acute phase). Administer two drops of dilute pilocarpine (0.1–0.125%), a parasympathomimetic in each eye. Miosis (constriction) will occur in Adie's pupil within 30 minutes (normal pupils will react only to ≈1% pilocarpine).

Pharmacologic pupil

General information

Follows administration of a mydriatic agent. The mydriatic agent may be "occult" when other care providers have not been alerted that this has been used on a patient (this should always be noted in the chart), or when health care personnel unwittingly inoculate agents, e.g. scopolamine, atropine[12]... into a patient's eye or into their own eye. May present with accompanying H/A, and if it is unknown that a mydriatic is involved, this may be misinterpreted e.g. as a warning of an expanding p-comm aneurysm.

A pharmacologically dilated pupil is very large (7–8 mm), and is larger than typical mydriasis due to third nerve compression (5–6 mm).

To differentiate pharmacologic pupil from a third nerve lesion: instill 1% pilocarpine (a parasympathomimetic) in both eyes (for comparison). A pharmacologic pupil does *not* constrict, whereas the normal side and a dilated pupil from a third nerve palsy will.

Agents

Drugs intentionally used by physicians to dilate the pupils (e.g. Mydriacyl, see below). For other mydriatics, see above.

Management

Option: admit and observe overnight, pupil should normalize.

Using mydriatic agents to produce pupillary dilatation

Indications: to improve the ability to examine the retina. NB: ability to follow bedside examination of pupils will be lost for duration of drug effect. This could mask pupillary dilatation from third nerve compression due to herniation. Always alert other caregivers and place a note in the chart to document that the pupil has been pharmacologically dilated (see above), including the agent(s) used and the time administered.

℞: 2 gtt of 0.5% or 1% tropicamide (Mydriacyl®) blocks the parasympathetic supply to pupil, and produces a mydriasis that lasts a couple hrs to half a day. This can be augmented with 1 gtt 2.5% phenylephrine ophthalmic (Mydfrin®, Neofrin®, Phenoptic® and others) which stimulates the sympathetics.

Oculomotor nerve compression

Third nerve compression may manifest initially with a mildly dilated pupil (5–6 mm). Possible etiologies include uncal herniation or expansion of a p-comm or basilar bifurcation aneurysm. However, within 24 hours, most of these cases will also develop an oculomotor palsy (with down and out deviation of the eye and ptosis). These pupils respond to mydriatics and to miotic agents (the latter helps differentiate this from a pharmacologic pupil, see above).

Although it is possible for a unilaterally dilated pupil alone to be the initial presentation in uncal herniation, in actuality almost all of these patients will have some other finding, e.g. alteration in mental status (confusion, agitation, etc.) before midbrain compression occurs (i.e. it would be rare for a person undergoing early uncal herniation with a dilating pupil to be awake, talking, appropriate and neurologically intact).

Table 32.1 Findings in Horner's syndrome

- miosis (constricted pupil)
- ptosis
- enophthalmos
- hyperemia of eye
- anhidrosis of half of face

Neuromuscular blocking agents (NMBAs)

Due to the absence of nicotinic receptors on the iris, non-depolarizing muscle blocking agents, such as pancuronium (Pavulon®) normally do not alter pupillary reaction to light[13] except in large doses where some of the first and second order neurons may be blocked.

Paradoxical pupillary reaction

Pupils constrict when light is removed.
1. congenital stationary night blindness
2. Best disease: autosomal dominant hereditary progressive macular dystrophy
3. optic nerve hypoplasia
4. retinitis pigmentosa

32.5.6 Horner's syndrome

General information

Horner's syndrome (**HS**) is caused by interruption of sympathetics to the eye and face anywhere along their path; see Pupilodilator (sympathetic) (p. 560). Unilateral findings on the involved side in a fully developed Horner's syndrome are shown in ▶ Table 32.1.

Miosis in HS

32

The miosis (pupillary constriction) in Horner's syndrome is only ≈ 2–3 mm. This will be accentuated by darkening the room, which causes the normal pupil to dilate.

Ptosis and enophthalmos

Ptosis is due primarily to paralysis of the superior and inferior tarsal muscles (weakness of the inferior tarsal muscle is technically called "inverse ptosis"). Enophthalmos is due to Müller's muscle paralysis, which also contributes a maximum of ≈ 2 mm to the ptosis. Ptosis in HS is partial, c.f. complete ptosis which is due to weakness of levator palpebra superioris which is not involved in Horner's syndrome.

Possible sites of disruption of sympathetics

General information

See also anatomy of 1st, 2nd, and 3rd order sympathetic neurons (p. 560).

1st order neuron (central neuron)

Interruption is often accompanied by other brainstem abnormalities. Etiologies of dysfunction: infarction from vascular occlusion (usually PICA), syringobulbia, intraparenchymal neoplasm.

2nd order neuron (preganglionic)

Etiologies of dysfunction: lateral sympathectomies, significant chest trauma, apical pulmonary neoplasms[14] (Pancoast tumor), high thoracic or cervical neuroblastoma.

3rd order neuron (postganglionic)

The most common type. Etiologies of dysfunction: neck trauma, carotid vascular disease/studies – e.g. carotid dissections (p. 1324) -, cervical bony abnormalities, migraine, skull base neoplasms, cavernous sinus lesions (e.g. meningioma). With involvement only of fibers on ICA, anhidrosis does not occur (i.e. sweating is preserved) on ipsilateral face since fibers to facial sweat glands travel with ECA.

Pharmacologic testing in Horner's syndrome

Establishing the diagnosis

If the diagnosis of Horner's syndrome is in doubt, the following may be used (not necessary when a pupil lag upon darkening the room can be demonstrated in the affected eye) (does *not localize* lesion as 1st order, etc.).

Cocaine. ℞: 1 gtt 4% *cocaine* OU (not the 10% solution that is commonly used in ENT procedures which will also anesthetize the sphincter pupillae, thus preventing miosis), repeat in 10 min. Observe pupils over 30 min. Cocaine blocks the NE re-uptake of postganglionics at the neuroeffector junction. In HS, no NE is released and cocaine will not dilate eye. If pupil dilates normally, no HS. Delayed dilatation occurs in partial HS.

Apraclonidine ophthalmic (Iopidine®) has essentially replaced cocaine for establishing diagnosis. It works like low-dose pilocarpine works with Adie's pupil. Iopidine causes the miotic pupil to dilate in Horner's syndrome due to denervation hypersensitivity in the pupilodilator muscle fibers.

Localizing the site of the lesion

First order HS usually is accompanied by other hypothalamic, brainstem, or medullary findings.

To differentiate a second from third-order: 1% *hydroxyamphetamine* (Paradrine®) releases NE from nerve endings at neuroeffector junction causing dilation of pupil except in 3rd order neuron lesions (injured postganglionics do not release NE).

32.6 Extraocular muscle (EOM) system

32.6.1 General information

Cr. N. III (oculomotor) innervates the ipsilateral medial rectus (MR), inferior rectus (IR), inferior oblique (IO), and superior rectus (SR). Cr. N IV (trochlear) innervates the ipsilateral superior oblique (SO), contralateral to the trochlear nucleus (p. 567). Cr. N. VI (abducens) innervates the ipsilateral lateral rectus (LR).

The frontal eye field is the cortical area that initiates voluntary (supranuclear) lateral saccadic eye movements ("pre-programmed", rapid, ballistic) to the *opposite* side, involved in suppressing reflexive saccades and generating voluntary, non-visual saccades. It is located in Brodmann's area 8 (in the frontal lobe, anterior to the primary motor cortex, ▶ Fig. 1.1). These corticobulbar fibers pass through the genu of the internal capsule to the paramedian pontine reticular formation (PPRF), which controls horizontal gaze, which sends fibers to the ipsilateral abducens/para-abducens (VI) nuclear complex, and via the medial longitudinal fasciculus (MLF) to the contralateral III nucleus to innervate the contralateral MR. Inhibitory fibers go to the ipsilateral third nerve to inhibit the antagonist MR muscle. Thus, the right PPRF controls lateral eye movements to right. 32

32.6.2 Internuclear ophthalmoplegia

Internuclear ophthalmoplegia (INO) is due to a lesion of the MLF (see above) rostral to the abducens nucleus. Findings in unilateral INO[15] (see ▶ Fig. 32.2 for illustration):

1. on attempting to look to the side contralateral to the INO:
   a) the eye ipsilateral to the lesion fails to ADDuct completely
   b) abduction nystagmus in the contralateral eye (monocular nystagmus) often with some weakness of ABDuction
2. convergence is *not* impaired in isolated MLF lesions (INO is not an EOM palsy)

The most common causes of INO:

1. MS: the most common cause of bilateral INO in young adults
2. brainstem stroke: the most common cause of unilateral INO in the elderly

32.6.3 Oculomotor (Cr. N. III) nerve palsy (OMP)

General information

The oculomotor nerve exits the brainstem ventrally and has two components: motor neurons which originate in the oculomotor nucleus, and more *peripherally situated* parasympathetic fibers which arise from the Edinger-Westphal nucleus. The nerve passes through the cavernous sinus and enters the superior orbital fissure where it divides into a superior division (innervating the superior rectus and the levator palpebrae superioris) and an inferior division (supplying the medial rectus, inferior rectus and inferior oblique). The parasympathetic fibers travel with the inferior division and branch

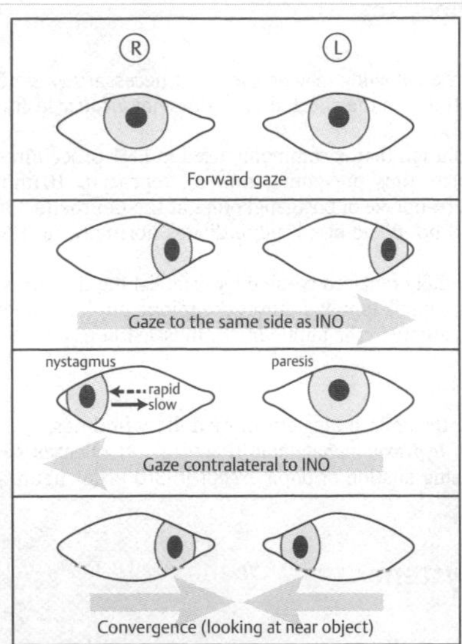

Fig. 32.2 Illustration of gaze findings with a left internuclear ophthalmoplegia

off to the ciliary ganglion where they synapse. Postganglionic fibers enter the posterior globe to innervate the ciliary muscle (relaxes the lens which "thickens" and accommodates for near vision) and the constrictor pupillae muscle.

Oculomotor nerve *motor* palsy causes ptosis with eye deviated "down & out." Nuclear involvement of 3rd nerve is rare. NB: 3rd nerve palsy alone can cause up to 3 mm exophthalmos (proptosis) from relaxation of the rectus muscles.

Also see Painful ophthalmoplegia (p.568) and Painless ophthalmoplegia (p.569). For brainstem syndromes, see Benedikt's syndrome (p.99), and Weber's syndrome (p.99). Also, see Anisocoria (p.561).

Non pupil-sparing oculomotor palsy

The rule of the pupil in third nerve palsy

Elucidated in 1958 by Rucker. In effect, states "Third nerve palsy due to *extrinsic* compression of the nerve will be associated with impaired pupillary constriction." However, it is often overlooked that in 3% the pupil is spared.[16]

Etiologies

Most cases are due to extrinsic compression of 3rd nerve. Etiologies include:

1. tumor: the most common tumors affecting 3rd nerve:
   a) chordomas
   b) clival meningiomas
2. vascular: the most common vascular lesions:
   a) aneurysms of p-comm artery (pupil sparing with aneurysmal oculomotor palsy occurs in $<$ 1%). ✱ Development of a new 3rd nerve palsy ipsilateral to a p-comm aneurysm may be a sign of expansion with the possibility of imminent rupture, and is traditionally considered an indication for urgent treatment
   b) aneurysms of the distal basilar artery or bifurcation (basilar tip)
   c) carotid-cavernous fistula (p. 1256): look for pulsatile proptosis
3. uncal herniation
4. cavernous sinus lesions: usually cause additional cranial nerve findings (V1, V2, IV, VI); see Cavernous sinus syndrome (p. 1401). Classically the third nerve palsy e.g. from enlarging cavernous aneurysm will *not* produce a dilated pupil because the sympathetics which dilate the pupil are also paralyzed[1 (p 1492)]

Pupil sparing oculomotor palsy (pupil reacts to light)

General information

Usually from intrinsic vascular lesions occluding vaso-nervorum causing central ischemic infarction. Spares parasympathetic fibers located peripherally in 3rd nerve in 62–83% of cases.[16]

Etiologies

Etiologies include:
1. diabetic neuropathy
2. atherosclerosis (as seen in chronic HTN)
3. vasculopathies: including giant cell arteritis (p. 195) (temporal arteritis)
4. chronic progressive ophthalmoplegia: usually bilateral
5. myasthenia gravis

Rarely, pupil-sparing OMP has been described following an intra-axial lesion, as in a midbrain infarction.[17]

Other causes of oculomotor palsy

Trauma, uncal herniation, laterally expanding pituitary adenomas, Lyme disease, cavernous sinus lesions: usually cause additional cranial nerve findings; see Multiple cranial nerve palsies (cranial neuropathies) (p. 1399).

Lesions within the orbit tend to affect 3rd nerve branches unequally. Superior division lesion → ptosis and impaired elevation; inferior division lesion → impairment of depression, adduction and pupillary reaction.

32.6.4 Trochlear nerve (IV) palsy

Anatomy: the trochlear nucleus lies ventral to the cerebral aqueduct at the level of the inferior colliculi. Trochlear nerve axons pass *dorsally* around the aqueduct and decussate internally just caudal to the inferior colliculi. The nerve innervates the superior oblique muscle which primarily depresses the adducted eye, but in primary gaze it intorts and secondarily abducts and depresses the globe (i.e. it moves the eye down & out).

Some unique features of the trochlear nerve:
1. the only cranial nerve to decussate internally (i.e. the trochlear nucleus is on the contralateral side to the nerve that exits and to the superior oblique it goes to)
2. the only cranial nerve to exit posteriorly on the brain stem
3. the only cranial nerve passing through the superior orbital fissure that does not pass through the annulus of Zinn (AKA annulus tendineus or annular tendon)

Trochlear palsy results in eye deviation "up and in." Patients tend to spontaneously tilt the head to the side *opposite* the IV palsy to "intort" the paretic eye and eliminate the diplopia. Diplopia is exacerbated when looking down (e.g. on descending stairs) especially when also looking inward, or when the examiner tilts the head *towards* the paretic side.

Isolated fourth nerve palsy is uncommon. It may occasionally occur with lesions of the cerebral peduncle or injury to the floor of the fourth ventricle near the aqueduct.

32.6.5 Abducens (VI) palsy

Produces a lateral rectus palsy. Clinically produces diplopia that is exaggerated with lateral gaze to the side of the palsy. Etiologies of isolated 6th nerve palsy include[18]:
1. vasculopathy: including diabetes and giant cell arteritis. Most cases resolve within 3 months (alternative cause should be sought in cases lasting longer)
2. increased intracranial pressure: palsy may occur with increased ICP even in the absence of direct compression of the nerve (a "false localizing" sign in this setting). Postulated to occur due to the fact that the VI nerve has a long intracranial course which may render it more sensitive to increased pressure. May be bilateral. Etiologies include:
   a) traumatically increased ICP
   b) increased ICP due to hydrocephalus (p. 592), e.g. from p-fossa tumor
   c) idiopathic intracranial hypertension (pseudotumor cerebri) (p. 766)

32

3. cavernous sinus lesions: cavernous carotid aneurysm (p. 1225), neoplasm (meningioma…), carotid cavernous fistula (p. 1256)
4. inflammatory:
   a) Gradenigo's syndrome (p. 570), involvement at Dorello's canal)
   b) sphenoid sinusitis: (involvement at Dorello's canal)
5. intracranial neoplasm: e.g. clivus chordoma, chondrosarcoma
6. pseudoabducens palsy: may be due to
   a) thyroid eye disease: the most common cause of chronic VI palsy. Will have positive forced duction test (eye cannot be moved by examiner)
   b) myasthenia gravis: responds to edrophonium (Tensilon®) test
   c) long-standing strabismus
   d) Duane's syndrome (p. 570)
   e) fracture of the medial wall of the orbit with medial rectus entrapment
7. following lumbar puncture (p. 1507): almost invariably unilateral
8. fracture through clivus (p. 884)
9. idiopathic

32.6.6 Multiple extraocular motor nerve involvement

Lesions in cavernous sinus (see below) involve cranial nerves III, IV, VI and V1 & V2 (ophthalmic and maxillary divisions of trigeminal nerve), and spare II and V3.

Superior orbital fissure syndrome: dysfunction of nerves III, IV, VI and V1.

Orbital apex syndrome: involves II, III, IV, VI and partial V1.

4th nerve palsy may result from a contrecoup injury in frontal head trauma.

32.6.7 Painful ophthalmoplegia

Definition

Pain and dysfunction of ocular motility (may be due to involvement of one or more of cranial nerves III, IV, V & VI).

32

Etiologies

1. intraorbital
   a) inflammatory pseudotumor (idiopathic orbital inflammation): see below
   b) contiguous sinusitis
   c) invasive fungal sinus infection producing orbital apex syndrome. Rhinocerebral *mucormycosis* (AKA zygomycosis): sinusitis with painless black palatal or nasal septal ulcer or eschar with hyphal invasion of blood vessels by fungi of the order Mucorales, especially rhizopus.[19] Usually seen in diabetic or immunocompromised patients, occasionally in otherwise healthy patients.[20] Often involves dural sinuses and may cause cavernous sinus thrombosis
   d) mets
   e) lymphoma
2. superior orbital fissure/anterior cavernous sinus
   a) Tolosa-Hunt syndrome: see below
   b) mets
   c) nasopharyngeal Ca
   d) lymphoma
   e) herpes zoster
   f) carotid-cavernous fistula
   g) cavernous sinus thrombosis
   h) intracavernous aneurysm
3. parasellar region
   a) pituitary adenoma
   b) mets
   c) nasopharyngeal Ca
   d) sphenoid sinus mucocele
   e) meningioma/chordoma
   f) apical petrositis (Gradenigo's syndrome): see below
4. posterior fossa
   a) p-comm aneurysm
   b) basilar artery aneurysm (rare)

5. miscellaneous
   a) diabetic ophthalmoplegia
   b) migrainous ophthalmoplegia
   c) cranial arteritis
   d) tuberculous meningitis: may cause ophthalmoplegia, usually incomplete, most often primarily oculomotor nerve

32.6.8 Painless ophthalmoplegia

Differential diagnosis:
1. chronic progressive ophthalmoplegia: pupil sparing, usually bilateral, slowly progressive
2. myasthenia gravis: pupil sparing, responds to edrophonium (Tensilon®) test
3. myositis: usually also produces symptoms in other organ systems (heart, gonads…)

32.7 Neurophthalmologic syndromes

32.7.1 Pseudotumor (of the orbit)

General information

AKA "chronic granuloma" (a misnomer, since true epithelioid granulomas are rarely found). An idiopathic inflammatory disease confined to the orbit that may mimic a true neoplasm. Lymphocytic infiltration of extraocular muscles. Usually unilateral.

Typically presents with rapid onset of proptosis, pain, and EOM dysfunction (painful ophthalmoplegia with diplopia). Often follows URI, may be associated with scleral inflammation. Most commonly involves the superior orbital tissues.

Differential diagnosis

See Orbital lesions (p. 1375) for list.

Key points for Graves' disease (GD): the histologic appearance of GD (hyperthyroidism) may be indistinguishable from pseudotumor. Involvement with GD is usually bilateral.

Treatment

Surgery tends to cause a flare up, and is thus usually best avoided.

Steroids are the treatment of choice. ℞: 50–80 mg prednisone q d. Severe cases may necessitate treatment with 30–40 mg/d for several months.

Radiation treatment with 1000–2000 rads may be needed for cases of reactive lymphocytic hyperplasia.

32.7.2 Tolosa-Hunt syndrome

Nonspecific inflammation in the region of the superior orbital fissure, often with extension into the cavernous sinus, sometimes with granulomatous features. A diagnosis of exclusion. May be a topographical variant of orbital pseudotumor (see above). Clinical diagnostic criteria:
1. painful ophthalmoplegia
2. involvement of any nerve traversing the cavernous sinus. The pupil is usually spared (frequently not the case with aneurysms, specific inflammation, etc.)
3. symptoms last days to weeks
4. spontaneous remission, sometimes with residual deficit
5. recurrent attacks with remissions of months or years
6. no systemic involvement (occasional N/V, due to pain?)
7. dramatic improvement with systemic steroids: 60–80 mg prednisone PO q day (slow taper), relief within about 1 day
8. occasional inflammation of rectus muscle from contiguous inflammation

32.7.3 Raeder's paratrigeminal neuralgia

Two essential components[21]:
1. unilateral oculosympathetic paresis (AKA partial Horner's syndrome (HS), this usually lacks anhidrosis, and in this syndrome, possibly ptosis also)

32

2. homolateral trigeminal nerve involvement (usually tic-like pain, but may be analgesia or masseter weakness; pain, if present, must be tic-like and does not include e.g. unilateral head, face or vascular pain)

Localizing value of syndrome: region adjacent to trigeminal nerve in middle fossa. The cause is often not determined, but may rarely be due to aneurysm[22] compressing V1 with sympathetics.

32.7.4 Gradenigo's syndrome

AKA apical petrositis. Mastoiditis with involvement of petrous apex (if pneumatized). Usually seen by ENT physicians. Classic triad:
1. abducens palsy: from inflammation of 6th nerve at Dorello's canal, which is where it enters the cavernous sinus just medial to the petrous apex
2. retro-orbital pain: due to inflammation of V1
3. draining ear

32.8 Miscellaneous neurophthalmologic signs

32

► **Corneal mandibular reflex.** Eliciting the corneal reflex produces a jaw jerk or contralateral jaw movement (ipsilateral pterygoid contraction). A primitive pontine reflex, may be seen in a variety of insults to the brain (trauma, intracerebral hemorrhage…).

► **Duane syndrome.** AKA retraction syndrome: paradoxical innervation causing co-contraction of the lateral and medial rectus muscles on attempted adduction with relaxation on abduction, produces mild enophthalmos with pseudoptosis. May be congenital (e.g. part of one of the following syndromes: acrorenal-ocular syndrome, Okihiro syndrome…).

► **Hippus.** Rhythmic, irregular pupillary oscillations, changing by ≥ 2 mm. May confuse examination when checking pupillary responses; record the *initial* response. May be normal. No localizing value.

► **Marcus Gunn phenomenon.** Not to be confused with Marcus Gunn pupil (p. 562). Opening the mouth causes opening of a ptotic eye (abnormal reflex between proprioception of pterygoid muscles and third nerve). Reverse Marcus Gunn phenomenon: normal eye that closes with opening the mouth. Seen only in patients with peripheral facial nerve injuries, and probably results from aberrant regeneration.

► **Ocular bobbing**[23]. Abrupt, spontaneous, conjugate downward eye deviation with slow return to midposition, 2 to 12 times per min. It is associated with bilateral paralysis of horizontal gaze, including to doll's-eyes and calorics. Most commonly seen with destructive lesions of the pontine tegmentum (usually hemorrhage, but also infarction, glioma, trauma), but has also been described with compressive lesions.[24] Atypical bobbing is similar except that horizontal gaze is preserved, and can be seen with cerebellar hemorrhage, hydrocephalus, trauma, metabolic encephalopathy…

► **Opsoclonus**[25]. (Rare.) Rapid, conjugate, irregular, non-rhythmic (differentiates this from nystagmus) eye movements vertically or horizontally, persist (attenuated) during sleep (opsochoria if dysconjugate). Usually associated with diffuse myoclonus (fingers, chin, lips, eyelid, forehead, trunk and LEs); also, malaise, fatigability, vomiting and some cerebellar findings. Often resolves spontaneously within 4 mos.

► **Oscillopsia.** Visual sensation that stationary objects are swaying side-to-side or vibrating.[26] Rarely the sole manifestation of Chiari I malformation[27] (often associated with downbeat nystagmus). Other causes include MS, or injury to both vestibular nerves; e.g. aminoglycoside ototoxicity,[28] bilateral vestibular neurectomies, see Dandy's syndrome (p. 572).

► **Pseudo von Grafe sign.** Lid retraction on downward gaze (true von Grafe sign is lid lag in hyperthyroidism) seen in aberrant nerve regeneration (inferior rectus innervation → activation of levator palpebrae).

► **Optic atrophy.** Chronic, progressive optic atrophy is due to a compressive lesion (aneurysm, meningioma, osteopetrosis…) until proven otherwise.

References

[1] Wilkins RH, Rengachary SS. Neurosurgery. New York 1985

[2] Pinel JF, Larmande P, Guegan Y, et al. Down-Beat Nystagmus: Case Report with Magnetic Resonance Imaging and Surgical Treatment. Neurosurgery. 1987; 21:736–739

[3] Williams DP, Troost BT, Rogers J. Lithium-Induced Downbeat Nystagmus. Arch Neurol. 1988; 45:1022–1023

[4] Sher NA, Wirtschafter J, Shapiro SK, et al. Unilateral Papilledema in 'Benign' Intracranial Hypertension (Pseudotumor Cerebri). JAMA. 1983; 250:2346–2347

[5] Horton JC. Wilbrand's knee of the primate optic chiasm is an artefact of monocular enucleation. Trans Am Ophthalmol Soc. 1997; 95:579–609

[6] Grzybowski A. Harry Moss Traquair (1875-1954), Scottish ophthalmologist and perimetrist. Acta Ophthalmol. 2009; 87:455–459

[7] Shin RK, Li TP. Visualization of Wilbrand's knee. Snowbird, UT 2013

[8] Lee JH, Tobias S, Kwon JT, Sade B, Kosmorsky G. Wilbrand's knee: does it exist? Surg Neurol. 2006; 66:11–7; discussion 17

[9] Zweckberger K, Unterberg AW, Schick U. Pre-chiasmatic transection of the optic nerve can save contralateral vision in patients with optic nerve sheath meningioms. Clin Neurol Neurosurg. 2013; 115:2426–2431

[10] Kawasaki A. Physiology, assessment, and disorders of the pupil. Curr Opin Ophthalmol. 1999; 10:394–400

[11] Walsh FB, Hoyt WF. Clinical Neuro-Ophthalmology. Baltimore 1969

[12] Nakagawa TA, Guerra L, Storgion SA. Aerosolized atropine as an unusual cause of anisocoria in a child with asthma. Pediatr Emerg Care. 1993; 9:153–154

[13] Wijdicks EF. Determining Brain Death in Adults. Neurology. 1995; 45:1003–1011

[14] Lepore FE. Diagnostic Pharmacology of the Pupil. Clin Neuropharmacol. 1985; 8:27–37

[15] Zee DS. Internuclear ophthalmoplegia: pathophysiology and diagnosis. Baillieres Clin Neurol. 1992; 1:455–470

[16] Trobe JD. Third nerve palsy and the pupil. Footnotes to the rule. Arch Ophthalmol. 1988; 106:601–602

[17] Breen LA, Hopf HC, Farris BK, Gutmann L. Pupil-Sparing Oculomotor Nerve Palsy due to Midbrain Infarction. Arch Neurol. 1991; 48:105–106

[18] Galetta SL, Smith JL. Chronic Isolated Sixth Nerve Palsies. Arch Neurol. 1989; 46:79–82

[19] DeShazo RD, Chapin K, Swain RE. Fungal Sinusitis. N Engl J Med. 1997; 337:254–259

[20] Radner AB, Witt MD, Edwards JE. Acute Invasive Rhinocerebral Zygomycosis in an Otherwise Healthy Patient: Case Report and Review. Clin Infect Dis. 1995; 20:163–166

[21] Mokri B. Raeder's Paratrigeminal Syndrome. Arch Neurol. 1982; 39:395–399

[22] Kashihara K, Ito H, Yamamoto S, et al. Raeder's Syndrome Associated with Intracranial Internal Carotid Artery Aneurysm. Neurosurgery. 1987; 20:49–51

[23] Fisher CM. Ocular Bobbing. Arch Neurol. 1964; 11:543–546

[24] Sherman DG, Salmon JH. Ocular Bobbing with Superior Cerebellar Artery Aneurysm: Case Report. J Neurosurg. 1977; 47:596–598

[25] Smith JL, Walsh FB. Opsoclonus - Ataxic Conjugate Movements of the Eyes. Arch Ophthalm. 1960; 64:244–250

[26] Brickner R. Oscillopsia: A new symptom commonly occurring in multiple sclerosis. Arch Neurol Psychiatry. 1936; 36:586–589

[27] Gingold SI, Winfield JA. Oscillopsia and Primary Cerebellar Ectopie: Case Report and Review of the Literature. Neurosurgery. 1991; 29:932–936

[28] Marra TR, Reynolds NC, Stoddard JJ. Subjective Oscillopsia ("Jiggling Vision") Presumably Due to Aminoglycoside Ototoxicity: A Report of Two Cases. J Clin Neuro Ophthalmol. 1988; 8:35–38

33 Neurotology

33.1 Dizziness and vertigo

33.1.1 Differential diagnosis of dizziness

► **Near syncope.** Some overlap with syncope; see Syncope and apoplexy (p. 1396)
1. orthostatic hypotension
2. cardiogenic hypotension
   a) arrhythmia
   b) valvular disease
3. vasovagal episode
4. hypersensitive carotid sinus; see Syncope and apoplexy (p. 1396)

► **Dysequilibrium**
1. multiple sensory deficits: e.g. peripheral neuropathy, visual impairment
2. cerebellar degeneration

► *Vertigo*. Sensation of movement (usually spinning)
1. inner ear dysfunction
   a) labyrinthitis
   b) Meniere's disease (see below)
   c) trauma: endolymphatic leak
   d) *drugs*: especially aminoglycosides
   e) **benign (paroxysmal) positional vertigo**[1]: AKA *cupulolithiasis*. Attacks of severe vertigo when the head is turned to certain positions (usually in bed). Due to calcium concretions in the semicircular canals. Self limited (most cases do not last > 1 year). No hearing loss
   f) syphilis
   g) vertebrobasilar insufficiency (p. 1305)
2. vestibular nerve dysfunction
   a) vestibular neuronitis: sudden onset of vertigo, gradual improvement
   b) compression:
      • meningioma
      • vestibular schwannoma: usually slowly progressive ataxia instead of severe vertigo. BAER latencies usually abnormal. CT or MRI usually abnormal
3. **disabling positional vertigo** : as described by Jannetta et al.,[2] *constant* disabling positional vertigo or dysequilibrium, causing ≈ constant nausea, no vestibular dysfunction nor hearing loss (tinnitus may be present). One possible cause is vascular compression of the vestibular nerve which may respond to microvascular decompression
4. brainstem dysfunction
   a) vascular disease; see Vertebrobasilar insufficiency (p. 1305): less distinct vestibular symptoms, prominent nonvestibular symptoms
   b) migraine: especially basilar artery migraine
   c) demyelinating disease: e.g. multiple sclerosis
   d) *drugs*: anticonvulsants, alcohol, sedatives/hypnotics, salicylates
5. dysfunction of cervical proprioceptors: as in cervical osteoarthritis

► **Poorly defined lightheadedness.** Mostly psychiatric. May also include:
1. hyperventilation
2. hypoglycemia
3. anxiety neurosis
4. hysterical

33.1.2 Vestibular neurectomy

General information

Complete loss of vestibular function from one side is thought to produce transient vertigo due to the mismatch of vestibular input from the two ears. Theoretically, a central compensatory mechanism (the "cerebellar clamp") results in the amelioration of symptoms. In cases of unilateral *fluctuating* vestibular dysfunction, this compensatory mechanism may be impaired. Unilateral selective vestibular neurectomy (SVN) may convert the fluctuating or partial loss to a complete cessation of input and facilitate compensation. Bilateral SVN is often complicated by oscillopsia (p.570) – AKA Dandy's syndrome, with difficulty in maintaining balance in the dark due to loss of the vestibulo-ocular reflex – and is to be avoided.

Indications

The two conditions for which SVN is most commonly employed are Meniere's disease (see below) and partial vestibular injury (viral or traumatic). SVN may be indicated in disabling cases refractory to medical or non-destructive surgical treatment when vestibular studies demonstrate continued or progressive uncompensated vestibular dysfunction.[3]

SVN preserves hearing and in Meniere's disease is > 90% effective in eliminating episodic vertiginous spells (≈ 80% success rate in non-Meniere's cases), but is unlikely to improve stability with rapid head movement.

Surgical approaches for SVN

1. retrolabyrinthine, AKA postauricular approach: anterior to sigmoid sinus. Primary choice in patients with Meniere's disease who have not had previous endolymphatic sac (ELS) procedures since it permits simultaneous SVN and decompression of the endolymphatic sac. Requires mastoidectomy with skeletonization of the semicircular canals and ELS. The dural opening is bounded anteriorly by the posterior semicircular canal, posteriorly by the sigmoid sinus. Watertight dural closure is difficult
2. retrosigmoid, AKA posterior fossa, AKA suboccipital approach: posterior to sigmoid sinus. The original approach plied by Dandy in pre-microsurgical era, usually sacrificed hearing, and occasionally facial nerve function. Better results today with microscopic techniques. Indicated for cases other than Meniere's disease where there is no need for identification of the ELS. Also the best approach for positive identification of eighth nerve
3. middle fossa (extradural) approach: the fibers of the vestibular division may be more segregated from the cochlear fibers in the IAC than in the CPA, thus permitting more complete section of the vestibular nerve. May be appropriate for failed response to SVN by the above approaches. Disadvantages: requires temporal lobe retraction, does not allow exposure of ELS, and higher morbidity and risk of damage to facial nerve[4] than retrolabyrinthine approach

Surgical considerations for selective vestibular neurectomy

(Also ▶ Fig. 1.7)

1. the vestibular nerve is in the superior half of the eighth nerve complex, and is slightly more *gray* in color than the cochlear division (due to less myelin[5]). They may be separated by a small vessel or by an indentation in the bundle
2. facial (VII) nerve:
   a) whiter than the VIII nerve complex
   b) lies anterior and superiorly to the VIII nerve
   c) EMG monitoring of the facial nerve is recommended
   d) direct stimulation confirms the identification
3. any vessels present on eighth nerve bundle must be preserved to save hearing (primarily, the artery of the auditory canal must be preserved)
4. if no plane of cleavage can be defined between vestibular & cochlear divisions, the superior half of the nerve bundle is divided
5. the endolymphatic sac lies ≈ midway between the posterior edge of the internal auditory meatus and the sigmoid sinus

33.2 Meniere's disease

33.2.1 General information

Key concepts

- increased endolymphatic pressure
- clinical triad: vertigo, tinnitus & fluctuating hearing loss
- surgical options for failure of medical management include endolymphatic shunt or selective vestibular neurectomy

33

Probably due to a derangement of endolymphatic fluid regulation (a consistent finding is endolymphatic hydrops: increased endolymphatic volume and pressure with dilatation of endolymph spaces), with resultant fistulization into the perilymphatic spaces.

33.2.2 Epidemiology

Incidence ≈ 1 per 100,000 population.[6] Most cases have onset between 30–60 years of age, rarely in youth or in the elderly. May become bilateral in 20%.

33.2.3 Clinical

Clinical triad

1. attacks of violent vertigo (due to vestibular nerve dysfunction): usually the earliest and the most disabling symptom. Nausea, vomiting, and diaphoresis are frequent concomitants. Severe attacks may cause prostration. Vertigo may persist even after complete deafness. Balance is normal between attacks
2. tinnitus: often described as resembling the sound of escaping steam, not a true "ringing"
3. fluctuating low frequency hearing loss: may fluctuate for a periods of weeks to years, and may progress to permanent deafness if untreated (a sensation of fullness in the ear is commonly described,[7] however, this is nonspecific and may occur with hearing loss for any reason)

Other clinical features

Drop attacks ("otolithic crises of Tumarkin") occasionally occur.

Attack duration: ≈ 5–30 minutes (some say 2–6 hours), with a "post-ictal" period of fatigue lasting several hrs.

Frequency: varies from one or two attacks a year to several times per week.

Two subtypes differ from classical form: vestibular Meniere's (episodic vertigo with normal hearing) and cochlear Meniere's (few vestibular symptoms).

Natural course of syndrome is characterized by periods of remission. Eventually the vertiginous attacks either progress in severity, or "burn out" (being replaced by constant unsteadiness[7]).

Differential diagnosis

Also see Differential diagnosis: Dizziness and vertigo (p. 572) for more details.

1. benign (paroxysmal) positional vertigo: AKA *cupulolithiasis*. Self limited (most cases last < 1 year). No hearing loss
2. disabling positional vertigo: *constant* disabling positional vertigo or dysequilibrium, ≈ constant nausea, no vestibular dysfunction nor hearing loss (tinnitus may be present)
3. vestibular schwannoma: usually slowly progressive ataxia instead of episodic severe vertigo. BAER latencies usually abnormal. CT or MRI usually positive
4. vestibular neuronitis: sudden onset of vertigo with gradual improvement
5. vertebrobasilar insufficiency (VBI) (p. 1305): less distinct vestibular symptoms, and prominence of nonvestibular symptoms

Diagnostic studies

1. electronystagmography (ENG) with bithermal caloric stimulation usually abnormal, may show blunted thermal responses
2. audiogram: low frequency hearing loss, fairly good preservation of discrimination and loudness recruitment, negative tone decay on impedance testing
3. BAER usually shows normal latencies
4. radiographic imaging (CT, MRI, etc.): no findings in Meniere's disease
5. in bilateral cases, a VDRL should be checked to R/O luetic disease

Treatment

Medical treatment

1. reduced intake of salt (strict salt restriction is as effective as any medication) and caffeine
2. diuretics: taken daily until ear fullness abates, then PRN ear pressure (usually once or twice weekly suffices)

a) acetazolamide: ℞ Diamox® sequels 500 mg p.o. q d × 1 week, increase to BID if symptoms persist. D/C if paresthesias develop. Do not use during 1st trimester of pregnancy
3. vestibular suppressants
a) diazepam (Valium®): probably the most effective
b) meclizine HCl (Antivert®): ℞ Adult dose for vertigo associated with the vestibular system (during attacks): 25–100 mg/day PO divided. Dose for motion sickness: 25–50 mg PO one hr prior to stimulus. Supplied: 12.5, 25 & 50 mg tabs. **Side effects:** drowsiness
4. vasodilators: postulated to be mediated by increased cochlear blood flow: inhalation of 5–10% CO_2 works well, but relief is short lived

Surgical treatment

Reserved for *incapacitating* cases *refractory* to medical management. When functional hearing exists, procedures that spare hearing are preferred because of high incidence of bilateral involvement. Procedures include:

1. endolymphatic shunting procedures: to mastoid cavity (Arenberg shunt) or to subarachnoid space. Reserved for cases with serviceable hearing. ≈ 65% success rate (see below). If symptoms are relieved ≥ 1 year, then a recurrence would be treated by shunt revision, if < 1 year then vestibular neurectomy
2. direct application of corticosteroids to the inner ear
3. nonselective vestibular ablation (in cases with nonserviceable hearing on the side of involvement)
a) surgical labyrinthectomy
b) middle ear perfusion with gentamicin
c) translabyrinthine section of the 8th nerve
4. selective vestibular neurectomy (p. 572), in cases with serviceable hearing

Outcome

Endolymph shunting procedures

Outcomes from 112 endolymphatic shunting procedures are shown in ▶ Table 33.1.

Neurectomy procedures

Vestibulocochlear nerve section (based on early posterior fossa surgery by Dandy; entire eighth nerve bundle was sectioned in 587 patients; all were deaf post-op): 90% relieved of vertigo, 5% unchanged and 5% worse; 9% incidence of facial paralysis (3% incidence of permanent paralysis). 33

Selective vestibular nerve section (sparing cochlear portion, 95 patients from Dandy): 10% had improved hearing, 28% unchanged, 48% worse, 14% deaf.

Retrolabyrinthine approach: in 32 patients with Meniere's syndrome (25 failed endolymph shunt) responding to survey, 85% had complete relief of vertigo, 6% improved, 9% no relief (one of whom responded to middle fossa neurectomy).[5]

Complications and untoward effects

Patients with little vestibular nerve function pre-op (determined by ENG) usually have little difficulty immediately following vestibular neurectomy; patients with more function may have a transient worsening post-op until they accommodate.

Among 42 patients undergoing retrolabyrinthine approach: none lost hearing as a result of surgery, no facial weakness, one CSF rhinorrhea requiring re-operation, and one meningitis with good outcome.[5]

Table 33.1 Outcome in 112 endolymphatic-subarachnoid shunts[7]

	Vertigo	Tinnitus	Hearing[a]	Ear pressure
improved	79 (70%)[b]	53 (47%)	19 (17%)	57 (51%)
stable	33 (29%)	49 (43%)	50 (45%)	24 (21%)
worse	(none)	10 (10%)	39 (35%)	31 (28%)

[a]improved hearing considered serviceable (50 dB pure tone, 70% speech discrimination); additional 4 patients had improved but non-serviceable hearing
[b]5 patients had recurrence of vertigo after 1–3 years

In post-op failures, check ENG. If any vestibular nerve function is demonstrated on operated side, then the nerve section was incomplete; consider re-operating.

33.3 Facial nerve palsy

33.3.1 Severity grading

Severity of facial palsy is often graded with the House and Brackmann scale (see ▶ Table 41.3).

33.3.2 Localizing site of lesion

Central facial palsy (AKA supranuclear facial palsy)

The cortical representation for facial movement occurs in the motor strip along the lateral aspect (just above the most inferior opercular portion of the precentral gyrus). The keys to differentiating central paralysis (due to *supranuclear* lesions) from peripheral facial palsy are that *central* palsies:

1. are confined primarily to the lower face due to some bilateral cortical representation of upper facial movement
2. may spare emotional facial expression[8] (e.g. smiling at a joke)

Nuclear facial palsy

The motor nucleus of the seventh nerve is located at the pontomedullary junction. Nuclear VII palsy results in paralysis of all VII nerve motor function. In nuclear facial palsies, other neurologic findings also often occur from involvement of adjacent neural structures by the underlying process (stroke, tumor...), e.g. in Millard-Gubler syndrome (p.99), there is ipsilateral abducens palsy + contralateral limb weakness. Tumors invading the floor of the 4th ventricle (e.g. medulloblastoma) may also cause nuclear facial palsy (from involvement of facial colliculus in the floor of 4th ventricle).

Facial nerve lesion

Motor fibers ascend within the pons and form a sharp bend ("internal genu") around the sixth nerve (abducens) nucleus, forming a visible bump in the floor of the 4th ventricle (facial colliculus). The seventh nerve exits from the brain stem at the ponto-medullary junction (▶ Fig. 2.6) where it may be involved in CPA tumors. It enters the supero-anterior portion of the internal auditory canal (▶ Fig. 1.7). The geniculate ganglion ("external genu") is located within the temporal bone. The first branch from the ganglion is the greater superficial petrosal nerve (GSPN) which passes to the pterygopalatine ganglion and innervates the nasal and palatine mucosa and the lacrimal gland of the eye; lesions proximal to this point produce a dry eye. The next branch is the branch to the stapedius muscle; lesions proximal to this point produce hyperacusis. Next, the chorda tympani joins the facial nerve bringing taste sensation from the anterior two-thirds of the tongue. Basal skull fractures may injure the nerve just proximal to this point. Travelling with the chorda tympani are fibers to the submandibular and sublingual glands. The facial nerve exits the skull at the stylomastoid foramen. It then enters the parotid gland, where it splits into the following branches to the facial muscles (cranial to caudal): temporal, zygomatic, buccal, mandibular, and cervical. Lesions within the parotid gland (e.g. parotid tumors) may involve some branches but spare others.

33.3.3 Etiologies

These etiologies produce primarily facial nerve palsy, also see Multiple cranial nerve palsies (cranial neuropathies) (p.1399). **Note:** 90–95% of all cases of facial palsy are accounted for by Bell's palsy, herpes zoster oticus, and trauma (basal skull fractures).[9]

1. Bell's palsy (p.577)
2. herpes zoster oticus (auris) (p.578)
3. trauma: basal skull fracture
4. birth:
   a) congenital
      - *bilateral facial palsy (facial diplegia) of Möbius syndrome (p.1399): unique in that it affects upper face more than lower face
      - *congenital facial diplegia may be part of facioscapulohumeral or myotonic muscular dystrophy
   b) traumatic

5. otitis media: with acute otitis media, facial palsy usually improves with antibiotics. With chronic suppurative otitis surgical intervention is required
6. central facial paralysis and nuclear facial paralysis: see Localizing site of lesion above
7. neoplasm: usually causes hearing loss, and (unlike Bell's palsy) *slowly progressive* facial paralysis
   a) most are either benign schwannomas of the facial or auditory nerve, or malignancies metastatic to the temporal bone. Facial neuromas account for ≈ 5% of peripheral facial nerve palsies[10]; the paralysis tends to be slowly progressive
   b) parotid tumors may involve some branches but spare others
   c) Masson's vegetant intravascular hemangioendothelioma (p.770)
8. *neurosarcoidosis (p.189): VII is the most commonly affected cranial nerve
9. diabetes: 17% of patients > 40 yrs old with peripheral facial palsy (PFP) have abnormal glucose tolerance tests. Diabetics have 4.5 times the relative risk of developing PFP than nondiabetics[11]
10. *stage II Lyme disease (p.334) [12]: facial diplegia is a hallmark
11. *Guillain-Barré syndrome: facial diplegia occurs in ≈ 50% of fatal cases
12. occasionally seen in Klippel-Feil syndrome
13. *isolated 4th ventricle (p.402): compression at the facial colliculus

* Items with an asterisk are often associated with facial *diplegia* (i.e. bilateral facial palsy), see also multiple cranial neuropathies (p.1399).

33.3.4 Bell's palsy

General information

Bell's palsy (BP), AKA idiopathic peripheral facial palsy (PFP), is the most common cause of facial paralysis (50–80% of PFPs). Incidence: 150–200/1-million/yr.

Etiology: by definition, PFP is called Bell's palsy when it is not due to known causes of PFP (e.g. infection, tumor or trauma) and there are no other neurological (e.g. involvement of other cranial nerves) or systemic manifestations (e.g. fever, diabetes, possibly hypertension[13]).[14] Thus, true BP is idiopathic, and is a diagnosis of exclusion. Most cases probably represent a viral inflammatory demyelinating polyneuritis[15] usually due to the herpes simplex virus.[16] Facial palsy due to Lyme disease can usually be recognized on clinical grounds.[17] Severity may be graded on the House & Brackmann grading scale (see ▶ Table 41.3).

Presentation

A viral prodrome is frequent: URI, myalgia, hypesthesia or dysesthesia of the trigeminal nerve, N/V, diarrhea... Paralysis may be incomplete and remain so (Type I); it is complete at onset in 50% (Type II), the remainder progress to completion in 1 week. Usually exhibits distal to proximal progression: motor branches, then chorda tympani (loss of taste and decreased salivation), then stapedial branch (hyperacusis), then geniculate ganglion (decreased tearing). Associated symptoms are shown in ▶ Table 33.2, and are usually, but not always, ipsilateral. Herpes zoster vesicles develop in 4% of patients 2–4 days after onset of paralysis; and in 30% of patients 4–8 days after onset. During the recovery phase excessive lacrimation may occur (aberrant nerve regeneration).

Evaluation

Patients with PFP should be examined at an early stage to optimize outcome.

Electrodiagnostics: EMG may detect re-innervation potentials, aids prognostication. Nerve conduction study: electrical stimulation of the facial nerve near the stylomastoid foramen while recording EMG in facial muscles (a facial nerve may continue to conduct for up to ≈ 1 week even after complete transection).

Table 33.2 Associated symptoms with Bell's palsy

Symptom	%
facial & retroauricular pain	60%
dysgeusia	57%
hyperacusis	30%
reduced tearing	17%

33

Management

General measures

Eye protection: protection of the eye is critical. Artificial tears during the day, eye ointment at night, avoid bright light (using dark glasses during the day).

Medical management

Steroids: prednisolone 25 mg p.o. BID × 10 days, started within 72 hours of onset of symptoms, improves the chances of complete recovery at 3 & 9 months.

Acyclovir: does *not* help (alone or in combination with prednisolone).[18]

Surgical management

Surgical decompression: controversial. The definitive study has not been done. Rarely utilized. Indications may include:

1. complete facial nerve degeneration without response to nerve stimulation (although this absence is also used as an argument against surgery[9])
2. progressively deteriorating response to nerve stimulation
3. no clinical nor objective (nerve testing) improvement after 8 wks (however, in cases where the diagnosis of Bell's palsy is felt to be certain, the active disease will have abated by ≈ 14 days after onset[9])

Prognosis

Essentially all cases show some recovery (if none by 6 mos, other etiologies should be sought). Extent of recovery: 75–80% of cases recover completely, 10% partial, remainder poor. If recovery begins by 10–21 d, tends to be complete; if not until 3–8 wks → fair, if not until 2–4 mos → poor recovery. If paralysis is complete at onset, 50% will have incomplete recovery. Cases of incomplete paralysis at onset that do not progress to complete paralysis → complete recovery; incomplete paralysis at onset that progresses to complete → incomplete recovery in 75%. A worse prognosis is associated with: more proximal involvement, hyperacusis, decreased tearing, age > 60 yrs, diabetes, HTN, psychoneuroses, and aural, facial or radicular pain.

33.3.5 Herpes zoster oticus facial paralysis

33

Symptoms are more severe than Bell's palsy, herpetic vesicles are usually present, and antibody titers to varicella-zoster virus rise. These patients have a higher risk of facial nerve degeneration.

33.3.6 Surgical treatment of facial palsy

General information

For cases with focal injury to the facial nerve (e.g. trauma, injury during surgery for CPA tumor…), dynamic reconstruction by nerve anastamoses are usually considered superior to static methods.[19] For nonfocal causes, e.g. Bell's palsy, only "static" methods may be applicable. A functional neural repair is not possible if the facial muscles have atrophied or fibrosed.

Surgical options

Surgical treatment options include:

1. for intracranial injury to facial nerve (e.g. during CPA tumor surgery): intracranial reapproximation (with or without graft) offers the best hope for the most normal facial reanimation
   a) timing
      - at time of tumor removal (for a divided facial nerve during removal of vestibular schwannoma[20,21,22]): the best result that can be achieved with this is House-Brackmann Grade III. The operation fails to produce good results in ≈ 33% of cases[22]
      - in delayed fashion, especially if the nerve was left in anatomic continuity
   b) techniques
      - direct reanastamosis: difficult due to the frail nature of the VII nerve (especially when it has been stretched by a tumor)
      - cable graft: e.g. using greater auricular nerve[23] or sural nerve

2. extracranial facial nerve anastomosis
   a) hypoglossal nerve (Cr. N. XII)-facial nerve anastomosis (see below)
   b) spinal accessory nerve (Cr. N. XI)-facial nerve anastomosis (see below)
   c) phrenic nerve-facial nerve anastamosis
   d) glossopharyngeal (Cr. N. IX)-facial nerve anastamosis
   e) crossface grafting (VII-VII): results have not been very good
3. "mechanical" or "static" means
   a) facial suspension: e.g. with polypropylene (Marlex®) mesh[24]
   b) eye closure techniques (protects the eye from exposure and reduced tearing)
      - tarsorrhaphy: partial or complete
      - gold weights in eyelid
      - stainless-steel spring in eyelid

Timing of surgery

If the facial nerve is known to be interrupted (e.g. transected during removal of vestibular schwannoma) then early surgical treatment is indicated. When the status of the nerve is unknown or if in continuity but not functioning, then several months of observation and electrical testing should be allowed for spontaneous recovery. Very late attempts at anastomosis have less chance for recovery due to facial muscle atrophy.

Hypoglossal nerve-facial nerve (XII-VII) anastomosis

General information

Cannot be used bilaterally in patients with facial diplegia or in those with other lower cranial nerve deficits (or potential for same). In spite of some suggestions to the contrary, sacrificing the XII nerve does create some morbidity (tongue atrophy with difficulty speaking, mastication and swallowing in ≈ 25% of cases, exacerbated when the facial muscles do not function on that side; aspiration may occur if vagus (Cr. N. X) dysfunction coexists with loss of XII).

Not as effective as it would theoretically seem possible. The resultant facial reanimation is often less than ideal (may permit mass movement). To avoid severe disappointment, the patient should thoroughly understand the likely side effects and that the facial movement will probably be much less than normal, often with poor voluntary control.

Usually performed in conjunction with anastamosis of the descendens hypoglossi to the distal hypoglossal nerve to try and reduce hemiatrophy of the tongue. Atrophy may also be reduced by using a "jump graft" without completely interrupting XII.[25]

33

Technique

Position: supine, head turned slightly to the opposite side. Skin incision: 6–8 cm incision from just above the mastoid process obliquely downward across the neck to 2 cm below the angle of the jaw. The platysma is opened, and the tip of the mastoid is exposed by incising the insertion of the SCM and using a periosteal elevator. Incise the deep fascia; avoid the parotid gland, which is retracted superiorly. Rongeur the anterior third of the mastoid process (wax any exposed air cells) and identify the facial nerve as it exits the stylomastoid foramen between the mastoid process and the styloid process. Retract the posterior belly of the digastric inferiorly to aid the exposure.

The SCM is retracted laterally until the carotid sheath is identified, revealing the hypoglossal nerve. It loops around the occipital artery at this level (where it gives off the descendens hypoglossi) to pass between the carotid artery and jugular vein. The nerve is freed proximally to the point where it enters the carotid sheath and distally to the submandibular triangle where it is sharply divided.

The facial nerve is divided at the stylomastoid foramen and is approximated to the proximal hypoglossal nerve. The descendens hypoglossi is divided as far distally as possible and is then anastomosed to the distal stump of the hypoglossal nerve.

Variations

1. interposition jump grafts: spares function in the XII nerve (to minimize glottic denervation, the incision of XII should be distal to the descendens hypoglossi[25])
   a) using cutaneous nerve jump graft[25]
   b) using muscle interposition jump graft[26]
2. mobilizing the intratemporal portion of VII out of the fallopian canal (as previously described[27]) and then anastamosing it using a bevelled cuts to a partially incised XII[28]

Outcome

Results are better if performed early, although good results can occur up to 18 mos after injury. In 22 cases, 64% had good results, 14% fair, 18% poor, and 1 patient had no evidence of reinnervation. In 59% of cases, evidence of reinnervation was seen by 3–6 mos, in the remaining patients with reinnervation improvement was noted by 8 mos.[29] Recovery of forehead movement occurs in only ≈ 30%. Return of tone precedes movement by ≈ 3 months.

Spinal accessory nerve-facial nerve (XI-VII) anastamosis

General information

First described in 1895 by Sir Charles Ballance.[30] Sacrifices some shoulder movement rather than use of tongue. Initial concerns about significant shoulder disability and pain resulted in the technique of using only the SCM branch of XI,[31] however these problems have not occurred in the majority of patients even with use of the major division.[32]

Technique

See reference.[32]

Skin incision: curves across the mastoid tip along the anterior margin of the SCM. Strip and remove the anterior third of the mastoid process (wax any exposed air cells), identify the facial nerve and divide it as close to its exit from the stylomastoid foramen as possible. Locate the XI nerve 3–4 cm below the mastoid tip, and divide it distal to the SCM division. Mobilize the free end and anastamose it to the distal stump of VII. Results in loss of trapezius function, which may not cause deficit even if done bilaterally. Alternatively, the SCM branch of XI may be used, sparing the trapezius function, however the shorter length may be difficult to work with and in some individuals there may only be multiple small branches to the SCM.

33.4 Hearing loss

Two anatomic types: conductive and sensorineural.

33.4.1 Conductive hearing loss

33

1. Patients tend to speak with normal or low volume voice
2. etiologies: anything that interferes with ossicular movement. Included:
   a) otitis media with middle ear effusion
   b) otosclerosis
3. clinical findings with unilateral hearing loss (see ▶ Table 33.3):
   a) *Weber test* will lateralize to side of hearing loss (Weber test: place a vibrating 256 or 512 Hz tuning fork on the center of the forehead; the sound will lateralize – sound louder – on the side of conductive hearing loss, or opposite to the side of SNHL)
   b) *Rinne test* will be abnormal (BC > AC) on the side of hearing loss, called a *negative* Rinne (Rinne test: place a vibrating 256 or 512 Hz tuning fork on the mastoid process, when sound is no longer heard, move the fork to just outside the ear to see if air conduction [AC] is > bone conduction [BC])
4. middle ear impedance measurements are abnormal

Table 33.3 Interpretation of Weber and Rinne test results

Weber	Rinne	Interpretation
nonlateralizing	AC > BC bilat	normal[a]
lateralizes to side A	normal bilaterally (AC > BC)	sensorineural hearing loss (SNHL) side B
lateralizes to side A	abnormal in side A (BC > AC)	conductive hearing loss side A
lateralizes to side A	abnormal in side B (BC > AC)	combined conductive + SNHL side B

[a]normal, or symmetric hearing loss

33.4.2 Sensorineural hearing loss (SNHL)

1. Patients tend to speak with loud voice
2. clinical findings with unilateral hearing loss (▶ Table 33.3):
   a) *Weber test* will lateralize to side of better hearing (Weber test: place a vibrating 256 or 512 Hz tuning fork on the center of the forehead; the sound will lateralize – sound louder – on the side of conductive hearing loss, or opposite to the side of SNHL)
   b) *Rinne test* will be normal (AC > BC), called a *positive* Rinne (Rinne test: place a vibrating 256 or 512 Hz tuning fork on the mastoid process, when sound is no longer heard, move the fork to just outside the ear to see if air conduction [AC] is > bone conduction [BC])
3. further divided into sensory or neural. Distinguished by otoacoustic emissions (only produced by a cochlea with functioning hair cells) or BSAERs
   a) sensory: loss of outer hair cells in the cochlea. Etiologies: cochlear damage (usually causes high-frequency hearing loss) from noise exposure, ototoxic drugs (e.g. aminoglycosides), senile cochlear degeneration, viral labyrinthitis. Speech discrimination may be relatively preserved
   b) neural: due to compression of the 8th cranial nerve. Etiologies: CP angle tumor (e.g. vestibular schwannoma). Typically much greater loss of word discrimination out of proportion to pure tone audiogram abnormalities

Sensory hearing loss may be distinguished from neural hearing loss by
1. otoacoustic emissions which are only produced by a cochlea with functioning hair cells
2. or BSAERs
3. an elevated stapedial reflex threshold out of proportion to PTA abnormalities is also highly diagnostic of a retrocochlear (neural) lesion

References

[1] Brandt T, Daroff RB. The Multisensory Physiological and Pathological Vertigo Syndromes. Ann Neurol. 1980; 7:195–203

[2] Jannetta PJ, Moller MB, Moller AR. Disabling Positional Vertigo. N Engl J Med. 1984; 310:1700–1705

[3] Arriaga MA, Chen DA. Vestibular Nerve Section in the Treatment of Vertigo. Contemp Neurosurg. 1997; 19:1–6

[4] McElveen JT, House JW, Hitselberger WE, et al. Retrolabyrinthine Vestibular Nerve Section: A Viable Alternative to the Middle Fossa Approach. Otolaryngol Head Neck Surg. 1984; 92:136–140

[5] House JW, Hitselberger WE, McElveen J, et al. Retrolabyrinthine Section of the Vestibular Nerve. Otolaryngol Head Neck Surg. 1984; 92:212–215

[6] Tarlov EC. Microsurgical Vestibular Nerve Section for Intractable Meniere's Disease. Clin Neurosurg. 1985; 33:667–684

[7] Glassock ME, Miller GW, Drake FD, et al. Surgical Management of Meniere's Disease with the Endolymphatic Subarachnoid Shunt. Laryngoscope. 1977; 87:1668–1675

[8] Shambaugh GE. In: Facial Nerve Decompression and Repair. Surgery of the Ear. Philadelphia: W. B. Saunders; 1959:543–571

[9] Adour KK. Diagnosis and Management of Facial Paralysis. N Engl J Med. 1982; 307:348–351

[10] Shambaugh GE, Clemis JD, Paparella MM, Schumrick DA. In: Facial Nerve Paralysis. Otolaryngology. Philadelphia: W. B. Saunders; 1973

[11] Adour KK, Wingerd J, Doty HE. Prevalence of Concurrent Diabetes Mellitus and Idiopathic Facial Paralysis (Bell's Palsy). Diabetes. 1975; 24:449–451

[12] Treatment of Lyme Disease. Med Letter. 1988; 30:65–66

[13] Abraham-Inpijn L, Devriese PP, Hart AAM. Predisposing Factors in Bell's Palsy: A Clinical Study with Reference to Diabetes Mellitus, Hypertension, Clotting Mechanism and Lipid Disturbance. Clin Otolaryngol. 1982; 7:99–105

[14] Devriese PP, Schumacher T, Scheide A, et al. Incidence, Prognosis and Recovery of Bell's Palsy: A Survey of About 1000 Patients (1974-1983). Clin Otolaryngol. 1990; 15:15–27

[15] Adour KK, Byl FM, Hilsinger RL, Kahn ZM, et al. The True Nature of Bell's Palsy: Analysis of 1000 Consecutive Patients. Laryngoscope. 1978; 88:787–801

[16] Adour KK, Bell DN, Hilsinger RL. Herpes simplex virus in idiopathic facial paralysis (Bell palsy). JAMA. 1975; 233:527–530

[17] Kuiper H, Devriese PP, de Jongh BM, Vos K, Dankert J. Absence of Lyme Borreliosis Among Patients With Presumed Bell's Palsy. Arch Neurol. 1992; 49:940–943

[18] Sullivan FM, Swan IR, Donnan PT, Morrison JM, Smith BH, McKinstry B, Davenport RJ, Vale LD, Clarkson JE, Hammersley V, Hayavi S, McAteer A, Stewart K, Daly F. Early treatment with prednisolone or acyclovir in Bell's palsy. N Engl J Med. 2007; 357:1598–1607

[19] Conley J, Baker DC. Hypoglossal-Facial Nerve Anastamosis for Reinnervation of the Paralyzed Face. Plast Reconstr Surg. 1979; 63:63–72

[20] Pluchino F, Fornari M, Luccarelli C. Intracranial Repair of Interrupted Facial Nerve in Course of Operation for Acoustic Neuroma by Microsurgical Technique. Acta Neurochir. 1986; 79:87–93

[21] Stephanian E, Sekhar LN, Janecka IP, Hirsch B. Facial Nerve Repair by Interposition Nerve Graft: Results in 22 Patients. Neurosurgery. 1992; 31:73–77

[22] King TT, Sparrow OC, Arias JM, O'Connor AF. Repair of Facial Nerve After Removal of Cerebellopontine Angle Tumors: A Comparative Study. J Neurosurg. 1993; 78:720–725

[23] Alberti PWRM. The Greater Auricular Nerve. Donor for Facial Nerve Grafts: A Note on its Topographical Anatomy. Arch Otolaryngol. 1962; 76:422–424

[24] Strelzow VV, Friedman WH, Katsantonis GP. Reconstruction of the Paralyzed Face With the Polypropylene Mesh Template. Arch Otolaryngol. 1983; 109:140–144

[25] May M, Sobol SM, Mester SJ. Hypoglossal-Facial Nerve Interpositional-Jump Graft for Facial Reanimation without Tongue Atrophy. Otolaryngol Head Neck Surg. 1991; 104:818–825

[26] Drew SJ, Fullarton AC, Glasby MA, et al. Reinnervation of Facial Nerve Territory Using a Composite Hypoglossal Nerve-Muscle Autograft-Facial Nerve

Bridge. An Experimental Model in Sheep. Clin Otolaryngol. 1995; 20:109–117
[27] Hitselberger WE, House WF, Luetje CM. In: Hypoglossal-Facial Anastamosis. Acoustic Tumors: Management. Baltimore: University Park Press; 1979:97–103
[28] Atlas MD, Lowinger DSG. A new technique for hypoglossal-facial nerve repair. Laryngoscope. 1997; 107:984–991
[29] Pitty LF, Tator CH. Hypoglossal-Facial Nerve Anastamosis for Facial Nerve Palsy Following Surgery for Cerebellopontine Angle Tumors. J Neurosurg. 1992; 77:724–731
[30] Duel AB. Advanced Methods in the Surgical Treatment of Facial Paralysis. Ann Otol Rhinol Laryngol. 1934; 43:76–88
[31] Poe DS, Scher N, Panje WR. Facial Reanimation by XI-VII Anastamosis Without Shoulder Paralysis. Laryngoscope. 1989; 99:1040–1047
[32] Ebersold MJ, Quast LM. Long-Term Results of Spinal Accessory Nerve-Facial Nerve Anastamosis. J Neurosurg. 1992; 77:51–54

Part XII

Primary Tumors of the Nervous and Related Systems: Tumors of Neuroepithelial Tissue

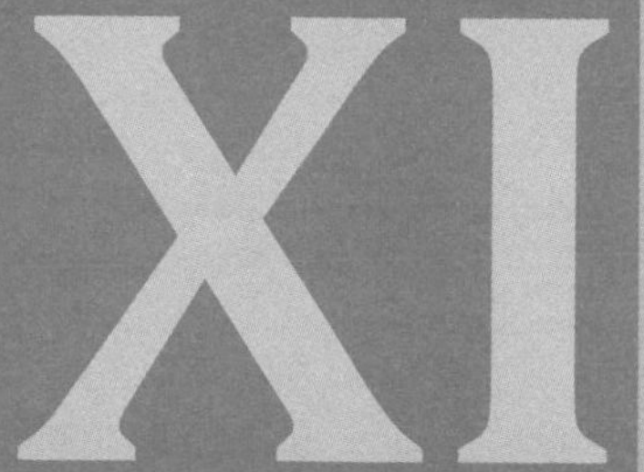

34 General Information, Classification and Tumor Markers

34.1 Classification of nervous system tumors

WHO classification of tumors of the nervous system

The 2007 WHO classification[1] identifies 7 categories of tumors of the nervous system (see ▶ Table 34.1) and a modified outline appears below[1,2,3,4,5] (along with the unofficial category "intracranial and/or intraspinal embryonal remnants", and pituitary adenomas (not part of the CNS)). Also to be considered: cysts (neurocysticercosis…), tumor-like masses (e.g. giant aneurysms), and local extension of regional tumors. Cytogenetic and molecular genetic information are playing an ever increasing role in the rapidly evolving classification of many brain tumors.

Table 34.1 Overview of WHO classification of nervous system tumors[3]

1. tumors of neuroepithelial tissue
2. tumors of cranial and paraspinal nerves
3. tumors of the meninges
4. lymphomas and hematopoietic neoplasms
5. germ cell tumors
6. tumors of the sellar region
7. metastatic tumors

Table 34.2 2007 WHO classification of tumors of the nervous system[1]

Tumor			ICD-O[a]
A. TUMORS OF NEUROEPITHELIAL TISSUE[b]			
I. Astrocytes ➞ astrocytic tumors[c] (p.612)			
1.	astrocytomas that are typically infiltrating (p.612) (lower grade tumors in this category tend to progress in malignancy)		
	a.	diffuse astrocytoma (WHO II[d]) (p.612). Variants:	9400/3
		• fibrillary	9420/3
		• protoplasmic	9410/3
		• gemistocytic	9411/3
	b.	anaplastic (malignant) astrocytoma (WHO III) (p.616)	9401/3
	c.	glioblastoma (WHO IV) (p.616) (formerly glioblastoma multiforme (GBM)). Variants:	9440/3
		• giant cell glioblastoma	9441/3
		• gliosarcoma	9442/3
	d.	gliomatosis cerebri (p.619)	9381/3
2.	more circumscribed lesions (these do *not* tend to progress to anaplastic astrocytoma and GBM)		
	a.	pilocytic astrocytoma (p.629)	9421/1
		• pilomyxoid astrocytoma (WHO II) (p.632)	9425/3
	b.	pleomorphic xanthoastrocytoma (PXA) (p.635)	9424/3
	c.	subependymal giant cell astrocytoma (p.607): associated with tuberous sclerosis	9384/1

Table 34.2 continued

Tumor			ICD-O[a]
II. Oligodendrocytes ➡ oligodendroglial tumors			
1.	oligodendroglioma (WHO II) (p. 638)		9450/3
2.	anaplastic oligodendroglioma (WHO III) (p. 639)		9451/3
III. Oligoastrocytic tumors (nee: mixed gliomas)			
1.	oligoastrocytoma (WHO II) (p. 641)		9382/3
2.	anaplastic (malignant) oligoastrocytoma (WHO III) (p. 641)		9382/3
IV. Ependymocytes ➡ ependymal tumors			
1.	ependymoma (WHO II) (p. 642). Variants:		9391/3
	a.	cellular (p. 642)	9391/3
	b.	papillary (p. 642)	9393/3
	c.	clear cell (p. 642)	9391/3
	d.	tanycytic (p. 642)	9391/3
2.	anaplastic (malignant) ependymoma (WHO III) (p. 643)		9392/3
3.	myxopapillary ependymoma: filum terminale only (WHO I) (p. 642)		9394/1
4.	subependymoma (WHO I) (p. 643)		9383/1
V. Choroid plexus tumors (p. 648)			
1.	choroid plexus papilloma		9390/0
2.	atypical choroid plexus papilloma		9390/1
3.	choroid plexus carcinoma		9390/3
VI. Other neuroepithelial tumors (p. 649)			
1.	astroblastoma		9430/3
2.	chordoid glioma of the 3rd ventricle		9444/1
3.	angiocentric glioma		9431/1
VII. neuronal and mixed neuronal-glial tumors (p. 651)			
1.	gangliocytoma		9492/0
2.	ganglioglioma (p. 651)		9505/1
3.	dysembryoplastic neuroepithelial tumor (DNT) (p. 646)		9413/0
4.	desmoplastic infantile astrocytoma/ganglioglioma (DIG) (p. 645)		9412/1
5.	dysplastic gangliocytoma of cerebellum (Lhermitte-Duclos) (p. 647)		9493/0
6.	anaplastic (malignant) ganglioglioma		9505/3
7.	central neurocytoma (p. 645)		9506/1
8.	extraventricular neurocytoma		9506/1
9.	cerebellar liponeurocytoma		9506/1
10.	papillary glioneuronal tumor		9509/1
11.	rosette-forming glioneuronal tumor of the 4th ventricle		9509/1
12.	paraganglioma (of the filum terminale)		8680/1

Table 34.2 continued

Tumor			ICD-O[a]
VIII. Pinealocytes → pineal parenchymal tumors (p. 659)			
1.	pineocytoma (pinealoma)		9361/1
2.	pineoblastoma		9362/3
3.	pineal parenchymal tumor of intermediate differentiation		9362/3
4.	papillary tumor of the pineal region		9395/3
IX. Embryonal tumors (p. 663)			
1.	medulloblastoma (p. 663). Variants:		9470/3
	a.	desmoplastic/nodular medulloblastoma (p. 664)	9471/3
	b.	anaplastic medulloblastoma	9474/3
	c.	large-cell medulloblastoma (p. 664)	9474/3
	d.	medulloblastoma with extensive nodularity	9471/3
2.	CNS primitive neuroectodermal tumors (PNET) (p. 663)		9473/3
	a.	CNS neuroblastoma	9500/3
	b.	CNS ganglioneuroblastoma	9490/3
	c.	medulloepithelioma	9501/3
	d.	ependymoblastoma (p. 666)	9392/3
3.	atypical teratoid/rhabdoid tumor (AT/RT) (p. 666)		9508/3
B. TUMORS OF CRANIAL, SPINAL AND PERIPHERAL NERVES			
I. Schwannoma (neurilemmoma, neurinoma) (vestibular schwannoma AKA acoustic neuroma)			**9560/0**
1.	cellular		9560/0
2.	plexiform		9560/0
3.	melanotic		9560/0
II. Neurofibroma (p. 604)			**9540/0**
1.	plexiform (p. 604)		9550/0
III. Perineurioma (p. 687)			**9571/0**
1.	perineurioma, NOS		9571/0
2.	malignant perineurioma		9571/3
IV. Malignant peripheral nerve sheath tumor (MPNST) (neurogenic sarcoma, anaplastic neurofibroma, "malignant schwannoma"). Variants:			**9540/3**
1.	epithelioid MPNST		9540/3
2.	MPNST with mesenchymal differentiation		9540/3
3.	melanotic MPNST		9540/3
4.	MPNST with glandular differentiation		9540/3

Table 34.2 continued

Tumor			ICD-O[a]
C. TUMORS OF THE MENINGES			
I. Tumors of meningothelial cells			
1.	meningioma (p. 690). Variants:		9530/0
	a.	meningothelial (WHO I)	9531/0
	b.	fibrous (fibroblastic) (WHO I)	9532/0
	c.	transitional (mixed) (WHO I)	9537/0
	d.	psammomatous (WHO I)	9533/0
	e.	angiomatous (WHO I)	9534/0
	f.	microcystic (WHO I)	9530/0
	g.	secretory (WHO I)	9530/0
	h.	lymphoplasmacyte-rich (WHO I)	9530/0
	i.	metaplastic (WHO I)	9530/0
	the following meningiomas exhibit more malignant behavior		
	j.	clear cell (intracranial) (WHO II)	9538/1
	k.	chordoid (WHO II)	9538/1
	l.	atypical meningioma (WHO II) (p. 693)	9539/1
	m.	papillary meningioma (WHO III)	9538/3
	n.	rhabdoid meningioma (WHO III) (p. 694)	9538/3
	o.	anaplastic (malignant) meningioma (WHO III) (p. 694)	9530/3
II. Mesenchymal, non-meningothelial tumors (p. 701)			
1.	lipoma, e.g. of corpus callosum (p. 260)		8850/0
2.	angiolipoma		8861/0
3.	hiberneuroma		8880/0
4.	liposarcoma (intracranial)		8850/3
5.	solitary fibrous tumor		8815/0
6.	fibrosarcoma		8810/3
7.	malignant fibrous histiocytoma		8830/3
8.	leiomyoma		8890/0
9.	leiomyosarcoma		8890/3
10.	rhabdomyoma		8900/0
11.	rhabdomyosarcoma		8900/3
12.	chondroma		9220/0
13.	chondrosarcoma		9220/3
14.	osteoma		9180/0

Table 34.2 continued

Tumor		ICD-O[a]
15.	osteosarcoma	9180/3
16.	osteochondroma	9210/0
17.	hemangioma	9120/0
18.	epithelioid hemangioendothelioma	9133/1
19.	hemangiopericytoma (p. 701)	9150/1
20.	anaplastic hemangiopericytoma	9150/3
21.	angiosarcoma	9120/3
22.	Kaposi sarcoma	9140/3
23.	Ewing sarcoma – PNET	9364/3
III. Primary melanocytic lesions		
1.	diffuse melanocytosis	8728/0
2.	melanocytoma	8728/1
3.	malignant melanoma (primary CNS) (p. 701)	8720/3
4.	meningeal melanomatosis	8728/3
IV. Other neoplasms related to the meninges		
1.	hemangioblastoma (p. 701)	9161/1
D. LYMPHOMAS AND HEMATOPOIETIC NEOPLASMS		
I. Malignant lymphoma (primary CNS lymphoma) (p. 710)		**9590/3**
II. Plasmacytoma		**9731/3**
III. Granulocytic sarcoma		**9930/3**
E. GERM CELL TUMORS		
I. Germinoma (p. 659)		**9064/3**
II. Embryonal carcinoma		**9070/3**
III. Endodermal sinus tumor (EST) (yolk sac tumor)		**9071/3**
IV. Choriocarcinoma		**9100/3**
V. Teratoma (from all 3 germ-cell layers) (p. 660)		**9080/1**
1.	mature	9080/0
2.	immature	9080/3
3.	teratoma with malignant transformation	9084/3
VI. Mixed germ cell tumors		9085/3
F. TUMORS OF THE SELLAR REGION		
I. Craniopharyngioma (p. 763). **Variants:**		**9350/1**
1.	adamantinomatous	9351/1
2.	papillary	9352/1

Table 34.2 continued

Tumor		ICD-O[a]
II. Adenohypophyseal cells ➡ pituitary adenoma[e] (p. 718)		**8272/0**
1.	prolactinoma[e] (p. 722)	8271/0
2.	ACTH secreting adenoma	
3.	growth-hormone secreting adenoma	
4.	thyrotropin (TSH) secreting adenoma (p. 726)	
5.	gonadotropin (LH and/or FSH) secreting adenoma	
III. Neurohypophysis and infundibulum (p. 727)		
1.	granular cell tumor (p. 727)	9582/0
2.	neurohypophyseal cells	9432/1
IV. Pituitary carcinoma (p. 718)		
V. Spindle cell oncocytoma of the adenohypophysis		**8291/0**
G. METASTATIC TUMORS (p. 800) **Those commonly involving brain include:**		
I. Lung cancer: especially small-cell (p. 802)		
II. Breast		
III. Melanoma (p. 803)		
IV. Renal cell (p. 805)		
V. Lymphoma		
VI. GI		
H. LOCAL EXTENSIONS FROM REGIONAL TUMORS[e]		
I. Paraganglioma (chemodectoma)		
1.	glomus jugulare tumor (p. 654)	
II. Notochord ➡ chordoma (p. 778)		
III. Carcinoma		
I. CYSTS AND TUMOR-LIKE LESIONS[e]		
I. Rathke's cleft cyst (p. 756)		
II. Ectodermal rests		
1.	epidermoid cyst (p. 761)	
2.	cholesteatoma (p. 761)	

Table 34.2 continued

Tumor	ICD-O[a]
III. Dermoid cyst (p. 760)	
IV. Colloid cyst of the third ventricle (p. 756)	
V. Neurenteric/enterogenous cyst (p. 290)	
VI. Neuroglial cyst	
VII. Hypothalamic neuronal hamartoma (p. 261)	
VIII. Nasal glial heterotopia	
IX. Plasma cell granuloma	
J. UNCLASSIFIED TUMORS[e]	

[a]ICD-O = morphology code of the International Classification of Diseases for Oncology (http://codes.iarc.fr). The extension after the slash is the "behavior code": /0 = benign, /1 = low or uncertain malignant potential or borderline malignancy, /2 = in situ lesions, /3 = malignant tumors
[b]represents a significant portion of what is usually considered to be primary brain tumors
[c]the term "glioma" is occasionally used to refer to all glial tumors (e.g. "low-grade glioma" is often used when discussing low-grade tumors of any glial lineage), although in its usual sense glioma (especially "high grade gliomas") refers only to astrocytic tumors
[d]"WHO II" means World Health Organization (WHO) grade II, "WHO III" means WHO grade III, etc.
[e]these tumors are not part of the 2007 WHO classification5]

34.2 Brain tumors – general clinical aspects

34.2.1 General information

For details of presentation, see sections below for supratentorial and infratentorial tumors. Most brain tumors present with:

- Progressive neurologic deficit (68%): usually motor weakness (45%).
- Headache: was a presenting symptom in 54% (see below).
- Seizures in 26%. Often focal in onset (due to cortical irritation in the area of the tumor), may generalize secondarily.

34.2.2 Focal neurologic deficits associated with brain tumors

In addition to nonfocal signs and symptoms (e.g. seizures, increased ICP…), as with any destructive brain lesion, tumors may produce progressive deficits related to the function of the involved brain. Some characteristic "syndromes":

1. frontal lobe: abulia, dementia, personality changes. Often nonlateralizing, but apraxia, hemiparesis or dysphasia (with dominant hemisphere involvement) may occur
2. temporal lobe: auditory or olfactory hallucinations, déja vu, memory impairment. Contralateral superior quadrantanopsia may be detected on visual field testing
3. parietal lobe: contralateral motor or sensory impairment, homonymous hemianopsia. Agnosias (with dominant hemisphere involvement) and apraxias may occur; see Clinical syndromes of parietal lobe disease (p. 97)
4. occipital lobe: contralateral visual field deficits, alexia (especially with corpus callosum involvement with infiltrating tumors)
5. posterior fossa: (see above) cranial nerve deficits, ataxia (truncal or appendicular)

34.2.3 Headaches with brain tumors

General information

Headache (H/A) may occur with or without elevated ICP. H/A are present equally in patients with primary or metastatic tumor (≈ 50% of patients[6]). Classically described as being worse in the morning (possibly due to hypoventilation during sleep), this may actually be uncommon.[6] Often exacerbated by coughing, straining, or (in 30%) bending forward (placing head in dependent position). Associated with nausea and vomiting in 40%, may be temporarily relieved by vomiting (possibly due to hyperventilation during vomiting). These features along with the presence of a focal neurologic deficit or seizure were thought to differentiate tumor H/A from others. However, H/A in 77% of brain tumor patients were similar to tension H/A, and in 9% were migraine-like.[6] Only 8% showed the "classic" brain tumor H/A, two-thirds of these patients had increased ICP.

Etiologies of tumor headache

The brain itself is not pain sensitive. H/A in the presence of brain tumor may be due to any combination of the following:

1. increased intracranial pressure (ICP): which may be due to
   a) tumor mass effect
   b) hydrocephalus (obstructive or communicating)
   c) mass effect from associated edema
   d) mass effect from associated hemorrhage
2. invasion or compression of pain sensitive structures:
   a) dura
   b) blood vessels
   c) periosteum
3. secondary to difficulty with vision
   a) diplopia due to dysfunction of nerves controlling extra-ocular muscles
      - direct compression of III, IV, or VI
      - abducens palsy from increased ICP, see diplopia (p.592)
      - internuclear ophthalmoplegia due to brainstem invasion/compression
   b) difficulty focusing: due to optic nerve dysfunction from invasion/compression
4. extreme hypertension resulting from increased ICP (part of Cushing's triad)
5. psychogenic: due to stress from loss of functional capacity (e.g. deteriorating job performance)

34.2.4 Supratentorial tumors

See reference.[7]

Signs and symptoms include:

1. those due to increased ICP (see below):
   a) from mass effect of tumor and/or edema
   b) from blockage of CSF drainage (hydrocephalus): less common in supratentorial tumors (classically occurs with colloid cyst, may also occur with entrapped lateral ventricle)
2. progressive focal deficits: includes weakness, dysphasia (which occurs in 37–58% of patients with left-sided brain tumors[8]): see below
   a) due to destruction of brain parenchyma by tumor invasion
   b) due to compression of brain parenchyma by mass and/or peritumoral edema and/or hemorrhage
   c) due to compression of cranial nerve(s)
3. headache: see below
4. seizures: not infrequently the first symptom of a brain tumor. Tumor should be aggressively sought in an idiopathic first time seizure in a patient > 20 years (if negative, the patient should be followed with repeat studies at later dates). Rare with posterior fossa tumors or pituitary tumors
5. mental status changes: depression, lethargy, apathy, confusion
6. symptoms suggestive of a TIA (dubbed "tumor TIA") or stroke, may be due to:
   a) occlusion of a vessel by tumor cells
   b) hemorrhage into the tumor: any tumor may hemorrhage, see Hemorrhagic brain tumors (p.1335)
   c) focal seizure
7. in the special case of pituitary tumors (p.718):
   a) symptoms due to endocrine disturbances
   b) pituitary apoplexy (p.720)
   c) CSF leak

Booking the case: Craniotomy for supratentorial tumor

Also see defaults & disclaimers (p.27). If awake craniotomy is required, see Booking the case: Awake craniotomy (p.1433).

1. position: (depends on location of tumor)
2. pre-op embolization (by neuroendovascular interventionalist) for some vascular tumors including some meningiomas

3. equipment:
   a) microscope
   b) ultrasonic aspirator
   c) image guidance system
4. blood availability: type and cross 2 U PRBC
5. post-op: ICU
6. consent (in lay terms for the patient – not all-inclusive):
   a) procedure: surgery through the skull to remove as much of the tumor as is safely possible
   b) alternatives: nonsurgical management, radiation therapy for some tumors
   c) complications: usual craniotomy complications (p. 28) plus inability to remove all of the tumor

34.2.5 Infratentorial tumors

Signs and symptoms

Seizures are rare (unlike the situation with supratentorial tumors, (seizures arise from irritation of cerebral cortex).

1. most posterior fossa tumors present with signs and symptoms of increased intracranial pressure (ICP) due to hydrocephalus (HCP). These include:
   a) headache: (see below)
   b) nausea/vomiting: due either to increased ICP from HCP, or from direct pressure on the vagal nucleus or the area postrema (so-called "vomiting center")
   c) papilledema: estimated incidence is ≈ 50–90% (more common when the tumor impairs CSF circulation)
   d) gait disturbance/ataxia
   e) vertigo
   f) diplopia: may be due to VI nerve (abducens) palsy which may occur with increased ICP in the absence of direct compression of the nerve
2. S/S indicative of mass effect in various locations within the p-fossa
   a) lesions in cerebellar *hemisphere* may cause: ataxia of the extremities, dysmetria, intention tremor
   b) lesions of cerebellar *vermis* may cause: broad based gait, truncal ataxia, titubation
   c) brainstem involvement usually results in multiple cranial nerve and long tract abnormalities, and should be suspected when nystagmus is present (especially rotatory or vertical)

Evaluation

Posterior fossa (infratentorial) tumors

See Posterior fossa lesions (p. 905) for differential diagnosis (includes non-neoplastic lesions as well.

In pediatric patients with a posterior fossa tumor, an MRI of the lumbar spine should be done pre-op to rule-out drop mets (post-op there may be artifact from blood).

In adults, most intraparenchymal p-fossa tumors will be metastatic, and work-up for a primary should be undertaken.

Treatment of associated hydrocephalus

In cases with hydrocephalus at the time of presentation, some authors advocate initial placement of VP shunt or EVD prior to definitive surgery (waiting ≈ 2 wks before surgery) because of possibly lower operative mortality.[9] Theoretical risks of using this approach include the following:

1. placing a shunt is generally a lifelong commitment, whereas not all patients with hydrocephalus from a p-fossa tumor will require a shunt
2. possible seeding of the peritoneum with malignant tumor cells e.g. with medulloblastoma. Consider placement of tumor filter (may not be justified given the high rate of filter occlusion and the low rate of "shunt metastases"[10])
3. some shunts may become infected prior to the definitive surgery
4. definitive treatment is delayed, and the total number of hospital days may be increased
5. upward transtentorial herniation (p. 303) may occur if there is excessively rapid CSF drainage

Either approach (shunting followed by elective p-fossa surgery, or semi-emergent definitive p-fossa surgery) is accepted. At Children's Hospital of Philadelphia, dexamethasone is started and the surgery is performed on the next elective operating day, unless neurologic deterioration occurs necessitating emergency surgery.[11]

Some surgeons place a ventriculostomy at the time of surgery. CSF is drained only after the dura is opened (to avoid upwards herniation) to help equilibrate the pressures between the infra- and supra-tentorial compartments. Post-op, the external ventricular drain EVD is usually set at a low height (≈ 10 cm above the EAM) for 24 hours, and is progressively raised over the next 48 hrs and should be D/C'd by ≈ 72 hrs post-op.

Booking the case: Craniotomy for infratentorial tumor

Also see defaults & disclaimers (p. 27) and retromastoid surgery for vestibular schwannomas (p. 681).

1. position: (typically either prone or park bench, depending on tumor type/location and surgeon preference)
2. pre-op embolization (by neuroendovascular interventionalist) for some vascular tumors such as hemangioblastoma
3. equipment:
   a) microscope
   b) ultrasonic aspirator
   c) image guidance system (optional)
4. blood availability: type and cross 2 U PRBC
5. post-op: ICU
6. consent (in lay terms for the patient – not all-inclusive):
   a) procedure: surgery through the skull remove as much of the tumor as is safely possible
   b) alternatives: nonsurgical management, radiation therapy for some tumors
   c) complications: usual craniotomy complications (p. 28) plus inability to remove all of the tumor, hydrocephalus, CSF leak

34.3 Pediatric brain tumors

34.3.1 General information

Among all childhood cancers, brain tumors are the second only to leukemias in incidence (20%), and are the most common solid pediatric tumor,[12] comprising 40–50% of all tumors.[13] Annual incidence: 2–5 cases per 100,000.

34.3.2 Types of tumors

The common pediatric brain tumors are gliomas (cerebellum, brain stem, and optic nerve), pineal tumors, craniopharyngiomas, teratomas, granulomas, and primitive neuroectodermal tumors (PNETs, primarily medulloblastoma).

Meningiomas: 1.5% of meningiomas occur in childhood and adolescence (usually between 10–20 years), comprising 0.4–4.6% of intracranial tumors[14(p 3263)]; see Meningiomas (p. 690).

34.3.3 Infratentorial vs. supratentorial

It has traditionally been taught that most pediatric brain tumors (≈ 60%) are infratentorial, and that these are ≈ equally divided among brain stem gliomas, cerebellar astrocytomas, and medulloblastomas. In reality, the ratio of supratentorial to infratentorial tumors is dependent on the specific age group studied, as illustrated in ► Table 34.3. ► Table 34.4 shows the breakdown for pooled data from 1350 pediatric brain tumors.

Astrocytomas are the most common supratentorial tumor in pediatrics as in adulthood.

34.3.4 Intracranial neoplasms during the first year of life

Brain tumors presenting during the first year of life is a different subset of tumors than those presenting later in childhood. In a busy neurosurgical unit in a children's hospital, they represented ≈ 8% of children admitted with brain tumors, an average of only ≈ 3 admissions per year.[17]

90% of brain tumors in *neonates* are of neuroectodermal origin, teratoma being the most common. Some of these tumors may be congenital.[18] Other supratentorial tumors include: astrocytoma,

Table 34.3 Location of pediatric brain tumors by age

Age	% Infratentorial
0–6 mos	27%
6–12 mos	53%
12–24 mos	74%
2–16 yrs	42%

Table 34.4 Incidence of pediatric brain tumors[a]

Tumor type	% of total
infratentorial tumors	**54%**
cerebellar astrocytomas (p. 630)	15%
medulloblastomas (p. 664)	14%
brain stem gliomas (p. 633)	12%
ependymomas (p. 642) [15]	9%
supratentorial benign astrocytomas	**13%**
[a]data pooled from 1350 pediatric brain tumors[16 (p 368)]	

choroid plexus tumors, ependymomas, and craniopharyngiomas. Posterior fossa tumors include medulloblastoma and cerebellar astrocytoma.

Many of these tumors escape diagnosis until they are very large in size due to the elasticity of the infant skull, the adaptability of the developing nervous system to compensate for deficits, and the difficulty in examining a patient with limited neurologic repertoire and inability to cooperate. The most common presenting manifestations are vomiting, arrest or regression of psychomotor development, macrocrania, poor feeding/failure to thrive. They may also present with seizures.

34

34.4 Medications for brain tumors

34.4.1 Steroid use in brain tumors

The beneficial effect of steroids in metastatic tumors is often much more dramatic than with primary infiltrating gliomas.

Dexamethasone (Decadron®) dose for brain tumors:

- for patients not previously on steroids:
  - adult: 10 mg IVP loading, then 6 mg PO/IVP q 6 hrs.[19,20] In cases with severe vasogenic edema, doses up to 10 mg q 4 hrs may be used
  - peds: 0.5–1 mg/kg IVP loading, then 0.25–0.5 mg/kg/d PO/IVP divided q 6 hrs. NB: avoid prolonged treatment because of growth suppressant effect in children
- for patients already on steroids:
  - for acute deterioration, a dose of approximately double the usual dose should be tried
  - see also "stress doses" (p. 146)

34.4.2 Prophylactic anticonvulsants with brain tumors

20–40% of patients with a brain tumor will have had a seizure by the time their tumor is diagnosed.[21] Antiepileptic drugs (AEDs) are indicated in these patients. 20–45% more will ultimately develop a seizure.[21] Prophylactic AEDs do not provide substantial benefit (reduction of risk > 25% for seizure-free survival) and there are significant risks involved. Practice guidelines for AED use with brain tumors is shown below. Prophylactic AEDs are not indicated for isolated posterior fossa tumors.

Practice guideline: Prophylactic anticonvulsants with brain tumors

Level I[21]: prophylactic AEDs should not be used routinely in patients with newly diagnosed brain tumors

Level II[21]: in patients with brain tumors undergoing craniotomy, prophylactic AEDs may be used, and if there has been no seizure, it is appropriate to taper off AEDs starting 1 week post-op

34.5 Chemotherapy for brain tumors

34.5.1 General information

General information is presented here. Chemotherapy for some specific tumors is also included in the section devoted to that tumor where appropriate. Some agents used for CNS tumors: see ▶ Table 34.5.[22,23]

34.5.2 Alkylating agents

Temozolomide (Temodar®) is a derivative of Dacarbazine (DTIC®) and is an oral alkylating agent. Temozolomide is a prodrug which undergoes rapid non-enzymatic conversion at physiologic pH to the active metabolite monomethyl triazenoimidazole carboxamide (MTIC). The cytotoxic effect of MTIC is associated with alkylation (adding an alkyl group, the smallest of which is a methyl group) of DNA at various sites primarily at the O6 and N7 positions on guanine. Some tumors can repair this damage via a protein (AGT) that is coded for by the O-6-methylguanine-DNA methyltransferase (MGMT) gene.

Table 34.5 Chemotherapeutic agents used for CNS tumors

Agent	Mechanism
nitrosoureas: BCNU (carmustine), CCNU (AKA lomustine), ACNU (nimustine)	DNA crosslinks, carbamoylation of amino groups
alkylating (methylating) agents: procarbazine, temozolomide (Temodar®) (p. 595)	DNA alkylation, interferes with protein synthesis
carboplatin, cisplatin	chelation via intrastrand crosslinks
nitrogen mustards: cyclophosphamide, isofamide, cytoxan	DNA alkylation, carbonium ion formation
vinca alkaloids: vincristine, vinblastine, paclitaxel	microtubule function inhibitors
epidophyllotoxins (ETOP-oside, VP16, teniposide, VM26)	topoisomerase II inhibitors
topotecan, irinotecan (CPT-11)	topoisomerase I inhibitors
tamoxifen	protein kinase C inhibitor at high doses
bevacizumab (Avastin®)	anti-VEGF antibody may be useful in vestibular neuromas
hydroxyurea bleomycin taxol (paxlitaxol) methotrexate cytosine, arabinoside corticosteroids: dexamethasone, prednisone fluorouracil (FU)	

34

34.5.3 Nitrosoureas

Excellent BBB penetration (see below). Significant hematopoietic, pulmonary and renal toxicity.

34.5.4 Blood-brain barrier (BBB) and chemotherapy agents

Traditionally, the BBB has been considered to be a major hindrance to the use of chemotherapy for brain tumors. In theory, the BBB effectively excludes many chemotherapeutic agents from the CNS, thereby creating a "safe haven" for some tumors, e.g. metastases. This concept has been challenged.[24] Regardless of the etiology, the response of most brain tumors to systemic chemotherapy is usually very modest, with a notable exception being a favorable response of oligodendrogliomas (p.640) and gliomas lacking MGMT activity. Considerations regarding chemotherapeutic agents in relation to the BBB include:

1. some CNS tumors may partially disrupt the BBB, especially malignant gliomas[25]
2. lipophilic agents (e.g. nitrosoureas) may cross the BBB more readily
3. selective intraarterial (e.g. intracarotid or intervertebral) injection[26]: produces higher local concentration of agents which increases penetration of the BBB, with lower associated systemic toxicities than would otherwise occur
4. the BBB may be iatrogenically disrupted (e.g. with mannitol) prior to administration of the agent
5. the BBB may be bypassed by intrathecal administration of agents via LP or ventricular access device, e.g. methotrexate for CNS lymphoma (p.713)
6. biodegradable polymer wafers containing the agent may be directly implanted

34.5.5 Imaging studies following surgical removal of tumor

At many academic centers, it is common to get a noncontrast CT scan within 6–12 hours of surgery to assess for acute complications (primarily blood – within brain or epidural or subdural hematoma, amount of pneumocephalus, hydrocephalus...).

Then to assess the extent of tumor removal, a post-op brain CT or MRI without and with contrast should either be obtained within 2–3 days,[27] or should be delayed at least ≈ 30 days. The *non*-contrast scan is important to help differentiate blood from enhancement. The contrast images demonstrates areas of enhancement, which may represent residual tumor. After ≈ 48 hours, contrast enhancement due to post-operative inflammatory vascular changes ensues, which may be difficult to differentiate from tumor. This usually subsides by ≈ 30 days,[28] but may persist for 6–8 weeks.[29] This recommendation regarding the timing of post-op imaging does not apply to pituitary tumors (p.718). The effect of steroids on contrast enhancement is controversial,[30,31] and may depend on many factors (including tumor type).

34.6 Intraoperative pathology consultations ("frozen section")

34.6.1 Accuracy of intraoperative pathology consultations

Accuracy of intraoperative pathologic diagnosis can be increased by:

- Providing the pathologist with information regarding: patient demographics, clinical history, imaging results, relevant previous pathologic diagnoses, and clinical impression
- Larger specimen sizes when possible
- Avoiding artifact created by excessive crushing or coagulation

Frozen section diagnoses should be considered preliminary. The final diagnosis differs from the frozen section in approximately 3–10 % of cases.[32,33,34] If the frozen section interpretation does not correlate with the clinical impression, direct discussion with the pathologist may be advisable.

34.6.2 Techniques for intraoperative tissue preparation

▶ **Touch preparation.** The specimen is gently "touched" with a glass slide which is then rapidly fixed, stained and dehydrated for examination. This technique is particularly useful for tumors with discohesive cells (e.g. lymphoma, pituitary adenoma).

▶ **Smear or squash preparation.** A small portion of specimen is smeared or compressed with moderate pressure between two glass slides, rapidly fixed, stained, and dehydrated for examination. This technique can be particularly useful for: multiple sclerosis (identifying histiocytes), visualizing long cell processes in gliomas, and identifying cytoplasmic inclusions or intranuclear pseudoinclusions).[35(p 5–6)] The cohesive nature often seen in tumors such as metastases and meningiomas is apparent, as are areas of necrosis.

► **Frozen section.** A portion of tissue is rapidly frozen in liquid nitrogen and cut into 4–6 micron sections, mounted on a slide, rapidly fixed, stained, and dehydrated for examination. Unlike touch and smear preparations, this allows more accurate assessment of lesion architecture, cellularity, and interface with adjacent brain tissue. Disadvantages include use of greater tissue with less available for permanent histology (important with small biopsies), as well as artifacts such as freezing ice crystal artifact (which, when present, suggests lesional tissue has been biopsied but limits interpretation of cellularity).[35(p 6)] When possible, some tissue should be preserved for processing without freezing to avoid artifacts.

At the time of frozen section interpretation, consideration for additional studies such as tissue cultures or flow cytometry should be entertained. With minute specimens, a discussion is warranted whether frozen section is required to preserve tissue for permanent studies.

34.6.3 Selected frozen section pitfalls or potential critical diagnoses

- Differentiating low grade gliomas from normal or reactive brain tissue can be challenging.[32,33] Increased cellularity (best evaluated at low power), nuclear atypia when present, and increased perineuronal satellitosis can be helpful, though not always readily observed.[35(p 72–3, p 174–7)]
  Pearl: Secondary structures of Scherer may be useful in identifying gliomas in challenging cases and include increased perineuronal and perivascular satellitosis (limited perineuronal satellitosis is normal) and accumulation of neoplastic cells in the subpial molecular layer with subpial tumor spread.[36]
- Metastasis vs Glioma: Usually not problematic on frozen section, except occasionally with markedly atypical gliomas with limited sampling.[32,33,34] In such rare cases immunohistochemistry is helpful.
- Astrocytoma vs oligodendroglioma: Usually not a critical distinction at the time of frozen section diagnosis. However, in part due to frozen section artifact imparted to the nuclei, oligodendrogliomas can be interpreted as astrocytomas in the frozen section room.[32] Smear preparations can at times be helpful due to decreased "frozen" artifact. Also, perineuronal satellitosis may in some cases be more pronounced in oligodendrogliomas.
  Pearl: The "fried egg" appearance in oligodendrogliomas is an artifact of formalin fixation for permanent sections and is NOT present on frozen sections, also hindering intraoperative interpretation.
- Glioma grading: Sampling bias, particularly in biopsy specimens, can lead to undergrading (i.e. mitotic figures underrepresented in the biopsy material, vascular proliferation or necrosis not present in the biopsy). However, overgrading of gliomas at the time of intraoperative consultation also can occur, including with low grade childhood gliomas such as pilocytic astrocytomas.[32] 34
- Radionecrosis vs recurrent glioblastoma: Despite the fact that a history of prior radiation therapy is usually know at the time of intraoperative consultation, differentiation of the two entities can at times be difficult.[32] Both lesions often are present simultaneously. Identifying obvious tumor cells and palisading necrosis suggests recurrent/residual glioblastoma. Radiation necrosis, which affects primarily white matter, is supported by large areas of geographic necrosis, sclerosis/hyalinization of vessels or fibrinoid necrosis of vessel walls, perivascular lymphocytes, calcifications, and the presence of macrophages.
- Ischemic infarct: May see ischemic red neuron change (if the biopsy includes gray matter), as well as histiocytes (similar to demyelinating lesions). Necrosis may mimic the center of ring enhancing lesions (such as glioblastoma or metastasis), though tumor necrosis will typically involve vessels and lack a macrophage response.[35(p 663–6)]
- Demyelinating lesions (e.g. tumefactive MS): Primarily affects white matter with discrete borders. Identifying histiocytes at the time of frozen section is critical for the diagnosis. The histiocytes can mimic astrocytes of gliomas on frozen section preparation; smear preparations are particularly helpful in the distinction.
- Lymphoma (PCNSL) and small cell carcinoma: Accurate frozen section diagnosis may be critical as both conditions typically require only biopsy unless there is significant mass effect. The two entities may resemble each other on frozen section as well as resembling astrocytomas, oligodendrogliomas, and other types of metastatic carcinomas.[32,33,34,35(p 395–7)] Touch preparations can be particularly useful in identifying PCNSL.
- Spindle cell tumor/meningioma: It has been demonstrated that at times distinguishing between meningioma and spindled cell lesions such as schwannomas can be difficult at the time of

intraoperative consultation.[32] Classic features of meningiomas (whorls, psammoma bodies, intranuclear pseudoinclusions) may be absent, and freeze artifact can create Antoni B appearing areas in meningiomas.[32] In addition, underdiagnosis of malignant meningiomas and sarcomas at the time of frozen section has been noted.[32,33]

- Spinal cord astrocytoma vs. ependymoma: On occasion these entities can be difficult to distinguish during intraoperative consultation, especially as most spinal cord biopsies for frozen interpretation are minute. Due to the critical surgical implications of the accuracy of the frozen section diagnosis for intramedullary spinal gliomas, a careful discussion should be had between the surgeon and pathologist at the time of intraoperative consultation (refer to section on tumors of the spine and spinal cord).

34.6.4 Tissue preparation for permanent sections

Tissue is processed overnight through a variety of alcohol/xylene steps to remove water. This allows for embedding into paraffin so that thin sections can be cut for slide mounting. The specimens are then rehydrated by essentially reversing the alcohol/xylene steps in preparation for staining, and then dehydrated again for permanent slide coverslipping. This produces better histology with fewer artifacts, allows for processing of larger specimen volumes for evaluation, and allows for application of special stains as needed.

► **Fresh specimens.** Tissue should be sent "fresh" (i.e. without preservatives such as formalin) when the following techniques are needed:
- electron microscopy
- flow cytometry: e.g. when lymphoma is suspected
- muscle
- cultures (typically: aerobic, anaerobic, acid fast and fungal) should be sent in situations where infection is a consideration

34.7 Select commonly utilized stains in neuropathology

34.7.1 Organism and special stains

1. Organism stains:
   - tissue Gram stains (Brown & Brenn, Brown & Hopps)
   - fungi (Periodic acic-Schiff: PAS, Gomori methenamine silver: GMS)
   - acid fast bacilli (Ziehl-Neelsen, Kinyoun, FITE)
2. Special stains:
   - luxol fast blue: stains myelin; absence of staining highlights demyelinating lesions. Presence within histiocytes demonstrates ingestion of myelin as seen in MS
   - trichrome and reticulin stain: Both delineate the sarcomatous component of gliosarcomas. A reticulin stain demonstrates the connective tissue around acini of the normal pituitary gland, a feature that is lost with pituitary adenomas

34

34.7.2 Immunohistochemical stains

General information

Staining patterns: An individual tumor may lack a marker that is typically representative of its type. ✱ Therefore, a positive stain is typically more significant than a negative stain.[37] General staining patterns[37] are shown in ► Table 34.6.

Glial fibrillary acidic protein (GFAP)

Polypeptide, MW = 49,000 Daltons. Stains intermediate filaments classically identified in astrocytes/astrocytic tumors. However, is also typically expressed in ependymomas, oligodendrogliomas (especially in minigemistocytes and gliofibrillary oligodendrocytes), and some choroid plexus papillomas.[38 (p 30-1),1 (p 56, 76, 83)] GFAP is only rarely found outside the CNS in such tissues as Schwann cells, epithelium of the lens, certain liver cells, chondrocytes, etc). ✱ It would be unusual for a metastatic lesion to demonstrate staining for GFAP. However, GFAP expression may be limited in certain subsets of GBM (e.g. small cell GBM).[1 (p 37)]

Table 34.6 Immunohistochemical staining patterns for nervous system tumor masses of epithelioid cells[a]

<table>
<tr><th>Neoplasm</th><th colspan="6">Immunohistochemical stain response[b,c]</th></tr>
<tr><th></th><th>GFAP</th><th>CAM5.2</th><th>EMA</th><th>S-100</th><th>CgA</th><th>Syn</th></tr>
<tr><td>oligodendroglioma</td><td>+</td><td rowspan="2">–</td><td>–</td><td rowspan="4">+</td><td rowspan="2">–</td><td>0</td></tr>
<tr><td>ependymoma</td><td>0</td><td rowspan="2">0</td><td>–</td></tr>
<tr><td>choroid plexus papilloma</td><td rowspan="8">–</td><td rowspan="5">+</td><td>0</td><td>+</td></tr>
<tr><td>chordoma</td><td rowspan="4">+</td><td rowspan="2">–</td><td rowspan="2">–</td></tr>
<tr><td>craniopharyngioma</td><td rowspan="2">–</td></tr>
<tr><td>carcinoma</td><td>0</td><td>0</td></tr>
<tr><td>pituitary adenoma</td><td rowspan="3">0</td><td rowspan="2">+</td><td rowspan="2">+</td></tr>
<tr><td>paraganglioma</td><td rowspan="2">0</td><td>–</td></tr>
<tr><td>meningioma</td><td>+</td><td rowspan="3">–</td><td rowspan="2">–</td></tr>
<tr><td>melanoma</td><td rowspan="2">–</td><td rowspan="2">–</td><td>+</td></tr>
<tr><td>hemangioblastoma</td><td>0</td><td>0</td><td>0</td></tr>
</table>

[a]modified from McKeever, P E, Immunohistochemistry of the Nervous System, in Dobbs, D J. Diagnostic Immunohistochemistry, Churchill Livingstone, NY, © 2002

[b]abbreviations: GFAP = glial fibrillary acidic protein, EMA = epithelial membrane antigen, CAM5.2 = cytokeratin CAM5.2, CgA = chromogranin A, syn = synaptophysin

[c]a "+" or a "–" sign indicates presence or absence of the stain respectively; "0" entries indicate that the stain is not decisive for that particular tumor

S-100 protein

A low molecular weight (21,000 Daltons) calcium-binding protein that stains a variety of tissues including glia, neurons, chondrocytes, stellate cells of the adenohypophysis, myoepithelial cells, etc.[37 (p 75)] Stains a variety of CNS neoplasms such as gliomas (though less specific than GFAP), PNET, ependymomas, chordomas, and craniopharyngiomas.[1,37] Primary uses in neuropathology include to support the diagnosis of metastatic melanoma, and, in the peripheral nervous system, to confirm the diagnosis of schwannoma or neurofibroma (less intense staining in the latter).[1 (p 156)] 34

Clinically has been measured in serum (see below).

Cytokeratins (high and low molecular weight)

A variety of stains (low (e.g. CAM 5.2) & high molecular weight keratin, CK7, CK20, etc.) which stain epithelial cells. Useful to distinguish metastatic carcinoma (positive staining) from primary CNS tumors (note: cytokeratins can be expressed in choroid plexus papillomas, and GBM can express cytokeratins in rare cases).[1 (p 39-40)] Different keratin staining combinations can be used to suggest possible sites of origin for metastatic tumors.

Epithelial membrane antigen (EMA)

Stains cell membranes in many carcinomas; useful to distinguish hemangioblastoma (negative) from metastatic renal cell carcinoma (positive). Also, meningiomas typically demonstrate positive staining, as do ependymomas.[1 (p 169)]

MIB-1 (AKA monoclonal mouse anti-human Ki-67 antibody)

The Ki-67 antigen is expressed in all phases of the cell cycle except G0. Available since the early 1990s, it is a valuable marker of cell proliferation but can only be used with fresh-frozen specimens. MIB-1 is a monoclonal antibody developed using recombinant parts of the Ki-67 protein as an immunogen, and can be used on paraffin-embedded sections of fixed tissue. Cells leaving the G0/G1-phase and entering the S-phase (performing DNA synthesis) stain positive with MIB-1 immunohistochemical stain. This stain can be used to compute a semi-quantitative score. A high MIB-1 labeling index denotes high mitotic activity which often correlates with degree of malignancy. Often used in lymphomas, endocrine tumors, carcinoids, etc. See also use in astrocytomas (p.617) and in meningiomas (p.694).

Neuroendocrine stains

Includes:

In neuropathology, utilized in central neurocytoma, medulloblastoma, PNET, pineocytoma, ganglion cell tumors, paragangliomas, and choroid plexus tumors.[37] Metastases that are positive for neuroendocrine stains include small-cell carcinoma of the lung (most common), malignant pheochromocytoma, and Merkel cell tumor.

Includes:

1. chromogranin: stains synaptic vesicles. Perhaps less commonly utilized than synaptophysin in primary CNS tumor
2. synaptophysin: stains synaptic vesicles; has higher sensitivity but lower specificity than chromogranin.[37 (p 200)] Often positive for central neurocytoma which typically lacks chromogranin staining.[1 (p 107)]
3. CD56 (Neural cell adhesion molecule): a family of glycoproteins present in nervous tissue as well as other tissues such as thyroid, liver, etc.[37 (p 142-3, 264)] Frequently used to confirm neuroendocrine differentiation.
4. neuron specific enolase (NSE): sensitive but not specific for neuronal or neuroendocrine differentiation despite its name (often referred to as "neuron non-specific enolase").[37 (p 338)] Due to this, it is less often utilized as a neuroendocrine marker.

Cluster of differentiation (CD) markers

A number of immunohistochemical stains that detect antigens on the surface of leukocytes, though many stain other cell types as well. Examples include:

- CD45: General leukocyte marker
- CD3 and CD5: T-cells
- CD20: B-cells
- CD38 and CD138: Plasma cells
- CD68: Histiocytes
- CD56 (Neural cell adhesion molecule): Classically stains natural killer cells, but also a neuroendocrine marker (see above)
- organism-specific immunohistochemical stains are available to detect certain organisms that infect the nervous system including HSV, CMV, and Toxoplasma gondii

34

Metastases that are positive for neuroendocrine stains include: small-cell carcinoma of the lung, malignant pheochromocytoma, Merkel cell tumor. Metastatic small-cell tumors to the brain staining positive for neuroendocrine stains are almost all due to lung primaries (all other primaries are a distant possibility).

34.7.3 Tumor markers used clinically

Human chorionic gonadotropin (hCG)

A glycoprotein, MW = 45,000. Secreted by placental trophoblastic epithelium. Beta chain (β-hCG) is normally present only in the fetus or in gravid or postpartum females, otherwise it indicates disease. Classically associated with choriocarcinoma (uterine or testicular), also found in patients with embryonal cell tumors, teratocarcinoma of testis, and others.

CSF β-hCG is 0.5–2% of serum β-hCG in non-CNS tumors. Higher levels are diagnostic of cerebral mets from uterine or testicular choriocarcinoma, or primary choriocarcinoma or embryonal cell carcinoma of pineal (p.658) or suprasellar region.

Alpha-fetoprotein

Alpha-fetoprotein (AFP) is a normal fetal glycoprotein (MW = 70,000) initially produced by the yolk sac, and later by the fetal liver. It is found in the fetal circulation throughout gestation, and drops rapidly during the first few weeks of life, reaching normal adult levels by age 1 yr. It is detectable only in trace amounts in normal adult males or nonpregnant females. It is present in amniotic fluid in normal pregnancies, and is detectable in maternal serum starting at ≈ 12–14 weeks gestation, increasing steadily throughout pregnancy until ≈ 32 weeks.[39]

Abnormally elevated serum AFP may occur in Ca of ovary, stomach, lung, colon, pancreas, as well as in cirrhosis or hepatitis and in the majority of gravid women carrying a fetus with an open neural tube defect; see Prenatal detection of neural tube defects (p. 290). Serum AFP > 500 ng/ml usually means primary hepatic tumor.

CSF-AFP is elevated in some pineal region germ-cell tumors (p. 659). 16–25% of patients with testicular tumors get cerebral mets and elevated CSF AFP levels are reported in some.

Carcinoembryonic antigen (CEA)

A glycoprotein, MW = 200,000. Normally present in fetal endodermal cells. Originally described in the early 1960s in the serum in patients with colorectal adeno-Ca, now known to be elevated in many malignant and nonmalignant conditions (including cholecystitis, colitis, diverticulitis, hepatic involvement from any tumor, with 50–90% of terminal patients having elevation).

CSF CEA: levels > 1 ng/ml are reported with leptomeningeal spread of lung Ca (89%), breast Ca (60–67%), malignant melanoma (25–33%), and bladder Ca. May be normal even in CEA secreting cerebral mets if they don't communicate with the subarachnoid space. Only carcinomatous meningitis from lung or breast Ca consistently elevates CSF CEA in the majority of patients.

S-100 protein

Serum S-100 protein levels rise after head trauma, and possibly after other insults to the brain. Levels may also be elevated in Creutzfeldt-Jakob disease.

References

[1] Louis DN, Ohgaki H, Wiestler OD, Cavenee WK, Bosman FT, Jaffe ES, Lakhani SR, Ohgaki H. WHO classification of tumors of the central nervous system. Lyon 2007

[2] Kleihues P, Cavenee WK. World Health Organization classification of tumors: Pathology and genetics of tumors of the nervous system. Lyon 2000

[3] Kleihues P, Louis DN, Scheithauer BW, Rorke LB, Reifenberger G, Burger PC, Cavenee WK. The WHO classification of tumors of the nervous system. J Neuropathol Exp Neurol. 2002; 61:215–25; discussion 226-9

[4] Kleihues P, Burger PC, Scheithauer BW. The new WHO classification of brain tumors. Brain Pathol. 1993; 3:255–268

[5] Escourolle R, Poirier J, Rubinstein LJ. Manual of Basic Neuropathology. 2nd ed. Philadelphia: W. B. Saunders; 1971

[6] Forsyth PA, Posner JB. Headaches in Patients with Brain Tumors: A Study of 111 Patients. Neurology. 1993; 43:1678–1683

[7] Mahaley MS, Mettlin C, Natarajan N, Laws ER, et al. National Survey of Patterns of Care for Brain-Tumor Patients. J Neurosurg. 1989; 71:826–836

[8] Whittle IR, Pringle A-M, Taylor R. Effects of Resective Surgery for Left-Sided Intracranial Tumors on Language Function: A Prospective Study. Lancet. 1998; 351:1014–1018

[9] Albright L, Reigel DH. Management of Hydrocephalus Secondary to Posterior Fossa Tumors. Preliminary Report. J Neurosurg. 1977; 46:52–55

[10] Berger MS, Baumeister B, Geyer JR, Milstein J, et al. The Risks of Metastases from Shunting in Children with Primary Central Nervous System Tumors. J Neurosurg. 1991; 74:872–877

[11] McLaurin RL, Venes JL. Pediatric Neurosurgery. Philadelphia 1989

[12] Allen JC. Childhood Brain Tumors: Current Status of Clinical Trials in Newly Diagnosed and Recurrent Disease. Ped Clin N Am. 1985; 32:633–651

[13] Laurent JP, Cheek WR. Brain Tumors in Children. J Pediatr Neurosci. 1985; 1:15–32

[14] Youmans JR. Neurological Surgery. Philadelphia 1990

[15] Duffner PK, Cohen ME, Freeman AI. Pediatric Brain Tumors: An Overview. Ca. 1985; 35:287–301

[16] Section of Pediatric Neurosurgery of the American Association of Neurological Surgeons. Pediatric Neurosurgery. New York 1982

[17] Jooma R, Hayward RD, Grant DN. Intracranial Neoplasms During the First Year of Life: Analysis of One Hundred Consecutive Cases. Neurosurgery. 1984; 14:31–41

[18] Wakai S, Arai T, Nagai M. Congenital Brain Tumors. Surg Neurol. 1984; 21:597–609

[19] Galicich JH, French LA. Use of Dexamethasone in the Treatment of Cerebral Edema Resulting from Brain Tumors and Brain Surgery. Am Pract Dig Treat. 1961; 12:169–174

[20] French LA, Galicich JH. The Use of Steroids for Control of Cerebral Edema. Clin Neurosurg. 1964; 10:212–223

[21] Glantz MJ, Cole BF, Forsyth PA, et al. Practice Parameter: Anticonvulsant Prophylaxis in Patients with Newly Diagnosed Brain Tumors. Report of the Quality Standards Subcommittee of the American Academy of Neurology. Neurology. 2000; 54:1886–1893

[22] Chicoine MR, Silbergeld DL. Pharmacology for Neurosurgeons. Part I. Anticonvulsants, Chemotherapy, Antibiotics. Contemp Neurosurg. 1996; 18:1–6

[23] Prados MD, Berger MS, Wilson CB. Primary Central Nervous System Tumors: Advances in Knowledge and Treatment. CA Cancer J Clin. 1998; 48:331–360

[24] Stewart DJ. A Critique of the Role of the Blood-Brain Barrier in the Chemotherapy of Human Brain Tumors. J Neurooncol. 1994:121–139

[25] Broadwell RD, Salcman M. In: The Blood Brain Barrier. Neurobiology of Brain Tumors. Baltimore: Williams and Wilkins; 1991:229–250

[26] Madajewicz S, Chowhan N, Tfayli A, et al. Therapy for Patients with High Grade Astrocytoma Using Intraarterial Chemotherapy and Radiation Therapy. Cancer. 2000; 88:2350–2356

[27] Barker FG, Prados MD, Chang SM, et al. Radiation Response and Survival Time in Patients with Glioblastoma Multiforme. J Neurosurg. 1996; 84:442–448

[28] Laohaprasit V, Silbergeld DL, Ojemann GA, Eskridge JM, Winn HR. Postoperative CT Contrast Enhancement Following Lobectomy for Epilepsy. J Neurosurg. 1990; 73:392–395

[29] Jeffries BF, Kishore PR, Singh KS, et al. Contrast Enhancement in the Posoperative Brain. Radiology. 1981; 139:409–413

[30] Gerber AM, Savolaine ER. Modification of Tumor Enhancement and Brain Edema in Computerized Tomography by Corticosteroids: Case Report. Neurosurgery. 1980; 6:282–284

[31] Hatam A, Bergström M, Yu ZY, et al. Effect of Dexamethasone Treatment in Volume and Contrast Enhancement of Intracranial Neoplasms. J Comput Assist Tomogr. 1983; 7:295–300

[32] Plesec TP, Prayson RA. Frozen section discrepancy in the evaluation of central nervous system tumors. Arch Pathol Lab Med. 2007; 131:1532–1540

[33] Shah AB, Muzumdar GA, Chitale AR, Bhagwati SN. Squash preparation and frozen section in intraoperative diagnosis of central nervous system tumors. Acta Cytol. 1998; 42:1149–1154

[34] Uematsu Y, Owai Y, Okita R, Tanaka Y, Itakura T. The usefulness and problem of intraoperative rapid diagnosis in surgical neuropathology. Brain Tumor Pathol. 2007; 24:47–52

[35] Burger PC. Smears and Frozen Sections in Surgical Neuropathology: A manual. PB Medical Publishing; 2009

[36] Scherer HB. Structural Developments in Gliomas. American Journal of Cancer. 1938; 34:333–351

[37] McKeever PE, Dabbs DJ. In: Immunohistochemistry of the Nervous System. Diagnostic Immunohistochemistry. New York: Churchill Livingstone; 2002:559–624

[38] Russell DS, Rubenstein LJ. Pathology of Tumours of the Nervous System. 5th ed. Baltimore: Williams and Wilkins; 1989

[39] Burton BK. Alpha-Fetoprotein Screening. Adv Pediatr. 1986; 33:181–196

35 Syndromes Involving Tumors

35.1 Neurocutaneous disorders

35.1.1 General information

Formerly called phakomatoses. Neurocutaneous disorders (NCD) are a group of conditions, each with unique neurologic findings and benign cutaneous lesions (NB: both skin and the CNS derive embryologically from ectoderm), usually with dysplasia of other organ systems (often including the eyes). With the exception of ataxia-telangiectasia (not discussed here) all exhibit autosomal dominant inheritance. There is also a high rate of spontaneous mutations. These syndromes should be kept in mind in a pediatric patient with a tumor, and other stigmata of these syndromes should be sought.

NCDs that are more likely to come to the attention of the neurosurgeon:

1. neurofibromatosis: see below
2. tuberous sclerosis (p.606)
3. von Hippel-Lindau disease (p.703)
4. Sturge Weber syndrome (p.608)
5. racemose angioma (Wyburn-Mason syndrome): midbrain and retinal AVMs

35.1.2 Neurofibromatosis

General information

Neurofibromatosis (NFT) is the most common of the NCDs. There are as many as 6 distinct types, the two most common of which (NF1 & NF2) are compared in ▶ Table 35.1 (variant forms also occur).

Table 35.1 Comparison of neurofibromatosis 1 & 2[1]

current designation →	Neurofibromatosis 1 (NF1) (p.604)	Neurofibromatosis 2 (NF2) (p.605)
alternate term	von Recklinghausen's	bilateral acoustic NFT AKA MISME syndrome
obsolete term	peripheral NFT	central NFT
U.S. prevalence	100,000 people	≈ 3000 people
incidence	1/3000 births	1 in 40,000
inheritance	AD	AD
sporadic occurrence	30–50%	>50%
gene locus	17 (17q11.2)	22 (22q12.2)
gene product	neurofibromin	schwannomin (merlin)
vestibular schwannomas (VS)	almost never bilateral	bilateral VSs are the hallmark
cutaneous schwannomas	no	70%
Lisch nodules	very common	not associated
cataracts	not associated	60–80%
skeletal anomalies	common	not associated
pheochromocytoma	occasional	not associated
MPNST[a]	≈ 2%	not associated
intellectual impairment	associated	not associated
associated medullary spinal cord tumors	astrocytoma	ependymoma

[a]malignant peripheral nerve sheath tumor

35

Schwannoma vs. neurofibroma

While similar in many ways, these tumors differ histologically. Schwannomas (nee: neurilemmomas) arise from schwann cells which produce myelin. Neurofibromas consist of neurites (axons or dendrites of immature or developing neurons), Schwann's cells, and fibroblasts within a collagenous or myxoid matrix. In contrast to schwannomas which displace axons (centrifugal), neurofibromas are unencapsulated and engulf the nerve of origin (centripetal). Neurofibromas may occur as solitary lesions, or, may be multiple as part of NF1 in the setting of which there is potential for malignant transformation. Both tumors have Antoni A (compact) and Antoni B (loose) fibers, but neurofibromas tend to have more Antoni B fibers. A patient ≤ 30 years of age with a vestibular schwannoma is at increased risk of having NF2.

Neurofibromatosis 1 (NF1 AKA von Recklinghausen's disease)

See reference.[2]

General information

More common than NF2, representing > 90% of cases of neurofibromatosis.

Clinical

Diagnostic criteria: see ▶ Table 35.2.[3]

Associated conditions

1. Schwann-cell tumors on any nerve (but bilateral VSs are virtually nonexistent)
2. spinal and/or peripheral-nerve neurofibromas
3. multiple skin neurofibromas
4. aqueductal stenosis (p. 258)
5. macrocephaly: secondary to aqueductal stenosis and hydrocephalus, increased cerebral white matter
6. intracranial tumors: hemispheric astrocytomas are the most common, solitary or multicentric meningiomas (usually in adults). Gliomas associated with NF1 are usually pilocytic astrocytomas. Brain stem astrocytomas include both contrast-enhancing pilocytic lesions and those that are non-enhancing and radiologically diffuse
7. unilateral defect in superior orbit → pulsatile exophthalmos
8. neurologic or cognitive impairment: 30–60% have mild learning disabilities
9. kyphoscoliosis (seen in 2–10%, often progressive which then requires surgical stabilization)
10. visceral manifestations from involvement of autonomic nerves or ganglia within the organ. Up to 10% of patients have abnormal gastrointestinal motility/neuronal intestinal dysplasia related to neuronal hyperplasia within submucosal plexus
11. ≈ 20% develop plexiform neurofibromas: tumors from multiple nerve fascicles that grow along the length of the nerve. Almost pathognomonic for NF1[4]
12. syringomyelia

35

Table 35.2 Diagnostic criteria for NF1[3]

Two or more of the following:
• ≥ 6 café au lait spots[a], each ≥ 5 mm in greatest diameter in prepubertal individuals, or ≥ 15 mm in greatest diameter in postpubertal patients • ≥ 2 neurofibromas of any type, or one plexiform neurofibroma (neurofibromas are usually not evident until age 10–15 yrs). May be painful • freckling (hyperpigmentation) in the axillary or intertriginous (inguinal) areas • optic glioma: see below • ≥ 2 Lisch nodules: pigmented iris hamartomas that appear as translucent yellow/brown elevations that tend to become more numerous with age • distinctive osseous abnormality, such as *sphenoid dysplasia* or thinning of long bone cortex with or without pseudarthrosis (e.g. of tibia or radius) • a first degree relative (parent, sibling or offspring) with NF1 by above criteria
[a]café au lait spots: hyperpigmented oval light brown skin macules (flat). May be present at birth, increase in number and size during 1st decade. Are present in > 99% of NF1 cases. Rare on face

13. malignant tumors that have increased frequency in NFT: neuroblastoma, ganglioglioma, sarcoma, leukemia, Wilm's tumor, breast cancer[5]
14. pheochromocytoma: is occasionally present
15. "unidentified bright objects" (UBOs) on brain or spinal MRI in 53–79% of patients (bright on T2WI, isointense on T1WI) that may be hamartomas, heterotopias, foci of abnormal myelination or low grade tumors.[6] Tend to resolve with age

Genetics

Simple autosomal dominant inheritance with variable expressivity but almost 100% penetrance after age 5 years. The NF1 gene is on chromosome 17q11.2 which codes for neurofibromin[7] (neurofibromin is a negative regulator of the Ras oncogene). Loss of neurofibromin as in NF1 results in elevation of growth-promoting signals. The spontaneous mutation rate is high, with 30–50% of cases representing new somatic mutations.[8]

Counselling: prenatal diagnosis is possible by linkage analysis only if there are 2 or more affected family members.[7] 70% of NF1 gene mutations can be detected using protein truncation analysis.

Management

1. optic gliomas
   a) unlike optic gliomas in the absence of NFT, these are rarely chiasmal (usually involving the nerve), are often multiple, and have a better prognosis
   b) most are non progressive, and should be followed ophthalmologically and with serial imaging (MRI or CT)
   c) surgical intervention probably does not alter visual impairment. Therefore, surgery is reserved for special situations (large disfiguring tumors, pressure on adjacent structures…)
2. other neural tumors in patients with NF1 should be managed in the same manner as in the general population
   a) focal, resectable, symptomatic lesions should be surgically removed
   b) intracranial tumors in NF1 may often be unresectable, and in these cases chemotherapy and/or radiation therapy may be appropriate, with surgery reserved for cases with increasing ICP
   c) when malignant degeneration is suspected (rare, but incidence of sarcomas and leukemias is increased), biopsy with or without internal decompression may be indicated

Neurofibromatosis 2 (NF2 AKA bilateral acoustic NFT)

See reference.[9]

General information

AKA MISME Syndrome (Multiple Inherited Schwannomas, Meningiomas, and Ependymomas).

Clinical

Diagnostic criteria: see ► Table 35.3.[10]

Other clinical features:

1. seizures or other focal deficits
2. skin nodules, dermal neurofibromas, café au lait spots (less common than in NF1)
3. multiple intradural spinal tumors are common (less common in NF1)[11]: including intramedullary (especially ependymomas) and extramedullary (schwannomas, meningiomas…)
4. retinal hamartomas

Table 35.3 Diagnostic criteria for NF2[10]

Definite diagnosis if either:
1. bilateral vestibular schwannomas (VS) on imaging (MRI or CT) or 2. a first degree relative (parent, sibling or offspring) with NF2 and either: a) unilateral VS at age < 30 years or b) any two of the following: meningioma, schwannoma (including spinal root), glioma (includes astrocytoma, ependymoma), posterior subcapsular lens opacity
Probable diagnosis if either: 1. unilateral VS at age < 30 and any of the following: meningioma, schwannoma, glioma, posterior subcapsular lens opacity or 2. multiple meningiomas and either of the following: schwannoma, glioma, or posterior lens opacity

5. antigenic nerve growth factor is increased (does not occur with NF1)
6. despite its name, is not associated with neurofibromas

Two subtypes[10]:
1. the more common, severe form with younger age of onset (2nd to 3rd decade), with rapid progression of hearing loss and multiple associated tumors
2. milder form, presents later in life, with slower deterioration in hearing and fewer associated tumors

Genetics

Autosomal dominant inheritance. NF2 is due to a mutation at chromosome 22q12.2 Which results in the inactivation of schwannomin (AKA merlin, a semi-acronym for moesin-, ezrin, and radixin-like proteins), a tumor suppression peptide. NF2 patients with nonsense and frameshift mutations are more likely to have intramedullary tumors (but not any other type of tumor) compared with other mutation types.

Management considerations

1. bilateral vestibular schwannomas:
   a) chance of preserving hearing is best when tumor is small. Thus, one should attempt to remove smaller tumor. If hearing is serviceable in that ear after surgery, then consider removing the second tumor, otherwise follow the second tumor as long as possible and perform a subtotal removal in an attempt to prevent total deafness
   b) stereotactic radiosurgery therapy may be a treatment option
2. most NF2 patients will become deaf at some time during their life
3. prior to surgery, obtain MRI of cervical spine to R/O intraspinal tumors that may cause cord injuries during other operations
4. NB: pregnancy may accelerate the growth of eighth nerve tumors

35.1.3 Tuberous sclerosis complex

General information

35

Key concepts

- most cases are due to spontaneous mutation. Inherited cases are autosomal dominant. Incidence: 1 in 6K-10K live births
- clinical triad: seizures, mental retardation and sebaceous adenomas; the full clinical triad is seen in < 1/3 of cases
- typical CNS finding: subependymal nodules ("tuber") – a hamartoma
- common associated neoplasm: subependymal giant cell astrocytoma
- 2 tumor suppressor genes: TSC1 (on chromosome 9q34) codes for hamartin, and TSC2 (on chromosome 16p13) encodes tuberlin
- CT shows intracerebral calcifications (usually subependymal)

Tuberous sclerosis complex (TSC), AKA Bourneville's disease, is a neurocutaneous disorder characterized by hamartomas of many organs including the skin, brain, eyes and kidneys. In the brain, the hamartomas may manifest as cortical tubers, glial nodules located subependymally or in deep white matter, or giant cell astrocytomas. Associated findings include pachygyria or microgyria.

Epidemiology/genetics/epigenetics

Incidence: 1 in 6,000–10,000 live births.[12] Point prevalence: 10.6 per 100,000 persons (from Rochester, MN[13]).

Autosomal dominant inheritance, however spontaneous mutation account for the majority of cases.[14] Two distinct tumor suppressor genes have been identified: TSC1 (located on chromosome 9q34) codes for hamartin, and TSC2 (on chromosome 16p13) codes for tuberlin. Only 1 gene needs to be affected to develop TSC. These proteins work together to inhibit activation of rapamycin (mTOR).

Genetic counseling for unaffected parents with one affected child: 1–2% chance of recurrence.

Pathology

Subependymal nodules ("tubers") are benign hamartomas that are almost always calcified, and protrude into the ventricles.

Subependymal giant cell astrocytoma (SEGA): a transformation lesion. Almost always located at the foramen of Monro. Occurs in 5–15% of patients with TSC.[15] Histology shows fibrillary areas alternating with cells containing generous amounts of eosinophilic cytoplasm. Areas of necrosis and abundant mitotic figures may be seen, but are not associated with the typical malignant aggressiveness that these features usually denote.[16]

Clinical

Diagnostic criteria are shown in ▶ Table 35.4.

In the infant, the earliest finding is of "ash leaf" macules (hypomelanotic, leaf shaped) that are best seen with a Wood's lamp. Infantile myoclonus may also occur.

In older children or adults, the myoclonus is often replaced by generalized tonic-clonic or partial complex seizures which occurs in 70–80%. Facial adenomas are not present at birth, but appear in > 90% by age 4 yrs (these are not really adenomas of the sebaceous glands, but are small hamartomas of cutaneous nerve elements that are yellowish-brown and glistening and tend to arise in a butterfly malar distribution usually sparing the upper lip).

Retinal hamartomas occur in ≈ 50% (central calcified hamartoma near the optic disc or a more subtle peripheral flat salmon-colored lesion). A distinctive depigmented iris lesion may also occur.

Evaluation

Plain skull x-rays

May show calcified cerebral nodules.

CT scan

See reference.[18]

Intracerebral *calcifications* are the most common (97% of cases) and characteristic finding. Primarily located subependymally along the lateral walls of the lateral ventricles or near the foramina of Monro.

Low density lesions that do not enhance are seen in 61%. Probably represent heterotopic tissue or defective myelination. Most common in occipital lobe.

Hydrocephalus (HCP) may occur even without obstruction. In the absence of tumor, HCP is usually mild. Moderate HCP usually occurs only in the presence of tumor.

Subependymal nodules are usually calcified, and protrude into the ventricle (**"candle guttering"** described the appearance on pneumoencephalography).

Table 35.4 Diagnostic criteria of tuberous sclerosis complex[17]
• TSC: diagnosis requires 2 major criteria, or 1 major and 2 minor criteria • Probable TSC: 1 major + 1 minor • Possible TSC: 1 major or 2 minor
Major criteria
• cutaneous manifestations: facial angiofibroma, ungual fibroma, > 3 hypomelanotic macules, shagreen patch • brain and eye lesions: cortical tuber, subependymal nodules, subependymal giant cell astrocytoma, multiple retinal nodular hamartomas • tumors in other organs: cardiac, rhabdomyoma, lymphangioleiomyomatosis, renal angiomyolipoma
Minor criteria
• rectal polyps • pits in dental enamel • bone cysts • migration abnormalities of cerebral white matter • gingival fibromas • nonrenal hamartomas • achromic retinal patches • confetti skin lesions • multiple renal cysts

Paraventricular tumors (mostly giant cell astrocytomas) see pathology) are essentially the *only* enhancing lesion in TSC.

MRI

Subependymal tubers are high on T2 and low on T1 and only ≈ 10% enhance.

Low signal in subependymal lesions may represent calcification. SEGA enhance intensely (enhancing subependymal lesion are almost always SEGAs).

Radial bands sign: abnormal signal intensity extending in a radial manner, representing cells of varying degrees of neuronal and astrocytic differentiation as well as difficult to classify cells.[19]

Treatment

Paraventricular tumors should be followed. Tubers grow minimally, but SEGA progress should be removed if they are symptomatic. A transcallosal approach or ventriculoscopic removal are options.

Infantile myoclonus may respond to steroids. Seizures are treated with AEDs.

Surgery for intractable seizures may be considered when a particular lesion is identified as a seizure focus. Better seizure control, not cure, is the goal in TSC.

Patients ≥ 3 years of age with increasing size of SEGA lesions have had sustained reduction of SEGA volume on everolimus.[20]

35.1.4 Sturge–Weber syndrome

General information

Key concepts

- cardinal signs: 1) localized cerebral cortical atrophy and calcifications, 2) ipsilateral port-wine facial nevus (usually in distribution of V1)
- contralateral seizures usually present
- plain skull films classically show "tram-tracking" (double parallel lines)

AKA encephalotrigeminal angiomatosis. A neurocutaneous disorder consisting of:

1. cardinal features:
   a) localized cerebral cortical atrophy and calcifications (especially cortical layers 2 and 3, with a predilection for the occipital lobes):
      - calcifications appear as curvilinear double parallel lines ("tram-tracking") on plain x-rays
      - cortical atrophy usually causes contralateral hemiparesis, hemiatrophy, and homonymous hemianopia (with occipital lobe involvement)

35

   b) ipsilateral port-wine facial nevus (nevus flammeus) usually in distribution of 1st division of trigeminal nerve (rarely bilateral)
2. other findings that may be present:
   a) ipsilateral exophthalmos and/or glaucoma, coloboma of the iris
   b) oculomeningeal capillary hemangioma
   c) convulsive seizures: contralateral to the facial nevus and cortical atrophy. Present in most patients starting in infancy
   d) retinal angiomas

Genetics

Most cases are sporadic. Other cases are suggestive of recessive inheritance, with chromosome 3 being implicated.

Treatment

Treatment is supportive. Anticonvulsants are used for seizures. Lobectomy or hemispherectomy may be needed for refractory seizures. XRT: complications are common and benefits are lacking. Laser surgery for the cutaneous nevus is disappointing; better results obtain from masking the nevus with a skin colored tattoo.

35.1.5 Neurocutaneous melanosis (NCM)

Background

1. a rare, congenital, nonheritable phakomatosis in which large or numerous congenital melanocytic nevi are associated with benign and/or malignant melanocytic tumors of the leptomeninges[21]
2. pathogenesis: neuroectodermal defect during morphogenesis involving melanoblasts of skin and pia mater originating from neural crest cells[21]

Clinical features

1. two-thirds of patients with NCM have giant congenital melanocytic nevi[21]: pigmented nevi that are large, hairy, or both. (The chances that nevi represents NCM is higher when the nevi are located on head, posterior neck or paravertebral)
2. one-third have numerous lesions without a single giant lesion[21]
3. virtually all have large cutaneous melanocytic (pigmented) nevi located on the posterior torso[22]
4. neurologic manifestations: usually before age 2 years. Signs of intracranial hypertension (lethargy, vomiting…), focal seizures, motor deficits or aphasia[21]
5. hydrocephalus: in almost 66%. Usually due to obstruction of CSF flow or reduced absorption as a result of thickened leptomeninges[21]

Clinical diagnostic criteria

See reference.[23]

1. large or multiple congenital melanocytic nevi with meningeal melanosis or melanoma
2. absence of cutaneous melanoma, except in patients with benign meningeal lesions (i.e. must rule out meningeal metastases from cutaneous melanoma)
3. no evidence of meningeal melanoma, except in patients with benign cutaneous lesions

Associated conditions

NCM is sometimes associated with

1. neurocutaneous syndromes[21]
   a) Sturge-Weber syndrome (p. 608)
   b) von Recklinghausen's neurofibromatosis (NF1) (p. 604)
2. posterior fossa cystic malformations: e.g. Dandy Walker malformation (p. 256); occurs in up to 10%. These cases have worse prognosis due to malignant transformation[21]
3. intraspinal lipoma and syringomyelia[21]

Diagnostic testing

1. MRI: T1 and T2 signal shortening produced by melanin. IV gadolinium may demonstrate enhancement of tumor-infiltrated meninges[21]
2. histological exam of CNS lesions shows leptomeningeal melanosis (benign) which develops from the melanocytes of the pia matter. Melanoma (malignant) occurs in 40–62% of cases but distinction has little prognostic significance because of the poor outcome of the symptomatic NCM patient even in the absence of melanoma[21]

Management

The benefit of resecting skin lesions is questionable in the presence of leptomeningeal lesions.[24] NCM appears refractory to radiation therapy and chemotherapy[24]

Neurosurgical involvement is usually limited to[23]:

1. shunting for hydrocephalus
2. palliative operative decompression if early in the course
3. biopsy for tissue diagnosis in questionable cases

Prognosis

1. when neurological signs are present, prognosis is poor regardless of whether or not malignancy is present
2. > 50% of patients die within 3 years after the first neurologic manifestation[21]

35

Table 35.5 Familial syndromes associated with CNS tumors

Syndrome	CNS tumor
von Hippel-Lindau (p. 703)	hemangioblastoma
tuberous sclerosis (p. 606)	subependymal giant cell astrocytoma
neurofibromatosis type I (p. 604)	optic glioma, astrocytoma, neurofibroma
neurofibromatosis type II (p. 605)	vestibular schwannoma, meningioma, ependymoma, astrocytoma
Turcot syndrome (BTP syndrome) (p. 610) [25]	GBM, AA, & medulloblastoma, pineoblastoma
Li-Fraumeni (p. 610)	astrocytoma, PNET
Cowden (p. 647)	meningiomas
Lhermitte-Duclos (p. 647)	

35.2 Familial tumor syndromes

35.2.1 General information

Several familial syndromes are associated with CNS tumors as shown in ▶ Table 35.5.

35.2.2 Turcot syndrome

A rare inherited disorder characterized by multiple colorectal neoplasms (carcinomas or benign adenomatous polyps) together with neuroepithelial tumors of the CNS (GBM, AA, MB, pineoblastoma, ganglioglioma & ependymoma).[12] Type 1: GBM without familial polyposis (but often with nonpolyposis colorectal cancer). Mean survival of Turcot patients with GBM is 27 months (longer than sporadic cases). Type 2: MB & familial adenomatous polyposis.

35.2.3 Li-Fraumeni syndrome

Rare (< 400 families identified) inherited autosomal dominant mutation of the TP53 tumor *suppressor* gene. Patients have increased incidence of multiple types of tumors, including: sarcoma & osteosarcoma, breast cancer, astrocytoma and PNET, adrenocortical carcinoma, leukemia.

35

References

[1] Burger PC, Scheithauer BW. AFIP Atlas of Tumor Pathology. Fourth series. Fascicle 7: Tumors of the Central Nervous System. Washington, D.C.: Armed Forces Institute of Pathology; 2007

[2] Riccardi VM. von Recklinghausen Neurofibromatosis. N Engl J Med. 1981; 305:1617–1627

[3] National Institutes of Health Consensus Development Conference. Neurofibromatosis: Conference Statement. Arch Neurol. 1988; 45:575–578

[4] Packer RJ, Gutmann DH, Rubenstein A, Viskochil D, Zimmerman RA, Vezina G, Small J, Korf B. Plexiform neurofibromas in NF1: toward biologic-based therapy. Neurology. 2002; 58:1461–1470

[5] Sharif S, Moran A, Huson SM, Iddenden R, Shenton A, Howard E, Evans DG. Women with neurofibromatosis 1 are at a moderately increased risk of developing breast cancer and should be considered for early screening. J Med Genet. 2007; 44:481–484

[6] Sevick RJ, Barkovich AJ, Edwards MS, Koch T, Berg B, Lempert T. Evolution of white matter lesions in neurofibromatosis type 1: MR findings. AJR Am J Roentgenol. 1992; 159:171–175

[7] Karnes PS. Neurofibromatosis: A Common Neurocutaneous Disorder. Mayo Clin Proc. 1998; 73:1071–1076

[8] Walker L, Thompson D, Easton D, Ponder B, Ponder M, Frayling I, Baralle D. A prospective study of neurofibromatosis type 1 cancer incidence in the UK. Br J Cancer. 2006; 95:233–238

[9] Martuza RL, Eldridge R. Neurofibromatosis 2: (Bilateral Acoustic Neurofibromatosis). N Engl J Med. 1988; 318:684–688

[10] Parry DM, Eldridge R, Kaiser-Kupfer MI, Bouzas EA, Pikus A, Patronas N. Neurofibromatosis 2 (NF2): clinical characteristics of 63 affected individuals and clinical evidence for heterogeneity. Am J Med Genet. 1994; 52:450–461

[11] Egelhoff JC, Bates DJ, Ross JS, Rothner AD, Cohen BH. Spinal MR Findings in Neurofibromatosis Types 1 and 2. AJNR. 1992; 13:1071–1077

[12] Hottinger AF, Khakoo Y. Neurooncology of familial cancer syndromes. J Child Neurol. 2009; 24:1526–1535

[13] Wiederholt WC, Gomez MR, Kurland LT. Incidence and Prevalence of Tuberous Sclerosis in Rochester, Minnesota, 1950 through 1982. Neurology. 1985; 35:600–603

[14] Logue LG, Acker RE, Sienko AE. Best cases from the AFIP: angiomyolipomas in tuberous sclerosis. Radiographics. 2003; 23:241–246

[15] Thiele EA. Managing epilepsy in tuberous sclerosis complex. J Child Neurol. 2004; 19:680–686

[16] Chow CW, Klug GL, Lewis EA. Subependymal Giant-Cell Astrocytoma in Children: An Unusual

Discrepancy Between Histological and Clinical Features. J Neurosurg. 1988; 68:880–883
[17] Roach ES, Gomez MR, Northrup H. Tuberous sclerosis complex consensus conference: revised clinical diagnostic criteria. J Child Neurol. 1998; 13:624–628
[18] McLaurin RL, Towbin RB. Tuberous Sclerosis: Diagnostic and Surgical Considerations. Pediat Neurosci. 1985; 12:43–48
[19] Bernauer TA. The radial bands sign. Radiology. 1999; 212:761–762
[20] Franz DN, Agricola K, Mays M, Tudor C, Care MM, Holland-Bouley K, Berkowitz N, Miao S, Peyrard S, Krueger DA. Everolimus for subependymal giant cell astrocytoma: 5-year final analysis. Ann Neurol. 2015. DOI: 10.1002/ana.24523
[21] Di Rocco F, Sabatino G, Koutzoglou M, Battaglia D, Caldarelli M, Tamburrini G. Neurocutaneous melanosis. Childs Nerv Syst. 2004; 20:23–28
[22] DeDavid M, Orlow SJ, Provost N, Marghoob AA, Rao BK, Wasti Q, Huang CL, Kopf AW, Bart RS. Neurocutaneous melanosis: clinical features of large congenital melanocytic nevi in patients with manifest central nervous system melanosis. J Am Acad Dermatol. 1996; 35:529–538
[23] McClelland S, III, Charnas LR, SantaCruz KS, Garner HP, Lam CH. Progressive brainstem compression in an infant with neurocutaneous melanosis and Dandy-Walker complex following ventriculoperitoneal shunt placement for hydrocephalus. Case report. J Neurosurg. 2007; 107:500–503
[24] Mena-Cedillos CA, Valencia-Herrera AM, Arroyo-Pineda AI, Salgado-Jimenez MA, Espinoza-Montero R, Martinez-Avalos AB, Perales-Arroyo A. Neurocutaneous melanosis in association with the Dandy-Walker complex, complicated by melanoma: report of a case and literature review. Pediatr Dermatol. 2002; 19:237–242
[25] Paraf F, Jothy S, Van Meir EG. Brain Tumor-Polyposis Syndrome: Two Genetic Diseases. J Clin Oncol. 1997; 15:2744–2758

36 Astrocytomas

36.1 Incidence, risk factors

Astrocytic tumors are the most common primary intra-axial brain tumor. The average annual age adjusted incidence from 2006 – 2010 was 5.17 per 100,000,[1] approximately 16,000 new cases/year in the U. S.

The best-established causes for brain tumors are syndromic (familial diseases…) and post-radiation therapy.

The controversy of cell phones as a risk factor: The substantial increase in the number of mobile phone subscriptions since the early 1990's has not been observed to be associated with increased incidence of brain tumor in the US.[2,3,4] Nonetheless, primarily due to lack of data for extremely long exposure (> 15 years), in May 2011, the WHO issued a warning of possible cancer risk in relation to the use of devices that emit nonionizing electromagnetic radiation, such as cellular phones.[5]

36.2 Classification and grading of astrocytic tumors

36.2.1 Classification by general morphology or behavior

In general
- Circumscribed vs. Diffuse
- Non-infiltrative vs. Infiltrative[6]
- Special vs. Ordinary

Detailed classification:
1. Infiltrating astrocytoma
   a) Diffuse astrocytoma (AKA low grade astrocytoma): WHO II. Genetic hallmark: frequent TP53 mutation. Histological variants:
      - fibrillary: the most common subtype
      - gemistocytic
      - protoplasmic: rare
   b) Mixed oligoastrocytoma WHO II
   c) Anaplastic astrocytoma WHO III
   d) Anaplastic oligoastrocytoma WHO III
   e) Glioblastoma multiforme WHO IV
2. Non-infiltrative astrocytoma
   a) Juvenile Pilocytic astrocytoma WHO I
   b) Subependymal giant cell astrocytoma (Tuberous Sclerosis) WHO I
   c) Desmoplastic infantile astrocytoma WHO I
   d) Pilomyxoid astrocytoma WHO II
3. Unique astrocytoma (unique variant that the prognosis does not conform to the grading):
   a) Pleomorphic xanthoastrocytoma WHO II
   b) Gemistocytic astrocytoma WHO II

In diffuse/infiltrative tumors, since complete surgical excision is rarely attainable, there is higher recurrence rate and poorer prognosis in general.

Special vs Ordinary:
- dividing tumors according to favorable or poor behavior is not considered to be a contemporary classification system
- Special – favorable outcome, younger age group, includes pilocytic astrocytoma, microcytic cerebellar and subependymal giant cell astrocytoma
- Ordinary – poorer outcome, includes in WHO Grade II-IV or St.Anne/Mayo Grade I-IV group

36.2.2 Grading and neuropathology

General information

The grading of astrocytomas has been historically fraught with disagreement, and a number of grading systems have been proposed over the years. The first system of Bailey and Cushing was a 3-tiered system, the Kernohan system was 4-tiered, and since then a number of 3-tiered systems like the

Ringertz system,[7] have been proposed. As a result, there is a lack of uniformity in, for example, what constitutes a glioblastoma from series to series over time. The current trend has been to use one of two different systems, the WHO definition or the St. Anne/Mayo system, both of which appear below.

Grading of astrocytomas remains controversial. Some special concerns:

1. sampling error: may have different degrees of malignancy in different areas
2. dedifferentiation (p. 615): tumors tend to progress in malignancy over months or years
3. histological criteria that affect prognosis include: cellularity, presence of giant cells, anaplasia, mitosis, vascular proliferation with or without endothelial proliferation, necrosis, and pseudopalisading[8]
4. in addition to histology, issues that affect clinical behavior (many of which are not factored into most grading systems) include:
   a) patient age
   b) extent of tumor
   c) topography: tumor location, especially in relation to critical structures

Obsolete grading systems

► **Ringertz's system.** The obsolete Ringertz's system developed three grades for astrocytoma malignancy.[7] Necrosis was used to divide the intermediate grade from the glioblastoma multi-forme. The Ringertz three-tiered grading system was more clinically correlated with the prognosis for astrocytomas.

► **Kernohan system.** The obsolete Kernohan system,[9] originally devised at the Mayo Clinic, divided these tumors into 4 grades (grade IV AKA glioblastoma multiforme) based on the degree of presence of a number of features such as anaplasia, nuclear pleomorphism, number of mitoses. The Kernohan system determined tumor grade according to the proportion of normal tissue remaining in the invading tumor and the type of invading edge of the tumor into normal tissue. Prognostically, this system distinguished only 2 clinically different groups (grades I/II, and grades III/IV) and is not used today. It is presented for completeness when reviewing older literature.

Current grading systems

The 2 main systems in use today are shown below, and differ primarily in the definition of Grade I.

► **WHO system.** The World Health Organization (WHO) system is shown in ► Table 36.1.[10] In the WHO system, grade I is reserved for special types of astrocytomas that are more circumscribed, including pilocytic astrocytomas, while the more typical astrocytic neoplasms are graded II through IV. The approximate equivalence to the Ringertz system, Kernohan grade, and St Anne-Mayo grading is also shown in ► Table 36.2.

Table 36.1 WHO classification of ("ordinary") astrocytic tumors

Designation	Criteria
II: diffuse astrocytoma	cytological atypia alone
III: anaplastic astrocytoma	anaplasia and mitotic activity
IV: glioblastoma (GBM)	also show microvascular proliferation and/or necrosis

Table 36.2 Approximate equivalence of Ringertz system, Kernohan grade (I-IV), and St Anne-Mayo grading to WHO system

Modified Ringertz	Kernohan	St. Anne-Mayo	WHO 2007[10]
			Grade I (e.g. pilocytic astrocytoma)
Astrocytoma (low grade)	I & II	Astrocytoma 1 & 2	Diffuse astrocytoma II
Anaplastic astrocytoma	III	Astrocytoma 3	Anaplastic astrocytoma III
Glioblastoma multiforme	IV	Astrocytoma 4	Glioblastoma multiforme IV

WHO 2007 Grading of astrocytomas for specific types of astrocytomas:

1. Grade I
   - Subependymal giant cell astrocytoma (SEGA)
   - Pilocytic astrocytoma
2. Grade II
   - Pilomyxoid astrocytoma
   - Diffuse astrocytoma
   - Pleomorphic xanthastrocytoma
3. Grade III – anaplastic astrocytoma
4. Grade IV
   - Glioblastoma
   - Giant cell glioblastoma
   - Gliosarcoma

► **St. Anne/Mayo grading system.** Grading systems such as those described above are very dependent upon subjective impression of histological findings. The classification system known as the St. Anne/Mayo (SA/M) system[11] addresses histological considerations, and is reproducible and prognostically significant.[12] It is restricted to "ordinary" astrocytomas, as grade has not been shown to correlate with clinical behavior in pilocytic or microcystic cerebellar astrocytomas. It is similar to the WHO system except that SA/M grade I astrocytomas are a very rare diffuse astrocytoma without atypia.[10]

The SA/M system assesses the presence or absence of 4 criteria (see ► Table 36.3) and then assigns a grade based on the number of criteria present (► Table 36.4). When the presence of any criteria is uncertain, it is considered to be absent.

The criteria tended to occur in a predictable sequence: nuclear atypia occurred in all grade 2 tumors, mitotic activity was seen in 92% of grade 3 tumors (and in none of the grade 2 tumors), necrosis and endothelial proliferation were restricted almost only to grade 4 tumors (they were seen in only 8% of grade 3 tumors).

The frequencies of occurrence among 287 "ordinary" astrocytomas were: grade 1 = 0.7% (a very rare tumor), grade 2 = 16%, grade 3 = 17.8%, and grade 4 = 65.5%.

Median survival was as follows[11]: (there were only two grade 1 patients, one survived 11 years and the other was still alive after 15 years), grade 2 = 4 years, grade 3 = 1.6 years, and grade 4 = 0.7 years (8.5 months).

► **Relative frequency of astrocytoma grades.** Glioblastoma comprise approximately 54% of all gliomas and about 6% of anaplastic astrocytoma. Less common ones like anaplastic oligodendroglioma and anaplastic oligoastrocytoma, together with the scarcer tumors such as anaplastic ependymoma and anaplastic ganglioglioma make up 7.2% of all gliomas.[1]

Table 36.3 St. Anne/Mayo criteria

- nuclear atypia: hyperchromatasia and/or obvious variation in size and shape
- mitoses: regardless of normal or abnormal configuration
- endothelial proliferation: vascular lumina are surrounded by "piled-up" endothelial cells (instead of the normal single layer). Does *not* include hypervascularity (which may occur in non-tumoral gliosis)
- necrosis: only when obviously present. Does *not* include pseudopalisading when seen alone

Table 36.4 St. Anne/Mayo grade

Grade	No. of criteria
1	0
2	1
3	2
4	3 or 4

Future directions of astrocytoma grading

Guideline for future WHO classification[13]: In order to align with new developments in glioma molecular genetics, a consensus was reached amongst world leaders in neuropathology. Guidelines for the next WHO classification were issued:

- diagnostic entities should be defined as narrowly as possible to optimize interobserver reproducibility, clinicopathological predictions and therapeutic planning
- diagnoses should be "layered" with histologic classification, WHO grade and molecular information listed below an "integrated diagnosis"
- determinations should be made for each tumor entity as to whether molecular information is required, suggested or not needed for its definition
- some pediatric entities should be separated from their adult counterparts
- input for guiding decisions regarding tumor classification should be solicited from experts in complementary disciplines of neuro-oncology
- entity-specific molecular testing and reporting formats should be followed in diagnostic reports. It is hoped that these guidelines will facilitate the forthcoming update of the fourth edition of the WHO classification of central nervous system tumors

Low-grade astrocytoma (WHO II) comments

AKA low-grade diffuse astrocytoma. Three histopathological types:

1. fibrillary astrocytoma: the most common histological subtype of Grade II
2. gemistocytic astrocytoma: particularly prone to progress to Grade II & IV
3. protoplasmic astrocytoma

These tumors tend to occur in children and young adults. Most present with seizures. There is a predilection for temporal, posterior frontal and anterior parietal lobes.[14] They demonstrate low degrees of cellularity and preservation of normal brain elements within the tumor. Calcifications are rare. Anaplasia and mitoses are absent (a single mitosis is allowed). Blood vessels may be slightly increased in number. The ultimate behavior of these tumors is usually not benign. The most important favorable prognosticator is young age. Poor prognosis is associated with findings of increased ICP, altered consciousness, personality change, significant neurologic deficits,[15] short duration of symptoms before diagnosis (suggesting rapid progression), and enhancement on imaging studies.

Dedifferentiation

The major cause of morbidity with low-grade astrocytomas is dedifferentiation to a more malignant grade. Low grade fibrillary astrocytomas tend to undergo malignant transformation more quickly (with six-fold increased rapidity) when diagnosed after age 45 years than when diagnosed earlier[16] (see ▶ Table 36.5). Gemistocytic astrocytomas tend to dedifferentiate more rapidly than fibrillary astrocytomas. > 60% of fibrillary astrocytomas have a mutation of the TP53 gene located on chromosome 17p; these tumors are more likely to dedifferentiate. Once dedifferentiation occurs, median survival is 2–3 years beyond that event. Genetic markers that correlate with a higher degree of malignant degeneration include[17,18]:

1. loss of heterozygosity on chromosomes 10 & 17
2. alteration in tumor suppressor genes at 9p, 13q, 19q & 22q
3. changes in epidermal growth factor receptor (EGRF) and platelet-derived growth factor (PDGF)
4. transformation of the p53 suppressor gene
5. isocitrate dehydrogenase (IDH) mutations (p. 616) – genetic aberrations that lead to epigenetic machinery dysfunction

Table 36.5 Dedifferentiation rate for low grade astrocytomas

	Patients diagnosed @ age < 45 yrs	Patients diagnosed @ age ≥ 45 yrs
mean time to dedifferentiation	44.2 ± 17 mos	7.5 ± 5.7 mos
time to death	58 mos	14 mos

Malignant astrocytomas (WHO III and IV) comments

This category encompasses anaplastic astrocytoma (AA) and glioblastoma (GBM). Although both are "malignant", AA and GBM have distinct differences. Among 1265 patients with malignant astrocytomas, the mean age was 46 yrs for AA, and 56 yrs for GBM. Mean duration of symptoms pre-op: 5.4 mos for GBM, and 15.7 mos for AA. Malignant astrocytomas may develop from low grade astrocytomas via dedifferentiation (see above), however they may also arise de novo.

Infratentorial glioblastoma (GBM) is rare, and often represents subarachnoid dissemination of a supratentorial GBM (used as an argument for irradiation in all patients with p-fossa GBM).[19]

Glioblastoma (multiforme) (WHO IV) comments

The most common primary brain tumor, it is also the most malignant astrocytoma. Current nomenclature omits "multiforme".[20]

Histological findings associated with GBM (not all may be present, and this list does not follow any of the standard grading systems above):

- gemistocytic astrocytes
- neovascularization with endothelial proliferation
- areas of necrosis
- pseudopalisading around areas of necrosis

36.3 Molecular genetics and epigenetics

36.3.1 Molecular pathways in the development of glioblastomas

Genome-wide profiling studies have shown remarkable genomic diversities among glioblastomas.[21,22] Molecular studies have helped identify at least 3 different pathways in the development of glioblastomas.[23]

- 1st pathway: **dysregulation of growth factor signaling through amplification and mutational activation of receptor tyrosine kinase (RTK) genes.** RTKs are a diverse group of transmembrane proteins that act as receptors for growth factors like epithelial growth factor (EGF), vascular endothelial growth factor (VEGF), platelet-derived growth factor (PDGF). They can also act as receptors for cytokines, hormones and other signaling pathways.
- 2nd pathway: the **activation of the phosphatidylinositol-3-OH kinase (PI3K)/AKT/mTOR**, which is an intracellular signaling pathway. It is essential in regulating cell survival.
- 3rd pathway: the **inactivation of the p53 and retinoblastoma (Rb) tumor suppressor** pathways.

36.3.2 Transcriptional silencing

O^6-Methylguanine-DNA methyltransferase (MGMT) Methylation: MGMT is an independent prognosticator for response of malignant gliomas to chemotherapy with alkylating chemotherapeutic agents (e.g. nitrosourea or temozolomide)[24] which damage tumor DNA by attaching an alkyl group to the guanine base. The MGMT gene is located on chromosome 10q26 and codes for a DNA repair enzyme that specifically removes the mutagenic alkyl O^6 methylguanine and restores guanine residues to their native state.[25,26] The loss of MGMT expression is likely to be caused by transcriptional silencing through hypermethylation of the CpG islands on the genome[27,28] and this hypermethylation phenomenon is frequently (45% to 75%) present in glioblastomas.

In short: Loss of MGMT expression makes alkylating agent (e.g.Temodar) more effective.

36

36.3.3 IDH 1/2 mutation

IDH1 Arg132 mutations and IDH2 Arg140 and Arg172 mutations accounting for > 90% of aberrations.[29,30] IDH1 and IDH2 mutations reduce the enzymatic capacity of these proteins to bind isocitrate, their substrate, and convert it into α-ketoglutarate (α-KG), generating carbon dioxide and replenishing NADH and NADPH as side products.[31] This is one of the irreversible steps in the tricarboxylic acid cycle important for cellular respiration. Mutant IDH1 (cytoplasmic) and IDH2 (mitochondrial) enzymes also show a modified enzymatic capacity to convert α-KG into 2-hydroxyglutarate (2-HG), a small onco-metabolite. Equally important, IDH1 and IDH2 mutations stratify individuals into molecular subtypes with distinct clinical outcomes – the mutations are associated with lower-grade astrocytomas, oligodendrogliomas (grade II/III) and secondary gliomas with better overall survival, progression-free survival and chemosensitivity than glioblastomas that are wild type for both genes.[29,30,31]

36.3.4 Primary vs. secondary glioblastoma

Primary vs. secondary glioblastoma[32]: First described in 1940 by German pathologist Scherer.

- primary glioblastoma: the majority of GBMs. Arise without evidence (clinical or histological) of a less malignant precursor. More common in older patients (mean age = 55 years) after a short (< 3 month) clinical history. Characterized by EGFR amplification (≈ 40% of cases) and/or overexpression (60%), PTEN mutations (30%), p16^{INK4a} deletion (30–40%), MDM2 amplification (< 10%), and/or overexpression (50%), and in 50–80% of cases, loss of heterozygosity (LOH) on the entire chromosome 10.
- secondary glioblastoma: develop by malignant degeneration of WHO grade II or III astrocytoma. Patients are younger (mean age = 40 years) and have a slower clinical course. Secondary glioblastomas are less frequent than primary glioblastomas. 60% have TP53 mutations (present in > 90% of the less malignant precursors). Malignant degeneration is characterized by allelic loss of chromosomes 19q and 10q. MGMT promoter methylation appears to occur with a higher frequency in secondary than in primary glioblastoma.[33,34] Genetic sequencing of 200 glioblastomas uncovered IDH1 and IDH2 as recurrently mutated in 5% of primary gliomas and a majority of about 60–90% of secondary gliomas.[29,30]

36.3.5 Subclassification of GBM

With the widespread use of molecular technology over the past two decades, considerable achievements have been made to identify the heterogeneity of glioblastoma, even though it is still under a single disease entity. Based on molecular genetic data from The Cancer Genome Atlas (TCGA) Research Network,[35] Verhaak et al used gene expression analysis to further sub-classify GBM into 4 subtypes: I. Classical, II. Mesenchymal, III. Proneural, and IV. Neural.[36]

36.4 Miscellaneous pathological features

► **Glial fibrillary acidic protein (GFAP).** Most astrocytomas stain positive for GFAP (astrocytomas that may not stain GFAP positive: some poorly differentiated gliomas, purely gemistocytic astrocytomas since fibrillary astrocytes are required to stain positive).

► **Cysts.** Gliomas may have cystic central necrosis, but may also have an associated cyst even without necrosis. When fluid from these cysts is aspirated it can be differentiated from CSF by the fact that it is usually xanthochromic and often clots once removed from the body (unlike e.g. fluid from a chronic subdural). Although they may occur with malignant gliomas, cysts are more commonly associated with pilocytic astrocytomas (p. 630).

► **MIB-1 index.** It has been suggested that a MIB-1 index ≥ 7–9% is indicative of an anaplastic tumor, while MIB-1 < 5% favors a low-grade tumor. However, variability between observers and institutions precludes using the MIB-1 index as a sole discriminant between grade II & III astrocytomas.[37]

36.5 Neuroradiological grading and findings

Astrocytomas typically arise in white matter (e.g. centrum semiovale) and traverse through white matter tracts (see below). See also MR-spectroscopy findings (p. 233).

► **CT scan & MRI grading.** Grading gliomas by CT or MRI is imprecise,[38] but may be used as a preliminary assessment (see ► Table 36.6). Neuroradiologic grading is *not* applicable to pediatric patients or special astrocytomas (e.g. pilocytic astrocytomas).

Table 36.6 Grading gliomas by CT or MRI

WHO grade	Typical radiographic findings	
II	CT: low density MRI: abnormal signal on T2WI	no enhancement with little or no mass effect
III	complex enhancement[a]	
IV	necrosis (ring enhancement)	

[a]however, some may not enhance

► **Low-grade gliomas.** Usually hypodense on CT. Most are hypointense on T1WI MRI, and show high intensity changes on T2WI that extend beyond the tumor volume. Most do not enhance on CT or MRI (although up to 40% do,[39] and these may have a worse prognosis). The UCSF preoperative grading system for low-grade infiltrating gliomas[40] assigns 1 point for the presence of each of 4 parameters shown in ► Table 36.7. The points are summed and the prognosis is shown in ► Table 36.8 (this scale needs to be validated at other institutions). Another study found poor prognosis associated with: age ≥ 40 years, tumor ≥ 6 cm dia, tumor crossing midline and the presence of neurologic deficit.[41]

► **Malignant gliomas.** Anaplastic astrocytomas (AA) may not enhance[42] (31% of highly anaplastic and 59% of moderately anaplastic astrocytomas do not enhance on CT[43]; MRI not studied). Calcifications and cysts occur in 10–20% of AA.[42] Most glioblastomas enhance, but some rare ones do not.[38,43]

► **Ring-enhancement with glioblastoma (GBM).** The nonenhancing center may represent necrosis or associated cyst (see above). The enhancing ring is cellular tumor, however, tumor cells also extend ≥ 15 mm beyond the ring.[44]

► **Positron emission tomography (PET) scan.** Low grade fibrillary astrocytomas appear as hypometabolic "cold" spots with fluorodeoxyglucose PET scans. Hypermetabolic "hot" spots suggest high-grade astrocytomas and help distinguish high grade glioma that do not enhance on MRI from lower grade (II) astrocytomas.

► **Angiographic appearance.** AAs usually appear as an avascular mass. Tumor blush and AV-shunting with early draining veins are more characteristic of GBM.

36.6 Spread

Gliomas may spread by the following mechanisms[45] (note: < 10% of recurrent gliomas recur away from the original site[46]):

1. tracking through white matter
   a) corpus callosum (CC)
      - through genu or body of CC → bilateral frontal lobe involvement ("butterfly glioma")
      - through splenium of CC → bilateral parietal or occipital lobes
   b) cerebral peduncles → midbrain involvement
   c) internal capsule → encroachment of basal ganglion tumors into centrum semiovale
   d) uncinate fasciculus → simultaneous frontal and temporal lobe tumors
   e) interthalamic adhesion → bilateral thalamic gliomas

Table 36.7 Preoperative grading of *low-grade* gliomas[40]

Item	Yes/No
age > 50 years	Yes = 1, No = 0
KPS[a] ≤ 80	Yes = 1, No = 0
located in eloquent brain[b]	Yes = 1, No = 0
maximal diameter > 4 cm	Yes = 1, No = 0

[a]KPS = Karnofsky performance score (p. 1358)
[b]for this study, eloquent brain is defined as any of: primary sensory or motor cortex, Wernicke's or Broca's area, basal ganglia/internal capsule, thalamus or primary visual cortex

Table 36.8 Sum of points from ► Table 36.7

Sum	5-year survival	5-year progression-free survival
0–1	97%	76%
2	81%	49%
3–4	56%	18%

2. CSF pathways (subarachnoid seeding): 10–25% frequency of meningeal and ventricular seeding by high grade gliomas[47]
3. rarely, gliomas may spread systemically

36.7 Multiple gliomas

Discussion of multiple gliomatous masses has to acknowledge the concept that astrocytoma is a multifocal disease, not a focal one. Some terms are probably artificial, e.g. since gliomatosis cerebri probably represents a diffuse infiltrating glial tumor with areas that may dedifferentiate into higher grade and then is called multicentric glioma.

Settings in which multiple gliomatous masses are encountered:
1. conventional glioma that has spread by one of the mechanisms previously described (see above)
2. gliomatosis cerebri: a diffuse, infiltrating astrocytoma that invades almost all of the cerebral hemispheres and brainstem. Usually low-grade,[39] areas of anaplasia and glioblastoma may also occur[48] and may present as focal mass.[49] Occurs most frequently in 1st 2 decades
3. multiple primary gliomas: some of the following terms are inconsistently used interchangeably: "multicentric", "multifocal", and "multiple." Reported range of occurrence is 2–20% of gliomas[50,51] (lower end of range ≈ 2–4% is probably more accurate, the higher end of the range is probably accounted for by infiltrative extension[52(p 3117)])
   a) commonly associated with neurofibromatosis and tuberous sclerosis
   b) rarely associated with multiple sclerosis and progressive multifocal leukoencephalopathy
4. meningeal gliomatosis: dissemination of glioma throughout the CSF, similar to carcinomatous meningitis (p. 811). Occurs in up to 20% of autopsies on patients with high-grade gliomas. May present with cranial neuropathies, radiculopathies, myelopathy, dementia, and/or communicating hydrocephalus

In a series of 25 patients with multicentric glioma,[53] glioblastoma was the most common pathology (48%), followed by anaplastic astrocytoma (20%), and glioblastoma with simultaneous AA (20%).

▶ **Treatment considerations for multiple gliomas.** There is little data available. In a nonrandomized study of 25 patients with multifocal glioma,[53] the 16 patients who underwent debulking did better than the 9 who did not. However, there was significant selection bias in choosing patients suitable for craniotomy.

Biopsy is generally required/recommended to confirm the diagnosis.

Σ

Once the diagnosis of multiple gliomatous masses has been ascertained, local therapies (e.g. surgery, interstitial radiation...) are impractical. Whole brain radiation and possibly chemotherapy are indicated. An exception would be to consider debulking tumor to prevent herniation in a patient deteriorating from mass effect.

36

36.8 Treatment

36.8.1 Low-grade astrocytomas (WHO grade II)

Treatment options

1. no treatment: follow serial neurologic exams and imaging studies, with intervention reserved for cases showing progression
2. radiation
3. chemotherapy
4. surgery
5. combinations of radiation and chemotherapy, with or without surgery

Analysis

No well-designed study has shown that *any* approach for supratentorial WHO grade II infiltrating astrocytomas in adults is clearly superior to any other. Some treatments may simply expose the patient to the risk of treatment side effects. The argument holds that these tumors are slow growing, and that until progression on imaging or malignant degeneration is documented, that it may be no worse to not treat the patient.[54] Although this view has been challenged,[55] a definitive study has yet to be performed. The following are associated with more aggressive tumors and should prompt consideration for some form of treatment:

1. extremely young patients, or patients > 50 yrs age; increasing age at diagnosis is associated with more rapid dedifferentiation (p. 615)
2. large tumors that enhance (tumor size is one of the most important prognosticators[56])
3. symptomatic patients, especially those with short clinical history
4. evidence of progression on imaging studies
5. Astrocytic/Astrocytic-dominant mixed glioma histology
6. Biopsy only without resection

Surgery for low grade gliomas

4 objectives in performing surgery for low grade gliomas[57]:

1. To obtain histological confirmation/molecular genetic analysis
2. To improve neurological condition
3. To reduce risk of tumor growth
4. To prevent malignant transformation

Surgery is the principal treatment for low-grade glioma in most circumstances. Although there is no randomized control trial (RCT) comparing tumor resection to biopsy alone in low-grade glioma, current opinion advocates early resection. A recent Norway study showed a significant lower overall survival in a center favoring watchful waiting approach. More aggressive excision is associated with better outcome[58,59,60] and later malignant transformation to anaplastic types.[59] Even in recurrent low-grade glioma, surgical resection is associated with a survival benefit.

Intraoperative Mapping and Awake Craniotomy

Complete resection is often not possible due to the infiltrative nature of low-grade gliomas and its frequent location near or at eloquent areas. Resection can be safely maximized by means of intraoperative mapping and awake-surgeries.[61] A meta-analysis of 8091 patients showed the use of intraoperative stimulation brain mapping achieved more gross total removal with less late severe neurological deficits, and is recommended as a standard for glioma surgery especially if eloquent areas are involved.[62] Multicentric gliomas, previously considered not resectable can also be resected with aid of awake intraoperative map-ping.[63] Despite this advances, the role of surgery remains limited for gliomatosis cerebri or very deep-seated lesions.

Surgery is the principal treatment in the following situations of low-grade astrocytomas:

1. surgical biopsy or partial resection is recommended *in almost all cases* to establish the diagnosis since clinical and radiographic data are not definitive[14]
2. pilocytic astrocytomas
   a) cerebellar tumors occurring in children & young adults (p. 630)
   b) supratentorial pilocytic astrocytomas
3. when herniation threatens from large tumors or tumor cysts
4. tumors causing obstruction of CSF flow
5. may help in seizure control with refractory seizures
6. in an attempt to delay adjuvant therapy and its side-effects in children (especially XRT in those < 5 yrs old)[14]
7. for prevention of malignant transformation

The role of surgery is limited in the following situations of low-grade astrocytomas:

1. disseminated (poorly circumscribed) tumors
2. multifocal tumors
3. location in eloquent brain

Adjuvant therapy for low-grade gliomas

▸ **Radiation therapy (XRT).** Early radiotherapy (54 Gy in fractions of 1.8 Gy) is recommended as adjuvant therapy and is shown to prolong median progression free survival from 3.4 to 5.3 years but does not affect overall survival.[64] In patients with the tumor radically resected, early RT did not prolong PFS and is recommended to be deferred until progression. Following incomplete resection, early RT significantly prolongs PFS and disease specific survival.[65] Two prospective trials found no difference in OS or PFS between different XRT doses (EORTC trial[56]: 45 Gy in 5 weeks vs. 59.4 Gy in 6.6 weeks; Intergroup study[66] 50.4 vs. 64.8 Gy). Side effects from WBXRT include: leukoencephalopathy and cognitive impairment; see Radiation injury and necrosis (p. 1560). The frequency of side effects may[66] or may not[67] be higher at higher XRT doses.

► **Chemotherapy** . Usually reserved for tumor progression. Temozolomide (Temodar®) may be effective in progressive WHO grade II astrocytomas (off label use).[68] Effectiveness of PCV (procarbazine, CCNU, and vincristine) was assessed by RTOG 9802. It showed no significant difference in 5-yr OS rates (RT + PCV versus RT: 72% versus 63%. But on post hoc analysis of survival for patients surviving to 2 years, RT + PCV group had higher 5-yr OS than RT alone.[69]

36.8.2 Malignant astrocytomas (WHO grades III and IV)

Surgery for newly diagnosed high-grade gliomas

The aim of surgery in high-grade gliomas is cytoreduction, to relieve mass effect, and to obtain adequate tissue for histological and molecular study. Cytoreductive surgery followed by external beam radiation and concurrent temozolomide has become the standard against which other treatments are compared.[70]

► **Extent of resection.** The extent of tumor removal and (in an inverse relationship) the volume of residual tumor on post-op imaging studies[71] have a significant effect on time to tumor progression and median survival.[72] It was demonstrated that excision for 97 percent or more was associated with increased survival time.[73] Whenever feasible, gross total resection of tumor with preservation of eloquent and critical structures should be the goal. Recent advances in tumor localization, intraoperative monitoring and mapping have allowed more effective and safer resection.

► **5-aminolevulinic-acid (5-ALA) guided resection.** In addition to techniques of stereotactic localization using preoperative imaging as well as intraoperative brain mapping, techniques to enhance visual identification of tumor intraoperatively may be used and include 5-aminolevulinic-acid (5-ALA). 5-ALA is metabolized into fluorescent porphyrins, which accumulate in malignant glioma cells. This property permits use of ultraviolet illumination during surgery as an adjunct to map out the tumor. This has been proven with RCT where use of 5-ALA leads to more complete resection (65% vs 36%, $p < 0.0001$), which translates into a higher 6-month progression free survival (41% vs 21.1%, $p = 0.0003$) but no effect on OS.[74]

Partial resection of a GBM carries significant risk of post-operative hemorrhage and/or edema (wounded glioma syndrome)with risk of herniation. Furthermore, the benefit of subtotal resection is dubious. Retrospective evidence suggested survival benefits in gross total resection but not with incomplete resection.[75] Therefore, surgical excision should only be considered when the goal of gross total removal is feasible.

As a result of the above, the following are usually not candidates for surgical debulking

1. extensive dominant lobe GBM
2. lesions with significant bilateral involvement (e.g. large butterfly gliomas)
3. elderly patients
4. Karnofsky score < 70 (in general, with infiltrating tumors, the neurologic condition on steroids is as good as it is going to get, and surgery rarely improves this)
5. multicentric gliomas

► **Stereotactic biopsy.** Due to sampling error, stereotactic biopsy may underestimate the occurrence of GBM by as much as 25%.

Indications for *stereotactic biopsy* (instead of initial resection) in suspected malignant astrocytomas[76]:

1. tumors located in eloquent or inaccessible areas of brain
2. patients in poor medical condition precluding general anesthesia
3. to ascertain a diagnosis when one is not definitely established (including when considering a more definitive operation). Some CNS lymphomas mimic GBM radiographically (and without immunostaining, some have also been mistaken pathologically) biopsy should be given serious consideration (to avoid operating on a lymphoma which may be best treated with XRT & intrathecal chemotherapy)

Technique: Yield of biopsy is highest when targets within the low density (necrotic) center and enhancing rim are chosen.[44]

Patients with left-sided tumors and dysphasia are at significant risk of worsening of language function following stereotactic biopsy (the risk of deterioration is low if there is no dysphasia before biopsy).[77]

Adjuvant therapy after cytoreductive surgery for newly diagnosed GBM (Stupp regimen)

Temozolomide is an oral alkylating agent that is given as a prodrug which undergoes rapid non-enzymatic conversion at physiologic pH to the active metabolite monomethyl triazenoimidazole carboxamide (MTIC). The cytotoxic effect of MTIC is associated with alkylation (methylation) of DNA at various sites including the O^6 and N^7 positions on guanine.

Cytoreductive surgery followed by the Stupp regimen has become the standard for newly diagnosed GBM.[70] Stupp regimen included concomitant chemoradiotherapy and adjuvant chemotherapy. Chemoradiotherapy started within six weeks after histological diagnosis of GBM. Radiotherapy in the Stupp regimen consists of fractionated focal irradiation at a dose of 2 Gy per fraction once daily five days per week over a period of six week, for a total dose of 60 Gy, with a 2-3 cm margin of clinical target volume. The is compared to the usual XRT regime for malignant gliomas of 50-60 Gy (usually 50 Gy to a margin 2-3 cm greater than the enhanced volume on MRI with a boost to the enhancing volume to bring the total to 60 Gy[42]). Concomitant chemotherapy consists of temozolomide 75 mg/m^2/day, 7 days per week till the end of radiotherapy. Four weeks later, six cycles of adjuvant chemotherapy starts. Each cycle consists of 5-days of temozolomide repeated every 28 days. The dose was 150 mg/m^2/day for first cycle and stepped up to 200 mg/m^2/day. The median survival was 14.6 months with the Stupp regimen compared to 12.1 months with radiotherapy alone with median survival benefit of 2.1 months. The five-year survival rate was 9.8% for the Stupp regimen in contrast to 1.9%.[78] Regardless of extent of resection and MGMT status, patients received the Stupp regimen had longer median survival. Patients with MGMT promoter region methylation had median survival time of 23.4 months compared to 12.6 months in the non-methylated group. In the MGMT unmethylated group, the Stupp regimen only improved median survival from 11.8 months to 12.6 months. Some groups do extend the adjuvant chemotherapy after the standard six-month regimen until tumor progression is observed, in one study this extended the median survival time from 16.5 months to 24.6 months.[79]

Side effects: Temozolomide may cause myelosuppression. It should not be given unless the neutrophil count $\geq 1.5 \times 10^9$/L and platelet count $\geq 100 \times 10^9$/L. For all patients with newly diagnosed GBM for concomitant temozolomide and radiotherapy, prophylaxis against Pneumocystis carinii pneumonia is required for the 42-day regimen.

► **Other treatment protocols for GBM.** Gliadel® wafer carmustine (BCNU) 7.7 mg in a 200 mg polifeprosan 20 hydrophobic polymer carrier (wafer) that can be applied to resection cavity after tumor excision. The wafers are degraded by hydrolysis and the drug is released over 2-3 wks. This exposes the tumor to 113 times the con-centration of BCNU compared to IV administration. Following tumor removal, up to 8 of the 1.4 cm × 1 mm (dime-sized) wafers are applied to the tumor resection bed at the time of surgery.

36

It increases median survival to 13.8 months compared with 11.6 months in placebo groups for newly diagnosed GBM.[80] It showed no survival benefit for recurrent dis-ease.[81] Side effects: seizures, cerebral edema, healing abnormalities, intracranial infection.

Some other regimens that have not proven to be successful for GBM:

- AVAglio: a phase III trial with addition of bevacizumab to the Stupp regimen for newly diagnosed GBM[82] and RTOG 0825 (another trial of similar design) showed improved PFS, but no significant improvement on OS.[83]
- CENTRIC: a phase III trial studied another antiangiogenic (cilengitide, an integrin inhib-itor) to the standard temozolomide and radiation therapy. There was no improvement in either PFS or OS.[17,84]
- RTOG 93-05: stereotactic radiosurgery followed by conventional chemoirradiation did not improved the median survival of GBM patient compared to those without stereotactic radiotherapy.[85]
- Brachytherapy has shown no significant benefit as an adjunct to EBRT in the initial treatment of malignant astrocytomas.[86]
- Whole brain XRT has not been shown to increase survival compared to focal XRT, and the risk of side effects is greater.[87]
- Combination chemotherapy of procarbazine, lomustine and vincristine (PCV) was used before the proven benefit of the Stupp regimen. But randomized trial did not show any benefit.[88]
- RTOG 0525: a phase 3 trial of dose-dense temozolomide at 100 mg/m^2 day 1-21 of a 28-day cycle showed no significant benefit over standard dosing for median OS or median PFS.[89]

Treatment protocols for anaplastic astrocytoma (WHO Grade III)

For newly diagnosed anaplastic astrocytoma, surgery followed by radiotherapy was the standard treatment with median OS 5.7 yrs. In a retrospective review, radiotherapy followed by chemoradiation, concurrent chemoradiation using temozolomide did not achieve better median OS nor PFS compared with radiotherapy alone.[90] On the other hand, temozolomide was approved by FDA in 1999 for anaplastic astrocytoma refractory to both a nitrosourea and procarbazine. The median duration of all response was 50 weeks, median PFS was 4.4 months and median OS was 15.9 months.[91,92]

36.8.3 Pseudoprogression

Since temozolomide has become the new standard of care in the treatment of GBM, there has been an increasing awareness of progressive contrast-enhancing areas on MRI that mimics tumor progression, typically seen ≤ 3 months after treatment. This phenomenon of pseudoprogression occurs in up to 28-60% of patients after XRT + temozolomide treatment. Histologically it resembles radiation necrosis and is believed to be associated with tumor kill by radiation. Increased tumor kill with chemotherapy results in more pseudoprogression. 91% in methylated MGMT patients vs. 41% in the unmethylated group.[93]

Management: The MRI findings usually improve without treatment,[94] and steroids may help control symptoms.

Diagnosis: There is no definitive diagnostic test. MR perfusion has been tried to distinguish pseudoprogression from true progression but is not reliable. DWI with higher apparent diffusion co-efficient (ADC), MR spectroscopy, and PET have also not achieved high sensitivity and specificity. Monitoring with serial MRIs and clinical exams seems to be an effective strategy.

36.8.4 Treatment for recurrent GBM

Less than 10% of recurrent gliomas recur away from the original tumor site.[46]

1. Surgery: reoperation extends survival by an additional 36 weeks in patients with GBM, and 88 weeks in AA[95,96] (duration of high quality survival was 10 weeks and 83 weeks respectively, and was lower with pre-op Karnofsky score < 70). In addition to Karnofsky score, significant prognosticators for response to repeat surgery include: age and time from the first operation to reoperation (shorter times → worse prognosis).[97] Morbidity is higher with reoperation (5-18%); the infection rate is ≈ 3 x that for first operation, wound dehiscence is more likely.
2. Chemotherapy
   a) temozolomide:
      - in a 2013 Cochrane review,[98] chemotherapy with temozolomide was not associated with extension of PFS nor OS

Table 36.9 Summary of systemic treatment for relapsed GBM

Endpoint	Bevacizumab[100]	Bevacizumab + irinotecan[100]	Temozolomide[99]	PCV[103]
6-months PFS, %	43	50	7-36	38
Median PFS, months	4.2	5.6	1.8-3.7	N/A
ORR, %	28	38	3-11	3.5
Median DoR, months	5.6	4.3	N/A	N/A
Median OS, months	9.3	8.9	N/A	N/A
12-month OS, %	38	38	14.8-28.6	N/A
Decrease dose of corticosteroid[a]	46.5%	30.2%	N/A	N/A
Improved or stabilized neurocognitive function	59%-97%[104]	N/A	N/A	N/A

[a] ≥ 50% corticosteroid dose reduction, relative to baseline

Table 36.10 Median survival for astrocytomas

Grade	Median survival
I	8–10 yrs
II	7–8 yrs
III	≈ 2–3 yrs
IV	<1 yr

Table 36.11 MGMT Promotor Methylation Survival Outcome

MGMT	Unmethylated	Methylated
Median OS (months)	12.2	18.2
2-year survival	7.8%	34.1%

- the RESCUE study looked at continuous dose-intense temozolomide at 50 mg/m²/day showed one year survival ranged 14.8–28.6% depended on the timing of progression and the start of dose-intense treatment[99]

b) bevacizumab (Avastin®) – a monoclonal antibody against VEGF. FDA approved in May, 2009 for progressive GBM following prior treatment based on two trials: the BRAIN study, AVF3708g[100] and NCI 06-C-0064E.[101] Given as 10 mg/kg every 2 weeks until disease progression. The reported 6-month PFS rate was 36.0%. The median response durations were 3.9 months and 4.2 months from the two trials. The median OS was 9.3 months.[102] Side effects: gastrointestinal perforations, wound healing complications, hemorrhage, fistula formation, arterial thromboembolic events, hypertension

Summary: For recurrent GBM, surgery is still the mainstay of treatment; in general, surgery is recommended only for patients with KPS ≥ 70.

36.9 Outcome

Survival with various grades of astrocytoma

In general, with “optimal treatment” the survival of the various grades of astrocytoma are approximately given in ▶ Table 36.10 (more details may be found in other sections – see also ▶ Table 36.13 and below for recursive partitioning analysis (RPA) for GBM).

Low-grade astrocytomas (WHO grade II)

For low grade infiltrating gliomas, see prognosis based on pre-op grading (▶ Table 36.7).

36

Malignant astrocytomas (WHO grades III & IV)

Prognostic indicators:

1. patient age: consistently found to be the most significant prognosticator, with younger patients faring better.
2. histological features
3. performance status, e.g. Karnofsky score (KPS) at presentation (p. 1358)
4. Mental Status changes and symptoms < 3 months portends a worse prognosis
5. MGMT Methylation status

MGMT Promotor Methylation Survival Outcome (▶ Table 36.11)[24]

Analysis of 206 patients for MGMT methylation: Median overall survival for MGMT methylation positive patients treated with temozolomide and RT was 21.7 month, RT only 15.3 months; no survival difference between treatments in patients with unmethylated MGMT.

Stupp Regime vs. radiotherapy alone, survival outcome[70,78]

EORTC – NCIC Trial, 573 patients, 5-year Follow-up (▶ Table 36.12)

Recursive partitioning analysis (RPA) with glioblastoma (▶ Table 36.13)[105]: RPA classification developed to compare survival categories and determine homogenous patient subsets. Useful for refining stratification and phase III study design. Can determine which patient subsets will benefit from specific treatments (and which may be spared unnecessary treatment).

Table 36.12 Stupp Regime vs. radiotherapy alone, survival outcome

Survival	RT	RT + TMZ
Median	12.1 months	14.6 months
2-year	10.9%	27.2%
3-year	4.4%	16.0%
4-year	3.0%	12.1%
5-year	1.9%	9.8%

Table 36.13 Recursive partitioning analysis (RPA) with glioblastoma

	Median survival		2-year survival	
RPA Class	Months	95% CI	%	95% CI
III	17	15-21	32	21-42
IV	15	13-16	19	15-24
V	10	9-12	11	7-16

The European Nomogram GBM Calculator[106]: http://www.eortc.be/tools/gbmcalculator. Data from randomized trials by EORTC and NCIC analyzed for the prediction of survival of GBM patients.

References

[1] Ostrom QT, Gittleman H, Farah P, Ondracek A, Chen Y, Wolinsky Y, Stroup NE, Kruchko C, Barnholtz-Sloan JS. CBTRUS statistical report: Primary brain and central nervous system tumors diagnosed in the United States in 2006-2010. Neuro Oncol. 2013; 15 Suppl 2:ii1–i56

[2] Inskip PD, Hoover RN, Devesa SS. Brain cancer incidence trends in relation to cellular telephone use in the United States. Neuro Oncol. 2010; 12:1147–1151

[3] Linet MS, Inskip PD. Cellular (mobile) telephone use and cancer risk. Rev Environ Health. 2010; 25:51–55

[4] Little MP, Rajaraman P, Curtis RE, Devesa SS, Inskip PD, Check DP, Linet MS. Mobile phone use and glioma risk: comparison of epidemiological study results with incidence trends in the United States. BMJ. 2012; 344

[5] World Health Organization. Electromagnetic fields and public health: mobile phones. 2011

[6] Berger MS, Leibel SA, Brunner JM, Finlay JL, Levin VA. In: Primary Cerebral Tumours. Cancer of the Nervous System. 2nd ed. Oxford: Oxford University Press; 2002:84–99

[7] Ringertz N. Grading of gliomas. Acta Pathol Microbiol Scand. 1950; 27:51–64

[8] Russell DS, Rubenstein LJ. Pathology of Tumours of the Nervous System. 5th ed. Baltimore: Williams and Wilkins; 1989:83–161

[9] Kernohan JW, Mabon RF, Svien HJ, et al. A Simplified Classification of the Gliomas. Proc Staff Meet Mayo Clin. 1949; 24:71–75

[10] Kleihues P, Louis DN, Wiestler OD, Burger PC, Scheithauer BW, Louis DN, Ohgaki H, Wiestler OD, Cavenee WK, Bosman FT, Jaffe ES, Lakhani SR, Ohgaki H. In: WHO grading of tumors of the central nervous system. WHO classification of tumors of the central nervous system. 4th ed. Lyon: International Agency for Research on Cancer; 2007:10–11

[11] Daumas-Duport C, Scheithauer B, O'Fallon J, Kelly P, et al. Grading of Astrocytomas: A Simple and Reproducible Method. Cancer. 1988; 62:2152–2165

[12] Kim TS, Halliday AL, Hedley-Whyte T, Convery K. Correlates of Survival and the Daumas-Duport Grading System for Astrocytomas. J Neurosurg. 1991; 74:27–37

[13] Louis DN, Perry A, Burger P, Ellison DW, Reifenberger G, von Deimling A, Aldape K, Brat D, Collins VP, Eberhart C, Figarella-Branger D, Fuller GN, Giangaspero F, Giannini C, Hawkins C, Kleihues P, Korshunov A, Kros JM, Beatriz Lopes M, Ng HK, Ohgaki H, Paulus W, Pietsch T, Rosenblum M, Rushing E, Soylemezoglu F, Wiestler O, Wesseling P. International Society Of Neuropathology–Haarlem consensus guidelines for nervous system tumor classification and grading. Brain Pathol. 2014; 24:429–435

[14] Berger MS, Apuzzo MLJ. In: Role of Surgery in Diagnosis and Management. Benign Cerebral Glioma. Park Ridge, Illinois: American Association of Neurological Surgeons; 1995:293–307

[15] Laws ER, Taylor WF, Clifton MB, et al. Neurosurgical Management of Low-Grade Astrocytoma of the Cerebral Hemispheres. J Neurosurg. 1984; 61:665–673

[16] Shafqat S, Hedley-Whyte ET, Henson JW. Age-Dependent Rate of Anaplastic Transformation in Low-Grade Astrocytoma. Neurology. 1999; 52:867–869

[17] Nutt CL, Stemmer-Rachamimov AO, Cairncross JG, Louis DN, Ali-Osman F. In: Molecular Pathology of Nervous System Tumors. Brain Tumors. Humana Press; 2005:33–54

[18] James CD, Ali-Osman F. In: Molecular Genetics of Tumors of the Central Nervous System. Brain Tumors. Humana Press; 2005:19–32.

[19] Kopelson G, Linggood R. Infratentorial Glioblastoma: The Role of Neuraxis Irradiation. Int J Radiation Oncology Biol Phys. 1982; 8:999–1003

[20] Louis DN, Ohgaki H, Wiestler OD, Cavenee WK, Bosman FT, Jaffe ES, Lakhani SR, Ohgaki H. WHO classification of tumors of the central nervous system. Lyon 2007

[21] Maher EA, Brennan C, Wen PY, Durso L, Ligon KL, Richardson A, Khatry D, Feng B, Sinha R, Louis DN, Quackenbush J, Black PM, Chin L, DePinho RA. Marked genomic differences characterize primary and secondary glioblastoma subtypes and identify two distinct molecular and clinical secondary glioblastoma entities. Cancer Res. 2006; 66:11502–11513

[22] Liang Y, Diehn M, Watson N, Bollen AW, Aldape KD, Nicholas MK, Lamborn KR, Berger MS, Botstein D, Brown PO, Israel MA. Gene expression profiling reveals molecularly and clinically distinct subtypes of glioblastoma multiforme. Proc Natl Acad Sci U S A. 2005; 102:5814–5819

[23] Furnari FB, Fenton T, Bachoo RM, Mukasa A, Stommel JM, Stegh A, Hahn WC, Ligon KL, Louis DN, Brennan C, Chin L, DePinho RA, Cavenee WK. Malignant astrocytic glioma: genetics, biology, and paths to treatment. Genes Dev. 2007; 21:2683–2710

[24] Hegi ME, Diserens AC, Gorlia T, Hamou MF, de Tribolet N, Weller M, Kros JM, Hainfellner JA, Mason W, Mariani L, Bromberg JE, Hau P, Mirimanoff RO, Cairncross JG, Janzer RC, Stupp R. MGMT gene silencing and benefit from temozolomide in glioblastoma. N Engl J Med. 2005; 352:997–1003

[25] Margison GP, Kleihues P. Chemical carcinogenesis in the nervous system. Preferential accumulation of O6-methylguanine in rat brain deoxyribonucleic acid during repetitive administration of N-methyl-N-nitrosourea. Biochem J. 1975; 148:521–525

[26] Goth R, Rajewsky MF. Persistence of O6-ethylguanine in rat-brain DNA: correlation with nervous system-specific carcinogenesis by ethylnitrosourea. Proc Natl Acad Sci U S A. 1974; 71:639–643

[27] Qian XC, Brent TP. Methylation hot spots in the 5' flanking region denote silencing of the O6-methylguanine-DNA methyltransferase gene. Cancer Res. 1997; 57:3672–3677

[28] Esteller M, Hamilton SR, Burger PC, Baylin SB, Herman JG. Inactivation of the DNA repair gene O6-methylguanine-DNA methyltransferase by promoter hypermethylation is a common event in primary human neoplasia. Cancer Res. 1999; 59:793–797

[29] Yan H, Parsons DW, Jin G, McLendon R, Rasheed BA, Yuan W, Kos I, Batinic-Haberle I, Jones S, Riggins GJ, Friedman H, Friedman A, Reardon D, Herndon J, Kinzler KW, Velculescu VE, Vogelstein B, Bigner DD. IDH1 and IDH2 mutations in gliomas. N Engl J Med. 2009; 360:765–773

[30] Parsons DW, Jones S, Zhang X, Lin JC, Leary RJ, Angenendt P, Mankoo P, Carter H, Siu IM, Gallia GL, Olivi A, McLendon R, Rasheed BA, Keir S, Nikolskaya T, Nikolsky Y, Busam DA, Tekleab H, Diaz LA, Jr, Hartigan J, Smith DR, Strausberg RL, Marie SK, Shinjo SM, Yan H, Riggins GJ, Bigner DD, Karchin R, Papadopoulos N, Parmigiani G, Vogelstein B, Velculescu VE, Kinzler KW. An integrated genomic analysis of human glioblastoma multiforme. Science. 2008; 321:1807–1812

[31] Yen KE, Bittinger MA, Su SM, Fantin VR. Cancer-associated IDH mutations: biomarker and therapeutic opportunities. Oncogene. 2010; 29:6409–6417

[32] Ohgaki H, Kleihues P. The definition of primary and secondary glioblastoma. Clin Cancer Res. 2013; 19:764–772

[33] Bello MJ, Alonso ME, Aminoso C, Anselmo NP, Arjona D, Gonzalez-Gomez P, Lopez-Marin I, de Campos JM, Gutierrez M, Isla A, Kusak ME, Lassaletta L, Sarasa JL, Vaquero J, Casartelli C, Rey JA. Hypermethylation of the DNA repair gene MGMT: association with TP53 G:C to A:T transitions in a series of 469 nervous system tumors. Mutat Res. 2004; 554:23–32

[34] Nakamura M, Watanabe T, Yonekawa Y, Kleihues P, Ohgaki H. Promoter methylation of the DNA repair gene MGMT in astrocytomas is frequently associated with G:C – > A:T mutations of the TP53 tumor suppressor gene. Carcinogenesis. 2001; 22:1715–1719

[35] Cancer Genome Atlas Research Network. Comprehensive genomic characterization defines human glioblastoma genes and core pathways. Nature. 2008; 455:1061–1068

[36] Verhaak RG, Hoadley KA, Purdom E, Wang V, Qi Y, Wilkerson MD, Miller CR, Ding L, Golub T, Mesirov JP, Alexe G, Lawrence M, O'Kelly M, Tamayo P, Weir BA, Gabriel S, Winckler W, Gupta S, Jakkula L, Feiler HS, Hodgson JG, James CD, Sarkaria JN, Brennan C, Kahn A, Spellman PT, Wilson RK, Speed TP, Gray JW, Meyerson M, Getz G, Perou CM, Hayes DN, Cancer Genome Atlas Research Network. Integrated genomic analysis identifies clinically relevant subtypes of glioblastoma characterized by abnormalities in PDGFRA, IDH1, EGFR, and NF1. Cancer Cell. 2010; 17:98–110

[37] Kleihues P, Louis DN, Scheithauer BW, Rorke LB, Reifenberger G, Burger PC, Cavenee WK. The WHO classification of tumors of the nervous system. J Neuropathol Exp Neurol. 2002; 61:215–25; discussion 226-9

[38] Kondziolka D, Lunsford LD, Martinez AJ. Unreliability of Contemporary Neurodiagnostic Imaging in Evaluating Suspected Adult Supratentorial (Low-Grade) Astrocytoma. J Neurosurg. 1993; 79:533–536

[39] Zee CS, Conti P, Destian S, et al. Apuzzo MLJ. In: Imaging Features of Benign Gliomas. Benign Cerebral Glioma. Park Ridge, Illinois: American Association of Neurological Surgeons; 1995:247–274

[40] Chang EF, Smith JS, Chang SM, Lamborn KR, Prados MD, Butowski N, Barbaro NM, Parsa AT, Berger MS, McDermott MM. Preoperative prognostic classification system for hemispheric low-grade gliomas in adults. J Neurosurg. 2008; 109:817–824

[41] Pignatti F, van den Bent M, Curran D, Debruyne C, Sylvester R, Therasse P, Afra D, Cornu P, Bolla M, Vecht C, Karim AB. Prognostic factors for survival in adult patients with cerebral low-grade glioma. J Clin Oncol. 2002; 20:2076–2084

[42] Narayan P, Olson JJ. Management of anaplastic astrocytoma. Contemp Neurosurg. 2001; 23:1–6

[43] Chamberlain MC, Murovic J, Levin VA. Absence of Contrast Enhancementon CT Brain Scans of Patients with Supratentorial Malignant Gliomas. Neurology. 1988; 38:1371–1373

[44] Greene GM, Hitchon PW, Schelper RL, et al. Diagnostic Yield in CT-Guided Stereotactic Biopsy of Gliomas. J Neurosurg. 1989; 71:494–497

[45] Scherer HJ. The Forms of Growth in Gliomas and their Practical Significance. Brain. 1940; 63:1–35

[46] Choucair AK, Levin VA, Gutin PH, et al. Development of Multiple Lesions During Radiation Therapy and Chemotherapy. J Neurosurg. 1986; 65:654–658

[47] Erlich SS, Davis RL. Spinal Subarachnoid Metastasis from Primary Intracranial Glioblastoma Multiforme. Cancer. 1978; 42:2854–2864

[48] Artigas J, Cervos-Navarro J, Iglesias JR, et al. Gliomatosis Cerebri: Clinical and Histological Findings. Clin Neuropathol. 1985; 4:135–148

[49] Wilson NW, Symon L, Lantos PL. Gliomatosis Cerebri: Report of a Case Presenting as a Focal Cerebral Mass. J Neurol. 1987; 234:445–447

[50] Barnard RO, Geddes JF. The Incidence of Multifocal Cerebral Gliomas: A Histological Study of Large Hemisphere Sections. Cancer. 1987; 60:1519–1531

[51] van Tassel P, Lee Y-Y, Bruner JM. Synchronous and Metachronous Malignant Gliomas: CT Findings. AJNR. 1988; 9:725–732

[52] Harsh GR, Wilson CB, Youmans JR. In: Nuroepithelial Tumors of the Adult Brain. Neurological Surgery. 3rd ed. Philadelphia: W. B. Saunders; 1990:3040–3136

[53] Salvati M, Caroli E, Orlando ER, Frati A, et al. Multicentric glioma: our experience in 25 patients and critical review of the literature. Neurosurg Rev. 2003; 26:275–279

[54] Cairncross JG, Laperriere NJ. Low-Grade Glioma: To Treat or Not to Treat? Arch Neurol. 1989; 46:1238–1239

[55] Shaw EG. Low-Grade Gliomas: To Treat or Not to Treat? A Radiation Oncologist's Viewpoint. Arch Neurol. 1990; 47:1138–1139

[56] Karim ABMF, Maat B, Hatlevoll R, et al. A randomized trial on dose-response in radiation therapy of low-grade cerebral glioma: European Organization for Research and Treatment of Cancer (EORTC) Study 22844. Int J Radiation Oncology Biol Phys. 1996; 36:549–556

[57] van den Bent MJ, Snijders TJ, Bromberg JE. Current treatment of low grade gliomas. Memo. 2012; 5:223–227

[58] McGirt MJ, Goldstein IM, Chaichana KL, Tobias ME, Kothbauer KF, Jallo GI. Extent of surgical resection of malignant astrocytomas of the spinal cord: outcome analysis of 35 patients. Neurosurgery. 2008; 63:55–60; discussion 60-1

[59] Capelle L, Fontaine D, Mandonnet E, Taillandier L, Golmard JL, Bauchet L, Pallud J, Peruzzi P, Baron MH, Kujas M, Guyotat J, Guillevin R, Frenay M, Taillibert S, Colin P, Rigau V, Vandenbos F, Pinelli C, Duffau H. Spontaneous and therapeutic prognostic factors in adult hemispheric World Health Organization Grade II gliomas: a series of 1097 cases: clinical article. J Neurosurg. 2013; 118:1157–1168

[60] Shaw EG, Berkey B, Coons SW, Bullard D, Brachman D, Buckner JC, Stelzer KJ, Barger GR, Brown PD, Gilbert MR, Mehta M. Recurrence following neurosurgeon-determined gross-total resection of adult supratentorial low-grade glioma: results of a prospective clinical trial. J Neurosurg. 2008; 109:835–841

[61] De Benedictis A, Moritz-Gasser S, Duffau H. Awake mapping optimizes the extent of resection for low-grade gliomas in eloquent areas. Neurosurgery. 2010; 66:1074–84; discussion 1084

[62] De Witt Hamer PC, Robles SG, Zwinderman AH, Duffau H, Berger MS. Impact of intraoperative stimulation brain mapping on glioma surgery outcome: a meta-analysis. J Clin Oncol. 2012; 30:2559–2565

[63] Terakawa Y, Yordanova YN, Tate MC, Duffau H. Surgical management of multicentric diffuse low-grade gliomas: functional and oncological outcomes: clinical article. J Neurosurg. 2013; 118:1169–1175

[64] van den Bent MJ, Afra D, de Witte O, Ben Hassel M, Schraub S, Hoang-Xuan K, Malmstrom PO, Collette L, Pierart M, Mirimanoff R, Karim AB. Long-term efficacy of early versus delayed radiotherapy for low-grade astrocytoma and oligodendroglioma in adults: the EORTC 22845 randomised trial. Lancet. 2005; 366:985–990

[65] Hanzely Z, Polgar C, Fodor J, Brucher JM, Vitanovics D, Mangel LC, Afra D. Role of early radiotherapy in the treatment of supratentorial WHO Grade II astrocytomas: long-term results of 97 patients. J Neurooncol. 2003; 63:305–312

[66] Shaw E, Arusell R, Scheithauer B, O'Fallon J, O'Neill B, Dinapoli R, Nelson D, Earle J, Jones C, Cascino T, Nichols D, Ivnik R, Hellman R, Curran W, Abrams R. Prospective randomized trial of low- versus high-dose radiation therapy in adults with supratentorial low-grade glioma: initial report of a North Central Cancer Treatment Group/Radiation Therapy Oncology Group/Eastern Cooperative Oncology Group study. J Clin Oncol. 2002; 20:2267–2276

[67] Laack NN, Brown PD, Ivnik RJ, Furth AF, Ballman KV, Hammack JE, Arusell RM, Shaw EG, Buckner JC. Cognitive function after radiotherapy for supratentorial low-grade glioma: a North Central Cancer Treatment Group prospective study. Int J Radiat Oncol Biol Phys. 2005; 63:1175–1183

[68] Quinn JA, Reardon DA, Friedman AH, Rich JN, Sampson JH, Provenzale JM, McLendon RE, Gururangan S, Bigner DD, Herndon JE, II, Avgeropoulos N, Finlay J, Tourt-Uhlig S, Affronti ML, Evans B, Stafford-Fox V, Zaknoen S, Friedman HS. Phase II trial of temozolomide in patients with progressive low-grade glioma. J Clin Oncol. 2003; 21:646–651

[69] Shaw EG, Wang M, Coons SW, Brachman DG, Buckner JC, Stelzer KJ, Barger GR, Brown PD, Gilbert MR, Mehta MP. Randomized trial of radiation therapy plus procarbazine, lomustine, and vincristine chemotherapy for supratentorial adult low-grade glioma: initial results of RTOG 9802. J Clin Oncol. 2012; 30:3065–3070

[70] Stupp R, Mason WP, van den Bent MJ, Weller M, Fisher B, Taphoorn MJ, Belanger K, Brandes AA, Marosi C, Bogdahn U, Curschmann J, Janzer RC, Ludwin SK, Gorlia T, Allgeier A, Lacombe D, Cairncross JG, Eisenhauer E, Mirimanoff RO. Radiotherapy plus concomitant and adjuvant temozolomide for glioblastoma. N Engl J Med. 2005; 352:987–996

[71] Grabowski MM, Recinos PF, Nowacki AS, Schroeder JL, Angelov L, Barnett GH, Vogelbaum MA. Residual tumor volume versus extent of resection: predictors of survival after surgery for glioblastoma. J Neurosurg. 2014; 121:1115–1123

[72] Keles GE, Anderson B, Berger MS. The Effect of Extent of Resection on Time to Tumor Progression and Survival in Patients with Glioblastoma Multiforme of the Cerebral Hemirsphere. Surg Neurol. 1999; 52:371–379

[73] Lacroix M, Abi-Said D, Fourney DR, Gokaslan ZL, Shi W, DeMonte F, Lang FF, McCutcheon IE, Hassenbusch SJ, Holland E, Hess K, Michael C, Miller D, Sawaya R. A multivariate analysis of 416 patients with glioblastoma multiforme: prognosis, extent of resection, and survival. J Neurosurg. 2001; 95:190–198

[74] Stummer W, Pichlmeier U, Meinel T, Wiestler OD, Zanella F, Reulen HJ. Fluorescence-guided surgery with 5-aminolevulinic acid for resection of malignant glioma: a randomised controlled multicentre phase III trial. Lancet Oncol. 2006; 7:392–401

[75] Kreth FW, Thon N, Simon M, Westphal M, Schackert G, Nikkhah G, Hentschel B, Reifenberger G, Pietsch T, Weller M, Tonn JC. Gross total but not incomplete resection of glioblastoma prolongs survival in the era of radiochemotherapy. Ann Oncol. 2013; 24:3117–3123

[76] Coffey RJ, Lunsford LD, Taylor FH. Survival After Stereotactic Biopsy of Malignant Gliomas. Neurosurgery. 1988; 22:465–473

[77] Thomson A-M, Taylor R, Fraser D, Whittle IR. Stereotactic Biopsy of Nonpolar Tumors in the Dominant Hemisphere: A Prospective Study of Effects on Language Functions. J Neurosurg. 1997; 89:923–926

[78] Stupp R, Hegi ME, Mason WP, van den Bent MJ, Taphoorn MJ, Janzer RC, Ludwin SK, Allgeier A, Fisher B, Belanger K, Hau P, Brandes AA, Gijtenbeek J, Marosi C, Vecht CJ, Mokhtari K, Wesseling P, Villa S, Eisenhauer E, Gorlia T, Weller M, Lacombe D, Cairncross JG, Mirimanoff RO. Effects of radiotherapy with concomitant and adjuvant temozolomide versus radiotherapy alone on survival in glioblastoma in a randomised phase III study: 5-year analysis of the EORTC-NCIC trial. Lancet Oncol. 2009; 10:459–466

[79] Roldan Urgoiti GB, Singh AD, Easaw JC. Extended adjuvant temozolomide for treatment of newly diagnosed glioblastoma multiforme. J Neurooncol. 2012; 108:173–177

[80] Westphal M, Ram Z, Riddle V, Hilt D, Bortey E. Gliadel wafer in initial surgery for malignant glioma: long-term follow-up of a multicenter controlled trial. Acta Neurochir (Wien). 2006; 148:269–75; discussion 275

[81] Hart MG, Grant R, Garside R, Rogers G, Somerville M, Stein K. Chemotherapy wafers for high grade glioma. Cochrane Database Syst Rev. 2011. DOI: 10.1002/14651858.CD007294.pub2

[82] Genentech Study Showed That Avastin Helped People with Newly Diagnosed Glioblastoma Live Longer without Their Disease Worsening When Added to Radiation and Chemotherapy. 2012

[83] Gilbert MR, Dignam J, Won M, Blumenthal DT, et al. RTOG 0825: Phase III double-blind placebo-controlled trial evaluating bevacizumab in patients with newly diagnosed glioblastoma. J Clin Oncol. 2013; 31

[84] Merck: Phase III Trial of Cilengitide Did Not Meet Primary Endpoint in Patients With Newly Diagnosed Glioblastoma. 2013

[85] Souhami L, Seiferheld W, Brachman D, Podgorsak EB, Werner-Wasik M, Lustig R, Schultz CJ, Sause W, Okunieff P, Buckner J, Zamorano L, Mehta MP, Curran WJ, Jr. Randomized comparison of stereotactic radiosurgery followed by conventional radiotherapy with carmustine to conventional radiotherapy with carmustine for patients with glioblastoma multiforme: report of Radiation Therapy Oncology Group 93-05 protocol. Int J Radiat Oncol Biol Phys. 2004; 60:853–860

[86] Sneed PK, McDermott MW, Gutin PH. Interstitial brachytherapy procedures for brain tumors. Semin Surg Oncol. 1997; 13:157–166

[87] Shapiro WR, Green SB, Burger PC, et al. Randomized Trial of Three Chemotherapy Regimens and Two Radiotherapy Regimens in Postoperative Treatment of Malignant Glioma: Brain Tumor Cooperative Group Trial 8001. J Neurosurg. 1989; 71:1–9

[88] Randomized trial of procarbazine, lomustine, and vincristine in the adjuvant treatment of high-grade astrocytoma: a Medical Research Council trial. J Clin Oncol. 2001; 19:509–518

[89] Gilbert MR, Wang M, Aldape KD, Stupp R, Hegi ME, Jaeckle KA, Armstrong TS, Wefel JS, Won M, Blumenthal DT, Mahajan A, Schultz CJ, Erridge S, Baumert B, Hopkins KI, Tzuk-Shina T, Brown PD, Chakravarti A, Curran WJ,Jr, Mehta MP. Dose-dense temozolomide for newly diagnosed glioblastoma: a randomized phase III clinical trial. J Clin Oncol. 2013; 31:4085–4091

[90] Shonka NA, Theeler B, Cahill D, Yung A, Smith L, Lei X, Gilbert MR. Outcomes for patients with anaplastic astrocytoma treated with chemoradiation, radiation therapy alone or radiation therapy followed by chemotherapy: a retrospective review within the era of temozolomide. J Neurooncol. 2013; 113:305–311

[91] Yung WK, Prados MD, Yaya-Tur R, et al. Multicenter phase II trial of temozolomide in patients with anaplastic astrocytoma or anaplastic oligoastrocytoma at first relapse. Temodal Brain Tumor Group. J Clin Oncol. 1999; 17:2762–2771

[92] Food and Drug Administration (FDA). Briefing book for the March 13, 2003 ODAC meeting regarding accelerated approval clinical phase 4 commitments NDA 21-029 Temodar® (temozolomide). 2003

[93] Brandes AA, Tosoni A, Spagnolli F, Frezza G, Leonardi M, Calbucci F, Franceschi E. Disease progression or pseudoprogression after concomitant radiochemotherapy treatment: pitfalls in neurooncology. Neuro Oncol. 2008; 10:361–367

[94] Brandsma D, Stalpers L, Taal W, Sminia P, van den Bent MJ. Clinical features, mechanisms, and management of pseudoprogression in malignant gliomas. Lancet Oncol. 2008; 9:453–461

[95] Harsh GR, Levin VA, Gutin PH, Wilson CB, et al. Reoperation for Recurrent Glioblastoma and Anaplastic Astrocytoma. Neurosurgery. 1987; 21:615–621

[96] Ammirati M, Galicich JH, Arbit E, et al. Reoperation in the Treatment of Recurrent Intracranial Malignant Gliomas. Neurosurgery. 1987; 21:607–614

[97] Brem H, Piantadosi S, Burger PC, et al. Placebo-Controlled Trial of Safety and Efficacy of Intraoperative Controlled Delivery by Biodegradable Polymers of Chemotherapy for Recurrent Gliomas. Lancet. 1995; 345:1008–1012

[98] Hart MG, Garside R, Rogers G, Stein K, Grant R. Temozolomide for high grade glioma. Cochrane Database Syst Rev. 2013; 4. DOI: 10.1002/14651858.CD007415.pub2

[99] Perry JR, Belanger K, Mason WP, Fulton D, Kavan P, Easaw J, Shields C, Kirby S, Macdonald DR, Eisenstat DD, Thiessen B, Forsyth P, Pouliot JF. Phase II trial of continuous dose-intense temozolomide in recurrent malignant glioma: RESCUE study. J Clin Oncol. 2010; 28:2051–2057

[100] Friedman HS, Prados MD, Wen PY, Mikkelsen T, Schiff D, Abrey LE, Yung WK, Paleologos N, Nicholas MK, Jensen R, Vredenburgh J, Huang J, Zheng M, Cloughesy T. Bevacizumab alone and in combination with irinotecan in recurrent glioblastoma. J Clin Oncol. 2009; 27:4733–4740

[101] Kreisl TN, Kim L, Moore K, Duic P, Royce C, Stroud I, Garren N, Mackey M, Butman JA, Camphausen K, Park J, Albert PS, Fine HA. Phase II trial of single-agent bevacizumab followed by bevacizumab plus irinotecan at tumor progression in recurrent glioblastoma. J Clin Oncol. 2009; 27:740–745

[102] Cohen MH, Shen YL, Keegan P, Pazdur R. FDA drug approval summary: bevacizumab (Avastin) as treatment of recurrent glioblastoma multiforme. Oncologist. 2009; 14:1131–1138

[103] Schmidt F, Fischer J, Herrlinger U, Dietz K, Dichgans J, Weller M. PCV chemotherapy for recurrent glioblastoma. Neurology. 2006; 66:587–589

[104] Henriksson R, Asklund T, Poulsen HS. Impact of therapy on quality of life, neurocognitive function and their correlates in glioblastoma multiforme: a review. J Neurooncol. 2011; 104:639–646

[105] Mirimanoff RO, Gorlia T, Mason W, Van den Bent MJ, Kortmann RD, Fisher B, Reni M, Brandes AA, Curschmann J, Villa S, Cairncross G, Allgeier A, Lacombe D, Stupp R. Radiotherapy and temozolomide for newly diagnosed glioblastoma: recursive partitioning analysis of the EORTC 26981/22981-NCIC CE3 phase III randomized trial. J Clin Oncol. 2006; 24:2563–2569

[106] Gorlia T, van den Bent MJ, Hegi ME, Mirimanoff RO, Weller M, Cairncross JG, Eisenhauer E, Belanger K, Brandes AA, Allgeier A, Lacombe D, Stupp R. Nomograms for predicting survival of patients with newly diagnosed glioblastoma: prognostic factor analysis of EORTC and NCIC trial 26981-22981/CE.3. Lancet Oncol. 2008; 9:29–38

37 Other Astrocytic Tumors

37.1 Pilocytic astrocytomas

37.1.1 General information

Key concepts

- a subgroup of astrocytomas with better prognosis (10-year survival: 94%) than infiltrating fibrillary or diffuse astrocytomas
- age ≤ 20 yrs in 75%, which is lower than for typical astrocytomas
- common locations: cerebellar hemisphere, optic nerve/chiasm, hypothalamus
- radiographic appearance: discrete appearing, contrast enhancing lesion, often cystic with mural nodule
- pathology: compacted and loose textured astrocytes with Rosenthal fibers and/or eosinophilic granular bodies
- danger of overgrading and overtreating if not recognized. Histology alone may be inadequate for diagnosis; knowledge of radiographic appearance is critical

Background and terminology

Pilocytic astrocytoma (PCA) is the currently recommended nomenclature for these tumors that have been previously referred to variously as cystic cerebellar astrocytomas, juvenile pilocytic astrocytomas, optic gliomas, and hypothalamic gliomas.[1(p 77–96)] However, since treatment decisions vary based on location and neural involvement, it is still helpful to discuss differences in management of these subtypes.

PCAs differ markedly from infiltrating fibrillary astrocytomas in terms of their ability to invade tissue and for malignant degeneration.

37.1.2 Location

PCAs arise throughout the neuraxis and are more common in children and young adults:

1. optic gliomas & hypothalamic gliomas:
   a) PCAs arising in the optic nerve are called optic gliomas (p. 631)
   b) when they occur in the region of the chiasm they cannot always be distinguished clinically or radiographically from so-called hypothalamic gliomas (p. 632) or gliomas of the third ventricular region
2. cerebral hemispheres: tends to occur in older patients (i.e. young adults) than optic nerve/hypothalamic lesions. These PCAs are potentially confused with fibrillary astrocytomas possessing more malignant potential. PCAs are often distinguished by a cystic component with an enhancing mural nodule (would be atypical for a fibrillary astrocytoma), & some PCAs have dense calcifications[1]
3. brainstem gliomas (p. 633): usually are fibrillary infiltrating type and only a small proportion are pilocytic. Those that are PCAs may comprise the majority of the prognostically favorable group described as "dorsally exophytic"[2]
4. cerebellum: formerly referred to as cystic cerebellar astrocytoma (p. 630)
5. spinal cord: PCAs may also occur here, but little information is available on these. Again, patients tend to be younger than with spinal cord fibrillary astrocytomas

37.1.3 Pathology

PCAs are composed of loosely knit tissue comprised of stellate astrocytes in microcystic regions containing eosinophilic granular bodies intermixed with regions of compact tissue consisting of elongated and fibrillated cells often associated with Rosenthal fiber formation[1] (Rosenthal fibers: sausage or corkscrew shaped cytoplasmic eosinophilic inclusion bodies consisting of glial filament aggregates resembling hyaline; stain bright red on Masson trichrome smears).

These latter two distinctive features facilitate the diagnosis. Another characteristic finding is that the tumors easily break through the pia to fill the overlying subarachnoid space. PCAs may also infiltrate into the perivascular spaces. Vascular proliferation is common. Multinucleated giant cells with peripherally located nuclei are common, especially in PCAs of the cerebellum or cerebrum. Mitotic figures may be seen, but are not as ominous as with fibrillary astrocytomas. Areas of necrosis may also be seen. In spite of well-demarcated margins grossly and on MRI, at least 64% of PCAs infiltrate the surrounding parenchyma, especially the white matter[3] (the clinical significance of this is uncertain, one study found no statistically significant decrease in survival[4]).

Differentiating from a diffuse or infiltrating fibrillary astrocytoma: Unless some of the distinctive findings described above are seen, pathology alone may not be able to differentiate. This may be especially problematic with small specimens obtained e.g. with stereotactic biopsy. Factors that suggest the diagnosis include young age, and knowledge of the radiographic appearance is often critical (see below).

Malignant degeneration: Malignant degeneration has been reported, often after many years. This may occur without radiation therapy (XRT),[5] although in most cases XRT had been administered.[6]

37.1.4 Radiographic appearance

On CT or MRI, PCAs are usually well circumscribed, 94% enhance with contrast[3] (unlike most low-grade fibrillary astrocytomas), frequently have a cystic component with a mural nodule, and have little or no surrounding edema. Although they may occur anywhere in the CNS, 82% are periventricular.[3] Calcifications are only occasionally present.[3] 4 main imaging patterns of cerebellar or cerebral PCAs are shown in ▶ Table 37.1.

37.1.5 Epidemiology

Usually presents during second decade of life (ages 10–20). 75% occur in age < 20 years.[7] No evidence of gender predilection.

37.1.6 Pilocytic astrocytoma of the cerebellum

General information

Key concepts

- often cystic, half of these have mural nodule
- usually presents during the second decade of life (ages 10–20 yrs)
- also, see Key concepts for pilocytic astrocytomas in general (p. 629)

Formerly referred to by the nonspecific and confusing term cystic cerebellar astrocytoma. One of the more common pediatric brain tumors (≈ 10%[8]), comprising 27–40% of pediatric p-fossa tumors.[9(p 367–74),10(p 3032)] They may also occur in adults, where the mean age is lower and the post-operative survival is longer than for fibrillary astrocytomas.[11]

Presentation

Signs and symptoms of pilocytic astrocytoma (PCA) of the cerebellum are usually those of any p-fossa mass, i.e. those of hydrocephalus or cerebellar dysfunction; see Posterior fossa (infratentorial) tumors (p. 592).

Table 37.1 Common imaging characteristics of cerebellar or cerebral PCAs

<table>
<tr><th>%</th><th colspan="2">Description</th></tr>
<tr><td>21%</td><td>nonenhancing cyst with enhancing mural nodule</td><td rowspan="2">over 66% are cystic with enhancing mural nodule</td></tr>
<tr><td>46%</td><td>enhancing cyst with enhancing mural nodule</td></tr>
<tr><td>16%</td><td colspan="2">mass with nonenhancing central area (necrosis)</td></tr>
<tr><td>17%</td><td colspan="2">solid mass with minimal or no cyst</td></tr>
</table>

Pathology

The classic "juvenile pilocytic astrocytoma" of the cerebellum is a distinctive entity with its macroscopic cystic architecture and microscopic spongy appearance.[1] For other microscopic findings, see above.

These tumors may be solid, but are more often cystic (hence the older term "cystic cerebellar astrocytoma"), and tend to be large at the time of diagnosis (cystic tumors: 4–5.6 cm dia; solid tumors: 2–4.8 cm dia). Cysts contain highly proteinaceous fluid (averaging ≈ 4 Hounsfield units higher density than CSF on CT[8]).

50% of cystic tumors have a mural nodule and a cyst lining of reactive, non-neoplastic cerebellar tissue or ependymal lining (non-enhancing on CT), whereas the remaining 50% lack a nodule and have a cyst wall of poorly cellular tumor[12] (enhances on CT).

Histological classification of Winston

The Winston classification system[13] is shown in ▶ Table 37.2. 72% of cerebellar PCAs tended to cluster with either Type A or B characteristics, 18% in his series had both, and 10% had neither.

Treatment guidelines

The natural history of these tumors is slow growth. Treatment of choice is surgical excision of the maximal amount of the tumor that can be removed without producing deficit. In some, invasion of brainstem or involvement of cranial nerves or blood vessels may limit resection. In tumors composed of a nodule with a true cyst, excision of the nodule is sufficient; the cyst wall is non-neoplastic and need not be removed. In tumors with a so-called "false cyst" where the cyst wall is thick and enhances (on CT or MRI), this portion must be removed also. Because of the high 5 and 10 year survival rates together with the high complication rate of radiation therapy over this time interval – see Radiation injury and necrosis (p. 1560) -, and the fact that many incompletely resected tumors enlarge minimally if at all over periods of 5, 10 or even 20 years, it is recommended to *not* radiate these patients post-op. Rather, they should be followed with serial CT or MRI and be re-operated if there is recurrence.[14] Radiation therapy is indicated for nonresectable recurrence (i.e. reoperation is preferred if possible) or for recurrence with malignant histology. Chemotherapy is preferable to XRT in younger patients.[15]

Also, see Posterior fossa (infratentorial) tumors (p. 592) for guidelines regarding hydrocephalus, etc.

Prognosis

Children with Winston Type A cerebellar PCAs had 94% 10-yr survival, whereas those with Type B had only 29% 10-yr survival.

Tumor recurrence is relatively common, and although it has been said that they generally occur within ≈ 3 yrs of surgery,[16] this is controversial and very late recurrences (violating Collins' law, which says that a tumor may be considered cured if it does not recur within a time period equal to the patient's age at diagnosis + 9 months) are well known.[14] Also, some tumors excised partially fail to show further growth, representing a form of cure.

About 20% of cases develop hydrocephalus requiring treatment following surgery.[17] So-called "drop metastases" are rare with PCAs.

37.1.7 Optic glioma

General information

Accounts for ≈ 2% of gliomas in adults, and 7% in children. The incidence is higher (≈ 25%) in neurofibromatosis (NFT) (p. 603).

Table 37.2 Classification of cerebellar astrocytoma
• Type A: microcysts, leptomeningeal deposits, Rosenthal fibers, foci of oligodendroglioma
• Type B: perivascular pseudorosettes, high cell density, mitosis, calcification
• common features of types A & B: hypervascularity, endothelial proliferation, parenchymal desmoplasia, pleomorphism

May arise in any of the following patterns:

1. one optic nerve (without chiasmal involvement)
2. optic chiasm: less commonly involved in patients with NFT than in sporadic cases
3. multicentric in both optic nerves sparing the chiasm: almost only seen in NFT
4. may occur in conjunction with or be part of a hypothalamic glioma (see below)

Pathology

Most are composed of low-grade (pilocytic) astrocytes. Rarely, a malignant chiasmal glioma occurs.

Presentation

Painless proptosis is an early sign in lesions involving one optic nerve. Chiasmal lesions produce variable and nonspecific visual defects (usually monocular) without proptosis. Large chiasmal tumors may cause hypothalamic and pituitary dysfunction, and may produce hydrocephalus by obstruction at the foramen of Monro. Gliosis of the optic nerve head may be seen on fundoscopy.

Evaluation

Plain x-rays: not usually helpful, although in some cases dilatation of the optic canal can be seen in optic canal views.

CT/MRI: CT scan is excellent for imaging structures within the orbit. MRI is helpful for demonstrating chiasmal or hypothalamic involvement. On CT or MRI, involvement of the optic nerve produces contrast enhancing fusiform enlargement of the nerve usually extending > 1 cm in length.

Treatment

Tumor involving a single optic nerve, sparing the chiasm, producing proptosis and visual loss should be treated with a transcranial approach with excision of the nerve from the globe all the way back to the chiasm (a transorbital (Kronlein) approach is not appropriate since tumor may be left in the nerve stump). In addition to the anticipated blindness in the involved eye, this may produce a junctional scotoma (p.730).

Chiasmal tumors are generally not treated surgically except for biopsy (especially when it is difficult to distinguish an optic nerve glioma from a hypothalamic glioma), CSF shunting, or to remove the rare exophytic component to try and improve vision.

Further treatment: Chemotherapy[15] (especially in younger patients) or XRT is used for chiasmal tumors, for multicentric tumors, post-op if tumor is found in the chiasmal stump end of the resected nerve, and for the rare malignant tumor. Typical XRT treatment planning is for 45 Gy given in 25 fractions of 1.8 Gy.

37.1.8 Hypothalamic glioma

Pilocytic astrocytomas of the hypothalamus and third ventricular region occur primarily in children. Radiographically, the lesion may have an intraventricular appearance. Many of these tumors have some chiasmal involvement and the distinction from optic nerve glioma cannot be made (see above).

37

May present with so-called "diencephalic syndrome", a rare syndrome seen in peds, usually caused by an infiltrating glioma of the anterior hypothalamus. Classically: cachexia (loss of subcutaneous fat) associated with hyperactivity, over-alertness and an almost euphoric affect. May also see: hypoglycemia, failure to thrive, macrocephaly.

When complete resection is not possible, further treatment may be needed as outlined under optic gliomas (above).

37.1.9 Pilomyxoid astrocytoma (PMA)

WHO grade II. Related to pilocytic astrocytomas (PCA) but more aggressive with greater tendency to recur and spread in CSF.[18] May be an infantile form of PCA with a case report of "maturation" to a typical PCA.[19] Typical onset in infancy (10 months).

Histologically: dominant mucoid matrix, monomorphic bipolar cells, and angiocentric cell arrangement. By definition, does not contain Rosenthal fibers.

May also occur in spinal cord, with a case report of extraneural peritoneal mets spread through a VP shunt.[20]

37.1.10 Brainstem glioma

General information

Key concepts

- not a homogeneous group. MRI can differentiate malignant from benign lesions
- trend: lower grade tumors tend to occur in the upper brainstem, and higher grade tumors in the lower brainstem/medulla
- usually presents with multiple cranial nerve palsies and long tract findings
- most are malignant, have poor prognosis, and are not surgical candidates
- role of surgery primarily limited to dorsally exophytic lesions and shunting

Brainstem gliomas (BSG) tend to occur during childhood and adolescence (77% are < 20 yrs old, they comprise 1% of adult tumors[21]). BSG are one of the 3 most common brain tumors in pediatrics – see Pediatric brain tumors (p. 593) – comprising ≈ 10–20% of pediatric CNS tumors.[2]

Presentation

See reference.[22]

Upper brainstem tumors tend to present with cerebellar findings and hydrocephalus, whereas lower brainstem tumors tend to present with multiple lower cranial nerve deficits and long tract findings. Due to their invasive nature, signs and symptoms usually do not occur until the tumor is fairly extensive in size.

Signs and symptoms:

1. gait disturbance
2. headache (p. 590)
3. nausea/vomiting
4. cranial nerve deficits: diplopia, facial asymmetry
5. distal motor weakness in 30%
6. papilledema in 50%
7. hydrocephalus in 60%, usually due to aqueductal obstruction (often late, except with periaqueductal tumors, e.g. below)
8. failure to thrive (especially in age ≤ 2 yrs)

Pathology

BSG is a heterogeneous group. There may be a tendency towards lower grade tumors in the upper brainstem (76% were low-grade) versus the lower brainstem (100% of the glioblastomas were in the medulla).[23] A cystic component is seen rarely. Calcifications are also rare. 4 growth patterns that can be identified by MRI[24] that may correlate with prognosis[25]:

1. diffuse: all are malignant (most are anaplastic astrocytomas, the rest are glioblastomas). On MRI these tumors extend into the adjacent region in vertical axis (e.g. medullary tumors extend into pons and/or cervical cord) with very little growth towards obex, remaining intraaxial
2. cervicomedullary: most (72%) are low-grade astrocytomas. The rostral extent of these tumors is limited to the spinomedullary junction. Most bulge into the obex of the 4th ventricle (some may have an actual exophytic component)
3. focal: extent limited to medulla (does not extend up into pons nor down into spinal cord). Most (66%) are low-grade astrocytomas
4. dorsally exophytic: may be an extension of "focal" tumors (see above). Many of these may actually be low grade gliomas including:
   a) pilocytic astrocytomas (p. 629)
   b) gangliogliomas (p. 651): very rare, only 13 cases reported as of 1984. Compared to other BSGs, these patients tend to be slightly older and the medulla is involved more frequently[26]

Evaluation

MRI

The diagnostic test of choice. MRI evaluates status of ventricles, gives optimal assessment of tumor (CT is poor in the posterior fossa) and detects exophytic component. T1WI: almost all are hypointense, homogeneous (excluding cysts). T2WI: increased signal, homogeneous (excluding cysts). Gadolinium enhancement is highly variable.[24]

CT

Most do not enhance on CT, except possibly an exophytic component. If there is marked enhancement, consider other diagnoses (e.g. high grade vermian astrocytoma).

Treatment

Surgery

Biopsy: should *not* be performed when the MRI shows a diffuse infiltrating brainstem lesion[27] (does not change treatment or outcome).

Treatment is usually non-surgical. Exceptions where surgery may be indicated:

1. tumors with a dorsally exophytic component[2]: see below these may protrude into 4th ventricle or CP angle, tend to enhance with IV contrast, tend to be lower grade
2. some success has been achieved with non-exophytic tumors that are *not* malignant astrocytomas (surgery in malignant astrocytomas is without benefit)[25] (detailed follow-up is lacking)
3. shunting for hydrocephalus

Dorsally exophytic tumors

These tumors are generally histologically benign (e.g. gangliogliomas) and are amenable to radical subtotal resection. Prolonged survival is possible, with a low incidence of disease progression at short-term follow-up.[2]

Surgical goals in exophytic tumors include:

1. enhanced survival by subtotal removal of exophytic component[28]: broad attachment to the floor of 4th ventricle is typical and usually precludes complete excision (although some "safe entry" zones have been described[29]). An ultrasonic aspirator facilitates debulking
2. establishing diagnosis: radiographic differentiation of exophytic brainstem gliomas tumors from other lesions (e.g. medulloblastoma, ependymoma and dermoids) may be difficult
3. tumors that demonstrate recurrent growth after resection remained histologically benign and were amenable to re-resection[2]

Complications of surgery generally consisted of exacerbation of pre-operative symptoms (ataxia, cranial nerve palsies…) which usually resolved with time.

Medical

No proven chemotherapeutic regimen. Steroids are usually administered. In pediatrics, there is some indication of response to Temodar® (temozolomide) (p. 595).

Radiation

Traditionally given as 45–55 Gy over a six week period, five days per week. When combined with steroids, symptomatic improvement occurs in 80% of patients.

Possible improved survival with so called "hyperfractionation" where multiple smaller doses per day are used.

Prognosis

Most children with malignant BSG will die within 6–12 months of diagnosis. XRT may not prolong survival in patients with grade III or IV tumors. A subgroup of children have a more slowly growing tumor and may have up to 50% five-year survival. Dorsally exophytic tumors comprised of pilocytic astrocytomas may have a better prognosis.

37.1.11 Tectal gliomas

General information

A topically defined diagnosis generally consisting of low-grade astrocytomas. Considered a benign subgroup of brainstem glioma. Because of location, tends to present with hydrocephalus. Was dramaticllay referred to as "the smallest tumor in the body that can lead to the death of the patient".[30] Focal neurologic findings are rare – diplopia, visual field deficits, nystagmus, Parinaud's syndrome (p. 99), ataxia, seizures… – and are often reversible after the hydrocephalus is corrected.

Epidemiology

Comprises ≈ 6% of surgically treated pediatric brain tumors.[31] Presents primarily in childhood. Median age of patients becoming symptomatic = 6–14 years.[31]

Pathology

Since many of these are not biopsied, meaningful statistical analysis is not possible. Pathologies identified include: WHO II diffuse astrocytoma, pilocytic astrocytomas, WHO II ependymoma, anaplastic astrocytoma, oligodendroglioma & oligoastrocytoma.

Radiographic evaluation

CT scan detects hydrocephalus, but may miss the tumor in ≈ 50%.[32] Calcification on CT has been described in 9–25%.[32,33]

MRI is the study of choice for diagnosis and follow-up. Typically appears as a mass projecting dorsally from the quadrigeminal plate. Isointense on T1WI, iso- or hyperintense on T2WI.[31,34] Enhancement with gadolinium occurs in 18% and is of uncertain prognostic significance.

Treatment

General information

Due to the indolent course, open surgery is not recommended. Options include:

1. VP shunt: the standard treatment for years. Long-term results are good with a functioning shunt
2. endoscopic third ventriculostomy: may avoid the need for a shunt. Endoscopic biopsy[35] may be done at the same time through the same burr hole if it is technically feasible (requires a dilated foramen of Monro, which is often present). Long-term results unknown
3. endoscopic aqueductoplasty (with or without stenting): an option for some. Long-term results unknown

Stereotactic radiosurgery: May be offered for tumor progression (criteria are not defined: radiographic progression may not be associated with clinical deterioration[34]). Dosing should be limited to ≤ 14 Gray at the 50–70% isodose line to avoid radiation-induced side effects.[36]

Prognosis

Tumor progression: described in 15–25%.

Follow-up: no accepted guidelines. Serial neurologic exams and MRIs every 6–12 months has been suggested.[31]

37.2 Pleomorphic xanthoastrocytoma (PXA)

37.2.1 General information

Key concepts

- low-grade glioma, possibly from subpial astrocytes → superficial location, > 90% supratentorial, most common in children or young adults
- mural nodule with cystic component in 25%, meninges involved in > 67%
- pathology: pleomorphic cells (xanthomatous (lipid laden) cells, fibrillary and giant multinucleated astrocytes). Usually circumscribed, occasionally invasive
- WHO grade II unless high mitotic index or necrosis, which is WHO grade III
- treatment: maximal safe resection. XRT or chemo ≈ only for grade III

A low-grade glioma thought to arise from subpial astrocytes which may explain their superficial location and abundance of reticulin fibers. Over 90% are supratentorial. Predilection for temporal lobes (50%), followed by parietal, occipital & frontal lobes. Most have a cystic component (may be multiloculated, but > 90% have a large, single cyst).

37.2.2 Epidemiology

≈ 1% of astrocytomas. Usually occurs in children or young adults (most are < 18 years age). No gender difference.

37.2.3 Clinical

Usual presentation: seizures. May also produce focal deficit or increased ICP.

37.2.4 Differential diagnosis

1. imaging: meningioma is also superficial with dural tail, may also resemble low grade fibrillary astrocytoma
2. pathology: may be confused with anaplastic astrocytoma

37.2.5 Pathology

WHO grade II (MIB is usually < 1%) unless there is a high mitotic index or necrosis which qualifies as WHO grade III "PXA with anaplastic features".[37] Compact, superficial tumor with marked cellular pleomorphism (fibrillary and giant multinucleated astrocytes, large xanthomatous (lipid laden) GFAP staining cells (bespeaking glial origin)), abundant reticulin and frequent perivascular chronic inflammatory cells. The reticulin fibers surround two cell types:

1. spindle cells: fusiform cell shape with elongate nuclei
2. pleomorphic cells: round cells with heterochromic, pleomorphic nuclei that may be mononucleated or multinucleated. Variable intracellular lipid content

Usually circumscribed, occasionally infiltrates cortex. Marked cellular pleomorphism may cause these tumors to be mistaken for anaplastic astrocytoma. Vascular proliferation and necrosis are absent,[38] most but not all lack mitotic figures. Some PXAs undergo anaplastic change.[39] There have also been several reported cases of malignant transformation to anaplastic astrocytoma or glioblastoma.[40]

37.2.6 Imaging

The cyst, when present, may partially enhance on CT or MRI. A mural nodule is present in 25%. May have "dural tail" (67% show leptomeningeal involvement, 13% show involvement of all 3 meningeal layers). Peritumoral edema may be mild to moderate, calcifications are rare.[41]

CT: solid portion of tumor is ill-defined and may be isodense to grey matter.

MRI: T1WI: hypointense cystic component with ill-defined isointense solid component that strongly enhances with gadolinium. T2WI: hyperintense cystic component with ill-defined isointense solid component.

37.2.7 Treatment

1. surgery: primary treatment
   a) gross total resection if it can be accomplished without unacceptable neurologic deficit, otherwise subtotal resection
   b) extent of resection: most strongly associated with recurrence free survival[42]
   c) incomplete resections should be followed since these tumors may grow very slowly over many years before retreatment is necessary, and repeat excision should be considered
2. radiation therapy: controversial
   a) literature suggests either no difference in overall survival or possibly a trend toward prolonged survival[38]
   b) considered with: residual disease, high mitotic index, or necrosis
3. chemotherapy: role not defined

37.2.8 Prognosis

Overall survival with gross total resection or subtotal resection, with or without radiation and chemotherapy: 5 years = 80%, 10 years = 71%.[37]

Extent of resection, mitotic index, and necrosis appear to be the best predictors of outcome.[41,42]

References

[1] Burger PC, Scheithauer BW. Atlas of Tumor Pathology. Tumors of the Central Nervous System. Washington, D.C.: Armed Forces Institute of Pathology; 1994

[2] Pollack IF, Hoffman HJ, Humphreys RP, Becker L. The Long-Term Outcome After Surgical Treatment of Dorsally Exophytic Brain-Stem Gliomas. J Neurosurg. 1993; 78:859–863

[3] Coakley KJ, Huston J, Scheithauer BW, Forbes G, Kelly PJ. Pilocytic Astrocytomas: Well-Demarcated Magnetic Resonance Appearance Despite Frequent Infiltration Histologically. Mayo Clin Proc. 1995; 70:747–751

[4] Hayostek CJ, Shaw EG, Scheithauer B, et al. Astrocytomas of the Cerebellum: A Comparative Clinicopathologic Study of Pilocytic and Diffuse Astrocytomas. Cancer. 1993; 72:856–869

[5] Bernell WR, Kepes JJ, Seitz EP. Late Malignant Recurrence of Childhood Cerebellar Astrocytoma. J Neurosurg. 1972; 37:470–474

[6] Schwartz AM, Ghatak NR. Malignant Transformation of Benign Cerebellar Astrocytoma. Cancer. 1990; 65:333–336

[7] Wallner KE, Gonzales MF, Edwards MSB, Wara WM, Sheline GE. Treatment of juvenile pilocytic astrocytoma. J Neurosurg. 1988; 69:171–176

[8] Zimmerman RA, Bilaniuk CT, Bruno LA, et al. CT of Cerebellar Astrocytoma. Am J Roentgenol. 1978; 130:929-933

[9] Section of Pediatric Neurosurgery of the American Association of Neurological Surgeons. Pediatric Neurosurgery. New York 1982

[10] Youmans JR. Neurological Surgery. Philadelphia 1990

[11] Ringertz N, Nordenstam H. Cerebellar Astrocytoma. J Neuropathol Exp Neurol. 1951; 10:343–367

[12] Gol A. Cerebellar Astrocytomas in Children. Am J Dis Child. 1963; 106:21–24

[13] Winston K, Gilles FH, Leviton A, et al. Cerebellar Gliomas in Children. J Natl Cancer Inst. 1977; 58:833–838

[14] Austin EJ, Alvord EC. Recurrences of Cerebellar Astrocytomas: A Violation of Collins' Law. J Neurosurg. 1988; 68:41–47

[15] Packer RJ, Lange B, Ater J, et al. Carboplatin and Vincristine for Recurrent and Newly Diagnosed Low-Grade Gliomas of Childhood. J Clin Oncol. 1993; 11:850–856

[16] Bucy PC, Thieman PW. Astrocytomas of the Cerebellum. A Study of Patients Operated Upon Over 28 Years Ago. Arch Neurol. 1968; 18:14–19

[17] Stein BM, Tenner MS, Fraser RAR. Hydrocephalus Following Removal of Cerebellar Astrocytomas in Children. J Neurosurg. 1972; 36:763–768

[18] Tihan T, Fisher PG, Kepner JL, Godfraind C, McComb RD, Goldthwaite PT, Burger PC. Pediatric astrocytomas with monomorphous pilomyxoid features and a less favorable outcome. J Neuropathol Exp Neurol. 1999; 58:1061–1068

[19] Ceppa EP, Bouffet E, Griebel R, Robinson C, Tihan T. The pilomyxoid astrocytoma and its relationship to pilocytic astrocytoma: report of a case and a critical review of the entity. J Neurooncol. 2007; 81:191–196

[20] Arulrajah S, Huisman TA. Pilomyxoid astrocytoma of the spinal cord with cerebrospinal fluid and peritoneal metastasis. Neuropediatrics. 2008; 39:243–245

[21] Packer RJ, Nicholson HS, Vezina LG, Johnson DL. Brainstem gliomas. Neurosurg Clin N Am. 1992; 3:863–879

[22] Laurent JP, Cheek WR. Brain Tumors in Children. J Pediatr Neurosci. 1985; 1:15–32

[23] Reigel DH, Scarff TB, Woodford JE. Biopsy of Pediatric Brain Stem Tumors. Childs Brain. 1979; 5:329–340

[24] Epstein FJ, Farmaer J-P. Brain-Stem Glioma Growth Patterns. J Neurosurg. 1993; 78:408–412

[25] Epstein F, McCleary EL. Intrinsic Brain-Stem Tumors of Childhood: Surgical Indications. J Neurosurg. 1986; 64:11–15

[26] Garcia CA, McGarry PA, Collada M. Ganglioglioma of the Brain Stem. Case Report. J Neurosurg. 1984; 60:431–434

[27] Albright AL, Packer RJ, Zimmerman R, et al. Magnetic Resonance Scans Should Replace Biopsies for the Diagnosis of Diffuse Brain Stem Gliomas: A Report from the Children's Cancer Group. Neurosurgery. 1993; 33:1026–1030

[28] Hoffman HJ, Becker L, Craven MA. A Clinically and Pathologically Distinct Group of Benign Brainstem Gliomas. Neurosurgery. 1980; 7:243–248

[29] Kyoshima K, Kobayashi S, Gibo H, Kuroyanagi T. A Study of Safe Entry Zones via the Floor of the Fourth Ventricle for Brain-Stem Lesions. J Neurosurg. 1993; 78:987–993

[30] Kernohan WJ, Armed Forces Institute of Pathology. In: Tumors of the central nervous system. Atlas of Tumor Pathology. Washington, DC 1952:19–42

[31] Stark AM, Fritsch MJ, Claviez A, Dorner L, Mehdorn HM. Management of tectal glioma in childhood. Pediatr Neurol. 2005

[32] Bognar L, Turjman F, Villanyi E, Mottolese C, Guyotat J, Fischer C, Jouvet A, Lapras C. Tectal plate gliomas. Part II: CT scans and MR imaging of tectal gliomas. Acta Neurochir (Wien). 1994; 127:48–54

[33] Pollack IF, Pang D, Albright AL. The long-term outcome in children with late-onset aqueductal stenosis resulting from benign intrinsic tectal tumors. J Neurosurg. 1994; 80:681–688

[34] Grant GA, Avellino AM, Loeser JD, Ellenbogen RG, Berger MS, Roberts TS. Management of intrinsic gliomas of the tectal plate in children. A ten-year review. Pediatr Neurosurg. 1999; 31:170–176

[35] Oka K, Kin Y, Go Y, Ueno Y, Hirakawa K, Tomonaga M, Inoue T, Yoshioka S. Neuroendoscopic approach to tectal tumors: a consecutive series. J Neurosurg. 1999; 91:964–970

[36] Kihlstrom L, Lindquist C, Lindquist M, Karlsson B. Stereotactic radiosurgery for tectal low-grade gliomas. Acta Neurochir Suppl. 1994; 62:55–57

[37] Fouladi M, Jenkins J, Burger P, Langston J, Merchant T, Heideman R, Thompson S, Sanford A, Kun L, Gajjar A. Pleomorphic xanthoastrocytoma: favorable outcome after complete surgical resection. Neurooncol. 2001; 3:184–192

[38] Kepes JJ, Rubinstein LJ, Eng LF. Pleomorphic Xanthoastrocytoma: A Distinctive Meningeal Glioma of Young Subjects with Relatively Favorable Prognosis. A Study of 12 Cases. Cancer. 1979; 44:1839–1852

[39] Weldon-Linne CM, Victor TA, Groothuis DR, Vick NA. Pleomorphic Xanthoastrocytoma: Ultrastructural and Immunohistochemical Study of a Case with a Rapidly Fatal Outcome Following Surgery. Cancer. 1983; 52:2055–2063

[40] Kumar S, Retnam TM, Menon G, Nair S, Bhattacharya RN, Radhakrishnan VV. Cerebellar hemisphere, an uncommon location for pleomorphic xanthoastrocytoma and lipidized glioblastoma multiformis. Neurol India. 2003; 51:246–247

[41] Pahapill PA, Ramsay DA, Del Maestro RF. Pleomorphic xanthoastrocytoma: case report and analysis of the literature concerning the efficacy of resection and the significance of necrosis. Neurosurgery. 1996; 38:822–8; discussion 828-9

[42] Giannini C, Scheithauer BW, Burger PC, Brat DJ, Wollan PC, Lach B, O'Neill BP. Pleomorphic xanthoastrocytoma: what do we really know about it? Cancer. 1999; 85:2033–2045

38 Oligodendroglial Tumors and Tumors of the Ependyma, Choroid Plexus, and Other Neuroepithelial Tumors

38.1 Oligodendroglial tumors

38.1.1 General information

Key concepts

- frequently presents with seizures
- predilection for the frontal lobes
- histology: classic features of "fried egg" cytoplasm (on permanent pathology) & "chicken wire" vasculature are unreliable. Calcifications are common
- grading: controversial. Recommendation: low grade and high grade
- recommended treatment: surgery for mass effect or low grade lesions (high-grade lesions are controversial). Chemotherapy for all (with or without surgery), XRT only for anaplastic transformation

38.1.2 Epidemiology

Oligodendroglioma (ODG) have long been thought to comprise only ≈ 2–4% of primary brain tumors[1,2] or 4–8% of cerebral gliomas[2]; but recent evidence indicates these tumors have been underdiagnosed (many are misinterpreted as fibrillary astrocytomas, especially the infiltrative portion of these tumors) and ODGs may represent up to 25–33% of glial tumors.[3,4] Ratio of male:female = 3:2. Primarily a tumor of adults: average age ≈ 40 years (peak between 26–46 years), but with a smaller earlier peak in childhood between 6–12 years.[5] CSF metastases reportedly occur in up to 10%, but 1% may be a more realistic estimate.[1] Spinal ODGs comprise only ≈ 2.6% of intramedullary tumors of the cord and filum.

38.1.3 Clinical

Classic presentation of ODG: a patient with seizures for many years prior to the diagnosis being made when they would present with an apoplectic event due to peritumoral intracerebral hemorrhage. This scenario is less common in the CT/MRI era.

Seizures are the presenting symptoms in ≈ 50–80% of cases.[1,5] The remainder of presenting symptoms are nonspecific for ODG, and are more often related to local mass effect and less commonly to ↑ ICP. Presenting symptoms are shown in ▶ Table 38.2.

38.1.4 Evaluation

Calcifications are seen in 28–60% of ODGs on plain radiographs,[1] and on 90% of CTs.

Table 38.1 Location of oligodendrogliomas

Location	%
supratentorial	**>90%**
frontal lobes	45%
hemisphere (outside frontal lobes)	40%
within third or lateral ventricle	15%
infratentorial + spinal cord	**<10%**

Table 38.2 Presenting symptoms in 208 oligodendrogliomas[1]

Symptom	%
seizures	57%
headache	22%
mental status changes	10%
vertigo/nausea	9%

Table 38.3 Features associated with low-grade and high-grade oligodendrogliomas

Feature	WHO II (low grade)	WHO III (high grade)
contrast enhancement on CT or MRI	absent	present
endothelial proliferation on histology	absent	present
pleomorphism (large variability in nuclear and cytoplasmic size and shape)	absent	present
tumor proliferation (evidenced by mitotic figures or high MIB-1 index[a])	absent	present
astrocytic component	absent	present

[a] for information on the MIB-1 index (p. 599)

38.1.5 Pathology

General information

73% of tumors have microscopic calcifications.[6] Isolated tumor cells consistently penetrate largely intact parenchyma, an associated solid tumor component may or may not be present.[4] The solid portion, when present, classically demonstrates lucent perinuclear halos giving a "fried egg" appearance (actually an artifact of *formalin* fixation, which is not present on frozen section and may make diagnosis difficult on frozen). A "chicken-wire" vascular pattern has also been described.[7] These features are felt to be unreliable, and cells with monotonous round nuclei (often in cellular sheets) with an eccentric rim of eosinophilic cytoplasm lacking obvious cell processes are more consistent features.[8]

16% of hemispheric ODGs are *cystic*[6] (cysts form from coalescence of microcysts from micro-hemorrhages, unlike astrocytomas which actively secrete fluid).

33–41% have a component of ependymal or neoplastic astrocytic cells (so called oligoastrocytomas or mixed gliomas[9] or collision tumors (p. 645)).

GFAP staining: Since most ODGs contain microtubules instead of glial filaments,[10] ODGs usually do not stain for GFAP (p. 598) although some do.[11] In mixed gliomas, the astrocytic component may stain for GFAP.

Grading

A work-in-progress. Historically, a number of attempts at grading ODGs have been proposed and then abandoned because of lack of prognostic significance (for a review, see reference[8]). For example, the system of Smith et al.[12] (see below) was based on 5 histopathologic features which have been shown not to be independent determinants of tumor progression (only pleomorphism has been shown to be statistically correlated with survival[8]). Necrosis does not appear to reliably predict a poor prognosis.[8]

For prognostic purposes, it is suggested that ODGs be stratified into *two groups*:

- oligodendroglioma (WHO grade II) or low grade
- anaplastic oligodendroglioma (WHO grade III) or high grade.[2,8]

Although there is not uniform agreement on the means for differentiating the two, the factors shown in ▶ Table 38.3 should be taken into account as they have been demonstrated to have prognostic significance. Using the spatial grading system for low grade gliomas, no ODGs are of the Type 1 tumor (solid tumor without infiltrative component).

Table 38.4 Smith grading of oligodendrogliomas

Grade	Nuclear to cytoplasm ratio	Maximal cell density	Pleomorphism	Endothelial proliferation	Necrosis
A	↓	↓	–	–	–
B	↑[a]	↑[a]	+[a]	–	–
C	↑	↑	+	+	–
D	↑	↑	+	+	+

↑ means high; ↓ means low; + means feature is present; – means feature is absent
[a]considered grade B if one or more of these are present

Smith grading system

See reference.[12]

Tumors composed of at least 51% oligodendroglial elements are graded on 5 histologic features:

1. maximal nuclear/cytoplasmic ratio: the normal oligodendroglial cell ratio is considered low (↓), anything above that is coded as high (↑)
2. maximal cell density: coded according to predominant appearance of sample. Cell density similar to white matter is low (↓), sheets of cells with little or no intervening extracellular neuropil is high (↑)
3. pleomorphism: coded according to predominant appearance of sample. Coded as present (+) if there is large variability in nuclear and cytoplasmic size and shape
4. endothelial proliferation: coded present (+) if 1 or more instance noted
5. necrosis: coded present (+) if 1 or more instance of coagulation necrosis and/or areas of debris filled with macrophages noted

Tumor grade is then determined from ▶ Table 38.4.

38.1.6 Treatment

General information

Σ

Recommendation (see text for details). Following an appropriate surgical procedure (if indicated), chemotherapy is the primary treatment modality. XRT is reserved for anaplastic transformation, if it should occur.[8]

Chemotherapy

Most ODGs respond to some form of chemotherapy, usually in < 3 mos, often with a reduction in size. The response is variable in degree and duration.[13] No pathological or clinical feature of high-grade ODGs has been identified that reliably predicts response to chemotherapy. However, allelic loss of chromosome 1p, and combined loss of chromosome arms 1p and 19q, are associated with response to chemo; and losses of both 1p and 19q were associated with longer tumor-free survival after chemo.[14]

The most experience is with PCV (procarbazine 60 mg/m^2 IV, CCNU AKA lomustine (CeeNU ®) 110 mg/m^2 PO, and vincristine 1.4 mg/m^2 IV, all given on a 29 day cycle repeated every 6 weeks).[15,16] Also studied: temozolomide for recurrent anaplastic oligoastrocytoma showed some efficacy.[17]

Surgery

Indications for surgery:

1. ODGs with significant mass effect regardless of grade: surgery decreases the need for corticosteroids, reduces symptoms and prolongs survival[8]

38

2. tumors without significant mass effect:
   a) *low-grade* ODGs and oligoastrocytoma: surgery is recommended for resectable lesions. Gross total removal should be attempted when possible (survival is improved even more than with astrocytomas[18]), but not at the expense of neurologic function
   b) *high-grade* ODGs: data for improved survival is less convincing, and some studies show no advantage of gross total removal over partially resected or biopsied-only high-grade lesions.[8] Older dogma was that aggressive removal leads to longer survival,[19] and results in fewer side effects than "partial debulking" operations[20]

Grossly, the tumor appears as a pink to red, friable mass. There may be a false plane of demarcation between tumor and what appears to be normal brain.

Postoperative radiation

Benefits of postoperative irradiation is controversial.[5] In a retrospective analysis with no set selection criteria, survival was better in patients receiving > 45 Gy.[21] In another series, no difference in 5 year survival following surgery was seen with or without XRT (amount of radiation not specified).[22] Radiation side effects of memory loss, dementia and personality changes are more common with the longer survival seen in many of these cases.[23]

38.1.7 Prognosis

Pure ODGs have a better prognosis than mixed oligoastrocytomas which are better than pure astrocytomas (an oligodendroglial component, no matter how small, confers a better prognosis).

With the Smith grading system (see above), median survival in 323 cases was as follows: grade A was 94 months, grades B & C were not statistically different and were 51 and 45 months respectively, and grade D was 17 months.

10 year survival of 10–30% has been quoted for tumors that are completely or predominantly ODGs.[21] As a group, median survival for surgically treated lesions is given as 35 months post-op (mean 52 months).[1]

The presence of calcifications is debated as a prognosticator; in one series, calcified ODG on plain films had a longer median survival of 108 months (vs. 58 months for non calcified).[1]

Frontal lobe ODGs survived longer than those in temporal lobes (37 months vs. 28 months postoperative survival),[1] possibly due to increased ease of radical resection with the former.

Chromosomal 1p loss (or combined 1p and 19q loss) is also associated with longer survival.[14,24]

38.2 Oligoastrocytic tumors

38.2.1 Molecular biology

May show changes typical for diffuse astrocytoma (TP53 mutation & LOH on 17p) or for ODG (LOH on 1p and 19q). No molecular genetic markers have been identified to distinguish oligoastrocytoma from either astrocytoma or ODG. Unlike ODG, the prognostic/therapeutic value of LOH on 1p is less clear.[24]

Oligoastrocytoma (WHO grade II)

Two distinct neoplastic cell types, 1 type resembles oligodendroglioma cells, and the other resembles cells in diffuse astrocytomas. Some cells may have features of both. The 2 cell types may be segregated or diffusely admixed.

38

Anaplastic oligoastrocytoma (WHO grade III)

Increased cellularity, nuclear atypia, pleomorphism, and high mitotic activity. Necrosis and microvascular proliferation may be present. Differentiating from GBM may be difficult since GMS may have areas resembling anaplastic ODG (the term "glioblastoma with oligodendroglioma component" is a disputed term suggested for these – unproven suggestion that survival may be better than for ordinary GBM[25]).

38.3 Ependymal tumors

38.3.1 Ependymoma

General information regarding intracranial and spinal ependymomas

Ependymomas arise from ependymal cells lining the cerebral ventricles and the central canal of the spinal cord. They may occur anywhere along the neuraxis, in pediatrics they are most common in the posterior fossa (see below), in adults they tend to be intraspinal (p. 788).

Epidemiology

- intracranial: comprises only ≈ 5–6% of intracranial gliomas, 69% occur in children,[26] comprise 9% of pediatric brain tumors.[27] Incidence of pediatric intracranial ependymomas: ≈ 200 cases/yr in the U.S.
- spinal: ≈ 60% of spinal cord gliomas (the most common primary intramedullary spinal cord glioma below the mid-thoracic region – see Intramedullary spinal cord tumors (p. 787) – 96% occur in adults,[26] especially those of filum terminale; see myxopapillary ependymoma below).

The mean age at diagnosis is shown in ▶ Table 38.5.

Ependymomas have the potential to spread via the CSF through the neuraxis (including to the spinal cord), a process known as "seeding", resulting in so-called "drop mets" in the spinal cord in 11%. The incidence is higher with higher grade.[27] Systemic spread occurs on rare occasion.

Pathology

Although they are usually circumscribed with a covering layer of ependyma, ependymomas may be invasive.

Classification is a work in progress. Ependymomas from different locations (p-fossa, supratentorial, spinal cord) are genetically distinct.[28] The World Health Organization (WHO) classification of ependymal tumors:

1. ependymoma (WHO II) – variants:
   a) cellular
   b) papillary: "classic lesion" occurring in brain or spinal cord. Can metastasize in up to 30% of cases. Dark, small nuclei. 2 cytoplasmic patterns:
      - differentiation along glial line: these form perivascular pseudorosettes (areas of radiating processes lacking nuclei surrounding blood vessels) which, when they occur, are diagnostic
      - cuboidal cells: these can form true rosettes (where the cytoplasmic processes extend to form a lumen-like structure with no central blood vessel – as if trying to recreate an ependymal lining e.g. of a ventricle). True rosettes are classically associated with ependymomas, however, perivascular pseudorosettes are more common
   c) clear cell
   d) tanycytic: rare. Tumor cells appear similar to "ependymoglia" or "tanycytes" (stretched cells present to a limited degree in the normal CNS). True rosettes are absent. No preference for age, sex or location within CNS.[29] Treatment of choice: gross total resection[29]
2. myxopapillary ependymoma: (WHO I) distinctive, occurs only in filum terminale. Papillary, with microcystic vacuoles and mucosubstance

Table 38.5 Mean age at diagnosis of ependymoma[26]

Location (in 101 patients)	All patients (yrs)	Children (yrs) (age < 15 yrs)
intracranial	17.5	5
infratentorial	14.5	4.5
supratentorial	22	6.5
intraspinal	40	
intramedullary	47	
cauda region	32	

3. **subependymomas:** (WHO I) typically occur in anterior lateral ventricles or posterior fourth ventricle, with prominent role of subependymal glial cells. Not uncommon at autopsy, rarely surgical. Classically do not enhance; see Ependymal and subependymal enhancement (p.1385)
4. anaplastic ependymomas: (WHO III) pleomorphism, multinucleation, giant cells, mitotic figures, vascular changes and areas of necrosis; the term ependymoblastoma has occasionally been used for more anaplastic lesions, but this term is best reserved for a distinct, rare childhood primitive neuroectodermal tumor (p.666). It is unclear if the degree of anaplasia has any effect on outcome

General information for intracranial ependymomas

Key concepts

- usually benign tumors, often fibrillary with epithelial appearance. Perivascular pseudorosettes or true rosettes may be seen in classic (papillary) form
- most often occur in the floor of the 4th ventricle, presenting with hydrocephalus (increased ICP) and cranial nerve VI & VII palsies
- evaluation: includes imaging the entire neuraxis (usually with enhanced MRI: cervical, thoracic, lumbar & brain) because of potential for seeding through CSF
- worse prognosis the younger the patient (especially age < 24 months)
- treatment: the best outcomes are associated with gross total removal (no enhancing tumor on post-op MRI) followed by XRT. XRT may be withheld for age < 3
- do LP ≈ 2 weeks post-op to send ≈ 10 cc of CSF for cytology for prognostication

Usually well circumscribed and benign (although anaplastic (malignant) ependymomas do occur), commonly arises in the floor of the fourth ventricle (60–70% are infratentorial, all of these occur near 4th ventricle,[26] they comprise 25% of tumors in region of 4th ventricle[30(p 2792)]). Children with p-fossa ependymomas often have anaplastic tumors with a higher risk of spread through the neuraxis. Supratentorial ependymomas are often cystic. Rarely occur outside the CNS in: mediastinum, lung or ovaries. Although not as malignant histologically as medulloblastomas, ependymomas have a worse prognosis due to their propensity to invade the obex which precludes complete removal.

Clinical

Symptoms

Mostly those of posterior fossa mass with increased ICP[30(p 2795)] (from hydrocephalus) and cranial nerve involvement.

Symptoms of increased ICP:

1. headache: 80%
2. N/V: 75%
3. ataxia or vertigo: 60%
4. seizures: only in ≈ 30% of supratentorial lesions; comprise only 1% of patients with intracranial tumors presenting with seizures

Signs

Cranial nerve involvement: invasion of the floor of the 4th ventricle may involve the facial colliculus producing facial nerve palsy (p.576) (involvement of internal genu of VII) and abducens palsy (from VI nucleus).

Evaluation

MRI: imaging study of choice. Image the entire craniospinal axis with and without contrast because of possibility of drop mets. Usually appears as a mass in the floor of fourth ventricle, often with obstructive hydrocephalus. May be difficult to distinguish from medulloblastoma (MBS) radiographically, see differentiating features (p.1365).

CT: not as detailed for evaluation of posterior fossa.

Myelogram: water-soluble contrast myelography is about as sensitive as gadolinium enhanced MRI in detecting "drop mets." Myelography also provides CSF for cytology for staging purposes.

Treatment

Surgical resection

Goal of surgery: maximal possible resection of intracranial portion without causing neurological deficits (since extent of resection is an important prognosticator). Gross total resection may not possible when invasion of the floor is extensive, or when tumor extends through the foramen of Luschka (bradycardia may prevent GTR).

2 weeks postoperatively, perform LP to look for "drop mets": 10 cc of CSF is sent for cytology to quantitate (if any) number of malignant cells (may be used to follow treatment). If LP is positive, then by definition there are drop mets. If negative, it is not as helpful (sensitivity is not high). CSF from an EVD is not as sensitive as LP.

Lesions in fourth ventricle region are approached via midline suboccipital craniectomy.

Radiation therapy (XRT)

Ependymomas rank 2nd only to medulloblastomas in radiosensitivity. XRT is administered after surgical excision (survival is improved with post-op XRT[26,31]: 50% survival time was 2 yrs longer with XRT than without,[26] and 5-year survival increased from 20–40% without XRT to 40–80% with XRT[31]), however, for patients age < 3 years, see below.

1. cranial XRT
   a) traditional therapy: 45–48 Gy to tumor bed[31] (recurrence treated with additional 15–20 Gy)[30(p 2797)]
   b) recent recommendations: 3-D conformal XRT with higher doses (59.4 Gy delivered to tumor bed + 1 cm margins)[32]
   c) intensity modulated proton beam therapy appears equivalent in terms of local control, but may be better at sparing normal tissue[33]
2. spinal XRT: most radiate only if drop mets or if positive CSF cytology (however, prophylactic spinal is controversial[34])
   a) low dose XRT to entire spinal axis (median dose = 30 Gy in one series[31])
   b) boost to any regions showing drop mets
3. XRT is undesirable in age < 3 due to side effects. XRT was avoided in ≈ 30% of patients < 3 years age with comparable survival when XRT was reserved for treatment failures.[35,36] This concept of selective XRT may be applicable to older children as well[37]

Chemotherapy

Role is very limited.

1. has little impact on newly diagnosed cases. Adjuvant chemo after XRT in patients > 3 years showed no benefit
2. may reduce vascularity of ependymomas which may facilitate GTR (sometimes in a second stage operation)
3. may be considered for infants < ≈ 3 years age to delay use of XRT (see above)
4. chemo at the time of recurrence may arrest tumor progression for short periods

Outcome

Operative mortality[30(p 2797)]: 20–50% in early series; more recently: 5–8%.

Operative morbidity: advise patients/families pre-op of the likelihood need for post-op gastric feeding tube (G-tube) and tracheostomy (these may be temporary).

Age: peds vs. adults: 5-year survival is 20–30% in the pediatric group,[27,38] compared with up to 80% in adults. Patients 24–35 months old did better (5-year survival = 73%) than those younger than 24 months (26% 5-YS) or those older than 36 months (36% 5-YS).[39]

Pathology: prognosis is worse with anaplastic ependymoma (WHO III) than with "standard" grade (WHO II).[40,41] However, excluding WHO III tumors, malignant features in an ependymoma do not necessarily portend a worse prognosis.[42]

Extent of resection: the risk of recurrence is highest following subtotal resection. Gross total resection (GTR) (surgical) of primary intracranial tumor followed by craniospinal XRT as outlined above yields 41% 5-year survival.

Treatment failure: WHO Grade II tumors tend to recur initially at the site of origin.[40] However, primary failure in 9–25% of patients is via drop mets.[39,43]

38.4 Neuronal and mixed glial tumors

38.4.1 Desmoplastic infantile astrocytoma/ganglioglioma

The former entities "desmoplastic cerebral astrocytoma of infancy" and "desmoplastic infantile ganglioglioma" have been combined to "desmoplastic infantile astrocytoma and ganglioglioma" (DIG).[44] A lesion with either astrocytic or dual glioneuronal differentiation. Prognosis is usually favorable.

38.4.2 Central neurocytoma

General information

Key concepts

- Rare, WHO Grade II neuronal tumor
- Primarily seen in young adults
- Gross total resection can be curative
- If MIB-1 labeling index > 2-4%, there is an increased risk of recurrence after subtotal resection
- If MIB-1 labeling is elevated, radiation therapy after subtotal resection can reduce the risk of recurrence

Central neurocytoma is a WHO Grade II neuronal tumor that constitutes 0.1-0.5% of brain tumors. These are generally attached to the septum pellucidum within the lateral ventricles or they are within the third ventricle. Incidence peaks in the 3rd decade, but they can also present in children and the elderly. No gender predominates. The most common presentation is with increased intracranial pressure and ventriculomegaly.[45,46]

Pathology

Central neurocytoma cells have small, round nuclei. Cells often have a "fried egg" appearance on H&E staining, which can mimic oligodendroglioma. There are two primary architectures: honeycomb (also mimicking oligodendroglioma) and fibrillary. Rosettes can also be seen. Immunohistochemisty is often positive for neuronal markers synaptophysin and Neu-N. When the diagnosis is not clear, electron microscopy is used to demonstrate neuronal features including: a prominent golgi apparatus, parallel microtubules, and dense core neurosecretory granules.[45,46]1p/19q deletion has not been reported in central neurocytoma, but it can be seen in extraventricular neurocytoma.[47]

Variants

1. Extraventricular neurocytomais a more rare subtype that may be located in the cerebral parenchyma, cerebellum, thalamus, brainstem, pineal region, and spinal cord. Tumor cells can be focally infiltrative into surrounding tissue. Pathology findings include vessel wall hyalinization and ganglionic differentiation. Immunohistochemistry is positive for synaptophysin in the cytoplasm and neuropil. Neu-N staining is often positive. Electron microscopy findings include round nuclei and neurosecretory granules, as in central neurocytoma. 1p and 19q deletions, in isolation or in combination, can be seen in extraventricular neurocytoma.[47]
2. Liponeurocytomais a lipid-laden neurocytoma that most often appears in the cerebellum. Rarely, similar tumors can also appear in the lateral ventricles. Some authors suggest the more inclusive name "Liponeurocytoma" should replace the separate WHO classification of "Cerebellar liponeurocytoma." Others contend that the supratentorial exceptions are central neurocytomas which contain neurocytes that underwent lipidization, instead of having actual adipose metaplasia.[48]

Imaging

CT scan: 25-50% of these tumors show calcifications. Tumors are usually iso- to hyperdense, with hypodense areas that represent cystic degeneration.[45]

MRI: Tumors appear heterogeneously isointense on T1 and hyperintense on T2. MR spectroscopy often shows a high glycine peak.[49]

Moderate to strong contrast enhancement shows on both CT and MR images.[46]

Treatment

1. Total resection is often curative. After gross total resection, radiation therapy is generally not necessary.[45]
2. Subtotal resection can be followed by stereotactic radiosurgery, especially if MIB-1 labeling is > 2-4%.[45,46,49,50]
3. Chemotherapy for recurrent and inoperable tumors has been reported with many agents, including: alkylating agents (carmustine, cyclophosphamide, ifosfamide, lomustine), platinum-based agents (carboplatin and cisplatin), etoposide, topotecan, and vincristine.[49,50]
4. After treatment, patients should have long-term follow-up imaging as surveillance for tumor recurrence.[46]

Prognosis

Total resection can be curative.[45,49] Recurrence risk after subtotal resection varies with the MIB-1 labeling index. In a 2004 study of neurocytomas with MIB-1 labeling > 2%, the 5-year local control rate after subtotal resection alone was 7%, but if subtotal resection was followed with radiation therapy it was 70%.[50] In a 2013 study, patients with MIB-1 labeling < 4% had no recurrence at 4 years after subtotal resection. If MIB-1 labeling was > 4% at subtotal resection, recurrence was found in 50% of patients at 2 years and 75% at 4 years.[49] Most local recurrences occur within 3-6 years. Recurrence is more common in extraventricular neurocytoma.[50]

38.4.3 Cerebellar liponeurocytoma

Née lipomatous medulloblastoma. Occurs exclusively in cerebellum of adults (mean age: 50 years). No gender preference.

Histology: clusters of neoplastic neurocytes with lipidization (resembling adipocytes) with background of small neoplastic cells with morphological features more suggestive of neurocytes. Synaptophysin (p.600) and MAP-2 immunostaining is consistent and diffuse, focal GFAP staining is common. Usually no mitotic figures. MIB-1 index 1–3%.

38.4.4 Dysembryoplastic neuroepithelial tumors (DNT) or (DNET)

See references.[51,52]

Epidemiology

Incidence: not accurately known because the diagnosis may be missed. Estimated range: 0.8–5% of all primary brain tumors. Typically occurs in children and young adults.

Most common locations: temporal or frontal. Parietal and especially occipital lobe involvement is rare. DNTs have been reported in the cerebellum, pons & basal ganglia.

Pathology

A WHO Grade I glioma. Thought to arise embryologically from the secondary germinal layer (which includes subependymal layer, cerebellar external granular layer, hippocampal dentate fascia & subpial granular layer).

Multinodularity at low-power is a key feature, and the primary constituent cells are oligodendrocytes and to a lesser extent, astrocytes that are often pilocytic. Occasionally difficult to differentiate from oligodendroglioma.

38

Two distinct forms[53] (do not appear to have different prognoses):

1. simple form: glioneural elements consisting of axon bundles perpendicular to the cortical surface, lined with oligodendroglial-like cells that are S-100 positive and GFAP negative. Normal appearing neurons floating in a pale eosinophilic matrix are scattered between these columns (no resemblance to ganglion cells, unlike gangliogliomas)
2. complex form: glioneural elements as described above in the simple form, with glial nodules scattered throughout. The glial component may mimic a low-grade fibrillary astrocytoma. Foci of cortical dysplasia occur

Clinical

Typically associated with longstanding medically intractable seizures, usually complex partial. Symptoms usually begin before age 20.

Imaging

Cortical lesions with no surrounding edema and no midline mass effect.

CT: hypodense with distinct margins. Deformity of overlying calvaria is common.

MRI: T1WI: hypointense. T2WI: hyperintense, septations may be seen. If there is enhancement, it is usually nodular.

PET scan: hypometabolic with [18F]-fluorodeoxyglucose. Negative [11C]-methionine uptake (unlike all other gliomas).

Outcome

Seizure control: usually improves after surgery. Degree of control seems to correlate with completeness of removal. Improvement in seizures correlates inversely with the duration of intractable seizures.

Recurrence/continued growth: recurrence after complete removal, or tumor growth after partial resection is rare. Adjuvant treatment (XRT, chemotherapy…) is of no benefit in these benign tumors. Mitoses or endothelial proliferation, seen on occasion, do not affect outcome. Malignant transformation is very rare.

38.4.5 Dysplastic gangliocytoma of cerebellum (Lhermitte-Duclos disease)

General information

AKA: ganglioneuroma of the cerebellum, purkinjoma, granular cell hypertrophy of the cerebellum, gangliocytoma dysplasticum, hamartoma of the cerebellum.

Rare (200 case reports[54]) cerebellar lesion with features of both a malformation and a low grade (WHO I) neoplasm that has the propensity to progress (enlarge) and recur after surgery. May be focal or diffuse. Diffuse enlargement of cerebellar folia.

Strongly associated with Cowden syndrome: AKA multiple hamartoma syndrome. Autosomal dominant. Incidence: 1 in 250,000 live births.[55] Associated with thyroid, breast & uterine Ca, mucosal neuromas & meningiomas.

Pathology

Derangement of normal laminar cellular architecture of the cerebellum with:
1. thickening of the outer molecular cell layer
2. loss of middle Purkinje cell layer
3. infiltration of inner granular cell layer with dysplastic ganglion cells

Clinical

Typically a middle aged *adult* with signs and symptoms of a cerebellar mass. May also present with hydrocephalus or may be an incidental finding.

Imaging

CT: hypo- to iso-dense, nonenhancing lesion with mass effect.

MRI: T1WI: hypo- to iso-intense. T2WI: hyperintense, heterogeneous. Nonenhancing. Characteristic striated appearance[56] (tiger stripes) due to widened cerebellar folia. May contain calcifications. DWI: hyperintense. ADC map: hypointense.

NB: in a child with MRI findings of Lhermitte-Duclos disease (LDD) (even if classic), a medulloblastoma is statistically more likely[57,58] (especially medulloblastoma with extensive nodularity[59] (MBEN)).

Treatment

Controversial. A few cases with a benign course have been described.[60] Shunting for hydrocephalus. Biopsy is recommended[58] particularly for pediatric cases to rule-out medulloblastoma. Surgical excision may be considered when there is significant mass effect.[61] Efficacy of XRT is unknown.

38.5 Choroid plexus tumors

38.5.1 General information

Most are histologically benign (choroid plexus papilloma (CPP), WHO I), although intermediate (atypical choroid plexus papilloma, WHO II) and malignant tumors (choroid plexus carcinoma (CPC), WHO III) may occur. Malignant degeneration from WHO I or II to grade III was seen in 2 out of 124 patients with 59 months mean follow-up.[62] All may produce drop mets in the CSF, but WHO III do so more commonly. Although usually slow growing, they sometimes grow rapidly.

Atypical CPP have more mitotic figures than CPP without frank signs of malignancy seen in CPC,[63] and up to 2 of the following 4 features may be observed: increased cellularity, nuclear pleomorphism, blurring of the papillary pattern, areas of necrosis.

38.5.2 Epidemiology

Prevalence: 0.4–1% of all intracranial tumors. 1.5–6% of tumors in peds.

Although they may occur at any age, 70% of patients are < 2 yrs old.[64] Some tumors occur in neonates, supporting the hypothesis that some of these are congenital.[65]

Location: in adults these tumors are usually infratentorial, whereas in children they tend to occur supratentorially (a reverse from the situation for most other tumors) in the lateral ventricle[65] with a predilection for the left side. See Intraventricular lesions (p. 1381) for differential diagnosis. They can be located anywhere there is choroid plexus, with the most frequent locations: the lateral or fourth ventricles, the CPA (from extension of choroid plexus through the foramen of Luschka).

38.5.3 Presentation

Most present with symptoms of increased ICP from hydrocephalus (H/A, N/V, craniomegaly), others may present with seizures, subarachnoid hemorrhage (with meningismus), or focal neurologic deficit (hemiparesis, sensory deficits, cerebellar signs, or cranial nerve palsies of III, IV and VI).

Hydrocephalus, which may result from: overproduction of CSF (although total removal of these tumors does not always cure the hydrocephalus – especially in patients with high CSF protein, hemorrhage from tumor or surgery, or ependymitis), obstruction of CSF outflow, or communicating hydrocephalus from CSF borne particulates.

38.5.4 Imaging

Brain MRI or CT without and with contrast usually demonstrates a densely enhancing multilobulated intraventricular mass classically with projecting "fronds." Hydrocephalus is common.

38.5.5 Treatment

General information

There is no role for chemotherapy or radiation for WHO I lesions. For choroid plexus carcinoma, chemotherapy benefits a subset of patients.[66]

Surgical treatment

Benign lesions may be cured surgically with total removal, and even the malignant tumors respond well to surgery. The operation may be difficult due to fragility of the tumor and bleeding from the choroidal arteries. However, persistence with a second and sometimes even third operation is recommended as 5-year survival rate of 84% can be achieved.[65] Post-operative subdural collections after transcortical tumor excision may occur, and may result from a persistent ventriculosubdural fistula, which may require subdural-peritoneal shunting.[64]

38.5.6 Recurrence

12 recurrences (6% of WHO I and 29% of WHO II patients) requiring neurosurgical intervention occurred in 124 complete resections with 59 months mean follow-up.[62]

38.6 Other neuroepithelial tumors

1. astroblastoma
2. chordoid glioma of the 3rd ventricle[67]: rare, benign tumor of adulthood. Solid, enhancing mass of the 3rd ventricle. Female:male ratio = 3:1. Mitotic activity is absent in most tumors. GFAP immunostaining is common, S100 reactivity is variable. Histologically similar appearing to chordoid meningioma, which lacks GFAP staining. Attachment to wall of 3rd ventricle (hypothalamus) may prevent total removal
3. angiocentric glioma

References

[1] Mork SJ, Lindegaard KF, Halvorsen TB, et al. Oligodendroglioma: Incidence and Biological Behavior in a Defined Population. J Neurosurg. 1985; 63:881–889

[2] Daumas-Duport C, Tucker M-L, Kolles H, et al. Oligodendrogliomas: Part II - A new grading system based on morphological and imaging criteria. J Neurooncol. 1997; 34:61–78

[3] Coons SW, Johnson PC, Scheithauer BW, et al. Improving Diagnostic Accuracy and Interobserver Concordance in the Classification and Grading of Primary Gliomas. Cancer. 1997; 79:1381–1393

[4] Daumas-Duport C, Varlet P, Tucker M-L, et al. Oligodendrogliomas: Part I - Patterns of Growth, Histological Diagnosis, Clinical and Imaging Correlations: A Study of 153 Cases. J Neurooncol. 1997; 34:37–59

[5] Chin HW, Hazel JJ, Kim TH, et al. Oligodendrogliomas. I. A Clinical Study of Cerebral Oligodendrogliomas. Cancer. 1980; 45:1458–1466

[6] Roberts M, German W. A Long Term Study of Patients with Oligodendrogliomas. J Neurosurg. 1966; 24:697–700

[7] Coons SW, Johnson PC, Pearl DK, Olafsen AG. The Prognostic Significance of Ki-67 Labeling Indices for Oligodendrogliomas. Neurosurgery. 1997; 41:878–885

[8] Fortin D, Cairncross GJ, Hammond RR. Oligodendroglioma: An Appraisal of Recent Data Pertaining to Diagnosis and Treatment. Neurosurgery. 1999; 45:1279–1291

[9] Hart MN, Petito CK, Earle KM. Mixed Gliomas. Cancer. 1974; 33:134–140

[10] Rutka JT, Murakami M, Dirks PB, et al. Role of Glial Filaments in Cells and Tumors of Glial Origin: A Review. J Neurosurg. 1997; 87:420–430

[11] Kros JM, Schouten WCD, Janssen PJA, et al. Proliferation of Gemistocytic Cells and Glial Fibrillary Acidic Protein (GFAP)-Positive Oligodendroglial Cells in Gliomas: A MIB-1/GFAP Double Labeling Study. Acta Neuropathol (Berl). 1996; 91:99–103

[12] Smith MT, Ludwig CL, Godfrey AD, et al. Grading of Oligodendrogliomas. Cancer. 1983; 52:2107–2114

[13] Cairncross JG, Macdonald D, Ludwin S, et al. Chemotherapy for Anaplastic Oligodendroglioma. J Clin Oncol. 1994; 12:2013–2021

[14] Cairncross JG, Ueki K, Zlatescu MC, et al. Specific Genetic Predictors of Chemotherapeutic Response and Survival in Patients with Anaplastic Oligodendrogliomas. J Natl Cancer Inst. 1998; 90:1473–1479

[15] Levin VA, Edwards MS, Wright DC, et al. Modified Procarbazine, CCNU and Vincristine (PCV-3) Combination Chemotherapy in the Treatment of Malignant Brain Tumors. Cancer Treat Rep. 1980; 64:237–244

[16] Glass J, Hochberg FH, Gruber ML, Louis DN, et al. The Treatment of Oligodendrogliomas and Mixed Oligodendroglioma-Astrocytomas with PCV Chemotherapy. J Neurosurg. 1992; 76:741–745

[17] Yung WK, Prados MD, Yaya-Tur R, et al. Multicenter phase II trial of temozolomide in patients with anaplastic astrocytoma or anaplastic oligoastrocytoma at first relapse. Temodal Brain Tumor Group. J Clin Oncol. 1999; 17:2762–2771

[18] Berger MS, Rostomily RC. Low Grade Gliomas: Functional Mapping Resection Strategies, Extent of Resection, and Outcome. J Neurooncol. 1997; 34:85–101

[19] Earnest F, Kernohan JW, Craig WM. Oligodendrogliomas: A Review of 200 Cases. Arch Neurol Psychiat. 1950; 63:964–976

[20] Ciric I, Ammirati M, Vick N, et al. Supratentorial Gliomas: Surgical Considerations and Immediate Postoperative Results. Neurosurgery. 1987; 21:21–26

[21] Gonzales M, Sheline GE. Treatment of Oligodendrogliomas With or Without Postoperative Radiation. J Neurosurg. 1988; 68:684–688

[22] Reedy DP, Bay JW, Hahn JF. Role of Radiation Therapy in the Treatment of Cerebral Oligodendroglioma. Neurosurgery. 1983; 13:499–503

[23] Taphoorn MJ, Heimans JJ, Snoek FJ, et al. Assessment of Quality of Life in Patients Treated for Low-Grade Glioma: A Preliminary Report. J Neurol Neurosurg Psychiatry. 1992; 55:372–376

[24] Smith JS, Perry A, Borell TJ, Lee HK, O'Fallon J, Hosek SM, Kimmel D, Yates A, Burger PC, Scheithauer BW, Jenkins RB. Alterations of chromosome arms 1p and 19q as predictors of survival in oligodendrogliomas, astrocytomas, and mixed oligoastrocytomas. J Clin Oncol. 2000; 18:636–645

[25] Kraus JA, Lamszus K, Glesmann N, Beck M, Wolter M, Sabel M, Krex D, Klockgether T, Reifenberger G, Schlegel U. Molecular genetic alterations in glioblastomas with oligodendroglial component. Acta Neuropathol (Berl). 2001; 101:311–320

[26] Mork SJ, Loken AC. Ependymoma: A Follow-Up Study of 101 Cases. Cancer. 1977; 40:907–915

[27] Duffner PK, Cohen ME, Freeman AI. Pediatric Brain Tumors: An Overview. Ca. 1985; 35:287–301

[28] Taylor MD, Poppleton H, Fuller C, Su X, Liu Y, Jensen P, Magdaleno S, Dalton J, Calabrese C, Board J, Macdonald T, Rutka J, Guha A, Gajjar A, Curran T, Gilbertson RJ. Radial glia cells are candidate stem cells of ependymoma. Cancer Cell. 2005; 8:323–335

[29] Kleihues P, Louis DN, Scheithauer BW, Rorke LB, Reifenberger G, Burger PC, Cavenee WK. The WHO classification of tumors of the nervous system. J Neuropathol Exp Neurol. 2002; 61:215–25; discussion 226-9

[30] Youmans JR. Neurological Surgery. Philadelphia 1982

[31] Shaw EG, Evans RG, Scheithauer BW, et al. Postoperative Radiotherapy of Intracranial Ependymoma in Pediatric and Adult Patients. Int J Radiation Oncology Biol Phys. 1987; 13:1457–1462

[32] Merchant TE, Mulhern RK, Krasin MJ, Kun LE, Williams T, Li C, Xiong X, Khan RB, Lustig RH, Boop FA, Sanford RA. Preliminary results from a phase II trial of conformal radiation therapy and evaluation of radiation-related CNS effects for pediatric patients with localized ependymoma. J Clin Oncol. 2004; 22:3156–3162

[33] MacDonald SM, Safai S, Trofimov A, Wolfgang J, Fullerton B, Yeap BY, Bortfeld T, Tarbell NJ, Yock T. Proton radiotherapy for childhood ependymoma: initial clinical outcomes and dose comparisons. Int J Radiat Oncol Biol Phys. 2008; 71:979–986

[34] Vanuytsel L, Brada M. The Role of Prophylactic Apinal Irradiation in Localized Intracranial Ependymoma. Int J Radiation Oncology Biol Phys. 1991; 21:825–830

[35] van Veelen-Vincent ML, Pierre-Kahn A, Kalifa C, Sainte-Rose C, Zerah M, Thorne J, Renier D. Ependymoma in childhood: prognostic factors, extent of

38

surgery, and adjuvant therapy. J Neurosurg. 2002; 97:827–835
[36] Grundy RG, Wilne SA, Weston CL, Robinson K, Lashford LS, Ironside J, Cox T, Chong WK, Campbell RH, Bailey CC, Gattamaneni R, Picton S, Thorpe N, Mallucci C, English MW, Punt JA, Walker DA, Ellison DW, Machin D. Primary postoperative chemotherapy without radiotherapy for intracranial ependymoma in children: the UKCCSG/SIOP prospective study. Lancet Oncol. 2007; 8:696–705
[37] Little AS, Sheean T, Manoharan R, Darbar A, Teo C. The management of completely resected childhood intracranial ependymoma: the argument for observation only. Childs Nerv Syst. 2009; 25:281–284
[38] Sutton LN, Goldwein J, Perilongo G, et al. Prognostic Factors in Childhood Ependymomas. Pediatr Neurosurg. 1990; 16:57–65
[39] Zacharoulis S, Ji L, Pollack IF, Duffner P, Geyer R, Grill J, Schild S, Jaing TH, Massimino M, Finlay J, Sposto R. Metastatic ependymoma: a multi-institutional retrospective analysis of prognostic factors. Pediatr Blood Cancer. 2008; 50:231–235
[40] Kawabata Y, Takahashi JA, Arakawa Y, Hashimoto N. Long-term outcome in patients harboring intracranial ependymoma. J Neurosurg. 2005; 103:31–37
[41] Tihan T, Zhou T, Holmes E, Burger PC, Ozuysal S, Rushing EJ. The prognostic value of histological grading of posterior fossa ependymomas in children: a Children's Oncology Group study and a review of prognostic factors. Mod Pathol. 2008; 21:165–177
[42] Ross GW, Rubinstein LJ. Lack of Histopathological Correlation of Malignant Ependymomas with Postoperative Survival. J Neurosurg. 1989; 70:31–36
[43] Foreman NK, Love S, Thorne R. Intracranial ependymomas: analysis of prognostic factors in a population-based series. Pediatr Neurosurg. 1996; 24:119–125
[44] Louis DN, Ohgaki H, Wiestler OD, Cavenee WK, Bosman FT, Jaffe ES, Lakhani SR, Ohgaki H. WHO classification of tumors of the central nervous system. Lyon 2007
[45] Patel DM, Schmidt RF, Liu JK. Update on the diagnosis, pathogenesis, and treatment strategies for central neurocytoma. J Clin Neurosci. 2013; 20:1193–1199
[46] Sharma MC, Deb P, Sharma S, Sarkar C. Neurocytoma: a comprehensive review. Neurosurg Rev. 2006; 29:270–85; discussion 285
[47] Agarwal S, Sharma MC, Sarkar C, Suri V, Jain A, Sharma MS, Ailawadhi P, Garg A, Mallick S. Extraventricular neurocytomas: a morphological and histogenetic consideration. A study of six cases. Pathology (Phila). 2011; 43:327–334
[48] Chakraborti S, Mahadevan A, Govindan A, Yasha TC, Santosh V, Kovoor JM, Ramamurthi R, Alapatt JP, Hedge T, Shankar SK. Supratentorial and cerebellar liponeurocytomas: report of four cases with review of literature. J Neurooncol. 2011; 103:121–127
[49] Kaur G, Kane AJ, Sughrue ME, Oh M, Safaee M, Sun M, Tihan T, McDermott MW, Berger MS, Parsa AT. MIB-1 labeling index predicts recurrence in intraventricular central neurocytomas. J Clin Neurosci. 2013; 20:89–93
[50] Rades D, Fehlauer F, Schild SE. Treatment of atypical neurocytomas. Cancer. 2004; 100:814–817
[51] Daumas-Duport C, Scheithauer BW, Chodkiewicz J-P, Laws ER, Vedrenne C. Dysembryoplastic Neuroepithelial Tumor: A Surgically Curable Tumor of Young Patients with Intractable Seizures. Neurosurgery. 1988; 23:545–556
[52] Daumas-Duport C, Varlet P, Bacha S, Beuvon F, Cervera-Pierot P, Chodkiewicz JP. Dysembryoplastic neuroepithelial tumors: nonspecific histological forms – a study of 40 cases. J Neurooncol. 1999; 41:267–280
[53] Adada B, Sayed K. Dysembryoplastic neuroepithelial tumors. Contemp Neurosurg. 2004; 26:1–5
[54] Robinson S, Cohen AR. Cowden disease and Lhermitte-Duclos disease: an update. Case report and review of the literature. Neurosurg Focus. 2006; 20
[55] Nelen MR, van Staveren WC, Peeters EA, Hassel MB, Gorlin RJ, Hamm H, Lindboe CF, Fryns JP, Sijmons RH, Woods DG, Mariman EC, Padberg GW, Kremer H. Germline mutations in the PTEN/MMAC1 gene in patients with Cowden disease. Hum Mol Genet. 1997; 6:1383–1387
[56] Meltzer CC, Smirniotopoulos JG, Jones RV. The striated cerebellum: an MR imaging sign in Lhermitte-Duclos disease (dysplastic gangliocytoma). Radiology. 1995; 194:699–703
[57] Chen KS, Hung PC, Wang HS, Jung SM, Ng SH. Medulloblastoma or cerebellar dysplastic gangliocytoma (Lhermitte-Duclos disease)? Pediatr Neurol. 2002; 27:404–406
[58] Someshwar S, Hogg JP, Nield LS. Lhermitte-Duclos disease or neoplasm? Applied Neurology. 2007; 3:37–39
[59] Suresh TN, Santosh V, Yasha TC, Anandh B, Mohanty A, Indiradevi B, Sampath S, Shankar SK. Medulloblastoma with extensive nodularity: a variant occurring in the very young-clinicopathological and immunohistochemical study of four cases. Childs Nerv Syst. 2004; 20:55–60
[60] Capone Mori A, Hoeltzenbein M, Poetsch M, Schneider JF, Brandner S, Boltshauser E. Lhermitte-Duclos disease in 3 children: a clinical long-term observation. Neuropediatrics. 2003; 34:30–35
[61] Carlson JJ, Milburn JM, Barre GM. Lhermitte-Duclos disease: case report. J Neuroimaging. 2006; 16:157–162
[62] Jeibmann A, Wrede B, Peters O, Wolff J, Paulus W, Hasselblatt M. Malignant progression in choroid plexus papillomas. J Neurosurg. 2007; 107:199–202
[63] Jeibmann A, Hasselblatt M, Gerss J, Wrede B, Egensperger R, Beschorner R, Hans VH, Rickert CH, Wolff JE, Paulus W. Prognostic implications of atypical histologic features in choroid plexus papilloma. J Neuropathol Exp Neurol. 2006; 65:1069–1073
[64] Boyd MC, Steinbok P. Choroid Plexus Tumors: Problems in Diagnosis and Management. J Neurosurg. 1987; 66:800–805
[65] Ellenbogen RG, Winston KR, Kupsky WJ. Tumors of the Choroid Plexus in Children. Neurosurgery. 1989; 25:327–335
[66] Wrede B, Liu P, Wolff JE. Chemotherapy improves the survival of patients with choroid plexus carcinoma: a metaanalysis of individual cases with choroid plexus tumors. J Neurooncol. 2007; 85:345–351
[67] Brat DJ, Scheithauer BW, Staugaitis SM, Cortez SC, Brecher K, Burger PC. Third ventricular chordoid glioma: a distinct clinicopathologic entity. J Neuropathol Exp Neurol. 1998; 57:283–290

39 Neuronal and Mixed Neuronal-Glial Tumors

39.1 Ganglioglioma

39.1.1 General information

Key concepts

- composed of two cell types: ganglion cells (neurons) and glial cells
- extremely rare (< 2% of intracranial neoplasms)
- seen primarily in the first 3 decades of life
- characterized by slow growth and a tendency to calcify

The term "ganglioglioma" was introduced in 1930 by Courville.[1] A tumor composed of two types of cells: ganglion cells (neurons) which may arise from primitive neuroblasts, and glial cells, usually astrocytic in any phase of differentiation.[2]

39.1.2 Epidemiology

Incidence

Typically quoted[3] as 0.3–0.6%. One series[4] found gangliogliomas in 1.3% of all brain tumors (including mets), or 3% of primary brain tumors. Considering only children and young adults, incidence ranges from 1.2–7.6% of brain tumors.[3]

Demographics

Occurs primarily in children and young adults (peak age of occurrence: 11 yrs).

39.1.3 Location

May occur in various parts of the nervous system (cerebral hemispheres, spinal cord, brainstem, cerebellum, pineal region, thalamus, intrasellar, optic nerve, and peripheral nerve have been reported[3]). Most occur above the tentorium, primarily in or near the 3rd ventricle, in the hypothalamus or in the temporal or frontal lobes.[5] Brainstem gangliogliomas (p. 633) occur rarely.

39.1.4 Pathology

Mixture of 2 types of neoplastic cells: neuronal (ganglion) and astrocytic (glial). Very slow growing.

Two major classifications: ganglioneuromas (less common, more benign; predominance of neuronal component) and gangliogliomas (preponderance of glial cells).

Grossly: white matter mass; well-circumscribed, firm, with occasional cystic areas and calcified regions. Most dissect easily from brain, but the solid portion may show an infiltrative tendency.[3]

Microscopically: ganglion cells must demonstrate nerve cell differentiation, e.g. Nissl substance and axons or dendrites. Pitfall: differentiating neoplastic neurons from neurons entrapped by an invading astrocytoma may be difficult. Also, neoplastic astrocytes may resemble neurons on light microscopy. 2 of 10 patients had areas of oligodendroglioma. One series found necrotic areas in 7 of 14 patients, minimal calcification, and Rosenthal bodies.[6] Suggested criteria for diagnosis[7]:

1. clusters of large cells potentially representing neurons (required for diagnosis)
2. no perineural clustering of glial cells around the suspected neoplastic neurons
3. fibrosis (desmoplasia)
4. calcification

Aggressive malignant changes in the glial component may dictate a poor outcome, although an "aggressive" background is not unusual and may not indicate malignancy.

39.1.5 Presentation

Most common presenting symptom was seizure, or a change in a pre-existing seizure pattern. Often, the seizures are difficult to control medically.

39.1.6 Radiologic Evaluation

Neuroradiologic findings are not specific for this tumor.

Plain skull x-ray: calcification was noted in 2 of 6 patients.[3]

CT: all of 10 patients had a low density lesion on non-contrast CT; 8 enhanced slightly with contrast; 5 of the 10 had calcification on CT.[4] 6 of the 10 were in temporal lobe (this predilection has been noted in many but not all series), and 4 were in frontal lobe. Frequently appears cystic on CT, but still may be found to be solid at operation. Mass effect rare (suggests slow growth).

MRI: high signal on T1WI, low signal on T2WI. Calcifications appear as low signal on both.[3]

Angiography: shows either an avascular or a minimally vascular mass.

39.1.7 Treatment

Recommendation is wide radical excision when possible (may be more limited in spinal cord and brainstem tumors). Close follow-up is recommended, and re-resection should be considered for recurrence. The role of XRT is unknown, and due to the deleterious effects together with the good long-term prognosis, it is not recommended initially but may be considered for recurrence.[8]

39.1.8 Prognosis

Russell and Rubinstein[9] first proposed that the grade of the astrocytic component of the tumor determines the prognosis. This has been supported by some case reports, but clinical series have not been able to correlate histology with outcome.[8] Thus, anaplasia is not significantly associated with a worse prognosis.[8]

The majority of patients did well and were asymptomatic after resection. 1 patient in a series of 10 died 3 days post-op from cerebral edema.

In 58 patients, 5-year survival was 89% and 10-year survival was 84%.[8] In 9 brainstem gangliogliomas, 5-year survival was 78%.

The value of radiation therapy is not known. Consider radiation when growth is evident on follow-up CT, or when infiltration is felt to occur at time of surgery.

1 patient had degeneration to glioblastoma when a recurrence was discovered 5 years after removal (this patient received radiation therapy).

The prognosis with following subtotal resection of brainstem gangliogliomas is better than for brainstem gliomas as a group.[5]

39.2 Paraganglioma

39.2.1 General information

AKA chemodectoma, AKA glomus tumors. ▶ Table 39.1 shows the designation of these tumors in various sites.

Table 39.1 Designation based on site of origin

Site	Designation
carotid bifurcation (most common)	carotid body tumors
auricular branch of vagus (middle ear)	glomus tympanicum
superior vagal ganglion (jugular foramen)	glomus jugulare
inferior vagal (nodose) ganglion (nasopharynx at skull base) (least common)	glomus intravagale (AKA glomus vagale)
adrenal medulla & sympathetic chain	pheochromocytoma

These tumors arise from paraganglion cells (not chemoreceptor cells as previously thought, therefore the term chemodectoma is losing favor). Slow growing tumors (< 2 cm in 5 years). Histologically benign (< 10% associated with lymph node involvement or distant spread). Most contain secretory granules on EM (mostly epinephrine & nor-epinephrine, and these tumors may occasionally secrete these catecholamines with risk of life-threatening HTN and/or cardiac arrhythmias).

Glomus tumors may occur in 2 patterns:

1. familial: non multicentric. Up to 50%
2. nonfamilial. may be multicentric (metachronous) 5%

39.2.2 Pheochromocytoma

General information

Located in the adrenal gland. May be sporadic, or as part of familial syndrome (von Hippel-Lindau disease (p. 703), MEN 2A & 2B, & neurofibromatosis). Consider genetic testing if age at diagnosis is < 50 years for mutations of VHL and other genetic abnormalities (RET, SDHS, SDHB, SDHC[10]).

Laboratory studies

1. fractionated plasma metanephrines: 96% sensitivity, 85% specificity.[11] More sensitive than serum catecholamines with sporadic elevations. Pheochromocytoma is ruled out if plasma normetanephrine (NMN) < 112 pg/ml and metanephrine (MN) < 61 pg/ml. Highly suspicious if NMN > 400 pg/ml or MN > 236 pg/ml
2. 24 hr urine collection for: total catecholamines (epinephrine and nor-epinephrine) and metanephrines (88% sensitivity, 99.7% specificity[12]). **Note:** testing for vanillylmandelic acid (VMA) is no longer done as it does not measure fractionated metanephrines.
3. where elevation is found, a clonidine suppression test can be done. Normal response consists of a fall in plasma catecholamines to ≤ 50% of baseline and below 500 pg/ml (there will be a reduction in essential hypertension, but no change with pheochromocytoma or other tumor production)

Imaging

Indicated when laboratory tests confirm pheochromocytoma.

MRI with contrast is preferred over CT.

CT may be used when MRI is contraindicated, but is less sensitive, especially for lesions < 1 cm diameter.

123I MIBG (iodine-123-meta-iodobenzylguanidine) scintigraphy detects extra-adrenal pheochromocytomas with 83–100% sensitivity, 95–100% specificity. If not available 131I MIBG may be used with 77–90% sensitivity, 95–100% specificity.

39.2.3 Carotid body tumors

General information

Possibly the most common paraganglioma (pheochromocytoma may be more common). Approximately 5% are bilateral; the incidence of bilaterality increases to 26% in familial cases (these are probably autosomal dominant).

Clinical

Usually present as painless, slow growing mass in upper neck. Large tumors may → cranial nerve involvement (especially vagus and hypoglossal). May also cause stenosis of ICA → TIAs or stroke.

Evaluation

1. carotid angiogram: demonstrates predominant blood supply (usually external carotid, with possible contributions from vertebral and thyrocervical trunk). May also detect bilateral lesions. Characteristic finding: splaying of bifurcation
2. MRI (or CT): evaluates extent, and assesses for intracranial extension

Treatment

Resection reported to carry a high complication rate, including stroke (8–20%) and cranial nerve injury (33–44%). Mortality rate is 5–13%.

39.2.4 Glomus tumors

General information

Glomus tumors may be subdivided into glomus jugulare and glomus tympanicum tumors. Glomus jugulare tumors arise from the jugular bulb (in the jugular foramen at the junction of the sigmoid sinus and jugular vein). Glomus tympanicum tumors are centered higher than glomus jugulare. Glomus tumors are rare (0.6% of all head and neck tumors), yet the glomus tympanicum is the most common neoplasm of the middle ear. Glomus jugulare tumors (GJT) arise from glomus bodies, usually in the area of the jugular bulb, and track along vessels. May have finger-like extension into the jugular vein (which may embolize during resection).[13] Most are slow growing, although rapidly growing tumors do occur.

Vascular supply: very vascular. Main feeders of GJT are from the external carotid (especially inferior tympanic branch of ascending pharyngeal artery, and branches of posterior auricular, occipital, and internal maxillary), with additional feeders from petrous portion of the ICA. Glomus tympanicum tumors feed from the auricular artery.

Epidemiology

Female:male ratio is 6:1. Bilateral occurrence is almost nonexistent.

Pathology

General information

Histologically indistinguishable from carotid body tumors. May invade locally, both through temporal bone destruction and especially along pre-existing pathways (along vessels, eustachian tube, jugular vein, carotid artery). Intradural extension is rare. Malignancy may occur, but is rare. These tumors rarely metastasize.

Secretory properties

These tumors usually possess secretory granules (even the functionally inactive tumors) and may actively secrete catecholamines (similar to pheochromocytomas, occurs in only 1–4% of GJT[14]). Norepinephrine will be elevated in functionally active tumors since glomus tumors lack the methyltransferase needed to convert this to epinephrine. Alternatively, serotonin and kallikrein may be released, and may produce a carcinoid-like syndrome (bronchoconstriction, abdominal pain and explosive diarrhea, violent H/A, cutaneous flushing, hypertension, hepatomegaly and hyperglycemia).[15] During surgical manipulation, these tumors may also release histamine and bradykinin, causing hypotension and bronchoconstriction.[16]

Clinical

Symptoms

Patients commonly present with hearing loss and pulsatile tinnitus. Dizziness is the third most common symptoms. Ear pain may also occur.

Signs

39

Hearing loss may be conductive (e.g. due to obstruction of the ear canal) or sensorineural due to invasion of the labyrinth often with accompanying vertigo (the eighth nerve is the most common cranial nerve involved). Various combinations of palsies of cranial nerves IX, X, XI & XII occur – see Jugular foramen syndromes (p. 100) – with occasional VII palsy (usually from involvement within the temporal bone). Ataxia and/or hydrocephalus can occur with massive lesions that cause brainstem compression. Occasionally patients may present with symptoms due to secretory products (see below).

Otoscopic exam → pulsatile reddish-blue mass behind eardrum (occasionally, lamentably biopsied by ENT physician with possible ensuing massive blood loss).

Differential diagnosis

See Cerebellopontine angle (CPA) lesions (p. 1365). The major differential is neurilemmomas (vestibular schwannomas), both enhance on CT. A cystic component and extrinsic compression of the jugular bulb are characteristic of neurilemmomas. Angiography will differentiate difficult cases.

Evaluation

Neurophysiologic testing

Audiometric and vestibular testing should be performed.

Imaging

1. CT or MRI used to delineate location and extent of tumor; CT is better for assessing bony involvement of the skull base
2. angiography: confirms diagnosis (helping to rule out vestibular schwannoma), and ascertains patency of contralateral jugular vein in event that jugular on side of tumor must be sacrificed; jugular bulb and/or vein are usually partially or completely occluded

Endocrine/laboratory studies

See also details (p. 653).

Classification

A number of classification schemes have been proposed. The modified Jackson classification is shown in ▶ Table 39.2.

Treatment

Surgical resection is usually simple and effective for small tumors confined to the middle ear. For larger tumors that invade and destroy bone, the relative role of surgery and/or radiation is not fully determined. With large tumors, surgery carries the risk of significant cranial nerve palsies.

Medical management

General information

For tumors that actively secrete catecholamines, medical therapy is useful for palliation or as adjunctive treatment before embolization or surgery. Alpha and beta blockers given before embolization or surgery blocks possibly lethal blood pressure lability and arrhythmias. Adequate blockade takes ≈ 2–3 weeks of alpha blocker and at least 24 hours of beta blocker therapy; in emergency, 3 days of treatment may suffice.

Alpha blockers

Reduce BP by preventing peripheral vasoconstriction.

1. phenoxybenzamine (Dibenzyline®): long acting; peak effect 1–2 hrs. Start with 10 mg PO BID and gradually increase to 40–100 mg per day divided BID
2. phentolamine (Regitine®): short acting. Usually used IV for hypertensive crisis during surgery or embolization.
   ℞: 5 mg IV/IM (peds: 1 mg) 1–2 hrs pre-op, repeat PRN before and during surgery

Table 39.2 Modified Jackson classification[17]

Type	Description	Intracranial extension
I	small; involves jugular bulb, middle ear & mastoid	none
II	extends under IAC	possible
III	extends into petrous apex	possible
IV	extends beyond petrous apex into clivus or infratemporal fossa	possible

Beta blockers

Reduces catecholamine induced tachycardia and arrhythmias (may also prevent hypotension that might occur if only alpha blockade is used). These drugs are not always needed, but when used 6 NB: these drugs must *not* be started before starting alpha-blockers (to prevent hypertensive crisis and myocardial ischemia).

1. propranolol (Inderal®): ℞: oral dose is 5–10 mg q 6 hrs. IV dose for use during surgery is 0.5–2 mg slow IVP
2. labetalol (Normodyne®) (p. 126): may have some efficacy in blocking α1 selective and β non-selective (potency < propranolol)

Serotonin, bradykinin, histamine release blockers

These agents may provoke bronchoconstriction that does not respond to steroids, but may respond to inhaled β-agonists or inhaled anticholinergics. Somatostatin may be used to inhibit release of serotonin, bradykinin, or histamines. Since this drug has a short half-life, it is preferable to give octreotide (p. 742) 100 mcg sub-Q q 8 hrs.

Radiation therapy

XRT may relieve symptoms and stop growth in spite of persistence of tumor mass. 40–45 Gy in fractions of 2 Gy has been recommended.[18] Lower doses of ≈ 35 Gy in 15 fractions of 2.35 Gy appear as effective and have fewer side effects.[19] Generally used as primary treatment only for large tumors or in patients too elderly or infirmed to undergo surgery. Some surgeons pretreat 4–6 mos pre-operatively with XRT to decrease vascularity[20] (controversial).

Embolization

1. generally reserved for large tumors with favorable blood supply (i.e. vessels that can be selectively embolized with no danger of particles passing thru to normal brain)
2. post-embolization tumor swelling may compress brainstem or cerebellum
3. may be used preoperatively to reduce vascularity. Performed 24–48 hours pre-op (not used prior to that, because of post-embolization edema)
4. caution with actively secreting tumors which may release vasoactive substances (e.g. epinephrine) upon infarction from the embolization
5. may also be used as primary treatment (± radiation) in patients who are not surgical candidates. In this case, is only palliative, as tumor will develop new blood supply
6. absorbable (Gelfoam®) and non-absorbable (Ivalon®) materials have been used

Surgical treatment

General information

The tumor is primarily extradural, with extremely vascular surrounding dura.

Suboccipital approach may cause dangerous bleeding and usually results in incomplete resection. Team approach by a neurosurgeon in conjunction with a neuro-otologist and possibly head and neck surgeon has been advocated.[21] This approach utilizes an approach to the skull base through the neck.

ECA feeders are ligated early, followed rapidly by draining veins (to prevent systemic release of catecholamines).

Sacrifice of the jugular vein (JV) is tolerated if the contralateral JV is patent (often, the ipsilateral JV will already be occluded).

Surgical complications and outcome

The most common complications are CSF fistula, facial nerve palsy, and varying degrees of dysphagia (from dysfunction of lower cranial nerves). Dysfunction of any of the cranial nerves VII thru XII can occur, and a tracheostomy should be performed if there is any doubt of lower nerve function, and a gastrostomy feeding tube may be needed temporarily or permanently. Lower cranial nerve dysfunction also predisposes to aspiration, the risk of which is also increased by impaired gastric emptying and ileus that may occur due to reduced cholecystokinin (CCK) levels post-op. Excessive blood loss can also occur.

Even after gross total tumor removal, recurrence rate may be as high as one third.[20,22]

39.3 Neuroblastomas

39.3.1 General information

Tumors arising from sympathetic ganglion.[23] May occur anywhere in the sympathetic nervous system, most commonly from adrenal gland (40%), followed by sympathetic ganglia of thoracic (15%), cervical (5%) and pelvic regions (5%). Neoplasms under this rubric include:

1. neuroblastomas: the most undifferentiated and aggressive in this group
2. ganglioneuroblastomas
3. ganglioneuromas

Note: Olfactory neuroblastomas are called esthesioneuroblastomas (p. 1388).

39.3.2 Presentation

May present with abdominal mass, local or radicular pain, or (with high thoracic or cervical tumors) Horner's syndrome. Spinal cord compression may occur from invasion through the neural foramen, and scoliosis may occur. Catecholamine precursors (homovanillic acid (HVA), vanillylmandelic acid (VMA) and dopamine) may be excreted and cause HTN (can be assayed in urine). Periorbital tumor metastases may produce raccoon's eyes (usually unilateral ecchymosis and proptosis). Many of the low-grade tumors regress spontaneously and never present.

References

[1] Courville CB. Ganglioglioma. Tumor of the Central Nervous System: Review of the Literature and Report of Two Cases. Arch Neurol Psychiatry. 1930; 24:439–491

[2] Rubinstein LJ. Tumors of the Central Nervous System. Atlas of Tumor Pathology, Second Series, Fascicle 6. Washington, DC: Armed Forces Institute of Pathology; 1972

[3] Demierre B, Stichnoth FA, Hori A, et al. Intracerebral Ganglioglioma. J Neurosurg. 1986; 65:177–182

[4] Kalyan-Raman UP, Olivero WC. Ganglioglioma: A Correlative Clinicopathological and Radiological Study of Ten Surgically Treated Cases with Follow-Up. Neurosurgery. 1987; 20:428–433

[5] Garcia CA, McGarry PA, Collada M. Ganglioglioma of the Brain Stem. Case Report. J Neurosurg. 1984; 60:431–434

[6] Sutton LN, Packer RJ, Rorke LB, et al. Cerebral Gangliogliomas During Childhood. Neurosurgery. 1983; 13:124–128

[7] Miller DC, Lang FF, Epstein FJ. Central Nervous System Gangliogliomas. Part 1: Pathology. J Neurosurg. 1993; 79:859–866

[8] Lang FF, Epstein FJ, Ransohoff J, et al. Central Nervous System Gangliogliomas. Part 2: Clinical Outcome. J Neurosurg. 1993; 79:867–873

[9] Russell DS, Rubenstein LJ. Ganglioglioma: A Case with a Long History and Malignant Evolution. J Neuropathol Exp Neurol. 1962; 21:185–193

[10] van Nederveen FH, Gaal J, Favier J, Korpershoek E, Oldenburg RA, de Bruyn EM, Sleddens HF, Derkx P, Riviere J, Dannenberg H, Petri BJ, Komminoth P, Pacak K, Hop WC, Pollard PJ, Mannelli M, Bayley JP, Perren A, Niemann S, Verhofstad AA, de Bruine AP, Maher ER, Tissier F, Meatchi T, Badoual C, Bertherat J, Amar L, Alataki D, Van Marck E, Ferrau F, Francois J, de Herder WW, Peeters MP, van Linge A, Lenders JW, Gimenez-Roqueplo AP, de Krijger RR, Dinjens WN. An immunohistochemical procedure to detect patients with paraganglioma and phaeochromocytoma with germline SDHB, SDHC, or SDHD gene mutations: a retrospective and prospective analysis. Lancet Oncol. 2009; 10:764–771

[23] Brodeur GM, Pritchard J, Berthold F, et al. Revisions of the international criteria for neuroblastoma diagnosis, staging, and response to treatment. J Clin Oncol. 1993; 11:1466–1477

[11] Kudva YC, Sawka AM, Young WF, Jr. Clinical review 164: The laboratory diagnosis of adrenal pheochromocytoma: the Mayo Clinic experience. J Clin Endocrinol Metab. 2003; 88:4533–4539

[12] de Jong WH, Eisenhofer G, Post WJ, Muskiet FA, de Vries EG, Kema IP. Dietary influences on plasma and urinary metanephrines: implications for diagnosis of catecholamine-producing tumors. J Clin Endocrinol Metab. 2009; 94:2841–2849

[13] Chretien PB, Engelman K, Hoye RC, et al. Surgical Management of Intravascular Glomus Jugulare Tumor. Am J Surg. 1971; 122:740–743

[14] Jackson CG, Harris PF, Glasscock MEI, et al. Diagnosis and Management of Paragangliomas of the Skull Base. Am J Surg. 1990; 159:389–393

[15] Farrior JB, Hyams VJ, Benke RH, Farrior JB. Carcinoid Apudoma Arising in a Glomus Jugulare Tumor: Review of Endocrine Activity in Glomus Jugulare Tumors. Laryngoscope. 1980; 90:110–119

[16] Jensen NF. Glomus Tumors of the Head and Neck: Anesthetic Considerations. Anesth Analg. 1994; 78:112–119

[17] Jackson CG, Glasscock ME, Nissen AJ, et al. Glomus Tumor Surgery: The Approach, Results, and Problems. Otolaryngol Clin North Am. 1982; 15:897–916

[18] Kim J-A, Elkon D, Lim M-L, Constable WC. Optimum Dose of Radiotherapy for Chemodectomas of the Middle Ear. Int J Radiation Oncology Biol Phys. 1980; 6:815–819

[19] Cummings BJ, Beale FA, Garrett PG, Harwood AR, et al. The Treatment of Glomus Tumors in the Temporal Bone by Megavoltage Radiation. Cancer. 1984; 53:2635–2640

[20] Spector GJ, Fierstein J, Ogura JH. A Comparison of Therapeutic Modalities of Glomus Tumors in the Temporal Bone. Laryngoscope. 1976; 86:690–696

[21] Schmidek HH, Sweet WH. Operative Neurosurgical Techniques. New York 1982

[22] Hatfield PM, James AE, Schulz MD. Chemodectomas of the Glomus Jugulare. Cancer. 1972; 30:1164–1168

40 Pineal Region and Embryonal Tumors

40.1 Pineal region tumors

40.1.1 General information

Key concepts

- wide variety of pathology: germ cell tumors (mostly germinomas, teratomas), astrocytomas,& pineal tumors (mostly pineoblastomas) account for most tumors
- since tumors may be of mixed cell types, CSF tumor markers (β-hCG, AFP...) are not as useful for diagnosis as they are for following response to treatment
- traditionally a test dose of XRT was employed, but there is a growing trend to obtain tissue diagnosis in all cases if possible before instituting treatment

Pineal region[1]: the area of the brain bounded dorsally by the splenium of the corpus callosum and the tela choroidea, ventrally by the quadrigeminal plate and midbrain tectum, rostrally by the posterior aspect of the 3rd ventricle, and caudally by the cerebellar vermis.

A striking feature is the diversity of lesions (neoplastic and nonneoplastic) that may occur in this location due to the variety of tissues and conditions normally present, as shown in ▶ Table 40.1.

40.1.2 Pineal cysts (PCs)

General information

Usually an incidental finding (i.e. not symptomatic), seen on ≈ 4% of MRIs[2] or on 25–40% of autopsies[3] (many are microscopic). The most common ones are intra-pineal glial-lined cysts with diameter < 1 cm. Etiology is obscure, PCs are nonneoplastic, and may be due to ischemic glial degeneration or due to sequestration of the pineal diverticulum. They have been regarded as benign, but

Table 40.1 Conditions giving rise to pineal region tumors

Substrate in pineal region	Tumor that may arise
pineal glandular tissue	pineocytomas and pineoblastomas
glial cells	astrocytomas (including pilocytic), oligodendrogliomas, glial cysts (AKA pineal cyst)
arachnoid cells	meningiomas, arachnoid cysts (non-neoplastic). Meningiomas characteristically displace the internal cerebral vein inferiorly
ependymal lining	ependymomas
sympathetic nerves	chemodectomas
rests of germ cells	germ cell tumors: choriocarcinoma, germinoma, embryonal carcinoma, endodermal sinus tumor (yolk sac tumor), and teratoma
absence of blood-brain barrier (BBB) in pineal gland	makes it a susceptible site for hematogenous metastases
remnants of ectoderm	epidermoid or dermoid cysts
Non neoplastic lesions that may mimic tumors	
vascular	vein of Galen aneurysm (p. 1255), AVM
infectious	cysticercosis (p. 371)

40

the natural history is not known with certainty.[4] PCs may contain clear, slightly xanthochromic, or hemorrhagic fluid. Rarely, they may enlarge, and like other pineal region masses, may become symptomatic by causing hydrocephalus by aqueductal compression,[5] gaze paresis[6] including Parinaud's syndrome (p.99), or hypothalamic symptoms.

Positional H/As have been attributed to PCs, the theory is that the cyst could intermittently compress the vein of Galen and/or sylvian aqueduct.[7] This remains unproven since asymptomatic compression of the vein of Galen and the quadrigeminal plate has been demonstrated on MRI.[8]

Imaging

May escape detection on CT because the cyst fluid density is often similar to CSF. MRI T1WI shows round or ovoid abnormality in region of pineal recess, signal varies with protein content (isointense or slightly hyperintense). T2WI occasionally show increased intensity.[4] Gadolinium occasionally enhances the cyst wall with a maximum thickness of 2 mm; irregularities of the wall with nodular enhancement suggests the lesion is not benign.

Epidermoid-dermoid cysts may also occur in the pineal region, and are larger and have different signal characteristics on MRI.

Management

Asymptomatic PCs < 2 cm diameter with typical appearance should be followed clinically and with annual imaging studies. Surgery to relieve symptoms or to obtain a diagnosis is suggested for symptomatic lesions or for ones that show changes on MRI.

Surgery options for patients with hydrocephalus:

1. CSF shunt: may not relieve gaze disturbance (from pressure on tectal plate)
2. cyst excision: relieves symptoms and establishes diagnosis. Low morbidity
3. stereotactic or endoscopic aspiration: may not get enough tissue for diagnosis
4. endoscopic third ventriculostomy (ETV) (p.1517): useful only for typical PC as it does not obtain tissue for pathology. A few cases of regression of PCs after ETV have been reported[9]

40.1.3 Pineal region neoplasms

General information

Tumors in this region are more common in children (3–8% of pediatric brain tumors) than in adults (≤ 1%).[10] Over 17 tumor types occur in this re-gion.[11] Germinoma is the most common tumor (21–44% in American/European population, 43–70% in Japan), followed by astrocytoma, teratoma and pineoblastoma.[12] Many tumors are of mixed cell type.

Germ cell tumors (GCT), ependymomas and pineal cell tumors metastasize easily through the CSF ("drop metastases").

Pineal gland tumors

Pineal cell tumors

A pineocytoma (AKA pinealcytoma) is a well differentiated neoplasm arising from pineal epithelium. Pineoblastoma (AKA pinealblastoma) is a malignant tumor that is considered a primitive neuroectodermal tumor (PNET) (p.666). Both can metastasize through the CSF, and both are radiosensitive.

Germ cell tumors (GCT)

When they arise in the CNS, GCTs occur in the midline in the suprasellar and/or pineal region (simultaneous suprasellar and pineal region lesions is diagnostic of a GCT, so-called synchronous germ cell tumors, comprise 13% of GCTs, and are highly sensitive to XRT[13]). In the pineal region, these tumors occur predominantly in males. In females, GCTs are more common in the suprasellar region.[14] Aside from benign teratomas, all intracranial GCTs are malignant and may metastasize via CSF and systemically. Types of GCTs:

1. germinomas: malignant tumors of primitive germ cells that occur in the gonads (called testicular seminomas in males, dysgerminomas in females) or in the CNS. Survival with these is much better than with nongerminomatous tumors
2. non-germinomatous germ cell tumors (NGGCT) include:
   a) embryonal carcinoma
   b) choriocarcinoma

Table 40.2 Occurrence of CSF tumor markers with pineal germ cell tumors[a]

Tumor	β-hCG[b]	AFP	PLAP[c]
choriocarcinoma	≈ 100%	–	–
germinoma	10–50%	–	+
embryonal carcinoma	–	+	–
yolk sac carcinoma	–	+	–
immature teratoma	–	+	–
mature teratoma	–	–	–

[a]adapted with permission from personal communication, Ashraf Samy Youssef, M.D., Ph.D.
[b]abbreviations: β-hCG = beta human chorionic gonadotropin, AFP = alpha-fetoprotein, PLAP = placental alkaline phosphatase
[c]elevated PLAP may also occur in serum

c) endodermal sinus tumor (EST) AKA yolk sac carcinoma: usually malignant
d) teratoma
  - mature
  - immature

Tumor markers

GCTs characteristically (but not always) give rise to tumor markers in the CSF; see Tumor markers used clinically (p. 600). Elevated CSF beta-human chorionic gonadotropin (β-hCG) is classically associated with choriocarcinomas, but also occurs with up to 50% of germinomas (which are more common). Alpha-fetoprotein (AFP) is elevated with endodermal sinus tumors, embryonal carcinoma and occasionally with teratomas. Elevated placental alkaline phosphatase (PLAP) in serum or CSF occurs with intracranial germinomas.[15] ▶ Table 40.2 summarizes these findings. When positive, tumor markers can be followed serially to assess treatment and to look for recurrence (they should be checked in serum and CSF). NB: tumor markers alone are not usually sufficient for making a definitive diagnosis of a pineal region tumor since many of these tumors are mixed cell type.

Pediatric

A breakdown of pediatric pineal region tumors in one series is shown in ▶ Table 40.3 (series A).

In 36 patients < 18 yrs age, 17 distinct histological tumor types were identified: 11 germinomas (the most common tumor), 7 astrocytomas, and the remaining 18 had 15 different tumors.[17]

Adult

GCTs and pineal cell tumors occur primarily in childhood and young adults. Thus, over the age of 40, a pineal region tumor is more likely to be a meningioma or a glioma. Series B in ▶ Table 40.3 includes both adult and pediatric patients.

Clinical

Almost all patients have hydrocephalus by the time of presentation, causing typical signs and symptoms of headache, vomiting, lethargy, memory disturbance, abnormally increasing head circumference in infants, and seizures. Parinaud's syndrome (p. 99), or the syndrome of the sylvian aqueduct, may be present. Precocious puberty may occur only in boys with choriocarcinomas or germinomas with syncytiotrophoblastic cells, due to luteinizing hormone-like effects of β-hCG secreted in the CSF. Suprasellar GCT: triad of diabetes insipidus, visual deficit and panhypopituitarism.[14]

Drop metastases from CSF seeding can produce radiculopathy and/or myelopathy.

Management

The optimal management strategy for pineal region tumors has yet to be determined.

" Test dose" radiation: Controversial (p. 662). This is giving way to the doctrine of obtaining histology in most cases (e.g. by stereotactic biopsy) because of the harmful effects of XRT and because 36–50% of pineal tumors are benign or radioresistant.[18] The concept was that if a pineal region

Table 40.3 Pineal region tumors

Tumor	Series A[a] (%)	Series B[b] (%)
germinoma	30	27
astrocytoma	19	26
pineocytoma	6	12
malignant teratoma	6	
unidentified germ-cell tumor	6	
choriocarcinoma	3	1.1
malignant teratoma/embryonal cell tumor	3	1.6
glioblastoma	3	
teratoma	3	4.3
germinoma/ectodermal sinus tumor	3	
dermoid	3	
embryonal cell tumor	3	
pineoblastoma	3	12
pineocytoma/pineoblastoma	3	
endodermal sinus tumor	3	
glial cyst (pineal cyst)[16]	3	2.7
arachnoid cyst	3	
metastases		2.7
meningioma		2.7
ependymoma		4.3
oligodendrogliomas		0.54
ganglioglioneuroma		2.7
lymphoma		2.7

[a]36 children ≤ 18 yrs[17]
[b]370 tumors in patients 3–73 yrs old[10]

tumor enhanced uniformly and had the classic appearance of a germinoma on MRI, a test dose of 5 Gy was given, and if the tumor would shrink then the diagnosis of germinoma was virtually certain and XRT was continued without surgery. This may needlessly expose a patient with benign or radio-resistant tumors to XRT.[10] "Trial XRT" should be avoided in tumors suspected of being teratomas or epidermoid cyst on MRI, and the response may be misleading in the relatively common situation of tumors with mixed cell types.

Management suggestions

1. get MRI of cervical, thoracic and lumbar spine to assess for drop mets
2. send for GCT markers (β-hCG, AFP, PLAP) (p. 660). Somewhat helpful, but not adequate for diagnosis: if negative for GCT markers, it may be a pineal cell tumor, or it may be a GCT without markers, see Tumor markers (p. 660); if positive, it can still be a mixed cell-type tumor:
   a) serum
   b) CSF (if able to safely obtain; LP is contraindicated with large intracranial mass and/or obstructive hydrocephalus; CSF may be obtained from EVD if placed)

3. obtain histology in most cases. Most often this involves a biopsy, which should be generous (to avoid missing other histologies in mixed cell tumors)
   a) if hydrocephalus: transventricular biopsy
   b) if no hydrocephalus:
      - open biopsy or
      - stereotactic biopsy or
      - ? by CACE (see below)
4. based on markers and histology:
   a) germinoma: XRT + chemo
   b) all other tumors: one option is resection followed by adjuvant therapy (usually not very helpful) – see Indications (p.662) for controversies

Hydrocephalus

Patients presenting acutely due to hydrocephalus may be best treated with external ventricular drainage (EVD). This permits control over the amount of CSF drained, prevents peritoneal seeding with tumor (a rare event[19]), and may avoid having a permanent shunt placed in the significant number of patients who will not need one after tumor removal (although ≈ 90% of patients with a pineal GCT require a shunt). Ventricular access, via EVD or Frazier burr hole (p.1450), in the post-op period is important in the event of acute hydrocephalus.

Stereotactic procedures

May be used to ascertain diagnosis (biopsy), or to treat symptomatic pineal region cysts.[20,21] Caution is advised since the pineal region has numerous vessels (vein of Galen, basal veins of Rosenthal, internal cerebral veins, posterior medial choroidal artery)[22] which may be displaced from their normal position. The complication rate of stereotactic biopsy is: ≈ 1.3% mortality, ≈ 7% morbidity, and 1 case of seeding in 370 patients, and the diagnostic rate is≈ 94%.[10] A shortcoming of stereotactic biopsy is that it may fail to disclose the histologic heterogeneity of some tumors.

Two main stereotactic trajectories: 1) anterolateral (low frontal) approach below the internal cerebral veins, and 2) posterolateral trans-parieto-occipital.[11] One study found that the trajectory correlated with complications, and they recommended the anterolateral approach.[23] However, the correlation of trajectory and complications was not born out in another study,[10] and they found that the complication rate was higher in firm tumors (pineocytomas, teratomas, and astrocytomas) and they recommend an open approach when the tumor appears difficult to penetrate on the first attempt at biopsy.

Stereotactic radiosurgery may be appropriate for treatment of some lesions.

Computer-assisted cisternal endoscopic approach (CACE)

Employs a supracerebellar infratentorial approach that permits visualization of neurovascular structures and avoids traversing brain parenchyma.[11]

Radiation treatment

For controversies regarding "test dose" XRT, see Management (p.660). Germinomas are very sensitive to radiation (and chemotherapy), and are probably best treated with these modalities and followed.

XRT is also utilized post-op for other malignant tumors. For highly malignant tumors or if there is evidence of CSF seeding, craniospinal XRT with a boost to the tumor bed is appropriate.

If possible, XRT is best avoided in the young child. Chemotherapy may be used for age < 3 yrs until the child is older when XRT is better tolerated.[14]

Surgical treatment of the tumor

Indications

Controversial. Some authors feel that most tumors (except germinomas, which are best treated with XRT) are amenable to open resection.[24] Others feel that resection should be limited to ≈ 25% of tumors which are[10]:

1. radioresistant (e.g. malignant nongerminoma GCTs): 35–50% of pineal region tumors (larger numbers occur in series not limited to pediatric patients)
2. benign (e.g. meningioma, teratomas…)
3. well encapsulated
4. NB: malignant germ cell tumors should be without evidence of metastases (those with metastases do not benefit from surgery on the primary tumor)
5. pineocytoma: recommendation is for surgical excision + SRS for any residual

Options

1. direct surgery: obtains generous tissue for biopsy. Curative for benign lesions. Not the optimum treatment for malignant tumors and germinomas without complications

2. biopsy followed by adjuvant therapy: the preferred management (p. 660) for malignancies and germinomatous germ cell tumors

Surgical approaches
Choice is aided by the pre-op MRI and includes:
1. most common approach: midline infratentorial-supracerebellar approach of Horsley and Krause as refined by Stein.[25] Cannot be used if the angle of the tentorium is too steep (best assessed on MRI). May be done in the sitting position – risk of air embolism (p. 1445) – or in the Concorde position (p. 1445)
2. occipital transtentorial: wide view. Risk of injury to occipital visual cortex or splenium of corpus callosum. Recommended for lesions centered at or superior to the tentorial edge or located above the vein of Galen or for rare cysts with superior extension. The occipital lobe is retracted laterally, and the tentorium is incised 1 cm lateral to the straight sinus
3. transventricular: indicated for large, eccentric lesions with ventricular dilatation. Usually via a cortical incision in the posterior portion of the superior temporal gyrus. Risks: visual defect, seizures, and on dominant side language dysfunction
4. lateral paramedian infratentorial
5. transcallosal: largely abandoned except for tumors extending into corpus callosum and third ventricle
6. paramedian infratentorial-supracerebellar approach may be used for cysts that do not extend superiorly or contralaterally[4]: avoids midline venous structures

Important surgical considerations:

The base of the pineal gland is the posterior wall of the 3rd ventricle. The splenium of the corpus callosum lies above, and the thalamus surrounds both sides. The pineal projects posteriorly and inferiorly into the quadrigeminal cistern. The deep cerebral veins are a major obstacle to operations in this region. Venous drainage of the pineal region must be preserved.

Surgical outcome

Mortality rate: 5–10%.[10] Postoperative complications include: new visual field deficits, epidural fluid collection, infection, and cerebellar ataxia.

40.2 Embryonal tumors

40.2.1 General information

A few words about PNETs

Initially, the term primitive neuroectodermal tumor (PNET) encompassed a wide variety of previously individually named tumors which all seemed to share certain pathologic features suggesting origin from a common progenitor cell in the subependymal matrix (primitive neuroectodermal cells) (although the actual cell of origin is unknown). They are histologically indistinguishable but genetically distinct.[26] Now, the recommendation is to call these "embryonal tumors",[27] but the term PNET is entrenched. These tumors include: retinoblastoma, pineoblastoma, neuroblastoma, esthesioneuroblastoma. Medulloblastoma (MB) is more than just a PNET of the posterior fossa (see below), as alterations involved in evolution of MBs such as beta-catenin and APC mutations are absent in pineoblastomas and supratentorial PNETs (sPNETs). At least some MBs originate from the external granular layer (EGL) of the cerebellum.

Embryonal tumors

Location: Embryonal tumors most commonly arise in the cerebellar vermis (medulloblastoma), but also occur in cerebrum, pineal, brainstem or spinal cord. Primary spinal cord PNETs are extremely rare (approximately 30 cases reported by 2007[28]). sPNETS have a worse prognosis than MB (see below).

Dissemination: Embryonal tumors (ETs) may disseminate via the CSF spontaneously,[29] or iatrogenically (following surgery or shunting, the latter is a rare cause of tumor dissemination[19]). Thus, all patients with ETs require spinal axis evaluation (gadolinium enhanced MRI is about as sensitive as water-soluble myelography) and cytologic examination of CSF. Prophylactic craniospinal XRT is indicated following surgical removal, but cranial XRT is avoided if at all possible before 3 years of age to avoid intellectual impairment and growth retardation; see Radiation injury and necrosis (p. 1560). Extraneural metastases can also occur.

Collin's law: AKA period of risk of recurrence (PRR) is often applied to children who have been treated for embryonal tumors (especially medulloblastoma) but may also be used with any tumor thought to arise from a gestational event. It states that PRR is equal to the age at diagnosis plus 9 months.[30] Patients that remain free of recurrence beyond the PRR have a much lower risk of recurrence, however recurrence beyond this time has been reported in a small number (≈ 1.4%) of cases,[31] and other tumors may occur e.g. as a result of induction by XRT used to treat the initial tumor.

40.2.2 Medulloblastoma (MB)

General information

Key concepts

- a small-cell embryonal tumor of the cerebellum found predominantly in children (peak: 1st decade). The most common pediatric brain malignancy
- usually arises in the cerebellar vermis in the region of the apex of the roof of the 4th ventricle (fastigium), often producing hydrocephalus
- brainstem invasion usually limits complete surgical excision
- all patients must be evaluated for "drop mets"

Epidemiology

In children: MBs comprise 15–20% of intracranial tumors,[32] 30- 55% of p-fossa tumors. MB is the most common malignant pediatric brain tumor.[33] MBs comprise < 1% of adult brain neoplasms. Peak incidence: during 1st decade. Median age at diagnosis: 5–7 years (75% are diagnosed by age 15). Male:female ratio is 2:1. Familial cancer syndromes that include MB: Gorlin syndrome, Turcot syndrome (p.610).

Pathology

All MB are WHO grade IV.[34]

Histologic subtypes[34]:

1. classic (90%): small, densely packed undifferentiated cells with hyperchromatic nuclei, scant cytoplasm (and inconstant cell clusters in Homer-Wright rosettes)[35] (sometimes called "blue tumor") (monotonous appearance)
2. desmoplastic (6%): similar to classic type with "glomeruli" AKA pale islands (collagen bundles and scattered, less cellular areas). Marked tendency for neuronal differentiation. More common in adults. Prognosis controversial: may be the same[36] or less aggressive[37] than classic MB
3. large cell (4%[38]): large, round, and/or pleomorphic nucleoli, higher mitotic activity. In the few case reports, all were male. More aggressive than classic. Resembles atypical teratoid/rhabdoid tumors of cerebellum, but has different phenotype and cytogenic features

Molecular biology

The molecular genetic alterations in MBs can be divided into 3 groups:

1. non-random chromosomal abnormalities: (e.g. consistent deletion of 17p markers) has been shown in 35–40%
2. information from gene profiling:
   a) ZIC and NSCL1 were the genes most closely correlated with MBs
   b) certain genes were associated with more favorable outcome (using 8 genes a pattern associated with 80% 5-year survival compared to 17% when the pattern was lacking)[26]
3. abnormalities in signal transduction pathways: e.g. neurotrophin signaling pathway (important in cerebellar development) or Sonic hedgehog (Shh)[39]

Seeding and metastases

≈ 10–35% have seeded the craniospinal axis at the time of diagnosis,[32] and extraneural mets occur in 5% of patients,[33] sometimes promoted by shunting[40] (although this is uncommon[19]).

Clinical

Clinical history is typically brief (6–12 weeks). MBs usually arise in the cerebellar vermis, at the apex of the roof of the 4th ventricle (fastigium in the region of the posterior medullary velum), which predisposes to early obstructive hydrocephalus. Usual presenting symptoms: H/A, N/V, and truncal & appendicular ataxia. Infants with hydrocephalus may present with irritability, lethargy, or progressive macrocrania.[41] Spinal drop mets may produce back pain, urinary retention or leg weakness. Common signs: papilledema, ataxia, nystagmus, EOM palsies.

Evaluation

Usually appears as a solid, IV-contrast-enhancing lesion on CT or MRI (however, a rare diffuse variant in children < 3 yrs, medulloblastoma with extensive nodularity[42] (MBEN), has been described). Most are located in the midline in the region of the 4th ventricle (laterally situated tumors are more common in adults). Most have hydrocephalus. Ependymoma (p. 1365) is the main entity to differentiate from on imaging.

CT: noncontrast → typically hyperdense (due to high cellularity), contrast → most enhance. 20% have calcifications.

MRI: T1WI → hypo- to isointense. T2WI → heterogeneous due to tumor cysts, vessels and calcifications.[35] Most enhance (including MBEN)

Spinal imaging: MRI with IV gadolinium or CT/myelography with water-soluble contrast should be done to rule-out "drop mets." Staging is done either pre-op or within 2–3 weeks of surgery.

Treatment

Stratification of patients into risk groups guides therapy (▶ Table 40.4).

MB are highly radiosensitive and moderately chemosensitive.

Treatment of choice: surgical debulking of as much tumor as possible (without causing neurological injury) followed by craniospinal XRT (radiation is necessary because of propensity to recur and to seed). Invasion of or attachment to the floor of the fourth ventricle (brainstem in the region of the facial colliculus) often limits excision. It is better to leave a small residual on the brain-stem (these patients do fairly well) than it is to chase every last remnant into the brain-stem (neurologic deficit is more likely with this).

Surgical exposure of midline cerebellar medulloblastomas requires opening of the foramen magnum, usually removal of the posterior arch of C1, and occasionally the arch of C2. Tumor spread with arachnoidal thickening ("sugar coating") may occur.

XRT: optimal irradiation dose: 35–40 Gy to whole craniospinal axis + 10–15 Gy boost to tumor bed (usually posterior-fossa) and to any spinal mets seen, all fractionated over 6–7 wks.[43,44] Reduce dosages by 20–25% for age < 3 yrs, or use chemotherapy instead. Lower dose radiation (25 Gy) to the neuraxis may provide acceptable control when confirmed gross total excision is achieved.[45]

Chemotherapy: there is no standardized chemotherapy regimen. Lomustine (CCNU), cisplatin and vincristine (VCR) are primarily used, but are usually reserved for recurrence, for poor risk patients (below), or for children < 3 yrs age. Significant survival advantage was shown in poor-risk children with adjuvant chemotherapy (5-year actuarial disease-free survival rate = 87%) compared to those without (33%). No difference was observed among standard risk patients.[46]

Shunts: 30–40% of children require permanent VP shunts following p-fossa resection. The risk of shunt-related seeding has been quoted as high as 10–20%,[32] but this is probably overestimated.[19] In the past, tumor filters were frequently used. They are less commonly used today because of the high incidence of obstruction.

Table 40.4 Risk stratification in medulloblastoma

Standard-risk patients
No residual tumor on post-op MRI and negative CSF results. 5-year survival is > 5%, and progression-free survival = 50%[48,49]
Poor-risk patients
Bulky residual tumor > 1.5 cm² post-op and dissemination in the brain, spine or CSF. Worse prognosis. 5-year disease-free survival is 35–50%[50]
Intermediate risk patients
An intermediate risk group probably exists, but has been poorly characterized

Prognosis

Poor prognosticators[47]

- younger age (especially if < 3 yrs)
- disseminated (metastatic) disease
- inability to perform gross-total removal (especially if residual > 1.5 cm^2 in patient with localized disease)
- histological differentiation along glial, ependymal, or neuronal lines

One stratification scheme is shown in ▶ Table 40.4.

The sex of the child is an important predictor for survival of MB; girls had a much better outcome.[51] Gene expression profiling is highly predictive of response to therapy, predicting outcome with much greater accuracy than current staging criteria.[26] The ability of multiple biological and clinical markers to predict outcomes for patients with MB is currently under investigation.[52,53]

Long-term survivors of MB are at significant risk for permanent endocrinologic, cognitive, and psychological sequelae of treatments. Infants and very young children with MB remain a difficult therapeutic challenge because they have the most virulent form of the disease and are at highest risk for treatment-related sequelae.

Most common site of recurrence is p-fossa.

Collins' law (p. 664) has also been used to define the period of risk of recurrence (PRR) but exceptions to the law have been reported.[31]

40.2.3 Supratentorial primitive neuroectodermal tumors

General information

Supratentorial primitive neuroectodermal tumor (sPNETs) are highly malignant lesions primarily affecting young children (65% occur in age < 5 years) and account for 2.5–6% of childhood brain tumors. Occur rarely in adults. No gender predilection. Histologically indistinguishable from medulloblastoma (MB), they have a distinct genetic profile, are more aggressive, and often respond poorly to MB-specific therapies (especially pineoblastomas). Overall survival rate for sPNETs is substantially lower than that for MBs, with an expected 3- year progression-free survival of approximately 50% for localized supratentorial PNETs.[54,55]

Ependymoblastoma

A highly cellular embryonal form of ependymal tumor.[56] Occurs most often in age < 5 yrs. Prognosis is poor, with median post-op survival ranging from 12–20 months, and almost 100% mortality rate at 3 yrs. As with other tumors in this category, there is a tendency for subarachnoid seeding.

40.2.4 Atypical teratoid/rhabdoid tumors (AT/RT)

A unique embryonal tumor of the CNS. Many of these tumors were probably previously misdiagnosed as MBs. Occurs primarily in infants and children (> 90% are < 5 years of age, with most age < 2 years). A minority are associated with primary renal rhabdoid tumor. 50% of AT/RTs occur in posterior fossa with a predilection for the cerebellopontine angle (CPA).

33% have CSF spread at presentation. Most patients die within 1 year of diagnosis.

Histopathology: some tumors are composed entirely of rhabdoid cells, others have a combination of rhabdoid and areas resembling PNET/MB. Other cell types include: malignant mesenchymal cells (usually spindle cells), malignant epithelial cells (glandular or squamous).

Molecular biology: AT/RT and the rhabdoid renal tumors have a deletion or monosomy of chromosome 22.

40.2.5 Esthesioneuroblastoma

General information

Esthesioneuroblastoma (ENB), originally described in 1924, AKA olfactory neuroblastoma, AKA olfactory esthesioneuroblastoma, AKA esthesioneurocytoma, AKA olfactory placode tumor.[57] A rare nasal neoplasm with an incidence 0.4 per 1,000,000 people.[58] Believed to arise from the olfactory neural crest cells in the upper nares, it is considered to be malignant. These tumors occur over a wide age range (3 to 90 years), with a bimodal peak between the second and third decade and a second peak in the sixth and seventh decades.

Imaging

MRI: isointense with brain on T1-weighted imaging and intermediate to high signal intensity on T2-weighted imaging and enhance heterogeneously with gadolinium. Signal characteristics may mimic meningioma. For higher stage lesions, the cribiform plate may be eroded, better seen on thin cut CT. The most important factor determining resectability is intracranial extension. Magnetic resonance aids in the distinction between extradural tumor, dural invasion, or parenchymal brain invasion. None of these are specific to this tumor.

Differential diagnosis

Includes SNUC, nasal melanoma, nasal squamous cell carcinoma, and meningioma.

Diagnosis

Endoscopic biopsy is typically performed in the otolaryngology office prior to surgery.

A clinical oncology exam should be performed, and if there is suspicion for metastatic disease a PET scan should be ordered which is sensitive for metastatic disease.

Clinical classification systems

The modified Kadish system[59] (which added category D to the original Kadish system[60]) is shown in ▶ Table 40.5. This classification appears to correlate with survival.[59] Alternative systems by Biller et al.[61] and Dulguerov and Calcaterra,[62] (see ▶ Table 40.5) attempt to subdivide the Kadish C classification, however the more popular modified Kadish system is more frequently used.

Pathologic grading

Hyams grading, a system used to define all upper respiratory tract carcinomas is utilized which assess nuclear pleomorphism, mitotic activity, rosette presence, necrosis, and summates these to produce Hyams 1–4 classification.[63] It has been shown in meta-analysis as well as large series that Hyams grade 1 and 2 predict benign disease course, as compared to Hyams 3 and 4 which predict poor disease course. It is recommended grading be performed in all cases.[64,65]

Treatment

Primary Treatment is controversial. Some institutions believe in upfront combined radiation therapy and chemotherapy prior to craniofacial resection. However most practice upfront surgery, which classically consisted of endoscopic resection with negative margins for Kadish A and B lesions, and for Kadish C and D lesions craniofacial resection which was bifrontal craniotomy with associated lateral rhinotomy. However, with the advent of endoscopic techniques the lateral rhinotomy is often replaced with a purely endoscopic approach unless there is inferior lateral orbital or maxillary involvement, in which case the lateral rhinotomy is frequently used. Finally, some institutions are now managing Kadish stages purely endoscopically unless they are unable to get negative margins at the time of surgery, then conversion to an open approach is performed or SRS is performed, however this is controversial.

Outcome

Median overall survival is typically 7.2 ± 0.7 years.[64]

Table 40.5 Clinical classification systems for esthesioneuroblastoma

Modified Kadish[59]	Biller et al.[61]	Dulguerov and Calcattera[62]
A: Confined to Nasal Cavity	T1: Nasal/Paranasal Sinuses	T1: Nasal/Paranasal Sinuses
B: Extends to Paranasal Sinus	T2: Periorbital/Anterior Fossa Extension	T2: Erosion of Cribiform Plate
C: Local Extension (orbit or cribriforms plate)	T3: Brain Involvement, Resectable Margins	T3: Periorbital/Anterior Fossa Extension
D: Distant Metastasis	T4: Unable to Obtain Negative Margins- Unresectable	T4: Brain Involvement

Mean progression free survival is 4.8 ± 0.7 years. The 5 and 10 year survivals are 63% and 40%.[64]

Population based analysis of the Surveillance Epidemiology and End Results (SEER) database confirm that Kadish staging, lymph node involvement, and age at diagnosis have significant prognostic value.[66] These findings have been confirmed in a large meta-analysis recently published by Kane et al., in 2010[65] Further, higher Hyams grading (grades 3 and 4) correlate with a poorer prognosis.[64,65]

Salvage treatment: For patients with recurrent disease, this typically occurs in 2 patterns: that of intracranial recurrence or those with distant metastasis.[67,68] Intracranial recurrence is typically treated with repeat transcranial resection, however stereotactic radiosurgery is a viable option.[67,68,69] In patients with distant metastasis, those with cervical lymph node metastasis should undergo modified radical neck dissection to understand the extant of disease. This typically leads to chemotherapy, of which platinum based therapies remain the standard of therapy at this time.[67,70,71]

References

[1] Ringertz N, Nordenstam H, Flyger G. Tumors of the Pineal Region. J Neuropathol Exp Neurol. 1954; 13:540–561

[2] Di Costanzo A, Tedeschi G, Di Salle F, Golia F, Morrone R, Bonavita V. Pineal Cysts: An Incidental MRI Finding? J Neurol Neurosurg Psychiatry. 1993; 56:207–208

[3] Hasegawa A, Ohtsubo K, Mori W. Pineal Gland in Old Age: Quantitative and Qualitative Morphological Study of 168 Human Autopsy Cases. Brain Res. 1987; 409:343–349

[4] Torres A, Krisht AF, Akouri S. Current Management of Pineal Cysts. Contemp Neurosurg. 2005; 27:1–5

[5] Maurer PK, Ecklund J, Parisi JE, Ondra S. Symptomatic Pineal Cysts: Case Report. Neurosurgery. 1990; 27:451–454

[6] Wisoff JH, Epstein F. Surgical Management of Symptomatic Pineal Cysts. J Neurosurg. 1992; 77:896–900

[7] Klein P, Rubinstein LJ. Benign Symptomatic Glial Cysts of The Pineal Gland: A Report of Seven Cases and Review of the Literature. J Neurol Neurosurg Psychiatry. 1989; 52:991–995

[8] Mamourian AC, Towfighi J. Pineal Cysts: MR Imaging. AJNR. 1986; 7:1081–1086

[9] Di Chirico A, Di Rocco F, Velardi F. Spontaneous regression of a symptomatic pineal cyst after endoscopic third-ventriculostomy. Childs Nerv Syst. 2001; 17:42–46

[10] Regis J, Bouillot P, Rouby-Volot F, et al. Pineal Region Tumors and the Role of Stereotactic Biopsy: Review of the Mortality, Morbidity, and Diagnostic Rates in 370 Cases. Neurosurgery. 1996; 39:907–914

[11] Youssef AS, Keller JT, van Loveren HR. Novel application of computer-assisted cisternal endoscopy for the biopsy of pineal region tumors: cadaveric study. Acta Neurochir (Wien). 2007; 149:399–406

[12] Oi S, Matsumoto S. Controversy pertaining to therapeutic modalities for tumors of the pineal region: a worldwide survey of different patient populations. Childs Nerv Syst. 1992; 8:332–336

[13] Sugiyama K, Uozumi T, Kiya K, Mukada K, Arita K, Kurisu K, Hotta T, Ogasawara H, Sumida M. Intracranial germ-cell tumor with synchronous lesions in the pineal and suprasellar regions: report of six cases and review of the literature. Surg Neurol. 1992; 38:114–120

[14] Hoffman HJ, Ostubo H, Hendrick EB, et al. Intracranial Germ-Cell Tumors in Children. J Neurosurg. 1991; 74:545–551

[15] Shinoda J, Yamada H, Sakai N, Ando T, Hirata T, Miwa Y. Placental alkaline phosphatase as a tumor marker for primary intracranial germinoma. J Neurosurg. 1988; 68:710–720

[16] Todo T, Kondo T, Shinoura N, Yamada R. Large Cysts of the Pineal Gland: Report of Two Cases. Neurosurgery. 1991; 29:101–106

[17] Edwards MSB, Hudgins RJ, Wilson CB, et al. Pineal Region Tumors in Children. J Neurosurg. 1988; 68:689–697

[18] Oi S, Matsuzawa K, Choi JU, Kim DS, Kang JK, Cho BK. Identical characteristics of the patient populations with pineal region tumors in Japan and in Korea and therapeutic modalities. Childs Nerv Syst. 1998; 14:36–40

[19] Berger MS, Baumeister B, Geyer JR, Milstein J, et al. The Risks of Metastases from Shunting in Children with Primary Central Nervous System Tumors. J Neurosurg. 1991; 74:872–877

[20] Stern JD, Ross DA. Stereotactic Management of Benign Pineal Region Cysts: Report of Two Cases. Neurosurgery. 1993; 32:310–314

[21] Musolino A, Cambria S, Rizzo G, Cambria M. Symptomatic Cysts of the Pineal Gland: Stereotactic Diagnosis and Treatment of Two Cases and Review of the Literature. Neurosurgery. 1993; 32:315–321

[22] Kelly PJ. Comment on Musolino A, et al.: Symptomatic Cysts of the Pineal Gland: Stereotactic Diagnosis and Treatment of Two Cases and Review of the Literature. Neurosurgery. 1993; 32:320–321

[23] Dempsey PK, Kondziolka D, Lunsford LD. Stereotactic Diagnosis and Treatment of Pineal Region Tumors and Vascular Malformations. Acta Neurochir. 1992; 116:14–22

[24] Kelly PJ. Comment on Regis J, et al.: Pineal Region Tumors and the Role of Stereotactic Biopsy: Review of the Mortality, Morbidity, and Diagnostic Rates in 370 Cases. Neurosurgery. 1996; 39:912–913

[25] Stein BM. The infratentorial supracerebellar approach to pineal lesions. J Neurosurg. 1971; 35:197–202

[26] Pomeroy SL, Tamayo P, Gaasenbeek M, Sturla LM, Angelo M, McLaughlin ME, Kim JY, Goumnerova LC, Black PM, Lau C, Allen JC, Zagzag D, Olson JM, Curran T, Wetmore C, Biegel JA, Poggio T, Mukherjee S, Rifkin R, Califano A, Stolovitzky G, Louis DN, Mesirov JP, Lander ES, Golub TR. Prediction of central nervous system embryonal tumour outcome based on gene expression. Nature. 2002; 415:436–442

[27] Louis DN, Ohgaki H, Wiestler OD, Cavenee WK, Bosman FT, Jaffe ES, Lakhani SR, Ohgaki H. WHO classification of tumors of the central nervous system. Lyon 2007

[28] Kumar R, Reddy SJ, Wani AA, Pal L. Primary spinal primitive neuroectodermal tumor: case series and review of the literature. Pediatr Neurosurg. 2007; 43:1–6

[29] Tomita T, McLone DG. Spontaneous Seeding of Medulloblastoma: Results of Cerebrospinal Fluid Cytology and Arachnoid Biopsy from the Cisterna Magna. Neurosurgery. 1983; 12:265–267

[30] Collins VP, Loeffler RK, Tivey H. Observations on growth rates of human tumors. Am J Roentgenol Radium Ther Nucl Med. 1956; 76:988–1000

[31] Sure U, Berghorn WJ, Bertalanffy H. Collins' law. Prediction of recurrence or cure in childhood medulloblastoma? Clin Neurol Neurosurg. 1997; 99:113–116

[32] Laurent JP, Cheek WR. Brain Tumors in Children. J Pediatr Neurosci. 1985; 1:15–32

[33] Allen JC. Childhood Brain Tumors: Current Status of Clinical Trials in Newly Diagnosed and Recurrent Disease. Ped Clin N Am. 1985; 32:633–651

[34] Eberhart CG, Kepner JL, Goldthwaite PT, Kun LE, Duffner PK, Friedman HS, Strother DR, Burger PC. Histopathologic grading of medulloblastomas: a

Pediatric Oncology Group study. Cancer. 2002; 94:552–560

[35] Blaser SI, Harwood-Nash DC. Neuroradiology of pediatric posterior fossa medulloblastoma. J Neurooncol. 1996; 29:23–34

[36] Pramanik P, Sharma MC, Mukhopadhyay P, Singh VP, Sarkar C. A comparative study of classical vs. desmoplastic medulloblastomas. Neurol India. 2003; 51:27–34

[37] Kleihues P, Louis DN, Scheithauer BW, Rorke LB, Reifenberger G, Burger PC, Cavenee WK. The WHO classification of tumors of the nervous system. J Neuropathol Exp Neurol. 2002; 61:215–25; discussion 226-9

[38] Giangaspero F, Rigobello L, Badiali M, et al. Large-cell medulloblastoma. Am J Surg Pathol. 1992; 16:687–693

[39] Corcoran RB, Scott MP. Oxysterols stimulate Sonic hedgehog signal transduction and proliferation of medulloblastoma cells. Proc Natl Acad Sci U S A. 2006; 103:8408–8413

[40] Kessler LA, Dugan P, Concannon JP. Systemic Metastases of Medulloblastoma Promoted by Shunting. Surg Neurol. 1975; 3:147–152

[41] Park TS, Hoffman HJ, Hendrick EB, et al. Medulloblastoma: Clinical Presentation and Management. J Neurosurg. 1983; 58:543–552

[42] Suresh TN, Santosh V, Yasha TC, Anandh B, Mohanty A, Indiradevi B, Sampath S, Shankar SK. Medulloblastoma with extensive nodularity: a variant occurring in the very young-clinicopathological and immunohistochemical study of four cases. Childs Nerv Syst. 2004; 20:55–60

[43] Merchant TE, Wang MH, Haida T, Lindsley KL, Finlay J, Dunkel IJ, Rosenblum MK, Leibel SA. Medulloblastoma: long-term results for patients treated with definitive radiation therapy during the computed tomography era. Int J Radiat Oncol Biol Phys. 1996; 36:29–35

[44] Packer RJ, Gajjar A, Vezina G, Rorke-Adams L, Burger PC, Robertson PL, Bayer L, LaFond D, Donahue BR, Marymont MH, Muraszko K, Langston J, Sposto R. Phase III study of craniospinal radiation therapy followed by adjuvant chemotherapy for newly diagnosed average-risk medulloblastoma. J Clin Oncol. 2006; 24:4202–4208

[45] Tomita T, McLone DG. Medulloblastoma in Childhood: Results of Radical Resection and Low-Dose Radiation Therapy. J Neurosurg. 1986; 64:238–242

[46] Packer RJ, Sutton LN, Goldwein JW, Perilongo G, Bunin G, Ryan J, Cohen BH, D'Angio G, Kramer ED, Zimmerman RA, et al. Improved survival with the use of adjuvant chemotherapy in the treatment of medulloblastoma. J Neurosurg. 1991; 74:433–440

[47] Gilbertson RJ. Medulloblastoma: signalling a change in treatment. Lancet Oncol. 2004; 5:209–218

[48] David KM, Casey AT, Hayward RD, Harkness WF, Phipps K, Wade AM. Medulloblastoma: is the 5-year survival rate improving? A review of 80 cases from a single institution. J Neurosurg. 1997; 86:13–21

[49] Albright AL, Wisoff JH, Zeltzer PM, Boyett JM, Rorke LB, Stanley P. Effects of medulloblastoma resections on outcome in children: a report from the Children's Cancer Group. Neurosurgery. 1996; 38:265–271

[50] Evans AE, Jenkins RD, Sposto R, et al. The Treatment of Medulloblastoma: Results of a Prospective Randomized Trial of Radiation Therapy With and Without CCNU, Vincristine, and Prednisone. J Neurosurg. 1990; 72:572–582

[51] Weil MD, Lamborn K, Edwards MS, Wara WM. Influence of a child's sex on medulloblastoma outcome. JAMA. 1998; 279:1474–1476

[52] Gajjar A, Hernan R, Kocak M, Fuller C, Lee Y, McKinnon PJ, Wallace D, Lau C, Chintagumpala M, Ashley DM, Kellie SJ, Kun L, Gilbertson RJ. Clinical, histopathologic, and molecular markers of prognosis: toward a new disease risk stratification system for medulloblastoma. J Clin Oncol. 2004; 22:984–993

[53] Ray A, Ho M, Ma J, Parkes RK, Mainprize TG, Ueda S, McLaughlin J, Bouffet E, Rutka JT, Hawkins CE. A clinicobiological model predicting survival in medulloblastoma. Clin Cancer Res. 2004; 10:7613–7620

[54] Reddy AT, Janss AJ, Phillips PC, Weiss HL, Packer RJ. Outcome for children with supratentorial primitive neuroectodermal tumors treated with surgery, radiation, and chemotherapy. Cancer. 2000; 88:2189–2193

[55] Hong TS, Mehta MP, Boyett JM, Donahue B, Rorke LB, Yao MS, Zeltzer PM. Patterns of failure in supratentorial primitive neuroectodermal tumors treated in Children's Cancer Group Study 921, a phase III combined modality study. Int J Radiat Oncol Biol Phys. 2004; 60:204–213

[56] Mork SJ, Rubinstein LJ. Ependymoblastoma. A Reappraisal of a Rare Embryonal Tumor. Cancer. 1985; 55:1536–1542

[57] Berger L, Luc G, Richard D. L'Esthesioneuroepitheliome Olfactif. Bull Assoc Franc Etude Cancer. 1924; 13:410–421

[58] Theilgaard SA, Buchwald C, Ingeholm P, Kornum Larsen S, Eriksen JG, Sand Hansen H. Esthesioneuroblastoma: a Danish demographic study of 40 patients registered between 1978 and 2000. Acta Otolaryngol. 2003; 123:433–439

[59] Chao KS, Kaplan C, Simpson JR, Haughey B, Spector GJ, Sessions DG, Arquette M. Esthesioneuroblastoma: the impact of treatment modality. Head Neck. 2001; 23:749–757

[60] Kadish S, Goodman M, Wang CC. Olfactory neuroblastoma. A clinical analysis of 17 cases. Cancer. 1976; 37:1571–1576

[61] Biller HF, Lawson W, Sachdev VP, Som P. Esthesioneuroblastoma: surgical treatment without radiation. Laryngoscope. 1990; 100:1199–1201

[62] Dulguerov P, Calcaterra T. Esthesioneuroblastoma: the UCLA experience 1970-1990. Laryngoscope. 1992; 102:843–849

[63] Hyams V. Tumors of the upper respiratory tract and ear. Washington, D.C.: Armed Forces Institute of Pathology; 1988

[64] Van Gompel JJ, Giannini C, Olsen KD, Moore E, Piccirilli M, Foote RL, Buckner JC, Link MJ. Long-term outcome of esthesioneuroblastoma: hyams grade predicts patient survival. J Neurol Surg B Skull Base. 2012; 73:331–336

[65] Kane AJ, Sughrue ME, Rutkowski MJ, Aranda D, Mills SA, Buencamino R, Fang S, Barani IJ, Parsa AT. Posttreatment prognosis of patients with esthesioneuroblastoma. J Neurosurg. 2010; 113:340–351

[66] Gardner G, Robertson JH. Hearing Preservation in Unilateral Acoustic Neuroma Surgery. Ann Otol Rhinol Laryngol. 1988; 97:55–66

[67] Dias FL, Sa GM, Lima RA, Kligerman J, Leoncio MP, Freitas EQ, Soares JR, Arcuri RA. Patterns of failure and outcome in esthesioneuroblastoma. Arch Otolaryngol Head Neck Surg. 2003; 129:1186–1192

[68] Gore MR, Zanation AM. Salvage Treatment of Local Recurrence in Esthesioneuroblastoma: A Meta-analysis. Skull Base. 2011; 21:1–6

[69] Van Gompel JJ, Carlson ML, Pollock BE, Moore EJ, Foote RL, Link MJ. Stereotactic radiosurgical salvage treatment for locally recurrent esthesioneuroblastoma. Neurosurgery. 2013; 72:332–9; discussion 339-40

[70] Foote RL, Morita A, Ebersold MJ, Olsen KD, Lewis JE, Quast LM, Ferguson JA, O'Fallon WM. Esthesioneuroblastoma: the role of adjuvant radiation therapy. Int J Radiat Oncol Biol Phys. 1993; 27:835–842

[71] Kim HJ, Cho HJ, Kim KS, Lee HS, Kim HJ, Jung E, Yoon JH. Results of salvage therapy after failure of initial treatment for advanced olfactory neuroblastoma. J Craniomaxillofac Surg. 2008; 36:47–52

41 Tumors of Cranial, Spinal and Peripheral Nerves

41.1 Vestibular schwannoma

41.1.1 General information

Key concepts

- Histologically benign tumor of cranial nerve VIII located in the cerebellopontine angle (CPA)
- Usually arises from inferior division (controversial) of the vestibular portion of the VIII nerve
- 3 most common early symptoms (clinical triad): hearing loss (insidious and progressive), tinnitus (high pitched) and dysequilibrium (true vertigo is uncommon)
- W/U: All patients: ✔ MRI (without & with contrast), ✔ audiometrics (pure tone audiogram and speech discrimination). In addition for small VSs (≤ 15 mm dia): ✔ ENG, ✔ VEMP, ✔ ABR
- Histology: comprised of Antoni A (narrow elongated bipolar cells) and Antoni B fibers (loose reticulated)
- Choice of management option (observation, surgery, XRT or chemotherapy (Avastin®)) depends heavily on tumor size, growth, hearing status, VII function and presence of NF2

Vestibular schwannoma (VS) is a histologically benign schwann-cell sheath tumor that usually arises from of the inferior division of the *vestibular nerve* (not the cochlear portion). VSs arise as a result of the loss of a tumor-suppressor gene on the long arm of chromosome 22 (in sporadic cases this is a somatic mutation; in neurofibromatosis Type 2 (NF2) this is either inherited or represents a new mutation that may then be transmitted to offspring).

Older terms included for reference, that should be avoided[1,2]): acoustic neuroma, acoustic neurinomas (neurinoma being obsolete term for schwannoma), neurilemoma or neurilemmoma.

41.1.2 Epidemiology

One of the most common intracranial tumors, comprising 8–10% of tumors in most series.[3] Annual incidence is probably about 1.5 cases per 100,000 population – over the past couple decades this estimate has increased and the typical size at diagnosis has decreased as a result of the proliferation of MRI scans.[4] In the US, annual incidence has been found to vary between 1.1 and 1.3 per 100,000 population between 2004 and 2007.[5] VSs typically become symptomatic after age 30. At least 95% are unilateral.

Neurofibromatosis Type 2

The incidence of vestibular schwannomas (VS) is increased in neurofibromatosis (NFT), with bilateral VS being pathognomonic of neurofibromatosis Type 2 (NFT2), see central NFT (p. 605). Any patient < 40 yrs old with unilateral VS should also be evaluated for NFT2. Cytologically, the VSs of NFT2 are identical to sporadic cases, however in NFT2 the tumors form grape-like clusters that may infiltrate the nerve fibers (unlike most sporadic VSs which *displace* the eighth nerve).

41.1.3 Pathology

Tumors are composed of Antoni A fibers (narrow elongated bipolar cells) and Antoni B fibers (loose reticulated). Verocay bodies are also seen, and consist of acellular eosinophilic areas surrounded by parallel arrangement of spindle shaped schwann cells (they are not a cell type).

41.1.4 Clinical

Symptoms

General information

Symptoms are shown in ▶ Table 41.1. The type of symptoms are closely correlated with tumor size. Most initially cause the triad of ipsilateral sensorineural hearing loss, tinnitus and balance difficulties. Larger tumors can cause facial numbness, weakness or twitching, and possibly brainstem symptoms. Rarely, large tumor may produce hydrocephalus. With current imaging modalities (CT and especially MRI), increasing numbers of smaller lesions are being detected.

Table 41.1 Symptoms in vestibular schwannoma (131 patients[3])

Symptom	%
hearing loss	98%
tinnitus	70%
dysequilibrium[a]	67%
H/A	32%
facial numbness	29%
facial weakness	10%
diplopia	10%
N/V	9%
otalgia	9%
change of taste	6%
[a]or vertigo	

Symptoms from 8th nerve compression

Unilateral sensorineural hearing loss, tinnitus and dysequilibrium are related to pressure on the eighth nerve complex in the IAC. These are the earliest symptoms, and by the time of diagnosis, virtually all tumors have caused otologic symptoms.

Hearing loss is insidious and progressive in most (c.f. the hearing loss in Meniere's disease which fluctuates), however 10% report sudden hearing loss (see below). 70% have a high frequency loss pattern, and word discrimination is usually affected (especially noticeable in telephone conversation).

The tinnitus is usually high pitched.

Unsteadiness manifests primarily as difficulty with balance; true vertigo occurs in < 20%.

Sudden hearing loss: The differential diagnosis for sudden hearing loss (SHL) is extensive.[6] *Idiopathic* SHL (i.e. no identified etiology: must rule out neoplasm, infection, autoimmune, vascular and toxic causes) occurs in an estimated 10 per 100,000 population.[7] 1% of patients with SHL will be found to have a VS, and SHL may be the presenting symptom in 1–14% of patients with VS.[8] SHL with VS is presumably due to an infarction of the acoustic nerve, or acute occlusion of the cochlear artery. Treatment options for SHL include:

1. steroids: e.g. prednisone 60 mg PO q d × 10 d then tapered[8]
2. famciclovir (Famvir®) 500 mg po TID × 10 d
3. ✖ heparin has been shown *not* to be of help
4. conservative treatment: rest, restriction of salt, alcohol and tobacco[9]
5. experimental: consideration may be given to thrombolytic therapy (p. 1286), e.g. rt-PA

Symptoms from 5th and 7th nerve compression

Otalgia, facial numbness and weakness, and taste changes occur as the tumor enlarges and compresses the fifth and seventh nerves. These symptoms usually do not occur until the tumor is > 2 cm. This highlights an interesting paradox: facial weakness is a rare or late occurrence, even though the 7th nerve is almost always distorted early; whereas facial numbness occurs sooner once trigeminal compression occurs (often in the presence of normal facial movement), despite the fact that the 5th nerve is farther away.[10] This may be due to the resiliency of motor nerves relative to sensory nerves.

Symptoms from compression of brainstem and other cranial nerves

Larger tumors cause brainstem compression (with ataxia, H/A, N/V, diplopia, cerebellar signs, and if unchecked, coma, respiratory depression and death) and lower cranial nerve (IX, X, XII) palsies (hoarseness, dysphagia…). Obstruction of CSF circulation by larger tumors (usually > 4 cm) may produce hydrocephalus with increased ICP.

Rarely, 6th nerve involvement may cause diplopia.

Signs

Hearing loss due to VIII involvement is the earliest cranial nerve finding. 66% of patients have no abnormal physical finding except for hearing loss (for other findings, see ▶ Table 41.2).

Since hearing loss is sensorineural, **Weber test** (p.580) will lateralize to the uninvolved side, and if there is enough preserved hearing, **Rinne test** (p.580) will be positive (i.e. normal; air conduction > bone conduction) on both sides.

Facial nerve (VII) dysfunction is uncommon before treatment. When present, it is usually graded clinically on the House and Brackmann scale (see ▶ Table 41.3).

Vestibular involvement causes nystagmus (may be central or peripheral) and abnormal electronystagmography (ENG) with caloric stimulation.

Table 41.2 Signs in 131 vestibular schwannomas (excluding hearing loss)[3]

Sign	%
abnormal corneal reflex	33
nystagmus	26
facial hypoesthesia	26
facial weakness (palsy)	12
abnormal eye movement	11
papilledema	10
Babinski sign	5

Table 41.3 Clinical grading of facial nerve function(House and Brackmann[11])

Grade	Function	Description
1	normal	normal facial function in all areas
2	mild dysfunction	1. gross: slight weakness noticeable on close inspection; may have very slight synkinesis 2. at rest: normal symmetry and tone 3. motion: a) forehead: slight to moderate movement b) eye: complete closure with effort c) mouth: slight asymmetry
3	moderate dysfunction	1. gross: obvious but not disfiguring asymmetry: noticeable but not severe synkinesis 2. motion: a) forehead: slight to moderate movement b) eye: complete closure with effort c) mouth: slightly weak with maximal effort
4	moderate to severe dysfunction	1. gross: obvious weakness and/or disfiguring asymmetry 2. motion: a) forehead: none b) eye: incomplete closure c) mouth: asymmetry with maximum effort
5	severe dysfunction	1. gross: only barely perceptible motion 2. at rest: asymmetry 3. motion: a) forehead: none b) eye: incomplete closure
6	total paralysis	no movement

Differential diagnosis

See Cerebellopontine angle (CPA) lesions (p. 1365). The major differentials are: meningioma, or neuroma of an adjacent cranial nerve (e.g. trigeminal).

41.1.5 Evaluation

General information

1. Brain MRI without and with contrast. FIESTA MRI if available. If MRI is contraindicated, then a CT scan without and with contrast
2. Temporal bone CT for detailed bony anatomy if surgery is contemplated
3. audiometric evaluation:
   a) pure tone audiogram (see below)
   b) speech discrimination evaluation (see below)
   c) patients with small VSs (≤ 15 mm dia) also get:
      - ENG: (p. 674) assesses *superior* vestibular nerve
      - VEMP: (p. 675) assesses *inferior* vestibular nerve
      - ABR: (p. 675) prognosticates chance of hearing preservation

Audiometric and audiologic studies

General information

Baseline studies are helpful for management treatment decisions and for later comparison and to assess the contralateral ear.

Pure tone audiogram (PTA)

May be useful as first-step screening test. Air conduction assesses the entire system, bone conduction assesses from the cochlea and proximally. PTA assesses the functionality of hearing (to help in treatment decision making) and acts as a baseline for future comparison. The pure tone average (also abbreviated PTA) is a single numerical score that is an *average* of the thresholds for frequencies across the audio spectrum (at 500, 1000 & 2000 Hz). On a standard audiogram, X's denote the left ear (AS) and O's denote the right ear (AD).

Progressive unilateral or *asymmetric* sensorineural hearing loss of high tones occurs in > 95% of VSs.[12] High-frequency hearing loss also happens to be the most common type of hearing loss with age or with noise induced sensorineural hearing loss, but is usually symmetrical. Only ≈ 1 in 1000 patients with asymmetric hearing have a VS.[1] Other causes of asymmetrical sensorineural hearing loss[13]: other CPA lesions (e.g. meningioma), inner ear lesions, intraaxial lesions (including 9 infarctions), multiple sclerosis. On hearing screening tests, an unexplained PTA difference from one ear to the other > 10–15 dB is suspicious and should be investigated further.

Speech discrimination evaluation

Speech discrimination is maintained in conductive hearing loss, moderately impaired in cochlear hearing loss, and worst with retrocochlear lesions. No longer used for diagnostic purposes; a score of 4% suggests a retrocochlear lesion, as does a score that is worse than would be predicted based on PTA testing (the speech recognition threshold should be similar to PTA thresholds below 4 kHz). Has found usefulness in determining serviceability of hearing and prognosticating for hearing preservation surgery. Open-set word recognition score (WRS ▶ Table 41.4) is a more sensitive measure of communication ability than PTA.

Table 41.4 Open-set word recognition score

Class	WRS%
I	70–100%
II	50–69%
III	1–49%
IV	0

Table 41.5 Gardener and Robertson modified hearing classification[a]

Class	Clinical utility	Description	Pure tone audiogram[b] (dB)	Speech discrimination[b]
I	serviceable	good-excellent	0–30	70–100%
II	serviceable	serviceable	31–50	50–59%
III	non-serviceable	non-serviceable	51–90	5–49%
IV	non-serviceable	poor	91-max	1–4%
V	non-serviceable	none	not testable	0

[a]modification[15] of the Silverstein and Norrell system[16]
[b] if PTA and speech discrimination score do not qualify in the same class, use the lower class

Table 41.6 American Academy of Otolaryngology-Head and Neck Surgery Foundation hearing classification system

Class	Clinical utility	Pure tone threshold (dB)[a]		Speech discrimination score[b] (%)
A	"useful"	≤ 30	AND	≥ 70
B	"useful"	> 30 AND ≤ 50	AND	≥ 50
C	"aidable"	> 50	AND	≥ 50
D	"nonfunctional"	any level		< 50

[a]average of pure tone hearing thresholds by air conduction at 0.5, 1, 2 & 3 kHz
[b]speech discrimination at 40 dB or maximum comfortable loudness

Definition of serviceable hearing

There are many definitions of what constitutes serviceable hearing. Also, even nonserviceable hearing can offer some benefit. If WRS is good (≥ 70%) but PTA is poor, a hearing aid may provide significant benefit.

Two commonly used scoring systems for hearing are shown here:

1. Modified **Gardener-Robertson** system for grading hearing: shown in ▶ Table 41.5. Class I patients may use a phone on that side, class II patients can localize sounds.
2. The American Academy of Otolaryngology – Head and Neck Surgery Foundation (AAO-HNS) hearing classification system[14]: shown in ▶ Table 41.6.

Some definitions of serviceable hearing (see text that follows for details):

1. AAO-HNS class A or B
2. "50/50 rule": Gardner-Robertson class I or II (pure tone audiogram threshold ≤ 50 dB and speech discrimination score ≥ 50%)
3. some prefer a 70/30 rule (70% WRS, 30 dB PTA)
4. in a patient with good hearing in the contralateral ear, a speech discrimination score (SDS) of < 70% in the affected ear is not considered good hearing; whereas if the contralateral ear is totally deaf, a SDS of ≥ 50% can be useful[17]

Additional tests that are helpful with small VSs (≤ 15 mm diameter)

The **ENG and VEMP** evaluate the superior and inferior division of the vestibular nerve (VN) respectively. The inferior VN is closer to the cochlear nerve than the superior VN (▶ Fig. 1.7), and small tumors (≤ 4 mm) of the inferior VN tend to be deeper and closer to the cochlear nerve than similar sized tumors of the superior division which tend to be more superficial and more easily removed.

Electronystagmography (ENG): Only tests the horizontal semicircular canal ∴ assesses the *superior* vestibular nerve which innervates it. Normally, each ear contributes an equal portion of the response. The ENG is considered abnormal if there is > 20% difference between the two sides. Response may be normal with a small tumor arising from the *inferior* division of vestibular nerve. NB: the vestibular nerve may continue to function until almost all of the nerve fibers are affected. Mnemonic for the directionality of the nystagmus (direction is classified based on the fast phase of the nystagmus). COWS (Cold Opposite, Warm Same). NB: this is different than caloric testing for brain death and is a source of confusion.

Vestibular evoked myogenic potential (VEMP): Assesses *inferior* vestibular nerve by imparting acoustic energy to the saccule.[18] Independent of hearing (can be done even with deafness from profound sensorineural hearing loss). Electrodes are placed on sternocleidomastoid muscle (SCM).

Auditory brainstem responses (ABR): AKA BAER (p. 240). The most common findings are prolonged I-III and I-V interpeak latencies. No longer used for diagnostic purposes (sensitivity is only ≈ 88–90% (i.e. will miss 10–12% of VSs) and specificity is only 85%. ABR is useful for prognostication – poor wave morphology correlates with lower chance of preserving hearing (even with good hearing).

Radiographic evaluation

MRI

Thin slice axial plane gadolinium enhanced MRI is the diagnostic procedure of choice with sensitivity close to 98% and almost 0% false positive rate. Characteristic findings: round or oval enhancing tumor centered on IAC. Large VSs (> 3 cm dia) may show cystic appearing areas on CT or MRI; in actuality these areas are usually solid. Adjacent trapped CSF cisterns may also give cystic appearance. In a pilot study, hyperintensity on T2 has been associated with soft and suckable tumors at the time of surgery[19] and a trend towards better VII function preservation.

FIESTA MRI (fast imaging employing steady state acquisition): uses CSF as the contrast agent (∴ does *not* use gadolinium), may improve visualization of the tumor and nerves.

CT scan

CT with IV contrast is second choice for imaging modality. If MRI is contraindicated and clinical suspicion of VS is strong but the CT is negative, small lesions may be visualized by introducing 3-4 ml of subarachnoid air via lumbar puncture, and scanning the patient with the affected side up (to trap air in region of IAC), non-filling of the IAC is indicative of an intracanalicular mass. Even with air contrast, CT was normal in 6% in Mayo series.[3]

Many VSs enlarge the ostium of the IAC (called trumpeting). Normal diameter of the IAC: 5-8 mm. 3-5% of VSs do not enlarge the IAC on CT (percentage is likely higher in small VSs vs. large ones).

Thin-cut temporal bone CT should be obtained for operative planning. Important features to identify:

- For middle fossa approach: bony coverage of Geniculate ganglion to identify dehiscence
- For translab approach:
  - Extent of pneumatization of the mastoid and position of sigmoid sinus. An anterior sinus with poorly pneumatized mastoids can indicate a tight space for this approach
  - Position of the jugular bulb. If high riding, can indicate a tight space in translab approach
- For retrosigmoid transmeatal approach: location and thickness of bone coverage over the posterior semicircular canal and vestibular aqueduct. The extent of peritubular air cells and retro facial air cells needs to be assessed in planning the approach and preventing CSF leaks.

41.1.6 Management

Management options

Management options include:

1. expectant management: follow symptoms, hearing (audiometrics) and tumor growth on serial imaging (MRI or CT). Intervention is performed for progression. Growth patterns observed:
   a) little or no growth: applies to most (83%) VSs confined within the IAC and 30% extending into CPA (see natural history of growth below)
   b) slow growth ≈ 2 mm/yr
   c) rapid growth: ≥ 10 mm/yr
   d) a few actually shrink[4]
2. radiation therapy (alone, or in conjunction with surgery)
   a) external beam radiation therapy (EBRT)
      - stereotactic radiation
      - stereotactic radiosurgery (SRS) (p. 1564): single dose
      - stereotactic radiotherapy (SRT) (p. 1564): fractionated

3. surgery: approaches include the following (see below for details)
   a) retrosigmoid (AKA suboccipital): may be able to spare hearing
   b) translabyrinthine (and its several variations): sacrifices hearing, may be slightly better for sparing VII
   c) middle fossa approach (extradural subtemporal): only for small lateral VSs
4. chemotherapy: some preliminary promise for progressive NF2-related vestibular schwannomas with bevacizumab (Avastin®), an anti-VEGF (vascular endothelial growth factor) monoclonal antibody (see below). Side effects: hemorrhage occurs in ≈ 7% due to vessel necrosis

Patient/tumor factors influencing management decisions

In addition to the usual factors involved in the decision process with brain tumors, e.g. the patient's general medical condition, age, natural history, etc., elements unique to VSs include: chances of preserving VII & V nerve function and hearing (in those with serviceable hearing) (all of which are related to tumor size), and the presence of NF2.

Specifics:

1. natural history of growth
   a) usual quoted range: ≈ 1–10 mm/yr. However this can be quite variable
   b) strictly intracanalicular tumors: only 17% grew outside the meatus (in 552 VSs over 3.6 years mean follow-up (230 were intrameatal at time of diagnosis, 322 had extrameatal extension)[4])
   c) extrameatal tumors (with extension into CP angle): 30% grew > 2 mm (in 522 VSs over 3.6 years mean follow-up[4])
   d) VSs that did not grow in the 5 years after diagnosis did not grow after that
   e) 6% actually decrease in size[20]
2. natural history of hearing function in untreated intracanalicular VSs in AAO-HNS Group A (► Table 41.6) patients[21]
   a) 50% deteriorated to a lower class over 4.6 years (loss of ≥ 10 dB PTA or ≥ 10% SDS)
   b) after 4.6 years of observation, the proportion of patients eligible for hearing preservation treatment (as determined by a word recognition score class I (70–100% SDS)) was reduced to 28% (a 44% reduction) and by AAO-HNS class A to 9% (a 53% reduction)
   c) the risk of losing hearing was not related to: age, gender, acoustic tumor size (all tumors were intracanalicular) or tumor sublocalization (fundus, central, porus)
   d) hearing loss was positively correlated to the absolute volumetric tumor growth rate (tumors that eventually expand out of the IAC have a faster rate and degree of hearing loss compared to tumors remaining in the IAC)
   e) the risk of losing hearing was significantly lower for patients with 100% word recognition score. Over 4.6 years observation, 89% remained in WRS class I (► Table 41.4) compared to only 43% for patients with only a small (1–10%) loss of WRS at diagnosis
3. size: as tumors exceed 15 mm diameter, treatment complications increase
   a) significantly lower chance for hearing preservation
   b) increased incidence of VII injury
4. presence of cysts: cystic tumors may display sudden and dramatic growth[4]
5. serviceable hearing: see Definition of serviceable hearing (p. 674)
6. hearing in contralateral ear

Management algorithm

- Small tumors (< 15 mm diameter) with perfect hearing (WRS 100%):
  Observe both radiographically (CT or MRI scan) plus serial hearing tests:
  - Scan: recommend treatment for growth > 2 mm between studies. Scan schedule guide:
    - Every 6 months × 2 years after diagnosis, then (if stable)
    - Annually until 5 years after diagnosis, then (if stable)
    - At years 7, 9 & 14 after diagnosis[4]
  - Annual audiology evaluations
    - Hearing deterioration (WRS < 100%) but no growth: see below
    - Rationale: in patients with small tumors and normal WRS, comparing the results of hearing preservation following surgery or SRS to the natural history, the conclusion is that *established tumor growth* should be the main determinant for treatment[17]
- Small tumors with serviceable hearing: management is very controversial
  - In general, patients with serviceable hearing but WRS < 100% have a 50% chance of preserving their serviceable hearing (50/50 rule or AAO-HNS class A or B) with either observation, SRS or microsurgical resection

  - Hearing preservation rates better than 50% have been reported for both microsurgery and radiosurgery in very selected patients (smaller tumors, located medially in the IAC, intact pre-op ABR amplitudes and latencies)
  - Decisions to try to beat the natural history (50% chance of hearing loss at 10 years) should be very individualized based on tumor factors (size, location) and patient's factors (ABR, age, co-morbidities, preferences)
  - Final management decisions are often dictated by non medical reasons (patient's perception, social situation, financial considerations, support system etc.)
- Medium size tumors (15-25 mm diameter)
  - Tumors > 15-20 mm should be treated.[4,17] This is mostly true for young patients
  - Close observation to establish growth is a valid option in older patients or patients with medical co-morbidities
  - Complication rate increases and facial outcome worsens with increasing tumor size
  - NF2 patients present a challenge and should be evaluated individually. In general the success rate in the management of their tumors is lower (higher cranial nerve deficit and higher recurrence rate).[22,23] Early management is considered more favorable for good outcome.[24] A retrospective study found significant hearing improvement and tumor shrinkage in > 50% of NF2 patients with progressive VS using bevacizumab (Avastin®) (see above)
- Large tumors (> 25 mm diameter): treatment is recommended
  - Microsurgical resection is favored to reduce mass effect and decompress the brainstem
  - SRS is also useful in larger tumors for older patients or those with significant co-morbidities

Selection options for intervention

Once treatment is elected (see algorithm above), the type of treatment must be selected.

Comparison of microsurgery vs. radiosurgery (SRS)

1. hearing preservation
   a) for patients with testable pre-operative hearing
      - summary: radiosurgery or stereotactic radiation appears to be better at preserving hearing than microsurgery. The difference is minor for tumors < 10 mm and very good pre-operative hearing (70% SDS, and 30 dB PTA). The advantage of radiation is more pronounced for larger tumors and greater pre-operative hearing loss. Details:
      - SRS: overall, at 3, 5, and 10 years, 81%, 77% and 66% of the patients maintained their GR hearing class (▶ Table 41.5). For patients receiving a tumor margin dose of 13 Gy or less, those same percentages were 93%, 87% and 87%.[25] Hearing preservation appears to be related to the radiation dose to the cochlea rather than to the tumor itself[26]
      - microsurgery: hearing preservation is significantly related to the tumor size and to the experience of the surgical team. Hearing preservation in Samii's series of 1000 VS[23] improved from 24% in the first 200 cases to 49% in later cases. Hearing preservation in microsurgery has improved with the use of direct cochlear nerve monitoring[27] compared to auditory brainstem responses monitoring only. Hearing preservation in patients with class A, small tumors and direct cochlear nerve monitoring (compound nerve action potential) was 91%.[28] With microsurgery, the durability of the hearing preservation is also excellent with only 15% of patients with class A hearing after surgery, and 33% of patients with class B hearing after surgery slipping one class at 5 years follow-up[29]
2. facial nerve preservation
   a) preservation has been excellent with both microsurgery and radiosurgery
   b) microsurgery: 98.5% overall[30] and 100% in tumors not touching the brainstem. Staged resection has been advocated by some to improve facial nerve preservation in giant VS (> 4–4.5 cm)[31]
   c) radiosurgery: 98% of patients.[25] The incidence of facial neuropathy has significantly decreased since the SRS dose was decreased to 12–13 Gy. Facial neuropathy in the recent series occurred in patients having received 18–20 Gy
3. trigeminal neuropathy (TGN)
   a) a complication classically feared in large tumors especially following SRS
   b) SRS: 7% incidence of TGN (mainly in patients receiving higher doses, i.e. 18 Gy). No patients who received a dose < 13 Gy developed TGN[25]
   c) microsurgery: post-op TGN is not reported in most series
4. tumor control (local control rates, LCR):
   a) tumor control has been a concern with radiosurgery and with the more recent decrease in dose from 18–20 Gy to 12–14 Gy, long term data are lacking
   b) microsurgery: tumor recurrence has been poorly studied. Quoted rates in the literature vary between 0.5% at 6 years[30] to 9.2%[32]

c) SRS: tumor recurrence requiring re-treatment at 5 years was 4%[25] but 18% of patients presented with transient increase in the size of the tumor ("pseudogrowth") at a mean of 8 months, with later regression in half and stabilization to the new size in the other half

Vertigo and dizziness

For patients with episodic vertigo or balance difficulties as the predominant symptom; also, see points under Selection options for intervention (p. 677):

1. remember: patients with VS are susceptible to other causes of vertigo as well, and patients should undergo ENG and functional balance assessment
2. vertigo that is due to the VS is often self-limited, and improves in 6–8 weeks to a reasonably tolerable level with no treatment (patients may do better with so-called "vestibular rehab")
3. residual dizziness and balance disturbances are common whether stereotactic radiosurgery (SRS) or microsurgery (MS) is used, but are typically less after MS
4. a recent study based on patient's reported vertigo intensity has shown that symptoms of vertigo are improved by any treatment versus observation (van Gompel et al[33])
5. after SRS: a minimum of 5-6 mos, and sometimes up to eighteen months may be required to produce beneficial effects. Symptoms are improved more rapidly after MS than with SRS
6. following MS: The severity of dizziness after MS depends on the pre-operative vestibular function on the affected side. If the ipsilateral vestibular function is absent pre-operatively, then patients will not suffer from dizziness or nausea post-op. if ipsilateral vestibular function is intact pre-op, then patients may be very dizzy and nauseated in particular for the first 24 hrs
7. conclusion:
   - observation may be the best choice for ≈ 20% of patients
   - when treatment is desired:
     - surgery is the best choice for most VSs producing vertigo
     - SRS may be the right choice for some, especially: elderly patients (> 70 yrs) with other health problems, for recurrence of VS, and for individual preference

Hydrocephalus

When hydrocephalus is present, it may require separate treatment with a CSF shunt – see Surgical considerations (p. 679) – and may possibly be done at the same time as surgery for the VS (if surgery for the VS is indicated).

41.1.7 Surgical treatment

Approaches

General information

Three basic surgical approaches:

1. those with possibility of hearing preservation
   a) middle fossa (MF): poor access to posterior fossa (see below)
   b) retrosigmoid (RS) (see below) AKA retrosigmoid-transmeatal approach
2. translabyrinthine (TL): non hearing preserving (see below)

Excellent results have been reported with each of these approaches. These guidelines assume that the surgical team is comfortable with all three approaches.

Decision algorithm for approach

The choice of approach is dictated by hearing salvageability and tumor size as follows:

1. salvageable hearing (▶ Table 41.7 for definition and guidelines)
   a) if tumor is intracanalicular (no extension beyond a few mm into the posterior fossa (CPA); note: differences of opinion exist regarding how much tumor in the CPA can be removed via MF): use the middle fossa approach. Note: some authors exclusively use the retrosigmoid approach for hearing preservation even for these tumors with excellent results
   b) if tumor extends > few mm into the posterior fossa: use the retrosigmoid approach (it is generally accepted that the cisternal part of the tumor is not well exposed by the middle fossa approach, especially regarding the ability to dissect tumor off the nerves)
2. non salvageable hearing (see ▶ Table 41.7 for definition and guidelines)
   a) Use translabyrinthine approach or retrosigmoid approach

Table 41.7 Hearing salvageability
Serviceable and unsalvageable hearing
Definition of serviceable hearing
A generous definition of serviceable hearing: PTA < 50 dB and SDS > 50%[a]
Unsalvageable hearing
Serviceable hearing is *unlikely* to be preserved post-op when 1. pre-op SDS < 75% 2. or pre-op PTA loss > 25 dB 3. or pre-op BAER has abnormal wave morphology 4. or tumor > 2–2.5 cm diameter
[a]see also other definitions of serviceable hearing (p. 674)

b) Either can be used irrespective of tumor size. Surgical team preference is the main deciding factor. Some influencing aspects:
   - a young patient with no cerebellar atrophy might favor a translab approach
   - an anteriorly situated sigmoid sinus and/or a high riding jugular bulb restrict the working space in the translab approach, and might favor a retrosigmoid approach

Surgical considerations

General information

The first surgical removal of a vestibular schwannoma was performed over a century ago in 1894.[34]

The facial nerve is pushed forward by the tumor in ≈ 75% of cases (range: 50–80%), but may occasionally be pushed rostrally, less often inferiorly, and rarely posteriorly. It may even continue to function while it is flattened to a mere ribbon on the tumor capsule surface.

Anesthesia with minimal muscle relaxants allows intra-op seventh nerve monitoring. In only ≈ 10% of large tumors is the cochlear nerve a separate band on the tumor capsule, in the remainder it is incorporated into the tumor.

Although total excision of tumor is usually the goal of surgery, facial nerve preservation must take precedence over degree of resection. Near total resection (very small sliver of tumor left on the facial nerve) or subtotal resection are all excellent options if the tumor is tightly adherent to the facial nerve or the brainstem. Both have excellent long term tumor control rate with either observation or post-op radiation.

If hydrocephalus is present, it used to be standard practice to place a CSF shunt and wait ≈ 2 weeks before the definitive operation.[35] While still acceptable, this is less commonly done at present, and shunting or EVD is often performed under the same anesthesia.

Large tumors may be approached by a staged surgical approach to debulk tumor and preserve facial nerve, or a planned subtotal resection followed by radiation. For tumors > 3 cm, such approach seems to lead to improved results of facial nerve function[36]

The extra anesthesia time involved in translab approach may be detrimental in the elderly.

Middle fossa approach

- indications:
  a) hearing preservation
  b) laterally placed tumors
  c) small tumors (usually < 2.5 cm)
- pros:
  a) allows drilling and exposure of the IAC all the way to the geniculate ganglion (good for laterally placed tumors)
  b) basically an extradural subtemporal operation
- cons:
  a) potential damage to temporal lobe with risk of seizures
  b) facial nerve is the most superficial nerve in this exposure and therefore the surgeon works "around" the facial nerve (possibility of injury)
- technique summary
  a) lumbar drain

Table 41.8 Pros & cons of translab approach

Disadvantages	Advantages
• sacrifices hearing (acceptable when hearing is already non-functional or unlikely to be spared by other approach) • may take longer than retrosigmoid approach • possibly higher rate of post-op CSF leak	• early identification of VII may result in higher preservation rate • less risk to cerebellum and lower cranial nerves • patients do not get as "ill" from blood in cisterna magna, etc. (essentially an extracranial approach)

b) usually straight incision, starting in front of the tragus, extending cephalad for 6 cm, held open with a self retaining retractor
c) the temporalis muscle is incised vertically (along the muscle fibers) along the most posterior aspect of the exposure, as well and reflected anteriorly
d) craniotomy: 4 cm × 3 cm
e) elevate the middle fossa dura, section the middle meningeal artery. Identify and preserve the greater superficial petrosal nerve (GSPN), arcuate eminence, V3, and true edge of the petrous bone (the false edge is the groove occupied by the superior petrosal sinus)
f) drill and expose the internal auditory canal all the way to Bill's bar (for tumors extending laterally)
g) localize the facial nerve with the nerve stimulator
h) open the IAC dura along the main axis of the IAC, avoiding VII
i) identify the vestibular, cochlear and facial nerves
j) dissect the tumor off the nerves

Translabyrinthine approach

Often preferred by neurotologists.

1. pros & cons: See ▶ Table 41.8
2. technique summary
   a) Position: supine head rotated to contralateral side, can be done either with pins or doughnut if it is anticipated that no retractors will be used
   b) Prep the abdomen for fat graft (almost always used)
   c) skin incision should be tailored to the location of the sigmoid sinus (observe location of the sigmoid sinus and pinna of the ear on the pre-op MRI). Usually smaller opening than retrosigmoid approach
      - does not require a craniotomy. For large tumors requiring an "extended translab", 1–2 cm of retrosigmoid dura should be exposed during the mastoidectomy to allow for retraction of the sigmoid sinus
      - dural opening along the IAC after identification of VII with stimulator
      - for large tumor: section the superior petrosal sinus and section the tentorium to gain better intradural exposure
      - closure requires fat graft

Booking the case: Translabyrinthine approach for vestibular schwannoma

Also see defaults & disclaimers (p. 27).

1. position: supine with shoulder roll
2. equipment:
   a) microscope
   b) high speed drill
   c) ultrasonic aspirator
3. some surgeons work with neurotologist to assist with the IAC and for follow-up
4. neuromonitoring: facial EMG (does not require EEG tech), SSEPs for tumors involving the brainstem (requires EEG tech)
5. post-op: ICU
6. consent (in lay terms for the patient – not all-inclusive):
   a) procedure: surgery through an incision behind the ear to remove a tumor growing inside the skull on the nerve to the ear. Possible need for post-op lumbar drain. Fat graft (≈ always used)

b) alternatives: nonsurgical management with follow-up MRIs, other surgical approaches, radiation (stereotactic radiosurgery)
c) complications: CSF leak with possible meningitis, loss of hearing in ipsilateral ear (if not already lost), paralysis of facial muscles on the side of surgery with possible need for surgical procedures to help correct (correction is often far from perfect), facial numbness, post-op balance difficulties/vertigo, brainstem injury with stroke

Retrosigmoid approach

AKA posterior fossa, AKA suboccipital approach.[37,38]

- pros:
  a) familiar to most neurosurgeons ∴ often preferred by neurosurgeons
  b) quick access to the tumor
  c) hearing preservation possible
  d) NOTE: this approach is very versatile. Samii[23] resected all his acoustic tumors via a retrosigmoid approach; he achieved a significant amount of brain relaxation and improved exposure by using in the sitting position, which is generally not used in the USA because of associated complications (p. 1445)
- cons:
  a) cerebellar retraction: not a problem for tumors < 4 cm, provided the craniotomy is sufficiently lateral and the cisterna magna and the CP angle cistern has been opened
  b) headaches: it has been suggested that headaches are more common following retrosigmoid craniotomy than after translabyrinthine craniotomy. Postulated mechanisms: purely extradural drilling in translab with no bone dust in subarachnoid space. More anterior skin incision in translab and less disruption of the suboccipital musculature and greater occipital nerve

Booking the case: Retrosigmoid craniotomy for vestibular schwannoma

Also see defaults & disclaimers (p. 27).

1. position: lateral decubitus with tumor side up
2. equipment:
   a) microscope
   b) ultrasonic aspirator
   c) image guided navigation system (if used) (may be helpful for placing skin incision and craniotomy more than for tumor localization)
3. some surgeons work with neurotologist to assist with the IAC and for follow-up
4. neuromonitoring: facial EMG (does not require EEG tech), BAERS, near field monitoring (CNAP: compound nerve action potential)
5. post-op: ICU
6. consent (in lay terms for the patient – not all-inclusive):
   a) procedure: surgery through an incision behind the ear to remove a tumor growing inside the skull on the nerve to the ear. Possible need for post-op lumbar drain. Possible fat graft (optional)
   b) alternatives: nonsurgical management with follow-up MRIs, other surgical approaches, radiation (stereotactic radiosurgery)
   c) complications: CSF leak with possible meningitis, loss of hearing in ipsilateral ear (if not already lost), paralysis of facial muscles on the side of surgery with possible need for surgical procedures to help correct (correction is often far from perfect), facial numbness post-op balance difficulties/vertigo, brainstem injury with stroke. Facial numbness (infrequent)

Technique summary

1. position: lateral decubitus with tumor side up, head in pins rotated (might need shoulder roll), zygomatic arch horizontal. 30° elevation of the head is paramount; see Posterior fossa (suboccipital) craniectomy, Lateral oblique position (p. 1446)
2. percutaneous lumbar drain (optional)

Table 41.9 Aids in localizing VII nerve origin[41]

- VII nerve originates in the pontomedullary sulcus near the lateral end of the sulcus, 1–2 mm anterior to the VIII nerve
- the pontomedullary sulcus ends just medial to the foramen of Luschka (extending from the lateral recess of the IV ventricle, ▶ Fig. 1.9)
- a tuft of choroid plexus usually extends out of the foramen of Luschka on the posterior surface of IX and X nerve, just inferior to the origin of VII
- the flocculus of the cerebellum projects from the lateral recess into the CPA just posterior to the origin of VII and VIII
- VII origin is 4 mm cephalad and 2 mm anterior to that of the IX nerve

3. incision is shaped like the pinna of the ear, 3 finger breaths behind the external auditory canal
4. the craniotomy has to be lateral enough to expose part of the sigmoid and part of the transverse sinuses and to allow a straight line of sight to the lateral end of the IAC
5. to prevent CSF leak, seal all bone edges with bone wax
6. dural opening along the lines of the craniotomy
7. exposure is enhanced by opening the cerebello-pontine angle cistern and the cisterna magna under the microscope and draining CSF (20–40 ml of CSF can also be drained via a lumbar subarachnoid catheter)
8. the petrosal vein is often sacrificed at the beginning of the procedure to allow the cerebellum to relax and fall back and to avoid tearing off the transverse sinus. Be careful not to coagulate the SCA that often runs with the petrosal vein
9. using the facial nerve stimulator, the posterior aspect of the tumor is inspected to make sure the facial nerve has not been pushed posteriorly
10. the thin layer of arachnoid that covers most tumors is identified. Vessels within the arachnoid may contribute to cochlear function and may be preserved by keeping them with the arachnoid
11. the plane between tumor and cerebellum may be followed to the brainstem, and occasionally to the VII nerve (this plane is harder to follow once bleeding from tumor debulking occurs)
12. to help locate the origin of the VII nerve at the brainstem see ▶ Table 41.9 and CPA anatomy in ▶ Fig. 1.9
13. the posterolateral tumor capsule is opened, and internal decompression is performed. The tumor is collapsed inward and the capsule is kept intact and is rolled laterally off of VII and is eventually removed. The most difficult area to separate VII from tumor is just proximal to the entrance to the porus acusticus. A general recommendation is to accept a subtotal or near total resection to preserve anatomic continuity of the facial nerve in cases where it is identified by stimulation but because it is so flattened it cannot be seen as a separate structure on the surface of the tumor.
14. after the extracanalicular portion of tumor is removed, the dura over the IAC is incised, and the IAC is drilled open and tumor is removed from this portion. To preserve hearing, the bony labyrinth must not be violated. The posterior semicircular canal (SCC) is the most vulnerable structure (▶ Fig. 41.1). The vestibule of the SCCs is also at risk but is less likely to be entered. The maximal amount of temporal bone drilling that can be accomplished without entering the posterior SCC can be determined from the pre-op CT. The operculum of the temporal bone, is a small step-off palpable with a nerve hook posteriorly from the porus acusticus. It marks the location of the vestibular aqueduct and is a good landmark for the posterior extent of the drilling in the retrosigmoid exposure of the IAC. Measuring the distance from the IAC to the posterior semicircular canal on a pre-op CT and measuring the thickness of the bone overlying the posterior semicircular canal are recommended for safe exposure of the IAC, in particular for hearing preservation. However, opening the labyrinth cannot always be avoided; and any opening should be plugged with bone-wax or muscle.[39] If the facial nerve is not intact and is not going to be grafted, then the IAC should be plugged, e.g. by bone wax covered with a small piece of hammered muscle (hammering makes the muscle sticky by activating extrinsic clotting factors) and Gelfoam®.

NB: *large tumors*: in some large tumors, the capsule may be adherent to the brainstem and so portions of tumor must be left; recurrence rate among these is ≈ 10–20%.[40] Large tumors may also involve V superiorly (sometimes VII is pushed up against V), and inferiorly may involve IX, X, and XI. The lower cranial nerves can usually be spared by dissecting them off of the tumor capsule, and protecting them with cottonoids.

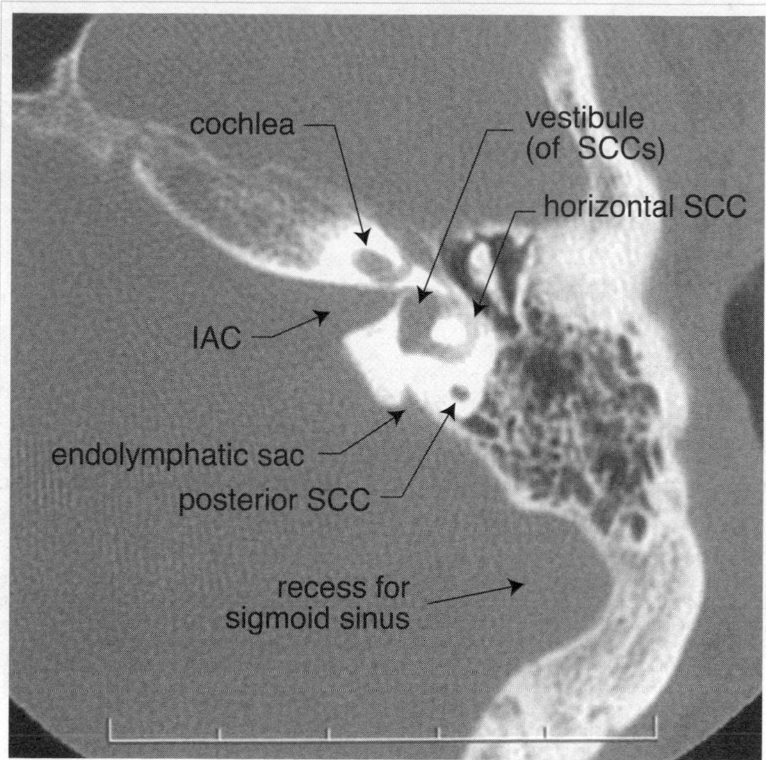

Fig. 41.1 Structures of the left temporal bone. CT scan (left petrous bone, axial slice) provided courtesy of Chris Danner, M.D.

Post-op care and care for complications

Cranial nerve and brainstem dysfunction

Facial nerve (VII)

If eye closure is impaired due to VII dysfunction: ℞ natural tears 2 gtts to affected eye q 2 hrs and PRN. Apply Lacrilube® to affected eye and tape it shut q hs. If there is complete VII palsy with little chance of early recovery, or if facial sensation (Vth nerve) is also impaired, tarsorrhaphy is performed within a few days.

Facial re-animation (e.g. hypoglossal-facial anastamosis) is performed after 1–2 months if VII was divided, or if no function returns after 1 year with an anatomically intact nerve.

Vestibular nerve (VIII)

Vestibular dysfunction is common post-op, nausea and vomiting due to this (and also intracranial air) is common. Balance difficulties due to this clear rapidly, however, ataxia from brainstem dysfunction may have a permanent component.

Lower cranial nerves

The combination of IX, X and XII dysfunction creates swallowing difficulties and creates a risk of aspiration.

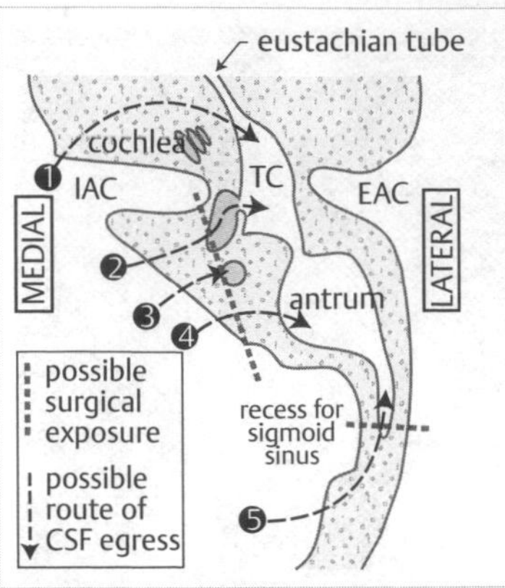

Fig. 41.2 Possible routes for CSF rhinorrhea following vestibular schwannoma surgery (see text) (right petrous bone, axial slice). Adapted from Surgical Neurology, Vol. 43, Nutik S L, Korol H W, Cerebrospinal Fluid Leak After Acoustic Neuroma Surgery, 553–7, 1995, with permission from Elsevier Science

Brainstem dysfunction

Brainstem dysfunction may occur from dissection of tumor off of the brainstem. This may produce ataxia, contralateral paresthesias in the body. Although there may be improvement, once present, there is often some permanent residual.

CSF fistula

Also, see CSF fistula (cranial) (p.384) for general information. CSF fistula may develop through the skin incision, the ear (CSF otorrhea) through a ruptured tympanic membrane, or via the eustachian tube and then through the nose (rhinorrhea) or down the back of the throat.

Rhinorrhea may occur through any of the following routes (circled numbers in ▶ Fig. 41.2):

- ① via the apical cells to the tympanic cavity (TC) or eustachian tube (the most common path)
- entry into the bony labyrinth – in order to reach the middle ear would require rupture e.g. of the oval window by overpacking bone wax into the labyrinth)
  - ② through the vestibule of the horizontal semicircular canal (SCC)
  - ③ through the posterior SCC (the posterior SCC is the most common area that is entered by drilling)
- ④ follows the perilabyrinthine cells and tracts to the mastoid antrum
- ⑤ through the mastoid air cells surgically exposed at the craniotomy site

Most leaks are diagnosed within 1 week of surgery, although 1 presented 4 years post-op.[42] They appear to be more common with more lateral unroofing of the IAC.[42] Meningitis complicates a CSF leak in 5–25% of cases, and usually develops within days of the onset of leak.[42] Hydrocephalus may promote the development of a CSF fistula.

Treatment: 25–35% of leaks stop spontaneously (one series reported 80%).[42] Treatment options include:

1. non-surgical:
   a) elevate HOB
   b) a percutaneous lumbar subarachnoid drain may be tried,[43,44] although some debate its efficacy,[38] and there is a theoretical risk of drawing bacteria into the CNS
2. surgical treatment for persistent leaks: In general, post-operative CSF leak (including rhinorrhea) is best addressed with immediate surgical re-exploration
   a) in the case of a translabyrinthine approach with absent ipsilateral hearing: to treat rhinorrhea, pack and permanently close the Eustachian tube via a trans tympanic membrane approach. This is very effective and avoids re-opening the surgical incision and removing the previously placed fat graft.
   b) if hearing is preserved (which excludes translab), every effort should be made to preserve the Eustachian tube function to preserve middle ear function. Re-explore the surgical field, re-wax the aircells and place additional fat graft, fascia, pericranium or other sealant over the exposed aircells. This aggressive management is the most definitive and rapid treatment, and avoids prolonged bed rest required by placing a lumbar drain and trying to control the leak in a conservative way
3. a CSF leak may be an indication of altered CSF hydrodynamics. Most of these patients demonstrate frank ventriculomegaly (hydrocephalus). In some patients the leak may function as a

Table 41.10 Cranial nerve preservation in retrosigmoid removal of VSs[a]

Size of tumor	Preserved function	
	VII nerve	VIII nerve
< 1 cm	95–100%	57%
1–2 cm	80–92%	33%
> 2 cm	50–76%	6%

[a]series of 135 VSs[48 (p 729)] and other sources[40 (p 3337),45]

pressure relief valve and thereby ameliorate the ventriculomegaly (i.e. there would be hydrocephalus if there wasn't a leak). Adjunctive CSF shunting is usually also necessary or the repair will be more likely to fail

Outcome and follow-up

Complete surgical removal was reported in 97–99% of cases.[45]

Surgical morbidity and mortality

Also see Post-op considerations for p-fossa cranis (p. 1451). Estimated frequency of some complications[46]: the most common complication is CSF leakage in 4–27%[42] (see above), meningitis in 5.7%, stroke in 0.7%, subsequent requirement for CSF shunt (for hydrocephalus or to treat leak) in 6.5%.

The mortality rate is ≈ 1% at specialized centers.[23,45,47]

Cranial nerve dysfunction

▶ Table 41.10 shows statistics of VII and VIII cranial nerve preservation following suboccipital removal of VSs in several combined groups of patients. For more details, see below.

Post-radiation cranial neuropathies generally appear 6–18 months following stereotactic radiosurgery (SRS),[49] and since more than half of these resolve within 3–6 months after the onset the recommendation is treat these with a course of corticosteroids.

Facial nerve (VII)

See ▶ Table 41.3 for the House and Brackmann grading scale. Grades 1–3 are associated with acceptable function. Facial nerve preservation is related to tumor size.

Surgery: With the use of modern facial nerve monitoring techniques, anatomical integrity of the facial nerve can be achieved in > 90% even for very large tumors and in close to 99% in medium size tumors.[50] In cases where the nerve is so flattened that tumor has to be left over the nerve to preserve its anatomical integrity, functional outcome of the facial nerve is nevertheless lower, especially with larger tumors. Excellent outcome (HB grade I-III) was only achieved in 75% of the patients with large tumors and 91% in medium size tumors.

SRS for tumors ≤ 3 cm diameter: With modern SRS dosimetry (12-13 Gy for patients with serviceable hearing and 13-14 Gy for patients with non serviceable hearing, the incidence of new facial nerve weakness was 4%.[51]

Vestibulo-acoustic nerve (VIII)

Patients with unilateral VS and Class I or II hearing (▶ Table 41.5) comprised ≈ 12% of cases in a large series.[52] Preservation of hearing is critically dependent on tumor size, with little chance of preservation with tumors > 1–1.5 cm diameter. Chances of preserving hearing may possibly be improved by intra-operative brainstem auditory evoked potential monitoring.[53] In centers treating large numbers of VSs, hearing *preservation* rates of 35–71% can be achieved with tumors < 1.5 cm[52,54] (although a range of 14–48% may be more realistic[55]). Hearing may rarely be improved post-op.[56]

SRS: for tumors ≤ 3 cm diameter,[57] hearing was preserved in 26% of 65 cases with pre-op pure tone threshold < 90 dB. Hearing loss has been correlated with increase in tumor size.[58] NB: there is a *high* rate of hearing loss at 1 year. SRT: useful hearing was preserved in 93%.[59]

Vestibular nerve function is rarely normal post-op. Attempts at "vestibular" sparing surgery have shown no better results than surgery not specifically addressing this issue. Most patients with unilateral loss of vestibular nerve function will learn to compensate to a significant degree with input from the contralateral side, if normal. Patients with ataxia as a result of brainstem injury from the tumor or the surgery will have more difficulties post-op. Some patients will seem to do well initially post-op with respect to vestibular nerve function, only to undergo a delayed deterioration several months post-op. These cases likely represent aberrant regeneration of the vestibular nerve fibers and may be extremely difficult to manage. Some experts advocate cutting the vestibular nerve, as for Meniere's disease (p. 573).

Trigeminal nerve (V)

Postoperative trigeminal nerve symptoms occur transiently in 22% and permanently in 11% following microsurgery, similar to the results of SRS.[60] New facial numbness occurred in 2% with SRT.[59]

Lower cranial nerves

Injuries to IX, X and XI occur infrequently following surgery on large tumors that distort the nerves and displace them inferiorly against the occipital bone.

Recurrence

Following microsurgery (MS)

Recurrence is highly dependent on extent of removal. However, recurrence can develop in tumors that were apparently totally removed, or when subtotal resection was performed. This can occur many years after treatment. Tumor progression rate following subtotal resection is ≈ 20%.[55] All patients should be followed with imaging (CT or MRI). In older series with up to 15 yrs follow-up, local control rate (LCR) after "total resection" is ≈ 94%. More recent series with MRI follow-up indicate recurrence rates of 7–11% (3–16 yrs follow-up).[55]

Use of EBRT

EBRT may improve LCR in incompletely resected tumors as shown in ▶ Table 41.11 (note: with the long survival expected with benign tumors, post XRT complications may occur).

Microsurgery vs. SRS

The long-term results for SRS using the current recommended dose of 14 Gy are still not known[34] (in spite of journal article titles suggesting otherwise[62]). In a non-randomized retrospective study[60] of VSs < 3 cm dia, the *short-term* LCR (median 24 mos follow-up) was 97% for microsurgery vs. 94% for stereotactic radiosurgery (SRS). However, for benign tumors, long-term follow-up is critical (possibly 5–10 years[49]), and this study *suggests* that the long-term LCR will be better for MS than SRS. SRS studies with long-term follow-up[63] are not directly comparable because in the cases with longest follow-up, higher radiation doses were used with a resultant higher incidence of radiation complications, and an anticipated better LCR.

Initially there may be temporary enlargement of the tumor accompanied by loss of central contrast enhancement following SRS in ≈ 5% of patients[64] (with up to 2% of patients showing actual initial tumor growth), and so the need for further treatment after SRS should be postponed until there is evidence of sustained growth.[65] Surgery should therefore be avoided during the interval from 6 to 18 months after SRS because this is time of maximum damage from the radiation.[65]

Although the numbers are small, there have been indications that the rate of VII nerve injury may be higher in patients undergoing microsurgery following SRS failure to achieve LCR compared to cases where microsurgery was the initial procedure,[66,67] however, this has been disputed.[65] Lastly, there is a potential for malignant transformation of VSs following SRS including triton tumors[68,69] (malignant neoplasms with rhabdoid features) or the induction of skull base tumors (which has been reported with external beam radiation[70]), as well as the risk of late arterial occlusion (the AICA lies near the surface of VSs), any of which may occur many years later.

Treatment for recurrence following microsurgery

Repeat surgery for recurrent VS is an option. One series of 23 patients[71] showed that 6 of 10 patients with moderate or normal VII function maintained at least moderate function after reoperation,

Table 41.11 Local control rates of surgery vs. surgery + EBRT for VSs[61]

Extent of surgical removal	Local control rate (LCR)	
	Surgery	Surgery + EBRT[a]
gross total	60/62 (97%)	no data
near total (90–99%)	14/15 (93%)	2/2 (100%)
subtotal (< 90%)	7/13 (54%)	17/20 (85%)[a]
biopsy only	no data	3/3 (100%)

[a]with doses < 45 Gy, LCR was 33%; with > 45 Gy LCR was 94%

3 patients had increased ataxia, and 1 patient had a cerebellar hematoma. The use of SRS has been endorsed by some for recurrence of VS following one or more MS procedures.[55] Using SRS for recurrent VSs resulted in worsening of facial nerve function in 23% of patients with Grade I-III function before SRS (median follow-up = 43 mos), and 14% developed new trigeminal symptoms.[55] 6% of patients developed tumor progression after SRS.

Hydrocephalus

May occur following treatment (MS or SRS) for VS, and may even occur years later. The increased CSF pressure may also predispose to development of a CSF fistula.

41.2 Tumors of peripheral nerves: Perineurioma

A nerve sheath tumor. Variants:

1. intraneural perineurioma: usually solitary lesion of adolescence or young adulthood, affecting primarily peripheral nerves (cranial nerve involvement is rare). Pseudo-onion bulb formation with cylindrical enlargement of the nerve over 2–10 cm. Mitotic activity is rare, MIB-1 labeling index is low. Chromosome 22 loss is characteristic,[72] no NF1 association. Treatment: conservative sampling of lesion, not resection
2. soft tissue perineurioma: uncommon. Only rarely can an associated nerve be identified. Almost exclusively benign, but malignant variety does occur. Female:male ratio = 4:1. In males, hands are often affected. Discrete, but not encapsulated, diameter = 1.5–20 cm. Treatment: gross total excision is curative

References

[1] National Institutes of Health Consensus Development Conference. Acoustic Neuroma: Consensus Statement. Bethesda, MD 1991

[2] Eldridge R, Parry D. Summary: Vestibular Schwannoma (Acoustic Neuroma) Consensus Development Conference. Neurosurgery. 1992; 30:962–964

[3] Harner SG, Laws ER. Clinical Findings in Patients with Acoustic Neuromas. Mayo Clin Proc. 1983; 58:721–728

[4] Stangerup SE, Caye-Thomasen P, Tos M, Thomsen J. The natural history of vestibular schwannoma. Otol Neurotol. 2006; 27:547–552

[5] Lau T, Olivera R, Miller T, Jr, Downes K, Danner C, van Loveren HR, Agazzi S. Paradoxical trends in the management of vestibular schwannoma in the United States. J Neurosurg. 2012; 117:514–519

[6] Jaffe B. Clinical Studies in Sudden Deafness. Adv Otorhinolaryngol. 1973; 20:221–228

[7] Byl F. Seventy-Six Cases of Presumed Sudden Hearing Loss Occurring in 1973: Prognosis and Incidence. Laryngoscope. 1977; 87:817–824

[8] Berenholz LP, Eriksen C, Hirsh FA. Recovery From Repeated Sudden Hearing Loss With Corticosteroid Use in the Presence of an Acoustic Neuroma. Ann Otol Rhinol Laryngol. 1992; 101:827–831

[9] Moskowitz D, Lee KJ, Smith HW. Steroid Use in Idiopathic Suden Sensorineuroal Hearing Loss. Laryngoscope. 1984; 94:664–666

[10] Tarlov EC. Microsurgical Vestibular Nerve Section for Intractable Meniere's Disease. Clin Neurosurg. 1985; 33:667–684

[11] House WF, Brackmann DE. Facial Nerve Grading System. Otolaryngol Head Neck Surg. 1985; 93:184–193

[12] Hardy DG, Macfarlane R, Baguley D, et al. Surgery for Acoustic Neurinoma: An Analysis of 100 Translabyrinthine Operations. J Neurosurg. 1989; 71:799–804

[13] Daniels RL, Swallow C, Shelton C, Davidson HC, Krejci CS, Harnsberger HR. Causes of unilateral sensorineural hearing loss screened by high-resolution fast spin echo magnetic resonance imaging: review of 1,070 consecutive cases. Am J Otol. 2000; 21:173–180

[14] Committee on Hearing and Equilibrium of the American Academy of Otolaryngology-Head and Neck Surgery Foundation. Guidelines for the evaluation of hearing preservation in acoustic neuroma (vestibular schwannoma). Otolaryngol Head Neck Surg. 1995; 113:179–180

[15] Gardner G, Robertson JH. Hearing Preservation in Unilateral Acoustic Neuroma Surgery. Ann Otol Rhinol Laryngol. 1988; 97:55–66

[16] Silverstein H, McDaniel A, Norrell H, Haberkamp T. Hearing Preservation After Acoustic Neuroma Surgery with Intraoperative Direct Eighth Cranial Nerve Monitoring: Part II. A Classification of Results. Otolaryngol Head Neck Surg. 1986; 95

[17] Stangerup SE, Caye-Thomasen P, Tos M, Thomsen J. Change in hearing during 'wait and scan' management of patients with vestibular schwannoma. J Laryngol Otol. 2008; 122:673–681

[18] Murofushi T, Matsuzaki M, Mizuno M. Vestibular evoked myogenic potentials in patients with acoustic neuromas. Arch Otolaryngol Head Neck Surg. 1998; 124:509–512

[19] Copeland WR, Hoover JM, Morris JM, Driscoll CL, Link MJ. Use of preoperative MRI to predict vestibular schwannoma intraoperative consistency and facial nerve outcome. J Neurol Surg B Skull Base. 2013; 74:347–350

[20] Bederson JB, von Ammon K, Wichmann WW, Yasargil MG. Conservative Treatment of Patients with Acoustic Tumors. Neurosurgery. 1991; 28:646–651

[21] Caye-Thomasen P, Dethloff T, Hansen S, Stangerup SE, Thomsen J. Hearing in patients with intracanalicular vestibular schwannomas. Audiol Neurootol. 2007; 12:1–12

[22] Asthagiri AR, Parry DM, Butman JA, Kim HJ, Tsilou ET, Zhuang Z, Lonser RR. Neurofibromatosis type 2. Lancet. 2009; 373:1974–1986

[23] Samii M, Matthies C. Management of 1000 Vestibular Schwannomas (Acoustic Neuromas): Surgical Management with an Emphasis on Complications and How to Avoid Them. Neurosurgery. 1997; 40:11–23

[24] Brackmann DE, Fayad JN, Slattery WH, III, Friedman RA, Day JD, Hitselberger WE, Owens RM. Early proactive management of vestibular schwannomas in neurofibromatosis type 2. Neurosurgery. 2001; 49:274–80; discussion 280-3

[25] Lobato-Polo J, Kondziolka D, Zorro O, Kano H, Flickinger JC, Lunsford LD. Gamma knife radiosurgery in younger patients with vestibular schwannomas. Neurosurgery. 2009; 65:294–300; discussion 300-1

[26] Timmer FC, Hanssens PE, van Haren AE, Mulder JJ, Cremers CW, Beynon AJ, van Overbeeke JJ, Graamans K. Gamma knife radiosurgery for vestibular schwannomas: results of hearing preservation in relation to the cochlear radiation dose. Laryngoscope. 2009; 119:1076–1081
[27] Danner C, Mastrodimos B, Cueva RA. A comparison of direct eighth nerve monitoring and auditory brainstem response in hearing preservation surgery for vestibular schwannoma. Otol Neurotol. 2004; 25:826–832
[28] Yamakami I, Yoshinori H, Saeki N, Wada M, Oka N. Hearing preservation and intraoperative auditory brainstem response and cochlear nerve compound action potential monitoring in the removal of small acoustic neurinoma via the retrosigmoid approach. J Neurol Neurosurg Psychiatry. 2009; 80:218–227
[29] Wang AC, Chinn SB, Than KD, Arts HA, Telian SA, El-Kashlan HK, Thompson BG. Durability of hearing preservation after microsurgical treatment of vestibular schwannoma using the middle cranial fossa approach. J Neurosurg. 2013; 119:131–138
[30] Samii M, Gerganov V, Samii A. Improved preservation of hearing and facial nerve function in vestibular schwannoma surgery via the retrosigmoid approach in a series of 200 patients. J Neurosurg. 2006; 105:527–535
[31] Patni AH, Kartush JM. Staged resection of large acoustic neuromas. Otolaryngol Head Neck Surg. 2005; 132:11–19
[32] Roche PH, Ribeiro T, Khalil M, Soumare O, Thomassin JM, Pellet W. Recurrence of vestibular schwannomas after surgery. Prog Neurol Surg. 2008; 21:89–92
[33] Van Gompel JJ, Patel J, Danner C, Zhang AN, Samy Youssef AA, van Loveren HR, Agazzi S. Acoustic neuroma observation associated with an increase in symptomatic tinnitus: results of the 2007-2008 Acoustic Neuroma Association survey. J Neurosurg. 2013; 119:864–868
[34] Pitts LH, Jackler RK. Treatment of Acoustic Neuromas. N Engl J Med. 1998; 339:1471–1473
[35] Ojemann RG. Microsurgical Suboccipital Approach to Cerebellopontine Angle Tumors. Clin Neurosurg. 1978; 25:461–479
[36] Porter RG, LaRouere MJ, Kartush JM, Bojrab DI, Pieper DR. Improved facial nerve outcomes using an evolving treatment method for large acoustic neuromas. Otol Neurotol. 2013; 34:304–310
[37] Rhoton AL, Jr. The cerebellopontine angle and posterior fossa cranial nerves by the retrosigmoid approach. Neurosurgery. 2000; 47:S93–129
[38] Ebersold MJ, Harner SG, Beatty CW, Harper CM, et al. Current Results of the Retrosigmoid Approach to Acoustic Neurinoma. J Neurosurg. 1992; 76:901–909
[39] Tatagiba M, Samii M, Matthies C, El Azm M, Schönmayr R. The Significance for Postoperative Hearing of Preserving the Labyrinth in Acoustic Neurinoma Surgery. J Neurosurg. 1992; 77:677–684
[40] Youmans JR. Neurological Surgery. Philadelphia 1990
[41] Rhoton AL. Microsurgical Anatomy of the Brainstem Surface Facing an Acoustic Neuroma. Surg Neurol. 1986; 25:326–339
[42] Nutik SL, Korol HW. Cerebrospinal Fluid Leak After Acoustic Neuroma Surgery. Surg Neurol. 1995; 43:553–557
[43] Symon L, Pell MF. Cerebrospinal Fluid Rhinorrhea Following Acoustic Neurinoma Surgery: Technical Note. J Neurosurg. 1991; 74:152–153
[44] Ojemann RG. Management of Acoustic Neuromas (Vestibular Schwannomas). Clin Neurosurg. 1993; 40:498–539
[45] Sekhar LN, Gormely WB, Wright DC. The Best Treatment for Vestibular Schwannoma (Acoustic Neuroma): Microsurgery or Radiosurgery? Am J Otol. 1996; 17:676–689
[46] Wiegand DA, Fickel V. Acoustic Neuromas. The Patient's Perspective. Subjective Assessment of Symptoms, Diagnosis, Therapy, and Outsome in 541 Patients. Laryngoscope. 1989; 99:179–187
[47] Gormley WB, Sekhar LN, Wright DC, et al. Acoustic Neuroma: Results of Current Surgical Management. Neurosurgery. 1997; 41:50–60
[48] Wilkins RH, Rengachary SS. Neurosurgery. New York 1985
[49] Flickinger JC, Kondziolka D, Pollock BE, Lunsford LD. Evolution in Technique for Vestibular Schwannoma Radiosurgery and Effect on Outcome. Int J Radiation Oncology Biol Phys. 1996; 36:275–280
[50] Samii M, Gerganov VM, Samii A. Functional outcome after complete surgical removal of giant vestibular schwannomas. J Neurosurg. 2010; 112:860–867
[51] Pollock BE, Driscoll CL, Foote RL, Link MJ, Gorman DA, Bauch CD, Mandrekar JN, Krecke KN, Johnson CH. Patient outcomes after vestibular schwannoma management: a prospective comparison of microsurgical resection and stereotactic radiosurgery. Neurosurgery. 2006; 59:77–85; discussion 77-85
[52] Glasscock ME, Hays JW, Minor LB, Haynes DS, Carrasco VN. Preservation of Hearing in Surgery for Acoustic Neuromas. J Neurosurg. 1993; 78:864–870
[53] Ojemann RG, Levine RA, Montgomery WM, et al. Use of Intraoperative Auditory Evoked Potentials to Preserve Hearing in Unilateral Acoustic Neuroma Removal. J Neurosurg. 1984; 61:938–948
[54] Brackmann DE, House JRIII, Hitselberger WE. Technical Modifications to the Middle Cranial Fossa Approach in Removal of Acoustic Neuromas. Los Angeles, CA 1993
[55] Pollock BE, Lunsford LD, Flickinger JC, Clyde BL, Kondziolka D. Vestibular Schwannoma Management. Part I. Failed Microsurgery and the Role of Delayed Stereotactic Radiosurgery. J Neurosurg. 1998; 89:944–948
[56] Shelton C, House WF. Hearing Improvement After Acoustic Tumor Removal. Otolaryngol Head Neck Surg. 1990; 103:963–965
[57] Hirsch A, Norén G. Audiological Findings After Stereotactic Radiosurgery in Acoustic Neuromas. Acta Otolaryngol (Stockh). 1988; 106:244–251
[58] Flickinger JC, Lunsford LD, Coffey RJ, Linskey ME, et al. Radiosurgery of Acoustic Neurinomas. Cancer. 1991; 67:345–353
[59] Selch MT, Pedroso A, Lee SP, Solberg TD, Agazaryan N, Cabatan-Awang C, DeSalles AA. Stereotactic radiotherapy for the treatment of acoustic neuromas. J Neurosurg. 2004; 101:362–372
[60] Pollock BE, Lunsford LD, Kondziolka D, et al. Outcome Analysis of Acoustic Neuroma Management: A Comparison of Microsurgery and Stereotactic Radiosurgery. Neurosurgery. 1995; 36:215–229
[61] Wallner KE, Sheline GE, Pitts LH, Wara WM, et al. Efficacy of Irradiation for Incompletely Excised Acoustic Neurilemomas. J Neurosurg. 1987; 67:858–863
[62] Kondziolka D, Lunsford LD, McLaughlin MR, Flickinger JC. Long-Term Outcomes After Radiosurgery for Acoustic Neuromas. N Engl J Med. 1998; 339:1426–1433
[63] Noren G, Hirsch A, Mosskin M. Long-Term Efficacy of Gamma Knife Radiosurgery in Vestibular Schwannomas. Acta Neurochir. 1993; 122
[64] Linskey ME, Lunsford LD, Flickinger JC. Neuroimaging of Acoustic Nerve Sheath Tumors After Stereotactic Radiosurgery. AJNR. 1991; 12:1165–1175
[65] Pollock BE, Lunsford LD, Kondziolka D, et al. Vestibular Schwannoma Management. Part II. Failed Radiosurgery and the Role of Delayed Microsurgery. J Neurosurg. 1998; 89:949–955
[66] Slattery WH, Brackmann DE. Results of Surgery Following Stereotactic Irradiation for Acoustic Neuromas. Am J Otol. 1995; 16:315–321

[67] Wiet RJ, Micco AG, Bauer GP. Complications of the Gamma Knife. Arch Otolaryngol Head Neck Surg. 1996; 122:414–416
[68] Yakulis R, Manack L, Murphy AI. Postradiation Malignant Triton Tumor: A Case Report and Review of the Literature. Arch Pathol Lab Med. 1996; 120:541–548
[69] Comey CH, McLaughlin MR, Jho HD, Martinez AJ, Lunsford LD. Death From a Malignant Cerebellopontine Angle Triton Tumor Despite Stereotactic Radiosurgery. J Neurosurg. 1998; 89:653–658
[70] Lustig LR, Jackler RK, Lanser MJ. Radiation-Induced Tumors of the Temporal Bone. Am J Otol. 1997; 18:230–235
[71] Beatty CW, Ebersold MJ, Harner SG. Residual and Recurrent Acoustic Neuromas. Laryngoscope. 1987; 97:1168–1171
[72] Emory TS, Scheithauer BW, Hirose T, Wood M, Onofrio BM, Jenkins RB. Intraneural perineurioma. A clonal neoplasm associated with abnormalities fo chromosome 22. Am J Clin Pathol. 1995; 103:696–704

42 Meningiomas

42.1 General information

Key concepts

- slow growing, extra-axial tumor, usually benign, arise from arachnoid (not dura)
- imaging (MRI or CT): classically broad based attachment on dura often with dural tail, typically enhance densely, may cause hyperostosis of adjacent bone
- MRI: isointense on T1WI, hypodense on T2WI
- 32% of incidentally discovered meningiomas do not grow over 3 years follow-up
- surgical indications: documented growth on serial imaging and/or symptoms referable to the lesion that are not satisfactorily controlled medically
- most (but not all) are cured if completely removed, which is not always possible
- most commonly located along falx, convexity, or sphenoid bone
- frequently calcified. Classic histological finding: psammoma bodies

Meningiomas are the most common primary intracranial tumors. They are usually slow growing, circumscribed (non-infiltrating), benign lesions. Histologically malignant (incidence: ≈ 1.7% of meningiomas[1]) and/or rapidly growing varieties are also described; a rapidly growing lesion that looks like a meningioma may be a hemangiopericytoma (p. 701). Actually arise from arachnoid cap cells (not dura). May be multiple in up to 8% of cases,[2] this finding is more common in neurofibromatosis. Occasionally forms a diffuse sheet of tumor (**meningioma en plaque**). This section considers intracranial meningiomas.

May occur anywhere that arachnoid cells are found (between brain and skull, within ventricles, and along spinal cord). Ectopic meningiomas may arise within the bone of the skull (primary intraosseous meningiomas)[3] and others occur in the subcutaneous tissue with no attachment to the skull. Most are asymptomatic (see below).

42.2 Epidemiology

As many as 3% of autopsies on patients > 60 yrs age reveals a meningioma.[4] Meningiomas account for 14.3–19% of primary intracranial neoplasms.[5] Incidence peaks at 45 years age. Female:male ratio is 1.8:1.

1.5% occur in childhood and adolescence, usually between 10–20 years age.[6(p 3263)] 19–24% of adolescent meningiomas occur in patients with neurofibromatosis type I (von Recklinghausen's).

42.3 Common locations

42.3.1 General information

▶ Table 42.1 lists common locations. Other locations include: CP-angle, clivus, planum sphenoidale and foramen magnum. ≈ 60–70% occur along the falx (including parasagittal), along sphenoid bone (including tuberculum sellae), or over the convexity. Childhood meningiomas are rare, 28% are intraventricular, and the posterior fossa is also a common site.

42.3.2 Sphenoid wing (or ridge) meningiomas

Three basic categories[8]:

1. lateral sphenoid wing (or pterional): behavior and treatment are usually similar to convexity meningioma
2. middle third (or alar)
3. medial (clinoidal): tend to encase the ICA and the MCA as well as cranial nerves in the region of the superior orbital fissure and the optic nerve. May compress brainstem. Total removal is often not possible

Table 42.1 Location of adult meningiomas (series of 336 cases[7])

Location	%
parasagittal	20.8
convexity	15.2
tuberculum sellae	12.8
sphenoidal ridge	11.9
olfactory groove	9.8
falx	8
lateral ventricle	4.2
tentorial	3.6
middle fossa	3
orbital	1.2
spinal	1.2
intrasylvian	0.3
extracalvarial	0.3
multiple	0.9

42.3.3 Parasagittal and falx meningiomas

Up to 50% invade the superior sagittal sinus (SSS). Grouped based on location along AP direction of SSS as:
1. anterior (ethmoidal plate to coronal suture): 33%. Most often present with H/A and mental status changes
2. middle (between coronal and lambdoidal sutures): 50%. Most often present as Jacksonian seizure and progressive monoplegia
3. posterior (lambdoidal suture to torcular Herophili): 20%. Most often present with H/A, visual symptoms, focal seizures, or mental status changes

Classification systems for the extent of SSS invasion include one by Bonnal and Brotchi,[9] and a more recent one by Sindou et al.[10] shown in ▶ Fig. 42.1.

Parasagittal meningiomas may originate at the level of the motor strip, and a common initial manifestation of these is a contralateral foot drop.[11]

42.3.4 Olfactory groove meningiomas

Presentation (usually asymptomatic until they are large) may include:
1. Foster Kennedy syndrome (p.99):anosmia (patient is usually unaware of this), ipsilateral optic atrophy, contralateral papilledema
2. mental status changes: often with frontal lobe findings (apathy, abulia…)
3. urinary incontinence
4. posteriorly located lesions may compress the optic apparatus causing visual impairment
5. large lesions may compress the fornix and cause short-term memory loss
6. seizure

The morbidity, mortality and difficulty in achieving total removal increase significantly for tumors > 3 cm in size.[12]

Pre-op MRA, CTA or angiogram may be helpful to assess location of anterior cerebral arteries relative to the tumor. 70–80% of these get the majority of their blood supply from the anterior ethmoidal artery, which is usually not embolized due to risk to ophthalmic artery (and blindness). If there are substantial middle meningeal feeders, these may be embolized, but the benefit tends to be small.

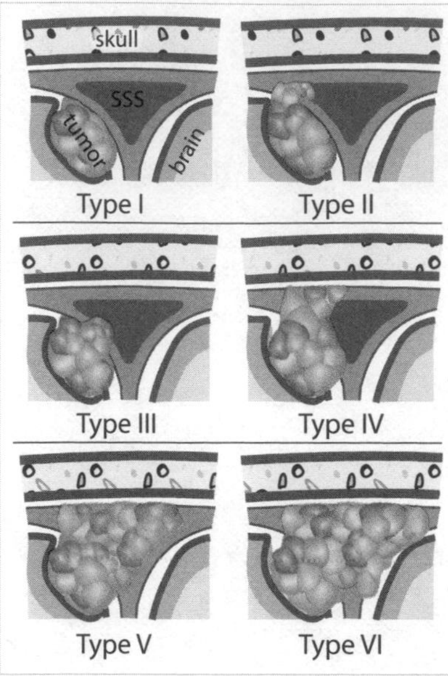

Fig. 42.1 Grading system for meningioma invasion of the superior sagittal sinus Modified from Sindou MP et al., J Neurosurg, 105: pp 514–25, 2006.
Shown: schematic coronal section through superior sagittal sinus (SSS).
Type I = attachment to lateral wall of sinus
Type II = invasion of lateral recess
Type III = invasion of lateral wall
Type IV = invasion of lateral wall and roof
Type V = total sinus occlusion, contralateral wall spared
Type VI = total sinus occlusion, invasion of all walls

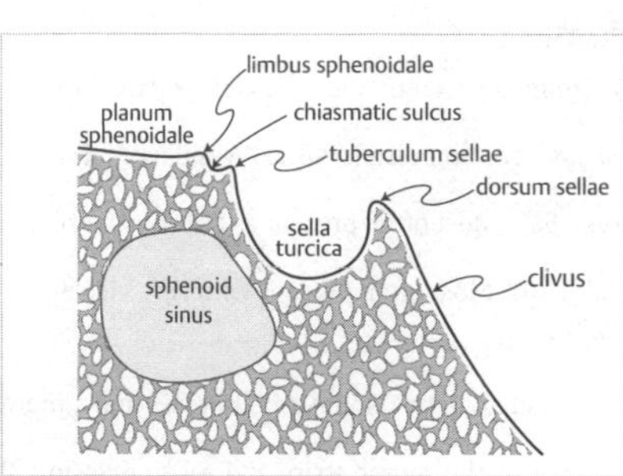

Fig. 42.2 Anatomic locations of planum sphenoidale and tuberculum sellae

42.3.5 Planum sphenoidale meningiomas

Arise from the flat part of the sphenoid bone (see ▶ Fig. 42.2) anterior to the chiasmatic sulcus in the posterior part of the anterior cranial fossa.

42.3.6 Tuberculum sellae meningiomas (TSM)

The site of origin of these tumors is only about 2 cm posterior to that of olfactory groove meningiomas.[12] The tuberculum sellae is the bony elevation between the chiasmatic sulcus and the sella turcica (see ▶ Fig. 42.2). By definition, the anterior margin of the chiasmatic sulcus (the limbus sphenoidale) is the demarcation between the anterior and middle cranial fossa. Therefore these tumors originate in the middle fossa (unlike planum sphenoidale meningiomas which are in the anterior fossa).

TSMs are notorious for producing visual loss (chiasmal syndrome = primary optic atrophy + bitemporal hemianopsia). When a TSM grows posteriorly into the sella turcica it may be mistaken for a pituitary macroadenoma (see ▶ Fig. 89.3 for MRI and differentiating features).

42.3.7 Foramen magnum meningiomas

As with any foramen magnum (FM) lesion (p. 1367); the neurologic symptoms and signs can be very confusing and often do not initially suggest a tumor in this location.

In the French Cooperative Study, there were 106 FM meningiomas,[13] 31% arose from the anterior lip, 56% were lateral, and 13% arose from the posterior lip of the FM. Most are intradural, but they can be extradural or a combination (the latter 2 have a lateral origin and are often invasive, which makes total removal more difficult).[14] They may be above, below, or on both sides of the vertebral artery.[14]

42.4 Pathology

Four critical histopathological variables:

1. grade see ▶ Table 42.2
2. histological subtype see ▶ Table 42.2
3. proliferation indices (p. 694)
4. brain invasion (p. 694)

There are a number of pathologic classification systems,[15,16(p 465),17] and transitional forms between the major types exist. More than one histological pattern may be seen in a given tumor. The WHO 2000 classification is shown in ▶ Table 42.2.

1. meningiomas with low risk of both recurrence and/or aggressive growth (WHO grade III)
   a) meningothelial or meningotheliomatous, AKA syncytial: the most common. Sheets of polygonal cells. Some use the term angiomatous for meningotheliomatous variety with closely packed blood vessels
   b) fibrous or fibroblastic: cells separated by connective tissue stroma. Consistency is more rubbery than meningotheliomatous or transitional
   c) transitional: intermediate between meningotheliomatous and fibrous. Cells tend to be spindle shaped, but areas of typical meningotheliomatous cells occur. Whorls, some of which are calcified (psammoma bodies)
   d) psammomatous: calcified meningothelial whorls
   e) angiomatous
   f) microcystic: AKA "humid" or vacuolated meningioma. The characteristic dilated extracellular spaces are usually empty, but occasionally contain substance that stains positive for PAS (? glycoprotein) or contain fat.[18] The cysts may coalesce and form grossly or radiologically visible cysts and may resemble astrocytomas
   g) secretory
   h) lymphoplasmacyte-rich
2. meningiomas with greater recurrence risk and/or aggressive growth include
   a) atypical meningioma: increased mitotic activity (1–2 mitotic figure/high-powered field), increased cellularity, focal areas of necrosis, giant cells. Cellular pleomorphism is not unusual

Table 42.2 WHO classification of meningiomas

WHO Grade	Meningiomas
WHO I	meningothelial fibrous (fibroblastic) transitional (mixed) psammomatous angiomatous microcystic secretory lymphoplasmacyte-rich metaplastic
WHO II	chordoid clear cell (intracranial) atypical
WHO III	papillary rhabdoid (see text) anaplastic

but is not significant in and of itself. Increasing atypia appears to correlate with increasing aggressiveness

b) rhabdoid meningiomas: usually have malignant features and behave aggressively. Behavior in the absence of malignant features is undetermined[19]

c) malignant meningiomas: AKA anaplastic, papillary or sarcomatous. Characterized by frequent mitotic figures, cortical invasion, rapid recurrence even after apparent total removal,[20] and, rarely, metastases (see below). Frequent mitotic figures (≥ 4 mitoses per high-power field) or the presence of papillary features are strong predictors of malignancy. May be more common in younger patients

Obsolete terms (in the current WHO classification) presented for context in older literature: metaplastic, myxomatous, xanthomatous (abundant cytoplasmic lipids; appear vacuolated), lipomatous, granular, chondroblastic, osteoblastic, melanotic. Angioblastic or (meningeal) hemangiopericytomas; true hemangiopericytomas are sarcomas (p. 701). (Others use the term "angioblastic" for tumors histologically similar to hemangioblastoma. Angioblastic meningiomas were felt to have more malignant clinical characteristics than other forms.[16(p 479–83)])

Proliferation indices

Due to variation between institutions and observers, it is advised that proliferation indices (e.g. Ki-67 or MIB-1) not be used as the sole discriminant for grading. However, these indices do correlate with prognosis (see ▶ Table 42.3). Adding the phrase "with high proliferative activity" is suggested for tumors with a very high index.[19]

42.4.1 Brain invasion

The presence of brain invasion increases the likelihood of recurrence to levels similar to atypical meningiomas (not anaplastic),[22] but is *not* an indicator of malignant grade. Brain invasion in atypical meningiomas does not dictate malignant behavior. Adding the phrase "with brain invasion" is suggested to denote higher risk of recurrence.[19]

42.4.2 Metastases

Very rarely a meningioma may metastasize outside the CNS. Most of these are angioblastic or malignant. Lung, liver, lymph nodes and heart are the most common sites.

42.4.3 Differential diagnosis/diagnostic considerations of meningioma

1. multiple meningiomas: suggests neurofibromatosis 2 (NF2)
2. pleomorphic xanthoastrocytoma (PXA) (p. 635): may mimic meningiomas since they tend to be peripherally located and may have a dural tail
3. Rosai-Dorfman disease: especially if extracranial lesions are also identified. A connective tissue disorder with sinus histiocytosis and massive painless lymphadenopathy (most have cervical lymphadenopathy). Usually in young adults. Isolated intracranial involvement is rare. MRI: dural-based enhancing mass with signal characteristics similar to meningioma, may have dural tail. Most common intracranial locations: cerebral convexities, parasagittal, suprasellar, cavernous sinus. Pathology: dense fibrocollagenous connective tissue with spindle cells and lymphocytic infiltration, stains for CD68 & S-100. Histiocytic proliferation without malignancy. Foamy histiocytes are characteristic. Surgery and immunosuppressive therapy not effective. Low-dose XRT may be the best option

Table 42.3 Ki-67 proliferation index in meningiomas[21d]

Description & WHO grade	Mean Ki-67 index[a]	Recurrence rate
Common meningioma (WHO grade I)	0.7%	9%
Atypical meningioma (WHO grade II)	2.1%	29%
Anaplastic meningioma (WHO grade III)	11%	50%

[a]not recommended for grading (see text)

42.5 Presentation

Symptoms depend on the location of the tumor, and some specific locations are associated with well-described symptom complexes.

Seizures may occur with supratentorial meningiomas as a result of irritation of the cerebral cortex.

Asymptomatic meningiomas

Meningiomas are the most common primary intracranial tumors, and most remain asymptomatic throughout the patient's life.[23] The routine use of CT & MRI for numerous indications inevitably results in the discovery of incidental (asymptomatic) meningiomas. In a population based study (the study population was middle class Caucasians and result may not be generalizable to other groups),[23] incidental meningiomas were seen in 0.9% of MRIs. In another series, 32% of primary brain tumors seen on imaging studies were meningiomas, and 39% of these were asymptomatic.[24] Of 63 cases followed for > 1 year with nonsurgical management, 68% showed no increase in size over an average follow-up of 36.6 mos, whereas 32% increased in size over 28 mos average follow-up.[24] Asymptomatic meningiomas with calcification seen on CT and/or hypointensity on T2WI MRI appeared to have a slower growth rate.[24]

Data is lacking to make evidence-based management guidelines. A suggestion is to obtain a follow-up imaging study 3–4 months after the initial study to rule-out rapid progression, and then repeat annually for 2–3 years. The development of symptoms would prompt performing a study at that time.

Treatment is indicated for lesions that produce symptoms that cannot be satisfactorily controlled medically, or for those that demonstrate significant continued growth on serial imaging studies. When surgery was performed, the perioperative morbidity rate was statistically significantly higher in patients > 70 years old (23%) than in those < 70 (3.5%).[24]

42.6 Evaluation

42.6.1 MRI

Occasionally may be isointense with brain on T1WI and T2WI, but most enhance with gadolinium. Brain edema may or may not be present. Calcifications appear as signal voids on MRI. Gives information regarding patency of dural venous sinuses (accuracy in predicting sinus involvement is ≈ 90%[25]). "Dural tail" is a common finding.[26]

42.6.2 CT

Appear as homogeneous, densely enhancing mass with broad base of attachment along dural border. Non-contrast Hounsfield numbers of 60–70 in a meningioma usually correlates with presence of psammomatous calcifications. There may be little cerebral edema, or it may be marked and may extend throughout the white matter of the entire hemisphere.

Intraventricular meningiomas: 50% produce extraventricular edema. On angio, these may falsely appear malignant.

Prostate cancer may mimic meningioma (prostate mets to brain are rare, but prostate frequently goes to bone, and may go to skull and can cause hyperostosis).

42.6.3 Angiography

Classic pattern: "comes early, stays late" (appears early in arterial phase, blush persists beyond venous phase). Meningiomas characteristically have *external* carotid artery feeders. Exceptions: low frontal median (e.g. olfactory groove) meningiomas which feed from the ICA (ethmoidal branches of the ophthalmic artery). Suprasellar meningiomas may also be fed by large branches of the ophthalmic arteries. Parasellar meningiomas tend to feed from the ICA. Secondary vascular supply may be derived from pial branches of the anterior, middle, and posterior cerebral arteries.

Artery of Bernasconi & Cassinari AKA artery of tentorium (a branch of the meningohypophyseal trunk) AKA the "Italian" artery: enlarged in lesions involving tentorium (e.g. tentorial meningiomas).

Angiography also gives information about occlusion of dural venous sinuses, especially for parasagittal/falx meningiomas. Oblique views are often best for evaluating patency of the superior sagittal sinus (SSS). Angiography can also help confirm diagnosis by the distinctive prolonged homogeneous tumor blush. Angiography also provides an opportunity for pre-op embolization (see below).

Pre-op embolization: Reduces the vascularity of these often bloody tumors, facilitating surgical removal. Timing of subsequent surgery is controversial. Some advocate waiting 7–10 days to permit tumor necrosis which simplifies resection.[27,28] Complications include: hemorrhage (intratumoral and SAH), cranial nerve deficits (usually transient), stroke from embolization through ICA or VA anastomoses, scalp necrosis, retinal embolus, and potentially dangerous tumor swelling. Some meningiomas (e.g. olfactory groove) are less amenable to embolization.

42.6.4 Plain x-rays

May show: calcifications within the tumor (in ≈10%), hyperostosis or blistering of the skull (including floor of frontal fossa with olfactory groove meningiomas), enlargement of vascular grooves (especially middle meningeal artery).

42.7 Treatment

42.7.1 General information

Surgery is the treatment of choice for symptomatic meningiomas. Incidental meningiomas with no brain edema or those presenting only with seizures that are easily controlled medically may be managed expectantly with serial imaging as meningiomas tend to grow slowly, and some may "burn out" and cease growing (p. 695).

Radiation therapy is considered for patients who are not surgical candidates, for some deep inaccessible tumors, for multiply recurrent meningiomas or for atypical or malignant meningiomas either after initial subtotal resection or after first recurrence.

42.7.2 Surgical technique

General information

These tumors are often very bloody. Preoperative embolization and autologous blood donation may be helpful for specific tumors. General principles of meningioma surgery[29]:

1. early interruption of the blood supply to the tumor
2. internal decompression (using ultrasonic aspirator, cautery loops…)
3. dissection of the tumor capsule from the brain by cutting and coagulating vascular and arachnoid attachments while infolding the tumor into the area of decompression with minimal retraction on adjacent brain
4. removal of attached bone and dura when possible

Position

As usual, the head should be elevated ≈ 30° above the right atrium.

For meningiomas involving the superior sagittal sinus (SSS)[30]:

- for tumors involving the anterior third of the SSS: supine semi-sitting position
- for tumors of the middle third of the SSS: lateral position with the side of the tumor *down*, the neck tilted 45° toward the upward shoulder
- for tumors of the posterior third of the SSS: prone position

Sinus involvement

Greenberg IMHO

Attempting to occlude or bypass the middle third of the superior sagittal sinus involved with meningioma is treacherous. Even in expert hands, there is significant risk of venous infarction/sinus occlusion with 8% morbidity and 3% mortality,[10] and complete removal is still not assured.[31] Venous drainage may occur through the dura adjacent to the sinus, in the skin, bone of the skull and even the tumor itself may participate. It is almost always preferable to leave residual tumor and consider treating it with radiation therapy than to cause a venous infarction.

Alternatives for treatment of dural sinus involvement include:

▶ **Superior sagittal sinus (SSS). If the tumor occludes the SSS**, it has been suggested that the sinus can be resected carefully preserving veins draining into the patent portions of the sinus. ✖ However, this should be undertaken with great trepidation since patients still not infrequently develop venous infarcts, probably as a result of loss of minimal sinus flow and venous channels in the dura. Before ligating the sinus, the lumen should be inspected for a tail of tumor within

partial occlusion of superior sagittal sinus:

1. anterior to the coronal suture, the sinus may usually be divided safely
2. posterior to the coronal suture (or, perhaps more accurately – posterior to the vein of Trolard), it must not be divided or else severe venous infarction will occur
   a) with superficial involvement (Type I, ▶ Fig. 42.1), tumor may be dissected off the sinus with care to preserve patency
   b) with extensive involvement:
      - sinus reconstruction: hazardous. Thrombosis rate using venous graft approaches 50%, and is close to 100% with artificial grafts (e.g. Gore-Tex) which should *not* be used
      - it may be best to leave residual tumor, and follow with CT or MRI. If the residual tumor grows, or if the Ki-67 score is high (p. 694), SRS may be used; SRS may also be used as initial treatment for tumors that are < 2.3–3 cm (p. 1564).

▶ **Transverse sinus (TS).** A patent dominant TS must not be suddenly occluded

Sphenoid wing, parasagittal or falx meningiomas (general principles)

Once tumor is exposed a partial internal debulking is performed. Then the point of attachment (to the falx or sphenoid bone) is peeled away using bipolar cautery to divide feeding vessels. Then the main portion of the tumor may be separated from brain, with the tumor being avascular once the vascular pedicle has been transected.

Parasagittal and falx meningiomas

The inferior portion of the tumor may adhere to branches of the anterior cerebral artery. Middle or posterior third tumors are exposed using a horseshoe incision based in the direction of the major scalp feeding vessels. The patient may be placed in a lateral position, or the sitting position may be used with doppler monitoring for air embolism (p. 1445). Anterior third tumors are approached using a bicoronal skin incision with the patient supine. For tumors that cross the midline, burr holes are placed to straddle the SSS. For managing superior sagittal sinus involvement, see above.

Since these tumors are often debulked from the inside, removal tends to be bloodier than meningiomas that can be removed in 1 piece. The ability to embolize these tumors pre-op is somewhat limited, but may be an adjunct. Technique: Cut through tumor leaving a thin layer on dura. Then remove the now relatively avascular part that impresses the brain. Then make an incision through the dura near the tumor; it tends to be bloody, but once you have control of both sides of the dura you can begin to excise the dura around the tumor (you may need to leave a cuff on SSS if it is involved).

Sphenoid wing meningiomas

A pterional craniotomy (p. 1453) is utilized. The neck is extended to allow gravity to retract the brain off of the floor of the skull.

Lateral sphenoid wing meningiomas: The approach to these tumors is often similar to convexity meningiomas. The height of the skin incision and bone opening should be high enough to encompass the tumor.

Medial sphenoid wing meningiomas: A lumbar drain is used. The head is turned 30° off the vertical. Aggressive extradural removal of sphenoid wing is performed. An FTOZ approach may provide additional exposure. The sylvian fissure is split widely. The ICA and MCA are often encased by tumor (look for the appearance of "grooves" on the surface of the tumor on MRI, which indicates vessels, e. g. MCA). To locate the ICA, identify MCA branches and follow them proximally into the tumor. The optic nerve is best identified at the optic canal. Avoid excessive retraction of the optic apparatus. The deep portion of the tumor often has numerous small parasitic vessels from the ICA (which makes this part very bloody), and may also invade the lateral wall of the cavernous sinus (which creates risk of cranial nerve deficits with attempted removal). Therefore, the recommendation is to leave some tumor behind and use radiosurgery to deal with it.

Olfactory groove meningiomas

Approached via a bifrontal craniotomy (preserving the periosteum to cover the frontal air sinus and floor of frontal fossa at the end of the case). Small tumors may be approached via unilateral craniotomy on the side with the most tumor).[6(p 3284)] For large tumors, a lumbar CSF drain will help with brain relaxation.[12] The head is rotated 20° to one side to facilitate dissection of the anterior cerebral arteries and optic nerve while preserving visualization of both sides of the tumor involvement.[32] The neck is slightly extended. The dura is opened low, and the superior sagittal sinus is ligated and divided at this location. Amputation of the frontal pole should be done if necessary to avoid excessive retraction. Vascular feeding arteries come through the floor of the frontal fossa in the midline. Initially, the anterior tumor capsule is opened and the tumor debulked from within heading towards the floor of the frontal fossa to interrupt the blood supply. The posterior capsule of the tumor is dissected carefully as this portion of the tumor may encase branches of the anterior cerebral artery, and/or optic nerves and chiasm. A large tumor with suprasellar extension usually displaces the optic nerve and chiasm *inferiorly*.[12] If necessary, the frontopolar branch and other small branches may be sacrificed without problem.[33] Post-op risks include CSF leak through the ethmoid sinuses.

Tuberculum sellae meningiomas

These tumors typically displace both optic nerves posteriorly and laterally.[12] Occasionally, the nerves are completely engulfed by tumor.

Cerebellopontine angle meningiomas

Usually arise from the meninges covering the petrous bone. May be divided into those that occur anterior to, and those that occur posterior to the IAC.

Foramen magnum meningiomas

Tumors arising from the posterior or posterolateral lip of the foramen magnum (FM) are removed relatively easily. Anterior and lateral FM tumors may be operated by the posterolateral approach, and for anterior tumors,[14] a transcondylar approach may alternatively be used.[34]

With meningiomas below the vertebral artery (VA), the lower cranial nerves are displaced superiorly with the VA. However, when the tumor is above the VA, the position of the lower cranial nerves cannot be predicted.[14]

Large tumors may adhere to or encase neurovascular structures, and these should be internally debulked and then dissected free.

Posterior suboccipital approach: Used for meningiomas arising from the posterior lip of the FM or slightly posterolateral.

The patient is positioned prone or three-quarter prone. Neck flexion should be kept to a minimum to avoid brainstem compression by the tumor.[35] The surgeon must remain vigilant for the PICA and vertebral arteries, which may be encased.

42.7.3 Radiation therapy (XRT)

Generally regarded as ineffective as primary modality of treatment. Many prefer not to use XRT for "benign" lesions. Efficacy of XRT in preventing recurrence is controversial (see below under Recurrence); some surgeons reserve XRT for malignant (invasive), vascular, rapidly recurring ("aggressive"), or non-resectable meningiomas.

For recurrent atypical or anaplastic meningioma with residual disease post-op, XRT with 55–60 Gy is recommended.

42.8 Outcome

5 year survival for patients with meningioma[36]: 91.3%.

Recurrence

The extent of surgical tumor removal is the most important factor in the prevention of recurrence. The Simpson grading system for the extent of meningioma removal is shown in ▶ Table 42.4. An often overlooked aspect of the Simpson grading system is that it refers exclusively to removal of intradural tumor, and thus leaving tumor e.g. in the sagittal sinus could still be compatible with complete removal. Recurrence after gross total tumor removal occurred in 11–15% of cases, but was 29% when removal is incomplete (length of follow-up not specified)[7]; 5-year recurrence rates of 37%

Table 42.4 Simpson grading system for removal of meningiomas[37]

Grade	Degree of removal
I	macroscopically complete removal with excision of dural attachment and abnormal bone (including sinus resection when involved)
II	macroscopically complete with endothermy coagulation (Bovie, or laser) of dural attachment
III	macroscopically complete without resection or coagulation of dural attachment or of its extradural extensions (e.g. hyperostotic bone)
IV	partial removal leaving tumor in situ
V	simple decompression (± biopsy)

[38]-85%[39] after partial resection are also quoted. The overall recurrence rate at 20 years was 19% in one series,[40] and 50% in another.[39] Malignant meningiomas have a higher recurrence rate than benign ones.

Value of XRT

A retrospective series of 135 non-malignant meningiomas followed 5–15 years post-op at UCSF revealed a recurrence rate of 4% with total resection, 60% for partial resection without XRT, and 32% for partial resection with XRT.[41] Mean time to recurrence was longer in the XRT group (125 mos) than in the non-XRT group (66 mos). These results suggest that XRT may be beneficial in partially resected meningiomas. Alternatively, one can follow these patients with CT or MRI and use XRT for documented progression.

In addition to the usual side effects of XRT – see Radiation injury and necrosis (p. 1560) – there is also a case report of a malignant astrocytoma developing after XRT was used to treat a meningioma.[42]

References

[1] Mahmood A, Caccamo DV, Tomecek FJ, Malik GM. Atypical and Malignant Meningiomas: A Clinicopathological Review. Neurosurgery. 1993; 33:955-963

[2] Sheehy JP, Crockard HA. Multiple Meningiomas: A Long-Term Review. J Neurosurg. 1983; 59:1–5

[3] Kulali A, Ilcayto R, Rahmanli O. Primary calvarial ectopic meningiomas. Neurochirurgia (Stuttg). 1991; 34:174–177

[4] Nakasu S, Hirano A, Shimura T, et al. Incidental Meningiomas in Autopsy Studies. Surg Neurol. 1987; 27:319–322

[5] Wara WM, Sheline GE, Newman H, et al. Radiation Therapy of Meningiomas. AJR. 1975; 123:453–458

[6] Youmans JR. Neurological Surgery. Philadelphia 1990

[7] Yamashita J, Handa H, Iwaki K, et al. Recurrence of Intracranial Meningiomas, with Special Reference to Radiotherapy. Surg Neurol. 1980; 14:33–40

[8] Cushing H, Eisenhardt L. In: Mengiomas of the Sphenoidal Ridge. A. Those of the Deep or Clinoidal Third. Meningiomas: Their Classification, Regional Behaviour, Life History, and Surgical End Results. Springfield, Illinois: Charles C Thomas; 1938:298–319

[9] Bonnal J, Brotchi J. Surgery of the superior sagittal sinus in parasagittal meningiomas. J Neurosurg. 1978; 48:935–945

[10] Sindou MP, Alvernia JE. Results of attempted radical tumor removal and venous repair in 100 consecutive meningiomas involving the major dural sinuses. J Neurosurg. 2006; 105:514–525

[11] Eskandary H, Hamzel A, Yasamy MT. Foot Drop Following Brain Lesion. Surg Neurol. 1995; 43:89–90

[12] Al-Mefty O, Sekhar LN, Janecka IP. In: Tuberculum Sella and Olfactory Groove Meningiomas. Surgery of Cranial Base Tumors. New York: Raven Press; 1993:507–519

[13] George B, Lot G, Velut S. Tumors of the Foramen Magnum. Neurochirurgie. 1993; 39:1–89

[14] George B, Lot G, Boissonnet H. Meningioma of the Foramen Magnum: A Series of 40 Cases. Surg Neurol. 1997; 47:371–379

[15] Zulch KJ. Histologic Typing or Tumors of the Central Nervous System. International Histological Classification of Tumors, no. 21. Geneva: World Health Organization; 1979

[16] Russell DS, Rubenstein LJ. Pathology of Tumours of the Nervous System. 5th ed. Baltimore: Williams and Wilkins; 1989

[17] Kleihues P, Burger PC, Scheithauer BW. The new WHO classification of brain tumors. Brain Pathol. 1993; 3:255–268

[18] Michaud J, Gagné F. Microcystic meningoma. Clinicopathologic Report of Eight Cases. Arch Pathol Lab Med. 1983; 107:75–80

[19] Kleihues P, Louis DN, Scheithauer BW, Rorke LB, Reifenberger G, Burger PC, Cavenee WK. The WHO classification of tumors of the nervous system. J Neuropathol Exp Neurol. 2002; 61:215–25; discussion 226-9

[20] Thomas HG, Dolman CL, Berry K. Malignant Meningioma: Clinical and Pathological Features. J Neurosurg. 1981; 55:929–934

[21] Kolles H, Niedermayer I, Schmitt C, Henn W, Feld R, Steudel WI, Zang KD, Feiden W. Triple approach for diagnosis and grading of meningiomas: histology, morphometry of Ki-67/Feulgen stainings, and cytogenetics. Acta Neurochir (Wien). 1995; 137:174–181

[22] Perry A, Scheithauer BW, Stafford SL, Lohse CM, Wollan PC. "Malignancy" in meningiomas: A clinicopathologic study of 116 patients with grading implications. Cancer. 1999; 85:2046–2056

[23] Vernooji MW, Ikram A, Tanghe HL, et al. Incidental findings on brain MRI in the general population. N Engl J Med. 2007; 357:1821–1828

[24] Kuratsu J-I, Kochi M, Ushio Y. Incidence and Clinical Features of Asymptomatic Meningiomas. J Neurosurg. 2000; 92:766–770

[25] Zimmerman RD, Fleming CA, Saint-Louis LA, et al. Magnetic Resonance of Meningiomas. AJNR. 1985; 6:149–157

[26] Taylor SL, Barakos JA, Harsh GR, Wilson CB. Magnetic Resonance Imaging of Tuberculum Sellae Meningiomas: Preventing Preoperative Misdiagnosis as Pituitary Macroadenoma. Neurosurgery. 1992; 31:621–627

[27] Chun JY, McDermott MW, Lamborn KR, Wilson CB, Higashida R, Berger MS. Delayed surgical resection reduces intraoperative blood loss for embolized meningiomas. Neurosurgery. 2002; 50:1231–5; discussion 1235-7

[28] Kai Y, Hamada J, Morioka M, Yano S, Todaka T, Ushio Y. Appropriate interval between embolization and surgery in patients with meningioma. AJNR Am J Neuroradiol. 2002; 23:139–142

[29] Ojemann RG. Management of Cranial and Spinal Meningiomas. Clin Neurosurg. 1992; 40:321–383

[30] Colli BO, Carlotti CG. Parasagittal meningiomas. Contemp Neurosurg. 2007; 29:1–8

[31] Heros RC. Meningiomas involving the sinus. J Neurosurg. 2006; 105:511–513

[32] Bogaev CA, Sekhar LN, Sekhar LN, Fessler RG. In: Ofactory groove and planum sphenoidale meningiomas. Atlas of Neurosurgical Techniques. New York: Thieme Medical Publishers, Inc.; 2006:608–617

[33] Ojemann RG, Schmidek HH, Sweet WH. In: Surgical Management of Olfactory Groove Meningiomas. Operative Neurosurgical Techniques. 3rd ed. Philadelphia: W.B. Saunders; 1995:393–401

[34] Hakuba A, Tsujimoto T, Sekhar LN, Janecka IP. In: Transcondyle Approach for Foramen Magnum Meningiomas. Surgery of Cranial Base Tumors. New York: Raven Press; 1993:671–678

[35] David CA, Spetzler R. Foramen Magnum Meningiomas. Clin Neurosurg. 1997; 44:467–489

[36] Mahaley MS, Mettlin C, Natarajan N, Laws ER, et al. National Survey of Patterns of Care for Brain-Tumor Patients. J Neurosurg. 1989; 71:826–836

[37] Simpson D. The recurrence of intracranial meningiomas after surgical treatment. J Neurol Neurosurg Psychiatry. 1957; 20:22–39

[38] Mirimanoff RO, Dosoretz DE, Lingood RM, et al. Meningioma: Analysis of Recurrence and Progression Following Neurosurgical Resection. J Neurosurg. 1985; 62:18–24

[39] Adegbite AV, Khan MI, Paine KWE, et al. The Recurrence of Intracranial Meningiomas After Surgical Treatment. J Neurosurg. 1983; 58:51–56

[40] Jaaskelainen J. Seemingly complete removal of histologically benign intracranial meningioma: late recurrence rate and factors predicting recurrence in 657 patients. A multivariate analysis. Surg Neurol. 1986; 26:461–469

[41] Barbaro NM, Gutin PH, Wilson CB, et al. Radiation Therapy in the Treatment of Partially Resected Meningiomas. Neurosurgery. 1987; 20:525–528

[42] Zuccarello M, Sawaya R, deCourten-Myers. Glioblastoma Occurring After Radiation Therapy for Meningioma: Case Report and Review of Literature. Neurosurgery. 1986; 19:114–119

43

43 Other Tumors Related to the Meninges

43.1 Mesenchymal, non-meningothelial tumors

43.1.1 Hemangiopericytoma

A sarcoma arising from pericytes (surrounding blood vessels). May metastasize (usually to bone, lung or liver). Occur ≈ anywhere (soft tissues, muscles, thoracic aorta, kidney, omentum...). May mimic meningioma on CT or MRI (MRS may help distinguish[1]). Recurrence is common, sometimes late. Neurosurgically relevant sites:
1. intracranial: includes intraventricular
2. spinal

Treatment: Surgery is primary treatment. XRT may reduce recurrence rate. Chemotherapy is used for metastases or for tumors failing local control measures.

43.1.2 Primary cerebral sarcoma

Rare. May result from sarcomatous change in preexisting tumor such as meningioma, glioblastoma, or oligodendroglioma.

43.2 Primary melanocytic lesions

Primary CNS melanoma

Probably arises from melanocytes in the leptomeninges. May spread through CSF pathways. May occasionally metastasize outside the CNS to produce systemic metastases.[2]

The peak age for this tumor is in the 4th decade (compared to the 7th decade for primary cutaneous melanoma).[3]

43.3 Hemangioblastoma

43.3.1 General information

Key concepts

- highly vascular well-circumscribed solid or cystic neoplasm of CNS or retina
- the most common primary intra-axial tumor in the adult posterior fossa
- may occur sporadically or as part of von Hippel-Lindau disease
- on imaging, may be solid, or cystic with enhancing mural nodule
- ✔ CBC: may be associated with erythrocytosis (polycythemia)

Hemangioblastomas[4(p 772–82)] (HGB) are histologically benign tumors. Intracranially, they occur almost exclusively in the p-fossa (hemangioblastomas are the most common *primary* intra-axial p-fossa tumor in adults). May occur in cerebellar hemisphere, vermis or brainstem. Less than 100 supratentorial cases have been reported. May also occur in spinal cord (p. 789) (1.5–2.5% of spinal cord tumors). Relationship and/or identity with angioblastic meningiomas is controversial. Also difficult to distinguish histologically from a renal cell carcinoma.

HGB may occur sporadically, but 20% occur as part of von Hippel-Lindau (VHL) disease (see below). Retinal HGB and/or angiomas occur in 6% of patients with cerebellar HGBs.

43.3.2 Hemangioblastomas (in general)

Epidemiology

HGB represent 1–2.5% of intracranial tumors. They comprise 7–12% of primary p-fossa tumors.[5] 5–30% of cases of cerebellar HGB and 80% of spinal HGB are associated with VHL (see above).

Sporadic cases tend to present in the 4th decade, whereas VHL cases present *earlier* (peak in 3rd decade). In sporadic cases, the HGB are solitary and originate in the cerebellum (83–95%), spinal cord (3–13%), medulla oblongata (2%)[6] or cerebrum (1.5%).[5] ≈ 30% of patients with cerebellar HGB have VHL.[7]

Presentation

S/S of cerebellar HGB are usually those of any p-fossa mass – H/A, N/V, cerebellar findings…; see Posterior fossa (infratentorial) tumors (p. 592) – and obstructive hydrocephalus may occur. HGB is rarely documented as a cause of apoplexy due to intracerebral hemorrhage (ICH) (lobar or cerebellar), however, some studies indicate that if cases of ICH are carefully examined, abnormal vessels consistent with HGB (and occasionally misidentified as AVM) may be found with surprising frequency (in spite of negative CT and/or angiography).[8]

Retinal HGBs tend to be located peripherally, and may hemorrhage and cause retinal detachment. Erythrocytosis may be due to erythropoietin liberated by the tumor.

Pathology

No report of malignant change. May spread thru CSF after surgery, but remain benign. No true capsule, but usually well circumscribed (narrow zone of infiltration). May be solid, or cystic with a mural nodule (70% of cerebellar lesions are cystic; nodules are very vascular, appear red, are often located near pial surface, and may be as small as 2 mm; cyst fluid is clear yellow with high protein). In cystic lesions, the cyst wall is lined with non-neoplastic compressed cerebellum. The cyst develops because the vessel walls are so thin that they leak water, proteins don't cross as readily.

Cardinal feature: numerous capillary channels, lined by a single layer of endothelium, surrounded by reticulin fibers (stains positive with reticulin stain). Macrophages stain PAS positive.

Three types of cells:

1. endothelial
2. pericytes: surrounded by basement membrane
3. stromal: polygonal. Foamy clear cytoplasm, often lipid laden. Origin controversial

Three types of HGB recognized[9]:

1. juvenile: thin walled capillaries & dilated vessels tightly packed
2. transitional: thin walled capillaries & dilated vessels intermingled with stromal cells, some of which are lipid laden (sudanophilic)
3. clear cell: neoplasm made up almost entirely of sheets of xanthoma cells with a rich vascular stroma

Cyst patterns[10]:

1. no associated cysts: 28%
2. peritumoral cyst alone: 51%
3. intratumoral cyst: 17%
4. peritumoral AND intratumoral cysts: 4%

Evaluation

Patients with a p-fossa HGB (radiologically suspected or histologically proven) should undergo MRI of entire neuraxis because of possibility of spinal HGBs (may be distant from p-fossa lesion; may suggest possibility of VHL).

CT: solid lesions are usually isodense with intense contrast enhancement. Cystic HGBs remain low density with contrast, with the nodule enhancing.

MRI: preferable to CT due to the tumor's predilection for the p-fossa. May show serpentine vascular signal voids, especially in the periphery of the lesion. Also, peripheral hemosiderin deposits may occur from previous hemorrhages.[5]

Vertebral angiography: usually demonstrates intense vascularity (most other tumors of the p-fossa are relatively avascular). May be required in HGBs where nodule is too small to be imaged on CT/MRI. 4 patterns: 1) vascular mural nodule on side of avascular cyst, 2) vascular lesion surrounding avascular cyst, 3) solid vascular mass, & 4) multiple, separate vascular nodules.

Labs: often discloses *polycythemia* (no hematopoietic foci within tumor). In cases with suggestive history, labwork to rule-out catecholamine production from pheochromocytoma may be indicated; see Endocrine/laboratory studies (p. 655).

Treatment

Surgery

Surgical treatment may be curative in cases of sporadic HGB, not in VHL.

Pre-operative embolization may help reduce the vascularity.

Cystic HGBs require removal of mural nodule (otherwise, cyst will recur). The cyst wall is not removed unless there is evidence of tumor within the cyst wall on MRI (typically thick-walled cysts) or visually at the time of surgery.[10] 5-ALA fluorescence may aid in visual localization of small hemangioblastomas within the cyst wall.[11]

Solid HGBs tend to be more difficult to remove. They are treated like AVMs (avoid piecemeal removal), working along margin and devascularizing blood supply. A helpful technique is to shrink the tumor by laying a length of bipolar forceps along tumor surface and coagulating. HGBs with attachment to floor of 4th ventricle may be hazardous to remove (cardio-respiratory complications).

Multiple lesions: if ≥ 0.8–1 cm diameter: may treat as in solitary lesion. Smaller and deeper lesions may be difficult to locate at time of surgery.

Cystic brainstem HGB: the solid nodule of the tumor is removed under the microscope by bipolaring and cutting the gliotic adhesions to the parenchyma. Removal of the cyst wall is not necessary. There is often a cleavage between the tumor and the floor of the fourth ventricle which facilitates tumor removal. To reduce bleeding, avoid piecemeal removal. Preserve large draining veins until the arterial feeders to the mural nodule have been isolated and resected.[12]

Radiation treatment

Effectiveness is dubious. May be useful to reduce tumor size or to retard growth, e.g. in patients who are not surgical candidates, for multiple small deep lesions, or for inoperable brainstem HGB. Does not prevent regrowth following subtotal excision.

43.3.3 von Hippel-Lindau disease (VHL)

General information

Key concepts

- disorder with hemangioblastomas (HGB) 1° of cerebellum, retina, brainstem & spinal cord, as well as renal cysts/tumors, pheochromocytomas (among others)
- autosomal dominant, due to inactivation of tumor suppressor gene on 3p25
- expression and age of onset are variable, but ≈ always manifests by age 60
- mean age of developing HGBs is at least 10 years younger than sporadic HGBs

A multisystem neoplastic disorder characterized by a tendency to develop hemangioblastomas (HGB) of the retina, brain and spinal cord, renal clear cell carcinoma (RCC), pheochromocytomas, endolymphatic sac tumors, and others[6,13] (retinal location is 2nd most common after cerebellar, ▶ Table 43.1). The variability of von Hippel-Lindau disease (VHL) has lead some to suggest the use of the term hemangioblastomatosis.

Epidemiology

Incidence: 1 in 31,000 to 36,000 live births. ≈ 30% of patients with cerebellar HGB have VHL.[7]

Genetics

Autosomal dominant inheritance with ≈ 95% penetrance at age 60 yrs.[6,16] 4% of VHL are asymptomatic carriers. The VHL gene is a tumor suppressor gene on chromosome 3p25, and biallelic inactivation is required for tumor development.[7] Most patients inherit a VHL gene (allele) with the germline mutation from the affected parent and a normal somatic (wild-type) VHL gene from the unaffected parent.

Subtypes of VHL

See reference.[17]

▶ **Type I.** May have any manifestation of VHL *except* pheochromocytoma

▶ **Type II.** Pheochromocytoma is characteristic

▶ **Type IIA.** Have low risk of renal cell Ca and neuroendocrine pancreatic tumor

Table 43.1 Associations with von Hippel-Lindau disease[a]

Common lesions	Frequency in VHL
hemangioblastomas	
• cerebellum (solid or cystic)	80%
• retina	41–59%
• brainstem	10–25%
• spinal cord	10–50%
pancreatic tumors or cysts	22–80%
renal clear cell Ca & cysts	14–60%
polycythemia	9–20% of intracranial HGBs
Rare lesions (pertinent to nervous system)	**Frequency in VHL**
supratentorial hemangioblastoma	3–6%
cystadenomas of the broad ligament	10% of ♀
papillary cystadenomas of epididymis	25–60% ♂
endolymphatic sac tumors	10–15%
adrenal medullary *pheochromocytoma* (tends to be bilateral)	7–24%

[a]see references[6,14,15] for more

► **Type IIB.** Higher risk of renal cell Ca and neuroendocrine pancreatic tumor

► **Type IIC.** Risk of pheochromocytoma only (without risk of HGB or RCC)

Diagnostic criteria

Suggested diagnostic criteria for VHL:
1. in 80% of patients with VHL there is a multigenerational family history, and only 1 manifestation (CNS HGB or visceral lesion) is necessary to make the diagnosis in these patients
2. if no family history (20% of VHL, many of these represent a de novo mutation): 2 manifestations including 1 CNS or retinal HGB are required[18]
3. genetic testing in uncertain cases (see below)

Tumors associated with VHL

1. cerebellar hemangioblastomas (HGB):
   a) prevalence: 44–72% of VHL patients
   b) mean age of diagnosis in VHL patients with cerebellar hemangioblastomas is at least 10 years younger than sporadic cerebellar hemangioblastomas
   c) cysts are commonly associated with cerebellar, brainstem and spinal HGBs
   d) cysts grow at a faster rate than the HGBs, ∴ symptoms related to mass effect are frequently secondary to the cysts
   e) cerebellar HGBs were located in the superficial, posterior and superior half of the cerebellar hemispheres[10]
   f) 93% of the cerebellar HGBs were located in the cerebellar hemispheres and 7% in the vermis
   g) the HGBs are also more frequently found in the superficial posterior half of the brainstem and the spinal cord
   h) the HGBs have multiple sequential growth and quiescent phases
2. spinal cord hemangioblastomas
   a) occur in 13–44% of VHL patients
   b) 90% are located rostrally within the cervical and thoracic cord. Almost all (96%) of the tumors are located in the posterior half of the spinal cord, 4% are located in the ventral half of the spinal cord. 1–3% are found in the lumbosacral nerve roots

c) by way of comparison, 80% of spinal cord HGB are associated with VHL, whereas only 5–31% of cerebellar HGB are associated with VHL
d) 95% of symptom-producing spinal HGBs are associated with syringomyelia

3. brainstem hemangioblastomas
   a) usually located in the posterior medulla oblongata usually around the obex and the region within the area postrema
4. pheochromocytomas (PCC): 20% of PCC are associated with VHL. PCC occur in 7–20% of families with VHL
5. endolymphatic sac tumors (ELST):
   a) locally invasive benign tumors that occur in 10–15% of VHL patients (30% of these will develop bilateral ELSTs – VHL is the only disease with bilateral ELSTs). Rarely metastasize
   b) presents with hearing loss in 95% (may be acute (86%) or insidious (14%), tinnitus (90%), vertigo or imbalance (66%), aural fullness (30%), and facial paresthesias (8%)
   c) mean age of onset of hearing loss: 22 years (range: 12–50)[19]
6. retinal hemangioblastomas[20]
   a) occur in > 50% of VHL patients. Mean age a presentation: 25 years
   b) frequently bilateral, multifocal and recurrent
   c) often asymptomatic. Visual symptoms occur with progressive growth, edema, retinal detachments and hard exudates
   d) typically located in the periphery and near or on the optic disc
   e) microangiomas measuring a few hundred microns without dilated feeding vessels may be located in the periphery
   f) retrobulbar HGB are rare (5.3% in NIH cohort)[21]
   g) severity of optic disease correlates with CNS and renal involvement
   h) early diagnosis and treatment with laser photocoagulation, and cryotherapy can prevent visual loss. Low dose external XRT may be an option for refractory cases
7. renal-cell carcinoma (RCC)[15,22,23,24,25,26,27,28]
   a) the most common malignant tumor in VHL. Usually a clear cell carcinoma
   b) lifetime risk for RCC in VHL: ≈ 70%.
   c) the growth rate of RCC is high variable
   d) RCC is the cause of death in 15–50% of patients
   e) metastases respond poorly to chemotherapy and radiation
   f) bilateral and multiple lesions are common
   g) partial nephrectomy or tumor enucleation is preferred to avoid/delay dialysis and transplantation
   h) nephron- or renal-sparing surgery recommended for tumors less < 3 cm
   i) promising techniques: cryo- and radiofrequency ablation of tumors < 3 cm
8. renal cysts[15,24,27,28,29]
   a) 50–70% of VHL patients have bilateral and multiple renal cysts
   b) rarely cause profound renal impairment
   c) chronic renal failure or renal hypertension not as common as with polycystic kidney disease
9. epididymal cystadenomas
   a) benign lesions that arise from the epididymal duct
   b) found in 10–60% of male VHL patients
   c) typically appear in the teenage years
   d) may cause infertility if bilateral
   e) may be multiple
10. broad ligament cystadenomas
   a) arise from the embryonic mesonephric duct
   b) true incidence unknown
   c) rarely reported and usually not recognized in women with VHL
11. pancreatic neuroendocrine tumors and cysts
   a) 35 to 70% of patients with VHL develop an endocrine tumor or cyst
   b) pancreatic cysts are generally asymptomatic and often multiple
   c) pancreatic neuroendocrine tumors are usually non-functional and 8% of them are malignant
   d) differential diagnosis: pancreatic islet cell tumors, MEN2

Treatment

Resection of individual CNS tumors is usually reserved until symptomatic to decrease the number of operations over a lifetime since the tumors in VHL are usually multiple, tend to recur, and the growth pattern is saltatory. Surgery is the treatment of choice for accessible *cystic* HGBs. For details, see Treatment, under Hemangioblastoma (p. 702).

Stereotactic radiosurgery (SRS)[30]: May provide local control rates of > 50% over 5 years. SRS has been recommended for asymptomatic HBG > 5 mm diameter if they are cystic or progressing in size during surveillance.[31] Cranial treatment plan: using a median dose of 22 Gy (range: 12–40 Gy) prescribed to the median 82% isodose line in 1–4 sessions. In cystic lesions, treatment is confined to the contrast enhancing mural nodule (the cyst wall is not treated). Spinal treatment plan: median dose of 21 Gy (range 20–25 Gy) prescribed to the median 77% isodose line in 1–3 sessions. Radiosurgery is usually contraindicated in hemangioblastomas with a cyst.

Surveillance

Because of the lifetime risk of developing tumors, regular surveillance is needed. Various protocols have been proposed,[33,34] including those by the NIH[15] and the Danish clinical recommendations.[35] The algorithm recommended by the VHL Family Alliance for patients with VHL and at-risk relatives is shown in ▶ Table 43.2. (Screening at-risk relatives can be stopped at age 60 years if no abnormalities have been detected.)

Individuals who do not carry the altered gene on DNA testing do not require surveillance.

Table 43.2 Health-care provider's surveillance guidelines for patients with or at risk for VHL[a]

Age	Surveillance
Any age	DNA testing for VHL marker is available to identify family members at risk
From birth	check for neurologic deficit, nystagmus, strabismus, white pupil... & refer to retinologist for abnormal findings. Newborn hearing screening
1 year	retina exam[b] (especially if positive for VHL mutation)
2–10 years	Annual: • PE[c] including orthostatic blood pressure measurement, neurologic exam, retina exam[b] • blood test or 24° urine for catecholamines & metanephrines (p. 653). If elevated: abdominal MRI or MIBG scan (p. 653) • abdominal U/S starting at age 8 Every 2–3 years: complete audiology exam. Annually if hearing loss, tinnitus or vertigo
11–19 years	Every 6 months: retina exam[b] Annual: • PE (including scrotal exam in males), neuro exam • 24° urine for catecholamines & metanephrines (p. 653). If elevated: abdominal MRI or MIBG scan (p. 653) • abdominal U/S (kidneys, pancreas & adrenals). If abnormal: abdominal MRI or CT (except in pregnancy) Every 1–2 years or if symptoms develop: • gadolinium MRI of brain & spine. Annually at onset of puberty or before and after pregnancy (only for emergencies during pregnancy) • complete audiology exam. If abnormal, or if tinnitus or vertigo at any time: MRI of IAC to look for ELST
≥ 20 years	Annual: • dilated retina exam[b] • PE (including scrotal exam in males), neuro exam • blood test or 24° urine for catecholamines & metanephrines (p. 653). If elevated: abdominal MRI or MIBG scan (p. 653) • check kidneys, pancreas & adrenals with abdominal U/S and at least every other year unenhanced/enhanced abdominal CT (not during pregnancy) Every 2 years: • (or before and after pregnancy, except for emergencies) gadolinium MRI of brain & spine • complete audiology exam. If abnormal, or if tinnitus or vertigo at any time: MRI of IAC to look for ELST
Prior to surgery or childbirth	• blood test or 24° urine for catecholamines & metanephrines (p. 653) to rule out pheochromocytoma

[a]adapted[32]
[b]indirect ophthalmoscope exam by retinologist familiar with VHL
[c]abbreviations: PE = physical exam by physician familiar with VHL, ELST = endolymphatic sac tumor

Prognosis

The lifespan of patients with VHL is decreased. 30–50% die of renal cell Ca (RCC). Metastases from RCC and neurologic complications from cerebellar HGB are the primary causes of death.

Metastases respond poorly to chemotherapy and XRT.

Resources

Genetic screening for VHL can be done at a few centers. Information for patients and families can be found at www.vhl.org/.

References

[1] Barba I, Moreno A, Martinez-Perez I, et al. Magnetic resonance spectroscipy of brain hemangiopericytomas: high myoinositol concentrations and discrimination from meningiomas. J Neurosurg. 2001; 94:55–60

[2] Savitz MH, Anderson PJ. Primary Melanoma of the Leptomeninges: A Review. Mt Sinai J Med. 1974; 41:774–791

[3] Gibson JB, Burrows D, Weir WP. Primary Melanoma of the Meninges. J Pathol Bacteriol. 1957; 74:419–438

[4] Wilkins RH, Rengachary SS. Neurosurgery. New York 1985

[5] Ho VB, Smirniotopoulos JG, Murphy FM, Rushing EJ. Radiologic-Pathologic Correlation: Hemangioblastoma. AJNR. 1992; 13:1343–1352

[6] Catapano D, Muscarella LA, Guarnieri V, Zelante L, D'Angelo VA, D'Agruma L. Hemangioblastomas of central nervous system: molecular genetic analysis and clinical management. Neurosurgery. 2005; 56:1215–21; discussion 1221

[7] Hottinger AF, Khakoo Y. Neurooncology of familial cancer syndromes. J Child Neurol. 2009; 24:1526–1535

[8] Wakai S, Inoh S, Ueda Y, et al. Hemangioblastoma Presenting with Intraparenchymatous Hemorrhage. J Neurosurg. 1984; 61:956–960

[9] Silver ML, Hennigar G. Cerebellar Hemangioma (Hemangioblastoma). A Clinicopathological Review of 40 Cases. J Neurosurg. 1952; 9:484–494

[10] Jagannathan J, Lonser RR, Smith R, DeVroom HL, Oldfield EH. Surgical management of cerebellar hemangioblastomas in patients with von Hippel-Lindau disease. J Neurosurg. 2008; 108:210–222

[11] Utsuki S, Oka H, Sato K, Shimizu S, Suzuki S, Fujii K. Fluorescence diagnosis of tumor cells in hemangioblastoma cysts with 5-aminolevulinic acid. J Neurosurg. 2009. DOI: 10.3171/2009.5.JNS08442

[12] Agrawal A, Kakani A, Vagh SJ, Hiwale KM, Kolte G. Cystic hemangioblastoma of the brainstem. J Neurosci Rural Pract. 2010; 1:20–22

[13] Glenn GM, Linehan WM, Hosoe S, Latif F, et al. Screening for von Hippel-Lindau Disease by DNA Polymorphism Analysis. JAMA. 1992; 267:1226–1231

[14] Wanebo JE, Lonser RR, Glenn GM, Oldfield EH. The natural history of hemangioblastomas of the central nervous system in patients with von Hippel-Lindau disease. J Neurosurg. 2003; 98:82–94

[15] Butman JA, Linehan WM, Lonser RR. Neurologic manifestations of von Hippel-Lindau disease. JAMA. 2008; 300:1334–1342

[16] Go RCP, Lamiell JM, Hsia YE, et al. Segregation and Linkage Analysis of von Hippel-Lindau Disease Among 220 Descendents from one Kindred. Am J Human Genet. 1984; 36:131–142

[17] Friedrich CA. Genotype-phenotype correlation in von Hippel-Lindau syndrome. Hum Mol Genet. 2001; 10:763–767

[18] Melmon KL, Rosen SW. Lindau's Disease. Review of the Literature and Study of a Large Kindred. Am J Med. 1964; 36:595–617

[19] Manski TJ, Heffner DK, Glenn GM, Patronas NJ, Pikus AT, Katz D, Lebovics R, Sledjeski K, Choyke PL, Zbar B, Linehan WM, Oldfield EH. Endolymphatic sac tumors. A source of morbid hearing loss in von Hippel-Lindau disease. JAMA. 1997; 277:1461–1466

[20] Chew EY. Ocular manifestations of von Hippel-Lindau disease: clinical and genetic investigations. Trans Am Ophthalmol Soc. 2005; 103:495–511

[21] Meyerle CB, Dahr SS, Wetjen NM, Jirawuthiworavong GV, Butman JA, Lonser RR, Oldfield E, Rodriguez-Coleman H, Wong WT, Chew EY. Clinical course of retrobulbar hemangioblastomas in von Hippel-Lindau disease. Ophthalmology. 2008; 115:1382–1389

[22] Niemela M, Lemeta S, Summanen P, Bohling T, Sainio M, Kere J, Poussa K, Sankila R, Haapasalo H, Kaariainen H, Pukkala E, Jaaskelainen J. Long-term prognosis of haemangioblastoma of the CNS: impact of von Hippel-Lindau disease. Acta Neurochir (Wien). 1999; 141:1147–1156

[23] Choyke PL, Glenn GM, Walther MM, Zbar B, Linehan WM. Hereditary renal cancers. Radiology. 2003; 226:33–46

[24] Meister M, Choyke P, Anderson C, Patel U. Radiological evaluation, management, and surveillance of renal masses in Von Hippel-Lindau disease. Clin Radiol. 2009; 64:589–600

[25] Maher ER, Kaelin WGJr. von Hippel-Lindau disease. Medicine (Baltimore). 1997; 76:381–391

[26] Hes FJ, Feldberg MA. Von Hippel-Lindau disease: strategies in early detection (renal-, adrenal-, pancreatic masses). Eur Radiol. 1999; 9:598–610

[27] Bisceglia M, Galliani CA, Senger C, Stallone C, Sessa A. Renal cystic diseases: a review. Adv Anat Pathol. 2006; 13:26–56

[28] Truong LD, Choi YJ, Shen SS, Ayala G, Amato R, Krishnan B. Renal cystic neoplasms and renal neoplasms associated with cystic renal diseases: pathogenetic and molecular links. Adv Anat Pathol. 2003; 10:135–159

[29] Bradley S, Dumas N, Ludman M, Wood L. Hereditary renal cell carcinoma associated with von Hippel-Lindau disease: a description of a Nova Scotia cohort. Can Urol Assoc J. 2009; 3:32–36

[30] Moss JM, Choi CY, Adler JR, Jr, Soltys SG, Gibbs IC, Chang SD. Stereotactic radiosurgical treatment of cranial and spinal hemangioblastomas. Neurosurgery. 2009; 65:79–85; discussion 85

[31] Chang SD, Meisel JA, Hancock SL, Martin DP, McManus M, Adler JR, Jr. Treatment of hemangioblastomas in von Hippel-Lindau disease with linear accelerator-based radiosurgery. Neurosurgery. 1998; 43:28–34; discussion 34-5

[32] VHL Family Alliance. VHL Handbook. Section 5: Suggested screening guidelines. 2009

[33] Constans JP, Meder F, Maiuri F, Donzelli R, Spaziante R, de Divitiis E. Posterior fossa hemangioblastomas. Surg Neurol. 1986; 25:269–275

[34] Hes FJ, van der Luijt RB. [Von Hippel-Lindau disease: protocols for diagnosis and periodical clinical monitoring. National Von Hippel-Lindau Disease Working Group]. Ned Tijdschr Geneeskd. 2000; 144:505–509

[35] Poulsen ML, Budtz-Jorgensen E, Bisgaard ML. Surveillance in von Hippel-Lindau disease (vHL). Clin Genet. 2009. DOI: 10.1111/j.1399-0004.2009.01281.x

Part XIII

Tumors Involving Non-Neural Origin: Metastases, Lymphomas, Chordomas

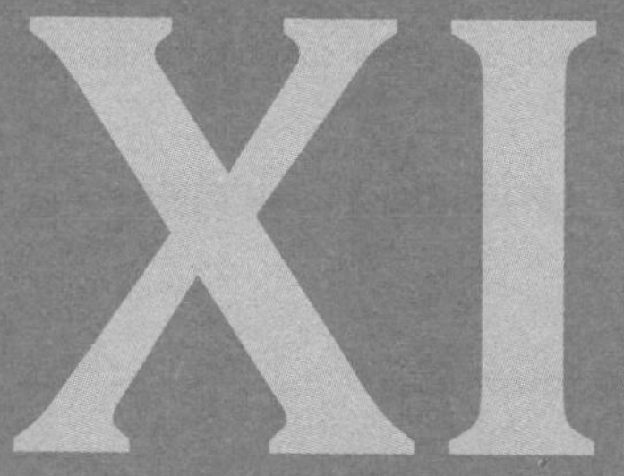

44 Lymphomas and Hematopoietic Neoplasms

44.1 CNS lymphoma

44.1.1 General information

44

Key concepts

- may be primary or secondary (pathologically identical)
- suspected with homogeneously enhancing lesion(s) in the central gray matter or corpus callosum (on MRI or CT) especially in AIDS patients
- may present with multiple cranial-nerve palsies
- diagnosis highly likely if tumor seen in conjunction with uveitis
- very responsive initially to steroids → short-lived disappearance(may produce "ghost tumors")
- treatment: usually XRT ± chemotherapy. Role of neurosurgery usually limited to biopsy and/or placement of ventricular access reservoir for chemotherapy
- risk factors: immunosuppression (AIDS, transplants), Epstein-Barr virus, collagen vascular diseases

CNS involvement with lymphoma may occur secondarily from a "systemic" lymphoma, or may arise primarily in the CNS. It is controversial whether most intracranial malignant lymphomas are primary[1] or secondary.[2]

44.1.2 Primary vs. secondary lymphoma

Secondary CNS lymphoma

Non CNS lymphoma is the fifth most common cause of cancer deaths in the U.S., 63% of new cases are non-Hodgkin's. Secondary CNS involvement usually occurs late in the course. Metastatic spread of systemic lymphoma to the cerebral *parenchyma* occurs in 1–7% of cases at autopsy.[3]

Primary CNS lymphoma

Older names include: reticulum cell sarcoma and microglioma[4] since they were thought to possibly arise from microglia which were considered part of the reticuloendothelial system.

A rare, malignant primary CNS neoplasm comprising 0.85–2% of all primary brain tumors and 0.2–2% of malignant lymphomas.[5] May occasionally metastasize outside the CNS.

44.1.3 Epidemiology

The incidence of primary CNS lymphoma (PCNSL) is rising relative to other brain lesions, and will likely exceed that of low-grade astrocytomas and approach meningiomas. This is in part due to the occurrence of PCNSL in AIDS and transplant patients, but the incidence has also increased in the general population over the past 20 years.[6]

Male:female ratio = 1.5:1 (based on literature review[7]).

Median age at diagnosis: 52 yrs[7] (younger among immunocompromised patients: ≈ 34 yrs).

Most common supratentorial locations: frontal lobes, then deep nuclei; periventricular also common. Infratentorially: cerebellum is the most common location.

44.1.4 Conditions with increased risk of primary CNS lymphomas (PCNSL)

1. collagen vascular disease
   a) systemic lupus erythematosus
   b) Sjögren's syndrome: an autoimmune connective tissue disorder
   c) rheumatoid arthritis
2. immunosuppression
   a) organ transplant recipients: related to chronic immunosuppression. Falls under category of post transplant lymphoproliferative disease (PTLD)[8]

b) severe-congenital immunodeficiency syndrome ("SCIDS")
c) AIDS[9,10]: CNS lymphoma occurs in ≈ 10% of AIDS patients, and is the first presentation in 0.6%
d) possibly increased incidence in the elderly due to reduced competency of immune system
3. Epstein-Barr virus[11] is associated with a broad spectrum of lymphoproliferative disorders, and is detectable in ≈ 30–50% of systemic lymphomas, however, it has been associated with almost 100% of PCNSL,[12] especially AIDS-related cases[13(p 317)]

44.1.5 Pathology

Characteristic sites: corpus callosum, basal ganglia, periventricular.

The neoplastic cells are identical to those of systemic lymphomas. Most are bulky tumors that are contiguous with the ventricles or meninges.

Histologic distinguishing features: tumor cells form cuffs around blood vessels which demonstrate multiplication of basement membranes (best demonstrated with silver reticulum stain).

Frozen section distorts the cells and may lead to a misdiagnosis of malignant glioma.[13(p 320)]

Immunohistochemical stains differentiates B-cell lymphomas from T-cell lymphomas (B-cell types are more common, especially in PCNSL and in AIDS).

EM shows absence of junctional complexes (desmosomes) that are usually present in epithelial derived tumors.

Intravascular lymphomatosis[14]: Formerly: (malignant) angioendotheliomatosis. A rare lymphoma with no solid mass in which malignant lymphoid cells are found in the lumen of small blood vessels in affected organs. CNS involvement is reported in most cases. Presentation is non specific: patients are often febrile, and may present with progressive multifocal cerebrovascular events (including stroke or hemorrhage), spinal cord or nerve root symptoms including cauda equina syndrome (p. 1050), encephalopathy or peripheral or cranial neuropathies.[15] Initial transient cerebral symptoms may mimic TIAs or seizures. The ESR is often elevated prior to initiation of steroids. Lymphoma cells may be seen in the CSF.

Painful skin nodules or plaques occur in ≈ 10% of cases, generally involving the abdomen or lower extremities, and these cases may be diagnosed with skin biopsy (differential diagnosis here includes angioendotheliomatosis, a benign capillary and endothelial cell disorder). Otherwise, diagnosis often requires brain biopsy (open or stereotactic), in which involved areas on imaging studies are targeted. Pathology: malignant lymphoid cells distend and occlude small arteries, veins and capillaries with little or no parenchymal extension.[13(p 324)] Treatment with combination chemotherapy can result in long-term remission in some patients, but early diagnosis before permanent damage occurs is critical (diagnosis is rarely made pre-mortem).

44.1.6 Presentation

General information

Presentation is similar with primary or secondary CNS lymphoma: the two most common manifestations are those due to epidural spinal cord compression and those of carcinomatous meningitis (multiple cranial nerve deficits) (p. 811). Seizures occur in up to 30% of patients.[1]

Symptoms

1. presents with non-focal non-specific symptoms in over 50% of patients; at time of presentation most commonly includes:
   a) mental status changes in one–third
   b) symptoms of increased ICP (H/A, N/V)
   c) generalized seizures in 9%
2. focal symptoms in 30–42% of cases:
   a) hemimotor or hemisensory symptoms
   b) partial seizures
   c) multiple cranial-nerve palsies (due to carcinomatous meningitis)
3. combination of focal and non-focal symptoms

Signs

1. non-focal in 16%:
   a) papilledema
   b) encephalopathy
   c) dementia

2. focal findings in 45% of cases:
   a) hemimotor or hemisensory deficits
   b) aphasia
   c) visual field deficits
3. combination of focal and non-focal signs

Uncommon but characteristic syndromes

1. uveocyclitis, coincident with (in 6% of cases) or preceding the diagnosis of (in 11% of cases) lymphoma
2. subacute encephalitis with subependymal infiltration
3. MS-like illness with steroid-induced remission

44.1.7 Evaluation

All patients should be assessed (history, physical, and if appropriate, laboratory tests) for any of the conditions associated with lymphoma (p.710). Since primary CNS lymphoma is less common than secondary involvement, any patient with CNS lymphoma should have work-up for occult systemic lymphoma including:
1. careful physical exam of all lymph nodes (LN)
2. evaluation of perihilar and pelvic LN (CXR, CT of chest & abdomen)
3. routine blood and urine testing
4. bone marrow biopsy
5. MRI of the entire spine
6. testicular ultrasound in males
7. ophthalmologic examination (including slit-lamp evaluation of both eyes) in all
   a) for possible uveitis
   b) ≈ 28% of patients with PCNSL will also have intraocular lymphoma. Often resistant to methotrexate, but responds to low dose ocular XRT (7–8 Gy)

44.1.8 Diagnostic tests

General information

On imaging (CT or MRI) 50–60% occur in one or more cerebral lobes (in grey or white matter). 25% occur in deep midline structures (septum pellucidum, basal ganglion, corpus callosum). 25% are infratentorial. 10–30% of patients have multiple lesions at the time of presentation. In contrast, systemic lymphomas that spread to the CNS tend to present with leptomeningeal involvement instead of parenchymal tumors.[16]

CT

Non-AIDS-related cases tend to enhance homogeneously, whereas AIDS-related cases often have a necrotic center and appear as *multifocal ring-enhancing* lesions[17] (the wall is thicker than with an abscess).

Non-AIDS related cases: CNS lymphomas should be suspected with homogeneously enhancing lesion(s) in the central gray or corpus callosum. 75% are in contact with ependymal or meningeal surfaces (this together with dense enhancement may produce a "pseudomeningioma pattern", however lymphomas lack calcifications and tend to be multiple).

60% are hyperdense to brain, only 10% are hypodense. Characteristically, >90% of these tumors enhance; this is densely homogeneous in over 70%. As a result, when rare non-enhancing cases occur it often leads to a delay in diagnosis.[18] The appearance of enhanced PCNSL on CT has been likened to "fluffy cotton balls." There may be surrounding edema[19] and there is usually mass effect.

There is an almost diagnostic tendency of rapid partial to complete resolution on CT (and even at the time of surgery) following the administration of steroids, earning the nickname of "ghost-cell tumor"[20,21] or disappearing tumor.

MRI

No pathognomonic feature. May be difficult to discern if tumor is located subependymally (signal characteristics similar to CSF); proton-weighted image may avoid this pitfall. Nonenhancing lymphoma (on MRI or CT) is rare[22] (some of these may enhance after XRT) but may be underreported. Bright on DWI (restricted diffusion), isointense to hypointense on ADC map.

CSF

Should only be obtained if no mass effect. Usually abnormal, but non-specific. Most common abnormalities are elevated protein (in > 80%), and increased cell count (in 40%). Cytology is positive for lymphoma cells (pre-operatively) in only 10% (sensitivity may be higher with leptomeningeal involvement as in non-AIDS patients than with parenchymal involvement commonly seen in AIDS). Repeating up to 3 LPs may increase yield. Although the diagnosis of lymphoma can be made from CSF, cells obtained in this manner are not adequate for detailed tissue typing which is possible with solid tissue from biopsy.

Angiography

Rarely helpful. 60% of cases show only an avascular mass. 30–40% show diffuse homogeneous staining or blush.

44.1.9 Treatment

Surgery

Surgical decompression with partial or gross total removal does not alter patient's prognosis. The main indications for surgery:

- Biopsy: obtain solid tissue to ascertain that the tumor is a lymphoma, and to determine the type of lymphoma. Stereotactic techniques are often well-suited for these often deep tumors.[23]

Radiation therapy

The standard treatment after tissue biopsy is whole-brain radiation therapy. Doses used tend to be lower than for other primary brain tumors. ≈ 40–50 Gy total are usually given in 1.8–3 Gy daily fractions.

Chemotherapy

General information

In *non-AIDS* cases, chemotherapy combined with XRT prolongs survival compared to XRT alone.[24]

Methotrexate (MTX)

The addition of intraventricular MTX (rather than just intrathecal via LP) delivered through a ventricular access device (6 doses of 12 mg twice a week, with IV leucovorin rescue) may result in even better survival.[25] In the event of an intrathecal MTX overdose (OD), interventions recommended[26]: ODs of up to 85 mg can be well tolerated with little sequelae; immediate LP with drainage of CSF can remove a substantial portion of the drug (removing 15 ml of CSF can eliminate ≈ 20–30% of the MTX within 2 hrs of OD). This can be followed by ventriculolumbar perfusion over several hours using 240 ml of warmed isotonic preservative-free saline entering through the ventricular reservoir and exiting through a lumbar subarachnoid catheter. For major OD of > 500 mg, add intrathecal administration of 2,000 U of carboxypeptidase G2 (an enzyme that inactivates MTX). In cases of MTX OD, systemic toxicity should be prevented by treating with IV dexamethasone and IV (not IT) leucovorin.

Rituximab

Available since 1997 for treatment of refractory systemic B-cell non-Hodgkins lymphoma. Intrathecally, may be more effective for CD33 + lymphomas.

44.1.10 Prognosis

With no treatment, median survival is 1.8–3.3 months following diagnosis.

With radiation therapy,[1] median survival is 10 months, with 47% 1-year median survival, and 16% 2-year median survival. 3-year survival is 8%, and 5-year survival is 3–4%. With intraventricular MTX, median time to recurrence was 41 mos.[25] Occasionally, prolonged survival may be seen.[27]

About 78% of cases recur, usually ≈ 15 months after treatment (late recurrences also are seen). Of these recurrences, 93% are confined to the CNS (often at another site if the original site responded well), and 7% are elsewhere.

In AIDS-related cases, the prognosis appears worse. Although complete remission occurs in 20–50% following XRT, the median survival is only 3–5 months,[28,29] usually related to AIDS-related opportunistic infection. However, neurologic function and quality of life improve in ≈ 75%.[28]

Although there are individual studies that show trends, there are no prognostic features that consistently correlate with survival.

44.2 Multiple myeloma

44.2.1 General information

Multiple myeloma (MM) (sometimes referred to simply as myeloma) is a neoplasm of a single clone of plasma cells characterized by proliferation of plasma cells in bone marrow, infiltration of adjacent tissues with mature and immature plasma cells, and the production of an immunoglobulin, usually monoclonal IgG or IgA (referred to collectively as M-protein[30]). Circulating pre-myeloma cells lodge in appropriate microenvironments (e.g. in bone marrow) where they differentiate and expand. Although MM is often referred to in the context of "metastatic lesions" to bone, it is also sometimes considered a primary bone tumor. If only a single lesion is identified, then it is referred to as a plasmacytoma (see below).

44.2.2 Epidemiology

In the U.S., incidence is ≈ 1–2 per 100,000 in caucasians, and is ≈ twice that in blacks. MM accounts for 1% of malignancies, and 10% of hematologic cancers. The peak age of occurrence is 60–70 yrs of age, with < 2% of patients being < 40 yrs old. Slightly more common in males. Monoclonal gammopathy without MM occurs in ≈ 0.15% of the population, and in long-term follow-up 16% of these develop MM with an annual rate of 0.18%.[31]

44.2.3 Presentation

General information

MM presents as a result of the following (underscored items are characteristic for MM):

1. proliferation of plasma cells: interferes with normal immune system function → increased ***susceptibility to infection***
2. bone involvement
   a) bone marrow involvement → destruction of hematopoietic capacity → normocytic normochromic *anemia*, leukopenia, thrombocytopenia
   b) bone resorption
      - → weakening of the bone → *pathologic fractures* (see below)
      - → *hypercalcemia* (present initially in 25% of MM patients, see below)
   c) swelling or local tenderness of bone
   d) *bone pain*: characteristically induced by movement, and absent at rest
   e) spinal involvement
      - invasion of spinal canal in ≈ 10% of cases → spinal cord compression → myelopathy
      - nerve root compression (radiculopathy)
3. overproduction of certain proteins by plasma cells. May lead to:
   a) hyperviscosity syndrome
   b) cryoglobulinemia
   c) amyloidosis
   d) *renal failure*: multifactorial, but monoclonal light chains play a role

Skeletal disease

MM involvement is by definition multiple, and is usually restricted to sites of red marrow: ribs, sternum, spine, clavicles, skull, or proximal extremities. Lesions of the spine and/or skull are the usual reasons for presentation to the neurosurgeon.

Bone resorption in MM is not due simply to mechanical erosion by plasma cells. Increased osteoclastic activity has been observed.

Plasma cell tumors of the skull involving the cranial vault usually do not produce neurologic symptoms. Cranial nerve palsies can arise from skull base involvement. Orbital involvement may produce proptosis (exophthalmos).

Neurologic involvement

Neurologic manifestations can occur as a result of:
1. tumor involvement of bone causing compression (see above)
   a) tumor in spine with compression of spinal cord or nerve roots
   b) tumor in skull with compression of brain or cranial nerves
2. deposition of amyloid within the flexor retinaculum of the wrist → carpal tunnel syndrome; the median nerve itself does not contain amyloid, and therefore responds well to surgical division of the transverse carpal ligament (p. 524)
3. diffuse progressive sensorimotor polyneuropathy: occurs in 3–5% of patients with MM
   a) about half are due to amyloidosis (p. 549)
   b) polyneuropathy can also occur without amyloidosis, especially in the rare osteosclerotic variant of MM
4. multifocal leukoencephalopathy has been described in MM[32]
5. hypercalcemia: may produce a dramatic encephalopathy with confusion, delirium or coma. Neurologic symptoms of hypercalcemia associated with MM are more common than in hypercalcemia of other etiologies
6. very rare: intraparenchymal metastases[33]

44.2.4 Evaluation

The diagnostic criteria for MM is shown in ▶ Table 44.1. Tests that may be used in evaluating patients with MM or suspected MM include:
1. 24 hour urine for kappa Bence-Jones protein present in 75%. (Note: Small proteins (comprised of light chains of immunoglobulins) found in the urine of ≈ 80% of patients with MM (may also occur in other conditions). Monoclonal proteins cannot be detected in the urine or serum of ≈ 1% of MM patients; two or more monoclonal bands are produced in ≈ 0.5–2.5% of patients with MM.[34])
2. bloodwork: serum protein electrophoresis (SPEP) and immune electrophoresis (IEP) (looking for IgG kappa band)
3. skeletal radiologic survey. Characteristic x-ray finding: multiple, round, "punched-out" (sharply demarcated) lytic lesions in the bones typically involved (see above). Osteosclerotic lesions are seen in < 3% of patients with MM. Diffuse osteoporosis may also be seen
4. CBC: anemia eventually develops in most patients with MM. It is usually of moderate severity (Hgb ≈ 7–10 gm%) with a low reticulocyte count
5. technetium-99 m nuclear bone scan is usually *negative* in untreated MM (due to rarity of spontaneous new bone formation) and is less sensitive than conventional radiographs. Therefore it is not usually helpful except perhaps to implicate etiologies other than MM to explain the observed findings. After treatment, bone scan may become positive as osteoblastic activity ensues ("flare" response)
6. serum creatinine: for prognostication
7. bone marrow biopsy: virtually all MM patients have "myeloma cells" (although sensitive, this is not specific and other diagnostic criteria should be sought)

44.2.5 Treatment

Many aspects of treatment fall into the purvey of the oncologist (see review[31]). Some aspects pertinent to neurosurgical care include:
1. XRT (p. 808): MM Is very radiosensitive. Focal XRT for pain due to readily identifiable bone lesions, may allow pathologic fractures to heal and is effective in spinal cord compression

Table 44.1 Criteria for diagnosis of MM[a]

1. Cytologic criteria a) marrow morphology: plasma cells and/or myeloma cells ≥ 10% of 1000 or more cells b) biopsy proven plasmacytoma
2. Clinical and laboratory criteria a) myeloma protein (M-component) in serum (usually > 3 gm/dl) or urine IEP b) osteolytic lesions on x-ray (generalized osteoporosis qualifies if marrow contains > 30% plasma or myeloma cells) c) myeloma cells in ≥ 2 peripheral blood smears
[a]diagnosis requires[35]: 1A & 1B, or 1A or 1B and 2A, 2B, or 2C

2. mobilization: immobilization due to pain and fear of pathologic compression fractures leads to further detrimental increases in serum calcium and weakness
3. pain control: mild pain often responds well to salicylates (contraindicated in thrombocytopenia). Local XRT is also effective (see below)
4. percutaneous kyphoplasty (p. 1011) may be used for some spine lesions (preferred over vertebroplasty because of reduced potential of spreading neoplasm)
5. therapy for hypercalcemia usually improves symptoms related to that derangement
6. bisphosphonates (p. 1122) inhibit bone resorption and rapidly reduces hypercalcemia. Pamidronate is currently preferred over older agents
7. bortezomib (Velcade®): the first proteasome inhibitor, indicated for treatment of refractory MM

44.2.6 Prognosis

Untreated MM has a 6 month median survival. Solitary plasmacytoma has a 50% 10-year survival. If there is an solitary site of involvement but M-protein is present (i.e. essentially a plasmacytoma except for the M-protein), elimination of the M-protein following XRT indicates a 50–60% chance of remaining free of MM, if the M-protein doesn't resolve, there is a high chance of developing MM.

44.3 Plasmacytoma

44.3.1 General information

A neoplasm of a single clone of plasma cells similar to multiple myeloma (see above) but meeting the following criteria:
1. there must be no other lesions on complete skeletal survey (*not* bone scan)
2. bone marrow aspirate must show no evidence of myeloma
3. and serum and urine electrophoresis should show no M-protein

MM will develop in 55–60% of patients with a solitary plasmacytoma in 5 years, and in 70–80% by 10 yrs.

44.3.2 Treatment

1. local XRT provides good local control rates
2. percutaneous kyphoplasty (p. 1011): preferred over vertebroplasty because of reduced potential of spreading neoplastic cells

References

[1] O'Neill BP, Illig JJ. Primary Central Nervous System Lymphoma. Mayo Clin Proc. 1989; 64:1005–1020
[2] Kawakami Y, Tabuchi K, Ohnishi R, et al. Primary Central Nervous System Lymphoma. J Neurosurg. 1985; 62:522–527
[3] Jellinger K, Radaszkiewicz T. Involvement of the Central Nervous System in Malignant Lymphomas. Virchows Arch (Pathol Anat). 1976; 370:345–362
[4] Helle TL, Britt RH, Colby TV. Primary Lymphoma of the Central Nervous System. J Neurosurg. 1984; 60:94–103
[5] Alic L, Haid M. Primary Lymphoma of the Brain: A Case Report and Review of the Literature. J Surg Oncol. 1984; 26:115–121
[6] Eby NL, Grufferman S, Flannelly CM, Scholf SC, Vogel FS, Burger PC. Increasing Incidence of Primary Brain Lymphoma in the U.S. Cancer. 1988; 62:2461–2465
[7] Murray K, Kun L, Cox J. Primary Malignant Lymphoma of the Central Nervous System: Results of Treatment of 11 Cases and Review of the Literature. J Neurosurg. 1986; 65:600–607
[8] Penn I. Development of Cancer as a Complication of Clinical Transplantation. Transplant Proc. 1977; 9:1121–1127
[9] Levy RM, Bredesen DE, Rosenblum ML. Neurological manifestations of the acquired immunodeficiency syndrome (AIDS): Experience at UCSF and review of the literature. J Neurosurg. 1985; 62:475–495
[10] Jean WC, Hall WA. Management of Cranial and Spinal Infections. Contemp Neurosurg. 1998; 20:1–10
[11] Hochberg FH, Miller G, Schooley RT, et al. Central-Nervous-System Lymphoma Related to Epstein-Barr Virus. N Engl J Med. 1983; 309:745–748
[12] MacMahon EME, Glass JD, Hayward SD, et al. Epstein-Barr Virus in AIDS-Related Primary Central Nervous System Lymphoma. Lancet. 1991; 338:969–973
[13] Burger PC, Scheithauer BW, Vogel FS. Surgical Pathology of the Nervous System and Its Coverings. 4th ed. New York: Churchill Livingstone; 2002
[14] Calamia KT, Miller A, Shuster EA, et al. Intravascular Lymphomatosis: A Report of Ten Patients with Central Nervous System Involvement and a Review of the Disease Process. Adv Exp Med Biol. 1999; 455:249–265
[15] Glass J, Hochberg FH, Miller DC. Intravascular Lymphomatosis. A Systemic Disease with Neurologic Manifestations. Cancer. 1993; 71:3156–3164
[16] So YT, Beckstead JH, Davis RL. Primary central nervous system lymphoma in acquired immune deficiency syndrome: A clinical and pathological study. Ann Neurol. 1986; 20:566–572
[17] Poon T, Matoso I, Tchertkoff V, et al. CT features of primary cerebral lymphoma in AIDS and non-AIDS patients. J Comput Assist Tomogr. 1989; 13:6–9
[18] DeAngelis LM. Cerebral Lymphoma Presenting as a Nonenhancing Lesion of Computed Tomographic/

Magnetic Resonance Scan. Ann Neurol. 1993; 33:308–311

[19] Enzmann DR, Krikorian J, Norman D, et al. Computed Tomography in Primary Reticulum Cell Sarcoma of the Brain. Radiology. 1979; 130:165–170

[20] Vaquero J, Martinez R, Rossi E, et al. Primary Cerebral Lymphoma: the 'Ghost Tumor'. J Neurosurg. 1984; 60:174–176

[21] Gray RS, Abrahams JJ, Hufnagel TJ, et al. Ghost-cell tumor of the optic chiasm; primary CNS lymphoma. J Clin Neuroophthalmol. 1989; 9:98–104

[22] DeAngelis LM. Cerebral lymphoma presenting as a nonenhancing lesion on computed tomographic/magnetic resonance scan. Ann Neurol. 1993; 33:308–311

[23] O'Neill BP, Kelly PJ, Earle JD, et al. Computer-Assisted Stereotactic Biopsy for the Diagnosis of Primary Central Nervous System Lymphoma. Neurology. 1987; 37:1160–1164

[24] DeAngelis LM, Yahalom J, Heinemann M-H, et al. Primary Central Nervous System Lymphomas: Combined Treatment with Chemotherapy and Radiotherapy. Neurology. 1990; 40:80–86

[25] DeAngelis LM, Yahalom J, Thaler HT, Kher U. Combined Modality Therapy for Primary CNS Lymphomas. J Clin Oncol. 1992; 10:635–643

[26] O'Marcaigh AS, Johnson CM, Smithson WA, et al. Successful Treatment of Intrathecal Methotrexate Overdose by Using Ventriculolumbar Perfusion and Intrathecal Instillation of Carboxypeptidase G2. Mayo Clin Proc. 1996; 71:161–165

[27] Hochberg FH, Miller DC. Primary Central Nervous System Lymphoma. J Neurosurg. 1988; 68:835–853

[28] Baumgartner JE, Rachlin JR, Beckstead JH, Levy RM, et al. Primary Central Nervous System Lymphomas: Natural History and Response to Radiation Therapy in 55 Patients with Acquied Immunodeficiency Syndrome. J Neurosurg. 1990; 73:206–211

[29] Formenti SC, Gill PS, Lean E, et al. Primary Central Nervous System Lymphoma in AIDS: Results of Radiation Therapy. Cancer. 1989; 63:1101–1107

[30] Keren DF, Alexanian R, Goeken JA, Gorevic PD, Kyle RA, Tomar RH. Guidelines for Clinical and Laboratory Evaluation of Patients with Monoclonal Gammopathies. Arch Pathol Lab Med. 1999; 123:106–107

[31] Bataille R, Harousseau J-L. Multiple Myeloma. N Engl J Med. 1997; 336:1657–1664

[32] McCarthy J, Proctor SJ. Cerebral Involvement in Multiple Myeloma. Case Report. J Clin Pathol. 1978; 31:259–264

[33] Norum J, Wist E, Dahil IM. Cerebral Metastases from Multiple Myeloma. Acta Oncol. 1991; 30:868–869

[34] Foerster J, Lee GR, Bithell TC, Foerster J, Athens JW, Lukens JN. In: Multiple Myeloma. Wintrobe's Clinical Hematology. 9th ed. Philadelphia: Lea and Febiger; 1993:2219–2249

[35] Costa G, Engle RL, Schilling A, et al. Melphalan and Prednisone: An Effective Combination for the Treatment of Multiple Myeloma. Am J Med. 1973; 54:589–599

45

45 Pituitary Tumors – General Information and Classification

45.1 General information

Key concepts

- most are benign adenomas arising from the anterior pituitary (adenohypophysis)
- presentation (see below): most commonly present due to hormonal effects (includes: hyperprolactinemia, Cushing's syndrome, acromegaly...), mass effect (most commonly: bitemporal hemianopsia from compression of optic chiasm), as an incidental finding, or infrequently with pituitary apoplexy (p. 720)
- work-up for a newly diagnosed intrasellar lesion: see ▶ Table 46.1
- prolactinoma is the only type for which medical therapy (DA agonists) may be the primary treatment in certain cases (p. 737). For other tumor types, options primarily consist of surgery (transsphenoidal or transcranial), or XRT
- post-op concerns include: diabetes insipidus, adrenal insufficiency, CSF leak

See also review of pituitary embryology & neuroendocrinology (p. 149).

45.2 General tumor types

45.2.1 Pituitary adenomas

Most primary pituitary tumors are benign adenomas which arise from the anterior pituitary gland (adenohypophysis). Adenomas may be classified by a number of schemes, including: by endocrine function (aided by immunostaining), by light microscopy (p. 727) with routine histological staining and by electron microscopic appearance.

Microadenoma: A pituitary tumor < 1 cm diameter. Currently, 50% of pituitary tumors are < 5 mm at time of diagnosis. These may be difficult to find at the time of surgery.

Macroadenomas: Tumors > 1 cm diameter.

45.2.2 Pituitary carcinoma

See reference.[1]

Rare (< 140 reports). Usually invasive and secretory (most common hormones: ACTH, PRL). Can metastasize, at which point prognosis is poor (66% 1-year mortality). Little improvement with further surgery, XRT, or chemotherapy.

45.2.3 Neurohypophyseal tumors

Neurohypophyseal tumors (tumors of the neurohypophysis i.e. the posterior pituitary) are rare; see Pituicytoma (p. 728).

45.3 Epidemiology

Pituitary tumors represent ≈ 10% of intracranial tumors (incidence is higher in autopsy series). They are most common in the 3rd and 4th decades of life, and affect both sexes equally. The incidence is increased in multiple endocrine adenomatosis or neoplasia (MEA or MEN) (especially type I: autosomal dominant inheritance with high penetrance, also involves pancreatic islet cell tumors (which may produce gastrin and hence Zollinger-Ellison syndrome) and parathyroids (hyperparathyroidism), and in which the pituitary tumors are usually nonsecretory).

45.4 Differential diagnosis of pituitary tumors

See differential diagnosis (p. 1371), which also includes non-neoplastic etiologies.

45.5 Clinical presentation of pituitary tumors

45.5.1 General information

Classically, pituitary tumors are divided into functional (or secreting), and non-functional (AKA endocrine-inactive, which are either nonsecretory, or else secrete products such as gonadotropin that do not cause endocrinologic symptoms).

In general, secreting tumors tend to present earlier as a result of symptoms caused by physiologic effects of excess hormones that they secrete[2] (this applies less e.g. to prolactinomas in males since the symptoms may be mild or unrecognized). Nonsecreting tumors usually do not present until they are sufficiently large enough to cause neurologic deficits by mass effect.

45.5.2 Presentation

General information

Presentation may be the result of: endocrine syndromes, mass effect, incidental finding (essentially only with macroadenomas), pituitary apoplexy.

Endocrinologic disturbance

Hormone oversecretion (secretory tumor)

≈ 65% of adenomas secrete an active hormone (48% prolactin, 10% GH, 6% ACTH, 1% TSH)[3]:

1. prolactin (PRL) (p. 722): can cause amenorrhea-galactorrhea syndrome in females), impotence in males Etiologies:
   a) prolactinoma (p. 722): neoplasia of pituitary lactotrophs
   b) stalk effect (p. 732): pressure on the pituitary stalk may reduce the inhibitory control over PRL secretion
2. growth hormone (GH): elevated GH is due to a pituitary adenoma > 95% of the time
   a) in adults: causes acromegaly (p. 725)
   b) in prepubertal children (before epiphyseal plate closure): produces pituitary gigantism (very rare)
3. corticotropin AKA adrenocorticotropic hormone (ACTH):
   a) Cushing's disease (endogenous hypercortisolism): see below
   b) Nelson syndrome (p. 724): can develop only in patients who have had an adrenalectomy
4. thyrotropin (TSH) (p. 726): secondary (central) hyperthyroidism
5. gonadotropins (luteinizing hormone (LH) and/or follicle stimulating hormone (FSH)): usually does not produce a clinical syndrome

Underproduction of pituitary hormones

May be caused by compression of the normal pituitary by large tumors. More common with non-secretory tumors than with secretory tumors. In order of sensitivity to compression(i.e. the order in which pituitary hormones become depressed from mass effect): GH, gonadotropins (LH & FSH), TSH, ACTH (mnemonic: Go Look For The Adenoma). Chronic deficiency of all pituitary hormones (panhypopituitarism) may produce pituitary cachexia (AKA Simmonds' cachexia).

✖ NB: selective reduction of a single pituitary hormone is very atypical with pituitary adenomas. May occur with autoimmune hypophysitis (p. 1373), which most commonly involves ACTH or ADH (causing DI[4] – see below)

1. Deficiency of specific hormones
2. growth hormone deficiency (note: growth hormone stimulation test (p. 736) is more sensitive and specific for GH deficiency than measuring basal GH levels):
   a) in children: produces growth delay
   b) in adults: produces vague symptoms with metabolic syndrome (decreased lean body mass, centripetal obesity, reduced exercise tolerance, impaired sense of well-being)
   c) hypogonadism: amenorrhea (women), loss of libido, infertility
3. hypothyroidism: cold intolerance, myxedema, entrapment neuropathies (e.g. carpal tunnel syndrome), weight gain, memory disturbance, integumentary changes (dry skin, coarse hair, brittle nails), constipation, increased sleep demand
4. hypoadrenalism: orthostatic hypotension, easy fatigability
5. diabetes insipidus: almost never seen pre-operatively with pituitary tumors (except possibly with pituitary apoplexy, see below). If DI is present, other etiologies should be sought, including:
   a) autoimmune hypophysitis (p. 1373)
   b) hypothalamic glioma
   c) suprasellar germ cell tumor

6. gonadotropin deficiency (hypogonadotrophic hypogonadism) with anosmia is part of Kallmann syndrome[5]

Mass effect (other than compression of the pituitary)

Because they tend to get to a larger size before detection, this is more common with nonfunctioning tumors. Of functional tumors, prolactinoma is the most likely to become large enough to cause mass effect (especially in males or non-menstruating females); ACTH tumor is least likely. Nonspecific symptoms include headaches. ✖ seizures are rarely attributable to pituitary adenomas and other etiologies should be sought. Mass effect may occur suddenly as a result of expansion with pituitary apoplexy (see below).

45

Structures commonly compressed and their manifestations include:

1. optic chiasm: classically produces **bitemporal hemianopsia** (non-congruous). May also cause decreasing visual acuity
2. involvement of third ventricle may produce obstructive hydrocephalus
3. cavernous sinus
   a) pressure on cranial nerves contained within (III, IV, V1, V2, VI): ptosis, facial pain, diplopia (below)
   b) occlusion of the cavernous sinus: proptosis, chemosis
   c) encasement of the carotid artery by tumor: may cause slight narrowing, but complete occlusion is rare
4. invasive adenomas (p. 721) infrequently present with CSF rhinorrhea[6] with invasive prolactinomas this may be precipitated by shrinkage resulting from medical treatment
5. macroadenomas may produce H/A possibly via increased intrasellar pressure

Pituitary apoplexy

General information

Key concepts

- due to expansion of a pituitary adenoma from hemorrhage or necrosis
- typical presentation: paroxysmal H/A with endocrinologic and/or neurologic deficit (usually ophthalmoplegia or visual loss)
- management: immediate administration of glucocorticoids, and transsphenoidal decompression within 7 days in most cases

Definition

Neurologic and/or endocrinologic deterioration due to sudden expansion of a mass within the sella turcica.

Etiology

Sudden intrasellar expansion may occur as a result of hemorrhage, necrosis[7,8] and/or infarction within a pituitary tumor and adjacent pituitary gland. Occasionally, hemorrhage occurs into a normal pituitary gland or Rathke's cleft cyst.[9]

Epidemiology

In Wilson's series, 3% of his patients with macroadenomas had an episode of pituitary apoplexy. In another series of 560 pituitary tumors, a high incidence of 17% was found (major attack in 7%, minor in 2%, asymptomatic in 8%).[10] It is common for apoplexy to be the initial presentation of a pituitary tumor.[11]

Clinical features of pituitary apoplexy

Patients often present with abrupt onset of H/A, visual disturbance, and loss of consciousness. Neurologic involvement includes:

1. visual disturbances: one of the most common findings. Includes:
   a) ophthalmoplegia (unilateral or bilateral): opposite the situation with a pituitary tumor, ophthalmoplegia occurs more often (78%) than visual pathway deficits (52–64%)[12]
   b) one of the typical field cuts (p. 730) seen in pituitary tumors

2. reduced mental status: due to ↑ ICP or hypothalamic involvement
3. cavernous sinus compression can cause venous stasis and/or pressure on any of the structures within the cavernous sinus
   a) trigeminal nerve symptoms
   b) proptosis
   c) ophthalmoplegia (Cr. N. III palsy is more common than VI)
   d) ptosis may be an early symptom[13,14]
   e) pressure on carotid artery
   f) compression of sympathetics within the cavernous sinus may produce a form of Horner's syndrome with unilateral ptosis, miosis, & anhidrosis limited to the forehead
   g) carotid artery compression may cause stroke or vasospasm
4. when hemorrhage breaks through the tumor capsule and the arachnoid membrane into the chiasmatic cistern, signs and symptoms of SAH may be seen
   a) N/V
   b) meningismus
   c) photophobia
5. increased ICP may produce lethargy, stupor or coma
6. hypothalamic involvement may produce
   a) hypotension
   b) thermal dysautoregulation
   c) cardiac dysrhythmias
   d) respiratory pattern disturbances
   e) diabetes insipidus
   f) altered mental status: lethargy, stupor or coma
7. suprasellar expansion can produce acute hydrocephalus

Evaluation

CT or MRI shows hemorrhagic mass in sella turcica and/or suprasellar region, often distorting the anterior third ventricle.

Cerebral angiography should be considered in cases where differentiating pituitary apoplexy from aneurysmal SAH is difficult.

Management of pituitary apoplexy

Pituitary function is consistently compromised, necessitating rapid administration of corticosteroids and endocrine evaluation.

In the absence of visual deficits, prolactinomas may be treated with bromocriptine.

Rapid decompression is required for: sudden constriction of visual fields, severe and/or rapid deterioration of acuity, or neurologic deterioration due to hydrocephalus. Surgery in ≤ 7 days of pituitary apoplexy resulted in better improvement in ophthalmoplegia (100%), visual acuity (88%) and field cuts (95%) than surgery after 7 days, based on a retrospective study of 37 patients.[15] Decompression is usually via a transsphenoidal route (transcranial approach may be advantageous in some cases). Goals of surgery:
1. to decompress the following structures if under pressure: optic apparatus, pituitary gland, cavernous sinus, third ventricle (relieving hydrocephalus)
2. obtain tissue for pathology
3. complete removal of tumor is usually not necessary
4. for hydrocephalus: ventricular drainage is generally required

45.6 Specific types of pituitary tumors

45.6.1 Invasive pituitary adenomas

About 5% of pituitary adenomas become locally invasive. The genetic make-up of these tumors may differ from more benign adenomas,[16] even though the histology is similar. Numerous classifications systems have been devised for invasive adenomas, Wilson's system[17] (modified from Hardy[18,19]) is shown in ► Table 45.1.

The clinical course is variable, with some tumors being more aggressive than others. Occasionally, these tumors grow to gigantic sizes (> 4 cm dia), and these are often very aggressive and follow a malignant course.[20]

At times, an adenoma may push the medial wall of the cavernous sinus ahead of it without actually perforating this dural structure (i.e. not actually invading the sinus).[21] This is difficult to

Table 45.1 Anatomic classification of pituitary adenoma (modified Hardy system)[17]

Extension
• **Suprasellar extension** 0: none A: expanding into suprasellar cistern B: anterior recesses of 3rd ventricle obliterated C: floor of 3rd ventricle grossly displaced • **Parasellar extension** D[a]: intracranial (intradural) E: into or beneath cavernous sinus (extradural)
Invasion/Spread
• **Floor of sella intact** I: sella normal or focally expanded; tumor < 10 mm II: sella enlarged; tumor ≥ 10 mm • **Sphenoid extension** III: localized perforation of sellar floor IV: diffuse destruction of sellar floor • **Distant spread** V: spread via CSF or blood-borne
[a]specify: 1) anterior, 2) middle, or 3) posterior fossa

reliably identify on MRI, and the most definitive sign of cavernous sinus invasion is carotid artery encasement.[22]

Presentation

1. visual system
   a) most present due to compression of the optic apparatus, usually producing gradual visual deficit (however, sudden blindness is not unheard of)
   b) extraocular muscle deficits may occur with cavernous sinus invasion, and usually develop after visual loss
   c) exophthalmos may occur with orbital invasion due to compromise of orbital venous drainage
2. hydrocephalus: suprasellar extension may obstruct one or both foramen of Monro
3. invasion of the skull base may lead to nasal obstruction. CSF rhinorrhea may occasionally be precipitated by tumor shrinkage in response to dopamine agonists (e.g. bromocriptine) as a result of uncovering areas of bone erosion. This carries the risk of ascending meningitis.[23]
4. tumors that secrete prolactin (p. 719) often present with findings of hyperprolactinemia and with these, the prolactin levels are usually > 1000 ng/ml (caution: giant invasive adenomas with very high PRL production may have a falsely low PRL level due to "hook effect" (p. 733)

45.6.2 Hormonally active pituitary tumors

Prolactinomas

The most common secretory adenoma. Arise from neoplastic transformation of anterior pituitary lactotrophs. See ▶ Table 46.4 for DDx of hyperprolactinemia.

Manifestations of prolonged hyperprolactinemia:

1. females: amenorrhea-galactorrhea syndrome (AKA Forbes-Albright syndrome, AKA Ahumada-del Castillo syndrome). Variants: oligomenorrhea, irregular menstrual cycles. 5% of women with primary amenorrhea will be found to have a PRL-secreting pituitary tumor.[24] Remember: pregnancy is the most common cause of secondary amenorrhea in females of reproductive potential. The galactorrhea may be spontaneous or expressive (only on squeezing the nipples)
2. males: impotence, decreased libido. Galactorrhea is rare (estrogen is also usually required). Gynecomastia is rare. Prepubertal prolactinomas may result in small testicles and feminine body habitus
3. either sex:
   a) infertility is common
   b) bone loss (osteoporosis in women, and both cortical and trabecular osteopenia in men) due to a relative estrogen deficiency, not due to the elevated prolactin itself

At the time of diagnosis, 90% of prolactinomas in women are microadenomas, vs. 60% for males (probably due to gender specific differences in symptoms resulting in earlier presentation in females). Some tumors secrete both PRL and GH.

Cushing's disease

General information and Cushing's syndrome

Cushing's syndrome (CS) is a constellation of findings caused by hypercortisolism. Cushing's disease (p. 723) – endogenous hypercortisolism due to hypersecretion of ACTH by an ACTH secreting pituitary adenoma – is just one cause of CS. The most common cause of CS is iatrogenic (administration of exogenous steroids). Possible etiologies of *endogenous* hypercortisolism are shown in ▶ Table 45.2. To determine the etiology of CS, see Dexamethasone suppression test (p. 734).

45

Conversion factors[25] for ACTH and cortisol between U.S. units and SI units are shown in Eq (45.1) and (45.2).

$$\text{ACTH}: 1\,\text{pg/ml} = 1\,\text{ng/liter} \tag{45.1}$$

$$\text{Cortisol}: 1\,\mu\text{g/dl} = 27.59\,\text{nmol/liter} \tag{45.2}$$

Ectopic ACTH secretion

Hypercortisolism may also be due to ectopic secretion of ACTH usually by tumors, most commonly small-cell carcinoma of the lung, thymoma, carcinoid tumors, pheochromocytomas, and medullary thyroid carcinoma. In addition to findings of Cushing's syndrome, patients are typically cachectic due to the malignancy which is usually rapidly fatal.

Prevalence of Cushing's disease

40 cases/million population. ACTH-producing adenomas comprise 10–12% of pituitary adenomas.[26] Cushing's disease is 9 times more common in women, whereas *ectopic* ACTH production is 10 times more common in males. Non-iatrogenic CS is 25% as common as acromegaly.

At the time of presentation, over 50% of patients with Cushing's disease have pituitary tumors < 5 mm in diameter, which are very difficult to image with CT or MRI. Most are basophilic, some (especially the larger ones) may be chromophobic. Only ≈ 10% are large enough to produce some mass effect, which may cause enlargement of the sella turcica, visual field deficit, cranial nerve involvement and/or hypopituitarism.

Clinical findings in Cushing's disease

Findings are those of Cushing's syndrome (hypercortisolism from any cause) include:

1. weight gain
   a) generalized in 50% of cases

Table 45.2 Causes of endogenous hypercortisolism

Site of pathology	Secretion product	Percent of cases	ACTH levels
pituitary corticotroph adenoma: Cushing's disease (p. 723)	ACTH	60–80%	slightly elevated[a]
ectopic ACTH production (p. 723); most are lung tumors, others: pancreas...		1–10%	very elevated
adrenal (adenoma or carcinoma)	cortisol	10–20%	low
hypothalamic or ectopic secretion of corticotropin-releasing hormone (CRH) producing hyperplasia of pituitary corticotrophs; pseudo-Cushing's state (p. 723)	CRH	rare	elevated

[a]ACTH may be normal or slightly elevated; normal ACTH levels in the presence of hypercortisolism are considered inappropriately elevated

   b) centripetal fat deposition in 50%: trunk, upper thoracic spine ("buffalo hump"), supraclavicular fat pad, neck, "dewlap tumor" (episternal fat), with round plethoric face ("moon facies") and slender extremities
2. hypertension
3. ecchymoses and purple striae, especially on flanks, breasts and lower abdomen
4. amenorrhea in women, impotence in men, reduced libido in both
5. hyperpigmentation of skin and mucous membranes: due to MSH cross-reactivity of ACTH. Occurs only with elevated ACTH, i.e. Cushing's disease (not Cushing's syndrome) or ectopic ACTH production (also below)
6. atrophic, tissue-paper thin skin with easy bruising and poor wound healing
7. psychiatric: depression, emotional lability, dementia
8. osteoporosis
9. generalized muscle wasting with complaints of easy fatigability
10. elevation of other adrenal hormones: androgens may produce hirsutism and acne
11. sepsis: associated with advanced Cushing's syndrome

Laboratory findings in Cushing's disease

1. hyperglycemia: diabetes or glucose intolerance
2. hypokalemic alkalosis
3. loss of diurnal variation in cortisol levels
4. normal or elevated ACTH levels
5. failure to suppress cortisol with low-dose (1 mg) dexamethasone test (p. 734)
6. elevated 24-hour urine free-cortisol
7. CRH levels will be low (not commonly measured)

Nelson's syndrome (or Nelson syndrome) (NS)

General information

Key concepts

- a rare condition that follows 10–30% of total bilateral adrenalectomies (TBA) performed for Cushing's disease; see indications for TBA (p. 743)
- classic triad: hyperpigmentation (skin & mucus membranes), abnormal ↑ ACTH, and progression of pituitary tumor (the last criteria is now controversial)
- treatment options: surgery (transsphenoidal or transcranial), XRT, medication

A rare condition that follows 10-30% of total bilateral adrenalectomies (TBA) performed for Cushing's disease; see indications for TBA (p. 743). NS is due to continued growth of corticotroph (ACTH-secreting) adenoma cells. Usually occurs 1–4 years after TBA (range: 2 mos-24 years).[26] Theoretical explanation (unproven)[27]: following TBA, hypercortisolism resolves, and CRH levels increase back to normal from the (reduced) suppressed state; corticotroph adenomas in patients with NS have an increased & prolonged response to CRH resulting in increased growth. Also, corticotrophs in NS and CD show reduced inhibition by glucocorticoids. It is controversial if some cases may be related to insufficient glucocorticoid replacement after TBA.[26]

Manifestations

See reference.[27]

1. hyperpigmentation (due to melanin stimulating hormone (MSH) cross reactivity of ACTH and actual increased levels of MSH due to increased proopiomelanocortin production). Often the earliest sign that Nelson's syndrome is developing. Look for linea nigra (midline pigmentation from pubis to umbilicus) and hyperpigmentation of scars, gingivae, and areolae. DDx of hyperpigmentation includes: primary adrenal insufficiency (high levels of ACTH), ectopic ACTH secretion, hemochromatosis (more bronze color), jaundice (yellowish)
2. tumor growth → increased mass effect (p. 720) or invasion: the most serious consequence. These corticotroph tumors are among the most aggressive of pituitary tumors.[28 (p 545)] May produce any of the problems associated with macroadenomas (optic nerve compression, cavernous sinus invasion, pituitary insufficiency, H/A, bony invasion…) as well as necrosis with precipitous intracranial hypertension[29]; see pituitary apoplexy (p. 720)

3. malignant transformation of the corticotroph tumor (very rare)
4. hypertrophy of adrenal tissue rests: may be located in the testes → painful testicular enlargement and oligospermia. Rarely the rests can secrete enough cortisol to normalize cortisol levels or even cause a recurrence of Cushing's disease despite the adrenalectomy

Evaluation
1. Laboratories
   a) ACTH > 200 ng/L (usually thousands of ng/L) (normal: usually < 54 ng/L)
   b) exaggerated ACTH response to CRH (not required for diagnosis)
   c) other pituitary hormones may be affected as with any macroadenoma causing mass effect (p. 720) and endocrine screening (p. 731) should be done
2. Formal visual field testing (p. 730): should be done in patients with suprasellar extension or in those being considered for surgery (as a baseline for comparison)

Treatment
See treatment (p. 739).

Acromegaly

General information

Key concepts

- abnormally high levels of growth hormone in an adult. > 95% of cases are due to a benign pituitary somatotroph adenoma, > 75% are > 10 mm at time of diagnosis
- effects include soft tissue and skeletal changes, cardiomyopathy, colon Ca
- work-up: endocrine tests (p. 730), cardiology consult, colonoscopy
- treatment (p. 741): surgery for most, and then if necessary, medical therapy (p. 741) and/or XRT (p. 745)
- suggested criteria for biochemical cure (p. 753): normal IGF-1, growth hormone level < 5 ng/ml, AND GH nadir of < 1 ng/ml after OGST (p. 736)

Incidence: 3 cases/1-million persons/year. > 95% of cases of excess GH result from a pituitary somatotroph adenoma. Growth hormone carcinoma is extremely rare. Ectopic GH secretion may occur uncommonly with: carcinoid tumor, lymphoma, pancreatic islet-cell tumor. By the time of diagnosis, > 75% of pituitary GH tumors are macroadenomas (> 10 mm dia) with cavernous sinus invasion and/or suprasellar extension.

25% of acromegalics have thyromegaly with normal thyroid studies. 25% of GH adenomas also secrete prolactin. Acromegaly occurs rarely as part of a genetic syndrome, including: multiple endocrine neoplasia type 1 (MEN 1), McCune-Albright syndrome, familial acromegaly, and Carney complex.[30]

Clinical
Elevated levels of GH in children before closure of the epiphyseal plates in the long bones produces gigantism. Usually presents in the teen years.

In adults, elevated GH levels produces acromegaly (age: usually > 50 yrs) with findings that may include[31,32] (also see ▶ Table 45.3):
1. skeletal overgrowth deformities
   a) increasing hand and foot size
   b) thickened heel pad
   c) frontal bossing
   d) prognathism
2. cardiovascular
   a) cardiac findings (structural and functional): arrhythmias, valvular disease, concentric myocardial hypertrophy
   b) hypertension (30%)
3. soft tissue swelling (includes macroglossia)
4. glucose intolerance
5. peripheral nerve entrapment syndromes (including carpal tunnel syndrome)

45

Table 45.3 Risks of long-term exposure to excess growth hormone (GH)[34]
Arthropathy
1. unrelated to age of onset or GH levels 2. usually with longstanding acromegaly 3. reversibility[a]: a) rapid symptomatic improvement b) bone & cartilage lesions irreversible
Peripheral neuropathy
1. intermittent anesthesias, paresthesias 2. sensorimotor polyneuropathy 3. impaired sensation 4. reversibility[a]: a) symptoms may improve b) onion bulbs (whorls) do not regress
Cardiovascular disease
1. cardiomyopathy a) reduced LV diastolic function b) increased LV mass and arrhythmias c) fibrous hyperplasia of connective tissue 2. HTN: exacerbates cardiomyopathic changes 3. reversibility[a]: may progress even with normal GH
Respiratory disease
1. upper airway obstruction: caused by soft tissue overgrowth and decreased pharyngeal muscle tone with sleep apnea in ≈ 50% 2. reversibility[a]: generally improves
Neoplasia
1. increased risk of malignancies (especially colon-Ca) & soft-tissue polyps 2. reversibility[a]: unknown
Glucose intolerance
1. occurs in 25% of acromegalics (more common with family history of DM) 2. reversibility[a]: improves
[a]reversibility with normalization of GH levels

6. debilitating headache
7. excessive perspiration (especially palmar hyperhidrosis)
8. oily skin
9. joint pain
10. sleep apnea
11. fatigue
12. colon cancer: risk is ≈ 2 × risk of general population[33]

Patients with elevated levels of GH (including partially treated cases) have 2–3 times the expected mortality rate,[34] primarily due to hypertension, diabetes, pulmonary infections, cancer, and cardiovascular disease (▶ Table 45.3). Soft-tissue swelling and nerve entrapment may be reversible with normalization of GH levels, however many disfiguring changes and health risks are permanent (▶ Table 45.3 for specifics).

Thyrotropin (TSH)-secreting adenomas

General information

Rare: comprise ≈ 0.5–1% of pituitary tumors.[3,35] Produces central (secondary) hyperthyroidism (note: central hyperthyroidism may also occur with pituitary resistance to thyroid hormones[36]): elevated circulating T3 and T4 levels, with elevated or inappropriately normal TSH[36] (TSH should be undetectable in primary hyperthyroidism). Up to 33% of tumors positive for TSH immunostaining are nonsecretory.[36] Many of these tumors are plurihormonal, but the secondary hormone is usually clinically silent. Most of these tumors are aggressive and invasive and are large enough at presentation to also produce mass effect (especially if prior thyroid ablative procedures have been done, which occurs in up to 60% of cases due to lack of recognition of pituitary abnormality[36,37]).

Clinical

Symptoms of hyperthyroidism: anxiety, palpitations (due to a-fib), heat intolerance, hyperhidrosis, and weight loss despite normal or increased intake. Signs: hyperactivity, lid lag, tachycardia, irregular rhythm when a-fib is present, hyperreflexia, tremor. Exophthalmos and infiltrative dermopathy (e.g. pretibial myxedema) are present only in Grave's disease.

45.6.3 Pathological classification of pituitary tumors

Light microscopic appearance of adenomas

Older classification system. Of limited usefulness. With newer techniques (EM, immunohistochemistry, radio-immuno assay…) many tumors previously considered nonsecretory have been found to have all the components necessary to secrete hormones.

In order of decreasing frequency:

1. chromophobe: most common (ratio of chromophobe to acidophil is 4-20:1). Originally considered "non-secretory", in actuality may produce prolactin, GH, or TSH
2. acidophil (eosinophilic): produce prolactin, TSH, or usually *GH*
3. basophil→ gonadotropins, β-lipotropin, or usually *ACTH → Cushing's disease*

Classification of adenomas based on secretory products

1. endocrine-active tumors: ≈ 70% of pituitary tumors produce 1 or 2 hormones that are measurable in the serum and cause defined clinical syndromes, these are classified based on their secretory product(s)
2. endocrine-inactive (nonfunctional) tumors[38] (**note:** a and b constitute the bulk of endocrine-inactive adenomas):
   a) null-cell adenoma
   b) oncocytoma
   c) gonadotropin-secreting adenoma
   d) silent corticotropin-secreting adenoma
   e) glycoprotein-secreting adenoma

Tumors of the neurohypophysis and infundibulum

General information

The most common tumors encountered in the posterior pituitary are metastases (owing to the rich blood supply).

Granular cell tumors

AKA (infundibular) granular cell tumor (GCT). WHO grade I. Obsolete terms: choristoma,[39] granular cell myoblastoma, pituicytoma (this term is now reserved for a circumscribed glial neoplasm – see below). Tumors with nests of large cells having granular, eosinophilic cytoplasm.

While rare, GCTs are the most common primary tumor of the neurohypophysis and pituitary stalk/infundibulum[40] with a predilection for the stalk (these result in suprasellar extension). GCTs have been identified in the gastrointestinal tract, genitourinary tract, orbital region as well as in other locations of the central nervous system with no connection to the pituitary gland or hypothalamus (e.g. spinal meninges[41]). Female:male ratio ≥ 2:1. Asymptomatic microscopic clusters of granular cells (tumorettes) are more common, with an incidence up to 17%.[42]

The most common presentation is with visual field deficits due to optic chiasm compression.[39] However, any symptom typical of a hormonally inactive sellar mass may occur.

Imaging: may appear radiographically identical to adenomas. Rarely considered in the differential diagnosis pre-op. Isodense on CT and isointense on T1WI MRI, dense homogeneous enhancement on CT & MRI.

Treatment: if GTC is suspected pre-op, a transcranial approach is preferred over transsphenoidal because of the vascularity which has prevented total resection in 60–70% of reported cases.[43] XRT may be considered for subtotal resection.[40]

Pituicytoma

Less favored alternate terms include posterior pituitary astrocytoma. Rare (mostly case reports). Circumscribed tumor with spindle cells, arising from the neurohypophysis or infundibulum.[44] WHO grade I. Reported only in adults.

Treatment: surgical excision. Subtotal removal may be followed by recurrence over several years.

References

[1] Ragel BT, Couldwell WT. Pituitary carcinoma: a review of the literature. Neurosurg Focus. 2004; 16

[2] Ebersold MJ, Quast LM, Laws ER, et al. Long-Term Results in Transsphenoidal Removal of Nonfunctioning Pituitary Adenomas. J Neurosurg. 1986; 64:713–719

[3] Biller BM, Swearingen B, Zervas NT. A decade of the Massachusetts General Hospital Neuroendocrine Clinical Center. J Clin Endocrinol Metab. 1997; 82:1668–1674

[4] Abe T, Matsumoto K, Sanno N, Osamura Y. Lymphocytic Hypophysitis: Case Report. Neurosurgery. 1995; 36:1016–1019

[5] Lieblich JM, Rogol AD, White BJ, Rosen SW. Syndrome of anosmia with hypogonadotropic hypogonadism (Kallmann syndrome): clinical and laboratory studies in 23 cases. Am J Med. 1982; 73:506–519

[6] Nutkiewicz A, DeFeo DR, Kohout RI, et al. Cerebrospinal Fluid Rhinorrhea as a Presentation of Pituitary Adenoma. Neurosurgery. 1980; 6:195–197

[7] Reid RL, Quigley ME, Yen SC. Pituitary Apoplexy: A Review. Arch Neurol. 1985; 42:712–719

[8] Cardoso ER, Peterson EW. Pituitary Apoplexy: A Review. Neurosurgery. 1984; 14:363–373

[9] Onesti ST, Wisniewski T, Post KD. Pituitary Hemorrhage into a Rathke's Cleft Cyst. Neurosurgery. 1990; 27:644–646

[10] Wakai S, Fukushima T, Teramoto A, Sano K. Pituitary Apoplexy: Its Incidence and Clinical Significance. J Neurosurg. 1981; 55:187–193

[11] Rovit RL, Fein JM. Pituitary Apoplexy, A Review and Reappraisal. J Neurosurg. 1972; 37:280–288

[12] Liu JK, Couldwell W. Pituitary apoplexy: Diagnosis and management. Contemp Neurosurg. 2003; 25:1–5

[13] Yen MY, Liu JH, Jaw SJ. Ptosis as the early manifestation of pituitary tumour. Br J Ophthalmol. 1990; 74:188–191

[14] Telesca M, Santini F, Mazzucco A. Adenoma related pituitary apoplexy disclosed by ptosis after routine cardiac surgery: occasional reappearance of a dismal complication. Intensive Care Med. 2009; 35:185–186

[15] Bills DC, Meyer FB, Laws ER,Jr, Davis DH, Ebersold MJ, Scheithauer BW, Ilstrup DM, Abboud CF. A retrospective analysis of pituitary apoplexy. Neurosurgery. 1993; 33:602–8; discussion 608-9

[16] Pei L, Melmed S, Scheithauer B, et al. Frequent Loss of Heterozygosity at the Retinoblastoma Susceptibility Gene (RB) Locus in Aggressive Pituitary Tumors: Evidence for a Chromosome 13 Tumor Suppressor Gene Other Than RB. Cancer Res. 1995; 55:1613–1616

[17] Wilson CB, Tindall GT, Collins WF. In: Neurosurgical Management of Large and Invasive Pituitary Tumors. Clinical Management of Pituitary Disorders. New York: Raven Press; 1979:335–342

[18] Hardy J, Kohler PO, Ross GT. In: Transsphenoidal Surgery of Hypersecreting Pituitary Tumors. Diagnosis and Treatment of Pituitary Tumors. New York: Excerpta Medica/American Elsevier; 1973:179–194

[19] Hardy J, Thompson RA, Green R. In: Transsphenoidal Surgery of Intracranial Neoplasm. Adv Neurol. New York: Raven Press; 1976:261–274

[20] Krisht AF. Giant Invasive Pituitary Adenomas. Contemp Neurosurg. 1999; 21:1–6

[21] Laws ER. Comment on Knosp E, et al.: Pituitary Adenomas with Invasion of the Cavernous Sinus Space: A Magnetic Resonance Imaging Classification Compared with Surgical Findings. Neurosurgery. 1993; 33

[22] Scotti G, Yu CY, Dillon WP, et al. MR Imaging of Cavernous Sinus Involvement by Pituitary Adenomas. AJR. 1988; 151:799–806

[23] Barlas O, Bayindir C, Hepgul K, Can M, Kiris T, Sencer E, Unal F, Aral F. Bromocriptine-induced cerebrospinal fluid fistula in patients with macroprolactinomas: report of three cases and a review of the literature. Surg Neurol. 1994; 41:486–489

[24] Amar AP, Couldwell WT, Weiss MH. Prolactinomas: Focus on Indications, Outcomes, and Management of Recurrences. Contemp Neurosurg. 1989; 21:1–6

[25] Esposito F, Dusick JR, Cohan P, et al. Early morning cortisol levels as a predictor of remission after transsphenoidal surgery for Cushing's disease. J Clin Endocrinol Metab. 2006; 91:7–13

[26] Banasiak MJ, Malek AR. Nelson syndrome: comprehensive review of pathophysiology, diagnosis, and management. Neurosurg Focus. 2007; 23

[27] Assie G, Bahurel H, Coste J, Silvera S, Kujas M, Dugue MA, et al. Corticotroph tumor progression after adrenalectomy in Cushing's Disease: a reappraisal of Nelson's syndrome. J Clin Endocrinol Metab. 2007; 49:381–386

[28] Bertagna X, Raux-Demay M-C, Guilhaume B, er al., Melmed S. In: Cushing's Disease. The Pituitary. 2nd ed. Malden, MA: Blackwell Scientific; 2002:496–560

[29] Kasperlik-Zaluska AA, Bonicki W, Jeske W, Janik J, et al. Nelson's syndrome - 46 years later: clinical experience with 37 patients. Zentralbl Neurochir. 2006; 67:14–20

[30] Cook DM. AACE Medical Guidelines for Clinical Practice for the diagnosis and treatment of acromegaly. Endocr Pract. 2004; 10:213–225

[31] Melmed S. Acromegaly. N Engl J Med. 1990; 322:966–977

[32] Melmed S. Medical progress: Acromegaly. N Engl J Med. 2006; 355:2558–2573

[33] Renehan AG, Shalet SM. Acromegaly and colorectal cancer: risk assessment should be based on population-based studies. J Clin Endocrinol Metab. 2002; 87:1909–1909

[34] Acromegaly Therapy Consensus Development Panel. Consensus Statement: Benefits Versus Risks of Medical Therapy for Acromegaly. Am J Med. 1994; 97:468–473

[35] Beck-Peccoz P, Brucker-Davis F, Persani L, Smallridge RC, Weintraub BD. Thyrotropin-secreting pituitary tumors. Endocr Rev. 1996; 17:610–638

[36] Clarke MJ, Erickson D, Castro MR, Atkinson JL. Thyroid-stimulating hormone pituitary adenomas. J Neurosurg. 2008; 109:17–22

[37] Beck-Peccoz P, Persani L. Medical management of thyrotropin-secreting pituitary adenomas. Pituitary. 2002; 5:83–88

[38] Wilson CB. Endocrine-Inactive Pituitary Adenomas. Clin Neurosurg. 1992; 38:10–31

[39] Cohen-Gadol AA, Pichelmann MA, Link MJ, Scheithauer BW, Krecke KN, Young WF, Jr, Hardy J, Giannini C. Granular cell tumor of the sellar and suprasellar region: clinicopathologic study of 11 cases and literature review. Mayo Clin Proc. 2003; 78:567–573

[40] Schaller B, Kirsch E, Tolnay M, Mindermann T. Symptomatic granular cell tumor of the pituitary gland: case report and review of the literature. Neurosurgery. 1998; 42:166–70; discussion 170-1

[41] Markesbery WR, Duffy PE, Cowen D. Granular cell tumors of the central nervous system. J Neuropathol Exp Neurol. 1973; 32:92–109

[42] Fuller GN, Wesseling P, Louis DN, Ohgaki H, Wiestler OD, Cavenee WK, Bosman FT, Jaffe ES, Lakhani SR, Ohgaki H. In: Granular cell tumors of the neurohypophysis. WHO classification of tumors of the central nervous system. 4th ed. Lyon: International Agency for Research on Cancer; 2007:241–242
[43] Gueguen B, Merland JJ, Riche MC, Rey A. Vascular Malformations of the Spinal Cord: Intrathecal Perimedullary Arteriovanous Fistulas Fed by Medullary Arteries. Neurology. 1987; 37:969–979
[44] Wesseling P, Brat DJ, Fuller GN, Louis DN, Ohgaki H, Wiestler OD, Cavenee WK, Bosman FT, Jaffe ES, Lakhani SR, Ohgaki H. In: Pituicytoma. WHO classification of tumors of the central nervous system. 4th ed. Lyon: International Agency for Research on Cancer; 2007:243–244

46 Pituitary Adenomas – Evaluation and Nonsurgical Management

46.1 Evaluation

46.1.1 History and physical

Directed to look for signs and symptoms of:

1. endocrine hyperfunction (see Functional pituitary tumors above), including:
   a) prolactin: amenorrhea (women), nipple discharge (primarily in women since estrogen is also required), impotence (males)
   b) thyroid: heat intolerance
   c) growth hormone: change in ring size or shoe size or coarsening of facial features, gigantism (children)
   d) cortisol: hyperpigmentation, Cushingoid features
2. endocrine deficits due to mass effect (p. 720) on pituitary
3. visual field deficit: bedside confrontational testing to rule-out visual field deficit (classically bitemporal hemianopsia, *see below*)
4. deficits of cranial nerves within cavernous sinus
   a) III, IV, VI: disorder of pupil and extraocular muscles
   b) V1, V2: reduced sensation in forehead, nose, upper lip and cheek

46.1.2 Diagnostic tests

Overview

Initial (screening) tests to work-up a patient presenting with a known or suspected pituitary mass are shown in ▶ Table 46.1. Further testing is indicated for abnormal results or for strong suspicion of specific syndromes (see indicated page for details).

Visual fields

Formal visual field testing: by perimetry with a tangent screen (using the small red stimulus since desaturation of color is an early sign of chiasmal compression) or by Goldman or automated Humphrey perimeter (the latter requires good cooperation from the patient to be valid).

Visual field deficit patterns

Depends in part on location of chiasm with respect to sella turcica: the chiasm is located above the sella in 79%, posterior to the sella turcica (postfixed chiasm) in 4%; in front of the sella (pre-fixed) in 5%[2(p 2135)]

1. compression of the optic chiasm:
   a) bitemporal hemianopsia (p. 560) that obeys the vertical meridian: classic visual field deficit associated with a pituitary tumor. Due to impingement on crossing nasal fibers in the chiasm
   b) other reported patterns that occur rarely: monocular temporal hemianopsia
2. optic nerve compression: more likely in patients with a postfixed chiasm
   a) loss of vision in the ipsilateral eye. If carefully sought, there is usually a superior outer (temporal) quadrantanopsia in the contralateral eye[2(p 2135)] (so-called junctional scotoma AKA "pie in the sky" defect) from compression of the anterior knee of Wilbrand (p. 1214); may also be an early finding even without a post-fixed chiasm
   b) may produce central scotoma or monocular reduction in visual acuity
3. compression of the optic tract: may occur with a pre-fixed chiasm. Produces homonymous hemianopsia

Initial endocrinologic evaluation (screening) modified)

See reference.[3]

Also, see ▶ Table 46.1. May give indication of tumor type, determines whether any hormones need to be replaced, and serves as a baseline for comparison following treatment. Includes clinical assessment for signs and symptoms, as well as laboratory tests. Screening tests should be checked in

Table 46.1 Summary of initial (screening) work-up for pituitary tumors

Evaluation		Rationale
✔ Formal visual fields (usually Humphrey visual fields (HVF))		• compression of optic chiasm → visual field deficit (usually bitemporal hemianopsia)
Endocrine screening	✔ 8 A.M. cortisol[a] & 24-hour urine free cortisol[a]	• cortisol ↑ in hypercortisolism (Cushing's syndrome) (p. 731) • cortisol ↓ in hypoadrenalism (primary or secondary)
	✔ free T4[b], TSH	**Hypothyroidism• T4 ↓ & TSH ↑ in primary hypothyroidism (this may cause thyrotroph hyperplasia in pituitary gland)** • T4 ↓ & TSH nl or ↓ in secondary hypothyroidism (as in hypopituitarism)
	(alternatively, total T4 may be used, if preferred[b])	**Hyperthyroidism (thyrotoxicosis)• T4 ↑ & TSH ↓ in primary hyperthyroidism** • T4 ↑ & TSH ↑ in TSH-secreting pituitary adenomas
	✔ prolactin	• ↑ or ↑ ↑ with prolactinoma
		• slight ↑ with stalk effect (usually < 90 ng/ml)
	✔ gonadotropins (FSH, LH) and sex steroids (♀: estradiol, ♂: testosterone)	• ↓ in hypogonadotrophic hypogonadism (from mass effect causing compression of the pituitary gland) • ↑ with gonadotropin secreting adenoma
	✔ insulin-like growth factor-1 (IGF-1) AKA somatomedin-C[b]	• ↑ in acromegaly • ↓ in hypopituitarism (one of the most sensitive markers)
	✔ fasting blood glucose	↓ in hypoadrenalism (primary or secondary)
✔ Radiographic studies. Either: • Brain MRI and pituitary MRI without & with contrast (test of choice), usually with protocol for navigation system. Some surgeons also get noncontrast brain CT to look at bony anatomy (esp. sphenoid sinus) • If MRI contraindicated: CT without & with contrast (with coronal reconstruction) + cerebral angiogram		

[a]8 A.M. cortisol is the best test for hypocortisolism (e.g. to look for pituitary insufficiency), 24-hour urine free cortisol is the best test for hypercortisolism (p. 731) [1] (e.g. to look for Cushing's syndrome)
[b]IGF-1 is the primary test for excess growth hormone (GH); direct measurement of GH is unreliable

all patients with pituitary tumors. Note: selective loss of a *single* pituitary hormone together with thickening of the pituitary stalk is strongly suggestive of autoimmune hypophysitis (p. 1373).

1. adrenal axis screening; see tests to assess cortisol **reserve** (p. 735)
   a) Cortisol levels normally peak between 7-8 AM. AM cortisol may normally be elevated slightly above the reference range. 8 AM cortisol level: better for detecting hypocortisolism.[1] Normal: 6-18 mcg/100 ml. Interpretation:
      - 8 AM cortisol < 6 mcg/100 ml: suggestive of adrenal insufficiency
      - 8 AM cortisol 6-14 mcg/100 ml: nondiagnostic
      - 8 AM cortisol > 14 mcg/100 ml: adrenal insufficiency is unlikely
   b) in questionable cases, including to distinguish pseudo-Cushing states from Cushing's syndrome (p. 734)
   c) 24-hour urine free cortisol: more accurate for hypercortisolism[1] (almost 100% sensitive and specific, false negative rare except in stress or chronic alcoholism). If not elevated several times above normal, at least 2 additional determinations should be made[4]
2. thyroid axis: the basis for thyroid screening is shown in ▶ Table 46.2
   a) screening: T4 level (total or free), thyroid-stimulating hormone (TSH) (AKA thyrotropin). Normal values: free T4 index is 0.8–1.5, TSH 0.4–5.5 mcU/ml, total T4 4–12 mcg/100 ml (NB: be sure to check both T4 *AND* TSH)
   b) further testing: thyrotropin-releasing hormone *(TRH) stimulation test* (indicated if T4 is low or borderline): check baseline TSH, give 500 mcg TRH IV, check TSH at 30 & 60 mins. Normal response: peak TSH twice baseline value at 30 mins. Impaired response with a low T4 indicates pituitary deficiency. Exaggerated response suggests primary hypothyroidism

Table 46.2 Basis for thyroid screening

Rationale	T_4	TSH
Primary hypothyroidism[a] (problem with thyroid gland itself)	↓	↑
• chronic primary hypothyroidism may produce secondary pituitary hyperplasia (pituitary pseudotumor) indistinguishable from adenoma on CT or MRI. Must be considered in any patient with a pituitary mass[7,8] • pathophysiology: loss of negative feedback from thyroid hormones causes increased TRH release from the hypothalamus producing secondary hyperplasia of thyrotrophic cells in the adenohypophysis (thyrotroph hyperplasia). The patient may present due to pituitary enlargement (visual symptoms, elevated PRL from stalk effect, enlarged sella turcica on x-rays...) • chronic stimulation from elevated TRH may rarely produce thyrotroph adenomas • labs: T_4 low or normal, TSH elevated (> 90–100 in patients presenting with thyrotroph hyperplasia), prolonged and elevated TSH response to TRH stimulation test (see text)		
Secondary hypothyroidism[a] (insufficient TSH stimulation of thyroid)	↓	↓ or nl
• pituitary hypothyroidism accounts for only ≈ 2–4% of all hypothyroid cases[9] • ≈ 23% of patients with chromophobe adenomas develop secondary hypothyroidism if untreated (pituitary compression causes reduced TSH) • labs: T_4 low, TSH low or normal, reduced response to TRH stimulation test (see text)		
Primary hyperthyroidism (problem with thyroid gland itself)	↑	↓
• etiologies: localized hyperactive thyroid nodule, circulating antibody that stimulates the thyroid, or diffuse thyroid hyperplasia (Graves' disease, AKA ophthalmic hyperthyroidism) • labs: T_4 elevated, TSH subnormal (usually *undetectable*)		
Secondary hyperthyroidism (central hyperthyroidism)	↑	↑ or nl

• etiologies
  ○ TSH-secreting pituitary adenoma (rare)
  ○ pituitary resistance to thyroid hormones (disrupts negative feedback loop)
• labs: T_4 elevated, TSH elevated or inappropriately normal		

[a] ✖Caution: replacing thyroid hormone with inadequate cortisol reserves (as may occur in panhypopituitarism) can precipitate adrenal crisis; see management (p. 738)

3. gonadal axis
   a) screening:
      - serum gonadotropins: FSH & LH
      - sex steroids: estradiol in women, testosterone in men (measure *total* testosterone)
   b) further testing: none dependable in differentiating pituitary from hypothalamic disorders
4. prolactin levels (PRL): for prolactin neurophysiology (p. 151)
   a) interpretation is shown in ▶ Table 46.3. See ▶ Table 46.4 for differential diagnosis of hyperprolactinemia. Prolactin level correlates with size of prolactinomas[5]: if PRL is < 200 ng/ml, ≈ 80% of tumors are microadenomas, and 76% of these will have normal PRL after surgery; if PRL > 200, only ≈ 20% are microadenomas
   b) blood samples should be obtained midmorning (i.e. not soon after awakening) and not after stress, breast stimulation, or physical examination, which may increase PRL levels
   c) be aware of the following when interpreting PRL levels:
      - because of variations in secretion (daily fluctuations can be as high as 30%) and intrinsic inaccuracies of radioimmunoassay, PRL levels should be rechecked if there is a reason to question a specific result
      - heterophilic antibodies (seen in individuals routinely exposed to animal serum products) can cause anomalous results
      - stalk effect: PRL is the only pituitary hormone primarily under inhibitory regulation (p. 151). Injury to or compression of the hypothalamus or pituitary stalk from surgery or compression by any type of tumor can cause modest elevation of PRL due to decrease in prolactin inhibitory factor (PRIF). Rule of thumb: the percent chance of an elevated PRL being due to a prolactinoma is equal to one half the PRL level. Persistent post-op PRL elevation may occur even with total tumor removal as a result of injury to stalk (usually ≤ 90 ng/ml; stalk effect doubtful if PRL > 150). For stalk effect, follow these patients, do not use bromocriptine

Table 46.3 Significance of prolactin levels[a]

PRL (ng/ml)	Interpretation	Situations observed in
3–30[b]	normal	non-pregnant female
10–400		pregnancy (▶ Table 46.4)
2–20		postmenopausal female
25[b]-150	moderate elevation	• prolactinoma • "stalk effect" (see text) • other causes[d]
> 150[c]	significant elevation	prolactinoma[d]

[a]Note: ectopic sites of prolactin secretion have rarely been reported (e.g. in a teratoma[10])
[b]normal values vary, use your lab's reference range
[c]some authors recommend 200 ng/ml as the cutoff for probable prolactinomas[11]
[d]for DDx of hyperprolactinemia see ▶ Table 46.4

Table 46.4 Differential diagnosis of elevated prolactin (PRL) level (hyperprolactinemia)[a]

1. pregnancy-related
   a) during pregnancy[b]: 10–400 ng/ml
   b) postpartum: PRL decreases ≈ 50% (to ≈ 100 ng/ml) in the first week postpartum, and is usually back to normal in 3 weeks
   c) in the lactating female: suckling increases PRL, which is critical for lactogenesis (once initiated, nonpregnant PRL levels can maintain lactation).
   First 2–3 months postpartum: basal PRL = 40–50 ng/ml, suckling → increases × 10–20. 3–6 months postpartum: basal PRL levels become normal or slightly elevated, and double with suckling. PRL should normalize by 6 months after weaning
2. pituitary adenoma
   a) prolactinoma: larger prolactin microadenomas and macroadenomas usually produce PRL > 100 ng/ml
   b) stalk effect (p. 732): rule of thumb, the percent chance of an elevated PRL being due to a prolactinoma is equal to one half the PRL level
   c) some tumors secrete both PRL and GH
3. drugs: dopamine receptor antagonists (e.g. phenothiazines, metoclopramide), oral contraceptives (estrogens), tricyclic antidepressants, verapamil, H2 antagonists (e.g. ranitidine), some SSRIs in particular paroxetine (Paxil®)[12]...
4. primary hypothyroidism: TRH, a prolactin releasing factor (PRF), (p. 151) will be elevated
5. empty sella syndrome (p. 766)
6. post-ictal (p. 467): PRL usually normalizes within 1–2 hrs after a seizure
7. breast or chest-wall trauma/surgery: usually ≤ 50 ng/ml
8. excessive exercise: usually ≤ 50 ng/ml
9. stress: in some cases the stress of having the blood test is enough to elevate PRL, anorexia nervosa
10. ectopic secretion: reported in renal cell or hepatocellular tumors, uterine fibroids, lymphomas
11. infiltrating hypothalamic tumors
12. renal failure
13. cirrhosis
14. macroprolactinemia: see text

[a]hyperprolactinemia from causes other than prolactinomas rarely exceeds 200 ng/ml
[b]always R/O pregnancy as a cause of amenorrhea & hyerprolactinemia in a female with reproductive potential

- "prolactin level > 200 ng/ml": if the lab reports the prolactin level as " > 200" (or some other high value) instead of an actual number, it usually indicates a very high prolactin level that exceeds the upper limits of the assay. Call the lab and ask them to determine the *actual* value. This usually requires the lab to run serial dilutions until the PRL is in a range that their assay can quantify (they may be able to do it with the specimen they have, or else the patient will need to have another blood draw). The reasons this is important: (1) treatment decisions: PRL > 500 usually indicates that surgery alone will not be able to normalize the PRL (p. 739); (2) to assess response to treatment: it is essential to know what value you are starting with to determine response to medication, surgery, XRT...
- hook effect: extremely high PRL levels may overwhelm the assay (the large numbers of PRL molecules prevent the formation of the necessary PRL-antibody-signal complexes for

radioimmunoassay) and produce falsely low results. Therefore, for large adenomas with a normal PRL level, have the lab perform several dilutions of the serum sample and re-run the PRL, especially in patients with clinical hyperprolactinemia
   - macroprolactinemia: a situation where prolactin molecules polymerize and bind to immunoglobulins. Prolactin in this form has reduced biologically activity but produces a laboratory finding of hyperprolactinemia. Clinical significance is controversial,[6] asymptomatic patients usually do not require treatment
5. growth hormone:
   a) IGF-1 (somatomedin-C) level (p. 736) is the recommended initial test (testing for elevated IGF-1 is extremely sensitive for acromegaly)
   b) checking a single random GH level may not be a reliable indicator (p. 736) and is therefore *not* recommended
6. neurohypophysis (posterior pituitary): deficits are rare with pituitary tumors
   a) screening: check adequacy of ADH by demonstrating concentration of urine with water deprivation
   b) further testing: measurement of serum ADH in response to infusion of hypertonic saline

Specialized endocrinologic tests

Cushing's syndrome

Tests for hypercortisolism

These tests are used to determine if *hypercortisolism* (Cushing's syndrome, CS) is present or not, regardless of etiology. Usually only needed if the screening 24-hr urine free cortisol (p. 731) is equivocal (the basis of these tests is shown in ▶ Table 46.5).

1. overnight *low-dose* dexamethasone (DMZ) suppression tests[13]:
   a) overnight low dose test: give DMZ 1 mg PO @ 11 P.M. and draw serum cortisol the next day at 8 A.M. Results:
      - cortisol < 1.8 mcg/dl (note: this is the currently accepted normal value; previously it was 5 mcg/dl): Cushing's syndrome is ruled out (except for a few patients with CS who suppress at low DMZ doses, possibly due to low DMZ clearance[14])
      - cortisol 1.8 -10 mcg/dl: indeterminate, retesting is necessary
      - cortisol > 10 mcg/dl: CS is probably present. False positives can occur in the so-called pseudo-Cushing's state where ectopic CRH secretion produces hyperplasia of pituitary corticotrophs that is clinically indistinguishable from pituitary ACTH producing tumors (requires further testing[14]). Seen in: 15% of obese patients, in 25% of hospitalized and chronically ill patients, in high estrogen states, in uremia, and in depression. The combined DMZ-CRH test can be used to identify this (see reference[14]). False positives also may occur in alcoholics or patients on phenobarbital or phenytoin due increased metabolism of DMZ caused by induced hepatic microsomal degradation
   b) 2 day low dose test (used when overnight test is equivocal): give DMZ 0.5 mg PO q 6 hrs for 2 days starting at 6 A.M.; 24 hr urine collections are obtained prior to test and on the 2nd day of DMZ administration. Normal patients suppress urinary 17-hydroxycorticosteroids (OHCS) to less than 4 mg/24 hrs, whereas ≈ 95% of patients with CS have abnormal response (higher amounts in urine)[14]
2. 11 PM salivary cortisol: this is the time of the usual cortisol nadir. Test must be run at NIH approved lab. Accuracy is as good as low-dose DMZ suppression test

Distinguishing Cushing's disease from ectopic ACTH secretion

These tests are used to distinguish primary Cushing's disease (CD) (pituitary ACTH hypersecretion) from ectopic ACTH production and adrenal tumors (may be required since 40% of CD patients have a normal MRI[1])

Table 46.5 Basis for biochemical tests in Cushing's syndrome (CS)

- normally, low DMZ doses suppress ACTH release through negative feedback on hypothalamic-pituitary axis, reducing urine and serum corticosteroids
- in ≥ 98% of cases of Cushing's syndrome, suppression occurs, but at a much higher threshold
- adrenal tumors and most (85–90%) cases of ectopic ACTH production (especially bronchial Ca) will not suppress even with high dose DMZ
- ACTH response to CRH is exaggerated in CS
- DMZ does not interfere with measurement of urinary and plasma cortisol and 17-hydroxycorticosteroids

1. random serum ACTH: if < 5 ng/L indicates ACTH independent CS (e.g. adrenal tumor). Not sensitive or specific due to variability of ACTH levels
2. abdominal CT: usually shows unilateral adrenal mass with adrenal tumors, or normal or bilateral adrenal enlargement in ACTH-dependent cases
3. *high-dose* dexamethasone (DMZ) suppression test: (NB: up to 20% of patients with CD do not suppress with high-dose DMZ. Phenytoin may also interfere with high-dose DMZ suppression[15])
   a) overnight high-dose test: obtain a baseline 8 A.M. plasma cortisol level
   b) then give DMZ 8 mg PO @ 11 P.M. and measure plasma cortisol level the next morning at 8 A.M.
   c) in 95% of CD cases plasma cortisol levels are reduced to < 50% of baseline, whereas in ectopic ACTH or adrenal tumors it will usually be unchanged
4. **metyrapone** (Metopirone®) test: performed on an inpatient basis. Give 750 mg metyrapone (suppresses cortisol synthesis) PO q 4 hrs for 6 doses. Most patients with CD will have a rise in 17-OHCS in urine of 70% above baseline, or an increase in serum 11-deoxycortisol 400-fold above baseline
5. corticotropin-releasing hormone (CRH) stimulation test: CD responds to exogenous CRH 0.1 mcg/kg IV bolus with even further increased plasma ACTH and cortisol levels; ectopic ACTH and adrenal tumors do not[16]
6. inferior petrosal sinus (IPS) sampling (or, cavernous sinus sampling is preferred by some): done by interventional neuroradiologist. Uses a microcatheter to measure ACTH levels on each side at baseline, and then at 2, 5 & 10 minutes after stimulation with IV CRH (with simultaneous peripheral ACTH levels at each interval). General information:
   a) IPS sampling is not needed when the following criteria of CD are met[17]:
      - ACTH-dependent Cushing's disease
      - suppression with high-dose dexamethasone test (see above)
      - visible pituitary adenoma on MRI
   b) may also determine likely side of a microadenoma within the pituitary (thus may be able to avoid bilateral adrenalectomy which requires lifelong gluco- and mineralo-corticoid replacement and risks Nelson's syndrome (p. 724) in 10–30%. 15–30%[1] of the time this test falsely lateralizes the tumor due to the communication through the circular sinus
   c) a baseline IPS ACTH to peripheral ACTH ratio > 1.4:1 is consistent with primary Cushing's disease
   d) a post CRH ratio > 3 is also consistent with primary Cushing's disease
   e) complication rate: 1–2%, includes puncture of the sinus wall

Assessing cortisol reserve

1. cosyntropin stimulation test[18]:
   a) draw a baseline cortisol level (fasting is not required; test can be performed at any time of day)
   b) give cosyntropin (Cortrosyn®) (a potent ACTH analogue) 1 ampoule (250 mcg) IM or IV
   c) then check cortisol levels at 30 mins (optional) and at 60 mins
   d) normal response: peak cortisol level > 18 mcg/dl AND an increment > 7 mcg/dl, or a peak > 20 mcg/dl regardless of the increment
   e) subnormal response: indicates adrenal insufficiency. In primary adrenal insufficiency, pituitary ACTH secretion will be elevated. In secondary adrenal insufficiency, chronically reduced ACTH causes adrenal atrophy and unresponsiveness to acute stimulation with this exogenous ACTH analogue
   f) normal response: rules out primary and overt secondary adrenal insufficiency, but may be normal in *mild* cases of reduced pituitary ACTH or *early* after pituitary surgery where adrenal atrophy has not occurred. In these cases further testing may be positive: see metyrapone test (p. 753) or ITT (see below)
2. insulin tolerance test (ITT): "gold standard" for assessing integrity of the hypothalamic-pituitary-adrenal axis. Cumbersome to do. Abnormal in 80% of CS. Assesses ACTH, cortisol & GH reserve
   a) rationale: an appropriate cortisol increment in response to insulin-induced hypoglycemia suggests patient will also be able to respond to other stresses (acute illness, surgery…)
   b) contraindications: seizure disorder, ischemic cardiac disease, untreated hypothyroidism
   c) pre-test preparation: D/C estrogen replacement for 6 weeks prior to test. Have 50 ml of D50 and 100 mg IV hydrocortisone available during test
   d) protocol: give regular insulin 0.1 U/kg IV push, and draw blood for glucose, cortisol and GH at 0, 10, 20, 30, 45, 60, 90 and 120 mins (monitor blood sugar by fingerstick during test, and give IV glucose if patient becomes symptomatic). If fingerstick blood sugar is not < 50 mg/dl by 30 minutes and patient is asymptomatic, give additional regular insulin 5 U IVP. There must be 2 specimens after adequate hypoglycemia

e) results:
   - if adequate hypoglycemia (< 40 mg/dl) was not accomplished: cortisol or GH deficiency cannot be diagnosed
   - normal: cortisol increment > 6 mcg/dl to a peak > 20
   - peak cortisol = 16–20: steroids needed only for stress
   - peak cortisol < 16: glucocorticoid replacement needed
   - Cushing syndrome: increment < 6

Acromegaly

For suspected acromegaly, the most useful test is an IGF-1 level.

1. insulin-like growth factor-1 (IGF-1) (formerly somatomedin-C) level: an excellent integrative marker of average GH secretion. Normal levels depend on age (peaking during puberty), gender, pubertal stage and lab. Typical fasting levels by age are shown in ▶ Table 46.6. Estrogen may suppress IGF-1 levels
2. growth hormone (GH): normal basal fasting level is < 5 ng/ml. In patients with acromegaly, GH is usually > 10 ng/ml but can be normal. Normal basal levels do not reliably distinguish normal patient from GH deficiency.[19] Furthermore, due to pulsatile secretion of GH, normal patients may have sporadic peaks up to 50 ng/ml.[20] Occasionally acromegaly may be present even with GH levels as low as 37 pg/ml.[21] ∴ random GH levels are not generally useful for diagnosing acromegaly (see above for IGF-1)
3. other tests used uncommonly
   a) oral glucose suppression test (OGST): less precise and more expensive than measuring IGF-1, however may be more useful than IGF-1 for monitoring initial response to therapy. GH levels are measured at 0, 30, 60, 90 & 120 minutes after a 75 gm oral glucose load. If the GH nadir is not < 1 ng/ml, the patient is acromegalic.[22,23] GH suppression may also be absent with liver disease, uncontrolled DM & renal failure. ✖ Relatively contraindicated in patients with DM and high glucose levels
   b) growth-hormone releasing hormone (GHRH) levels: may help diagnose ectopic GH secretion in a patient with proven acromegaly with no evidence of pituitary tumor on imaging. If an extrapituitary source is suspected, chest and abdominal CT and/or MRI should also be obtained[24]
   c) GHRH stimulation test: results may be discordant in up to 50% of patients with acromegaly[22] and is thus rarely used (as of this writing, pharmaceutical production of GHRF has been discontinued)
4. octreotide scan: SPECT imaging 4 and 24 hours after injection with 6.5 mCi of indium-111 OctreoScan, a somatostatin receptor imaging agent

Radiographic evaluation

General information

≈ 50% of pituitary tumors causing Cushing's syndrome are too small to be imaged on CT or MRI (therefore endocrinologic testing is required to prove the pituitary origin). See differential diagnosis of intrasellar lesions (p. 1371); some are indistinguishable radiographically.

Table 46.6 Normal IGF-1 by age

Age (yrs)	Level (ng/ml)
1–5	49–327
6–8	52–345
9–11	74–551
12–15	143–996
16–20	141–903
21–39	109–358
40–54	87–267
> 54	55–225

Normal AP diameter of pituitary gland: female of childbearing age (≈ 13–35 yrs): ≤ 11 mm, for all others normal is ≤ 9 mm. (Note: pituitary glands in adolescent girls may be physiologically enlarged (mean height: 8.2 ± 1.4 mm) as a result of hormonal stimulation of puberty.[25])

Skull x-ray

A lateral skull x-ray may help define the bony anatomy of the sphenoid sinus in cases where transsphenoidal surgery is contemplated (currently, CT scan is usually employed).

MRI

Imaging test of choice for pituitary tumors.

Ordering MRI:

- typical order on initial workup: brain MRI and pituitary MRI without and with contrast (pituitary protocol includes thin coronal cuts through sella showing cavernous sinus and optic chiasm) with image navigation protocol (e.g. BrainLab™, or Stealth™…)
- if you are hunting for a microadenoma, then a dynamic MRI increases the chances that you might catch the tumor at a time when it enhances differentially from the gland.
- for follow-up of macroadenomas: routine coronal & sagittal pituitary MRI without & with contrast suffices

46

Findings: Information about invasion of cavernous sinus, and about location and/or involvement of para-sellar carotids. MRI may fail to demonstrate tumor in 25–45% of cases of Cushing's disease.[26] 3 T vs. 1.5 T MRI: based on 5 cases of Cushing's disease, a 3 T MRI showed the adenoma more clearly in 2 cases, in 1 case it showed the tumor on the correct side opposite to where the 1.5 T MRI showed it, and in 2 cases neither 1.5 T nor 3 T MRI could show the microadenoma).[27]

Microadenoma: 75% are low signal on T1WI, and high signal on T2WI (but 25% can behave in any way, including completely opposite to above). Enhancement is very time-dependent. Imaging must be done with 5 minutes of contrast administration to see a discrete microadenoma. Initially, gadolinium enhances the normal pituitary (no blood brain barrier) but *not* the pituitary tumor. After ≈ 30 minutes, the tumor enhances about the same. Dynamic MRI scans have been used to increase the sensitivity (contrast is injected while the MRI scanner is running).

Neurohypophysis: normally is high signal on T1WI[28] (possibly due to phospholipids). Absence of this "bright spot" often correlates with diabetes insipidus as may occur with autoimmune hypophysitis (p. 1373), however, failure to image the bright spot is not uniformly abnormal.

Deviation of the pituitary stalk may also indicate the presence of a microadenoma. Normal thickness of the pituitary stalk is approximately equal to basilar artery diameter. Thickening of stalk is usually NOT adenoma, differential diagnosis for a thickened stalk: lymphoma, autoimmune hypophysitis (p. 1373), granulomatous disease, hypothalamic glioma.

CT

Generally superseded by MRI. May be appropriate when MRI is contraindicated (e.g. pacemaker). When done, should include direct coronal imaging, or coronal reconstructions from thin-cut axial CT. If MRI cannot be done, consider also cerebral angiography to demonstrate parasellar carotid arteries and to R/O aneurysm as a possibility.

Calcium in pituitary usually signifies hemorrhage or infarction within tumor.

Angiography

Sometimes used in cases considered for transsphenoidal surgery (e.g. as a complement to CT) to localize the parasellar carotids (note: MRI provides this information, and evaluates invasion of cavernous sinuses, usually obviating the need for angiography).

46.2 Management/treatment recommendations

46.2.1 General information

See treatment of pituitary apoplexy (p. 720). For large invasive adenomas, see below.

Note: Prolactinoma is the only pituitary tumor for which medical therapy (dopamine agonist) is the primary treatment modality (in certain cases).

Hormone replacement therapy (HRT)

HRT may be required for patients with documented endocrine deficits pre-op or post-op in cases where pituitary function is not normal. Critical issues:

1. corticosteroids
   a) indications: inadequate cortisol reserve as demonstrate by failing a cosyntropin stimulation test; failure to achieve a peak cortisol level > 18 mcg/dl in response to cosyntropin (p. 735)
   b) may start cortisol immediately after bloodwork for cosyntropin test is drawn (do not need to wait for test results) – then, when test results available, continue or stop therapy based on test results
   c) ℞ physiologic replacement dose: cortisol 20 mg po q AM and 10 mg po q 4 PM. Stress doses may be needed (p. 146) in some situations
2. thyroid hormone replacement
   a) ✖ thyroid replacement can precipitate adrenal crisis if started before cortisol in a patient with adrenal insufficiency (as may occur in panhypopituitarism)
      - ∴ do a cosyntropin stimulation test (p. 735) and start cortisol
      - thyroid replacement may be initiated after 1 full day of cortisol.
        ℞: start with synthroid 125 mcg/d
   b) although there are warnings not to do surgery on a hypothyroid patient, the reality is that it takes 3–4 weeks for adequate replacement and hypothyroid patients frequently undergo surgery before then with no untoward effect
3. testosterone replacement: may increase intratumoral levels of estradiol which may promote tumor growth ∴ wait for stabilization of tumor before starting

46.2.2 Management of large, invasive adenomas

See reference.[29]

1. prolactinomas
   a) dopamine agonists (DA) (p. 739) unless there is unstable deficit
   b) for unstable deficit, or if the tumor does not respond to DAs: debulk the tumor transsphenoidally and then rechallenge with DA therapy
2. tumors secreting growth hormone or ACTH: an aggressive surgical approach is indicated with these tumors since the secretion product is harmful and effective medical adjuvants are lacking
   a) pre-treat invasive GH-secreting tumors with somatostatin analogue therapy before surgery to reduce surgical risks (general and cardiac)
   b) elderly patients or tumors > 4 cm diameter: debulk tumor transsphenoidally and/or adjuvant therapy (XRT and/or medications)
   c) young age and size < 4 cm: radical surgery (may utilize a cranio-orbito-zygomatic skull base approach; may be curative)
3. nonfunctional adenomas
   a) elderly patient: expectant management is an option, with intervention for signs of progression (radiographic or neurologic)
   b) central tumor or elderly patient with progression: transsphenoidal tumor debulking and/or XRT (residual tumor in the region of the cavernous sinus may show little or no change over several years, and with these nonfunctional tumors, there is less harm in following them than if there is a harmful secretion product)
   c) parasellar tumor and/or young age: radical surgery A (often not curative)

46.2.3 Hormonally inactive macroadenomas – management

General information

Due to poor response rates to medication, when treatment is indicated, surgery and/or XRT are usually the initial treatment of choice (see below for XRT).

Medical management of hormonally inactive macroadenomas

Bromocriptine has been tried with mild reductions in tumor size in only ≈ 20% of patients. The poor results are probably due to the paucity of dopaminergic receptors on cell membranes in these tumors. Octreotide reduces tumor volume in ≈ 10% of cases. These agents have been used pre-op in some cases to try to decrease tumor size for surgery.

Follow-up recommendations for medically managed hormonally inactive macroadenomas

For *asymptomatic microadenomas* (< 1 cm dia), recommend: F/U pituitary MRI at years 1, 2, 5 and ± 10 (can stop F/U after 10 and possibly 5 years if no growth).

For tumors *> 1 cm*, recommend: check visual fields, pituitary bloodwork (to R/O pituitary insufficiency) and pituitary MRI at years 0.5, 1, 2 & 5, and any time symptoms develop.

Gonadotropin-secreting tumors

Rarely, a non-functional tumor may secrete gonadotropins (FSH, LH). This does not produce a clinical syndrome. Normal and neoplastic pituitary gonadotrophs have gonadotropin-releasing hormone (GnRH) receptors, and may respond to long-acting GnRH agonists (by down-regulating receptors) or GnRH antagonists, but significant reductions in tumor size does not occur.

Surgical indications for hormonally inactive pituitary macroadenomas

1. tumors causing symptoms by mass effect: visual field deficit (classically: bitemporal hemianopsia, panhypopituitarism
2. some surgeons recommend surgery for macroadenomas that elevate the chiasm even in the absence of endocrine abnormalities or visual field deficit because of the possibility of injury to the optic apparatus (see below for *invasive* pituitary macroadenomas)
3. acute and rapid visual or other neurologic deterioration. May represent ischemia of the chiasm, or tumor hemorrhage/infarction causing expansion (*pituitary apoplexy*). The major danger is blindness (hypopituitarism, while concerning, can be treated with replacement therapy). Visual loss usually requires *emergent* decompression. Some surgeons feel that a transcranial approach is necessary, but transsphenoidal decompression is usually satisfactory[29,30]
4. to obtain tissue for pathological diagnosis in questionable cases
5. Nelson's syndrome (p. 724)
   a) surgery (transsphenoidal or transcranial): the primary treatment. The aggressiveness of the tumor sometimes requires total hypophysectomy
   b) XRT (possibly SRS) is used following subtotal excision
   c) medical therapy is usually ineffective. Agents that could be considered include[31]: dopamine agonists, valproic acid, somatostatin analogues, rosiglitazone, and serotonin agonists

46.2.4 Prolactinomas – management

General information

1. prolactin level (PRL) < 500 ng/ml in tumors that are not extensively invasive (see below for invasive tumors): PRL may be normalized with surgery
2. PRL > 500 ng/ml: the chances of normalizing PRL surgically are very low.[32] Algorithm:
   a) if no acute *progression* (worsening vision…), an initial attempt at purely medical control should be made as the chances of normalizing PRL surgically with pre-op levels > 500 ng/ml are very low[32] (these tumors may shrink dramatically with bromocriptine)
   b) response should be evident by 4–6 weeks (significant decrease in PRL, improvement of visual deficits, or shrinkage on MRI)
   c) if tumor *not* controlled medically (≈ 18% will not respond to bromocriptine): surgery followed by reinstitution of medical therapy may normalize PRL

Medical management with Dopamine agonists

Dopamine Agonists

Side effects[33]: (may vary with different preparations) nausea, H/A, fatigue, orthostatic hypotension with dizziness, cold induced peripheral vasodilatation, depression, nightmares and nasal congestion. Side effects are more troublesome during the first few weeks of treatment. Tolerance may be improved by bedtime dosing with food, slow dose escalation, sympathomimetics for nasal congestion, and acetaminophen 1–2 hrs before dosing to reduce H/A. Psychosis and vasospasm are rare side effects that usually necessitates discontinuation of the drug.

Drug info: Bromocriptine (Parlodel®)

A semi-synthetic ergot alkaloid that binds to dopamine receptors (dopamine agonist) on normal and tumor lactotrophs, inhibiting synthesis and secretion of PRL and other cell processes resulting in decreased cell division and growth. Bromocriptine lowers prolactin level regardless of the whether the source is an adenoma or normal pituitary (e.g. as a result of stalk effect) to < 10% of pretreatment values in most patients. It also frequently reduces the tumor size in 6–8 weeks in 75% of patients with macroadenomas, but only as long as therapy is maintained and only for tumors that actually produce prolactin. Only ≈ 1% of prolactinomas continue to grow while the patient is on bromocriptine. Prolactinomas may enlarge rapidly upon discontinuation of the drug. However, permanent normoprolactinemia can occur (see below).

Pregnancy issues: bromocriptine can restore fertility. Continued therapy during pregnancy is associated with a 3.3% incidence of congenital anomalies and 11% spontaneous abortion rate which is the same as for the general population. Estrogen elevation during pregnancy stimulates hyperplasia of lactotrophs and some prolactinomas, but the risk of symptomatic enlargement of microadenomas and totally intrasellar macroadenomas is < 3%, vs. 30% risk for macroadenomas.[34]

46

Prolonged treatment with bromocriptine may reduce the chances of surgical cure if this should be chosen at a later date. With a microadenoma, one year of bromocriptine may reduce the surgical cure rate by as much as 50%, possibly due to induced fibrosis.[35] Thus, it is suggested that if surgery is to be done that it be done in the first 6 months of bromocriptine therapy. Shrinkage of large tumors due to bromocriptine may cause CSF rhinorrhea.[36] **Side effects :** see above.

℞: start with 1.25 mg (half of a 2.5 mg tablet) PO q hs (nighttime dosing reduces some side effects) (vaginal administration is an alternative). Add additional 2.5 mg per day as necessary (based on PRL levels), making a dosage change every 2–4 weeks for microadenomas, or every 3–4 days for macroadenomas causing mass effect. Initial recheck of prolactin level after about 4 weeks at a reasonable dose to verify response. ✱ To shrink large tumors or for extremely high PRL levels, higher doses are usually needed initially (e.g. 7.5 mg TID for ≈ 6 mos), and then lower doses may be able to maintain normal levels (typical maintenance dosage: 5–7.5 mg daily (range: 2.5–15 mg) which may be given as a single dose or divided TID). **Supplied:** 2.5 mg scored tabs; 5 mg capsules.

Drug info: Cabergoline (Dostinex®)

An ergot alkaline derivative that is a selective D2 dopamine agonist (bromocriptine (see above) affects both D2 and D1 receptors).[37] The elimination half-life is 60–100 hrs which usually permits dosing 1–2 times weekly. Control of PRL and resumption of ovulatory cycles may be better than with bromocriptine.[38] **Side effects :** (see above) H/A and GI symptoms are reportedly less problematic than with bromocriptine. ✖ Cardiac valve disease[39] (incidence-rate ratio, 4.9; 95% CI) affecting the mitral, aortic, and tricuspid valves possibly leading to regurgitation (the drug activates 5-HT2B receptors which induces prolonged mitogenic effects in fibromyoblasts, which may lead to valvular fibroplasia) which has not been observed at doses used for prolactinomas (is associated with doses used for Parkinson's disease which are > 10 × pituitary doses): recommendation: do not discontinue cabergoline for this reason if dose is < 2 mg/wk. ✖ Contraindications: eclampsia or pre-eclampsia, uncontrolled HTN. Dosage should be reduced with severe hepatic dysfunction.

℞: Start with 0.25 mg PO twice weekly, and increase each dose by 0.25 mg every 4 weeks as needed to control PRL (up to a maximum of 3 mg per week). Typical dose is 0.5–1 mg twice weekly. Some combine the total dose and give it once weekly. Initial recheck of prolactin level after about 4 weeks to verify response. **Supplied:** 0.5 mg scored tablets.

Drug info: Pergolide (Permax®)

A long-acting ergot alkaloid dopamine agonist that reduces PRL levels for > 24 hrs. Not available in the U.S. for use in humans. Once daily dosing improves compliance. **Side effects :** ✖ Withdrawn due to risk of cardiac valve disease (see cabergoline (Dostinex®) above).

℞ Start with 0.05 mg PO q hs, and increase by 0.025–0.05 increments (up to a maximum of ≈ 0.25 mg/d) until desired PRL levels are achieved.

Response to medical treatment

Treatment response to DA is assessed with serial prolactin levels as shown in ▶ Table 46.7. It is uncommon for a prolactinoma to enlarge without an increase in prolactin level.[5]

Discontinuation of dopamine agonists: Long-term therapy with DA agonists has some cytocidal effect on pituitary tissue. In an early report, discontinuation of treatment after 24 months was associated with > 95% recurrence rate.[40] Recent literature suggests a 20–30% chance of normoprolactinemia off medication in select patients.[41]

Recommendations[41]: if response to DA agonist is satisfactory, treat for 1–4 years (microadenomas: check prolactin yearly, macroadenomas are more likely to grow and should be checked more often). Microadenomas or macroadenomas that are no longer visible on MRI are candidates for DA agonist withdrawal. For microadenomas: discontinue the drug; for macroadenomas: slowly taper the drug then discontinue. Recurrence rate is highest during 1st year, ∴ check prolactin levels and clinical symptoms every 3 months during the 1st year. Long-term follow up is required, especially for macroadenomas.

46.2.5 Acromegaly – management

See references.[23,42,43]

Surgery

Surgery is the primary treatment modality for acromegaly when treatment is indicated.
1. asymptomatic elderly patients do not require treatment since there is little evidence that intervention alters life expectancy in this group
2. if no contraindications, *surgery* (usually transsphenoidal) is currently the best initial therapy (worse prognosis with macroadenomas) providing more rapid reduction in GH levels and decompression of neural structures (e.g. optic chiasm) and improves the efficacy of subsequent somatostatin analogues.[43] Surgery is not recommended for elderly patients
3. medical therapy (p. 741); reserved for:
   a) patients not cured by surgery (reoperation doesn't work very often for acromegaly). Note: the definition of "biochemical cure" with acromegaly is not standardized (p. 754), surgery is still helpful for those "not cured" and improves efficacy of other therapies; IGF-1 may take months to normalize after surgery
   b) or for those who cannot tolerate surgery (e.g. due to cardiomyopathy, severe hypertension, airway obstruction…, these contraindications may improve with medical therapy and then surgery can be reconsidered)
   c) or for recurrence after surgery or XRT
4. XRT (p. 745): for failure of medical therapy. Not recommended as initial treatment. NB: some practitioners use XRT for surgical failure, and employ medical therapy while waiting for XRT to have an effect. GH levels decline very slowly after XRT, see details & side effects (p. 739)

Medical therapy

Overview

1. dopamine agonists (DAs): although not mentioned in the AACE guidelines,[22] it may be worth trying a DA to see if the tumor responds (≈ 20% respond). If responsive, DAs are especially well suited for GH tumors that cosecrete PRL
   a) bromocriptine: (see below) although it benefits only a minority, a first line drug since it is cheaper than pegvisomant or octreotide and is given PO
   b) cabergoline (see above)
   c) pergolide (see above)
   d) others: lisuride, depo-bromocriptine (bromocriptine-LAR)

Table 46.7 Prolactin level with DA agonist treatment

PRL level (ng/ml)	Recommendation
< 20	maintain
20–50	reassess dose
> 50	consider surgery

2. somatostatin analogues: indications: as initial medical therapy, or if no response to DAs, some also use this pre-op to improve surgical success rate
   a) octreotide & octreotide-LAR (see below)
   b) lanreotide, lanreotide SR & long-acting aqueous gel lanreotide (Autogel)
3. GH antagonists: pegvisomant (see below) considered for failures to above (not a primary therapy)
4. combination therapy: may be more effective than individual drugs. Pegvisomant or octreotide + dopamine agonist if no response to 1 drug alone

Specific agents

Drug info: Bromocriptine (Parlodel®)

Neoplastic somatotrophs may respond fortuitously to dopamine agonists and reduce growth hormone (GH) secretion. Bromocriptine lowers GH levels to < 10 ng/ml in 54% of cases, to < 5 ng/ml in only ≈ 12%. Tumor shrinkage occurs in only < 20%. Higher doses are usually required than for prolactinomas. If effective, the drug may be continued but should be periodically withdrawn to assess the GH level; see **Side effects** (p. 739). Estimated annual cost: $3,200 in the U.S.

℞ For growth hormone tumors that respond to bromocriptine, the usual dosage is 20–60 mg/d in divided doses (higher doses are unwarranted). The maximal daily dose is 100 mg.

Drug info: Octreotide (Sandostatin®)

A somatostatin analogue that is 45 times more potent than somatostatin in suppressing GH secretion but is only twice as potent in suppressing insulin secretion, has a longer half-life (≈ 2 hrs after SQ injection, compared to ≈ minutes for somatostatin), and does not result in rebound GH hypersecretion. GH levels are reduced in 71%, IGF-1 levels are reduced in 93%. 50–66% have normal GH levels, 66% achieve normal IGF-1 levels. Tumor volume reduces significantly in about 30% of patients. Many symptoms including H/A usually improve within the first few weeks of treatment. Annual cost to the patient: at least ≈ $7,800 in the U.S. Usually given in combination with bromocriptine.

After 50 mcg SQ injection, GH secretion is suppressed within 1 hr, nadirs at 3 hrs, and remains reduced for 6–8 hrs (occasionally up to 12 hrs). **Side effects:** reduced GI motility and secretion, diarrhea, steatorrhea, flatulence, nausea, abdominal discomfort (all of these usually remit in 10 days), clinically insignificant bradycardia in 15%, cholesterol *cholelithiasis* (in 10–25%) or bile sludge. Asymptomatic stones require no treatment and routine ultrasonography is not required. Mild hypothyroidism or worsening of glucose intolerance may occur.

℞: Start with 50–100 mcg SQ q 8 hrs. Increase up to a maximum of 1500 mcg/d (doses > 750 mcg/d are rarely needed). Average dose required is 100–200 mcg SQ q 8 hrs.

Sandostatin LAR Depot: long acting release (LAR) form given by IM injection. ℞: give a test dose of *short acting* octreotide SQ in the office, and if no reaction (e.g. N/V...) begin LAR injections with 20 mg IM q 4 weeks, increase to 30 mg if GH > 5 mU/L just before 4th dose. Control can achieved in some patients with dosing q 8–12 weeks.[44]

Drug info: Pegvisomant (Somavert®)

A genetically engineered competitive GH-receptor antagonist. Treatment for ≥ 12 mos results in normal IGF-1 levels in 97% of patients.[45] No change in pituitary tumor size has been observed.[46] Indications: failure of somatostatin in patient with GH secreting adenoma (patient is switched to pegvisomant, it is not added to regimen). **Side effects:** significant but reversible liver function abnormalities occur in < 1%. Serum GH increases, probably as a result of loss of negative feedback on IGF-1 production. Antibodies to GH occured in 17%, but tachyphylaxis was not observed

℞: 5–40 mg/d SQ (dose must be titrated to keep IGF-1 in the normal range, to avoid GH deficiency conditions).

46.2.6 Cushing's disease – management

Management algorithm

1. if pituitary MRI shows a mass: transsphenoidal surgery
2. if pituitary MR is negative (up to 40% of patients with Cushing's disease have negative MRI): perform inferior petrosal sinus (IPS) sampling (p. 735)
   a) if IPS sampling is positive: surgery
   b) if IPS sampling is negative: look for extra-pituitary source of ACTH (abdominal CT)
3. if pituitary surgery is performed but biochemical cure – see criteria (p. 753) – is not obtained with surgery:
   a) unlike acromegaly, a partial reduction is not helpful to the patient
   b) consider re-exploration if pituitary source is still suspected
   c) stereotactic radiosurgery or medical therapy (see below)
   d) adrenalectomy in appropriate patients (see below)

Transsphenoidal surgery

Transsphenoidal surgery is the treatment of choice for most (medical therapy is inadequate as initial therapy since there is no effective pituitary suppressive medication). Cure rates are ≈ 85% for microadenomas (i.e. tumors ≤ 1 cm dia), but are lower for larger tumors. Even with microadenomas, *hemihypophysectomy* on the side of the tumor is usually required for cure (the tumor is difficult to completely extirpate) with attendant increased risk of CSF leak. If this fails, consideration should then be for *total hypophysectomy*. Failure of total hypophysectomy prompts consideration for bilateral adrenalectomy (total hypophysectomy virtually eliminates risk of Nelson's syndrome following adrenalectomy – see below).

Stereotactic radiosurgery

Often normalizes serum cortisol levels. Useful for: recurrence after surgery, inaccessible tumors (e.g. cavernous sinus)[47]...

Adrenalectomy

Total bilateral adrenalectomy (TBA) corrects hypercortisolism in 96–100%[31] (unless there is an extra-adrenal remnant), but lifelong gluco- and mineralo-corticoid replacement are required and up to 30% develop Nelson's syndrome (p. 724); incidence reduced by total hypophysectomy or possibly by pituitary XRT.

Indications: continued hypercortisolism with:

1. non-resectable pituitary adenoma
2. failure of medical therapy to control symptoms after transsphenoidal surgery
3. life-threatening Cushing's disease (CD)
4. CD with no evidence of pituitary tumor; testing should include high-dose DMZ suppression test (p. 735) and/or inferior petrosal sinus sampling (p. 735)

Follow-up after TBA to rule-out Nelson's syndrome: there is no standardized regimen. Suggestion: check serum ACTH levels q 3–6 months × 1 year, q 6 months × 2 years, q year thereafter. A pituitary MRI is done if an ACTH level is > 100 ng/L, otherwise, annual MRIs are sufficient[48] × 3 years and then if ACTH levels remain low, get an MRI every other year.

Medical therapy

For patients who fail surgical therapy or for whom surgery cannot be tolerated, medical therapy and/or radiation are utilized. Occasionally may be used for several weeks prior to planned surgery to control significant manifestations of hypercortisolism, e.g. diabetes, HTN, psychiatric disturbances... (p. 723).

Ketoconazole (Nizoral®)[33]: an antifungal agent that blocks adrenal steroid synthesis. The initial drug of choice. Over 75% of patients have normalization of urinary free cortisol and 17-hydroxycorticosteroid levels. **Side effects:** reversible elevations of serum hepatic transaminase (in 15%), GI discomfort, edema, skin rash. Significant hepatotoxicity occurs in 1 of 15,000 patients. Watch ▶ Table 8.2.

℞ Start with 200 mg PO BID. Adjust dosage based on 24-hr urine free cortisol and 17-hydroxycorticosteroid levels. Usual maintenance doses 400–1200 mg daily in divided doses (maximum of 1600 mg daily).

Aminoglutethimide (Cytadren®)[33]: inhibits the initial enzyme in the synthesis of steroids from cholesterol. Normalizes urinary free cortisol in ≈ 50% of cases. **Side effects:** dose-dependent reversible effects include sedation, anorexia, nausea, rash and hypothyroidism (due to interference with thyroid hormone synthesis).

℞ Start with 125–250 mg PO BID. Effectiveness may diminish after several months and dose escalation may be needed. Generally do not exceed 1000 mg/d.

Metyrapone (Metopirone®): inhibits 11-β-hydroxylase (involved in one of the final steps of cortisol synthesis) may be used alone or in combination with other drugs. Normalizes mean daily plasma cortisol in ≈ 75%. **Side effects:** lethargy, dizziness, ataxia, N/V, primary adrenal insufficiency, hirsutism and acne.

℞ Usual dose range is 750–6000 mg/d usually divided TID with meals. Initial effectiveness may diminish with time.

Mitotane (Lysodren®): related to the insecticide DDT. Inhibits several steps in glucocorticoid synthesis, and is cytotoxic to adrenocortical cells (adrenolytic agent). 75% of patients enter remission after 6–12 months of treatment, and the medication may sometimes be discontinued (however hypercortisolism may recur). **Side effects:** may be limiting, and include anorexia, lethargy, dizziness, impaired cognition, GI distress, hypercholesterolemia, adrenal insufficiency (which may necessitate supernormal doses of glucocorticoids for replacement due to induced glucocorticoid degradation).

℞ Start with 250–500 mg PO q hs, and escalate dose slowly. Usual dose range is 4–12 gm/d usually divided TID-QID. Initial effectiveness may diminish with time.

Cyproheptadine (Periactin®): a serotonin receptor antagonist that corrects the abnormalities of Cushing's disease in a small minority of patients, suggesting that some cases of "pituitary" Cushing's disease are really due to a hypothalamic disorder. Combined therapy with bromocriptine may be more effective in some patients. **Side effects:** sedation & hyperphagia with weight gain usually limit usefulness.

℞ Usual dosage range: 8–36 mg/d divided TID.

46.2.7 Thyrotropin (TSH)-secreting adenomas – management

General information

1. transsphenoidal surgery has been the traditional first-line treatment.[49] These tumors may be fibrous and difficult to remove[50]
2. for incomplete resection: post-op XRT is employed
3. if hyperthyroidism persists: medical therapy is added with agents including octreotide, bromocriptine (more effective for tumors that co-secrete PRL), and oral cholecystographic agents (which inhibit conversion of T4 to T3) e.g. iopanoic acid

Medical therapy

Normal and neoplastic anterior hypophyseal thyrotroph cells possess somatostatin receptors and most respond to octreotide (see below). Occasionally, beta-blockers or low-dose antithyroid drugs (e.g. Tapazole® (methimazole) ≈ 5 mg PO TID for adults) may additionally be required.

Octreotide (Sandostatin®)

Doses required are usually < than with acromegaly. TSH levels decline by > 50% in 88% of patients, and become normal in ≈ 75%. T4 and T3 levels decrease in almost all, with 75% becoming normal. Tumor shrinkage occurs in ≈ 33%.

℞ Start with 50–100 mcg SQ q 8 hrs. Titrate to TSH, T4 and T3 levels.

46.3 Radiation therapy for pituitary adenomas

46.3.1 General information

Conventional EBXRT usually consists of 40–50 Gy administered over 4–6 weeks.

46.3.2 Side effects

Radiation injury to the remaining normal pituitary results in hypocortisolism, hypogonadism, or hypothyroidism in 40–50% of patients after 10 years. It may also injure the optic nerve and chiasm

Table 46.8 Recurrence rate of pituitary tumors removed transsphenoidally[a]

Extent of removal	Post-op XRT?	Recurrence rate
subtotal	no	50%
gross total		21%
subtotal	yes	10%
gross total		0

[a]108 macroadenomas, 6 mos to 14 years follow-up[52]

(possibly causing blindness), cause lethargy, memory disturbances, cranial nerve palsies, and tumor necrosis with hemorrhage and apoplexy. Cure rates but also complications are higher after proton beam therapy.

46

46.3.3 Recommendation

Radiation therapy should *not* be routinely used following surgical removal. Follow patient with yearly MRI. Treat recurrence with repeat operation. Consider radiation if recurrence cannot be removed and tumor continues to grow.

46.3.4 Sellar radiation therapy for nonfunctional pituitary tumors

In one series of 89 *nonfunctioning* pituitary tumors ranging 0.5–5 cm diameter (mean = 2 cm) not totally resected because of involvement of cavernous sinus (or other inaccessible sites), half were treated with radiation therapy (XRT). The recurrence rate was neither lower (and was actually higher) nor later in the XRT group.[51] However, another series of 108 pituitary macroadenomas found the recurrence rates shown in ▶ Table 46.8 which tend to favor radiation therapy.

When used, doses of 40 or 45 Gy in 20 or 25 fractions, respectively, is recommended.[53] The oncocytic variant of null cell pituitary tumors appears to be more radioresistant than the nononcocytic undifferentiated cell adenoma.[53]

46.3.5 Sellar radiation therapy for acromegaly

Not the preferred initial treatment. Works better with lower initial GH levels. In most patients, GH levels begin to fall during the first year after XRT, dropping by ≈ 50% after 2 years, and decrease gradually thereafter, reaching ≤ 10 ng/ml in 70% of patients after 10 years. It takes up to 20 years for 90% of patients to achieve GH levels < 5 ng/ml. During this latency period, patients are exposed to unacceptably high levels of GH (octreotide may be used while waiting). Patients are also still at risk for radiation side effects mentioned above. Options include: EBRT, stereotactic radiosurgery (about equally effective). Estimated cost: $20,000.

46.3.6 Sellar radiation therapy for Cushing's disease

XRT corrects hypercortisolism in 20–40%, and produces some improvement in another 40%. Improvement may not be seen for 1–2 yrs post treatment.

References

[1] Chandler WF. Treatment of disorders of the pituitary gland: pearls and pitfalls from 30 years of experience. Clin Neurosurg. 2008; 56:18–22

[2] Walsh FB, Hoyt WF. Clinical Neuro-Ophthalmology. Baltimore 1969

[3] Tindall GT, Barrow DL. Current Management of Pituitary Tumors: Part I. Contemp Neurosurg. 1988; 10:1–6

[4] Watts NB. Cushing's Syndrome: An Update. Contemp Neurosurg. 1995; 17:1–7

[5] Gillam MP, Molitch ME, Lombardi G, Colao A. Advances in the treatment of prolactinomas. Endocr Rev. 2006; 27:485–534

[6] Olukoga AO. Macroprolactinemia is clinically important. J Clin Endocrinol Metab. 2002; 87:4833–4834

[7] Bilaniuk LT, Moshang T, Cara J, et al. Pituitary Enlargement Mimicking Pituitary Tumor. J Neurosurg. 1985; 63:39–42

[8] Atchison JA, Lee PA, Albright L. Reversible Suprasellar Pituitary Mass Secondary to Hypothyroidism. JAMA. 1989; 262:3175–3177

[9] Watanakunakorn C, Hodges RE, Evans TC. Myxedema. A Study of 400 Cases. Arch Intern Med. 1965; 116:183–190

[10] Kallenberg GA, Pesce CM, Norman B, et al. Ectopic Hyperprolactinemia Resulting From an Ovarian Teratoma. JAMA. 1990; 263:2472–2474
[11] Randall RV, Scheithauer BW, Laws ER, et al. Pituitary Adenomas Associated with Hyperprolactinemia. Mayo Clin Proc. 1985; 60:753–762
[12] Cowen PJ, Sargent PA. Changes in plasma prolactin during SSRI treatment: evidence for a delayed increase in 5-HT neurotransmission. J Psychopharmacol. 1997; 11:345–348
[13] Tyrell JB, Aron DC, Forsham PH, Greenspan FS. In: Glucocorticoids and Adrenal Androgens. Basic and Clinical Endocrinology. 3rd ed. Norwalk: Appleton and Lange; 1991:323–362
[14] Yanovski JA, Cutler GB, Chrousos GP, Nieman LK. Corticotropin-releasing sormone stimulation following low-dose dexamethasone administration: A new test to distinguish Cushing's syndrome from pseudo-Cushing's states. JAMA. 1993; 269:2232–2238
[15] McCutcheon IE, Oldfield EH, Barrow DL, Selman W. In: Cortisol: Regulation, Disorders, and Clinical Evaluation. Neuroendocrinology. Baltimore: Williams and Wilkins; 1992:117–173
[16] Chrousos GP, Schulte HM, Oldfield EH, et al. The Corticotropin-Releasing Factor Stimulation Test: An Aid in the Evaluation of Patients with Cushing's Syndrome. N Engl J Med. 1984; 310:622–626
[17] Esposito F, Dusick JR, Cohan P, et al. Early morning cortisol levels as a predictor of remission after transsphenoidal surgery for Cushing's disease. J Clin Endocrinol Metab. 2006; 91:7–13
[18] Watts NB, Tindall GT. Rapid assessment of corticotropin reserve after pituitary surgery. JAMA. 1988; 259:708–711
[19] Abboud CF. Laboratory Diagnosis of Hypopituitarism. Mayo Clin Proc. 1986; 61:35–48
[20] Melmed S. Acromegaly. N Engl J Med. 1990; 322:966–977
[21] Dimaraki EV, Jaffe CA, DeMott-Friberg R, Chandler WF, Barkan AL. Acromegaly with apparently normal GH secretion: implications for diagnosis and follow-up. J Clin Endocrinol Metab. 2002; 87:3537–3542
[22] Cook DM. AACE Medical Guidelines for Clinical Practice for the diagnosis and treatment of acromegaly. Endocr Pract. 2004; 10:213–225
[23] Melmed S. Medical progress: Acromegaly. N Engl J Med. 2006; 355:2558–2573
[24] Frohman LA. Ectopic hormone production by tumors: growth hormone-releasing factor. Neuroendocrine Perspect. 1984; 3:201–224
[25] Peyster RG, Hoover ED, Viscarello RR, et al. CT Appearance of the Adolescent and Preadolescent Pituitary Gland. AJNR. 1983; 4:411–414
[26] Watson JC, Shawker TH, Nieman LK, et al. Localization of Pituitary Adenomas by Using Intraoperative Ultrasound in Patients with Cushing's Disease and No Demonstrable Pituitary Tumor on Magnetic Resonance Imaging. J Neurosurg. 1998; 89:927–932
[27] Kim LJ, Lekovic GP, White WL, Karis J. Preliminary Experience with 3-Tesla MRI and Cushing's Disease. Skull Base. 2007; 17:273–277
[28] Kucharczyk W, Davis DO, Kelly WM, et al. Pituitary adenomas: high-resolution MR imaging at 1.5 T. Radiology. 1986; 161:761–765
[29] Krisht AF. Giant Invasive Pituitary Adenomas. Contemp Neurosurg. 1999; 21:1–6
[30] Wilson CB. Endocrine-Inactive Pituitary Adenomas. Clin Neurosurg. 1992; 38:10–31
[31] Banasiak MJ, Malek AR. Nelson syndrome: comprehensive review of pathophysiology, diagnosis, and management. Neurosurg Focus. 2007; 23
[32] Barrow DL, Mizuno J, Tindall GT. Management of Prolactinomas Associated with Very High Serum Prolactin Levels. J Neurosurg. 1988; 68:554–558
[33] Blevins LS. Medical Management of Pituitary Adenomas. Contemp Neurosurg. 1997; 19:1–6
[34] Molitch ME. Pregnancy and the hyperprolactinemic woman. N Engl J Med. 1985; 312:1364–1370
[35] Landolt AM, Osterwalder V. Perivascular Fibrosis in Prolactinomas: Is it Increased by Bromocriptine? J Clin Endocrinol Metab. 1984; 58:1179–1183
[36] Barlas O, Bayindir C, Hepgul K, Can M, Kiris T, Sencer E, Unal F, Aral F. Bromocriptine-induced cerebrospinal fluid fistula in patients with macroprolactinomas: report of three cases and a review of the literature. Surg Neurol. 1994; 41:486–489
[37] Cabergoline for Hyperprolactinemia. Med Letter. 1997; 39:58–59
[38] Webster J, Piscitelli G, Polli A, et al. A Comparison of Cabergoline and Bromocriptine in the Treatment of Hyperprolactinemic Amenorrhea. N Engl J Med. 1994; 331:904–909
[39] Schade R, Andersohn F, Suissa S, Haverkamp W, Garbe E. Dopamine agonists and the risk of cardiac-valve regurgitation. N Engl J Med. 2007; 356:29–38
[40] Johnston DG, Hall K, Kendall-Taylor P, Patrick D, Watson M, Cook DB. Effect of dopamine agonist withdrawal after long-term therapy in prolactinomas. Studies with high-definition computerised tomography. Lancet. 1984; 2:187–192
[41] Schlechte JA. Long-term management of prolactinomas. J Clin Endocrinol Metab. 2007; 92:2861–2865
[42] Acromegaly Therapy Consensus Development Panel. Consensus Statement: Benefits Versus Risks of Medical Therapy for Acromegaly. Am J Med. 1994; 97:468–473
[43] Colao A, Attanasio R, Pivonello R, et al. Partial surgical removal of growth hormone-secreting pituitary tumors enhances the response to somatostatin analogs in acromegaly. J Clin Endocrinol Metab. 2006; 91:85–92
[44] Turner HE, Thornton-Jones VA, Wass JA. Systematic dose-extension of octreotide LAR: the importance of individual tailoring of treatment in patients with acromegaly. Clin Endocrinol (Oxf). 2004; 61:224–231
[45] van der Lely AJ, Hutson RK, Trainer PJ, Besser GM, Barkan AL, Katznelson L, Klibanski A, Herman-Bonert V, Melmed S, Vance ML, Freda PU, Stewart PM, Friend KE, Clemmons DR, Johannsson G, Stavrou S, Cook DM, Phillips LS, Strasburger CJ, Hackett S, Zib KA, Davis RJ, Scarlett JA, Thorner MO. Long-term treatment of acromegaly with pegvisomant, a growth hormone receptor antagonist. Lancet. 2001; 358:1754–1759
[46] Pegvisomant (Somavert) for acromegaly. Med Letter. 2003; 45:55–56
[47] Sheehan JM, Vance ML, Sheehan JP, Ellegala DB, Laws ER, Jr. Radiosurgery for Cushing's disease after failed transsphenoidal surgery. J Neurosurg. 2000; 93:738–742
[48] Assie G, Bahurel H, Coste J, Silvera S, Kujas M, Dugue MA, et al. Corticotroph tumor progression after adrenalectomy in Cushing's Disease: a reappraisal of Nelson's syndrome. J Clin Endocrinol Metab. 2007; 49:381–386
[49] Clarke MJ, Erickson D, Castro MR, Atkinson JL. Thyroid-stimulating hormone pituitary adenomas. J Neurosurg. 2008; 109:17–22
[50] Sanno N, Teramoto A, Osamura RY. Long-term surgical outcome in 16 patients with thyrotropin pituitary adenoma. J Neurosurg. 2000; 93:194–200
[51] Ebersold MJ, Quast LM, Laws ER, et al. Long-Term Results in Transsphenoidal Removal of Nonfunctioning Pituitary Adenomas. J Neurosurg. 1986; 64:713–719
[52] Ciric I, Mikhael M, Stafford T, et al. Transsphenoidal Microsurgery of Pituitary Macroadenomas with Long-Term Follow-Up Results. J Neurosurg. 1983; 59:395–401
[53] Breen P, Flickinger JC, Kondziolka D, Martinez AJ. Radiotherapy for Nonfunctional Pituitary Adenoma: Analysis of Long-Term Tumor Control. J Neurosurg. 1998; 89:933–938

47 Pituitary Adenomas – Surgical Management, Outcome, and Recurrence Management

47.1 Surgical treatment for pituitary adenomas

47.1.1 Medical preparation for surgery

1. stress dose steroids: given to all patients during and immediately after surgery
2. hypothyroidism: ideally, hypothyroid patients should have > 4 weeks of replacement to reverse hypothyroidism, however:
   a) ✖ do not replace thyroid hormone until the adrenal axis is assessed; giving thyroid replacement to a patient with hypoadrenalism can precipitate adrenal crisis. If hypoadrenal, begin cortisol replacement first, may begin thyroid hormone replacement after 24 hours of cortisol
   b) surgery is done frequently on patients with hypothyroidism and appears to be tolerated well in the vast majority of cases

47.1.2 Surgical approaches – overview

1. transsphenoidal: an extra-arachnoid approach, requires no brain retraction, no external scar (aside from where a fat graft is procured, if used). Usually the procedure of choice. Indicated for microadenomas, macroadenomas without significant extension laterally beyond the confines of the sella turcica, patients with CSF rhinorrhea, and tumors with extension into sphenoid air sinus
   a) sublabial
   b) trans-nares: an alotomy may be used to enlarge the exposure through the nares if necessary
2. transethmoidal approach[1 (p 343–50)]
3. transcranial approaches:
   a) indications: most pituitary tumors are operated by the transsphenoidal technique (see above), even if there is significant suprasellar extension. However, a craniotomy may be indicated for the following[2]:
      - minimal enlargement of the sella with a large suprasellar mass, especially if the diaphragma sellae is tightly constricting the tumor (producing a "cottage loaf" tumor) and the suprasellar component is causing chiasmal compression[3 (p 124)]
      - extrasellar extension into the middle fossa that is larger than the intrasellar component
      - unrelated pathology may complicate a transsphenoidal approach: rare, e.g. a parasellar aneurysm
      - unusually fibrous tumor that could not be completely removed on a previous transsphenoidal approach
      - recurrent tumor following a previous transsphenoidal resection
   b) choices of approach
      - subfrontal: provides access to both optic nerves. May be more difficult in patients with prefixed chiasm
      - frontotemporal (pterional): places optic nerve and sometimes carotid artery in line of vision of tumor. There is also incomplete access to intrasellar contents. Good access for tumors with significant lateral extrasellar extension
      - ✖ subtemporal: usually not a viable choice. Poor visualization of optic nerve/chiasm and carotid. Does not allow total removal of intrasellar component

47.1.3 Transsphenoidal surgery

Booking the case: Transsphenoidal surgery

Also see defaults & disclaimers (p. 27) and pre-op orders (p. 751).

1. position: supine, horseshoe head rest or (especially if image guided navigation is used) pin headholder
2. equipment:
   a) microscope
   b) C-arm (if used)
   c) image guided navigation system (if used)

d) endoscopy cart for cases performed endoscopically (surgeon preference)
3. instrumentation: transsphenoidal instrument set (usually includes speculum, curettes, long instruments including bipolars)
4. some surgeons use ENT to perform the approach and closure and for follow-up
5. post-op: ICU
6. consent (in lay terms for the patient – not all-inclusive):
   a) procedure: removal of pituitary tumor through the nose, possible placement of fat graft from abdomen
   b) alternatives: surgery through the skull (trans-cranial), radiation
   c) complications: CSF leak with possible meningitis, problems with pituitary hormones which may sometimes be permanent (which would require lifetime replacement therapy), injury to optic nerve with visual loss, injury to carotid artery with possible bleeding and/or stroke

Technique

47

General information

For pre- and post-op orders, see below.

Details of the surgery are beyond the scope of this text, see references.[3,4,5,6]

Intraoperative disasters

Usually related to loss of landmarks.[3] Can be minimized using intraoperative navigation or fluoroscopy to verify location.

- injury of carotid artery:
  - typically injured in lateral aspect of opening. Bone may be dehiscent over the ICA
  - signaled by profuse arterial bleeding
  - can usually be packed off, if fat/fascia graft from thigh or abdomen is available it may be used; otherwise use e.g. woven surgical)
  - the operation is halted, and a STAT post-op arteriogram must be done
  - if a pseudoaneurysm or site of injury is identified angiographically, it must be eliminated before a potentially lethal hemorrhage; accomplished either by endovascular techniques or by surgical trapping with clips above and below
- opening through the clivus and erroneous biopsy of the pons
- opening through the floor of the frontal fossa with injury to the olfactory nerves and entry into inferior frontal lobes

Overview of the procedure

1. lumbar drain: may be used with some macroadenomas to inject fluid in order to help bring the tumor down (see below), also may be used for post-op CSF drainage following transsphenoidal repair of CSF fistula
2. medications (in addition to pre-op meds, see below): intraoperatively 100 mg hydrocortisone IV q 8 hrs
3. positioning
   a) elevate thorax 10–15°: reduces venous pressure
   b) head stabilization: if image-guided navigation is to be used, the head is placed in a Mayfield headholder or a headband with registration array is attached and the head is placed on a horseshoe head rest. If no image guidance, a horseshoe headrest may be used
   c) position option 1: surgeon standing to right of patient
      - shoulder-roll
      - top of head canted slightly to left
      - neck position: For microscope: extend neck slightly with the head in either a Mayfield head-holder or on a horseshoe headrest. For endoscope: do not extend neck (more comfortable for holding instruments)
      - ET tube positioned down and to patient's *left* (to get it out of the way)
      - microscope: observer's eyepiece on the *left*
   d) position option 2: surgeon standing above patient's head: head pointing straight up towards ceiling, neck slightly extended
   e) abdomen or right thigh is prepped for fat graft
4. C-arm fluoro: image-guided navigation can eliminate the need for fluoro. Orient the C-arm for a true lateral by aligning the mandibular rami and/or by superimposing the floor of the left and

right frontal fossae. If this proves difficult, lay a Penfield 4 on the nasion oriented from lateral canthus to lateral canthus, then aim the fluoro to shoot "down the barrel" of the Penfield 4

5. after approach to floor of sella is complete (see below), outline the upper and lower boundaries of the sella using image navigation or for fluoro using an instrument (e.g. suction tip) – obtain hard-copy of images for documentation purposes
6. opening the sellar floor:
   a) starting the opening: open *exactly* in the midline using the nasal septum as a landmark (NB: the septum of the sphenoid sinus is unreliable as a midline indicator, and often curves inferiorly towards one of the carotid arteries).
      - macroadenomas may have thinned the bone to the point that it just flakes off
      - otherwise, use a bayoneted chisel or high-speed diamond burr to start the opening
   b) use a Kerrison rongeur to expand the opening. ✖ CAUTION: stay away from the extreme lateral sella to avoid entering the cavernous sinus or injuring the carotid artery
7. coagulate the dura centrally in an "X" pattern (*NOT* "+" pattern) with bipolar cautery. Macroadenomas may cause yellowish discoloration of the dura directly over the tumor
8. consider aspirating through dura with a 20 gauge spinal needle to R/O large venous sinus (dura often has bluish discoloration), aneurysm, or empty sella
9. incise the dura in the "X" pattern in the midline with a #11 scalpel on a bayonetted handle
10. tumor removal for **macroadenoma**:
    a) gently bring tumor into the field with ring curettes, and remove with pituitary rongeurs or aspirate with suction. Some tumors are very fibrous and may be difficult to remove
    b) do not *pull* on the lateral component of the tumor with pituitary rongeur due to risk of injuring carotid artery
    c) if the suprasellar component will not come down, it may be brought down by having the anesthesiologist inject 5 ml aliquots of saline into a lumbar drain while monitoring blood pressure and pulse[3 (p 135),7]
    d) once the tumor is debulked internally, try to develop a plane between the tumor capsule and the pituitary. A good place to start looking is inferiorly where the dura can be separated from the tumor capsule and then followed on the surface. Sometimes the tumor capsule cannot be removed due to severe bleeding
    e) complete tumor removal is often not possible, and the goal of the surgery then is "containment"
    f) endoscopic techniques and image guided navigation may be employed to assist in removal of macroadenomas
11. tumor removal for microadenoma
    a) if the side of the tumor is known, begin exploration of the gland on that side by making incision with #11 blade and using a dissector to try and locate the tumor (like a "grain of rice in a blueberry")
    b) for Cushing's disease, if no tumor is identified on pre-op MRI[8]:
       - intraoperative ultrasound may help localize tumor in ≈ 70% of cases[9] but a specialized U/S probe is required
       - if IPS sampling showed a lateralizing ACTH gradient: start with a paramedian incision on the side of the higher ACTH gradient; if no adenoma is encountered, the contralateral paramedian and then midline incisions are used to explore the gland
       - if IPS sampling and MRI do not suggest tumor location: the gland is explored sequentially with 2 paramedian incisions and then a midline incision
       - if the adenoma cannot be found, a hemihypophysectomy is performed on the side of higher ACTH levels if IPS sampling shows a lateralizing gradient, or on the side with more suspicious tissue on frozen section. Total hypophysectomy is not routinely performed[8]
    c) most adenomas are purplish-grey and easily aspirated, however some may be more fibrous. The normal pituitary gland is firm and rubbery (the adenohypophysis is orange-pink, the neurohypophysis is a whitish-grey), and normally does not curette very easily
    d) use image guidance or fluoro to determine approximate location of diaphragma sellae. Do not go cephalad to this to avoid a CSF leak, to avoid entering the circular venous sinus in the dura here and to avoid trauma to the optic chiasm
12. after removal of macroadenoma, check depth of tumor bed on fluoro or image guidance, and make sure it correlates with approximate tumor volume on MRI
13. the sella may be packed in a number of ways,[6] one method:
    a) if CSF leak occurs: place muscle or fat in defect within sella. Some recommend against the use of muscle because it always putrefies.[3(p 129)] Do not overpack to avoid recreating mass effect with the graft

47

b) recreate the floor of the sella using nasal cartilage placed within the sella. Alternatively, a nonporous Medpor® polyethylene transsphenoidal sellar implant (Porex Surgical Products http://www.porexsurgical.com) may be used
c) if CSF leak occurs pack sphenoid sinus with fat from abdomen (option: fat with fascia on surface)
d) fibrin glue may optionally be used to help hold any of these components in place

Approach to sphenoid sinus for microscopic removal
Often done by ENT co-surgeon. One method:
1. insert temporary speculum into nose. For this discussion, the right nares will be described
2. use endoscope to locate middle concha. Follow this posteriorly to identify os into sphenoid sinus which is usually located posterior to and slightly above the posterior extent of the middle concha
3. inject local anesthetic with epinephrine to blanch mucosa
4. insert sickle knife into os with sharp side facing the septum (medially) and incise the mucosa as the knife is drawn outward
5. use a Freer to dissect the thusly created mucosal flaps off the medial septum (pull one up, the other down)
6. break through the posterior part of the septum so that both sides of the floor of the sphenoid sinus are exposed. Cartilage or bone from this step is saved to use later in reconstructing the floor of the sella if desired
7. open the floor of the sphenoid and take it all the way to the right os (you will probably not see the left os)
8. place the Hardy speculum or equivalent
9. strip mucosa off the walls of the sphenoid sinus using a Blakely and *slow* pulling motion

Endoscopic tumor removal
There is no proof that removal is superior to microscopic approach through a speculum.

Advantages over microscopic removal: Visualization is better, especially within tumor bed.

Disadvantages: less familiarity with use of endoscopes by most neurosurgeons compared to ENT surgeons. Lack of 3D visualization (may be overcome using 3D endoscopes). Need for single handed technique (may be overcome by having assistant hold endoscope, or using an endoscope holder e.g. Mitaka), need for a binasal approach (if it is desired to use two hands for the actual surgery).

47.1.4 Peri-operative complications

1. hormonal imbalance:
   a) acute post-op concerns:
      - alterations in ADH: transient abnormalities are common – see typical post-op patterns (p. 752) – including DI. DI lasting > 3 mos is uncommon
      - cortisol deficiency → hypocortisolism → Addisonian crisis if severe
   b) long-term: hypopituitarism in ≈ 5% (retrospective series[10])
      - TSH deficiency → hypothyroidism → (rarely) myxedema coma if severe
      - adrenal insufficiency
      - deficiency of sex hormones → hypogonadotrophic hypogonadism
2. secondary empty sella syndrome (chiasm retracts into evacuated sella → visual impairment)
3. hydrocephalus with coma[11]: may follow removal of tumors with suprasellar extension (transsphenoidally or transcranially). Consider ventriculostomy placement if hydrocephalus is present (even if not symptomatic). Possible etiologies:
   a) traction on the attached 3rd ventricle
   b) cerebral edema due to vasopressin release from manipulation of the pituitary and/or stalk
   c) tumor edema following resection
4. infection
   a) pituitary abscess[12,13]
   b) meningitis
5. CSF rhinorrhea (fistula): 3.5% incidence[14]
6. carotid artery rupture: rare. May occur intraoperatively (see above) or in delayed fashion after surgery, often ≈ day 10 post-op (due to breakdown of fibrin around carotid, or possibly due to rupture of a pseudoaneurysm created at surgery)
7. entry into cavernous sinus with possible injury of any structure within
8. nasal septal perforation

47.1.5 Frontotemporal (pterional) approach

A right sided approach is usually employed (less risk to dominant hemisphere). Exceptions: when the left eye is the side of worse vision; if there is predominant left sided tumor extension; if there is other pathology on the left (e.g. aneurysm).

Positioning is that same as for ACoA aneurysm with the ▶ Fig. 94.5. The frontal lobe is elevated, and the temporal tip is gently retracted posteriorly. Bridging veins to the temporal tip must be coagulated to avoid rupture, as for any pterional approach. The approach is similar to that for an ACoA aneurysm (i.e. more emphasis is placed on frontal lobe elevation than on temporal tip retraction), except that unlike ACoA aneurysm, exposure of the ICA is not needed because proximal control is not necessary.

The tumor capsule can usually be seen between the two optic nerves. The capsule is coagulated with bipolar cautery, and is incised. The tumor is then debulked from within. By staying within the capsule, risk of injury to the pituitary stalk and optic chiasm is minimized. Significant amounts of tumor can be removed by aspiration if it is soft and suckable.

✖ Caution: the blood supply to the optic chiasm is from the inferior aspect. Skeletonizing the chiasm or attempting to tease away tumor adherent to it may worsen vision.

47.1.6 Peri-operative management

Pre-op orders

1. Polysporin® ointment (PSO) applied in both nostrils the night before surgery
2. antibiotics, one of the following regimens may be used:
   a) chloramphenicol 500 mg IVPB at 11 PM & 6 AM
      OR
   b) chloramphenicol 500 mg PO at MN & IV at 6 AM; ampicillin 1 gm PO at MN & IV at 6 AM
      OR
   c) Unasyn® 1.5 gm (1 gm ampicillin + 0.5 gm sulbactam) IVPB at MN & 6 AM
3. steroids, either:
   a) hydrocortisone sodium succinate (Solu-Cortef®) 50 mg IM at 11 PM & 6 AM. On call to OR: hang 1 L D5LR + 20 mEq KCl/l + 50 mg Solu-Cortef at 75 ml/hr
      OR
   b) hydrocortisone 100 mg PO at MN & IV at 6 AM
4. intra-op: continue 100 mg hydrocortisone IV q 8 hrs

Post-op orders

1. intake & output (I's & O's) q 1 hr; urine specific gravity (SG) q 4° and anytime urine output (UO) > 250 ml/hr
2. activity: BR with HOB @ 30°.
3. diet: ice chips PRN. Patient is not to drink through a straw (to avoid negative pressure on sphenoid sinus with risk of aggravating CSF fistula)
4. no incentive spirometry (to avoid negative pressure on sphenoid sinus with risk of aggravating CSF fistula)
5. *IVF*: base IV D5 1/2 NS + 20 mEq KCl/L at appropriate rate (75–100 ml/hr)
   PLUS: replace UO > base IV rate ml for ml with 1/2 NS.
   NB: if patient receives significant fluids intra-operatively, then they may have an appropriate post-op diuresis, in which case consider replacing only ≈ 2/3 of UO > base IV rate with 1/2 NS
6. meds
   a) antibiotics: continue chloramphenicol 500 mg IVPB q 6 hr (also continue ampicillin if used pre-op), change to PO when tolerated, D/C when nasal packing removed
   b) steroids (some surgeons routinely use post-op steroids until the adequacy of endogenous steroids is established, especially with Cushing's disease, see below). Either:
      - hydrocortisone 50 mg IM/IV q 6 hrs, on POD #2 change to prednisone 5 mg PO q 6 hrs × 1 day, then 5 mg PO BID, D/C on POD#6
        OR
      - hydrocortisone 50 mg IM/IV/PO BID, taper 10 mg/dose/day to physiologic dose of 20 mg q AM and 10 mg q PM until adrenal axis assessed
   c) *diabetes insipidus* (DI): patients are placed on "DI watch" (monitoring U.O. and serum and urine labs) see below for typical patterns.
      Diagnostic criteria: U.O. > 250 ml/hr × 1–2 hrs, *and* SG < 1.005 (usually < 1.003) (dilute urine), often with elevation of serum Na^+

If DI develops, attempt to keep up with fluid loss with IVF (see above); if rate is too high for IV or PO replacement (> 300 cc/hr × 4 hrs or > 500 cc/hr × 2 hrs), check urine S.G. and if < 1.005 then give a vasopressin preparation (see below, or see ▶ Table 5.7). ✖ Caution: danger of over-treating in case of triphasic response (see below), therefore use
EITHER:
- 5 U aqueous vasopressin (Pitressin®) IVP/IM/SQ q 6 hrs PRN
  OR
- desmopressin (DDAVP®) injection SQ/IV titrated to UO. Usual adult dose: 0.5–1 ml (2–4 mcg) daily in 2 divided doses
  AVOID
- ✖ avoid tannate oil suspension, because it is a long acting preparation (and may overtreat) and has erratic absorption
  THEN: when nasal packs out, EITHER
- intranasal DDAVP (100 mcg/ml): range 0.1–0.4 ml (10–40 mcg) intranasally BID (typically 0.2 ml BID) PRN
  OR
- clofibrate (Atromid S®) 500 mg PO QID (does not always work)

47

7. labs: renal profile with osmolarity q 6 hrs, 8 A.M. serum cortisol
8. nasal packs: remove on post-op day 3–6

Urinary output: patterns of postoperative diabetes insipidus

Manage diabetes insipidus (DI) as described above in post-op orders. Post-op DI generally follows one of three patterns[15]; see Diabetes insipidus for details (p. 120):
1. transient DI: lasts until ≈ 12–36 hrs post-op then normalizes
2. "prolonged" DI: lasts months, or rarely may be permanent
3. "**triphasic** response" (least common). 3 stages:
   a) DI (short duration): due to injury to posterior pituitary
   b) normalization or SIADH-like picture: due to release of ADH from neuron endings form hypothalamus. It is during this phase that there is a risk of severe iatrogenic hyponatremia from overtreatment initiated during the initial DI phase
   c) DI (long-term)

Discontinuation of steroids post-op

Simple management schemes

Some surgeons do not routinely assess ACTH reserve post-op for patients that were not hypocortisolemic pre-op:
- taper and stop hydrocortisone 24–48 hrs post-op. Then, check 6 AM serum cortisol level 24 hrs after discontinuing hydrocortisone and interpret the results as shown in ▶ Table 47.1.[16]
- If there is any question about reserve, the patient can be discharged on hydrocortisone 50 mg PO q AM and 25 mg PO q 4:00 PM until adrenal reserve can be formally assessed (see below)

Assessment of postoperative ACTH (corticotropin) reserve

Simple assessment protocol for patients who go home on hydrocortisone and were not on it pre-op.
- taper hydrocortisone over 2–3 weeks down to 20 mg po q AM and 10 mg q 4 PM (a little higher than maintenance to provide for some stress coverage) for several days
- then hold the PM dose and check an 8 AM serum cortisol the next day

Table 47.1 Interpretation of 6 AM cortisol levels

6 AM cortisol	Interpretation	Management
≥ 9 mcg/dl	normal	no further tests or treatment
3–9 mcg/dl	possible ACTH deficiency	place patient on hydrocortisone[a] (p. 144)
≤ 3 mcg/dl	ACTH deficient	

[a]perform cosyntropin stimulation test (p. 735) 1 month post-op; D/C steroids if normal; if subnormal, then permanent replacement required

- to avoid adrenal insufficiency in patients with incompetent reserve: as soon as the blood is drawn have the patient take their morning dose and resume regular dosing until the test results are available
- If this 8 AM cortisol shows any significant adrenal function, then taper the patient off hydrocortisone

Metyrapone (Metopirone®) test

This test more accurately assesses the hypothalamic-pituitary-adrenal axis and is useful if there is suspicion of reduced reserve of pituitary ACTH production. Metyrapone inhibits 11-β-hydroxylation in the adrenal cortex, reducing production of cortisol and corticosterone with concomitant increase of serum 11-deoxycortisol precursors and its 17-OHCS metabolites which appear in the urine. In response, a normal pituitary increases ACTH production.

1. All patients should have a cosyntropin stimulation test (p. 735) first to rule-out primary adrenal insufficiency .
2. ✖ Do not do this test if there is known primary adrenal insufficiency.
3. ✖ Do not do this test as an outpatient.
4. **Test protocol**
   a) give 2–3 grams metyrapone PO at midnight
   b) check serum 11-deoxycortisol level the next morning
   c) a normal response is a 11-deoxycortisol level > 7 mcg/dl
   d) CAUTION: in patients with very little reserve, the reduced cortisol may provoke adrenal insufficiency (this test is safer than the higher doses used for urinary 17-OHCS testing)

Postoperative CT/MRI scan

A study using CT in 12 patients with macroadenomas following transsphenoidal surgery without radiation therapy demonstrated that the maximal height of the pituitary "mass" did not return to normal immediately post-op (even with total tumor removal), rather a period of 3–4 months was required.[17]

Σ

The optimal timing of the initial post-op CT or MRI to function as a baseline to rule-out future recurrence after transsphenoidal surgery is ≈ 3–4 months post-op.

47.2 Outcome following transsphenoidal surgery

47.2.1 General information

In a series of 108 macroadenomas, gross total removal was unusual in tumors with > 2 cm suprasellar extension.[14]

47.2.2 Visual deficit

In cases with compression of the optic apparatus, there can be significant improvements in vision following surgery.[14,18]

47.2.3 Biochemical outcome

Prolactinomas

In a series of 108 macroadenomas, endocrinologic cure was attained in 25% of prolactin-secreting tumors.[14]

Acromegaly

Criteria of biochemical cure

The criteria for biochemical cure of acromegaly is not standardized. There may be a discord between IGF-1 levels and mean GH levels.[19] Many use a GH cutoff level; range of levels described: < 2.5–5 ng/ml. Others feel that an elevated IGF-1 represents lack of cure even if GH < 5. However, normal IGF-1 levels may not be mandatory.[20] Still others require a normal IGF-1 AND a normal response to an oral glucose suppression test (OGST) (p. 736).

Low GH levels that do not also suppress to < 1 ng/ml after an OGST are considered controlled but not cured (even with normal IGF-1 levels).[21] If asymptomatic, expectant management with close follow-up is recommended.[21]

Σ

Biochemical cure criteria for acromegaly is not standardized. Recommendation[21]:
1) IGF-1 levels within age-matched reference range
2) basal (morning) serum GH level < 5 ng/ml, AND GH nadir < 1 ng/ml in OGST

47

Outcome with acromegaly

Transsphenoidal surgery results in biochemical cure in 85% of cases with adenomas < 10 mm diameter, no evidence of local invasion, and random GH levels < 40 ng/ml pre-op. Overall, ≈ 50% of *all* acromegalics undergoing transsphenoidal surgery had a biochemical cure.[22] Only 30% of macroadenomas and very few with marked suprasellar extension have surgical cure. Patients not cured with surgery require lifelong medical suppression. These tumors may also recur years later after apparent cure. Patients should be monitored every 6–12 months for recurrence.[21]

Cushing's disease

There are numerous methodologies for determining biochemical cure for Cushing's disease. One difficulty is that exogenous steroids are often given post-op to avoid potential hypoadrenalism or Addisonian crisis or for nausea. Some options:

1. immediate post-op early morning cortisol levels[8]:
   a) all steroids are withheld post-op (including dexamethasone as an antiemetic) unless biochemical and/or clinical evidence of hypocortisolism (clinical signs: nausea, anorexia, H/A, arthralgias). ✖ Requires close monitoring and administration of steroids if symptoms develop
   b) serum ACTH and cortisol levels are drawn between 6–9:00 AM on post-op days 1 & 2
   c) early remission defined as a *lowest* cortisol level ≤ 140 nmol/L (≤ 5 mcg/dl)
      - 97% (31/32) patients with early remission had sustained remission with mean follow-up of 32 months
      - only 12.5% (1/8) without early remission showed evidence of sustained remission
      - this has been used to select patients for possible early re-exploration
      - early ACTH levels usually drop, but do not consistently become subnormal and are not reliable in predicting sustained remission[8]
2. provocative tests
   a) overnight low-dose dexamethasone suppression test: an AM cortisol level on post-op day 3 that is ≤ 8 mcg/dl after an overnight 1 mg dexamethasone suppression test is predictive of sustained remission in 97%[23]
   b) CRH stimulation test[24]
3. measurements usually conducted 3 days to 2 weeks post-op following 24 hours of steroid cessation after initial post-op coverage with glucocorticoids
   a) 24-hour urinary free cortisol
   b) serum cortisol: the criteria of a cortisol level < 50 nmol/l (< 1.8 mcg/dl)[25,26,27] is probably too stringent[28,29,8]
   c) serum ACTH

The overall remission rate since 1980 is 64–93%, with the highest rates (86–98%) in patients with noninvasive microadenomas identifiable on MRI.[8]

Following effective treatment, all of the following usually improve but may not normalize:

1. HTN and hyperglycemia: within ≈ 1 year
2. osteoporosis related to CD: over ≈ 2 years
3. psychiatric symptoms

Thyrotropin (TSH)-secreting adenomas

Following debulking, small amounts of residual tumor may continue to produce sufficient TSH for hyperthyroidism to persist.[30] Following surgery + XRT, only ≈ 40% achieve a cure (defined as no residual tumor at surgery or on imaging, and normal free T3 with TSH levels at or below normal).

47.3 Management of recurrent pituitary adenomas

Recurrence incidence: ≈ 12%, with most recurring 4–8 years post-op (in the same series[14]).

For tumors demonstrating significant regrowth or symptoms following initial resection, consideration for re-resection may be given. Once the tumor is debulked, consideration should be given to XRT, either immediately following the second operation, or, if recurrence after a second operation then almost certainly after a third debulking.

References

[1] Schmidek HH, Sweet WH. Operative Neurosurgical Techniques. New York 1982

[2] Wilson CB. Endocrine-Inactive Pituitary Adenomas. Clin Neurosurg. 1992; 38:10–31

[3] Powell M, Lightman SL. Management of Pituitary Tumours: A Handbook. New York 1996

[4] Hardy J. Transsphenoidal Hypophysectomy. J Neurosurg. 1971; 34:582–594

[5] Kern EB, Pearson BW, McDonald TJ, et al. The Transseptal Approach to Lesions of the Pituitary and Parasellar Region. Laryngoscope. 1979; 89S:1–34

[6] Spaziante R, de Divitiis E, Cappabianca P. Reconstruction of the Pituitary Fossa in Transsphenoidal Surgery: An Experience of 140 Cases. Neurosurgery. 1985; 17:453–458

[7] Zhang X, Fei Z, Zhang J, et al. Management of Nonfunctioning Pituitary Adenomas with Suprasellar Extension by Transsphenoidal Microsurgery. Surg Neurol. 1999; 52:380–385

[8] Esposito F, Dusick JR, Cohan P, et al. Early morning cortisol levels as a predictor of remission after transsphenoidal surgery for Cushing's disease. J Clin Endocrinol Metab. 2006; 91:7–13

[9] Watson JC, Shawker TH, Nieman LK, et al. Localization of Pituitary Adenomas by Using Intraoperative Ultrasound in Patients with Cushing's Disease and No Demonstrable Pituitary Tumor on Magnetic Resonance Imaging. J Neurosurg. 1998; 89:927–932

[10] Fatemi N, Dusick JR, Mattozo C, McArthur DL, Cohan P, Boscardin J, Wang C, Swerdloff RS, Kelly DF. Pituitary hormonal loss and recovery after transsphenoidal adenoma removal. Neurosurgery. 2008; 63:709–18; discussion 718-9

[11] Decker RE, Chalif DJ. Progressive Coma After the Transsphenoidal Decompression of a Pituitary Adenoma with Marked Suprasellar Extension: Report of Two Cases. Neurosurgery. 1991; 28:154–158

[12] Domingue JN, Wilson CB. Pituitary Abscesses. J Neurosurg. 1977; 46:601–608

[13] Robinson B. Intrasellar Abscess After Transsphenoidal Pituitary Adenectomy. Neurosurgery. 1983; 12:684–686

[14] Ciric I, Mikhael M, Stafford T, et al. Transsphenoidal Microsurgery of Pituitary Macroadenomas with Long-Term Follow-Up Results. J Neurosurg. 1983; 59:395–401

[15] Verbalis JG, Robinson AG, Moses AM. Postoperative and Post-Traumatic Diabetes Insipidus. Front Horm Res. 1985; 13:247–265

[16] Watts NB, Tindall GT. Rapid assessment of corticotropin reserve after pituitary surgery. JAMA. 1988; 259:708–711

[17] Teng MMH, Huang CI, Chang T. The Pituitary Mass After Transsphenoidal Hypophysectomy. AJNR. 1988; 9:23–26

[18] Cohen AR, Cooper PR, Kupersmith MJ, et al. Visual Recovery After Transsphenoidal Removal of Pituitary Adenoma. Neurosurgery. 1985; 17:446–452

[19] Turner HE, Thornton-Jones VA, Wass JA. Systematic dose-extension of octreotide LAR: the importance of individual tailoring of treatment in patients with acromegaly. Clin Endocrinol (Oxf). 2004; 61:224–231

[20] Ayuk J, Clayton RN, Holder G, Sheppard MC, Stewart PM, Bates AS. Growth hormone and pituitary radiotherapy, but not serum insulin-like growth factor I concentrations, predict excess mortality in patients with acromegaly. J Clin Endocrinol Metab. 2004; 89:1613–1617

[21] Cook DM. AACE Medical Guidelines for Clinical Practice for the diagnosis and treatment of acromegaly. Endocr Pract. 2004; 10:213–225

[22] Davis DH, Laws ER, Ilstrup DM, et al. Results of Surgical Treatment for Growth Hormone-Secreting Pituitary Adenomas. J Neurosurg. 1993; 79:70–75

[23] Chen JC, Amar AP, Choi S, Singer P, Couldwell WT, Weiss MH. Transsphenoidal microsurgical treatment of Cushing's disease: postoperative assessment of surgical efficacy by application of an overnight low-dose dexamethasone suppression test. J Neurosurg. 2003; 98:967–973

[24] Nishizawa S, Oki Y, Ohta S, Yokota N, et al. What can predict postoperative "endocrinological cure" in Cushing's disease? Neurosurgery. 1999; 45: 239–244

[25] Trainer PJ, Lawrie HS, Verhelst J, et al. Transsphenoidal resection in Cushing's disease: undetectable serum cortisol as the definition of successful treatment. Clinical Endocrinology (Oxf). 1993; 38:73–78

[26] Rees DA, Hanna FW, Davies JS, Mills RG, Vafidis J, Scanlon MF. Long-term follow-up results of transsphenoidal surgery for Cushing's disease in a single centre using strict criteria for remission. Clinical Endocrinology (Oxf). 2002; 56:541–551

[27] Yap LB, Turner HE, Adams CB, Wass JA. Undetectable postoperative cortisol does not always predict long-term remission in Cushing's disease: A single centre audit. Clinical Endocrinology (Oxf). 2002; 56:25–31

[28] Simmons NE, Alden TD, Thorner MO, Laws ER. Serum cortisol response to transsphenoidal surgery for Cushing disease. J Neurosurg. 2001; 95:1–8

[29] Rollin GA, Ferreira NP, Junges M, Gross JL, Czepielewski MA. Dynamics of serum cortisol levels after transsphenoidal surgery in a cohort of patients with Cushing's disease. J Clin Endocrinol Metab. 2004; 89:1131–1139

[30] Sanno N, Teramoto A, Osamura RY. Long-term surgical outcome in 16 patients with thyrotropin pituitary adenoma. J Neurosurg. 2000; 93:194–200

48 Cysts and Tumor-Like Lesions

48.1 Rathke's cleft cyst

Rathke's cleft cyst (RCC) are nonneoplastic lesions that are thought to be remnants of Rathke's pouch. They are primarily intrasellar, and are found incidentally in 13–23% of necropsies.[1] The adenohypophysis arises from proliferation of the anterior wall of Rathke's pouch, and so RCC have a similar lineage to pituitary adenomas and are rarely found together.[2] RCC are often discussed in contrast to craniopharyngiomas (**CP**) (see above). Some features are compared in ▶ Table 48.1.

RCC usually appear as low-density cystic lesions on CT. One half show capsular enhancement. MRI appearance is variable.[3] Rule of thumb: a lesion with a nodule in the sella is usually a RCC.

48.2 Colloid cyst

48.2.1 General information

48

Key concepts

- slow-growing benign tumor comprising < 1% of intracranial tumors
- classically occurs in the anterior 3rd ventricle, blocking foramina of Monro → obstructive hydrocephalus involving only the lateral ventricles (≈ pathognomonic)
- enhances minimally or not at all on CT/MRI
- natural history: risk of sudden death has been described, but is controversial
- treatment, when indicated, is surgical. Main options: transcallosal, transcortical/transventricular (only if hydrocephalus), ventriculoscopic

AKA neuroepithelial cysts. Comprise 2% of gliomas, and about 0.5–1% of all intracranial tumors.[4] Usual age of diagnosis: 20–50 yrs.

48.2.2 Pathogenesis

Origin: unknown. Implicated structures include: paraphysis (evagination in roof of third ventricle, rudimentary in humans), diencephalic ependyma in the recess of the postvelar arch, ventricular neuroepithelium.

Comprised of a fibrous epithelial-lined wall filled with either mucoid or dense hyloid substance. A slow growing, benign tumor.

Most commonly found in the third ventricle in the region of the foramina of Monro, but may be seen elsewhere, e.g. in septum pellucidum.[5]

48.2.3 Clinical signs and symptoms

Symptoms are shown in ▶ Table 48.2. Signs are shown in ▶ Table 48.3, most commonly presents either with signs of intermittent acute intracranial hypertension (classically attributed to movement of the cyst on its pedicle causing episodic obstruction of the foramina of Monro, rarely born out at

Table 48.1 Comparison of craniopharyngioma to Rathke's cleft cyst

Feature	Craniopharyngioma	Rathke's cleft cyst
site of origin	anterior superior margin of pituitary	pars intermedia of pituitary
cell lining	stratified squamous epithelium	single layer cuboidal epithelium
cyst contents	cholesterol crystals	resembles motor oil
surgical treatment	total removal is the goal	partial excision and drainage[3]
cyst wall	thick	thin

Table 48.2 Symptoms of colloid cyst at presentation[a]

Symptom	No.	%
headache	26	68%
gait disturbance	18	47%
disturbed mentation	14	37%
vomiting (± nausea)	14	37%
blurred vision	9	24%
incontinence	5	13%
dizziness	5	13%
tinnitus	5	13%
seizures	4	10%
acute deterioration	4	10%
diplopia	3	8%
"drop attacks"	1	
diabetes insipidus	1	
asymptomatic	1	

[a]38 patients, pre-CT era[4]

Table 48.3 Signs at presentation[a]

Sign	No.	%
papilledema	18	47%
gait disturbance	12	32%
normal exam	10	26%
hyperreflexia	9	24%
Babinski reflex	8	21%
incoordination	5	13%
nystagmus	5	13%
tremor	4	10%
hyporeflexia	3	8%
6th nerve palsy	2	5%

[a]38 patients with colloid cysts, pre-CT era[4]

operation) or with chronic hydrocephalus (from chronic obstruction). Most cysts < 1 cm diameter do not produce hydrocephalus and are asymptomatic.

► **Sudden death.** A high rate of sudden death has been reported with colloid cysts (20% in pre-CT era[6]) but is probably overestimated. The obsolete theory was that these tumors are mobile and thus could shift position and acutely block CSF flow with resultant herniation. Progressive obstruction from tumor growth does often produce chronic hydrocephalus, and it is possible that at some point the brain may decompensate in some cases. Changes in CSF dynamics resulting from procedures (LP, ventriculography…) may have also contributed.[7] Another proposed mechanism is disturbance of hypothalamic-mediated cardiovascular reflex control.[7]

48.2.4 Evaluation

Imaging (MRI or CT) demonstrates the tumor usually located in the anterior 3rd ventricle. Here, it often blocks both foramina of Monro causing almost pathognomonic hydrocephalus involving only the lateral ventricles (sparing the 3rd and 4th). Differential diagnosis includes basilar artery aneurysms, hamartomas, primary or secondary neoplasm, and xanthogranulomas.[8]

MRI: usually the optimal imaging technique. However, there are cases where cysts are isointense on MRI and CT is superior[9] (scrutinize the midline T1WI MRI images). When the lesion is identifiable, MRI clearly demonstrates the location of the cyst and relation to nearby structures, usually obviating an angiogram. MRI appearance: variable. Usually hyperintense on T1WI, hypointense on T2WI. Some data suggests that symptomatic patients are more likely to display T2 hyperintense cysts on MRI, indicating higher water content which may reflect a propensity for continued cyst expansion.[10] Enhancement: minimal, sometimes involving only capsule.

CT scan: findings are variable. Most are hyperdense (however, iso- and hypo-dense colloid cysts occur), and about half enhance slightly. Density may correlate with viscosity of contents, hyperdense cysts were harder to drain percutaneously.[11] CT is usually not quite as good as MRI, especially with isodense cysts. These tumors calcify only rarely.

48

✖ LP: *contraindicated* prior to placement of shunt due to risk of herniation.

48.2.5 Treatment

General information

Optimal treatment remains controversial. Initially, shunting without treating the cyst was advocated.[12] The nature of the obstruction (both foramina of Monro) requires *bilateral* ventricular shunts (or, unilateral shunt with fenestration of the septum pellucidum). Presently, one form or another of direct surgical treatment is usually recommended for some or all of the following reasons:

1. to prevent shunt dependency
2. to reduce the possibility of tumor progression
3. since the mechanism of sudden neurologic deterioration may be due to factors such as cardiovascular instability from hypothalamic compression and not due to hydrocephalus

Surgical treatment

Management options

Also see Approaches to the third ventricle (p. 1461).

1. transcallosal approaches: not dependent on dilated ventricles. Higher incidence of venous infarction or forniceal injury (see below)
2. transcortical approach (p. 1466): higher incidence of post-op seizures (≈ 5%). Not feasible with normal sized ventricles (e.g. in patient with VP shunt)
3. stereotactic drainage: see below
4. ventriculoscopic removal: see below

A meta-analysis of 1278 patients comparing endoscopic and various microsurgical techniques found that the microsurgical group had a significantly greater extent of resection (96.8% vs 58.2%), lower rates of recurrence (1.48% vs 3.91%), and lower rates of reoperation than the endoscopic group (0.38% vs 3.0%). Both groups had similar rates of mortality (1.4% vs 0.6%) and shunt dependency (6.2% vs 3.9%). Overall, the complication rate was lower in the endoscopic group than in the microsurgical group (10.5% vs 16.3%). Within the microsurgery group, the transcallosal approach had a lower overall morbidity rate (14.4%) than the transcortical approach (24.5%).[13]

Using natural history for treatment decisions

A review of 58 asymptomatic patients (average age 57 yr) with incidentally discovered colloid cysts of the third ventricle with mean follow up of 79 months demonstrated the incidence of symptomatic worsening at 2, 5, and 10 year follow up to be 0%,0%, and 8%, respectively. Of the 34 patients who obtained follow up imaging, 32 demonstrated no change in cyst size or ventricular caliber. The average age of these patients was significantly higher than that of the patients undergoing surgery for symptomatic lesions (57 vs 41) and thus may reflect a patient cohort with differing natural histories.[14]

NB: Many "asymptomatic" patients may have headaches at diagnosis. Careful evaluation of headache etiology (i.e. posttraumatic, migrainous, tension, etc) should be undertaken to determine whether the headaches are due to the colloid cyst or if the cyst is asymptomatic.

Pollock et al.[10]reviewed 155 patients with newly diagnosed colloid cysts, performing a recursive partitioning analysis, and divided patients into three classes as shown in ▶ Table 48.4.

Additionally, a significantly greater number Class III patients had hyperintense cyst contents on T2 weighted imaging (44% vs 13%) and that symptomatic patients were more likely to have increased T2 signal (44% vs 8%) compared to asymptomatic counterparts. The authors suggest that asymptomatic patients with low T2 signal containing cysts may reflect a group with low potential for cyst expansion and development of cyst related symptoms (even in the presence of ventriculomegaly) – thus they may represent a population that may be safely managed in a nonoperative fashion.[10] Nevertheless, most surgeons would recommend surgery for a patient with ventriculomegaly and symptoms such as headache even if they may not be definitely related.

48

Transcallosal approach

Access to the 3rd ventricle via either the foramen of Monro or by interfornicial approach. Since colloid cysts tend to occur exactly at the foramen of Monro, it is *rarely* necessary to enlarge the foramen to locate the tumor. See Transcallosal approach to lateral or third ventricle (p. 1462).

Stereotactic drainage of colloid cysts

May be useful,[15] especially in patients with normal ventricles from shunting, but the contents may be too viscous,[16] and the tough capsule may make blind penetration difficult. Total or even subtotal aspiration may not require further treatment in some patients; however, recurrence rate is higher than with surgical removal.[17]

Early morbidity was relatively high from this procedure (not widely reported in literature) possibly from vascular injury or mechanical trauma; this has improved. May be more feasible with intraoperative ventriculography[18] or with a ventriculoscope[19] (some say this is the initial procedure of choice,[20] with craniotomy reserved for treatment failures).

Two features that correlate with *unsuccessful* stereotactic aspiration[21]:

1. high viscosity: correlates with hyperdensity on CT (low viscosity correlated with hypo- or isodense CT appearance; no MRI finding correlated with viscosity)
2. deflection of the cyst from tip of aspirating needle due to small size

Table 48.4 Classes of colloid cyst based on recursive partitioning analysis

Class	Age	Cyst diameter	Ventricles	Symptomatic patients /% of total)	Treatment options
I	> 50 yrs	< 10 mm	Normal	12%	May be monitored clinically and with serial imaging (CT or MRI)
II	> 50 yrs	< 10 mm	Ventriculomegaly	50%	If asymptomatic, may be monitored clinically and with serial imaging (CT or MRI)
III	< 50 yrs	> 10 mm	Ventriculomegaly	85%	Surgical removal is recommended

Stereotactic technique[22]:
1. insertion point of stereotactic needle is just anterior to right coronal suture
2. start with sharp-tipped 1.8 mm probe, and advance to 3–5 mm beyond target site (to accommodate for displacement of cyst wall)
3. use a 10 ml syringe and apply 6–8 ml of negative aspiration pressure
4. if this does not yield any material, repeat with a 2.1 mm probe
5. although complete cyst evacuation is desirable, if this cannot be accomplished an acceptable goal of aspiration is re-establishment of patency of the ventricular pathways (may be verified by injecting 1–2 cc of iohexol)

48.3 Epidermoid and dermoid tumors

48.3.1 General information

AKA epidermoid or dermoid cysts.

Both are usually developmental, benign tumors that may arise when retained ectodermal implants are trapped by two fusing ectodermal surfaces. The growth rate of these tumors is linear, like skin (rather than exponential, as with neoplastic tumors).

They may occur in the following locations:

48

1. calvaria: skull involvement (p. 776) occurs when ectodermal rests are included in the developing cranium, epidural extension may occur with growth
2. intracranial: the most common sites include
   a) suprasellar: commonly produce bitemporal hemianopsia and optic atrophy, and only occasionally pituitary (endocrine) symptoms (including DI)
   b) sylvian fissure: may present with seizures
   c) cerebellopontine angle (CPA): may produce trigeminal neuralgia, especially in young patient
   d) basilar-posterior fossa: may produce lower cranial nerve findings, cerebellar dysfunction, and/or corticospinal tract abnormalities
   e) within the ventricular system: occur within the 4th ventricle more commonly than any other
3. scalp
4. within the spinal canal:
   a) most arise in the thoracic or upper lumbar spine
   b) epidermoids of the lower lumbar spine may occur iatrogenically following LP; see Lumbar puncture (p. 1504)
   c) dermoids of the spinal canal are usually associated with a dermal sinus tract (p. 270) and may produce recurrent bouts of spinal meningitis.

48.3.2 Comparison of dermoids and epidermoids

Distinguishing features between the two tumors are shown in ▶ Table 48.5.

Table 48.5 Comparison of epidermoids and dermoid

Feature	Epidermoid	Dermoid
Frequency	0.5–1.5% of brain tumors	0.3% of brain tumors
Lining	stratified squamous epithelium	also include dermal appendage organs (hair follicles and sebaceous glands)
Contents	keratin, cellular debris, and cholesterol, occasional hair	same as epidermoids, plus hair and sebum
Location	more common laterally (e.g. CP angle)	more commonly near midline
Associated anomalies	tend to be isolated lesions	associated with other congenital anomalies in up to 50% of cases
Meningitis	may have recurrent aseptic meningitis, including Mollarets meningitis (p. 762)	may have repeated bouts of bacterial meningitis

48.3.3 Epidermoid cysts

General information

Key concepts

- usually arise from ectoderm trapped within or displaced into the CNS
- predilection for: CP angle, 4th ventricle, suprasellar region, spinal cord
- sometimes AKA cholesteatoma (not to be confused with cholesterol granuloma)
- grow at linear rate (unlike exponential rate of true neoplasms)
- imaging: CSF-like mass (hi-signal on DWMRI is the best test to differentiate)
- may produce aseptic meningitis (Mollaret's meningitis is one form)
- treatment: surgical excision. XRT has no role

AKA cholesteatoma (not cholesterol granuloma, (see below), AKA pearly tumor, AKA ectodermal inclusion cyst (see ▶ Table 48.5 for comparison to dermoids). Although epidermoids and cholesteatomas are histologically identical (both arise from epithelium entrapped in an abnormal location, epidermoids are intradural, cholesteatomas are extradural), the term cholesteatoma is most often used to describe the lesion in the middle ear where the entrapped epithelium usually arises from chronic middle ear infections which lead to a retraction pocket (rarely, may instead be congenital).

▶ **May arise from any of the following**[23]:
1. displaced dorsal midline ectodermal cell rests trapped during neural tube closure between gestational weeks 3–5
2. multipotential embryonic cell rests
3. epithelial cell rests carried to the CPA with the developing otic vesicle
4. epidermal cells displaced into CNS, e.g. by LP – see Lumbar puncture (p. 1504) – or repeated percutaneous cranial subdural taps[24]

Epidemiology

Epidermoids comprise 1% of intracranial tumors556, and ≈ 7% of CPA tumors. Peak age of occurrence: 40 years. No gender difference.

Histology

Epidermoids are lined by stratified squamous epithelium, and contain keratin (from desquamated epithelium), cellular debris, and cholesterol.[25] Growth occurs at a linear rate like normal skin, unlike the exponential growth of true neoplasms.[26] The cyst contents may be liquid or may have a flaky consistency. They tend to spread along normal cleavage planes and surround vital structures (cranial nerves, ICA...). Bony destruction occurs in a minority, usually with larger tumors. Rare degeneration to squamous cell cancer[27] primarily in cases of repeated recurrences after multiple surgeries.

Distinction from cholesterol granuloma

Epidermoid cysts are sometimes mistakenly equated with cholesterol granulomas,[28] possibly because of the similarity between the terms cholesteatoma and cholesterol granuloma. However, these are distinct lesions.[29] Cholesterol granulomas usually occur following chronic inflammation (usually in pneumatized portions of the temporal bone: petrous apex, mastoid air cells, middle ear space). Some differences are delineated in ▶ Table 48.6.

Presentation

1. may present as any mass lesion in the same location
2. CPA lesions can produce V, VII or VIII neuropathies
3. recurrent episodes of aseptic meningitis caused by rupture of the cyst contents, which may also lead to hydrocephalus.
   a) Symptoms include fever and meningeal irritation.

Table 48.6 Characteristics of epidermoid & cholesteatoma vs. cholesterol granuloma

Feature	Epidermoid	Cholesteatoma	Cholesterol granuloma
origin	ectodermal cells in abnormal location		chronic inflammatory cells surrounding cholesterol crystals (? from breakdown of RBC membranes)
	(within CNS, intradural)	(within ear, extradural)	
precursor	usually congenital, occasionally acquired, e.g. after LP (p. 1507)	usually acquired (following chronic infection ? due to epithelial cells from tympanic membrane), occasionally congenital	chronic middle ear infection or idiopathic hemotympanum
symptoms	vary depending on location	chronic hearing loss, ear drainage, pain or numbness around ear	usually involve vestibular or cochlear dysfunction
Imaging (may not reliably distinguish among these)	**CT**: low density; no enhancement; bone erosion in only 33% **MRI**: T1WI: intensity slightly > CSF; T2WI: tumor & CSF similar hi intensity		**CT**: homogeneous & isodense; rim enhancement; extensive destruction of petrous bone **MRI**: increased signal on both T1WI and T2WI
gross appearance	pearly white		brown (from hemosiderin)
Microscopic pathology[32]	hyperkeratotic cyst lined with stratified squamous epithelium		fibroblastic proliferation, hemosiderin-laden macrophages, cholesterol clefts, giant cell reaction
ideal treatment	aggressive near-total excision		subtotal resection followed by drainage & restoration of pneumatization[33]

b) CSF shows pleocytosis, hypoglycorrhachia, elevated protein, and negative cultures. Cholesterol crystals may be seen and can be recognized by their amorphous birefringent appearance.
c) Mollaret's meningitis is a rare variant of aseptic meningitis which includes the finding of large cells in the CSF that resemble endothelial cells (which may be macrophages564) that may be seen in some patients with epidermoid cysts[30,31]

Imaging

MRI ▶ Fig. 48.1: mimics CSF on T1WI (low signal, may be slightly > CSF) and T2WI (high signal). Tumors are usually also high signal on T2WI, but most enhance with contrast on T1WI (epidermoids do not enhance). An epidermoid may pass from the posterior fossa through the incisura to the middle fossa.

Diffusion weighted imaging (DWI) is the best test to differentiate epidermoids from CSF (e.g. as in similar appearing arachnoid cyst). Epidermoids show intense signal on DWI as a result of restriction of water movement.

Treatment

Caution when removing epidermoid cysts to minimize spilling contents as they are quite irritating and may cause severe chemical meningitis (Mollaret's meningitis, see above). Berger[23] advocates intraoperative irrigation with hydrocortisone (100 mg/L of LR) to reduce the risk of post-op communicating hydrocephalus. Peri-operative IV steroids and copious saline irrigation during surgery may provide similar results. The tumor is not in the cyst wall, and the surgical plan is generally to remove as much as possible but to leave capsule adherent to critical structures such as brainstem and blood vessels as the morbidity of removal is high and a small residual does not preclude satisfactory outcome.

In spite of adequate removal, it is not unusual to see persistent brainstem distortion on post-op imaging.[29] Post-op radiation is not indicated as the tumor is benign and XRT does not prevent recurrence.[34]

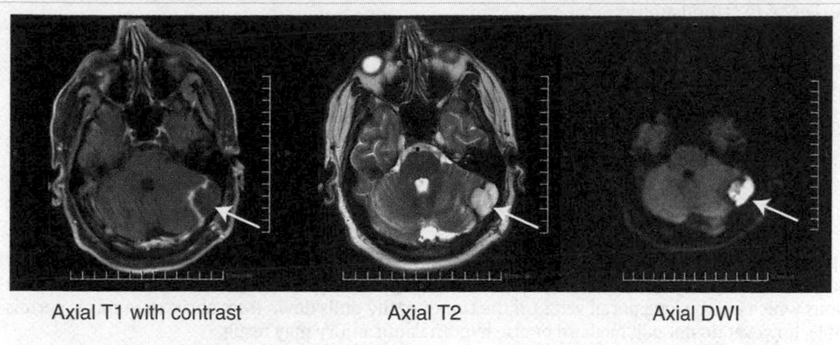

Fig. 48.1 MRI demonstrating left cerebellopontine angle epidermoid. Note that the CSF is dark on the DWI

48.4 Craniopharyngioma

48.4.1 General information

Craniopharyngiomas (**CP**) are tumors that develop from residual cells of Rathke's pouch (p. 149), and tend to arise from the anterior superior margin of the pituitary. They are lined with stratified squamous epithelium. Some CP may arise primarily within the third ventricle.[35] Almost all CP have solid and cystic components; fluid in the cysts varies, but usually contains cholesterol crystals. CP do not undergo malignant degeneration; but difficulty in cure makes them malignant in behavior.[36(p 905–15)] CP are distinct from Rathke's cleft cyst, but share some similarities (see below).

Calcification: microscopically 50%. Plain x-ray: 85% in childhood, 40% in adults.

48.4.2 Epidemiology

Incidence: 2.5–4% of all brain tumors; about 50% occur in childhood (9% of Matson's series). Peak incidence: age 5–10 yrs.

48.4.3 Anatomy

Arterial supply: usually small feeders from ACA and A-comm, or from ICA and P-comm (do not receive blood from PCA or BA-bifurcation unless blood supply of floor of third ventricle is parasitized).

48.4.4 Surgical treatment

Pre-op endocrinologic evaluation

As for pituitary tumor (p. 730). Hypoadrenalism may be corrected rapidly, but hypothyroidism takes longer; either condition can increase surgical mortality.

Approach

Usually via large right frontotemporal flap as low as possible along base of frontal fossa (lateral sphenoid wing rongeured/drilled). Approach to tumor is extra-axial, whether subfrontal or frontotemporal. *All* tumors should be aspirated (even if they appear solid radiographically). Then, with microscope, possible approaches include:

1. subchiasmatic: through space between optic nerves and anterior to chiasm. It was thought that a "prefixed chiasm" (i.e. congenitally short optic nerves with chiasm unusually close to the planum sphenoidale) was more common in patients with CP, making this approach more difficult. However, in reality the chiasm is probably bowed anteriorly by the tumor within the third ventricle giving the illusion of a prefixed chiasm in most cases
2. opticocarotid (between right ICA and right optic nerve/tract)
3. lamina terminalis (tumor often needs to be brought down and removed subchiasmatically)[35,37]

4. lateral to carotid artery
5. transfrontal-transsphenoidal: drill off tuberculum sellae

Alternative approaches to frontotemporal
1. pure transsphenoidal: if dark fluid is aspirated with no CSF evident, it is possible to leave a stent from the tumor cavity to the sphenoid air-sinus to permit continued drainage
2. transcallosal: strictly for tumors limited to the third ventricle
3. a combined subfrontal/pterional approach capitalizes on the advantages of each (head is positioned with slight lateral rotation)

Spare the following structures: small arterial feeders to *undersurface* of the chiasm (major supply) and tract; at least a remnant of pituitary stalk (recognized by unique pattern of longitudinal striations which are the long portal veins). If the tumor easily pulls down from above then this is permissible, however do not pull too hard or else hypothalamic injury may result.

Post-op

1. steroids: these patients are all considered hypo-adrenal. Give hydrocortisone in physiologic doses (for mineralocorticoid activity) in addition to dexamethasone (glucocorticoid that treats edema) taper. Taper steroids slowly to avoid aseptic (chemical) meningitis
2. diabetes insipidus (DI) (p. 752): often shows up early. May be part of a "triphasic response." Best managed initially with fluid replacement. If necessary, use short acting vasopressin (prevents iatrogenic renal shutdown if a SIADH-like phase develops during vasopressin therapy)

48

48.4.5 Radiation

Controversial. **Side effects:** include endocrine dysfunction, optic neuritis, dementia. Post-op XRT probably helps prevent regrowth when residual tumor is left behind,[38] however, in pediatric cases it may be best to postpone XRT (to minimize deleterious effect on IQ), recognizing that reoperation may be necessary for recurrence.

48.4.6 Outcome

5–10% mortality in most series, most from hypothalamic injury (unilateral hypothalamic lesions are rarely clinically evident; bilateral injuries may produce hyperthermia and somnolence; damage to anterior osmoreceptors may → loss of thirst sensation). Five year survival is ≈ 55–85% (range from 30–93% has been reported).

48.4.7 Recurrence

Most recurrences are in < 1 year, few > 3 yrs (very delayed recurrence usually follow what was thought to be "total" removal). Morbidity/mortality is higher with re-operation.

References

[1] Maggio WW, Cail WS, Brookeman JR, et al. Rathke's Cleft Cyst: Computed Tomographic and Magnetic Resonance Imaging Appearances. Neurosurgery. 1987; 21:60–62

[2] Nishio S, Mizuno J, Barrow DL, Takei Y, Tindall GT. Pituitary Tumors Composed of Adenohypophysial Adenoma and Rathke's Cleft Cyst Elements: A Clinicopathological Study. Neurosurgery. 1987; 21:371–377

[3] Voelker JL, Campbell RL, Muller J. Clinical, Radiographic, and Pathological Features of Symptomatic Rathke's Cleft Cysts. J Neurosurg. 1991; 74:535–544

[4] Little JR, MacCarty CS. Colloid Cysts of the Third Ventricle. J Neurosurg. 1974; 39:230–235

[5] Ciric I, Zivin I. Neuroepithelial (Colloid) Cysts of the Septum Pellucidum. J Neurosurg. 1975; 43:69–73

[6] Guner M, Shaw MDM, Turner JW, et al. Computed Tomography in the Diagnosis of Colloid Cyst. Surg Neurol. 1976; 6:345–348

[7] Ryder JW, Kleinschmidt BK, Keller TS. Sudden Deterioration and Death in Patients with Benign Tumors of the Third Ventricle Area. J Neurosurg. 1986; 64:216–223

[8] Tatter SB, Ogilvy CS, Golden JA, Ojemann RG, Louis DN. Third ventricular xanthogranulomas clinically and radiologically mimicking colloid cysts. Report of two cases. J Neurosurg. 1994; 81:605–609

[9] Mamourian AC, Cromwell LD, Harbaugh RE. Colloid Cyst of the Third Ventricle: Sometimes More Conspicuous on CT Than MR. AJNR. 1998; 19:875–878

[10] Pollock BE, Schreiner SA, Huston J, III. A theory on the natural history of colloid cysts of the third ventricle. Neurosurgery. 2000; 46:1077–81; discussion 1081-3

[11] El Khoury C, Brugieres P, Decq P, Cosson-Stanescu R, Combes C, Ricolfi F, Gaston A. Colloid cysts of the third ventricle: are MR imaging patterns predictive of difficulty with percutaneous treatment? AJNR Am J Neuroradiol. 2000; 21:489–492

[12] Torkildsen A. Should Extirpation be Attempted in Cases of Neoplasm in or Near the Third Ventricle of the Brain? Experiences with a Palliative Method. J Neurosurg. 1948; 5:249–275

[13] Sheikh AB, Mendelson ZS, Liu JK. Endoscopic versus microsurgical resection of colloid cysts: a systematic review and meta-analysis of 1,278 patients. World Neurosurg. 2014; 82:1187–1197

[14] Pollock BE, Huston J, III. Natural history of asymptomatic colloid cysts of the third ventricle. J Neurosurg. 1999; 91:364–369
[15] Bosch DA, Rahn T, Backlund EO. Treatment of Colloid Cyst of the Third Ventricle by Stereotactic Aspiration. Surg Neurol. 1978; 9:15–18
[16] Rivas JJ, Lobato RD. CT-Assisted Stereotaxic Aspiration of Colloid Cysts of the Third Ventricle. J Neurosurg. 1985; 62:238–242
[17] Mathiesen T, Grane P, Lindquist C, von Holst H. High Recurrence Rate Following Aspiration of Colloid Cysts in the Third Ventricle. J Neurosurg. 1993; 78:748–752
[18] Musolino A, Fosse S, Munari C, et al. Diagnosis and Treatment of Colloid Cysts of the Third Ventricle by Stereotactic Drainage. Report on Eleven Cases. Surg Neurol. 1989; 32:294–299
[19] Apuzzo MLJ, Chandrasoma PT, Zelman V, Giannotta SL, et al. Computed Tomographic Guidance Stereotaxis in the Management of Lesions of the Third Ventricular Region. Neurosurgery. 1984; 15:502–508
[20] Apuzzo MLJ. Comment on Garrido E, et al.: Cerebral Venous and Sagittal Sinus Thrombosis After Transcallosal Removal of a Colloid Cyst of the Third Ventricle: Case Report. Neurosurgery. 1990; 26
[21] Kondziolka D, Lunsford LD. Stereotactic Management of Colloid Cysts: Factors Predicting Success. J Neurosurg. 1991; 75:45–51
[22] Hall WA, Lunsford LD. Changing Concepts in the Treatment of Colloid Cysts. An 11-Year Experience in the CT Era. J Neurosurg. 1987; 66:186–191
[23] Berger MS, Wilson CB. Epidermoid Cysts of the Posterior Fossa. J Neurosurg. 1985; 62:214–219
[24] Gutin PH, Boehm J, Bank WO, Edwards MS, Rosegay H. Cerebral convexity epidermoid tumor subsequent to multiple percutaneous subdural aspirations. Case report. J Neurosurg. 1980; 52:574–577
[25] Fleming JFR, Botterell EH. Cranial Dermoid and Epidermoid Tumors. Surg Gynecol Obstet. 1959; 109:57–79
[26] Alvord EC. Growth Rates of Epidermoid Tumors. Ann Neurol. 1977; 2:367–370
[27] Link MJ, Cohen PL, Breneman JC, Tew JM, Jr. Malignant squamous degeneration of a cerebellopontine angle epidermoid tumor. Case report. J Neurosurg. 2002; 97:1237–1243
[28] Sabin HI, Bardi LT, Symon L. Epidermoid Cysts and Cholesterol Granulomas Centered on the Posterior Fossa: Twenty Years of Diagnosis and Management. Neurosurgery. 1987; 21:798–803
[29] Altschuler EM, Jungreis CA, Sekhar LN, Jannetta PJ, et al. Operative Treatment of Intracranial Epidermoid Cysts and Cholesterol Granulomas: Report of 21 Cases. Neurosurgery. 1990; 26:606–614
[30] Abramson RC, Morawetz RB, Schlitt M. Multiple Complications from an Intracranial Epidermoid Cyst: Case Report and Literature Review. Neurosurgery. 1989; 24:574–578
[31] Szabo M, Majtenyi C, Gusea A. Contribution to the Background of Mollaret's Meningitis. Acta Neuropathol. 1983; 59:115–118
[32] Friedman I. Epidermoid Cholesteatoma and Cholesterol Granuloma: Experimental and Human. Ann Otol Rhinol Laryngol. 1959; 68:57–79
[33] Chang P, Fagan PA, Atlas MD, Roche J. Imaging destructive lesions of the petrous apex. Laryngoscope. 1998; 108:599–604
[34] Keville FJ, Wise BL. Intracranial Epidermoid and Dermoid Tumors. J Neurosurg. 1959; 16:564–569
[35] Klein HJ, Rath SA. Removal of Tumors of the III Ventricle Using Lamina Terminalis Approach: Three Cases of Isolated Growth of Craniopharyngiomas in the III Ventricle. Childs Nerv Syst. 1989; 5:144–147
[36] Wilkins RH, Rengachary SS. Neurosurgery. New York 1985
[37] Patterson RH, Denylevich A. Surgical Removal of Craniopharyngiomas by a Transcranial Approach through the Lamina Terminalis and Sphenoid Sinus. Neurosurgery. 1980; 7:111–117
[38] Manaka S, Teramoto A, Takakura K. The Efficacy of Radiotherapy for Craniopharyngioma. J Neurosurg. 1985; 62:648–656

49 Pseudotumor Cerebri and Empty Sella Syndrome

49.1 Pseudotumor cerebri

49.1.1 General information

Key concepts

- papilledema and symptomatic ICP elevation > 20 cm H_2O in the absence of intracranial mass or infection. Often associated with dural sinus thrombosis
- a preventable cause of (often permanent) blindness from optic atrophy
- more common in obese females of childbearing age than general population
- recommended work-up:
  - preferred imaging studies: ✔ brain MRI (without & with contrast) and MRV. Imaging should be normal (allowed exception: slit-like ventricles)
  - ✔ LP. Findings: opening pressure (> 25 cm H_2O) & normal CSF analysis
  - ✔ ophthalmologic eval: test visual fields, acuity, and check for papilledema
- usually self-limited, recurrence is common, chronic in some patients
- risk of blindness is not reliably correlated to duration of symptoms, papilledema, H/A, Snellen visual acuity, or number of recurrences
- treatment for patients failing medical management (weight loss, Diamox...):
  - optic nerve sheath fenestration (ONSF) is best for visual loss without H/A
  - CSF shunt may be better than ONSF for H/A associated with visual loss

49

Pseudotumor cerebri (PTC) AKA idiopathic intracranial hypertension (IIH), AKA benign intracranial hypertension, (plus numerous other obsolete terms[1]) is a condition (or perhaps a heterogeneous group of conditions) characterized by increased intracranial pressure with no evidence of intracranial mass, hydrocephalus, infection (e.g. meningitis, especially chronic ones such as fungal meningitis), or hypertensive encephalopathy. Some, but not all, authors exclude patients with intracranial hypertension in the presence of dural sinus thrombosis. PTC is thus a diagnosis of *exclusion*. There is a juvenile and an adult form.

In general, the term pseudotumor cerebri is preferred (what was old is new!) because it encompases cases where there is a known etiology as well as idiopathic cases (the concept of "secondary idiopathic intracranial hypertension" is an oxymoron).

49.1.2 Epidemiology

1. female:male ratio reported ranges from 2:1 to 8:1 (no gender difference in juvenile form)
2. obesity is reported in 11–90% of cases, and is not as prevalent in men[2]
3. incidence among obese women of childbearing years[3,4]: 19–21/100,000, (whereas incidence in general population[1]: 1–2/100,000)
4. peak incidence in 3rd decade (range: 1–55 years). 37% of cases are in children, 90% of these are age 5–15 years. Very rare in infancy
5. frequently self limited (recurrence rate: 9–43%)
6. severe visual deficits develop in 4–12%, unrelated to duration of symptoms, degree of papilledema, headache, visual obscuration, and number of recurrences.[5] Perimetry is the best means to detect and follow visual loss

49.1.3 Pathogenesis

Pathogenesis is not fully understood. Increased cerebral edema & brain water content, increased venous pressure & cerebral blood volume, and reduced CSF absorption have all been demonstrated. Theories that also explain the high prevalence in obese females:

1. mechanical theory: obesity → ↑ intraabdominal pressure → ↑ central venous pressure → ↑ CSF resorption → ↑ ICP (however, other studies have indicated that elevated venous pressure may actually be an epiphenomenon to a primary increase in ICP[6])
2. hormonal theory: adipocytes convert androstenedione → estrone → ↑ CSF production

Table 49.1 Modified Dandy's criteria for PT
• signs & symptoms of increased ICP • no localizing signs other than Cr. N VI palsy[a] in an otherwise awake and alert patient • increased CSF pressure without chemical or cytological abnormalities • normal to small ventricles and no intracranial mass
[a] may result from ↑ ICP (p. 567)

49.1.4 Diagnostic criteria

Modified Dandy's criteria are shown in ▶ Table 49.1.

More specifically, four diagnostic criteria[7]:

1. CSF pressure: > 20 cm H_20 (pressures > 40 are not uncommon). Some recommend that the pressure should be > 25 to exclude normals.[8] **Note:** Diurnal variations in CSF pressure may occasionally cause a falsely low (i.e. normal) reading. ∴ If clinical suspicion is high, an LP at a different time of day or continuous ICP monitoring may be required.
2. CSF composition: normal glucose and cell count. Protein is normal, or in ≈ two thirds of cases it is low (< 20 mg%)
3. symptoms & signs are those of elevated ICP alone (i.e. papilledema & H/A) with no focal findings. Allowed exception: abducens nerve palsy which may be due to increased ICP (p. 567)
4. normal radiologic studies of the brain (CT or MRI) with the allowed exceptions of:
   a) the occasionally seen slit ventricles (the incidence may be no higher in PTC than in age-matched controls[9]) or empty sella
   b) infantile form may have generous ventricles and large fluid spaces over brain
   c) intra-orbital abnormalities may be seen: see below

49

49.1.5 Clinical

Symptoms

See references.[7,10]

1. classic (major) symptoms
   a) H/A (the most common symptom): 94–99%. Typically retro-ocular and pulsatile. May ↑ with eye movement. Severity does *not* correlate with degree of CSF pressure elevation. Occasionally worse in A.M.
   b) nausea: 32% (actual vomiting is less common)
   c) visual loss (PTC below):
      - transient visual obscuration (TVO)
      - permanent afferent visual pathway injury
   d) diplopia (more common in adult, usually due to VI nerve palsy): 30%
2. minor symptoms[11]
   a) neck stiffness: 30–50%
   b) tinnitus (the causal relationship with IIH has been demonstrated by resolution of these symptoms with reduction of CSF pressure): up to 60%. Usually pulse synchronous. Described as rushing noise. May be unilateral (in these, may be reduced by ipsilateral jugular vein compression + ipsilateral head rotation)
   c) ataxia: 4–11%
   d) acral paresthesias: 25%
   e) retrobulbar eye pain on eye movements
   f) arthralgia: 11–18%
   g) dizziness: 32%
   h) fatigue
   i) reduced olfactory acuity

Signs

Signs are generally restricted to visual system.

Conspicuously *absent*: altered level of consciousness in spite of high ICP

1. eye findings – also PTC below
   a) papilledema:
      - present in almost ≈ 100%

 - idiopathic intracranial hypertension without papilledema (**IIHWOP**)[12]: a variant of IIH. Visual loss tends not to occur
 - usually bilateral, occasionally unilateral[13]
 - may be mild (subtle nerve fiber elevation)

b) abducens nerve (Cr. N. VI) palsy: 20%; a false localizing sign (p. 567). The esotropia ranges from < 5 prism diopters dysconjugate angle in primary gaze to > 50[14]

c) visual acuity: relatively insensitive assessment of visual function

d) visual field defect: 9%.
 - early changes: peripheral fields & nasal quadrant defect
 - enlarged blind spot (66%) and concentric constriction of peripheral fields (blindness is very rare at presentation)

2. infantile form may have only enlarging OFC, frequently self limited, usually requires only follow-up without specific treatment

▶ **Note.** Worsening of any of the above symptoms with postural changes that increase ICP (bending over, Valsalva maneuver…) is characteristic in idiopathic intracranial hypertension.

Visual loss in PTC

General information

Quoted range of occurrence in PTC: 48–68% (lower numbers generally come from population based samples). A prospective study found changes by Goldman perimetry in 96% of 50 patients.[15] The only parameter associated with worsening vision is recent weight gain.

49

Pathomechanics

Increased ICP is transmitted along optic nerve sheath → circumferential compression of the retinal ganglion cell axons at the level of the lamina cribrosa.[14]

Manifestations

1. transient visual obscurations (TVO): graying or blacking out of vision. Lasts ≈ 1 second. Uni- or bi-lateral. Typically occur with eye movement, bending over or valsalva maneuver. Directly proportional to severity of papilledema. Frequency of TVOs parallels ICP elevation, but doesn't correlate with permanent visual loss
2. visual loss in PTC may occur early or late, may be sudden or gradually progressive, and is not reliably correlated to duration of symptoms, papilledema, H/A, Snellen visual acuity, or number of recurrences. It may escape detection until profound.
   a) early: usually constriction of fields and loss of color (∴ perimetry is the best test for following vision in PTC)
   b) late: central vision is affected. Findings include: concentric constrictions, enlargement of the blind spot, inferior nasal defects, arcuate defects, cecocentral scotomas…

49.1.6 Associated conditions

General information

Some cases of PTC are idiopathic (IIH). However, often what is considered "IIH" may actually be secondary to some other condition (e.g. transverse sinus thrombosis, see below). Many conditions cited as being associated with PTC may be coincidental. Four criteria suggested to establish a cause-effect relationship are shown in ▶ Table 49.2.[10]

▶ Table 49.3 shows a scale[16] to rank the likelihood of association between various conditions and IIH based on the number of the criteria met in ▶ Table 49.2.

Other conditions not included in this list that meet minimal criteria but are unconfirmed in case-control studies[1] include:

1. other drugs: isotretinoin (Accutane®), trimethoprim-sulfamethoxazole, cimetidine, tamoxifen
2. systemic lupus erythematosus (SLE)

Table 49.2 Criteria for causality of PTC by another condition[10]
• meets Dandy's criteria (▶ Table 49.1) • the condition should be proven to increase ICP • treatment of the condition should improve the IIH • properly controlled studies should show an association between the condition and IIH

Table 49.3 Conditions that may be associated with PTC[16]

Proven association
Meets 4 criteria from ▸ Table 49.2
• obesity
Likely association
Meets 3 criteria from ▸ Table 49.2
• drugs: keprone, lindane • hypervitaminosis A
Probable association
Meets 2 criteria from ▸ Table 49.2
• steroid withdrawal[a] • thyroid replacement in children • ketoprofen & indomethacin in Bartter syndrome • hypoparathyroidism • Addison's disease[a] • uremia • iron deficiency anemia • drugs: tetracycline, nalidixic acid, Danazol, lithium, amiodarone, phenytoin, nitrofurantoin, ciprofloxacin, nitroglycerin
Possible association
Meets 1 criterion from ▸ Table 49.2
• menstrual irregularity • oral contraceptive use[b] • Cushing's syndrome • Vitamin A deficiency • minor head trauma • Behçet syndrome
Unlikely association
Meets none of the criteria in ▸ Table 49.2
• hyperthyroidism • steroid use • immunization
Unsupported association
• pregnancy • menarche
[a]may respond to steroids [b]may be associated with dural sinus thrombosis, see text

49

Conditions that may be related by virtue of increased pressure in the dural sinuses (see below):
1. otitis media with petrosal extension (so-called otitic hydrocephalus)
2. radical neck surgery with resection of the jugular vein
3. hypercoagulable states

Venous hypertension and sinovenous abnormalities

Venous hypertension has often been proposed as a unifying underlying cause of PTC. Abnormalities of the dural sinuses, including thrombosis, stenosis,[17] obstruction, or elevated pressure (reaching levels as high as 40 mm Hg) have been demonstrated in a number of studies. While these findings may underlie a significant number of cases, they may in actuality be epiphenomena (e.g. venous hypertension may be due to compression of the transverse sinuses by elevated intracranial pressure[6]), and it is unlikely that such abnormalities will explain all cases.

Bilateral sinovenous stenosis was seen (using a sophisticated but sensitive test of elliptic-centric-ordered 3-D gadolinium-enhanced MRI venography) in 27 of 29 patients with PTC and in only 4 of 59 controls.[17]

49.1.7 Differential diagnosis

1. true mass lesions: tumor, cerebral abscess, subdural hematomas, rarely gliomatosis cerebri may be undetectable on CT and will be misdiagnosed as PTC
2. cranial venous outflow impairment (some authors consider these as IIH)[18]
   a) dural sinus thrombosis (p. 1308)
   b) congestive heart failure
   c) superior vena cava syndrome
   d) unilateral or bilateral jugular vein or sigmoid sinus[19] obstruction
   e) hyperviscosity syndromes
   f) Masson's vegetant intravascular hemangioendothelioma[20]: an uncommon, usually benign lesion that may rarely involve the neuraxis (including intracranial occurrence). Not definitely neoplastic. Organizing thrombi develop endothelialized projections into the vessel lumen. Must be distinguished from other conditions such as angiosarcoma
3. Chiari I malformation (CIM): may produce findings similar to PTC. 6% of PTC patients have significant tonsillar ectopia, and ≈ 5% of patient with CIM have papilledema[14]
4. infection (CSF will be abnormal in most of these): encephalitis, arachnoiditis, meningitis (especially basal meningitis or granulomatous infections, e.g. syphilitic meningitis, chronic cryptococcal meningitis), chronic brucellosis
5. inflammatory conditions: e.g. neurosarcoidosis (p. 189), SLE
6. vasculitis: e.g. Behçet's syndrome
7. metabolic conditions: e.g. lead poisoning
8. pseudopapilledema (anomalous elevation of the optic nerve head) associated with hyperopia and drusen. Retinal venous pulsations are usually present. Especially deceptive when a patient with migraines has pseudopapilledema: treat the H/A
9. malignant hypertension: may produce H/A & bilateral optic disc edema which can be indistinguishable from papilledema. May also produce hypertensive encephalopathy (p. 194). Check BP in all PTC suspects
10. meningeal carcinomatosis
11. Guillain-Barré syndrome (p. 184): CSF protein is usually elevated
12. following head trauma

49.1.8 Evaluation recommendations

Overview

Most tests are intended to rule out conditions that may mimic (or produce) PTC:
1. cerebral imaging: cerebral CT or MRI (see below) scan without and with contrast
2. LP:
   a) measure opening pressure (**OP**) with patient in lateral decubitus position
   b) CSF analysis to rule-out infection (e.g. fungus, TB or Lyme disease), inflammation (e.g. sarcoidosis, SLE) or neoplasm (e.g. carcinomatous meningitis)
      - protein/glucose
      - cell count
      - routine & fungal cultures
      - cytology if suspicion of carcinomatous meningitis
3. routine labs: CBC, electrolytes, PT/PTT
4. W/U for sarcoidosis or SLE if other findings suggestive (e.g. cutaneous nodules, hypercoagulable state…)
5. neuro-ophthalmologic evaluation is recommended. Includes: visual field testing using quantitative perimetry, with evaluation of size of blind spot, slit-lamp examination ± fundus photographs
6. check BP to R/O malignant HTN → hypertensive encephalopathy (p. 770)

CT

CT without and with IV contrast is usually adequate to R/O intracranial mass as a possible cause of intracranial hypertension, but may miss cases of dural sinus thrombosis. MRI & MRV are preferred.

MRI

Intracranial abnormalities are usually absent or minimal (slit ventricles, empty sella in 30–70%). However, intraorbital findings may be more substantial and include[14]:
1. flattening of the posterior sclera: occurs in 80%
2. enhancement of the prelaminar optic nerve: in 50%
3. distention of the perioptic subarachnoid space: in 45%
4. vertical tortuosity of the orbital optic nerve: in 40%
5. intraocular protrusion of the prelaminar optic nerve: in 30%

Venography

MR venography (MRV) has largely replaced conventional venography to rule out dural sinus or venous thrombosis.

49.1.9 Treatment and management

Natural history

Spontaneous resolution is common, sometimes within months, but usually after ≈ 1 year. Papilledema persists in ≈ 15%. *Permanent* visual loss occurs in 2–24% (depending on criteria used and degree to which it is sought). Persistent H/A may occur in some. Recurs in ≈ 10% after initial resolution.[14]

Interventions

Overview

Studies are often difficult to interpret especially since spontaneous remission is common.
1. all patients must have repeated thorough ophthalmologic exams (see above)
2. stop possible offending drugs
3. weight loss: a weight loss of 6% usually results in complete resolution of papilledema.[21] However, resolution may be too slow for acutely threatened vision. Weight loss is also associated with reduction of other health risks of obesity. Symptoms recur if the weight is regained
   a) dieting: uncontrolled studies[22] suggest that this is effective, but is it rarely accomplished or sustained
   b) bariatric surgery: gastric bypass, laparoscopic banding…
4. treatment of asymptomatic PTC patients is controversial as there is no reliable predictor for visual loss. Close follow up with serial formal visual field evaluation is necessary. Intervention is recommended in unreliable patients, or whenever visual fields deteriorate. It is possible to lose vision without H/A or papilledema
5. most cases remit by 6–15 weeks, however relapse is common
6. medical treatment
   a) fluid and salt restriction
   b) diuretics (slows CSF production) – see below
   c) if ineffective, add steroids (options: dexamethasone (Decadron®) 12 mg/day, prednisone 40–60 mg/day, or methylprednisolone 250 mg IV q 6 hrs). May ↑ CSF resorption in cases of inflammation or venous thrombosis. Can be used as temporizing agents for patients awaiting surgery. A reduction in symptoms should occur by 2 weeks, after which time the steroid should be tapered over 2 weeks. Long-term use is not recommended due to, among other things, associated weight gain
7. *surgical therapy*[23 (p 250–3)] only for cases refractory to above, or where visual loss is progressive or is severe initially or unreliable patient:
   a) serial LPs until remission (25% remit after 1st LP[24]): remove up to 30 ml to halve OP, perform qod until OP < 20 cm H_20, then decrease to q wk (no patient who had remission by 2nd LP had OP > 350 on 1st LP). Use a large gauge needle (e.g. 18 Ga) which may help promote a post-LP CSF leak into subcutaneous tissues. LPs may be difficult in obese patients. Revisions may be required in up to 50%. **Side effects:** include sciatica from nerve root irritation, acquired cerebellar tonsillar herniation (p. 418), spinal H/A (from intracranial hypotension)
   b) Shunts: see below
   c) optic nerve sheath fenestration: see below
   d) older treatment less commonly practiced today: subtemporal decompression (advocated by Dandy) or suboccipital decompression. Usually bilateral silver-dollar size craniectomies under

temporalis muscle to floor of middle fossa, open dura, cover brain with absorbable sponge, close fascia and muscle watertight, anticonvulsants were started due to risk of post-op seizures
8. interventional procedures: venous sinus stenting may be considered for refractory cases.[25]
9. patients should be followed at least two years (with repeat imaging, e.g. MRI) to R/O occult tumor

Diuretics

1. carbonic anhydrase (CA) inhibitors:
   a) *acetazolamide* (Diamox®): ℞ start at 125–250 mg PO q 8–12 hrs, or long acting Diamox Sequels® 500 mg PO BID. Increase by 250 mg/day until symptoms improve, side effects occur, or 2 gm/day reached. **Side effects:** (in high doses): acral paresthesias, nausea, metabolic acidosis, altered taste, renal calculi, drowsiness. Rare: Stevens-Johnson syndrome, toxic epidermal necrolysis, agranulocytosis. ✖ Contraindicated with allergy to sulfa or a history of renal calculi
   b) methazolamide (Neptazane®): better tolerated but less effective. ℞ 50–100 mg PO BID-TID. This branded product is no longer on the market. **Side effects:** similar to acetazolamide
   c) topiramate (Topamax®): anticonvulsant with secondary inhibition of CA. ℞ 200 mg PO BID. **Side effects:** Similar to acetazolamide, but can be used in sulfa allergic patients
2. *furosemide* (Lasix®)
   a) start: 160 mg per day in adults, adjust per symptoms and eye exam (not to CSF pressure)
   b) if ineffective, double (320 mg/day)
   c) monitor K^+ levels and supplement as needed

49

Shunts

1. lumbar shunt: usually lumboperitoneal; see insertion technique (p. 1517). May be difficult in obese patient. May need a horizontal-vertical valve (p. 418) to prevent H/A from intracranial hypotension. Alternative: lumbopleural shunt
2. other shunts may be used, especially when arachnoiditis precludes use of lumbar subarachnoid space, e.g.:
   a) VP shunt: often difficult since the ventricles are frequently small or slit-like.[26] Stereotactic techniques may make this more technically feasible
   b) cisterna magna shunt: may shunt to vascular system

Optic nerve sheath fenestration (ONSF)

See references.[27,28,29]

Generally better for protection of vision and reversal of papilledema than for other symptoms (e.g. H/A). Performed via medial or less commonly a lateral orbitotomy or transconjunctival medial approach. May reverse or stabilize visual deterioration[30] and sometimes (but not always) lowers ICP (by continued CSF filtration) and may protect the contralateral eye (if not, contralateral ONSF must be performed). Has succeeded in cases where visual loss progressed after LP shunting,[31] possibly due to poor communication between orbital and intracranial subarachnoid spaces. **Side effects:** potential adverse include: pupillary dysfunction, peripapillary hemorrhage, chemosis, chorioretinal scarring,[32] diplopia (usually self-limited) from medial rectus disruption. Repeat fenestration is needed in 0–6%.[14]

Management recommendations for specific situations

Weight loss should be attempted in all.

1. PTC patients with H/A and no visual loss: medical therapy to control ↑ ICP and H/A. ONSF *not* recommended. Shunting is an option if medical management fails
2. PTC with visual loss without H/A:
   a) mild visual loss: acetazolamide 500–1500 mg/d, follow-up q 2 weeks
   b) moderate visual loss: acetazolamide 2000–3000 mg/d, follow-up q week
   c) severe visual loss, moderate visual loss that doesn't respond to acetazolamide, or optic disc at risk:
      - methylprednisolone 250 mg IV q 6 hrs + acetazolamide 1000 mg PO BID
      - if no improvement: ONSF. Consider shunt if ICP > 300 mm H_2O
   d) PTC with visual loss AND H/A: for patients with surgical indications, either surgical procedure is appropriate. Shunting may relieve both problems simultaneously. ONSF may be more reliable to relieve the visual problems (the failure rate may be lower than the shunt malfunction rate) but is not as good for the H/A

3. IIHWOP: symptomatic treatment for H/A, diuretics
4. PTC in children and adolescents:
   a) may be seen with withdrawal of steroids used for asthma
   b) search for and correction of underlying etiology (offending drugs listed above, hypercalcemia, cancer…)
   c) acetazolamide has been used with success
5. PTC in pregnancy:
   a) women who first present with PTC during pregnancy: resolution of PTC following delivery is common
   b) women who become pregnant during therapy:
      - 1st trimester: observation, limitation of weight gain, serial LPs. ✖ Acetazolamide should be avoided because of teratogenicity
      - 2nd & 3rd trimester: acetazolamide has been used safely, but involvement of high-risk obstetrician specialist is advised
6. pseudopapilledema (associated with drusen, etc., in the absence of intracranial hypertension): no interventions.[14] Reassurance and H/A management are employed

49.2 Empty sella syndrome

49.2.1 General information

Empty sella syndrome (ESS) can be "primary" or "secondary."

49.2.2 Primary empty sella syndrome

General information

Occurs in the absence of prior treatment of a pituitary tumor (medical, surgical or XRT). Herniation of the arachnoid membrane into the sella turcica[33] which can act as a mass, probably as a result of repeated CSF pulsation. The sella can become enlarged (see Sella turcica (p. 216), for normal dimensions) and the pituitary gland may become compressed against the floor.

Frequent association: female sex (female:male ratio = 5:1), obesity and HTN. The frequency of intrasellar arachnoid herniation is higher in patients with pituitary tumors and in those with increased intracranial pressure for any reason – including idiopathic intracranial hypertension (p. 766) – than in the general population.

These patients usually present with symptoms that do not suggest an intrasellar abnormality including: headache (the most common symptom), dizziness, seizures… Occasionally patients may develop CSF rhinorrhea,[34] deterioration of vision (acuity or field deficit resulting from kinking of optic chiasm due to herniation into the sella), or amenorrhea-galactorrhea syndrome.

Clinically evident endocrine disturbances are rare with primary ESS, however up to 30% have abnormal pituitary function tests, most commonly reduced growth hormone secretion following stimulation. Mild elevation of prolactin (PRL) and reduction of ADH may occur, probably from compression of the stalk. These patients show a normal PRL rise with TRH stimulation (whereas patients with prolactinomas do not).

Treatment

Surgical treatment is usually not indicated, except in the case of CSF rhinorrhea. In this setting, it is necessary to determine if there is increased ICP, and if so, if there is an identifiable cause. Simple shunting for hydrocephalus runs the risk of producing tension pneumocephalus from air drawn in through the former leak site. This may necessitate transsphenoidal repair with simultaneous external lumbar drainage, to be converted to a permanent shunt shortly thereafter. Hyperprolactinemia may be treated e.g. with bromocriptine (p. 740) if it interferes with gonadal function.

49.2.3 Secondary empty sella syndrome

Entities associated with secondary empty sella syndrome:
1. following trauma[35]
2. after successful transsphenoidal removal or XRT for a pituitary tumor[35]
3. any cause of increased intracranial pressure, including: idiopathic intracranial hypertension (pseudotumor cerebri), Chiari malformation

Often presents with visual deterioration due to herniation of the optic chiasm into the empty sella. There may be hypopituitarism from the underlying cause.

Visual deterioration may be treated with chiasmapexy (propping up the chiasm) usually by transsphenoidal approach and packing the sella with fat, muscle or cartilage. May be done endoscopically.[36] Appears to be better for improving visual field deficits than loss of visual acuity.[37]

References

[1] Radhakrishnan K, Ahlskog JE, Garrity JA, Kurland LT. Idiopathic Intracranial Hypertension. Mayo Clin Proc. 1994; 69:169–180

[2] Digre KB, Corbett JJ. Pseudotumor Cerebri in Men. Arch Neurol. 1988; 45:866–872

[3] Durcan FJ, Corbett JJ, Wall M. The Incidence of Pseudotumor Cerebri: Population Studies in Iowa and Louisiana. Arch Neurol. 1988; 45:875–877

[4] Radhakrishnan K, Ahlskog JE, Cross SA, Kurland LT, et al. Idiopathic Intracranial Hypertension (Pseudotumor Cerebri): Descriptive Epidemiology in Rochester, Minn, 1976 to 1990. Arch Neurol. 1993; 50:78–80

[5] Rush JA. Pseudotumor Cerebri: Clinical Profile and Visual Outcome in 63 Patients. Mayo Clin Proc. 1980; 55:541–546

[6] King JO, Mitchell PJ, Thomson KR, Tress BM. Manometry combined with cervical puncture in idiopathic intracranial hypertension. Neurology. 2002; 58:26–30

[7] Ahlskog JE, O'Neill BP. Pseudotumor Cerebri. Ann Int Med. 1982; 97:249–256

[8] Corbett JJ, Mehta MP. Cerebrospinal fluid pressure in normal obese subjects and patients with pseudotumor cerebri. Neurology. 1983; 33:1386–1388

[9] Jacobson DM, Karanjia PN, Olson KA, Warner JJ. Computed Tomography Ventricular Size has no Predictive Value in Diagnosing Pseudotumor Cerebri. Neurology. 1990; 40:1454–1455

[10] Giuseffi V, Wall M, Siegel PZ, Rojas PB. Symptoms and disease associations in idiopathic intracranial hypertension (pseudotumor cerebri): a case-control study. Neurology. 1991; 41:239–244

[11] Round R, Keane JR. The minor symptoms of increased intracranial hypertension: 101 patients with benign intracranial hypertension. Neurology. 1988; 38:1461–1464

[12] Wang SJ, Silberstein SD, Patterson S, Young WB. Idiopathic intracranial hypertension without papilledema: a case control study in a headache center. Neurology. 1998; 51:245–249

[13] Sher NA, Wirtschafter J, Shapiro SK, et al. Unilateral Papilledema in 'Benign' Intracranial Hypertension (Pseudotumor Cerebri). JAMA. 1983; 250:2346–2347

[14] Bejjani GK, Cockerham KP, Pless M, Rothfus WE. Idiopathic intracranial hypertension. Contemp Neurosurg. 2002; 24:1–8

[15] Wall M, George D. Idiopathic Intracranial Hypertension: A Prospective Study of 50 Patients. Brain. 1991; 114:155–180

[16] Digre KB. Epidemioligy of idiopathic intracranial hypertension. 1992

[17] Farb RI, Vanek I, Scott JN, Mikulis DJ, Willinsky RA, Tomlinson G, TerBrugge KG. Idiopathic intracranial hypertension: The prevalence and morphology of sinovenous stenosis. Neurology. 2003; 60:1418–1424

[18] Johnston I, Hawke S, Halmagyi M, Teo C. The Pseudotumor Syndrome: Disorders of Cerebrospinal Fluid Circulation Causing Intracranial Hypertension Without Ventriculomegaly. Arch Neurol. 1991; 48:740–747

[19] Powers JM, Schnur JA, Baldree ME. Pseudotumor Cerebri due to Partial Obstruction of the Sigmoid Sinus by a Cholesteatoma. Arch Neurol. 1986; 43:519–521

[20] Wen DY, Hardten DR, Wirtschafter JD, et al. Elevated Intracranial Pressure from Cerebral Venous Obstruction by Masson's Vegetant Intravascular Hemangioendothelioma. J Neurosurg. 1991; 75:787–790

[21] Johnson LN, Krohel GB, Madsen RW, March GA,Jr. The role of weight loss and acetazolamide in the treatment of idiopathic intracranial hypertension (pseudotumor cerebri). Ophthalmology. 1998; 105:2313–2317

[22] Newberg B. Pseudotumor Cerebri Treated by Rice/Reduction Diet. Arch Intern Med. 1974; 133:802–807

[23] Wilkins RH, Rengachary SS. Neurosurgery. New York 1985

[24] Weisberg LA. Benign Intracranial Hypertension. Medicine (Baltimore). 1975; 54:197–207

[25] Higgins JN, Owler BK, Cousins C, Pickard JD. Venous sinus stenting for refractory benign intracranial hypertension. Lancet. 2002; 359:228–230

[26] Hahn FJ, McWilliams FE. The Small Ventricle in Pseudotumor Cerebri: Demonstration of the Small Ventricle in Benign Intracranial Hypertension. CT. 1978; 2:249–253

[27] Brourman ND, Spoor TC, Ramocki JM. Optic Nerve Sheath Decompression for Pseudotumor Cerebri. Arch Ophthalmol. 1988; 106:1384–1390

[28] Sergott RC, Savino PJ, Bosley TM. Modified Optic Nerve Sheath Decompression Provides Long-Term Visual Improvement for Pseudotumor Cerebri. Arch Ophthalmol. 1988; 106:1384–1390

[29] Corbett JJ, Nerad JA, Tse D, et al. Optic Nerve Sheath Fenestration for Pseudotumor Cerebri: The Lateral Orbitotomy Approach. Arch Ophthalmol. 1988; 106:1391–1397

[30] Kelman SE, Heaps R, Wolf A, Elman MJ. Optic Nerve Decompression Surgery Improves Visual Function in Patients with Pseudotumor Cerebri. Neurosurgery. 1992; 30:391–395

[31] Kelman SE, Sergott RC, Cioffi GA, et al. Modified Optic Nerve Decompression in Patients with Functioning Lumboperitoneal Shunts and Progressive Visual Loss. Ophthalmology. 1991; 98:1449–1453

[32] Spoor TC, Ramocki JM, Madion MP, et al. Treatment of Pseudotumor Cerebri by Primary and Secondary Optic Nerve Sheath Decompression. Am J Ophthalmol. 1991; 112:177–185

[33] Kaufman B. The "empty" sella turcica - A manifestation of the intrasellar subarachnoid space. Radiology. 1968; 90:931–941

[34] Perani D, Scotti G, Colombo N, Sterzi R, Castelli A. Spontaneous CSF rhinorrhea through the lamina cribrosa associated with primary empty sella. Ital J Neurol Sci. 1984; 5:167–172

[35] Lee WM, Adams JE. The Empty Sella Syndrome. J Neurosurg. 1968; 28:351–356

[36] Alvarez Berastegui GR, Raza SM, Anand VK, Schwartz TH. Endonasal endoscopic transsphenoidal chiasmapexy using a clival cranial base cranioplasty for visual loss from massive empty sella following macroprolactinoma treatment with bromocriptine: case report. J Neurosurg. 2015:1–7

[37] Fouad W. Review of empty sella syndrome and its surgical mangement. Alexandria Journal of Medicine. 2011; 47:139–147

50 Tumors and Tumor-Like Lesions of the Skull

50.1 Skull tumors

50.1.1 General information

See Skull lesions (p. 1376) for differential diagnosis and evaluation (including non-neoplastic lesions). Considering only tumors, the differential diagnosis includes:

1. benign tumors
   a) osteoma: see below
   b) hemangioma: see below
   c) dermoid and epidermoid tumors: see below
   d) chondroma: occur mainly in conjunction with the basal synchondroses
   e) meningioma
   f) aneurysmal bone cyst
2. malignant tumors: malignancy is suggested by a single large or multiple (> 6) small osteolytic lesions with margins that are ragged, undermined and lacking sclerosis[1]
   a) bone metastases to the skull. Common ones include:
      - prostate
      - breast
      - lung
      - kidney
      - thyroid
      - lymphoma
      - multiple myeloma/plasmacytoma (p. 714)
   b) chondrosarcoma
   c) osteogenic sarcoma
   d) fibrosarcoma

50.1.2 Osteoma

General information

Osteomas are the most common primary bone tumor of the calvaria. They are benign, slow-growing lesions, that occur commonly in the cranial vault, mastoid and paranasal air sinuses, and the mandible. Lesions within air sinuses may present as recurrent sinusitis. More common in females, highest incidence is in 6th decade. Triad of Gardner's syndrome: multiple cranial osteomas (of calvaria, sinuses, and mandible), colonic polyposis, and soft-tissue tumors.

See Localized increased density or hyperostosis of the calvaria (p. 1379) for differential diagnosis.

Pathology

Consists of osteoid tissue within osteoblastic tissue, surrounded by reactive bone. Difficult to distinguish from fibrous dysplasia.

Radiographic evaluation

Skull x-ray: round, sclerotic, well demarcated, homogeneous dense projection. Usually arise from outer table of skull (inner table less common). May be compact or spongy (spongy osteoma may be radiolucent). Unlike meningiomas, diploë are preserved and vascular channels are not increased.

Osteomas are "hot" on nuclear bone scan.

Treatment

Asymptomatic lesions may simply be followed. Surgery may be considered for cosmetic reasons, or if pressure on adjacent tissues produces discomfort. Lesions involving only the outer table may be removed leaving the inner table intact.

50.1.3 Hemangioma

General information

Comprise ≈ 7% of skull tumors.[1] These benign tumors commonly occur in the skull (discussed here) and spine (p. 794). Two types: cavernous (most common) and capillary (rare).

Radiographic evaluation

Skull x-ray: characteristically shows a circular lucency with honeycomb or trabecular pattern (seen in ≈ 50% of cases) or radial trabeculations producing a sunburst pattern (seen in ≈ 11% of cases).[1] Sclerotic margins are evident in only ≈ 33%.

CT: hypodense lesion with sclerotic spaced trabeculations. Nonenhancing.

Bone scan: typically hot.

Treatment

Accessible lesions may be cured by en bloc excision or curettage. The gross appearance is of a hard, blue-domed mass beneath the pericranium. Radiation may be considered for inaccessible tumors.

50.1.4 Epidermoid and dermoid tumors of the skull

General information

See also epidermoids and dermoids in general (p. 776).

50

Dermoids and epidermoids are benign inclusion cysts of ectoderm that may involve skull and underlying dural venous structures or brain. They may become infected. Primary skull involvement is rare and occurs when ectodermal rests are entrapped in the developing skull which causes these tumors to arise within the diploë and expand both inner and outer tables. Because they are not neoplastic, they grow at a linear rate (instead of exponential). Usually midline.

Epidermoid tumors contain only the outer layer of skin, and are therefore lined with stratified squamous epithelium and the resultant byproduct, keratin.

Dermoid tumors contain all elements of skin including hair follicles (which may produce hair in the tumor) sweat glands (sebaceous glands (apocrine) and sweat glands (eccrine)).[2]

Teratomas are true neoplasms and may also contain bone, cartilage, teeth and nails.

Presentation

These lesions may present as a result of mass effect from continued growth.

They may rupture (more common with dermoids than epidermoids), and can cause chemical meningitis (from the irritating properties of fat and or keratin), or, if infected, bacterial meningitis.

Radiographic evaluation

1. skull x-ray: these osteolytic lesions have well-defined, sclerotic margins
2. some imaging is required to evaluate possible intracranial involvement
   a) CT: the lesions are hypodense (keratin contains fats), and non-enhancing
   b) MRI: like CSF they are low intensity on T1WI and high signal on T2WI, but unlike CSF they are high signal on DWI > MRI (p. 762)

Treatment

Treatment is surgical. Radiation and chemotherapy are not indicated.

When possible, the goal is to avoid rupture during removal in order to avoid chemical and/or bacterial meningitis.

Bone margins are curetted. Search must be made for a tract leading to the intracranial cavity which must be followed if found. Preparation for dural sinus repair must be made for lesions overlying the sagittal sinus (including torcular Herophili).

Endoscopic surgery may be an option for some skull base lesions.

50.1.5 Langerhans cell histiocytosis

General information

Histiocytic disorders may be classified as follows:
1. malignant (true histiocytic lymphoma)
2. reactive (benign histiocytosis)
3. Langerhans cell histiocytosis (LCH)
   a) unifocal: nee eosinophilic granuloma: rare (1/1200 new cases/yr in US). More common in children. Slowly progressing disease. May occur in bone, skin, lungs or stomach.
   b) multifocal unisystem: seen mostly in children. Fever, bone & skin lesions
   c) multifocal multisystem: nee Letterer-Siwe disease (a fulminant, malignant lymphoma of infancy).[3] Hand-Schüller-Christian triad: DI (from invasion of pituitary stalk), exophthalmos (from intraorbital tumor) and lytic bone lesions (particularly of cranium).

This section deals with unifocal Langerhans cell histiocytosis, formerly AKA eosinophilic granuloma.

Clinical

Generally a condition of youth, 70% of patients are < 20 yrs age. In a series of 26 patients,[3] age range was 18 mos-49 yrs (mean: 16 yrs).

Most common presenting symptom: *tender*, enlarging skull mass (> 90%). May be asymptomatic and incidentally discovered on skull x-ray obtained for other reasons. Blood tests were normal in all except 1 who had eosinophilia of 23%.

Parietal bone was the most common site (42%), frontal bone next (31%)[3] (some series show frontal bone was the most common).

Evaluation

Skull x-rays

Classic radiographic finding: round or oval non-sclerotic punched out skull lesion with sharply defined margins, involving both inner and outer tables (the disease begins in diploic space), often with beveled edges. A central bone density is occasionally noted (rare, but diagnostic). No abnormal vascularity of adjacent bone. No periosteal reaction. Differentiate from hemangioma by absence of sunburst appearance.

CT scan

Characteristic appearance of a soft tissue mass within area of bony destruction having a central density.[4] Differentiate from epidermoid which has dense surrounding sclerosis.

Pathology

Gross: pinkish gray to purple lesion extending out of bone and involving pericranium. Dural involvement occurs in only 1 of 26 patients, but with no dural penetration.

Microscopic: numerous histiocytes, eosinophils, and multinucleated cells in a reticulin fiber network. No evidence that this is a result of an infection.

Treatment

Tendency toward spontaneous regression, however, most single lesions are treated by curettage. Multiple lesions are usually associated with extracalvarial bony involvement and are often treated with chemotherapy and/or low dose radiation therapy. Very radiosensitive.

Outcome

After a mean 8 years follow-up, 8 patients (31%) developed additional lesions, 5 of these were ≤ 3 yrs age (all of 5 patients < 3 yrs age)[3] (may suggest a form of multifocal LCH, thus young patients should be followed closely). Recurrences were local in one case, and in others involved other bones (including the skull, femur, lumbar spine) or brain (including the hypothalamus, presenting with diabetes insipidus and growth delay).

50.1.6 Chordoma

General information

Key concepts

- primary malignant tumor, usually of clivus or sacrum, with high recurrence rate
- histology: characteristic physaliphorous cells (containing intracellular mucin)
- generally slow-growing and radioresistant
- treatment of choice: wide en bloc resection when possible (piecemeal removal carries risk of inducing metastases), proton-beam radiation may help

Rare tumors (incidence of ≈ 0.51 cases/million) of the remnant of the primitive notochord (which normally differentiates into the nucleus pulposus of the intervertebral disks). Can arise anywhere along the neuraxis where there is remnant of notochord, however, cases tend to cluster at the two ends of the primitive notochord: 35% cranially[5] in the spheno-occipital region (clivus), and 53%[5] in the spine at the sacrococcygeal region.[6] Less commonly, they may occur in the spine above the sacrum.[7] They represent less than 1% of intracranial tumors and 3% of primary spine tumors.[8] The metastatic rate is low (5–20%),[9] but there is a high recurrence rate of 85% following surgery, and therefore aggressive RTX is usually employed post-op.

Pathology

50 Histologically, these tumors are considered low-grade malignancies. However, their behavior is more malignant because of the difficulty of total removal, a high recurrence rate, and the fact that they can metastasize (usually late). They are slow growing, locally aggressive and osseodestructive. Metastases occur in about 10% of sacral tumors, usually late and after multiple resections, and most often to lung, liver and bone. Malignant transformation into fibrosarcoma or malignant fibrous histiocytoma is rare. Physaliphorous cells are distinctive, vacuolated cells on histology that probably represent cytoplasmic mucus vacuoles seen ultrastructurally.

Radiographic appearance

Usually lytic with frequent calcifications.[10] Enhances on CT with contrast.[10] Rarely, may appear as a sclerotic vertebra[11] ("ivory vertebra").

Cranial chordomas

Peak incidence of cranial chordomas is 50–60 years of age. These tumors are rare in patients < 30 years of age.[12] Male:female distribution is ≈ equal.

Differential diagnosis: Primarily between other cartilaginous tumors of the skull base; see differential diagnosis of other foramen magnum region tumors (p. 1367):

1. chondrosarcomas
2. chondromas

Presentation: Usually produces cranial nerve palsies (usually oculomotor or abducens nerve).

Spinal chordomas

General information

Occur primarily in the sacrococcygeal region. Unlike cranial chordomas, sacrococcygeal chordomas show a male predominance,[5] and these patients tend to be older. May also arise in C2. Chordomas constitute over 50% of primary bone tumors of the sacrum. May produce pain, sphincter disturbance or nerve root symptoms from local nerve root compression. It may occasionally extend cephalad into the lumbar spinal canal. It is usually confined anteriorly by the presacral fascia, and only rarely invades the wall of the rectum.[13] A firm fixed mass may be palpable between the rectum and the sacrum on rectal exam.

Evaluation

Characteristic radiographic findings: centrally located destruction of several sacral segments, with an anterior soft-tissue mass that occasionally has small calcifications. CT and MRI show the bony destruction. This is usually difficult to see on plain x-rays. MRI also shows the soft-tissue mass.

Open or CT guided percutaneous *posterior* biopsy can confirm the diagnosis. Transrectal biopsy should be avoided because of the potential of rectal spread of tumor.[14]

Chest CT and bone scan: to R/O mets for staging purposes.

Treatment

Surgery

Wide en-bloc excision with postoperative radiation is usually the best option, although this may also be only temporarily effective. Decompression is best avoided since entering the mass serves to spread tumor (surgically induced metastases) which will then regrow. Chordomas located in C2 are usually not amenable to en bloc resection.[15]

Sacral chordomas: The particulars of the surgical procedure are highly dependent on the extent of the lesion. These tumors may spread through the gluteal musculature, and if significant muscular excision is required, then a pedicle based rectus abdominis flap may be employed. A diverting colostomy may be required if it is necessary to resect the rectum or if a cephalic sacral resection is anticipated.[16]

For chordomas caudal to the third sacral segment, most agree that a posterior approach is satisfactory. For more rostral lesions, some advocate a combined anterior-posterior approach. However, a posterior approach has been also been used for these.[16]

Adverse effects of sacrectomy: if S2 nerve roots are the most caudal nerve roots spared, there is ≈ 50% chance of normal bladder and bowel control.[16] If S1 or more cephalic roots are the most caudad nerve roots spared, most will have impaired bladder control and bowel problems.[16]

Radiation therapy (XRT)

Best results were obtained with en bloc excision (even if marginal), sometimes combined with high-dose XRT[7,17] (conventional XRT did not prevent recurrence when incorporated with palliative or debulking surgery[7], but it did lengthen the interval to recurrence[17]). Early radiation was associated with longer survival.[18] Higher XRT doses can be used in the sacrococcygeal region (4500–8000 rads) than in the cervical spine (4500–5500 rads) because of concerns of radiation injury to the spinal cord. IMRT and stereotactic radiosurgery have also been used.[15]

Proton beam therapy, alone[9] or combined with high-energy x-ray (photon) therapy[19,20] may be more effective than conventional XRT alone. However, proton beam therapy requires travel to one of a very limited number of facilities with a cyclotron (in the U.S.: Boston, or Loma Linda, California) which may be difficult to arrange for what is typically ≈ 7 weeks of fractionated treatments.

Chemotherapy

Imatinib (Gleevec®) (a tyrosine kinase inhibitor) has some antitumor effect in chordoma.[21]

Outcome

Median survival is 6.3 years.[15]

50.2 Non-neoplastic skull lesions

50.2.1 General information

Includes:

1. osteopetrosis (p. 1401)
2. Paget's disease of the skull
3. hyperostosis frontalis interna (see below)
4. fibrous dysplasia (p. 780)

50.2.2 Hyperostosis frontalis interna

General information

See differential diagnosis (p. 1379). Hyperostosis frontalis interna (HFI) is a benign irregular nodular thickening of the inner table of the frontal bone that is almost always bilateral. The midline is spared at the insertion of the falx. Unilateral cases have been reported,[22] and in these cases one must R/O other etiologies such as meningioma, calcified epidural hematoma, osteoma, fibrous dysplasia, an epidural fibrous tumor,[23] or Paget's disease.

50

Epidemiology

The incidence of HFI in the general population is ≈ 1.4–5%.[22] HFI is more common in women (female: male ratio may be as high as 9:1) with an incidence of 15–72% in elderly women. A number of possible associated conditions have been described (most are unproven), the majority of which are metabolic, earning it the alias of metabolic craniopathy. Associated conditions include:

1. Morgagni's syndrome (AKA Morgagni-Stewart-Morel syndrome): headache, obesity, virilism and neuropsychiatric disorders (including mental retardation)
2. endocrinologic abnormalities
   a) acromegaly (p.725) [24] (elevated growth hormone levels)
   b) hyperprolactinemia[24]
3. metabolic abnormalities
   a) hyperphosphatemia
   b) obesity
4. diffuse idiopathic skeletal hyperostosis (DISH) (p.1129)

Clinical

HFI may present without symptoms as an incidental finding on radiographic evaluation for other reasons. Many signs and symptoms have been attributed to HFI including: hypertension, seizures, headache, cranial nerve deficits, dementia, irritability, depression, hysteria, fatigability and mental dullness. The incidence of headache may be statistically higher in patients with HFI than in the general population.[25]

Evaluation

50

Blood tests to R/O some of the above noted conditions may be indicated in appropriate cases: check growth hormone, prolactin, phosphate, alkaline phosphatase (to R/O Paget's disease).

Plain skull x-ray shows thickening of the frontal bone with characteristic sparing of the midline. Spread to parietal and occipital bone occasionally occurs.

CT demonstrates the lesion which usually causes 5–10 mm of bone thickening, but as much as 4 cm has been reported.

Bone scan: usually shows moderate uptake in HFI (generally not as intense as with bone mets). Also, indium-111 leukocyte scan (commonly used to detect occult infection) will show accumulation in HFI (a false positive).[26,27]

Treatment

In spite of a large number of published descriptive works in the medical literature primarily in the early and mid-20th century, little has been written about treatment of cases where symptoms are suspected to be due to HFI. In one report, removal of the thickened bone was accomplished without evidence of dural adhesions, and with improvement in the presenting hysteria.[22]

Surgical technique

One technique described consists of using the craniotome to excise the thickened portion of the bone (a plain skull x-ray may be used to make a template), and then the thickened bone is thinned down with a high-speed drill, and the bone flap is then replaced. Alternatively, a cranioplasty with methylmethacrylate or custom-made implant fabricated using CT data may be performed.

50.2.3 Fibrous dysplasia

General information

Usually a benign condition in which normal bone is replaced by fibrous connective tissue (malignant transformation occurs in < 1%). Does not appear to be heritable. Most lesions occur in the ribs or craniofacial bones, especially the maxilla.

Patterns of involvement

1. monostotic: most common
2. polyostotic: 25% with this form have > 50% of the skeleton involved with associated fractures and skeletal deformities

3. as part of McCune-Albright syndrome (endocrine dysfunction, café au lait spots which tend to occur on one side of the midline and tend to be more jagged than those seen in neurofibromatosis (p. 604), fibrous dysplasia, and precocious puberty primarily in females) and its variants

Clinical

Clinical manifestations of the fibrous dysplasia (FD) lesions include:

1. incidental finding (i.e. asymptomatic)
2. local pain
3. local swelling (rarely marked distortion resembling aneurysmal bone cyst may occur) or deformity
4. may predispose to pathologic fractures when they occur in long bones
5. cranial nerve involvement: including loss of hearing when the temporal bone is involved as a result of obliteration of the external auditory canal
6. seizures
7. serum alkaline phosphatase is elevated in about 33%, calcium levels are normal
8. darkened hair pigmentation overlying skull lesions
9. spontaneous scalp hemorrhages
10. rarely associated with Cushing's syndrome, acromegaly

3 forms of the FD lesions:

1. cystic (the lesions are not actually cysts in the strict sense): widening of the diplöe usually with thinning of the outer table and little involvement of the inner table. Typically occurs high in calvaria
2. sclerotic: usually involves skull base (especially sphenoid bone) and facial bones
3. mixed: appearance is similar to cystic type with patches of increased density within the lucent lesions

Ground glass appearance on x-rays is due to the thin spicules of woven bone.

Treatment

There is no cure for FD. Local procedures (mostly orthopedic) are used for deformities or bone pain that is refractory to other treatment. Neurosurgical involvement may be required for skull lesions producing refractory pain or neurologic symptoms. Calvarial lesions may be treated with curettage and cranioplasty. Calcitonin may be used for widespread lesions with bone pain and/or high serum alkaline phosphatase levels.

References

[1] Thomas JE, Baker HL. Assessment of Roentgeno graphic Lucencies of the Skull: A Systematic Approach. Neurology. 1975; 25:99–106

[2] Smirniotopoulos JC, Chiechi MV. Teratomas, dermoids, and epidermoids of the head and neck. Radiographics. 1995; 15:1437–1455

[3] Rawlings CE, Wilkins RH. Solitary Eosinophilic Granuloma of the Skull. Neurosurgery. 1984; 15:155–161

[4] Mitnick JS, Pinto RS. CT in the Diagnosis of Eosinophilic Granuloma. J Comput Assist Tomogr. 1980; 4:791–793

[5] O'Neill P, Bell BA, Miller JD, Jacobson I, Guthrie W. Fifty Years of Experience with Chordomas in Southeast Scotland. Neurosurgery. 1985; 16:166–170

[6] Heffelfinger MJ, Dahlin DC, MacCarty CS, et al. Chordomas and Cartilaginous Tumors at the Skull Base. Cancer. 1973; 32:410–420

[7] Boriani S, Chevalley F, Weinstein JN, et al. Chordoma of the Spine Above the Sacrum. Treatment and Outcome in 21 Cases. Spine. 1996; 21:1569–1577

[8] Wright D. Nasopharyngeal and Cervical Chordoma - Some Aspects of the Development and Treatment. J Laryngol Otol. 1967; 81:1335–1337

[9] Hug EB, Loredo LN, Slater JD, et al. Proton Radiation Therapy for Chordomas and Chondrosarcomas of the Skull Base. J Neurosurg. 1999; 91:432–439

[10] Meyer JE, Lepke RA, Lindfors KK, et al. Chordomas: Their CT Appearance in the Cervical, Thoracic and Lumbar Spine. Radiology. 1984; 153:693–696

[11] Schwarz SS, Fisher WS, Pulliam MW, Weinstein ZR. Thoracic Chordoma in a Patient with Paraparesis and Ivory Vertebral Body. Neurosurgery. 1985; 16:100–102

[12] Wold LE, Laws ER. Cranial Chordomas in Children and Young Adults. J Neurosurg. 1983; 59:1043–1047

[13] Azzarelli A, Quagliuolo V, Cerasoli S, et al. Chordoma: Natural History and Treatment Results in 33 Cases. J Surg Oncol. 1988; 37:185–191

[14] Mindell ER. Current Concepts Review. Chordoma. J Bone Joint Surg. 1981; 63A:501–505

[15] Jiang L, Liu ZJ, Liu XG, Ma QJ, Wei F, Lv Y, Dang GT. Upper cervical spine chordoma of C2-C3. Eur Spine J. 2009; 18:293–298; discussion 298-300

[16] Samson IR, Springfield DS, Suit HD, Mankin HJ. Operative Treatment of Sacrococcygeal Chordoma. A Review of Twenty-One Cases. J Bone Joint Surg. 1993; 75:1476–1484

[17] Klekamp J, Samii M. Spinal Chordomas - Results of Treatment Over a 17-Year Period. Acta Neurochir (Wien). 1996; 138:514–519

[18] Cheng EY, Özerdemoglu RA, Transfeldt EE, Thompson RC. Lumbosacral Chordoma. Prognostic Factors and Treatment. Spine. 1999; 24:1639–1645

[19] Suit HD, Goitein M, Munzenrider J, et al. Definitive Radiation Therapy for Chordoma and Chondrosarcoma of Base of Skull and Cervical Spine. J Neurosurg. 1982; 56:377–385
[20] Rich TA, Schiller A, Mankin HJ. Clinical and Pathologic Review of 48 Cases of Chordoma. Cancer. 1985; 56:182–187
[21] Magenau JM, Schuetze SM. New targets for therapy of sarcoma. Curr Opin Oncol. 2008; 20:400–406
[22] Hasegawa T, Ito H, Yamamoto S, et al. Unilateral Hyperostosis Frontalis Interna: Case Report. J Neurosurg. 1983; 59:710–713
[23] Willison CD, Schochet SS, Voelker JL. Cranial Epidural Fibrous Tumor Associated with Hyperostosis: A Case Report. Surg Neurol. 1993; 40:508–511
[24] Fulton JD, Shand J, Ritchie D, McGhee J. Hyperostosis frontalis interna, acromegaly and hyperprolactinemia. Postgrad Med J. 1990; 66:16–19
[25] Bavazzano A, Del Bianco PL, Del Bene E, Leoni V. A statistical evaluation of the relationships between headache and internal frontal hyperostosis. Res Clin Stud Headache. 1970; 3:191–197
[26] Floyd JL, Jackson DE, Carretta R. Appearance of Hyperostosis Frontalis Interna on Indium-111 Leukocyte Scans: Potential Diagnostic Pitfall. J Nucl Med. 1986; 27:495–497
[27] Oates E. Spectrum of Appearance of Hyperostosis Frontalis Interna on In-111 Leukocyte Scans. Clin Nucl Med. 1988; 13:922–923

50

51 Tumors of the Spine and Spinal Cord

51.1 General information

15% of primary CNS tumors are intraspinal (the intracranial:spinal ratio for astrocytomas is 10:1; for ependymomas it's 3–20:1).[1] There is disagreement over the prevalence, prognosis, and optimal treatment. Most primary CNS spinal tumors are benign (unlike the case with intracranial tumors). Most present by compression rather than invasion.[2]

51.2 Compartmental locations of spinal tumors

May be classified into 3 groups based on the compartment involved. Although metastases may be found in each area, they are most commonly extradural. Frequencies quoted below are from a general hospital, extradural lesions are less common in neurosurgical clinics because many of these tumors are managed by oncologists without requiring neurosurgical involvement.

1. extradural (ED) (55%): arise outside cord in vertebral bodies or epidural tissues
2. intradural extramedullary (ID-EM) (40%): arise in leptomeninges or roots. Primarily meningiomas and neurofibromas (together = 55% of ID-EM tumors)
3. intramedullary spinal cord tumors (IMSCT) (p. 787), 5%: arise in SC substance. Invade and destroy tracts and grey matter

51.2.1 Spinal lymphoma

Lymphoma may occur in any of or all 3 compartments.

1. epidural
   a) metastatic or secondary lymphoma: the most common form of spinal lymphoma. Spinal involvement occurs in 0.1–10% of patients with non-Hodgkin's lymphoma
   b) primary spinal epidural non-Hodgkin's lymphoma: rare. Completely epidural with no bony involvement. The existence of this entity is controversial, and some investigators feel that it represents extension of undetected retroperitoneal or vertebral body lymphoma. May have a better prognosis than secondary lymphoma[3]
2. intramedullary
   a) secondary (p. 789)
   b) primary: very rare (see below)

51

51.3 Differential diagnosis: spine and spinal cord tumors

51.3.1 General information

See also Myelopathy (p. 1407) for a list including not only tumors but also *nonneoplastic* causes of spinal cord dysfunction (e.g. spinal meningeal cyst, epidural hematoma, transverse myelitis…).

51.3.2 Extradural spinal cord tumors (55%)

Arise in vertebral bodies or epidural tissues

1. metastatic: comprise the majority of ED tumors
   a) most are osteolytic (cause bony destruction): see Spinal epidural metastases (p. 814). Common ones include:
      - lymphoma: most cases represent spread of systemic disease (secondary lymphoma); some cases may be primary (see below)
      - lung
      - breast
      - prostate
   b) metastases that may be osteoblastic:
      - in men: prostate Ca is the most common
      - in women: breast Ca is the most common
2. primary spinal tumors (very rare)
   a) chordomas (p. 778)
   b) osteoid osteoma (p. 792)
   c) osteoblastoma (p. 792)

d) **aneurysmal bone cyst (ABC)**: an expansile tumor-like osteolytic lesion consisting of a highly vascular honeycomb of blood-filled cavities separated by connective tissue septa, surrounded by a thin cortical bone shell which may expand. Comprise 15% of spine tumors.[4] Etiology is controversial. May arise from preexisting tumor (including: osteoblastoma, giant cell tumor, fibrous dysplasia, chondrosarcoma) or following acute fracture. In spine, there is a tendency to involve primarily the posterior elements. Peak incidence is in 2nd decade of life. Treatment usually consists of intralesional curettage. High recurrence rate (25–50%) if not completely excised
e) chondrosarcoma: a malignant tumor of cartilage. Lobulated tumors with calcified areas
f) osteochondroma (chondroma): benign tumors of bone that arise from mature hyaline cartilage. Most common during adolescence. An enchondroma is a similar tumor arising within the medullary cavity
g) vertebral hemangioma (p. 794)
h) **giant cell tumors (GCT)** of bone: AKA osteoclastoma (p. 797)
i) giant cell (reparative) granuloma: AKA solid variant of ABC.[5] Related to GCT. Occurs primarily in mandible, maxilla, hands and feet, but there are case reports of spine involvement.[5,6] Not a true neoplasm – more of a reactive process. Treatment: curettage. Recurrence rate: 22–50%, treated with re-excision
j) brown tumor of hyperparathyroidism
k) osteogenic sarcoma: rare in spine

3. miscellaneous
   a) plasmacytoma (p. 716)
   b) multiple myeloma (p. 714)
   c) **unifocal Langerhans cell histiocytosis (LHC), nee eosinophilic granuloma**: osteolytic defect with progressive vertebral collapse; LHC is one cause of **vertebra plana** (p. 1392). C-spine is the most commonly affected region. Individual LHCs associated with systemic conditions (Letterer-Siwe or Hand-Schüller-Christian disease) are treated with biopsy and immobilization. Collapse or neurologic deficit from compression may require decompression and/or fusion. Low-dose RTX may also be effective[7,8]
   d) Ewing's sarcoma: aggressive malignant tumor with a peak incidence during 2nd decade of life. Spine mets are more common than primary spine lesions. Treatment is mostly palliative: radical excision followed by RTX (very radiosensitive) and chemotherapy[9]
   e) chloroma: focal infiltration of leukemic cells
   f) angiolipoma: ≈ 60 cases reported in literature
   g) neurofibromas (p. 786): most are intradural, but some are extradural, usually dilate neural foramen (dumbbell tumors)
   h) Masson's vegetant intravascular hemangioendothelioma (p. 770) [10]

51

51.3.3 Intradural extramedullary spinal cord tumors (40%)

1. meningiomas: usually intradural, but may be partly or, in 15% wholly extradural see below
2. neurofibromas: usually intradural, but may be partly or wholly extradural
3. many lipomas are extramedullary with intramedullary extension
4. miscellaneous: only ≈ 4% of spinal metastases involve this compartment

51.3.4 Intramedullary spinal cord tumors (5%)

1. astrocytoma (p. 789): 30%
2. ependymoma (p. 788): 30%, including myxopapillary ependymoma (p. 789)
3. miscellaneous: 30%, includes:
   a) malignant glioblastoma
   b) dermoid. In addition to the general population, dermoids present in a delayed fashion following ≈ 16% of myelomeningocele (MM) closures.[11] An iatrogenic etiology has been debated,[12] however a case of a congenital dermoid in a newborn with MM[13] indicates that the origin is not always from incompletely excised dermal elements at the time of MM closure
   c) epidermoid
   d) teratoma
   e) lipoma
   f) hemangioblastoma (p. 789)
   g) neuroma (very rare intramedullary)
   h) syringomyelia (not neoplastic)
4. extremely rare tumors
   a) lymphoma

b) oligodendroglioma
c) cholesteatoma
d) intramedullary metastases: comprises only ≈ 2% of spinal mets
e) solitary fibrous tumors of the spinal cord: recognized in 1996. Probable mesenchymal origin. May also occur extramedullary (less common). Treatment is complete surgical excision. Prognosis is unclear.[14]

51.4 Intradural extramedullary spinal cord tumors

51.4.1 Spinal meningiomas

See reference.[15]

Epidemiology

Peak age: 40–70 years. Female:male ratio = 4:1 overall, but the ratio is 1:1 in the lumbar region. 82% thoracic, 15% cervical, 2% lumbar. 90% are completely intradural, 5% are extradural, and 5% both intra- and extra-dural. 68% are lateral to the spinal cord, 18% posterior, 15% anterior. Multiple spinal meningiomas occur rarely.

Clinical

Symptoms

Signs prior to surgery (only 1 of 174 patients was intact)[15]:

1. motor
   a) pyramidal signs only: 26%
   b) walks with aid: 41%
   c) antigravity strength: 17%
   d) flexion-extension with gravity removed: 6%
   e) paralysis: 9%
2. sensory
   a) radicular: 7%
   b) long tract: 90%
3. sphincter deficit: 51%

Outcome

Recurrence rate with complete excision is 7% with a minimum of 6 years follow-up (relapses occurred from 4 to 17 years post-op).[15]

51.4.2 Spinal schwannomas

General information

Key concepts

- slow growing benign tumors
- most (75%) arise from the dorsal (sensory) rootlets
- early symptoms are often radicular
- recurrence is rare after total excision (except in neurofibromatosis)

Table 51.1 Symptoms of spinal meningiomas

	At onset	At time of first surgery
local or radicular pain	42%	53%
motor deficits	33%	92%
sensory symptoms	25%	61%
sphincter disturbance		50%

51

Incidence: 0.3–0.4/100,000/yr. Most occur sporadically and are solitary, but they may also be associated with neurofibromatosis (p. 603) primarily type 2 (NF2), but can occur with type 1.

Configurations

Most are entirely intradural, but 8–32% may be completely extradural,[16,17] 1–19% are a combination, 6–23% are dumbbell, and 1% are intramedullary.

Dumbbell tumors. Definition: tumors that develop an "hourglass" shape as a result of an anatomic barrier encountered during growth. Not all dumbbell tumors are Schwannomas, e.g. neuroblastoma (p. 603). Most have a contiguous intraspinal, foraminal (usually narrower) and extraforaminal components (widening of the neural foramen is a characteristic finding, can be recognized even on plain films, and speaks to the longstanding benign nature of the lesion). The waist may also be due to a dural constriction.

Asazuma et al.[18] classification system for dumbbell spinal Schwannomas is shown in ▶ Fig. 51.1.

Type I tumors are intradural and extradural and are restricted to the spinal canal. The constriction occurs at the dura.

Type II are all extradural, and are subclassified as: IIa do not extend beyond the neural foramen, IIb = inside spinal canal + paravertebral, IIc = foraminal + paravertebral.

Type IIIa are intradural and extradural foraminal, IIIb are intradural and extradural paravertebral.

Type IV are extradural and intravertebral. Type V are extradural and extralaminar with laminar invasion. Type VI show multidirectional bone erosion.

Craniocaudal spread: IF & TF designate the number of intervertebral foramina and transverse foramina involved, respectively (e.g. IF stage 2 = 2 foramens).

Schwannomas involving C1 & C2: May involve vertebral arteries and require additional caution.

Clinical

51

Patients typically present with local pain.

Neurologic deficits develop late. Tumors may cause radiculopathy (from nerve root compression), myelopathy (from spinal cord compression), radiculomyelopathy (from compression of both), or cauda equina syndrome (for tumors below conus medullaris).

Pathology

Composed of Antoni A (compact, interwoven bundles of long, spindly Schwann cells) and Antoni B tissue (sparse areas of Schwann cells in a loose eosinophilic matrix).

Surgical approaches

See reference.[19]

Posterior approaches: Types I, IIa IIIa, some upper cervical IIIb and some VI are generally amenable to a posterior approach. IIa & IIIa usually require total facetectomy for complete removal.[18] Reconstruction with instrumentation may be needed if substantial posterior disruption occurs.

Anterior and combined anterior/posterior approaches: Asazuma et al.[18] recommend a combined approach for Type IIb, IIc and IIIb lesions where the extraforaminal extension is large (viz. beyond the vertebral arteries). Reconstruction with instrumentation was required for some tumors (≈ 10% of all patients treated) which were type IV (2 patients), IIIb (1 pt) and VI (1 pt).

Nerve sacrifice

It is usually possible to preserve some fascicles of the nerve root, although sometimes section of the entire nerve root is required. New deficits may not occur since involved fascicles are often nonfunctional, and adjacent roots may compensate. The risk for motor deficit is higher for schwannomas than for neurofibromas, for cervical vs. lumbar tumors, and for cervical tumors with extradural extension.

Outcome

Recurrence is rare following gross total excision, except in the setting of NF2.

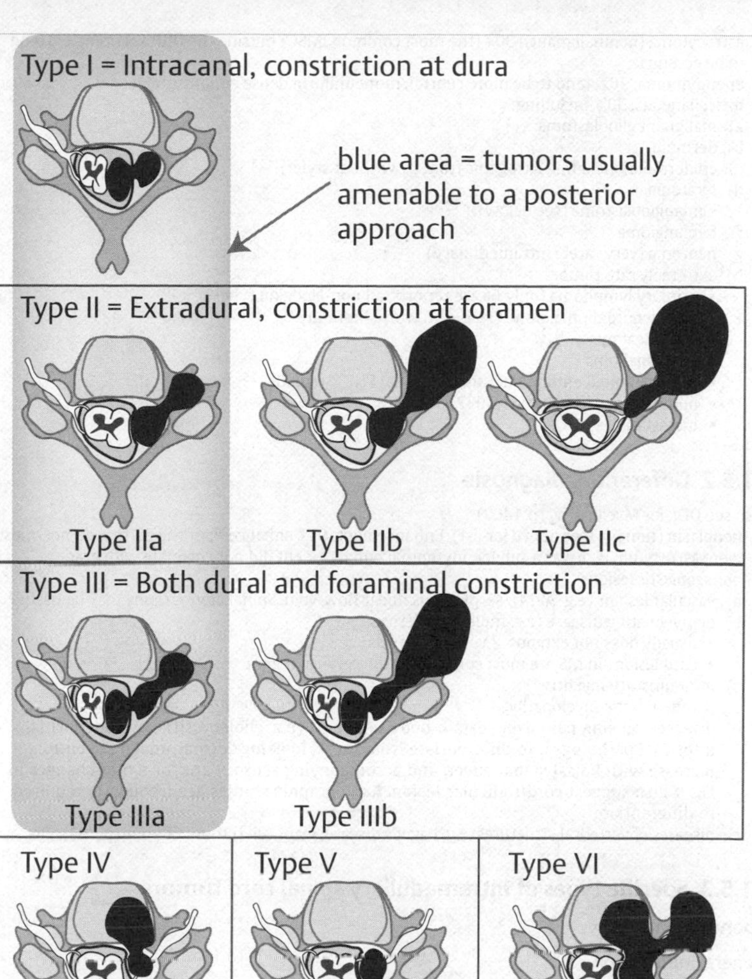

Fig. 51.1 Classification of dumbbell spinal tumors (Modified with permission from Asazuma T, Yoshiaki T, Hirofumi M, et al.: Surgical strategy for cervical dumbbell tumors based on a three-dimensional classification. Spine 29 (1): E10–4, 2003)

51.5 Intramedullary spinal cord tumors

51.5.1 Types of intramedullary spinal cord tumors

The following list excludes metastases (see below) and lipomas (of questionable neoplastic origin,[20] and most are actually extramedullary intradural, see below). **Note:** in pediatrics, astrocytoma and ependymoma constitute 90% of intramedullary spinal cord tumors (IMSCT).

1. astrocytoma (nonmalignant): 30% (the most common IMSCT outside the filum terminale[2]) tend to be eccentric
2. ependymoma: 30%, tend to be more central, more uniform dense enhancement
3. miscellaneous: 30%, including:
   a) malignant glioblastoma
   b) dermoid
   c) epidermoid (including iatrogenic from LP without stylet)[21,22]
   d) teratoma
   e) hemangioblastoma (see below)
   f) hemangioma
   g) neuroma (very rarely intramedullary)
   h) extremely rare tumors
      - primary lymphoma (only 6 case reports, all non-Hodgkin type[23])
      - oligodendroglioma, only 38 cases in world literature[24]
      - cholesteatoma
      - paraganglioma
      - primary spinal embryonal tumor ("spinal PNET") (p. 663) [25]
      - pilomyxoid astrocytoma (p. 632)
      - metastasis

51.5.2 Differential diagnosis

Also see DDx for Myelopathy (p. 1407).

1. neoplasm (tumor): (see above for list). Enhancement: 91% enhance[26]; of the 9% that do not, most were astrocytomas, 1 was a subependymoma; enhancement did not correlate with grade
2. *nonneoplastic* lesions
   a) vascular lesions (e.g. AVM): serpiginous linear flow-void. Spinal angiography may be useful[2]
   b) demyelinating disease (e.g. multiple sclerosis):
      - usually does not extend > 2 vertebral levels
      - cord lesions in MS are most common in the cervical region
   c) inflammatory myelitis
   d) paraneoplastic myelopathy
   e) diseases causing pain over certain body segments (e.g. cholecystitis, pyelonephritis, intestinal pathology). To differentiate from these, look for dermatomal distribution, increase with Valsalva maneuver, and accompanying sensory and/or motor changes in LEs which suggest cord/radicular lesion. Radiographic studies are frequently required to differentiate
   f) diseases of vertebral structures, e.g. Paget's disease, giant cell tumors of bone (p. 797), etc.

51.5.3 Specific types of intramedullary spinal cord tumors

Ependymoma

General information

Key concepts

- the most common glioma of lower cord, conus and filum (most ependymomas in conus and filum are myxopapillary ependymomas). More common in adults
- evaluation: includes imaging the entire neuraxis (usually with enhanced MRI: cervical, thoracic, lumbar & brain) because of potential for seeding through CSF
- associated cysts are common
- treatment: surgical excision (most are encapsulated)

The most common glioma of the lower spinal cord, conus and filum (below). Slow-growing. Benign. Slight male predominance; slight peak in 3rd to 6th decade. Over 50% in filum, next most common location is cervical. Histologically: papillary, cellular, epithelial, or mixed (in filum, myxopapillary ependymoma is most common, see below). Cystic degeneration in 46%. May expand spinal canal in filum.[27] Usually encapsulated and minimally vascular (papillary: may be highly vascular; may cause SAH). Symptoms present > 1 yr prior to diagnosis in 82% of cases.[28]

Myxopapillary ependymoma

Ependymomas of the conus medullaris and the filum terminale are usually of the myxopapillary subtype. WHO grade I. Usually solitary. Histology: papillary, with microcystic vacuoles, mucosubstance; connective tissue. No anaplasia, but CSF dissemination occurs rarely (can seed intracranially following removal of spinal tumor[29]). Denovo intracranial lesions also occur rarely. Rare reports of systemic mets.[1] Outside the CNS, may occur in sacrococcygeal subcutaneous tissues from heterotopic rests of ependymal cells.[30]

Surgical removal of filum tumors consists of coagulating and dividing the filum terminale just above and below the lesion – see Distinguishing features of the filum terminale intraoperatively (p.273) - and excising it in total. The filum is first cut *above* the lesion to prevent retraction upwards.

Astrocytoma

Uncommon in first year. Peak: 3rd – 5th decade. Male:female = 1.5:1. The ratio of low-grade:high-grade = 3:1 in all ages.[27] Occurs at all levels, thoracic most common, then cervical. 38% are cystic; cyst fluid usually has high protein.

Dermoid and epidermoid

Epidermoids are rare before late childhood. Slight female predominance. Cervical and upper thoracic rare; conus common. Usually ID-EM, but conus/cauda equina may have IM component (completely IM lesions rare).

Lipoma

May occur in conjunction with spinal dysraphism, see Lipomyeloschisis (p.269). The following considers lipomas that occur in the absence of spinal dysraphism.

Peak occurrence: 2nd, 3rd and 5th decade. Technically hamartomas. No sex predominance. Usually ID-EM (a sub-type is truly IM and essentially replaces the cord[31]), cervicothoracic region is the most common location. NB: unlike other IMSCT's, most common symptom is ascending mono- or para-paresis (c.f. pain). Sphincter disturbance is common with low lesions. Local subcutaneous masses or dimples are frequent. Malis recommends early subtotal removal at about 1 year age in asymptomatic patient.[31] Superficial extrasacral removal is inadequate, as patients then develop dense scarring intraspinally leading to fairly rapid severe neurological damage with poor salvageability even after the definitive procedure.

Hemangioblastoma

Usually non-infiltrating, well demarcated, may have cystic caps. 33% of patients with spinal hemangioblastoma will have von Hippel-Lindau disease (p.703). Cannot incise nor core because of vascularity. Requires microsurgical approach similar to AVM, possibly with intraoperative hypotension.

Metastases

Most spinal mets are extradural, Intramedullary metastases are rare,[32] accounting for 3.4% of symptomatic metastatic spinal cord lesions.[33] Primaries include: small-cell lung Ca,[34] breast Ca, malignant melanoma, lymphoma and colon Ca.[33,35] Ca rarely presents first as an intramedullary spinal met.

51.5.4 Presentation

1. pain: the most common complaint. Almost always present in filum tumors (exception: lipomas).[21] Possible pain patterns:
   a) radicular: increases with Valsalva maneuver and spine movement. Suspect SCT if dermatome is unusual for disk herniation
   b) local: stiff neck or back, Valsalva maneuver increases pain.
      * *Pain during recumbency ("nocturnal pain") is classic for SCT*
   c) medullary (as in syrinx): oppressive, burning, dysesthetic, non-radicular, often bilateral, unaffected by Valsalva maneuver
2. motor disturbances
   a) weakness is 2nd or 3rd most common complaint. Usually follows sensory symptoms temporally
   b) children present most frequently with gait disturbances

51

c) syringomyelic syndrome: suggests IMSCT. Findings: UE segmental weakness, decreased DTR, dissociative anesthesia (see below)
d) long-tract involvement → clumsiness and ataxia (distinct from weakness)
e) atrophy, muscle twitches, fasciculations
3. non-painful sensory disturbances
a) dissociated sensory loss: decreased pain and temperature, preserved light touch, as in Brown-Séquard syndrome (p. 947). There is disagreement whether this is common[2] or uncommon[36] in IMSCT. ± non-radicular dysesthesias (early), with upward extension[37]
b) paresthesias: either radicular or "medullary" distribution
4. sphincter disturbances
a) usually urogenital (anal less common) → difficulty evacuating, retention, incontinence, and impotence. Early in conus/cauda equina lesions, especially lipomas (pain not prominent)
b) sphincter dysfunction common in age < 1 yr due to frequency of lumbosacral lesions (dermoids, epidermoids, etc.)
5. miscellaneous symptoms:
a) scoliosis or torticollis
b) SAH
c) visible mass over spine

Time course of symptoms

Onset usually insidious, but abruptness occurs (benign lesions in children occasionally progress in hours). The onset is often erroneously attributed to coincidental injury. Temporal progression has been divided into 4 stages[38]:
1. pain only (neuralgic)
2. Brown-Séquard syndrome
3. incomplete transectional dysfunction
4. complete transectional dysfunction

51

Note: 78% (of 23) ependymomas, 74% (of 42) gliomas, all 7 dermoids, and 50% (of 8) lipomas reached the latter 2 stages before diagnosis (not affected by location in cross-sectional nor longitudinal dimension of SC (excludes conus lesions – more frequently diagnosed in 1st stage) (a pre-CT study).

51.5.5 Diagnosis

It is usually difficult to distinguish IMSCT, ID-EM and ED on clinical grounds.[2] Schwannomas often start with radicular symptoms that later progress to cord involvement. Most IMSCTs are located posteriorly in cord which may cause sensory findings to predominate early.[20]

Diagnostic studies

MRI: mainstay of diagnosis. Ependymomas enhance intensely and are often associated with hemorrhage and cysts. Cord edema may mimic a cyst.

Plain radiographs: vertebral body destruction, enlarged intervertebral foramina, or increases in interpedicular distances suggests ED SCT.

Lumbar puncture: Elevated protein is the most common abnormality[1] seen in ≈ 95%. The reported range with primary IMSCT's is 50–2,240 mg%. Glucose is normal except with meningeal tumor. SCT can cause complete block, indicated by:
- Froin's syndrome: clotting (due to fibrinogen) and xanthochromia of CSF
- Queckenstedt's test (failure of jugular vein compression to increase CSF pressure, which it normally does in the absence of block)
- barrier to flow of myelographic contrast media

Myelography (p. 818): classically shows fusiform cord widening (may be normal early). Distinct from ED tumors which produce hourglass deformity (with incomplete block) or paintbrush effect (with complete block), or ID-EM tumors which produce a capping effect with a sharp cutoff (meniscus sign).

CT: some IMSCTs enhance with IV contrast. Myelo-CT distinguishes IMSCT from ID-EM (poor in differentiating IMSCT subtypes).

Spinal angiography: rarely indicated, except in hemangioblastoma (may be suspected on myelography or MRI by linear serpiginous structures). MRI often obviates this test.

51.5.6 Management

General information

Asymptomatic lesions may be followed since there is significant risk of neurologic deficit with surgery. For symptomatic lesions, surgery should be performed as soon as possible (generally not as an emergency) after diagnosis since surgical results correlate with the preoperative neurologic condition, and it makes no sense to follow the patient as they develop progressive neurologic deficit[39] (some of which may be irreversible).

Astrocytomas: For low grade lesions, if a plane can be developed between the tumor and spinal cord (when it can, it usually consists of a thin gliotic layer traversed by small blood vessels and adhesions[20]), an attempt at total excision is an option.[40] For high grade astrocytomas or for low-grade astrocytomas without a plane of separation, biopsy alone or biopsy plus limited excision is recommended.[40]

For high-grade lesions, post-op RTX (± chemotherapy) is recommended.[40] RTX is not supported following radical resection of low grade gliomas.[40]

Ependymomas: An attempt at gross total removal should be attempted. XRT is not recommended following gross total removal.[40]

51.5.7 Technical surgical considerations

1. position: usually prone, well padded and also securely taped to avoid undesirable movement if MEP monitoring is to be used. Other options include: lateral oblique, sitting
2. if a cystic component is suspected, partial aspiration with a 25 Ga needle once the spinal cord is exposed will decrease the pressure (avoid total aspiration which makes it more difficult to locate the tumor).[41] If the cyst forms a "cap" at either end of the tumor, the dura does not need to be opened over the cyst as drainage can be accomplished with removal of tumor
3. adjunctive options include:
   a) intraoperative spinal cord monitoring (SSEP, and motor evoked potentials (MEPs)[42]): SEPs almost always degrade with the initial myelotomy and do not correlate well with motor outcome[43] (which is critical)[44,45] (e.g. it is not unusual for SEPs to be lost during the initial myelotomy without correlation with outcome) and postoperative motor deficit may occur in spite of unaltered intraoperative SEPs[42,43] and conversely SEPs may be lost without motor deficit. However, proof of improved outcomes with MEP monitoring is also lacking[44]
   b) intraoperative ultrasound: also controversial,[45] favored by some experts. Astrocytomas are usually iso-echoic with spinal cord, whereas ependymomas are usually hyperechoic
4. a myelotomy is performed either in the midline or just to one side of the dorsal midline to avoid the posteromedian vein. Alternatively, if the tumor is known to be very superficial off the midline (which may be confirmed by ultrasound), entry may be made there. Tumors may cause distortion and displacement of the midline – look for dorsal root entry zones on both sides to identify the midline as the midpoint between root entry zones
5. 6–0 silk sutures are placed through the pial edge to gently retract the spinal cord open. Standard sized (i.e. non-micro) bayonet forceps can be used to gently spread tissues
6. copious irrigation is used whenever bipolar cautery is employed on the tumor/spinal cord, to minimize transference of heat to the spinal cord. Monopolar cautery should not be used[41]
7. either laser or ultrasonic aspiration (USA) are used to debulk tumor from within until the glial-tumor interface is reached. Charring from laser may make it more difficult to recognize the glial/tumor interface than USA, and the laser tends to be slower when debulking larger tumors
8. watertight dural closure is critical

51.5.8 Prognosis

No well designed studies give long term functional results with microsurgery, laser and radiotherapy. Better results occur with lesser initial deficits.[20] Recurrence depends on totality of removal, and on growth pattern of the specific tumor.

Table 51.2 Key concepts in surgical removal of IMSCT

- in almost all cases, IMSCTs should be debulked from within using ultrasonic aspirator or laser (to avoid manipulation of neural tissue), and no attempt should be made initially to develop a plane between tumor and spinal cord (even for ependymomas, which of the 3 most common IMSCTs is the only one that actually has such a plane)
- if MEPs are monitored: it is suggested that tumor removal should be discontinued if the amplitudes drop to ≤ 50% of baseline

Ependymoma: total extirpation improves functional outcome, and myxopapillary ependymomas fare better than the "classic" type.[28] Best functional outcome occurs with modest initial deficits, symptoms < 2 years duration,[46] and total removal. Survival is independent of extent of excision.

Astrocytomas: radical removal rarely possible (cleavage plane unusual even with microscope). Long term functional results poorer than ependymomas. There is 50% recurrence rate in 4–5 yrs.

51.6 Primary bone tumors of the spine

51.6.1 General information

Types of tumors.

1. metastatic: the most common malignancy of spine
   a) common osteolytic metastatic tumors (p. 814) include:
      - lung
      - breast
      - prostate
      - lymphoma: most cases represent spread of systemic disease (secondary lymphoma), however some may be primary (p. 783)
      - plasmacytoma (p. 714)
      - multiple myeloma (p. 714)
      - Langerhans cell histiocytosis: see differentiating features (p. 784)
   b) metastases that may be osteoblastic:
      - in men: prostate Ca is the most common
      - in women: breast Ca is the most common
   c) Ewing's sarcoma (p. 784)
   d) chloroma: focal infiltration of leukemic cells
2. primary spinal tumors (very rare)
   a) benign
      - vertebral hemangioma (p. 784)
      - osteoid osteoma (p. 792)
      - osteoblastoma (p. 792)
      - aneurysmal bone cyst (p. 784): cavity of highly vascular honeycomb surrounded by a thin cortical shell which may expand
      - osteochondroma (chondroma) (p. 784)
      - giant cell tumors of bone (p. 797): AKA osteoclastoma. Almost always benign with pseudomalignant behavior
   b) malignant
      - chondrosarcoma (p. 784)
      - chordomas (p. 778)
      - osteogenic sarcoma: rare in spine

51

51.6.2 Osteoid osteoma and osteoblastoma

General information

Key concepts

- both are benign bone tumors
- histologically identical, differentiation depends on size (≤ 1 cm = osteoid osteoma, > 1 cm = osteoblastoma)
- can occur in the spine and may cause neurologic symptoms (esp. osteoblastoma)
- high cure rate with complete excision

Two types of benign osteoblastic lesions of bone: osteoid osteoma (OO) and benign osteoblastoma (BOB), see ▶ Table 51.3. They are indistinguishable histologically, and must be differentiated based on size and behavior.

Characteristically cause night pain and pain relieved by aspirin (see Clinical below).

Osteoblastoma is a rare, benign, locally recurrent tumor with a predilection for spine, that may rarely undergo sarcomatous change (to osteosarcoma,[48] only a handful of known cases of this). More vascular than OO.[49]

Table 51.3 Comparison of osteoid osteoma and benign osteoblastoma[47]

	Osteoid osteoma	Benign osteoblastoma
percent of primary bone tumors	3.2%	
percent of primary vertebral tumors	1.4%	
percent that occur in spine	10%	35%
size limitations	≤1 cm	>1 cm
growth pattern	confined, self limiting	more extensive, may extend into spinal canal
potential for malignant change?	no	rare
location within spine (83 patients)		
• % in cervical spine	27%	25%
• % in thoracic spine		35%
• % in lumbar region	59%	35%
location within vertebra (81 patients)		
• lamina only	33%	16%
• pedicle only	15%	32%
• articular facet only	19%	0
• vertebral body (VB) only	7%	5%
• transverse process only	6%	8%
• spinous process	5%	5%
• >1 element of neural arch	6%	19%
• combined posterior elements & VB	0	11%

Differential diagnosis

Lesions with similar symptoms and increased uptake on radionuclide bone scan:
1. benign osteoblastoma
2. osteoid osteoma: more pronounced sclerosis of adjacent bone than BOB
3. osteogenic sarcoma: rare in spine
4. aneurysmal bone cyst (p.784): typically trabeculae in central, lucent region
5. unilateral pedicle/laminar necrosis

Clinical

See ▸ Table 51.4 for signs and symptoms. Tenderness confined to vicinity of the lesion occurs in ≈ 60%. 28% of patients with BOB presented with myelopathy. OO presented with neurologic deficit in only 22%.

Evaluation

Bone scans are a very sensitive means for detecting these lesions. Once localized, CT or MRI may better define the lesion in that region.

Caution regarding needle biopsy: if the lesion turns out to be osteosarcoma, the contaminated needle tract can result in worse prognosis.

Osteoid osteoma

Radiolucent area with or without surrounding density, often isolated to pedicle or facet. May not show up on tomograms.

Table 51.4 Signs and symptoms in 82 patients[47]

Finding	Osteoid osteoma	Benign osteoblastoma
pain on presentation	100%	100%
pain increased by motion	49%	74%
pain increased by Valsalva	17%	36%
nocturnal pain	46%	36%
pain relieved by aspirin	40%	25%
radicular pain	50%	44%
scoliosis	66%	36%
neurologic abnormalities	22%	54%
myelopathy	0	28%
weakness	12%	51%
atrophy	9%	15%

Osteoblastoma

Most are expansile, destructive lesions, with 17% having moderate sclerosis. 31% have areas of ↑ density, 20% surrounded by calcified shell. Often a contralateral spondylolysis.[48]

Treatment

51

In order to obtain a cure, these lesions must be ***completely*** excised. The role of radiation therapy is poorly defined in these lesions, but is probably ineffective.[48]

Osteoid osteoma

Cortical bone may be hardened and thickened, with granulomatous mass in underlying cavity.

Osteoblastoma

Hemorrhagic, friable, red to purple mass well circumscribed from adjacent bone. Complete excision → complete pain relief in 93%. Curettage only → pain relief, with more likely recurrence. Recurrence rate with total excision is ≈ 10%.

51.6.3 Osteosarcoma

The most common primary bone cancer. More common in children, usually occurring near the ends of long bones, but also in the mandible, pelvis, and rarely in the spine.[50] Spinal osteosarcoma usually occurs in the lumbosacral region in males in their 40 s, sometimes arising from areas of osteoblastoma or Paget's disease. If a percutaneous biopsy reveals osteosarcoma, the contaminated needle tract can increase the difficulty of subsequent surgery. Poor prognosis, median survival = 10 months.[50]

51.6.4 Vertebral hemangioma

General information

Key concepts

- the most common primary spine tumor. Benign
- rarely symptomatic (< 1.2%), symptoms more commonly from compression fracture, disc herniation, and rarely neural compression from bone expansion

- MRI: small lesions are hyperintense on T1WI and T2WI. Larger ones may be hypointense. CT or X-ray: striations (corduroy pattern) or "honeycomb" appearance. Bone scan: usually do not have increased uptake
- treatment: incidental lesions require no routine follow-up. Biopsy when mets are a strong consideration. Treatment options (when indicated): XRT, embolization, vertebroplasty (better than kyphoplasty), surgery

Vertebral hemangiomas (VH), AKA spinal hemangioma, cavernous hemangioma, or hemangiomatous angioma. Benign lesions of the spine. The most common primary tumor of the spine (10–12% of primary spinal bone tumors). Estimated incidence: 9–12%.[51,52] 70% are solitary, 30% are multiple (up to 5 levels may be involved, often noncontiguous). Lumbar and lower thoracic spine are the most common locations, cervical and sacral lesions are rare. Lesions involve only the vertebral bodies in ≈ 25%, posterior spinal arch in ≈ 25%, and both areas in ≈ 50%. Occasional cases of purely extradural lesions have been described.[53] Intramedullary lesions are even less common.[54] Typically found in post-pubertal females.

Malignant degeneration does not occur. Mature thin-walled blood vessels of varying sizes replace normal marrow, producing hypertrophic sclerotic bony trabeculations oriented in a rostral-caudal direction in one of two forms: cavernous (venous) or capillary (difference in subtype carries no prognostic significance).

Presentation

1. incidental: most VH are asymptomatic, these require no follow-up (see below)
2. symptomatic: only 0.9–1.2% are symptomatic. There may be a hormonal influence (unproven) that may cause symptoms to increase with pregnancy (could also be due to increased blood volume and/or venous pressure)[55] or to vary with the menstrual cycle and may explain why symptoms rarely occur before puberty
   a) pain: occasionally VH may present with pain localized to the level of involvement with no radiculopathy. However, pain is more often due to other pathology (compression fracture, herniated disc, spinal stenosis…) rather than the VH itself
   b) progressive neurologic deficit: this occurs rarely, and usually takes the form of thoracic myelopathy. Deficit may be caused by the following mechanisms
      - subperiosteal (epidural) growth of tumor into the spinal canal
      - expansion of the bone (cortical "blistering") with widening of the pedicles and lamina producing a "bony" spinal stenosis
      - compression by vessels feeding or draining the lesion
      - compression fracture of the involved vertebra (very rare)[56]
      - spontaneous hemorrhage producing spinal epidural hematoma[57] (also very rare)
      - spinal cord ischemia due to "steal"

Evaluation

Plain x-rays: classically show coarse vertically oriented striations (corduroy pattern) or a "honeycomb" appearance. At least ≈ one-third of the VB must be involved to produce these findings on plain x-ray (see ▶ Fig. 51.2 for demonstration of this finding on sagittal CT).

Bone scan: VH are usually *not* hot (unless a compression fracture has occurred), which may help distinguish VH from metastatic disease (which usually light up).

CT: diagnostic procedure of choice. "Polka-dot sign"[58]: multiple high density dots within the bone represents cross-sections through thickened trabeculae (▶ Fig. 51.3).

MRI: small hemangiomas are focal, round, and hyperintense on T1WI and T2WI. More extensive lesions can be hypointense. MRI may help distinguish lesions that tend *not* to evolve (mottled increased signal on T1WI and T2WI, possibly due to adipose tissue) from those that tend to be symptomatic (isointense on T1WI, hyperintense on T2WI).

Spinal angiography: also may help distinguish nonevolutive (normal or slight increased vascularity compared to adjacent bone) from symptomatic (moderate to marked hypervascularity) lesions. Therapeutic: if the feeding artery does not also supply the anterior spinal artery, it may be embolized preoperatively or sacrificed at surgery.

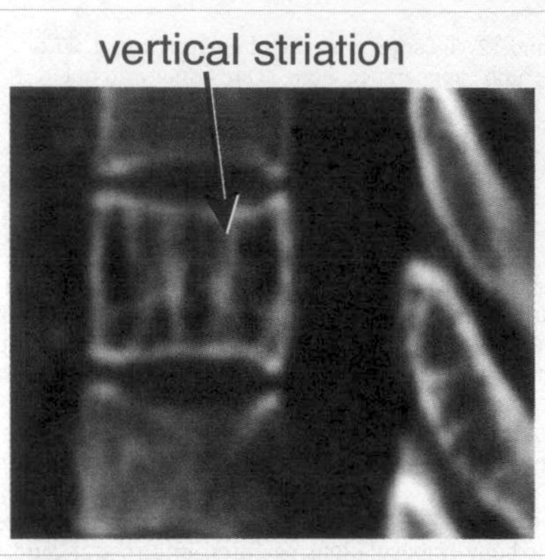

Fig. 51.2 Vertebral hemangioma. Vertical striations seen on sagittal CT reconstruction bone windows.

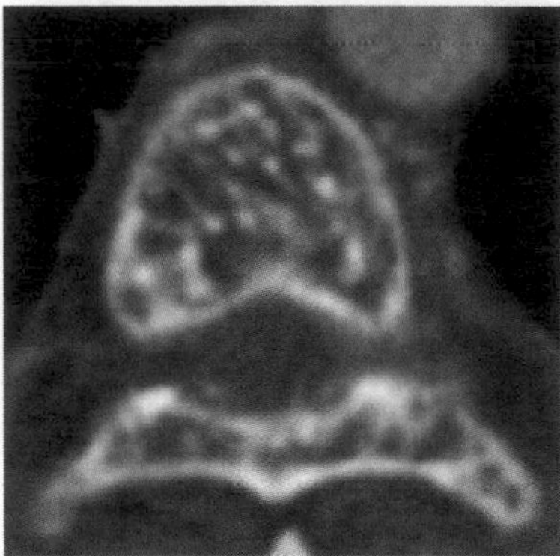

Fig. 51.3 Vertebral hemangioma. Axial CT bone windows demonstrating "polka-dot sign".

Treatment

See reference.[51]

Management guidelines:

1. asymptomatic VH require no routine follow-up or evaluation unless pain or neurologic deficit develop, which are rare occurrences in incidentally discovered VH
2. biopsy: may be indicated in cases where diagnosis is uncertain (e.g. when metastases are a strong consideration). In spite of highly vascular nature, there have been no reported bleeding complications with CT guided biopsy
3. those presenting with pain or neurologic deficit
   a) radiation therapy: may be used alone for painful lesions, preoperatively as a surgical adjunct, or post-op following incomplete removal. VH are radiosensitive and undergo sclerotic obliteration. Total dosage should be ≤ 40 Gy to reduce risk of radiation myelopathy. Improvement in pain may take months to years, and no radiographic evidence of response may occur
   b) embolization: provides more rapid relief of pain than RTX, can also be used pre-op as surgical adjunct. Risks spinal cord infarction if major radicular artery – e.g. artery of Adamkiewicz (p. 87) – is embolized
   c) vertebroplasty (p. 1011): may be better than kyphoplasty for VH because kyphoplasty destroys the trabecular bone
   d) surgery: for painful lesions that fail to respond to above measures, or for lesions with progressive neurologic deficit (see below)

Table 51.5 Recommendations for surgical management of VH[a] [51]

VH involvement	Approach	Post-op RTX?
posterior elements only	radical excision via posterior approach	not for total excision
VB involvement with anterior canal compression (with or without ST in canal)	anterior corpectomy with strut graft	
VB involved but no expansion, ST in lateral canal	laminectomy with removal of soft-tissue	follow serial CT, give RTX if VB expansion or ST expansion
extensive involvement of anterior and posterior vertebral elements with circumferential bone expansion, no ST compression	laminectomy	either RTX, or close follow-up with CT and RTX for ST recurrence or progressive VB expansion
extensive anterior and posterior involvement with ST in anterior canal	anterior corpectomy with strut graft	

[a]abbreviations: VB = vertebral body, ST = soft-tissue component of VH, RTX = radiation treatment

Surgical treatment

For surgical indications, see above. Recommendations for surgical management are shown in ▶ Table 51.5.

Major risks of surgery: blood loss, destabilization of the spine, neurologic deficit (during surgery, or postoperatively usually from epidural hematoma). Recurrence rate is 20–30% after subtotal resection, usually within 2 yrs. Patients with subtotal resection should have RTX which lowers recurrence rate to ≈ 7%.

51.6.5 Giant cell tumors of bone

AKA osteoclastoma (cells arise from osteoclasts). In the same general category as aneurysmal bone cysts. Typically arise in adolescence. Most common in knees and wrists. Those that come to the attention of the neurosurgeon generally arise in the skull (especially the skull base, and in particular the sphenoid bone), or in the vertebral column (≈ 4% occur in sacrum).

Pathology

Lytic with bony collapse. Almost always benign with pseudomalignant behavior (recurrence is common, and pulmonary mets can occur).

Evaluation

Soft tissues are best evaluated with MRI. Spine CT is critical to assess degree of bony destruction and for surgical planning purposes.

Work-up includes chest CT because of possibility of pulmonary mets.

Treatment

Intratumoral curettage, possibly aided by pre-op embolization. Recurrence rate with this treatment (even if resection is subtotal) is only ≈ 20%. Role of RTX is controversial[7] because of the possibility of malignant degeneration (therefore use RTX only for non-resectable recurrence). Use of osteoclast inhibiting drugs – bisphosphonates, e.g. pamidronate (p. 1122) -, has met with some success following subtotal resection.

For gross residual disease after resection, re-resection is a consideration.

Cryosurgery with liquid nitrogen has been employed in long bones. Its use is limited in neurosurgical cases because of risk of injury to adjacent neural structures (brain, spinal cord) and cryotherapy induced fractures, although it has been described for use in the sacrum.[59]

Close follow-up is required due to propensity for recurrence. MRI or CT initially q 3 months is suggested.

References

[1] Kopelson G, Linggood RM, Kleinman GM, et al. Management of Intramedullary Spinal Cord Tumors. Radiology. 1980; 135:473–479

[2] Adams RD, Victor M. In: Intraspinal Tumors. Principles of Neurology. 2nd ed. New York: McGraw-Hill; 1981:638–641

[3] Lyons MK, O'Neill BP, Kurtin PJ, Marsh WR. Diagnosis and Management of Primary Spinal Epidural Non-Hodgkin's Lymphoma. Mayo Clin Proc. 1996; 71:453–457

[4] Liu JK, Brockmeyer DL, Dailey AT, Schmidt MH. Surgical management of aneurysmal bone cysts of the spine. Neurosurg Focus. 2003; 15

[5] Suzuki M, Satoh T, Nishida J, Kato S, Toba T, Honda T, Masuda T. Solid variant of aneurysmal bone cyst of the cervical spine. Spine. 2004; 29:E376–E381

[6] Neviaser JS, Eisenberg SH. Giant cell reparative granuloma of the cervical spine; case report. Bull Hosp Joint Dis. 1954; 15:73–78

[7] Dunn EJ, Davidson RI, Desai S, The Cervical Spine Research Society Editorial Committee. In: Diagnosis and Management of Tumors of the Cervical Spine. The Cervical Spine. 2nd ed. Philadelphia: JB Lippincott; 1989:693–722

[8] Menezes AH, Sato Y. Primary Tumors of the Spine in Children - Natural History and Management. Concepts Pediatr Neurosurg. 1990; 10:30–53

[9] Grubb MR, Currier BL, Pritchard DJ, et al. Primary Ewing's Sarcoma of the Spine. Spine. 1994; 19:309–313

[10] Porter DG, Martin AJ, Mallucci CL, et al. Spinal Cord Compression Due To Masson's Vegetant Intravascular Hemangioendothelioma: Case Report. J Neurosurg. 1995; 82:125–127

[11] Scott RM, Wolpert SM, Bartoshesky LE, Zimbler S, Klauber GT. Dermoid tumors occurring at the site of previous myelomeningocele repair. J Neurosurg. 1986; 65:779–783

[12] Storrs BB. Are dermoid and epidermoid tumors preventable complications of myelomeningocele repair? Pediatr Neurosurg. 1994; 20:160–162

[13] Ramos E, Marlin AE, Gaskill SJ. Congenital dermoid tumor in a child at initial myelomeningocele closure: an etiological discussion. J Neurosurg Pediatrics. 2008; 2:414–415

[14] Metellus P, Bouvier C, Guyotat J, Fuentes S, Jouvet A, Vasiljevic A, Giorgi R, Dufour H, Grisoli F, Figarella-Branger D. Solitary fibrous tumors of the central nervous system: clinicopathological and therapeutic considerations of 18 cases. Neurosurgery. 2007; 60:715–22; discussion 722

[15] Solero CL, Fornari M, Giombini S, Lasio G, Oliveri G, Cimino C, Pluchino F. Spinal meningiomas: review of 174 operated cases. Neurosurgery. 1989; 25:153–160

[16] Seppala MT, Haltia MJ, Sankila RJ, Jaaskelainen JE, Heiskanen O. Long-term outcome after removal of spinal schwannoma: a clinicopathological study of 187 cases. J Neurosurg. 1995; 83:621–626

[17] Conti P, Pansini G, Mouchaty H, Capuano C, Conti R. Spinal neurinomas: retrospective analysis and long-term outcome of 179 consecutively operated cases and review of the literature. Surg Neurol. 2004; 61:34–43; discussion 44

[18] Asazuma T, Toyama Y, Maruiwa H, Fujimura Y, Hirabayashi K. Surgical strategy for cervical dumbbell tumors based on a three-dimensional classification. Spine. 2004; 29:E10–E14

[19] Gottfried ON, Binning MJ, Schmidt MH. Surgical Approaches to Spinal Schwannomas. Contemp Neurosurg. 2005; 27:1–8

[20] Stein B. Intramedullary Spinal Cord Tumors. Clin Neurosurg. 1983; 30:717–741

[21] Stern WE. Localization and Diagnosis of Spinal Cord Tumors. Clin Neurosurg. 1977; 25:480–494

[22] DeSousa AL, Kalsbeck JE, Mealey J, et al. Intraspinal Tumors in Children. A Review of 81 Cases. J Neurosurg. 1979; 51:437–445

[23] Hautzer NW, Aiyesimoju A, Robitaille Y. Primary Spinal Intramedullary Lymphomas: A Review. Ann Neurol. 1983; 14:62–66

[24] Alvisi C, Cerisoli M, Giuloni M. Intramedullary Spinal Gliomas: Long Term Results of Surgical Treatment. Acta Neurochir. 1984; 70:169–179

[25] Kumar R, Reddy SJ, Wani AA, Pal L. Primary spinal primitive neuroectodermal tumor: case series and review of the literature. Pediatr Neurosurg. 2007; 43:1–6

[26] White JB, Miller GM, Layton KF, Krauss WE. Nonenhancing tumors of the spinal cord. J Neurosurg Spine. 2007; 7:403–407

[27] Dorwart RH, LaMasters DL, Watanabe TJ, Newton TH, Potts DG. In: Tumors. Computed Tomography of the Spine and Spinal Cord. San Anselmo: Clavadal Press; 1983:115–131

[28] Mork SJ, Loken AC. Ependymoma: A Follow-Up Study of 101 Cases. Cancer. 1977; 40:907–915

[29] Tzerakis N, Georgakoulias N, Kontogeorgos G, Mitsos A, Jenkins A, Orphanidis G. Intraparenchymal myxopapillary ependymoma: case report. Neurosurgery. 2004; 55

[30] Helwig EB, Stern JB. Subcutaneous sacrococcygeal myxopapillary ependymoma. A clinicopathologic study of 32 cases. Am J Clin Pathol. 1984; 81:156–161

[31] Malis LI. Intramedullary Spinal Cord Tumors. Clin Neurosurg. 1978; 25:512–539

[32] Smaltino F, Bernini FP, Santoro S. Computerized Tomography in the Diagnosis of Intramedullary Metastases. Acta Neurochir. 1980; 52:299–303

[33] Edelson RN, Deck MDF, Posner JB. Intramedullary Spinal Cord Metastases. Neurology. 1972; 22:1222–1231

[34] Murphy KC, Feld R, Evans WK, et al. Intramedullary Spinal Cord Metastases from Small Cell Carcinoma of the Lung. J Clin Onc. 1983; 1:99–106

[35] Jellinger K, Kothbauer P, Sunder-Plassmann, et al. Intramedullary Spinal Cord Metastases. J Neurol. 1979; 220:31–41

[36] Stein B. Surgery of Intramedullary Spinal Cord Tumors. Clin Neurosurg. 1979; 26:473–479

[37] Sebastian PR, Fisher M, Smith TW, et al. Intramedullary Spinal Cord Metastasis. Surg Neurol. 1981; 16:336–339

[38] Nittner K, Olivecrona H, Tonnis W. Handbuch der Neurochirurgie. New York: Springer-Verlag; 1972:1–606

[39] Post KD, Stein BM, Schmidek HH, Sweet WH. In: Surgical Management of Spinal Cord Tumors and Arteriovenous Malformations. Operative Neurosurgical Techniques. 3rd ed. Philadelphia: W.B. Saunders; 1995:2027–2048

[40] Nadkarni TD, Rekate HL. Pediatric Intramedullary Spinal Cord Tumors: Critical Review of the Literature. Childs Nerv Syst. 1999; 15:17–28

[41] Greenwood J. Surgical Removal of Intramedullary Tumors. J Neurosurg. 1967; 26:276–282

[42] Morota N, Deletis V, Constantini S, et al. The Role of Motor Evoked Potentials During Surgery for Intramedullary Spinal Cord Tumors. Neurosurgery. 1997; 41:1327–1336

[43] Kothbauer P, Deletis V, Epstein FJ. Intraoperative Spinal Cord Monitoring for Intramedullary Surgery: An Essential Adjunct. Pediatric Neurosurgery. 1997; 26:247–254

[44] Albright AL. Intraoperative Spinal Cord Monitoring for Intramedullary Surgery: An Essential Adjunct? Pediatric Neurosurgery. 1998; 29

[45] Albright AL. Pediatric Intramedullary Spinal Cord Tumors. Childs Nerv Syst. 1999; 15:436–437

[46] Guidetti B, Mercuri S, Vagnozzi R. Long-Term Results of the Surgical Treatment of 129 Intramedullary Spinal Gliomas. J Neurosurg. 1981; 54:323–330

[47] Janin Y, Epstein JA, Carras R, et al. Osteoid Osteomas and Osteoblastomas of the Spine. Neurosurgery. 1981; 8:31–38

[48] Amacher AL, Eltomey A. Spinal Osteoblastoma in Children and Adolescents. Childs Nerv Syst. 1985; 1:29–32

[49] Lichtenstein L, Sawyer WR. Benign Osteoblastoma. J Bone Joint Surg. 1964; 46A:755–765

[50] Shives TC, Dahlin DC, Sim FH, Pritchard DJ, Earle JD. Osteosarcoma of the spine. J Bone Joint Surg Am. 1986; 68:660–668
[51] Fox MW, Onofrio BM. The Natural History and Management of Symptomatic and Asymptomatic Vertebral Hemangiomas. J Neurosurg. 1993; 78:36–45
[52] Healy M, Herz DA, Pearl L. Spinal Hemangiomas. Neurosurgery. 1983; 13:689–691
[53] Richardson RR, Cerullo LJ. Spinal Epidural Cavernous Hemangioma. Surg Neurol. 1979; 12:266–268
[54] Cosgrove GR, Bertrand G, Fontaine S, et al. Cavernous Angiomas of the Spinal Cord. J Neurosurg. 1988; 68:31–36
[55] Tekkök IH, Açikgöz B, Saglam A, Önol B. Vertebral Hemangioma Symptomatic During Pregnancy - Report of a Case and Review of the Literature. Neurosurgery. 1993; 32:302–306
[56] Graham JJ, Yang WC. Vertebral Hemangioma with Compression Fracture and Paraparesis Treated with Preoperative Embolization and Vertebral Resection. Spine. 1984; 9:97–101
[57] Kosary IA, Braham J, Shacked I, Shacked R. Spinal Epidural Hematoma due to Hemangioma of Vertebra. Surg Neurol. 1977; 7:61–62
[58] Persaud T. The polka-dot sign. Radiology. 2008; 246:980–981
[59] Marcove RC, Sheth DS, Brien EW, Huvos AG, Healey JH. Conservative surgery for giant cell tumors of the sacrum. The role of cryosurgery as a supplement to curettage and partial excision. Cancer. 1994; 74:1253–1260

52 Cerebral Metastases

52.1 General information

Key concepts

- brain metastases are the most common brain tumor seen clinically
- at the time of onset of neurologic symptoms, 70% will be multiple on MRI
- with solitary brain lesions in a patient with a history of cancer, biopsy should almost always be done since 11% of these lesions will not be mets
- although median survival with maximal treatment is only 8 months (similar to GBM), long-term survivors do occur

52.2 Metastases to the brain

Cerebral metastases are the most common brain tumor seen clinically, comprising slightly more than half of brain tumors (if one considers only imaging studies, they comprise ≈ 30%). In the U.S., the annual incidence of new cases of metastases is up to 170,000,[1] compared to 17,000 for primary brain tumors. 15–30% of patients with cancer (Ca) develop cerebral mets.[2] In patients with no Ca history, a cerebral met was the presenting symptom in 15%; of these, 43-60% will have an abnormal chest x-ray (**CXR**)[3,4] (showing either a bronchogenic primary or other mets to lung).

In 9% of cases, a cerebral met is the only detectable site of spread. Cerebral mets occur in only 6% of pediatric cancers.

The route of metastatic spread to the brain is usually hematogenous, although local extension can also occur.

52

Solitary mets

- CT (p. 806): at the time of *neurologic* diagnosis, 50% are solitary on CT[5,6]
- MRI: if the same patients have an MRI, < 30% will be solitary[7]
- on autopsy: mets are solitary in one–third of patients with brain mets, and 1–3% of solitary mets occur in the brain stem[8]

Increasing incidence of cerebral mets: May be due to a number of factors:
1. increasing length of survival of cancer patients[9] as a result of improvements in treatment of systemic cancer
2. enhanced ability to diagnose CNS tumors due to availability of CT and/or MRI
3. many chemotherapeutic agents used systemically do not cross the blood-brain barrier (BBB) well, providing a "haven" for tumor growth there
4. some chemotherapeutic agents may transiently weaken the BBB and allow CNS seeding with tumor

52.3 Metastases of primary CNS tumors

52.3.1 Spread via CSF pathways

CNS tumors that more commonly spread via CSF pathways include the following (when these tumors spread to the spinal cord, they are often called "drop mets"):
1. high grade gliomas (p. 619) (10–25%)
2. primitive neuroectodermal tumors (PNET), especially medulloblastoma (p. 664)
3. ependymoma (p. 642) (11%)
4. choroid plexus tumors (p. 648)
5. pineal region tumors
   a) germ cell tumors (p. 659)
   b) pineocytoma and pineoblastoma (p. 659)
6. rarely:
   a) oligodendrogliomas (p. 638) (≈ 1%)
   b) hemangioblastomas (p. 701)
   c) primary CNS melanoma (p. 701)

52.3.2 Extraneural spread

Although most CNS tumors do not spread systemically, there is some potential for extraneural spread with the following tumors:

1. medulloblastoma (cerebellar-PNET): the most common primary responsible for extraneural spread. May spread to lung, bone marrow, lymph nodes, abdomen
2. meningioma: rarely goes to heart or lungs
3. malignant astrocytomas rarely metastasize systemically
4. ependymomas
5. pineoblastomas
6. meningeal sarcomas
7. choroid plexus tumors
8. tumors that spread through CSF pathways (see above) may spread via a CSF shunt (e.g. to peritoneum with VP shunt or hematogenously with a VA shunt), however, this risk is probably quite small[10]

52.4 Location of cerebral mets

Intracranial metastases may be either parenchymal (≈ 75%) or may involve the leptomeninges in a carcinomatous meningitis (p. 811). 80% of solitary metastases are located in the cerebral hemispheres.

The highest incidence of parenchymal mets is posterior to the Sylvian fissure near the junction of temporal, parietal, and occipital lobes (presumably due to embolic spread to terminal MCA branches).[11] Many tend to arise at the gray/white-matter interface.

The cerebellum is a common site of intracranial mets, and is the location in 16% of cases of solitary brain mets. It is the most common p-fossa tumor in adults, thus "a solitary lesion in the posterior fossa of an adult is considered a metastasis until proven otherwise." Spread to the posterior fossa may be via the spinal epidural venous plexus (Batson's plexus) and the vertebral veins.

52.5 Primary cancers in patients with cerebral metastases

52.5.1 General information

Accurately ascertaining the source of cerebral metastases in the U.S. is difficult because of lack of detailed coding.[12] In over 2,700 adults with a primary cancer undergoing autopsy at Sloan-Kettering, the sources of cerebral metastases are shown in ▶ Table 52.1. Sources of brain metastases in pediatrics is shown in ▶ Table 52.2.

In adults, lung and breast Ca together account for > 50% of cerebral mets.

In patients with a metastatic brain tumor as the initial presentation (i.e. undiagnosed primary) compared to patients with a known primary, there is about the same number of brain lesions, but there was an increased frequency of extracranial mets.[14] In up to 26% of cases, the primary tumor was never identified.[14]

The autopsy incidence of cerebral mets for various types of primary cancers at Sloan-Kettering Cancer Center is shown in ▶ Table 52.3.

Table 52.1 Sources of cerebral mets in adults (autopsy data)

Primary	%
lung Ca	44%
breast	10%
kidney (renal cell)[a]	7%
GI	6%
melanoma[b]	3%
undetermined	10%

[a] a rare tumor that metastasizes frequently to brain (in 20–25% of cases)
[b] 16% in older series[13]

Table 52.2 Sources of cerebral mets in peds
neuroblastoma
rhabdomyosarcoma
Wilm's tumor

Table 52.3 Autopsy incidence of cerebral mets for given primary cancers

Primary	% with cerebral mets
lung	**21%**
breast	**9%**
melanoma	**40%**
lymphoma	**1%**
• Hodgkin's	0
• non-Hodgkin's	2%
GI	**3%**
• colon	5%
• gastric	0
• pancreatic	2%
GU	**11%**
• kidney (renal)	21%
• prostate[a]	0
• testes	46%
• cervix	5%
• ovary	5%
osteosarcoma	**10%**
neuroblastoma	**5%**
head and neck	**6%**

[a]uncommon, but does occur

52

52.5.2 Lung cancer

The lungs are the most common source of cerebral mets, and these are usually multiple. The lung primary may be so small as to render it occult.

Necropsy demonstrates cerebral mets in up to 50% of patients with small-cell lung Ca (SCLC) and non-squamous, non-small-cell lung Ca.[15]

Small-cell lung cancer (SCLC)

AKA "oat cell" Ca. A neuroendocrine tumor. 95% arise in proximal airways, usually in mainstem or lobar bronchi. Typically younger (27–66 years) than other lung Ca. Strongly associated with cigarette smoking. Median survival: 6–10 months. Considered a systemic disease. Staged in 1 of 2 categories:

1. limited: confined to an area of the chest that can be encompassed by a single radiation port
2. extensive: metastasis outside the thorax or intrathoracic disease that cannot be contained in a single radiation port

Although SCLC comprises only ≈ 20% of primary lung cancers, it is more likely to produce cerebral mets than other bronchogenic cell types (brain mets are found in 80% of patients who survive 2 yrs after diagnosis of SCLC).[9]

Treatment

Very radiosensitive.

No identified brain mets: prophylactic cranial irradiation (PCI) with WBXRT reduces the incidence of symptomatic brain mets and increases survival (disease-free & overall).[16,17] Typically 25 Gy in 10 fractions.

Brain mets: surgical resection considered for immediately life-threatening large lesions, XRT is used otherwise. Multiple SCLC brain lesions: XRT (initial treatment 30 Gy in 10 fractions) + chemotherapy.

Treatment of primary: usually not resected. Treated with chemotherapy ± XRT.

Recurrent brain mets after failure of initial treatment: 20 Gy in 10 fractions.

Non-small-cell lung cancer (NSCLC)

Includes: adenocarcinoma (the most common NSCLC), large cell, squamous cell, bronchoalveolar. Retrospective analysis of patients with NSCLC completely resected from lung found a 6.8% first recurrence rate in the brain.[15] Staged with typical TNM system. Prognosis better than SCLC.

Treatment of lung primary:

1. grades I, II, IIIA: resection
2. higher grades (e.g. distal mets, excluding single brain met): XRT + chemotherapy

Staging studies for known lung primary

1. PET scan: can detect small malignancies. Useful in NSCLC to determine eligibility of resection of primary. Not useful in initial evaluation of SCLC
2. chest CT: usually includes adrenals and liver (thus abdomen and pelvis CT not necessary)
3. bone scan
4. brain: CT or MRI

When metastatic lung cancer is the suspected source of a newly diagnosed brain lesion, the lung lesion should be biopsied (if technically feasible) to rule out SCLC before obtaining tissue from the cerebral mass.

52

52.5.3 Melanoma

General information

Melanoma: the 5th most common cancer in men, 7th in women. Incidence is increasing. Most common sites of origin of melanoma metastases: skin, retina, brain – primary CNS melanoma (p. 701) –, nail bed. The primary site cannot be identified in up to ≈ 14% of cases.[18] Extremely difficult to locate primary sites: intraocular, GI mucosa.

Brain mets are found in 10–70% of patients with metastatic melanoma in clinical studies, and in 70–90% on autopsy of patients who died from melanoma. Patients with melanoma who have neurosurgical lesions typically presented 14 months after primary lesion was identified. Once cerebral mets of melanoma are detected, median survival is ≤ 6 months[19,20,21] and the mets contributed to the death in 94% of cases.[22] A small group with survival > 3 yrs had a single surgically treated met in the absence of other visceral lesions.

Evaluation

Metastatic melanoma to the brain classically causes pia/arachnoid involvement on imaging. Hemorrhagic involvement is common.

CT: lesions may be slightly hyperdense to brain on unenhanced CT due to melanin. Enhancement is less constant than for other mets (e.g. bronchogenic Ca).

MRI: decreased signal on T2WI surrounded by intense halo of edema. Enhancing T1WI lesions in a patient with melanoma is highly suggestive of melanoma metastases.

Systemic work-up: systemic disease determines ultimate survival after treatment of melanoma mets to the brain in 70% of patients. ∴ search for systemic mets should be done, including: CT of chest/abdomen/pelvis & bone scan. PET scan may be more sensitive for detecting metastatic spread than CT when there are clinical signs that the tumor has spread[23]; *except for the brain*, where brain MRI is more sensitive than CT or PET.

Treatment

▶ **Surgical indications**

1. patients with 1-4 CNS metastases that can be completely resected when systemic disease is absent or slowly progressive: long-term survival is possible
2. patients with intracranial mets that cannot be completely removed or with uncontrolled systemic disease may be surgical candidates for the following:
   a) for symptomatic relief: e.g. lesion causing painful pressure
   b) life-threatening lesion: e.g. large p-fossa lesion with 4th ventricle compression
   c) for hemorrhagic lesion causing symptoms by mass effect from the clot

▶ **Whole-brain radiation therapy (WBXRT).** Melanoma is typically radioresistant. WBXRT provides 2–3 month survival benefit and may be considered for palliation in patients with multiple mets that preclude complete excision or SRS.

▶ **Stereotactic radiosurgery (SRS).** Considered for ≤ 4 lesions all ≤ 3 cm diameter that are surgically inaccessible, with limited or quiescent systemic involvement. Relative contraindications: hemorrhagic lesions, lesions with significant mass effect surrounding edema.

▶ **Chemotherapy**

1. alkylating agents:
   a) dacarbazine formerly the gold-standard treatment for melanoma. About equally as effective as its newer orally administered analog temozolomide (Temodar®). Response rate: 10–20%
   b) Fotemustine appeared promising in phase II trials but only 6% responded in phase III (vs. 0% for dacarbazine)[24]
2. immunotherapy:
   a) ipilimumab: monoclonal antibody against cytotoxic T lymphocyte antigen-4 (CTLA-4) antigen. More effective in patients who do not require corticosteroids
   b) interleukin-2 (IL-2): has shown minimal activity in brain mets, and trials have usually excluded patients with untreated or uncontrolled brain mets due to risk of cerebral edema and hemorrhage from capillary leak[25,26,27]
3. BRAF inhibitors (BRAFi): inhibits BRAF kinase (a protein that participates in regulation of cell division & differentiation) – useful in tumors with BRAF oncogene mutation (as opposed to BRAF wildtype) which is common in melanoma
   a) dabrafenib: phase II trial (NCT01266967)[28]
   b) vemurafenib: promising results in heavily treated patients. Phase II trial (NCT01378975)[29]
4. anti-PD-1 drug (monoclonal antibody to PD-1 programmed cell death receptor): pembrolizumab (Keytruda) approved for advanced or unresectable melanoma not responding to other drugs[30]

Suggested algorithm for patients with metastatic melanoma to the brain (adapted,[31] see ▶ Fig. 52.1). Patients with **Karnofsky performance scale (KPS) score** (p. 1358) **< 70** are likely to be poor surgical candidates.

Some key points:

1. patients with rapidly progressive systemic disease: treat the systemic disease first, before the brain mets
2. patients without systemic disease and 1-4 mets are candidates for surgery (based on the article by Bindal et al.[32]) if they are all accessible and can all be removed. SRS is an alternative

Outcome

1. In a patient with a single brain met (any type) and good Karnofsky performance score (> 70) and no evidence of extracranial disease, surgery + XRT had a median survival of 40 weeks vs. 15 weeks for XRT alone.[33,34]
2. For melanoma, retrospective studies have shown a benefit of treatment with either surgery or SRS only when all brain lesions are completely treated (selection bias possible in these studies)[34,35,36,37]
3. Predictors of poor outcome in melanoma:
   a) > 3 brain mets[20]
   b) development of brain mets after the diagnosis of extracranial disease[20]
   c) elevated lactate dehydrogenase > 2 × normal[21]

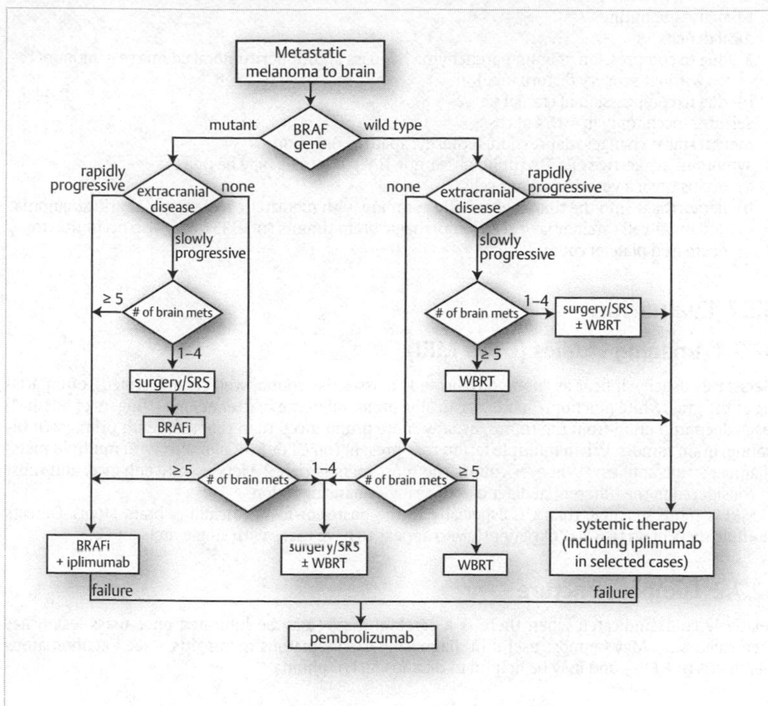

Fig. 52.1 Suggested algorithm for patients with metastatic melanoma to the brain (adapted[31])

d) presence of bone metastases[21]
e) multiple brain mets and extensive visceral disease[38]

52.5.4 Renal-cell carcinoma

AKA hypernephroma. Usually associated with spread to lungs, lymph nodes, liver, bone (high affinity for bone), adrenals, and contralateral kidney before invading the CNS (thus, this tumor rarely presents as isolated cerebral metastases). Look for hematuria, abdominal pain, and/or abdominal mass on palpation or CT. Response to XRT is only ≈ 10%.

52.5.5 Esophageal cancer

Median survival is 4.2 months based on a review of 26 cases.[39] Solitary brain met with good Karnofsky score and surgical treatment may indicate a better prognosis.

52.6 Clinical presentation

As with most brain tumors, signs and symptoms are usually slowly progressive compared to those from vascular events (ischemic or hemorrhagic infarcts) which tend to be sudden in onset and slowly resolve, or electrical events (seizures) which tend to be sudden in onset and rapidly resolve. There are no findings that would allow differentiation of a metastatic tumor from a primary neoplasm on clinical grounds.

Signs and symptoms include:

1. those due to increased ICP from mass effect and/or blockage of CSF drainage (hydrocephalus):
   a) headache (H/A): the most common presenting symptom, occurs in ≈ 50%

52

   b) nausea/vomiting
2. focal deficits:
   a) due to compression of brain parenchyma by mass and/or peritumoral edema (e.g. monoparesis without sensory disturbance)
   b) due to compression of cranial nerve
3. seizures: occur only in ≈ 15% of cases
4. mental status changes: depression, lethargy, apathy, confusion
5. symptoms suggestive of a TIA (dubbed "tumor TIA") or stroke, may be due to:
   a) occlusion of a vessel by tumor cells
   b) hemorrhage into the tumor, especially common with metastatic melanoma, choriocarcinoma, and renal-cell carcinoma[40]; see Hemorrhagic brain tumors (p. 1335). May also occur due to decreased platelet count

52.7 Evaluation

52.7.1 Imaging studies (CT or MRI)

Metastases usually appear as "non-complicated" masses (i.e. round, well circumscribed), often arising at the gray/white junction. Characteristically, profound white matter edema ("fingers of edema") reach deep into brain from the tumor, usually more pronounced than that seen with primary (infiltrating) brain tumors. When multiple lesions are present (on CT or MRI of brains with multiple mets) Chamber's rule applies: "Whoever counts the most mets is right." Mets usually enhance, and must be considered in the differential diagnosis of a ring-enhancing lesion.

MRI is more sensitive than CT, especially in the posterior-fossa (including brain stem). Detects multiple mets in up to ≈ 20% of patients who appear to have cases with single mets on CT.[2]

52.7.2 Lumbar puncture

Relatively contraindicated when there is a cerebral mass (may be indicated once mass lesion has been ruled out). May be most useful in diagnosing carcinomatous meningitis – see Carcinomatous meningitis (p. 811) – and may be helpful in diagnosing lymphoma.

52

52.7.3 Metastatic work-up for patients with suspected brain metastases

When metastatic disease is suspected based on imaging or on surgical tissue, a search for a primary site and assessment for other lesions may be considered since it may provide alternative sites for tissue for histologic diagnosis, and it may guide treatment (e.g. widely disseminated metastases may preclude aggressive therapy). Metastatic work-up should include:
1. CT of the chest (more sensitive than CXR), abdomen and pelvis. Evaluates for primary and additional mets (to lung, adrenals, liver... CT has superseded CXR
2. radionuclide bone scan: for patients with bone pain or bone lesions or for tumors that tend to produce osseous metastases (especially: prostate, breast, kidney, thyroid & lung)
3. mammogram in women
4. prostate specific antigen (PSA) in men
5. PET scan: can detect small malignancies

Cancer of unknown primary site (CUP) : If the metastatic work-up (see above) is negative, the pathology of a metastatic brain lesion as determined by biopsy may implicate specific primary sites.

Small-cell carcinoma metastatic to the brain is most likely from the lung. These tumors stain positive for neuroendocrine stains (p. 600).

Adenocarcinoma: lung is the most common primary. Other sources: GI (mostly colon), breast. The primary site may remain occult even after extensive evaluation in up to 88%.[41] Immunostaining has been tried to identify the primary site but has not been found to be widely useful.

52.8 Management

52.8.1 General information

With optimal treatment, median survival of patients with cerebral mets is still only ≈ 26–32 weeks, therefore management is mostly palliative. Also see Outcome (p. 810) for comparison of various treatments.

52.8.2 Confirming the diagnosis

NB: 11% of patients with abnormalities on brain CT or MRI with a history of cancer (within past 5 yrs) do not have cerebral metastases.[33] Differential diagnoses include: primary brain tumor (glioblastoma, low grade astrocytoma), abscess, and nonspecific inflammatory reaction. If non-surgical treatment (e.g. chemotherapy or RTX) is being contemplated, the diagnosis should be confirmed by biopsy in almost all cases.

52.8.3 Management decisions

Prognostication

This is critical since many treatment decisions depend on overall prognosis.

RTOG RPA: Radiation Therapy Oncology Group recursive partitioning analysis classification[42] (see ▶ Table 52.4; from 1200 patients with one or more brain metastases undergoing XRT). Conclusion: the specific tumor type, length of time since diagnosis, etc. are not as important prognostically as the Karnofsky Performance Scale (KPS) score (p. 1358).

The applicability of RPA to melanoma mets to the brain is controversial (it has been both validated[43] and disputed[37]).

RPA Class 3 patients have been shown to be unlikely to benefit from any of numerous treatment modalities studied. Class 1 are more likely to benefit. Most patients are Class 2, and benefit is unclear.

Management algorithm

▶ Table 52.5 shows a summary of management suggestions (details appear in following sections).

Also, surgical excision may be considered for patients with completely resectable brain mets who are candidates for chemotherapy with interleukin-2 (IL-2) for systemic disease (e.g. for renal-cell Ca or melanoma) since this drug in some case reports produces significant cerebral edema if there are cerebral mets as well.

52.8.4 Medical management

Initial treatment

1. anticonvulsants: e.g. Keppra® (levetiracetam): start with 500 mg PO or IV q 12 hours. Generally not needed for posterior fossa lesions
2. corticosteroids: many symptoms are due to peritumoral edema (which is primarily vasogenic), and respond to steroids within 24–48 hrs. This improvement is not permanent, and prolonged steroid administration may produce side effects; see Possible deleterious side effects of steroids (p. 594).
   ℞ typical dose for a patient with significant symptoms who is not already on steroids: dexamethasone (Decadron®) 10–20 mg IV, followed by 6 mg IV q 6 hrs for 2–3 days, after which it is converted to ≈ 4 mg PO QID. Once symptoms are controlled, this is tapered to ≈ 2–4 mg PO TID as long as symptoms do not worsen
3. H2 antagonists (e.g. ranitidine 150 mg PO q 12 hrs) or proton pump inhibitor (omeprazole)

Table 52.4 RPA Classification for patients with brain mets

RPA class	Description	Median survival (mos)[a]
1	• KPS[b] ≥ 70 and • age < 65 years and • controlled[c] or absent primary tumor with the brain the only site of metastasis	7
2	• all others[d]	4
3	• KPS < 70	2

[a]for patients undergoing XRT
[b]KPS = Karnofsky Performance Scale score (p. 1358)
[c]controlled = stable disease over 3 months observation
[d]i.e. not RPA class 1 or 3

Table 52.5 Management suggestions for cerebral metastases[a]

Clinical situation		Management
unknown primary or unconfirmed diagnosis		stereotactic biopsy for ≈ all patients if surgical excision is not a consideration
uncontrolled widespread systemic cancer & obviously short life expectancy and/or poor performance status, Karnofsky (p. 1358) ≤ 70		(biopsy as indicated above) + WBXRT or no treatment
Stable systemic disease & KPS > 70		
solitary met	symptomatic, large, or accessible lesion	surgical excision + WBXRT
	asymptomatic, small, or inaccessible lesion	WBXRT ± SRS boost
multiple mets	single large lesion that is life threatening or producing mass effect	surgery for the large lesion + WBXRT for the rest
	≤ 3 lesions: symptomatic & can all be removed	surgery + WBXRT or SRS + WBXRT
	≤ 3 lesions: cannot all be removed	WBXRT or SRS + WBXRT
	> 3 lesions: with no mass effect requiring surgery	WBXRT[44]

[a]adapted.[45] Abbreviations: WBXRT = whole brain radiation therapy, SRS = stereotactic radiosurgery

Chemotherapy

See discussion of Limitations of chemotherapy in the brain (p. 595). If multiple lesions of known small-cell Ca are detected on cerebral imaging, treatment of choice is radiation plus chemotherapy.

52

52.8.5 Radiation therapy

General information

NB: not all brain lesions in cancer patients are mets (see above).

In patients not considered for surgery, steroids and radiation may be palliative. H/A are usually reduced, and in ≈ 50% of cases symptoms improve or completely resolve.[46] This does not result in local control for the majority of these patients and they frequently succumb from progressive brain disease.

"Radiosensitivity" of various metastatic tumors to whole brain radiation therapy (WBXRT) are shown in ▶ Table 52.6.

The usual dose is 30 Gy in 10 fractions given over 2 weeks. With this dose, 11% of 1-yr survivors and 50% of 2-yr survivors develop severe dementia.

Prophylactic cranial irradiation

Prophylactic cranial irradiation after resection of small-cell lung carcinoma (SCLC) reduces relapses in brain, but does not affect survival.[47]

Post-op radiation therapy

WBXRT is usually recommended following craniotomy for metastatic disease,[48] especially with SCLC where "micro-metastases" are presumed to be present throughout brain. (**Note**: some centers do not routinely administer post-op WBXRT (except for very radiosensitive tumors such as SCLC) but instead follow patients with serial imaging studies and administer XRT only when metastases are documented.)

Optimal dose is controversial. Early reports recommended 30–39 Gy over 2–2.5 weeks (3 Gy fractions) with or without surgery.[49] This is acceptable in patients not expected to live long enough to get long-term radiation effects. Recent recommendations are for smaller daily fractions of 1.8–2.0 Gy to reduce neurotoxicity.[50] These low doses are also associated with a higher rate of recurrent brain metastases.[51] Since 50 Gy are needed to achieve > 90% control of micrometastases, some use 45–50 Gy WBXRT, plus a boost to the tumor bed to bring the total treatment up to 55 Gy, all with low fractions of 1.80–2.0 Gy.[52]

Table 52.6 "Radiosensitivity" of brain metastases to WBXRT

Radiosensitivity	Tumor
Radiosensitive[33]	• small-cell lung Ca • germ-cell tumors • lymphoma • leukemia • multiple myeloma
Moderately sensitive	• breast
Moderately resistant	• colon • non small-cell lung cancer
Highly resistant[a]	• thyroid • renal cell (10% respond) • malignant melanoma • sarcoma • adenocarcinoma
[a]SRS may be better than WBXRT for these	

Stereotactic radiosurgery

Inconsistent in its ability to reduce tumor size. Some retrospective studies show results comparable to surgery.[53] Others do not.[54] Does not obtain tissue for histological analysis, and generally cannot be used for lesions > 3 cm. Also, see Stereotactic radiosurgery (p. 811).

52.8.6 Surgical management

Solitary lesions

Indications favoring surgical excision of a solitary lesion:

1. primary disease quiescent
2. lesion accessible
3. lesion is symptomatic or life-threatening
4. primary tumor known to be relatively radioresistant (excision is rarely indicated for untreated brain metastases from SCLC because of its radiosensitivity)
5. for recurrent SCLC following XRT
6. diagnosis unknown: alternatively consider biopsy, e.g. stereotactic biopsy

Surgical resection in patients with progressive systemic disease and/or significant neurologic deficit is probably unjustified.[55] Also, in newly diagnosed cancer patients, craniotomy may delay systemic treatment for weeks and the ramifications of this need to be considered.

Multiple lesions

Patients with multiple metastases generally have much worse survival than those with solitary lesions.[50] Multiple metastases are usually treated with XRT without surgery. However, if total excision of *all* mets is feasible, then even multiple mets may be removed with survival similar to those having a single met removed[32] (also see ▸ Table 52.5 for summary). If only incomplete excision is possible (i.e. cannot remove all mets, or portions of 1 or more must be left behind) then there is no improvement in survival with surgery, and XRT alone is recommended. The mortality of removing > 1 met at a single sitting is not statistically significantly higher than removing a single met.

Situations where surgery may be indicated for multiple mets[56]:

1. one particular and accessible lesion is clearly symptomatic and/or life threatening (life-threatening lesions include p-fossa and large temporal lobe lesions). This is palliative treatment to reduce the symptom/threat from that particular lesion
2. multiple lesions that can all be completely removed (see above)
3. no diagnosis (e.g. no identifiable primary): consider stereotactic biopsy

Stereotactic biopsy

Considered for:

1. lesions not appropriate for surgery. Includes cases with no definite diagnosis and:
   a) deep lesions
   b) multiple small lesions
2. patients not candidates for surgical resection
   a) poor medical condition
   b) poor neurologic condition
   c) active or widespread systemic disease
3. to ascertain a diagnosis
   a) when another diagnosis is possible: e.g. no other sites of metastases, long interval between primary cancer and detection of brain mets…
   b) especially if nonsurgical treatment modalities are planned (see above)

Intra-operative considerations for surgical removal

Most lesions present themselves on the surface of the brain or through the dura. For lesions not visible on the surface nor palpable immediately beneath the surface, intra-operative ultrasound or stereotactic techniques may be used to localize the lesion.

Metastases usually have a well defined border, thus a plane of separation from normal brain may be exploited, often allowing gross total removal.

52.9 Outcome

52.9.1 General information

▶ Table 52.7 lists factors associated with better survival regardless of treatment. Also, the prognosis gets worse as the number of mets increases.[45] Median survival even with best treatment in some studies is only ≈ 6 months. To put this into perspective, this is worse than with glioblastoma.

52

52.9.2 Natural history

By the time that neurologic findings develop, median survival among untreated patients is ≈ 1 month.[57]

52.9.3 Steroids

Using steroids alone (to control edema) doubles survival[58] to 2 mos (**Note:** this is based largely on pre-CT era data, and the tumors were therefore probably larger than in current studies[59]).

52.9.4 Whole brain radiation therapy (WBXRT)

WBXRT + steroids increases survival to 3–6 mos.[32] 50% of deaths are due to progression of intracranial disease.

52.9.5 Surgery ± WBXRT

Recurrence of tumor was significantly less frequent and more delayed with the use of post-op WBXRT.[48] Length of survival was unchanged with supplemental use of WBXRT. There is also an

Table 52.7 Factors associated with better prognosis for brain mets (with any treatment)

- Karnofsky score[a] (KPS) > 70
- age < 60 yrs
- metastases to brain only (no systemic mets)
- absent or controlled primary disease
- > 1 yr since diagnosis of primary
- the fewer the number of brain mets
- female gender

[a]the KPS (p. 1358) is probably the most important predictor; those with a score of 100 had median survival > 150 weeks

additional loss of cognitive function in many cases, and patients are rarely independent after WBXRT.

In 33 patients treated with surgical resection of single mets and post-op WBXRT[60]: median survival was 8 months; with 44% 1-yr survival. If no evidence of systemic Ca, 1-yr survival is 81%. If systemic Ca is present (active or inactive), 1-yr survival is 20%. Patients with solitary mets and no evidence of active systemic tumor have the best prognosis.[46,55] With total removal, no recurrence nor new parenchymal mets occurred within 6 months, and the major cause of death was progression of Ca outside the CNS. A randomized trial verified the improved longevity and quality of survival of patients with solitary mets undergoing surgical excision plus WBXRT vs. WBXRT alone (40 weeks vs. 15 weeks median survival).[33] The surgical mortality was 4% (≈ same as 30-day mortality in the RTX-only group). More patients treated with WBXRT alone die of their brain mets than those who underwent surgery. Following total removal and post-op WBXRT, 22% of patients will have recurrent brain tumor at 1 year.[50] This is better than surgery without XRT (with reported failure rates of 46%[50] and 85%[51]).

52.9.6 Stereotactic radiosurgery (SRS)

There has not been a randomized study to compare surgery to SRS. *Retrospective* studies suggest that SRS may be comparable to surgery.[53,61] However, a prospective (non-randomized, retrospectively matched) study[54] found a median survival of 7.5 mos with SRS vs. 16.4 mos with surgery, and a higher mortality from cerebral disease in the SRS group (with the mortality due to the SRS treated lesions and not new lesions). A local control rate of ≈ 88% has been reported, with one study also recommending WBXRT following the SRS for better regional control.[62]

Actuarial control rates at 1 year following SRS + WBXRT were 75–80% and appear to be similar to surgery + WBXRT.[45] However, SRS was unreliable in reducing tumor size.

52.9.7 Multiple mets

Patients with multiple mets that were totally removed have a survival that is similar to those having single mets surgically removed[32] (see above).

52.10 Carcinomatous meningitis

52.10.1 General information

Carcinomatous meningitis (CM) AKA (lepto)meningeal carcinomatosis (LMC). Found in up to 8% of patients autopsied with systemic cancer. CM may be the presenting finding in up to 48% of patients with cancer (before the diagnosis cancer is known). Most common primaries: breast, lung, then melanoma.[63 (p 610–2)] Always include ***lymphomatous meningitis*** in the differential diagnosis; see CNS lymphoma (p. 710).

52.10.2 Clinical

Simultaneous onset of findings in multiple levels of neuraxis. Multiple cranial nerve findings are frequent (in up to 94%, most common: VII, III, V & VI), usually progressive. Most frequent symptoms: H/A, mental status changes, lethargy, seizure, ataxia. Non-obstructive hydrocephalus is also common. Painful radiculopathies can occur with "drop mets."

52.10.3 Diagnosis

Lumbar puncture

Perform only after mass lesion has been ruled out with cranial CT or MRI. Although the initial LP may be normal, CSF is eventually abnormal in > 95%.

CSF should be sent for:

1. cytology to look for malignant cells (requires ≈ 10 ml for adequate evaluation for CM). Repeat if negative (45% positive on first study, 81% eventually positive after up to 6 LPs). May need to pass CSF through a millipore filter
2. bacterial and fungal cultures (including unusual organisms, e.g. cryptococcus)
3. tumor markers: carcinoembryonic antigen, alpha-fetoprotein

52

4. protein/glucose: elevated protein is the most common abnormality. Glucose may be as low as ≈ 40 mg% in about a third of patients

MRI

Contrast enhanced MRI is more sensitive in showing meningeal enhancement.[64]

CT

May show (mild) ventricular dilatation, enhancement of basal cisterns. Sulcal enhancement may also occur with involvement of the convexities.

Myelography

Spinal seeding ("drop mets") will produce filling defects on myelography.

52.10.4 Survival

Untreated: < 2 months. With radiation therapy + chemotherapy: median survival is 5.8 mos (range 1–29). Chemotherapy may be given intrathecally. About half of patients die of CNS involvement, and half die of systemic disease.

References

[1] Johnson JD, Young B. Demographics of brain metastasis. Neurosurg Clin N Am. 1996; 7:337–344

[2] Mintz AP, Cairncross JG. Treatment of a Single Brain Metastasis. The Role of Radiation Following Surgical Excision. JAMA. 1998; 280:1527–1529

[3] Voorhies RM, Sundaresan N, Thaler HT. The Single Supratentorial Lesion: An Evaluation of Preoperative Diagnosis. J Neurosurg. 1980; 53:364–368

[4] Patchell RA, Posner JB. Neurologic Complications of Systemic Cancer. Neurol Clin. 1985; 3:729–750

[5] Zimm S, Galen L, Wampler GL, et al. Intracerebral Metastases in Solid-Tumor Patients: Natural History and Results of Treatment. Cancer. 1981; 48:384–394

[6] DeAngelis LM. Management of Brain Metastases. Cancer Invest. 1994; 12:156–165

[7] Davis PC, Hudgins PA, Peterman SB, Hoffman JC. Diagnosis of Cerebral Metastases: Double-Dose Delayed CT versus Contrast-Enhanced MR Imaging. AJNR. 1991; 12:293–300

[8] Weiss HD, Richardson EP. Solitary Brainstem Metastasis. Neurology. 1978; 28:562–566

[9] Nugent JL, Bunn PA, Matthews MJ, et al. CNS Metastses in Small-Cell Bronchogenic Carcinoma: Increasing Frequency and Changing Pattern with Lengthening Survival. Cancer. 1979; 44:1885–1893

[10] Berger MS, Baumeister B, Geyer JR, Milstein J, et al. The Risks of Metastases from Shunting in Children with Primary Central Nervous System Tumors. J Neurosurg. 1991; 74:872–877

[11] Kindt GW. The Pattern of Location of Cerebral Metastatic Tumors. J Neurosurg. 1964; 21:54–57

[12] Gavrilovic IT, Posner JB. Brain metastases: epidemiology and pathophysiology. J Neurooncol. 2005; 75:5–14

[13] Vieth RG, Odom GL. Intracranial Metastases and their Neurosurgical Treatment. J Neurosurg. 1965; 23:375–383

[14] Agazzi S, Pampallona S, Pica A, Vernet O, Regli L, Porchet F, Villemure JG, Leyvraz S. The origin of brain metastases in patients with an undiagnosed primary tumour. Acta Neurochir (Wien). 2004; 146:153–157

[15] Figlin RA, Piantadosi S, Feld R, et al. Intracranial Recurrence of Carcinoma After Complete Resection of Stage I, II, and III Non-Small-Cell Lung Cancer. N Engl J Med. 1988; 318:1300–1305

[16] Auperin A, Arriagada R, Pignon JP, Le Pechoux C, Gregor A, Stephens RJ, Kristjansen PE, Johnson BE, Ueoka H, Wagner H, Aisner J. Prophylactic cranial irradiation for patients with small-cell lung cancer in complete remission. Prophylactic Cranial Irradiation Overview Collaborative Group. N Engl J Med. 1999; 341:476–484

[17] Slotman B, Faivre-Finn C, Kramer G, Rankin E, Snee M, Hatton M, Postmus P, Collette L, Musat E, Senan S. Prophylactic cranial irradiation in extensive small-cell lung cancer. N Engl J Med. 2007; 357:664–672

[18] Solis OJ, Davis KR, Adair LB, et al. Intracerebral Metastatic Melanoma: CT Evaluation. Comput Tomogr. 1977; 1:135–143

[19] Zakrzewski J, Geraghty LN, Rose AE, Christos PJ, Mazumdar M, Polsky D, Shapiro R, Berman R, Darvishian F, Hernando E, Pavlick A, Osman I. Clinical variables and primary tumor characteristics predictive of the development of melanoma brain metastases and post-brain metastases survival. Cancer. 2011; 117:1711–1720

[20] Davies MA, Liu P, McIntyre S, Kim KB, Papadopoulos N, Hwu WJ, Hwu P, Bedikian A. Prognostic factors for survival in melanoma patients with brain metastases. Cancer. 2011; 117:1687–1696

[21] Staudt M, Lasithiotakis K, Leiter U, Meier F, Eigentler T, Bamberg M, Tatagiba M, Brossart P, Garbe C. Determinants of survival in patients with brain metastases from cutaneous melanoma. Br J Cancer. 2010; 102:1213–1218

[22] Sampson JH, Carter JH, Friedman AH, Seigler HF. Demographics, Prognosis, and Therapy in 702 Patients with Brain Metastases from Malignant Melanoma. J Neurosurg. 1998; 88:11–20

[23] Swetter SM, Carroll LA, Johnson DL, Segall GM. Positron emission tomography is superior to computed tomography for metastatic detection in melanoma patients. Ann Surg Oncol. 2002; 9:646–653

[24] Avril MF, Aamdal S, Grob JJ, Hauschild A, Mohr P, Bonerandi JJ, Weichenthal M, Neuber K, Bieber T, Gilde K, Guillem Porta V, Fra J, Bonneterre J, Saiag P, Kamanabrou D, Pehamberger H, Sufliarsky J, Gonzalez Larriba JL, Scherrer A, Menu Y. Fotemustine compared with dacarbazine in patients with disseminated malignant melanoma: a phase III study. J Clin Oncol. 2004; 22:1118–1125

[25] Guirguis LM, Yang JC, White DE, Steinberg SM, Liewehr DJ, Rosenberg SA, Schwartzentruber DJ. Safety and efficacy of high-dose interleukin-2 therapy in patients with brain metastases. J Immunother. 2002; 25:82–87

[26] Lochead R, McKhann G, Hankinson T, et al. High dose systemic interleukin-2 for metastatic melanoma in patients with treated brain metastases. J Immunother. 2004; 27

[27] Majer M, Jensen RL, Shrieve DC, Watson GA, Wang M, Leachman SA, Boucher KM, Samlowski WE. Biochemotherapy of metastatic melanoma in patients with or without recently diagnosed brain metastases. Cancer. 2007; 110:1329–1337

[28] ClinicalTrials.gov identifier: NCT 01266967. A Study of GSK 2118436 in BRAF Mutant Metastatic Melanoma to the Brain (Break MB). 2014

[29] ClinicalTrials.gov identifier: NCT 01378975. A Study of Vemurafenib in Metastatic Melanoma Patients With Brain Metastases. 2015

[30] U.S. Food and Drug Administration (FDA), . FDA approves Keytruda for advanced melanoma. 2014

[31] Carlino MatteoS, Fogarty GeraldB, Long GeorginaV. Treatment of Melanoma Brain Metastases: A New Paradigm. The Cancer Journal. 2012; 18:208–212

[32] Bindal RK, Sawaya R, Leavens ME, Lee JJ. Surgical Treatment of Multiple Brain Metastases. J Neurosurg. 1993; 79:210–216

[33] Patchell RA, Tibbs PA, Walsh JW, Young B, et al. A Randomized Trial of Surgery in the Treatment of Single Metastases to the Brain. N Engl J Med. 1990; 322:494–500

[34] Vecht CJ, Haaxma-Reiche H, Noordijk EM, Padberg GW, Voormolen JH, Hoekstra FH, Tans JT, Lambooij N, Metsaars JA, Wattendorff AR, et al. Treatment of single brain metastasis: radiotherapy alone or combined with neurosurgery? Ann Neurol. 1993; 33:583–590

[35] Sampson JH, Carter JH, Jr, Friedman AH, Seigler HF. Demographics, prognosis, and therapy in 702 patients with brain metastases from malignant melanoma. J Neurosurg. 1998; 88:11–20

[36] Fife KM, Colman MH, Stevens GN, Firth IC, Moon D, Shannon KF, Harman R, Petersen-Schaefer K, Zacest AC, Besser M, Milton GW, McCarthy WH, Thompson JF. Determinants of outcome in melanoma patients with cerebral metastases. J Clin Oncol. 2004; 22:1293–1300

[37] Eigentler TK, Figl A, Krex D, Mohr P, Mauch C, Rass K, Bostroem A, Heese O, Koelbl O, Garbe C, Schadendorf D. Number of metastases, serum lactate dehydrogenase level, and type of treatment are prognostic factors in patients with brain metastases of malignant melanoma. Cancer. 2011; 117:1697–1703

[38] Gupta G, Robertson AG, MacKie RM. Cerebral metastases of cutaneous melanoma. Br J Cancer. 1997; 76:256–259

[39] Song Z, Lin B, Shao L, Zhang Y. Brain metastases from esophageal cancer: clinical review of 26 cases. World Neurosurg. 2014; 81:131–135

[40] Kondziolka D, Bernstein M, Resch L, et al. Significance of Hemorrhage into Brain Tumors: Clinicopathological Study. J Neurosurg. 1987; 67:852–857

[41] Shildt RA, Kennedy PS, Chen TT, Athens JW, O'Bryan RM, Balcerzak SP. Management of patients with metastatic adenocarcinoma of unknown origin: a Southwest Oncology Group study. Cancer Treat Rep. 1983; 67:77–79

[42] Gaspar L, Scott C, Rotman M, Asbell S, Phillips T, Wasserman T, McKenna WG, Byhardt R. Recursive partitioning analysis (RPA) of prognostic factors in three Radiation Therapy Oncology Group (RTOG) brain metastases trials. Int J Radiat Oncol Biol Phys. 1997; 37:745–751

[43] Morris SL, Low SH, A'Hern RP, Eisen TG, Gore ME, Nutting CM, Harrington KJ. A prognostic index that predicts outcome following palliative whole brain radiotherapy for patients with metastatic malignant melanoma. Br J Cancer. 2004; 91:829–833

[44] Nieder C, Andratschke N, Grosu AL, Molls M. Recursive partitioning analysis (RPA) class does not predict survival in patients with four or more brain metastases. Strahlenther Onkol. 2003; 179:16–20

[45] Pollock BE. Management of Patients with Multiple Brain Metastases. Contemp Neurosurg. 1999; 21:1–6

[46] Horton J. Treatment of Metastases to the Brain. 1984

[47] Jackson DV, Richards F, Cooper MR, et al. Prophylactic Cranial Irradiation in Small Cell Carcinoma of the Lung: A Randomized Study. JAMA. 1977; 237:2730–2733

[48] Patchell RA, Tibbs PA, Regine WF, Dempsey RJ, Mohiuddin M, Kryscio RJ, Markesbery WR, Foon KA, Young B. Postoperative radiotherapy in the treatment of single metastases to the brain: a randomized trial. JAMA. 1998; 280:1485–1489

[49] Kramer S, Hendrickson F, Zelen M, et al. Therapeutic Trials in the Management of Metastatic Brain Tumors by Different Time/Dose Fraction Schemes. Natl Cancer Inst Monogr. 1977; 46:213–221

[50] DeAngelis LM, Mandell LR, Thaler HT, et al. The Role of Postoperative Radiotherapy After Resection of Single Brain Metastases. Neurosurgery. 1989; 24:798–804

[51] Smalley SR, Schray MF, Laws ER, O'Fallon JR. Adjuvant Radiation Therapy After Surgical Resection of Solitary Brain Metastasis: Association with Pattern of Failure and Survival. Int J Radiation Oncology Biol Phys. 1987; 13:1611–1616

[52] Shaw E. Comment on DeAngelis L M, et al.: The Role of Postoperative Radiotherapy After Resection of Single Brain Metastases. Neurosurgery. 1989; 24:804–805

[53] Sills AK. Current treatment approaches to surgery for brain metastases. Neurosurgery. 2005; 57:S24–32; discusssion S1-4

[54] Bindal AK, Bindal RK, Hess KR, Shiu A, Hassenbusch SJ, Shi WM, Sawaya R. Surgery versus Radiosurgery in the Treatment of Brain Metastasis. J Neurosurg. 1996; 84:748–754

[55] Smalley SR, Laws ER, O'Fallon JR, Shaw EG, Schray MF. Resection for Solitary Brain Metastasis: Role of Adjuvant Radiation and Prognostic Variables in 229 Patients. J Neurosurg. 1992; 77:531–540

[56] Tobler WD, Sawaya R, Tew JM. Successful Laser-assisted Excision of a Metastatic Midbrain Tumor. Neurosurgery. 1986; 18:795–797

[57] Markesbery WR, Brooks WH, Gupta GD, et al. Treatment for Patients with Cerebral Metastases. Arch Neurol. 1978; 35:754–756

[58] Ruderman NB, Hall TC. Use of Glucocorticoids in the Palliative Treatment of Metastatic Brain Tumors. Cancer. 1965; 18:298–306

[59] Posner JB. Surgery for Metastases to the Brain. N Engl J Med. 1990; 322:544–545

[60] Galicich JH, Sundaresan N, Thaler HT. Surgical Treatment of Single Brain Metastasis: Evaluation of Results by CT Scanning. J Neurosurg. 1980; 53:63–67

[61] Alexander E, Moriarty TM, Davis RB, et al. Stereotactic Radiosurgery for the Definitive Noninvasive Treatment of Brain Metastases. J Natl Cancer Inst. 1995; 87:34–40

[62] Fuller BG, Kaplan ID, Adler J, Cox RS, Bagshaw MA. Stereotactic Radiosurgery for Brain Metastases: The Importance of Adjuvant Whole Brain Irradiation. Int J Radiation Oncology Biol Phys. 1992; 23:413–418

[63] Wilkins RH, Rengachary SS. Neurosurgery. New York 1985

[64] Sze G, Soletsky S, Bronen R, Krol G. MR Imaging of the Cranial Meninges with Emphasis on Contrast Enhancement and Meningeal Carcinomatosis. AJNR. 1989; 10:965–975

53 Spinal Epidural Metastases

53.1 General information

Key concepts

- suspected in a cancer patient with back pain that persists in recumbency
- occurs in ≈ 10% of all cancer patients
- 80% of primary sites: lung, breast, GI, prostate, melanoma and lymphoma
- many treatments reduce pain. Surgery + XRT in selected cases increases chances of preserving ambulation & produces a modest improvement in survival
- if no neurologic compromise or bony instability, usual treatment: biopsy (CT- or fluoro-guided) followed by XRT (surgical indications ▶ Table 53.4)
- surgery not helpful for: total paralysis > 8 hrs, loss of ambulation > 24 hrs, and not recommended for prognosis < 3–4 months survival, poor medical condition (poor PFTs...), or radiosensitive tumor

Spinal epidural metastases (SEM) occur in up to 10% of cancer patients at some time,[1] and are the most common spinal tumor. 5–10% of malignancies present initially with cord compression.[2] For other etiologies of spinal cord compression, see items marked with a dagger (†) under Myelopathy (p. 1407).

Routes of metastasis to spine:

1. arterial
2. venous: via spinal epidural veins (Batson's plexus[3])
3. perinervous (direct spread)

The usual route of spread is hematogenous dissemination to the vertebral body with erosion back through pedicles and subsequent extension into the epidural space (i.e. *anterior* epicenter). Less commonly may initially metastasize to lateral or posterior aspect of canal. Most metastases (mets) are epidural, only 2–4% are intradural, and only 1–2% are intramedullary. Distribution between cervical, thoracic and lumbar spine is proportional to the length of the segment, thus the thoracic spine is the most common site (50–60%).

53.2 Primary tumors that metastasize to the spine

▶ Table 53.1 shows primary tumor types that give rise to SEM. The majority are common primaries that tend to metastasize to bone (lung, breast, prostate, renal-cell and thyroid). Rare tumors that may go to bone include the myxoid subtype of liposarcoma[4] (17% of these patients develop bone mets, 5-year median survival is 16%).

53.3 Presentation

Pain: the most common initial symptom. Occurs in up to 95% of patients with SEM.[6,7] Types of pain:

1. local pain: typically aching, experienced at the level of involvement. Increased pain with *recumbency* (especially at night) is characteristic
2. radicular: tends to be sharp or shooting, referred into dermatome of the involved nerve root. Commonly bilateral in thoracic region
3. mechanical: usually exacerbated by movement

Neck-flexion, straight-leg-raising, coughing, sneezing, or straining may also aggravate the pain.

Motor or autonomic dysfunction: the second most common presentation. Up to 85% of patients have weakness at the time of diagnosis. Leg stiffness may be an early symptom. Bladder dysfunction (urinary urgency, hesitancy or retention) is the most common autonomic manifestation; others include constipation or impotence.

Sensory dysfunction: anesthesia, hypesthesia, or paresthesias usually occur with motor dysfunction. Cervical or thoracic cord involvement may produce a sensory level.

Table 53.1 Sources of spinal epidural metastases causing cord compression

Site of primary	Series A	Series B[a]	Series C[b]
lung	17%	14%	31%
breast	16%	21%	24%
prostate	11%	19%	8%
kidney (renal-cell)	9%		1%
unknown site	9%	5%	2%
sarcoma	8%		2%
lymphoma	6%	12%	6%
GI tract	6%		9%
thyroid	6%		
melanoma	2%		4%
others (including multiple myeloma)	13%	29%[c]	13%

[a]series B: retrospective study of 58 patients undergoing MRI evaluation for SEM[1]
[b]series C: 75 patients with SEM out of 140 patients evaluated prospectively for back pain[5]
[c]in series B, "other" includes GI, GU, skin, ENT, CNS

Other presentations: pathologic fracture. Bone metastases can sometimes produce hypercalcemia (a medical emergency).

The greater the neurologic deficit when treatment is initiated, the worse the chances for recovery of lost function. 76% of patients have weakness by the time of diagnosis.[1] 15% are paraplegic on initial presentation, and < 5% of these can ambulate after treatment. Median time from onset of symptoms to diagnosis is 2 months.[8]

53.3.1 Metastases to the upper cervical spine

For differential diagnosis, see Foramen magnum lesions (p. 1367), and Axis (C2) vertebra lesions (p. 1391).

Metastases to the C1–2 region comprise only ≈ 0.5% of spinal mets.[9] They typically present initially with suboccipital and posterior cervical pain, and as the lesion progresses patients develop a characteristic pain that makes it difficult to sit up (some will hold their heads in their hands to stabilize it). Possibly as a result of the capacious spinal canal at this level, only ≈11–15% of patients present with neurologic symptoms. 15% develop spinal cord compression,[10] and quadriplegia from atlantoaxial subluxation occurred in ≈ 6%.[10]

Anterior approaches for stabilization at this location are difficult. Pathologic fractures due to osteoblastic types of tumors (e.g. prostate, some breast) may heal with radiation treatment and immobilization. For others, good pain relief and stabilization may be achieved with radiation followed by posterior fusion.[10]

53.4 Evaluation and management of epidural spinal metastases

53.4.1 General information

There is no difference in outcome between lesions above or below the conus; thus spinal cord, conus medullaris, or cauda equina mets are considered together here as epidural spinal cord compression (ESCC). Features that help distinguish conus lesions from cauda equina are shown in ▶ Table 53.2

53.4.2 Grading function

There is prognostic significance in the presenting neurologic condition. Grading scales such as that of Brice and McKissock (▶ Table 53.3) have been proposed, but are not widely used. The ASIA grading scale is more commonly applied.

Table 53.2 Features distinguishing conus lesions from cauda equina lesions with metastases[11]

	Conus medullaris lesions	Cauda equina lesions
spontaneous pain	rare; when present, is usually bilateral & symmetric in perineum or thighs	may be most prominent symptom; severe; radicular type; in perineum, thighs & legs, back or bladder
sensory deficit	saddle; bilateral; usually symmetric; sensory dissociation	saddle; no sensory dissociation; may be unilateral & asymmetric
motor loss	*symmetric*; not marked; fasciculations may be present	*asymmetric*; more marked; atrophy may occur; fasciculations rare
autonomic symptoms (including bladder dysfunction, impotency...)	prominent early	late
reflexes	only ankle jerk absent (preserved knee jerk)	ankle jerk & knee jerk may be absent
onset	sudden and bilateral	gradual and unilateral

Table 53.3 Grading spinal cord function with spinal metastases (Brice & McKissock)[12]

Group	Grade	Description
1	mild	patient able to walk
2	moderate	able to move legs, but not antigravity
3	severe	slight residual motor and sensory function
4	complete	no motor, sensory, or sphincter function below level of lesion

53

53.4.3 Diagnostic tests

MRI in evaluating SEM

MRI without and with contrast is the diagnostic test of choice in most situations.

MRI findings in spinal epidural metastases:

1. vertebral mets are slightly hypointense compared to normal bone marrow on T1WI, and are slightly hyperintense on T2WI
2. axial cuts typically show lesion involving the posterior vertebral body with invasion into one or both pedicles
3. when myelopathy or radiculopathy are present, there is usually tumor extension into the spinal canal (may not occur in lesions presenting only with local pain)
4. DWI images may help differentiate osteoporotic compression fracture from pathologic fracture[13]

Plain x-rays

Most spinal mets are osteolytic, but at least 50% of the bone must be eroded before plain x-rays will be abnormal.[14] Not very specific. Possible findings: pedicle erosion (defect in "owl's eyes" AKA "winking owl sign" on LS or thoracic spine AP view) or widening, pathological compression fracture, vertebral body (VB) scalloping, VB *sclerosis*, osteoblastic changes (may occur with prostate Ca, Hodgkin's disease, occasionally with breast Ca, and rarely with multiple myeloma)

Plain CT in evaluating SEM

Very good for bone detail. Often helpful for surgical planning. By itself, has low sensitivity for spinal cord compression by tumor. Sensitivity is increased with intrathecal contrast (CT-myelogram).

CT-myelogram (CT-myelo)

Indicated when MRI cannot be done (contraindications, unavailability...).

Advantages over MRI:
- Can obtain CSF (when performing LP to inject contrast) for cytological study
- Excellent bony detail
- Can be performed in patients with pacemaker/AICD, claustrophobia...

Disadvantages of myelography over MRI[1]:
- Invasive
- May require second procedure (C1–2 puncture) if there is a complete block (providers proficient in this technique are becoming fewer)
- Risk of neurologic deterioration from LP in patient with complete block
- Cannot detect lesions that do not cause bony destruction or distortion of the spinal subarachnoid space
- Up to 20% of patients with SEM have at least two sites of cord compression, MRI can evaluate region between two complete blocks, myelography cannot
- Cannot demonstrate paraspinal lesions
- Does not image spinal cord parenchyma

Positron emission tomography (PET) scan

PET scan using [18F]-fluorodeoxyglucose may be used for whole-body work-up for bone mets in patients with known cancer.[15] Sensitivity is high, but spatial resolution and specificity are low, so often must be used with CT and/or MRI.

Metastatic work-up for patients with suspected spine metastases

- CT of chest, abdomen and pelvis: assess tumor burden, staging, prognostication (which factors into decisions regarding surgery). Has superseded CXR to rule out lung lesion (primary or other mets)
- bone scan: looks for other sites of skeletal involvement
- serum prostate specific antigen (PSA) in males
- mammogram in females
- for multiple myeloma (p. 715)
- careful physical exam of lymph nodes

53.4.4 Management algorithm

General information

Management is dependent on the degree and rapidity of neurologic involvement.[11] Patients may be categorized into one of the three groups that follows which outlines the subsequent steps. In a patient with suspected spine mets, the goals of management are:
- Assessment of neurologic involvement and timeline of neurologic changes.
- Delineate the degree of spinal involvement
- Determine a histologic diagnosis: this affects management
- Preserve or restore neurologic function
- Preserve or restore spinal stability
- Control pain

The tools that are employed in the assessment and stabilization phase are listed under diagnostic tests above. The section that follows discusses the rapidity with which they are implemented.

A metastatic work-up (p. 817) is undertaken as time permits (a preliminary work-up, e.g. CXR and physical exam, may be all that can be initially obtained for patients in Group I, whereas more complete work-up can be done in others).

Group I – rapid progression or severe deficit

Signs / symptoms

Signs/symptoms of new or progressive (hours to days) cord compression (e.g. urinary urgency, ascending numbness). These patients have a high risk of rapid deterioration and require immediate evaluation.

Management

1. dexamethasone (DMZ) (Decadron®): reduces pain in 85%, may produce transient neurologic improvement. Optimal dose is not known. No difference was found comparing 100 mg IV bolus to 10 mg.[16] Suggestion: 10 mg IV or PO q 6 hrs × 72 hrs, followed by lower dose of 4–6 mg q 6 hrs. Steroids may temporarily mask lymphoma (on imaging and at surgery), however, in this group the benefit of giving steroids usually outweighs this pitfall
2. radiographic evaluation
   a) STAT *MRI* (above)
   b) *plain x-rays* of entire spine: 67–85% will be abnormal (see above)
   c) if time permits, plain CT scan through involved levels and at least 2 levels above and below to evaluate bone for surgical planning
   d) **emergency** myelogram: indicated if MRI cannot be done (include possible C1–2 puncture on the consent). Start with a so-called "blockogram" to R/O complete block: instill small volume of contrast, e.g. iohexol (Omnipaque™) (p. 219) via LP and run the dye all the way up the spinal column; CSF is usually xanthochromic with complete block, see Froin's syndrome (p. 790)
      - if there is not a complete block: withdraw 10 cc of CSF and send for *cytology*, protein & glucose. One may then inject more contrast to complete the study
      - if complete block: do *not* remove CSF (pressure shifts via LP caused neurologic deterioration in ≈ 14% of patients with complete block,[17] whereas there was no deterioration after C1–2 puncture). In some cases, contrast can be "squeezed" past a "complete" block by injecting 5–10 ml of room air through a millipore filter,[18] alternatively, perform a lateral C1–2 puncture (p. 1511) and instill water soluble contrast to delineate the superior extent of the lesion
      - with myelography, epidural lesions classically produce hourglass deformity with smooth edges if block is incomplete, or paintbrush effect (feathered edges) if block is complete, unlike the sharp margins (capping or meniscus sign) of intradural extramedullary lesion, or fusiform cord widening of intramedullary tumors
      - *bone scan* if time permits. Abnormal in ≈ 66% of patients with spine mets
3. treatment based on results of radiographic evaluation
   a) if no epidural mass: treat primary tumor (e.g. systemic **chemotherapy**). Local radiation therapy (XRT) to bony lesion if present. Analgesics for pain
   b) if epidural lesion, either surgery *or* start XRT (usually 30–40 Gy in 10 treatments over 7–10 d with ports extending 2 levels above and below lesion). XRT is usually as effective as laminectomy with fewer complications; for further discussion see Treatment for SEM (p. 819). Thus, *surgery* instead of XRT is considered only for the indications shown in ▶ Table 53.4
   c) **urgency** of treatment (surgery or XRT) is based on degree of block and rapidity of deterioration:
      - if > 80% block or rapid progression of deficit: emergency treatment ASAP (if treating with XRT instead of surgery, continue DMZ next day at 24 mg IV q 6 hrs x 2 days, then taper during XRT over 2 wks)
      - if < 80% block: treatment on "routine" basis (for XRT, continue DMZ 4 mg IV q 6 hrs, taper during treatment as tolerated)

53

Table 53.4 Indications for surgery for spinal metastases

Indications
1. unknown primary and no tissue diagnosis (CT guided needle biopsy is an option for accessible lesions). NB: lesions such as spinal epidural abscess can be mistaken for metastases[21] 2. spinal instability 3. deficit due to spinal deformity or compression by bone rather than by tumor (e.g. due to compression fracture with collapse and retropulsed bone) 4. radio-resistant tumors (e.g. renal-cell carcinoma, melanoma...) or progression during XRT (usual trial: at least 48 hrs, unless significant or rapid deterioration) 5. recurrence after maximal XRT 6. rapid neurologic deterioration
Relative contraindications
1. very radiosensitive tumors (multiple myeloma, lymphoma...) not previously radiated 2. total paralysis (Brice and McKissock group 4) > 8 hours duration, or inability to walk (B&M group > 1) for > 24 hrs duration (after this, there is essentially no chance of recovery and surgery is not indicated) 3. expected survival: ≤ 3–4 months 4. multiple lesions at multiple levels 5. patient unable to tolerate surgery: for patients with lung lesions, check PFTs

Group II – mild and stable signs and symptoms

Signs / symptoms

Mild and stable signs/symptoms of cord compression (e.g. isolated Babinski), or either plexopathy or radiculopathy without evidence of cord compression. Admit and evaluate within 24 hrs.

Management

1. for suspected ESCC, manage as in Group I except on less emergent basis. Use low dose dexamethasone (DMZ) unless radiographic evaluation shows > 80% block or if suspicion of lymphoma is high and tissue will be obtained relatively soon
2. for radiculopathy alone (radicular pain, weakness or reflex changes in one myotome or sensory changes in one dermatome): if plain x-rays show bony lesion then 70–88% will have ESCC on myelography. If the plain film is normal, only 9–25% will have ESCC. Obtain MRI or myelogram and manage as for suspected ESCC
3. for plexopathy (brachial or lumbosacral): pain is the most common early symptom, distribution not limited to single dermatome, commonly referred to elbow or ankle. May mask coexistent radiculopathy, distinguish by EMG (denervation of paraspinal muscles occurs in radiculopathy) or presence of proximal signs and symptoms (Horner's syndrome in cervical region, ureteral obstruction in lumbar region). Management:
   a) MRI is initial diagnostic procedure (CT if MRI unavailable): C4 through T4 for brachial plexopathy, L1 through pelvis for lumbosacral plexopathy
   b) if CT shows bony lesion or paraspinal mass (with negative CT, plain films and bone scan are rarely helpful; however, if done, and plain x-ray shows malignant appearing bony lesion, or if bone scan shows vertebral abnormality, perform MRI or myelogram within 24 hrs) (give dexamethasone if ESCC suspected or MRI/myelogram delayed). Management as in Group I based on degree of block, XRT ports extended laterally to include any mass shown on CT
   c) if no bony nor paraspinal lesion on MRI/CT, primary treatment of plexus tumor; analgesics for pain

Group III – pain without neurologic involvement

Signs / symptoms

Back pain without neuro signs/symptoms. Can be evaluated as outpatient over several days (modify based on ability of patient to travel, reliability, etc.).

53

53.4.5 Treatment for SEM

Treatment goals and outcome

No treatment for SEM significantly prolongs life. Treatment goals are palliative: pain control, preservation of spinal stability, and maintenance of sphincter control and ability to ambulate.

The most important factor affecting prognosis, regardless of treatment modality, is ability to walk at the time of initiation of therapy. Loss of sphincter control is a poor prognosticator and is usually irreversible.

The main decision is between surgery + post-op XRT, or XRT alone. As yet, no chemotherapy has been found to be useful for SEM (may help with primary). Surgery alone appears least effective for pain control (36%, compared to 67% for surgery + XRT, and 76% for XRT alone).[19] Surgery has the attendant complications of anesthetic risk, post-op pain, wound problems in 11% (further complicated by radiation),[19] and mortality in 5–6% after laminectomy and 10% after anterior approach with stabilization.[20] Therefore, surgery appears best reserved for situations described in ▶ Table 53.4 .

Medical therapy

Chemotherapy is ineffective for SEM.

Bisphosphonates reduce the risk of vertebral compression fractures (VCF) by ≈ 50%, but the effect seems to abate after ≈ 2–3 years.

Promising agents undergoing trials include: denosumab, a RANK ligand (RANKL) inhibitor (p. 1011) that may counteract RANKL which is overexpressed in response to lytic bony metastases.[22] The efficacy seems better than the bisphosphonates.

Vertebroplasty/kyphoplasty

Vertebroplasty/kyphoplasty (p. 1011) reduces pain associated with pathologic fractures in up to 84% [23] with an associated increase in functional outcome.[24] Kyphoplasty appears to offer comparable pain relief to vertebroplasty with lower rates of cement leakage.[24]

Relative contraindication: spinal cord compression. Unless the diagnosis has already been verified, a biopsy should be taken through one of the pedicles prior to injecting PMMA.

Radiation therapy

Radiosensitive tumors: ▶ Table 52.6 lists radiosensitivity of metastatic tumors (to brain or spine). Other radiosensitive tumors that metastasize to the spine include: myxoid liposarcoma.[25]

Treatment[26]: Dose: range = 25–40 Gy. Typical plan: 30 Gy delivered in 3 Gy fractions over 10 days (2 working weeks) to ports extending at least 1 vertebral level above and below the extent of the lesion. Timing: for initial treatment, try to start XRT within 24 hours of diagnosis; for post-op XRT, within about 14 days following surgery.

There is a theoretical risk of radiation induced edema causing or accelerating neurologic deterioration. This has not been borne out by experimental studies with the usual small daily fractions utilized. Deterioration is more likely to be due to tumor progression.[27] The spinal cord is usually the dose limiting structure in treating SEM.

Increased doses are being made possible with the application of the added precision of stereotactic radiosurgery techniques to spinal metastases.[28]

Surgical treatment

See ▶ Table 53.4 for indications for surgery.

Pre-op embolization by interventional radiologist may facilitate resection with less blood loss for highly vascular tumors such as: renal-cell, thyroid, and hepatocellular. Blood supply is through the intercostal arteries, and care must be taken to avoid embolizing vessels providing significant blood supply to the spinal cord, especially the artery of Adamkiewicz (p. 87).

Approaches

Laminectomy alone is *poor* for spinal metastases when the pathology is *anterior* to the cord because of poor access to the tumor and the destabilizing effect of laminectomy when metastatic involvement of the vertebral body is significant.[29,30]

Deterioration in one of the 3 major criteria (pain, continence, ambulation) occurred in 26% of patients treated with *laminectomy* alone, 20% of laminectomy + XRT, and 17% of XRT alone (roughly comparable). There is a 9% incidence of spinal instability[19] following laminectomy *without* stabilization.

In a randomized controlled trial by Patchell et al.,[31] approaches directed at the location of the tumor (e.g. costotransversectomy, transthoracic approach…) with stabilization where necessary, produced better results than simple laminectomy, and surgery + XRT was superior to XRT alone (see ▶ Table 53.5). This study found a modest increase in survival, but more significant maintenance or regaining of lost ambulation. However, operative mortality with anterior decompression and stabilization was ≈ double (10%) that of laminectomy with (5%) or without (6%) stabilization in a literature review.[20]

Table 53.5 Comparing surgery + XRT to XRT alone[31]

Result	XRT	Surgery + XRT
Ambulatory after treatment	57%	84%
Days ambulatory after treatment	13	122
Ambulatory after treatment when nonambulatory before treatment	19%	62%
Mean survival (days)	100	126

Solitary spinal metastases with indolent tumors (e.g. renal cell Ca) may be candidates for attempted cure with en bloc resection (total spondylectomy).[32,33]

Laminectomy is still appropriate with isolated involvement of the posterior elements. For anterior pathology, if the posterior elements are intact, a transthoracic approach with corpectomy and stabilization (e.g. with methylmethacrylate and Steinmann pins,[34] or with cage graft and lateral plate) followed by XRT improves neurologic function in ≈ 75% and pain in ≈ 85%. A posterolateral approach (e.g. costotransversectomy) may be used for anterolateral tumor.[35] Combining a corpectomy and removal of the pedicle and posterior elements destabilizes the spine, therefore posterior instrumentation prior to performing the corpectomy is required, followed by cage graft.[36,37,38,39,40,41,42] To access a VB via a costotransversectomy, the rib of the like numbered VB and the one below need to be removed.

References

[1] Godersky JC, Smoker WRK, Knutzon R. Use of MRI in the Evaluation of Metastatic Spinal Disease. Neurosurgery. 1987; 21:676–680

[2] Livingston KE, Perrin RG. The neurosurgical management of spinal metastases causing cord and cauda equina compression. J Neurosurg. 1978; 49:839–843

[3] Batson OV. The Function of the Vertebral Veins and Their Role in the Spread of Metastases. Ann Surg. 1940; 112

[4] Schwab JH, Boland P, Guo T, Brennan MF, Singer S, Healey JH, Antonescu CR. Skeletal metastases in myxoid liposarcoma: an unusual pattern of distant spread. Ann Surg Oncol. 2007; 14:1507–1514

[5] Rodichok LD, Ruckdeschel JC, Harper GR, et al. Early Detection and Treatment of Spinal Epidural Metastases: The Role of Myelography. Ann Neurol. 1986; 20:696–702

[6] Bach F, Larsen BH, Rhode K, et al. Metastatic spinal cord compression. Occurrence, symptoms, clinical presentations and prognosis in 398 patients with spinal cord compression. Acta Neurochir (Wien). 1990; 107:37–43

[7] Helwig-Larsen S, Sorensen PS. Symptoms and signs in metastatic spinal cord compression: a study from first symptom until diagnosis in 153 patients. Eur J Cancer. 1994; 30A:396–398

[8] Levack P, Graham J, Collie D, et al. Don't wait for a sensory level: listen to the symptoms: a prospective audit of the delays in diagnosis of malignant cord compression. Clin Oncol (R Coll Radiol). 2002; 14:472–480

[9] Sherk HH. Lesions of the Atlas and Axis. Clin Orthop. 1975; 109:33–41

[10] Nakamura M, Toyama Y, Suzuki N, Fujimura Y. Metastases to the upper cervical spine. J Spinal Disord. 1996; 9:195–201

[11] Portenoy RK, Lipton RB, Foley KM. Back Pain in the Cancer Patient: An Algorithm for Evaluation and Management. Neurology. 1987; 37:134–138

[12] Brice J, McKissock W. Surgical Treatment of Malignant Extradural Spinal Tumors. Br Med J. 1965; 1:1341–1344

[13] Li KC, Poon PY. Sensitivity and specificity of MRI in detecting spinal cord compression and in distinguishing malignant from benign compression fractures of vertebrae. Magn Reson Imaging. 1988; 6:547–556

[14] Gabriel K, Schi D. Metastatic spinal cord compression by solid tumors. Semin Neurol. 2004; 24:375–383

[15] Francken AB, Hong AM, Fulham MJ, et al. Detection of unsuspected spinal cord compression in melanoma patients by 18F-fluorodeoxyglucose-positron emission tomography. Eur J Surg Oncol. 2005; 31:197–204

[16] Vecht CJ, Haaxma-Reiche H, van Putten WL, et al. Initial bolus of conventional versus high-dose dexamethasone in metastatic spinal cord compression. Neurology. 1989; 39:1255–1257

[17] Hollis PH, Malis LI, Zappulla RA. Neurological Deterioration After Lumbar Puncture Below Complete Spinal Subarachnoid Block. J Neurosurg. 1986; 64:253–256

[18] Lee Y-Y, Glass JP, Wallace S. Myelography in Cancer Patients: Modified Technique. AJR. 1985; 145:791–795

[19] Findlay GFG. Adverse Effects of the Management of Malignant Spinal Cord Compression. J Neurol Neurosurg Psychiatry. 1984; 47:761–768

[20] Witham TF, Khavkin YA, Gallia GL, et al. Surgery insight: current management of epidural spinal cord compression from metastatic spine disease. Nat Clin Pract Neurol. 2006; 2:87–94

[21] Danner RL, Hartman BJ. Update of Spinal Epidural Abscess: 35 Cases and Review of the Literature. Rev Infect Dis. 1987; 9:265–274

[22] Mundy GR. Metastasis to bone: causes, consequences and therapeutic opportunities. Nat Rev Cancer. 2002; 2:584–593

[23] Fourney DR, Schomer DF, Nader R, Chlan-Fourney J, Suki D, Ahrar K, Rhines LD, Gokaslan ZL. Percutaneous vertebroplasty and kyphoplasty for painful vertebral body fractures in cancer patients. J Neurosurg. 2003; 98:21–30

[24] Bouza C, Lopez-Cuadrado T, Cediel P, Saz-Parkinson Z, Amate JM. Balloon kyphoplasty in malignant spinal fractures: a systematic review and meta-analysis. BMC Palliat Care. 2009; 8. DOI: 10.1186/1472-684X-8-12

[25] Reitan JB, Kaalhus O. Radiotherapy of liposarcomas. Br J Radiol. 1980; 53:969–975

[26] Faul CM, Flickinger JC. The use of radiation in the management of spinal metastases. J Neurooncol. 1995; 23:149–161

[27] Rubin P. Extradural Spinal Cord Compression by Tumor: Part I. Experimental Production and Treatment Trials. Radiology. 1969; 93:1243–1248

[28] Rock JP, Ryu S, Yin FF, Schreiber F, Abdulhak M. The evolving role of stereotactic radiosurgery and stereotactic radiation therapy for patients with spine tumors. J Neurooncol. 2004; 69:319–334

[29] Onimus M, Schraub S, Bertin D, et al. Surgical Treatment of Vertebral Metastasis. Spine. 1986; 11:883–891

[30] Cooper PR, Errico TJ, Martin R, Crawford B, DiBartolo T. A Systematic Approach to Spinal Reconstruction After Anterior Decompression for Neoplastic Disease of the Thoracic and Lumbar Spine. Neurosurgery. 1993; 32:1–8

[31] Patchell RA, Tibbs PA, Regine WF, Payne R, Saris S, Kryscio RJ, Mohiuddin M, Young B. Direct decompressive surgical resection in the treatment of spinal cord compression caused by metastatic cancer: a randomized trial. Lancet. 2005; 366:643–648

[32] Fourney DR, Abi-Said D, Rhines LD, et al. Simultaneous anterior-posterior approach to the thoracic and lumbar spine for the radical resection of tumors followed by reconstruction and stabilization. J Neurosurg. 2001; 94:232–244

[33] Sakaura H, Hosono N, Mukai Y, et al. Outcome of total en bloc spondylectomy for solitary metastasis of the thoracolumbar spine. J Spinal Disord. 2004; 17:297–300

[34] Sundaresan N, Galicich JH, Lane JM, et al. Treatment of Neoplastic Epidural Cord Compression by Vertebral Body Resection and Stabilization. J Neurosurg. 1985; 63:676–684
[35] Overby MC, Rothman AS. Anterolateral Decompression for Metastatic Epidural Spinal Cord Tumors: Results of a Modified Costrotransversectomy Approach. J Neurosurg. 1985; 62:344–348
[36] Shaw B, Mansfield FL, Borges L. One-Stage Posterolateral Decompression and Stabilization for Primary and Metastatic Vertebral Tumors in the Thoracic and Lumbar Spine. J Neurosurg. 1989; 70:405–410
[37] Akeyson EW, McCutcheon IE. Single-stage posterior vertebrectomy and replacement combined with posterior instrumentation for spinal metastasis. J Neurosurg. 1996; 85:211–220
[38] Fourney DR, Abi-Said D, Lang FF, et al. Use of pedicle screw fixation in the management of malignant spinal disease: experience in 100 consecutive cases. J Neurosurg. 2001; 94:25–37
[39] Wang JC, Boland P, Mitra N, et al. Single-stage posterolateral transpedicular approach for resection of epidural metastatic spine tumors involving the vertebral body with circumferential reconstruction: results in 140 patients. J Neurosurg Spine. 2004; 1:287–298
[40] Hunt T, Shen FH, Arlet V. Expandable cage placement via a posterolateral approach in lumbar spine reconstructions: technical note. J Neurosurg Spine. 2006; 5:271–274
[41] Snell BE, Nasr FF, Wolfla CE. Single-stage thoracolumbar vertebrectomy with circumferential reconstruction and arthrodesis: surgical technique and results in 15 patients. Neurosurgery (Operative Neurosurgery). 2006; 58:263–269
[42] Sciubba DM, Gallia GL, McGirt MJ, et al. Thoracic kyphotic deformity reduction with a distractible titanium cage via an entirely posterior approach. Neurosurgery. 2007; 60:223–231

Part XIV

Head Trauma

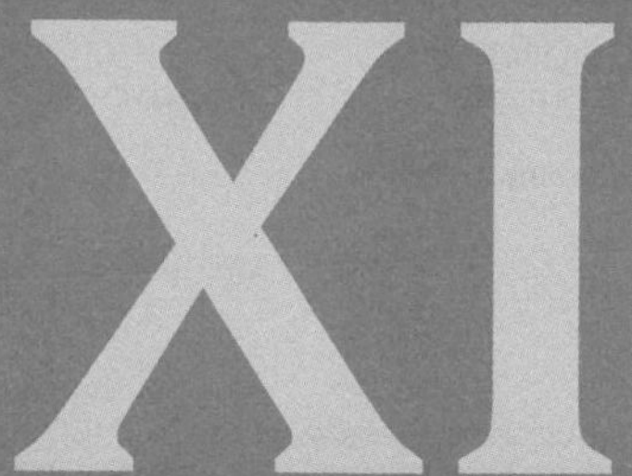

54 General Information, Grading, Initial Management

54.1 General information

54.1.1 Introduction

56–60% of patients with GCS score ≤ 8 have 1 or more other organ system injured.[1] 25% have "surgical" lesions. There is a 4–5% incidence of associated spine fractures with significant head injury (mostly C1 to C3).

When a detailed history is unavailable, remember: the loss of consciousness may have *preceded* (and possibly have caused) the trauma. Therefore, maintain an index of suspicion for e.g. aneurysmal SAH, hypoglycemia, etc. in the differential diagnosis of the causes of trauma and associated coma.

Brain injury from trauma results from two distinct processes:

1. primary brain injury: occurs at time of trauma (cortical contusions, lacerations, bone fragmentation, diffuse axonal injury, and brainstem contusion)
2. secondary injury: develops subsequent to the initial injury. Includes injuries from intracranial hematomas, edema, hypoxemia, ischemia (primarily due to elevated intracranial pressure (ICP) and/or shock), vasospasm

Since impact damage cannot be influenced by the treating neurosurgeon, intense interest has focused on reducing secondary injuries, which requires good general medical care and an understanding of intracranial pressure (p. 856).

54.1.2 Delayed deterioration

≈ 15% of patients who do not initially exhibit signs of significant brain injury may deteriorate in a delayed fashion, sometimes referred to as patients who "talk and deteriorate" or when more lethal, patient who "talk and die".[2] Etiologies:

1. ≈ 75% will exhibit an intracranial hematoma
   a) may be present on initial evaluation and can then worsen
   b) may develop in a delayed fashion
      - delayed epidural hematoma (EDH) (p. 894)
      - delayed subdural (SDH) (p. 898)
      - delayed traumatic contusions (p. 892)
2. posttraumatic diffuse cerebral edema (p. 848)
3. hydrocephalus
4. tension pneumocephalus
5. seizures
6. metabolic abnormalities, includes:
   a) hyponatremia
   b) hypoxia: etiologies include pneumothorax, MI, CHF…
   c) hepatic encephalopathy
   d) hypoglycemia: including insulin reaction
   e) adrenal insufficiency
   f) drug or alcohol withdrawal
7. vascular events
   a) dural sinus thrombosis (p. 1308)
   b) carotid (or rarely, vertebral) artery dissection (p. 1324)
   c) SAH: due to rupture of aneurysm (spontaneous or posttraumatic) or carotid-cavernous fistula (CCF) (p. 1256)
   d) cerebral embolism: including fat embolism syndrome (p. 835)
8. meningitis
9. hypotension (shock)

54.2 Grading

Despite many (valid) criticisms, the initial post-resuscitation Glasgow Coma Scale (GCS) score (▶ Table 18.1) remains the most widely used and perhaps best replicated scale employed in for the assessment of head trauma. Problems with this type of scale is that it is an ordinal scale that is non parametric (i.e. does not represent precise measurements of discrete quantities), it is non-linear, and it is not an interval scale, so that for example, a decrease of 2 points in one parameter is not necessarily equal to a decrease in 2 points of another.[3] Thus, performing mathematical manipulations (e.g. adding components, or calculating mean values), while often done, is not statistically sound.[4]

There are a number schemes to stratify the severity of head injury. Any such categorization is arbitrary and will be imperfect. A simple system based only on GCS score is as follows:

- GCS 14–15 = mild
- GCS 9–13 = moderate
- GCS ≤ 8 = severe

An example of a more involved system[3] incorporates other factors in addition to the GCS score as shown in ▶ Fig. 54.1.

54.3 Transfer of trauma patients

It is sometimes necessary for a neurosurgeon to accept a trauma patient in transfer from another institution that is not equipped to handle major neurologic injuries, or to transfer patients to other facilities for a variety of reasons. ▶ Table 54.1 lists factors that should be assessed and stabilized (if possible) prior to transfer. These items should also be evaluated in trauma patients on whom a neurosurgeon is consulted in his or her own E/R as well as in patients with other CNS abnormalities besides trauma (e.g. SAH).

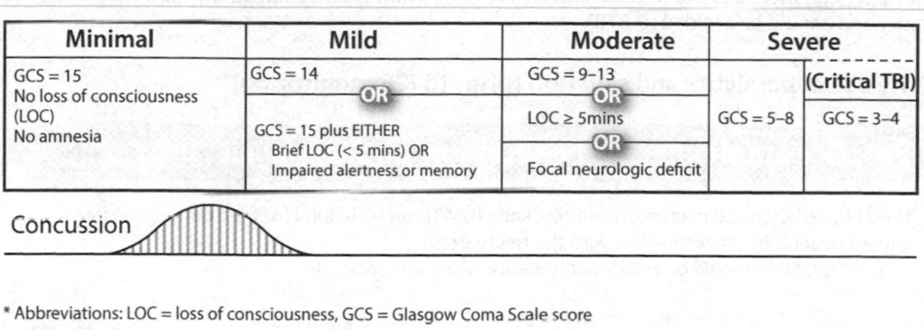

Minimal	Mild	Moderate	Severe	
				(Critical TBI)
GCS = 15 No loss of consciousness (LOC) No amnesia	GCS = 14 OR GCS = 15 plus EITHER Brief LOC (< 5 mins) OR Impaired alertness or memory	GCS = 9–13 OR LOC ≥ 5mins OR Focal neurologic deficit	GCS = 5–8	GCS = 3–4

Concussion

* Abbreviations: LOC = loss of consciousness, GCS = Glasgow Coma Scale score

Fig. 54.1 Categorization of head injury severity

Table 54.1 Factors to assess in head injured patients

Clinical concern	Items to check	Steps to remedy
hypoxia or hypoventilation	ABG, respiratory rate	intubate any patient who has hypercarbia, hypoxemia, or is not localizing
hypotension or hypertension	BP, Hgb/Hct	transfuse patients with significant loss of blood volume
anemia	Hgb/Hct	transfuse patients with significant anemia
seizures	electrolytes, AED levels	correct hyponatremia or hypoglycemia; administer AEDs when appropriate[a]
infection or hyperthermia	WBC, temperature	LP if meningitis is possible and no contraindications (p. 1504)
spinal stability	spine x-rays	spine immobilization (spine board, cervical collar & sandbags...); patients with locked facets should be reduced if possible before transfer

[a]see Seizures (p. 440), as well as Posttraumatic seizures (p. 462)

54.4 Management in E/R

54.4.1 General measures

Blood pressure and oxygenation

Practice guideline: IBP and oxygenation

Level II[5]: monitor BP and avoid hypotension (SBP < 90 mm Hg)
Level III[5]: monitor oxygenation and avoid hypoxia (PaO_2 < 60 mm Hg or O_2 saturation < 90%)

Hypotension

Hypotension (shock) is rarely attributable to head injury except:
- in terminal stages (i.e. with dysfunction of medulla and cardiovascular collapse)
- in infancy, where enough blood can be lost intracranially or into the subgaleal space to cause shock
- where enough blood has been lost from scalp wounds to cause hypovolemia (exsanguination)

Hypotension (defined as a single SBP < 90 mm Hg) doubles mortality, hypoxia (apnea or cyanosis in the field, or PaO_2 < 60 mm Hg on ABG) also increases mortality,[6] and the combination of both triples mortality and increases the risk bad outcome. SBP < 90 mm Hg may impair CBF and exacerbate brain injury and should be avoided (p. 870).

Early use of paralytics and sedation (prior to ICP monitoring)

Practice guideline: Early sedation and paralysis

Level III[7]: sedation and neuromuscular blockade (NMB) can be helpful for transporting the head-injured patient, but they interfere with the neuro exam
Level III[7]: NMB should be used when sedation alone is inadequate

54

The routine use of sedatives and paralytics in neurotrauma patients may lead to a higher incidence of pneumonia, longer ICU stays, and possibly sepsis.[8] These agents also impair neurologic assessment.[7,9] Use should therefore be reserved for cases with clinical evidence of intracranial hypertension (see ▶ Table 54.2), for intubation, or where use is necessary for transport or to permit evaluation of the patient (e.g. to get a combative patient to hold still for a CT scan).[10]

Intubation and hyperventilation

Indications for *intubation* in trauma; also see **Practice guideline: Intubation – indications** (p. 827):
1. depressed level of consciousness (patient cannot protect airway): usually GCS ≤ 7
2. need for hyperventilation (HPV): see below
3. severe maxillofacial trauma: patency of airway tenuous or concern for inability to maintain patency with further tissue swelling and/or bleeding
4. need for pharmacologic paralysis for evaluation or management

Table 54.2 Clinical signs of IC-HTN[a]

1. pupillary dilatation (unilateral or bilateral)
2. asymmetric pupillary reaction to light
3. decerebrate or decorticate posturing (usually contralateral to blown[b] pupil)
4. progressive deterioration of the neurologic exam not attributable to extracranial factors

[a]Items 1-3 represent clinical signs of herniation. The most convincing clinical evidence of IC-HTN is the witnessed evolution of 1 or more of these signs. IC-HTN may produce a bulging fontanelle in an infant.
[b] "blown pupil": fixed & dilated pupil

Practice guideline: Intubation – indications

Level III[11]: secure the airway (usually by endotracheal intubation) in patients with GCS ≤ 8 who are unable to maintain their airway or who remain hypoxic despite supplemental O_2

Cautions regarding intubation:
1. if basal skull fracture through cribriform plate is possible, avoid nasotracheal intubation (to avoid intracranial entry of tube). Use orotracheal intubation
2. prevents assessment of patient's ability to verbalize[9] e.g. for determining Glasgow Coma Scale score. This ability should be noted (none, unintelligible, inappropriate, confused, or oriented) prior to intubation
3. risk of pneumonia: see **Practice guideline: Antibiotics for intubation** (p. 827) regarding antibiotics

Practice guideline: Antibiotics for intubation

Level II[12]: periprocedural antibiotics for endotracheal intubation reduce the risk of pneumonia, but do not alter length of stay or mortality

Hyperventilation (HPV)

Practice guideline: Early/prophylactic hyperventilation

Level II[13]: prophylactic hyperventilation ($PaCO_2 \leq 25$ mm Hg) is not recommended

Level III

- hyperventilation (HPV) before ICP monitoring is established should be reserved as a temporizing measure[13] for patients with signs of transtentorial herniation (see ▶ Table 54.2) or progressive neurologic deterioration not attributable to extracranial causes[7]
- HPV should be avoided during the first 24 hrs after TBI (when CBF is often dangerously decreased) [13]

1. since HPV may exacerbate cerebral ischemia, **HPV should not be used prophylactically** (p. 872)
2. prior to ICP monitoring, HPV should only be used briefly when CT or clinical signs of IC-HTN are present[10] (see ▶ Table 54.2 for clinical signs)
   a) when appropriate indications are met: HPV to *$PaCO_2$ = 30–35 mm* Hg
   b) HPV should not be used to the point that $PaCO_2 < 30$ mm Hg (this further reduces CBF but does not necessarily reduce ICP)
3. acute alkalosis increases protein binding of calcium (decreases ionized Ca^{++}). Patients being *hyperventilated* may develop ionized hypocalcemia with tetany (despite normal total [Ca])

Mannitol in E/R

Practice guideline: Early use of mannitol

Level III[7,14]: the use of mannitol before ICP monitoring is established should be reserved for patients who are adequately volume-resuscitated with signs of transtentorial herniation (see ▶ Table 54.2) or progressive neurologic deterioration not attributable to extracranial causes

Indications in E/R, see also more details (p. 873):
1. evidence of intracranial hypertension (see ▶ Table 54.2)
2. evidence of mass effect (focal deficit, e.g. hemiparesis)

54

3. sudden deterioration prior to CT (including pupillary dilatation)
4. after CT, if a lesion that is associated with increased ICP is identified
5. after CT, if going to O.R.
6. to assess "salvageability": in patient with no evidence of brainstem function, look for return of brainstem reflexes

Contraindications:
1. prophylactic administration is *not* recommended due to its volume-depleting effect. Use only for appropriate indications (see above)
2. hypotension or hypovolemia: hypotension can negatively influence outcome.[10] Therefore, when intracranial hypertension (IC-HTN) is present, first utilize sedation and/or paralysis, and CSF drainage. If further measures are needed, fluid resuscitate the patient before administering mannitol. Use hyperventilation in hypovolemic patients until mannitol can be given
3. relative contraindication: mannitol may slightly impede normal coagulation
4. CHF: before causing diuresis, mannitol transiently increases intravascular volume. Use with caution in CHF, may need to pre-treat with furosemide (Lasix®)

℞: bolus with 0.25–1 gm/kg over < 20 min (for average adult: ≈ 350 ml of 20% solution). Peak effect occurs in ≈ 20 minutes (p. 873) (for follow-up dosing).

Prophylactic antiepileptic drugs (AEDs)

Practice guideline: Prophylactic anticonvulsants after TBI

Level II[15,16,17]: prophylactic phenytoin, carbamazepine, phenobarbital or valproate[18] do not prevent late PTS

Level II: AEDs[17] (e.g. phenytoin, valproate, or carbamazepine[15,16,18]) may be used to decrease the incidence of early PTS (within 7 days of TBI) in patients at high risk of seizures after TBI (see ▸ Table 54.3), however, this does not improve outcome

Routine use of prophylactic antiepileptic drugs (AEDs) in traumatic brain injury (TBI) is ineffective in preventing the late development of posttraumatic seizures (PTS) i.e. epilepsy, and has been shown to not be useful except in certain circumstances.[15,16]

See details on using (p. 463) and discontinuing (p. 463) prophylactic AEDs following TBI. ▸ Table 54.3 reiterates the markers for patients at increased risk of early PTSs.

54.4.2 Neurosurgical exam in trauma

General information

It is not possible to outline a physical exam that is universally applicable. Major trauma must be assessed rapidly, often under chaotic circumstances, and must be individualized based on patient's medical stability, type of injury, degree of combativeness, use of pharmacologic paralytics (p. 826), the needs of other caregivers attending to other organ injuries, the need to triage in the event of multiple patients requiring simultaneous attention…

The following describes some features that should be assessed under certain circumstances with the understanding that this *must be individualized*. This addresses only craniospinal injuries, and assumes that general systemic injuries (internal bleeding, myocardial and/or pulmonary

Table 54.3 Conditions with increased risk of posttraumatic seizures

1. acute subdural, epidural, or intracerebral hematoma SDH, EDH or ICH
2. open-depressed skull fracture with parenchymal injury
3. seizure within the first 24 hrs after injury
4. Glasgow Coma Scale score < 10
5. penetrating brain injury
6. history of significant alcohol abuse
7. ± cortical (hemorrhagic) contusion on CT

contusion…) as well as orthopedic injuries (long bone and pelvic fractures…) will be treated by other members of a "trauma team." Although organized here in outline form, the most efficient order of examination is usually dictated by circumstances unique to each situation.

General physical condition (oriented towards neuro assessment)

1. visual inspection of cranium:
   a) evidence of basal skull fracture (p. 884):
      - raccoon's eyes: periorbital ecchymoses
      - Battle's sign: postauricular ecchymoses (around mastoid air sinuses)
      - CSF rhinorrhea/otorrhea (p. 387)
      - hemotympanum or laceration of external auditory canal
   b) check for facial fractures
      - LeFort fractures (p. 887): palpate for instability of facial bones, including zygomatic arch
      - orbital rim fracture: palpable step-off
   c) periorbital edema, proptosis
2. cranio-cervical auscultation
   a) auscultate over carotid arteries: bruit may be associated with indicate carotid dissection
   b) auscultate over globe of eye: bruit may indicate traumatic carotid-cavernous fistula CCF; see Carotid-cavernous fistula (p. 1256)
3. physical signs of trauma to spine: bruising, deformity
4. evidence of seizure: single, multiple, or continuing (status epilepticus)

Neurologic exam

1. cranial nerve exam
   a) optic nerve function (p. 836)
      - if conscious: serial quantitation of vision in each eye is important.[19] A Rosenbaum near vision card is ideal (see inside back cover), otherwise use any printed material. If patient cannot see this, check if they can count fingers. Failing this, check for hand motion vision and lastly light perception. Children may develop transient cortical blindness lasting 1–2 days, usually after a blow to the back of the head
      - if unconscious: check for afferent pupillary defect (p. 562), best demonstrated with swinging flashlight test (p. 561). Indicates possible optic nerve injury
      - funduscopic exam: check for papilledema, pre-retinal hemorrhages, retinal detachment, or retinal abnormalities suggestive of anterior optic nerve injury. If a detailed exam is required, pharmacologic dilatation with mydriatics (p. 563) may be employed, however, this precludes pupillary exam for a variable period of time, and should be undertaken advisedly
   b) pupil: size in ambient light; reaction to light (direct & consensual)
   c) VII: check for peripheral VII palsy (p. 884) (facial asymmetry of unilateral upper and lower facial muscles)
   d) VI: abducens palsy (p. 567) following trauma may occur as a result of ↑ ICP or with clival fractures (p. 884)
2. level of consciousness/mental status
   a) Glasgow coma scale for quantitating level of consciousness in poorly responsive patient (see ▶ Table 18.1)
   b) check orientation in patient able to communicate
3. motor exam (assesses motor tracts from motor cortex through spinal cord)
   a) if patient is cooperative: check motor strength in all 4 extremities
   b) if uncooperative: check for appropriate movement of all 4 extremities to noxious stimulus (differentiate voluntary movement from posturing or stereotypical spinal cord reflex). This also assesses sensation in an unresponsive patient
   c) if any doubt about integrity of spinal cord: also check "resting" tone of anal sphincter on rectal exam, evaluate voluntary sphincter contraction if patient can cooperate, check anal wink with pinprick, and assess bulbocavernosus reflex (p. 943) (see Neurological assessment, for details)
4. sensory exam
   a) cooperative patient:
      - check pinprick on trunk and in all 4 extremities, touch on major dermatomes (C4, C6, C7, C8, T4, T6, T10, L2, L4, L5, S1, sacrococcygeal)
      - check posterior column function: joint position sense of LEs

b) uncooperative patient: check for central response to noxious stimulus (e.g. grimace, vocalization…, as opposed to flexion-withdrawal which could be a spinal cord mediated reflex)

5. reflexes
   a) muscle stretch ("deep tendon") reflexes if patient is not thrashing: e.g. preserved reflex indicates that a flaccid limb is due to CNS injury and not nerve root injury (and vice versa)
   b) check plantar reflex for upgoing toes (Babinski sign)
   c) in suspected spinal cord injury: the anal wink and bulbocavernosus reflex are checked on the rectal exam (see above)

54.4.3 Indications for CT and admission criteria for TBI

General information

Numerous stratagems have been devised to determine what studies should be ordered for which patients. Patients with trivial injuries rarely need a CT scan, and those with severe head injuries obviously need one. Most of the effort centers around identifying the patient who appears to have a minor head injury but may be harboring or apt to develop a significant intracranial injury. An optimal protocol has not been developed, and a rigorous prospective application and further refinement of published systems is sadly lacking. In view of this state of affairs, the following is presented as a guideline.

Patients may be stratified into one of three groups based on the likelihood of intracranial injury as outlined in the following sections.[20,21]

Category 1. Low risk for intracranial injury

Criteria

Possible findings are shown in ▶ Table 54.4.

In this group, there is an extremely low likelihood of intracranial injury (**ICI**) (incidence of ICI: ≤ 8.5 in 10,000 cases with 95% confidence level[20]).

Management recommendations

CT scan is not usually indicated. Plain SXRs are *not* recommended: 99.6% of SXRs in this group are normal. Linear non-displaced skull fractures in this group require *no treatment*, although in-hospital observation (at least overnight) may be considered.

Patients in this group who meet Criteria for observation at home shown in ▶ Table 54.5 may be managed with observation at home with written head-injury discharge instructions, e.g. as illustrated ▶ Table 54.6.

54

Category 2. Moderate risk for intracranial injury

Criteria

Possible findings are shown in ▶ Table 54.7

Management recommendations

1. head CT scan (unenhanced): clinical grounds alone may miss important lesions in this group.[22] 8–46% of patients with minor head injury (MHI) have an intracranial lesion (the most frequent finding was hemorrhagic contusion)[23]
2. SXR (p. 833): not recommended unless CT scan not available. Useless if normal. A SXR is helpful only if positive (a clinically unsuspected depressed skull fracture might be important)
3. observation
   a) at home, if the patient meets the criteria outlined in ▶ Table 54.5. Provide caregiver with written head-injury discharge instructions (sometimes called "subdural precautions"), as shown in ▶ Table 54.6

Table 54.4 Findings with low risk of ICI

- asymptomatic
- H/A
- dizziness
- scalp hematoma, laceration, contusion, or abrasion
- no moderate nor high risk criteria (see ▶ Table 54.7 and ▶ Table 54.8, no loss of consciousness, etc.)
- no history of loss of consciousness

Table 54.5 Criteria for observation at home

1. Head CT scan not indicated, or CT scan normal if indicated[22] 2. initial GCS ≥ 14 3. no high risk criteria 4. no moderate risk criteria except loss of consciousness 5. patient is now neurologically intact (amnesia for the event is acceptable) 6. there is a responsible, sober adult that can observe the patient 7. patient has reasonable access to return to the hospital E/R if needed 8. no "complicating" circumstances (e.g. no suspicion of domestic violence, including child abuse)

Table 54.6 Sample discharge instructions for head injuries

Seek medical attention for any of the following: 1. a change in level of consciousness (including difficulty in awakening) 2. abnormal behavior 3. increased headache 4. slurred speech 5. weakness or loss of feeling in an arm or leg 6. persistent vomiting 7. enlargement of one or both pupils (the black round part in the middle of the eye) that does not get smaller when a bright light is shined on it 8. seizures (convulsions or fits) 9. significant increase in swelling at injury site Do not take sedatives or pain medication stronger than acetaminophen (paracetamol in some countries) for 48 hours. Do not take aspirin or other anti-inflammatory medications because of interference with platelet function and theoretical increased risk of bleeding

Table 54.7 Findings with moderate risk of ICI

1. history of change or loss of consciousness on or after injury 2. progressive H/A 3. EtOH or drug intoxication 4. posttraumatic seizure 5. unreliable or inadequate history 6. age < 2 yr (unless trivial injury) 7. vomiting 8. posttraumatic amnesia 9. signs of basilar skull fracture 10. multiple trauma 11. serious facial injury 12. possible skull penetration or depressed fracture 13. suspected child abuse 14. significant subgaleal swelling[21]

b) in-hospital observation to rule-out neurologic deterioration if patient does not meet criteria in ▶ Table 54.5 (including cases where CT scan is not done).

Managing patients with in-hospital observation and only getting a CT scan in cases of deterioration (GCS score ≤ 13) is as sensitive as CT in detecting intracranial hematomas,[23,24,25,26,27] but is less cost effective than routinely performing an early CT scan and discharging patients who have a normal CT and no other indication for hospitalization[23]

Category 3. High risk for intracranial injury

Criteria

Possible findings are shown in ▶ Table 54.8.

Management recommendations

1. admit to hospital
2. STAT unenhanced head CT scan
3. if there are focal findings on neurologic examination

54

Table 54.8 Findings with high risk of ICI

- depressed level of consciousness not clearly due to EtOH, drugs, metabolic abnormalities, postictal, etc.
- focal neurological findings
- decreasing level of consciousness
- penetrating skull injury or depressed fracture

   a) notify operating room to be on standby
   b) if CT scan or MRI is not available, consider emergency burr holes (p. 836)
4. determine if intracranial monitor (p. 858) is indicated
5. SXR usually not recommended: a fracture is rarely surprising, and a SXR is inadequate for assessing for intracranial injury. A SXR is possibly useful for localizing a radio-opaque penetrating foreign body (knife blade, bullet…) for the O.R.

Other risk factors

Occipital vs. frontal fractures

Patients with occipital fractures may be at higher risk of significant intracranial injury (ICI). May be related to the fact that in forward trauma, one may protect oneself with the outstretched arms. Furthermore, the facial bones and air sinuses exert an impact absorbing effect. In 210 patients with facial fractures,[28] the highest incidence of ICI was seen in those with upper facial fractures. Those with mandibular and midfacial region fractures (without upper facial involvement) had a lower likelihood of ICI, and those with mandibular region trauma only were least likely to have ICI.

54.5 Radiographic evaluation

54.5.1 CT scans in trauma

General information

An unenhanced (i.e. non-contrast) CT scan of the head usually suffices for patients seen in the emergency department presenting after trauma or with a new neurologic deficit. Enhanced CT or MRI may be appropriate after the unenhanced CT, but are not usually required emergently (exceptions include: significant brain edema due to suspected neoplasm that is not demonstrated without contrast).

The main emergent conditions to rule out (and brief descriptions):

54

1. blood (hemorrhages or hematomas):
   a) extra-axial blood: surgical lesions are usually ≥ 1 cm maximal thickness
      - epidural hematoma (EDH) (p. 892): usually biconvex and often due to arterial bleeding. May cross dural barriers (unlike SDH) such as falx, tentorium
      - subdural hematoma (SDH) (p. 891): usually crescentic, usually due to venous bleeding. May cover larger surface area than EDH (dural adherence to inner table limits extension of EDH). Chronology of SDH: acute = high density, subacute ≈ isodense, chronic ≈ low density
   b) subarachnoid blood (SAH): Trauma is the most common cause of SAH. Unlike aneurysmal SAH where blood is thickest near the circle of Willis, traumatic SAH (tSAH) usually appears as high density spread thinly over convexity and filling sulci or basal cisterns. However, when the history of trauma is not clear, an arteriogram may be indicated to R/O a ruptured aneurysm (that might have precipitated the trauma in some cases)
   c) intracerebral hemorrhage (ICH): increased density in brain parenchyma
   d) hemorrhagic contusion (p. 891): often "fluffy" inhomogeneous high-density areas within brain parenchyma, usually adjacent to bony prominences (frontal and occipital poles, sphenoid wing). Typically less well defined than primary ICH
   e) intraventricular hemorrhage (p. 1192): present in ≈ 10% of severe head injuries.[29] Associated with poor outcome; may be a marker for severe injury rather than the cause of the poor outcome. Use of intraventricular rt-PA has been reported for treatment[30]
2. hydrocephalus: enlarged ventricles may sometimes develop following trauma
3. cerebral swelling: obliteration of basal cisterns (p. 921), compression of ventricles and sulci…
4. evidence of cerebral anoxia: loss of gray-white interface, signs of swelling
5. skull fractures:
   a) basal skull fractures (including temporal bone fracture)
   b) orbital blow-out fracture
   c) calvarial fracture (CT may miss some linear nondisplaced skull fractures)

- linear vs. stellate
- open vs. closed
- diastatic (separation of sutures)
- depressed vs. nondepressed: CT helps assess need for surgery

6. ischemic infarction: findings are usually minimal or subtle if < 24 hrs since stroke
7. pneumocephalus: may indicate skull fracture (basal or open convexity)
8. shift of midline structures (due to extra- or intra-axial hematomas or asymmetric cerebral edema): shift can cause altered levels of consciousness (p. 921)

Indications for initial brain CT

1. presence of any moderate[31] or high risk criteria (▸ Table 54.7 and ▸ Table 54.8) which include: GCS ≤ 14, unresponsiveness, focal deficit, amnesia for injury, altered mental status (including those that are significantly inebriated), deteriorating neuro status, signs of basal or calvarial skull fracture
2. assessment prior to general anesthesia for other procedures (during which neurologic exam cannot be followed in order to detect delayed deterioration)

Follow-up CT

Routine follow-up CT (when there is no indication for urgent follow-up CT, see below):

1. many facilities perform a repeat head CT at 24 hours for patients who are clinically stable but had findings on initial head CT of: traumatic SAH, small SDH or EDH, intraparenchymal contusions
2. for patients with *severe* head injuries:
   a) for *stable* patients, follow-up CTs are usually obtained between day 3 to 5, (some recommend at 24 hrs also) and again between day 10 to 14
   b) some recommend routine follow-up CT several hours after the "time zero" CT (i.e. initial CT done within hours of the trauma) to rule-out delayed EDH (p. 894), SDH (p. 898), or traumatic contusions (p. 891) [32]
3. for patients with mild to moderate head injuries:
   a) for those with an abnormal initial CT, the CT scan is usually repeated prior to discharge
   b) stable patients with mild head injury and normal initial CT do not require follow-up CT

Urgent follow-up CT: performed for neurological deterioration (loss of 2 or more points on the GCS, development of hemiparesis or new pupillary asymmetry), persistent vomiting, worsening H/A, seizures or unexplained rise in intracranial pressure (**ICP**) in patients with an ICP monitor.

54.5.2 Spine films

54

1. cervical spine: must be cleared radiographically from the cranio-cervical junction down through and including the C7-T1 junction. Spinal injury precautions (cervical collar...) are continued until the C-spine is cleared. The steps in obtaining adequate films are outlined in *Spine injuries*, Radiographic evaluation and initial C-spine immobilization (p. 952)
2. thoracic and lumbosacral LS-spine films should be obtained based on physical findings and on mechanism of injury; see *Spine injuries*, Radiographic evaluation and initial C-spine immobilization (p. 952)

54.5.3 Skull x-rays

A skull fracture increases the probability of a surgical intracranial injury (ICI) (in a comatose patient it is a 20-fold increase, in a conscious patient it is a 400-fold increase[33,34]). However, significant ICI can occur with a normal skull x-ray (SXR) SXR (SXR was normal in 75% of minor head injury patients found to have intracranial lesions on CT, attesting to the insensitivity of SXRs[23]). SXRs affect management of only 0.4–2% of patients in most reports.[20]

A SXR may be helpful in the following:

1. in patients with moderate risk for intracranial injury (▸ Table 54.7) by detecting an unsuspected depressed skull fracture (however, most of these patients will get a CT scan, which obviates the need for SXR)
2. if a CT scan cannot be obtained, a SXR may identify significant findings such as pineal shift, pneumocephalus, air-fluid levels in the air sinuses, skull fracture (depressed or linear)... (however, sensitivity for detecting ICI is very low)
3. with penetrating injuries: helps in visualization of some metallic objects

54.5.4 MRI scans in trauma

Usually not appropriate for acute head injuries. This is due to longer acquisition time, less access to patient during study, increased difficulty in supporting patient (requires special non-magnetic ventilators, cannot use most IV pumps...) and MRI is less sensitive than CT for detecting acute blood.[35] There were no *surgical* lesions demonstrated on MRI that were not evident on CT in one study.[36] There may be some additional benefit in combining CT with an MRI performed directly in the emergency department.[37]

MRI may be helpful later after the patient is stabilized, e.g. to evaluate brainstem injuries, small white matter changes,[38] e.g. punctate hemorrhages in the corpus callosum seen in diffuse axonal injury (p.848)... Spinal MRI is indicated in patients with spinal cord injuries.

Rapid sequence MRI may be useful for follow-up in pediatrics to minimize radiation exposure.

54.5.5 Arteriogram in trauma

Cerebral arteriogram (p.911): useful with non missile penetrating trauma.

54.6 Admitting orders for minor or moderate head injury

54.6.1 General information

Traditionally, mild head injury has been defined as GCS ≥ 13. However, the increased frequency of both surgical lesions and CT scan abnormalities in patients with GCS = 13 suggests that they would be better classified with the moderate rather than mild head injuries.[22] See Indications for CT and admission criteria for TBI (p.830) for admitting criteria.

54.6.2 Admitting orders for minor head injury (GCS ≥ 14)

1. activity: BR with HOB elevated 30–45°
2. neuro checks q 2 hrs (q 1 hr if more concerned; consider ICU for these patients). Contact physician for neurologic deterioration
3. NPO until alert; then clear liquids, advance as tolerated
4. isotonic IVF (e.g. NS + 20 mEq KCl/L) run at maintenance (p.870): ≈ 100 cc/hr for average size adult (peds: 2000 cc/m²/d). **Note:** the concept of "running the patient dry" is considered obsolete
5. mild analgesics: acetaminophen (PO, or PR if NPO), codeine if necessary
6. anti-emetic: give infrequently to avoid excessive sedation, avoid phenothiazine anti-emetics (which lower the seizure threshold); e.g. use trimethobenzamide (Tigan®) 200 mg IM q 8 hrs PRN for adults

54.6.3 Admitting orders for moderate head injury (GCS 9–13)

1. orders as for minor head injury (see above) except patient is kept NPO in case surgical intervention is needed (including ICP monitor)
2. for GCS = 9–12 admit to ICU. For GCS = 13, admit to ICU if CT shows any significant abnormality (hemorrhagic contusions unless very small, rim subdural...)
3. patients with normal or near-normal CTs should improve within hours. Any patient who fails to reach a GCS of 14–15 within 12 hrs should have a repeat CT at that time[31]

54.7 Patients with associated severe systemic injuries

54.7.1 Intraabdominal injuries

Diagnostic peritoneal lavage (DPL) looking for bloody fluid or FAST (focused abdominal sonogram for trauma) are often used by trauma surgeons to assess for intra-abdominal hemorrhage. If negative and the patient is hemodynamically stable, the patient should be taken for cranial CT (with DPL – if the initial fluid is not bloody, the remainder of the lavage fluid may be collected for quantitative analysis as the head CT is being done).

Patients with grossly positive DPL or positive FAST and/or hemodynamic instability may need to be rushed to the O.R. for emergent laparotomy by trauma surgeons without benefit of cerebral CT. Neurosurgical management is difficult in these patients, and must be individualized. These guidelines are offered:

✖ CAUTION: many patients with severe trauma may be in DIC (either due to systemic injuries, or directly related to severe head injury possibly because the brain is rich in thromboplastin[39]). Operating on patients in DIC is usually disastrous (p. 167). At the least, check a PT/INR/PTT

1. if GCS > 8 (which implies at least localizing)
   a) operative neurosurgical intervention is probably not required
   b) utilize good neuroanesthesia techniques (elevate head of bed, judicious administration of IV fluids, avoiding prophylactic hyperventilation…)
   c) obtain a head CT scan immediately post-op
2. if patient has focal neurologic deficit, an exploratory burr-hole should be placed in the O.R. simultaneously with the treatment of other injuries. Placement is guided by the pre-op deficit (p. 836)
3. if there is severe head injury (GCS ≤ 8) without localizing signs, or if initial burr hole is negative, or if there is no pre-op neuro exam, then
   a) measure the ICP: insert a ventriculostomy catheter (if the lateral ventricle cannot be entered after 3 passes, it may be completely compressed or it may be displaced, and an intraparenchymal fiber-optic monitor or subarachnoid bolt should be used)
      - normal ICP: unlikely that a surgical lesion exists. Manage ICP medically and, if a IVC was inserted, with CSF drainage
      - elevated ICP (≥ 20 mm Hg): inject 3–4 cc of air into ventricles through IVC, then obtain portable intraoperative AP skull x-ray (intra-operative pneumoencephalogram) to determine if there is any midline shift. If there is mass effect with ≥ 5 mm of midline shift is explored[40] with burr-hole(s) on the side opposite the direction of shift. If no mass effect, intracranial hypertension is managed medically and with CSF drainage
   b) routine use of exploratory burr holes for children with GCS = 3 has been found not to be justified[41]

54.7.2 Fat embolism syndrome

General information

Most often seen after a long bone fracture (usually femoral, but may include clavicular, tibial, and even isolated skull fracture). Although almost all patients have pulmonary fat emboli at autopsy, the syndrome is usually mild or subclinical, only ≈ 10–20% of cases are severe, and the fulminant form leading to multiple organ failure is rare. Clinical findings usually appear within 12–72 hrs of injury, and do not always include the complete classic clinical triad of:

- acute respiratory failure (including hypoxemia, tachypnea, dyspnea) with diffuse pulmonary infiltrates (usually seen as bilateral fluffy infiltrates). May be the only manifestation of fat emboli in up to 75% of cases
- global neurologic dysfunction: may include confusion (PaO_2 usually not low enough to account for these changes[42]), lethargy, seizures
- petechial rash: seen ≈ 24–72 hrs after the fracture, usually over thorax

Other possible findings include:

- pyrexia
- retinal fat emboli

There is no specific test for fat embolism syndrome (FES). The following have been proposed, but have poor sensitivity and specificity: fat globules in the urine (positive in ≈ one-third[43]) and serum, serum lipase activity. In cases of unexplained neurologic or pulmonary abnormalities, it may be possible to diagnose FES if on bronchoalveolar lavage[44] > 5% of cells in the washings staining for neutral fat with red oil O. Nonspecific tests include ABG (findings: hypoxemia, hypocarbia from hyperventilation, respiratory alkalosis).

Treatment

Pulmonary support with oxygen, and mechanical ventilation if necessary including use of PEEP. The use of steroids is controversial. Ethyl alcohol (to decrease serum lipase activity) and heparin have not been shown to be of benefit. Early operative fixation of long bone fractures may reduce the incidence of FES.[45]

54

Outcome

Usually related more to the underlying injuries. Although FES itself is usually compatible with good recovery, 10% mortality is usually quoted.

54.7.3 Indirect optic nerve injury

General information

≈ 5% of head trauma patients manifest an associated injury to some portion of the visual system. Approximately 0.5–1.5% of head trauma patients will sustain indirect injury (as opposed to penetrating trauma) to the optic nerve, most often from an ipsilateral blow to the head (usually frontal, occasionally temporal, rarely occipital).[19] The optic nerve may be divided into 4 segments: intraocular (1 mm in length), intraorbital (25–30 mm), intracanalicular (10 mm), and intracranial (10 mm). The intracanalicular segment is the most common one damaged with closed head injuries. Funduscopic abnormalities visible on initial exam indicates anterior injuries (injury to the intraocular segment (optic disc) or the 10–15 mm of the intraorbital segment immediately behind the globe where the central retinal artery is contained within the optic nerve), whereas posterior injuries (occurring posterior to this but anterior to the chiasm) takes 4–8 weeks to show signs of disc pallor and loss of the retinal nerve fiber layer.

Treatment

See reference.[19]

No prospective study has been carried out. Optic nerve decompression has been advocated for indirect optic nerve injury, however, the results are not clearly better than expectant management with the exception that documented *delayed* visual loss appears to be a strong indication for surgery. Transethmoidal is the accepted route, and is usually done within 1–3 weeks from the trauma.[46] The use of "megadose steroids" may be appropriate as an adjunct to diagnosis and treatment.

54.7.4 Post-traumatic hypopituitarism

Trauma is a rare cause of hypopituitarism. It may follow closed head injury (with or without basilar skull fracture) or penetrating trauma.[47] In 20 cases in the literature[48] all had deficient growth hormone and gonadotropin, 95% had corticotropin deficiency, 85% had reduced TSH, 63% had elevated PRL. Only 40% had transient or permanent DI.

54.8 Exploratory burr holes

54.8.1 General information

In a trauma patient, the clinical triad of altered mental status, unilateral pupillary dilatation with loss of light reflex, and contralateral hemiparesis is most often due to upper brainstem compression by uncal transtentorial herniation which, in the majority of trauma cases, is due to an extraaxial intracranial hematoma. Furthermore, the prognosis of patients with traumatic herniation is poor. Outcome may possibly be improved slightly by increasing the rapidity with which decompression is undertaken, however, an upper limit of salvageability is probably still only ≈ 20% satisfactory outcome.

Burr holes are primarily a *diagnostic tool*, as bleeding cannot be controlled and most acute hematomas are too congealed to be removed through a burr hole. However, if the burr hole is positive, it is possible that modest decompression may be performed, and then the definitive craniotomy can be undertaken incorporating the burr hole(s).

With widespread availability of quickly accessible CT scanning, exploratory burr holes are infrequently indicated.

54.8.2 Indications

1. clinical criteria: based on deteriorating neurologic exam. Indications in E/R (rare): patient dying of rapid transtentorial herniation (see below) or brainstem compression that does not improve or stabilize with mannitol and hyperventilation.[49]
   a) indicators of transtentorial herniation/brainstem compression:
      - sudden drop in Glasgow Coma Scale (GCS) score
      - one pupil fixes and dilates

   - paralysis or decerebration develops (usually contralateral to blown pupil)
 b) recommended situations where criteria should be applied:
   - neurologically stable patient undergoes *witnessed* deterioration as described above
   - awake patient undergoes same process in transport, and changes are well documented by competent medical or paramedical personnel
2. other criteria
 a) some patients needing emergent surgery for systemic injuries (e.g. positive peritoneal lavage + hemodynamic instability) where there is not time for a brain CT (p. 834)

54.8.3 Management

Controversial. The following should serve only as guidelines:

1. if patient fits the above criteria (emergent operation for systemic injuries or deterioration with failure to improve with mannitol and hyperventilation), and CT scan cannot be performed and interpreted immediately, then treatment should not wait for CT scan
 a) in general, if the O.R. can be immediately available, burr holes are preferably done there (equipped to handle craniotomy, better lighting and sterility, dedicated scrub nurse…) especially in older patients (> 30 yrs) not involved in MVAs (below). This may more rapidly diagnose and treat extraaxial hematomas in herniating patients, although no difference in outcome has been proven
 b) if delay in getting to the O.R. is foreseen, emergency burr holes in the E/R should be performed
2. placement of burrhole(s) as outlined under Technique below

54.8.4 Technique

Position

Shoulder roll, head turned with side to be explored up. Three pin skull-fixation used if concern about possible aneurysm or AVM (to allow for retractors and increased stability) or if additional stability is desired (e.g. with unstable cervical fractures), otherwise a horse-shoe head-holder suffices and saves time and makes it easier to turn the head to access to the other side if needed.

Choice of side for initial burr hole

Start with a temporal burr hole (see below) on the side:

1. ipsilateral to a blown pupil. This will be on the correct side in > 85% of epidurals[50] and other extra-axial mass lesions[51]
2. if both pupils are dilated, use the side of the *first* dilating pupil (if known)
3. if pupils are equal, or it is not known which side dilated first, place on side of obvious external trauma
4. if no localizing clues, place hole on *left* side (to evaluate and decompress the dominant hemisphere)

54

Approach

Burr holes are placed along a path that can be connected to form a "trauma flap" if a craniotomy becomes necessary (▶ Fig. 54.2). The "trauma flap" is so-called because it provides wide access to most of the cerebral convexity permitting complete evacuation of acute blood clot and control of most bleeding.

First outline the trauma flap with a skin marker:

1. start at the zygomatic arch < 1 cm anterior to the tragus (spares the branch of the facial nerve to the frontalis muscle and spares the anterior branch of the superficial temporal artery(STA))
2. proceed superiorly and then curve posteriorly at the level of top of the pinna
3. 4–6 cm behind the pinna it is taken superiorly
4. 1–2 cm ipsilateral to the midline (sagittal suture) curve anteriorly to end behind the hairline

Burr hole locations

1. first (temporal) burrhole: over middle cranial fossa (#1 in ▶ Fig. 54.2) just superior to the zygomatic arch. Provides access to middle fossa (the most common site of epidural hematoma) and usually allows access to most convexity subdural hematomas, as well as proximity to middle meningeal artery in region of pterion

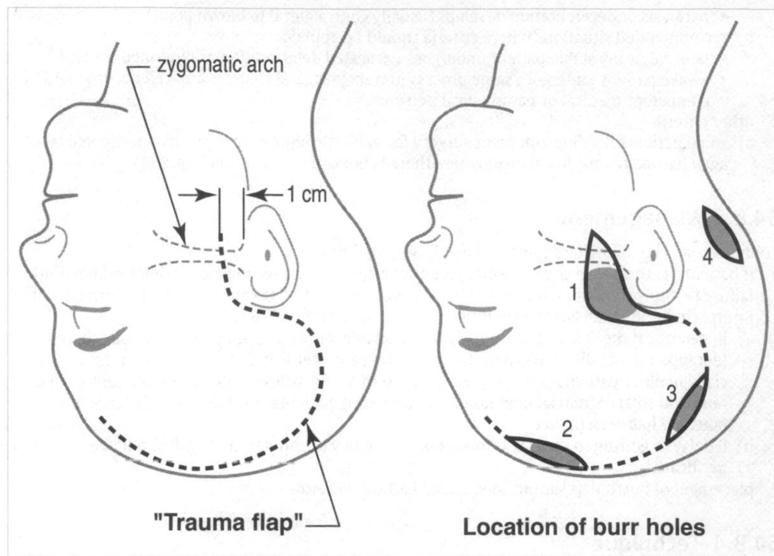

Fig. 54.2 Technique to convert burrhole(s) into trauma flap (adapted[51,52])

2. if no epidural hematoma, the dura is opened if it has bluish discoloration (suggests subdural hematoma(SDH)) or if there is a strong suspicion of a mass lesion on that side
3. if completely negative, usually perform temporal burr hole on contralateral side
4. if negative, further burr holes should be undertaken if a CT cannot now be done
5. proceed to ipsilateral frontal burr hole (#2 in ▶ Fig. 54.2)
6. subsequent burr holes may be placed at parietal region (#3 in ▶ Fig. 54.2) and lastly in posterior fossa (#4 in ▶ Fig. 54.2)

Literature

In 100 trauma patients undergoing transtentorial herniation or brainstem compression as outlined above,[51] exploratory burr holes (bilateral temporal, frontal and parietal, done in the O.R.) were positive in 56%. Lower rates in younger patients (< 30 yrs) and those in MVAs (as opposed to falls or assaults). SDH was the most common extraaxial mass lesion (alone and unilateral in 70%, bilateral in 11%, and in combination with EDH or ICH in > 9%).

When burr holes were positive, the first burr hole was on the correct side 86% of the time when placed as suggested above. Six patients had significant extraaxial hematomas missed with exploratory burr holes (mostly due to incomplete burr hole exploration). Only 3 patients had the above neurologic findings as a result of intraparenchymal hematomas.

Outcome

Mean follow-up: 11 mos (range: 1–37). 70 of the 100 patients died. No morbidity or mortality was directly attributable to the burr holes. Four patients with good outcome and 4 with moderate disability had positive burr holes.

References

[1] Saul TG, Ducker TB. Effect of Intracranial Pressure Monitoring and and Aggressive Treatment on Mortality in Severe Head Injury. J Neurosurg. 1982; 56:498–503
[2] Reilly PL, Adams JH, Graham DI. Patients with Head Injury Who Talk and Die. Lancet. 1975; 2:375–377
[3] Stein SC, Narayan RK, Wilberger JE, Povlishock JT. In: Classification of Head Injury. Neurotrauma. New York: McGraw-Hill; 1996:31–41
[4] Price DJ. Is Diagnostic Severity Grading for Head Injuries Possible? Acta Neurochir. 1986; Suppl 36:67–69
[5] Brain Trauma Foundation, Povlishock JT, Bullock MR. Blood pressure and oxygenation. J Neurotrauma. 2007; 24:S7–13
[6] Chesnut RM, Marshall LF, Klauber MR, et al. The Role of Secondary Brain Injury in Determining Outcome from Severe Head Injury. J Trauma. 1993; 34:216–222
[7] The Brain Trauma Foundation. The American Association of Neurological Surgeons. The Joint Section on Neurotrauma and Critical Care. Initial management. J Neurotrauma. 2000; 17:463–469
[8] Hsiang JK, Chesnut RM, Crisp CD, et al. Early, Routine Paralysis for Intracranial Pressure Control in Severe Head Injury: Is It Necessary? Crit Care Med. 1994; 22:1471–1476
[9] Marion DW, Carlier PM. Problems with Initial Glasgow Coma Scale Assessment Caused by Prehospital Treatment of Patients with Head Injuries: Results of a National Survey. J Trauma. 1994; 36:89–95
[10] Bullock R, Chesnut RM, Clifton G, et al. Guidelines for the Management of Severe Head Injury. 1995
[11] The Brain Trauma Foundation. The American Association of Neurological Surgeons. The Joint Section on Neurotrauma and Critical Care. Resuscitation of blood pressure and oxygenation. J Neurotrauma. 2000; 17:471–478
[12] Brain Trauma Foundation, Povlishock JT, Bullock MR. Infection prophylaxis. J Neurotrauma. 2007; 24:S26–S31
[13] Brain Trauma Foundation, Povlishock JT, Bullock MR. Hyperventilation. J Neurotrauma. 2007; 24: S87–S90
[14] Brain Trauma Foundation, Povlishock JT, Bullock MR. Hyperosmolar therapy. J Neurotrauma. 2007; 24:S14–S20
[15] Bullock R, Chesnut RM, Clifton G, et al. In: The role of anti-seizure prophylaxis following head injury. Guidelines for the Management of Severe Head Injury.The Brain Trauma Foundation (New York), The American Association of Neurological Surgeons (Park Ridge, Illinois), and The Joint Section of Neurotrauma and Critical Care; 1995
[16] Chang BS, Lowenstein DH. Antiepileptic drug prophylaxis in severe traumatic brain injury. Report of the Quality Standards Subcommittee of the American Academy of Neurology. Neurology. 2003; 60:10–16
[17] Brain Trauma Foundation, Povlishock JT, Bullock MR. Antiseizure prophylaxis. J Neurotrauma. 2007; 24:S83–S86
[18] The Brain Trauma Foundation. The American Association of Neurological Surgeons. The Joint Section on Neurotrauma and Critical Care. Role of antiseizure prophylaxis following head injury. J Neurotrauma. 2000; 17:549–553
[19] Kline LB, Morawetz RB, Swaid SN. Indirect Injury of the Optic Nerve. Neurosurgery. 1984; 14:756–764
[20] Masters SJ, McClean PM, Arcarese JS, et al. Skull X-Ray Examination After Head Trauma. N Engl J Med. 1987; 316:84–91
[21] Arienta C, Caroli M, Balbi S. Management of Head-Injured Patients in the Emergency Department: A Practical Protocol. Surg Neurol. 1997; 48:213–219
[22] Stein SC, Ross SE. The Value of Computed Tomographic Scans in Patients with Low-Risk Head Injuries. Neurosurgery. 1990; 26:638–640
[23] Ingebrigtsen R, Romner B. Routine Early CT-Scan is Cost Saving After Minor Head Injury. Acta Neurol Scand. 1996; 93:207–210
[24] Duus BR, Lind B, Christensen H, Nielsen OA. The Role of Neuroimaging in the Initial Management of Patients with Minor Head Injury. Ann Emerg Med. 1994; 23:1279–1283
[25] Feuerman T, Wackym PA, Gade GF, Becker DP. Value of Skull Radiography, Head Computed Tomographic Scanning, and Admission for Observation in Cases of Minor Head Injury. Neurosurgery. 1988; 22:449–453
[26] Schacford SR, Wald SR, Ross SE, et al. The Clinical Utility of Computed Tomographic Scanning and Neurologic Examination in the Management of Patients with Minor Head Injuries. J Trauma. 1992; 33:385–394
[27] Stein SC, Ross SE. Mild Head Injury: A Plea for Routine Early CT Scanning. J Trauma. 1992; 33:11–13
[28] Lee KF, Wagner LK, Lee YE, et al. The Impact-Absorbing Effects of Facial Fractures in Closed-Head Injuries. J Neurosurg. 1987; 66:542–547
[29] Le Roux PD, Haglund MM, Newell DW, Grady MS, Winn HR. Intraventricular Hemorrhage in Blunt Head Trauma: An Analysis of 43 Cases. Neurosurgery. 1992; 31:678–685
[30] Grabb PA. Traumatic intraventricular hemorrhage treated with intraventricular recombinant-tissue plasminogen activator: technical case report. Neurosurgery. 1998; 43:966–969
[31] Stein SC, Ross SE. Moderate Head Injury: A Guide to Initial Management. J Neurosurg. 1992; 77:562–564
[32] Young HA, Gleave JRW, Schmidek HH, Gregory S. Delayed Traumatic Intracerebral Hematoma: Report of 15 Cases Operatively Treated. Neurosurgery. 1984; 14:22-25
[33] Jennett B, Teasdale G. Management of Head Injuries. Philadelphia: Davis; 1981
[34] Dacey RG, Alves WM, Rimel RW, Jane JA, et al. Neurosurgical Complications After Apparently Minor Head Injury: Assessment of Risk in a Series of 610 Patients. J Neurosurg. 1986; 65:203–210
[35] Snow RB, Zimmerman RD, Gandy SE, Deck MDF. Comparison of Magnetic Resonance Imaging and Computed Tomography in the Evaluation of Head Injury. Neurosurgery. 1986; 18:45–52
[36] Wilberger JE, Deeb Z, Rothfus W. Magnetic Resonance Imaging After Closed Head Injury. Neurosurgery. 1987; 20:571–576
[37] Kesterson L, Benzel EC, Marchand EP, et al. Magnetic Resonance Imaging in Acute Cranial and Cervical Spine Trauma. Neurosurgery. 1990; 26
[38] Levin HS, Amparo EG, Eisenberg HM, et al. Magnetic Resonance Imaging After Closed Head Injury in Children. Neurosurgery. 1989; 24:223–227
[39] Kaufman HH, Hui K-S, Mattson JC, et al. Clinicopathological Correlations of Disseminated Intravascular Coagulation in Patients with Head Injury. Neurosurgery. 1984; 15:34–42
[40] Becker DP, Miller JD, Ward JD, et al. The Outcome from Severe Head Injury with Early Diagnosis and Intensive Management. J Neurosurg. 1977; 47:491–502
[41] Johnson DL, Duma C, Sivit C. The Role of Immediate Operative Intervention in Severely Head-Injured Children with a Glasgow Coma Scale Score of 3. Neurosurgery. 1992; 30:320–324
[42] Fabian TC, Hoots AV, Stanford DS, Patterson CR, et al. Fat Embolism Syndrome: Prospective Evaluation in 92 Fracture Patients. Crit Care Med. 1990; 18:42–46

[43] Dines DE, Burgher LW, Okazaki H. The Clinical and Pathologic Correlation of Fat Embolism Syndrome. Mayo Clin Proc. 1975; 50:407–411
[44] Chastre J, Fagon JY, Soler P, Fichelle A, et al. Bronchoalveolar Lavage for Rapid Diagnosis of the Fat Embolism Syndrome in Trauma Patients. Ann Intern Med. 1990; 113:583–588
[45] Riska EB, Myllynen P. Fat Embolism in Patients with Multiple Injuries. J Trauma. 1982; 22:891–894
[46] Niho S, Niho M, Niho K. Decompression of the Optic Canal by the Transethmoidal Route and Decompression of the Superior Orbital Fissure. Can J Ophthalmol. 1970; 5:22–40
[47] Vance ML. Hypopituitarism. N Engl J Med. 1994; 330:1651–1662
[48] Edwards OM, Clark JDA. Post-Traumatic Hypopituitarism: Six Cases and a Review of the Literature. Medicine (Baltimore). 1986; 65:281–290
[49] Mahoney BD, Rockswold GL, Ruiz E, Clinton JE. Emergency Twist Drill Trephination. Neurosurgery. 1981; 8:551–554
[50] McKissock W, Taylor JC, Bloom WH, et al. Extradural Hematoma: Observations on 125 Cases. Lancet. 1960; 2:167–172
[51] Andrews BT, Pitts LH, Lovely MP, et al. Is CT Scanning Necessary in Patients with Tentorial Herniation? Neurosurgery. 1986; 19:408–414
[52] Mayfield FH, McBride BH, Coates JB, Meirowsky AM. In: Differential Diagnosis and Treatment of Surgical Lesions. Neurological Surgery of Trauma. Washington D.C.: Office of the Surgeon General; 1965:55–64

55 Concussion, High Altitude Cerebral Edema, Cerebrovascular Injuries

55.1 Concussion

55.1.1 General information

Key concepts

- A traumatic biomechanically induced complex pathophysiologic process affecting the brain with no identifiable structural abnormalities on imaging studies
- Concussion is a subset of mild TBI (mTBI) and is therefore not equivalent to mTBI
- Indicators of concussion: post-traumatic alterations in any of: orientation, balance, speed of reaction, and/or impaired verbal learning and memory in a patient with GCS 13–15[1]
- Does not require loss of consciousness (LOC) or even a direct blow to the head
- Grading scales have been abandoned in favor of experienced assessment assisted by various "sideline" tools

Concussion occurs in a subset of patient with mild traumatic brain injury (mTBI; ► Fig. 54.1). It is considered "mild" because it is usually not life-threatening by itself. While most victims recover completely, effects of concussion can be serious, and in some instances, may be lifelong.

Much of the discussion in this chapter relates to concussion in sports which, is the largest source of data on the subject, and generalization to other types of trauma must be done circumspectly.

There has been a move away from grading scales for concussion, and the current recommendation is for the diagnosis to be determined in the judgement of an experienced examiner with the assistance of various assessment tools, ideally with the availability of pre-injury baseline metrics for comparison.

Concussion can occur without a direct blow to the head, e.g. with violent shaking of the torso and head. Concussion symptoms can present soon after an insult or in a delayed fashion.

The subject may not be aware that they have sustained a concussion.

55.1.2 Epidemiology

Incidence: 1.6–3.8 million concussions occur per year in the United States from sports and recreational activities. It is estimated that 50% of concussions go unreported.[2]

55.1.3 Concussion genetics

There is no clear evidence to support a genetic predisposition to concussion. Apolipoprotein E4, Apo E G-219T promoter and tau exon 6 have been studied in small retrospective and prospective trials without definitive association.[2,3]

55.1.4 Concussion – definition

There is no universally accepted definition for concussion.[4] Of the many contemporary definitions,[2,3,4,5,6,7] most key elements are contained in the Concussion in Sport Group 2012 consensus definition[3] summarized below. However, opinions differ e.g. whether there is any long-term effect of concussion or if that necessitates a different diagnosis.

Definition: Concussion is a complex pathophysiological process affecting the brain resulting in alteration of brain function, that is induced by nonpenetrating biomechanical forces, without identifiable abnormality in standard structural imaging.

The Concussion in Sport Group[3] elaborates on this definition as follows:

- Results in a graded set of neurological symptoms that may or may not involve loss of consciousness (LOC).
- Symptom onset is usually rapid, short-lived and resolves spontaneously. Manifestations may include transient deficits in balance, coordination, memory/cognition, strength, or alertness.

55

- May result in neuropathological changes, but the acute clinical symptoms largely reflect a functional disturbance rather than a structural injury.
- Resolution of the clinical and cognitive features typically follows a sequential course.
- Typically associated with grossly normal standard structural neuroimaging studies.

55.1.5 Concussion versus mTBI

- Concussion and mTBI are not interchangeable. Concussion may be thought as a subcategory of mTBI on the less severe end of the brain injury spectrum, though with similar clinical symptoms[2,5,6,8] (see ▶ Fig. 57.2).
- A major difference between the two is that mTBI may demonstrate abnormal structural imaging (such as cerebral hemorrhage/contusion) and concussion, by definition, must have normal imaging studies. mTBI is part of an injury severity spectrum primarily based on GCS score. TBI is evaluated 6 hours after injury and differentiated into mild, moderate and severe; see Grading (p. 824). Concussion is evaluated directly after the insult and based on a clinical diagnosis aided by a multitude of standardized assessment tools. To include concussion under the full spectrum of traumatic brain injury then it must fall at the low end of mTBI and overlap with the subset of "minimal" injury. Most mTBIs with negative imaging can be considered concussions but the majority of sports concussions cannot be classified as mTBI.[5,8]

55.1.6 Risk factors for concussion

- History of previous concussion increases risk for further concussion
- Being involved in an accident: bicyclist, pedestrian or motor vehicle collision
- Combat soldier
- Victim of physical abuse
- Falling (especially pediatrics or elderly)
- Males are diagnosed with sports-related concussion more than females (due to increased number of male participation in sports studied) but females have a higher risk overall when compared to males who play in the same sport. (i.e. soccer and basketball)[7]
- Participating in sports with high risk of concussion:
  - American football
  - Australian rugby
  - Ice hockey
  - Boxing
  - *Soccer is the highest risk for females
- (For contrast, sports with the lowest risk of concussion: baseball, softball, volleyball & gymnastics)
- BMI > 27 kg/m^2 and less than 3 hours of training per week increase risk of sports-related concussion[7]

55

55.1.7 Diagnosis

Triggers

Findings suggestive of concussion are listed in ▶ Table 55.1. The diagnosis of concussion should be considered when any of these findings occur following trauma. In pre-verbal children, findings may include those in ▶ Table 55.2.

General diagnostic information

Clinical evaluation

No physiologic measure has been identified that can detect the underlying changes that lead to the manifestations of concussion. Therefore the diagnosis relies on: self-reporting of abnormal function (symptoms), observed physiologic abnormalities (signs) including assessment of cognitive dysfunction,[11] sometimes with the assistance of imaging tests to rule out a structural substrate.

A clinical diagnosis of concussion is made if there are abnormal findings in balance, coordination, memory/cognition, strength, reaction speed or alertness after a traumatic insult to the head. Findings include confusion, amnesia, headache, drowsiness or LOC (LOC is *not* a requirement for diagnosing concussion,[6] patients themselves may be unaware whether or not they experienced LOC[4]). Frequent neurobehavioral features of concussion are shown in ▶ Table 55.1. In children who may not be able to verbalize their symptoms, evidence of concussion may include findings in ▶ Table 55.2. Positive imaging findings would necessitate a more severe diagnosis such as cerebral contusion

Table 55.1 Possible findings in concussion[2,9,10]

Physical	Cognitive	Emotional	Sleep
• vacant stare or befuddled expression • dazed or stunned • headache or pressure sensation in the head • nausea • vomiting • fatigue • "seeing stars" • photophobia • phonophobia • ringing in the ears (tinnitus) • delayed verbal & motor responses: • difficulty focusing attention • inability to perform normal activities • speech alterations: slurred or incoherent, disjointed or incomprehensible statements • incoordination stumbling • any period of LOC, paralytic coma, unresponsiveness to stimuli	• feeling like being in a fog • slow to answer questions or follow instructions • easy distractibility • disorientation (e.g. walking in the wrong direction) • unaware of date, time or place • memory deficits: amnesia for the event • repeatedly asking same question that has been answered	• exaggerated emotionality: inappropriate crying • distraught appearance • irritability • nervousness	• drowsiness • insomnia • hypersomnia • difficulty falling asleep or staying asleep

Table 55.2 Concussion findings in children

Listlessness and easy fatigability, change in sleeping patterns Irritability Appearing dazed Balance impairment Excessive crying Change in eating habits Loss of interest in favorite toys

55

Approach

- Take a concussion specific symptom survey including inquiries about: H/A, N/V, light sensitivity, tinnitus, feeling like being in a fog, sleep disturbances
- History of diagnoses that might have an impact on the assessment or on a current concussion
  - History of prior concussions
  - H/A history
  - ADD/HD
  - Learning disabilities
  - Medications (prescribed and other) that might affect alertness or cognition
- Perform a good general neurological exam
- Include a concussion specific neuro exam
  - Check orientation
  - Assess for amnesia and impaired verbal memory
  - Balance: Romberg test (look for significant sway or breaking stance), single leg stance
  - Eye movements: optokinetic nystagmus (OKN), smooth pursuit
  - Simultaneous task performance: e.g. snap fingers while walking
- Include assessment aides ("sideline tools") as appropriate (see below)

Assessment aids

- There is no single validated assessment tool for diagnosis of concussion.[4] It is primarily a *clinical* diagnosis that is ideally made by certified healthcare providers who are familiar with the patient based on a detailed history and physical examination and a continuum of evaluation from the sideline to the clinic (diagnosis is ideally within made within 24 hours of injury)[2,3,4,5,6,7]

- Diagnosis may be aided by concussion assessment tools such as the SCAT3, ImPACT™.
  ✖ No test has shown high validity on independent testing, and no test should be used as the sole method of diagnosing concussion or for determining suitability for return to play. Athletes have also learned to "game" some baseline tests to avoid removal from play after possible concussion
- SCAT3 (Sports Concussion Assessment Tool – 3rd Edition)[12]: Derived from the 2012 Zurich Conference.[3] The SCAT has become the most commonly used standardized tool for sideline assessment of sport concussion. The sensitivity and specificity of concussion assessment tools change over the course of a concussion so a tool designed for sideline use (i.e. SCAT3) is not appropriate for office use.
  - SCAT3™ is a trademarked tool developed by the Concussion in Sports Group for use only by medical professionals for assessing sports-related concussion.
  - It can be found at http://bjsm.bmj.com/content/47/5/259.full.pdf.
  - To be used in athletes of 13 years or older (for 12 and younger, use Child SCAT3[13])
  - Is a multimodal assessment tool with 8 sections that includes self-reported symptoms and evaluation of functional domains such as cognition, memory, balance, gait and motor skills
  - Takes 8–10 min to administer
  - A "normal" SCAT3 does *not* rule out concussion
  - It has not been validated
- Other types of sports concussion assessment tools (many can be viewed on YouTube):
  - Neurocognitive testing (may take up to 20 minutes to administer)
  - SAC (Standardized Assessment of Concussion)[14]: a neurocognitive test that includes tests of immediate memory, delayed recall, serial 7's, digit span
  - ImPACT™ (Immediate Post-Concussion Assessment and Cognitive Testing): a widely used commercially produced computer test (https://www.impacttest.com). Independent validation studies have yielded conflicting results and results can diverge from observations[15]
  - PCSS (Post-Concussive Symptom Scale)
  - CSI (Concussion Symptom Inventory)
  - BESS (Balance Error Scoring System): the subject stands in each of various standardized positions for 20 seconds each, and the number of errors are recorded (breaking stance, opening eyes, taking hands off hip…).
  - SOT (Sensory Organization Test)
  - "Concussion Quick Check" app for mobile devices produced by the AAN
  - King-Devick eye movement testing: only takes 2–3 minutes to administer. On printed cards or tablet computer (http://kingdevicktest.com/for-concussions/).
- Formal neuropsychological testing: it is recommended that this be reserved for patients with prolonged cognitive symptoms
- Concussion serum biomarkers: no moiety has been identified that can reliably diagnose concussion on serum or saliva testing. Neuron-specific enolase, S100, and cleaved tau protein have been studied for prognostication after mTBI and concussion. S100 has demonstrated only a 33.3% sensitivity for postconcussive symptoms and 93% sensitivity for an Extended Glasgow Outcome Scale < 5 at 1 month. Another study involving pediatric patients with mTBI showed no difference in levels of neuron-specific enolase or S100B in asymptomatic and symptomatic children. A prospective study found no significant correlation between cleaved tau protein and postconcussive syndrome in patients with mTBI[16]

On-site/sideline evaluation

Any individual suspected of having a concussion (displaying ANY findings in ▶ Table 55.1) should be removed from the activity (for athletes, stopped from playing) and assessed by a licensed healthcare provider trained in the evaluation and management of concussions with attention to excluding a cervical spine injury.[2,3] If no provider is available, return to the activity is not permitted and urgent referral to a physician should be arranged.

After ruling out emergency issues, the provider should perform a concussion assessment (may employ standardized tools such as SCAT3™ or other methodologies).

The patient should not be left alone, and serial evaluations for signs of deterioration should be made over the following few hours.

For return to play guidelines, see below.

55.1.8 Indications for imaging or other diagnostic testing

Imaging in concussion is typically used to rule out more serious traumatic injuries.

Indications[4] for CT or MRI imaging:

- Adults with or without LOC or amnesia
  - Focal neurologic deficit
  - GCS < 15
  - Severe headache
  - Coagulopathy
  - Vomiting
  - Age > 65 years old
  - Seizures
- Peds
  - LOC > 60 secs
  - Evidence of skull fracture
  - Focal neurologic deficit

Other imaging studies:

- Diffusion Tensor Imaging (DTI): used to quantify white matter tract integrity throughout the brain with 4 types of analysis methods – voxel analysis, region of interest (ROI) analysis, histogram analysis, and tractography. There is no strong consensus regarding the best method for utilizing DTI for diagnosis or prognosis in the *individual* patient but multiple studies have shown *group* differences in DTI parameters between mTBI and control patients.[8]
- Functional MRI (fMRI): consists of 2 types (task-based fMRI and resting state fMRI) and is based on the blood oxygen level dependent (BOLD) effect, in which specialized MRI sequences measure/detect regions of increased oxygen rich blood flow to areas of upregulated neuronal activity. Both task-based and resting state fMRI modalities have shown *group* differences between mTBI and control patients (specifically in frontal lobe dysfunction) but further studies need to be completed on both a single time point and longitudinal basis before these techniques can be widely adopted for individual diagnosis and therapeutic guidance.[8]
- Imaging studies that are currently used primarily in concussion research: positron emission tomography (PET), single photon emission CT (CT-SPECT), MR-spectroscopy (MRS).

Quantitative EEG (QEEG) is another research tool for concussion that assesses brain activity, patterns of cortical activation and neuronal networks. The concept is that post-concussion studies are compared to baseline. Currently undergoing proof of concept evaluation.

55.1.9 Acute pathophysiology

Biomechanical force results in unregulated ionic (K^+ efflux, Na^+/Ca^{2+} influx) flux and unrestricted hyperacute glutamate release from sublethal mechanoporation of lipid membranes at the cellular level. This triggers voltage/ligand gated ion channels causing a cortical spreading depression-like state that is thought to be the substrate behind immediate postconcussive symptoms. Subsequently, ATP-dependent ionic pumps are extensively upregulated to restore cellular homeostasis causing widespread intracellular energy reserve depletion and an increase in ADP. Cells then pass into a state of impaired metabolism (energy crisis) that can last up to 7–10 days and may be associated with alterations in CBF. This impaired metabolic state is associated with vulnerability to repeat injury as well as behavioral and spatial learning impairments. Cells also undergo cytoskeletal damage, axonal

Table 55.3 Physiologic perturbations and their proposed corresponding symptomology[17]

Pertubation	Symptom
Ionic influx →	Migraine headache, photophobia, phonophobia
Energy Crisis →	Vulnerability to second injury
Axonal injury →	Impaired cognition, slowed processing, slowed reaction time
Impaired neurotransmission →	Impaired cognition, slowed processing, slowed reaction time
Protease activation, altered cytoskeletal proteins, cell death →	chronic atrophy, persistent impairments

55

dysfunction, and altered neurotransmission with the as yet unproven impression that each of these pathologic processes correlate with a separate symptomology.[17]

55.1.10 Post concussion syndrome (PCS)

Occurs in 10%-15% of concussed individuals. As with most concussion related pathologies, there are multiple definitions of PCS. An amalgam of some definitions is as follows: Patients having ≥ 3 symptoms including headache, fatigue, dizziness, irritability, difficulty concentrating, memory difficulty, insomnia, and intolerance to stress, emotion, or alcohol, and symptoms must begin within 4 weeks of injury and remain for ≥ 1 month after onset of symptoms.[16,18] In one retrospective study, the following conclusions were reached[18]:

- > 80% of PCS patients had at least 1 previous concussion
- average number of previous concussions was 3.4
- median duration of PCS was 6 months
- 50% of patients were < 18 years of age
- LOC does not increase the risk for PCS

55.1.11 Prevention of concussion

- The AAN guidelines conclude that protective headgear in rugby is "highly probable" to decrease the incidence of concussion.[7] However, the AMSSM (American Medical Society for Sports Medicine) hold that there is no clear evidence that soft or hard helmets reduce the severity or incidence of concussion (in football, lacrosse, hockey, soccer, and rugby).[2,3] Biomechanical studies have shown helmets reduced impact forces on the brain but this has not translated into concussion prevention.[3]
- There is insufficient data to determine whether one type of football helmet protects better than another in preventing concussions[3,7]
- No significant evidence that a mouthpiece protects against concussion[3,7]

55.1.12 Management of concussion and post-concussion syndrome

Return to Play (RTP)

- No system of return to play (RTP) guidelines has been rigorously tested and proven to be scientifically sound
- After sustaining a concussion, athletes should not return to play the same day.[2,3,4,5,6,7] Prohibited by some state laws.
- ✖ a symptomatic player should not return to competition.
- If there is any uncertainty: "When in doubt, sit them out"
- Evaluation should proceed in a stepwise fashion. A player needs to be completely asymptomatic both at rest and with provocative exercise before full clearance is given.[3] There is no standardized RTP protocol. Each player's progression should be individualized.[2] Generally, the athlete's level of activity should be gradually increased over 24 hour increments from light aerobic activity to full contact practice. The athlete is evaluated after each progression. If postconcussive symptoms occur then the player is dropped back to the previous asymptomatic level and then allowed another attempt at progression after a 24-hour rest period. 80–90% of concussions resolve within 7–10 days. This recovery time may be longer for children or adolescents.[3]
- The CDC endorses a graded 5-step return to play for student athletes[19] as shown in ▶ Table 55.4. The athlete should move to the next step only if they have no new symptoms. If symptoms return or new ones develop, then medical attention should be sought and, after clearance the student can return to the previous step.

Contraindications for return to play are shown in ▶ Table 55.5.

Management of post-concussive syndrome

An extremely complicated topic, partly because of potential for litigation and the fact that symptoms are often vague and nonspecific and there may be no objective findings to corroborate subjective symptoms.

Most symptoms from concussion resolve within 7–10 days and do not require treatment. The most common exception to this is post-traumatic headache, the most common subtype being acute post-traumatic migraine.

55

Table 55.4 5-step return to play progression

Step	Description
Baseline	Athlete is back to regular school activities without symptoms
1	Light aerobic activity: only to increase heart rate for 5–10 minutes. No weight lifting
2	Moderate activity: increase heart rate with body or head movement. May include moderate intensity weight training (less time and intensity than their typical routine)
3	Heavy, non-contact activity: may include running, high-intensity stationary biking, regular weight training, non-contact sports-specific drills
4	Practice & full contact: in controlled practice
5	Competition

Table 55.5 Cerebral contraindications for return to contact sports

1. persistent postconcussion symptoms
2. permanent CNS sequelae from head injury (e.g. organic dementia, hemiplegia, homonymous hemianopsia)
3. hydrocephalus
4. spontaneous SAH from any cause
5. symptomatic (neurologic or pain producing) abnormalities about the foramen magnum (e.g. Chiari malformation)

Typical symptoms include: H/A, dizziness, insomnia, exercise intolerance, depression, irritability, anxiety, memory loss, difficulty concentrating, fatigue, light or noise hypersensitivity.

Patients with protracted symptoms may require more directed treatment.

- Psychological and neuropsychological involvement is often employed.
- Pharmacologic treatment: there are no evidence based studies of the utility of medications for post-concussive symptoms (aside form H/A).
- Intractable headaches: occurs in ≈ 15% of concussions
  - Expert neurology consultation is usually required for difficult to control headaches
  - The first line drugs are OTC medications
  - Triptans are usually employed for nonresponders
  - Third line drugs includ Ketorolac or DHE-45 (dihydroergotamine)
  - Steroids may be beneficial for some
  - Avoid: narcotics, butalbital/caffeine preparations (Fioricet, Esgic…), beta blockers and calcium channel blockers

55

55.1.13 Second impact syndrome (SIS)

A rare condition described primarily in athletes who sustain a second head injury while still symptomatic from an earlier one. Classically, the athlete walks off the field under their own power after the second injury, only to deteriorate to coma within 1–5 minutes and then, due to vascular engorgement, develops malignant cerebral edema that is refractory to all treatment and progresses to herniation. Mortality: 50–100%.

A syndrome compatible with SIS was first described by Schneider[20] in 1973, and was later dubbed the "second impact syndrome of catastrophic head injury" in 1984.[21] Although it is contended that SIS is rare (if it exists at all) and may be overdiagnosed,[22] its apparent predilection for teens and children still warrants extra precaution following concussion.

55.1.14 Chronic traumatic encephalopathy (CTE)

There is limited evidence-based research involving the pathophysiology and natural history of CTE. Thought to be a distinct neurodegenerative disease (tauopathy) associated with repetitive brain trauma, not limited to athletes with reported concussions, and can only be diagnosed postmortem with a pathology-confirmed analysis. Small studies have shown that there is a variable age of onset with variable behavioral, mood, and cognitive deficits present at the time of death (92% symptomatic at time of death).[10,16]

See section about CTE (p. 924) for further details.

55.2 Other TBI definitions

55.2.1 Contusion

A contusion is a TBI with CT findings that may include:
- low attenuation areas: representing associated edema
- high attenuation areas (AKA "hemorrhagic contusions"): usually produce less mass effect than their apparent size. Most common in areas where sudden deceleration of the head causes the brain to impact on bony prominences (e.g. temporal, frontal and occipital poles). These areas may progress (or "blossom" in neuroradiological jargon) to frank parenchymal hemorrhages. Surgical decompression may sometimes be considered if herniation threatens (p.891).

55.2.2 Contrecoup injury

(French: "counter blow") in addition to the potential injury to the brain directly under the point of impact, the force imparted to the head may cause the brain to be thrust against the skull directly opposite the blow. May result in contusions typically in locations described above.

55.2.3 Other definitions

Posttraumatic brain swelling

This term encompasses two distinct processes:
1. increased cerebral blood volume: may result from loss of cerebral vascular autoregulation (p.856). This hyperemia may sometimes occur with extreme rapidity, in which case it has sometimes been referred to as diffuse or "malignant cerebral edema"[23] which carries close to 100% mortality and may be more common in children. Management consists of aggressive measures to maintain ICP < 20 mm Hg and CPP > 60 mm Hg.[24] CPP ≥ 70 mm Hg is generally recommended, see ICP treatment threshold (p.866).
2. true cerebral edema: classically at autopsy these brains "weep fluid".[25] Both vasogenic and cytotoxic cerebral edema (p.90) can occur within hours of head injury[25,26] and occasionally may be treated with decompressive craniectomy (p.891).

Diffuse axonal injury (DAI) (AKA diffuse axonal shearing)

A *primary* lesion of rotational acceleration/deceleration head injury.[27] In its severe form, hemorrhagic foci occur in the corpus callosum and dorsolateral rostral brain stem with microscopic evidence of diffuse injury to axons (axonal retraction balls, microglial stars, and degeneration of white matter fiber tracts). Often cited as the cause of loss of consciousness in patients rendered immediately comatose following head injury in the absence of a space occupying lesion on CT[28] (although DAI may also be present with subdural[29] or epidural hematomas[30]).

55

May be diagnosed clinically when loss of consciousness (coma) lasts > 6 hours in absence of evidence of intracranial mass or ischemia. May be graded as shown in ▶ Table 55.6.

55.3 High-altitude cerebral edema

Acute high-altitude sickness (AHAS) is a systemic disorder that affects individuals usually within 6–48 hrs after ascent to high altitudes. Acute mountain sickness (AMS) is the most common form of AHAS, with symptoms of nausea, headache, anorexia, dyspnea, insomnia and fatigue[31]

Table 55.6 Grading DAI

DAI grade	Description
mild	coma > 6–24 hrs, followed by mild-to-moderate memory impairment, mild-to-moderate disabilities
moderate	coma > 24 hrs, followed by confusion & long-lasting amnesia. Mild-to-severe memory, behavioral and cognitive deficits
severe	coma lasting months with flexor and extensor posturing. Cognitive, memory, speech, sensorimotor and personality deficits. Dysautonomia may occur

and is often assessed using the Lake Louise system.[32] The incidence is ≈ 25% at 7,000 feet, and ≈ 50% at 15,000 feet. Other symptoms of AHAS include edema of feet and hands, and pulmonary edema (HAPE = high altitude pulmonary edema). Ocular findings include retinal hemorrhages,[33] nerve fiber layer infarction, papilledema and vitreous hemorrhage.[34] Cerebral edema (HACE = high altitude cerebral edema), usually associated with pulmonary edema, may occur in severe cases of AHAS. Symptoms of HACE include: severe headache, mental dysfunction (hallucinations, inappropriate behavior, reduced mental status), and neurologic abnormalities (ataxia, paralysis, cerebellar findings).

The unproven "tight-fit" hypothesis postulated that individuals with less compliant CSF systems (smaller ventricles and CSF spaces) were more vulnerable to AMS.[35] A small study of 10 volunteers[36] analyzing CT scans before ascent and symptoms showed a trend that supports the hypothesis.

Prevention: gradual ascent, 2–4 day acclimatization at intermediate altitudes (especially to include sleeping at these levels), avoidance of alcohol or hypnotics.

Treatment of cerebral edema: immediate descent and oxygen (6–12 L/min by NC or face-mask) are recommended. Dexamethasone 8 mg PO or IV followed by 4 mg q 6 hrs may help temporize.

55.4 Traumatic cervical artery dissections

55.4.1 General information

Cervical arterial dissections are a subset of cervical cerebrovascular injuries as shown below.

Cervical cerebrovascular injuries:

- penetrating injury (p. 1017)
- traumatic dissection: the subject of this chapter
  - due to blunt trauma
  - due to stretching: e.g. from neck hyperextension or therapeutic spinal manipulation
  - iatrogenic: dissection caused by intimal tear from angiography catheters
- traumatic compression or occlusion
  - kinking from malalignment: e.g. with cervical fracture-dislocation
  - compression by bone fragments: e.g. by fractures through foramen transversarium

This chapter deals with traumatic cervical artery dissections. There is significant overlap with spontaneous cerebrovascular arterial dissections (p. 1322), however, features that are more pertinent to post-traumatic dissections are covered here.

Optimal screening, diagnostic and treatment methods are controversial. A 13% mortality rate is considered low. Nearly one-third of patients are not treatable.

55.4.2 Epidemiology

Incidence: 1–2% of blunt trauma patients[37] (among those who stayed > 24 hrs in a trauma hospital the incidence was 2.4%[37]).

55

55.4.3 Risk factors

Traumatic risk factors for blunt cerebrovascular injury (BCVI) are shown in ▶ Table 55.7. Risk factors not directly related to the type of trauma include fibromuscular dysplasia, where dissections may follow minor injuries because of increased susceptibility. BCVI can occur even in the absence of identifiable risk factors.[37]

55.4.4 Presentation

Signs and symptoms of BCVI are shown in ▶ Table 55.8.

55.4.5 Evaluation of patients with risk factors or signs/symptoms of BCVI

The following is an adaptation of the guidelines of the Western Trauma Association flow chart[39] (including footnotes!) into an outline format. Their recommendations are based on observational studies and expert opinion (no Class I data was available).

NB: CTA on scanners with ≥ 16 detectors (16-slice multidetector CT angiography, (16MD-CTA) have an accuracy near 99%[40] & equivalent predictive value to cerebral angiogram. MRA[41,42] and

Table 55.7 Traumatic risk factors for BCVI[38,39]
• high energy transfer mechanism associated with: ◦ displaced mid face fracture: LeForte fracture type II or III (p. 887) ◦ basilar skull fracture involving carotid canal
• TBI consistent with DAI and GCS < 6
• cervical vertebral body or transverse foramen fracture, subluxation, or ligamentous injury at any level
• any fracture involving C1–3
• near hanging with anoxic brain injury
• clothesline-type injury or seat belt abrasion with significant cervical swelling, pain, or mental status changes

Table 55.8 Signs & symptoms of BCVI[39]
• arterial hemorrhage from neck/nose/mouth (? go to O.R.)
• cervical bruit in pt. < 50 yrs old
• expanding cervical hematoma
• focal neurologic deficit: TIA, Horner's syndrome, hemiparesis, VBI
• neurologic deficit inconsistent with head CT
• stroke on CT or MRI

ultrasound[43,44] are not considered adequate for BCVI screening. If unavailable, then catheter angiography should be employed.

1. 16MD-CTA should be obtained as follows:
   a) emergently in patients with signs/symptoms of BCVI (► Table 55.8)
   b) *asymptomatic* patients with risk factors (► Table 55.7) for BCVI:
      - if the presence of BCVI would alter therapy (e.g. no contraindication to heparin) then MDCTA should be done within 12 hours if possible
      - if heparin is contraindicated due to associated injuries, timing of MDCTA is determined by patient stability
2. if the MDCTA is equivocal, or if it is negative but clinical suspicion remains high: a catheter arteriogram should be done (otherwise, if negative: stop)
3. grading: if the MDCTA or the arteriogram shows positive findings (p. 1324):
   a) the injury is graded using the scale shown in ► Table 55.9 [45] (sometimes referred to as the "Denver grading scale")
   b) proceed with grade-based management (see below)

55

55.4.6 Management of documented BCVI

Antiplatelet therapy is as effective in preventing stroke as anticoagulation for cerebrovascular dissection.[46,47]

Grade specific therapy

- Grade I & II
  - Most resolve on their own
  - Even though there might be a slight benefit of heparin over aspirin for low grade injuries, due to the low overall risk the general trend is to treat these with aspirin
- Grade III
  - Anticoagulate with heparin. Rationale: heparin and aspirin are roughly equivalent for Grade III, however, most will need to be restudied in 7-10 days
  - Repeat angiogram or 16MD-CTA 7-10 days post-injury. See below for subsequent management
- Grade IV: endovascular occlusion to prevent embolization
- Grade V: highly lethal injury
  - accessible lesions should be considered for urgent surgical repair (anecdotal)
  - inaccessible lesions (the majority): incomplete transection may be amenable to endovascular stenting with concurrent antithrombotics; complete transections should be ligated (or occluded endovascularly)

Table 55.9 BCVI grading scale,[45] "Denver grading scale"

Grade	Description
I	luminal irregularity with < 25% stenosis
II	≥ 25% luminal stenosis or intraluminal thrombus or raised intimal flap
III	pseudoaneurysm
IV	occlusion
V	transection with free extravasation

For Grade III repeat MDCTA or angiography 7–10 days post injury to assess healing.[48] Results:
- lesion healed: discontinue anticoagulation
- non-healed lesions:
  - consider endovascular stenting "with caution" for severe luminal narrowing or expanding pseudoaneurysm (controversial: results have been mixed – favorable[46] and unfavorable[49])
  - transition from heparin to aspirin (75–150 mg/d) alone
  - repeat MDCTA or angiography 3 months post injury (rationale: most heal with canalization in 6 wks). Results:
    - healed lesion: consider discontinuing aspirin
    - non-healed: optimal drug and duration is not known. Recommendation[39]: lifelong antiplatelet therapy with either aspirin or clopidogrel. Dual therapy is used for acute coronary syndromes and following angioplasty (± stenting) but is not recommended in patients who have had a stroke or TIA[50]

Heparinization:

When anticoagulation is employed, perform a baseline PTT and then begin heparin drip 15 U/kg/hr IV. Repeat PTT after 6 hours, and titrate to PTT = 40–50 seconds.

Trauma contra-indications to anticoagulation: patients that are actively bleeding, have potential for bleeding, or in whom the consequences of bleeding are severe. Specific examples include: liver and spleen injuries, major pelvic fractures, and intracranial hemorrhage.

Dissection-related anticoagulation risks include: extension of the medial hemorrhage (with possible SAH), and intracerebral hemorrhage (conversion of pale infarct to hemorrhagic).

55.4.7 Carotid artery blunt injuries

General information

See general information related to cerebral arterial dissections and spontaneous dissections (p. 1322). For evaluation and management, see above.

This section considers blunt (i.e. nonpenetrating) specifically related to ICA dissection. Neck hyperextension with lateral rotation is a common mechanism of injury, and is thought to stretch the ICA over the transverse processes of the upper cervical spine. In posttraumatic dissection, ischemic symptoms are the most common.[51]

Etiologies:
1. following MVAs: the most common etiology
2. attempted strangulation[52]
3. spinal manipulation therapy: VA dissections are more common than ICA

Most carotid dissections start ≈ 2 cm distal to the ICA origin.

Clinical

The risk of stroke with various ICA dissection grades is shown in ▸ Table 55.10. The risk of stroke increases with increasing grade for ICA injuries. This does not hold true for VA injuries.

Grade I injuries: 70% heal with or without heparin. 25% will persist. 4–12% will progress to more severe grade. Data suggests that anticoagulation reduces the risk of progression.[38]

Grade II: ≈ 70% progress to more severe grade even with heparin therapy.

Grade III & IV: most persist.

55

Table 55.10 Risk of stroke with ICA dissection

Grade[a]	Description	Stroke risk
I	stenosis < 25%	3%
II	stenosis > 25%	11%
III	pseudoaneurysm	44%
IV	occlusion	uniformly lethal

[a]for grading, see ▶ Table 55.9

Table 55.11 Time to presentation after non-penetrating trauma

Time	%
0–1 hours	6–10% of cases
1–24 hours	57–73%
after 24 hours	17–35%

Initially, there may be no neurologic sequelae, however, progressive thrombosis, intramural hemorrhage or embolic phenomenon may develop in a delayed fashion. The distribution of time delays following trauma to time of presentation are shown in ▶ Table 55.11 (the majority are evident within the 1st 24 hours).

Management

See Management of documented BCVI (p. 849).

Outcome

Natural history is not well known. Many patients with minor symptoms may not present and presumably do well. In one series, 75% of patients returned to normal, 16% had a minor deficit, and 8% had a major deficit or died.[53]

55

55.4.8 Vertebral artery blunt injuries

General information

See anatomy of vertebral artery segments (p. 80).

Blunt vertebral artery injury (BVI) is very rare, being found in 0.5–0.7% of patients with blunt injuries with aggressive screening.[54] It may produce vertebrobasilar insufficiency (VBI) or posterior circulation stroke. Fractures through the foramen transversarium, facet fracture-dislocation, or vertebral subluxation are frequently identified in patients with BVI[38,55,56] (overall incidence increases to 6% in the presence of cervical fracture or ligamentous injury[54]).

Etiologies

While motor vehicle accidents are the most common mechanism of injury, any trauma that can injure the C-spine can cause BVI (diving accidents, spinal manipulation…).

1. automobile accidents
2. spinal manipulation therapy (SMT): including chiropractic[57] or similar, which comprise 11 of 15 case reports reviewed by Caplan et al.[58] VA dissections were independently associated with SMT within 30 days in multivariate analysis (odds ratio = 6.62, 95% CI 1.4 to 30)[59]
3. sudden head turning
4. direct blows to the back of the neck[58]

Stroke from BVI

The Denver grade of the dissection in BVI does not correlate with risk of stroke or mortality (as it does with ICA dissection).[60] Unlike with carotid injuries, there is rarely a premonitory "warning" TIA. Time from injury to stroke: mean 4 days (range: 8 hours -12 days).

Evaluation

When BVI is identified, it is critical to assess the status of the contralateral VA.

Practice guideline: Vertebral artery blunt injuries

Evaluation

Level I[61]

- Patients meeting the "Denver Screening Criteria" (symptoms shown in ► Table 55.8 or risk factors shown in ► Table 55.7) should undergo 16MD-CTA to screen for BVI

Level III[61]

- Catheter angiogram is recommended in select patients after blunt cervical trauma if 16MD-CTA is not available especially if concurrent endovascular intervention is a consideration.
- MRI is recommended for BVI after blunt cervical trauma in patients with incomplete SCI or vertebral subluxation injuries.

Treatment

Practice guideline: Vertebral artery blunt injuries

Treatment

Level III[61]

- No specific guidelines were made among treatment options (anticoagulation, antiplatelet therapy, or no treatment)
- The role of endovascular therapy for BVI has not been defined

Strokes were more frequent in patients with BVI who were not treated initially with IV heparin despite an asymptomatic BVI.[38] However, based on historical controls, it is not clear if either screening or treatment improves overall outcome.[54]

Recommendations: treat all BVI with aspirin. Restudy chronic occlusion in 3 months.

Treatment options include endovascular stenting when amenable. This can restore near-normal flow, but long-term results are lacking.[62] Also, stenting requires ≥ ≈3 months of antiplatelet therapy which is contraindicated in some situations.

Outcome

Overall mortality with unilateral BVI ranges from 8-18%[60] which is lower than with ICA dissections (17-40%). Bilateral VA dissection appears highly fatal.

References

[1] Carney N, Ghajar J, Jagoda A, Bedrick S, Davis-O'Reilly C, du Coudray H, Hack D, Helfand N, Huddleston A, Nettleton T, Riggio S. Concussion guidelines step 1: systematic review of prevalent indicators. Neurosurgery. 2014; 75 Suppl 1:S3–15

[2] Harmon KG, Drezner JA, Gammons M, Guskiewicz KM, Halstead M, Herring SA, Kutcher JS, Pana A, Putukian M, Roberts WO. American Medical Society for Sports Medicine position statement: concussion in sport. Br J Sports Med. 2013; 47:15–26

[3] McCrory P, Meeuwisse WH, Aubry M, Cantu B, Dvorak J, Echemendia RJ, Engebretsen L, Johnston K, Kutcher JS, Raftery M, Sills A, Benson BW, Davis GA, Ellenbogen RG, Guskiewicz K, Herring SA, Iverson GL, Jordan BD, Kissick J, McCrea M, McIntosh AS, Maddocks D, Makdissi M, Purcell L, Putukian M, Schneider K, Tator CH, Turner M. Consensus statement on concussion in sport: the 4th International Conference on Concussion in Sport held in Zurich, November 2012. Br J Sports Med. 2013; 47:250–258

[4] Scorza KA, Raleigh MF, O'Connor FG. Current concepts in concussion: evaluation and management. Am Fam Physician. 2012; 85:123–132
[5] McCrory P, Meeuwisse WH, Echemendia RJ, Iverson GL, Dvorak J, Kutcher JS. What is the lowest threshold to make a diagnosis of concussion? Br J Sports Med. 2013; 47:268–271
[6] Putukian M, Raftery M, Guskiewicz K, Herring S, Aubry M, Cantu RC, Molloy M. Onfield assessment of concussion in the adult athlete. Br J Sports Med. 2013; 47:285–288
[7] Giza CC, Kutcher JS, Ashwal S, Barth J, Getchius TS, Gioia GA, Gronseth GS, Guskiewicz K, Mandel S, Manley G, McKeag DB, Thurman DJ, Zafonte R. Summary of evidence-based guideline update: evaluation and management of concussion in sports: report of the Guideline Development Subcommittee of the American Academy of Neurology. Neurology. 2013; 80:2250–2257
[8] Yuh EL, Hawryluk GW, Manley GT. Imaging concussion: a review. Neurosurgery. 2014; 75 Suppl 4: S50–S63
[9] Kelly JP, Rosenberg JH. Diagnosis and Management of Concussion in Sports. Neurology. 1997; 48:575–580
[10] Putukian M, Kutcher J. Current concepts in the treatment of sports concussions. Neurosurgery. 2014; 75 Suppl 4:S64–S70
[11] Carney N, Ghajar J, Jagoda A, Bedrick S, Davis-O'Reilly C, du Coudray H, Hack D, Helfand N, Huddleston A, Nettleton T, Riggio S. Executive summary of Concussion guidelines step 1: systematic review of prevalent indicators. Neurosurgery. 2014; 75 Suppl 1:S1–S2
[12] SCAT3. Br J Sports Med. 2013; 47
[13] Child SCAT3. Br J Sports Med. 2013; 47
[14] McCrea M, Kelly JP, Kluge J, et al. Standardized Assessment of Concussion in Football Players. Neurology. 1997; 48:586–588
[15] Broglio SP, Ferrara MS, Macciocchi SN, Baumgartner TA, Elliott R. Test-Retest Reliability of Computerized Concussion Assessment Programs. Journal of Athletic Training. 2007; 42:509–514
[16] Saigal R, Berger MS. The long-term effects of repetitive mild head injuries in sports. Neurosurgery. 2014; 75 Suppl 4:S149–S155
[17] Giza CC, Hovda DA. The new neurometabolic cascade of concussion. Neurosurgery. 2014; 75 Suppl 4:S24–S33
[18] Tator CH, Davis H. The postconcussion syndrome in sports and recreation: clinical features and demography in 138 athletes. Neurosurgery. 2014; 75 Suppl 4:S106–S112
[19] Centers for Disease Control and Prevention. Brain Injury Basics - Returning to Sports and Activities. 2015
[20] Schneider RC. Head and Neck Injuries in Football. Baltimore: Williams & Wilkins; 1973
[21] Saunders RL, Harbaugh RE. Second Impact in Catastrophic Contact-Sports Head Trauma. JAMA. 1984; 252:538–539
[22] McCrory PR, Berkovic SF. Second Impact Syndrome. Neurology. 1998; 50:677–683
[23] Bruce DA, Alavi A, Bilaniuk L, et al. Diffuse Cerebral Swelling Following Head Injuries in Children: The Syndrome of "Malignant Brain Edema". J Neurosurg. 1981; 54:170–178
[24] Juul N, Morris GF, Marshall SB, et al. Intracranial Hypertension and Cerebral Perfusion Pressure: Influence on Neurological Deterioration and Outcome in Severe Head Injury. J Neurosurg. 2000; 92:1–6
[25] Kimelberg H. Current Concepts of Brain Edema. J Neurosurg. 1995; 83:1051–1059
[26] Bullock R, Maxwell W, Graham D. Glial Swelling Following Cerebral Contusion: An Ultrastructural Study. J Neurol Neurosurg Psychiatry. 1991; 54:427–434
[27] Gennarelli TA, Thibault LE, Adams JH, et al. Diffuse Axonal Injury and Traumatic Coma in the Primate. Ann Neurol. 1982; 12:564–574
[28] Adams JH, Graham DI, Murray LS, Scott G. Diffuse Axonal Injury Due to Nonmissile Head Injury in Humans: An Analysis of 45 Cases. Ann Neurol. 1982; 12:557–563
[29] Sahuquillo-Barris J, Lamarca-Ciuro J, Vilalta-Castan J, Rubio-Garcia E, et al. Acute Subdural Hematoma and Diffuse Axonal Injury After Severe Head Trauma. J Neurosurg. 1988; 68:894–900
[30] Lamarca-Ciuro J, Vilalta-Castan J, et al. Epidural Hematoma and Diffuse Axonal Injury. Neurosurgery. 1985; 17:378–379
[31] Montgomery AB, Mills J, Luce JM. Incidence of Acute Mountain Sickness at Intermediate Altitude. JAMA. 1989; 261:732–734
[32] Roach RC, Bartsch P, Hackett PH, Oelz O. The Lake Louise Acute Mountain Sickness scoring system. Burlington: Queen City Printers; 1993
[33] Butler FK, Harris DJ, Reynolds RD. Altitude Retinopathy on Mount Everest, 1989. Ophthalmology. 1992; 99:739–746
[34] Frayser R, Houston CS, Bryan AC, et al. Retinal Hemorrhage at High Altitude. N Engl J Med. 1970; 282:1183–1184
[35] Ross RT. The random nature of cerebral mountain sickness. Lancet. 1985; 1:990–991
[36] Wilson MH, Milledge J. Direct measurement of intracranial pressure at high altitude and correlation of ventricular size with acute mountain sickness: Brian Cummins' results from the 1985 Kishtwar expedition. Neurosurgery. 2008; 63:970–4; discussion 974-5
[37] Stein DM, Boswell S, Sliker CW, Lui FY, Scalea TM. Blunt cerebrovascular injuries: does treatment always matter? J Trauma. 2009; 66:132–43; discussion 143-4
[38] Biffl WL, Moore EE, Elliott JP, Ray C, Offner PJ, Franciose RJ, Brega KE, Burch JM. The devastating potential of blunt vertebral arterial injuries. Ann Surg. 2000; 231:672–681
[39] Biffl WL, Cothren CC, Moore EE. Western Trauma Association critical decisions in trauma: Screening for and treatment of blunt cerebrovascular injuries. J Trauma. 2009; 67:1150–1153
[40] Eastman AL, Chason DP, Perez CL, McAnulty AL, Minei JP. Computed tomographic angiography for the diagnosis of blunt cervical vascular injury: is it ready for primetime? J Trauma. 2006; 60:925–9; discussion 929
[41] Miller PR, Fabian TC, Croce MA, Cagiannos C, Williams JS, Vang M, Qaisi WG, Felker RE, Timmons SD. Prospective screening for blunt cerebrovascular injuries: analysis of diagnostic modalities and outcomes. Ann Surg. 2002; 236:386–93; discussion 393-5
[42] Biffl WL, Ray CE, Jr, Moore EE, Mestek M, Johnson JL, Burch JM. Noninvasive diagnosis of blunt cerebrovascular injuries: a preliminary report. J Trauma. 2002; 53:850–856
[43] Cogbill TH, Moore EE, Meissner M, Fischer RP, Hoyt DB, Morris JA, Shackford SR, Wallace JR, Ross SE, Ochsner MG, et al. The spectrum of blunt injury to the carotid artery: a multicenter perspective. J Trauma. 1994; 37:473–479
[44] Mutze S, Rademacher G, Matthes G, Hosten N, Stengel D. Blunt cerebrovascular injury in patients with blunt multiple trauma: diagnostic accuracy of duplex Doppler US and early CT angiography. Radiology. 2005; 237:884–892
[45] Biffl WL, Moore EE, Offner PJ, Brega KE, Franciose RJ, Burch JM. Blunt carotid arterial injuries: implications of a new grading scale. J Trauma. 1999; 47:845–853
[46] Edwards NM, Fabian TC, Claridge JA, Timmons SD, Fischer PE, Croce MA. Antithrombotic therapy and endovascular stents are effective treatment for blunt carotid injuries: results from longterm follow-up. J Am Coll Surg. 2007; 204:1007–13; discussion 1014-5
[47] Markus HS, Hayter E, Levi C, Feldman A, Venables G, Norris J. Antiplatelet treatment compared with anticoagulation treatment for cervical artery dissection (CADISS): a randomised trial. Lancet Neurol. 2015; 14:361–367
[48] Biffl WL, Ray CE, Jr, Moore EE, Franciose RJ, Aly S, Heyrosa MG, Johnson JL, Burch JM. Treatment-

related outcomes from blunt cerebrovascular injuries: importance of routine follow-up arteriography. Ann Surg. 2002; 235:699–706; discussion 706-7

[49] Cothren CC, Moore EE, Ray CE, Jr, Ciesla DJ, Johnson JL, Moore JB, Burch JM. Carotid artery stents for blunt cerebrovascular injury: risks exceed benefits. Arch Surg. 2005; 140:480–5; discussion 485-6

[50] Hermosillo AJ, Spinler SA. Aspirin, clopidogrel, and warfarin: is the combination appropriate and effective or inappropriate and too dangerous? Ann Pharmacother. 2008; 42:790–805

[51] Anson J, Crowell RM. Cervicocranial Arterial Dissection. Neurosurgery. 1991; 29:89–96

[52] Biller J, Hingtgen WL, Adams HP, et al. Cervicocephalic Arterial Dissections: A Ten-Year Experience. Arch Neurol. 1986; 43:1234–1238

[53] Hart RG, Easton JD. Dissections of Cervical and Cerebral Arteries. Neurol Clin North Am. 1983; 1:255–282

[54] Berne JD, Norwood SH. Blunt Vertebral Artery Injuries in the Era of Computed Tomographic Angiographic Screening: Incidence and Outcomes From 8292 Patients. J Trauma. 2009. DOI: 10.1097/TA.0b013e31818888c7

[55] Louw JA, Mafoyane NA, Small B, Neser CP. Occlusion of the vertebral artery in cervical spine dislocations. J Bone Joint Surg Br. 1990; 72:679–681

[56] Willis BK, Greiner F, Orrison WW, Benzel EC. The incidence of vertebral artery injury after midcervical spine fracture or subluxation. Neurosurgery. 1994; 34:435–41; discussion 441-2

[57] Mas JL, Henin D, Bousser MG, Hauw JJ. Dissecting Aneurysm of the Vertebral Artery and Cervical Manipulation: A Case Report with Autopsy. Neurology. 1989; 39:512–515

[58] Caplan LR, Zarins CK, Hemmati M. Spontaneous Dissection of the Extracranial Vertebral Arteries. Stroke. 1985; 16:1030–1038

[59] Smith WS, Johnston SC, Skalabrin EJ, Weaver M, Azari P, Albers GW, Gress DR. Spinal manipulative therapy is an independent risk factor for vertebral artery dissection. Neurology. 2003; 60:1424–1428

[60] Fusco MR, Harrigan MR. Cerebrovascular dissections: a review. Part II: blunt cerebrovascular injury. Neurosurgery. 2011; 68:517–30; discussion 530

[61] Harrigan MR, Hadley MN, Dhall SS, Walters BC, Aarabi B, Gelb DE, Hurlbert RJ, Rozzelle CJ, Ryken TC, Theodore N. Management of vertebral artery injuries following non-penetrating cervical trauma. Neurosurgery. 2013; 72 Suppl 2:234–243

[62] Lee YJ, Ahn JY, Han IB, Chung YS, Hong CK, Joo JY. Therapeutic endovascular treatments for traumatic vertebral artery injuries. J Trauma. 2007; 62:886–891

56 Neuromonitoring

56.1 General information

This section considers neuromonitoring instrumentation that can be done primarily at the patient's bedside, and therefore does not include CT perfusion studies, PET scans.... The bulk of neuromonitoring literature deals with intracranial pressure (ICP). Other parameters that can be monitored include: jugular venous oxygen monitoring (p. 865), regional CBF (p. 866), brain tissue oxygen tension (p. 865), and brain metabolites (pyruvate, lactate, glucose...) (p. 866).

The role of adjunctive monitoring is currently unknown. Unanswered questions include: should neuromonitoring be disease specific (e.g. is SAH different from TBI), which monitors provide additional unique information, what are the critical values of the monitored entity, and what interventions should be undertaken to correct abnormalities?

56.2 Intracranial pressure (ICP)

56.2.1 Background

Intracranial pressure (ICP) is discussed in this section on trauma because of the close relationship between elevated ICP and brain damage from head injury. However, factors involved in diagnosing and treating intracranial hypertension (IC-HTN) also may pertain (with modifications) to brain tumors, dural venous thrombosis, etc.

56.2.2 Cerebral perfusion pressure (CPP) and cerebral autoregulation

Secondary brain injury (i.e. following the initial trauma) is attributable in part to cerebral ischemia; see Secondary injury (p. 824). The critical parameter for brain function and survival is not actually ICP, rather it is adequate cerebral blood flow (CBF) to meet $CMRO_2$ demands; see discussion of CBF & $CMRO_2$ (p. 1264). CBF is difficult to quantitate, and can only be measured continuously at the bedside with specialized equipment and difficulty.[1] However, CBF depends on cerebral perfusion pressure (CPP), which is related to ICP (which is more easily measured) as shown in Eq (56.1).

$$\begin{gathered}\{\text{cerebral perfusion pressure}\} = \{\text{mean arterial pressure}^*\} - \{\text{intracranial pressure}\} \\ \text{or, expressed in symbols} \\ CPP = MAP^* - ICP\end{gathered} \tag{56.1}$$

*note: the actual pressure of interest is the mean carotid pressure (MCP) which may be approximated as the MAP with the transducer zeroed ≈ at the level of the foramen of Monro.[2]

56

As ICP becomes elevated, CPP is reduced at any given MAP. Normal adult CPP is > 50 mm Hg. Cerebral autoregulation is a mechanism whereby over a wide range, large changes in systemic BP produce only small changes in CBF. Due to autoregulation, CPP would have to drop below 40 in a normal brain before CBF would be impaired.

In the head injured patient, older recommendations were to maintain CPP ≥ 70 mm Hg due to increased cerebral vascular resistance.[3] However, recent evidence suggests that elevated ICP (≥ 20 mm Hg) may be more detrimental than changes in CPP (as long as CPP is > 60 mm Hg[4])[5] (higher levels of CPP were not protective against significant ICP elevations[5]).

56.2.3 ICP principles

The following are approximations to help simplify understanding ICP (these are only models, and as such are not entirely accurate):

1. *normal* intracranial constituents (and approximate volumes):
   a) brain parenchyma (which also contains extracellular fluid): 1400 ml
   b) cerebral blood volume (CBV): 150 ml
   c) cerebrospinal fluid (CSF): 150 ml
2. these volumes are contained in an inelastic, completely closed container (the skull)

3. pressure is distributed evenly throughout the intracranial cavity (in reality, pressure gradients exist[6,7])
4. the modified **Monro-Kellie** doctrine[8] states that the sum of the intracranial volumes (CBV, brain, CSF, and other constituents (e.g. tumor, hematoma...)) is constant, and that an increase in any one of these must be offset by an equal decrease in another. The mechanism: there is a pressure equilibrium in the skull. If the pressure from one intracranial constituent increases (as when that component increases in volume), it causes the pressure inside the skull (ICP) to increase. When this increased ICP exceeds the pressure required to force one of the other constituents out through the foramen magnum (FM) (the only true effective opening in the intact skull) that other component will decrease in size via that route until a new equilibrium is established. The cranio-spinal axis can buffer small increases in volume with no change or only a slight increase in ICP. If the expansion continues, then the new equilibrium will be at a higher ICP. The result:
   a) at pressures slightly above normal, if there is no obstruction to CSF flow (obstructive hydrocephalus), CSF can be displaced from the ventricles and subarachnoid spaces and exit the intracranial compartment via the FM
   b) intravenous blood can also be displaced through the FM via the IJVs
   c) as pressure continues to rise, arterial blood is displaced and CPP decreases, eventually producing diffuse cerebral ischemia. At pressures equal to mean arterial pressure, arterial blood will be unable to enter the skull through the FM, producing complete cessation of blood flow to the brain, with resultant massive infarction
   d) increased brain edema, or an expanding mass (e.g. hematoma) can push brain parenchyma downward into the foramen magnum (cerebral herniation) although brain tissue cannot actually exit the skull

56.2.4 Normal ICP

The normal range of ICP varies with age. Values for pediatrics are not well established. Guidelines are shown in ▶ Table 56.1.

56.2.5 Intracranial hypertension (IC-HTN)

General information

Traumatic IC-HTN may be due any of the following (alone or in various combinations):
1. cerebral edema
2. hyperemia: the normal response to head injury.[10] Possibly due to vasomotor paralysis (loss of cerebral autoregulation). May be more significant than edema in raising ICP (p.901)[11]
3. traumatically induced masses
   a) epidural hematoma
   b) subdural hematoma
   c) intraparenchymal hemorrhage (hemorrhagic contusion)
   d) foreign body (e.g. bullet)
   e) depressed skull fracture
4. hydrocephalus due to obstruction of CSF absorption or circulation
5. hypoventilation (causing hypercarbia → vasodilatation)
6. systemic hypertension (HTN)
7. venous sinus thrombosis
8. increased muscle tone and valsalva maneuver as a result of agitation or posturing → increased intrathoracic pressure → increased jugular venous pressure → reduced venous outflow from head
9. sustained posttraumatic seizures (status epilepticus)

Table 56.1 Normal ICP

Age group	Normal range (mm Hg)
adults and older children[a]	< 10–15
young children	3–7
term infants[b]	1.5–6

[a]the age of transition from "young" to "older" child is not precisely defined
[b]may be subatmospheric in newborns[9]

56

A *secondary increase in ICP* is sometimes observed 3–10 days following the trauma, and may be associated with a worse prognosis.[12] Possible causes include:

1. delayed hematoma formation
   a) delayed epidural hematoma (p. 894)
   b) delayed acute subdural hematoma (p. 898)
   c) delayed traumatic intracerebral hemorrhage[13] (or hemorrhagic contusions) with perilesional edema: usually in older patients, may cause sudden deterioration. May become severe enough to require evacuation (p. 892)
2. cerebral vasospasm[14]
3. severe adult respiratory distress syndrome (ARDS) with hypoventilation
4. delayed edema formation: more common in pediatric patients
5. hyponatremia

Clinical presentation – Cushing's triad

The classic clinical presentation of IC-HTN (regardless of cause) is Cushing's triad which is shown in ▶ Table 56.2. However, the full triad is only seen in ≈ 33% of cases of IC-HTN.

Patients with significant ICP elevation due to trauma, brain masses (tumor) or hydrocephalus (but paradoxically not with pseudotumor cerebri) will usually be obtunded.

CT scan and elevated ICP

Whereas CT findings may be correlated with a risk of IC-HTN, no combination of CT findings has been shown to allow accurate estimates of actual ICP. 60% of patients with closed head injury and an abnormal CT will have IC-HTN.[15] (**Note:** "abnormal" CT: demonstrates hematomas (EDH, SDH or ICH), contusions,[15] compression of basal cisterns (p. 921), herniation or swelling.[16,17])

Only 13% of patients with a *normal* CT scan will have IC-HTN.[15] However, patients with a normal CT AND 2 or more risk factors identified in ▶ Table 56.3 will have ≈ 60% risk of IC-HTN. If only 1 or none are present, ICP will be increased in only 4%.

56.2.6 ICP monitoring

Indications for ICP monitoring

Practice guideline: Indications for ICP monitoring

For salvageable patients with severe traumatic brain injury (GCS ≤ 8 after cardiopulmonary resuscitation)

Level II[17]: with an abnormal admitting brain CT(**note**: abnormal" CT: demonstrates hematomas (EDH, SDH or ICH), contusions,[15] compression of basal cisterns (p. 921), herniation or swelling[16,17])

Level III[17]: with a *normal* admitting brain CT, but with ≥ 2 of the risk factors for IC-HTN in ▶ Table 56.3

56

1. ✱ neurologic criteria: see **Practice guideline: Indications for ICP monitoring** (p. 858)
   a) some centers monitor patients who don't follow commands. Rationale: patients who follow commands (GCS ≥ 9) are at low risk for IC-HTN, and one can follow sequential neurologic exams in these patients and institute further evaluation or treatment based on neurologic deterioration
   b) some centers monitor patients who don't localize, and follow neuro exam on others

Table 56.2 Cushing's triad with elevated ICP

1. hypertension
2. bradycardia
3. respiratory irregularity

Table 56.3 Risk factors for IC-HTN with a normal CT

- age > 40 yrs
- SBP < 90 mm Hg
- decerebrate or decorticate posturing on motor exam (unilateral or bilateral)

2. multiple systems injured with altered level of consciousness (especially where therapies for other injuries may have deleterious effects on ICP, e.g. high levels of PEEP or the need for large volumes of IV fluids or the need for heavy sedation)
3. with traumatic intracranial mass (EDH, SDH, depressed skull fracture…)
   a) a physician may choose to monitor ICP in some of these patients[16,18]
   b) post-op, subsequent to removal of the mass
4. non-traumatic indications for ICP monitoring:
   a) some centers monitor ICP in patients with acute fulminant liver failure with an INR > 1.5 and Grade III of IV coma. A recent study shows that a *subarachnoid bolt* may be inserted after administration of factor VII 40 mcg/kg IV over 1–2 minutes (the bolt is inserted as soon as possible (usually within 15 minutes and no more than 2 hours after administration)) without significant risk of hemorrhage. All patients were treated with hypothermia; other ICP treatment measures were used for refractory IC-HTN

Contraindications (relative)

1. "awake" patient: monitor usually not necessary, can follow neuro exam
2. coagulopathy (including DIC): frequently seen in severe head injury. If an ICP monitor is essential, take steps to correct coagulopathy (FFP, platelets…) and consider *subarachnoid bolt* or *epidural monitor* (an IVC or intraparenchymal monitor is contraindicated). See recommended range of PT or INR (p. 157).

Duration of monitoring

D/C monitor when ICP normal × 48–72 hrs after withdrawal of ICP therapy. Caution: IC-HTN may have delayed onset (often starts on day 2–3, and day 9–11 is a common second peak especially in peds). Also see delayed deterioration (p. 824). Avoid a false sense of security imparted by a normal early ICP.

Complications of ICP monitors

General information

▶ Table 56.4 for a summary of complication rates for various types of monitors.[3]

1. infection: see below
2. hemorrhage[3]: overall incidence is 1.4% for all devices (see ▶ Table 56.4 for breakdown). The Angioma Alliance[21] definition of hemorrhage: acute or subacute symptoms (any of: headache, seizure, impaired consciousness, or new/worsened focal neurological deficit referable to the anatomic location of the CM) accompanied by radiological, pathological, surgical, or rarely only cerebrospinal fluid evidence of recent extra- or intralesional hemorrhage. This definition does not include either an increase in CM diameter without other evidence of recent hemorrhage, nor the presence of a hemosiderin halo. Risk of significant hematoma requiring surgical evacuation is ≈ 0.5–2.5%[15,22,23]
3. malfunction or obstruction: with fluid coupled devices, higher rates of obstruction occur at ICPs > 50 mm Hg
4. malposition: 3% of IVCs require operative repositioning

56

Table 56.4 Complication rates with various types of ICP monitors

Monitor type	Bacterial colonization[a]	Hemorrhage	Malfunction or obstruction
IVC	ave: 10–17% range[19,20]: 0–40%	1.1%	6.3%
subarachnoid bolt	ave: 5% range: 0–10%	0	16%
subdural	ave: 4% range: 1–10%	0	10.5%
parenchymal	ave: 14% (two reports, 12% & 17%)	2.8%	9–40%

[a]some studies report this as infection, but do not distinguish between clinically significant infection and colonization of ICP monitor

Infection with ICP monitors

Colonization of the monitoring device is much more common than clinically significant infection (ventriculitis or meningitis). See ▶ Table 56.4 for colonization rates. Fever, leukocytosis and CSF pleocytosis have low predictive value (CSF cultures are more helpful). Range of reported infection rates: 1–27%.[24]

Practice guideline: Infection prophylaxis with ICP monitors

Level III[25]: neither prophylactic antibiotics nor routine ventricular catheter exchange is recommended to reduce infection

Identified risk factors for infection include[20,24,26,27]:

1. intracerebral, subarachnoid or intraventricular hemorrhage
2. ICP > 20 mm Hg
3. duration of monitoring: contradictory results in literature. One prospective study in 1984 found an increased risk with monitor duration > 5 days (infection risk reaches 42% by day #11).[22,26] Another found no correlation with monitoring duration.[28] A retrospective analysis[20] found a non-linear increase of risk during the first 10–12 days after which the rate diminished rapidly
4. neurosurgical operation: including operations for depressed skull fracture
5. irrigation of system
6. leakage around IVCs
7. open skull fractures (including basilar skull fractures with CSF leak)
8. other infections: septicemia, pneumonia

Factors *not* associated with increased incidence of infection:

1. insertion of IVC in neuro intensive care unit (instead of O.R.)
2. previous IVC
3. drainage of CSF
4. use of steroids

Treatment of infection

Removal of device if at all possible (if continued ICP monitoring is required consideration may be given to inserting a monitor at another site) and appropriate antibiotics.

Types of monitors

56

1. intraventricular catheter (IVC): AKA external ventricular drainage (EVD), connected to an external pressure transducer via fluid-filled tubing. The standard by which others are judged (also below; **note**: other options for IVCs utilize transducers tipped with fiberoptic or strain gauge devices which are located within the intraventricular catheter; in this discussion, "IVC" does not refer to this type)
   a) advantages:
      - most accurate (can be recalibrated to minimize measurement drift)[29]
      - lower cost
      - in addition to measuring pressure, allows therapeutic CSF drainage (may help reduce ICP directly, and may drain particulate matter, e.g. blood breakdown products after SAH, that could occlude arachnoid granulations[30])
   b) disadvantages
      - may be difficult to insert into compressed or displaced ventricles
      - obstruction of the fluid column (e.g. by blood clot, or by coaptation of the ependymal lining on the catheter as the ventricle collapses with drainage) may cause inaccuracy
      - some effort is required to check and maintain function, e.g. IVC problems (p. 862) and IVC trouble shooting (p. 863)
      - transducer must be consistently maintained at a fixed reference point relative to patient's head (must be moved as HOB is raised/lowered)
2. intraparenchymal monitor (e.g. Camino labs or Honeywell/Phillips[31,32]): similar to IVC but more expensive. Some are subject to measurement drift,[33,34] others may not be[35]
3. *less accurate* monitors
   a) subarachnoid screw (bolt): risk of infection 1%, rises after 3 days. At high ICPs (often when needed most) surface of brain may occlude lumen → false readings (usually lower than actual, may still show ≈ normal waveform)

b) subdural: may utilize a fluid coupled catheter (e.g. Cordis Cup catheter), fiberoptic tipped catheter, or strain gauge tipped catheter
c) epidural: may utilize a fluid coupled catheter, or fiberoptic tipped catheter (e.g. Ladd fiberoptic). Accuracy is questionable
d) in infants, one can utilizing an open anterior fontanelle (AF):
   - fontanometry[36]: probably not very accurate
   - applanation principle: may be used in suitable circumstances (viz.: if the fontanelle is concave with the infant upright, and convex when flat or head down) to estimate the ICP within 1 cm H_2O.[9] The infant is placed supine, and the AF is visualized and palpated while the head is raised and lowered. When the AF is flat, the ICP equals atmospheric pressure, and ICP can be estimated in cm H_2O as the distance from the AF to the point where the venous pressure is 0 (for a recumbent infant, the midpoint of the clavicle usually suffices). If the AF is not concave with the infant erect, then this method cannot be used because either the ICP exceeds the distance from the AF to the venous zero point, or the scalp may be too thick

Conversion factors: between mm Hg and cm H_2O are shown in Eq (56.2) and Eq (56.3) (the density of mercury is 13.6 times that of water, and CSF is fairly close to water).

$$1 \text{ mm Hg [torr]} = 1.36 \text{ cm } H_2O \tag{56.2}$$

$$1 \text{ cm } H_2O = 0.735 \text{ mmHg [torr]} \tag{56.3}$$

Intraventricular catheter (IVC)

Insertion technique

For technique to place catheter in frontal horn, see Kocher's point (p. 1512). The right side is usually used unless specific reasons to use the left are present (e.g. blood clot in right lateral ventricle which might occlude IVC).

Set-up

▶ Fig. 56.1 shows a typical external ventricular drainage (EVD) system/ ventriculostomy ICP monitor. Not every system will have the same components (some may have less and some may have more). Note that the effect of having an opening on the top of the drip chamber (through an air-filter) is the same as having the drip nozzle open to air, and therefore as long as this filter is not wet or plugged the pressure in the IVC is regulated by the height of the nozzle (as read on the pressure scale; note that the "0" is level with the nozzle).

The external auditory canal (EAC) is often used as a convenient external landmark for "0" (approximates the level of the foramen of Monro). In ▶ Fig. 56.1 the drip chamber is illustrated at 8 cm above the EAC.

Normal functioning of the IVC system

The system should be checked for proper functioning at least every 2–4 hours, and any time there is a change in: ICP (increase or decrease), neuro exam, or CSF output (for systems open to drainage).

1. check for presence of good waveform with respiratory variations and transmitted pulse pressures
2. IVCs: to check for patency, open the system to drain and lower the drip chamber below level of head and observe for 2–3 drops of CSF (normally do not allow more than this to drain)
3. for systems open to drainage:
   a) volume of CSF in drip chamber should be indicated every hour with a mark on a piece of tape on the drip chamber, and the volume should increase with time unless ICP is less than the height of the drip chamber (in practice, under these circumstances the system would usually not be left open to drainage).
      NB: the maximum expected output from a ventriculostomy would be ≈ 450–700 ml per day in a situation where none of the produced CSF is absorbed by the patient. This is not commonly encountered. A typical amount of drainage would be ≈ 75 ml every 8 hrs
   b) drip chamber should be emptied into drainage bag regularly (e.g. q 4 or 8 hours) and any time the chamber begins to get full (record volume)

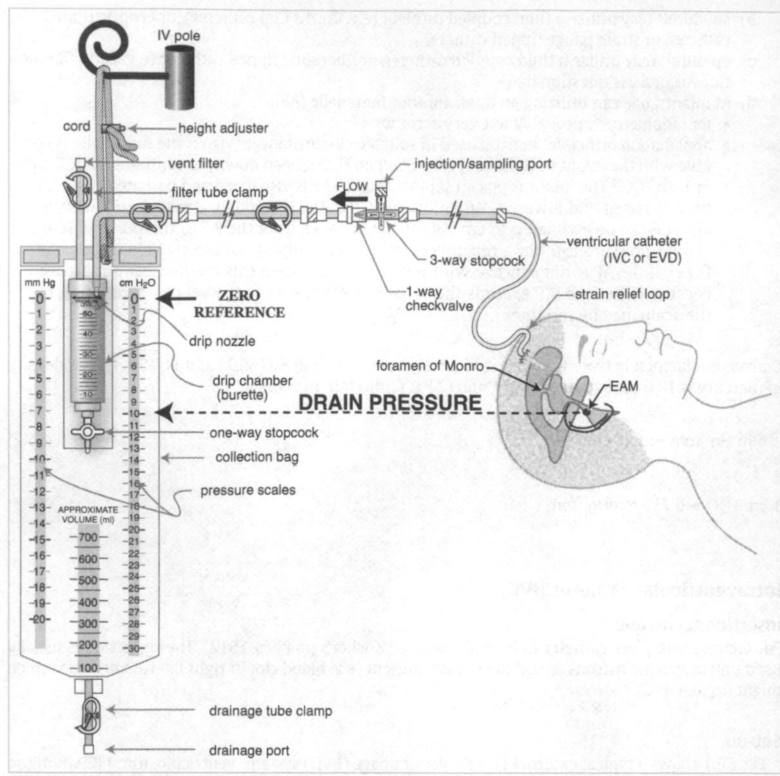

Fig. 56.1 Medtronic® ventricular drainage system/ICP monitor

4. in cases where there is a question whether the monitor is actually reflecting ICP, lowering the HOB towards 0° should increase ICP. Gentle pressure on both jugular veins simultaneously should also cause a gradual rise in ICP over 5–15 seconds that should drop back down to baseline when the pressure is released

56

IVC problems

The following represents some of the error or pitfalls that commonly occur with external ventricular drainage. Some also apply to ICP monitoring in general.

1. air filter on drip chamber gets wet (prevents air from passing through filter)
   a) result: fluid cannot drain freely into drip chamber (the pressure is no longer regulated by the height of the drip nozzle)
      - if the outflow from the drip chamber is clamped, then no flow at all is possible
      - if the clamp on the drip chamber outlet is open, then the pressure is actually regulated by the height of the nozzle in the *collection bag* and not the nozzle in the drip chamber
   b) solution: if a fresh filter is available, then replace the wet one. Otherwise one must improvise (with the risk of exposing the system to contamination): e.g. replace the wet filter with a filter from an IV set, or with a sterile gauze taped over the opening
2. air filter on collection bag gets wet: this will make it difficult to empty the drip chamber into the bag

a) this is not usually an urgent problem unless the drip chamber is full and the collection bag is distended tensely with air
b) the filter will dry out with time and will usually start to work again
c) if it is necessary to empty the drip chamber before the filter is dry, then using sterile technique insert a needle into the bag drainage port and decompress the bag of fluid and air
3. improper connections: a pressurized irrigation bag with or without heparinized solution should *never* be connected to an ICP monitor
4. changing position of head of bed: must move drip chamber up or down to keep it level with the same external landmarks (e.g. level of auditory canal):
a) when open to drainage, this will assure the correct pressure will be maintained
b) when opened to pressure transducer, will maintain correct zero
5. when open to drain, pressure reading from transducer is not meaningful: the pressure cannot exceed the height of the drip chamber in this situation (because at that point, fluid will drain off), and the opening to the "atmosphere" in the drip chamber will dampen the waveform
6. drip chamber falls to floor:
a) overdrainage, possible seizures and/or subdural hematoma formation
b) solution: securely tape chamber to pole, bed-rail…, check position regularly

IVC troubleshooting

See also IVC problems above.

▶ **IVC no longer works:**
1. manifestation of problem:
a) dampening or loss of normal waveform
b) no fluid drains into drip chamber (applies only when catheter has been opened to drain)
2. possible causes:
a) occlusion of catheter proximal to transducer
• slide clamp closed or stopcock closed
• catheter occluded by brain particles, blood cells, protein
b) IVC pulled out of ventricle
• test: temporarily lower drip nozzle and watch for 2–3 drops CSF
• solution:
c) verify all clamps are open
d) flush no more than 1.5 ml of non-bacteriostatic saline (AKA preservative-free saline) with very gentle pressure into ventricular catheter (NB: in elevated ICP the compliance of the brain is abnormally low and small volumes can cause large pressure changes)
• if no return then brain or clot is probably plugging catheter. If it is known that the ventricles are ≈ completely collapsed then the IVC may be OK and CSF should still drain over time. Otherwise this is a non-functioning catheter, and if a monitor/drain is still indicated then a new catheter may need to be inserted (CT may be considered first if the status of the ventricles is not known). If catheter is clotted by intraventricular hemorrhage, rt-PA may sometimes be used (p. 1344) [37]

▶ **ICP waveform dampened:**
1. possible causes:
a) occlusion of catheter proximal to transducer: see above
b) IVC pulled out of ventricle: no fluid will drain
c) air in system:
• solution: allow CSF to drain and expel air
• caution: do not allow excessive amount of CSF to drain (may allow obstruction of catheter, subdural formation…). Do not inject fluid to flush air into brain
d) following decompressive craniectomy: due to the fact that the monitor is no longer in a closed space, this is a normal finding in this setting

Types of ICP waveforms

Normal waveforms

The normal ICP waveform (as occurs with normal blood pressure and in the absence of IC-HTN) as illustrated in ▶ Fig. 56.2 is rarely seen since ICP is usually monitored only when it is elevated. The origin of the variations seen in the normal tracing is somewhat in dispute. One explanation describes these two types of waveforms[38]:

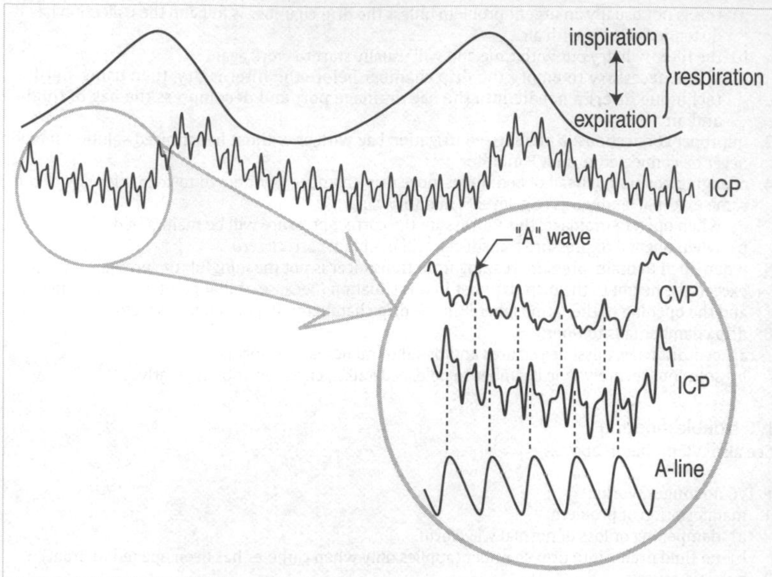

Fig. 56.2 Normal ICP waveform

1. small pulsations transmitted from the systemic blood pressure to the intracranial cavity
   a) large (1–2 mm Hg) peak corresponding to the arterial systolic pressure wave, with a small dicrotic notch
   b) this peak is followed by smaller and less distinct peaks
   c) followed by a peak corresponding to the central venous "A" wave from the right atrium
2. blood pressure pulsations are superimposed on slower respiratory variations. During expiration, the pressure in the superior vena cava increases which reduces venous outflow from the cranium causing an elevation in ICP. This may be reversed in a mechanically ventilated patients, and is opposite to that in the lumbar subarachnoid space which follows the pressure in the *inferior* vena cava

Pathological waveforms

As ICP rises and cerebral compliance decreases, the venous components disappear and the arterial pulses become more pronounced. In right atrial cardiac insufficiency, the CVP rises and the ICP waveform takes on a more "venous" or rounded appearance and the venous "A" wave begins to predominate.

A number of "pressure waves" that are more or less pathologic have been described. Currently, this classification is not considered to be of great clinical utility, with more emphasis being placed on recognizing and successfully treating elevations of ICP. Plateau waves will rarely be seen because they are usually aborted at the onset by instituting treatments outlined herein (p. 866). A brief description of some of these waveforms is included here for general information[39]:

1. Lundberg A waves AKA plateau waves (of Lundberg, ▶ Fig. 56.3): ICP elevations ≥ 50 mm Hg for 5–20 minutes. Usually accompanied by a simultaneous increase in MAP (it is debated whether the latter is cause or effect)
2. Lundberg B waves AKA pressure pulses: amplitude of 10–20 mm Hg is lower than A waves. Variation with types of periodic breathing. Last 30 secs – 2 mins
3. Lundberg C waves: frequency of 4–8/min. Low amplitude C waves (AKA Traube-Hering waves) may sometimes be seen in the normal ICP waveform. High amplitude C-waves may be pre-terminal, and may sometimes be seen on top of plateau waves

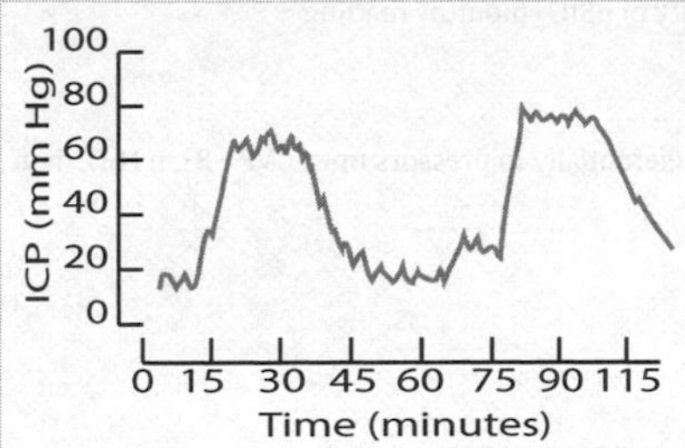

Fig. 56.3 Plateau waves (Lundberg A waves)

56.3 Adjuncts to ICP monitoring

56.3.1 Jugular venous oxygen monitoring

Indications for SjVOs or $pBtO_2$ monitoring include the need for augmented hyperventilation (PCO_2 = 20-25) to control ICP. Parameters related to oxygen content of the blood in the jugular veins are global in nature and are insensitive to focal pathology. Requires retrograde placement of catheter near to the origin of the internal jugular vein at the base of the skull. Parameters that can be measured:

1. jugular venous oxygen saturation ($SjVO_2$): measured continuously with special fiberoptic catheter. Normal $SjVO_2$: ≥ 60%. Desaturations to < 50% suggest ischemia. Multiple desaturations (< 50%), or sustained (≥ 10 minutes) or profound desaturation episodes are associated with poor outcome.[40,41] Sustained desaturations should prompt an evaluation for correctable etiologies: kinking of jugular vein, anemia, increased ICP, poor catheter position, CPP < 60 mm Hg, vasospasm, surgical lesion, $PaCO_2$ < 28 mm Hg. High $SjVO_2$ > 75% may indicate hyperemia or infarcted tissue and is also associated with poor outcome[42]
2. jugular vein oxygen content (CVO_2). Requires intermittent sampling of blood
3. arterial-jugular venous oxygen content difference ($AVdO_2$)[43]: $AVdO_2$ > 9 ml/dl (vol%) probably indicates global cerebral ischemia,[44,45] while values < 4 ml/dl indicate cerebral hyperemia[46] ("luxury perfusion" in excess of the brain's metabolic requirement[45])

56.3.2 Brain tissue oxygen tension monitoring ($pBtO_2$)

Indications for SjVOs or $pBtO_2$ monitoring include the need for augmented hyperventilation (PCO_2 = 20-25) to control ICP. Monitored e.g. with Licox® probe. The likelihood of death increases with longer times of brain tissue oxygen tension ($p_{Bt}O_2$) < 15 mm Hg or even a brief drop of $pBtO_2$ < 6.[47] Initial $pBtO_2$ < 10 mm Hg for > 30 minutes correlates with increased risk of death or bad outcome.[48] Also, see **Practice guideline: Brain oxygen monitoring** (p.867).

Probe placement:

1. TBI: assumed to be a diffuse process, often placed on *least* injured side
2. SAH: placed in vascular distributions at greatest risk of vasospasm
   a) ACA (with ACA or a-comm aneurysm): standard frontal placement (≈ 2–3 cm off midline on appropriate side)
   b) MCA (with ICA or MCA aneurysm): 4.5–5.5 cm off midline
   c) ACA-MCA watershed area: 3 cm lateral to midline
3. ICH: usually placed near the site of the hemorrhage

Effect of $pBtO_2$ monitoring/intervention on outcome: no randomized studies

1. in TBI[49]: goal was to maintain $pBtO_2$ > 25 mm Hg. Adding $pBtO_2$ monitoring resulted in improved outcome. May have been result of increased attentiveness ("Hawthorne effect")
2. in SAH[50]: a moving correlation coefficient (ORx) between CPP and $pBtO_2$ was used to label high ORx as disturbed autoregulation, and this value on post SAH days 5 & 6 had predictive value for delayed infarction

Management suggestions for $pBtO_2$ < 15–20 mmHg:

1. consider jugular venous O_2 saturation monitor or lactate microdialysis monitor for confirmation

56

2. consider CBF study to determine generalizability of $pBtO_2$ monitor reading
3. treatment: proceed to each tier as needed
   a) tier 1
      - keep body temperature < 37.5 C
      - increase CPP to > 60 mmHg (use fluids preferentially to pressors until CVP > 8 cm H_2O, then use pressors)
   b) tier 2
      - increase FiO_2 to 60%
      - increase $paCO_2$ to 45–50 mmHg
      - transfuse PRBCs until Hgb > 10 g/dl
   c) tier 3
      - increase FiO_2 to 100%
      - consider increasing PEEP to increase PaO_2 if FiO_2 is at 100%
      - decrease ICP to < 10 mmHg (drain CSF, mannitol, sedation…)

56.3.3 Bedside monitoring of regional CBF (rCBF)

Thermal diffusion flowmetry permits continuous rCBF monitoring by assessing thermal convection due to tissue blood flow. The probe tip is inserted into the *white matter* of the brain. Commercially available systems include Hemedex® monitoring system (Codman) utilizing the QFLOW 500® probe which is ✖ not MRI compatible.

Probe placement: issues similar to those discussed for $pBtO_2$ (see above).

Readout:

1. K value (thermal conduction): range for white matter is 4.9–5.8 mW/cm-°C (the monitor suppresses CBF readings if the K value is outside this range)
   a) K < 4.9: the probe tip is probably out of the brain tissue or white matter – the probe should be *advanced* 1–2 mm
   b) K > 5.8 the tip is probably too deep, near a blood vessel, or in the ventricle or epidural or subdural space – the probe should be *retracted* 1–2 mm
2. CBF
   a) normal white matter: 18–25 ml/100g-min
      - white matter CBF < 15: may indicate vasospasm or ischemia
      - white matter CBF < 10: may indicate infarction
   b) normal gray matter: 67–80 ml/100g-min

Observational data: in a small study of SAH (n=5) and TBI (n=3)[51] there was good correlation between rCBF and $pBtO_2$ 91% of the time. Monitoring was not possible 36% of the time due to patient fever (wherein the system prevents monitoring).

56.3.4 Cerebral microdialysis

Compounds assayed include: lactate, pyruvate, lactate/pyruvate ratio, glucose, glutamate, urea and electrolytes including K^+ & calcium. Some observational data:

56

1. lactate levels increase during episodes of $SjVO_2$ desaturation[52]
2. decreased extracellular glucose was associated with increased mortality[53]

56.4 Treatment measures for elevated ICP

56.4.1 General information

This section presents a general protocol for treating documented (or sometimes clinically suspected) intracranial hypertension (IC-HTN). Guidelines promulgated by the Brain Trauma Foundation[3,54,55,56] are generally followed. Unless otherwise stated, guidelines are for adult patients (≥ 18 years age).

56.4.2 Treatment thresholds

Intracranial pressure treatment thresholds

The optimal ICP at which to begin treatment is not known. Various cutoff values are used at different centers above which treatment measures for intracranial hypertension (IC-HTN) are initiated.

Although 15, 20 and 25 have been quoted, the Brain Trauma Foundation guideline is ICP > 20 mm Hg[57] as shown in **Practice guideline: ICP treatment threshold** (p. 867). ✖ Caution: patients can herniate even at ICP < 20[58] (depends on location of intracranial mass).

Rationale: There is high mortality and worse outcome[5] among patients with ICP persistently > 20 compared to 20% in those where ICP could be kept < 20.[59] Better control may be possible by treating early rather than waiting and trying to control higher ICPs or when plateau waves occur.[60]

Practice guideline: ICP treatment threshold

Level II[57]: treatment for IC-HTN should be initiated for ICP > 20 mm Hg

Level III[57]: the need for treatment should be based on ICP in combination with clinical examination & brain CT findings

Cerebral perfusion pressure (CPP)

The optimal value for CPP has yet to be determined. The threshold for ischemia is in the range of CPP < 50–60 mm Hg. Because of deleterious systemic effects, paradigms of maintaining CPP > 70 mm Hg have been superseded. **Practice guideline: Cerebral perfusion pressure issues** (p. 867) outlines current recommendations regarding CPP.

Practice guideline: Cerebral perfusion pressure issues

Level II[61]: ✖ avoid aggressive use of fluids and pressors to maintain CPP > 70 mm Hg (because of risk of adult respiratory distress syndrome (ARDS))

Level III[61]: ✖ avoid CPP < 50 mm Hg

Level III[61]: ancillary monitoring of CBF, oxygenation or metabolism assists CPP management

Brain oxygenation parameters

Suggestions for treatment thresholds are shown in **Practice guideline: Brain oxygen monitoring** (p. 867). It remains to be determined which interventions are useful to achieve this, and whether this improves outcome.

Practice guideline: Brain oxygen monitoring

Level III[62]: jugular venous O_2 saturation < 50% or brain tissue oxygen tension ($pBtO_2$) < 15 mm Hg are treatment thresholds

56

56.4.3 ICP management protocol: Quick reference summary

► Table 56.5 summarizes a protocol for control of IC-HTN (below for details).

Dosages are given for an average adult, unless specified as mg/kg. Treatment may be initiated prior to insertion of a monitor if there is acute neurologic deterioration or clinical signs of IC-HTN, but continued treatment requires documentation of persistent IC-HTN.

For persistent IC-HTN consider "second tier" therapies (p. 871).

Temporary measures which may be used to quickly treat an acute ICP crisis are shown in ► Table 56.6.

Table 56.5 Summary of measures to control IC-HTN[a] Goals: keep ICP < 20 mm Hg, and CPP ≥ 50 mm Hg[57,61]

Step	Rationale/Remedy
GENERAL MEASURES (should be utilized routinely)	
elevate HOB to 30–45°	↓ ICP by enhancing venous outflow, but also reduces mean carotid pressure → no net change in CBF
keep neck straight, avoid neck constrictions (tight trach tape, tight cervical collar...)	constriction of jugular venous outflow causes ↑ ICP
avoid arterial hypotension (SBP < 90 mm Hg)	• Hypotension reduces CBF • ℞: normalize intravascular volume, use pressors if needed
control hypertension if present	• ℞: nicardipine if not tachycardic • ℞: beta-blocker if tachycardic (labetalol, esmolol...) • ✖ avoid overtreatment → hypotension
avoid hypoxia (PaO_2 < 60 mm Hg or O_2 sat < 90%)	hypoxia may cause further ischemic brain injury ℞: maintain airway and adequate oxygenation
ventilate to normocarbia ($PaCO_2$ = 35–40 mm Hg)	✖ avoid prophylactic hyperventilation (p. 872)
light sedation: e.g. codeine 30–60 mg IM q 4 hrs PRN	(same as heavy sedation, see below)
controversial: prophylactic hypothermia. If used, hold at target temp > 48 hrs	Hypothermia → ↓ $CMRO_2$ – efficacy not rigorously proven (p. 872)
unenhanced head CT scan for ICP problems[b]	rule out surgical condition
SPECIFIC MEASURES FOR IC-HTN	
proceed to successive steps if documented IC-HTN persists – each step is ADDED to the previous measure)	
heavy sedation (e.g. fentanyl 1–2 ml or MSO4 2–4 mg IV q 1 hr) and/or paralysis (e.g. vecuronium 8–10 mg IV)	reduces elevated sympathetic tone and HTN induced by movement, tensing abdominal musculature...
drain 3–5 ml CSF if IVC present	reduces intracranial volume
hyperventilate to $PaCO_2$ = 30–35 mm Hg ("blows off" CO_2)	CO_2 is a potent vasodilator Hyperventilation → ↓ $PaCO_2$ → ↓ CBV → ↓ ICP ✖ hyperventilation also → ↓ CBF
mannitol 0.25–1 gm/kg, then 0.25 mg/kg q 6 hrs, increase dose if IC-HTN persists & serum osmol ≤ 320 (NB: skip this step if hypovolemia or hypotension)	Mannitol → initially ↑ plasma volume & ↑ serum tonicity which draws fluid out of brain → ↓ intracranial volume, may also improve rheologic properties of blood. ✖ Mannitol is an osmotic diuretic, and eventually → ↓ plasma volume
if there is "osmotic room" (i.e. serum osmol < 320) bolus with 10–20 ml of 23.4% hypertonic saline (HS)	some patients refractory to mannitol will respond to HS
Augmented hyperventilation to ↓ $PaCO_2$ to 25–30 mm Hg	Due to risk of cerebral ischemia from ↓ CBF, monitor $SjVO_2$ (p. 865) or CBF if possible
If IC-HTN persists, consider unenhanced head CT[b] & EEG[c]. Proceed to "second tier" therapy (p. 871)	

[a]see text for details (p. 870). As IC-HTN subsides, carefully withdraw treatment
[b]if IC-HTN persists, and especially for a sudden unexplained rise in ICP or loss of previously controlled ICP, give strong consideration to repeating cranial CT to rule out a surgical condition, i.e. "clot" (SDH, EDH, or ICH) or hydrocephalus
[c]EEG to rule-out subclinical status epilepticus which is a rare cause of sustained IC-HTN

Table 56.6 Measures to treat an acute ICP crisis[a]

Step	Rationale
Verify basics: check airway, neck position… (see general measures in ▶ Table 56.5). For resistant or sudden IC-HTN, consider STAT unenhanced head CT	
be sure patient is sedated and paralyzed (▶ Table 56.5)	(▶ Table 56.5)
drain 3–5 ml CSF if IVC present	↓ intracranial volume
mannitol[b] 1 gm/kg IV bolus or 10–20 ml of 23.4% saline	↑ plasma volume → ↑ CBF → ↓ ICP, also ↑ serum osmolality → ↓ extracellular brain water
hyperventilate with Ambu® bag (✖ do not reduce $PaCO_2$ < 25 mm Hg)	"blow off" (reduce) $PaCO_2$ → ↓ CBV → ↓ ICP. ✖ CAUTION: due to reduced CBF, use for no more than several minutes (p. 872)
pentobarbital[c] 100 mg slow IV or thiopental 2.5 mg/kg IV over 10 minutes	sedates, ↓ ICP, treats seizures, may be neuroprotective ✖ also myocardial depressant → ↓ MAP

[a]for measures to treat ICP that is trending up over a longer period, see ▶ Table 56.5 or information starting
[b]skip this step and go to hyperventilation if hypotensive, volume depleted, or if serum osmolality > 320 mOsm/L
[c]the availability of pentobarbital in the U.S. has been reduced, and other sedatives may need to be substituted (p. 876)

56.4.4 ICP management protocol details

Goals of therapy

1. keep ICP ≤ 20 mm Hg (prevents "plateau waves" from compromising cerebral blood-flow (CBF) and causing cerebral ischemia and/or brain death[30])
2. keep CPP ≥ 50 mm Hg.[61] The primary goal is to control ICP, simultaneously, CPP should supported by maintaining adequate MAP[63] (no study shows any deleterious effect on ICP, morbidity or mortality as a result of normalizing intravascular volume or inducing systemic hypertension to achieve the desired CPP).

Surgical treatment

1. Traumatic Intracranial masses should be treated as indicated. See surgical indications for subdural (p. 895), epidural (p. 893) or intraparenchymal (p. 891) hematoma or posterior fossa mass lesions (p. 905)
2. patients with hemorrhagic contusions ("pulped brain") showing progressive deterioration may benefit from surgical excision of portions of the contused brain tissue especially if not eloquent brain (p. 871)
3. decompressive craniectomy may be considered for IC-HTN that cannot be controlled medically

56

General care

Major goals

1. avoid hypoxia (pO_2 < 60 mm Hg)
2. avoid hypotension (SBP ≤ 90 mm Hg): 67% positive-predictive value (PPV) for poor outcome (79% PPV when combined with hypoxia)[64]

Details of general treatment measures

1. prophylaxis against steroid ulcers (if steroids are used) and Cushing's (stress) ulcers (seen in severe head injury and in increased ICP, accompanied by hypergastrinemia)[65,66,67,68,69] for all patients including peds; see Prophylaxis for stress ulcers (p. 129).
   a) elevating gastric pH: titrated antacid and/or H2 antagonist (e.g. ranitidine 50 mg IV q 8 hrs) or proton pump inhibitor. See discussion of potential increased mortality as a result of increased gastric pH (p. 129)
   b) sucralfate

2. aggressive control of fever (fever is a potent stimulus to increase CBF, and may also increase plateau waves)[30]
3. arterial line for BP monitoring and frequent ABGs
4. CVP or PA line if high doses of mannitol are needed (goal: keep patient euvolemic)
5. IV fluids
   a) choice of fluids:
      - isolated head injury: IVF of choice is isotonic (e.g. NS + 20 mEq KCl/L)
      - avoid hypotonic solutions (e.g. lactated ringers) which may impair cerebral compliance[70]
   b) fluid volume:
      - provide adequate fluid resuscitation to avoid hypotension
      - normalization of intravascular fluid volume is not detrimental to ICP
      - although fluid restriction reduces the amount of mannitol needed to control ICP,[71] the concept of "running patients dry" is obsolete[72]
      - if mannitol is required, patient should be maintained at euvolemia
      - also exercise caution in restricting fluids following SAH; see Cerebral salt wasting (p. 118)
      - if injuries to other systems are present (e.g. perforated viscus), they may dictate fluid management
   c) pressors (e.g. dopamine) are preferable to IV fluid boluses in head injury

Measures to lower ICP

General measures that should be routine

1. positioning:
   a) elevate HOB 30–45° (see below)
   b) keep head midline (to prevent kinking jugular veins)
2. light sedation: codeine 30–60 mg IM q 4 hrs PRN, or lorazepam (Ativan®) 1–2 mg IV q 4–6 hrs PRN
3. avoid hypotension (SBP < 90 mm Hg): normalize intravascular volume, support with pressors if needed
4. control HTN; in ICH, aim for patient's baseline, see Initial management of ICH (p. 1339)
5. prevent hyperglycemia: (aggravates cerebral edema) usually present in head injury,[73,74] may be exacerbated by steroids
6. intubation: for GCS ≤ 8 or respiratory distress. Give IV lidocaine first (below) and antibiotics (p. 827)
7. avoid hyperventilation: keep $PaCO_2$ at the low end of eucapnia (35 mm Hg)
8. prophylactic hypothermia: non-statistically significant trend suggests reduced mortality.[75] Maintain target temperature for > 48 hours

Measures to use for documented IC-HTN

First, check General measures that should be routine above. Proceed to each step if IC-HTN persists.

56

1. heavy sedation and/or paralysis when necessary (also assists treatment of HTN) e.g. when patient is agitated, or to blunt the elevation of ICP that occurs with certain maneuvers such as moving the patient to CT table. Caution: with heavy sedation or paralysis, the ability to follow the neurologic exam is lost (follow ICPs)
   a) for heavy sedation (intubation recommended to avoid respiratory depression → elevation of $PaCO_2$ → ↑ ICP): e.g. one of the following:
      - MSO4: ℞ 2–4 mg/hr IV drip
      - fentanyl: ℞ 1–2 ml IV q 1 hr (or 2–5 mcg/kg/hr IV drip)
      - sufentanil: ℞ 10–30 mcg test dose, then 0.05 -2 mcg/kg/hr IV drip
      - midazolam (Versed®): ℞ 2 mg test dose, then 2–4 mg/hr IV drip
      - propofol drip (p. 106): 0.5 mg/kg test dose, then 20–75 mcg/kg/min IV drip ✖ avoid high-dose propofol (do not exceed 83 mcg/kg/min)
      - "low dose" pentobarbital (adult: 100 mg IV q 4 hrs; peds: 2–5 mg/kg IV q 4 hrs)
   b) paralysis (intubation mandatory): e.g. vecuronium 8–10 mg IV q 2–3 hrs
2. CSF drainage (when IVC is being utilized to measure ICP): 3–5 ml of CSF should be drained with the drip chamber at ≤ 10 cm above EAC. Works immediately by removal of CSF (reducing intracranial volume) and possibly by allowing edema fluid to drain into ventricles[76] (latter point is controversial)
3. "osmotic therapy" when there is evidence of IC-HTN:
   a) *mannitol* (also see below) 0.25–1 gm/kg bolus (over < 20 mins) followed by 0.25 gm/kg IVP (over 20 min) q 6 hrs PRN ICP > 20. Recent literature suggests that 1.4 gm/kg initial dose is more effective. May "alternate" with:

furosemide (Lasix®) (also see below): adult 10–20 mg IV q 6 hrs PRN ICP > 20. Peds: 1 mg/kg, 6 mg max IV q 6 hrs PRN ICP > 20
b) keep patient euvolemic to slightly hypervolemic
c) if IC-HTN persists and serum osmolarity is < 320 mOsm/L, increase mannitol up to 1 gm/kg, and shorten the dosing interval
d) if ICP remains refractory to mannitol, consider hypertonic saline, either continuous 3% saline infusion or as bolus of 10–20 ml of 23.4% saline (D/C after ≈ 72 hours to avoid rebound edema)
e) hold osmotic therapy if serum osmolarity is ≥ 320 mOsm/L (higher tonicity may have no advantage and risks renal dysfunction; see below) or SBP < 100

4. hyperventilation (HPV) to $PaCO_2$ = 30–35 mm Hg (for details, see below)
   a) ✖ do not use prophylactically
   b) ✖ avoid aggressive HPV ($PaCO_2 \leq 25$ mm Hg) at all times
   c) use only for
      - short periods for acute neurologic deterioration
      - or chronically for documented IC-HTN unresponsive to sedation, paralytics, CSF drainage and osmotic therapy
   d) avoid HPV during the first 24 hrs after injury if possible
5. ✖ steroids: the routine use of glucocorticoids is not recommended for treatment of patients with head injuries (see below)

"Second tier" therapy for persistent IC-HTN

If IC-HTN remains refractory to the above measures, and especially if there is loss of previously controlled ICP, strong consideration should be given to repeating a head CT to rule out a surgical condition before proceeding with "second tier" therapies which are either effective but with significant risks (e.g. high-dose barbiturates), or are unproven in terms of benefit on outcome. Also consider an EEG to rule-out subclinical status epilepticus (seizures that are not clinically evident); see treatment measures for status epilepticus (p. 471); some medications are effective for both seizures and IC-HTN, e.g. pentobarbital, propofol…

1. high dose barbiturate therapy (p. 875): initiate if ICP remains > 20–25 mm Hg
2. hyperventilate to $PaCO_2$ = 25–30 mm Hg. Monitoring $SjVO_2$, $AVdO_2$, and/or CBF is recommended (see below)
3. hypothermia[77,78]: patients must be monitored for a drop in cardiac index, thrombocytopenia, elevated creatinine clearance, and pancreatitis. Avoid shivering which raises ICP[78]
4. decompressive surgery:
   a) decompressive craniectomy removal of portion of calvaria.[79] Controversial (may enhance cerebral edema formation[80]). Craniectomy decreased ICP to < 20 mm Hg in 85%[81] regardless of pupillary response to light, timing of craniectomy, brain shift and age. Outcomes were improved when IC-HTN responded.[81,82,17] Further randomized trials are indicated. Early decompressive craniectomy may be considered in patients undergoing emergent surgery (for fracture, EDH, SDH…).[83] Flap must be at least 12 cm in diameter, and duraplasty is mandatory. Also, see Hemicraniectomy for malignant MCA territory infarction (p. 1303)
   b) removal of large areas of contused hemorrhagic brain (makes room immediately; removes region of disrupted BBB). If contused, consider temporal tip lobectomy (no more than 4–5 cm on dominant side, 6–7 cm on non-dominant) (total temporal lobectomy[84] is probably too aggressive) or frontal lobectomy. Has not shown great therapeutic promise
5. lumbar drainage: showing some promise. Watch for "cerebral sag"
6. hypertensive therapy

Adjunctive measures

1. *lidocaine*: 1.5 mg/kg IVP (watch for hypotension, reduce dose if necessary) at least one minute before endotracheal intubation or suctioning. Blunts the rise in ICP as well as tachycardia and systemic HTN (based on patients with brain tumors undergoing intubation under light barbiturate-nitrous oxide anesthesia; extrapolation to trauma patients is unproven)[85]
2. high frequency (jet) ventilation: consider if high levels of positive end-expiratory pressure (PEEP) are required[86] (NB: patients with reduced lung compliance, e.g. pulmonary edema, transmit more of PEEP through lungs to thoracic vessels and may raise ICP). PEEP ≤ 10 cm H_2O does not cause clinically significant increases in ICP.[87] Higher levels of PEEP > 15–20 are not recommended. Also, rapid elimination of PEEP may cause a sudden increase in circulating blood volume which may exacerbate cerebral edema and also elevate ICP

Details of some measures employed in treating increased ICP

Elevating head of bed (HOB)

Seemingly simple, but there is still some controversy. Early data obtained from dog studies indicated that keeping the HOB at 30–45° optimized the trade-off between the following two factors as the HOB is elevated: reducing ICP (by enhancing venous outflow and by promoting displacement of CSF from the intracranial compartment to the spinal compartment) and reducing the arterial pressure (and thus CPP) at the level of the carotid arteries. Some studies showed a deleterious effect from elevating the HOB and were used to justify nursing these patients with HOB flat.[2]

Recent data[88] indicate that although mean carotid pressure (MCP) is reduced, the ICP is also reduced and the CBF is unaffected by elevating the HOB to 30°. The onset of action of raising the HOB is immediate.

Prophylactic hypothermia

Practice guideline: Prophylactic hypothermia

Level III[75]: prophylactic hypothermia:

- improves the chances of having a moderate to good outcome – 4–5 on the Glasgow Outcome Score▶ Table 88.5 – at the end of the follow-up period when target temperatures of 32–35° C (91.4–95° F) were used (**note**: no clear relationship was found for cooling duration or rewarming rate)
- showed a non-significant trend suggesting that it lowers *mortality* when the target temperature is maintained for > 48 hrs (**note**: the actual target temperature and rewarming rate did not influence mortality)

Hyperventilation

Intraarterial carbon dioxide ($PaCO_2$) is the most potent cerebrovascular vasodilator, the effect of which is probably mediated by changes in pH caused by the rapid diffusion of CO_2 across the BBB.[89] Hyperventilation (HPV) lowers ICP by reducing $PaCO_2$ which causes cerebral vasoconstriction, thus reducing the cerebral (intracranial) blood volume (CBV).[90] Of concern, vasoconstriction also lowers cerebral blood flow (CBF) which could produce focal ischemia in areas with preserved cerebral autoregulation as a result of shunting.[91,92] However, ischemia does not necessarily follow as the O_2 extraction fraction (OEF) may also increase, up to a point.[93]

Practice guideline: Hyperventilation for ICP management[a]

Level I[94]: in the absence of IC-HTN, chronic prolonged hyperventilation (HPV) ($PaCO_2 \le 25$ mm Hg) should be avoided

56

Level II[95]: prophylactic hyperventilation ($PaCO_2 \le 25$ mm Hg) is not recommended

Level III

- HPV may be necessary for brief periods when there is acute neurologic deterioration, or for longer periods if there is IC-HTN refractory to sedation, paralysis, CSF drainage and osmotic diuretics[94]
- HPV should be avoided ≤ 24 hrs after head injury[95]
- if HPV is used, jugular venous oxygen saturation ($SjVO_2$) (p. 865) or $PbrO_2$ (p. 865) should be measured to monitor brain O_2 delivery[95]

[a]See also **Practice guideline: Early/prophylactic hyperventilation** (p. 827).

✖ Hyperventilation (HPV), is to be used in moderation only in specific situations[3] (see below). Prophylactic HPV may actually be associated with a *worse* outcome[96] (**note**: prophylactic HPV implies cases where there are no clinical signs of IC-HTN and where IC-HTN unresponsive to other measures has not been documented by ICP monitoring). When indicated, use HPV only to $PaCO_2$ = 30–35 mm Hg (see Caveats for hyperventilation below). CBF in severe head trauma patients is already about half of normal during the first 24 hrs after injury (typically < 30 cc/100 g/min during the first 8 hours, and may be < 20 during the first 4 hours in patients with the worst injuries).[97,98,99,100] In one study,

Table 56.7 Summary of recommendations for $PaCO_2$ following head trauma (see text for details)

$PaCO_2$ (mm Hg)	Description
35–40	normocarbia. Use routinely
30–35	hyperventilation. Do not use prophylactically. Use only as follows: briefly for clinical evidence of IC-HTN (neurologic deterioration) or chronically for documented IC-HTN unresponsive to other measures
25–30	augmented hyperventilation. A second tier treatment. Use only when other methods fail to control IC-HTN. Additional monitoring recommended to R/O cerebral ischemia
<25	aggressive hyperventilation. No documented benefit. Significant potential for ischemia

the use of HPV to $PaCO_2 = 30$ mm Hg within 8–14 hrs of severe head injury did not impair global cerebral metabolism,[93] but focal changes were not studied. Hyperventilation to $PaCO_2 < 30$ mm Hg further reduces CBF, but does not consistently reduce ICP and may cause loss of cerebral autoregulation.[45] If carefully monitored, there may be occasion to use this. There are no studies showing any improvement in outcome with aggressive HPV ($PaCO_2 \le 25$ mm Hg) which can cause diffuse cerebral ischemia.[45] A summary of the ranges of $PaCO_2$ and the recommendations is shown in ▶ Table 56.7.

Reducing $PaCO_2$ from 35 to 29 mm Hg lowers ICP 25–30% in most patients. Onset of action: ≤ 30 seconds. Peak effect at ≈ 8 mins. Duration of effect is occasionally as short as 15–20 mins. Effect may be blunted by 1 hour (based on patients with intracranial tumors), after which it is difficult to return to normocarbia without rebound elevation of ICP.[101,102] Thus, HPV must be weaned slowly.[30]

Indications for hyperventilation (HPV)

1. HPV for brief periods (minutes) at the following times
   a) prior to insertion of ICP monitor: if there are clinical signs of IC-HTN (▶ Table 54.2)
   b) after insertion of a monitor: if there is a sudden increase in ICP and/or acute neurologic deterioration, HPV may be used while evaluating patient for a treatable condition (e.g. delayed intracranial hematoma)
2. HPV for longer periods: when there is documented IC-HTN unresponsive to sedation, paralytics, CSF drainage (when available) and osmotic diuretics
3. HPV may be appropriate for IC-HTN resulting primarily from hyperemia (p. 901)

Caveats for hyperventilation

1. avoid during the first 5 days after head injury if possible (especially first 24 hrs)
2. do not use prophylactically (i.e. without appropriate indications, see above)
3. If documented IC-HTN is unresponsive to other measures, hyperventilate only to $PaCO_2 = 30$–35 mm Hg
4. if prolonged HPV to $PaCO_2$ of 25–30 mm Hg is deemed necessary, consider monitoring $SjVO_2$, $AVdO_2$, or CBF to rule-out cerebral ischemia (p. 865)
5. do not reduce $PaCO_2 < 25$ mm Hg (except for very brief periods of a few minutes)

56

Mannitol

Practice guideline: Mannitol in severe traumatic brain injury

Level II[103,104]

mannitol is effective for control of IC-HTN after severe TBI(**note:** current information did not allow recommendations regarding hypertonic saline to be made[104]

- intermittent boluses may be more effective than continuous infusion
- effective doses range from 0.25–1 gm/kg body weight
- avoid hypotension (SBP < 90 mm Hg) which may result from the diuretic effect of mannitol which can lead to ↓ circulating fluid volume

Level III[103]

- indications: signs of transtentorial herniation or progressive neurological deterioration not attributable to systemic pathology
- euvolemia should be maintained (hypovolemia should be avoided) by fluid replacement. An indwelling urinary catheter is essential
- serum osmolarity should be kept < 320 mOsm when there is concern about renal failure

No controlled clinical trial has been conducted to show the benefits of mannitol over placebo.[3] The exact mechanism(s) by which mannitol provides its beneficial effects is still controversial, but probably includes some combination of the following

1. lowering ICP
   a) immediate plasma expansion[105,106,107]: reduces the hematocrit and blood viscosity (improved rheology) which increases CBF and O_2 delivery. This reduces ICP within a few minutes, and is most marked in patients with CPP < 70 mm Hg
   b) osmotic effect: increased serum tonicity draws edema fluid from cerebral parenchyma. Takes 15–30 minutes until gradients are established.[105] Effect lasts 1.5–6 hrs, depending on the clinical condition[108,109,3]
2. supports the microcirculation by improving blood rheology (see above)
3. possible free radical scavenging[110]

With bolus administration, onset of ICP lowering effect occurs in 1–5 minutes; peaks at 20–60 minutes. When urgent reduction of ICP is needed, an initial dose of 1 gm/kg should be given over 30 minutes. When long-term reduction of ICP is intended, the infusion time should be lengthened to 60 minutes[111] and the dose reduced (e.g. 0.25–0.5 gm/kg q 6 hrs). A large previous dose reduces the effectiveness of subsequent doses[71]; thus it is desirable to *use the smallest effective dose* (small frequent doses may be preferable, e.g. 0.25 mg/kg q 2–3 hrs; also results in fewer peaks as mannitol "troughs" are smoothed out). Titrating to ICP (instead of dosing at regular intervals) results in less mannitol being given.[71,112] The effectiveness of mannitol may be synergistically enhanced when combined with the use of loop acting diuretics (e.g. furosemide, see below),[113] and alternating these medications has been suggested.[71]

Cautions with mannitol

1. mannitol opens the BBB, and mannitol that has crossed the BBB may draw fluid into the CNS (this may be minimized by repeated bolus administration vs. continuous infusion[106,114]) which can aggravate vasogenic cerebral edema.[115] Thus, when it is time to D/C mannitol, it should be tapered to prevent ICP rebound[111]
2. caution: corticosteroids + phenytoin + mannitol may cause hyperosmolar nonketotic state with high mortality[30]
3. excessively vigorous bolus administration may → HTN and if autoregulation is defective → increased CBF which may promote herniation rather than prevent it[116]
4. high doses of mannitol carries the risk of acute renal failure (acute tubular necrosis), especially in the following[10,117]: serum osmolarity > 320 mOsm/L, use of other potentially nephrotoxic drugs, sepsis, pre-existing renal disease
5. large doses prevents diagnosing DI by use of urinary osmols or SG (p. 121)
6. because it may further increase CBF,[118] the use of mannitol may be deleterious when IC-HTN is due to hyperemia (p. 901)

56

Furosemide

The use of furosemide (Lasix®) has been advocated, but little data exists to support this.[3] Loop acting diuretics may reduce ICP[119] by reducing cerebral edema[120] (possibly by increasing serum tonicity), and may also slow the production of CSF.[121] They also act synergistically with mannitol[122] (above).

℞: 10–20 mg IV q 6 hrs, may be alternated with mannitol such that the patient receives one or the other q 3 hrs. Hold if serum osmolarity > 320 mOsm/L.

Hypertonic saline (HS)

May reduce ICP in patients refractory to mannitol,[123,124] although no improvement in outcome over mannitol has been demonstrated.[124,125] Potentially deleterious effect on stroke penumbra in animal studies. Studies[126,127] are not adequate to make recommendations regarding use.[104]

℞: Continuous infusion: 3% saline at 25–50 ml/hr may be given through a peripheral IV. Bolus: 10–20 ml of 7.5–23.4% saline must be given through a central line. HS should be discontinued after ≈ 72 hours to avoid rebound edema.[124] Hold if serum osmolarity > 320 mOsm/L.

Steroids

Practice guideline: Glucocorticoids in severe head injury

Level I[128]: the use of glucocorticoids (steroids) is not recommended for improving outcome or reducing ICP in patients with severe TBI (except in patients with known depletion of endogenous adrenal hormones[129,130]). High-dose methylprednisolone is associated with increased mortality and is contraindicated[128]

Although glucocorticoids reduce vasogenic cerebral edema (e.g. surrounding brain tumors) and may be effective in lowering ICP in pseudotumor cerebri, they have little effect on cytotoxic cerebral edema which is the more prevalent derangement following trauma; see Cerebral edema (p. 90).

Significant side effects may occur with steroids[131] including coagulopathies, hyperglycemia[132] with its undesirable effect on cerebral edema – see Possible deleterious side effects of steroids (p. 594) – and increased incidence of infection (due to immunosuppression). High-dose methylprednisolone is associated with increased mortality.[133]

Non-glucocorticoid steroids (e.g. 21-aminosteroids, AKA lazaroids, including tirilazad[134,135]) and the synthetic glucocorticoid triamcinolone[136] have also failed to show overall benefit.

High-dose barbiturate therapy

Practice guideline: Barbiturates in severe head injury

Level II[137]: ✖ prophylactic use of barbiturates for burst suppression EEG is not recommended

Level II[137]: high-dose barbiturates are recommended for IC-HTN refractory to maximal medical and surgical ICP lowering therapy. Patients should be hemodynamically stable before and during treatment

Theoretical benefits of barbiturates in head injury derive from vasoconstriction in normal areas (shunting blood to ischemic brain tissue), decreased metabolic demand for O_2 ($CMRO_2$) with accompanying reduction of CBF, free radical scavenging, reduced intracellular calcium, and lysosomal stabilization.[138] There is little question that barbiturates lower ICP, even when other treatments have failed,[139] but regarding outcome, studies have shown both benefits[140,141] and lack of same.[142,143] A subgroup of patients with preserved vasoreactivity may benefit from the use of barbiturates[144]; and when reserved for use in patients who failed to respond sufficiently to other measures, barbiturates have been shown to lower ICP.[145] Patients that do respond have a lower mortality (33%) than those in whom ICP control could not be accomplished (75%).[141]

The limiting factor for therapy is usually *hypotension* due to barbiturate induced reduction of sympathetic tone[146 (p 354)] (causing peripheral vasodilatation) and direct mild myocardial depression. Hypotension occurs in ≈ 50% of patients in spite of adequate blood volume and use of dopamine.[147]

NB: the ability to follow the neurologic exam is lost with high-dose barbiturates, and one must follow ICP.

"Barbiturate coma" vs. high-dose therapy: If barbiturates are given until there is burst suppression on EEG, this is considered true "barbiturate coma." This results in near maximal reductions in $CMRO_2$ and CBF.[3] However, most regimens should technically be called "high dose intravenous therapy" since they simply try to establish target serum barbiturate levels (e.g. 3–4 mg% for pentobarbital), even though there is poor correlation between serum level, therapeutic benefit, and systemic complications.[3]

Adjunctive measures to administration of high-dose barbiturates:

1. consider a Swan-Ganz (PA) catheter placed during the first hour of loading dose
2. high-dose barbiturates often causes paralytic ileus: therefore NG tube to suction & IV hyperalimentation are usually needed

Indications

The use of barbiturates should be reserved for situations where the ICP cannot be controlled by the previously outlined measures,[141] as there is evidence that *prophylactic* barbiturates do not favorably alter outcome, and are associated with significant side effects, mostly hypotension,[147] that can cause neurologic deterioration.

Choice of agents

A number of agents have been studied, however, there is inadequate data to recommend one drug over another. The most information is available on pentobarbital (see below). Alternative agents which have not been as well studied: thiopental (see below), phenobarbital (p.451) & propofol (p.877).

Drug info: Pentobarbital (Nembutal®)

Pentobarbital has a fast onset (full effects within ≈ 15 minutes), short duration of action (3–4 hrs), and a half-life of 15–48 hrs.

Protocols for pentobarbital therapy in adults

There are many protocols. A simple one from a randomized clinical trial[145]:

1. loading dose:
   a) pentobarbital 10 mg/kg IV over 30 minutes
   b) then 5 mg/kg q 1 hr × 3 doses
2. maintenance: 1 mg/kg/hr

A more elaborate protocol:

1. *loading dose*: pentobarbital 10 mg/kg/hr IV over 4 hrs as follows:
   a) *FIRST HOUR*: 2.5 mg/kg slow IVP q 15 min × 4 doses (total: 10 mg/kg in first hr), follow BP closely
   b) *next 3 hours*: 10 mg/kg/hr continuous infusion (put 2500 mg in 250 ml of appropriate IVF, run at K ml/hr × 3 hrs (K = patient's weight in kg))
2. maintenance: 1.5 mg/kg/hr infusion (put 250 mg in 250 ml IVF and run at 1.5 × K ml/hr)
3. check serum pentobarbital level 1 hr after loading dose completed; usually 3.5–5.0 mg%
4. check serum pentobarbital level q day thereafter
5. if level ever > 5 mg% and ICP acceptable, reduce dose
6. baseline brain stem auditory evoked response (BAER) early in treatment. May be omitted on clinical grounds. Repeat BAER if pentobarbital level ever > 6 mg%. Reduce dose if BAER deteriorates (NB: hemotympanum may interfere with BAER)
7. goal: ICP < 24 mm Hg and pentobarbital level 3–5 mg%. Consider discontinuing pentobarbital due to ineffectiveness if ICP still > 24 with adequate drug levels × 24 hrs
8. if ICP < 20 mm Hg, continue treatment × 48 hrs, then taper dose. Backtrack if ICP rises

Neuro function takes ≈ 2 days off pentobarbital to return ▶ Table 56.8). If is desired to perform a brain death exam, the pentobarbital level needs to be ≈ ≤ 10 mcg/ml before the exam is valid.

Table 56.8 CNS effects of various pentobarbital levels[a]

Degree of CNS depression	mg%	mcg/ml
level for valid brain death exam	≤ 1	≤ 10
sedated, relaxed, easily aroused	0.05–0.3	0.5–3
heavy sedation, difficult to arouse, respiratory depression	2	20
"coma" level (burst suppression occurs in most patients)	5	50

[a]levels reported are for intolerant patients; there is significant variability between patients and tolerant patients may not be sedated even at levels as high as 100 mcg/ml

Drug info: Thiopental (Pentothal®)

May be useful when a rapidly acting barbiturate is needed (e.g. intra-op) or when large doses of pentobarbital are not available. One of many protocols follows (note: thiopental has not been as well studied for this indication, but is theoretically similar to pentobarbital[148,149]):

1. loading dose: thiopental 5 mg/kg (range: 3–5) IV over 10 minutes → transient burst suppression (< 10 minutes) and blood thiopental levels of 10–30 mcg/ml. Higher doses (≈ 35 mg/kg) have been used in the absence of hypothermia to produce longer duration burst suppression for cardiopulmonary bypass
2. follow with continuous infusion of 5 mg/kg/hr (range: 3–5) for 24 hours
3. may need to rebolus with 2.5 mg/kg as needed for ICP control
4. after 24 hours, fat stores become saturated, reduce infusion to 2.5 mg/kg/hr
5. titrate to control ICP or use EEG to monitor for electrocerebral silence
6. "therapeutic" serum level: 6–8.5 mg/dl

Drug info: Propofol (Diprivan®)

Level II[137]: propofol may control ICP after several hours of dosing, but it does not improve mortality or 6 month outcome. ✖ Caution: high-dose propofol (total dose > 100 mg/kg for > 48 hrs) can cause significant morbidity (see propofol infusion syndrome).

℞: 0.5 mg/kg test dose, then 20–75 mcg/kg/min infusion. Increase by 5–10 mcg/kg/min q 5–10 minutes PRN ICP control (do not exceed 83 mcg/kg/min = 5 mg/kg/hr).

Side effects: include Propofol Infusion Syndrome (p. 133). Use with caution at doses > 5 mg/kg/hr or at any dose for > 48 hrs.

References

[1] Sioutos PJ, Orozco JA, Carter LP, et al. Continuous Regional Cerebral Cortical Blood Flow Monitoring in Head-Injured Patients. Neurosurgery. 1995; 36:943–950

[2] Rosner MJ, Coley IB. Cerebral Perfusion Pressure, Intracranial Pressure, and Head Elevation. J Neurosurg. 1986; 65:636–641

[3] Bullock R, Chesnut RM, Clifton G, et al. Guidelines for the Management of Severe Head Injury. 1995

[4] Unterberg AW, Kienning KL, Hartl R, et al. Multimodal Monitoring in Patients with Head Injury: Evaluation of the Effects of Treatment on Cerebral Oxygenation. J Trauma. 1997; 42:S32–S37

[5] Juul N, Morris GF, Marshall SB, et al. Intracranial Hypertension and Cerebral Perfusion Pressure: Influence on Neurological Deterioration and Outcome in Severe Head Injury. J Neurosurg. 2000; 92:1–6

[6] Yano M, Ikeda Y, Kobayashi S, et al. Intracranial Pressure in Head-Injured Patients with Various Intracranial Lesions is Identical Throughout the Supratentorial Intracranial Compartment. Neurosurgery. 1987; 21:688–692

[7] Takizawa H, Gabra-Sanders T, Miller JD. Analysis of Changes in Intracranial Pressure and Pressure-Volume Index at Different Locations in the Craniospinal Axis During Supratentorial Epidural Balloon Inflation. Neurosurgery. 1986; 19:1–8

[8] Mokri B. The Monro-Kellie hypothesis: applications in CSF volume depletion. Neurology. 2001; 56:1746–1748

[9] Welch K. The Intracranial Pressure in Infants. J Neurosurg. 1980; 52:693–699

[10] Mendelow AD, Teasdale GM, Russell T, et al. Effect of Mannitol on Cerebral Blood Flow and Cerebral Perfusion Pressure in Human Head Injury. J Neurosurg. 1985; 63:43–48

[11] Bruce DA, Alavi A, Bilaniuk L, et al. Diffuse Cerebral Swelling Following Head Injuries in Children: The Syndrome of "Malignant Brain Edema". J Neurosurg. 1981; 54:170–178

[12] Unterberg A, Kiening K, Schmiedek P, Lanksch W. Long-Term Observations of Intracranial Pressure After Severe Head Injury. The Phenomenon of Secondary Rise of Intracranial Pressure. Neurosurgery. 1993; 32:17–24

[13] Young HA, Gleave JRW, Schmidek HH, Gregory S. Delayed Traumatic Intracerebral Hematoma: Report of 15 Cases Operatively Treated. Neurosurgery. 1984; 14:22–25

[14] Taneda M, Kataoka K, Akai F, et al. Traumatic Subarachnoid Hemorrhage as a Predictable Indicator of Delayed Ischemic Symptoms. J Neurosurg. 1996; 84:762–768

[15] Narayan RK, Kishore PRS, Becker DP, et al. Intracranial Pressure: To Monitor or Not to Monitor? A Review of Our Experience with Severe Head Injury. J Neurosurg. 1982; 56:650–659

[16] The Brain Trauma Foundation. The American Association of Neurological Surgeons. The Joint Section on Neurotrauma and Critical Care. Indications for intracranial pressure monitoring. J Neurotrauma. 2000; 17:479–491

[17] Brain Trauma Foundation, Povlishock JT, Bullock MR. Indications for intracranial pressure monitoring. J Neurotrauma. 2007; 24:S37–S44

[18] Bullock R, Chesnut RM, Clifton G, et al. In: Indications for intracranial pressure monitoring. Guidelines for the Management of Severe Head Injury. The Brain Trauma Foundation (New York), The American Association of Neurological Surgeons (Park Ridge, Illinois), and The Joint Section of Neurotrauma and Critical Care; 1995

[19] Smith RW, Alksine JF. Infections Complicating the Use of External Ventriculostomy. J Neurosurg. 1976; 44:567–570

[20] Holloway KL, Barnes T, Choi S, et al. Ventriculostomy Infections: The Effect of Monitoring Duration

and Catheter Exchange in 584 Patients. J Neurosurg. 1996; 85:419–424
[21] Al-Shahi Salman R, Berg MJ, Morrison L, Awad IA. Hemorrhage from cavernous malformations of the brain: definition and reporting standards. Angioma Alliance Scientific Advisory Board. Stroke. 2008; 39:3222–3230
[22] Paramore CG, Turner DA. Relative Risks of Ventriculostomy Infection and Morbidity. Acta Neurochir. 1994; 127:79–84
[23] Maniker AH, Vaynman AY, Karimi RJ, Sabit AO, et al. Hemorrhagic complications of external ventricular drainage. Operative Neurosurgery. 2006; 59:419–425
[24] Lozier AP, Sciacca RR, Romanoli M, et al. Ventriculostomy-related infection: a critical review of the literature. Neurosurgery. 2002; 51:170–182
[25] Brain Trauma Foundation, Povlishock JT, Bullock MR. Infection prophylaxis. J Neurotrauma. 2007; 24:S26–S31
[26] Mayhall CG, Archer NH, Lamb VA, Spadora AC, Baggett JW, Ward JD, Narayan RK. Ventriculostomy-related infections. A prospective epidemiologic study. N Engl J Med. 1984; 310:553–559
[27] Lyke KE, Obasanjo OO, Williams MA, et al. Ventriculitis complicating use of intraventricular catheters in adult neurosurgical patients. Clin Infect Dis. 2001; 33:2028–2033
[28] Winfield JA, Rosenthal P, Kanter R, et al. Duration of intracranial pressure monitoring does not predict daily risk of infections complications. Neurosurgery. 1993; 33:424–431
[29] Brain Trauma Foundation, Povlishock JT, Bullock MR. Intracranial pressure monitoring technology. J Neurotrauma. 2007; 24:S45–S54
[30] Ropper AH. Raised Intracranial Pressure in Neurologic Disease. Sem Neurology. 1984; 4:397–407
[31] Sundbarg G, Nordstrom C-H, Messetter K, et al. A Comparison of Intraparenchymatous and Intraventricular Pressure Recording in Clinical Practice. J Neurosurg. 1987; 67:841–845
[32] Crutchfield JS, Narayan RK, Robertson CS, Michael LH. Evaluation of a Fiberoptic Intracranial Pressure Monitor. J Neurosurg. 1990; 72:482–487
[33] Ostrup RC, Luerssen TG, Marshall LF, et al. Continuous Monitoring of Intracranial Pressure with a Miniaturized Fiberoptic Device. J Neurosurg. 1987; 67:206–209
[34] Piek J, Bock WJ. Continuous Monitoring of Cerebral Tissue Pressure in Neurosurgical Practice - Experience with 100 Patients. Intens Care Med. 1990; 16:184–188
[35] Gopinath SP, Robertson CS, Contant CF, et al. Clinical Evaluation of a Miniature Strain-Gauge Transducer for Monitoring Intracranial Pressure. Neurosurgery. 1995; 36:1137–1141
[36] Salmon JH, Hajjar W, Bada HS. The Fontogram: A Noninvasive Intracranial Pressure Monitor. Pediatrics. 1977; 60:721–725
[37] Grabb PA. Traumatic intraventricular hemorrhage treated with intraventricular recombinant-tissue plasminogen activator: technical case report. Neurosurgery. 1998; 43:966–969
[38] Hamer J, Alberti E, Hoyer S, Wiedemann K. Factors Influencing CSF Pulse Waves. J Neurosurg. 1977; 46:36–45
[39] Lundberg N. Continuous Recording and Control of Ventricular Fluid Pressure in Neurosurgical Practice. Acta Psych Neurol Scand. 1960; 36S:1–193
[40] Cruz J. On-Line Monitoring of Global Cerebral Hypoxia in Acute Brain Injury. Relationship to Intracranial Hypertension. J Neurosurg. 1993; 79:228–233
[41] Sheinberg M, Kanter MJ, Robertson CS, et al. Continuous Monitoring of Jugular Venous Oxygen Saturation in Head-Injured Patients. J Neurosurg. 1992; 76:212–217
[42] Cormio M, Valadka AB, Robertson CS. Elevated jugular venous oxygen saturation after severe head injury. J Neurosurg. 1999; 90:9–15
[43] Robertson CS, Narayan RK, Gokaslan ZL, et al. Cerebral Arteriovenous Oxygen Difference as an Estimate of Cerebral Blood Flow in Comatose Patients. J Neurosurg. 1989; 70:222–230
[44] Gotoh F, Meyer JS, Takagi Y. Cerebral Effects of Hyperventilation in Man. Arch Neurol. 1965; 12:410–423
[45] Obrist WD, Langfitt TW, Jaggi JL, et al. Cerebral Blood Flow and Metabolism in Comatose Patients with Acute Head Injury. Relationship to Intracranial Hypertension. J Neurosurg. 1984; 61:241–253
[46] Pickard JD, Czosnyka M. Management of Raised Intracranial Pressure. J Neurol Neurosurg Psychiatry. 1993; 56:845–858
[47] Valadka AB, Gopinath SP, Contant CF, Uzura M, Robertson CS. Relationship of brain tissue PO2 to outcome after severe head injury. Crit Care Med. 1998; 26:1576–1581
[48] van den Brink WA, van Santbrink H, Steyerberg EW, Avezaat CJ, Suazo JA, Hogesteeger C, Jansen WJ, Kloos LM, Vermeulen J, Maas AI. Brain oxygen tension in severe head injury. Neurosurgery. 2000; 46:868–76; discussion 876-8
[49] Stiefel MF, Spiotta A, Gracias VH, Garuffe AM, Guillamondegui O, Maloney-Wilensky E, Bloom S, Grady MS, LeRoux PD. Reduced mortality rate in patients with severe traumatic brain injury treated with brain tissue oxygen monitoring. J Neurosurg. 2005; 103:805–811
[50] Jaeger M, Schuhmann MU, Soehle M, Nagel C, Meixensberger J. Continuous monitoring of cerebrovascular autoregulation after subarachnoid hemorrhage by brain tissue oxygen pressure reactivity and its relation to delayed cerebral infarction. Stroke. 2007; 38:981–986
[51] Jaeger M, Soehle M, Schuhmann MU, Winkler D, Meixensberger J. Correlation of continuously monitored regional cerebral blood flow and brain tissue oxygen. Acta Neurochir (Wien). 2005; 147:51–6; discussion 56
[52] Goodman JC, Valadka AB, Gopinath SP, Uzura M, Robertson CS. Extracellular lactate and glucose alterations in the brain after head injury measured by microdialysis. Crit Care Med. 1999; 27:1965–1973
[53] Vespa PM, McArthur D, O'Phelan K, Glenn T, Etchepare M, Kelly D, Bergsneider M, Martin NA, Hovda DA. Persistently low extracellular glucose correlates with poor outcome 6 months after human traumatic brain injury despite a lack of increased lactate: a microdialysis study. J Cereb Blood Flow Metab. 2003; 23:865–877
[54] Bullock R, Chesnut RM, Clifton G, et al. Guidelines for the Management of Severe Head Injury. J Neurotrauma. 1996; 13:639–734
[55] Bullock R, Chestnut R, Ghajar J, et al. Guidelines for the management of severe traumatic brain injury. J Neurotrauma. 2000; 17:449–454
[56] Brain Trauma Foundation, Povlishock JT, Bullock MR. Blood pressure and oxygenation. J Neurotrauma. 2007; 24:S7–13
[57] Brain Trauma Foundation, Povlishock JT, Bullock MR. Intracranial pressure thresholds. J Neurotrauma. 2007; 24:S55–S58
[58] Marshall LF, Barba D, Toole BM, Bowers SA. The oval pupil: clinical significance and relationship to intracranial hypertension. J Neurosurg. 1983; 58:566–568
[59] Miller JD, Butterworth JF, Gudeman SK, et al. Further Experience in the Management of Severe Head Injury. J Neurosurg. 1981; 54:289–299
[60] Saul TG, Ducker TB. Effect of Intracranial Pressure Monitoring and and Aggressive Treatment on Mortality in Severe Head Injury. J Neurosurg. 1982; 56:498–503
[61] Brain Trauma Foundation, Povlishock JT, Bullock MR. Cerebral perfusion thresholds. J Neurotrauma. 2007; 24:S59–S64
[62] Brain Trauma Foundation, Povlishock JT, Bullock MR. Brain oxygen monitoring and thresholds. J Neurotrauma. 2007; 24:S65–S70
[63] Bouma GJ, Muizelaar JP. Relationship between Cardiac Output and Cerebral Blood Flow in Patients with Intact and with Impaired Autoregulation. J Neurosurg. 1990; 73:368–374

[64] The Brain Trauma Foundation. The American Association of Neurological Surgeons. The Joint Section on Neurotrauma and Critical Care. Hypotension. J Neurotrauma. 2000; 17:591–595
[65] Larson DE, Farnell MB. Upper Gastrointestinal Hemorrhage. Mayo Clin Proc. 1983; 58:371–387
[66] Grosfeld JL, Shipley F, Fitzgerald JF, et al. Acute Peptic Ulcer in Infancy and Childhood. Am Surgeon. 1978; 44:13–19
[67] Curci MR, Little K, Sieber WK, et al. Peptic Ulcer Disease in Childhood Reexamined. J Ped Surg. 1976; 11:329–335
[68] Krasna IH, Schneider KM, Becker JM. Surgical Management of Stress Ulcerations in Childhood. J Ped Surg. 1971; 6:301–306
[69] Chan K-H, Lai ECS, Tuen H, et al. Prospective Double-Blind Placebo-Controlled Randomized Trial on the Use of Ranitidine in Preventing Postoperative Gastroduodenal Complications in High-Risk Neurosurgical Patients. J Neurosurg. 1995; 82:413–417
[70] Shackford SR, Zhuang J, Schmoker J. Intravenous Fluid Tonicity: Effect on Intracranial Pressure, Cerebral Blood Flow, and Cerebral Oxygen Delivery in Focal Brain Injury. J Neurosurg. 1992; 76:91–98
[71] Garretson HD, McGraw CP, O'Connor C, Howard G, et al. Ishii S, Nagai H, Brock M. In: Effectiveness of Fluid Restriction, Mannitol and Furosemide in Reducing ICP. Intracranial Pressure V. Berlin: Springer-Verlag; 1983:742–745
[72] Ward JD, Moulton RJ, Muizelaar PJ, Marmarou AM, Wirth FP, Ratcheson RA. In: Cerebral Homeostasis. Neurosurgical Critical Care. Baltimore: Williams and Wilkins; 1987:187–213
[73] De Salles AAF, Muizelaar JP, Young HF. Hyperglycemia, Cerebrospinal Fluid Lactic Acidosis, and Cerebral Blood Flow in Severely Head-injurred Patients. Neurosurgery. 1987; 21:45–50
[74] Kaufman HH, Bretaudiere J-P, Rowlands BJ, et al. General Metabolism in Head Injury. Neurosurgery. 1987; 20:254–265
[75] Brain Trauma Foundation, Povlishock JT, Bullock MR. Prophylactic hypothermia. J Neurotrauma. 2007; 24:S21–S25
[76] Cao M, Lisheng H, Shouzheng S. Resolution of Brain Edema in Severe Brain Injury at Controlled High and Low ICPs. J Neurosurg. 1984; 61:707–712
[77] Metz C, Holzschuh M, Bein T, et al. Moderate Hypothermia in Patients with Severe Head Injury: Cerebral and Extracerebral Effects. J Neurosurg. 1996; 85:533–541
[78] Mild therapeutic hypothermia to improve the neurologic outcome after cardiac arrest. N Engl J Med. 2002; 346:549–556
[79] Polin RS, Shaffrey ME, Bogaev CA, et al. Decompressive Bifrontal Craniectomy in the Treatment of Severe Refractory Posttraumatic Cerebral Edema. Neurosurgery. 1997; 41:84–94
[80] Cooper PR, Hagler H, Clark W, Shulman K, Marmarou A. Intracranial Pressure IV. New York: Springer Verlag; 1980:277–279
[81] Aarabi B, Hesdorffer DC, Ahn ES, Aresco C, Scalea TM, Eisenberg HM. Outcome following decompressive craniectomy for malignant swelling due to severe head injury. J Neurosurg. 2006; 104:469–479
[82] Timofeev I, Kirkpatrick PJ, Corteen E, Hiler M, Czosnyka M, Menon DK, Pickard JD, Hutchinson PJ. Decompressive craniectomy in traumatic brain injury: outcome following protocol-driven therapy. Acta Neurochir Suppl. 2006; 96:11–16
[83] Holland M, Nakaji P. Craniectomy: Surgical indications and technique. Operative Techniques in Neurosurgery. 2004; 7:10–15
[84] Nussbaum ES, Wolf AL, Sebring L, Mirvis S. Complete Temporal Lobectomy for Surgical Resuscitation of Patients with Transtentorial Herniation Secondary to Unilateral Hemispheric Swelling. Neurosurgery. 1991; 29:62–66
[85] Hamill JF, Bedford RF, Weaver DC, et al. Lidocaine before Endotracheal Intubation: Intravenous or Laryngotracheal? Anesthesiology. 1981; 55:578–581
[86] Hurst JM, Saul TG, DeHaven CB, et al. Use of High Frequency Jet Ventilation during Mechanical Hyperventilation to Reduce ICP in Patients with Multiple Organ System Injury. Neurosurgery. 1984; 15:530–534
[87] Cooper KR, Boswell PA, Choi SC. Safe Use of PEEP in Patients with Severe Head Injury. J Neurosurg. 1985; 63:552–555
[88] Feldman Z, Kanter MJ, Robertson CS, Contant CF, et al. Effect of Head Elevation on Intracranial Pressure, Cerebral Perfusion Pressure, and Cerebral Blood Flow in Head-Injured Patients. J Neurosurg. 1992; 76:207–211
[89] Raichle ME, Plum F. Hyperventilation and cerebral blood flow. Stroke. 1972; 3:566–575
[90] Grubb RL, Raichle ME, Eichling JO, et al. The Effects of Changes in PaCO2 on Cerebral Blood Volume, Blood Flow, and Vascular Mean Transit Time. Stroke. 1974; 5:630–639
[91] Darby JM, Yonas H, Marion DW, Latchaw RE, et al. Local 'Inverse Steal' Induced by Hyperventilation in Head Injury. Neurosurgery. 1988; 23:84–88
[92] Fleischer AS, Patton JM, Tindall GT. Monitoring Intraventricular Pressure Using an Implanted Reservoir in Head Injured Patients. Surg Neurol. 1975; 3:309–311
[93] Diringer MN, Yundt K, Videen TO, et al. No Reduction in Cerebral Metabolism as a Result of Early Moderate Hyperventilation Following Severe Traumatic Brain Injury. J Neurosurg. 2000; 92:7–13
[94] Bullock R, Chesnut RM, Clifton G, et al. In: The use of hyperventilation in the acute management of severe traumatic brain injury. Guidelines for the Management of Severe Head Injury.The Brain Trauma Foundation (New York), The American Association of Neurological Surgeons (Park Ridge, Illinois), and The Joint Section of Neurotrauma and Critical Care; 1995
[95] Brain Trauma Foundation, Povlishock JT, Bullock MR. Hyperventilation. J Neurotrauma. 2007; 24: S87–S90
[96] Muizelaar JP, Marmarou A, Ward JD, et al. Adverse Effects of Prolonged Hyperventilation in Patients with Severe Head Injury: A Randomized Clinical Trial. J Neurosurg. 1991; 75:731–739
[97] Bouma GJ, Muizelaar JP, Choi SC, et al. Cerebral Circulation and Metabolism After Severe Traumatic Brain Injury: The Elusive Role of Ischemia. J Neurosurg. 1991; 75:685–693
[98] Bouma GJ, Muizelaar JP, Stringer WA, et al. Ultra Early Evaluation of Regional Cerebral Blood Flow in Severely Head Injured Patients using Xenon Enhanced Computed Tomography. J Neurosurg. 1992; 77:360–368
[99] Fieschi C, Battistini N, Beduschi A, et al. Regional Cerebral Blood Flow and Intraventricular Pressure in Acute Head Injuries. J Neurol Neurosurg Psychiatry. 1974; 37:1378–1388
[100] Schroder ML, Muizelaar JP, Kuta AJ. Documented Reversal of Global Ischemia Immediately After Removal of an Acute Subdural Hematoma. Neurosurgery. 1994; 80:324–327
[101] James H, Langfitt T, Kumar V, et al. Treatment of Intracranial Hypertension; Analysis of 105 Consecutive Continuous Recordings of ICP. Acta Neurochir. 1977; 36:189–200
[102] Lundberg N, Kjallquist A. A Reduction of Increased ICP by Hyperventilation, a Therapeutic Aid in Neurological Surgery. Acta Psych Neurol Scand (Suppl). 1958; 139:1–64
[103] Bullock R, Chesnut RM, Clifton G, et al. In: The use of mannitol in severe head injury. Guidelines for the Management of Severe Head Injury.The Brain Trauma Foundation (New York), The American Association of Neurological Surgeons (Park Ridge, Illinois), and The Joint Section of Neurotrauma and Critical Care; 1995
[104] Brain Trauma Foundation, Povlishock JT, Bullock MR. Hyperosmolar therapy. J Neurotrauma. 2007; 24:S14–S20

[105] Barry KG, Berman AR. Mannitol Infusion. Part III. The Acute Effect of the Intravenous Infusion of Mannitol on Blood and Plasma Volume. N Engl J Med. 1961; 264:1085–1088

[106] James HE. Methodology for the Control of Intracranial Pressure with Hypertonic Mannitol. Acta Neurochir. 1980; 51:161–172

[107] McGraw CP, Howard G. The Effect of Mannitol on Increased Intracranial Pressure. Neurosurgery. 1983; 13:269–271

[108] Cruz J, Miner ME, Allen SJ, et al. Continuous Monitoring of Cerebral Oxygenation in Acute Brain Injury: Injection of Mannitol During Hyperventilation. J Neurosurg. 1990; 73:725–730

[109] Marshall LF, Smith RW, Rauscher LA, Shapiro HM. Mannitol Dose Requirements in Brain-Injured Patients. J Neurosurg. 1978; 48:169–172

[110] Takagi H, Saito T, Kitahara T, Ishii S, Nagai H, Brock M. In: The Mechanism of the ICP Reducing Effect of Mannitol. ICP V. Berlin: Springer-Verlag; 1993:729–733

[111] Node Y, Yajima K, Nakazawa S, Ishii S, Nagai H, Brock M. In: A Study of Mannitol and Glycerol on the Reduction of Raised Intracranial Pressure on Their Rebound Phemonenon. Intracranial Pressure V. Berlin: Springer-Verlag; 1983:738–741

[112] Smith HP, Kelly DL, McWhorter JM. Comparison of Mannitol Regimens in Patients with Severe Head Injury Undergoing Intracranial Monitoring. J Neurosurg. 1986; 65:820–824

[113] Pollay M, Roberts PA, Fullenwider C, Stevens FA, Ishii S, Nagai H, Brock M. In: The Effect of Mannitol and Furosemide on the Blood-Brain Osmotic Gradient and Intracranial Pressure. Intracranial Pressure V. Berlin: Springer-Verlag; 1983:734–736

[114] Cold GE. Cerebral Blood Flow in Acute Head Injury: The Regulation of Cerebral Blood Flow and Metabolism During the Acute Phase of Head Injury, and Its Significance for Therapy. Acta Neurochir. 1990; Suppl 49:1–64

[115] Kaufmann AM, Cardoso ER. Aggravation of Vasogenic Cerebral Edema by Multiple Dose Mannitol. J Neurosurg. 1992; 77:584–589

[116] Ravussin P, Abou-Madi M, Archer D, et al. Changes in CSF Pressure After Mannitol in Patients With and Without Elevated CSF Pressure. J Neurosurg. 1988; 69:869–876

[117] Feig PU, McCurdy DK. The Hypertonic State. N Engl J Med. 1977; 297:1444–1454

[118] Muizelaar JP, Lutz HA, Becker DP. Effect of Mannitol on ICP and CBF and Correlation with Pressure Autoregulation in Severely Head-Injured Patients. J Neurosurg. 1984; 61:700–706

[119] Cottrell JE, Robustelli A, Post K, et al. Furosemide- and Mannitol-Induced Changes in Intracranial Pressure and Serum Osmolality and Electrolytes. Anesthesiology. 1977; 47:28–30

[120] Tornheim PA, McLaurin RL, Sawaya R. Effect of Furosemide on Experimental Cerebral Edema. Neurosurgery. 1979; 4:48–52

[121] Buhrley LE, Reed DJ. The Effect of Furosemide on Sodium-22 Uptake into Cerebrospinal Fluid and Brain. Exp Brain Res. 1972; 14:503–510

[122] Marion DW, Letarte PB. Management of Intracranial Hypertension. Contemp Neurosurg. 1997; 19:1–6

[123] Doyle JA, Davis DP, Hoyt DB. The use of hypertonic saline in the treatment of traumatic brain injury. J Trauma. 2001; 50:367–383

[124] Ogden AT, Mayer SA, Connolly ES. Hyperosmolar agents in neurosurgical practice: The evolving role of hypertonic saline. Neurosurgery. 2005; 57:207–215

[125] Vialet R, Albanese J, Thomachot L, Antonini F, Bourgouin A, Alliez B, Martin C. Isovolume hypertonic solutes (sodium chloride or mannitol) in the treatment of refractory posttraumatic intracranial hypertension: 2 mL/kg 7.5% saline is more effective than 2 mL/kg 20% mannitol. Crit Care Med. 2003; 31:1683–1687

[126] Shackford SR, Bourguignon PR, Wald SL, Rogers FB, Osler TM, Clark DE. Hypertonic saline resuscitation of patients with head injury: a prospective, randomized clinical trial. J Trauma. 1998; 44:50–58

[127] Qureshi AI, Suarez JI, Castro A, Bhardwaj A. Use of hypertonic saline/acetate infusion in treatment of cerebral edema in patients with head trauma: experience at a single center. J Trauma. 1999; 47:659–665

[128] Brain Trauma Foundation, Povlishock JT, Bullock MR. Steroids. J Neurotrauma. 2007; 24:S91–S95

[129] Bullock R, Chesnut RM, Clifton G, et al. In: The role of glucocorticoids in the treatment of severe head injury. Guidelines for the Management of Severe Head Injury.The Brain Trauma Foundation (New York), The American Association of Neurological Surgeons (Park Ridge, Illinois), and The Joint Section of Neurotrauma and Critical Care; 1995

[130] The Brain Trauma Foundation. The American Association of Neurological Surgeons. The Joint Section on Neurotrauma and Critical Care. Role of steroids. J Neurotrauma. 2000; 17:531–535

[131] Braughler JM, Hall ED. Current Application of "High-Dose" Steroid Therapy for CNS Injury: A Pharmacological Perspective. J Neurosurg. 1985; 62:806–810

[132] Lam AM, Winn HR, Cullen BF, et al. Hyperglycemia and Neurologic Outcome in Patients with Head Injury. J Neurosurg. 1991; 75:545–551

[133] Roberts I, Yates D, Sandercock P, et al. Effects of intravenous corticosteroids on death within 14 days in 10,008 adults with clinically significant head injury (MRC CRASH trial): randomized placebo controlled trial. Lancet. 2004; 364

[134] Doppenberg EMR, Bullock R. Clinical neuro-protection trials in severe traumatic brain injury: lessons from previous studies. J Neurotrauma. 1997; 14:71–80

[135] Marshall LF, Maas AL, Marshall SB, et al. A multicenter trial on the efficacy of using tirilazad mesylate in cases of head injury. J Neurosurg. 1998; 89:519–525

[136] Grumme T, Baethmann A, Kolodziejczyk D, et al. Treatment of patients with severe head injury by triamcinolone: a prospective, controlled multicenter clinical trial of 396 cases. Res Exp Med (Berl). 1995; 195:217–229

[137] Brain Trauma Foundation, Povlishock JT, Bullock MR. Anesthetics, analgesics, and sedatives. J Neurotrauma. 2007; 24:S71–S76

[138] Lyons MK, Meyer FB. Cerebrospinal Fluid Physiology and the Management of Increased Intracranial Pressure. Mayo Clin Proc. 1990; 65:684–707

[139] Shapiro HM, Wyte SR, Loeser J. Barbiturate Augmented Hypothermia for Reduction of Persistent Intracranial Hypertension. J Neurosurg. 1979; 40:90–100

[140] Marshall LF, Smith RW, Shapiro HM. The Outcome with Aggressive Treatment in Severe Head Injuries. Part II: Acute and Chronic Barbiturate Administration in the Management of Head Injury. J Neurosurg. 1979; 50:26–30

[141] Rea GL, Rockswold GL. Barbiturate Therapy in Uncontrolled Intracranial Hypertension. Neurosurgery. 1983; 12:401–404

[142] Ward JD, Becker DP, Miller JD, et al. Failure of Prophylactic Barbiturate Coma in the Treatment of Severe Head Injury. J Neurosurg. 1985; 62:383–388

[143] Schwartz M, Tator C, Towed D, et al. The University of Toronto Head Injury Treatment Study: A Prospective Randomized Comparison of Pentobarbital and Mannitol. Can J Neurol Sci. 1984; 11:434–440

[144] Nordstrom C-H, Messeter K, Sundbarg G, et al. Cerebral Blood Flow, Vasoreactivity, and Oxygen Consumption During Barbiturate Therapy in Severe Traumatic Brain Lesions. J Neurosurg. 1988; 68:424–431

[145] Eisenberg HM, Frankowski RF, Contant CF, Marshall LF, et al. High-Dose Barbiturate Control of Elevated Intracranial Pressure in Patients with Severe Head Injury. J Neurosurg. 1988; 69:15–23

[146] Gilman AG, Goodman LS, Gilman A. Goodman and Gilman's The Pharmacological Basis of Therapeutics. New York 1980

[147] Ward JD, Becker DP, Miller JD, et al. Failure of Prophylactic Barbiturate Coma in the Treatment of Severe Head Injury. J Neurosurg. 1985; 62:383–388

[148] Boarini DJ, Kassell NF, Coester HC. Comparison of Sodium Thiopental and Methohexital for High-Dose Barbiturate Anesthesia. J Neurosurg. 1984; 60:602–608

[149] Spetzler RF, Martin N, Hadley MN, et al. Microsurgical Endarterectomy Under Barbiturate Protection: A Prospective Study. J Neurosurg. 1986; 65:63–73

57 Skull Fractures

57.1 General information

Classified as either closed (simple fracture) or open (compound fracture).

Diastatic fractures extend into and separate sutures. More common in young children.[1]

57.2 Linear skull fractures over the convexity

90% of pediatric skull fractures are linear and involve the calvaria.

▶ Table 57.1 shows some differentiating features to distinguish linear skull fractures. See also Indications for CT and admission criteria for TBI (p. 830).

By themselves, linear skull fractures over the convexity rarely require surgical intervention.

57.3 Depressed skull fractures

For special considerations in pediatrics, see Depressed skull fractures (p. 915) in pediatrics section.

57.3.1 Indications for surgery

See **Practice guideline: Surgical management of depressed skull fractures** (p. 882). Some additional observations regarding surgery to elevate a depressed skull fracture in an adult:

1. consider surgery for depressed skull fractures with deficit referable to underlying brain
2. ✖ more conservative treatment is recommended for fractures overlying a major dural venous sinus (**note:** exception: depressed fractures overlying and depressing one of the dural sinuses may be dangerous to elevate, and if the patient is neurologically intact, and no indication for operation (e.g. CSF leak mandates surgery) may be best managed conservatively).

Practice guideline: Surgical management of depressed skull fractures

Indications for surgery

Level III[2]:

1. open (compound) fractures
   a) surgery for fractures depressed > thickness of calvaria and those not meeting criteria for nonsurgical management listed below
   b) nonsurgical management may be considered if
      - there is no evidence (clinical or CT) of dural penetration (CSF leak, intradural pneumocephalus on CT...)
      - and no significant intracranial hematoma
      - and depression is < 1 cm
      - and no frontal sinus involvement
      - and no wound infection or gross contamination
      - and no gross cosmetic deformity
2. closed (simple) depressed fractures: may be managed surgically or nonsurgically

Timing of surgery

Level III[2]: early surgery to reduce risk of infection

Surgical methods

Level III[2]:

1. elevation and debridement are recommended
2. option: if there is no evidence of wound infection, primary bone replacement
3. antibiotics should be used for all compound depressed fractures

Table 57.1 Differentiating linear skull fractures from normal *plain* film findings			
Feature	**Linear skull fracture**	**Vessel groove**	**Suture line**
density	dark black	grey	grey
course	straight	curving	follows course of known suture lines
branching	usually none	often branching	joins other suture lines
width	very thin	thicker than fracture	jagged, wide

There is no evidence that elevating a depressed skull fracture will reduce the subsequent development of posttraumatic seizures,[3] which are probably more related to the initial brain injury.

57.3.2 Surgical treatment for depressed skull fractures

General information

Booking the case: Craniotomy for depressed skull fracture

Also see defaults & disclaimers (p. 27).
1. position: (depends on location of the fracture)
2. post-op: ICU
3. blood: type & screen (for severe fractures: type and cross 2 U PRBC)
4. consent (in lay terms for the patient – not all-inclusive):
   a) procedure: surgery in the area of the skull fracture to bone fragments that may have been displaced, to repair the covering of the brain, to remove any foreign material that can be identified and any permanently damaged brain tissue (i.e. dead brain tissue), remove any blood clot and stop any bleeding identified, possible placement of intracranial pressure monitor. If a large opening has to be left in the skull, it may require surgery to correct in a number of months (3 or more)
   b) alternatives: nonsurgical management
   c) complications – usual craniotomy complications (p. 28) – plus any permanent brain injury that has already occurred is not likely to recover, seizures may occur (with or without the surgery), hydrocephalus, infection (including delayed infection/abscess)

Technical considerations of surgery

Surgical goals (modified[4])
1. debridement of skin edges
2. elevation of bone fragments
3. repair of dural laceration
4. debridement of devitalized brain
5. reconstruction of the skull
6. skin closure

57

Techniques
1. with open (compound) contaminated fractures, it may be necessary to excise depressed bone. In these cases or when air sinuses are involved, to minimize the risk of infecting the flap, some surgeons follow the patient for 6–12 months to rule out infection before performing a cosmetic cranioplasty. There has been no documented increase in infection with replacement of bone fragments; soaking the fragments in povidone-iodine has been recommended[4]
2. elevating the bone may be facilitated by drilling burr holes around the periphery and either using rongeurs or craniotome to excise the depressed portion
3. in cases where laceration of a major dural sinus is suspected and surgery is mandated, adequate preparation must be made for dural sinus repair[5]; NB: the SSS is often to the right of the sagittal suture (p. 61)

a) prepare for massive blood loss
b) have small Fogarty catheter ready to temporarily occlude sinus
c) have dural shunt ready (Kapp-Gielchinsky shunt, if available, has an inflatable balloon at both ends)
d) prep out saphenous vein area for vein graft
e) bone fragments that may have lacerated sinus should be removed last

57.4 Basal skull fractures

57.4.1 General information

Most basal (AKA basilar) skull fractures (BSF) are extensions of fractures through the cranial vault.

Severe basilar skull fractures may produce shearing injuries to the pituitary gland.

BSF, especially those involving the clivus, may be associated with traumatic aneurysms. This rarely occurs in pediatrics.[6]

57.4.2 Some specific fracture types

Temporal bone fractures

General information

Although often mixed, there are two basic types of temporal bone fractures:
- longitudinal fracture: more common (70–90%). Usually through petro-squamosal suture, parallel to and through EAC. Can often be diagnosed on otoscopic inspection of the EAC. Usually passes between cochlea and semicircular canals (SCC) sparing the VII and VIII nerves, but may disrupt the ossicular chain
- transverse fracture: perpendicular to EAC. Often passes through cochlea and may place stretch on geniculate ganglion, resulting in VIII and VII nerve deficits respectively

Posttraumatic facial palsy

Posttraumatic unilateral peripheral facial nerve palsy may be associated with transverse petrous bone fractures as noted above.

Management

Management is often complicated by multiplicity of injuries (including head injury requiring endotracheal intubation) making it difficult to determine the time of onset of facial palsy. Guidelines:
1. regardless of time of onset:
   a) steroids (glucocorticoids) are often utilized (efficacy unproven)
   b) consultation with ENT physician is usually indicated
2. immediate onset of unilateral peripheral facial palsy: facial EMG (AKA electroneuronography[7] or ENOG) takes at least 72 hrs to become abnormal. These cases are often followed and are possible candidates for surgical VII nerve decompression if no improvement occurs with steroids (timing of surgery is controversial, but is usually not done emergently)
3. delayed onset of unilateral peripheral facial palsy: follow serial ENOGs, if continued nerve deterioration occurs while on steroids, and activity on ENOG drops to less than 10% of the contralateral side, surgical decompression may be considered (controversial, thought to improve recovery from ≈ 40% to ≈ 75% of cases)

Clival fractures

See reference.[8]

3 categories (75% are longitudinal or transverse):
1. longitudinal: may be associated with injuries of vertebrobasilar vessels including:
   a) dissection or occlusion: may cause brain stem infarction
   b) traumatic aneurysms
2. transverse: may be associated with injuries to the anterior circulation
3. oblique

Clival fractures are highly lethal. May be associated with:
1. cranial nerve deficits: especially III through VI; bitemporal hemianopsia
2. CSF leak

3. diabetes insipidus
4. delayed development of traumatic aneurysms[9]

Occipital condyle fractures

These are considered in the section on Spine fractures (p. 966).

57.4.3 Radiographic diagnosis

BSF appear as linear lucencies through the skull base.

CT scan with multiplanar projections is the most sensitive means for directly demonstrating BSF. Plain skull x-rays and clinical criteria (see below) may also be able to make the diagnosis.

Indirect radiographic findings (on CT or plain films) that suggest BSF include: pneumocephalus (diagnostic of BSF in the absence of an open fracture of the cranial vault), air/fluid level within or opacification of air sinus with fluid (suggestive).

57.4.4 Clinical diagnosis

Some of these signs may take several hours to develop. Signs include:
1. CSF otorrhea or rhinorrhea
2. hemotympanum or laceration of external auditory canal
3. postauricular ecchymoses (Battle's sign)
4. periorbital ecchymoses (raccoon's eyes) in the absence of direct orbital trauma, especially if bilateral
5. cranial nerve injury:
   a) VII and/or VIII: usually associated with temporal bone fracture
   b) olfactory nerve (Cr. N. I) injury: often occurs with anterior fossa BSF and results in anosmia, this fracture may extend to the optic canal and cause injury to the optic nerve (Cr. N. II)
   c) VI injury: can occur with fractures through the clivus (see below)

57.4.5 Management

NG tubes

✖ Caution: cases have been reported with BSF where an NG tube has been passed intracranially through the fracture[10,11,12] and is associated with fatal outcome in 64% of cases. Possible mechanisms include: a cribriform plate that is thin (congenitally or due to chronic sinusitis) or fractured (due to a frontal basal skull fracture or a comminuted fracture through the skull base).

Suggested contraindications to blind placement of an NG tube include: trauma with possible basal skull fracture, ongoing or history of previous CSF rhinorrhea, meningitis with chronic sinusitis.

Prophylactic antibiotics

The routine use of prophylactic antibiotics is controversial. This remains true even in the presence of a CSF fistula; see CSF fistula (cranial) (p. 384). However, most ENT physicians recommend treating fractures through the nasal sinuses as open contaminated fractures, and they use broad spectrum antibiotics (e.g. ciprofloxacin) for 7–10 days.

57

Treatment of the BSF

Most do not require treatment by themselves. However, conditions that may be associated with BSF which may require specific management include:
1. "traumatic aneurysms" (p. 1227)[13]
2. posttraumatic carotid-cavernous fistula (p. 1256)
3. CSF fistula: operative treatment may be required for persistent CSF rhinorrhea; see CSF fistula (cranial) (p. 384)
4. meningitis or cerebral abscess: may occur with BSF into air sinuses (frontal or mastoid) even in the absence of an identifiable CSF leak. May even occur many years after the BSF was sustained; see Post craniospinal trauma meningitis / post-traumatic meningitis (p. 318)
5. cosmetic deformities
6. posttraumatic facial palsy (below)

57.5 Craniofacial fractures

57.5.1 Frontal sinus fractures

General information

Frontal sinus fractures account for 5–15% of facial fractures.

In the presence of a frontal sinus fracture, intracranial air (pneumocephalus) on CT even without a clinically evident CSF leak, must be presumed to be due to dural laceration (although it could also be due to a basal skull fracture, below).

Anesthesia of the forehead may occur due to supratrochlear and/or supraorbital nerve involvement.

The risks of posterior wall fractures are not immediate, but may be delayed (some even by months or years) and include:

1. brain abscess
2. CSF leak with risk of meningitis
3. cyst or mucocele formation: injured frontal sinus mucosa has a higher predilection for mucocele formation than other sinuses.[14] Mucoceles may also develop as a result of frontonasal duct obstruction due to fracture or chronic inflammation. Mucoceles are prone to infection (mucopyocele) which can erode bone and expose dura with risk of infection

Anatomic considerations of the frontal sinus

The frontal sinus begins to appear around age 2 yrs, and becomes radiographically visible by age 8 as it extends above the superior orbital rim.[15] The sinus is lined with respiratory epithelium, the mucous secretion of which drains through the frontonasal duct medially and inferiorly into the middle nasal meatus.

Surgical considerations

Indications

Linear fractures of the anterior wall of the frontal sinus are treated expectantly.

Indications for exploration of posterior wall fractures is *controversial.*[16] Some argue that a few mm of displacement, or that CSF fistula that resolves may not require exploration. Others vehemently disagree.

Technique

In the presence of a traumatic forehead laceration, the frontal sinus may be exposed through judicious incorporation of the laceration in a forehead incision. Without such a laceration, either a bicoronal (souttar) skin incision or a butterfly incision (through the lower part of the eyebrows, crossing the midline near the glabella) is used.

In the presence of pneumocephalus, if no obvious dural laceration is found the dural undersurface of the frontal lobes should be checked for leaks. Extradural inspection and repair is rarely indicated; the act of lifting the dura off the floor of the frontal fossa in the region of the ethmoid sinuses often creates lacerations.[17] Intradural repair is accomplished using a graft (fascia lata is most desirable; periosteum is thinner but is often acceptable) which is held in place with sutures and must extend all the way back to the ridge of the sphenoid wing (fibrin glue may be a helpful adjunct).

57 A periosteal flap is placed across the floor of the frontal fossa to help isolate the dura from the frontal sinus and to prevent CSF fistula.

Dealing with frontal sinus

✖ Simple packing of the sinus (with bone wax, Gelfoam®, muscle or fat) increases the possibility of infection or mucocele formation.

The rear wall of the sinus is removed (so-called cranialization of the frontal sinus). The sinus is then exenterated (mucosa is stripped from sinus wall down to the nasofrontal duct, the mucosa is inverted over itself in the region of the duct and is packed down into the duct, temporalis muscle plugs are then packed into the frontonasal ducts[16]), then the bony wall of the sinus is drilled with a diamond burr to remove tiny remnants of mucosa found in the surface of bone that may proliferate and form a mucocele.[14] If there is any remnant of sinus, it may then be packed with abdominal fat that fills all corners of the cavity. Post-op risks related to frontal sinus injury include: infection, mucocele formation and CSF leak.

57.5.2 LeFort fractures

Complex fractures through inherently weak "cleavage planes" resulting in an unstable segment ("floating face"). Shown in ► Fig. 57.1 (usually occur as variants of this basic scheme).

- LeFort I: *transverse* AKA transmaxillary fracture. Fracture line crosses pterygoid plate and maxilla just above the apices of the upper teeth. May enter maxillary sinus(es)
- LeFort II: *pyramidal*. Fracture extends upward across inferior orbital rim and orbital floor to medial orbital wall, then across nasofrontal suture. Often from downward blow to the nasal area
- LeFort III: *craniofacial dislocation*. Involves zygomatic arches, zygomaticofrontal suture, nasofrontal suture, pterygoid plates, and orbital floors (separating maxilla from cranium). Requires significant force, therefore often associated with other injuries, including brain injuries

57.6 Pneumocephalus

57.6.1 General information

AKA (intra)cranial aerocele, AKA pneumatocele, is defined as the presence of intracranial gas. It is critical to distinguished this from tension pneumocephalus which is gas under pressure (see below). The gas may be located in any of the following compartments: epidural, subdural, subarachnoid, intraparenchymal, intraventricular.

57.6.2 Etiologies of pneumocephalus

Anything that can cause a CSF leak can produce associated pneumocephalus (p. 386).

1. skull defects
   a) post neurosurgical procedure
      - craniotomy: risk is higher when patient is operated with surgery in the sitting position[18]
      - shunt insertion[19,20]
      - burr-hole drainage of chronic subdural hematoma[21,22]: incidence is probably < 2.5%[22] although higher rates have been reported
   b) posttraumatic
      - fracture through air sinus (frontal, ethmoid…): including basal skull fracture
      - open fracture over convexity (usually with dural laceration)
   c) congenital skull defects: including defect in tegmen tympani[23]
   d) neoplasm (osteoma,[24] epidermoid,[25] pituitary tumor): usually caused by tumor erosion through floor of sella into sphenoid sinus
2. infection
   a) with gas-producing organisms
   b) mastoiditis

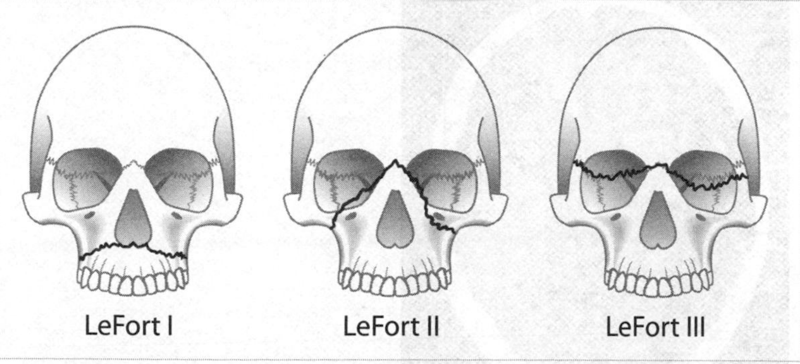

Fig. 57.1 LeFort fractures

3. post invasive procedure:
   a) lumbar puncture
   b) ventriculostomy
   c) spinal anesthesia[26]
4. spinal trauma (LP could be included here as well)
5. barotrauma[27]: e.g. with scuba diving (possibly through a defect in the tegmen tympani)
6. may be potentiated by a CSF drainage device in the presence of a CSF leak[28]

57.6.3 Presentation

H/A in 38%, N/V, seizures, dizziness, and obtundation.[29] An intracranial succussion splash is a rare (occurring in ≈ 7%) but pathognomonic finding. Tension pneumocephalus may additionally cause signs and symptoms just as any mass (may cause focal deficit or increased ICP).

57.6.4 Differential diagnosis (things that can mimic pneumocephalus)

Although intracranial low-density on CT may be associated with epidermoid, lipoma, or CSF, nothing is as intensely black as air. This can often be better appreciated on bone-windows than on soft-tissue windows.

57.6.5 Tension pneumocephalus

Intracranial gas can develop elevated pressure in the following settings:
1. when nitrous oxide anesthesia is not discontinued prior to closure of the dura[30]; see nitrous oxide, N_2O (p. 105)
2. when a "ball-valve" effect occurs due to an opening to the intracranial compartment with soft tissue (e.g. brain) that may permit air to enter but prevent exit of air or CSF
3. when trapped room temperature air expands with warming to body temperature: a modest increase of only ≈ 4% results from this effect[31]
4. in the presence of continued production by gas-producing organisms

57.6.6 Diagnosis

Pneumocephalus is most easily diagnosed on CT[32] which can detect quantities of air as low as 0.5 ml. Air appears dark black (darker than CSF) and has a Hounsfield coefficient of –1000. One characteristic finding with bilateral pneumocephalus is the Mt. Fuji sign in which the two frontal poles appear peaked and are surrounded by and separated by air, resembling the silhouette of the twin peaks of Mt. Fuji[22] (see ▸ Fig. 57.2). Intracranial gas may also be evident on plain skull x-rays.

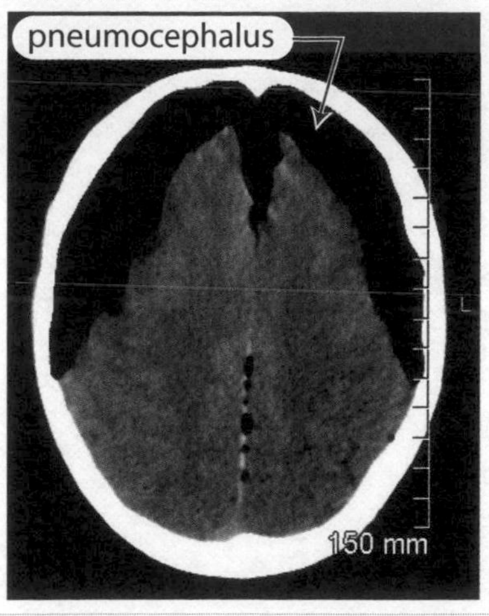

Fig. 57.2 Mt. Fuji sign with bilateral pneumocephalus. Axial noncontrast CT scan

57

Since simple pneumocephalus usually does not require treatment, it is critical to differentiate it from tension pneumocephalus, which may need to be evacuated if symptomatic. It may be quite difficult to distinguish the two; brain that has been compressed e.g. by a chronic subdural hematoma may not expand immediately post-op and the "gas gap" may mimic the appearance of gas under pressure.

57.6.7 Treatment

When pneumocephalus is due to gas-producing organisms, treatment of the primary infection is initiated and the pneumocephalus is usually followed.

Treatment of non-infectious simple pneumocephalus depends on the whether or not the presence of a CSF leak is suspected. If there is no leak the gas will be resorbed with time, and if the mass effect is not severe it may simply be followed. If a CSF leak is suspected, management is as with any CSF fistula, see CSF fistula (cranial) (p. 384).

Treatment of significant or symptomatic post-op pneumocephalus by breathing 100% O_2 via a nonrebreather mask increases the rate of resorption[33] (100% FiO_2 can be tolerated for 24–48 hours without serious pulmonary toxicity[34]).

Tension pneumocephalus producing significant symptoms must be evacuated. The urgency is similar to that of an intracranial hematoma. Dramatic and rapid improvement may occur with the release of gas under pressure. Options include placement of new twist drill or burr holes, or insertion of a spinal needle through a pre-existing burr hole (e.g. following a craniotomy).

References

[1] Mealey J, Section of Pediatric Neurosurgery of the American Association of Neurological Surgeons. In: Skull Fractures. Pediatric Neurosurgery. 1st ed. New York: Grune and Stratton; 1982:289–299

[2] Bullock MR, Chesnut RM, Ghajar J, et al. Surgical management of depressed cranial fractures. Neurosurgery. 2006; 58:S56–S60

[3] Jennett B. Epilepsy after Non-Missile Head Injuries. 2nd ed. London: William Heinemann; 1975

[4] Raffel C, Litofsky NS, Cheek WR, Marlin AE, McLone DG, Reigel DH, Walker ML, American Society of Pediatric Neurosurgeons Section of Pediatric Neurosurgery of the A.A.N.S.. In: Skull fractures. Pediatric Neurosurgery: Surgery of the Developing Nervous System. 3rd ed. Philadelphia: W.B. Saunders; 1994:257–265

[5] Kapp JP, Gielchinsky I, Deardourff SL. Operative Techniques for Management of Lesions Involving the Dural Venous Sinuses. Surg Neurol. 1977; 7:339–342

[6] Buckingham MJ, Crone KR, Ball WS, Tomsick TA, Berger TS, Tew JM. Traumatic Intracranial Aneurysms in Childhood: Two Cases and a Review of the Literature. Neurosurgery. 1988; 22:398–408

[7] Esslen E, Miehlke A. In: Electrodiagnosis of Facial Palsy. Surgery of the Facial Nerve. 2nd ed. Philadelphia: W. B. Saunders; 1973:45–51

[8] Feiz-Erfan I, Ferreira MAT, Rekate HL, Petersen SR. Longitudinal clival fracture: A lethal injury survived. BNI Quarterly. 2001; 17

[9] Meguro K, Rowed DW. Traumatic aneurysm of the posterior inferior cerebellar artery caused by fracture of the clivus. Neurosurgery. 1985; 16:666–668

[10] Seebacher J, Nozik D, Mathieu A. Inadvertend Intracranial Introduction of a Nasogastric Tube. A Complication of Severe Maxillofacial Trauma. Anesthesia. 1975; 42:100–102

[11] Wyler AR, Reynolds AF. An Intracranial Complication of Nasogastric Intubation: Case Report. J Neurosurg. 1977; 47:297–298

[12] Baskaya MK. Inadvertend Intracranial Placement of a Nasogastric Tube in Patients with Head Injuries. Surg Neurol. 1999; 52:426–427

[13] Benoit BG, Wortzman G. Traumatic Cerebral Aneurysms: Clinical Features and Natural History. J Neurol Neurosurg Psychiatry. 1973; 36:127–138

[14] Donald PJ. The Tenacity of the Frontal Sinus Mucosa. Otolaryngol Head Neck Surg. 1979; 87:557–566

[15] El-Bary THA. Neurosurgical Management of the Frontal Sinus. Surg Neurol. 1995; 44:80–81

[16] Robinson J, Donald PJ, Pitts LH, Wagner FC. In: Management of Associated Cranial Lesions. Craniospinal Trauma. New York: Thieme Medical Publishers, Inc.; 1990:59–87

[17] Lewin W. Cerebrospinal Fluid Rhinorrhea in Closed Head Injuries. Br J Surgery. 1954; 17:1–18

[18] Lunsford LD, Maroon JC, Sheptak PE, et al. Subdural Tension Pneumocephalus: Report of Two Cases. J Neurosurg. 1979; 50:525–527

[19] Little JR, MacCarty CS. Tension Pneumocephalus After Insertion of Ventriculoperitoneal Shunt for Aqueductal Stenosis: Case Report. J Neurosurg. 1976; 44:383–385

[20] Pitts LH, Wilson CB, Dedo HH, Anderson RE. Pneumocephalus Following Ventriculoperitoneal Shunt: Case Report. J Neurosurg. 1975; 43:631–633

[21] Caron J-L, Worthington C, Bertrand G. Tension Pneumocephalus After Evacuation of Chronic Subdural Hematoma and Subsequent Treatment with Continuous Lumbar Subarachnoid Infusion and Craniostomy Drainage. Neurosurgery. 1985; 16:107–110

[22] Ishiwata Y, Fujitsu K, Sekino T, et al. Subdural Tension Pneumocephalus Following Surgery for Chronic Subdural Hematoma. J Neurosurg. 1988; 68:58–61

[23] Dowd GC, Molony TB, Voorhies RM. Spontaneous Otogenic Pneumocephalus: Case Report and Review of the Literature. J Neurosurg. 1998; 89:1036–1039

[24] Mendelsohn DB, Hertzanu Y, Friedman R. Frontal Osteoma with Spontaneous Subdural and Intracerebral Pneumatacele. J Laryngol Otol. 1984; 98:543–545

[25] Clark JB, Six EG. Epidermoid Tumor Presenting as Tension Pneumocephalus. J Neurosurg. 1984; 60:1312–1314

[26] Roderick L, Moore DC, Artru AA. Pneumocephalus with Headache During Spinal Anesthesia. Anesthesiology. 1985; 62:690–692

[27] Goldmann RW. Pneumocephalus as a Consequence of Barotrauma: Case Report. JAMA. 1986; 255:3154–3156

[28] Black PM, Davis JM, Kjellberg RN, et al. Tension Pneumocephalus of the Cranial Subdural Space: A Case Report. Neurosurgery. 1979; 5:368–370

[29] Markham TJ. The Clinical Features of Pneumocephalus Based on a Survey of 284 Cases with Report of 11 Additional Cases. Acta Neurochir. 1967; 15:1–78

[30] Raggio JF, Fleischer AS, Sung YF, et al. Expanding Pneumocephalus due to Nitrous Oxide Anesthesia: Case Report. Neurosurgery. 1979; 4:261–263
[31] Raggio JF. Comment on Black P M, et al.: Tension Pneumocephalus of the Cranial Subdural Space: A Case Report. Neurosurgery. 1979; 5
[32] Osborn AG, Daines JH, Wing SD, et al. Intracranial Air on Computerized Tomography. J Neurosurg. 1978; 48:355–359
[33] Gore PA, Maan H, Chang S, Pitt AM, Spetzler RF, Nakaji P. Normobaric oxygen therapy strategies in the treatment of postcraniotomy pneumocephalus. J Neurosurg. 2008; 108:926–929
[34] Klein J. Normobaric pulmonary oxygen toxicity. Anesth Analg. 1990; 70:195–207

58 Traumatic Hemorrhagic Conditions

58.1 Posttraumatic parenchymal injuries

58.1.1 Cerebral edema

Surgical decompression is occasionally an option; see **Practice guideline: Posttraumatic cerebral edema** (p. 891).

Practice guideline: Posttraumatic cerebral edema

Indications and timing for surgery

Level III[1]: bifrontal decompressive craniectomy within 48 hrs of injury is a treatment option for patients with diffuse, medically refractory posttraumatic cerebral edema and associated IC-HTN

58.1.2 Diffuse injuries

Patients with severe diffuse injuries occasionally may be considered for decompressive craniectomy; see **Practice guideline: Diffuse injuries** (p. 891).

Practice guideline: Diffuse injuries

Indications for surgery

Level III[1]: decompressive craniectomy is an option for patients with refractory IC-HTN and diffuse parenchymal injury with clinical and radiographic evidence for impending transtentorial herniation

58.2 Hemorrhagic contusion

58.2.1 General information

AKA traumatic intracerebral hemorrhage (TICH). The definition is not uniformly agreed upon. Often considered as high density areas on CT (some exclude areas < 1 cm diameter[2]). TICH usually produce much less mass effect than their apparent size. Most commonly occur in areas where sudden deceleration of the head causes the brain to impact on bony prominences (e.g. temporal, frontal and occipital poles) in coup or contrecoup fashion.

TICH often enlarge and/or coalesce with time as seen on serial CTs. They also may appear in a delayed fashion (below). Surrounding low density may represent associated cerebral edema. CT scans months later often show surprisingly minimal or no encephalomalacia.

58.2.2 Treatment

Practice guideline: Surgical management of TICH

- Level III[1]: Indications for surgical evacuation for TICH:
  - progressive neurological deterioration referable to the TICH, medically refractory IC-HTN, or signs of mass effect on CT
  - or TICH volume > 50 cm^3 cc or ml
  - or GCS = 6–8 with frontal or temporal TICH volume > 20 cm^3 with midline shift (MLS) ≥ 5 mm (p. 921) and/or compressed basal cisterns on CT (p. 921)
- nonoperative management with intensive monitoring and serial imaging: may be used for TICH without neurologic compromise and no significant mass effect on CT and controlled ICP

58

58.2.3 Delayed traumatic intracerebral hemorrhage (DTICH)

TICH demonstrated in patients on imaging that was not evident on initial admitting CT scan.

Incidence of DTICH in patients with GCS ≤ 8: ≈ 10%[3,4] (reported incidence varies with resolution of CT scanner,[5] timing of scan, and definition). Most DTICH occur within 72 hrs of the trauma.[4] Some patients seem to be doing well and then present with an apoplectic event (although DTICH accounted only for 12% of patients who "talk and deteriorate"[6]).

Factors that contribute to formation of DTICH include local or systemic coagulopathy, hemorrhage into an area of necrotic brain softening, coalescence of extravasated microhematomas.[7]

Treatment is the same as for TICH (see above).

Outcome for patients with DTICH described in the literature is generally poor, with a mortality ranging from 50–75%.[7]

58.3 Epidural hematoma

58.3.1 General information

Incidence of epidural hematoma (EDH): 1% of head trauma admissions (which is ≈ 50% the incidence of acute subdurals). Ratio of male:female = 4:1. Usually occurs in young adults, and is rare before age 2 yrs or after age 60 (perhaps because the dura is more adherent to the inner table in these groups).

Dogma was that a temporoparietal skull fracture disrupts the middle meningeal artery as it exits its bony groove to enter the skull at the pterion, causing arterial bleeding that gradually dissects the dura from the inner table resulting in a delayed deterioration. Alternate hypothesis: dissection of the dura from the inner table occurs first, followed by bleeding into the space thus created.

Source of bleeding: 85% = arterial bleeding (the middle meningeal artery is the most common source of middle fossa EDHs). Many of the remainder of cases are due to bleeding from middle meningeal vein or dural sinus.

70% occur laterally over the hemispheres with their epicenter at the pterion, the rest occur in the frontal, occipital, and posterior fossa (5–10% each).

58.3.2 Presentation with EDH

"Textbook" presentation (< 10%-27% have this classic presentation[8]):
- brief posttraumatic loss of consciousness (LOC): **from initial impact**
- followed by a "lucid interval" for several hours
- then, obtundation, contralateral hemiparesis, ipsilateral pupillary dilatation as a result of mass effect from hematoma

Deterioration usually occurs over a few hours, but may take days and rarely, weeks (longer intervals may be associated with venous bleeding).

Other presenting findings: H/A, vomiting, seizure (may be unilateral), hemi-hyperreflexia + unilateral Babinski sign, and elevated CSF pressure (LP is seldom used any longer). Bradycardia is usually a late finding. In peds, EDH should be suspected if there is a 10% drop in hematocrit after admission.

Contralateral hemiparesis is not uniformly seen, especially with EDH in locations other than laterally over the hemisphere. Shift of the brain stem away from the mass may produce compression of the opposite cerebral peduncle on tentorial notch which can produce ipsilateral hemiparesis (so called Kernohan's phenomenon or Kernohan's notch phenomenon),[9] a false localizing sign.

58

60% of patients with EDH have a dilated pupil, 85% of which are *ipsilateral*.

No initial loss of consciousness occurs in 60%. No lucid interval in 20%. NB: a lucid interval may also be seen in other conditions (including subdural hematoma).

58.3.3 Differential diagnosis

- subdural hematoma
- a posttraumatic disorder described by Denny-Brown consisting of a "lucid interval" followed by bradycardia, brief periods of restlessness and vomiting, without intracranial hypertension or mass. Children especially may have H/A, and may become drowsy and confused. Theory: a form of vagal syncope. CT must be done to rule-out EDH.

58.3.4 Evaluation

Plain skull x-rays

Usually not helpful. No fracture is identified in 40% of EDH. In these cases the patient's age was almost always < 30 yrs.

CT scan in EDH

"Classic" CT appearance occurs in 84% of cases: high density biconvex (lenticular) shape adjacent to the skull. In 11% the side against the skull is convex and that along the brain is straight, and in 5% it is crescent shaped (resembling subdural hematoma).[10] An EDH may cross the falx (distinct from SDH which is limited to one side of the falx) but is usually limited by skull sutures. EDH usually has uniformly density, sharply defined edges on multiple cuts, high attenuation (undiluted blood), contiguous with inner table, usually confined to small segment of calvaria. Mass effect is frequent. Occasionally, an epidural may be isodense with brain and may not show up unless IV contrast is given.[10] Mottling of density has been described as a finding in hyperacute EDH.[11]

58.3.5 Mortality with EDH

Overall: 20–55% (higher rates in older series). Optimal diagnosis and treatment within few hours results in 5–10% estimated mortality (12% in a recent CT era series[12]). Mortality without lucid interval double that with. Bilateral Babinski's or decerebration pre-op → worse prognosis. Death is usually due to respiratory arrest from uncal herniation causing injury to the midbrain.

20% of patients with EDH on CT also have ASDH at autopsy or operation. Mortality with both lesions concurrently is higher, reported range: 25–90%.

58.3.6 Treatment of EDH

Medical

CT may detect small EDHs and can be used to follow them. However, in most cases, EDH is a surgical condition (below).

Nonsurgical management may be attempted in the following:

Small (≤ 1 cm maximal thickness) subacute or chronic EDH,[13] with minimal neurological signs/symptoms (e.g. slight lethargy, H/A) and no evidence of herniation. Although medical management of p-fossa EDHs has been reported, these are more dangerous and surgery is recommended.

In 50% of cases there will be a slight transient increase in size between days 5–16, and some patients required emergency craniotomy when for signs of herniation occurred.[14]

Management

Management includes: admit, observe (in monitored bed if possible). Optional: steroids for several days, then taper. Follow-up CT: in 1 wk if clinically stable. Repeat in 1–3 mos if patient becomes asymptomatic (to document resolution). Prompt surgery if signs of local mass effect, signs of herniation (increasing drowsiness, pupil changes, hemiparesis…) or cardiorespiratory abnormalities.

Surgical

Surgical indications and timing

See also more details (p. 893). EDH in pediatric patients is riskier than adults since there is less room for clot. The threshold for surgery in pediatrics should be very low.

58

Practice guideline: Surgical management of EDH

Indications for surgery

Level III[15]:

1. EDH volume > 30 cm³ should be evacuated regardless of GCS
2. EDH with the all of the following characteristics can be managed nonsurgically with serial CT scans and close neurological observation in a neurosurgical center:
   a) volume < 30 cm³
   b) and thickness < 15 mm

c) and with midline shift (MLS) < 5 mm (p. 921)
d) and GCS > 8
e) and no focal neurologic deficit

Timing of surgery

Level III[15]: it is strongly recommended that patients with an acute EDH and GCS < 9 and anisocoria undergo surgical evacuation ASAP

(Note: Volume of a lens = 1.6 to 2 × r^2t = 0.4 to 0.5 × d^2t ≈ (A × B × T)/2 as in an ellipsoid, 1/2 the products of the height times the AP diameter and the thickness T. For a 1.5 cm thick EDH to be < 30 cc it would have to have a diameter (not radius) < 6.3-7 cm. For a 1 cm thick EDH to be < 30 cc, it would have to have a diameter < 7.7 – 8.6 cm.)

Booking the case: Craniotomy for acute EDH/SDH

Also see defaults & disclaimers (p. 27).

1. position: (depends on location of bleed, usually supine)
2. blood: type & screen (for severe SDH: T & C 2 U PRBC)
3. post-op: ICU
4. consent (in lay terms for the patient – not all-inclusive):
   a) procedure: surgery through the skull to remove blood clot, stop any bleeding identified, possible placement of intracranial pressure monitor
   b) alternatives: nonsurgical management
   c) complications: usual craniotomy complications (p. 28) plus further bleeding which may cause problems (especially in patients taking blood thinners, antiplatelet drugs including aspirin, or those with coagulation abnormalities or previous bleeds) and may require further surgery, any permanent brain injury that has already occurred is not likely to recover, hydrocephalus

Surgical technical issues

Evacuation is performed in the O.R. unless the patient herniates in E/R and access to OR is not within acceptable timeframe. Objectives:

1. clot removal: lowers ICP and eliminates focal mass effect. Blood is usually thick coagulum, thus exposure must provide access to most of clot. Craniotomy permits more complete evacuation of hematoma than e.g. burr holes[15]
2. hemostasis: coagulate bleeding soft tissue (dural veins & arteries). Apply bone wax to intra-diploic bleeders (e.g. middle meningeal artery). Also requires large exposure
3. prevent reaccumulation: (some bleeding may recur, and dura is now detached from inner table) place dural tack-up sutures to edges of craniotomy and use central "tenting" suture

58.3.7 Special cases of epidural hematome

Delayed epidural hematoma (DEDH)

58

Definition: an EDH that is not present on the initial CT scan, but is found on subsequent CT. Comprise 9–10% of all EDHs in several series.[16,17]

Theoretical risk factors for DEDH include the following (NB: many of these risk factors may be incurred *after* the patient is admitted following a negative initial CT):

1. lowering ICP either medically (e.g. osmotic diuretics) and/or surgically (e.g. evacuating contralateral hematoma) which reduces tamponading effect
2. rapidly correcting shock (hemodynamic "surge" may cause DEDH)[18]
3. coagulopathies

Observation agrees with what one would predict based on the above in that DEDH tend to occur in patients with severe head injury and associated systemic injuries. However, DEDH have been reported in *mild* head injury (GCS > 12) infrequently.[19] Presence of a skull fracture has been identified as a common feature of DEDH.[19]

Key to diagnosis: high index of suspicion. Avoid a false sense of security imparted by an initial "nonsurgical" CT. 6 of 7 patients in one series improved or remained unchanged neurologically despite enlarging EDH (most eventually deteriorate). 1 of 5 with an ICP monitor did not have a heralding increase in ICP. May develop once an intracranial lesion is surgically treated, as occurred in 5 of 7 patients within 24 hrs of evacuation of another EDH. 6 of 7 patients had known skull fractures in the region where the delayed EDH developed,[17] but none of 3 had a skull fracture in another report.[18]

Posterior fossa epidural hematoma

Comprise ≈ 5% of EDH.[20,21] More common in 1st two decades of life. Although as many as 84% have occipital skull fractures, only ≈ 3% of children with occipital skull fractures develop p-fossa EDH. The source of bleeding is usually not found, but there is a high incidence of tears of the dural sinuses. Cerebellar signs are surprisingly lacking or subtle in most. See surgical indications (p. 905). Overall mortality is ≈ 26% (mortality was higher in patients with an associated intracranial lesion).

58.4 Acute subdural hematoma

58.4.1 General information

The magnitude of **impact damage**, as opposed to secondary damage (p. 824), is usually much higher in acute subdural hematoma (ASDH) than in epidural hematomas, which generally makes this lesion much more lethal. There is often associated underlying brain injury, which may be less common with EDH. Symptoms may be due to compression of the underlying brain with midline shift, in addition to parenchymal brain injury and possibly cerebral edema.[22,23]

Two common causes of traumatic ASDH:

1. accumulation around parenchymal laceration (usually frontal or temporal lobe). There is usually severe underlying primary brain injury. Often no "lucid interval." Focal signs usually occur later and are less prominent than with EDH
2. surface or bridging vessel torn from cerebral acceleration-deceleration during violent head motion. With this etiology, primary brain damage may be less severe, a lucid interval may occur with later rapid deterioration

ASDH may also occur in patients receiving anticoagulation therapy,[24,25] usually with, but sometimes without, a history of trauma (the trauma may be minor). Receiving anticoagulation therapy increases the risk of ASDH 7-fold in males and 26-fold in females.[24]

58.4.2 CT scan in ASDH

Crescentic mass of increased density adjacent to inner table. Edema is often present.

Locations:

- Usually over convexity
- Interhemispheric
- Layering on tentorium
- in p-fossa

Changes with time on CT (see ▶ Table 58.1):isodense after ≈ 2 wks, only clues may be obliteration of sulci and lateralizing shift, the latter may be absent if bilateral. Subsequently becomes hypodense to brain (p. 898). Membrane formation begins by about 4 days after injury.[26]

Table 58.1 ASDH density changes on CT with time

Category	Time frame	Density on CT
acute	1 to 3 days	hyperdense
subacute	4 days to 2 or 3 wks	≈ isodense
chronic	usually > 3 wks and < 3–4 mos	hypodense (approaching density of CSF)
	after about 1–2 months	may become lenticular shaped (similar to epidural hematoma) with density > CSF, < fresh blood

Differences from EDH: SDH is more diffuse, less uniform, usually *concave* over brain surface, often less dense (from mixing with CSF), and bridging subdural veins (from brain surface to the skull) may be seen (cortical vein sign).

58.4.3 Treatment

Indications for surgery

Level III surgical indications are shown in **Practice guideline: Surgical management of ASDH** (p. 896). Other factors that should be considered:

1. presence of anticoagulants or platelet inhibitors: patients in good neurologic condition may be better served by reversing these agents prior to operating (to increase the safety of surgery)
2. location of hematoma: in general, a SDH high over the convexity is less threatening than a temporal/parietal SDH of the same volume that also has MLS
3. patient's baseline level of function, DNR status…
4. while the guidelines suggest evacuating SDH < 10 mm thick in some circumstances, clots that are smaller than this may not be causing problems but may simply be an epiphenomenon

Practice guideline: Surgical management of ASDH

Indications for surgery

Level III[27]:

1. ASDH with thickness > 10 mm or midline shift (MLS) > 5 mm (on CT) should be evacuated regardless of GCS
2. ASDH with thickness < 10 mm and MLS < 5 mm (see text regarding the evacuation of ASDH < 10 mm thick) should undergo surgical evacuation if:
   a) GCS drops by ≥ 2 points from injury to admission
   b) and/or the pupils are asymmetric or fixed and dilated
   c) and/or ICP is > 20 mm Hg
3. monitor ICP in all patients with ASDH and GCS < 9

Timing of surgery

Level III[27]: ASDH meeting surgical criteria should be evacuated ASAP (for issues regarding timing of surgery, see text)

Surgical methods

Level III[27]: ASDH meeting the above criteria for surgery should be evacuated via craniotomy with or without bone flap removal and duraplasty (a large craniotomy flap is often required to evacuate the thick coagulum and to gain access to possible bleeding sites).

Timing of surgery

Timing of surgery for ASDH is a matter of controversy. As a general principle, when surgery for ASDH is indicated it should be done as soon as possible.

58

"Four hour rule"

This "rule" was based on a 1981 series of 82 patients with ASDH,[28] which held that:

1. patients operated within 4 hrs of injury had 30% mortality, compared to 90% mortality if surgery was delayed > 4 hrs
2. functional survival (Glasgow Outcome Scale ≥ 4, see ▶ Table 88.5) rate of 65% could be achieved with surgery within 4 hrs
3. other factors related to outcome in this series included:
   a) post-op ICP: 79% of patients with functional recovery had post-op ICPs that didn't exceed 20 mm Hg, whereas only 30% of patients who died had ICP < 20 mm Hg
   b) initial neuro exam
   c) age was *not* a factor in this study (ASDH tend to occur in older patients than EDH)

However, a subsequent study of 101 patients with ASDH found a delay to surgery (delays > 4 hours from the injury) showed a nonstatistically-significant trend where mortality increased from 59% to 69% and functional survival decreased (Glasgow Outcome Scale ≤ 4, see ▶ Table 88.5) from 26% to 16%.[29]

Booking the case: Acute subdural hematoma

Same as for acute epidural hematoma (p. 894).

Technical considerations

One may start with a small linear dural opening to effect clot removal and enlarge it as needed and only if brain swelling seems controllable. The actual bleeding site is often not identified at the time of surgery.

58.4.4 Morbidity and mortality with ASDH

Mortality Range: 50–90% (a significant percentage of this mortality is from the underlying brain injury, and not the ASDH itself).

Mortality is traditionally thought to be higher in aged patients (60%), and is 90–100% in patients on anticoagulants.[25]

In a series of 101 patients with ASDH, functional recovery was 19%.[29] Postoperative seizures occurred in 9%, and did not correlate with outcome. The following variables were identified as strongly influencing outcome:

- mechanism of injury: the worst outcome was with motorcycle accidents, with 100% mortality in unhelmeted patients, 33% in helmeted
- age: correlated with outcome only > 65 yrs age, with 82% mortality and 5% functional survival in this group (other series had similar results[30])
- neurologic condition on admission: the ratio of mortality to functional survival rate related to the admission Glasgow Coma Scale (**GCS**) is shown in ▶ Table 58.2
- postoperative ICP: patients with peak ICPs < 20 mm Hg had 40% mortality, and no patient with ICP > 45 had a functional survival

Of all the above factors, only the time to surgery and postoperative ICP can be directly influenced by the treating neurosurgeon.

58.4.5 Special cases of acute subdural hematoma

Interhemispheric subdural hematoma

General information

Subdural hematoma along the falx between the two cerebral hemispheres (older term: interhemispheric scissure).

May occur in children,[31] possibly associated with child abuse.[32]

In adults, a consequence of: head trauma in 79–91%, ruptured aneurysm[33] in ≈ 12%, surgery in the vicinity of the corpus callosum, and rarely spontaneously.[34]

Incidence is unknown. Spontaneous cases should be investigated for possible underlying aneurysm. Occasionally may be bilateral, sometimes may be delayed (see below)

Table 58.2 Outcome as related to admission GCS

Admission GCS	Mortality	Functional survival
3	90%	5%
4	76%	10%
5	62%	18%
6 & 7	51%	44%

Most often are asymptomatic, or may present with the so-called "falx syndrome" – paresis or focal seizures contralateral to the hematoma. Other presentations: gait ataxia, dementia, language disturbance, oculomotor palsies.

Treatment

Controversial. Small asymptomatic cases may be managed expectantly. Surgery should be considered for progressive neurological deterioration with larger lesions. Approached through a parasagittal craniotomy. ✖ Surgery for these lesions can be treacherous – there is risk of venous infarction and one often finds they are dealing with a superior sagittal sinus injury.

Outcome

Reported mortality: 25–42%. Mortality is higher in the presence of altered levels of consciousness. Mortality rate may actually be lower (24%) than with all-comers.[34] This is significantly lower than SDH in other sites (see above).

Delayed acute subdural hematoma (DASDH)

DASDHs have received less attention than delayed epidural or intraparenchymal hematomas. Incidence is ≈ 0.5% of operatively treated ASDHs.[7]

Definition: ASDH not present on an initial CT (or MRI) that shows up on a subsequent study. Indications for treatment are the same as for ASDH. Neurologically stable patients with a small DASDH and medically controllable ICP are managed expectantly.

Infantile acute subdural hematoma

General information

Infantile acute subdural hematoma (IASDH) is often considered as a special case of SDH. Roughly defined as an acute SDH in an infant due to minor head trauma without initial loss of consciousness or cerebral contusion,[35] possibly due to rupture of a bridging vein. The most common trauma is a fall backwards from sitting or standing. The infants will often cry immediately and then (usually within minutes to 1 hour) develop a generalized seizure. Patients are usually < 2 yrs old (most are 6–12 mos, the age when they first begin to pull themselves up or walk).[36]

These clots are rarely pure blood, and are often mixed with fluid. 75% are bilateral or have contralateral subdural fluid collections. It is speculated that IASDH may represent acute bleeding into a preexisting fluid collection.[36]

Skull fractures are rare. In one series, retinal and preretinal hemorrhages were seen in all 26 patients.[35]

Treatment

Treatment is guided by clinical condition and size of hematoma. Minimally symptomatic cases (vomiting, irritability, no altered level of consciousness and no motor disturbance) with liquefied hematoma may be treated with percutaneous subdural tap, which may be repeated several times as needed. Chronically persistent cases may require a subduroperitoneal shunt.

More symptomatic cases with high density clot on CT require craniotomy. A subdural membrane similar to those seen in adult chronic SDH is not unusual.[36] *Caution*: these patients are at risk of developing intraoperative hypovolemic shock.

Outcome

8% morbidity and mortality rate in one series.[35] Much better prognosis than ASDH of all ages probably because of the absence of cerebral contusion in IASDH.

58.5 Chronic subdural hematoma

58.5.1 General information

Originally termed "pachymeningitis hemorrhagica interna" by Virchow[37] in 1857. Chronic subdural hematomas (CSDH) generally occur in the elderly, with the average age being ≈ 63 yrs; exception: subdural collections of infancy (p. 903). Head trauma is identified in < 50% (sometimes rather trivial trauma can produce these lesions). Other risk factors: alcohol abuse, seizures, CSF shunts, coagulopathies (including therapeutic anticoagulation[25]), and patients at risk for falls (e.g. with hemiplegia from previous stroke). CSDHs are bilateral in ≈ 20–25% of cases.[38,39]

Hematoma thickness tends to be larger in older patients due to a decrease in brain weight and increase in subdural space with age.[40]

Classically CSDHs contains dark "motor oil" fluid which does not clot.[41] When the subdural fluid is clear (CSF), the collection is termed a subdural hygroma (p. 902).

58.5.2 Pathophysiology

Many CSDH probably start out as acute subdurals. Blood within the subdural space evokes an inflammatory response. Within days, fibroblasts invade the clot, and form neomembranes on the inner (cortical) and outer (dural) surface. This is followed by ingrowth of neocapillaries, enzymatic fibrinolysis, and liquefaction of blood clot. Fibrin degradation products are reincorporated into new clots and inhibit hemostasis. The course of CSDH is determined by the balance of plasma effusion and/or rebleeding from the neomembranes on the one hand and reabsorption of fluid on the other.[42,43]

58.5.3 Presentation

Patients may present with minor symptoms of headache, confusion, language difficulties (e.g. word-finding difficulties or speech arrest, usually with dominant hemisphere lesions), or TIA-like symptoms (p. 1398). Or, they may develop varying degrees of coma, hemiplegia, or seizures (focal, or less often generalized). Often, the diagnosis may be unexpected prior to imaging.

58.5.4 Treatment

Overall management

1. seizure prophylaxis: used by some. It may be safe to discontinue after a week or so if there are no seizure. If late seizure occurs with or without prior use of AEDs, longer-term therapy is required
2. coagulopathies (including iatrogenic anticoagulation) should be reversed
3. surgical evacuation of hematoma indications as follows
   a) symptomatic lesions: including focal deficit, mental status changes…
   b) or subdurals with maximum thickness greater than ≈ 1 cm
   c) or progressive increase in size on serial imaging (CT or MRI scans)

Surgical considerations

Booking the case: Craniotomy: for chronic subdural

Also see defaults & disclaimers (p. 27).
1. position: (usually supine), horseshoe headrest
2. post-op: ICU
3. consent (in lay terms for the patient – not all-inclusive):
   a) procedure: surgery through the skull to remove blood clot, stop any bleeding identified, placement a drainage tube to allow further fluid to drain after surgery for a day or so
   b) alternatives: nonsurgical management
   c) complications: usual craniotomy complications (p. 28) plus further bleeding which may cause problems (especially in patients taking blood thinners, antiplatelet drugs including aspirin, or those with coagulation abnormalities or previous bleeds) and may require further surgery, hydrocephalus

Surgical options

There is not uniform agreement on the best method to treat CSDHs. For details of techniques (burr holes, whether or not to use subdural drain…) see below.
1. placing two burr holes, and irrigating through and through with tepid saline until the fluid runs clear
2. single "large" burr hole with irrigation and aspiration: see below

3. single burr hole drainage with placement of a subdural drain, maintained for 24–48 hrs (removed when output becomes negligible)
4. twist drill craniostomy: see below (note that small "twist drill" drainage without subdural drain has higher recurrence rate than e.g. burr holes)
5. formal craniotomy with excision of subdural membrane (may be necessary in cases which persistently recur after above procedures, possibly due to seepage from the subdural membrane). Still a safe and valid technique.[44] *No* attempt should be made to remove the deep membrane adherent to the surface of brain

Techniques that promote continued drainage after the immediate procedure and that may thus reduce residual fluid and prevent reaccumulation:
1. use of a subdural drain: (see below)
2. using a generous burr hole under the temporalis muscle: (see below)
3. bed-rest restriction with the head of the bed flat (1 pillow is permitted) with mild overhydration for 24–48 hours post-op (or if a drain is used, until 24–48 hours after it is removed). May promote expansion of the brain and expulsion of residual subdural fluid. Allowing patients to sit up to 30–40° immediately post-op was associated with higher radiographic recurrence rate (2.3% for those kept flat, vs. 19% for those who sat up) but usually did not require reoperation[45]
4. some advocate continuous lumbar subarachnoid infusion when the brain fails to expand, however there are possible complications[46]

Twist drill craniostomy for chronic subdurals

This method is thought to decompress the brain more slowly and avoids the presumed rapid pressure shifts that occurs following other methods, which may be associated with complications such as intraparenchymal (intracerebral) hemorrhage. May even be performed at the bedside under local anesthesia.

A 0.5 cm incision is made in the scalp in the rostral portion of the hematoma, and then a twist drill hole is placed at a 45° angle to the skull, aimed in the direction of the longitudinal axis of the collection. If the drill does not penetrate the dura, this is done with an 18 Ga. spinal needle. A ventricular catheter is inserted into the subdural space, and is drained to a standard ventriculostomy drainage bag maintained 20 cm *below* the level of the craniostomy site[47,48,49] (below). The patient is kept flat in bed (see above). Serial CTs assess the adequacy of drainage. The catheter is removed when at least ≈ 20% of the collection is drained and when the patient shows signs of improvement, which occurs within a range of 1–7 days (mean of 2.1 days). Some include a low pressure shunt valve in the system to prevent reflux of fluid or air.

Burr holes for chronic subdural hematomas

To prevent recurrence, the use of *small* burr holes (without a subdural drain) is not recommended. A generous (> 2.5 cm diameter – it is recommended that one actually measure this) subtemporal craniectomy should be performed, and bipolar coagulation is used to shrink the edges of the dura and subdural membrane back to the full width of the bony opening (do not try to separate these two layers as this may promote bleeding). This allows continued drainage of fluid into the temporalis muscle where it may be resorbed. A piece of Gelfoam® may be placed over the opening to help prevent fresh blood from oozing into the opening.

Subdural drain

Use of a subdural drain is associated with a decrease in need for repeat surgery from 19% to 10%.[50] If a subdural drain is used, a closed drainage system is recommended. Difficulties may occur with ventriculostomy catheters because the holes are small and are restricted to the tip region (so-designed to keep choroid plexus from plugging the catheter when inserted into the ventricles when used as intended as a CSF shunt), especially with thick "oily" fluid (on the positive side, slow drainage may be desirable). The drainage bag is maintained ≈ 50–80 cm below the level of the head.[49,51] An alternative is a small Jackson-Pratt® drain using "thumb-print" indentation of the suction bulb which provides good drainage with a self-contained one-way valve (however, there may be a risk of excessive negative pressure with overcompression of the bulb).

Post-op, the patient is kept flat (see above). Prophylactic antibiotics may be given until ≈ 24–48 hrs following removal of the drain, at which time the HOB is gradually elevated. CT scan prior to removal of the drain (or shortly after removal) may be helpful to establish a baseline for later comparison in the event of deterioration.

There is a case report of administration of urokinase through a subdural drain to treat reaccumulation of clot following evacuation.[52]

58.5.5 Outcome

General information

There is clinical improvement when the subdural pressure is reduced to close to zero, which usually occurs after ≈ 20% of the collection is removed.[49]

Patients who have high subdural fluid pressure tend to have more rapid brain expansion and clinical improvement than patients with low pressures.[51]

Residual subdural fluid collections after treatment are common, but clinical improvement does not require complete resolution of the fluid collection on CT. CTs showed persistent fluid in 78% of cases on post-op day 10, and in 15% after 40 days,[51] and may take up to 6 months for complete resolution. Recommendation: do *not* treat persistent fluid collections evident on CT (especially before ≈ 20 days post-op) unless it increases in size on CT or if the patient shows no recovery or deteriorates.

76% of 114 patients were successfully treated with a single drainage procedure using a twist drill craniostomy with subdural ventricular catheter, and 90% with one or two procedures.[47] These statistics are slightly better than twist drill craniostomy with aspiration alone (i.e. no drain).

Complications of surgical treatment

Although these collections often appear innocuous, severe complications may occur, including:

1. seizures (including intractable status epilepticus)
2. intracerebral hemorrhage (ICH): occurs in 0.7–5%.[53] Very devastating in this setting: one-third of these patients die and one third are severely disabled (also, see below)
3. failure of the brain to re-expand and/or reaccumulation of the subdural fluid
4. tension pneumocephalus
5. subdural empyema: may also occur with untreated subdurals[54]

In 60% of patients ≥ age 75 yrs (and in no patients < 75 yrs), rapid decompression is associated with hyperemia in the cortex immediately beneath the hematoma, which may be related to the complications of ICH or seizures.[53] All complications are more common in elderly or debilitated patients.

Overall mortality with surgical treatment for CSDH is 0–8%.[53] In a series of 104 patients treated mostly with craniostomy,[55] mortality was ≈ 4%, all of which occurred in patients > 60 yrs old and were due to accompanying disease. Another large personal series reported 0.5% mortality.[56] Worsening of neurologic status following drainage occurs in ≈ 4%.[55]

58.6 Spontaneous subdural hematoma

58.6.1 General information

Occasionally patients with no identifiable trauma will present with severe H/A with or without associated findings (nausea, seizures, lethargy, focal findings including possible ipsilateral hemiparesis[57]...) and CT or MRI discloses a subdural hematoma that may be acute, subacute or chronic in appearance. The onset of symptoms is often sudden.[57]

58.6.2 Risk factors

Risk factors identified in a review of 21 cases in the literature[58] include:

1. hypertension: present in 7 cases
2. vascular abnormalities: arteriovenous malformation (AVM), aneurysm[59]
3. neoplasm
4. infection: including meningitis, tuberculosis
5. substance abuse: alcoholism, cocaine[60]
6. hypovitaminosis: especially vitamin C deficiency[37]
7. coagulopathies, including:
   a) iatrogenic (anticoagulation e.g. with warfarin)
   b) Ginkgo biloba (GB) extract: EGb761 and LI1379. Contains ginkgolides (especially Type B) which are inhibitors of platelet activating factor (PAF) at high concentrations,[61] also cause

vasodilation and decreased blood viscosity. There have been case reports showing temporal relationship of hemorrhage to intake of GB,[62] especially at higher doses over long periods of time. However, no consistent alteration was demonstrable in 29 measurable coagulation/clotting variables after 7 days[63] (bleeding time was mildly prolonged in some case reports[62,64]). Some individuals may possibly be more susceptible to the supplement, and there may be as-yet uncharacterized interactions with other entities (such as alcohol, aspirin...) but studies so far have been unrevealing[65]

c) factor XIII deficiency (protransglutaminase).[66,67] In peds: history may include report of bleeding from umbilical cord at birth. Check factor XIII levels as coagulation parameters may be normal or only slightly elevated

8. seemingly innocuous insults (e.g. bending over) or injuries resulting in no direct trauma to the head (e.g. whiplash injuries)
9. intracranial hypotension: spontaneous, after epidural anesthesia, lumbar puncture, or VP shunt[68,69]

58.6.3 Etiology

The bleeding site was determined in 14 of the 21 cases, and was *arterial* in each, typically involving a cortical branch of the MCA in the area of the sylvian fissure[58] where there is a large number of branches to a wide cortical area.

Possible mechanisms for arterial rupture in idiopathic acute subdural hematoma (ASDH) include tears occur secondary to sudden head movements or trivial head trauma of the following[70,71]:

1. small artery at perpendicular branch point off a cortical artery
2. small artery connecting the dura and cortex
3. adhesions between cortical artery and dura

58.6.4 Treatment

As for traumatic SDH. If symptomatic and/or > ≈ 1 cm thick, surgical evacuation is the treatment of choice. For subacute to chronic subdurals, burr-hole evacuation is usually adequate (see above). For acute SDH, a craniotomy is usually required, and should expose the sylvian fissure to identify bleeding point(s). Microsurgical repair of arterial wall has been described.[71]

58.7 Traumatic subdural hygroma

58.7.1 General information

From the Greek hygros meaning wet. AKA traumatic subdural effusion, AKA hydroma. Excess fluid in the subdural space (may be clear, blood tinged, or xanthochromic and under variable pressure) is almost always associated with head trauma, especially alcohol-related falls or assaults.[72] Skull fractures were found in 39% of cases. Distinct from chronic subdural hematoma, which is usually associated with underlying cerebral contusion, and usually contains darker clots or brownish fluid ("motor oil" fluid), and may show membrane formation adjacent to inner surface of dura (hygromas lack membranes).

"Simple hygroma" refers to a hygroma without significant accompanying conditions. "Complex hygroma" refers to hygromas with associated significant subdural hematoma, epidural hematoma, or intracerebral hemorrhage.

58.7.2 Pathogenesis

58

Mechanism of formation of hygroma is probably a tear in the arachnoid membrane with resultant CSF leakage into the subdural compartment. Hygroma fluid contains pre-albumin, which is also found in CSF but not in subdural hematomas. The most likely locations of arachnoid tears are in the sylvian fissure or the chiasmatic cistern. Another possible mechanism is post-meningitis effusion (especially influenza meningitis).

May be under high pressure. May increase in size (possibly due to a flap-valve mechanism) and exert mass effect, with the possibility of significant morbidity. Cerebral atrophy was present in 19% of patients with simple hygromas.

58.7.3 Presentation

▶ Table 58.3 shows clinical findings of subdural hygromas. Many present without focal findings. Complex hygromas usually present more acutely and require more urgent treatment.

Table 58.3 Major clinical features of traumatic subdural hygromas[72]

Type of hygroma	Simple	Complex	Total
number of patients	66	14	80
spontaneous eye opening	74%	57%	71%
disorientation or stupor	65%	57%	64%
mental status change without focal signs	52%	50%	51%
neurological plateau with deficit or delayed deterioration	42%	7%	36%
seizures (usually generalized)	36%	43%	38%
hemiparesis	32%	21%	30%
neck stiffness	26%	14%	24%
anisocoria (maintained light reflex)	15%	7%	14%
headache	14%	14%	14%
alert (no mental status change)	8%	0%	6%
hemiplegia	6%	14%	8%
comatose (responsive to pain only)	3%	43%	10%

58.7.4 Imaging

On CT, the density of the fluid is similar to that of CSF.

Signal characteristics on MRI follow those of CSF.

58.7.5 Treatment

Asymptomatic hygromas do not require treatment. Recurrence following simple burr-hole drainage is common. Many surgeons maintain a subdural drain for 24–48 hrs post-op. Recurrent cases may require either a craniotomy to locate the site of CSF leak (may be very difficult), or a subdural-peritoneal shunt may be placed.

58.7.6 Outcome

Outcome may be more related to accompanying injuries than to the hygroma itself.

5 of 9 patients with complex hygromas and subdural hematoma died. For simple hygromas, morbidity was 20% (12% for decreased mental status without focal findings, 32% if hemiparesis/plegia was present).

58.8 Extraaxial fluid collections in children

58.8.1 Differential diagnosis

1. benign subdural collection in infants (see below)
2. chronic *symptomatic* extraaxial fluid collections or effusions (see below)
3. cerebral atrophy: should not contain xanthochromic fluid with elevated protein
4. "external hydrocephalus": ventricles often enlarged, fluid is CSF (p. 400)
5. normal variant of enlarged subarachnoid spaces and interhemispheric fissure
6. acute subdural hematoma: high density (fresh blood) on CT (occasionally these will appear as low density collections in children with low hematocrits). Will usually be unilateral (the others above are usually bilateral). These lesions may occur as birth injuries, and typically present with seizures, pallor, tense fontanelle, poor respirations, hypotension, and retinal hemorrhages
7. "craniocerebral disproportion" (head too large for the brain)[73]: extracerebral spaces enlarged up to 1.5 cm in thickness and filled with CSF-like fluid (possibly CSF), ventricles at upper limits of normal, deep sulci, widened interhemispheric fissure, normal intracranial pressure. Patients are developmentally normal. May be the same as benign extra-axial fluid of infancy (see below). Making this diagnosis with certainty is difficult in first few months of life

58.8.2 Benign subdural collections of infancy

General information

Benign subdural collections (or effusions) of infancy,[74,75] are perhaps better characterized by the term benign extra-axial fluid collections of infancy, since it is difficult to distinguish whether they are subdural or subarachnoid.[76] They appear on CT as peripheral hypodensities over the frontal lobes in infants. Imaging may also show dilatation of the interhemispheric fissure, cortical sulci,[77] and sylvian fissure. Ventricles are usually normal or slightly enlarged, with no evidence of transependymal absorption. Brain size is normal. Transillumination is increased over both frontal regions. The fluid is usually clear yellow (xanthochromic) with high protein content. The etiology of these is unclear, some cases may be due to perinatal trauma. They are more common in term infants than preemies. Must be differentiated from external hydrocephalus (p. 400).

Presentation

Mean age of presentation is ≈ 4 months.[76]

May show: signs of elevated intracranial pressure (tense or large fontanelle, accelerated head growth crossing percentile curves), developmental delay usually as a result of poor head control due to the large size (Carolan et al. feel that developmental delay without macrocrania runs counter to the concept of "benign" collections[76]), frontal bossing, jitteriness. The poor head control may lead to positional flattening. Other symptoms, such as seizures (possibly focal) are indicative of symptomatic collections (see below). Large collections in the absence of macrocrania are more suggestive of cerebral atrophy.

Treatment

Most cases gradually resolve spontaneously, often within 8–9 months. A single subdural tap (p. 1504) for diagnostic purposes (to differentiate from cortical atrophy and to rule out infection) may be done, and may accelerate the rate of disappearance. Repeat physical exams with OFC measurements should be done at ≈ 3–6 month intervals. Head growth usually parallels or approaches normal curves by ≈ 1–2 yrs age, and by 30–36 months orbital-frontal head circumference (OFC) approaches normal percentiles for height and weight. They usually catch up developmentally as OFCs normalize.

58.8.3 Symptomatic chronic extraaxial fluid collections in children

General information

Variously classified as hematomas (chronic subdural hematoma), effusions, or hygromas, with differing definitions associated with each. Since the appearance on imaging and the treatment is similar, Litofsky et al. proposed that they all be classified as extraaxial fluid collections.[78] The difference between these lesions and "benign" subdural effusions (see above) may simply be the degree of clinical manifestation.

Etiologies

The following etiologies were listed in a series of 103 cases[78]:

1. 36% were thought to be the result of trauma (22 were victims of child abuse)
2. 22% followed bacterial meningitis (post-infectious)
3. 19 occurred after placement or revision of a shunt (p. 425)
4. no cause could be identified in 17 patients

Other causes include[73]:

1. tumors: extracerebral or intracerebral
2. post-asphyxia with hypoxic brain damage and cerebral atrophy
3. defects of hemostasis: vitamin K deficiency…

Signs and symptoms

Symptoms include: seizure (26%), large head (22%), vomiting (20%), irritability (13%), lethargy (13%), headache (older children), poor feeding, respiratory arrest…

Signs include: full fontanelle (30%), macrocrania (25%), fever (17%), lethargy (13%), hemiparesis (12%), retinal hemorrhages, coma, papilledema, developmental delay…

Evaluation

CT/MRI usually shows ventricular compression and obliteration of the cerebral sulci, unlike with benign subdural collections. The "cortical vein sign" (p. 401) helps distinguish this from external hydrocephalus.

Treatment

Options include:

1. observation: follow-up with serial OFC measurements, ultrasound and CT/MRI
2. serial percutaneous subdural taps (p. 1504): some patients require as many as 16 taps.[79] Some series show good results and others show low success rate[80,81]
3. burr hole drainage: may include long-term external drainage. Simple burr hole drainage may not be effective with severe craniocephalic disproportion as the brain will not expand to obliterate the extra-axial space
4. subdural-peritoneal shunt: unilateral shunt is usually adequate even for bilateral effusions[78,81,82] (recent recommendations: no study is required to demonstrate communication between the 2 sides[78,83]). An extremely low pressure system should be utilized. The general practice is to remove the shunt after 2–3 months of drainage (once the collections are obliterated) to reduce the risk of associated mineralization of the dura and arachnoid and possible risk of seizures (these shunts are easily removed at this time, but may be more difficult to remove at a later date)[84]

Other recommendations:

At least one percutaneous tap should be performed to rule-out infection.

Many authors recommend observation for the patient with no symptoms or with only enlarging head and developmental delay.

58.9 Traumatic posterior fossa mass lesions

Less than 3% of head injuries involve traumatic mass lesions of the posterior fossa.[85] Epidural hematomas constitute the majority of these (p. 894). Other entities (subdural hematoma, intraparenchymal hematoma[86]) comprise the small remainder. See **Practice guideline: Surgical management of traumatic posterior fossa mass lesions** (p. 905) for surgical management recommendations. Any of these can cause hydrocephalus.[85]

Practice guideline: Surgical management of traumatic posterior fossa mass lesions

Indications for surgery

Level III[87]: symptomatic posterior fossa mass lesions or those with mass effect on CT should be surgically removed. **Note:** mass effect on CT: defined as dislocation, compression or obliteration of the 4th ventricle; compression or loss of basal cisterns (p. 921) or the presence of obstructive hydrocephalus

- asymptomatic lesions without mass effect on CT may be managed with close observation and serial imaging

Timing of surgery

Level III[87]: p-fossa mass lesions meeting surgical criteria should be evacuated ASAP due to the potential for rapid deterioration

Surgical methods

Level III[87]: suboccipital craniectomy is the recommended procedure

Most parenchymal hemorrhages managed nonsurgically were < 3 cm diameter.

References

[1] Bullock MR, Chesnut RM, Ghajar J, et al. Surgical management of traumatic parenchymal lesions. Neurosurgery. 2006; 58:S25–S46

[2] Lipper MH, Kishore PRS, Girevendulis AK, et al. Delayed Intracranial Hematoma in Patients with Severe Head Injury. Neuroradiology. 1979; 133:645–649

[3] Cooper PR, Maravilla K, Moody S, Clark WK. Serial Computerized Tomographic Scanning and the Prognosis of Severe Head Injury. Neurosurgery. 1979; 5:566–569

[4] Gudeman SK, Kishore PR, Miller JD, Girevendulis AK. The Genesis and Significance of Delayed Traumatic Intracerebral Hematoma. Neurosurgery. 1979; 5:309–313

[5] Young HA, Gleave JRW, Schmidek HH, Gregory S. Delayed Traumatic Intracerebral Hematoma: Report of 15 Cases Operatively Treated. Neurosurgery. 1984; 14:22–25

[6] Rockswold GL, Leonard PR, Nagib M. Analysis of Management in Thirty-Three Closed Head Injury Patients Who "Talked and Deteriorated". Neurosurgery. 1987; 21:51–55

[7] Cohen TI, Gudeman SK, Narayan RK, Wilberger JE, Povlishock JT. In: Delayed Traumatic Intracranial Hematoma. Neurotrauma. New York: McGraw-Hill; 1996:689–701

[8] McKissock W, Taylor JC, Bloom WH, et al. Extradural Hematoma: Observations on 125 Cases. Lancet. 1960; 2:167–172

[9] Kernohan JW, Woltman HW. Incisura of the Crus due to Contralateral Brain Tumor. Arch Neurol Psychiatr. 1929; 21

[10] Tsai FY, Teal JS, Hieshima GB. Neuroradiology of Head Trauma. Baltimore: University Park Press; 1984

[11] Greenberg JJ, Cohen WA, Cooper PR. The "hyperacute" extraaxial intracranial hematoma: computed tomographic findings and clinical significance. Neurosurgery. 1985; 17:48–56

[12] Rivas JJ, Lobato RD, Sarabia R, et al. Extradural Hematoma: Analysis of Factors Influencing the Courses of 161 Patients. Neurosurgery. 1988; 23:44–51

[13] Kaye EM, Cass PR, Dooling E, et al. Chronic Epidural Hematomas in Childhood: Increased Recognition and Nonsurgical Management. Pediat Neurol. 1985; 1:255–259

[14] Pang D, Horton JA, Herron JM, et al. Nonsurgical Management of Extradural Hematomas in Children. J Neurosurg. 1983; 59:958–971

[15] Bullock MR, Chesnut RM, Ghajar J, et al. Surgical management of acute epidural hematomas. Neurosurgery. 2006; 58:S7–15

[16] Piepmeier JM, Wagner FC. Delayed Post-Traumatic Extracerebral Hematoma. J Trauma. 1982; 22:455–460

[17] Borovich B, Braun J, Guilburd JN, et al. Delayed Onset of Traumatic Extradural Hematoma. J Neurosurg. 1985; 63:30–34

[18] Bucci MN, Phillips TW, McGillicuddy JE. Delayed Epidural Hemorrhage in Hypotensive Multiple Trauma Patients. Neurosurgery. 1986; 19:65–68

[19] Riesgo P, Piquer J, Botella C, et al. Delayed Extradural Hematoma After Mild Head Injury: Report of Three Cases. Surg Neurol. 1997; 48:226–231

[20] Zuccarello M, Pardatscher K, Andrioli GC, Fiore DL, Iavicoli R, Cervellini P. Epidural hematomas of the posterior cranial fossa. Neurosurgery. 1981; 8:434–437

[21] Roda JM, Giminez D, Perez-Higueras A, et al. Posterior Fossa Epidural Hematomas: A Review and Synthesis. Surg Neurol. 1983; 19:419–424

[22] Aoki N, Oikawa A, Sakai T. Symptomatic Subacute Subdural Hematoma Associated with Cerebral Hemispheric Swelling and Ischemia. Neurol Res. 1996; 18:145–149

[23] Nishio M, Akagi K, Abekura M, Matsumoto K. [A Case of Traumatic Subacute Subdural Hematoma Presenting Symptoms Arising from Cerebral Hemisphere Edema]. No Shinkei Geka. 1998; 26:425–429

[24] Wintzen AR, Tijssen JGP. Subdural Hematoma and Oral Anticoagulation Therapy. Ann Neurol. 1982; 39:69–72

[25] Kawamata T, Takeshita M, Kubo O, et al. Management of Intracranial Hemorrhage Associated with Anticoagulant Therapy. Surg Neurol. 1995; 44:438–443

[26] Munro D, Merritt HH. Surgical Pathology of Subdural Hematoma: Based on a Study of One Hundred and Five Cases. Arch Neurol Psychiatry. 1936; 35:64–78

[27] Bullock MR, Chesnut RM, Ghajar J, et al. Surgical management of acute subdural hematomas. Neurosurgery. 2006; 58:S16–S24

[28] Seelig JM, Becker DP, Miller JD, et al. Traumatic Acute Subdural Hematoma: Major Mortality Reduction in Comatose Patients Treated within Four Hours. N Engl J Med. 1981; 304:1511–1518

[29] Wilberger JE, Harris M, Diamond DL. Acute Subdural Hematoma: Morbidity, Mortality, and Operative Timing. J Neurosurg. 1991; 74:212–218

[30] Howard MA, Gross AS, Dacey RG, Winn HR. Acute Subdural Hematomas: An Age-Dependent Clinical Entity. J Neurosurg. 1989; 71:858–863

[31] Houtteville JP, Toumi K, Theoron J, Derlon JM, Benazza A, Hubert P. Interhemispheric subdural hematoma: seven cases and review of the literature. Br J Neurosurg. 1988; 2:357–367

[32] Duhaime A-C, Gennarelli TA, Thibault LE, Bruce DA, et al. The Shaken Baby Syndrome: A Clinical, Pathological, and Biomechanical Study. J Neurosurg. 1987; 66:409–415

[33] Fein JM, Rovit RL. Interhemispheric subdural hematoma secondary to hemorrhage from a calloso-marginal artery aneurysm. Neuroradiology. 1970; 1:183–186

[34] Rapana A, Lamaida E, Pizza V, et al. Inter-hemispheric scissure, a rare location for a traumatic subdural hematoma, case report and review of the literature. Clin Neurol Neurosurg. 1997; 99:124–129

[35] Aoki N, Masuzawa H. Infantile Acute Subdural Hematoma. J Neurosurg. 1984; 61:273–280

[36] Ikeda A, Sato O, Tsugane R, Shibuya N, et al. Infantile Acute Subdural Hematoma. Childs Nerv Syst. 1987; 3:19–22

[37] Scott M. Spontaneous Nontraumatic Subdural Hematomas. JAMA. 1949; 141:596–602

[38] Robinson RG. Chronic Subdural Hematoma: Surgical Management in 133 Patients. J Neurosurg. 1984; 61:263–268

[39] Wakai S, Hashimoto K, Watanabe N, et al. Efficacy of Closed-System Drainage in Treating Chronic Subdural Hematoma: A Prospective Comparative Study. Neurosurgery. 1990; 26:771–773

[40] Fogelholm R, Heiskanen O, Waltimo O. Influence of Patient's Age on Symptoms, Signs, and Thickness of Hematoma. J Neurosurg. 1975; 42:43–46

[41] Weir BK, Gordon P. Factors Affecting Coagulation, Fibrinolysis in Chronic Subdural Fluid Collection. J Neurosurg. 1983; 58:242–245

[42] Labadie EL, Sawaya R. In: Fibrinolysis in the Formation and Growth of Chronic Subdural Hematomas. Fibrinolysis and the Central Nervous System. Philadelphia: Hanley and Belfus; 1990:141–148

[43] Drapkin AJ. Chronic Subdural Hematoma: Pathophysiological Basis of Treatment. Br J Neurosurg. 1991; 5:467–473

[44] Hamilton MG, Frizzell JB, Tranmer BI. Chronic Subdural Hematoma: The Role for Craniotomy Reevaluated. Neurosurgery. 1993; 33:67–72

[45] Abouzari M, Rashidi A, Rezaii J, Esfandiari K, Asadollahi M, Aleali H, Abdollahzadeh M. The role of postoperative patient posture in the recurrence of traumatic chronic subdural hematoma after burr-hole surgery. Neurosurgery. 2007; 61:794–7; discussion 797

[46] Caron J-L, Worthington C, Bertrand G. Tension Pneumocephalus After Evacuation of Chronic Subdural Hematoma and Subsequent Treatment with Continuous Lumbar Subarachnoid Infusion and

Craniostomy Drainage. Neurosurgery. 1985; 16:107–110
[47] Camel M, Grubb RL. Treatment of Chronic Subdural Hematoma by Twist-Drill Craniostomy with Continuous Catheter Drainage. J Neurosurg. 1986; 65:183–187
[48] Hubschmann OR. Twist Drill Craniostomy in the Treatment of Chronic and Subacute Hematomas in Severely Ill and Elderly Patients. Neurosurgery. 1980; 6:233–236
[49] Tabaddor K, Shulman K. Definitive Treatment of Chronic Subdural Hematoma by Twist-Drill Craniostomy and Closed-System Drainage. J Neurosurg. 1977; 46:220–226
[50] Lind CR, Lind CJ, Mee EW. Reduction in the number of repeated operations for the treatment of subacute and chronic subdural hematomas by placement of subdural drains. J Neurosurg. 2003; 99:44–46
[51] Markwalder T-M, Steinsiepe KF, Rohner M, et al. The Course of Chronic Subdural Hematomas After Burr-Hole Craniostomy and Closed-System Drainage. J Neurosurg. 1981; 55:390–393
[52] Arginteanu MS, Byun H, King W. Treatment of a recurrent subdural hematoma using urokinase. J Neurotrauma. 1999; 16:1235–1239
[53] Ogasawara K, Koshu K, Yoshimoto T, Ogawa A. Transient Hyperemia Immediately After Rapid Decompression of Chronic Subdural Hematoma. Neurosurgery. 1999; 45:484–489
[54] Dill SR, Cobbs CG, McDonald CK. Subdural Empyema: Analysis of 32 Cases and Review. Clin Inf Dis. 1995; 20:372–386
[55] Ernestus R-I, Beldzinski P, Lanfermann H, Klug N. Chronic Subdural Hematoma: Surgical Treatment and Outcome in 104 Patients. Surg Neurol. 1997; 48:220–225
[56] Sambasivan M. An Overview of Chronic Subdural Hematoma: Experience with 2300 Cases. Surg Neurol. 1997; 47:418–422
[57] Talalla A, McKissock W. Acute 'Spontaneous' Subdural Hemorrhage: An Unusual Form of Cerebrovascular Accident. Neurology. 1971; 21:19–25
[58] Hesselbrock R, Sawaya R, Means ED. Acute Spontaneous Subdural Hematoma. Surg Neurol. 1984; 21:363–366
[59] Korosue K, Kondoh T, Ishikawa Y, Nagao T, et al. Acute Subdural Hematoma Associated with Nontraumatic Middle Meningeal Artery Aneurysm: Case Report. Neurosurgery. 1988; 22:411–413
[60] Keller TM, Chappell ET. Spontaneous acute subdural hematoma precipitated by cocaine abuse: case report. Surg Neurol. 1997; 47:12–4; discussion 14–5
[61] Koch E. Inhibition of platelet activating factor (PAF)-induced aggregation of human thrombocytes by ginkgolides: considerations on possible bleeding complications after oral intake of Ginkgo biloba extracts. Phytomedicine. 2005; 12:10–16
[62] Rowin J, Lewis SL. Spontaneous bilateral subdural hematomas associated with chronic Ginkgo biloba ingestion. Neurology. 1996; 46:1775–1776
[63] Kohler S, Funk P, Kieser M. Influence of a 7-day treatment with Ginkgo biloba special extract EGb 761 on bleeding time and coagulation: a randomized, placebo-controlled, double-blind study in healthy volunteers. Blood Coagul Fibrinolysis. 2004; 15:303–309
[64] Vale S. Subarachnoid haemorrhage associated with Ginkgo biloba. Lancet. 1998; 352
[65] Wolf HR. Does Ginkgo biloba special extract EGb 761 provide additional effects on coagulation and bleeding when added to acetylsalicylic acid 500 mg daily? Drugs R D. 2006; 7:163–172
[66] Albanese A, Tuttolomondo A, Anile C, Sabatino G, Pompucci A, Pinto A, Licata G, Mangiola A. Spontaneous chronic subdural hematomas in young adults with a deficiency in coagulation factor XIII. Report of three cases. J Neurosurg. 2005; 102:1130–1132
[67] Vural M, Yarar C, Durmaz R, Atasoy MA. Spontaneous Acute Subdural Hematoma and Chronic Epidural Hematoma in a Child with F XIII Deficiency. J Emerg Med. 2008. DOI: 10.1016/j.jemermed.2007.11.041
[68] de Noronha RJ, Sharrack B, Hadjivassiliou M, Romanowski CA. Subdural haematoma: a potentially serious consequence of spontaneous intracranial hypotension. J Neurol Neurosurg Psychiatry. 2003; 74:752–755
[69] Chung SJ, Lee JH, Kim SJ, Kwun BD, Lee MC. Subdural hematoma in spontaneous CSF hypovolemia. Neurology. 2006; 67:1088–1089
[70] McDermott M, Fleming JF, Vanderlinden RG, Tucker WS. Spontaneous arterial subdural hematoma. Neurosurgery. 1984; 14:13–18
[71] Matsuyama T, Shimomura T, Okumura Y, Sakaki T. Acute subdural hematomas due to rupture of cortical arteries: a study of the points of rupture in 19 cases. Surg Neurol. 1997; 47:423–427
[72] Stone JL, Lang RGR, Sugar O, et al. Traumatic Subdural Hygroma. Neurosurgery. 1981; 8:542–550
[73] Strassburg HM. Macrocephaly is Not Always Due to Hydrocephalus. J Child Neurol. 1989; 4:S32–S40
[74] Briner S, Bodensteiner J. Benign Subdural Collections of Infancy. Pediatrics. 1980; 67:802–804
[75] Robertson WC, Chun RWM, Orrison WW, et al. Benign Subdural Collections of Infancy. J Pediatr. 1979; 94
[76] Carolan PL, McLaurin RL, Towbin RB, Towbin JA, Egelhoff JC. Benign Extraaxial Collections of Infancy. Pediatr Neurosci. 1986; 12:140–144
[77] Mori K, Handa H, Itoh M, Okuno T. Benign Subdural Effusion in Infants. J Comput Assist Tomogr. 1980; 4:466–471
[78] Litofsky NS, Raffel C, McComb JG. Management of Symptomatic Chronic Extra-Axial Fluid Collections in Pediatric Patients. Neurosurgery. 1992; 31:445–450
[79] McLaurin RL, Isaacs E, Lewis HP. Results of Nonoperative Treatment in 15 Cases of Infantile Subdural Hematoma. J Neurosurg. 1971; 34:753–759
[80] Herzberger E, Rotem Y, Braham J. Remarks on Thirty-Three Cases of Subdural Effusions in Infancy. Arch Dis Childhood. 1956; 31:44–50
[81] Moyes PD. Subdural Effusions in Infants. Can Med Assoc J. 1969; 100:231–234
[82] Aoki N, Miztani H, Masuzawa H. Unilateral Subdural-Peritoneal Shunting for Bilateral Chronic Subdural Hematomas in Infancy. J Neurosurg. 1985; 63:134–137
[83] Aoki N. Chronic Subdural Hematoma in Infancy. Clinical Analysis of 30 Cases in the CT Era. J Neurosurg. 1990; 73:201–205
[84] Johnson DL. Comment on Litofsky N S, et al.: Management of Symptomatic Chronic Extra-Axial Fluid Collections in Pediatric Patients. Neurosurgery. 1992; 31
[85] Karasawa H, Furuya H, Naito H, Sugiyama K, Ueno J, Kin H. Acute hydrocephalus in posterior fossa injury. J Neurosurg. 1997; 86:629–632
[86] d'Avella D, Servadei F, Scerrati M, Tomei G, Brambilla G, Angileri FF, Massaro F, Cristofori L, Tartara F, Pozzati E, Delfini R, Tomasello F. Traumatic intracerebellar hemorrhage: clinicoradiological analysis of 81 patients. Neurosurgery. 2002; 50:16–25; discussion 25-7
[87] Bullock MR, Chesnut RM, Ghajar J, et al. Surgical management of posterior fossa mass lesions. Neurosurgery. 2006; 58:S47–S55

59 Gunshot Wounds and Non-Missile Penetrating Brain Injuries

59.1 Gunshot wounds to the head

59.1.1 General information

Gunshot wounds to the head (GSWH) account for the majority of penetrating brain injuries, and comprise ≈ 35% of deaths from brain injury in persons < 45 yrs old. GSWH are the most lethal type of head injury, ≈ two-thirds die at the scene, and GSWH ultimately are the proximal cause of death in > 90% of victims.[1]

59.1.2 Primary injury

Primary injury from GSWH results from a number of factors including:
1. injury to soft tissue
   a) direct scalp and/or facial injuries
   b) soft tissue and bacteria may be dragged intracranially, the devitalized tissue may also then support growth of the bacteria
   c) pressure waves of gas combustion may cause injury if the weapon is close
2. comminuted fracture of bone: may injure subjacent vascular and/or cortical tissue (depressed skull fracture). May act as secondary missiles
3. cerebral injuries from missile
   a) direct injury to brain tissue in path of bullet, exacerbated by
      - fragmentation of bullet
      - ricochet off bone
      - deviations of the bullet from a straight path as it travels: tumbling (forward rotation – pitch), yaw (rotation about vertical axis), rotation (spin), nutation
      - deformation of bullet at impact: e.g. mushrooming
   b) injury to tissue by shock waves, cavitation
4. coup + contrecoup injury from missile impact on head (may cause injuries distant from bullet path)

Because of the complexities of ballistics (some of which are described above) there is often more damage distally than at the entry site even though the bullet slows (losing kinetic energy).

Extent of primary injury is related to *impact velocity*:
- *impact* velocity > 100 m/s: causes explosive intracranial injury that is uniformly fatal (NB: impact velocity is less than muzzle velocity)
- non-bullet missiles (e.g. grenade fragments) are considered low velocity
- low *muzzle* velocity bullets (≈ < 250 m/s): as with most handguns. Tissue injury is caused primarily by laceration and maceration along a path slightly wider than missile diameter
- high *muzzle* velocity bullets (≈ 600–750 m/s): from military weapons and hunting rifles. Causes additional damage by shock waves and temporary cavitation (tissue pushed away from the missile causes a conical cavity of injury that may exceed bullet diameter many-fold, and causes low-pressure region which may draw surface debris into the wound)

59.1.3 Secondary injury

Cerebral edema occurs similar to closed head injury. ICP may rise rapidly within minutes (higher ICPs result from higher impact velocities). Cardiac output may also fall initially. Together, ↑ ICP and ↓ MAP adversely effect cerebral perfusion pressure.

Other common complicating factors include: DIC, intracranial hemorrhage from lacerated blood vessels.

59

59.1.4 Late complications

Late complications include:
1. cerebral abscess: migration of bullet may be a tip-off (see below). Usually associated with retained contaminated material (bullet, bone, skin…) but may also result from persistent communication with nasal sinuses

2. traumatic aneurysm[2]
3. seizures
4. fragment migration
   a) migration of a bullet: often indicates abscess[3] or, less commonly, a hematoma cavity. May also migrate within the ventricles
   b) intraventricular fragments may migrate and cause obstructive hydrocephalus[4]
5. lead toxicity: more of an issue with bullet in disc space (p. 1017)

59.1.5 Evaluation

Physical exam

Exam should describe visible entrance and exit wounds. In through-and-through missile wounds of the skull, the entrance wound is typically smaller than the exit wound due to bullet mushrooming. Entrance wounds may be especially small with direct contact of the muzzle to the head. At surgery or autopsy, the entrance wound will typically show beveling of the inner table, whereas exit wounds have a beveled outer table.

Imaging

AP and lateral skull x-rays

This is one situation where skull x-rays still may provide useful information, as they are less susceptible to artifact from the bullet than the CT scan. Helps to localize metal and bone fragments, and to help identify entrance/exit sites (omit if time not available)

Head CT scan without contrast

The main assessment tool. Demonstrates location of bone and metal. Delineates bullet trajectory: assesses if bullet passed through ventricles and how many quadrants of the hemisphere have been traversed. Shows amount of blood in brain and assesses intracranial hematomas (epidural, subdural or intraparenchymal).

Angiography in GSWH

Rarely performed emergently. When done, usually performed on ≈ day 2–3.

Indications for angiography[5]:
- unexpected delayed hemorrhage
- a trajectory that would likely involve named vessels in a salvageable patient
- large intraparenchymal hemorrhages in a salvageable patient

59.1.6 Management

Initial management

General measures

1. CPR as required; endotracheal intubation if stuporous or airway compromised
2. additional injuries (e.g. chest wounds) identified and treated appropriately
3. usual precautions taken for spine injury
4. fluids as needed to replace estimated blood loss which may be variable: exercise restraint to avoid excessive hydration (to minimize cerebral edema)
5. pressors to support MAP during and after fluid resuscitation

Treatment specific to the injury

Neurological assessment as rapidly as possible and as thoroughly as time permits.

The Glasgow Coma Scale is still the most widely used grading system and allows better comparison between series than specialized scales for GSWHs.

Decision by experienced neurosurgeon regarding the ultimate treatment of the patient will determine appropriate steps to be taken. Patients with little CNS function (in the absence of shock) are unlikely to benefit from craniotomy. Supportive measures are indicated in most cases (for possibility of organ donation, opportunity for family to adjust to situation, and requirements for observation period to determine actual brain death).

In patients considered for further treatment, rapid deterioration at any point with signs of herniation requires immediate surgical intervention. As time permits, the following should be undertaken:

1. initial steps
   a) control bleeding from scalp and associated wounds (hemostats on scalp vessels)
   b) shave scalp to identify entrance/exit sites, and to save time in the O.R.
2. medical treatment (similar to closed head injury)
   a) assume ICP is elevated:
      - elevate HOB 30–45° with head midline (avoids kinking jugular veins)
      - mannitol (1 gm/kg bolus) as blood pressure tolerates
      - hyperventilate to $PaCO_2 = 30–35$ mm Hg if indications are met (p. 873)
      - steroids: (unproven efficacy) 10 mg dexamethasone IVP
   b) prophylaxis against GI ulcers: H2 antagonist (e.g. ranitidine 50 mg IVPB q 8 hrs) or proton pump inhibitor, NG tube to suction
   c) begin anticonvulsants (does not reduce incidence of late seizures)
   d) antibiotics: generally used although no controlled study demonstrates efficacy in preventing meningitis or abscess. Most organisms are sensitive to penicillinase resistant agents, e.g. *nafcillin*, recommended for ≈ 5 days
   e) tetanus toxoid administration

Surgical treatment

Indications for surgery are controversial. Some authors suggest that better outcome might occur with more aggressive management, and that poor outcome may be a self-fulfilling prophecy.[6] Patients with minimal neurologic function, e.g. fixed pupils, decorticate or decerebrate posturing… (when not in shock and with good oxygenation) should *not* be operated upon, because the chance of meaningful recovery is close to zero. Patients with less severe injuries should be considered for urgent operation.

Goals of surgery

1. debridement of devitalized tissue: less tissue is injured in civilian GSWH, but elevated ICP post-op may imply more vigorous debridement was needed, especially of non-eloquent brain (e.g. temporal tips)
2. evacuation of hematomas: subdural, intraparenchymal…
3. removal of *accessible* bone fragments
4. retrieval of bullet fragment for forensic purposes (note: everyone who handles the fragments may be subpoenaed to testify as to the "chain of evidence"). Large intact fragments should be sought as they tend to migrate (**note:** risk of infection and seizures due to retained bullet fragments is not high in civilian GSWH, therefore only accessible fragments should be sought and removed)
5. obtaining hemostasis
6. watertight dural closure (usually requires graft)
7. separation of intracranial compartment from air sinuses traversed by bullet
8. identification of entry and exit wounds for forensic purposes; see Evaluation (p. 909)

Surgical technique

Some key points of surgical technique[7 (p 2098–104)]:

- positioning and draping should make both entry and exit wounds accessible
- devitalized tissue around the entry & exit wounds should be excised
- fractured bone should be excised by a circumferential craniectomy (craniotomy may be used in some civilian GSWH, the entry site within the craniotomy should be rongeured or drilled back to clean bone)
- air sinuses that are traversed should have the mucosa exenterated, and are then packed with muscle, and covered with a graft (e.g. periosteum or fascia lata) to separate them from intracranial compartment
- the dura is opened in a stellate fashion
- pulped brain is removed from within using suction and bipolar in an enlarging cone until healthy tissue is encountered (further injury to deep midline structures should be avoided, here, stay within bullet tract)
- contralateral fragments with no exit wound should only be removed if accessible
- intraventricular fragments can present significant risk. Ventriculoscopy (if available) may be well suited for removing these
- dural closure should be watertight; grafts of pericranium, temporalis fascia, or fascia lata grafts may be used; avoid dura substitutes

- cranioplasty should be delayed 6–12 months to reduce risk of infection
- a post-op CSF fistula that persists > 2 weeks should be repaired

ICP monitoring

ICP is often elevated after surgical debridement[6] and monitoring may be warranted.

Outcome

Prognostic factors:
1. level of consciousness is the most important prognostic factor: ≈ 94% of patients who are comatose with inappropriate or absent response to noxious stimulus on admission die, and half the survivors are severely disabled[8]
2. as initially espoused by Cushing, the path of the bullet is also an important prognosticator. Especially *poor prognosis* is associated with:
   a) bullets that cross the midline
   b) bullets that pass through the geographic center of the brain
   c) bullets that enter or traverse the ventricles
   d) the more lobes traversed by the bullet
3. hematomas seen on CT are poor prognostic findings
4. suicide attempts are more likely to be fatal

59.2 Non-missile penetrating trauma

59.2.1 General information

This section deals with penetrating injuries to the brain (and to some extent to the spinal cord) excluding missile injuries, i.e. gunshot wounds (p. 908). Includes trauma from: knives, arrows, lawn darts… Injury to neural tissue tends to be more limited than with missiles because many of the associated injurious aspects of the missile are absent (p. 908).

59.2.2 Arrow injuries

As a result of the lower velocity (e.g. 58 m/s) compared to firearms and the sharp tip, injury is usually limited to tissue directly incised by the arrowhead.[9]

59.2.3 Cases with foreign body still embedded

In penetrating trauma, it is usually not appropriate to remove any protruding part of the foreign body until the patient is in the operating room, unless it cannot be avoided. If possible, it is helpful to have another identical object for comparison in planning extrication of the embedded object.[10] To minimize extending the trauma to the CNS, the protruding object should be stabilized in some way during transportation and evaluation. Intraoperatively, devices such as the Greenberg retractor may be used to stabilize the object during preparation and the initial approach.

59.2.4 Indications for pre-op angiography

1. object passes in region of large named artery
2. object passes near dural sinuses
3. visible evidence of arterial bleeding: angiography is not appropriate if hemorrhage cannot be controlled

59.2.5 Surgical techniques

It is impossible to give details to cover every situation. Some guidelines:
1. empiric antibiotic coverage is appropriate; see Meningitis post craniospinal trauma (p. 318). Take cultures from the wound and the foreign body to guide later antibiotic therapy
2. optimal control can usually be gained by performing a craniotomy up to and if possible around the object, such that removing the bone flap will not disturb the object. The last remnants of bone may then be removed with a rongeur

3. if at all possible open the dura before removing the object, since removal with the dura closed does not allow adequate control of any bleeding from the brain
4. removal of the object ideally should follow the entry trajectory if possible
5. although gunshot wounds are not sterile as once thought, they are probably less contaminated than penetrating wounds. One should debride any easily accessible impacted bone and other extracranial tissue and material along the track

59.2.6 Post-op care

1. a course of antibiotics are usually appropriate since infection is common
2. consider a post-op arteriogram to rule-out traumatic aneurysm

References

[1] Kaufman HH. Civilian Gunshot Wounds to the Head. Neurosurgery. 1993; 32:962–964

[2] Kaufman HH, Moake JL, Olson JD, et al. Delayed Intracerebral Hematoma due to Traumatic Aneurysm caused by a Shotgun Wound: A Problem in Prophylaxis. Neurosurgery. 1980; 6:181–184

[3] DesChamps GT, Jr, Morano JU. Intracranial bullet migration - a sign of brain abscess: case report. J Trauma. 1991; 31:293–295

[4] Sternbergh WC, Jr, Watts C, Clark K. Bullet within the fourth ventricle. Case report. J Neurosurg. 1971; 34:805–807

[5] Miner ME. Comment on Benzel EC, et al. Civilian Craniocerebral Gunshot Wounds. Neurosurgery. 1991; 29

[6] Kaufman HH, Makela ME, Lee KF, et al. Gunshot Wounds to the Head: A Perspective. Neurosurgery. 1986; 18:689–695

[7] Youmans JR. Neurological Surgery. Philadelphia 1990

[8] Benzel EC, Day WT, Kesterson L, Willis BK, et al. Civilian Craniocerebral Gunshot Wounds. Neurosurgery. 1991; 29:67–72

[9] Karger B, Sudhues H, Kneubuehl BP, Brinkmann B. Experimental arrow wounds: ballistics and traumatology. J Trauma. 1998; 45:495–501

[10] Salvino CK, Origitano TC, Dries DJ, Shea JF. Transoral Crossbow Injury to the Cervical Spine: An Unusual Case of Penetrating Cervical Spine Injury. Neurosurgery. 1991; 28:904–907

60 Pediatric Head Injury

60.1 General information

75% of children hospitalized for trauma have a head injury. Although most pediatric head injuries are mild and involve only evaluation or brief hospital stays, CNS injuries are the most common cause of pediatric traumatic death.[1] The overall mortality for all pediatric head injuries requiring hospitalization has been reported between 10–13%,[2] whereas the mortality associated with severe pediatric head injury presenting with decerebrate posturing has been reported as high as 71%.[3]

Differences between adult and pediatric head injury:

1. epidemiology:
   a) children often have milder injuries than adults
   b) lower chance of a surgical lesion in a comatose child than in an adult[4]
2. types of injury: injuries peculiar to pediatrics
   a) birth injuries: skull fractures, cephalhematoma (see below), subdural or epidural hematomas, brachial plexus injuries (p. 550)
   b) perambulator/walker injuries
   c) child abuse (see below): shaken baby syndrome…
   d) injuries from skateboarding, scooters…
   e) lawn darts
   f) cephalhematoma: see below
   g) leptomeningeal cysts, AKA "growing skull fractures" (p. 915)
3. response to injury
   a) responses to head injury of older adolescent are very similar to adults
   b) "malignant cerebral edema": acute onset of severe cerebral swelling (probably due to hyperemia[5,6]) following some head injuries, especially in young children (may not be as common as previously thought[7])
   c) posttraumatic seizures: more likely to occur within the 1st 24 hrs in children than in adults (p. 462) [8]

60.2 Management

60.2.1 Imaging studies

Indications for CT are shown below.

When not contraindicated, rapid sequence MRI may be used (avoids additional radiation in the growing child), especially for follow-up imaging.

Practice guideline: Imaging in minor pediatric head injury

- Recommendations[9]: CT scan for children with neurologic or cognitive dysfunction, or suspicion of a depressed or basilar skull fracture.
- Recommendations[9]: when a CT scan is not done in a child ≤ 1 year age meeting the above criteria (e.g. because of sedation concerns), a skull film may be considered.

Based mostly on prospective trials (not randomized) or large case series.

Definitions: pediatrics = ages 1 month – 17 years of age. Minor head injury: GCS ≥ 13 (excludes: suspicion or proof of child abuse, patients requiring hospitalization for other reasons).

≈ 22% of those with a history of loss of consciousness (LOC) > 5 mins have a brain injury, whereas 92% without LOC > 5 mins will have no brain injury.[9]

60.2.2 Home observation

Practice guideline: Home observation in minor pediatric head injury

Recommendations[9]: a child with GCS = 14–15 and normal CT scan can be considered for home observation if neurologically stable (these patients are at near zero risk of having an occult brain injury).

Based mostly on prospective trials (not randomized) or large case series.

Definitions: pediatrics = ages 1 month – 17 years of age. Minor head injury: GCS ≥ 13 (excludes: suspicion or proof of child abuse, patients requiring hospitalization for other reasons).

60.3 Outcome

As a group, children fare better than adults with head injury.[10] However, very young children do not do as well as the school-age child.[11]

All aspects of neuropsychological dysfunction following head injury may not always be related to the trauma, as children who get injured may have pre-existing problems that increase their propensity to get hurt[12] (this is controversial[13]).

60.4 Cephalhematoma

60.4.1 General information

Accumulation of blood under the scalp. Occurs almost exclusively in children.

Two types:

1. subgaleal hematoma: may occur without bony trauma, or may be associated with linear nondisplaced skull fracture (especially in age < 1 yr). Bleeding into loose connective tissue separates galea from periosteum. May *cross sutures*. Usually starts as a small localized hematoma, and may become huge (with significant loss of circulating blood volume in age < 1 year, transfusion may be necessary). Inexperienced clinicians may suspect CSF collection under the scalp which does not occur. Usually presents as a soft, fluctuant mass. These do *not* calcify
2. subperiosteal hematoma (some refer to this as cephalhematoma): most commonly seen in the newborn (associated with parturition, may also be associated with neonatal scalp monitor[14,15]). Bleeding elevates periosteum, extent is *limited by sutures*. Firmer and less ballotable than subgaleal hematoma[16(p 312)]; scalp moves freely over the mass. 80% reabsorb, usually within 2–3 weeks. Occasionally may calcify

Infants may develop jaundice (hyperbilirubinemia) as blood is resorbed, occasionally as late as 10 days after onset.

60.4.2 Treatment

Treatment beyond analgesics is almost never required, and most usually resolve within 2–4 weeks. Avoid the temptation of percutaneously aspirating these as the risk of infection exceeds the risk of following them expectantly, and in the newborn removal of the blood may make them anemic. Follow serial hemoglobin and hematocrit in large lesions. If a subperiosteal hematoma persists > 6 weeks, obtain a skull film. If the lesion is calcified, surgical removal may be indicated for cosmetic reasons (although with most of these the skull will return to normal contour in 3–6 months.[16(p 315)]

60.5 Skull fractures in pediatric patients

60.5.1 General information

This section deals with some special concerns of skull fractures in pediatrics. Also see Child abuse (p. 916).

60.5.2 Posttraumatic leptomeningeal cysts (growing skull fractures)

General information

Posttraumatic leptomeningeal cysts (PTLMC) (sometimes just traumatic leptomeningeal cysts) AKA growing skull fractures are not to be confused with arachnoid cysts (AKA leptomeningeal cysts, which are not posttraumatic). PTLMC consists of a fracture line that widens with time. Although usually asymptomatic, the cyst may cause mass effect with neurologic deficit.

PTLMCs were first described in 1816,[17] and are *very* rare, occurring in 0.05–0.6% of skull fractures.[18,19] Usually requires both a widely separated fracture AND a dural tear. Mean age at injury: < 1 year, over 90% occur before age 3 years[20] (formation may require the presence of a rapidly growing brain[21]) although rare adult cases have been described[22,23,17] (a total of 5 cases in the literature as of 1998[17]). PTLMC rarely occur > 6 mos out from the injury. Some children may develop a skull fracture that seems to grow during the initial few weeks, that is *not* accompanied by a subgaleal mass, and that heal spontaneously within several months; the term "pseudogrowing fracture" has been suggested for these.[24]

Presentation

Most often presents as scalp mass (usually subgaleal), although there are reports of presentation with head pain alone.[22]

Diagnosis

Radiographic findings: progressive widening of fracture and scalloping (or saucering) of edges.

Screening for development of PTLMC

If early growth of a fracture line with no subgaleal mass is noted, repeat skull films in 1–2 months before operating (to rule-out pseudogrowing fracture). In young patients with separated skull fractures (the width of the initial fracture is rarely mentioned), consider obtaining follow-up skull film 6–12 mos post-trauma. However, since most PTLMCs are brought to medical attention when the palpable mass is noticed, routine follow-up x-rays may not be cost-effective.

Treatment

Treatment of true PTLMC is surgical, with dural closure mandatory. Since the dural defect is usually larger than the bony defect, it may be advantageous to perform a craniotomy around the fracture site, repair the dural defect, and replace the bone.[23] Pseudogrowing fractures should be followed with x-rays and operated only if expansion persists beyond several months or if a subgaleal mass is present.

60.5.3 Depressed skull fractures in pediatrics

See reference.[25]

General information

Most common in frontal and parietal bones. One third are closed, and these tend to occur in younger children (3.4 ± 4.2 yrs, vs. 8.0 ± 4.5 yrs for compound fractures) as a result of the thinner, more deformable skull. Open fractures tended to occur with MVAs, closed fractures tended to follow accidents at home. Dural lacerations are more common in compound fractures.

Simple depressed skull fractures

There was no difference in outcome (seizures, neurologic dysfunction or cosmetic appearance) in surgical vs. nonsurgical treatment in 111 patients < 16 yrs age. In the younger child, remodelling of the skull as a result of brain growth tends to smooth out the deformity.

Indications for surgery for pediatric simple depressed skull fracture:

1. definite evidence of dural penetration
2. persistent cosmetic defect in the older child after the swelling has subsided
3. ± focal neurologic deficit related to the fracture (this group has a higher incidence of dural laceration, although it is usually trivial)

"Ping-pong ball" fractures

See reference.[26]

A green-stick type of fracture → caving in of a focal area of the skull as in a crushed area of a ping-pong ball. Usually seen only in the newborn due to the plasticity of the skull.

Indications for surgery

No treatment is necessary when these occur in the temporoparietal region in the absence of underlying brain injury as the deformity will usually correct as the skull grows.

- radiographic evidence of intraparenchymal bone fragments
- associated neurologic deficit (rare)
- signs of increased intracranial pressure
- signs of CSF leak deep to the galea
- situations where the patient will have difficulty getting long-term follow-up

Technique

Frontally located lesions may be corrected for cosmesis by a small linear incision behind the hairline, opening the cranium adjacent to the depression, and pushing it back out e.g. with a Penfield #3 dissector.

60.6 Nonaccidental trauma (NAT)

60.6.1 General information

AKA Child abuse. At least 10% of children < 10 yrs age that are brought to E/R with alleged accidents are victims of child abuse.[27] The incidence of accidental head trauma of significant consequence below age 3 is low, whereas this is the age group in which battering is highest.[28]

There are no findings that are pathognomonic for child abuse. Factors which raise the index of suspicion include:

1. retinal hemorrhage (see below)
2. bilateral chronic subdural hematomas in a child < 2 yrs age (p.904)
3. skull fractures that are multiple (see below) or those that associated with intracranial injury
4. significant neurological injury with minimal signs of external trauma

60.6.2 Shaken baby syndrome

Vigorous shaking of a child produces violent whiplash-like angular acceleration-decelerations of the head (the infant head is relatively large in proportion to the body, and the neck muscles are comparatively weak)[29] which may lead to significant brain injury. Some researchers believe that shaking alone may be inadequate to produce the severe injuries seen, and that impact is often also involved.[30]

Characteristic findings include retinal hemorrhages (see below), subdural hematomas (bilateral in 80%) and/or subarachnoid hemorrhage (SAH). There are usually few or no external signs of trauma (including cases with impact, although findings may be apparent at autopsy). In some cases there may be finger marks on the chest, multiple rib fractures and/or pulmonary compression ± parenchymal lung hemorrhage. Deaths in these cases are almost all due to uncontrollable intracranial hypertension. There may also be injury to the cervicomedullary junction.[31]

60.6.3 Retinal hemorrhage (RH) in child abuse

"In a traumatized child with multiple injuries and an inconsistent history, the presence of RH is pathognomonic of battering".[28] However, RH may also occur in the absence of any evidence of child abuse. 16/26 battered children < 3 yrs age had RH on funduscopy, whereas 1/32 non-battered traumatized children with head injury had RH (the single false positive: traumatic parturition, where the incidence of RH is 15–30%).

Differential diagnosis of etiologies of retinal hemorrhage:

1. child abuse (including "shaken baby syndrome", see above)
2. benign subdural effusion in infants (p.904)
3. acute high altitude sickness (p.848)
4. acute increase in ICP: e.g. with a severe seizure (may be similar to Purtscher's retinopathy – see below)

5. Purtscher's retinopathy[32]: loss of vision following major trauma (chest crush injuries, airbag deployment[33]...), pancreatitis, childbirth or renal failure, among others. Posterior pole ischemia with cotton-wool exudates and hemorrhages around the optic disc due to microemboli of possibly fat, air, fibrin clots, complement-mediated aggregates or platelet clumps. No known treatment

60.6.4 Skull fractures in child abuse

A series comparing 39 cases of skull fracture from documented child abuse to 95 cases of probable accidental injury[27] showed the following:

1. the parietal bone was the most common site of fracture in both groups (≈ 90%)
2. depression of skull fractures was frequently missed clinically due to overlying hematoma
3. clinical features in patients with skull fractures did not reliably differentiate child abuse from trauma (retinal hemorrhages (RH) were seen in 1 child abuse and 1 accidental trauma patient: note that RH is more common in "shaken child" syndrome which is not commonly associated with skull fractures)
4. 3 characteristics more frequently seen after child abuse than after other trauma:
   a) multiple fractures
   b) bilateral fractures
   c) fractures that cross sutures

References

[1] Ward JD, Narayan RK, Wilberger JE, Povlishock JT. In: Pediatric Head Injury. Neurotrauma. New York: McGraw-Hill; 1996:859–867
[2] Zuccarello M, Facco E, Zampieri P, et al. Severe Head Injury in Children: Early Prognosis and Outcome. Childs Nerv Syst. 1985; 1:158–162
[3] Bruce DA, Raphaely RC, Goldberg AI, et al. Pathophysiology, Treatment and Outcome following Severe Head Injury in Children. Childs Brain. 1979; 5:174–191
[4] Alberico AM, Ward JD, Choi SC, et al. Outcome After Severe Head Injury: Relationahip to Mass Lesions, Diffuse Injury, and ICP Course in Pediatric and Adult Patients. J Neurosurg. 1987; 67:648–656
[5] Bruce DA, Alavi A, Bilaniuk L, et al. Diffuse Cerebral Swelling Following Head Injuries in Children: The Syndrome of "Malignant Brain Edema". J Neurosurg. 1981; 54:170–178
[6] Humphreys RP, Hendrick EB, Hoffman HJ. The Head Injured Child Who "Talks and Dies". Childs Nerv Syst. 1990; 6:139–142
[7] Muizelaar JP, Marmarou AM, DeSalles AA, et al. Cerebral Blood Flow in Severely Head-Injured Children: Part I. Relationship with GCS Score, Outcome, ICP, and PVI. J Neurosurg. 1989; 71:63–71
[8] Hahn YS, Fuchs S, Flannery AM, Barthel MJ, McLone DG. Factors Influencing Posttraumatic Seizures in Children. Neurosurgery. 1988; 22:864–867
[9] Health Policy & Clinical Effectiveness Program. Evidence Based Clinical Practice Guideline for Management of Children with Mild Traumatic Head Injury. Cincinnati, Ohio 2000
[10] Luerson TG, Klauber MR, Marshall LF. Outcome from Head Injury Related to Patient's Age: A Longitudinal Prospective Study of Adult and Pediatric Head Injury. J Neurosurg. 1988; 68:409–416
[11] Kriel RL, Krach LE, Panser LA. Closed Head Injury: Comparison of Children Younger and Older Than 6 Years of Age. Pediatr Neurol. 1989; 5:296–300
[12] Bijur PE, Haslum M, Golding J. Cognitive and Behavioral Sequelae of Mild Head Injury in Children. Pediatrics. 1990; 86:337–344
[13] Pelco L, Sawyer M, Duffielf G, et al. Premorbid Emotional and Behavioral Adjustment in Children with Mild Head Injury. Brain Inj. 1992; 6:29–37
[14] Listinsky JL, Wood BP, Ekholm SE. Parietal Osteomyelitis and Epidural Abscess: A Delayed Complication of Fetal Monitoring. Pediatr Radiol. 1986; 16:150–151
[15] Kaufman HH, Hochberg J, Anderson RP, et al. Treatment of Calcified Cephalhematoma. Neurosurgery. 1993; 32:1037–1040
[16] Matson DD. Neurosurgery of Infancy and Childhood. 2nd ed. Springfield: Charles C Thomas; 1969
[17] Britz GW, Kim K, Mayberg MR. Traumatic Leptomeningeal Cyst in an Adult: A Case Report and Review of the Literature. Surg Neurol. 1998; 50:465–469
[18] Ramamurthi B, Kalyanaraman S. Rationale for Surgery in Growing Fractures of the Skull. J Neurosurg. 1970; 32:427–430
[19] Arseni CS. Growing Skull Fractures of Children. A Particular Form of Post-Traumatic Encephalopathy. Acta Neurochir. 1966; 15:159–172
[20] Lende R, Erickson T. Growing Skull Fractures of Childhood. J Neurosurg. 1961; 18:479–489
[21] Gadoth N, Grunebaum M, Young LW. Leptomeningeal Cyst After Skull Fracture. Am J Dis Child. 1983; 137:1019–1020
[22] Halliday AL, Chapman PH, Heros RC. Leptomeningeal Cyst Resulting from Adulthood Trauma: Case Report. Neurosurgery. 1990; 26:150–153
[23] Iplikciglu AC, Kokes F, Bayar A, Buharali Z. Leptomeningeal Cyst. Neurosurgery. 1990; 27:1027–1028
[24] Sekhar LN, Scarff TB. Pseudogrowth in Skull Fractures of Childhood. Neurosurgery. 1980; 6:285–289
[25] Steinbok P, Flodmark O, Martens D, Germann ET. Management of Simple Depressed Skull Fractures in Children. J Neurosurg. 1987; 66:506–510
[26] Loeser JD, Kilburn HL, Jolley T. Management of depressed skull fracture in the newborn. J Neurosurg. 1976; 44:62–64
[27] Meservy CJ, Towbin R, McLaurin RL, et al. Radiographic Characteristics of Skull Fractures Resulting from Child Abuse. AJR. 1987; 149:173–175
[28] Eisenbrey AB. Retinal Hemorrhage in the Battered Child. Childs Brain. 1979; 5:40–44
[29] Caffey J. On the Theory and Practice of Shaking Infants. Its Potential Residual Effects of Permanent Brain Damage and Mental Retardation. Am J Dis Child. 1972; 124:161–169
[30] Duhaime A-C, Gennarelli TA, Thibault LE, Bruce DA, et al. The Shaken Baby Syndrome: A Clinical, Pathological, and Biomechanical Study. J Neurosurg. 1987; 66:409–415
[31] Hadley MN, Sonntag VKH, Rekate HL, Murphy A. The Infant Whiplash-Shake Injury Syndrome: A Clinical and Pathological Study. Neurosurgery. 1989; 24:536–540
[32] Buckley SA, James B. Purtscher's retinopathy. Postgrad Med J. 1996; 72:409–412
[33] Shah GK, Penne R, Grand MG. Purtscher's retinopathy secondary to airbag injury. Retina. 2001; 21:68–69

61

61 Head Injury: Long-Term Management, Complications, Outcome

61.1 Airway management

Practice guideline: Timing of tracheostomy

Level II[1]: early tracheostomy reduces the number of days of mechanical ventilation but does not affect mortality or incidence of pneumonia

Practice guideline: Timing of extubation

Level III[1]: early extubation for patients meeting extubation criteria does not increase the risk of pneumonia

61.2 Deep-vein thrombosis (DVT) prophylaxis

Also see further details about thromboembolism (p. 167) in neurosurgical patients. The risk of developing DVT is ≈ 20% in untreated severe TBI.[2] See also **Practice guideline: DVT prophylaxis in severe TBI** (p. 918).

Practice guideline: DVT prophylaxis in severe TBI

Level III[3]:

- unless contraindicated, graduated compression stockings or intermittent compression boots are recommended until patients are ambulatory
- low molecular weight heparin (LMWH) (p. 164) or low-dose unfractionated heparin in conjunction with mechanical measures lowers the DVT risk, but a trend suggests they increase the risk of expansion of intracranial hemorrhage (**note:** there is insufficient evidence: to support use of one pharmacologic agent over another, or to define the optimal dose or timing of agents[3]

61.3 Nutrition in the head-injured patient

61.3.1 Summary of recommendations (see text for details)

Practice guideline: Nutrition

Level II[4]: full caloric replacement should be attained by post-trauma day 7

Σ

1. by post-trauma day 7, replace the following (enterally or parenterally):
   a) non-paralyzed patients: 140% of predicted basal energy expenditure (BEE)
   b) paralyzed patients: 100% of predicted BEE
2. provide ≥ 15% of calories as protein
3. nutritional replacement should begin within 72 hrs of head injury in order to achieve goal #1 by day 7
4. the enteral route is preferred (IV hyperalimentation is preferred if higher nitrogen intake is desired or if there is decreased gastric emptying)

61.3.2 Caloric requirements

Rested comatose patients with isolated head injury have a metabolic expenditure that is 140% of normal for that patient (range: 120–250%).[5,6,7,8] Paralysis with muscle blocker or barbiturate coma reduced this excess expenditure in most patients to ≈ 100–120% of normal, but some remained elevated by 20–30%.[9] Energy requirements rise during the first 2 weeks after injury, but it is not known for how long this elevation persists. Mortality is reduced in patients who receive full caloric replacement by day 7 after trauma[10] (a beneficial effect with an earlier goal of replacement by 3 days post-trauma was not found[11]). Since it generally takes 2–3 days to get nutritional replacement up to speed whether the enteral or parenteral route is utilized,[8] it is recommended that nutritional supplementation begin within 72 hrs of head injury.

61.3.3 Enteral vs. IV hyperalimentation

Caloric replacement that can be achieved is similar between enteral or parenteral routes.[12] The enteral route is preferred because of reduced risk of hyperglycemia, infection and cost.[13] IV hyperalimentation may be utilized if higher nitrogen intake is desired or if there is decreased gastric emptying. No significant difference in serum albumin, weight loss, nitrogen balance, or final outcome was found between enteral and parenteral nutrition.[12]

Estimates of basal energy expenditure (BEE) can be obtained from the Harris-Benedict equation,[14] shown in Eq (61.1), (61.2) and (61.3), where W is weight in kg, H is height in cm, and A is age in years.

$$\text{Males}: \text{BEE} = 66.47\ 13.75 \times W\ 5.0 \times H - 6.76 \times A \tag{61.1}$$

$$\text{Females}: \text{BEE} = 65.51\ 9.56 \times W\ 1.85 \times H - 4.68 \times A \tag{61.2}$$

$$\text{Infants}: \text{BEE} = 22.1\ 31.05 \times W\ 1.16 \times H \tag{61.3}$$

61.3.4 Enteral nutrition

Isotonic solutions (such as Isocal® or Osmolyte®) should be used at full strength starting at 30 ml/hr. Check gastric residuals q 4 hrs and hold feedings if residuals exceed ≈ 125 ml in an adult. Increase the rate by ≈ 15–25 ml/hr every 12–24 hrs as tolerated until the desired rate is achieved.[15] Dilution is not recommended (may slow gastric emptying), but if it is desired, dilute with normal saline to reduce free water intake.

Cautions:

NG tube feeding may interfere with absorption of phenytoin; see phenytoin (PHT, Dilantin®) (p. 446). Reduced gastric emptying may be seen following head-injury[16] (NB: some may have temporarily elevated emptying) as well as in pentobarbital coma, patients may need IV hyperalimentation until the enteric route is usable. Others have described better tolerance of enteral feedings using jejunal administration.[17]

61.3.5 Nitrogen balance

A normal subject fed a protein-free diet for 3 days will excrete 85 mg of nitrogen/kg/d. These loses increase with injury. The rise in urinary N is due primarily to an increase in urea (comprises 80–90% of urinary N). This is thought to represent an increase in mobilization and breakdown of amino acids, which are felt to originate mainly from skeletal muscle.[18] Some of this represents a primary reaction to injury in which certain vital organs seem to be maintained at the expense of less active organs, and a significantly higher nitrogen balance cannot be achieved by increasing the amount of calories supplied as protein beyond a certain level.[12,15] Catabolism of protein yields 4 kcal/g (compared to 1 kcal/g for carbohydrates and 9 kcal/g for fat), and in the non-injured adult normally supplies only ≈ 10% of energy needs.[19]

As an estimate, for each gram of N excreted (mostly in the urine, however, some is also lost in the feces), 6.25 gm of protein have been catabolized. It is recommended that at least 15% of calories be supplied as protein. The percent of calories consumed (PCC) derived from protein can be calculated from Eq (61.4), where N is nitrogen in grams, and BEE is the basal energy expenditure[5] (see Eq (61.1), (61.2) and (61.3)).

$$\text{PCC (from protein)} = \frac{\text{N (gm N)} \times \frac{6.25\text{ gm protein}}{\text{gm N}} \times \frac{4.0\text{ kcal}}{\text{gm protein}}}{\text{BEE}} \times 100 \tag{61.4}$$

Thus, to supply PCC (protein) = 15% once the BEE is known, use Eq (61.5). Some enteral formulations include Magnacal® (PCC = 14%) and TraumaCal® (PCC = 22%).

$$\text{N (gm N)} = 0.006 \times \text{BEE} \tag{61.5}$$

61.4 Posttraumatic hydrocephalus

61.4.1 General information

Hydrocephalus was found in 40% of 61 patients with severe head injury (GCS = 3–8) and in 27% of 34 patients with moderate head injury (GCS = 9–13).[20] Hydrocephalus developed by 4 weeks after injury in 58% and by 2 months in 70%.[20] There was no statistically significant relationship between posttraumatic hydrocephalus and age, the presence of SAH, or type of lesion (focal or diffuse). Posttraumatic hydrocephalus was associated with worse outcome.[20]

Hydrocephalus after traumatic subarachnoid hemorrhage

Incidence of clinically **symptomatic** hydrocephalus within 3 months of traumatic subarachnoid hemorrhage (tSAH) is ≈ 12%.[21] In this series of 301 tSAH patients, multivariate analysis showed the risk of developing hydrocephalus increased with age, intraventricular hemorrhage, blood thickness ≥ 5 mm, and diffuse distribution of blood (vs. focal distribution). There was *no* correlation with gender, admission GCS score, basal location of tSAH, or use of decompressive craniectomy.[21] NB: this is potentially confusing, univariate analysis shows the risk of hydrocephalus increases with increasing severity of TBI.

61.4.2 Differentiating true hydrocephalus from hydrocephalus ex vacuo

Delayed ventricular enlargement months to years after TBI may instead be due to atrophy (hydrocephalus ex vacuo) secondary to diffuse axonal injury, and may not represent true hydrocephalus. It may not be possible to accurately differentiate these two conditions, and the decision to shunt may therefore be difficult (similar to the dilemma in patients with NPH vs. atrophy).

61.4.3 Indications for surgical treatment

Factors favoring hydrocephalus, for which shunt should be considered:
1. elevated pressure on 1 or more LPs
2. papilledema on funduscopic exam
3. symptoms of headache/pressure
4. findings of "transependymal absorption" on CT or T2WI MRI (p. 406)
5. ± patient's whose neurologic recovery seems worse than expected
6. provocative tests have been recommended (p. 255) [22]

Patients with enlarged ventricles who are asymptomatic and are doing well following their head injury should be managed expectantly.

61.5 Outcome from head trauma

61.5.1 Age

In general, the degree of recovery from closed head injury is better in infants and young children than in adults. In adults, decerebrate posturing or flaccidity with loss of pupillary or oculovestibular reflex is associated with a poor outcome in most cases, these findings are not as ominous in pediatrics.

61.5.2 Outcome prognosticators

General information

The frequency of poor outcome from closed head injury is increased with persistent ICP > 20 mm Hg after hyperventilation, increasing age, impaired or absent pupillary light response or eye movement, hypotension (SBP < 90), hypercarbia, hypoxemia, or anemia.[23] This is probably due at least in part to the fact that some of these are markers for significant injury to other body systems. One of the most important predictors for poor outcome is the presence of a mass lesion requiring surgical removal.[24] High ICP during the first 24 hrs is also a poor prognosticator.

Obliteration of basal cisterns on CT

The status of the basal cisterns (BCs) is evaluated on axial CT scan at the level of the midbrain (▶ Fig. 61.1) where they are divided into 3 limbs[25] (1 posterior limb = quadrigeminal cistern, 2 lateral limbs = posterior portion of the ambient cisterns). **Note:**"basal cisterns" in the trauma literature are a subset of the perimesencephalic cisterns (p. 1232). Possible findings:

1. open: all 3 limbs open
2. partially closed: 1 or 2 limbs obliterated
3. completely closed: 3 limbs obliterated

Compression or absence of the BCs carries a threefold risk of increased ICP, and the status of the BCs correlates with outcome.[25]

In a study of 218 patients with GCS ≤ 8, the BCs were classified on initial CT (within 48 hrs of admission) as: absent, compressed, normal, or not visualized (quality of CT too poor to tell).[26] The relationship of the BCs to outcome is shown in ▶ Table 61.1.

18 patients had a shift of brain structures > 15 mm associated with absent BCs, all of them died. The status of the BCs were more important within each GOS score than across scores. Also, see ▶ Table 58.3 for further information on CT.

Midline shift (MLS)

The presence of MLS correlates with a worse outcome. For the purpose of standardizing measurements in trauma, MLS is defined at the level of the foramen of Monro[25] as shown in ▶ Fig. 61.2, and is calculated using Eq (61.6).

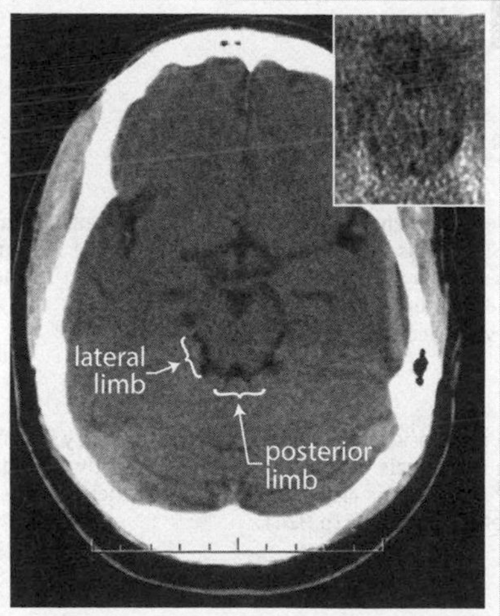

Fig. 61.1 Basal cisterns CT demonstrating *open* basal cisterns (inset: example of ≈ complete obliteration of BCs)

Table 61.1 Correlation of GOS[a] with basal cisterns

Basal cisterns	Outcome[a]				
	Mortality	Vegetative	Severe disability	Moderate disability	Good
	(GOS 1)	(GOS 2)	(GOS 3)	(GOS 4)	(GOS 5)
normal	22%	6%	16%	21%	35%
compressed	39%	7%	18%	17%	19%
absent	77%	2%	6%	4%	11%
not-visualized	68%	0%	11%	9%	12%

[a]GOS = Glasgow outcome scale, see ▶ Table 88.4

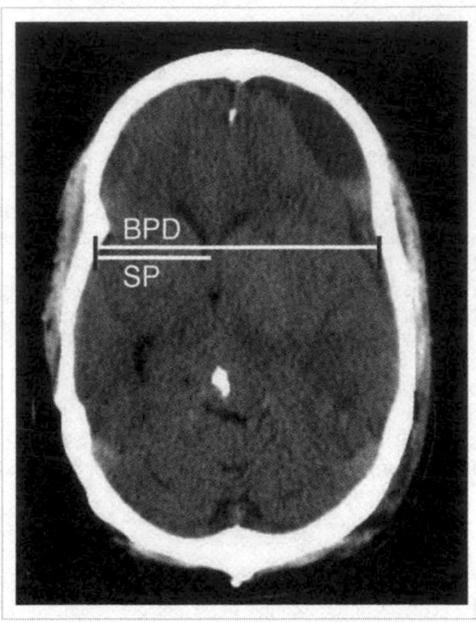

Fig. 61.2 Measurement of midline shift (axial non-contrast CT of a brain with a left-sided acute-on-chronic subdural hematoma)

$$\text{midline shift (MLS)} = \frac{\text{BPD}}{2} - \text{SP} \qquad (61.6)$$

where the midline is found by dividing the biparietal diameter (BPD) (the width of intracranial compartment at this location) by 2, and subtracting SP (the distance from the inner table to the septum pellucidum on the side of the shift). Measurements may be inaccurate if the vertical axis of the patient's head is not parallel to the long axis of the CT scanner.

Midline shift may be associated with altered levels of consciousness (p. 298).

Apolipoprotein E (apoE) ε4 allele

The presence of this genotype portends a worse prognosis following traumatic brain injury.[27] Furthermore, the incidence of severe brain injury in individuals with the apoE-4 allele greatly exceeds the rate of the allele in the general population.[28] This allele is also a risk factor for Alzheimer's disease (see below) as well as for chronic traumatic encephalopathy (p. 924).

61.6 Late complications from traumatic brain injury

61.6.1 General information

Long term complications include:
1. posttraumatic seizures (p. 462)
2. communicating hydrocephalus: incidence ≈ 3.9% of severe head injuries
3. posttraumatic syndrome (or postconcussive syndrome): see below
4. hypogonadotropic hypogonadism (p. 836) [29]
5. chronic traumatic encephalopathy (p. 924)
6. Alzheimer's disease (AD): head injury (especially if severe) promotes the deposition of amyloid proteins, especially in individuals possessing the apolipoprotein E (apoE) ε4 allele,[28] which may be related to the development of AD[30,31,32]

61.6.2 Postconcussive syndrome

General information

Variously defined collection of symptoms (see below) that is usually considered as a possible sequelae to minor head trauma (although some of these features can certainly be seen following more serious head trauma). Loss of consciousness is *not* a prerequisite to the development of the syndrome.

Controversy exists over the relative contribution of actual organic dysfunction vs. psychological factors (including conversion reaction, secondary gain which may be for attention, financial reward, drug seeking…). Furthermore, the presence of some of these symptoms can undoubtedly lead to the development of others (e.g. headache can cause difficulty concentrating and thus poor job performance and thence depression).

Presentation

A paradox has been noted by clinicians that the complaints following minor head injury seem out of proportion when considered in the context of the frequency of complaints after serious head injury. It has also been noted that patients with early post-traumatic complaints generally improve with time, whereas the late development of symptoms is often associated with a more protracted and fulminant course.

Symptoms commonly considered part of this syndrome include the following (with headache, dizziness and memory difficulties being the most frequent):
1. somatic
   a) headache
   b) dizziness or light-headedness
   c) visual disturbances: blurring is a common complaint
   d) anosmia
   e) hearing difficulties: tinnitus, reduced auditory acuity
   f) balance difficulties
2. cognitive
   a) difficulty concentrating
   b) dementia: more common with multiple brain injuries than with a single concussion (p. 924)
      - loss of intellectual ability
      - memory problems: usually impairs short-term memory more than long-term
   c) impaired judgement
3. psychosocial
   a) emotional difficulties: including depression, mood swings (emotional lability), euphoria/giddiness, easy irritability, lack of motivation, abulia
   b) personality changes
   c) loss of libido
   d) disruption of sleep/wake cycles, insomnia
   e) easy fatigability
   f) intolerance to light (photophobia) and/or loud (or even moderate) noise
   g) increased rate of job loss and divorce (may be related to any of above)

Virtually any symptom can be ascribed to the condition. Other symptoms that may be described by patients which are generally not included in the definition:
1. fainting (vaso-vagal episodes): may need to rule out posttraumatic seizures, as well as other causes of syncope

2. altered sense of taste
3. dystonia[33]

Treatment

Treatment for symptoms attributed to this syndrome tends to be more supportive and reassuring than anything else. Often times these patients obtain treatment from primary care physicians, neurologists, physiatrists, and/or psychiatrists/psychologists. Neurosurgical involvement in the continuing care for these patients is usually at the discretion of the individual physician based on his or her practice patterns. Recovery follows a highly variable course.

Early follow-up care (consisting mainly of reassurance, providing information and neuropsychological assessment and counselling) was found to reduce post-concussion symptoms at 6 months in patients with post-traumatic amnesia lasting ≥ 1 hour or those who required hospitalization, but had no benefit in those not requiring hospitalization or having amnesia < 1 hr.[34]

Some symptoms may need to be evaluated for possible correctable late complications (seizures, hydrocephalus, CSF leak…). Alves and Jane[35] perform a head CT, MRI, BAER and neuropsychological battery if symptoms after minor head injury persist > 3 months. An EEG may be appropriate in cases where there is a question of seizures. If all studies are negative, "the authors tell the patient (and the lawyer) that there is no objective evidence for disease and that psychiatric evaluation is warranted." Non-correctable abnormalities on these studies prompt reassurance that significant symptoms should subside by 1 year, and that no specific treatment, other than psychological counselling, is helpful.

61.6.3 Chronic traumatic encephalopathy

General information

Often described in retired boxers, chronic traumatic encephalopathy (CTE) encompasses a spectrum of symptoms that range from mild to a severe form AKA dementia pugilistica,[36] or punch drunk syndrome (among others). Symptoms involve motor, cognitive and psychiatric systems. CTE is distinct from post-traumatic dementia (which may follow a single closed head injury) or from post-traumatic Alzheimer's syndrome. Although generally accepted, not all authorities agree that repeated concussions have any long-term sequelae.[37]

There are some similarities with Alzheimer's disease (AD), including the presence of neurofibrillary tangles having similar microscopic characteristics (the main difference is that they tend to be more superficial in CTE than in AD[38]) and the development of amyloid angiopathy with the attendant risk of intracerebral hemorrhage.[39] EEG changes occur in one-third to one-half of professional boxers (diffuse slowing or low-voltage records).

Neuropathology

Findings include:
1. cerebral and cerebellar atrophy
2. neurofibrillary degeneration of cortical and subcortical areas
3. deposition of β-amyloid protein
   a) forming diffuse amyloid plaques
   b) in a subset of CTE patients this involves the vessel walls giving rise to cerebral amyloid angiopathy

Clinical

Clinical features of CTE are shown in ▶ Table 61.2 [36] and include[36]
1. cognitive: mental slowing and memory deficits (dementia)
2. personality changes: explosive behavior, morbid jealousy, pathological intoxication with alcohol, and paranoia
3. motor: cerebellar dysfunction, symptoms of Parkinson's disease, pyramidal tract dysfunction

Grading scales have been devised to rank patients as having probable, possible, and improbable CTE.

The chronic brain injury scale (CBIS) assesses involvement of motor, cognitive, and psychological axes as shown in ▶ Table 61.3.

Table 61.2 CTE of boxing[a]

Motor	Cognitive	Psychiatric
Early (≈ 57%)		
dysarthria tremors mild incoordination especially non-dominant hand	decreased complex attention	emotional lability euphoria/hypomania irritability, suspiciousness ease of aggression & talkativeness
Middle (≈ 17%)		
parkinsonism increased dysarthria, tremors, and incoordination	slowed mental speed mild deficits in memory, attention & executive ability	magnified personality decreased spontaneity paranoid, jealous inappropriate violent outbursts
Late (< 3%)		
pyramidal signs prominent parkinsonism prominent dysarthria, tremors & ataxia	prominent slowness of thought/speech amnesia attention deficits executive dysfunction	cheerful/silly decreased insight paranoid, psychotic disinhibited, violent possible Klüver-Bucy

[a]in professional boxers with ≥ 20 bouts

Table 61.3 Chronic brain injury scale

Grade involvement of each of the following axes separately:	Scoring for each axis:
• motor • cognitive • psychological	• 0 = none • 1 = mild • 2 = moderate • 3 = severe
Sum total points	**Severity**
0	normal
1 – 2	mild
3 – 4	moderate
> 4	severe

Risk factors for dementia pugilistica in boxing:

See reference.[36]

- risk increases with length of boxing career, especially > 10 yrs
- age at retirement: risk goes up after age 28 yrs
- number of bouts: especially ≥ 20 (more important than the number of knock-outs)
- boxing style: increased risk among poorer performers, those known as sluggers rather than "scientific" boxers, those known to be hard to knock out or known to take a punch and keep going
- age at examination: long latency causes increased prevalence with age
- and possibly, the number of head blows
- risk increases in patients with the apolipoprotein E (apo E) ε4 allele (as in Alzheimer's disease) as shown in ▶ Table 61.4
- professional boxers (more risk than amateurs)

Table 61.4 Odds ratio for developing Alzheimer's disease

Head injury	Apo E ε4 allele	Odds ratio
–	–	1
–	+	2
+	–	1
+	+	10

Neuro-imaging

The most common finding is cerebral atrophy. A cavum septum pellucidum (CSP) is observed in 13% of boxers.[40] CSP in this setting probably represents an acquired condition[41] and correlates with cerebral atrophy.

References

[1] Brain Trauma Foundation, Povlishock JT, Bullock MR. Infection prophylaxis. J Neurotrauma. 2007; 24:S26–S31

[2] Kaufman HH, Slatterwhite T, McConnell BJ, et al. Deep vein thrombosis and pulmonary embolism in head-injured patients. Angiology. 1983; 34:627–638

[3] Brain Trauma Foundation, Povlishock JT, Bullock MR. Deep vein thrombosis prophylaxis. J Neurotrauma. 2007; 24:S32–S36

[4] Brain Trauma Foundation, Povlishock JT, Bullock MR. Nutrition. J Neurotrauma. 2007; 24:S77–S82

[5] Clifton GL, Robertson CS, Grossman RG, et al. The Metabolic Response to Severe Head Injury. J Neurosurg. 1984; 60:687–696

[6] Young B, Ott L, Norton J, et al. Metabolic and Nutritional Sequelae in the Non-Steroid Treated Head Injury Patient. Neurosurgery. 1985; 17:784–791

[7] Deutschman CS, Konstantinides FN, Raup S, et al. Physiological and Metabolic Response to Isolated Closed Head Injury. J Neurosurg. 1986; 64:89–98

[8] Bullock R, Chesnut RM, Clifton G, et al. Guidelines for the Management of Severe Head Injury. 1995

[9] Clifton GL, Robertson CS, Choi SC. Assessment of Nutritional Requirements of Head Injured Patients. J Neurosurg. 1986; 64:895–901

[10] Rapp RP, Young B, Twyman D, et al. The Favorable Effect of Early Parenteral Feeding on Survival in Head Injured Patients. J Neurosurg. 1983; 58:906–912

[11] Young B, Ott L, Twyman D, et al. The Effect of Nutritional Support on Outcome from Severe Head Injury. Neurosurgery. 1987; 67:668–676

[12] Hadley MN, Grahm TW, Harrington T, et al. Nutritional Support and Neurotrauma: A Critical Review of Early Nutrition in Forty-Five Acute Head Injury Patients. Neurosurgery. 1986; 19:367–373

[13] The Brain Trauma Foundation. The American Association of Neurological Surgeons. The Joint Section on Neurotrauma and Critical Care. Nutrition. J Neurotrauma. 2000; 17:539–547

[14] Harris JA, Benedict FG. Biometric Studies of Basal Metabolism in Man. Washington, D.C. 1919

[15] Clifton GL, Robertson CS, Contant CF, et al. Enteral Hyperalimantation in Head Injury. J Neurosurg. 1985; 62:186–193

[16] Ott L, Young B, Phillips R, et al. Altered Gastric Emptying in the Head-Injured Patient: Relationship to Feeding Intolerance. J Neurosurg. 1991; 74:738–742

[17] Grahm TW, Zadrozny DB, Harrington T. Benefits of Early Jejunal Hyperalimantation in the Head-Injured Patient. Neurosurgery. 1989; 25:729–735

[18] Gadisseux P, Ward JD, Young HF, Becker DP. Nutrition and the Neurosurgical Patient. J Neurosurg. 1984; 60:219–232

[19] Duke JH, Jorgensen SB, Broell JR, et al. Contribution of Protein to Caloric Expenditure Following Injury. Surgery. 1970; 68:168–174

[20] Poca MA, Sahuquillo J, Mataro M, Benejam B, Arikan F, Baguena M. Ventricular enlargement after moderate or severe head injury: a frequent and neglected problem. J Neurotrauma. 2005; 22:1303–1310

[21] Tian HL, Xu T, Hu J, Cui YH, Chen H, Zhou LF. Risk factors related to hydrocephalus after traumatic subarachnoid hemorrhage. Surg Neurol. 2008; 69:241–6; discussion 246

[22] Marmarou A, Foda MA, Bandoh K, Yoshihara M, Yamamoto T, Tsuji O, Zasler N, Ward JD, Young HF. Posttraumatic ventriculomegaly: hydrocephalus or atrophy? A new approach for diagnosis using CSF dynamics. J Neurosurg. 1996; 85:1026–1035

[23] Miller JD, Butterworth JF, Gudeman SK, et al. Further Experience in the Management of Severe Head Injury. J Neurosurg. 1981; 54:289–299

[24] Stablein DM, Miller JD, Choi SC, et al. Statistical Methods for Determining Prognosis in Severe Head Injury. Neurosurgery. 1980; 6:243–248

[25] Bullock MR, Chesnut RM, Ghajar J, et al. Appendix II: Evaluation of relevant computed tomographic scan findings. Neurosurgery. 2006; 58

[26] Toutant SM, Klauber MR, Marshall LF, et al. Absent or Compressed Basal Cisterns on First CT Scan: Ominous Predictor of Outcome in Severe Head Injury. J Neurosurg. 1984; 61:691–694

[27] Friedman G, Froom P, Sazbon L, et al. Apolipoprotein E-e4 Genotype Predicts a Poor Outcome in Survivors of Traumatic Injury. Neurology. 1999; 52:244–248

[28] Nicoll JAR, Roberts GW, Graham DI. Apolipoprotein E e4 Allele Is Associated with Deposition of Amyloid ß-Protein Following Head Injury. Nature Med. 1995; 1:135–137

[29] Clark JDA, Raggatt PR, Edward OM. Hypothalamic Hypogonadism Following Major Head Injury. Clin Endocrin. 1988; 29:153–165

[30] Mayeux R, Ottman R, Tang MX, et al. Genetic Susceptibility and Head Injury as Risk Factors for Alzheimer's Disease Among Community-Dwelling Elderly Persons and Their First Degree Relatives. Ann Neurol. 1993; 33:494–501

[31] Roberts GW, Gentleman SM, Lynch A, et al. ß Amyloid Protein Deposition in the Brain After Severe Head Injury: Implications for the Pathogenesis of Alzheimer's Disease. J Neurol Neurosurg Psychiatry. 1994; 57:419–425

[32] Mayeux R, Ottman R, Maestre G, et al. Synergistic Effects of Traumatic Head Injury and Apolipoprotein-e4 in Patients with Alzheimer's Disease. Neurology. 1995; 45:555–557

[33] Lee MS, Rinne JO, Ceballos-Bauman A, et al. Dystonia After Head Trauma. Neurology. 1994; 44:1374–1378

[34] Wade DT, Crawford S, Wenden FJ, et al. Does Routine Follow Up After Head Injury Help? A Randomized Controlled Trial. J Neurol Neurosurg Psychiatry. 1997; 62:478–484

[35] Alves WM, Jane JA, Youmans JR. In: Post-Traumatic Syndrome. Neurological Surgery. 3rd ed. Philadelphia: W. B. Saunders; 1990:2230–2242

[36] Mendez MF. The Neuropsychiatric Aspects of Boxing. Int'l J Psychiatry in Medicine. 1995; 25:249–262

[37] Parkinson D. Evaluating Cerebral Concussion. Surg Neurol. 1996; 45:459–462

[38] Hof PR, Bouras C, Buee L, et al. Differential Distribution of Neurofibrillary Tangles in the Cerebral Cortex of Dementia Pugilistica and Alzheimer's Disease Cases. Acta Neuropathol. 1992; 85:23–30

[39] Jordan BD, Kanik AB, Horwich MS, et al. Apolipoprotein E e4 and Fatal Cerebral Amyloid Angiopathy Associated with Dementia Pugilistica. Ann Neurol. 1995; 38:698–699

[40] Jordan BD, Jahre C, Hauser WA, et al. CT of 338 Active Professional Boxers. Radiology. 1992; 185:509–512

[41] Jordan BD, Jahre C, Hauser WA. Serial Computed Tomography in Professional Boxers. J Neuroimaging. 1992; 25:249–262

Part XV

Spine Trauma

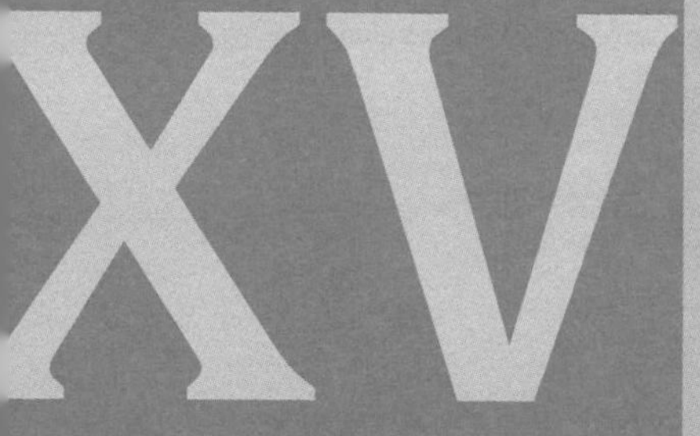

62

62 General Information, Neurologic Assessment, Whiplash and Sports-Related Injuries, Pediatric Spine Injuries

62.1 Introduction

20% of patients with a major spine injury will have a second spinal injury at another level, which may be noncontiguous. These patients often have simultaneous but unrelated injuries (e.g. chest trauma, TBI…). Injuries directly associated with spinal cord injuries include arterial dissections (carotid and/or vertebral arteries).

62.2 Terminology

62.2.1 Spinal stability

Many definitions have been proposed. A conceptual definition of clinical stability from White and Panjabi[1]: the ability of the spine under physiologic loads to limit displacement so as to prevent injury or irritation of the spinal cord and nerve roots (including cauda equina) and, to prevent incapacitating deformity or pain due to structural changes.

Biomechanical stability refers to the ability of the spine ex vivo to resist forces.

Predicting spinal stability is often difficult, and to this end various models have been developed, none of which is perfect. See models of stability for cervical spine injuries (p. 987), and thoracolumbar fractures (p. 1002).

62.2.2 Level of injury

There is disagreement over what should be defined as "the level" of a spinal cord injury. Some define the "level" of a spinal cord injury as the lowest level of completely *normal* function (thus a patient would be termed a C5 quadriplegic even with minor C6 motor function). However, most sources define the "level" as the most caudal segment with motor function that is at least 3 out of 5 and if pain and temperature sensation is present.

62.2.3 Completeness of lesion

Categorization is important for treatment decisions and prognostication.

Incomplete lesion

Definition: any residual motor or sensory function more than 3 segments below the level of the injury.[2] Look for signs of preserved long-tract function.

Signs of incomplete lesion:

1. sensation (including position sense) or voluntary movement in the LEs in the presence of a cervical or thoracic spinal cord injury
2. "sacral sparing": preserved sensation around the anus, voluntary rectal sphincter contraction, or voluntary toe flexion
3. an injury does *not* qualify as incomplete with preserved sacral reflexes alone (e.g. bulbocavernosus)

Types of incomplete lesion:

1. central cord syndrome (p. 944)
2. Brown-Séquard syndrome (cord hemisection) (p. 947)
3. anterior cord syndrome (p. 946)
4. posterior cord syndrome (p. 947): rare

Complete lesion

No preservation of any motor and/or sensory function more than 3 segments below the level of the injury in the absence of spinal shock. About 3% of patients with complete injuries on initial exam will develop some recovery within 24 hours. Recovery is essentially zero if the spinal cord injury remains complete beyond 72 hours.

Spinal shock

This term is often used in two completely different senses:

1. hypotension (shock) that follows spinal cord injury (SBP usually ≈ 80 mm Hg). See Hypotension (p. 950) for treatment. Caused by multiple factors:
   a) interruption of sympathetics: implies spinal cord injury above T1
      - loss of vascular tone (vasoconstrictors) below level of injury
      - leaves parasympathetics relatively unopposed causing *bradycardia*
   b) loss of muscle tone due to skeletal muscle paralysis below level of injury results in venous pooling and thus a relative hypovolemia
   c) blood loss from associated wounds → true hypovolemia
2. transient loss of all neurologic function (including segmental and polysynaptic reflex activity and autonomic function) below the level of the SCI[3,4] → flaccid paralysis and areflexia
   a) Duration: may abate in as little as 72 hours, but typically persists 1–2 weeks, occasionally several months
   b) Accompanied by loss of the bulbocavernosus reflex
   c) Spinal cord reflexes immediately above the injury may also be depressed on the basis of the Schiff-Sherrington phenomenon
   d) When spinal shock resolves, there will be spasticity below the level of the lesion and return of the bulbocavernosus reflex
   e) A poor prognostic sign

62.3 Whiplash-associated disorders

62.3.1 General information

"Whiplash" was initially a lay term, which is currently defined as a traumatic injury to the soft tissue structures in the region of the cervical spine (including: cervical muscles, ligaments, intervertebral discs, facet joints...) due to hyperflexion, hyperextension, or rotational injury to the neck in the absence of fractures, dislocations, or intervertebral disc herniation.[5] It is the most common non-fatal automobile injury.[6] Symptoms may start immediately, but more commonly are delayed several hours or days. In addition to symptoms related to the cervical spine, common associated complaints include headaches, cognitive impairment, and low back pain.

62.3.2 Clinical grading

A proposed clinical classification system of WAD is shown in ▶ Table 62.1.[7]

62.3.3 Evaluation and treatment

A consensus[8] regarding diagnosis and management of these injuries is shown in ▶ Table 62.2 and ▶ Table 62.3. Keep in mind that conditions such as occipital neuralgia may occasionally follow whiplash type injuries and should be treated appropriately (▶ Table 62.3).

Table 62.1 Clinical grading of WAD severity

Grade		Description
	0	no complaints, no signs[a]
	1	neck pain or stiffness or tenderness, no signs
Whiplash	2	above symptoms with reduced range of motion or point tenderness
	3	above symptoms with weakness, sensory deficit, or absent deep tendon reflexes
	4	above symptoms with fracture or dislocation[a]

[a]the definition of whiplash excludes these patients[5]

Table 62.2 Evaluation of WAD

Grade 1 patients with normal mental status and physical exam do not require plain radiographs on presentation
Grade 2 & 3 patients: C-spine x-rays, possibly with flexion-extension views. Special imaging studies (MRI, CT, myelography...) are not indicated
Grade 3 & 4: these patients should be managed as suspected spinal cord injury; see Initial management of spinal cord injury (p. 949), and sections that follow

Table 62.3 Treatment of WAD[8][a]

Whiplash is usually a benign condition requiring little treatment and usually resolves in days to a few weeks in most cases.

Recommendation	**Grade**		
	1	2	3
Range of motion exercises	should be started immediately for all		
Encourage early return to regular activities	immediately	ASAP	
Cervical collars and rest[b]	no	not for > 72 hrs	not for > 96 hrs
Passive modality therapies: heat, ice, massage, TENS, ultrasound, relaxation techniques, acupuncture, and work alteration	no	optional if symptoms last > 3 wks	
Medications: optional use of NSAIDs and non-narcotic analgesics? (recommended for ≤ 3 wks)	no	yes	yes. Limited narcotics may also occasionally be needed
Surgery	no	no	only for progressive neurologic deficit or persisting arm pain

✖ ***Not*** recommended: cervical pillows and soft collars, bed rest, spray and stretch exercises, muscle relaxant medication, TENS, reflexology, magnetic necklaces, herbal remedies, homeopathy, OTC medications (except NSAIDs, see above), and intra-articular, intrathecal, or trigger point steroid injections

[a]excluding patients with fractures, dislocations, or spinal cord injuries
[b]soft foam collars are generally discouraged; if they are to be used, the narrow part should be placed in front to avoid neck extension[5]

62.3.4 Outcome

In a study of 117 patients < 56 years of age having WAD due to automobile accidents (excluding those with cervical fractures, dislocations, or injuries elsewhere in the body) conducted in Switzerland[9] (where all medical costs were paid by the state and there was no opportunity for litigation and no compensation for pain and suffering, although there was the possibility of permanent disability), the recovery rate was as shown in ▶ Table 62.4. Of the 21 patients with continued symptoms at 2 yrs, only 5 were restricted with respect to work (3 reduced to part-time work, 2 on disability). Patients with persistent symptoms were older, had more varied complaints on initial exam, had a more rotated or inclined head position at the time of impact, had a higher incidence of pretraumatic headaches, and had a higher incidence of certain pre-existing findings (such as radiologic evidence of cervical osteoarthritis). The amount of damage to the automobile and the speed of the cars had little relationship to the degree of injury, and outcome was not influenced by gender, vocation, or psychological factors.

Table 62.4 Recovery of patients with WAD

Time (mos)	Percent recovered
3	56%
6	70%
12	76%
24	82%

62.4 Pediatric spine injuries

62.4.1 General information

Spinal cord injury is fairly uncommon in children, with the ratio of head injuries to spinal cord injuries being ≈ 30:1 in pediatrics. Only ≈ 5% of spinal cord injuries occur in children. Due to ligamentous laxity together with a high head to body weight ratio, immaturity of paraspinal muscles and the underdeveloped uncinate processes, these tend to involve ligamentous rather than bony injuries, see SCIWORA (p.999). There is also the potential for physeal (growth plate) separation in young children, which may have good potential to heal. The cervical spine is the most vulnerable segment (with subaxial injuries being fairly uncommon), with 42% of injuries occurring here, 31% thoracic, and 27% lumbar. The fatality rate is higher with pediatric spine injuries than with adults (opposite to the situation with head injury), with the cause of death more often related to other severe injuries than to the spinal injury.[10]

62.4.2 Evaluation

Practice guidelines for diagnostic workup is shown below (see Practice guideline: Evaluation of pediatric C-spine injuries (p.934)).

62.4.3 Pediatric cervical spine injuries and mimics

General information

See pediatric C-spine anatomy (p.214). In the age group ≤ 9 yrs, 67% of cervical spine injuries occur in the upper 3 segments of the cervical spine (occiput-C2).[11]

Synchondroses

Normal synchondroses (p.215) may be mistaken for fractures, especially the dentocentral synchondrosis of the atlas (p.214) which may be mistaken for an odontoid fracture. Conversely, actual fractures may occur through synchondroses.[12,13] Recommended treatment for fractures through synchondroses: the tendency for synchondroses to fuse suggests that emergency reduction followed by external immobilization be attempted. Internal immobilization/fusion should be reserved for persistent instability.[13]

Pseudospread of the atlas

See reference.[14]

Pseudospread of the atlas (defined as > 2 mm total overlap of the two C1 lateral masses on C2 on AP open-mouth view) is present in most children 3 mos to 4 yrs age. Prevalence is 91–100% during the second year of life. Youngest example at 3 mos, oldest at 5.75 yrs. Normal total offset is typically 2 mm during the first year, 4 mm during the second, 6 mm during the third, and decreasing thereafter. The maximum is 8 mm. Trauma is not a contributing factor.

Pseudospread is probably a result of disproportionate growth of the atlas on the axis. This could be misdiagnosed as a *Jefferson fracture* (p.971), which rarely occurs prior to the teen-ages (owing to lower weight of children, more flexible necks, increased plasticity of skull, and shock absorbing synchondroses of C1).

Neck rotation can also sometimes simulate the appearance of a Jefferson fracture.

When suspicion of fracture is high: CT scan through C1 can resolve the issue of whether or not there is a fracture.

Pseudosubluxation

Either anterior displacement of C2 (axis) on C3 and/or significant angulation at this level. Seen in children (up to age 10 yrs) on lateral C-spine x-ray after trauma. Up to age 10 yrs, flexion and extension are centered at C2–3; this moves down to C4–5 or C5–6 after age 10. C2 normally moves forward on C3 up to 2–3 mm in peds.[15] When the head is flexed, displacement is expected; may be exacerbated by spasm.[16] Does not represent pathological instability. Fractures and dislocations are unusual in children, and when they do occur, they resemble those in adults.

10 cases reported between ages 4–6 yrs[17]: pain was not uncommon. In each case, either the head or neck was flexed (sometimes minimally); the pseudosubluxation corrected when x-ray was repeated with head in true neutral position.

Recommendation: treat patient for soft-tissue injury and not for subluxation.

Treatment

Practice guideline: Evaluation of pediatric C-spine injuries

Level I[18]

- Use CT to assess the condyle-C1 interval (CCI) for pediatric patients with potential atlanto-occipital dislocation (AOD)

Level II[18]:

- Do not perform C-spine imaging in children > 3 years age with trauma who are:
  - alert
  - neurologically intact
  - without posterior midline cervical tenderness (with no distracting pain)
  - not hypotensive without explanation
  - not intoxicated
- Do not perform C-spine imaging in children < 3 years age with trauma who meet all of the following conditions:
  - have a GCS > 13
  - are neurologically intact
  - have no cervical midline tenderness (without distracting injury)
  - are not intoxicated
  - do not have unexplained hypotension
  - were not in a motor vehicle collision, a fall > 10 feet, or non-accidental trauma (NAT) as the known or suspected mechanism of injury
- Obtain cervical spine x-rays or high-resolution cervical CT in pediatric trauma victims who do not meet either set of criteria above
- Obtain 3-position CT with C1-2 motion analysis to confirm and classify the diagnosis for children suspected of having atlantoaxial rotatory fixation (AARF)

Level III[18]:

- children < 8 yrs age: when restrained, immobilize with thoracic elevation or an occipital recess (allows more neutral alignment due to the relatively large head)
- children < 7 yrs age with injuries of the C2 synchondrosis (p. 215): closed reduction and halo immobilization
- patients with AARF:
  - acute AARF (< 4 weeks duration) that does not reduce spontaneously: reduction with manipulation or halter traction
  - chronic AARF (> 4 weeks duration): reduction with halter or tong/halo traction
  - recurrent or irreducible AARF: internal fixation and fusion
- for isolated cervical spine ligamentous injuries and unstable or irreducible fractures of dislocations with associated deformity: consider primary operative treatment
- for cervical spine injuries that fail non-operative management: operative treatment

Level III[19]:

- children < 8 yrs age: immobilize with thoracic elevation or an occipital recess (allows more neutral alignment due to the relatively large head)

- children < 7 yrs age with injuries of the C2 dentocentral synchondrosis (p. 215): closed reduction and halo immobilization
- consider: primary operative treatment for isolated C-spine ligamentous injuries with associated deformity

62.5 Cervical bracing

62.5.1 Soft collars

Soft (sponge rubber) collar: does not immobilize the cervical spine to any significant degree. Its function is primarily to remind the patient to reduce neck movements.

62.5.2 Rigid cervical collars

Inadequate for stabilizing upper and mid-cervical spine and for preventing rotation.

Common rigid collars:

- Miami J collar & Aspen collar: have removable pads
- Philadelphia collar: no removable pads. Feels hotter to wear

62.5.3 Poster braces

Distinguished from cervicothoracic orthoses (see below) by the lack of straps under the axilla. Includes the four poster brace. Generally good for preventing flexion at midcervical levels.

62.5.4 Cervicothoracic orthoses

Cervicothoracic orthoses (CTO) incorporate some form of body vest to immobilize the cervical spine. The following are presented in increasing degree of immobilization.

Guilford brace: essentially a ring around the occiput and chin connected by two posts to anterior and posterior thoracic pads.

SOMI brace: acronym for Sternal Occipital Mandibular Immobilizer. Good for bracing against flexion (especially upper cervical spine). Inadequate for hyper-extension type injuries because of weak occipital support. Has special forehead attachment to allow patient to eat comfortably without mandibular support.

"Yale brace": a sort of extended Philadelphia collar. The most effective CTO for bracing against flexion-extension and rotation. Major shortcoming is poor prevention of lateral bending (only ≈ 50% reduced).

62.5.5 Halo-vest brace

Can immobilize the upper or lower cervical spine, not very good for mid-cervical spine (due to snaking of the midcervical spine). Unable to provide adequate distraction support following vertebral body resection when patient assumes upright position (i.e. it is *not* a portable cervical traction device). Overall reduction of flexion/extension as well as lateral bending is ≈ 90–95%, rotation is reduced by 98%. See placement (p. 958).

62.6 Follow-up schedule

After initial management (surgical or nonsurgical) of cervical spine problems (stable or unstable) the follow-up schedule shown in ▶ Table 62.5 is suggested to permit recognition of problems in time for treatment[1] (start with 3 weeks and keep doubling the interval to 1 year).

62.7 Sports-related cervical spine injuries

62.7.1 General information

Any of the spine injuries described in this book can be sports-related. This section considers some injuries peculiar to sports.

62

Table 62.5 Sample follow-up cervical spine clinic visit schedule

Time post-op	Agenda
7–10 d	(for post-op patients only) wound check, D/C sutures/staples if used
4-6 weeks	AP & lateral C-spine x-ray in brace
10-12 weeks	• AP & lateral C-spine x-rays with flexion/extension views out of brace • if x-rays look good and patient is doing well, begin weaning brace
6 months	• AP & lateral C-spine x-rays with flexion/extension views • some surgeons release patients at this time if they are doing well
1 year (optional)	• AP & lateral C-spine x-rays with flexion/extension views • release patient if they are doing well

Table 62.6 Sports-related spinal cord injuries

Type	Description
I	permanent SCI
II	transient SCI without radiographic abnormality
III	radiologic abnormality without neurologic deficit

Bailes et al.[20] classified sports-related spinal cord injuries (SCI) as shown in ▶ Table 62.6. Type I injures may be complete or may have features of any of the incomplete SCI syndromes (often in mixed or partial forms). Type II injuries include spinal concussion, spinal neuropraxia (see below), and the burning hands syndrome (see below), all in the absence of radiographic abnormalities and all with complete resolution of symptoms. Patients should be carefully evaluated, and return to competition should not be allowed in the presence of neurologic deficit, radiographically demonstrated injury, certain congenital C-spine abnormalities, and possibly for "repeat offenders" (p.937). Type III injuries are the most common. Unstable injuries should be treated appropriately (p.997).

62.7.2 Football-related cervical spine injuries

General information

✖ Football players with suspected C-spine injury should not have their helmet removed in the field (p.949).

Terminology

The following terms probably originated as locker-room jargon for various cervical spine-related injuries usually sustained in playing football. Medical definitions have subsequently been retro-fitted to them. As a result, the precise definitions may not be uniformly agreed upon. Although the semantics may differ, it is more important from a diagnostic and therapeutic standpoint to distinguish nerve root injuries, brachial plexus injuries, and spinal cord injuries.

1. cervical cord neuropraxia[21] (CCN): sensory changes which may involve numbness, tingling or burning. May or may not be associated with motor symptoms of weakness or complete paralysis. Typically lasts < 15 mins (although may persist up to 48 hrs), involves all 4 extremities in 80% of cases. Narrowing of the sagittal diameter of the cervical spinal canal is felt to be a contributory factor. With resumption of contact activities, recurrence rate is ≈ 56%, with higher risks of recurrence among those with narrower canal diameters. Evaluation should include cervical MRI. Torg[21] feels that uncomplicated cases of CCN (no spinal instability and no MRI evidence of cord defect or edema) have a low risk of permanent injury and does not recommend activity restrictions
2. "stinger" or "burner": distinct from the burning hands syndrome. Unilateral. burning dysesthetic pain radiating down one arm from the shoulder, sometimes associated with weakness involving the C5 or C6 nerve roots. Usually follows a tackle. May result from downward traction on the upper trunk of the brachial plexus (when the shoulder is forcefully depressed with the neck

flexed to the contralateral side) or by direct nerve root compression in the neural foramina (not a SCI)
3. burning hands syndrome[22]: similar to a stinger, but bilateral. Probably represents a *SCI*; possibly a mild variant of a central cord syndrome (p. 944)
4. other neurologic injuries include: vascular injury to carotid or vertebral arteries. Usually related to intimal dissection (p. 1018) following a direct blow to the neck or by extreme movements. Symptoms are those of a TIA or stroke

Spear tackler's spine

Rule changes in 1976 banned spearing (the practice of using the football helmet as a battering ram to tackle an opponent) and resulted in a reduction of the number of football-related occurrences of cervical spine fractures and quadriplegia.[23]

Four characteristics of spear tackler's spine:
1. cervical spinal stenosis
2. loss of normal cervical lordosis: as a result, the stress of axial loading is more likely to be imparted to the vertebral bodies, rather than being absorbed by the cervical musculature and ligaments, increasing the risk of burst fractures and quadriplegia
3. evidence of pre-existing traumatic abnormalities
4. documented spear-tackler's technique

Suggested management:

The athlete is removed from competition until the cervical lordosis returns and the player learns to use other tackling techniques. This tackling technique has been banned since 1976.

62.7.3 Return to play and pre-participation guidelines

Return to play (RTP) and pre-participation evaluation guidelines related to the cervical spine are shown in ▶ Table 62.7 (modified[24]). These are just guidelines, and do not insure safety. Clinical judgement must always be employed.

Table 62.7 C-spine-related contraindications for participation in contact sports[a]

Condition[b]			C.I.[c]
		Congenital[d]	
1.	odontoid abnormalities (serious injury may result from atlanto-axial instability)		
	a.	complete aplasia (rare)	absolute
	b.	hypoplasia (seen in conjunction with achondroplasia and spondyloepiphyseal dysplasia)	absolute
	c.	os odontoideum (probably of traumatic origin)	absolute
2.	atlanto-occipital fusion (partial or complete fusion of atlas to occiput): sudden onset of symptoms & sudden death have been reported		absolute
3.	Klippel-Feil anomaly (congenital fusion of 2 or more cervical vertebrae)[e]		
	a.	Type I: mass fusion of C-spine to upper T-spine	absolute
	b.	Type II: fusion of only 1 or 2 interspaces	
		• associated with limited ROM, occipitocervical anomalies, instability, disc disease or degenerative changes	absolute
		• associated with full ROM and none of the above	none
		Acquired	
1.	cervical spinal stenosis[f]		
	a.	asymptomatic	none
	b.	with one episode of cord neuropraxia	relative

Table 62.7 continued

Condition[b]			C.I.[c]
	c.	cord neuropraxia + MRI evidence of cord defect or edema	absolute
	d.	cord neuropraxia + ligamentous instability, symptoms or neurologic findings > 36 hrs, or multiple episodes	absolute
2.	spear tackler's spine (see text)		absolute
3.	spina bifida occulta: rare, incidental x-ray finding		none
Post-traumatic upper cervical spine			
1.	atlantoaxial instability (ADI > 3 mm adults, > 4 mm peds)		absolute
2.	atlantoaxial rotatory fixation (may be associated with disruption of transverse ligament)		absolute
3.	fractures		
	a.	healed, pain-free, full ROM, & no neurologic findings with any of the following fractures: nondisplaced Jefferson fracture; odontoid fracture; or lateral mass fracture of axis	none
	b.	all others	absolute
4.	post-surgical atlantoaxial fusion		absolute
Post-traumatic subaxial cervical spine			
1.	ligamentous injuries: > 3.5 mm subluxation, or > 11° angulation on flexion-extension views		absolute
2.	fractures		
	a.	healed, stable fractures listed here with normal exam: VB compression fracture without posterior involvement; spinous process fractures	none
	b.	VB fractures with sagittal component or posterior bony or ligamentous involvement	absolute
	c.	comminuted fracture with displacement into spinal canal	absolute
	d.	lateral mass fracture producing facet incongruity	absolute
3.	intervertebral disc injury		
	a.	healed herniated disc treated conservatively	none
	b.	S/P ACDF with solid fusion, no symptoms, normal exam and full pain-free ROM	none
	c.	chronic herniated disc with pain, neuro findings or ↓ ROM, or acute herniated disc	absolute
4.	S/P fusion		
	a.	stable one-level fusion	none
	b.	stable two-level fusion	relative
	c.	fusion > 2 levels	absolute

[a]organized contact sports includes[24]: boxing, football, ice hockey, lacrosse, rugby & wrestling
[b] see also cranial-related (and craniocervical) conditions (p. 1151) (e.g. Chiari I malformation...)
[c]C.I. = contraindications, classified as absolute, relative (i.e. uncertain) or none
[d]congenital abnormalities may have particular relevance to Special Olympics
[e]NB: Klippel-Feil may be associated with abnormalities in other organ systems (e.g. cardiac) which may impact on participation in contact sports (p. 271)
[f] Pavlov ratio (p. 1088) has a low positive predictive value for injuries in contact sports and is therefore not a useful screening test (i.e. an asymptomatic Pavlov ratio < 0.8 is not a contraindication to participation)

62.8 Neurological assessment

62.8.1 General information

Evaluation of the level of the lesion requires familiarity with the following concepts about the relationship between the bony spinal canal and the spinal cord and nerves (▶ Fig. 62.1).

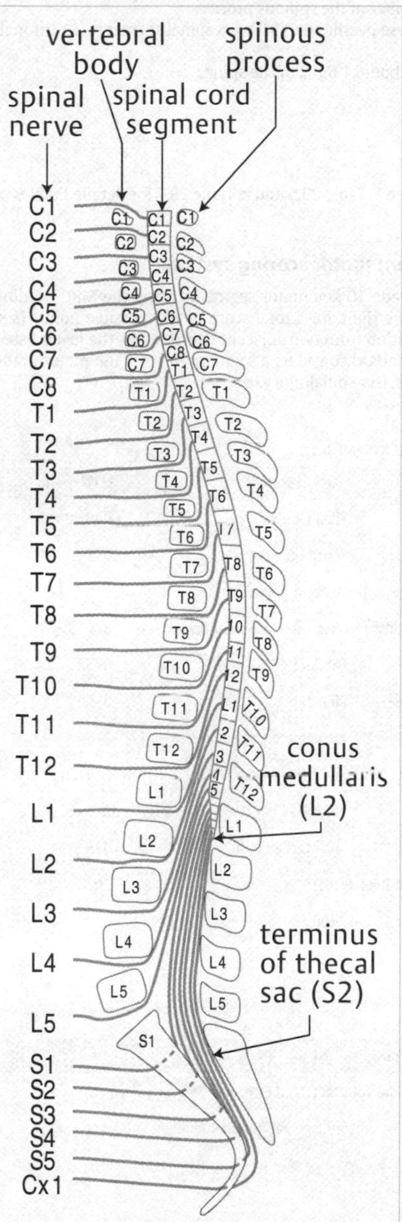

Fig. 62.1 Relationship between spinal cord, nerve roots, and bony spine

1. since there are 8 pairs of cervical nerves and only 7 cervical vertebra
   a) cervical nerves 1 through 8 exit *above* the pedicles of their like-numbered vertebra
   b) thoracic, lumbar and sacral nerves exit *below* the pedicles of their like-numbered vertebra
2. due to disproportionately greater growth of the spinal column than the spinal cord during development, the following relationships of the spinal *cord* to the vertebral column exist:
   a) to determine which segment of the cord underlies a given vertebra:
      - from T2 through T10: add 2 to the number of the spinous process
      - for T11, T12 and L1, remember that these overlie the 11 lowest spinal segments (L1 through L5, S1 through S5, and Coxygeal-1)
   b) the conus medullaris in the adult lies at about L1 or L2 of the spine

62.8.2 Motor level assessment

General information

The following tables are for rapid assessment (see ▶ Table 29.5 and ▶ Table 29.7 for detailed tables of motor innervation).

ASIA (American Spinal Injury Association) motor scoring system

A system[25,26] that may be rapidly applied to grade 10 key motor segments using the MRC Grading Scale (▶ Table 29.2) from 0–5 on the left and the right, for a total score of 100 possible points (see ▶ Table 62.8). NB: most muscles receive innervation from two adjacent spinal levels, the levels listed in ▶ Table 62.8 are the *lower* of the two. The standard considers a segment intact if the motor grade is fair (≥ 3). For additional information, see www.asia-spinalinjury.org.

Table 62.8 Key muscles for motor level classification (EXTREMITIES)

RIGHT grade	Segment	Muscle	Action to test	LEFT grade
0–5	C5	biceps	flex elbow	0–5
0–5	C6	wrist extensors	cock up wrist	0–5
0–5	C7	triceps	extend elbow	0–5
0–5	C8	flexor digitorum profundus	flex middle distal phalanx	0–5
0–5	T1	hand intrinsics	abduct little finger	0–5
0–5	L2	iliopsoas	flex hip	0–5
0–5	L3	quadriceps	straighten knee	0–5
0–5	L4	tibialis anterior	dorsiflex foot	0–5
0–5	L5	EHL	dorsiflex big toe	0–5
0–5	S1	gastrocnemius	plantarflex foot	0–5
50		← TOTAL POSSIBLE POINTS →		50
		GRAND TOTAL: 100		

Table 62.9 Axial muscle evaluation[27]

Level	Muscle	Action to test
C4	diaphragm	tidal volume (TV), FEV1, and vital capacity (VC)
T2–9 T9–10 T11–12	intercostals upper abdominals lower abdominals	use sensory level, abdominal reflexes, & Beevor's sign

More detailed motor evaluation

Table 62.10 Skeletal muscles and their major spinal innervation (major contributing segment is shown in boldface)

Segment	Muscle	Action to test	Reflex
C1–4	neck muscles		
C3, 4, 5	diaphragm	inspiration, TV, FEV1, VC	
C5, 6	deltoid	abduct arm > 90°	
C5, 6	biceps	elbow flexion	biceps
C6, 7	extensor carpi radialis	wrist extension	supinator
C7, 8	triceps, extensor digitorum	elbow and finger extension	triceps
C8, T1	flexor digitorum profundus	grasp (flex distal phalanges)	
C8, T1	hand intrinsics	abduct little finger, adduct thumb	
T2–9	intercostals[a]		
T9,10	upper abdominals[a]	Beevor's sign[b]	abdominal cutaneous reflex[c]
T11,12	lower abdominals[a]		
L2, 3	iliopsoas, adductors	hip flexion	cremasteric reflex[d]
L3, 4	quadriceps	knee extension	infrapatellar (knee jerk)
L4, 5	medial hamstrings, tibialis anterior	ankle dorsiflexion	medial hamstrings
L5, S1	lateral hamstrings, posterior tibialis, peroneals	knee flexion	
L5, S1	extensor digitorum, EHL	great toe extension	
S1, 2	gastrocs, soleus	ankle plantarflexion	achilles (ankle jerk)
S2, 3	flex digitorum, flex hallucis		
S2, 3, 4	bladder, lower bowel, anal sphincter	clamp down during rectal exam	anal cutaneous reflex[e], bulbocavernosus & priapism

[a]also use sensory level to help evaluate these segments
[b]Beevor's sign: used to assess abdominal musculature for level of lesion. Patient lifts head off of bed by flexing neck; if lower abdominal muscles (below ≈ T9) are weaker than upper abdominal musculature, then umbilicus moves cephalad. Not helpful if both upper and lower abdominals are weak
[c]the abdominal cutaneous reflex: scratching one quadrant of abdomen with sharp object causes contraction of underlying abdominal musculature, causing umbilicus to migrate toward that quadrant. Upper abdominal reflex: T8–9. Lower abdominal reflex: T10–12. This is a cortical reflex (i.e. reflex loop ascends to cortex, and then descends to abdominal muscles). The presence of this response indicates an incomplete lesion for cord injuries above the lower thoracic level
[d]cremasteric reflex: L1–2 superficial reflex
[e]**anal-cutaneous reflex**: AKA anal wink. Normal reflex: mild noxious stimulus (e.g. pinprick) applied to skin in region of anus results in involuntary anal contraction. **bulbocavernosus (BC) reflex**: see section 62.8.5

62

Table 62.11 Key sensory landmarks	
Level	**Dermatome**
C2	occipital protuberance
C3	supraclavicular fossa
C4	top of acromioclavicular joint
C5	Lateral side of antecubital fossa
C6	thumb, dorsal surface, proximal phalanx
C7	middle finger, dorsal surface, proximal phalanx
C8	little finger, dorsal surface, proximal phalanx
T1	medial (ulnar) side of antecubital fossa
T2	apex of axilla
T3	third intercostal space (IS)
T4	fourth IS (nipple line)
T5	fifth IS (midway between T6 & T8)
T6	sixth IS (xiphoid process)
T7	seventh IS (midway between T6 & T8)
T8	eighth IS (midway between T6 & T10)
T9	ninth IS (midway between T8 & T10)
T10	tenth IS (umbilicus)
T11	eleventh IS (midway between T10 & T12)
T12	inguinal ligament at mid-point
L1	half the distance between T12 & L2
L2	mid-anterior thigh
L3	medial femoral condyle
L4	medial malleolus
L5	dorsum of foot at 3rd MTP (metatarsal phalangeal) joint
S1	lateral heel
S2	popliteal fossa in the mid-line
S3	ischial tuberosity
S4–5	perianal area (taken as 1 level)

62.8.3 Sensory level assessment (dermatomes and sensory nerves)

ASIA standards[25]

28 key points identified in ▶ Table 62.11 are scored separately for pinprick and light touch on the left & right side using the grading scale shown in ▶ Table 62.12, for a maximum possible total of 112 points for pinprick (left & right) and 112 points for light touch (left & right).

Table 62.12 Sensory grading scale

Grade	Description
0	absent
1	impaired (partial or altered appreciation)
2	normal
NT	not testable

NB: regarding the “C4 cape” AKA “bib” region across the upper chest and back: sensory segments “jump” from C4 to T2 with the intervening levels distributed exclusively on the UEs (▶ Fig. 1.14). The location of this transition is not constant from person to person.

62.8.4 Rectal exam

1. external anal sphincter is tested by insertion of the examiner's gloved finger
   a) perceived sensation is recorded as present or absent. Any sensation felt by the patient indicates that the injury is sensory incomplete
   b) record resting sphincter tone and any voluntary sphincter contraction
2. bulbocavernosus (BC) reflex (p. 941); see also below: Absence suggests the presence of spinal shock, and it may not be possible to declare a suprasacral SCI as complete because there might be spinal shock which could transiently suppress spinal cord function

62.8.5 Bulbocavernosus (BC) reflex

A polysynaptic spinal cord mediated reflex relayed via S2-S4 nerve roots. Contraction of anal sphincter in response to squeezing the glans penis in males, or to tugging on the Foley catheter in either sex is a normal response (must be differentiated from the movement of the Foley catheter balloon).

Loss of reflex can occur with:

1. spinal shock: the BC reflex may be lost with spinal shock as can occur with suprasacral injuries. Reportedly, the return of the BC reflex may be the earliest clinical indicator that spinal shock has subsided.
2. injuries involving the cauda equina or conus medullaris

Presence of BC reflex used to be taken as an indication of an incomplete injury, but its presence alone is no longer considered to have a good prognosis for recovery.

62.8.6 Additional sensory exam

The following elements are considered optional but it is recommended that they be graded as absent, impaired or normal:

1. position sense: test index finger and great toe on both sides
2. awareness of deep pressure/deep pain

62.8.7 ASIA impairment scale

The ASIA impairment scale*[25] is shown in ▶ Table 62.13 (a modified Frankel Neurological Performance scale[28]).

* NB: this scale indicates the completeness of spinal cord injury and is distinct from the other ASIA grading scales; see also motor and sensory scoring (p. 940).

62.9 Spinal cord injuries

62.9.1 Complete spinal cord injuries

See definition of complete vs. incomplete spinal cord injury (p. 930).

In addition to loss of voluntary movement, sphincter control and sensation below the level of the injury, there may be priapism. Hypotension and bradycardia (p. 931) (spinal shock) may also present.

Table 62.13 ASIA impairment scale

Class	Description
A	Complete: no motor or sensory function preserved
B	Incomplete: sensory but no motor function preserved below the neurologic level (includes sacral segments S4–5)
C	Incomplete: motor function preserved below the neurologic level (more than half of key muscles below the neurologic level have a muscle strength grade < 3)[a]
D	Incomplete: motor function preserved below the neurologic level (more than half of key muscles below the neurologic level have a muscle strength grade ≥ 3)
E	Normal: Sensory & motor function normal

[a]for muscle strength grading see ▶ Table 29.2

62.9.2 Bulbar-cervical dissociation

Occurs as a result of spinal cord injury at or above ~ C3 (includes SCI from atlanto-occipital and atlantoaxial dislocation). Bulbar-cervical dissociation produces immediate pulmonary and, often, cardiac arrest. Death results if CPR is not instituted within minutes. Patients are usually quadriplegic and ventilator dependent (phrenic nerve stimulation may eventually allow independence from ventilator).

62.9.3 Incomplete spinal cord injuries

Central cord syndrome

General information

Key concepts

- disproportionately greater motor deficit in the upper extremities than lower
- usually results from hyperextension injury in the presence of osteophytic spurs
- surgery is often employed for ongoing compression, usually on a non-emergency basis except for rare cases of progressive deterioration

Originally described by Schneider et al.[29] in 1954. Central cord syndrome (CCS) is the most common type of incomplete spinal cord injury syndrome. Usually seen following acute hyperextension injury in an older patient with pre-existing acquired stenosis as a result of bony hypertrophy (anterior spurs) and infolding of redundant ligamentum flavum (posteriorly), sometimes superimposed on congenital spinal stenosis. Translational movement of one vertebra on another may also contribute. A blow to the upper face or forehead is often disclosed on history, or is suggested on exam (e.g. lacerations or abrasions to face and/or forehead). This often occurs in relation to a motor vehicle accident or to a forward fall, often while intoxicated. Younger patients may also sustain CCS in sporting injuries; see burning hands syndrome (p. 1421). CCS may occur with or without cervical fracture or dislocation.[30] CCS may be associated with acute traumatic cervical disc herniation. CCS may also occur in rheumatoid arthritis.

Pathomechanics

Theory: the centermost region of the spinal cord is a vascular watershed zone which renders it more susceptible to injury from edema. Long tract fibers passing through the cervical spinal cord are somatotopically organized such that cervical fibers are located more medially than the fibers serving the lower extremities (▶ Fig. 1.13).

Presentation

See reference.[29]

The clinical syndrome is somewhat similar to that seen in syringomyelia.

1. motor: weakness of upper extremities with lesser effect on lower extremities
2. sensory: varying degrees of disturbance below level of lesion may occur
3. myelopathic findings: sphincter dysfunction (usually urinary retention)

Hyperpathia to noxious and non-noxious stimuli is also common, especially in the proximal portions of the upper extremities, and is often delayed in onset and extremely distressing to the patient.[31] Lhermitte's sign occurs in ≈ 7% of cases.

Natural history

There is often an initial phase of improvement (characteristically: LEs recover first, bladder function next, UE strength then returns with finger movements last; sensory recovery has no pattern) followed by a plateau phase and then late deterioration.[32] 90% of patients are able to walk with assistance within 5 days.[33] Recovery is usually incomplete, and the amount of recovery is related to the severity of the injury and patient age.[34]

If CCS results from hematomyelia with cord destruction (instead of cord contusion), then there may be extension (upward or downward).

Evaluation

Findings: young patients tend to have disc protrusion, subluxation, dislocation or fractures.[33] Older patients tend to have multi-segmental canal narrowing due to osteophytic bars, discs, and inbuckling of ligamentum flavum.[33]

C-spine x rays: may demonstrate congenital narrowing, superimposed osteophytic spurs, traumatic fracture/dislocation. Occasionally, AP narrowing alone without spurs may be seen.[30] Plain x-rays will fail to demonstrate canal narrowing due to: thickening or inbuckling of ligamentum flavum, hypertrophy of facet joints, and poorly calcified spurs.[30]

Cervical CT scan: also helpful in diagnosing fractures and osteophytic spurs. Not as good as MRI for assessing status of discs, spinal cord and nerves.

MRI: discloses compromise of anterior spinal canal by discs or osteophytes (when combined with plain C-spine x-rays, it increases the ability to differentiate osteophyte from traumatic disc herniation). Also good for evaluating ligamentum flavum. T2WI may show spinal cord edema acutely,[35] and can detect hematomyelia. MRI is poor for identifying fractures.

Treatment

The indications, timing and best treatment method for CCS remains controversial.

Practice guideline: Acute traumatic central cord injuries (ATCCS)

Level III[34,36]

- ICU management of patients with acute traumatic central cord syndrome, especially for those with severe neurologic deficits (because of possible cardiac, pulmonary & BP disturbances)
- medical management to include the following: cardiac, hemodynamic and respiratory monitoring and maintainence of MAP 85–90 mm Hg (use BP augmentationif necessary) for the 1st week after injury to improve spinal cord perfusion
- early reduction of fracture-dislocation injuries
- surgical decompression of the compressed spinal cord, particularly if the compression is focal and anterior. Unresolved: the role of surgery in ATCCS with long segment cord compression or with spinal stenosis without bony injury[36] (see text for details)

Indications for surgery

1. continued compression of the spinal cord[37 (p 1010)] that correlates with the level of deficit with any of the following:
   a) persistent significant motor deficit following a varying period of recovery (below)
   b) deterioration of function
   c) continued significant dysesthetic pain
2. instability of the spine

Improvement has been shown in short and long-term follow-up with subacute decompression of the offending lesion.[33] Nonsurgical treatment results in a longer period of pain and weakness in many cases.

Timing of surgery: A perennial point of controversy. Classic teaching was that early surgery for this condition is *contraindicated* because this may worsen the deficit. In the absence of spinal instability, traditional management consisted of bed rest in a soft collar for ≈ 3–4 weeks, with consideration for surgery after this time, or else gradual mobilization in the same collar for an additional 6 weeks. However, the basis for this recommendation was at least in part derived from an early report of only 8 patients with CCS, 2 of which underwent surgery, with 1 being worse post-op (the operation consisted of laminectomy, opening the dura, sectioning the dentate ligament, and manipulation of the spinal cord in order to inspect the anterior spinal canal).[29] It is presently felt that there is no solid evidence that early decompressive surgery (without cord manipulation) is actually harmful, but there is also no evidence that it is helpful, either. There may be good justification for early surgery in the rare patient who is improving and then deteriorates,[38] however, great restraint must be used in avoiding what would be an inappropriate operation in many patients.[39] Surgery may improve the rate and degree of recovery in selected patients.[40] Surgery has been recommended for patients with gross spinal instability or for patients with significant persistent cord compression (e.g. by osteophytic spurs) who fail to progress consistently after an initial period of improvement,[35] often within 2–3 weeks following the trauma. Better results occur with decompression within the first few weeks or months rather than very late (e.g. ≥ 1–2 years).[37 (p 1010)]

Σ

There is no role for surgery without ongoing compression or instability. The rare patient with ongoing compression undergoing documented *progressive deterioration* should be decompressed ASAP. Patients that are improving should be followed and decompression can be done electively for ongoing compression. There is controversy regarding timing of surgery for stable CCS and ongoing compression: while Class I or II data are lacking, there seems to be a trend to decompress these patients as soon as they are medically stable without an arbitrary waiting period.

Technical considerations: The most rapid procedure to decompress the cord is often a multi-level laminectomy. This is frequently accompanied by dorsal migration of the spinal cord which may be seen on MRI.[32] With myelopathy, fused patients fare better than those that are just decompressed without fusion. Fusion may be accomplished posteriorly (e.g. with lateral mass screws and rods) at the time of decompression, or anteriorly (e.g. multi-level discectomy, or corpectomy with strut graft and anterior cervical plating) at the same sitting as the laminectomy or staged at a later date.

Prognosis

In patients with cord contusion without hematomyelia, ≈ 50% will recover enough LE strength and sensation to ambulate independently, although typically with significant spasticity. Recovery of UE function is usually not as good, and fine motor control is usually poor. Bowel and bladder control often recovers, however bladder spasticity is common. Elderly patients with this condition generally do not fare as well as younger patients, with or without surgical treatment (only 41% over age 50 become ambulatory, versus 97% for younger patients[41]).

Anterior cord syndrome

General information

AKA anterior spinal artery syndrome. Cord infarction in the territory supplied by the anterior spinal artery. Some say this is more common than central cord syndrome.

May result from occlusion of the anterior spinal artery, or from anterior cord compression, e.g. by dislocated bone fragment, or by traumatic herniated disc.

Presentation

1. paraplegia, or (if higher than ≈ C7) quadriplegia
2. dissociated sensory loss below lesion:
   a) loss of pain and temperature sensation (spinothalamic tract lesion)
   b) preserved two-point discrimination, joint position sense, deep pressure sensation (posterior column function)[42]

Evaluation

It is vital to differentiate a non-surgical condition (e.g. anterior spinal artery occlusion) from a surgical one (e.g. anterior bone fragment). This requires one or more of: myelography, CT, or MRI.

Treatment

Surgical intervention is indicated for patients with evidence of cord compression (e.g. by large central disc herniation) or for spinal instability (ligamentous or bony).

Prognosis

The worst prognosis of the incomplete injuries. Only ≈ 10–20% recover functional motor control. Sensation may return enough to help prevent injuries (burns, decubitus ulcers…).

Brown-Séquard syndrome

General information

Spinal cord hemisection. First described in 1849 by Brown-Sequard.[43]

Etiologies

Usually a result of penetrating trauma, it is seen in 2–4% of traumatic spinal cord injuries.[44] Also may occur with radiation myelopathy, cord compression by spinal epidural hematoma, large cervical disc herniation[45,46,47] (rare), spinal cord tumors, spinal AVMs, cervical spondylosis, and spinal **cord** herniation (p. 1150).

Presentation

Classical findings (rarely found in this pure form):

1. *ipsilateral* findings:
   a) motor paralysis (due to corticospinal tract lesion) below lesion
   b) loss of posterior column function (proprioception & vibratory sense)
2. *contralateral* findings: dissociated sensory loss
   a) loss of pain and temperature sensation inferior to lesion beginning 1–2 segments below (spinothalamic tract lesion)
   b) preserved light (crude) touch due to redundant ipsilateral and contralateral paths (anterior spinothalamic tracts)

Prognosis

This syndrome has the best prognosis of any of the incomplete spinal cord injuries. ≈ 90% of patients with this condition will regain the ability to ambulate independently as well as anal and urinary sphincter control.

Posterior cord syndrome

AKA contusio cervicalis posterior. Relatively rare. Produces pain and paresthesias (often with a burning quality) in the neck, upper arms, and torso. There may be mild paresis of the UEs. Long tract findings are minimal.

References

[1] White AA, Panjabi MM. In: The Problem of Clinical Instability in the Human Spine: A Systematic Approach. Clinical Biomechanics of the Spine. 2nd ed. Philadelphia: J.B. Lippincott; 1990:277–378

[2] Waters RL, Adkins RH, Yakura J, Sie I. Profiles of Spinal Cord Injury and Recovery After Gunshot Injury. Clin Orthop. 1991; 267:14–21

[3] Atkinson PP, Atkinson JLD. Spinal Shock. Mayo Clin Proc. 1996; 71:384–389

[4] Chesnut RM, Narayan RK, Wilberger JE, Povlishock JT. In: Emergency Management of Spinal Cord Injury. Neurotrauma. New York: McGraw-Hill; 1996:1121–1138

[5] Hirsch SA, Hirsch PJ, Hiramoto H, Weiss A. Whiplash Syndrome: Fact or Fiction? Orthop Clin North Am. 1988; 19:791–795

[6] Riley LH, Long D, Riley Jr. LH. The Science of Whiplash. Medicine (Baltimore). 1995; 74:298–299

[7] Spitzer WO, LeBlanc FE, Dupuis M, et al. Scientific Approach to the Assessment and Management of Activity-Related Spinal Disorders: A Monograph for Clinicians: Report of the Quebec Task Force on Spinal Disorders. Chapter 3: Diagnosis of the Problem (The Problem of Diagnosis). Spine. 1987; 12:S16–S21

[8] Spitzer WO, Skovron ML, Salmi LR, et al. Scientific Monograph of the Quebec Task Force on Whiplash-Associated Disorders: Redefining "Whiplash" and Its Management. Spine. 1995; 20:1S–73S

[9] Radanov BP, Sturzenegger M, Di Stefano G. Long-Term Outcome After Whiplash Injury. Medicine (Baltimore). 1995; 74:281–297

62

[10] Hamilton MG, Myles ST. Pediatric Spinal Injury: Review of 61 Deaths. J Neurosurg. 1992; 77:705–708
[11] Hamilton MG, Myles ST. Pediatric Spinal Injury: Review of 174 Hospital Admissions. J Neurosurg. 1992; 77:700–704
[12] Mandabach M, Ruge JR, Hahn YS, et al. Pediatric axis fractures: early halo immobilization, management and outcome. Pediatric Neurosurgery. 1993; 19:225–232
[13] Garton HJL, Park P, Papadopoulos SM. Fracture dislocation of the neurocentral synchondroses of the axis. Case illustration. J Neurosurg. 2002; (Spine 3) 96
[14] Suss RA, Zimmerman RD, Leeds NE. Pseudospread of the Atlas: False Sign of Jefferson Fracture in Young Children. AJR. 1983; 140:1079–1082
[15] Bailey DK. The Normal Cervical Spine in Infants and Children. Radiology. 1952; 59:712–719
[16] Townsend EH, Rowe ML. Mobility of the Upper Cervical Spine in Health and Disease. Pediatrics. 1952; 10:567–574
[17] Jacobson G, Bleeker HH. Pseudosubluxation of the Axis in Children. Am J Roentgenol. 1959; 82:472–481
[18] Rozzelle CJ, Aarabi B, Dhall SS, Gelb DE, Hurlbert RJ, Ryken TC, Theodore N, Walters BC, Hadley MN. Management of pediatric cervical spine and spinal cord injuries. Neurosurgery. 2013; 72 Suppl 2:205–226
[19] Section on Disorders of the Spine and Peripheral Nerves of the American Association of Neurological Surgeons and the Congress of Neurological Surgeons. Management of pediatric cervical spine and spinal cord injuries. Neurosurgery. 2002; 50 Supplement:S85–S99
[20] Bailes JE, Hadley MN, Quigley MR, Sonntag VKH, Cerullo LJ. Management of Athletic Injuries of the Cervical Spine and Spinal Cord. Neurosurgery. 1991; 29:491–497
[21] Torg JS, Corcoran TA, Thibault LF, et al. Cervical Cord Neuropraxia: Classification, Pathomechanics, Morbidity, and Management Guidelines. J Neurosurg. 1997; 87:843–850
[22] Maroon JC. "Burning Hands" in Football Spinal Cord Injuries. JAMA. 1977; 238:2049–2051
[23] Cantu RC, Mueller FO. Catastrophic Spine Injuries in Football. J Spinal Disord. 1990; 3:227–231
[24] Torg JS, Ramsey-Emrhein JA. Management Guidelines for Participation in Collision Activities with Congenital, Developmental, or Post-Injury Lesions Involving the Cervical Spine. Clin Sports Med. 1997; 16:501–531
[25] American Spinal Injury Association. International Standards for Neurological Classification of Spinal Cord Injury, Revised 2000. 6th ed. Chicago, IL: American Spinal Injury Association; 2000
[26] Ditunno JF, Jr. New spinal cord injury standards, 1992. Paraplegia. 1992; 30:90–91
[27] Lucas JT, Ducker TB. Motor Classification of Spinal Cord Injuries with Mobility, Morbidity and Recovery Indices. Am Surg. 1979; 45:151–158
[28] Frankel HL, Hancock DO, Hyslop G, et al. The Value of Postural Reduction in the Initial Management of Closed Injuries of the Spine with Paraplegia and Tetraplegia. Part I. Paraplegia. 1969; 7:179–192
[29] Schneider RC, Cherry G, Pantek H. The Syndrome of Acute Central Cervical Spinal Cord Injury. J Neurosurg. 1954; 11:546–577
[30] Epstein N, Epstein JA, Benjamin V, Ransohoff J. Traumatic Myelopathy in Patients With Cervical Spinal Stenosis Without Fracture or Dislocation: Methods of Diagnosis, Management, and Prognosis. Spine. 1980; 5:489–496
[31] Merriam WF, Taylor TKF, Ruff SJ, McPhail MJ. A Reappraisal of Acute Traumatic Central Cord Syndrome. J Bone Joint Surg. 1986; 68B:708–713
[32] Levi L, Wolf A, Mirvis S, Rigamonti D, et al. The Significance of Dorsal Migration of the Cord After Extensive Cervical Laminectomy for Patients with Traumatic Central Cord Syndrome. J Spinal Disord. 1995; 8:289–295
[33] Chen TY, Lee ST, Lui TN, et al. Efficacy of Surgical Treatment in Traumatic Central Cord Syndrome. Surg Neurol. 1997; 48:435–440
[34] Section on Disorders of the Spine and Peripheral Nerves of the American Association of Neurological Surgeons and the Congress of Neurological Surgeons. Management of acute central spinal cord injuries. Neurosurgery. 2002; 50 Supplement:S166–S172
[35] Massaro F, Lanotte M, Faccani G. Acute Traumatic Central Cord Syndrome. Acta Neurol (Napoli). 1993; 15:97–105
[36] Aarabi B, Hadley MN, Dhall SS, Gelb DE, Hurlbert RJ, Rozzelle CJ, Ryken TC, Theodore N, Walters BC. Management of acute traumatic central cord syndrome (ATCCS). Neurosurgery. 2013; 72 Suppl 2:195–204
[37] Rothman RH, Simeone FA. The Spine. Philadelphia 1992
[38] Fox JL, Wener L, Drennan DC, Manz HJ, Won DJ, Al-Mefty O. Central spinal cord injury: magnetic resonance imaging confirmation and operative considerations. Neurosurgery. 1988; 22:340–347
[39] Ducker TB. Comment on Fox J L, et al.: Central spinal cord injury: magnetic resonance imaging confirmation and operative considerations. Neurosurgery. 1988; 22:346–347
[40] Bose B, Northrup BE, Osterholm JL, et al. Reanalysis of Central Cervical Cord Injury Management. Neurosurgery. 1984; 15:367–372
[41] Penrod LE, Hegde SK, Ditunno JF. Age Effect on Prognosis for Functional Recovery in Acute, Traumatic Central Cord Syndrome. Arch Phys Med Rehabil. 1990; 71:963–968
[42] Schneider RC. The Syndrome of Acute Anterior Spinal Cord Injury. J Neurosurg. 1955; 12:95–122
[43] Brown-Sequard CE. De la transmission des impressions sensitives par la moelle epiniere. C R Soc Biol. 1849; 1
[44] Roth EJ, Park T, Pang T, Yarkony GM, Lee MY. Traumatic Cervical Brown-Sequard and Brown-Sequard Plus Syndromes: The Spectrum of Presentations and Outcomes. Paraplegia. 1991; 29:582–589
[45] Rumana CS, Baskin DS. Brown-Sequard Syndrome Produced By Cervical Disc Herniation: Case Report and Literature Review. Surg Neurol. 1996; 45:359–361
[46] Kobayashi N, Asamoto S, Doi H, Sugiyama H. Brown-Sequard syndrome produced by cervical disc herniation: report of two cases and review of the literature. Spine J. 2003; 3:530–533
[47] Kim JT, Bong HJ, Chung DS, Park YS. Cervical disc herniation producing acute Brown-Sequard syndrome. J Korean Neurosurg Soc. 2009; 45:312–314

63 Management of Spinal Cord Injury

63.1 General information

The major causes of death in spinal cord injury (SCI) are aspiration and shock.[1] Initial survey under ATLS protocol: assessment of airway takes precedence, then breathing, then circulation & control of hemorrhage ("ABC's"). This is followed by a brief neurologic exam.

NB: other injuries (e.g. abdominal injuries) may be masked below the level of SCI.

Any of the following patients should be treated as having a SCI until proven otherwise:

1. all victims of significant trauma
2. trauma patients with loss of consciousness
3. minor trauma victims with complaints referable to the spine (neck or back pain or tenderness) or spinal cord (numbness or tingling in an extremity, weakness, paralysis)
4. associated findings suggestive of SCI include
   a) abdominal breathing
   b) priapism (autonomic dysfunction)

Trauma patients are triaged as follows:

1. no history of significant trauma, completely alert, oriented and free of drug or alcohol intoxication with no complaints referable to the spine: most may be cleared clinically without the need for C-spine x-rays; see Radiographic evaluation (p.952)
2. significant trauma, but no strong evidence of spine or spinal cord injury: the emphasis here is in ruling-out a bony lesion and preventing injury
3. patients with neurologic deficit: the emphasis here is to define the skeletal injury and to take steps to prevent further cord injury and loss of function and minimize or reverse the present deficit. The pros and cons of the high-dose methylprednisolone protocol (p.951) should be weighed if a neurologic deficit is identified

63.2 Management in the field

1. Spine immobilization prior to and during extrication from vehicle and transport to prevent active or passive movements of the spine.
   a) For possible C-spine injuries in football players, see ▶ Table 63.1 for the National Athletic Trainers' Association (NATA) guidelines for helmet removal. When CPR is necessary it takes precedence. Caution with intubation (see below)
   b) place patient on back-board

Table 63.1 NATA helmet removal guidelines[a]

✖ NB: do not remove the helmet in the field.
• most injuries can be visualized with the helmet in place • neurological exam can be done with the helmet in place • the patient may be immobilized on a spine board with the helmet in place • the facemask can be removed with special tools to access the airway • hyperextension must be avoided following removal of the helmet and shoulder pads
In a controlled setting (usually after x-rays) the helmet and shoulder-pads are removed together as a unit to avoid neck flexion or extension
Possible indications for removal of helmet
• face mask cannot be removed in a reasonable amount of time • airway cannot be established even with face mask removed • life threatening hemorrhage under the helmet that can be controlled only by removal • helmet & strap do not hold head securely so that immobilizing the helmet does not adequately immobilize the spine (e.g. poor fitting or damaged helmet) • helmet prevents immobilization for transportation in an appropriate position • certain situations where the patient is unstable (M.D. decision)
[a]for more details, see http://www.nata.org

c) sandbags on both sides of the head with a 3 inch strip of adhesive tape from one side of the back-board to the other across the forehead immobilizes the spine as well as a rigid orthosis[2] but allows movement of the jaw and access to the airway
d) a rigid cervical collar (e.g. Philadelphia collar) may be used to supplement

2. maintain blood pressure, see below under Hypotension (p. 950)
   a) pressors treat the underlying problem (SCI is essentially a traumatic sympathectomy). Dopamine is the agent of choice, and is preferred over fluids (except as necessary to replace losses); see Cardiovascular agents for shock (p. 127) for pressors. ✖ Avoid phenylephrine (see below)
   b) fluids as necessary to replace losses
   c) military anti-shock trousers (MAST): immobilizes lower spine, compensates for lost muscle tone in cord injuries (prevents venous pooling)
3. maintain oxygenation (adequate FIO_2 and adequate ventilation)
   a) if no indication for intubation: use NC or face mask
   b) intubation: may be required for airway compromise or for hypopnea. In SCI, hypopnea may be due to: paralyzed intercostal muscles, paralysis of diaphragm (phrenic nerve = C3, 4 & 5). Hypopnea may also be due to depressed LOC in TBI
   c) caution with intubation with uncleared C-spine
      - use chin lift (not jaw thrust) without neck extension
      - nasotracheal intubation may avoid movement of C-spine but patient must have spontaneous respirations
      - avoided tracheostomy or cricothyroidotomy if possible (may compromise later anterior cervical spine surgical approaches)
4. brief *motor* exam to identify possible deficits (also to document delayed deterioration); ask patient to:
   a) move arms
   b) move hands
   c) move legs
   d) move toes

63.3 Management in the hospital

63.3.1 Stabilization and initial evaluation

1. immobilization: maintain backboard/head-strap (see above) to facilitate transfers to CT table, etc. Log-roll patient to turn. Once studies are completed, remove patient from backboard ASAP (early removal from board reduces risk of decubitus ulcers)
2. *hypotension* (spinal shock): maintain SBP ≥ 90 mm Hg. Spinal cord injuries cause hypotension by a combination of factors (p. 931) which may further injure spinal cord[3] or other organ systems
   a) pressors if necessary: dopamine is agent of choice (✖ avoid phenylephrine: non-inotropic and possible reflex increase in vagal tone → bradycardia)
   b) careful hydration (abnormal hemodynamics → propensity to pulmonary edema)
   c) atropine for bradycardia associated with hypotension
3. oxygenation (see above)
4. NG tube to suction: prevents vomiting and aspiration, and decompresses abdomen which can interfere with respirations if distended (paralytic ileus is common, and usually lasts several days)
5. indwelling (Foley) urinary catheter: for I's & O's and to prevent distension from urinary retention
6. DVT prophylaxis: see below
7. temperature regulation: vasomotor paralysis may produce poikilothermy (loss of temperature control), this should be treated as needed with cooling blankets
8. electrolytes: hypovolemia and hypotension cause increased plasma aldosterone which may lead to hypokalemia
9. more detailed neuro evaluation (p. 939). Patients may be stratified using the ASIA impairment scale (▸ Table 62.13)
   a) focused history: key questions should center on:
      - mechanism of injury (hyperflexion, extension, axial loading…)
      - history suggestive of loss of consciousness
      - history of weakness in the arms or legs following the trauma
      - occurrence of numbness or tingling at any time following the injury
   b) palpation of the spine for point tenderness, a "step-off", or widened interspinous space

c) motor level assessment
   - skeletal muscle exam (can localize dermatome)
   - rectal exam for voluntary anal sphincter contraction
d) sensory level assessment
   - sensation to pinprick (tests spinothalamic tract, can localize dermatome): be sure to test sensation in face also (spinal trigeminal tract can sometimes descend as low as ≈ C4)
   - light (crude) touch: tests anterior cord (anterior spinothalamic tract)
   - proprioception/joint position sense (tests posterior columns)
e) evaluation of reflexes
   - muscle stretch reflexes: usually absent initially in cord injury
   - abdominal cutaneous reflexes
   - cremasteric reflex
   - sacral: bulbocavernosus (p. 941), anal-cutaneous reflex
f) examine for signs of autonomic dysfunction
   - altered patterns of perspiration (abdominal skin may have low coefficient of friction above lesion, and may seem rough below due to lack of perspiration)
   - bowel or bladder incontinence
   - priapism: persistent penile erection

10. radiographic evaluation: see below
11. medical management specific to spinal cord injury:
    a) methylprednisolone (see below)
    b) experimental/investigational drugs: none of these agents shown to have unequivocal benefit in man: naloxone, DMSO, Lazaroid®. Tirilazad mesylate (Freedox®) was less beneficial than methylprednisolone[4]

63.3.2 General information

Practice guideline: Assessment of SCI in the hospital

Clinical Assessment

Level III[5]: the ASIA international standards for neurological and functional assessment of spinal cord injury (SCI) is recommended (p. 940)

Functional outcome assessment

Level II[5]: the Functional Impairment Measure™ (FIM™) is recommended (see ▶ Table 88.7)
Level III[5]: the modified Barthel index is recommended (▶ Table 88.6)

Practice guideline: In-hospital critical care management of SCI

Level III[6]: monitor patients with acute SCI (especially those with severe cervical level injuries) in an ICU or similar monitored setting
Level III[6]: cardiac, hemodynamic & respiratory monitoring after acute SCI is recommended
Level III[7]: hypotension (SBP < 90 mm Hg) should be avoided or corrected ASAP
Level III[7]: maintain MAP at 85–90 mm Hg for the first 7 days after SCI to improve spinal cord perfusion

63.3.3 Methylprednisolone

Practice guideline: Methylprednisolone in SCI

Level I[8]
- Methylprednisolone (MP) for the treatment of acute SCI is not recommended.
- GM-1 ganglioside (Sygen) for the treatment of acute SCI is not recommended.

MP is not FDA approved for use in treating acute SCI. There is no Class I or II evidence of benefit supporting this use of MP. Class III data that had been used to advocate its use, but the benefits were likely due to random chance and/or selection bias.[8] Conversely, there is Class I, II and III level evidence that high dose steroids are associated with harmful side effects and even death.[8] Use of high-dose MP among spine surgeons has shown a steady decline,[9] however, it was still used by as many as 56% of respondents to one survey.[9]

63.3.4 Hypothermia for spinal cord injury

The position statement of the joint sections of the AANS and the CNS is that there is not enough evidence to recommend for or against local or systemic hypothermia for acute SCI, and that it should be noted that systemic hypothermia is associated with medical complications in TBI.[10]

63.3.5 Deep-vein thrombosis in spinal cord injuries

General information

Also see Thromboembolism in neurosurgery (p. 167). Incidence of DVT may be as high as 100% when 125I-fibrinogen is used.[11] Overall mortality from DVT is 9% in SCI patients.

Practice guideline: DVT in patients with cervical SCI

Prophylaxis

Level I[12]:

- prophylactic treatment of venous thromboembolism (VTE) in patients with severe motor deficits due to SCI. Choices include:
  - LMW heparin, rotating beds, adjusted dose heparin, or some combination of these measures
  - or, low-dose heparin + pneumatic compression stockings or electrical stimulation

Level II[12]:

- early administration of VTE prophylaxis (within 72 hours)
- treat for 3 months
  - ✖ low-dose heparin should not be used alone
  - ✖ oral anticoagulation should not be used alone

Level III[12]:

- vena cava interruption filters should not be used for routine prophylaxis; they may be used for select patients who fail anticoagulation or are not candidates for anticoagulation

Diagnosis

Level III[12]:

- duplex doppler ultrasound, impedance plethysmography, venography, and the clinical examination are recommended as diagnostic tests for DVT in patients with SCI

Prophylaxis

A study of 75 patients found titrating dose of SQ heparin q 12 hrs to a PTT of 1.5 times control resulted in lower incidence of thromboembolic events (DVT, PE) than "mini-dose" heparin (5000 U SQ q 12 hrs) (7% vs. 31%).[13] Heparin can cause thrombosis, thrombocytopenia and chronic therapy may produce osteoporosis; see heparin (p. 164).

63.4 Radiographic evaluation and initial C-spine immobilization

63.4.1 Clinical criteria to rule-out cervical spine instability

There is almost no chance of a significant occult cervical spine injury[14,15] in a trauma patient who met all of the criteria in the Practice Guideline below. (**Note:** Although reports of bony or ligamentous abnormalities have be described as possibly occurring in these patients, there has been no report of a patient who had neurologic injury as a result of these abnormalities.)

Practice guideline: Radiographic evaluation in awake, asymptomatic trauma patients

Level I[16] & Level II[17,18]: radiographic studies are not indicated in patients who meet all of the following (these are basically the NEXUS criteria[19]):

- no mental status changes (and no evidence of alcohol or drugs). Note: altered mental status can include GCS ≤ 14; disorientation to person, place, time or events; inability to remember 3 objects at 5 minutes; delayed response to external stimuli. Evidence of alcohol or drugs includes information from the history, physical findings (slurred speech, ataxia, odor of alcohol on the breath) or positive blood or urine tests
- no neck pain or posterior midline tenderness (and no distracting pain)
- no focal neurologic deficit (on motor or sensory exam)
- do not have significant associated injuries that detract/distract from their evaluation

Cervical immobilization may be discontinued without cervical spine imaging in these patients.

The Canadian C-Spine Rule (CCR) was found to be more sensitive & specific,[20] but the EAST has not embraced it as of this writing.[17]

63.4.2 Cervical immobilization

General information

Cervical collars should be removed as soon as it can be determined that it is safe to do so. The benefits from early collar removal include: reduction of skin breakdown,[21] fewer days of mechanical ventilation,[22] shorter ICU stays,[22] reduction of ICP.[23,24]

Guidelines

Guidelines for "clearing" the cervical spine and removing the cervical collar are shown in **Practice guideline: Cervical immobilization in trauma patients** (p. 953).

Practice guideline: Cervical immobilization in trauma patients

A cervical collar is not needed in trauma patients who meet these criteria

- Asymptomatic patients as in **Practice guideline: Radiographic evaluation in asymptomatic trauma patients** (p. 953): patients who are alert, without neurologic deficit or distracting injury who have *no neck pain* or tenderness and full ROM of the cervical spine (Level II[17])
- Penetrating brain trauma: unless the trajectory suggests direct cervical spine injury (Level III[17])
- **Level III**[25] & **Level III**[17]: Patients who are awake *with* neck pain or tenderness and normal cervical CT scan after either (these tests are performed in the absence of an identifiable fracture or obviously unstable dislocation to rule-out ligamentous or other soft-tissue injury that might be occult and unstable)
  - normal & adequate dynamic flexion-extension C-spine x-rays
  - or a normal cervical MRI is obtained. **Note:** AANS/CNS guidelines from 2002 recommended getting the MRI within 48 hours.[25] MRI is usually employed in this setting when the patient is unable to co-operate for flex-ext x-rays; see MRI findings and issues related to timing (p. 957), etc.

In *obtunded* patients with normal cervical CT scan and gross movement of all 4 extremities

- ✖ flexion-extension C-spine x-rays should *not* be performed (Level II[17])
- options:
  - maintain cervical collar until a clinical exam can be performed[17]

- remove the collar on the basis of the normal CT scan alone[17] (the incidence of ligamentous injury with negative CT is < 5%, and the incidence of clinically significant injury is unknown but is much < 1%[17])
- obtain cervical MRI (AANS/CNS guidelines from 2002 recommended getting the MRI within 48 hours[25]) :
  - Level III[17]: the risk and benefit of cervical MRI in addition to CT is unclear, and must be individualized
  - Level II[17]: If the MRI is normal, the collar may be safely removed

63.4.3 Minimum radiographic evaluation

General information

There is controversy regarding what constitutes a minimum radiographic evaluation of the cervical spine in multiple trauma patient. No imaging modality is 100% accurate.

Asymptomatic patients – meeting criteria outlined in **Practice guideline: Radiographic evaluation in awake, asymptomatic trauma patients** (p. 953) – may be considered to have a stable cervical spine and *no* radiographic studies of the cervical spine are indicated.[17,25] Factors associated with increased risk of failing to recognize spinal injuries include: decreased level of consciousness (due to injury or drugs/alcohol), multiple injuries, technically inadequate x-rays (p. 1019).[26]

Primary imaging recommendations

Practice guideline: Radiographic imaging in trauma patients who are obtunded or unevaluable

Includes unresponsive patients or unreliable exam (altered mental status, distracting pain or injuries)

- Level I[18]
  - high-quality computed tomography (CT) imaging is the modality of choice
    ✖ if high-quality CT imaging is available, routine 3-view cervical spine x-rays are not recommended
  - if high-quality CT imaging is not available, 3-view cervical spine x-rays (AP, lateral and open-mouth odontoid view) are recommended. Supplement with CT when available if needed to further define areas that are suspicious or poorly visualized on plain x-rays
- Level II[18]
  - if high-quality CT imaging is normal but the index of suspicion is high, further management should fall to physicians trained in the diagnosis and treatment of spine injuries
- Level III[18]
  - if high-quality CT imaging is normal, options include:
    - continue cervical immobilization until asymptomatic
    - obtain cervical MRI within 48 hours of injury and, if normal, D/C cervical immobilization*
    - D/C cervical immobilization at the discretion of the treating physician
      ✖ the routine use of dynamic imaging (flexion-extension) is of marginal benefit and is not recommended in this situation

* limited and conflicting Class II & III medical evidence

CT scan, while extremely sensitive for bony injuries, is not adequate for assessing soft tissues (e.g. traumatic disc herniation, spinal cord contusion…) or ligamentous injuries (may require flexion-extension x-rays (see below) and/or MRI).

When CT scan is not appropriate/available as the initial radiographic exam

When CT cannot be done, the following guidelines are offered:

See **X-rays**, C-Spine (p.212) for normal vs. abnormal findings. ▶ Table 63.2 lists some indicators that should alert the reviewer that there may be significant C-spine trauma (they do *not* indicate definite instability by themselves).

1. cervical spine: must be cleared radiographically from the cranio-cervical junction down through and including the C7-T1 junction (incidence of pathology at C7-T1 junction may be as high as 9%[27]):
   a) lateral portable C-spine x-ray while in rigid collar: this study by itself will miss ≈ 15% of injuries[28]
   b) if all 7 cervical vertebra *AND* the C7-T1 junction are adequately visualized and are normal, and if the patient has no neck pain or tenderness and is neurologically intact (neurologically intact implies patient is alert, not drugged/intoxicated, & able to report pain reliably), then remove the cervical collar and complete the remainder of the cervical spine series (AP and open-mouth odontoid (OMO) view). Lateral, AP, and OMO views together detect essentially all unstable fractures in neurologically intact patients[29] (although the AP view rarely provides unique information[30]). In a severely injured patient, limitation to an AP and lateral view usually suffices for the *acute* (but not complete) evaluation[31]
   c) if the above studies are normal, but there is neck pain, tenderness or neurologic findings (there may be a spinal cord injury even with normal plain films), or if the patient is unable to reliably verbalize neck pain or cannot be examined for neurologic deficit, then further studies are indicated, which may include any of the following:
      - oblique views (some authors include oblique views in a "minimal" evaluation,[31] others do not[29]): demonstrates the neural foramina – may be blocked with a unilateral locked facet (p.992) -, shows a different projection of the uncinate processes than the AP view, and helps assess the integrity of the articular masses and lamina (the lamina should align like shingles on a roof)[31]
      - flexion-extension views: see below
      - CT scan: helpful in identifying bony injuries, especially in areas difficult to visualize on plain radiographs. However, CT cannot exclude significant soft-tissue or ligamentous injury[32]
      - MRI: utility is limited to specific situation (p.957) and the accuracy has not been determined
      - polytomograms: becoming less available
      - pillar view: devised to demonstrate the cervical articular masses en face (reserved for cases of suspected of having articular mass fracture)[33]: the head is rotated to one side (requires that the upper cervical spine injury has been excluded by previous radiographs), the x-ray tube is off centered 2 cm from midline in the opposite direction and the beam is angled 25° caudad, centered at the superior margin of the thyroid cartilage

Table 63.2 Radiographic signs of C-spine trauma (modified[34])

Soft tissues
• retropharyngeal space > 7 mm, or retrotracheal space > 14 mm (adult) or 22 mm (peds), see ▶ Table 12.2 for details) • displaced prevertebral fat stripe • tracheal deviation & laryngeal dislocation
Vertebral alignment
• loss of lordosis • acute kyphotic angulation • torticollis • widened interspinous space (flaring) • axial rotation of vertebra • discontinuity in contour lines (p.212)
Abnormal joints
• ADI: > 3 mm (adult) or > 4 mm (peds) (see ▶ Table 12.1 for details) • narrowed or widened disc space • widening of apophyseal joints

   d) if subluxation is present at any level and is ≤ 3.5 mm and the patient is neurologically intact (neurologically intact implies patient is alert, not drugged/intoxicated, and able to report pain reliably), then obtain flexion-extension films (see below)
      - if no pathologic movement, may discontinue cervical collar
      - even if no instability is demonstrated, may need delayed films once pain and muscle spasms have resolved to reveal instability
   e) if *lower* C-spine (and/or cervical-thoracic junction) are not well visualized
      - repeat lateral C-spine x-ray with caudal traction on the arms (if not contraindicated based on other injuries, e.g. to shoulders)
      - if still not visualized, then obtain a "swimmer's" (Twining) view: the x-ray tube is positioned above the shoulder furthest from the film, and aimed towards the axilla closest to the film with the tube angled 10–15° toward the head while the arm is elevated above the head
      - if still not visualized: CT scan through non-visualized levels (CT is poor for evaluating alignment and for fractures in the horizontal plane, thin cuts with reconstructions ameliorates this shortcoming)
   f) see questions regarding stability of the subaxial spine (p.987)
   g) patients with C-spine fractures or dislocations should have daily C-spine x-rays during initial traction or immobilization
2. thoracic and lumbosacral LS-spine: AP and lateral x-rays for all trauma patients who:
   a) were thrown from a vehicle, or fell ≥ 6 feet to the ground
   b) complain of back pain
   c) are unconscious
   d) are unable to reliably describe back pain or have altered mental status preventing adequate exam (including inability to verbalize regarding back pain/tenderness)
   e) have an unknown mechanism of injury, or other injuries that cast suspicion of spine injury
3. reminder: when abnormalities of questionable vintage are identified, a bone scan may be helpful to distinguish an old injury from an acute one (less useful in the elderly; in an adult, a bone scan will become "hot" within 24–48 hrs of injury, and will remain hot for up to a year; in the elderly, the scan may not become hot for 2–3 weeks and can remain so for over a year)
4. if a bony abnormality is identified or if there is a level of neurologic deficit ascribable to a specific spinal level, either a CT or MRI scan through that area should be done if possible

Flexion-extension cervical spine x-rays

Purpose: to disclose occult ligamentous instability.

Rationale: It is possible to have a purely ligamentous injury involving the posterior ligamentous complex without any bony fracture (p.991). Lateral flexion-extension views help detect these injuries, and also evaluate other injuries (e.g. compression fracture) for stability. For patients with limited flexion due to paraspinal muscle spasm (sometimes resulting from pain), a rigid collar should be prescribed, and if the pain persists 2–3 weeks later[35] the flexion-extension films should be repeated.

Options: a cervical MRI done within 48–72 hours of the trauma (may be more sensitive with STIR sequences or equivalent) may identify ligamentous or other soft-tissue injury, especially in patients who cannot cooperate for flexion-extension x-rays.

✖ Contraindications

- the patient must be cooperative and free of mental impairment (i.e. no head injury, street or prescription drugs, alcohol…)
- there should not be any subluxation > 3.5 mm at any level on cross-table C-spine x-rays, which is a marker for possible instability (p.991)
- patient must be neurologically intact (if there is any degree of spinal cord injury, proceed instead first with imaging studies, e.g. MRI)
- F/E x-rays are no longer recommended in obtunded patients due to a low yield, poor cost-effectiveness, and they may be dangerous[17]

Technique

The patient should be sitting, and is instructed to flex the head slowly, and to stop if it becomes painful. Serial x-rays are taken at 5–10° increments (or followed under fluoro with spot films at the end of movement), and if normal, the patient may be encouraged to flex further. This is repeated until evidence of instability is seen, or the patient cannot flex further because of pain or limitation of motion. The process is then repeated for extension.

Findings

Normal flexion-extension views demonstrate slight anterior subluxation distributed over all cervical levels with preservation of the normal contour lines (▶ Fig. 12.1). Abnormal findings include: "flaring" of the spinous processes, see exaggerated widening (p. 214).

Emergent MRI (or myelogram)

General information

Indications for *emergent* MRI in spinal cord injury (SCI) are listed below.

When an MRI cannot be performed, a *myelogram* is required (employing intrathecal contrast with CT to follow) ✖ Caution: cervical myelogram in patients with cervical spine injuries usually requires C1–2 puncture to achieve adequate dye concentration in the cervical region without dangerous extension of the neck or tilting of the patient as required when dye is injected via LP. Furthermore, pressure shifts from LP exacerbates deficit in 14% of cases with complete block.[36]

Indications

1. incomplete SCI (to check for R/O soft tissue compressing cord) with normal alignment: to check for soft tissue compressing cord
2. neurologic deterioration (worsening deficit or rising level) including after closed reduction
3. neurologic deficit not explained by radiographic findings, including:
   a) fracture level different from level of deficit
   b) no bony injury identified: further imaging is done to R/O soft tissue compression (disc herniation, hematoma…) that would require surgery
   c) always keep in mind the possibility of arterial dissection in this setting (p. 1322)

MRI (non-emergent)

General information

MRI may be used to identify potentially unstable occult ligamentous or soft tissue injury. Note: abnormal signal on MRI is not always associated with instability on flexion-extension x-rays.[37] It has been recommended that this MRI should be done within 48 hours[25] or 72 hrs[38] of injury. MRI is not reliable for identifying osseous injury.

Indications for non-emergent MRI (modified):

See reference[39]

1. inconclusive cervical spine radiography, including questionable fractures
2. significant midline paraspinal tenderness and patient unable to have flexion-extension x-rays
3. obtunded or comatose patients

T2WI and STIR are the most helpful sequences. Significant abnormal findings:

1. ventral signal abnormalities with prevertebral swelling
2. dorsal signal abnormalities. Abnormal signal limited to the interspinous is probably not as unstable as when it extends into the ligamentum flavum.[39] These patients were treated with rigid collars or Minerva jackets for 1–3 months, and one that was felt to be very unstable underwent fusion
3. disc disruption indicated by abnormal signal intensity within the disc, increased disc height, or frank disc protrusions

63.5 Traction/reduction of cervical spine injuries

63.5.1 General information

Purpose

To reduce fracture-dislocations, maintain normal alignment and/or immobilize the cervical spine to prevent further spinal cord injury. Reduction decompresses the spinal cord and roots, and may facilitate bone healing.

63

Practice guidelines

Practice guideline: Initial closed reduction in fracture/dislocation cervical SCI

Level III[40,41]

- early closed reduction of C-spine fracture/dislocation injuries with craniocervical traction to restore anatomic alignment in awake patients
- ✖ *not* recommended: closed reduction in patients with an additional rostral injury
- patients with C-spine fracture-dislocation who cannot be examined during attempted closed reduction, or before open posterior reduction, should undergo cervical MRI before attempted reduction (see note below). The presence of a significant herniated disc in this setting is a relative indication for anterior decompression (e.g. by an anterior cervical discectomy and fusion – ACDF) before reduction
- cervical MRI is also recommended for patients who fail attempts at closed reduction (see note below).

Controversies

1. the rapidity with which reduction should be done[1]
2. whether MRI should be done prior to attempted closed reduction (prereduction MRI (p. 958), will show disrupted or herniated discs in 33–50% of patients with facet subluxation. These findings do not seem to significantly influence outcome after closed-reduction in awake patients; ∴ the usefulness of prereduction MRI in this setting is uncertain)
   a) in intact patients, to R/O a condition that might cause worsening of neurologic condition with reduction (e.g. traumatic disc herniation) – must be balanced against risks of transferring patients to MRI
   b) in patients with neurologic deficit (complete or partial SCI)

✖ Contraindications

1. atlantooccipital dislocation (p. 963): traction may worsen deficit. If immobilization with tongs/halo is desired, use no more than ≈ 4 lbs
2. types IIA or III hangman's fracture (p. 973)
3. skull defect/fracture at anticipated pin site: may necessitate alternate pin site
4. use with caution in pediatric age group (do not use if age ≤ 3 yrs)
5. very elderly patients
6. demineralized skull: some elderly patients, osteogenesis imperfecta…
7. patients with an additional rostral injury
8. patients with movement disorders: constant motion may cause pin erosion through the skull

63.5.2 Application of tongs or halo ring

General information

Supplies: gloves, local anesthetic (typically 1% lidocaine with epinephrine), betadine ointment. Optional equipment: razor or hair clipper, scalpel.

Choice of device: a number of cranial "tongs" are available. Crutchfield tongs require predrilling holes in the skull. Gardner-Wells tongs are the most common tongs in use. If, after the acute stabilization, the later use of halo-vest immobilization is anticipated, a halo ring may be used for the initial cervical traction, and then converted to vest traction at the appropriate time (e.g. post-fusion).

Preparation: placed with patient supine on a gurney or bed. Option: shave hair around proposed pin sites (see below). Betadine skin prep, then infiltrate local anesthetic. Option: incise skin with scalpel (prevents pins from driving in surface contaminants).

Gardner-Wells tongs

Pin sites: the pins are placed in the temporal ridge (above the temporalis muscle), 2–3 fingerbreadths (3–4 cm) above pinna. Place directly above external acoustic meatus for *neutral* position traction; 2–3 cm posterior for *flexion* (e.g. for locked facets); 2–3 cm anterior for *extension*.

One pin has a central spring-loaded force-indicator. Tighten pins until the indicator protrudes 1 mm beyond the flat surface. Retighten the pins daily until indicator protrudes 1 mm for 1 or 2 days only, then stop.

Halo ring

Supplies (in addition to above): optional paddle AKA "spoon" to support the head beyond the edge of the bed, traction adapter (called a "traction bail" from the circular handle on a baille, the old French word for bucket). Read all of this (including pointers) before starting

1. ring size: choose an appropriately sized ring that leaves a ≈ 1–2 cm gap between the scalp and the ring all the way around
2. ring position: generally placed at or just below the widest portion of the skull (the "equator"), but the front should be ≈ 1 cm above the orbital rim and the back should be ≈ 1 cm above the pinna.[42] The ring is usually stabilized with temporary pins that have plastic discs where they contact the skull
3. pin sites: choose the threaded holes in the ring that place the pins as perpendicular to the skull as possible as follows
   a) anterior pins: above the *lateral* two–thirds of the orbit
   b) posterior pins: just behind the ears
   c) in pediatrics, additional pins may be placed to further distribute the load on the thinner skull
4. pin insertion: the pins are gradually brought close to the scalp which is then anesthetized with local anesthetic. Pins are then sequentially tightened, starting with any pin then going to the kitty-corner pin, then a third pin and finally its opposite. Most halos provide some type of torque wrench to permit approximately 8 in-lb of torque for most adults; 2–5 in-lb for peds
5. placement pointers
   a) the cervical collar is left in place until traction/immobilization is established
   b) try to place the halo as level from left to right as possible. While a skewed placement can be compensated for when attaching the vest, it looks bad
   c) prior to penetrating the forehead skin for anterior pins, have the patient close their eyes and hold them closed as the pins are advanced (this avoids "pinning the eyes open")
   d) avoid placing pins in the temporalis muscle or the temporal squamosa
   e) do not place pins above the medial third of the orbit to avoid the supraorbital and supratrochlear nerves, and to reduce theorist of penetrating the relatively thin anterior wall of the frontal sinus

Application of traction

For traction, transfer to a bed with ortho headboard with the tongs or halo ring in place. Tie a rope to tongs/halo and feed through a pulley at the head of bed. Slight flexion or extension is achieved by changing the height of the pulley relative to the patient's long axis.

X-rays: lateral C-spine x-rays *immediately* after application of traction and at regular intervals and after every change in weights and every move from bed. Check alignment and rule-out overdistraction at any level and atlanto-occipital dislocation; BDI should be ≤ 12 mm (p. 963).

Weight: if there is no malalignment and traction is being used just to stabilize the injury and to compensate for ligamentous instability, use 5 lbs for the upper C-spine or 10 lbs for lower levels. See information on reducing locked facets (p. 992). May remove cervical collar once patient is in traction with adequate reduction or stabilization.

Post-placement care

Pin tightening: pins are re-torqued in 24 hours. Some authors do one additional tightening the day after that. Avoid further tightenings which can penetrate the skull

Pin care: clean (e.g. half strength hydrogen peroxide), then apply povidone-iodine ointment. Frequency: in hospital: q shift. At home following discharge: twice daily.

Alternatively, simple cleaning with soap and water twice daily is acceptable.

Application of halo vest

For vest placement (i.e. patients not remaining in traction) once the halo ring is placed (see above) it needs to be attached to the vest by posts. The mechanism varies between manufacturers. If possible, have the patient in a cotton T-shirt prior to placing the vest (this may require cutting the neck opening to accommodate the ring).

The vest should be snug, but too tight so as to restrict respirations. Shoulder straps should be contacting the shoulders (the vest will tend to ride up when the patient is sitting). Most vests come with a wrench that is taped to the vest for emergency removal e.g. for cardiopulmonary resuscitation.

Reduction of locked facets

63

See Practice guideline: Initial closed reduction in fracture/dislocation cervical SCI (p.958) for background information and Reduction of locked facets (p.992) for technique.

Complications

1. skull penetration by pins. May be due to:
   a) pins torqued too tightly
   b) pins placed over thin bone: temporal squamosa or over frontal sinus
   c) elderly patients, pediatric patients, or those with an osteoporotic skull
   d) invasion of bone with tumor: e.g. multiple myeloma
   e) fracture at pin site
2. reduction of cervical dislocations may be associated with neurologic deterioration which is usually due to retropulsed disc[43] and requires immediate investigation with MRI or myelogram/CT
3. overdistraction from excessive weight (especially with upper cervical spine injuries), may also endanger supporting tissues
4. caution with C1-C3 injury, especially with posterior element fracture (traction may pull fragments in towards canal)
5. infection:
   a) osteomyelitis in pin sites: risk is reduced with good pin care
   b) subdural empyema (p.327): rare[44,45]

63.6 Indications for emergency decompressive surgery

63.6.1 Cautions and contraindications

✖ Caution: laminectomy in the face of acute spinal cord injury has been associated with neurologic deterioration in some cases. When emergency decompression is indicated, it is usually combined with a stabilization procedure.

Contraindications to emergent operation

- *complete* spinal cord injury ≥ 24 hrs (no motor or sensory function below level of lesion) in the absence of spinal shock (i.e. the deficit is attributable to a complete spinal cord injury and not a temporary condition due to spinal shock). Bulbocavernosus reflex is generally used as a guide to the presence of spinal shock (see Bulbocavernosus reflex)
- medically unstable patient
- central cord syndrome (p.944): controversial

63.6.2 Modified recommendations of Schneider

See reference.[46]

In patients with *complete* spinal cord lesions, no study has demonstrated improvement in neurologic outcome with either open decompression or closed reduction.[47] In general, surgery is reserved for *incomplete* lesions – possibly excluding central cord syndrome (p.944) – with extrinsic compression, who, following maximal possible reduction of subluxation show:

1. progression of neurologic signs
2. complete subarachnoid block by Queckenstedt test or radiographically (on myelography or MRI)
3. compression of spinal cord (on CT/myelogram, CT, or MRI) e.g. by bone fragments or soft tissue elements (e.g. traumatic disc herniation)
4. necessity for decompression of a vital cervical root
5. compound fracture or penetrating trauma of the spine
6. acute anterior spinal cord syndrome (p.946)
7. non-reducible fracture-dislocations from locked facets causing spinal cord compression

References

[1] Chesnut RM, Narayan RK, Wilberger JE, Povlishock JT. In: Emergency Management of Spinal Cord Injury. Neurotrauma. New York: McGraw-Hill; 1996:1121–1138

[2] Podolsky SM, Baraff LJ, Simon RR, et al. Efficacy of Cervical Spine Immobilization Methods. J Trauma. 1983; 23:687–690

[3] Meguro K, Tator CH. Effect of Multiple Trauma on Mortality and Neurological Recovery After Spinal Cord or Cauda Equina Injury. Neurol Med Chir. 1988; 28:34–41

[4] Bracken MB, Shepard MJ, Holford TR, et al. Administration of Methylprednisolone for 24 or 48 Hours or Tirilazad Mesylate for 48 Hours in the Treatment of Acute Spinal Cord Injury. JAMA. 1997; 277:1597–1604

[5] Section on Disorders of the Spine and Peripheral Nerves of the American Association of Neurological Surgeons and the Congress of Neurological Surgeons. Clinical assessment after acute cervical spinal cord injury. Neurosurgery. 2002; 50 Supplement:S21–S29

[6] Section on Disorders of the Spine and Peripheral Nerves of the American Association of Neurological Surgeons and the Congress of Neurological Surgeons. Management of acute spinal cord injuries in an intensive care unit or other monitored setting. Neurosurgery. 2002; 50 Supplement:S51–S57

[7] Section on Disorders of the Spine and Peripheral Nerves of the American Association of Neurological Surgeons and the Congress of Neurological Surgeons. Blood pressure management after acute spinal cord injury. Neurosurgery. 2002; 50 Supplement:S58–S62

[8] Hurlbert RJ, Hadley MN, Walters BC, Aarabi B, Dhall SS, Gelb DE, Rozzelle CJ, Ryken TC, Theodore N. Pharmacological therapy for acute spinal cord injury. Neurosurgery. 2013; 72 Suppl 2:93–105

[9] Schroeder GD, Kwon BK, Eck JC, Savage JW, Hsu WK, Patel AA. Survey of Cervical Spine Research Society members on the use of high-dose steroids for acute spinal cord injuries. Spine (Phila Pa 1976). 2014; 39:971–977

[10] Resnick DK, Kaiser MG, Fehlings M, McCormick PC. Hypothermia and human spinal cord injury: Position statement and evidence based recommendations from the AANS/CNS Joint Section on Disorders of the Spine and the AANS/CNS Joint Section on Trauma. 2007

[11] Hamilton MG, Hull RD, Pineo GF. Venous Thromboembolism in Neurosurgery and Neurology Patients: A Review. Neurosurgery. 1994; 34:280–296

[12] Dhall SS, Hadley MN, Aarabi B, Gelb DE, Hurlbert RJ, Rozzelle CJ, Ryken TC, Theodore N, Walters BC. Deep venous thrombosis and thromboembolism in patients with cervical spinal cord injuries. Neurosurgery. 2013; 72 Suppl 2:244–254

[13] Green D, Lee MY, Ito VY, et al. Fixed- vs Adjusted-Dose Heparin in the Prophylaxis of Thromboembolism in Spinal Cord Injury. JAMA. 1988; 260:1255–1258

[14] Bachulis BL, Hynes GD, et al. Clinical indications for cervical spine radiographs in the traumatized patient. Am J Surg. 1987; 153:473–478

[15] Harris MB, Waguespack AM, Kronlage S. 'Clearing' Cervical Spine Injuries in Polytrauma Patients: Is It Really Safe to Remove the Collar? Orthopedics. 1997; 20:903–907

[16] Section on Disorders of the Spine and Peripheral Nerves of the American Association of Neurological Surgeons and the Congress of Neurological Surgeons. Radiographic assessment of the cervical spine in asymptomatic trauma patients. Neurosurgery. 2002; 50 Supplement:S30–S35

[17] Como JJ, Diaz JJ, Dunham CM, et al. Practice management guidelines for identification of cervical spine injuries following trauma: update from the Eastern Association for the Surgery of Trauma Practice Management Guidelines Committee. J Trauma. 2009; 67:651–659

[18] Ryken TC, Hadley MN, Walters BC, Aarabi B, Dhall SS, Gelb DE, Hurlbert RJ, Rozzelle CJ, Theodore N. Radiographic assessment. Neurosurgery. 2013; 72 Suppl 2:54–72

[19] Hoffman JR, Mower WR, Wolfson AB, Todd KH, Zucker MI. Validity of a set of clinical criteria to rule out injury to the cervical spine in patients with blunt trauma. National Emergency X-Radiography Utilization Study Group. N Engl J Med. 2000; 343:94–99

[20] Stiell IG, Clement CM, McKnight RD, Brison R, Schull MJ, Rowe BH, Worthington JR, Eisenhauer MA, Cass D, Greenberg G, MacPhail I, Dreyer J, Lee JS, Bandiera G, Reardon M, Holroyd B, Lesiuk H, Wells GA. The Canadian C-spine rule versus the NEXUS low-risk criteria in patients with trauma. N Engl J Med. 2003; 349:2510–2518

[21] Chendrasekhar A, Moorman DW, Timberlake GA. An evaluation of the effects of semirigid cervical collars in patients with severe closed head injury. Am Surg. 1998; 64:604–606

[22] Stelfox HT, Velmahos GC, Gettings E, Bigatello LM, Schmidt U. Computed tomography for early and safe discontinuation of cervical spine immobilization in obtunded multiply injured patients. J Trauma. 2007; 63:630–636

[23] Hunt K, Hallworth S, Smith M. The effects of rigid collar placement on intracranial and cerebral perfusion pressures. Anaesthesia. 2001; 56:511–513

[24] Mobbs RJ, Stoodley MA, Fuller J. Effect of cervical hard collar on intracranial pressure after head injury. ANZ J Surg. 2002; 72:389–391

[25] Section on Disorders of the Spine and Peripheral Nerves of the American Association of Neurological Surgeons and the Congress of Neurological Surgeons. Radiographic assessment of the cervical spine in symptomatic trauma patients. Neurosurgery. 2002; 50 Supplement:S36–S43

[26] Walter J, Doris P, Shaffer M. Clinical Presentation of Patients with Acute Cervical Spine Injury. Ann Emerg Med. 1984; 13:512–515

[27] Nichols CG, Young DH, Schiller WR. Evaluation of Cervicothoracic Junction Injury. Ann Emerg Med. 1987; 16:640–642

[28] Shaffer M, Doris P. Limitation of the Cross Table Lateral View in Detecting Cervical Spine Injuries: A Retrospective Analysis. Ann Emerg Med. 1981; 10:508–513

[29] MacDonald RL, Schwartz ML, Mirich D, et al. Diagnosis of Cervical Spine Injury in Motor Vehicle Crash Victims: How Many X-Rays Are Enough? J Trauma. 1990; 30:392–397

[30] Holliman C, Mayer J, Cook R, et al. Is the AP Radiograph of the Cervical Spine Necessary in Evaluation of Trauma? Ann Emerg Med. 1990; 19:483–484

[31] Harris JH. Radiographic Evaluation of Spinal Trauma. Orthop Clin North Am. 1986; 17:75–86

[32] Tehranzedeh J, Bonk T, Ansari A, Mesgarzdeh M. Efficacy of Limited CT for Non-Visualized Lower Cervical Spine in Patients with Blunt Trauma. Skeletal Radiol. 1994; 23:349–352

[33] Miller MD, Gehweiler JA, Martinez S, et al. Significant new observations on cervical spine trauma. AJR. 1978; 130:659–663

[34] Clark WM, Gehweiler JA, Laib R. Twelve Significant Signs of Cervical Spine Trauma. Skeletal Radiol. 1979; 3:201–205

[35] Wales L, Knopp R, Morishima M. Recommendations for Evaluation of the Acutely Injured Spine: A

Clinical Radiographic Algorithm. Ann Emerg Med. 1980; 9:422–428
[36] Hollis PH, Malis LI, Zappulla RA. Neurological Deterioration After Lumbar Puncture Below Complete Spinal Subarachnoid Block. J Neurosurg. 1986; 64:253–256
[37] Horn EM, Lekovic GP, Feiz-Erfan I, Sonntag VK, Theodore N. Cervical magnetic resonance imaging abnormalities not predictive of cervical spine instability in traumatically injured patients. J Neurosurg Spine. 2004; 1:39–42
[38] Schuster R, Waxman K, Sanchez B, Becerra S, Chung R, Conner S, Jones T. Magnetic resonance imaging is not needed to clear cervical spines in blunt trauma patients with normal computed tomographic results and no motor deficits. Arch Surg. 2005; 140:762–766
[39] Benzel EC, Hart BL, Ball PA, Baldwin NG, Orrison WW, Espinosa MC. Magnetic resonance imaging for the evaluation of patients with occult cervical spine injury. J Neurosurg. 1996; 85:824–829
[40] Section on Disorders of the Spine and Peripheral Nerves of the American Association of Neurological Surgeons and the Congress of Neurological Surgeons. Initial closed reduction of cervical spine fracture-dislocation injuries. Neurosurgery. 2002; 50 Supplement:S44–S50
[41] Gelb DE, Aarabi B, Dhall SS, Hurlbert RJ, Rozzelle CJ, Ryken TC, Theodore N, Walters BC, Hadley MN. Treatment of subaxial cervical spinal injuries. Neurosurgery. 2013; 72 Suppl 2:187–194
[42] Botte MJ, Byrne TP, Abrams RA, Garfin SR. Halo Skeletal Fixation: Techniques of Application and Prevention of Complications. J Am Acad Orthop Surg. 1996; 4:44–53
[43] Robertson PA, Ryan MD. Neurological Deterioration After Reduction of Cervical Subluxation: Mechanical Compression by Disc Material. J Bone Joint Surg. 1992; 74B:224–227
[44] Garfin SR, Botte MJ, Triggs KJ, Nickel VL. Subdural Abscess Associated with Halo-Pin Traction. J Bone Joint Surg. 1988; 70A:1338–1340
[45] Dill SR, Cobbs CG, McDonald CK. Subdural Empyema: Analysis of 32 Cases and Review. Clin Inf Dis. 1995; 20:372–386
[46] Schneider RC, Crosby EC, Russo RH, et al. Traumatic Spinal Cord Syndromes and Their Management. Clin Neurosurg. 1972; 20:424–492
[47] Wagner FC, Chehrazi B. Early Decompression and Neurological Outcome in Acute Cervical Spinal Cord Injuries. J Neurosurg. 1982; 56:699–705

64 Occiptoatlantoaxial Injuries (Occiput to C2)

64.1 Atlanto-occipital dislocation

64.1.1 General information

See Occiptoatlantoaxial-complex anatomy (p. 68) for relevant anatomy.

Atlanto-occipital dislocation (AOD) AKA craniocervical junction dislocation. Disruption of the stability of the craniocervical junction (which results from *ligamentous* injuries). Probably underdiagnosed, may be present in ≈ 1% of patients with "cervical spine injuries"[1] (definition of cervical spine injuries not specified), found in 8–19% of fatal cervical spine injury autopsies.[2,3] More than twice as common in pediatrics as adults, possibly owing to the flatter (i.e. less cupped) condyles in peds, the higher ratio of cranium to body weight, and increased ligamentous laxity. Patients usually either have minimal neurological deficit or exhibit bulbar-cervical dissociation (BCD) (p. 944). Some may exhibit cruciate paralysis (p. 1419). Most mortality results from anoxia due to respiratory arrest as a result of BCD.

Classification

See reference.[4]

For illustration, see ► Fig. 64.1.

► **Type I.** Anterior dislocation of occiput relative to the atlas

► **Type II.** Longitudinal dislocation (distraction)

► **Type III.** Posterior dislocation of occiput

Combinations (e.g. anterior-distracted AOD[5]) may also occur.

Practice guideline: Diagnosis of atlanto-occipital dislocation

Level I[6]

- In pediatric patients, CT to assess the condyle-C1 interval (CCI) is recommended to diagnose AOD

Level III[6]

- In pediatric patients, CCI measured on CT has the highest sensitivity and specificity for AOD. The utility in adults has not been reported
- A lateral cervical spine x-ray is recommended to diagnose AOD. If it is desired to employ a radiologic method of measurement, the BAI-BDI method is recommended (see ► Table 64.1). Prevertebral soft tissue swelling in the upper cervical spine on an otherwise nondiagnostic x-ray should be followed with a cervical CT to rule out AOD

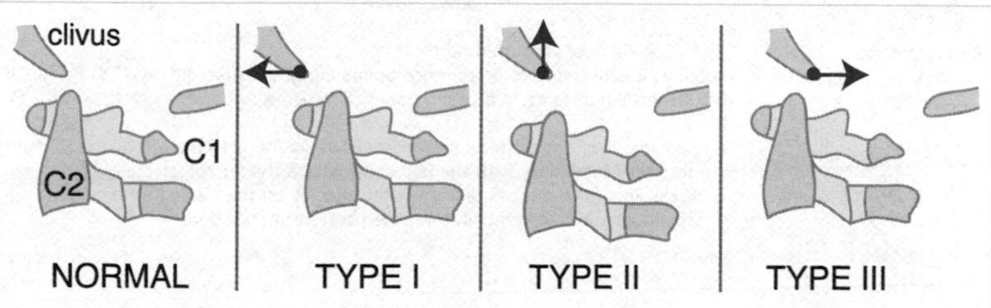

Fig. 64.1 Classification of atlanto-occipital dislocation

Table 64.1 Radiographic evaluation of atlanto-occipital dislocation (AOD)

Method	Comments	Normal Values	
		Plain X-ray	CT
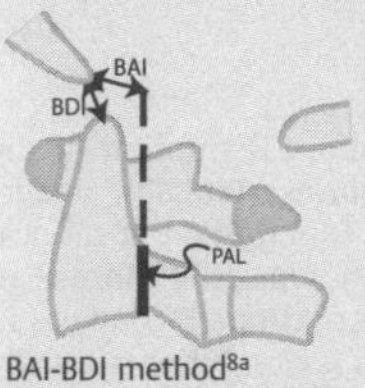 BAI-BDI method[8a] Both BAI & BDI should be measured in adults.	BAI[9] (basion-axial interval) = distance from basion (inferior tip of the clivus) to rostral extension of posterior axial line (PAL) (the posterior cortical margin of the body of C2). AKA Harris line. Better for *anterior* or *posterior* AOD	Adults: -4 ≤ BAI ≤ 12 mm. Normal: BAI & BDI each ≤ 12 mm	May be used,[10] but was not reliably reproducible on CT[11]
		Peds: 0–12 mm (BAI should never be negative)	
	BDI (basion-dental interval) = distance from basion to the closest point on the tip of the dens. Better for *distracted* AOD	Adult: ≤ 12 mm (range: 2–15 mm) (mean: 7.5 ±þ4.3)	Adult: < 8.5 mm (range: 1.4–9 mm)[11]
		Peds: unreliable in age < 13 yrs because of variable age of ossification and fusion of the odontoid tip (os)	Peds[12b]: < 10.5 mm (95th percentile). With os[c]: < 9.5 mm. Without os[c]: < 11.5 mm
Atlanto-occipital interval (AOI) 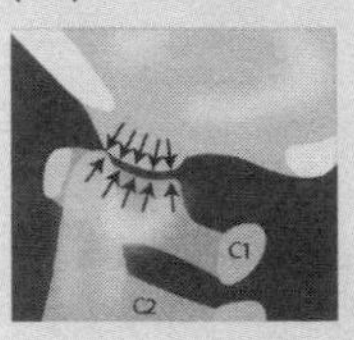	AKA condylar gap.[13] Distance between occipital condyle and superior articular surface of C1 measured on lateral x-ray or sagittal CT reconstructions thru O-C1 junction. Pang[14] averaged the interval between the condyle and C1 at 4 equidistant points on sagittal and 4 on coronal images (8 points total)	Adult[d]: ≤ 2 mm[13]	Adult:: < 1.4 mm (95th percentile) (based on single measurement)[11]
		Peds: ≤ 5 mm (for all of 5 equally spaced measurements[15])	Peds: < 2.5 mm (single measure),[12] or < 4.0 mm (average of 8 measurements in 2 planes)[16]
Powers' ratio & Dublin measure 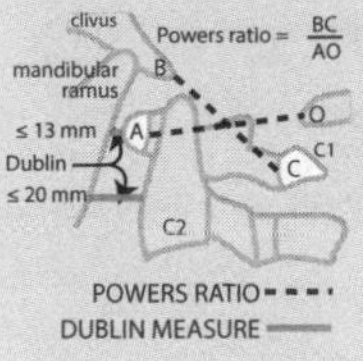	Powers' ratio: cannot be used with fractures of C1 or foramen magnum. Only for *anterior* AOD (see text). Requires identification of 4 reference points: B = basion, A = anterior arch of C1, C = posterior arch of C1, O = opisthion[e]	Adult: < 1 (range: 0.5–1.2) (95th percentile = 0.6–0.9) (see text for details)	Same as plain x-ray[11]
		Peds: < 0.9[f]	
	Dublin measure[17] 25% sensitive[18]	Mandible to anterior atlas: ≤ 13 mm. Posterior mandible to dens: ≤ 20 mm	
X-Line method 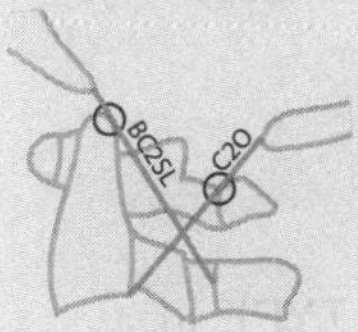	AKA occipital-axial lines method.[18] Requires identification of 6 reference points and 2 lines (sensitivity 75%).[18] Uses a 6 ft target-film distance in a sitting patient[19] which is not always practical in the E/R[5] • C2O line: from the posteroinferior corner of axis body to the opisthionΔ. Should intersect tangentially with the highest point on the C1 spinolaminar line • BC2SL line: from the basion to a point midway on the C2 spinolaminar line. Should intersect tangentially with the posterosuperior dens		

Table 64.1 continued

Method	Comments	Normal Values	
		Plain X-ray	CT
MRI 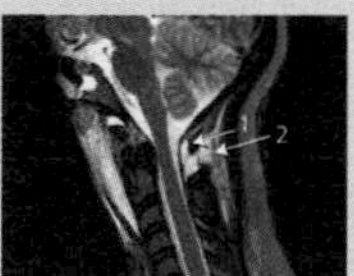	Abnormal MRI findings include: abnormal high signal on T2WI in the occipitoatlantal joints or in the posterior occipitoatlantal (O-C1) ligaments. Very sensitive (≈ 100%) but not specific for *unstable* AOD. The figure at left shows abnormal signal in the posterior O-C1 ligaments (arrow 1) and in the ligamentum flavum and soft tissues (arrow 2).		

[a]original study of lateral x-ray in a supine patient with a target-film distance of 40 in. (1 m). The sensitivity of the BAI-BDI method for AOD is good when all landmarks can be identified, but still may only be ≈ 75%[10]
[b]for this study, peds is defined up to the age of 10 years, by age ≈ 8–10 years the C-Spine reaches adult proportions (not necessarily size)
[c]os = ossiculum terminale (p. 981)
[d]the articular process of C1 is often obscured by the tip of the mastoid process on plain films
[e]the opisthion cannot be identified in ≈ 56% of lateral C-spine x-rays[9]
[f]could not be measured in many peds cases often due to lack of ossification (usually of posterior C1 arch)

64.1.2 Clinical presentation

1. may be neurologically intact, therefore must be ruled-out in any major trauma
2. bulbar-cervical dissociation (p. 944)
3. may have lower cranial nerve deficits (as well as VI palsies) ± cervical cord injury
4. worsening neurologic deficit with the application of cervical traction: check lateral C-spine films immediately after applying traction (p. 959)

64.1.3 Radiographic evaluation

Numerous methodologies have been devised to radiographically diagnose AOD. Most utilize *surrogate markers* for the end-point of interest: viz. instability of the occipital-cervical junction. None are completely reliable.[7] Measurements on CT scans are more accurate than plain radiographs (land marks are easier to identify, no magnification or rotation error) – however, normal values differ from plain radiographs. Some methods are shown in ▶ Table 64.1. The BAI-BDI method and the AOI method are recommended.

A helpful rule-of-thumb: the inferior tip of the clivus should point directly to tip of dens (this may be obscured on x-ray).

Additional CT clues: there may be blood in the basal cisterns (an indirect sign). On thin-cut axial CT, there may be one or more slices showing no bone at all due to the gap between the occiput and C1.

64.1.4 Technical suggestions for radiographic evaluation

1. X-rays: verify that the film is a true lateral (e.g. check alignment of the two mandibular rami as well as of the posterior clinoids)
2. CT: sensitivity, specificity, and positive/negative predictive values of most of the these measures improves when sagittal CT reconstructions are used instead of plain radiographs[20] (relevant landmarks could be identified in > 99% of CTs, vs. 39–84% on x-ray)

Powers' ratio[1]: distance **BC** (basion to posterior arch of atlas) is divided by distance **AO** (opisthion to anterior arch of atlas), see ▶ Table 64.1. Interpretation is shown in ▶ Table 64.2.

✖ Cannot be used with any fracture involving the atlas or the foramen magnum, or with congenital anatomic abnormalities. Applies only to *anterior* AOD (i.e. not for posterior or distracted AOD).

64.1.5 Management

Initial management

If AOD is suspected, immediately immobilize the neck with halo orthosis or with sandbags. ✖ Do not apply cervical traction in an attempt to reduce AOD because there is a 10% risk of neurologic deterioration with the use of traction in AOD.

64

Table 64.2 Powers' ratio

Ratio BC/AO	Interpretation	Comment
< 0.9	normal	1 standard deviation below the lowest case of AOD
≥ 0.9 and < 1	"grey zone" (indeterminate)	included 7% of normals and no cases of AOD
≥ 1	AOD	encompassed all AOD cases

Table 64.3 Grading & management of AOD[10]

Grade	Definition	Management
I	no abnormal CT criteria[a] with only moderately abnormal MRI (high signal in posterior ligaments or occipitoatlantal joints)	external orthosis (halo or collar)
II	≥ 1 abnormal CT criteria[a] or grossly abnormal MRI findings in occipitoatlantal joints, tectorial membrane, or alar or cruciate ligaments	surgical stabilization

[a]CT criteria used: Power's ratio, BAI-BDI, X-line

Subsequent management

Controversial whether operative fusion vs. prolonged immobilization (4–12 months) with halo brace is required. However, posterior occipitocervical fusion is usually recommended (p. 1138).

Practice guideline: Treatment of atlanto-occipital dislocation

Level III[6]
- internal fixation & arthrodesis (fusion) using one of a variety of methods
- ✖ CAUTION: traction is not recommended in the management of AOD

Horn et al.[10] suggest that patients be grouped and then managed as shown in ▶ Table 64.3.

In infants: reduce in the OR and fuse (usually with transarticular screws).

64.1.6 Prognosis

The most important predictor of outcome is the severity of neurologic injuries at the time of presentation.[10] Among AOD patients who survived the initial injury, those with severe TBI and brainstem dysfunction or complete bulbar-cervical dissociation all had poor outcome.[10] Those with incomplete SCI or nonsevere TBI may improve.

64.2 Occipital condyle fractures

64.2.1 General information

Key concepts

- uncommon (0.4% of trauma patients)
- may present with lower cranial nerve deficits which may be delayed in onset (e.g. hypoglossal nerve palsy), mono-, para-, or quadriparesis or plegia
- W/U: ✔ CT scan with reconstructions (rarely detected on plain x-rays)

- Tx: usually treated with rigid collar. Indications for occipitocervical fusion or halo immobilization: craniocervical misalignment (occipital-C1 interval > 2.0 mm)

Occipital condyle fractures (OCF) were first described in 1817 by Bell.[21]

Rare. Incidence: 0.4% (in a series of 24,745 consecutive trauma patients surviving to the E/R[22]).

64.2.2 Diagnosis

Clinical suspicion of occipital condyle fracture (OCF) should be raised by the presence of ≥ 1 of the following[23]:

- blunt trauma with high energy
- craniocervical injuries
- altered consciousness
- occipital pain or tenderness
- impaired cervical movement
- lower cranial nerve palsies
- retropharyngeal soft-tissue swelling

Practice guideline: Diagnosis of occipital condyle fractures

Level II[24]

- CT to establish the diagnosis of occipital condyle fracture (OCF)

Level III[24]

- MRI to assess the integrity of the ligaments of the craniocervical complex

64.2.3 Classification

A widely used classification system is that of Anderson & Montesano[25] as shown in ▶ Table 64.4.

Maserati et al.[22] classified patients simply on the basis of whether craniocervical misalignment was present or absent on CT with reconstructions (they defined craniocervical misalignment as an occipital condyle-C1 interval > 2.0 mm). They felt other classification systems were superfluous as they did not affect outcome in their retrospective review (see Treatment below).

64.2.4 Treatment

Controversial. Lower cranial nerve deficits often develop in untreated cases of OCF, and may resolve or improve with external immobilization. Anderson & Montesano Types I & II have been treated with or without external immobilization (cervical collar or, occasionally, halo) without obvious difference. External immobilization × 6–8 weeks is suggested for Type III fractures because of the higher risk of delayed deficits.

Table 64.4 Anderson & Montesano classification of occipital condyle fractures

Type	Description
I	comminuted from impact: may occur from axial loading
II	extension of linear basilar skull fracture[26]
III	*avulsion* of condyle fragment (traction injury): may occur during rotation, lateral bending, or a combination of mechanisms. Considered unstable by many

Practice guideline: Treatment of occipital condyle fractures

Level III[24]:
- For OCF with associated atlanto-occipital ligamentous injury or evidence of instability: halo vest immobilization or occipitocervical stabilization (fusion).
- For bilateral OCFs, consider halo vest instead of a collar to provide increased immobilization.
- External cervical immobilization for all other OCFs.

64.2.5 Outcome

In a retrospective review of 100 patients with OCF,[22] 3 patients underwent occipitocervical fusion (p.1474) for craniocervical misalignment (2) or unrelated C1–2 fracture (1). The remainder (without craniocervical misalignment) were treated with a rigid collar and delayed clinical & radiographic follow-up. None of their unoperated patients had neurologic deficit, and none developed delayed instability, malalignment, or neurologic deficit (regardless of their classification on the other systems in use).

64.3 Atlantoaxial subluxation/dislocation

64.3.1 General information

Lower morbidity and mortality than atlantooccipital dislocation.[27] See Occiptoatlantoaxial-complex anatomy (p.68) for relevant anatomy.

Types of atlantoaxial subluxation:
1. rotatory: (see below) usually seen in children after a fall or minor trauma
2. anterior: more ominous (see below)
3. posterior: rare. Usually from erosion of odontoid. Unstable. Requires fusion

64.3.2 Atlantoaxial rotatory subluxation

General information

Key concepts

- typically seen in children
- associations: trauma, RA, respiratory tract infections in peds (Grisel syndrome)
- often present with cock-robin head position (tilt, rotation, sl. flexion)
- classification: Fielding & Hawkins (▶ Table 64.5)
- Tx: early traction often successful. Treat infection in Grisel syndrome. Subluxation unreducible in traction may need transoral release then posterior fusion

Table 64.5 Fielding & Hawkins classification of rotatory atlantoaxial subluxation

Type	Description		AD(mm)	Comment
	TAL[a]	facet injury		
I	intact	bilateral	≤3	dens acts as pivot
II	injured	unilateral	3.1–5	intact joint acts as pivot
III	injured	bilateral	>5	rare. Very unstable
IV	incompetence of the odontoid with *posterior* displacement			rare. Very unstable

[a]TAL = transverse atlantal ligament, AD = anterior displacement of C1 on C2

Rotational deformity at the atlanto-axial junction is usually of short duration and easily corrected. Rarely, the atlantoaxial joint locks in rotation (AKA atlantoaxial rotatory fixation[28]). Usually seen in children. May occur spontaneously (with rheumatoid arthritis[29] or with congenital dens anomalies), following major or minor trauma (including neck manipulation or even with neck rotation while yawning[28]), or with an infection of the head or neck including upper respiratory tract (known as Grisel syndrome[30]: inflammation may cause mechanical and chemical injury to the facet capsules and/or transverse atlantal ligament (TAL)).

The vertebral arteries (VA) may be compromised in excessive rotation, especially if it is combine with anterior displacement.

Mechanism of subluxation

The dislocation may be at the occipito-atlantal and/or the atlanto-axial articulations.[31] The mechanism of the irreducibility is poorly understood. With an intact TAL, rotation occurs without anterior displacement. If the TAL is incompetent as a result of trauma or infection, there may also be anterior displacement with more potential for neurologic injury. Posterior displacement occurs only rarely.[28]

Classification

The Fielding and Hawkins classification[28] is shown in ▶ Table 64.5.

Clinical findings

Patients are usually young. Neurologic deficit is rare. Findings may include: neck pain, headache, torticollis – characteristic "cock robin" head position with ~ 20° lateral tilt to one side, 20° rotation to the other, and slight (≈ 10°) flexion, see DDx (p. 1390) -, reduced range of motion, and facial flattening.[28] Although the patient cannot reduce the dislocation, they can increase it with head rotation towards the subluxed joint with potential injury to the high cervical cord.

Brainstem and cerebellar infarction and even death may occur with compromise of circulation through the VAs.[32]

Radiographic evaluation

X-rays : Findings (may be confusing) include:

- pathognomonic finding on AP C-spine x-ray in severe cases: frontal projection of C2 with simultaneous oblique projection of C1.[33 (p 124)] In less severe cases, the C1 lateral mass that is forward appears larger and closer to the midline than the other
- asymmetry of the atlantoaxial joint that is not correctable with head rotation, which may be demonstrated by persistence of asymmetry on open mouth odontoid views with the head in neutral position and then rotated 10–15° to each side
- the spinous process of the axis is tilted in one direction and rotated to the other (may occur in torticollis of any etiology)

CT scan: Demonstrates rotation of the atlas.[31]

MRI: May assess the competence of the transverse ligament.

Treatment

Grisel's syndrome

Appropriate antibiotics for causative pathogen with traction (see below) and then immobilization for the subluxation as follows[30]: Fielding (▶ Table 64.5) Type I: soft collar, Type II: Philadelphia collar or SOMI, Type III or IV: halo. After 6–8 weeks of immobilization, check stability with flexion-extension x-rays. Surgical fusion for residual instability

Traction

If treated within the first few months[34] the subluxation can usually be reduced with gentle traction (in children start with 7–8 lbs and gradually increase up to 15 lbs over several days, in adults start with 15 lbs and gradually increase up to 20). If the subluxation is present > 1 month, traction is less successful. Active left-right neck rotation is encouraged in traction.

If reducible, immobilization in traction or halo is maintained × 3 months[28] (range: 6–12 weeks).

Surgical fusion

Subluxation that cannot be reduced or that recurs following immobilization should be treated by surgical arthrodesis after 2–3 weeks of traction to obtain maximal reduction. The usual fusion is C1 to C2 (p.1479) unless other fractures or conditions are present.[28] Fusion may be performed even if the rotation between C1 & C2 is not completely reduced. For irreducible fixation, a staged procedure can be done with anterior transoral release of the atlantoaxial complex (the exposure is taken laterally to expose the atlantoaxial joints which must be done carefully to avoid injury to the VAs, soft tissue is carefully removed from the joints and the atlantodental interval, no attempt at reduction was made at the time of this 1st stage) followed by gradual skull traction and then a second stage posterior C1–2 fusion[34]

64.3.3 Anterior atlantoaxial subluxation (AAS)

See reference.[27]

General information

One third of patients with AAS have neurologic deficit or die. For relevant anatomy, see Occiptoatlantoaxial-complex anatomy (p.68).

Subluxation may be due to:

1. disruption (rupture) of the transverse (atlantal) ligament (TAL): the atlantodental interval (ADI) (see below) will be increased
   a) attachment points of the TAL may be weakened in rheumatoid arthritis (p.1479)
   b) trauma: may cause anatomic or functional ligament disruption (see below)
2. incompetence of the odontoid process: ADI will be normal
   a) odontoid fracture
   b) congenital hypoplasia, e.g. Morquio syndrome (p.1151)

Presentation

Neck pain is common. There are no specific patterns to the pain that is characteristic.

"V" shaped pre-dens space

See reference.[35]

Widening of the upper space between the anterior arch of C1 and the odontoid seen on lateral C-spine flexion x-ray. It is not known if this increased mobility represents elongation or laxity of the transverse ligament and/or the posterior ligamentous complex. This may also be a normal finding in flexion in peds.

True subluxation will result in malalignment between C1 and C2. The key differentiating feature is whether the ADI is increased or normal, as indicated above.

Evaluation and classification

Both CT & MRI are recommended to evaluate fractures, TAL & its bony attachments.

Assessing the integrity of the transverse ligament

1. disruption of the TAL may be inferred from *indirectly* from
   a) Rule of Spence: on open-mouth odontoid x-ray, if the total overhang of both C1 lateral masses on C2 is ≥ 7 mm
   b) atlantodental interval (ADI) (p.213): > 3 mm in adults, > 4 mm in peds
2. MRI may be able to image the TAL directly. Findings of disruption (axial MRI): high signal within TAL on gradient-echo MRI, loss of continuity of TAL, blood at insertion site[36]
3. CT demonstrates bony injuries in regions of TAL insertion on C1 tubercles

Classification of TAL disruption

See reference.[37]

► **Type I.** Anatomic disruption. Tear of TAL itself. Rare (the odontoid usually fractures before the TAL tears). Unlikely to heal. Requires surgical stabilization

▸ **Type II.** Physiologic disruption. Detachment of the tubercle of C1 to which TAL is attached (▸ Fig. 1.12) as may occur in comminuted C1 lateral mass fractures. 74% chance of healing with immobilization (halo recommended[37])

Treatment

- For TAL disruption: One approach is to fuse all Type I TAL injuries, and those Type II TAL injuries that are still unstable after 3–4 months of immobilization.[37] Fusion is also recommended with irreducible subluxations. If C1 is intact, a C1–2 fusion is usually adequate. For situations involving C1 fractures, see below.
- For odontoid fractures with intact TAL managed as outlined (p.979)

64.4 Atlas (C1) fractures

64.4.1 General information

Acute C1 fractures account for 3–13% of cervical spine fractures.[38] 56% of 57 patients had isolated C1 fractures; 44% had combination C1–2 fractures; 9% had additional non-contiguous C-spine fractures. 21% had associated head injuries.[38]

64.4.2 Classification of C1 fractures

See reference.[39]

Type I: fractures involving a single arch (31–45% of C1 fractures)
Type II: burst fracture (37–51%): the classic Jefferson fracture (see below)
Type III: lateral mass fractures of the atlas (13–37%)

64.4.3 Jefferson fracture

Described by Sir Geoffrey Jefferson.[40] Classically a four-point (burst) fracture of the C1 ring,[41] but the term is now often used to include the more common three or two-point fractures,[42] the latter through the C1 arches (thinnest portion). Usually from *axial* load (a "blow-out" fracture). 41% chance of an associated C2 fracture.

In pediatrics, it is critical to differentiate a C1 fracture from the normal synchondroses (p.214) and from pseudospread of the atlas (p.933). A fracture may also occur through the unfused synchondroses.

64.4.4 Stability

To reiterate: stability of the occiptoatlantoaxial complex is primarily due to ligaments, with little contribution from bony articulations; see Occiptoatlantoaxial-complex anatomy (p.68). ✱ Integrity of transverse ligament (TAL) is the most important determinant of stability (see Assessing the integrity of the transverse ligament above).

Jefferson fractures are unstable, however, there is usually no neurologic deficit for isolated Jefferson fractures (due to the large canal diameter at this level, plus the tendency for fragments to be forced outwards away from spinal cord).

64.4.5 Clinical

Neurologic deficit is rare. 3 of 25 patients with Jefferson fractures sustained neurologic injuries (1 complete injury, 2 central cord syndromes) in one series.

64.4.6 Evaluation

Thin cut high-resolution CT is the diagnostic test of choice. It is critical to evaluate from C1 through C3 to delineate details of the C1 fracture and to assess for associated C2 injury.

MRI may be able to assess the integrity of the TAL, but images are often difficult to interpret for this.

64.4.7 Treatment

Treatment options depend heavily on the status of the TAL. Practice guidelines are shown here. Specifics are delineated in ▶ Table 64.6.[43] When external immobilization is employed, it is used for 8–16 weeks (mean = 12).

Practice guideline: Treatment of isolated atlas fractures

Level III[44]: for isolated atlas fractures:
- treatment is based on the fracture type and integrity of transverse atlantal ligament
- if the transverse ligament is intact: cervical immobilization alone
- if the transverse ligament is disrupted: either (note: disruption of the TAL may be anatomic or physiologic; see text for details)
  a) cervical immobilization alone
  b) or, surgical fixation and fusion

Fusion options when surgery is indicated[37]:
1. unilateral ring or anterior C1 arch fractures: C1–2 fusion
2. multiple ring fractures or posterior C1 arch fractures: occipital-cervical fusion

Surgical options: 1. fusion A. unilateral ring..., B. multiple ring... 2. Surgical options that do not involve arthrodesis include: posterior C1 screw placement, anterior transoral screw/plate placement.

64.4.8 Outcome

In many series,[38,45] treatment without surgery results in satisfactory outcome when the TAL is not disrupted.

64.5 Axis (C2) fractures

64.5.1 General information

Acute fractures of the axis represent ≈ 20% of cervical spine fractures. Neurological injury is uncommon, and occurs in < 10% of cases. Most injuries may be treated by rigid immobilization.

Steele's rule of thirds: each of the following occupies one-third of the area of the canal at the level of the atlas: dens, space, spinal cord.[46]

64.5.2 Types of C2 fractures

1. odontoid fractures (p.978): type II odontoid fracture is the most common injury of the axis
2. hangman's fracture: see below
3. miscellaneous C2 fractures (p.982)

Table 64.6 Treatment options for isolated C1 fractures

Fracture type	Treatment options
anterior or posterior arch	collar or SOMI
anterior AND posterior arch (burst)	
• stable (TAL[a] intact)	collar or SOMI, halo
• unstable (TAL disrupted)	halo, C1–2 stabilization & fusion
lateral mass fractures	
• comminuted fracture	collar or SOMI, halo
• transverse process fracture	collar or SOMI

[a]abbreviations: TAL = transverse atlantal ligament

64.5.3 Hangman's fracture

General information

Key concepts

- bilateral fracture through the pars interarticularis of C2 with traumatic subluxation of C2 on C3, most often due to hyperextension + axial loading
- most are stable with no neurologic deficit
- classification: Levine system (▶ Table 64.7). Critical dividing line: disruption of C2–3 disc (Types II and higher) which may render the fracture unstable
- W/U: ✓ cervical CT with sagittal & coronal recons for all. ✓ Cervical MRI to assess C2–3 disc disruption (Levine II). ✓ CTA for dissection if fx passes thru foramen transversarium (consider for all C2 fractures – see ▶ Table 55.7)
- most do well with non-halo immobilization x 8–14 weeks. Esceptions: severe/unstable fractures (p. 975) or those that do not remain aligned in brace

AKA traumatic spondylolisthesis of the axis (a term first used in 1964[47]).

Description: bilateral fracture through the pars interarticularis (isthmus) of the pedicle of C2 (▶ Fig. 64.2; the configuration of C2 is unique, and the distinction between the pars and the pedicle is ambiguous). There is often anterior subluxation of C2 on C3.

The term "hangman's fracture" (HF) was coined by Schneider et al.[48] although the mechanism of most modern HFs (hyperextension and *axial loading*, from MVAs or diving accidents) differs from that sustained in judicial hangings (where submental placement of the knot results in hyperextension and distraction[49]). Some cases may be due to forced flexion or compression of the neck while in extension.

Pediatrics: rare in children < 8 years old where the forces tend to fracture the incompletely fused odontoid, see epiphyseal fracture (p. 214). In pediatrics, consider pseudosubluxation in the differential diagnosis (p. 934).

Usually *stable*. Deficit is rare. Nonunion is rare. 90% heal with immobilization only. Operative fusion is rarely needed. Fractures of C2 that do not go through the isthmus are not true hangman's fractures and may require different management (p. 982).

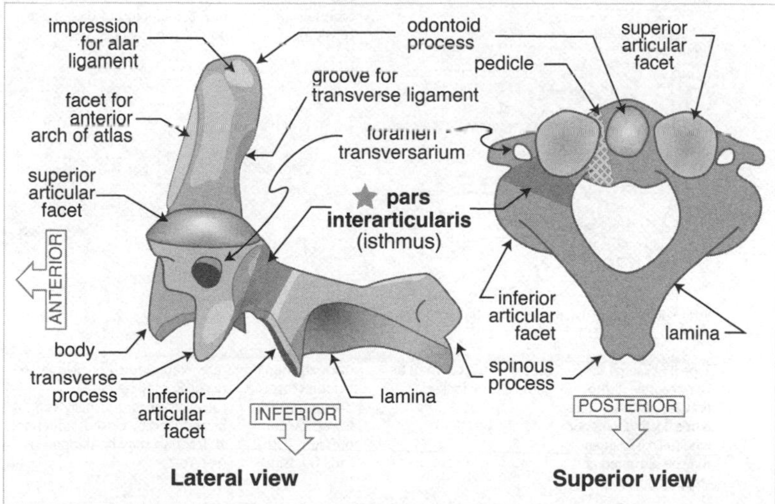

Fig. 64.2 Anatomy of axis (C2). The pars interarticularis is shown in dark blue

Classification

Levine/Effendi classification

The system of Effendi et al.[50] as modified by Levine[51] and others (▶ Table 64.7) is widely used in grading adult HF (not applicable to peds). Angulation is measured as the angle between the inferior endplates of C2 and C3. Anterior subluxation of C2 on C3 > 3 mm (Type II) is a surrogate marker for C2–3 disc disruption which can be evaluated more directly with cervical MRI.

Grading system of Frances et al.

The grading system[54] is shown in ▶ Table 64.8.

The methodology of measurements is depicted in ▶ Fig. 64.3.

Levine/Francis correlation

In a series of 340 axis fractures,[55] the most common fracture type was Type I in the Levine system (72%) and Grade I in the Francis system (65%); and there was a close correlation as follows:

Levine Type I ≈ Francis Grade I

Levine Type III ≈ Francis Grade IV

Table 64.7 Levine classification of hangman's fractures (modified Effendi system)[a]

Type	Description	Radiographic Findings	Mechanism	Comment
I	vertical pars fx just posterior to the VB	≤ 3 mm subluxation of C2 on C3 & *no* angulation	axial loading & extension	stable on flexion/extension x-rays. Neurologic deficit rare
I A	fx lines on each side are not parallel. Fx may pass thru *foramen transversarium* on one side	fx line may not be visible on x-ray. *Anterior* C2 VB may be subluxed 2–3 mm anteriorly on C3 & the C2 VB may appear elongated.	may be hyperextension + lateral bending	"atypical hangman's fracture".[52] Spinal canal may be narrowed. 33% incidence of paralysis
II	vertical fx thru pars. *Disruption of C2–3 disc* & posterior longitudinal ligament	subluxation of C2 on C3 > 3 mm and/or angulation[b]. Slight anterior compression of C3 possible	axial loading & extension with rebound flexion	may lead to early instability. Neurologic deficit rare. Usually reduces with traction
IIA	oblique fx (usually anterior-inferior to posterior superior) 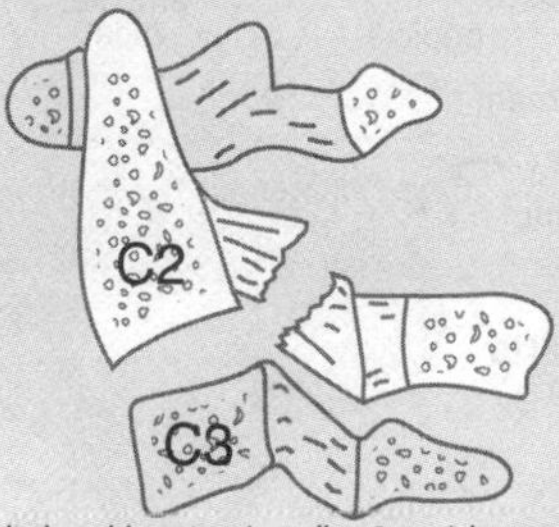 little subluxation (usually ≤ 3 mm) but more angulation (can be > 15°)		flexion distraction (posterior arch fails in tension)	rare (< 10%). Unstable. ✖ Traction → increased angulation & widening of disc space ∴ *do not use* traction
III	Type II + bilateral C2–3 facet capsule disruption. C2 posterior arch is free floating. Anterior longitudinal ligament may be disrupted or stripped off C3	facets of C2/C3 may be subluxed or locked	unclear, may be flexion (capsule disruption) followed by compression (isthmus fracture)	rare. Neurologic deficit may occur & may be fatal. Facet dislocation usually cannot be reduced by closed reduction. ✖ Traction may be dangerous (see text)

[a]Effendi et al.,[50] Levine and Edwards,[51] Sonntag and Dickman[27] and Levine[53]

[b]amount of angulation was not specified in original article, but > 10° has been suggested by some

Other fracture types

Not all fractures fit into one or both of these classification systems.[56] Example: coronally oriented fracture extending through the posterior C2 vertebral body.

Presentation

Most (≈ 95%) are neurologically intact, those few with deficits are usually minor (paresthesias, monoparesis...) and many recover within one month.[54] Almost all conscious patients will have cervical pain usually in the upper posterior cervical region, and occipital neuralgia is not uncommon.[57] There is a high incidence of associated head injury and there will be other associated C-spine injuries – e.g. C1 fracture (see above) or clay shoveler's fracture (p. 988) – in ≈ one third, with most occurring in the upper 3 cervical levels. There are usually external signs of injury to the face and head associated with the hyperextending and axial force.

Evaluation

Cervical CT: with sagittal & coronal reconstructions should be done to fully assess the fracture.

CTA: should be done to evaluate the vertebral arteries if fracture extends through foramen transversarium (especially Levine Type IA) and in patients with symptoms suggestive of stroke. Some

Table 64.8 Francis grading[a] system for hangman's fracture

Grade	Angulation θ	Displacement
I	< 11°	d < 3.5 mm
II	> 11°	
III	< 11°	d > 3.5 mm and d/b < 0.5
IV	> 11°	
V		disc disruption

[a]see ▶ Fig. 64.3 for definitions

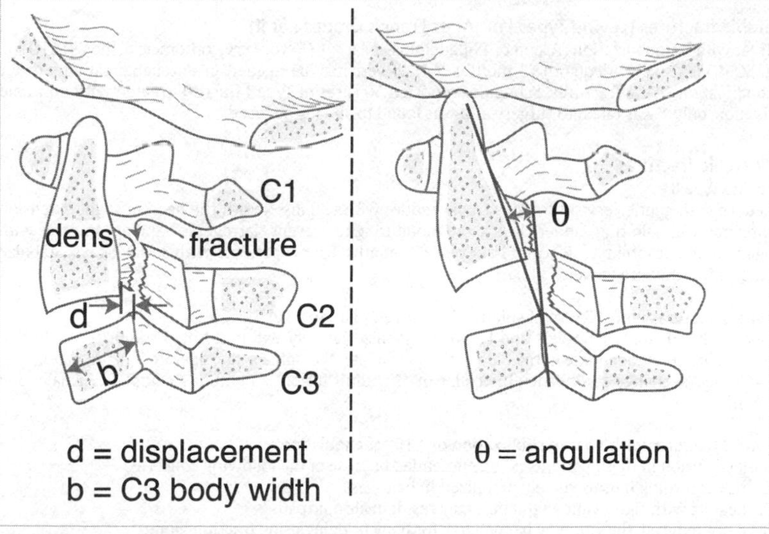

Fig. 64.3 Grading system of Francis

recommend CTA for all C2 fractures – ▶ Table 55.7). Angiography or MRA may be done as an alternative to CTA.

✱ MRI: cervical MRI should be done to look for C2–3 disc disruption (a marker for instability (Levine grade II) which usually requires surgical stabilization). Findings may include abnormal increased signal intensity on MRI (best seen on sagittal FLAIR images or T2WI).

X-Rays: lateral C-spine x-rays show the fracture in 95% of cases. Also demonstrates C2 angulation and/or subluxation. Most fractures pass through the pars or the transverse foramen,[54] 7% go through the body of C2 (p. 982). Instability can usually be identified as marked anterior displacement of C2 on C3 (guideline[54]: unstable if displacement exceeds 50% of the AP diameter of C3 vertebral body), excessive angulation of C2 on C3, or by excessive motion on flexion-extension films.

Patients suspected of having Levine Type I fractures and are neurologically intact should have physician-supervised flexion-extension x-rays to rule out a reduced type II fracture.

Treatment

General information

Nonsurgical management produces adequate reduction in 97–100% and results in a fusion rate of 93–100%[27,58,59] if the external immobilization is adequately maintained for 8–14 weeks[60] (average time for healing is ≈ 11.5 weeks[54]). Specific treatment depends on the reliability of the patient and the degree of stability as described below. Most cases do well with non-halo immobilization.[59] Practice guidelines are shown here, and details follow.

Practice guideline: Management of isolated hangman's fracture

Level III[61,62]

- hangman's fractures may initially be managed with external immobilization in most cases (halo or collar)
- surgical stabilization should be considered in cases of:
  a) severe angulation of C2 on C3 (Levine II, Francis II & IV)
  b) disruption of the C2–3 disc space (Levine II, Francis V)
  c) or inability to establish or maintain alignment with external immobilization

Stable fractures (Levine Types I or IA, or Francis Grades I or II)

Treat with immobilization (Aspen or Philadelphia collar[63 (p 2326)] or cervicothoracic orthosis (CTO) (e. g. SOMI) is usually adequate) × 3 months.[53] Halo-vest may be needed in unreliable patients or for combination C1-C2 fractures. Schneider reported 50 cases of Type I fracture treated with non-halo fixation, only 1 was taken to surgery and was found to already be fused.

Unstable fractures

Levine Type II

Reduce with gentle *cervical traction* (most reduce with ≤ 30 lbs[53]) with the head in slight extension (preferably in halo ring) under close x-ray monitoring to prevent "iatrogenic hanging" in cases with ligamentous instability.[54] Place in halo vest × 3 months. Follow patients with serial x-rays. Stabilize surgically if fracture moves.

Type II fractures with ≤ 5 mm of subluxation and angulation < 10°

Once reduced, apply halo-vest and begin to mobilize (usually within 24 hrs of injury). Verify that immobilization is adequate in the halo with upright lateral C-spine x-ray, operate if inadequate. After 8–12 weeks, change to Philadelphia collar or CTO until fusion is definitely complete (usually 3–4 months).

Type II fractures with > 5 mm subluxation or ≥ 10° of angulation

Surgical fusion in these patients is recommended because of the following concerns:

1. risk of settling if immediately mobilized in halo-vest
2. healing with significant angulation may result in chronic pain
3. if not reduced, the gap may be too large for bony bridging using traction alone

Alternatively, cervical traction can be maintained for ≈ 4 weeks and then reduction should be reassessed 1 hour after removing weight from traction, and if stable, again 24 hours after mobilizing in a halo vest. If unstable, return to traction and repeat trial at 5 & 6 weeks. If still unstable at 6 weeks, surgical fusion is recommended.[53]

Levine Type IIA

✖ Traction will accentuate the deformity.[53] Fractures should be reduced by immediate placement in halo vest (bypassing traction) with extension and *compression* applied. Halo-vest immobilization × 3 months produces ≈ 95% union rate.

Levine Type III

✖ Reduction with traction may be dangerous with locked facets. ORIF is recommended.[27] MRI prior to surgery is recommended to assess the C2–3 disc. Can follow ORIF with halo-vest for the fracture, or can fuse at the same time as ORIF.

Surgical treatment

Indications

Few patients have indications for surgical treatment of HF, and include those with:

1. inability to reduce the fracture (includes most Levine Type III & some Type II)
2. failure of external immobilization to prevent movement at fracture site
3. traumatic C2–3 disc herniation with compromise of the spinal cord[64]
4. established non-union: evidenced by movement on flexion-extension film (p. 956) [54]; all failures of nonoperative treatment had displacement > 4 mm[27]

Hangman's fractures likely to need surgery[55]:

1. Levine Type II or III
2. or Francis grade II, IV or V
3. or if either:
   a) anterior displacement of C2 VB > 50% of the AP diameter of the C3 VB
   b) or if angulation produces widening of either the anterior or posterior borders of the C2–3 disc space > the height of the normal C3–4 disc below

Surgical options

1. fusion techniques:
   a) posterior approach: if the fracture is not transfixed (osteosynthesis – see below) then a C1–2 fusion is required. This depends on the integrity of the C2–3 disc and facet joint capsules, otherwise a C1–3 fusion is required. Occasionally the occiput is incorporated as well. Options for C1–2 fusion:
      - C1–2 wiring and fusion
      - C1–2 lateral mass screws/rods (p. 1481)
   b) anterior C2–3 discectomy[54] with fusion. Optional anterior plating or zero-profile graft/plate. Performed via a transverse anterior cervical incision midway between the angle of the jaw and the thyroid cartilage[58,64]
      - preserves more motion by excluding C1
      - this approach is also recommended for established non-union[54]
      - not optimal for Levine Type III requiring ORIF for locked facets
      - also used when at least a partial reduction cannot be achieved
      - technique: for special considerations for approach to the C2–3 junction, see the section on operative techniques
2. osteosynthesis: screw placement from posterior approach through the C2 pedicle across the fracture fragment.[53 (p 443)] Reduction must be achieved before the screw holes are drilled.[65] The technique for C2 pedicle screws (p. 1481) is used. The posterior fracture fragment may be overdrilled with a 3.5 mm drill. A "top hat" is placed in the hole and a 2.7 mm drill is used to drill the VB. Screw length: 30–35 mm for average adults. Alternatively, a lag screw may be used (with 20 mm unthreaded)

Treatment endpoint

Plain x-rays should show trabeculation across the fracture site or interbody fusion of C2 to C3. Flexion-extension lateral radiographs should show no movement at the fracture site.

64

64.5.4 Odontoid fractures

General information

Key concepts

- 10–15% of C-spine fx. Can occur in older patients with minor trauma (GLF), or in younger patients typically following MVA, falls from a height, skiing...
- may be fatal at time of injury, most survivors are intact. Neck pain is common
- classification: Anderson & D'Alonzo (▶ Table 64.9). Type II (at base) is the most common
- Tx: surgery is considered for: Type II if age > 50 yrs, Type IIA, or Type II & III if displacement ≥ 5 mm or if alignment cannot be maintained with halo

Significant force is required to produce an odontoid fracture in a young individual, and is usually sustained in a motor vehicle accident (MVA), a fall from a height, a skiing accident, etc. In patients > 70 years age, simple ground level falls (GLF) with head trauma may produce the fracture. Odontoid fractures comprise ≈10–15% of all cervical spine fractures.[66] They are easily missed on initial evaluation, especially since significant associated injuries are frequent and may mask symptoms. Pathologic fractures can also occur, e.g. with metastatic involvement (p. 1391).

Flexion is the most common mechanism of injury, with resultant anterior displacement of C1 on C2 (atlantoaxial subluxation). Extension only occasionally produces odontoid fractures, usually associated with posterior displacement.

Signs and symptoms

The frequency of fatalities at the time of the accident resulting directly from odontoid fractures is unknown, it has been estimated as being between 25–40%.[67] 82% of patients with Type II fractures in a review of 7 reports in the literature were neurologically intact, 8% had minor deficits of scalp or limb sensation, and 10% had significant deficit (ranging from monoparesis to quadriplegia).[68] Type III fractures are rarely associated with neurologic injury.

Common symptoms are high posterior cervical pain, sometimes radiating in the distribution of the greater occipital nerve (occipital neuralgia). Almost all patients with high posterior cervical pain will also have paraspinal muscle spasm, reduced range of motion of the neck, and tenderness to palpation over the upper cervical spine. A very suggestive finding is the tendency to support the head with the hands when going between the upright and supine position. Paresthesias in the upper extremities and slight exaggeration of muscle stretch reflexes may also occur. Myelopathy may develop in patients with non-union (p. 980).

Classification

The most widely used classification system of Anderson and D'Alonzo[69] is shown in ▶ Fig. 64.4 and ▶ Table 64.9.

Type I fractures are due to avulsion of the attachment of the alar ligament. They are very rare. Although long considered to be a stable injury, they may not occur as an isolated fracture and may

Table 64.9 Anderson and D'Alonzo classification of odontoid fractures

Type	Characteristics	Stability
I	through tip (above transverse ligament), rare	unstable[a]
II	through base of neck the most common dens fracture (may be best seen on AP x-ray)	usually *unstable*
IIA	similar to type II, but with large bone chips at fracture site,[70] comprise ≈ 3% of type II odontoid fractures. Diagnosed by plain radiographs and/or CT	usually *unstable*
III	through body of C2 (usually involves marrow space). May involve superior articular surface	usually stable

[a]controversial, see text

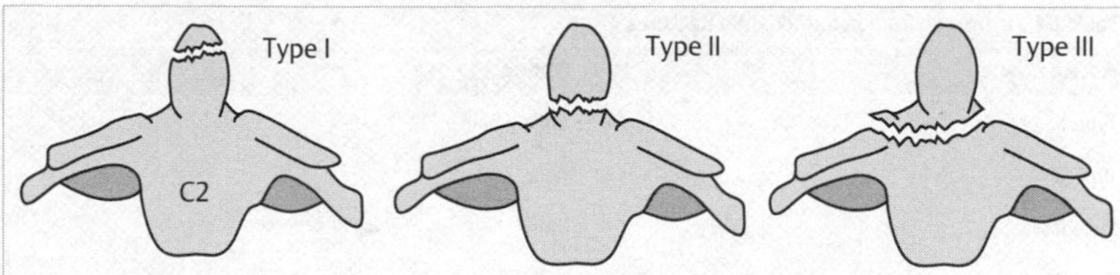

Fig. 64.4 Major types of odontoid fractures (AP view)

be a manifestation of atlanto-occipital dislocation.[71] Also, it may be a marker for possible disruption of the transverse ligament[72] which may result in atlanto-axial instability.

► **Imaging pearl.** A type III odontoid fracture may be misinterpreted as type II on sagittal CT reconstructions because the fracture appears to lie above the VB. Always check the coronal reconstruction which more readily demonstrates the relationship of the fracture to the VB.

Treatment

Practice guidelines

Practice guidelines are shown below. Details appear in the following sections.

Practice guideline: Management of isolated odontoid fractures

- Level II[62]: isolated Type II odontoid fractures in adults ≥ 50 years age should be considered for surgical stabilization & fusion
- Level III[62]
  - Nondisplaced type I, II & III fractures may be managed initially with external cervical immobilization, recognizing that type II odontoid fractures have a higher rate of nonunion
  - Type II & III: consider surgical fixation for:
    a) dens displacement ≥ 5 mm
    b) or Type IIA fracture (comminution of fracture)
    c) or inability to maintain or achieve alignment with external immobilization
  - For surgical intervention, either an anterior or posterior approach may be used

Immobilization

For those not meeting surgical indications, 10–12 weeks of immobilization as suggested in ► Table 64.10 is recommended. There is no Class I medical evidence comparing immobilization options.

Halo vest: fusion rate = 72%,[73] appears superior to a SOMI. If a halo is used, obtain supine and upright lateral C-spine x-rays in the halo. If there is movement at the fracture site, then surgical stabilization is recommended.

Rigid collar[73,74]: fusion rate = 53%.

In patients who are poor surgical candidates, there is theoretical and anecdotal rationale to consider calcitonin therapy (p. 1010) in conjunction with a rigid cervical orthosis.[75]

Type I

So rare that meaningful analysis is difficult. If there is associated atlanto-axial instability, surgical fusion may at times be necessary.

Type II

General information

Treatment remains controversial. No agreement has been reached after many attempts to identify factors that will predict which type II fractures are most likely to heal with immobilization and

Table 64.10 Immobilization for odontoid fractures

Fracture Type	Option
Type I	collar, halo
Type II[a]	halo, collar[a]
Type IIA[a]	halo[a]
Type III[a]	collar, halo[a]
[a]consider surgery for these, use indicated brace when surgery not deemed appropriate	

which will require operative fusion. Critical review of the literature reveals a paucity of well designed studies. A wide range of nonunion rates with immobilization alone (5–76%) is quoted: 30% is probably a reasonable estimate for overall nonunion rate, with 10% nonunion rate for those with displacement < 6 mm.[73] Possible key factors in predicting nonunion include:

1. degree of displacement: probably the most important factor
   a) some authors feel that displacement > 4 mm increases nonunion[69,76]
   b) some authors use ≥ 6 mm as the critical value, citing a 70% nonunion rate[60] in these regardless of age or direction of displacement
2. age:
   a) children < 7 yrs old almost always heal with immobilization alone
   b) some feel that there is a critical age above which the nonunion rate increases, and the following ages have been cited: age > 40 yrs (possibly ≈ doubling the nonunion rate),[76] age > 55 yrs,[77] age > 65 yrs,[78] yet others do not support increasing age as a factor[73]

Indications for surgery for odontoid Type II fractures

Given the above, there can be no hard and fast rules. The following is offered as a guideline (also, above).

✱ Surgical treatment (instead of external immobilization) is recommended for odontoid Type II fractures in patients ≥ 7 years age with any of the following:

1. displacement ≥ 5 mm
2. instability at the fracture site in the halo vest (see below)
3. age ≥ 50 years: increases nonunion rate (with halo) 21-fold[79]
4. nonunion (see ▶ Table 64.11 for radiographic criteria) including firm fibrous union,[80] especially if accompanied by myelopathy[57]
5. disruption of the transverse ligament: associated with delayed instability[37]

Surgical options

1. odontoid compression screw (p. 1480): appropriate for acute type II fractures with transverse ligament intact and attached
2. C1–2 arthrodesis (p. 1479): for options including wiring/fusion, transarticular screws, halifax clamps…

Type IIA

Early surgery is recommended for all type IIA fractures.[70]

Type III

≈ 90% heal with external immobilization (and analgesics) if adequately maintained for 8–14 weeks.[60] Halo-vest brace is probably best,[74] fusion rate ≈ 100% in 1 series.[73] Rigid collar: fusion rate = 50–70%; if used, monitor the patient with frequent C-spine x-rays to rule-out nonunion.

Surgical treatment options

See Atlantoaxial fusion (C1–2 arthrodesis) (p. 1479) and Anterior odontoid screw fixation (p. 1476) for surgical options and operative details.

Nonunion

The radiographic criteria for nonunion are shown in ▶ Table 64.11.

Table 64.11 Radiographic criteria of nonunion of odontoid fractures

- defect in the dens with contiguous sclerosis of both fragments (vascular pseudarthrosis)
- defect in the dens with contiguous resorption of both fragments (rarefying osteitis or atrophic pseudarthrosis)
- defect in the dens with definite loss of cortical continuity
- movement of dens fragment demonstrated on flexion-extension x-rays

The most common symptom of nonunion is continued high posterior cervical pain beyond the time that the brace is removed. Late myelopathy can develop in as many as 77% of mobile nonunions[67,81] as a result of motion and soft tissue proliferation around the unstable fracture site.

Os odontoideum

General information

A separate bone ossicle of variable size with *smooth* cortical borders separated from a foreshortened odontoid peg, occasionally may fuse with the clivus. May mimic Type 1 or 2 odontoid fracture. Etiology is debated with evidence to support both of the following (diagnosis & treatment do not depend on which etiologic theory is correct):

1. congenital: developmental anomaly (nonunion of dens to body of axis). However, does not follow known ossification centers (▸ Fig. 12.4) and has been demonstrated in 9 patients with previously normal odontoid processes[82]
2. acquired: postulated to represent an old nonunion fracture or injury to vascular supply of developing odontoid[82,83]

True os odontoideum is rare. Ossiculum terminale: nonunion of the apex at the secondary ossification center, is more common.

Two anatomic types:

1. orthotopic: ossicle moves with the anterior arch of C1
2. dystopic: ossicle is functionally fused to the basion. May sublux anterior to the C1 arch

Presentation

Main groups identified in the literature[84]:

1. occipitocervical/neck pain
2. myelopathy: further subdivided[82]
   a) transient myelopathy: common following trauma
   b) static myelopathy
   c) progressive myelopathy
3. intracranial signs or symptoms: from vertebrobasilar ischemia
4. incidental finding

Most patients are neurologically intact and present with atlantoaxial instability which may be discovered incidentally. Many symptomatic and asymptomatic patients have been reported with no new problems over many years of follow-up.[85] Conversely, cases of precipitous spinal cord injury after seemingly minor trauma have been reported.[86]

Σ

The natural history is variable, and predictive factors for deterioration, especially in asymptomatic patients, have not been identified.[87]

Evaluation

Practice guideline: Diagnosis of os odontoideum

Level III[88]

- recommended: the following plain C-spine x-rays: AP, open-mouth odontoid, lateral (static & flexion-extension) with or without tomography (CT or plain) and/or MRI of craniocervical junction

It is critical to R/O C1–2 instability. However, myelopathy does not correlate with the degree of C1–2 instability. An AP canal diameter < 13 mm does correlate with the presence of myelopathy.

Treatment

Regardless of whether os odontoideum is congenital or an old non-union fracture, immobilization is unlikely to result in fusion. Therefore, when treatment is elected, surgery – usually atlantoaxial arthrodesis (p. 1479) – is required.

64

Practice guideline: Management of os odontoideum

Level III[88]

- patients without neurologic signs or symptoms:
  - may be followed with clinical & radiographic surveillance
  - or posterior C1–2 fusion may be done
- patients with neurologic signs or symptoms or C1–2 instability: posterior C1–2 internal fixation and fusion
- if surgery is done: post-op halo immobilization is recommended (e.g. following posterior wiring & fusion) unless rigid internal instrumentation is used
- for patients with irreducible cervicomedullary compression and/or evidence of associated occipitoatlantal instability: occipital-cervical fusion ± C1 laminectomy
- for patients with irreducible cervicomedullary compression, consider ventral decompression

64.5.5 Miscellaneous C2 fractures

Comprise ≈ 20% of C2 fractures.[27] Includes fractures of spinous process, lamina, facets, lateral mass or C2 vertebral body. Fractures of spinous process or lamina may be treated with Philadelphia collar or cervicothoracic orthosis (CTO). Fractures which compromise the anterior or middle columns (i.e. fractures of facets, C2 body, or lateral mass) requires CTO or halo-vest if nondisplaced, or halo if displaced.

Practice guideline: Management of fractures of the axis (C2) body

Level III[61,62]:

- fractures may initially be managed with external immobilization in most cases (halo or collar)
- surgical stabilization should be considered in cases of:
  a) severe ligamentous instability
  b) or inability to establish or maintain alignment with external immobilization
- evaluate for vertebral artery injury in cases of comminuted fracture of the axis body

64.6 Combination C1–2 injuries

64.6.1 General information

Combination C1–2 injuries are relatively common and may imply more significant structural and mechanical injury than isolated C1 or C2 fractures. The frequency of C2 fractures in C1–2 combination injuries is shown in ▶ Table 64.12. 5–53% of patients with Type II or III odontoid fractures and 6–26% of hangman's fractures have an associated C1 fracture.[89]

Table 64.12 Accompanying C2 injuries

Injury	%
Type II dens fracture	40%
Type III dens fracture	20%
hangman's fracture	12%
other	28%

Table 64.13 Treatment options for combination C1-C2 injuries

Injury	Treatment options
C1 + hangman's	
• stable	collar, halo, surgery[a]
• unstable (C2–3 angulation ≥ 11°)	halo, surgery
C1 + Type II odontoid fracture	
• stable (ADI[a] < 5 mm)	collar, halo, surgery
• unstable (ADI ≥ 5 mm)	halo, surgery
C1 + Type III odontoid fracture	halo
C1 + miscellaneous C2	collar, halo

[a]abbreviations: ADI = atlantodental interval; surgery = surgical fixation & fusion

64

64.6.2 Treatment

Practice guideline: Treatment of combination atlas and axis fractures

Level III[89]

1. recommended: base treatment primarily on the type of C2 injury
2. recommended: external immobilization of most C1–2 fractures
3. consider surgical stabilization for these situations. **Note**: loss of integrity of the C1 ring may necessitate modification of the surgical technique; these injuries are potentially unstable: see Axis (C2) fractures (p. 972):
   a) C1-Type II odontoid combination fractures with an ADI ≥ 5 mm
   b) C1-hangman's combination fractures with C2–3 angulation ≥ 11°

Treatment options are summarized in ▶ Table 64.13.[89]

64.6.3 Outcome

Only 1 nonunion (C1 + Type II odontoid, treated initially with halo). No new neuro deficits.

References

[1] Powers B, Miller MD, Kramer RS, et al. Traumatic Anterior Atlanto-Occipital Dislocation. Neurosurgery. 1979; 4:12–17

[2] Alker GJ, Leslie EV. High Cervical Spine and Craniocervical Junction Injuries in Fatal Traffic Accidents: A Radiological Study. Orthop Clin North Am. 1978; 9:1003–1010

[3] Bucholz RW, Burkhead WZ, Graham W, Petty C. Occult Cervical Spine Injuries in Fatal Traffic Accidents. J Trauma. 1979; 19:768–771

[4] Traynelis VC, Marano GD, Dunker RO, et al. Traumatic Atlanto-Occipital Dislocation. Case Report. J Neurosurg. 1986; 65:863–870

[5] Harris JH, Jr, Carson GC, Wagner LK, Kerr N. Radiologic diagnosis of traumatic occipitovertebral dissociation: 2. Comparison of three methods of detecting occipitovertebral relationships on lateral radiographs of supine subjects. AJR Am J Roentgenol. 1994; 162:887–892

[6] Theodore N, Aarabi B, Dhall SS, Gelb DE, Hurlbert RJ, Rozzelle CJ, Ryken TC, Walters BC, Hadley MN. The diagnosis and management of traumatic atlanto-occipital dislocation injuries. Neurosurgery. 2013; 72 Suppl 2:114–126

[7] Przybylski GJ, Clyde BL, Fitz CR. Craniocervical junction subarachnoid hemorrhage associated with atlanto-occipital dislocation. Spine. 1996; 21:1761–1768

[8] Section on Disorders of the Spine and Peripheral Nerves of the American Association of Neurological Surgeons and the Congress of Neurological Surgeons. Diagnosis and management of traumatic atlanto-occipital dislocation injuries. Neurosurgery. 2002; 50 Supplement:S105–S113

[9] Harris JH, Carson GC, Wagner LK. Radiologic diagnosis of traumatic occipitovertebral dissociation: 1. Normal occipitovertebral relationships on lateral radiographs of supine subjects. AJR Am J Roentgenol. 1994; 162:881–886

[10] Horn EM, Feiz-Erfan I, Lekovic GP, Dickman CA, Sonntag VK, Theodore N. Survivors of occipitoatlantal dislocation injuries: imaging and clinical correlates. J Neurosurg Spine. 2007; 6:113–120

[11] Rojas CA, Bertozzi JC, Martinez CR, Whitlow J. Reassessment of the craniocervical junction: normal values on CT. AJNR Am J Neuroradiol. 2007; 28:1819–1823

[12] Bertozzi JC, Rojas CA, Martinez CR. Evaluation of the pediatric craniocervical junction on MDCT. AJR Am J Roentgenol. 2009; 192:26–31
[13] Werne S. Studies in spontaneous atlas dislocation. Acta Orthop Scand Suppl. 1957; 23:1–150
[14] Pang D, Nemzek WR, Zovickian J. Atlanto-occipital dislocation: part 1-normal occipital condyle-C1 interval in 89 children. Neurosurgery. 2007; 61:514–21; discussion 521
[15] Kaufman RA, Carroll CD, Buncher CR. Atlantooccipital junction: standards for measurement in normal children. AJNR Am J Neuroradiol. 1987; 8:995–999
[16] Pang D, Nemzek WR, Zovickian J. Atlanto-occipital dislocation–part 2: The clinical use of (occipital) condyle-C1 interval, comparison with other diagnostic methods, and the manifestation, management, and outcome of atlanto-occipital dislocation in children. Neurosurgery. 2007; 61:995–1015; discussion 1015
[17] Dublin AB, Marks WM, Weinstock D, Newton TH. Traumatic dislocation of the atlanto-occipital articulation (AOA) with short-term survival. With a radiographic method of measuring the AOA. J Neurosurg. 1980; 52:541–546
[18] Lee C, Woodring JH, Goldstein SJ, Daniel TL, Young AB, Tibbs PA. Evaluation of traumatic atlantooccipital dislocations. AJNR Am J Neuroradiol. 1987; 8:19–26
[19] Wholey MH, Bruwer AJ, Baker HL. The lateral roentgenogram of the neck; with comments on the atlanto-odontoid-basion relationship. Radiology. 1958; 71:350–356
[20] Dziurzynski K, Anderson PA, Bean DB, Choi J, Leverson GE, Marin RL, Resnick DK. A blinded assessment of radiographic criteria for atlanto-occipital dislocation. Spine. 2005; 30:1427–1432
[21] Bell CL. Surgical Observations. Middlesex Hosp J. 1817; 4
[22] Maserati MB, Stephens B, Zohny Z, Lee JY, Kanter AS, Spiro RM, Okonkwo DO. Occipital condyle fractures: clinical decision rule and surgical management. J Neurosurg: Spine. 2009; 11:388–395
[23] Section on Disorders of the Spine and Peripheral Nerves of the American Association of Neurological Surgeons and the Congress of Neurological Surgeons. Occipital condyle fractures. Neurosurgery. 2002; 50 Supplement:S114–S119
[24] Theodore N, Aarabi B, Dhall SS, Gelb DE, Hurlbert RJ, Rozzelle CJ, Ryken TC, Walters BC, Hadley MN. Occipital condyle fractures. Neurosurgery. 2013; 72 Suppl 2:106–113
[25] Anderson PA, Montesano PX. Morphology and treatment of occipital condyle fractures. Spine. 1988; 13:731–736
[26] Jacoby CG. Fracture of the occipital condyle. AJR Am J Roentgenol. 1979; 132
[27] Sonntag VKH, Dickman CA, Rea GL, Miller CA, . In: Treatment of Upper Cervical Spine Injuries. Spinal Trauma: Current Evaluation and Management. American Association of Neurological Surgeons; 1993:25–74
[28] Fielding JW, Hawkins RJ. Atlanto-Axial Rotatory Fixation. (Fixed Rotatory Subluxation of the Atlanto-Axial Joint). J Bone Joint Surg. 1977; 59A:37–44
[29] Lourie H, Stewart WA. Spontaneous atlantoaxial dislocation: a complication of rheumatic disease. N Engl J Med. 1961; 265:677–681
[30] Wetzel FT, La Rocca H. Grisel's syndrome. Clin Orthop. 1989:141–152
[31] Fielding JW, Stillwell WT, Chynn KY, Spyropoulos EC. Use of computed tomography for the diagnosis of atlanto-axial rotatory fixation. J Bone Joint Surg. 1978; 60A:1102–1104
[32] Schneider RC, Schemm GW. Vertebral artery insufficiency in acute and chronic spinal trauma. With special reference to the syndrome of acute central cervical spinal cord injury. J Neurosurg. 1961; 18:348–360
[33] Banna M. In: Spinal Fractures and Dislocations. Clinical Radiology of the Spine and the Spinal Cord. Rockville, Maryland: Aspen Systems Corporation; 1985:102–159
[34] Govender S, Kumar KP. Staged reduction and stabilisation in chronic atlantoaxial rotatory fixation. J Bone Joint Surg Br. 2002; 84:727–731
[35] Bohrer SP, Klein MD, Martin W. "V" shaped predens space. Skeletal Radiol. 1985; 14:111–116
[36] Dickman CA, Mamourian A, Sonntag VK, Drayer BP. Magnetic resonance imaging of the transverse atlantal ligament for the evaluation of atlantoaxial instability. J Neurosurg. 1991; 75:221–227
[37] Dickman CA, Greene KA, Sonntag VK. Injuries involving the transverse atlantal ligament: classification and treatment guidelines based upon experience with 39 injuries. Neurosurgery. 1996; 38:44–50
[38] Hadley MN, Dickman CA, Browner CM, et al. Acute Traumatic Atlas Fractures: Management and Long-Term Outcome. Neurosurgery. 1988; 23:31–35
[39] Landells CD, Van Peteghem PK. Fractures of the atlas: classification, treatment and morbidity. Spine. 1988; 13:450–452
[40] Jefferson G. Fractures of the atlas vertebra: report of four cases, and a review of those previously recorded. Br J Surg. 1920; 7:407–422
[41] Papadopoulos SM, Rea GL, Miller CA. In: Biomechanics of Occipito-Atlanto-Axial Trauma. Spinal Trauma: Current Evaluation and Management. American Association of Neurological Surgeons; 1993:17–23
[42] Alker GJ, Oh YS, Leslie EV, et al. Postmortem Radiology of Head and Neck Injuries in Fatal Traffic Accidents. Radiology. 1975; 114:611–617
[43] Section on Disorders of the Spine and Peripheral Nerves of the American Association of Neurological Surgeons and the Congress of Neurological Surgeons. Isolated fractures of the atlas in adults. Neurosurgery. 2002; 50 Supplement: S120–S124
[44] Ryken TC, Aarabi B, Dhall SS, Gelb DE, Hurlbert RJ, Rozzelle CJ, Theodore N, Walters BC, Hadley MN. Management of isolated fractures of the atlas in adults. Neurosurgery. 2013; 72 Suppl 2:127–131
[45] Levine AM, Edwards CC. Fractures of the atlas. J Bone Joint Surg Am. 1991; 73:680–691
[46] Spence KF, Decker S, Sell KW. Bursting Atlantal Fracture Associated with Rupture of the Transverse Ligament. J Bone Joint Surg. 1970; 52A:543–549
[47] Garber J. Abnormalities of the atlas and axis vertebrae: Congenital and traumatic. J Bone Joint Surg Am. 1964; 46A:1782–1791
[48] Schneider RC, Livingston KE, Cave AJE, Hamilton G. 'Hangman's Fracture' of the Cervical Spine. J Neurosurg. 1965; 22:141–154
[49] Wood-Jones F. The Ideal Lesion Produced by Judicial Hanging. Lancet. 1913; 1
[50] Effendi B, Roy D, Cornish B, Dussault RG, Laurin CA. Fractures of the Ring of the Axis: A Classification Based on the Analysis of 131 Cases. J Bone Joint Surg. 1981; 63B:319–327
[51] Levine AM, Edwards CC. The Management of Traumatic Spondylolisthesis of the Axis. J Bone Joint Surg. 1985; 67A:217–226
[52] Starr JK, Eismont FJ. Atypical hangman's fractures. Spine. 1993; 18:1954–1957
[53] Levine AM, The Cervical Spine Research Society Editorial Committee. In: Traumatic Spondylolisthesis of the Axis: "Hangman's Fracture". The Cervical Spine. 3rd ed. Philadelphia: Lippincott-Raven; 1998:429–448
[54] Francis WR, Fielding JW, Hawkins RJ, Pepin J, et al. Traumatic Spondylolisthesis of the Axis. J Bone Joint Surg. 1981; 63B:313–318
[55] Greene KA, Dickman CA, Marciano FF, et al. Acute axis fractures. Analysis of management and outcome in 340 consecutive cases. Spine. 1997; 22:1843–1852
[56] Burke JT, Harris JH, Jr. Acute injuries of the axis vertebra. Skeletal Radiol. 1989; 18:335–346
[57] The Cervical Spine Research Society Editorial Committee. The Cervical Spine. Philadelphia 1989
[58] Tuite GF, Papadopoulos SM, Sonntag VKH. Caspar plate fixation for the treatment of complex hangman's fractures. Neurosurgery. 1992; 30:761–765

[59] Coric D, Wilson JA, Kelly DL. Treatment of Traumatic Spondylolisthesis of the Axis with Nonrigid Immobilization: A Review of 64 Cases. J Neurosurg. 1996; 85:550–554
[60] Sonntag VKH, Hadley MN. Nonoperative Management of Cervical Spine Injuries. Clin Neurosurg. 1988; 34:630–649
[61] Section on Disorders of the Spine and Peripheral Nerves of the American Association of Neurological Surgeons and the Congress of Neurological Surgeons. Isolated fractures of the axis in adults. Neurosurgery. 2002; 50 Supplement:S125–S139
[62] Ryken TC, Hadley MN, Aarabi B, Dhall SS, Gelb DE, Hurlbert RJ, Rozzelle CJ, Theodore N, Walters BC. Management of isolated fractures of the axis in adults. Neurosurgery. 2013; 72 Suppl 2:132–150
[63] Youmans JR. Neurological Surgery. Philadelphia 1982
[64] Hadley MN. Comment on Tuite G F, et al.: Caspar plate fixation for the treatment of complex hangman's fractures. Neurosurgery. 1992; 30:761–765
[65] ElMiligui Y, Koptan W, Emran I. Transpedicular screw fixation for type II Hangman's fracture: a motion preserving procedure. Eur Spine J. 2010; 19:1299–1305
[66] Husby J, Sorensen KH. Fracture of the Odontoid Process of the Axis. Acta Orthop Scand. 1974; 45:182–192
[67] Crockard HA, Heilman AE, Stevens JM. Progressive myelopathy secondary to odontoid fractures: clinical, radiological, and surgical features. J Neurosurg. 1993; 78:579–586
[68] Przybylski GJ. Management of Odontoid Fractures. Contemp Neurosurg. 1998; 20:1–6
[69] Anderson LD, D'Alonzo RT. Fractures of the Odontoid Process of the Axis. J Bone Joint Surg. 1974; 56A:1663–1674
[70] Hadley MN, Browner CM, Liu SS, Sonntag VKH. New Subtype of Acute Odontoid Fractures (Type IIA). Neurosurgery. 1988; 22:67–71
[71] Scott EW, Haid RW, Peace D. Type I Fractures of the Odontoid Process: Implications for Atlanto-Occipital Instability: Case Report. J Neurosurg. 1990; 72:488–492
[72] Naim-ur-Rahman, Jamjoom ZA, Jamjoom AB. Ruptured transverse ligament: an injury that is often forgotten. Br J Neurosurg. 2000; 14:375–377
[73] Hadley MN, Dickman CA, Browner CM, Sonntag VKH. Acute Axis Fractures: A Review of 229 Cases. J Neurosurg. 1989; 71:642–647
[74] Polin RS, Szabo T, Bogaev CA, et al. Nonoperative Management of Types II and III Odontoid Fractures: The Philadelphia Collar versus the Halo Vest. Neurosurgery. 1996; 38:450–457
[75] Darakchiev BJ, Bulas RV, Dunsker S. Use of Calcitonin for the Treatment of an Odontoid Fracture: Case Report. J Neurosurg. 2000; (Spine 1) 93:157–160
[76] Apuzzo MLJ, Heiden JS, Weiss MH, et al. Acute Fractures of the Odontoid Process. An Analysis of 45 Cases. J Neurosurg. 1978; 48:85–91
[77] Ekong CEU, Schwartz ML, Tator CH, et al. Odontoid Fracture: Management with Early Mobilization Using the Halo Device. Neurosurgery. 1981; 9:631–637
[78] Dunn ME, Seljeskog EL. Experience in the Management of Odontoid Process Injuries: An Analysis of 128 Cases. Neurosurgery. 1986; 18:306–310
[79] Lennarson PJ, Mostafavi H, Traynelis VC, Walters BC. Management of type II dens fractures: a case-control study. Spine. 2000; 25:1234–1237
[80] Bohler J. Anterior Stabilization for Acute Fractures and Non-Unions of the Dens. J Bone Joint Surg. 1982; 64:18–28
[81] Paridis GR, Janes JM. Posttraumatic Atlanto-Axial Instability: The Fate of the Odontoid Process Fracture in 46 Cases. J Trauma. 1973; 13:359–367
[82] Fielding JW, Hensinger RN, Hawkins RJ. Os Odontoideum. J Bone Joint Surg. 1980; 62A:376–383
[83] Ricciardi JE, Kaufer H, Louis DS. Acquired Os Odontoideum Following Acute Ligament Injury. J Bone Joint Surg. 1976; 58A:410–412
[84] Clements WD, Mezue W, Mathew B. Os odontoideum: congenital or acquired? That's not the question. Injury. 1995; 26:640–642
[85] Spierings EL, Braakman R. The management of os odontoideum. Analysis of 37 cases. J Bone Joint Surg Br. 1982; 64:422–428
[86] Menezes AH, Ryken TC. Craniovertebral abnormalities in Down's syndrome. Pediatr Neurosurg. 1992; 18:24–33
[87] Section on Disorders of the Spine and Peripheral Nerves of the American Association of Neurological Surgeons and the Congress of Neurological Surgeons. Os odontoideum. Neurosurgery. 2002; 50 Supplement:S148–S155
[88] Rozzelle CJ, Aarabi B, Dhall SS, Gelb DE, Hurlbert RJ, Ryken TC, Theodore N, Walters BC, Hadley MN. Os odontoideum. Neurosurgery. 2013; 72 Suppl 2:159–169
[89] Section on Disorders of the Spine and Peripheral Nerves of the American Association of Neurological Surgeons and the Congress of Neurological Surgeons. Management of combination fractures of the atlas and axis in adults. Neurosurgery. 2002; 50 Supplement:S140–S147

65 Subaxial (C3 through C7) Injuries / Fractures

65.1 Classification systems

65.1.1 General information

Various systems have been proposed to help assess stability and/or guide management. The Allen-Ferguson system (p.987) is based on the mechanism of injury. Attempts at quantifying biomechanical stability include the White and Panjabi system (p.987) and the more recent subaxial injury classification (SLIC) (see below). Measurements for spine injuries are based on methods outlined by Bono et al.[1]

Practice guideline: Subaxial cervical spine injury classification

Level I[2]

- Use the Subaxial Injury Classification (SLIC) and severity scale for SCI (see section 65.1.2)
- Classify the stability and fracture pattern using the Cervical Spine Injury Severity Score (CSISS): the CSISS is somewhat complicated and may be better suited to clinical trials than daily practice (see reference[2])

65.1.2 Spine Trauma Study Group subaxial cervical spine injury classification (SLIC)

▶ **General information.** The subaxial injury classification (SLIC)[3] is shown in (▶ Table 65.1) and assesses injuries to the disco-ligamentous complex (DLC) in addition to neurologic and bony injuries. Inter-rater reliability intraclass correlation coefficient is 0.71.

Table 65.1 Subaxial injury classification (SLIC)[3]

Injury (rate *the most severe injury* at that level)	Points
Morphology	
No abnormality	0
Simple compression (compression fx, endplate disruption, sagittal or coronal plane VB fx.)	1
Burst fracture	2
Distraction (perched facet, posterior element fx.)	3
Rotation/translation (facet dislocation, teardrop fx., advanced compression injury, bilateral pedicle fx., floating lateral mass (p. 994). Guidelines: relative axial rotation ≥ 11°[4] or any translation not related to degenerative causes	4
Discoligamentous complex (DLC)	
Intact	0
Indeterminate (isolated interspinous widening with < 11° relative angulation & no abnormal facet alignment, ↑ signal on T2WI MRI in ligaments...)	1
Disrupted (perched or dislocated facet, < 50% articular apposition, facet diastasis > 2 mm, widened anterior disc space, ↑ signal on T2WI MRI through entire disc...)	2
Neurologic status	
Intact	0
Root injury	1
Complete spinal cord injury	2
Incomplete spinal cord injury	3
• Continuous cord compression with neuro deficit	+ 1

► **DLC integrity**[3] . The DLC includes: anterior longitudinal ligament (the strongest component of the anterior DLC), posterior longitudinal ligament, ligamentum flavum, facet capsule (the strongest component of the posterior DLC), interspinous and supraspinous ligaments. The DLC is the hardest SLIC parameter to evaluate. Largely inferred indirectly from MRI findings. Healing is less predictable than bone healing in the adult. More data needs to be accrued before this parameter can be reliably quantified.

► **Management based on the total SLIC score is shown in ► Table 65.2.**

► **A given injury can be described using the SLIC as follows:**
1. spinal level
2. *SLIC morphology* (from ► Table 65.1): use the most severe injury type at this level
3. description of bony injury: e.g. fracture or dislocation of transverse process, pedicle, endplate, superior or inferior articular process, lateral mass…
4. *SLIC DLC status* (from ► Table 65.1) with descriptors: e.g. herniated disc…
5. *SLIC neurologic status* (from ► Table 65.1)
6. confounders: e.g. presence of ankylosing spondylitis, DISH, osteoporosis, previous surgery, degenerative disease…

65.1.3 Cervical spine injury classification on the basis of mechanism of trauma

A modification of the Allen-Ferguson system[5] divides cervical spine fracture/dislocations into 8 major groups based on the dominant loading force and neck position at the time of injury as shown in ► Table 65.3. Grades of severity within each group are described, and any of these fractures may also be associated with damage from rotatory loads.

Details on some of these fracture types are provided in following sections.

65.1.4 Stability model of White and Panjabi

Guidelines for determination of clinical instability (p.930) of the subaxial cervical spine published by White and Panjabi[6(p 314)] are shown in ► Table 65.4. In general, all else being equal, compromise of

Table 65.2 Management based on total SLIC score

SLIC score	Management
1–3	non surgical
4	not specified
≥5	surgical

Table 65.3 Examples of types of cervical spine injuries[a]

Major loading force	Acting alone	With compression	With distraction
Flexion (p.989)	unilateral or bilateral facet dislocation (p.992)	• anterior VB fx. with kyphosis • disruption of interspinous ligament • teardrop fx (p.989)	• torn posterior ligaments (may be occult) • dislocated or locked facets (p.992)
Extension[b] (p.994)	fractured spinous process and possibly lamina[b]	fracture through lateral mass or facet[b], including horizontalization of facet (p.994)	disruption of ALL with retrolisthesis of superior vertebrae on inferior one[b]
Neutral position		burst fracture (p.989)	complete ligamentous disruption (very unstable)

[a]abbreviations: ALL = anterior longitudinal ligament; VB = vertebral body, fx = fracture; numbers in parentheses are page numbers for that topic
[b]any of the extension injuries may produce SCIWORA in young patients, or central cord syndrome in the presence of stenosis

Table 65.4 Guidelines for diagnosing clinical instability of the mid & lower C-spine[6]

Item	Points[a]
anterior elements[b] destroyed or unable to function	2
posterior elements[b] destroyed or unable to function	2
positive stretch test[c]	2
spinal cord damage	2
nerve root damage	1
abnormal disc narrowing	1
developmentally narrow spinal canal, either • sagittal diameter < 13 mm, OR • Pavlov ratio[d] < 0.8	1
dangerous loading anticipated[e]	1
Radiographic criteria	
neutral position x-rays	
• sagittal plane displacement > 3.5 mm or 20%	2
• relative sagittal plane angulation > 11°	2
OR	
flexion-extension x-rays	
• sagittal plane translation > 3.5 mm or 20%	2
• sagittal plane rotation > 20°	2
Unstable if total ≥ 5	

[a]if there is inadequate information for any item, add half of the value for that item to the total
[b]in the C-spine, posterior elements = anatomic components posterior to the posterior longitudinal ligament
[c]stretch test: apply incremental cervical traction loads of 10 lbs q 5 mins up to 33% body wt. (65 lbs max). Check X-ray and neuro exam after each ≈. Positive if ≈ in separation > 1.7 mm or ≈ angle > 7.5° on x-ray or change in neuro exam. This test is contraindicated if obvious instability
[d]Pavlov ratio = the ratio of (distance from the midlevel of the posterior VB to the closest point on the spinolaminar line): (the AP diameter of the middle of the VB)
[e]e.g. heavy laborers, contact sports athletes, motorcyclists

anterior elements produces more instability in extension, whereas compromise of the posterior elements produces more instability in flexion (important in patient transfers and immobilization). NB: certain conditions such as ankylosing spondylitis (p. 1123) may cause an otherwise stable injury to be unstable.

Stretch test: The cervical stretch test may be helpful in cases where stability is difficult to determine based on other factors. It may also be useful in detecting instability in cases such as an athlete with no obvious bony or ligamentous disruption. It is performed by applying graduated cervical traction with the patient lying supine on an x-ray table. Serial neurologic exams and lateral radiographs are performed as outlined in the footnote of ▶ Table 65.4.

65.2 Clay shoveler's fracture

Avulsion of spinous processes (usually C7) first described in Perth, Australia (pathomechanics: during the throwing phase of shoveling, clay may stick to the shovel jerking the trapezius and other muscles which are attached to cervical spinous processes).[7] Can also occur with: whiplash injury,[8] injuries that jerk the arms upwards (e.g. catching oneself in falling), neck hyperflexion, or a direct blow to the spinous process.

This fracture is stable, and by itself poses little risk. If the patient is intact, they should have further study (flexion-extension C-spine x-rays or CT scan through the affected level) to R/O other occult fractures. A rigid collar is used PRN pain.

65.3 Vertical compression injuries

In order to apply a purely compressive force to the cervical spine without flexion or extension, reversal of the normal cervical lordosis is required, as may occur in a slightly flexed posture. Burst fractures are the most common result, with the possibility of retropulsion of bone into the spinal canal with neurologic deficit.

65.4 Flexion injuries of the subaxial cervical spine

65.4.1 General information

Constitute up to 15% of cervical spine trauma. Common causes include: MVAs, falls from a height, and diving into shallow water.[9]

65.4.2 Compression flexion injuries

The classic diving injury is the prototypical example. Posterior element fractures occur in up to 50% of compression flexion injuries.[10] Although flexion-compression injuries do distract the posterior elements to some degree, most do not produce posterior ligamentous injuries. Subtypes of compression-flexion fractures include: teardrop fractures (see below), quadrangular fractures (p.991).

Treatment: mild cervical compression fractures without neurologic deficit or retropulsion of bone into the spinal canal are usually treated with a rigid orthosis until x-rays show healing has occurred (usually 6–12 wks). Stability is assessed with flexion-extension views (p.956) before completely discontinuing the brace. More severe compression fractures heal in a halo brace with ≈ 90% rate of ankylosing fusion.

65.4.3 Teardrop fractures

General information

Originally described by Schneider & Kahn.[11] Results from hyperflexion or axial loading at the vertex of the skull with the neck flexed (eliminating the normal cervical lordosis)[12] (often mistakenly attributed to hyperextension because of the retrolisthesis). Two forces are involved: 1) compression of the anterior column, and 2) tension on DLC. There are varying degrees of severity. In its most severe form, the injury consists of complete disruption of all of the ligaments, the facet joints and the intervertebral disk[13] and ≥ 3 mm of posterior displacement of the body into the canal. As originally described, an important feature is displacement of the inferior margin of the fractured vertebral body posteriorly into the spinal canal.[11] Usually unstable.

Seen in ≈ 5% of patients in a large series of patients with x-ray evidence of cervical spine trauma.[14] Patients are often quadriplegic, although some may be intact and some may have anterior cervical cord syndrome (p.947).

Findings

Possible associated injuries and radiographic findings include[13,15]:

1. a small chip of bone (the "teardrop") just beyond the anterior inferior edge of the involved vertebral body (VB) on lateral cervical spine film
2. often associated with a fracture through the sagittal plane of the VB (sagittal split) which can almost always be seen on AP view (may be midline or off-center). Thin cut CT scan is more sensitive
3. a large triangular fragment of the anterior inferior VB
4. other fractures through the vertebral body may also occur
5. the fractured vertebrae is usually displaced *posteriorly* on the vertebra below (easily appreciated on oblique x-rays, ► Fig. 65.1). However, cases without retrolisthesis are also described[10]
6. the fractured body is often wedged anteriorly (kyphosis), and may also be wedged possibly laterally
7. disruption of the facet joints which may be appreciated as separation of the joints on lateral x-ray, often unmasked by cervical traction

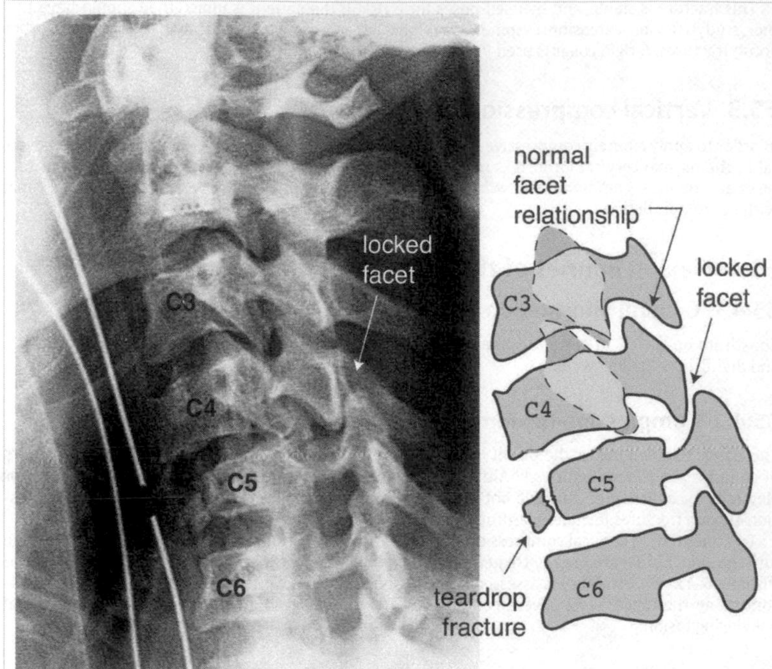

Fig. 65.1 Unilateral locked facets (left C4 on C5) & C5 teardrop fracture (p. 989). 60° LAO C-spine x-ray on left, and schematic on right (sagittally oriented VB fracture through C5 seen on CT scan, not shown). Note the anterior subluxation of C4 on C5, and the slight retrolisthesis of C5 on C6

8. prevertebral soft-tissue swelling, see for measurements (p. 214)
9. narrowing of the intervertebral disc below the fracture (indicating disruption)

Distinguishing between teardrop fracture and avulsion fracture

Rationale: Teardrop fractures must be distinguished from a simple avulsion fracture which may also result in a small chip of bone off the anterior inferior VB, usually pulled off by traction of the anterior longitudinal ligament (ALL) in hyperextension. Although there may be disruption of the ALL in these cases, it does not usually cause instability.

Methodology: In a patient with a small bone chip off of the inferior anterior VB, a "teardrop" fracture needs to be ruled-out. Determine if the following criteria are met:

- neurologically intact (because of the need for cooperation, this includes mental status, and excludes the inebriated or concussed patient)
- size of bone fragment is small
- no malalignment of vertebral bodies
- no evidence of VB fracture in sagittal plane on AP C-spine x-rays or on CT
- no posterior element fracture on x-ray or CT
- no prevertebral soft tissue swelling (p. 214) at level of fragment
- and no loss of vertebral body height or disc space height

If the above criteria are met, obtain flexion-extension C-spine x-rays (p. 956). If no abnormal movement, discharge patient in rigid collar (e.g. Philadelphia collar), and repeat the films in 4–7 days (i.e. after the pain has subsided to be certain that alignment is not being maintained by cervical muscle spasm from pain), D/C collar if 2nd set of films is normal.

If the patient does not meet the above criteria, treat them as an unstable fracture and obtain a CT scan through the fractured vertebra to evaluate for associated fractures (e.g. sagittal plane fracture that may not be apparent on plain x-ray).

MRI assesses the integrity of the disc and gives some information about the posterior ligaments.

65.4.4 Treatment of teardrop fracture

If the disc and ligaments are intact (determined by MRI) then an option is to employ a halo brace until the fragment is healed (perform flexion-extension x-rays after removing the halo to rule-out persistent instability). Alternatively, surgical stabilization may be performed, especially if ligamentous or disc injury is seen on MRI. When the injury is primarily posterior due to disruption of the posterior ligaments and facet joints, and if there is no anterior compromise of the spinal canal, then posterior fusion suffices (p.998). Severe injuries with canal compromise often require a combined anterior decompression and fusion (performed first) followed by posterior fusion using either a modified Bohlman triple-wire technique or lateral mass screws and rods.

65.4.5 Quadrangular fractures

See reference.[16]

Four features:

1. oblique vertebral body (VB) fracture passing from anterior-superior cortical margin to inferior end plate
2. posterior subluxation of superior VB on the inferior VB
3. angular kyphosis
4. disruption of disc and anterior and posterior ligaments

Treatment:

May require combined anterior and posterior fusion.

65.5 Distraction flexion injuries

65.5.1 General information

Ranges from hyperflexion sprain (mild, see below) to minor subluxation (moderate) to bilateral locked facets (severe, see below). Posterior ligaments are injured early and are usually evidenced by widening of the interspinous distance (p.214).

65.5.2 Hyperflexion sprain

A purely ligamentous injury that involves disruption of the posterior ligamentous complex without bony fracture. May be missed on plain lateral C-spine x-rays if they are obtained in normal alignment; requires flexion-extension views (p.956). Instability may be concealed when films are obtained shortly after the injury if spasm of the cervical paraspinal muscles splints the neck and prevents true flexion.[17] For patients with limited flexion, a rigid collar should be prescribed, and if the pain persists 1–2 weeks later the films should be repeated (including flexion-extension).

Radiographic signs of hyperflexion sprain[18] (x-rays may also be normal):

1. kyphotic angulation
2. anterior rotation and/or slight (1–3 mm) subluxation
3. anterior narrowing and posterior widening of the disc space
4. increased distance between the posterior cortex of the subluxed vertebral body and the anterior cortex of the articular masses of the subjacent vertebra
5. anterior and superior displacement of the superior facets (causing widening of the facet joint)
6. fanning (abnormal widening) of the interspinous space on lateral C-spine x-ray, or increased interspinous distance on AP; see Interspinous distances (p.214)

65.5.3 Subluxation

Cadaver studies have shown that horizontal subluxation > 3.5 mm of one vertebral body on another, or > 11° of angulation of one vertebral body relative to the next indicates ligamentous instability[19,20] (▶ Table 65.4). Thus, if subluxation of ≤ 3.5 mm on plain films is seen, and there is no neuro deficit, obtain flexion-extension films; see Flexion-extension cervical spine x-rays (p. 956). If no abnormal movement, remove cervical collar.

65.5.4 Locked facets

General information

Severe flexion injuries can result in locked facets (AKA "sprung" facets AKA "jumped" facets) with reversal of the normal "shingled" relationship between facets (normally the inferior facet of the level above is posterior to the superior facet of the level below). Involves disruption of facet capsule. Facets that have not completely locked but have had significant ligamentous disruption allowing distraction just short of the point of locking are known as "perched facets."

Flexion + rotation → unilateral locked facets. Hyperflexion → bilateral locked facets.

Unilateral locked facets

25% of patients are neurologically intact, 37% have root deficit, 22% have incomplete cord injuries, and 15% are complete quadriplegics.[21]

Bilateral locked facets

Occurs with disruption of ligaments of apophyseal joints, ligamentum flavum, longitudinal and interspinous ligaments, and the anulus. Rare. Most common at C5–6 or C6–7. 65–87% have complete quadriplegia, 13–25% incomplete, ≤ 10% are intact. Adjacent fractures (VB, facet, lamina, pedicle…) occur in 40–60%.[5,22] Nerve root deficits may also occur.

Diagnosis

Sagittal CT: usually the optimal manner to identify locked facets.

C-spine x-rays: both unilateral (ULF) and bilateral locked facets (BLF) will produce subluxation (ULF → rotatory subluxation).

BLF: usually produces > 50% subluxation on lateral C-spine x-ray.

ULF:

1. AP: spinous processes above the subluxation rotate to the same side as the locked facet (with respect to those below)
2. lateral: "bow-tie sign" (visualization of left & right facets at the level of the injury instead of the normal superimposed position[21]). Subluxation may be seen. Disruption of the posterior ligamentous complex may produce widening of the interspace between spinous processes
3. oblique (▶ Fig. 65.1): may demonstrate the locked facet which will be seen blocking the neural foramen (use ≈ 60° LAO for left locked facet, 60° RAO for right; LAO = left anterior oblique, RAO = right anterior oblique: e.g. with RAO the patient is angled with the right shoulder closer to the film)

Axial CT: "naked facet sign": the articular surface of the facet will be seen with the appropriate articulating mate either absent or on the wrong side of the facet (▶ Fig. 65.2). With ULF, CT also demonstrates the rotation of the level above anteriorly on the level below on the side of the locked facet.

MRI: the best test to rule-out traumatic disc herniation (found in 80% of BLF).[23]

Treatment

Practice guidelines

See Practice guideline: Initial closed reduction in fracture/dislocation cervical SCI (p. 958).

Closed reduction of locked facets

✖ Contraindicated if traumatic disc herniation is demonstrated on MRI. Patients who cannot be assessed neurologically may be done using SSEP/MEP monitoring. Two methods of closed reduction:

1. traction: more commonly employed in the U.S.
   a) initial weight (in lbs) ≈ 3 × cervical vertebral level, increase in 5–10 lb increments usually at 10–15 minute intervals until desired alignment is attained (assess neurologic exam (or SSEP/MEP) and lateral C-spine x-ray or fluoroscopy after each ≈ to avoid overdistraction)
   b) end points (i.e. stop the procedure):

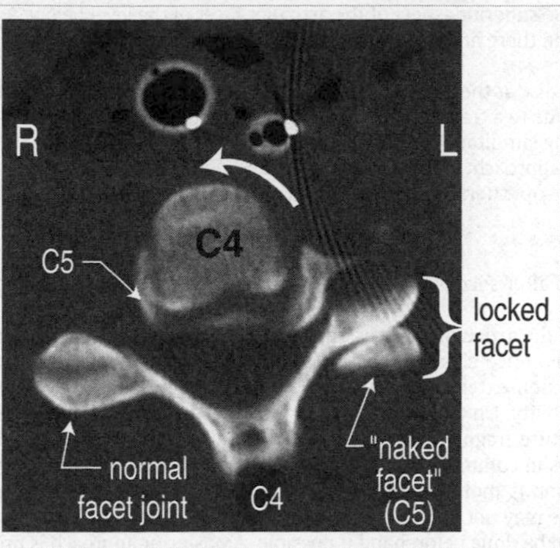

Fig. 65.2 Locked facet (left C4–5). (CT scan). Note the rotation of the C4 vertebral body on C5 (curved arrow)

- do not exceed 10 lbs per vertebral level (some say 5 lbs/level) under most circumstances. This is a guideline – you are trying to avoid overdistraction at the index level and at normal levels
- distraction of perched/locked facet or desired reduction is achieved
- if occipitocervical instability develops
- if any disc space height exceeds 10 mm (overdistraction)
- if any neurologic deterioration or deterioration of SSEP/MEP

c) with unilateral locked facets, one may add gentle manual torsion *towards* the side of the locked facets. With bilateral locked facets, one may add gentle manual posterior tension (e.g. with a rolled towel under the occiput)

d) once the facets are perched or distracted, gradual reduction of the weights will usually result in reduction – verify with x-ray (placing the neck in slight extension, e.g. with small shoulder roll, may help maintain the reduction)

2. manipulation (usually under anesthesia): less commonly employed,[21] more frequently used in Europe. Involves manually applying axial traction and sagittal angulation sometimes with rotation and direct pressure at the fracture level under fluoroscopy

Paraspinal muscle relaxation (but not enough to cause obtundation) may assist in reduction. Use IV diazepam (Valium®) and/or narcotic. General anesthesia may be used in difficult cases (with SSEP/MEP monitoring).

Once reduction is achieved, the patient is left in 5–10 lbs of traction for stabilization.

Disadvantage of closed reduction

1. fails to reduce ≈ 25% of cases of BLF
2. risks overdistraction at higher levels or worsening of other fractures
3. neurologic worsening following closed reduction may occur with traumatic disc herniation[22,24] and should be evaluated immediately with MRI and if confirmed treated with prompt discectomy
4. adds time and potentially pain to the patient's care, especially since many will go on to have surgical fusion anyway

Following closed reduction, the need for internal (operative) stabilization vs. external stabilization (i. e. bracing) may be addressed (below).

Open reduction and fixation is usually required if reduction is not achieved. Closed reduction is often more difficult with bilateral locked facets than with unilateral.

Open reduction of locked facets

1. posterior approach: the most common approach. Although rare, still subjects the patient to risk of deterioration from traumatically herniated disc. Therefore a pre-op MRI should be done if

possible. Often requires drilling of the superior aspect of the articular facet of the level below. A foraminotomy is recommended when there are root symptoms to visualize and decompress the root
2. anterior approach: by removing the disc at the subluxed level and exploring the anterior epidural space, the risk of worsening deficit due to a traumatic herniated disc is theoretically reduced. Reduction may be achieved by adding simultaneous manual traction
3. combined anterior/posterior (360°) approach: using anterior plate and posterior lateral mass screws/rods eliminates need for post-op external immobilization

Stabilization

Surgical fusion is commonly performed after successful closed reduction, failed closed reduction, or following open reduction.

If there are fracture fragments about the articular surfaces, there may be satisfactory healing with halo vest immobilization (for 3 months) once closed reduction is achieved.[25] Frequent x-rays are needed to rule-out redislocation.[26] Flexion-extension x-rays are obtained upon halo removal and surgery is required for continued instability. Up to 77% of patients with unilateral or bilateral facet dislocation (with or without facet fracture fragments) will have a poor anatomic result with halo vest alone (although late instability was uncommon), suggesting that surgery should be considered for all of these patients.[27] Surgical fusion is more clearly indicated in cases without facet fracture fragments (ligamentous instability alone may not heal) or if open reduction is required.

If surgery is indicated, an MRI should be done beforehand if possible. A posterior approach is preferred if there are no anterior masses (such as traumatic disc herniation or large osteophytic spurs), if subluxation of the bodies is > one-third the VB width (suggesting severe posterior ligamentous injury), or for fractures of the posterior elements. A posterior approach is mandatory if there is an unreducible dislocation. See also Options for posterior approach (p. 998).

65.6 Extension injuries of the subaxial cervical spine

65.6.1 Extension injury without bony injury

Extension injuries can produce spinal cord injury (SCI) without evidence of bony injury. Injury patterns include central cord syndrome (p. 944) usually in an older adult with cervical spondylosis, and SCIWORA (see below) usually in young children. Middle aged adults with hyperextension dislocations that reduce spontaneously immediately may present with SCI and no bony abnormality on x-ray, but there may be rupture of the anterior longitudinal ligament ALL and/or intervertebral disc on MRI or autopsy. Extension forces may also be associated with carotid artery dissections (p. 1324).

65.6.2 Minor extension injuries

Results from extension acting alone. Includes spinous process and lamina fractures. By themselves, are stable.

65.6.3 Extension compression injury

This is the most common mechanism of lateral mass/facet fractures (see below).

65.6.4 Lateral mass and facet fractures of the cervical spine

General information

Often results from extension combined with compression.

Classification of cervical lateral mass and facet fractures

4 patterns identified in lateral mass and facet fractures[28] are shown in ▶ Table 65.5.

Anterior subluxation of the fractured vertebra was observed in 77% of whole lateral-mass fractures.[28]

Horizontal facet or separation fracture of the articular mass

Extension combined with compression and rotation may produce fracture of one pedicle and ipsilateral lamina which permits the detached articular mass ("floating" lateral mass) to rotate forward to

Table 65.5 Classification of cervical lateral mass & facet fractures[28]

Designation	Diagram	Description
separation fracture	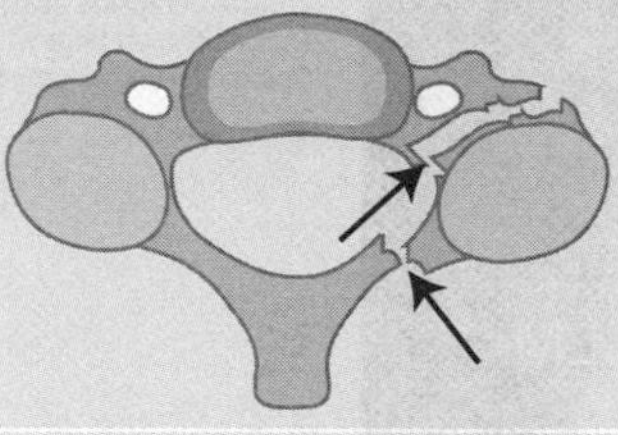	fractures through lamina and ipsilateral pedicle. Permits *horizontalization* of facet[29] (see text)
comminuted fracture	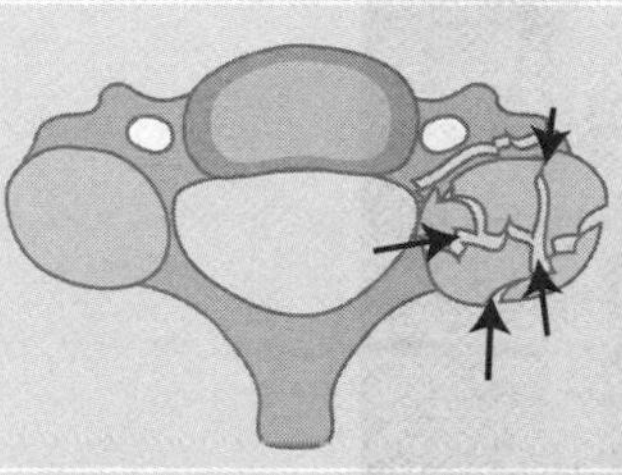	multiple fractures. Often associated with lateral angulation deformity
split fracture	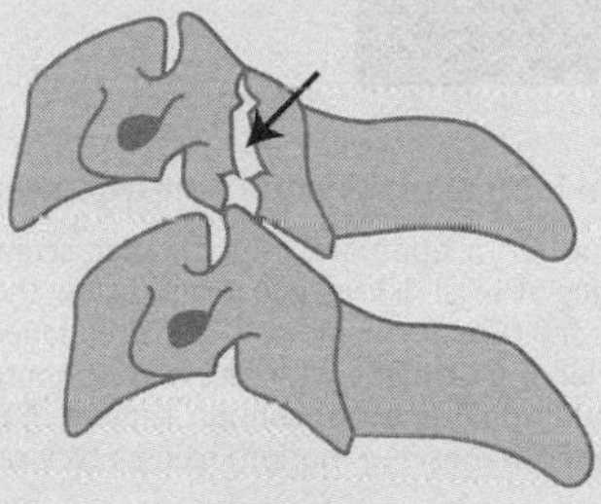	coronally oriented vertical fracture in 1 lateral mass, with invagination of the superior articular facet of the level below
traumatic spondylolysis	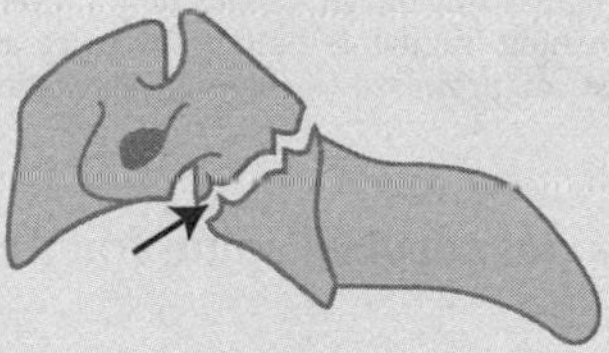	*bilateral* horizontal fractures through pars interarticularis, separating anterior spinal elements from posterior

a more horizontal orientation[29] (horizontalization of the facet) (▶ Table 65.5). May be associated with rupture of the anterior longitudinal ligament (ALL) and fissure of the disc at one or two levels. Neuro deficit is common. Unstable.

Failure of nonoperative treatment

A study of *CT scans* of 26 ***unilateral*** cervical facet fractures[30] identified the risk factors shown below for failure of nonoperative treatment (▶ Fig. 65.3 for illustration of the measurement definitions): where the fracture fragment (FF) height was defined as the maximum tip-to-tip cephalocaudal height on sequential sagittal reconstructions.

Nonoperative management is likely to fail if FF is:

1. > 1 cm, or
2. > 40% of LM (the height of the intact contralateral lateral mass at the same level, defined as the maximum tip-to-tip cephalocaudal height on sequential sagittal reconstructions)

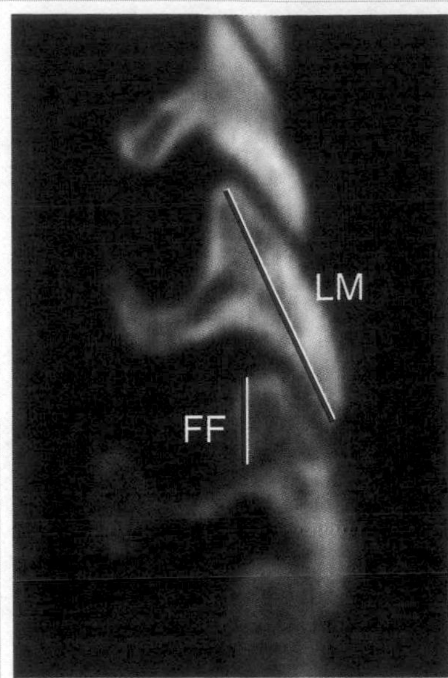

Fig. 65.3 Facet fracture fragment measurements. Sagittal reconstructed CT. FF = fracture fragment height, LM = lateral mass height (measured on the contralateral side at the same level as the fracture, (not as shown here which just illustrates the technique used to measure LM)

Surgical treatment of cervical lateral mass and facet fractures

Most cases can be treated with a posterior approach using fixation screws (lateral mass screws or pedicle screws[28]) and rods extending at least 1 level above and below the level of fracture (usually omitting a screw on the side of the fracture at the index level). Simultaneous neural decompression is performed when needed. Additional treatment with an anterior approach may be required for release of rigid deformity or for additional anterior column support.[28] Some separation fractures may be candidates for osteosynthesis (to preserve motion) using a cervical pedicle screw[28] that traverses the fracture.

An anterior approach is an alternative. Advantage: usually only 1 level needs to be fused. Disadvantages: decompression of compressing fragments cannot always be accomplished and requires disrupting an area that may not be compromised (if there is subluxation, the anterior column is probably compromised).

65.7 Treatment of subaxial cervical spine fractures

65.7.1 General information

Practice guideline: Treatment of subaxial cervical spine fractures or dislocations

Level III[31]

- closed or open reduction of subaxial fractures or dislocations with the goal of decompression of the spinal cord and restoration of the spinal canal
- stable immobilization either by internal fixation or by external immobilization to facilitate early patient mobilization and rehabilitation. If surgical treatment is employed, either anterior or posterior fixation is acceptable when a particular approach for decompression of the spinal cord is not required
- treatment with prolonged bed rest in traction if more contemporary treatment options are not available
- for patients with ankylosing spondylitis

- routine use of CT and MRI is recommended even after minor trauma
- when surgical stabilization is required, posterior long segment instrumentatin and fusion or a combined anterior/posterior procedure (360° fusion). Anterior standalone instrumentation and fusion procedures are associated with a failure rate of up to 50% in these patients

65.7.2 Management overview

Management of some specific types of C-spine fractures is covered in the corresponding preceding sections. For injuries not specifically addressed, general management principles are as follows[6]:

1. immobilize and reduce externally (if possible): may use traction × 0–7 days
2. determine if there is an indication for decompression as soon as practical (clinical conditions permitting), and decompress if needed. Although controversial, the following are generally accepted indications for *acute* decompression in patients without complete spinal cord injury:
   a) radiographic evidence of bone or foreign material in the spinal canal with associated spinal cord symptoms
   b) complete block on CT, myelogram or MRI
   c) clinical judgement: e.g. a progressive incomplete spinal cord injury where the surgeon believes that decompression would be beneficial
3. ascertain stability of the injury (see ▸ Table 65.4)
   a) stable fractures: treat in non-halo orthosis for 1–6 weeks (p. 935)
   b) unstable fractures: all of the following choices are appropriate, with little evidence (based on long-term spinal stability) to recommend one scheme over another in most cases
      - traction × 7 weeks, followed by orthosis × 8 weeks
      - halo × 11 weeks, followed by orthosis × 4 weeks
      - surgical fusion, followed by orthosis × 15 weeks
      - surgical fusion with internal immobilization (lateral mass screws & rods…) ± orthosis for short period of time (≈ several weeks)

65.7.3 Surgical treatment

In patients with complete spinal cord lesions

Operating on a patient with a complete cord injury (ASIA A and not in spinal shock) does not result in significant recovery of neurologic function.[32] If there is ongoing spinal cord compression and the bulbocavernosus reflex is absent, the patient may be in spinal shock–operate at the earliest time that is safe to do so at your institution. However, aggressive non-surgical reduction of traumatic subluxation should be pursued.

The primary goal of surgery in this setting is spinal stabilization, allowing the patient to be placed in a sitting position for improved pulmonary function, for psychological benefit, and to allow initiation of rehabilitation. Although the spine will fuse spontaneously in many cases (taking ≈ 8–12 weeks), surgical *stabilization* expedites the mobilization process and reduces the risk of delayed kyphotic angulation deformity. Early surgery may lead to further neurological injury, and should be delayed until the patient has stabilized medically and neurologically. In most cases, performing surgery within 4–5 days (if the patient is otherwise stable) is probably early enough to help reduce pulmonary complications.

In patients with incomplete lesions

Patients with incomplete cord injuries who have compromise of the spinal canal (by bone, disc, unreducible subluxation or hematoma) and either do not improve with nonoperative therapy or deteriorate neurologically should undergo surgical decompression and stabilization.[32] This may facilitate some further return of spinal cord function. An exception may be the central cord syndrome (p. 944).

Anterior or posterior?

The choice of technique depends to a large degree on the *mechanism* of injury, as the treatment should tend to counteract the instability, and ideally should not compromise structures that are still functioning. Instrumentation (wires/cables, lateral mass screws & rods, clamps…) immobilize the area of instability while bony fusion is occurring. In the absence of bony fusion, all mechanical devices will eventually fail, and so it becomes a "race" between fusion and instrument failure. Extensive injuries (including teardrop fractures (p. 989) and compression burst fractures) may require a combined anterior and posterior approach (staged, or in a single sitting; anterior decompression precedes posterior fusion).

Posterior immobilization and fusion

Indications: The procedure of choice for most *flexion* injuries. Useful when there is minimal injury to the vertebral bodies and in the absence of anterior compression of the spinal cord and nerves. Including: posterior ligamentous instability, traumatic subluxation, unilateral or bilateral locked facets, simple wedge compression fractures.

The most common technique consists of open or closed reduction, followed by lateral mass screws & rods (p. 972). Interlaminar Halifax clamps are an alternative.[33] Although successes have been reported using methylmethacrylate,[34] it does not bond to bone and weakens with age, and thus its use in the setting of traumatic injury is *discouraged.*[35]

Choice of posterior technique: If the anterior weight-bearing column is significantly damaged, or if there is absence or compromise of the lamina or spinous processes, then either a combined anterior-posterior approach is needed or posterior rigid instrumentation (e.g. lateral mass screw-plate or rod fixation) with fusion is recommended.[36]

Anterior approach

Does not depend on integrity of posterior elements to achieve stability.

Indications:

1. fractured vertebral body with bone retropulsed into spinal canal (burst fracture)
2. most *extension* injuries
3. severe fractures of posterior elements that preclude posterior stabilization and fusion
4. may be used for traumatic subluxation of the cervical spine

Usually consists of:

1. corpectomy: decompresses the neural elements (if necessary) and removes fractured and structurally compromised bone
   a) decompression usually requires wide corpectomy, at least ≈ 16 mm (palpate anterior surface of vertebral body to determine width; note position of vertebral arteries on pre-op CT). NB: it is suggested to take the corpectomy no wider than 3 mm lateral to the medial edge of the longus coli muscle, this leaves ~ 5 mm margin of safety to the foramen transversarium[37]
   b) if decompression is not needed, ≈ 12 mm corpectomy suffices (i.e. about the width of a half-inch cottonoid)
2. AND
   a) strut graft fusion: replaces the involved body or bodies with either:
      • bone (usually iliac crest, rib or fibula, either homologous or cadaveric)
      • or synthetic cage (e.g. titanium or PEEK)
   b) usually accompanied with compression plates
   c) usually followed with external immobilization
   d) corpectomy of > 1 level, or presence of injury to posterior elements is usually an indication for augmentation with posterior instrumentation

Complications of surgical treatment

1. hardware problems
   a) anterior cage problems
      • cage displacement/extrusion
      • cage subsidence/telescoping into endplace
      • vertebral body fracture
   b) problems with plating
      • screw pull-out, loosening or breakage
      • fatigue fracture of plate
      • screw injury: nerve root, spinal cord or vertebral artery
2. inadequate post-operative immobilization
   a) improper brace selected
   b) poor patient compliance with immobilization device
3. failure of graft to take (nonunion)

4. judgmental error
   a) failure to incorporate all unstable levels
   b) improper surgical approach

65.8 Spinal cord injury without radiographic abnormality (SCIWORA)

65.8.1 General information

Although spinal cord injuries are uncommon in children, there is a subgroup of these in which no radiographic evidence of bony or ligamentous disruption can be demonstrated (including on dynamic flexion-extension x-rays). This is attributed to the normally increased elasticity of the spinous ligaments and paravertebral soft-tissue in the young population[38] and has been dubbed SCIWORA (an acronym for "Spinal Cord Injury Without Radiographic Abnormality"). The age range of children with SCIWORA is 1.5–16 years, it has a much higher incidence in age ≤ 9 yrs.[39] The spinal cord may undergo contusion, transection, infarction, stretch injuries, or meningeal rupture. Additional etiologies include: blunt abdominal trauma with disruption of blood flow from the aorta or segmental branches, traumatic disc herniation. There may be an increased risk of SCIWORA among young children with asymptomatic Chiari I malformation.[40]

54% of children with SCIWORA had a delay between injury (at which time some children experience transient numbness, paresthesias, Lhermitte's sign, or a feeling of total body weakness) and the onset of *objective* sensorimotor dysfunction ("latent period") ranging from 30 minutes to 4 days.

Practice guideline: Diagnosis of SCIWORA

Level III[41]

- MRI of the region of suspected injury
- radiographic screening of entire spine
- assess spinal stability with flexion-extension x-rays in the acute setting and at a late follow-up, even if MRI is negative for extraneural injury

✖ *not* recommended: spinal angiography or myelography

65.8.2 Radiographic evaluation

In addition to plain films and flexion-extension films (to identify overt instability which would require surgical fusion), should include MRI which may show increased signal within the spinal cord parenchyma on T2WI. There were no intraspinal space occupying lesions in 13 patients studied with myelography/CT.[38]

65.8.3 Management

Practice guideline: Management of SCIWORA

Level III[41]

- external immobilization of the injured spinal segment for up to 12 weeks
- early discontinuation of external immobilization for patients who become asymptomatic and are confirmed to have no instability on flexion-extension x-rays
- avoidance of "high-risk" activities for up to 6 months after SCIWORA

Surgical intervention, including laminectomy, has shown no benefit in the few cases where it has been tried.[43]

Due to a 20% rate of repeat injury (some due to trivial trauma, and some without identifiable trauma) within 10 weeks of the original trauma when treated with only a rigid collar and restriction

Table 65.6 Treatment protocol for SCIWORA (modified[42])
• admit patient to hospital (helps emphasize seriousness of injury) • BR with rigid cervical collar until flexion-extension films are normal • MRI of cervical spine to document presence of spinal cord injury • detailed discussion with patient and family about seriousness of injury and rationale for treatment outlined here • immobilization in Guilford brace for 3 months[a] • prohibition of contact and noncontact sports • regular follow-up visits for monitoring condition and compliance • liberalize activities at 3 months if flexion-extension films are normal
[a]this represents an extremely conservative recommendation, a less restrictive recommendation is immobilization for 1–3 weeks[43]; see **Practice guideline: SCIWORA** (p. 999).

of contacts sports (both for 2 months), more aggressive measures were initially recommended (▶ Table 65.6).

References

[1] Bono CM, Vaccaro AR, Fehlings M, et al. Measurment techniques for lower cervical spine injuries: consensus statement of the Spine Trauma Study Group. Spine. 2006; 31:603–609

[2] Aarabi B, Walters BC, Dhall SS, Gelb DE, Hurlbert RJ, Rozzelle CJ, Ryken TC, Theodore N, Hadley MN. Subaxial cervical spine injury classification systems. Neurosurgery. 2013; 72 Suppl 2:170–186

[3] Vaccaro AR, Hulbert RJ, Patel AA, Fisher C, Dvorak M, Lehman RAJr, Anderson P, Harrop J, Oner FC, Arnold P, Fehlings M, Hedlund R, Madrazo I, Rechtine G, Aarabi B, Shainline M. The subaxial cervical spine injury classification system: a novel approach to recognize the importance of morphology, neurology, and integrity of the disco-ligamentous complex. Spine. 2007; 32:2365–2374

[4] White AA, III, Panjabi MM. Update on the evaluation of instability of the lower cervical spine. Instr Course Lect. 1987; 36:513–520

[5] Allen BL, Ferguson RL, Lehmann TR, O'Brien RP. A Mechanistic Classification of Closed, Indirect Fractures and Dislocations of the Lower Cervical Spine. Spine. 1982; 7:1–27

[6] White AA, Panjabi MM. In: The Problem of Clinical Instability in the Human Spine: A Systematic Approach. Clinical Biomechanics of the Spine. 2nd ed. Philadelphia: J.B. Lippincott; 1990:277–378

[7] Hall RDM. Clay-Shoveller's Fracture. J Bone Joint Surg. 1940; 22:63–75

[8] Gershon-Cohen J, Budin E, Glauser F. Whiplash Fractures of Cervicodorsal Spinous Processes. JAMA. 1954; 155:560–561

[9] Abitbol J-J, Kostuik JP, The Cervical Spine Research Society Editorial Committee. In: Flexion Injuries to the Lower Cervical Spine. The Cervical Spine. 3rd ed. Philadelphia: Lippincott-Raven; 1998:457–464

[10] Fuentes J-M, Bloncourt J, Vlahovitch B, Castan P. La Tear Drop Fracture: Contribution à l'étude du Mécanisme et des Lésions Ostéo-Disco-Ligamentaires. Nirochirurgie. 1983; 29:129–134

[11] Schneider RC, Kahn EA, Arbor A. Chronic Neurologic Sequelae of Acute Trauma to the Spine and Spinal Cord. The Significance of Acute Flexion or Teardrop Cervical Fracture-Dislocation of the Cervical Spine. J Bone Joint Surg. 1956; 38A

[12] Torg JS, Vegso JJ, Sennett B. The national football head and neck injury registry: 14-year report of cervical quadriplegia (1971-1984). Clin Sports Med. 1987; 6:61–72

[13] Harris JH, Edeiken-Monroe B, Kopaniky DR. A Practical Classification of Acute Cervical Spine Injuries. Orthop Clin North Am. 1986; 17:15–30

[14] Gehweiler JA, Clark WM, Schaaf RE, Powers B, et al. Cervical Spine Trauma: The Common Combined Conditions. Radiology. 1979; 130

[15] Gehweiler JA, Osborne RL. The Radiology of Vertebral Trauma. Philadelphia: W. B. Saunders; 1980

[16] Favero KJ, VanPeteghem PK. The Quadrangular Fragment Fracture: Roentgenographic Features and Treatment Protocol. Clin Orthop. 1989; 239:40–46

[17] Webb JK, Broughton RBK, McSweeney T, et al. Hidden Flexion Injury of the Cervical Spine. J Bone Joint Surg. 1976; 58B:322–327

[18] Fazl M, LaFebvre J, Willinsky RA, et al. Posttraumatic Ligamentous Disruption of the Cervical Spine, an Easily Overlooked Diagnosis: Presentation of Three Cases. Neurosurgery. 1990; 26:674–677

[19] White AA, Johnson RM, Panjabi MM, et al. Biomechanical Analysis of Clinical Stability in the Cervical Spine. Clin Orthop. 1975; 109:85–96

[20] White AA, Southwick WO, Panjabi MM. Clinical Instability in the Lower Cervical Spine - A Review of Past and Current Concepts. Spine. 1976; 1:15–27

[21] Andreshak JL, Dekutoski MB. Management of Unilateral Facet Dislocations: A Review of the Literature. Orthopedics. 1997; 20:917–926

[22] Payer M, Schmidt MH. Management of traumatic bilateral locked facets of the subaxial cervical spine. Contemp Neurosurg. 2005; 27:1–4

[23] Rizzolo SJ, Piazza MR, Cotler JM, Balderston RA, Schaefer D, Flanders A. Intervertebral disc injury complicating cervical spine trauma. Spine. 1991; 16:S187–S189

[24] Doran SE, Papadopoulos SM, Ducker TB, et al. Magnetic Resonance Imaging Documentation of Coexistent Traumatic Locked Facets of the Cervical Spine and Disc Herniation. J Neurosurg. 1993; 79:341–345

[25] Sonntag VKH. Management of Bilateral Locked Facets of the Cervical Spine. Neurosurgery. 1981; 8:150–152

[26] Glasser JA, Whitehall R, Stamp WG, Jane JA. Complications Associated with the Halo Vest. J Neurosurg. 1986; 65:76–79

[27] Sears W, Fazl M. Prediction of Stability of Cervical Spine Fracture Managed in the Halo Vest and Indications for Surgical Intervention. J Neurosurg. 1990; 72:426–432

[28] Kotani Y, Abumi K, Ito M, Minami A. Cervical spine injuries associated with lateral mass and facet joint fractures: New classification and surgical treatment with pedicle screw fixation. Eur Spine J. 2005; 14:69–77

[29] Roy-Camille R, Saillant G. Osteosynthese des fractures du rachis cervical. Actual Chir Orthop Hop R Poincarré Mason, Paris. 1970; 8:175–194

[30] Spector LR, Kim DH, Affonso J, Albert TJ, Hilibrand AS, Vaccaro AR. Use of computed tomography to predict failure of nonoperative treatment of unilateral facet fractures of the cervical spine. Spine (Phila Pa 1976). 2006; 31:2827–2835

[31] Gelb DE, Aarabi B, Dhall SS, Hurlbert RJ, Rozzelle CJ, Ryken TC, Theodore N, Walters BC, Hadley MN. Treatment of subaxial cervical spinal injuries. Neurosurgery. 2013; 72 Suppl 2:187–194

[32] Sonntag VKH, Hadley MN. Nonoperative Management of Cervical Spine Injuries. Clin Neurosurg. 1988; 34:630–649
[33] Aldrich EF, Crow WN, Weber PB, Spagnolia TN. Use of MR Imaging-Compatible Halifax Interlaminar Clamps for Posterior Cervical Fusion. J Neurosurg. 1991; 74:185–189
[34] Branch CL, Kelly DL, Davis CH, McWhorter JM, et al. Fixation of Fractures of the Lower Cervical Spine Using Methylmethacrylate and Wire: Technique and Results in 99 Patients. Neurosurgery. 1989; 25:503–513
[35] Cooper PR. Comment on Branch C L, et al.: Fixation of Fractures of the Lower Cervical Spine Using Methylmethacrylate and Wire. Neurosurgery. 1989; 25:512–513
[36] McGuire RA, The Cervical Spine Research Society Editorial Committee. In: Cervical Spine Arthrodesis. The Cervical Spine. 3rd ed. Philadelphia: Lippincott-Raven; 1998:499–508
[37] Vaccaro A, Ring D, Seuderi G, Garfin S. Vertebral artery location in relation to the vertebral body as determined by two-dimensional computed tomography evaluation. Spine. 1994; 19
[38] Pang D, Wilberger JE. Spinal Cord Injury without Radiographic Abnormalities in Children. J Neurosurg. 1982; 57:114–129
[39] Hamilton MG, Myles ST. Pediatric Spinal Injury: Review of 174 Hospital Admissions. J Neurosurg. 1992; 77:700–704
[40] Bondurant CP, Oró JJ. Spinal Cord Injury without Radiographic Abnormality and Chiari Malformation. J Neurosurg. 1993; 79:833–838
[41] Rozzelle CJ, Aarabi B, Dhall SS, Gelb DE, Hurlbert RJ, Ryken TC, Theodore N, Walters BC, Hadley MN. Spinal cord injury without radiographic abnormality (SCIWORA). Neurosurgery. 2013; 72 Suppl 2:227–233
[42] Pollack IF, Pang D, Sclabassi R. Recurrent Spinal Cord Injury without Radiographic Abnormalities in Children. J Neurosurg. 1988; 69:177–182
[43] Madsen JR, Freiman T. Cervical Spinal Cord Injury in Children. Contemp Neurosurg. 1998; 20:1–5

66 Thoracic, Lumbar and Sacral Spine Fractures

66.1 Assessment and management of thoracolumbar fractures

66.1.1 General information

A widely used model for thoracolumbar spine stability is the 3-column model of Denis (see below). See also the more recently proposed TLICS system (p. 1006).

66.1.2 Three column model

General information

66

Denis' 3 column model of the spine (▶ Fig. 66.1) attempts to identify *CT* criteria of instability of *thoracolumbar* spine fractures.[1] This model has generally good predictive value, however, any attempt to create "rules" of instability will have some inherent inaccuracy.

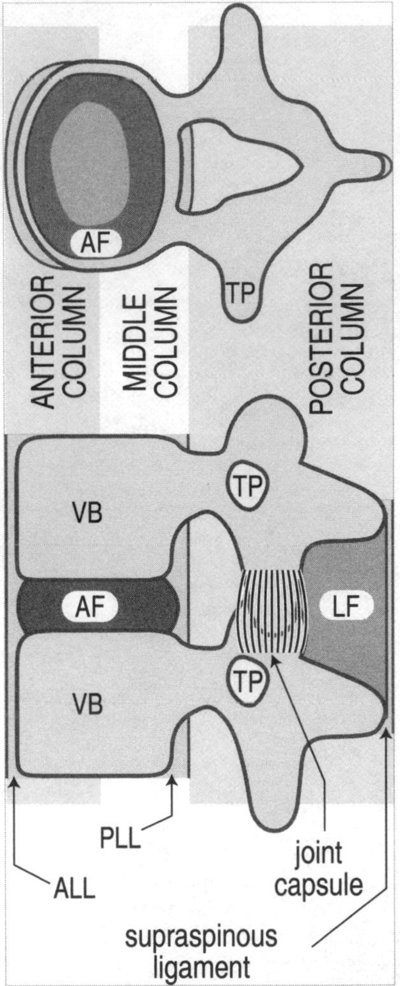

Fig. 66.1 Three column model of the spine (TP = transverse process, see text for other abbreviations) (Adapted from Spine, Denis F, Vol. 8, pp. 317–31, 1983, with permission)

Definitions

- anterior column: anterior half of disc and vertebral body (VB) (includes anterior anulus fibrosus (AF)) plus the anterior longitudinal ligament (ALL)
- middle column: posterior half of disc and vertebral body (includes posterior wall of vertebral body and posterior AF), posterior longitudinal ligament (PLL), & the pedicles
- posterior column: posterior bony complex (posterior arch) with interposed posterior ligamentous complex (supraspinous and interspinous ligament, facet joints and capsule, and ligamentum flavum (LF)). Injury to this column alone does *not* cause instability

Classification into major and minor injuries

Minor injuries

Involve only a part of a column and do not lead to acute instability (when not accompanied by major injures). Includes:

1. fracture of transverse process: usually neurologically intact except in two areas:
   a) L4–5 → lumbosacral plexus injuries (there may be associated renal injuries, check U/A for blood)
   b) T1–2 → brachial plexus injuries
2. fracture of articular process or pars interarticularis
3. isolated fractures of the spinous process: in the TL spine: these are usually due to direct trauma. Often difficult to detect on plain x-ray
4. isolated laminar fracture: rare. Should be stable

Major injuries

The McAfee classification describes 6 main types of fractures.[2] A simplified system with four categories follows (also see ▶ Table 66.1):

Type 1: Compression fracture: compression failure of anterior column. Middle column *intact* (unlike the 3 other major injuries below) acting as a fulcrum,

1. 2 subtypes:
   a) anterior: most common between T6-T8 and T12-L3
      - lateral x-ray: wedging of the VB anteriorly, no loss of height of posterior VB, no subluxation
      - CT: spinal canal intact. Disruption of anterior end-plate
   b) lateral (rare)
2. clinical: no neurologic deficit

Type 2: Burst fracture: pure axial load → compression of vertebral body → compression failure of anterior and middle columns. Occur mainly at TL junction, usually between T10 and L2

1. 5 subtypes; L5 burst fractures may constitute a rare subtype (p. 1006)
   a) fracture of both end-plates: seen in lower lumbar region (where axial load → increased extension, unlike T-spine where axial load → flexion)
   b) fracture of superior end-plate: the most common burst fracture. Seen at TL junction. Mechanism = axial load + flexion
   c) fracture of inferior end-plate: rare

Table 66.1 Column failure in the four major types of thoracolumbar spine injuries

Fracture type	Column		
	Anterior	Middle	Posterior
compression	compression	intact	intact, or distraction if severe
burst	compression	compression	intact
seat-belt	intact or mild compression of 10–20% of anterior VB	distraction	
fracture-dislocation	compression, rotation, shear	distraction, rotation, shear	

[a]adapted[1] with permission

   d) burst rotation: usually midlumbar. Mechanism = axial load + rotation
   e) burst lateral flexion: mechanism = axial load + lateral flexion
2. radiographic evaluation
   a) lateral x-ray: cortical fracture of posterior VB wall, loss of posterior VB height, retropulsion of bone fragment from end plate(s) into canal
   b) AP x-ray: increase of interpediculate distance (IPD), vertical fracture of lamina, splaying of facet joints: ↑ IPD indicates failure of *middle* column
   c) CT: demonstrates break in posterior wall of VB with retropulsed bone in spinal canal (average: 50% obstruction of canal area), increase in IPD with splaying of posterior arch (including facets)
   d) MRI: compromise of anterior canal by bone fragment; possible cord compression usually with fragments occupying > 50% of the canal diameter
   e) MRI or myelogram: compression in spinal canal
3. clinical: depends on level (thoracic cord more sensitive and less room in canal than conus region), the impact at the time of disruption, and the extent of canal obstruction
   a) ≈ 50% intact at initial examination (half of these recalled leg numbness, tingling, and/or weakness initially after trauma that subsided)
   b) of patients with deficits, only 5% had *complete* paraplegia

Type 3: Seat-belt fracture (**some call this a flexion-distraction fracture, but that term is also used for a subtype of fracture-dislocation**): flexion across a fulcrum anterior to the anterior column (e.g. seat belt) → compression of anterior column & distraction failure of both middle and posterior columns. May be bony or ligamentous

1. 4 subtypes
   a) Chance fracture (named for G. Q. Chance, 1948): one level, totally through bone
   b) one level, through ligaments
   c) two level, through bone in middle column, through ligament in anterior and posterior columns
   d) two level, through ligament in all 3 columns
2. radiographic evaluation
   a) plain x-ray: ↑ interspinous distance, pars interarticularis fractures, and horizontal split of pedicles and transverse process. No subluxation
   b) CT: axial cuts are poor for this type (most of fracture is in plane of axial CT cuts). Sagittal and coronal reconstructions demonstrate well. May demonstrate pars fracture
3. clinical: no neurologic deficit

Type 4: Fracture-dislocation: failure of all 3 columns due to compression, tension, rotation or shear → subluxation or dislocation

1. x-ray: occasionally, may be reduced when imaged. Look for other markers of significant trauma (multiple rib fractures, unilateral articular process fractures, spinous process fractures, horizontal laminar fractures)
2. 3 subtypes
   a) flexion rotation: posterior and middle columns totally ruptured, anteriorly compressed → anterior wedging
      - lateral x-ray: subluxation or dislocation. Preserved posterior VB wall. Increased interspinous distance
      - CT: rotation and offset of VBs with → canal diameter. Jumped facets
      - clinical: 25% neurologically intact. 50% of those with deficits were complete paraplegics
   b) shear: all 3 columns disrupted (including ALL)
      - when trauma force directed posteriorly to anteriorly (more common) VB above shears forward fracturing the posterior arch (→ free floating lamina) and the superior facet of the inferior vertebra
      - clinical: all 7 cases were complete paraplegics
   c) flexion distraction
      - radiographically resemble seat-belt type with addition of subluxation, or with compression of anterior column > 10–20%
      - clinical: neurologic deficit (incomplete in 3 cases, complete in 1)

Associated injuries

In addition to the above, associated injuries include: vertebral end-plate avulsion, ligamentous injuries, and hip and pelvic fractures. Thoracolumbar fractures may be associated with hemodynamic instability as a result of hemothorax or aortic injury. Fractures of the transverse processes may be associated with abdominal trauma (e.g. renal injuries at L4–5).

Stability and treatment of thoracolumbar spine fractures

Minor injuries

Isolated thoracolumbar transverse process fractures (as demonstrated on spinal CT) do not require intervention or consultation of a spine service.[3,4]

Major spine injuries

Denis categorized the instability as:

- 1st degree: mechanical instability
- 2nd degree: neurological instability
- 3rd degree: both mechanical & neurological instability

Anterior column injury

Isolated anterior column injuries are usually stable and are treated as outlined in ▶ Table 66.2

The following exceptions may be *unstable* (1st degree) and often require surgery[1,5]:

Unstable compression fractures

1. a single compression fracture with:
   a) loss of > 50% of height with angulation (particularly if the anterior part of the wedge comes to a point)
   b) excessive kyphotic angulation at one segment (various criteria are used, none are absolute. Values quoted: > 30°, > 40°)
2. 3 or more contiguous compression fractures
3. neurologic deficit (generally does not occur with pure compression fracture)
4. disrupted posterior column or more than minimal middle column failure
5. progressive kyphosis: risk of progressive kyphosis is increased when loss of height of anterior vertebral body is > 75%. Risk is higher for lumbar compression fractures than thoracic

Middle column failure

These are unstable (often requiring surgery) with the following exceptions which should be stable (stable injuries may be treated as outlined in ▶ Table 66.2.

Stable middle column fractures

- above T8 if the ribs and sternum are intact (provides anterior stabilization)
- below L4 if the posterior elements are intact
- Chance fracture (anterior column compression, middle column distraction)
- anterior column disruption with minimal middle column failure

Posterior column disruption

Not *acutely* unstable unless accompanied by failure of the middle column (posterior longitudinal ligament and posterior anulus fibrosus). However, *chronic* instability with kyphotic deformity may develop (especially in children).

Seat-belt type injuries without neurologic deficit

No immediate danger of neurologic injury. Treat most with external immobilization in extension (e.g. Jewett hyperextension brace or molded TLSO).

Table 66.2 Treatment of stable anterior or middle column thoracolumbar spine injuries
• treat initially with analgesics and recumbency (bed-rest) for comfort × 1–3 weeks • diminution of pain is a good indication to commence mobilization with or without external immobilization (corset or Boston brace or extension TLSO × ≈ 12 weeks) depending on the degree of kyphosis • vertebroplasty (± kyphoplasty) may be an option (p. 1011) • serial x-rays to rule-out progressive deformity

Fracture-dislocation

Unstable. Treatment options:

1. surgical decompression and stabilization: usually needed in cases with
   a) compression with > 50% loss of height with angulation
   b) or, kyphotic angulation > 40° (or > 25%)
   c) or, neurologic deficit
   d) or, desire to shorten length of time of bedrest
2. prolonged bedrest: an option if none of the above are present

When vertebral body resection (vertebral corpectomy) is performed, options to access: transthoracic or transabdominal approach (or combined), transpedicular (for thoracic spine), lateral (retroperitoneal/retropleural) approach. Fracture and compression usually occurs at the superior margin of vertebral body, thus start resection at the *inferior* disc interspace. Followed by strut graft (cage or bone: iliac crest or fibula or tibia). Posterior instrumentation is usually required; see Spinal instrumentation (p. 1007).

Burst fractures

Not all burst fractures are alike. Some burst fractures may eventually cause neurologic deficit (even if no deficit initially). Middle column fragments in canal endanger the neuro elements. Criteria have been proposed to differentiate mild burst fractures from severe ones. No system is uniformly accepted. Recommendations.[1,6]

Surgical indications for burst fractures: burst fracture with any of the following:

- anterior vertebral body height ≤ 50% of the posterior height
- residual canal diameter ≤ 50% of normal (note: retropulsed bone in the canal is often resorbed with either bracing or surgery and is therefore controversial as an isolated indication for surgery[7,8])
- kyphotic angulation ≥ 20°
- when the increased interpediculate distance usually present on the initial film widens further on AP x-ray when standing in brace/cast
- neurologic deficit (incomplete)
- progressive kyphosis

Common surgical options for burst or severe compression fractures:

1. If instrumentation alone is needed
   a) can place pedicle screws in 2 levels above and 2 levels below the fracture
   b) if the index level can be included (i.e. if the pedicles are intact enough to accept shorter screws), similar biomechanical stability can be achieved by placing screws at the index level (the fractured level) and then just 1 above and 1 below[9]
2. If decompression of the spinal canal and/or anterior support is needed, corpectomy and strut graft (e.g. with expandable cage) with percutaneous pedicle screws may be used. Approaches:
   a) from posterior approach e.g. laminectomy with transpedicular approach and impacting bone anteriorly out of canal with a mallet and reverse angled Scoville curette, or
   b) lateral corpectomy and removal of bone from canal

For those not undergoing surgery (i.e. when surgery is not required or is contraindicated), an option is to treat with recumbency from 1–6 weeks (the duration depending on pain and degree of deformity).[6] Avoid early ambulation → further axial loading (even in cast). When appropriate, begin ambulation in an orthosis (e.g. molded thoracolumbar sacral orthosis (TLSO) or a Jewett brace) and follow patient for 3–5 months with serial x-rays to detect progressive collapse or angulation which may need further intervention. L5 burst fractures may be an exception to the usual management (see below).

66.1.3 Thoracolumbar injury classification and severity score (TLICS)

The TLICS system has been proposed to simplify classification and discussion of thoracolumbar fractures.[10,11] Points are assigned as shown in ▶ Table 66.3. The scores are summed, and management guidelines are given in ▶ Table 66.4.

Neurologic deficit, especially when partial, favors surgery.

Table 66.3 Thoracolumbar injury classification & severity score (TLICS)

Category	Finding	Points
Radiographic findings	compression fx	1
	burst component or lateral angulation > 15°	1
	distraction injury	2
	translational/rotational injury	3
Neurologic status	intact	0
	root injury	2
	complete SCI	2
	incomplete SCI	3
	cauda equina syndrome	3
Integrity of posterior ligamantous complex	intact	0
	undetermined	2
	definite injury	3
	TLICS = Total Points →	

Table 66.4 Management based on TLICS

TLICS	Management
≤ 3	nonoperative candidates
4	"grey zone" may be considered for operative or nonoperative management
≥ 5	surgical candidates

66.2 Surgical treatment

66.2.1 Ligamentotaxis

May work with fragments retropulsed into the anterior canal if the PLL is intact (may not be the case with middle column failure), distraction may be able to "pull" the fragments back into their normal position (ligamentotaxis) although this is not assured.[12] Ligamentotaxis has a better chance of succeeding if performed within 48 hours of injury. From a posterior approach with laminectomy: intraoperative ultrasound may demonstrate residual canal fragments,[13] and if needed the fragments may be impacted anteriorly out of the canal, e.g. using tamps such as Sypert spinal impactors. It is important not to overdistract to avoid neural injury.

66.2.2 Choice of surgical approach

The posterior approach is preferred when there is not a specific need to go from the front.

66.2.3 Spinal instrumentation

Anterior instrumentation of the lower lumbar spine is difficult, and is usually not recommended below ≈ L4.

66.2.4 Burst fractures

Choice of approach

Surgical considerations: a posterior approach is preferred if there is a dural tear, whereas a burst fracture with partial deficit and canal compromise may be treated more effectively from an anterior approach.[2] A small progression in angular deformity may occur when posterior stabilization is performed alone (since the injury to the anterior column is not corrected), but by itself usually does not require intervention.

For a posterior approach

In ideal situation (good bone quality, pedicle screw placement goes well (i.e. no fracture, no breach), and non-smoking patient) then one can fuse/rod one above and one below the fracture (using pedicle screws; longer constructs are needed with laminar hooks). With a short segment fusion like this, approximately 10° of lordosis be lost with time, therefore, one should try to overcorrect a little to accommodate the anticipated settling. If the patient does not meet the above criteria (e.g. poor bone quality), an option is to "rod long, fuse short" (e.g. rod 2 levels above and below the fracture but fuse only 1 level above and below) and then to remove the hardware when the fusion is solid (e.g. at 8–12 months) – this avoids fusing a nonpathologic segment just to get a better anchor. Junctional deterioration to the point that further surgery is needed often occurs at 3 years when 4 segments are fused, whereas it occurs at 8–9 years when only 3 levels are fused. Fusing across critical levels (i.e. thoracolumbar junction with T11 or L1 compression fractures) requires that the fusion incorporate 2–3 levels on each side of the junction (the forces of the long segment of the relatively immobile thoracic spine with the lumbar spine at the T-L junction increase the risk of nonunion).

For thoracic fractures that are not severe and do not require decompression, an option is to place pedicle screws and rods (which can be done percutaneously) without placing any graft. The concept is that the ribs anteriorly and the screws/rods posteriorly provide adequate stabilization while the fractured VB heals. The hardware can be removed electively once the fusion is solid (usually at 8–12 months). This is more commonly practiced in Europe than the U.S.

66.2.5 Wound infections

Postoperative wound infections with spinal instrumentation are usually due to Staph. aureus. With titanium hardware it may respond to debridement of devitalized tissue (e.g. onlay bone graft) and thorough washout (typically with 3 L of antibiotic irrigation flushed into the wound using a pulse lavage device – avoiding direct irrigation of any exposed dura) without removal of instrumentation, followed by antibiotics.[2] Persistent infection may respond to. If this inadequate, removal of instrumentation may occasionally be required.

66.3 Osteoporotic spine fractures

66.3.1 General information

Osteoporosis is defined as a condition of skeletal fragility as a result of low bone mass, microarchitectural deterioration of bone, or both.[14] It is found most commonly in post-menopausal white females, and is rare prior to menopause. Lifetime risk of symptomatic vertebral body (VB) osteoporotic compression fractures is 16% for women, and 5% for men. There are ≈ 700,000 VB compression fractures per year in the U.S.

These patients are often found to have significant VB compression fractures on plain films after presenting with back pain following a seemingly minor fall. CT often shows an impressive appearing amount of bone retropulsed into the canal.

66.3.2 Risk factors

Factors that increase the risk of osteoporosis include:

1. weight < 58 kg
2. cigarette smoking[15]
3. low-trauma VB fracture in the patient or a first degree relative
4. drugs
   a) heavy alcohol consumption
   b) AEDs (especially phenytoin)

c) warfarin
d) steroid use:
• bone changes can be seen with 7.5 mg/d of prednisone for > 6 months
• VB fractures occur in 30–50% of patients on prolonged glucocorticoids
5. postmenopausal female
6. males undergoing androgen deprivation therapy (e.g. for prostate Ca). Orchiectomy or ≥ 9 doses of gonadotropin-releasing hormone agonists had a 1.5 fold increase in risk of all fractures[16]
7. physical inactivity
8. low calcium intake
9. low serum levels of vitamin D (which decreases calcium absorption – see below). Lab: serum 25-hydroxyvitamin D [25(OH)D], AKA calcidiol is the best indicator of vitamin D status ▶ Table 66.5

Factors that protect against osteoporosis include impact exercise and excess body fat.

66.3.3 Diagnostic considerations

To differentiate osteoporotic compression fractures from other pathologic fractures, see Pathologic fractures of the spine (p. 1391).

Pre-fracture diagnosis

1. measuring bone fragility is not possible
2. the best correlate with bone fragility is radiographic measurement of bone mineral density (BMD) using DEXA scan (see below)
3. patients with low-trauma fractures or fragility fractures are considered osteoporotic even if their BMD are greater than these cutoffs

DEXA scan (dual energy x-ray absorptiometry): the preferred way to measure BMD
1. proximal femur: BMD measurement in this location is the best predictor for future fractures
2. LS spine: best location to assess response to treatment (need AP *and* lateral views, since AP often overestimates BMD because of superimposition of overlying posterior elements and aortic calcifications)
3. forearm BMD may be used if hip or spine are unsuitable

Interpretation of DEXA scan results:
1. findings are reported as
a) T-score: norms for healthy *young adults*
b) Z-score: norms of subjects of *same age* and sex as the patient
2. diagnostic criteria: WHO definitions (with a normal distribution 1 SD below the mean is the lowest 25th percentile, 2 SD below is 2.5th percentile)
a) normal: > –1 standard deviations (SD)
b) osteopenia: from –1 to –2.5 SD
c) osteoporosis: < than –2.5 SD[17]

Post-fracture considerations
1. other causes of pathologic fracture, especially neoplastic (e.g. multiple myeloma, metastatic breast cancer) should be ruled out

Table 66.5 Serum 25-hydroxyvitamin D levels

ng/ml[a]	nmol/L[a]	Interpretation
< 10–11	< 25–27.5	vit D deficiency → rickets (in peds) and osteomalacia (adults)
< 10–15	< 25–37.5	inadequate for bone and overall health
≥ 15	≥ 37.5	adequate for bone and overall health
consistently > 200	consistently > 500	potentially toxic → hypercalcemia & hyperphosphatemia

[a] 1 ng/ml = 2.5 nmol/L

2. younger patients with osteoporosis require evaluation for a remediable cause of the osteoporosis (hyperthyroidism, steroid abuse, hyperparathyroidism, osteomalacia, Cushing's syndrome)

66.3.4 Treatment

See references.[18,19,20,21]

Prevention of osteoporosis

High calcium intake during childhood may increase peak bone mass. Weight-bearing exercise in adulthood helps slow calcium loss from bones. Also effective: estrogen (see below), bisphosphonates (alendronate and risedronate), and raloxifene.

Treating established osteoporosis

66

Drugs that increase bone formation include:
1. intermittent low-dose parathyroid hormone: still experimental
2. sodium fluoride: 75 mg/d increases bone mass but did *not* significantly reduce the fracture rate. 25 mg PO BID of a delayed-release formulation (Slow Fluoride®) reduced fracture rate but may make bone more fragile and could increase risk of hip fractures. Fluoride increases demand for Ca^{++}, therefore supplement with 800 mg/d Ca^{++} and 400 IU/d vitamin D. Not recommended for use > 2 yrs

Drugs that reduce bone resorption are less effective on cancellous bone (found mainly in the spine and at the end of long bones[19]). Improvement in spine bone mineral density accounts for only a small part of the observed reduction in the risk of vertebral fracture.[22] Medications include:
1. estrogen: cannot be used in men. Studies of estrogen hormone replacement therapy (HRT) have shown increased vertebral bone mass by > 5% and decreased rate of vertebral fractures by 50%. Also relieves post-menopausal symptoms and reduces risk of CAD. However, because HRT increases the risk of breast cancer[23] and of breast cancer recurrence[24] as well as DVT, its use has diminished substantially
2. calcium: current recommendation for postmenopausal women: 1,000-1,500 mg/d taken with meals[25]
3. vitamin D or analogues: promote calcium absorption from the GI tract. Typically administered with calcium therapy (either calcium or vitamin D alone are less effective). Vitamin D 400–800 IU/d is usually sufficient. If urinary Ca^{++} remains low, high dose vitamin D (50,000 IU q 7–10 d) may be tried. Since high-dose formulations have been discontinued in the U.S., analogues such as calcifediol (Calderol®) 50 mcg/d or calcitriol (Rocaltrol®) up to 0.25 mcg/d may be tried with Ca^{++} supplement. Serum levels of 25-hydroxyvitamin D [25(OH)D], AKA calcidiol is the best indicator of vitamin D status. The significance of vitamin D levels are shown in ▶ Table 66.5.[25] With high dose vitamin D or analogues, monitor serum and urinary Ca^{++}
4. calcitonin: a hormone synthesized by the thyroid gland which decreases bone resorption by osteoclasts. May be derived from a number of sources, salmon is one of the more common ones. The skeletal response is maximal during the first 18–24 months of therapy. Benefit in preventing fractures is less well established[21]
   a) parenteral salmon calcitonin (Calcimar®, Miacalcin®): indicated for patients for whom estrogen is contraindicated. Expensive ($1,500–3,000/yr) and must be given IM or sub-Q. 30–60% of patients develop antibodies to the drug which negates its effect. ℞: 0.5 ml (100 U) of calcitonin (given with calcium supplements to prevent hyperparathyroidism) SQ q d
   b) intranasal forms (Miacalcin nasal spray): less potent (works better in older women > 5 yrs post menopause). 200–400 IU/d given in one nostril (alternate nostrils daily) plus Ca^{++} 500 mg/d and vitamin D
5. bisphosphonates: carbon-substituted analogues of pyrophosphate have a high affinity for bone and inhibit bone resorption by destroying osteoclasts. Not metabolized. Remain bound to bone for several weeks
   a) etidronate (Didronel®), a 1st generation drug. Not FDA approved for osteoporosis. May reduce rate of VB fractures, not confirmed on F/U. Possible increased risk of hip fractures due to inhibition of bone mineralization may not occur with 2nd & 3rd generation drugs listed below. ℞ 400 mg PO daily × 2 wks followed by 11–13 weeks of Ca^{++} supplementation
   b) alendronate (Fosamax®): can cause esophageal ulcers. ℞ Prevention: 5 mg PO daily; treatment 10 mg PO daily; taken upright with water on an empty stomach at least 30 minutes before eating or drinking anything else. Once weekly dosing of 35 mg for prevention and 70 mg for treatment.[21,26] Taken concurrently with 1000–1500 mg/d Ca^{++} and 400/d IU of vitamin D

c) risedronate (Actonel®): ℞ Prevention or treatment: 5 mg PO daily, or 35 mg once/week[26] on an empty stomach (as for alendronate, see above)

6. estrogen analogues:
   a) tamoxifen (Nolvadex®), an estrogen antagonist for breast tissue but an estrogen agonist for bone, has a partial agonist effect on uterus associated with an increased incidence of endometrial cancer
   b) raloxifene (Evista®): similar to tamoxifen but is an estrogen antagonist for uterus.[27] Decreases the effect of warfarin (Coumadin®).
   ℞: 60 mg PO q d. **Supplied:** 60 mg tablets
7. RANK ligand (RANKL) inhibitors: RANKL binds to RANK receptors and stimulates precursor cells to mature into osteoclasts and inhibits their apoptosis.[28] Agents undergoing investigation include denosumab (Prolia®) 60 mg SQ q 6 months appears more effective than alendronate[29]

Treatment of osteoporotic vertebral compression fractures

66

Patients rarely have neurologic deficit. They are also usually fragile elderly women who usually do not tolerate large surgical procedures well, and the rest of their bones are also osteoporotic which are poor for internal fixation.

Management consists primarily of analgesics and bed rest followed by progressive mobilization, often in an external brace (often not tolerated well). Surgery is rarely employed. In cases where pain control is difficult to obtain or where neural compression causes deficit, limited bony decompression may be considered. Percutaneous vertebroplasty (see below) is a newer option.

Typical time course of conservative treatment:

1. initially, severe pain may require hospital or subacute care facility admission for adequate pain control utilizing
   a) sufficient pain medication
   b) bed rest for about 7–10 days (DVT prophylaxis recommended)
2. begin physical therapy (PT) after ≈ 7–10 days as patient tolerates (prolonged bed rest can promote "disuse osteoporosis")
   a) pain control as patient is mobilized may be enhanced by a *lumbar brace* which may work by reducing movement which causes repetitive "microfractures"
   b) discharge from the hospital with lumbar brace for outpatient PT
3. pain subsides on the average after 4–6 weeks (range 2–12 weeks)

Vertebral body augmentation

Percutaneous vertebroplasty (PVP)

Transpedicular injection of polymethylmethacrylate (PMMA) AKA "methylmethacrylate cement" into the compressed bone with the following goals (note: PMMA injection is FDA approved for treatment of compression fractures due to osteoporosis or tumor, but not for trauma as PMMA would prevent healing of the fracture):

1. to shorten the duration of pain (sometimes providing pain relief within minutes to hours). Remember: the natural history is that pain will eventually diminish in essentially all of these patients. Mechanism of pain relief may be due to stabilization of bone and/or due to disruption of nerve pain transmission by heat released during the exothermic curing of the cement
2. to try and stabilize the bone: may prevent progression of kyphosis

Randomized studies published in 2009 found no benefit in vertebroplasty over a sham procedure at 1 month[30] or at any time up to 6 months post-procedure.[31] NB: kyphoplasty (see below) was not studied; use with metastatic spine tumors was also not evaluated. Patient selection issues may make these results more or less applicable to a specific patient.

Kyphoplasty

Similar to PVP, except first, a balloon is inserted into the compressed VB through the pedicle. The balloon is inflated and then deflated and removed. PMMA is injected into the thusly created defect. Potential benefits of this over vertebroplasty: there may be some restoration of height, and there may be less tendency for PMMA extravasation/embolization (due to the cavity creation and the thicker PMMA used). In the (industry sponsored) randomized non-blinded FREE study[32] there was a significant positive difference in pain reduction and quality of life improvement in the kyphoplasty group compared to the nonoperated group at 1 month that diminished by 1-year post-op.

Indications

1. painful osteoporotic compression fractures:
   a) usually do not treat fractures producing < 5–10% loss of height
   b) severe pain that interferes with patient activity
   c) failure to adequately control pain with oral pain medication
   d) ✱ pain localized to fracture level
   e) acute fractures: procedure is not effective for healed fractures. In questionable cases, look for changes on STIR MRI (see below)
2. levels: FDA approved for use from T5 through L5, however has been used off-label (primarily for tumor, e.g. multiple myeloma) from T1 through sacrum, and has been described (for tumor) in the cervical spine from an anterior approach
3. vertebral hemangiomas that cause vertebral collapse or neurologic deficit as a result of extension into the spinal canal (not for incidental hemangiomas) (p. 795): the first indication for PVP[33]
4. osteolytic metastases and multiple myeloma[34]: pain relief and stabilization
5. pathologic compression fractures[35] from metastases: PVP does not give as rapid pain relief as with osteoporotic compression fractures (it may actually be necessary to increase pain meds for 7–10 days post PVP)
6. pedicle screw salvage when pedicle fractures or screws strip during pedicle screw placement

Contraindications

1. coagulopathy
2. completely healed fractures (no edema on MRI or cold on bone scan)
3. active infections: sepsis, osteomyelitis, discitis and epidural abscess
4. spinal instability
5. focal neurologic exam: may indicate herniated disc, retropulsed fragment in canal. Get CT or MRI to rule these out
6. relative contraindications:
   a) fractures > 80% loss of VB height (technically challenging)
   b) acute burst fractures
   c) significant canal compromise from tumor or retropulsed bone
   d) partial or total destruction of the posterior VB wall: not an absolute contraindication
7. iodine allergy: there is a small risk of a balloon rupturing with spill of the iodinated contrast used to fill the balloons prior to injecting the PMMA. Options include: iodine allergy prep (p. 221), use of gadolinium instead of iodinated contrast

Complications

Complication = rate: 1–9%. Lowest when used to treat osteoporotic compression fractures, higher with vertebral hemangiomas, highest with pathological fractures

1. methacrylate leakage:
   a) into soft tissues: usually of little consequence
   b) into spinal canal: symptomatic spinal cord compression is very rare
   c) into neural foramen: may cause radiculopathy
   d) into disc space
   e) venous: can get into spinal venous plexus or vena cava with ≈ 0.3–1% risk of clinically significant methycrylate pulmonary embolism (PE)[36]
2. radiculopathy: 5–7% incidence. Some cases may be due to heat released during cement curing. Often treated conservatively: steroids, pain meds, nerve block…
3. pedicle fracture
4. rib fracture
5. transverse process fracture
6. anterior penetration with needle: puncture of great vessels, pneumothorax…
7. increased incidence of future VB compression fractures at adjacent levels

Management of some associated developments

1. chest pain
   a) get rib x-rays
   b) VQ scan if indicated
2. patient starts coughing during injection: fairly common. May be reaction to rib pain or to odor of PMMA, may also indicate solvent in lungs. Stop injecting
3. back pain: take x-ray to rule-out new fracture or PMMA in veins
4. neurologic symptoms: get CT scan

Pre-procedure evaluation

1. plain x-rays: minimum requirement, most practitioners get MRI or bone scan
2. CT: helps rule-out *bony* compromise of spinal canal which may indicate increased risk of leakage for PMMA into canal during procedure
3. MRI: not mandatory, may be helpful in some cases
   a) short tau inversion recovery (STIR) images demonstrate bone edema indicative of acute fractures (not as good for differentiating pathology)[37]
   b) MRI can also disclose neurologic compression by *soft* tissue (e.g. tumor)
4. patients with multiple compression fractures: consider getting bone scan and perform PVP in the VB near the level of pain that lights up the most (↑ activity on bone scan correlates strongly with good outcome from PVP)

Booking the case: Kyphoplasty

Also see default values (p. 27).

1. position: prone
2. anesthesia: may be done under general, or under MAC
3. equipment: 2 C-arms for bi-plane fluoro
4. implants:
   a) kyphoplasty set
   b) iodinated contrast from radiology to fill balloons
5. consent (in lay terms for the patient – not all-inclusive):
   a) procedure: insertion of a needle into the fractured/abnormal bone, sometimes getting a biopsy as well, and then inflating a balloon in the bone to try and bring it back to a more normal size and then to inject a liquid cement which will then harden inside the bone to strengthen it
   b) alternatives: nonsurgical management, open surgery, in cases of tumor sometimes radiation therapy can be done
   c) complications: leakage of cement which can compress nerves and may need to be removed surgically if possible, rib fracture (from positioning), injury to large blood vessel or lung by the needle, failure to achieve the desired pain relief

66

Procedure

1. pain medication
   a) remember, this procedure is done with the patient lying on their stomach and is usually performed on frail, elderly females who smoke. Therefore use caution to avoid oversedation and respiratory compromise
   b) sedation and pain medication
   c) use of local anesthetic during needle placement
   d) additional pain medication just prior to injection
2. use bi-plane fluoro to pass needle through the pedicle to enter VB – see Percutaneous pedicle screws (p. 1495) – and place tip ≈ 1/2 to 2/3 of the way through the VB
3. test inject with contrast, e.g. iohexol (Omnipaque 300) (p. 219); do digital subtraction study if equipment is available. For kyphoplasty, the balloon is inflated at this time
   a) a little venous enhancement is acceptable
   b) if you visualize vena cava
      - do not pull needle back (the fistula has already been created)
      - push needle in a little further, or
      - push some gelfoam (soaked in contrast) through the needle, or
      - inject a very small amount of PMMA under visualization and allow it to set to block the fistula
4. inject PMMA (that has been opacified with tantalum or barium-sulfate) under fluoroscopic visualization until:
   a) 3–5 cc injected (minimal compression fractures accept more cement, sometimes up to ≈ 8 cc). No correlation between amount of PMMA injected and pain relief[34]
   b) PMMA approaches posterior VB wall. Stop if cement ever: enters disc space, vena cava, pedicle, or spinal canal

Post-procedure

1. PVP is often an outpatient procedure, but sometimes overnight admission is used
2. watch for
   a) chest or back pain (may indicate rib fracture)
   b) fever: may be reaction to cement
   c) neurologic symptoms
3. activity
   a) gradual mobilization after ≈ 2 hours
   b) ± physical therapy
   c) ± short term use of external brace (most centers do not use)
4. institute medical treatment for osteoporosis: remember the patient with fragility fractures by definition has osteoporosis with risk of future fractures

66.4 Sacral fractures

66.4.1 General information

Uncommon. Usually caused by shear forces. Identified in 17% of patients with pelvic fractures[38] (∴ keep in mind that neurologic deficits in patients with pelvic fractures may be due to associated sacral fractures). Neurologic injuries occur in 22–60%.[38]

The sacrum below S2 is not essential to ambulation or support of the spinal column, but may still be unstable since pressure to the area may occur when supine or sitting.

66.4.2 Classification

Three characteristic clinical presentations based on zone of involvement[38,39] as shown in ▶ Table 66.6.

Table 66.6 Classification of sacral fractures

Zone I	Zone II	Zone III Vertical	Zone III Transverse
Zone I: Region of ala sparing the central canal and neural foramina. Occasionally associated with partial L5 root injury possibly as a result of entrapment of the L5 root between the upwardly migrated fracture fragment and the transverse process of the L5 vertebra	Zone II: Region of sacral foramina (sparing the central canal). A vertical fracture which may be associated with unilateral L5, S1 and/or S2 nerve root involvement (producing sciatica). Bladder dysfunction is rare	Zone III: Region of sacral canal. Frequently associated with sphincter dysfunction (occurs only with bilateral root injuries) and saddle anesthesia. Subdivided[38]:	
		Vertical: almost always associated with pelvic ring fracture	Transverse (horizontal): rare. Often due to a direct blow to the sacrum as in a fall from a great height. Marked displacement of fracture fragment can produce severe deficit[a] (bowel & bladder incontinence)

[a] significant deficit is rare in fractures at or below S4

66.4.3 Treatment

In one series,[40] all 35 fractures were treated without surgery, and only 1 patient with a complete cauda equina syndrome did not improve. Others feel that surgery may have a useful role[38]:

1. operative reduction and internal fixation of unstable fractures may aid in pain control and promote early ambulation
2. decompression and/or surgical reduction/fixation may possibly improve radicular or sphincter deficits

Some observations[38]:

1. reduction of the ala may promote L5 recovery with Zone I fractures
2. Zone II fractures with neurologic involvement may recover with or without surgical reduction and fixation
3. horizontal Zone III with severe deficit: controversial. Reduction & decompression does not ensure recovery, which may occur with nonoperative management

References

[1] Denis F. The Three Column Spine and Its Significance in the Classification of Acute Thoracolumbar Spinal Injuries. Spine. 1983; 8:817–831

[2] Chedid MK, Green C. A Review of the Management of Lumbar Fractures With Focus on Surgical Decision-Making and Techniques. Contemp Neurosurg. 1999; 21:1–5

[3] Hommick A, Lavery R, Nicastro O, Livingston DH, Hauser CJ. Isolated thoracolumbar transverse process fractures: call physical therapy, not spine. J Trauma. 2007; 63:1292–1295

[4] Bradley LH, Paullus WC, Howe J, Litofsky NS. Isolated transverse process fractures: spine service management not needed. J Trauma. 2008; 65:832–6; discussion 836

[5] Hitchon PW, Jurf AA, Kernstine K, Torner JC. Management options in thoracolumbar fractures. Contemp Neurosurg. 2000; 22:1–12

[6] Hitchon PW, Torner JC, Haddad SF, Follett KA. Management Options in Thoracolumbar Burst Fractures. Surg Neurol. 1998; 49:619–627

[7] Klerk LWL, Fontijne PJ, Stijnen T, et al. Spontaneous remodeling of the spinal canal after conservative management of thoracolumbar burst fractures. Spine. 1998; 23:1057–1057

[8] Dai LY. Remodeling of the spinal canal after thoracolumbar burst fractures. Clin Orthop. 2001; 382:119–119

[9] Baaj AA, Reyes PM, Yaqoobi AS, Uribe JS, Vale FL, Theodore N, Sonntag VK, Crawford NR. Biomechanical advantage of the index-level pedicle screw in unstable thoracolumbar junction fractures. J Neurosurg Spine. 2011; 14:192–197

[10] Vaccaro AR, Zieller SC, Hulbert RJ, et al. The thoracolumbar injury severity score: a proposed treatment algorithm. Journal of Spinal Disorders Tech. 2005; 18:209–215

[11] Vaccaro AR, Lehman RA, Jr, Hurlbert RJ, Anderson PA, Harris M, Hedlund R, Harrop J, Dvorak M, Wood K, Fehlings MG, Fisher C, Zeiller SC, Anderson DG, Bono CM, Stock GH, Brown AK, Kuklo T, Oner FC. A new classification of thoracolumbar injuries: the importance of injury morphology, the integrity of the posterior ligamentous complex, and neurologic status. Spine. 2005; 30:2325–2333

[12] Bose B, Osterholm JL, Northrup BE, et al. Management of Lumbar Translocation Injuries: Case Reports. Neurosurgery. 1985; 17:958–961

[13] Blumenkopf B, Daniels T. Intraoperative Ultrasonography (IOUS) in Thoracolumbar Fractures. J Spinal Disord. 1988; 1:86–93

[14] Consensus Development Conference. Prophylaxis and Treatment of Osteoporosis. Am J Med. 1991; 90:107–110

[15] Daniell HW. Osteoporosis of the Slender Smoker: Vertebral Compression Fracture and Loss of Metacarpal Cortex in Relation to Postmenopausal Cigarette Smoking and Lack of Obesity. Arch Int Med. 1976; 136:298–304

[16] Shahinian VB, Kuo YF, Freeman JL, Goodwin JS. Risk of fracture after androgen deprivation for prostate cancer. N Engl J Med. 2005; 352:154–164

[17] Kanis JA, Melton J, Christiansen C, et al. The Diagnosis of Osteoporosis. J Bone Miner Res. 1994; 9:1137–1141

[18] Choice of Drugs for Postmenopausal Osteoporosis. Med Letter. 1992; 34:101–102

[19] Riggs BL, Melton LJ. The Prevention and Treatment of Osteoporosis. N Engl J Med. 1992; 327:620–627

[20] Khosla S, Riggs BL. Treatment Options for Osteoporosis. Mayo Clin Proc. 1995; 70:978–982

[21] Drugs for Prevention and Treatment of Postmenopausal Osteoporosis. Med Letter. 2000; 42:97–100

[22] Cummings SR, Karpf DB, Harris F, Genant HK, Ensrud K, LaCroix AZ, Black DM. Improvement in spine bone density and reduction in risk of vertebral fractures during treatment with antiresorptive drugs. Am J Med. 2002; 112:281–289

[23] Rossouw JE, Anderson GL, Prentice RL, LaCroix AZ, Kooperberg C, Stefanick ML, Jackson RD, Beresford SA, Howard BV, Johnson KC, Kotchen JM, Ockene J. Writing Group for the Women's Health Initiative Investigators. Risks and benefits of estrogen plus progestin in healthy postmenopausal women: principal results From the Women's Health Initiative randomized controlled trial. JAMA. 2002; 288:321–333

[24] Holmberg L, Anderson H. Data monitoring committees. HABITS (hormonal replacement therapy after breast cancer–is it safe?), a randomised comparison: trial stopped. Lancet. 2004; 363:453–455

[25] Office of Dietary Supplement - National Institutes of Health. Dietary supplement fact sheet: Vitamin D. 2009

[26] Once-A-Week Risedronate (Actonel). Med Letter. 2002; 44:87–88

[27] Raloxifene for Postmenopausal Osteoporosis. Med Letter. 1998; 40:29–30

[28] Bell NH. RANK ligand and the regulation of skeletal remodeling. J Clin Invest. 2003; 111:1120–1122

[29] McClung MR, Lewiecki EM, Cohen SB, Bolognese MA, Woodson GC, Moffett AH, Peacock M, Miller PD, Lederman SN, Chesnut CH, Lain D, Kivitz AJ,

66

Holloway DL, Zhang C, Peterson MC, Bekker PJ. Denosumab in postmenopausal women with low bone mineral density. N Engl J Med. 2006; 354:821–831

[30] Kallmes DF, Comstock BA, Heagerty PJ, Turner JA, Wilson DJ, Diamond TH, Edwards R, Gray LA, Stout L, Owen S, Hollingworth W, Ghdoke B, Annesley-Williams DJ, Ralston SH, Jarvik JG. A randomized trial of vertebroplasty for osteoporotic spinal fractures. N Engl J Med. 2009; 361:569–579

[31] Buchbinder R, Osborne RH, Ebeling PR, Wark JD, Mitchell P, Wriedt C, Graves S, Staples MP, Murphy B. A randomized trial of vertebroplasty for painful osteoporotic vertebral fractures. N Engl J Med. 2009; 361:557–568

[32] Wardlaw D, Cummings SR, Van Meirhaeghe J, Bastian L, Tillman JB, Ranstam J, Eastell R, Shabe P, Talmadge K, Boonen S. Efficacy and safety of balloon kyphoplasty compared with non-surgical care for vertebral compression fracture (FREE): a randomised controlled trial. Lancet. 2009; 373:1016–1024

[33] Deramond H, Depriester C, Galibert P, Le Gars D. Percutaneous Vertebroplasty with Polymehtylmethacrylate. Radiol Clin North Am. 1998; 36:533–546

[34] Cotten A, Dewatre F, Cortet B, Assaker R, Leblond D, Duquesnoy B, Chastanet P, Clarisse J. Percutaneous vertebroplasty for osteolytic metastases and myeloma: effects of the percentage of lesion filling and the leakage of methyl methacrylate at clinical follow-up. Radiology. 1996; 200:525–530

[35] Fourney DR, Schomer DF, Nader R, Chlan-Fourney J, Suki D, Ahrar K, Rhines LD, Gokaslan ZL. Percutaneous vertebroplasty and kyphoplasty for painful vertebral body fractures in cancer patients. J Neurosurg. 2003; 98:21–30

[36] Choe DH, Marom EM, Ahrar K, et al. Pulmonary embolism of polymethyl methacrylate during percutaneous vertebroplasty and kyphoplasty. Am J Roentgenol. 2004; 183:1097–1102

[37] Bendok BR, Halpin RJ, Rubin MN, Boco T, Przybylo JH, Liu JC. Percutaneous vertebroplasty. Contemp Neurosurg. 2004; 26:1–6

[38] Gibbons KJ, Soloniuk DS, Razack N. Neurological injury and patterns of sacral fractures. J Neurosurg. 1990; 72:889–893

[39] Denis F, Davis S, Comfort T. Sacral fractures: An important problem. Retrospective analysis of 236 cases. Clin Orthop. 1988; 227:67–81

[40] Sabiston CP, Wing PC. Sacral fractures: classification and neurologic implications. J Trauma. 1986; 26:1113–1115

67 Penetrating Spine Injuries and Long Term Management / Complications

67.1 Gunshot wounds to the spine

67.1.1 General information

Most are due to assaults with handguns. Distribution: cervical 19–37%, thoracic 48–64%, and lumbosacral 10–29% (roughly proportional to lengths of each segment). Spinal cord injury due to civilian GSWs are primarily due to direct injury from the bullet (unlike military weapons which may create injury from shock waves and cavitation). Steroids are not indicated (p. 951).

67.1.2 Indications for surgery

1. injury to the cauda equina (whether complete or incomplete) if nerve root compression is demonstrated[1]
2. neurologic deterioration: suggesting possibility of spinal epidural hematoma
3. compression of a nerve root
4. CSF leak
5. spinal instability: very rare with isolated GSW to the spine
6. to remove a copper jacketed bullet: copper can cause intense local reaction[2]
7. incomplete lesions: very controversial. Some series show improvement with surgery,[3] others show no difference from unoperated patients
8. debridement to reduce the risk of infection: more important for *military* GSW where there is massive tissue injury, not an issue for most civilian GSW except in cases where the bullet has traversed GI or respiratory tract
9. vascular injuries
10. surgery for late complications:
    a) migrating bullet
    b) lead toxicity[4] (plumbism): absorption of lead from a bullet occurs only when it lodges in joints, bursae, or *disc space*. Findings include: anemia, encephalopathy, motor neuropathy, nephropathy, abdominal colic
    c) late spinal instability: especially after surgery

67

67.2 Penetrating trauma to the neck

67.2.1 General information

Most often, injuries to the soft-tissues of the neck fall into the purvey of general/trauma surgeons and/or vascular surgeons. However, depending on local practice patterns, neurosurgeons may participate in care of these injuries, or they may get involved by virtue of associated spinal injuries (p. 1017).

The mortality rate for penetrating injury to the neck is ≈ 15%, with most early deaths due either to asphyxiation from airway compromise, or exsanguination externally or into the chest or upper airways. Late death is usually due to cerebral ischemia or complications from spinal cord injury.

67.2.2 Vascular injuries

Venous injuries occur in ≈ 18% of penetrating neck wounds, and arterial injuries in ≈ 12%. Of the cervical arteries, the common carotid is most usually involved, followed by the ICA, the ECA, and then the vertebral artery. Outcome probably correlates most closely with neurologic condition on admission, regardless of treatment.

Vertebral artery (VA): the majority of injuries are penetrating. Due to the proximity of other vessels, the spinal cord and nerve roots, injuries are rarely isolated to the VA. 72% of documented VA injuries had no related physical findings on exam.[5]

67.2.3 Classification

Trauma surgeons have traditionally divided penetrating injuries of the neck into 3 zones,[6] and although definitions vary, the following is a general scheme[7]:

Zone I: inferiorly from the head of the clavicle to include the thoracic outlet

Zone II: from the clavicle to the angle of the mandible

Zone III: from the angle of the mandible to the base of the skull

67.2.4 Evaluation

Neurologic examination: global deficits may be due to shock or hypoxemia due to asphyxiation. Cerebral neurologic deficits are usually due to vascular injury with cerebral ischemia. Local findings may be related to cranial nerve injury. Unilateral UE deficits may be due to nerve root or brachial plexus involvement. Median or ulnar nerve dysfunction can occur from compression by a pseudoaneurysm of the proximal axillary artery. Spinal cord involvement may present with complete injury, or with an incomplete spinal cord injury syndrome (p. 944). Shock due to spinal cord injury is usually accompanied by bradycardia (p. 931), as opposed to the tachycardia seen with hypovolemic shock.

67

Cervical spine x-rays: assesses trajectory of injury and integrity C-spine.

Angiography: indicated in most cases if the patient is stable (especially for zone I or III injuries, and for zone II patients with no other indication for exploration, or for patients with penetration of the posterior triangle or wounds near the transverse processes where the VA may be injured). Patients actively hemorrhaging need to be taken to the OR without pre-op angiography. Angiographic abnormalities include:

1. extravasation of blood
   a) expanding hematoma into soft tissues: may compromise airway
   b) pseudoaneurysm
   c) AV fistula
   d) bleeding into airways
   e) external bleeding
2. intimal dissection, with
   a) occlusion, or
   b) luminal narrowing (including possible "string sign")
3. occlusion by soft tissue or bone

67.2.5 Treatment

Airway

Stable patients without airway compromise should not have "prophylactic" intubation to protect the airway. Immediate intubation is indicated for hemodynamically unstable patients or for airway compromise. Options:

- endotracheal: preferred
- cricothyroidotomy: if endotracheal intubation cannot be performed (e.g. due to tracheal deviation or patient agitation) or if there is evidence of cervical spine injury and manipulation of the neck is contraindicated, then cricothyroidotomy is performed with placement of a #6 or 7 cuffed endotracheal tube (followed by a standard tracheostomy in the OR once the patient is stabilized)
- awake nasotracheal: may be considered in the setting of possible spinal injury

Indications for surgical exploration

Surgical exploration has been advocated for all wounds that pierce the platysma and enter the anterior triangles of the neck,[8] however, 40–60% of these explorations will be negative. Although a selective approach may be based on angiography, false negatives have resulted in some authors recommending exploration of all zone II injuries.[9]

Surgical treatment for vascular injuries

Endovascular techniques may be suitable for select cases, especially for patients who are already in the endovascular suite for angiography. However, patients who are actively bleeding usually end up in the O.R. with an open procedure.

Carotid artery: choices are primary repair, interposition grafting, or ligation. Patients in coma or those with severe strokes caused by vascular occlusion of the carotid artery are poor surgical candidates for vascular reconstruction due to a high mortality rate ≥ 40%,[7] however the outcome with ligation is worse. Repair of injuries is recommended in patients with no or only minor neurologic deficit. ICA ligation is recommended for bleeding that cannot be controlled and was used for extravasation of dye at the base of the skull in 1 patient.[10]

Vertebral artery: injuries are more often managed by ligation than by direct repair,[11] especially when bleeding occurs during exploration. Less urgent conditions (e.g. AV fistula) requires knowledge of the patency of the contralateral VA and the ability to fill the ipsilateral PICA from retrograde flow through the BA before ligation can considered (arteriographic anomalies contraindicate ligation in 15% of cases). Proximal occlusion may be accomplished with an anterior approach after the sternocleidomastoid is detached from the sternum. The VA is the normally the first branch of the subclavian artery. Alternatively, endovascular techniques may be used, e.g. detachable balloons for proximal occlusion, or thrombogenic coils for pseudoaneurysms. Distal interruption may also be required, and this necessitates surgical exposure and ligation. Optimal management of a thrombosed injured VA in a foramen transversarium is unknown, and may require arterial bypass if ligation is not a viable option.

67.3 Delayed cervical instability

67.3.1 General information

Definition (adapted[12]): cervical instability that is not recognized until beyond 20 days after the injury (p. 930). The instability itself may be delayed, or the recognition may be delayed.

67.3.2 Etiologies

Reasons for delayed cervical instability:

1. inadequate radiologic evaluation[13]
   a) incomplete studies (e.g. must see all the way down to C7-T1 junction)
   b) suboptimal studies: motion artifact, incorrect positioning… Etiologies include: poor patient cooperation as a result of agitation/intoxication, portable films, poor technique…
2. abnormality missed on x-ray
   a) overlooked fracture, subluxation
   b) injury failed to be demonstrated despite sufficiently adequate x-rays[12]; see recommendations of extent of radiologic workup (p. 1088)
      - type of fracture not demonstrated on the radiographs obtained
      - patient positioning (e.g. supine) may reduce some malalignment
      - spasm of cervical muscles may reduce and/or stabilize the injury
      - microfractures
3. inadequate models: some findings may be judged to be stable using certain models, but in the long-run may prove to be unstable (there is no perfect model for instability)

67.3.3 Indications for additional studies

Further studies or repeat x-rays several weeks after the trauma should be considered in patients with neurologic deficit, persistent pain, significant degenerative changes when the original films were suboptimal, subluxations < 3 mm, or when surgery is contemplated.[14]

67.4 Delayed deterioration following spinal cord injuries

Etiologies include:

1. posttraumatic syringomyelia (p. 1148). Latency to symptoms: 3 mos-34 yrs
2. subacute progressive ascending myelopathy (SPAM): rare. Median time of occurrence: 13 days post injury (range: 4–86 days).[15] Signal changes extending to ≥ 4 levels above the original injury
3. unrecognized spinal instability[16]: mean delay in diagnosis was 20 days
4. tethered spinal cord: may be due to scar tissue at site of injury
5. delayed spinal epidural hematoma (SEH): most symptomatic SEH occur within 72 hours of surgery, however longer delays have been reported[17]
6. apoptosis of neurons, oligodendrogliocytes, and astrocytes[18]: initiated during the acute phase, deterioration occurs during the chronic phase of SCI (months to years after SCI)
7. glial scar formation: mass effect as well as release of factors that may damage surviving neurons[19(p 43–5)]

67

67.5 Chronic management issues with spinal cord injuries

67.5.1 Overview

Most of the following topics are treated elsewhere in this manual, but are pertinent to spinal cord injured (SCI) patients, and reference to the specific section is made.

- autonomic hyperreflexia: see below
- ectopic bone, includes para-articular heterotopic ossification: ossification of some joints that occurs in 15–20% of paralyzed patients
- osteoporosis and pathologic fracture (p. 1009)
- spasticity (p. 1528)
- syringomyelia (p. 1144)
- deep vein thrombosis (p. 952): see below
- shoulder-hand syndrome: possibly sympathetically maintained

67.5.2 Respiratory management problems in spinal cord injuries

In attempting to wean high level SCI patients from a ventilator, it may be helpful to change tube feedings to Pulmonaid® which lowers the CO_2 load.

Patients with cervical SCIs are more prone to pneumonia due to the fact that most of the effort in a normal cough originates in the abdominal muscles which are paralyzed.

67.5.3 Autonomic hyperreflexia

General information

Key concepts

- exaggerated autonomic response to normally innocuous stimuli
- in spinal cord injury, occurs only in patients with lesions above ≈ T6
- patients complain of pounding headache, flushing and diaphoresis above lesion
- can be life threatening, requires rapid control of hypertension and a search for an elimination of offending stimuli

AKA autonomic dysreflexia. Autonomic hyperreflexia[20,21] (AH) is an exaggerated autonomic response (sympathetic usually dominates) secondary to stimuli that would only be mildly noxious under normal circumstances. It occurs in ≈ 30% of quadriplegic and high paraplegic patients (reported range is as high as 66–85%), but does not occur in patients with lesions below T6 (only patients with lesions above the origin of the splanchnic outflow are prone to develop AH, and the origin is usually T6 or below). It is rare in first 12–16 weeks post-injury.

During attacks, norepinephrine (NE) (but not epinephrine) is released. Hypersensitivity to NE may be partially due to subnormal resting levels of catecholamines. Homeostatic responses include vasodilatation (above the level of the injury) and bradycardia (however, sympathetic stimulation may also cause tachycardia).

Stimuli sources

Stimulus sources causing episodes of autonomic hyperreflexia:

1. bladder: 76% (distension 73%, UTI 3%, bladder stones…)
2. colorectal: 19% (fecal impaction 12%, administering enema or suppository 4%)
3. decubitus ulcers/skin infection: 4%
4. DVT
5. miscellaneous: tight clothing or leg bag straps, procedures such as cystoscopy or debriding decubitus ulcers, case report of suprapubic tube

Presentation

1. paroxysmal HTN: 90%
2. anxiety
3. diaphoresis

4. piloerection
5. pounding H/A
6. ocular findings:
   a) mydriasis
   b) blurring of vision
   c) lid retraction or lid lag
7. erythema of face, neck and trunk: 25%
8. pallor of skin below the lesion (due to vasoconstriction)
9. pulse rate: tachycardia (38%) or mild elevation over baseline, bradycardia (10%)
10. "splotches" over face and neck: 3%
11. muscle fasciculations
12. increased spasticity
13. penile erection
14. Horner's syndrome
15. triad seen in 85%: cephalgia (H/A), hyperhidrosis, cutaneous vasodilatation

Evaluation

In the appropriate setting (e.g. a quadriplegic patient with an acutely distended bladder), the symptoms are fairly diagnostic.

Many features are also common to pheochromocytoma. Studies of catecholamine levels have been inconsistent, however they can be mildly elevated in AH. The distinguishing feature of AH is the presence of hyperhidrosis and flushing of the face in the presence of pallor and vasoconstriction elsewhere on the body (which would be unusual for a pheochromocytoma).

Treatment

1. immediately elevate HOB (to decrease ICP), check BP q 5 min
2. treatment of choice: identify and eliminate the offending stimulus
   a) make sure bladder is empty (if catheterized check for kinks or sediment plugs). Caution: irrigating bladder may exacerbate AH (consider suprapubic aspiration)
   b) check bowels (avoid rectal exam, may exacerbate). Palpate abdomen or check abdominal x-ray (AH from this usually resolves spontaneously without manual disimpaction)
   c) check skin and toenails for ulceration or infection
   d) remove tight apparel
3. HTN that is extreme or that does not respond quickly may require treatment to prevent seizures and/or cerebral hemorrhage/hypertensive encephalopathy. Caution must be used to prevent hypotension following the episode. Agents used include: sublingual nifedipine[22] 10 mg SL, IV phentolamine – alpha cholinergic blocker (p. 655) – or nicardipine (p. 126).
4. consider diazepam (Valium®) 2–5 mg IVP (@ < 5 mg/min). Relieves spasm of skeletal and smooth muscle (including bladder sphincter). Is also anxiolytic

Prevention

Good bowel/bladder and skin care are the best preventative measures.

Prophylaxis in patients with recurrent episodes:

- *phenoxybenzamine* (Dibenzyline®): an alpha blocker. Not helpful during the acute crisis. May not be as effective for alpha stimulation from sympathetic ganglia as with circulating catecholamines.[23] The patient may also develop hypotension after the sympathetic outflow subsides. Thus this is used only for resistant cases (note: will not affect sweating which is mediated by acetylcholine).
  ℞ Adult: wide range quoted in literature: average 20–30 mg PO BID
- beta-blockers: may be necessary in addition to α-blockers to avoid possible hypotension from β_2-receptor stimulation (a theoretical concern)
- phenazopyridine (Pyridium®): a topical anesthetic that is excreted in the urine. May decrease bladder wall irritation, however, the primary cause of irritation should be treated if possible.
  ℞ Adult: 200 mg PO TID after meals. **Supplied** : 100, 200 mg tabs.
- "radical measures" such as sympathectomy, pelvic or pudendal nerve section, cordectomy, or intrathecal alcohol injection have been advocated in the past, but are rarely necessary and may jeopardize reflex voiding
- prophylactic treatment prior to procedures may employ use of anesthetics even in regions rendered anesthetic by the cord injury. Nifedipine 10 mg SL has also been used effective for AH during cystoscopy and prophylactically[22]

References

[1] Robertson DP, Simpson RK. Penetrating Injuries Restricted to the Cauda Equina: A Retrospective Review. Neurosurgery. 1992; 31:265–270
[2] Messer HD, Cereza PF. Copper Jacketed Bullets in the Central Nervous System. Neuroradiology. 1976; 12:121–129
[3] Benzel EC, Hadden TA, Coleman JE. Civilian Gunshot Wounds to the Spinal Cord and Cauda Equina. Neurosurgery. 1987; 20:281–285
[4] Linden MA, Manton WI, Stewart RM, et al. Lead Poisoning from Retained Bullets. Pathogenesis, Diagnosis, and Management. Ann Surg. 1982; 195:305–313
[5] Reid JDS, Weigelt JA. Forty-Three Cases of Vertebral Artery Trauma. J Trauma. 1988; 28:1007–1012
[6] Monson DO, Saletta JD, Freeark RJ. Carotid Vertebral Trauma. J Trauma. 1969; 9:987–989
[7] Perry MO, Rutherford RB. In: Injuries of the Brachiocephalic Vessels. Vasc Surg. 4th ed. Philadelphia: W.B. Saunders; 1995:705–713
[8] Fogelman MJ, Stewart RD. Penetrating Wounds of the Neck. Am J Surg. 1956; 91:581–596
[9] Meyer JP, Barrett JA, Schuler JJ, Flanigan DP. Mandatory versus Selective Exploration for Penetrating Neck Trauma. A Prospective Assessment. Arch Surg. 1987; 122:592–597
[10] Ledgerwood AM, Mullins RJ, Lucas CE. Primary Repair vs Ligation for Carotid Artery Injuries. Arch Surg. 1980; 115:488–493
[11] Meier DE, Brink BE, Fry WJ. Vertebral Artery Trauma: Acute Recognition and Treatment. Arch Surg. 1981; 116:236–239
[12] Herkowitz HN, Rothman RH. Subacute Instability of the Cervical Spine. Spine. 1984; 9:348–357
[13] Walter J, Doris P, Shaffer M. Clinical Presentation of Patients with Acute Cervical Spine Injury. Ann Emerg Med. 1984; 13:512–515
[14] Delfini R, Dorizzi A, Facchinetti G, et al. Delayed Post-Traumatic Cervical Instability. Surg Neurol. 1999; 51:588–595
[15] Planner AC, Pretorius PM, Graham A, Meagher TM. Subacute progressive ascending myelopathy following spinal cord injury: MRI appearances and clinical presentation. Spinal Cord. 2008; 46:140–144
[16] Levi AD, Hurlbert RJ, Anderson P, Fehlings M, et al. Neurologic deterioration secondary to unrecognized spinal instability following trauma - a multicenter trial. Spine. 2006; 41:451–458
[17] Parthiban CJKB, Majeed SA. Delayed spinal extradural hematoma following thoracic spine surgery and resulting in paraplegia: a case report. 2008
[18] Liu XZ, Xu HM, Hu R, Du C, et al. Neuronal and glial apoptosis after traumatic spinal cord injury. J Neurosci. 1997; 17:5395–5406
[19] Liverman CT, Altevogt BM, Joy JE, Johnson RT. Spinal cord injury: progress, promise and priorities. Washington, D.C. 2005
[20] Erickson RP. Autonomic Hyperreflexia: Pathophysiology and Medical Management. Arch Phys Med Rehabil. 1980; 61:431–440
[21] Kewalramani LS, Orth MS. Autonomic Dysreflexia in Traumatic Myelopathy. Am J Phys Med. 1980; 59:1–21
[22] Dykstra DD, Sidi AA, Anderson LC. The Effect of Nifedipine on Cyctoscopy-Induced Autonomic Hyperreflexia in Patients with High Spinal Cord Injuries. J Urol. 1987; 138:1155–1157
[23] Sizemore GW, Winternitz WW. Autonomic Hyper-Reflexia - Suppression with Alpha-Adrenergic Blocking Agents. N Engl J Med. 1970; 282

67

Part XVI

Spine and Spinal Cord

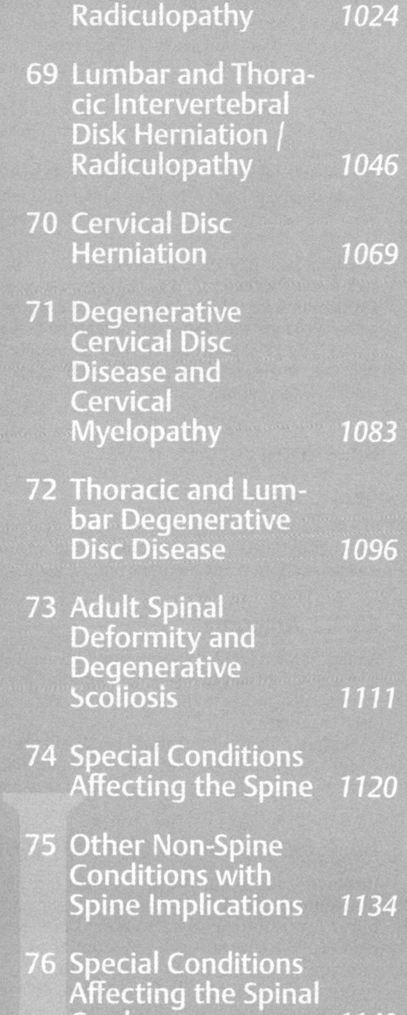

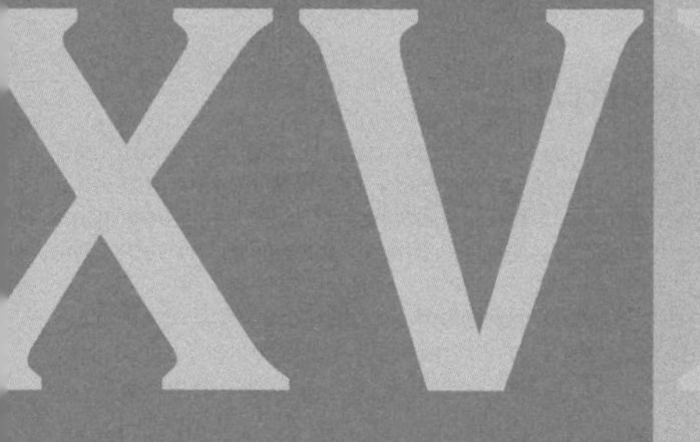

68 Low Back Pain and Radiculopathy

68.1 General information

Key concepts

See reference.[1]

- low back pain is common, and in ≈ 85% of cases no specific diagnosis can be made
- initial assessment is geared to detecting "red flags" (indicating potentially serious pathology), and in the absence of these, imaging studies and further testing of patients is usually not helpful during the first 4 weeks of low back symptoms
- relief of discomfort is usually best achieved with nonprescription pain meds and/or spinal manipulation
- while activities may need to be modified, bed rest beyond 4 days may be more harmful than helpful, and patients are encouraged to return to work or their normal daily activities as soon as possible
- 89–90% of patients with low back problems will improve within 1 month even without treatment (including patients with sciatica from disc herniation)

Low back pain (LBP) is extremely prevalent, and is the second most common reason for people to seek medical attention.[2] After the common cold, it is the number two cause for loss of time at work. LBP accounts for ≈ 15% of all sick leave from work, and is the most common cause of disability for persons < 45 yrs age.[3] Estimates of lifetime prevalence range from 60–90%, and the annual incidence is 5%.[4] Only 1% of patients will have nerve-root symptoms, and only 1–3% have lumbar disc herniation. The prognosis for most cases of LBP is good, and improvement usually occurs with little or no medical intervention.

68.2 Intervertebral disc

68.2.1 General information

The function of the intervertebral disc is to permit stable motion of the spine while supporting and distributing loads under movement. The intervertebral disc has been characterized as the largest nonvascularized structure in the human body, which imparts some unique attributes to it.

68.2.2 Anatomy

Anulus fibrosus (anulus may alternatively be spelled annulus, but fibrosus is the only correct spelling and is distinct from fibrosis)[5]: the multilaminated ligament that encompasses the periphery of the disc space. Attaches to the end-plate cartilage and ring apophyseal bone. Blends centrally with the nucleus pulposus.

Nucleus pulposus: the central portion of the disc. A remnant of the notocord.

Capsule[5]: combined fibers of the anulus fibrosus and the posterior longitudinal ligament (this term is useful because these 2 structures may not be distinguishable on imaging studies).

68.3 Nomenclature for disc pathology

Historically, the terminology for lumbar disc pathology has been contentious and nonstandardized. A committee tasked to standardize the nomenclature has issued version 2.0 of their recommendations.[6] Some of these standardizations are useful primarily for consistency related to radiographic reports and for research, and may not be as useful for day-to-day clinical practice A subset of the recommendations is shown in ▶ Table 68.1.

Degenerated disc: (see ▶ Table 68.1 for definition) some reports indicate that these can cause radicular pain possibly by an inflammatory mechanism,[7] but this is not universally accepted.

Vacuum disc: gas in the disc space (empty space on imaging), usually indicates disc degeneration, *not* infection.

Table 68.1 Nomenclature for lumbar disc pathology[6]

Term	Description
anular tears AKA anular fissures	separations between anular fibers, avulsions of fibers from their VB insertions, or breaks through fibers that extend radially, transversely, or concentrically
degeneration	desiccation, fibrosis, narrowing of the disc space, diffuse bulging of the anulus beyond the disc space, extensive fissuring (numerous anular tears), mucinous degeneration of the anulus, defects & sclerosis of endplates, & osteophytes at the vertebral apophyses
degenerative disc disease	clinical syndrome of symptoms related to degenerative changes in the intervertebral disc (described above), also often considered to encompass degenerative changes outside the disc as well
bulging disc	generalized displacement of disc material (arbitrarily defined as > 50% or 180°) beyond the peripheral limits of the disc space[a]. Not considered a form of herniation. May be a normal finding, not usually symptomatic
herniation	localized displacement of disc material (< 50% or 180°) beyond the limits of the intervertebral disc space[a]
	focal: < 25% of the disc circumference
	broad-based: 25–50% of the disc circumference
	protrusion: the fragment does not have a "neck" that is narrower than the fragment in any dimension
	extrusion: the fragment has a "neck" that is narrower than the fragment in at least 1 dimension. 2 subtypes a) sequestration: the fragment has lost continuity with the disc of origin (AKA free fragment) b) migration: the fragment is displaced away from the site of extrusion, regardless of whether sequestered or not
	intravertebral herniation (AKA Schmorl's node (p. 1060): disc herniates in the cranio-caudal direction through the cartilaginous end-plate into the VB

Table 68.2 Modic's classification

Modic Type	Intensity changes		Description	
	T1WI	T2WI		
1[a]	↓	↑	bone marrow edema associated with acute or subacute inflammation	
2	↑	iso or ↑	chronic changes	replacement of bone marrow by fat
3	↓	↑		reactive osteosclerosis

[a]Type 1 Modic changes disappear on STIR images (the signal characteristics mimic CSF/water). Back pain in this group may respond to fusion (p. 1036).

68.4 Vertebral body marrow changes

Associated with degenerative or inflammatory changes. Modic's classification[8] of MRI characteristics is shown in ▶ Table 68.2.

68.5 Clinical terms

▶ **Radiculopathy.** Dysfunction of a nerve root; signs and symptoms may include: pain in the distribution of that nerve root, dermatomal sensory disturbances, weakness of muscles innervated by that nerve root, and hypoactive muscle stretch reflexes of the same muscles

► **Mechanical low back pain** (p. 1024). AKA "musculoskeletal" back pain (both non-specific terms). The most common form of low back pain. May result from strain of the paraspinal muscles and/or ligaments, irritation of facet joints... Excludes anatomically identifiable causes (e.g. tumor, disc herniation...)

► **Sciatica.** Pain along the course of the sciatic nerve, usually resulting from nerve root compromise (the sciatic nerve is comprised of nerve roots L1 through L5)

68.6 Disability, pain and outcome determinations

Disability scales for low back pain have been developed to assess outcomes for research purposes. Some widely used measures include:

1. visual analogue scale: used for any type of pain. The patient is asked to mark their pain level on a line divided into segments with sequential labels 0 (no pain) to 10 (the worst pain)
2. Oswestry disability index (ODI)[9]: a categorical ordinal scale that is used for low back pain. There are 4 English versions in wide use,[10] version 2.0[11] is recommended.[10]
   It consists 10 questions related to activities of daily living. Each item is scored 0–5 (5 being the most disability) and the total is multiplied by 2% to obtain the final score (range: 0–100%). The interpretation of the final score is shown in ► Table 68.3. A score > 45% is essentially completely disabled. A score in the teens is very functional
3. Roland–Morris disability questionnaire[12]
4. Short Form 36 (SF36)[13]

68.7 Differential diagnosis of low back pain

The differential diagnosis of low back pain (p. 1024) overlaps with that of myelopathy. In ≈ 85% of cases of LBP no specific diagnosis can be made,[14] however, serious and/or dangerous conditions can usually be reliably ruled out.

68.8 Initial assessment of the patient with back pain

68.8.1 Background

Initial assessment consists of a history and physical exam focused on identifying serious underlying conditions such as: fracture, tumor, infection or cauda equina syndrome (p. 1050). Serious conditions presenting as low back problems are relatively rare.

68.8.2 History

The following information has been found to be helpful in identifying patients with serious underlying conditions such as cancer and spinal infection.[1] ► Table 68.4 shows the sensitivity and specificity of some features of the history for various conditions.

1. age
2. history of cancer (especially malignancies that are prone to skeletal metastases: prostate, breast, kidney, thyroid, lung, lymphoma/myeloma)
3. unexplained weight loss

Table 68.3 Oswestry disability index score

Score	Interpretation
0–20%	minimal disability: can cope with most daily activities
21–40%	moderate disability: pain and difficulty with sitting, lifting & standing. The patient may be disabled from work
41–60%	severe disability: pain is the main problem, but other areas are affected
61–80%	crippled: back pain impinges on all aspects of the patient's life
81–100%	these patients are either bed-bound or else are exaggerating their symptoms

Table 68.4 Sensitivity and specificity of historical findings in patients with low back problems[1]

Condition	History	Sensitivity	Specificity
cancer	age ≥ 50 yrs	0.77	0.71
	previous Ca	0.31	0.98
	unexplained weight loss	0.15	0.94
	failure to improve after conservative therapy × 1 month	0.31	0.90
	any of the above	1.00	0.60
	pain > 1 month	0.50	0.81
spinal osteomyelitis	IV drug abuse, UTI, or skin infection	0.40	NA
compression fracture	age ≥ 50 yrs	0.84	0.61
	age ≥ 70yrs	0.22	0.96
	trauma	0.30	0.85
	steroid use	0.06	0.995
HLD	sciatica	0.95	0.88
spinal stenosis	pseudoclaudication	0.60	NA
	age ≥ 50 yrs	0.90[a]	0.70
ankylosing spondylitis	positive response to 4 out of 5 of the following	0.23	0.82
	age at onset ≤ 40 yrs	1.00	0.07
	pain not relieved when supine	0.80	0.49
	AM back stiffness	0.64	0.59
	pain ≥ 3 mos duration	0.71	0.54

[a]estimate

4. immunosuppression: from steroids, organ transplant medication, or HIV
5. prolonged use of steroids
6. duration of symptoms
7. responsiveness to previous therapy
8. pain that is worse at rest
9. history of skin infection: especially furuncle
10. history of IV drug abuse
11. UTI or other infection
12. pain radiating below the knee
13. persistent numbness or weakness in the legs
14. history of significant trauma. In a young patient: usually involves MVA, a fall from a height, or a direct blow to the back. In an older patient: minor falls, heavy lifting or even a severe coughing episode can cause a fracture especially in the presence of with osteoporosis
15. findings consistent with cauda equina syndrome (p. 1050):
    a) bladder dysfunction (usually urinary retention, or overflow incontinence) or fecal incontinence
    b) saddle anesthesia (p. 1050)
    c) unilateral or bilateral leg weakness or pain
16. psychological and socioeconomic factors may influence the patient's report of symptoms (p. 1033), and one should inquire about:
    a) work status
    b) typical job tasks
    c) educational level

d) pending litigation
e) worker's compensation or disability issues
f) failed previous treatments
g) substance abuse
h) depression

68.8.3 Physical examination

Less helpful than the history in identifying patients who may be harboring conditions such as cancer, but may be more helpful in detecting spinal infections.

1. spinal infection (p. 349): findings that suggest this as a possibility (but are also common in patients without infection)
   a) fever: common in epidural abscess and vertebral osteomyelitis, less common in discitis
   b) vertebral tenderness
   c) very limited range of spinal motion
2. findings of possible neurologic compromise: the following physical findings will identify most cases of clinically significant nerve root compromise due to L4–5 or L5-S1 HLD which comprise > 90% of cases of radiculopathy due to HLD; limiting the exam to the following might not detect the much less common upper lumbar disc herniations, which may be difficult to detect on PE (p. 1057)
   a) dorsiflexion strength of ankle and great toe: weakness suggests L5 and some L4 dysfunction
   b) achilles reflex: diminished reflex suggests S1 root dysfunction
   c) light touch sensation of the foot:
      - diminished over medial malleolus and medial foot: suggests L4 nerve root involvement
      - diminished over dorsum of foot: suggests L5
      - diminished over lateral malleolus and lateral foot: suggests S1
   d) straight leg raising (SLR); also check for crossed SLR (p. 1048)

68.8.4 "Red flags" in the history and physical exam for low back problems

Based upon the above history and physical exam, the findings in ▶ Table 68.5 would suggest the possibility of a serious underlying condition as the cause of the low back problem. Also, thoracic region pain is relatively uncommon and should raise the index of suspicion.

68.8.5 Special diagnostic tests

For patients without features suggesting a serious underlying condition, special diagnostic tests are not needed during the first month of symptoms. This covers approximately 95% of patients with low back problems.[1]

Table 68.5 "Red flags" for patients with low back problems

Condition	Red flags
cancer or infection	1. age > 50 or < 20 yrs 2. history of cancer 3. unexplained weight loss 4. immunosuppression (see text) 5. UTI, IV drug abuse, fever or chills 6. back pain not improved with rest
spinal fracture	1. history of significant trauma (see text) 2. prolonged use of steroids 3. age > 70 yrs
cauda equina syndrome or severe neurologic compromise	1. acute onset of urinary retention or overflow incontinence 2. fecal incontinence or loss of anal sphincter tone 3. saddle anesthesia 4. global or progressive weakness in the LEs

68.9 Radiographic evaluation

68.9.1 General information

Diagnosing lumbar spinal stenosis or herniated intervertebral disc is usually helpful only in potential surgical candidates.[15] This includes patients with appropriate clinical syndromes who have not responded satisfactorily to adequate non-surgical treatment over a sufficient period of time, and who have no medical contraindications to surgery. Radiologic confirmation of these diagnoses usually requires CT, myelography, MRI, or some combination (see below). NB: myelography,[16] CT,[17] or MRI[18] may also show bulging or herniated lumbar discs (HLD) or spinal stenosis in *asymptomatic* patients (e.g. 24% of asymptomatic patients have herniated discs on MRI and 4% have spinal stenosis; these numbers become 36% and 21% respectively in patients 60–80 years old).[19] Thus, these tests must be interpreted in light of clinical findings, and the anatomic level and side should correspond to the history, examination, and/or other physiologic data. Diagnostic radiology is of limited benefit as the initial evaluation in the majority of spinal disorders.[20]

In the absence of red flags for serious conditions, imaging studies are not recommended in the first month of symptoms.[1] For patients who have had previous back surgery, MRI with contrast is probably the best test. Myelography (with or without CT) is invasive and has increased risk of complications, and is therefore indicated only in situations where MRI cannot be done or is inadequate, and the possibility of surgery is anticipated.

68

Σ

Patients for whom radiographic imaging is recommended are those with:

1. suspected *benign* conditions with symptoms persisting > 4 weeks of great enough severity to consider surgery, including:
   a) back related leg symptoms and clinically specific signs of nerve root compromise
   b) a history of neurogenic claudication (p. 1100) or other finding suggestive of lumbar spinal stenosis
   c) symptoms related to spinal deformity/imbalance, especially positional back pain that increases with time spent upright
2. red flags: physical examination or other test results suggesting other serious conditions affecting the spine (e.g. cauda equina syndrome, fracture, infection, tumor, or other mass lesions or defects)

Recommendations for use of MRI and discography to select patients for **fusion** are shown in the Practice Guideline (p. 1029).

Practice guideline: MRI and discography for patient selection for lumbar fusion*

1. **Level II**[21]:
   a) MRI is recommended as the initial diagnostic test
   b) normal appearing discs on MRI should not be considered for discography or treatment
   c) lumbar discography should not be used as a stand-alone test
   d) to consider a disc level for treatment, if discography is used, there should be a concordant pain response[a] and associated abnormalities on MRI[b]
2. **Level III**[21]: discography should be reserved for equivocal MRI findings, especially at levels adjacent to unequivocally abnormal levels

Notes:

* see also recommendations on use of facet injections (p. 1036)

[a] concordant pain response: pain identical or very similar to the patient's usual pain complaints (NB: discography can produce severe LBP in patients with no prior complaints[22,23])

[b] abnormal disc morphology on MRI: loss of T2WI signal intensity ("black disc"), disc space collapse, Modic changes (see ▶ Table 68.2), and high-intensity zones (these findings also frequently occur in asymptomatic patients[24])

68.9.2 Plain lumbosacral x-rays

General information

Unexpected findings occurred in only 1 in 2500 adults < 50 years age.[25] Diagnosis of surgical conditions of disc herniation and spinal stenosis cannot be made from plain films (although they may be inferred, further study would be required). Various congenital abnormalities of uncertain significance may be identified (e.g. spina bifida occulta), and evidence of degenerative changes (including osteophytes) are as frequent in symptomatic as in asymptomatic patients. Gonadal radiation is significant. Seldom indicated during pregnancy.

Recommendation

Not recommended for routine evaluation of patients with acute low back problems during the first month of symptoms unless a "red flag" is present (see below). Reserve LS x-rays for patients with a likelihood of having spinal malignancy, infection, inflammatory spondylitis, or clinically significant fracture. In these cases, plain x-rays are often just a starting point, and further study (CT, MRI…) may be indicated even if the plain x-rays are normal. "Red flags" for these conditions include the following:

- age > 70 years, or < 20 yrs
- systemically ill patients
- temp > 100°F (or > 38° C)
- history of malignancy
- recent infection
- patients with neurologic deficits suggesting possible cauda equina syndrome (saddle anesthesia, urinary incontinence or retention, LE weakness) (p. 1050)
- heavy alcohol or IV drug abusers
- diabetics
- immunosuppressed patients (including prolonged treatment with corticosteroids)
- recent urinary tract or spinal surgery
- *recent* trauma: any age with significant trauma, or > 50 yrs old with mild trauma
- unrelenting pain at rest
- persistent pain for more than ≈ 4 weeks
- unexplained weight loss

When spine x-rays are indicated, AP and lateral views are usually adequate.[26] Obliques and coned-down L5-S1 views more than double the radiation exposure, and add information in only 4–8% of cases,[27] and can be obtained in specific instances where warranted (e.g. to diagnose spondylolysis when spondylolisthesis is found on the lateral film).

68.9.3 MRI

Unless contraindicated, noncontrast MRI is the initial diagnostic test of choice for diagnosing most cases of disc herniation and spinal stenosis. Specificity and sensitivity for HLD are on the same order as CT/myelography, which is better than myelography alone.[1,28,29]

Advantages:

- Provides the most information about soft tissues (intervertebral discs, spinal cord, inflammation…) of any available diagnostic test
- provides information regarding tissue outside of the spinal canal, e.g. extreme lateral disc herniation (p. 1058), tumors…
- non-invasive and does not utilize ionizing radiation

Disadvantages:

- patients in severe pain or with claustrophobia may have difficulty holding still
- dose not visualize bone well
- poor for studying blood early (e.g. spinal epidural hematoma)
- expensive
- interpretation with scoliosis is more difficult, may be partially compensated by contouring visualization plane through center of canal
- a number of contraindications: see Contraindications to MRI (p. 230)

Findings:

In addition to demonstrating herniated lumbar disc (HLD) outside of the disc interspace compressing nerve root or thecal sac, MRI can demonstrate signal changes within the interspace suggestive of *disc degeneration*[30] (loss of signal intensity on T2WI, loss of disc space height) and is useful in diagnosing infections and tumors.

68.9.4 Lumbosacral CT

If technically adequate images can be obtained (e.g. good quality scanner, images not obscured by artifact from patient movement or obesity), CT can demonstrate most spine pathology. For HLD, sensitivity is 80–95%, and specificity is 68–88%.[31,32] However, even some large disc herniations will be missed with plain CT. CT studies for HLD tend to be less satisfactory in the elderly. When MRI is an option, the main utility of CT is for imaging bone to assess fractures or to demonstrate details of bony anatomy for surgery.

Disc material has density (Hounsfield units) ≈ twice that of the thecal sac. Associated findings with herniated disc include:
- loss of epidural fat (normally seen as low density in the anterolateral canal)
- loss of normal "convexity" of thecal sac (indentation by herniated disc)

Advantages:
- excellent bony detail
- non-invasive
- outpatient evaluation
- evaluates paraspinal soft tissue (e.g. to rule out tumor, paraspinal abscess…)
- advantages over MRI: faster scanning (significant in patients who have difficulty laying still for long time), less expensive, less claustrophobic, fewer contraindications, see Contraindications to MRI (p. 230)

68

Disadvantages:
- involves ionizing radiation (x-rays)
- sensitivity is significantly lower than MRI or myelogram/CT

68.9.5 Myelography

With water soluble intrathecal contrast introduced via lumbar puncture, sensitivity (62–100%) and specificity (83–94%)[33,34,35,36] are similar to CT for detection of HLD. Usually combined with post myelographic CT scan (myelogram/CT), which increases the sensitivity and especially the specificity.[37] A herniated disk in the large space between thecal sac and posterior border of vertebral bodies at L5-S1 (insensitive space) may not be seen on myelography alone (CT or MRI are usually better at demonstrating this).

Advantages:
1. evaluates cauda equina better than noncontrast CT
2. provides "functional" information about degree of stenosis (a high-degree block will allow flow of dye only after certain position changes)
3. when combined with CT, may demonstrate some anatomy obscured by metal artifact on MRI in patients with prior instrumentation

Disadvantages:
1. may miss pathology outside of the dura (including far laterally herniated disc), sensitivity is improved with post-myelographic CT
2. invasive
   a) drugs e.g. warfarin must be stopped, and sometimes bridged to heparin
   b) with occasional side effects (post LP H/A, N/V, rare seizures)
3. iodine allergic patients
   a) requires iodine allergy prep
   b) may still be risky (especially in severely iodine allergic patients)

Findings:

HLD produces extradural filling defect at the level of the intervertebral disc. Massive disc herniation or severe lumbar stenosis may produce a total or near total block. In some cases of HLD, the finding may be very subtle and may consist of a cut-off of the filling (with contrast) of the nerve root sleeve (compared to normal nerve(s) on contralateral side or at other levels). Another subtle finding may be a "dual shadow" on lateral view.

68.9.6 Bone scan

See Bone scan for low back problems (p. 1032).

68.9.7 Discography

Injection of water-soluble contrast agent directly into the nucleus pulposus of the intervertebral disc being studied by percutaneous needle access through Kambin's trianglein an awake patient. Results of the test depend on volume of dye accepted into the disc, the pressure needed to inject the dye, the configuration of the dye (including leakage from the confines of the disc space) on radiographic imaging (plain x-rays produce the so-called "discogram", CT scan is often also be utilized), and reproduction of the patient's pain on injection. Some of the basis for performing a discogram is to identify levels that may produce "discogenic pain" or "painful disc syndrome" (p. 1032), a controversial point. When the pain produced mimics the patient's presenting pain, the pain is said to be "concordant."

Critique:

Invasive. Interpretation is equivocal, and complications may occur (disc space infection, disc herniation, and significant radiation exposure with CT-discography). May be abnormal in asymptomatic patients[22,23] (as any of the above tests may be) although the false positive rate may not be quite this high.[38] See **Practice guideline: MRI and discography for patient selection for lumbar fusion** (p. 1029) for recommendations.

68.10 Electrodiagnostics for low back problems

If the diagnosis of radiculopathy seems likely on clinical grounds, electrophysiologic testing is not recommended.[1]

1. needle EMG (p. 242): can assess acute and chronic nerve root dysfunction, myelopathy and myopathy, and may be useful for patients with suspicion of other conditions (e.g. neuropathy) or when a reliable strength exam is not possible. Reduced recruitment may be seen within the first several days of onset, however, spontaneous activity takes 10–21 days to develop (p. 242) (∴ less helpful in the first ≈ 3 weeks). Also, not usually helpful with normal muscle strength exam. Accuracy is highly operator dependent and improves with knowledge about imaging studies and clinical information.[39] See findings in radiculopathy (p. 243).
2. H-reflex (p. 243): measures sensory conduction through nerve roots. Use is limited to assessing S1 radiculopathy.[40] Correlates with achilles reflex.
3. SSEPs (p. 239): assesses afferent fibers which travel in peripheral nerve and the posterior column of the spinal cord. May be abnormal in conditions affecting the dorsal columns with impaired joint position and proprioception (e.g. cervical spondylotic spinal myelopathy)
4. nerve conduction studies (including NCVs): helps identify acute and chronic entrapment neuropathies that may mimic radiculopathy
5. ✖ not recommended for assessing acute low back problems[1]
   a) F-wave response (p. 243): measures motor conduction through nerve roots, used to assess proximal neuropathies
   b) surface EMG: assesses acute and chronic recruitment patterns during static or dynamic tasks using surface (instead of needle) electrodes

68.11 Bone scan for low back problems

Description: injection of a radiolabeled compound (usually technetium-99m) that is taken up by metabolically active bone. A gamma camera localizes regions of uptake. Total radiation dose is ≈ to a set of lumbar spine x-rays.[1] Contraindicated during pregnancy. Breast feeding must be briefly suspended following a bone scan due to presence of radiotracer in the breast milk.

A moderately sensitive test which may be used in evaluating low back pain when spinal tumor,[41] infection,[42] or occult fracture is suspected from "red flags" (see ▸ Table 68.5) on history or examination, or results of lab tests or plain x-rays. Not very specific, but may locate occult lesions and help differentiate these conditions from degenerative changes. A positive bone scan suggesting one of these conditions usually must be confirmed by other diagnostic tests or procedures (no studies have compared bone scans to CT or MRI).

Low yield in patients with longstanding low back problems and normal plain x-rays and laboratory tests (especially ESR or CRP).[41]

SPECT scans may provide additional information to a bone scan.

68.12 Thermography for low back problems

✖ Not recommended.[1] Did not accurately predict absence or presence of nerve root compression seen at surgery,[43] and may be positive in a significant percentage of asymptomatic patients.[44]

68.13 Psychosocial factors

Although some patients with chronic LPB (> 3 months duration) may have started off with a diagnosable condition, psychological and socioeconomic factors (such as depression, secondary gain…) may come to play a significant role in perpetuating or amplifying pain. Psychological factors, especially elevated hysteria or hypochondriasis scales on the Minnesota Multiphasic Personality Inventory (MMPI) were found to be a better predictor of outcome than findings on radiographic imaging in one study.[39] A screening scale of 5 factors has been proposed[45] (positive findings in any 3 suggests psychological distress):

1. These items are potentially reliable[46]
   a) pain on simulated axial loading: press on top of head
   b) inconsistent performance: e.g. difficulty tolerating straight leg raising (SLR) while supine, but no difficulty when sitting
   c) overreaction during the physical exam
2. These items may not be reliable[46]
   a) inappropriate tenderness that is superficial or widespread
   b) motor or sensory abnormalities not corresponding to anatomic boundaries (e.g. for sensation: dermatomes, peripheral nerve distribution…)

However, the usefulness of this information is limited, and no effective interventions have been identified to address these factors. Therefore the AHCPR panel was unable to recommend specific assessment tools or interventions.[1]

68.14 Treatment

68.14.1 General information

An initial period of nonsurgical management (below) is indicated except in the following circumstances where urgent surgery is indicated:

Situations where conservative treatment is not indicated:

- symptoms of cauda equina syndrome: urinary retention, saddle anesthesia... (p. 1050)
- progressive neurologic deficit, or profound motor weakness
- a relative indication for proceeding to urgent surgery without conservative management is severe pain that cannot be sufficiently controlled with adequate pain medication (rare)

If specific diagnoses such as herniated intervertebral lumbar disc or symptomatic lumbar stenosis are made, surgical treatment for these conditions may be considered if the patient fails to improve satisfactorily. In cases where no specific diagnosis can be made, management consists of conservative treatment and following the patient to rule out the possible development of symptoms suggestive of a more serious diagnosis that may not have initially been evident.

68.14.2 "Conservative" treatment

This term has regrettably come to be used for non-surgical management. With minor modification, similar approaches can be used for mechanical low back pain, as well as for acute radiculopathy from disc herniation.

Recommendations (based on AHCPR findings[1] in the absence of "red flags"; note: some key literature citations are given here, primarily those from the better studies that support the Agency for

Health Care Policy and Research [AHCPR] panel recommendations. However, refer to Bigos et al.[1] for full analysis and list of references):

1. activity modifications: no studies were found that met the panels review criteria for adequate evidence. However, the following information was felt to be useful:
   a) bed rest: for 2–3 days maximum
      - the theoretical objective is to reduce symptoms by reducing pressure on the nerve roots and/or intradiscal pressures which is lowest in the supine semi-Fowler position,[47] and also to reduce movements which are experienced as painful by the patient
      - deactivation from prolonged bed rest (> 4 days) appears to be worse for patients (producing weakness, stiffness, and increased pain) than a gradual return to normal activities[48]
      - recommendations: the majority of patients with low back problems will not require bed rest. Bed rest for 2–4 days may be an option for those with severe initial radicular symptoms, however, this may be no better than watchful waiting[49] and may be harmful[50]
   b) activity modification
      - the goal is to achieve a tolerable level of discomfort while continuing sufficient physical activity to minimize disruption of daily activities
      - risk factors: although there is not agreement on their exact role, the following were identified as having an increased incidence of low back problems. Jobs requiring heavy or repetitive lifting, total body vibration (from vehicles or industrial machinery), asymmetric postures, or postures sustained for long periods (including prolonged sitting)
      - recommendations: temporarily limit heavy lifting, prolonged sitting, and bending or twisting of the back. Establish activity goals to help focus attention on expected return to full functional status

68

   c) exercise (may be part of a *physical therapy* program):
      - during the 1st month of symptoms, low-stress aerobic exercise can minimize debility due to inactivity. In the first 2 weeks, utilize exercises that minimally stress the back: walking, bicycling, or swimming
      - conditioning exercises for trunk muscles (especially back extensors, and possibly abdominal muscles) are helpful if symptoms persist (during the first 2 weeks, these exercises may aggravate symptoms)
      - there is no evidence to support stretching of back muscles, or to recommend back-specific exercise machines over traditional exercise
      - recommended exercise quotas that are gradually escalated results in better outcome than having patients simply stop when pain occurs[51]
2. analgesics:
   a) for the initial short-term period, acetaminophen (APAP) or NSAIDs (p. 137) may be used. In one study[52] of acute LBP, NSAIDs did not add any benefit to APAP + standard education (see below)
   b) stronger analgesics – mostly opioids (p. 138) – may be required for severe pain, usually severe radicular pain. For non-specific back pain, there was no earlier return to full activity than with NSAIDs or APAP.[1] Opioids should not be used > 2–3 weeks, at which time NSAIDs should be instituted unless contraindicated
3. muscle relaxants
   a) the therapeutic objective is to reduce pain by relieving muscle spasm. However, muscle spasms have not been proven to cause pain, and the most commonly used muscle relaxants have no peripheral effect on muscle spasm
   b) probably more effective than placebo, but have not been shown to be more effective than NSAIDs, and their use in combination with NSAIDs has not been shown to be more effective than use of NSAIDs alone
   c) potential for side effects: drowsiness (in up to 30%). Most manufacturers recommend use for < 2–3 weeks. Agents such as chlorzoxazone (Parafon Forte® and others) may be associated with risk of serious and potentially fatal hepatotoxicity[53]
4. education: (may be provided as part of a *physical therapy* program)
   a) explanation of the condition to the patient[54] in understandable terms, and positive reassurance that the condition will almost certainly subside[55] have been shown to be more effective than many other forms of treatment
   b) proper posture, sleeping positions, lifting techniques… should be conveyed to the patient. Formal "back school" seems to be marginally effective.[56] There may be some early benefit, but long-term efficacy could not be shown.[57] The quality and expense of such programs varies widely[1]
5. spinal manipulation therapy (SMT): defined as manual therapy in which loads are applied to the spine using long or short lever methods with the selected joint being taken to its end range of

voluntary motion, followed by application of an impulse loading (may be part of a *physical therapy* program)
   a) may be helpful for patients with acute low back problems without radiculopathy when used in the first month of symptoms (efficacy after 1 month is unproven) for a period not to exceed 1 month. One study[52] found no added benefit to APA + standard education
   b) there is insufficient evidence to recommend SMT in the presence of radiculopathy
   c) SMT should not be used in the face of severe or progressive neurologic deficit until serious conditions have been ruled out
   d) ✖ reports of arterial dissection: especially vertebral artery (p. 1325) and stroke, myelopathy & subdural hematoma with *cervical* SMT and cauda equina syndrome with lumbar SMT[58,59,60] and the uncertainty of benefits have led to the questioning of the use of SMT[58] (especially cervical)
6. epidural injections:
   a) epidural (cortico)steroid injections (ESI): there is no evidence that this is effective in treating acute radiculopathy.[61] Most studies that show benefit are retrospective and noncontrolled. Prospective studies yield varied results.[62] Some improvement at 3 & 6 weeks may occur (but no functional benefit, and no change in the need for surgery), with no benefit at 3 months.[63] The response in chronic back pain is poor in comparison to acute pain. ESI may be an option for *short-term* relief of radicular pain when control on oral medications is inadequate or for patients who are not surgical candidates
   b) there is no evidence to support the use of epidural injections of steroids, local anesthetics and/or opioids for LBP without radiculopathy
   c) reports on efficacy with conditions such as lumbar spinal stenosis are conflicting,[62] relief is almost uniformly temporary (4–6 weeks with initial injection, shorter times with subsequent ones)

✖ *Not* recommended by the AHCPR panel[1] for treatment of acute low back problems in the absence of "red flags" (▶ Table 68.5):
1. medications
   a) oral steroids: no difference was found at one week and 1 year after randomization to receive 1 week therapy with oral dexamethasone or placebo[64]
   b) colchicine: conflicting evidence shows either some[65] or no[66] therapeutic benefit. Side effects of N/V and diarrhea were common[1]
   c) antidepressant medications: most studies of these medications were for chronic back pain. Some methodologically flawed studies failed to show benefits when compared to placebo for chronic (not acute) LBP[67]
2. physical treatments
   a) TENS (transcutaneous electrical nerve stimulation): *not* statistically significantly better than placebo, and added no benefit to exercise alone[68]
   b) traction (including pelvic traction): not demonstrated to be effective.[69] One possible explanation for lack of benefit is that due to the sizable paraspinal muscles and ligaments (as compared to the cervical spine) the amount of weight required to distract the intervertebral disc space is approximately ≥ 2/3 of the patient's body weight, which is painful and/or pulls the patient to the foot of the bed
   c) physical agents and modalities: including heat (including diathermy), ice, ultrasound. Benefit is insufficiently proven to justify their cost, however, self-administered home programs for application of heat or cold may be considered. Ultrasound and diathermy should not be used in pregnancy
   d) lumbar corsets and support belts: not proven beneficial for acute back problems. Prophylactic use has been advocated to reduce time lost from work by individuals doing frequent lifting as part of their job, but this is controversial[70]
   e) biofeedback: has not been studied for acute back problems. Primarily advocated for chronic LBP, where effectiveness is controversial[71]
3. injection therapy
   a) trigger point and ligamentous injections: the theory that trigger points cause or perpetuate LBP is controversial and disputed by many experts. Injections of local anesthetic are of equivocal efficacy (saline may be as effective[72]) and are mildly invasive
   b) (zygapophyseal) facet joint injections: theoretical basis is that there exists a "facet syndrome" producing LBP which is aggravated by spine extension, with no nerve root tension signs (p. 1047). No studies have adequately investigated injections for pain < 3 months duration. For chronic LBP, neither the agent nor the location (intrafacet or pericapsular) made a significant difference in outcomes[73,74]

c) epidural injections in the absence of radiculopathy: see above
d) acupuncture: no studies were found that evaluated the use in acute back problems. All randomized clinical trials found were for patients with chronic LBP, and even the best studies were felt to be mediocre and contradictory. Meta-analysis found acupuncture was more effective in relieving chronic LBP than sham or no treatment,[75] but there was no comparison to other therapies

Practice guideline: Injection therapy for low-back pain

Therapeutic recommendations

Level III[76]: lumbar epidural injections or trigger point injections are not recommended for long-term relief of chronic LBP. These techniques or facet injections may be used to provide temporary relief in select patients

Diagnostic recommendations

Level III[76]: lumbar facet injections

- may predict the response to radiofrequency facet ablation
- ✖ not recommended as a diagnostic tool to predict the response to lumbar fusion

68.14.3 Surgical treatment

Indications for surgery for herniated lumbar disc

See the section on **herniated lumbar discs** (p. 1049).

Indications for fusion for chronic LBP without stenosis or spondylolisthesis

Very controversial.

Practice guideline: Lumbar fusion for LBP without stenosis or spondylolisthesis

Level I[77]: lumbar fusion is recommended for carefully selected patients with disabling LBP due to one- or two-level degenerative disease without stenosis or spondylolisthesis (in the primary quoted study[78] patients had chronic LBP for ≥ 2 years and had radiologic evidence of disc degeneration at L4-L5, L5-S1, or both, and had failed best medical management)

Level III[77,79]: an intensive course of PT and cognitive therapy is recommended as an option for patients with LBP in whom conventional medical management has failed

Practice guideline: Choice of fusion technique

Level II[80]: for ALIF or ALIF + instrumentation, the addition of a posterolateral fusion is not recommended (the demonstrated benefit does not outweigh the additional time and blood loss involved)

Level III[80]:

- either a posterolateral fusion or an interbody fusion (PLIF, TLIF or ALIF) are options for patients with LBP due to DDD at 1 or 2 levels
- an interbody graft is an option to improve fusion rates and functional outcome (caution: the improvement in fusion rate and outcome is marginal, and interbody fusion is associated with an increased complication rate, especially with combined approaches, e.g. 360° fusion)

✖ the use of multiple approaches (anterior + posterior) is not recommended as a routine option for LBP without deformity

Surgical treatment options

The type of surgical procedure chosen is tailored to the specific condition identified. Examples are shown in ▶ Table 68.6. Discussion of some options is also provided below.

Lumbar spinal fusion

Although there is no consensus on the indications,[81] lumbar spinal fusion (LSF) is accepted treatment for fracture/dislocation or instability resulting from tumor or infection.

For degenerative spine disease, practice parameters have been developed and are included herein. Pain associated with Modic type 1 changes (see ▶ Table 68.2) may respond to stabilization procedures, the other Modic types do not exhibit this association.

Practice guideline: Lumbar fusion for disc herniation

Level III[82]:
1. lumbar fusion is *not* routinely recommended following disc excision in patients with HLD or 1st time recurrent HLD causing radiculopathy
2. lumbar fusion is a potential adjunct to disc excision in cases of a HLD or recurrent HLD:
   a) with evidence of preoperative lumbar spinal deformity or instability
   b) in patients with chronic axial LBP associated with radiculopathy

Instrumentation as an adjunct to fusion

Practice guideline: Pedicle screw fixation

Level III[83]: pedicle screw fixation is recommended as a treatment option for patients with LBP treated with posterolateral fusion who are at high risk for fusion failure (routine use of pedicle screws is discouraged because of conflicting evidence of benefit, together with considerable evidence of increased cost and complications)

The use of instrumentation increases the fusion rate.[84] Hardware used in the absence of fusion will eventually fatigue, especially in the region of the lumbar lordosis. Therefore, instrumentation must be viewed as a temporary internal stabilizing measure while awaiting the fusion process to complete.

68.15 Chronic low back pain

Rarely can an anatomic diagnosis be made in patients with chronic LBP ≥ 3 months duration.[85] Also, see Psychosocial factors (p. 1033). Patients with chronic pain syndromes (CPS) refer to their problems with affective or emotional terms with a higher frequency than those with acute pain.[86] The

Table 68.6 Surgical options for low back problems

Condition	Surgical treatment options
"routine" HLD or initial recurrence of HLD	• standard discectomy and microdiscectomy are of similar efficacy • ✖ intradiscal procedures: nucleotome, laser disc decompression are not recommended (p. 1052)
foraminal or far lateral HLD	• partial or total facetectomy (p. 1059) • extracanal approach (p. 1059) • endoscopic techniques
lumbar spinal stenosis	• simple decompressive laminectomy • laminectomy plus fusion: may be indicated for patients with degenerative spondylolisthesis, stenosis and radiculopathy, adult degenerative scoliosis (ADS), or instability

Table 68.7 Chances of patients going back to work

Time out of work	Chances of getting back to work
<6 mos	50%
1 yr	20%
2 yrs	<5%

amount of time that a patient has been out of work due to low back problems is related to the chances of the patient getting back to work as shown in ▶ Table 68.7.

68.16 Coccydynia

68.16.1 General information

Pain and tenderness around the coccyx. A symptom, not a diagnosis. Typically, discomfort is experienced on sitting or on rising from sitting. More common in females, possibly due to a more prominent coccyx. The condition is unusual enough in males that in the absence of local trauma, strong consideration should be given to an underlying condition.

68

68.16.2 Etiologies

For differential diagnosis, see Acute low back pain (p.1416). Better accepted etiologies include[87]:

1. local trauma (may be associated with fracture or dislocation):
   a) 25% of patients give a history of a fall
   b) 12% had repetitive trauma (rowing machine, prolonged bicycle riding…)
   c) 12% started with parturition
   d) 5% started following a surgical procedure (half of which were in the lithotomy position)
2. idiopathic: excluding traumatic cases, no etiology can be identified in most cases
3. neoplasms
   a) chordoma
   b) giant cell tumor
   c) intradural schwannoma
   d) perineural cyst
   e) intra-osseous lipoma
   f) carcinoma of the rectum
   g) sacral hemangioma[88]
   h) pelvic metastases (e.g. from prostate cancer)
4. prostatitis

Controversial etiologies include[87,89]:

1. local pressure over a prominent coccyx
2. referred pain:
   a) spinal disease
      - herniated lumbosacral disc
      - cauda equina syndrome
      - arachnoiditis
   b) pelvic/visceral disease
      - pelvic inflammatory disease (PID)
      - perirectal abscess
      - perirectal fistula
      - pilonidal cyst
3. inflammation of the various ligaments attached to the coccyx
4. neurosis or frank hysteria

Histological evaluation of the coccyx has not helped delineate the cause, even though avascular necrosis has been suggested.[90]

68.16.3 Evaluation

MRI: effective for detecting soft tissue masses, including presacral masses

CT scan: no characteristic finding in coccydynia findings. Very sensitive for detecting bony pathology (fracture, destructive lesion…).

Sacrococcygeal films are often performed to rule-out a bony destructive lesion. Often, the question of a fracture will be raised, and many times cannot be definitely ruled-in or out based on this study. There may or may not be any significance of such a fracture.

Nuclear bone scans were not helpful in 50 patients with coccydynia.[87]

68.16.4 Treatment

Numerous treatments have been proposed, and some are offered here for historical purposes[87] (and to dissuade casual attempts to effect a "new" cure that in reality has already been tried):
1. plaster jackets
2. hot baths (sitz baths), heating pads
3. massage therapy
4. XRT
5. psychotherapy

Most cases resolve within ≈ 3 months of conservative management consisting of NSAIDs, mild analgesics, and measures to reduce pressure on the coccyx (e.g. a rubber ring ("doughnut") sitting cushion, lumbar supports to maintain sitting lumbar lordosis to shift weight from coccyx to posterior thighs).[91]

Management recommendations for refractory cases[87,91]
1. local injection: 60% respond to corticosteroid + local anesthetic (40 mg Depo-Medrol® in 10 cc of 0.25% bipuvicaine). Recommended as initial treatment; response should be achieved by 2 injections
2. manipulation of the coccyx: usually under general anesthesia. ≈ 85% successful when combined with local injection
3. ± physiotherapy (diathermy & ultrasound): found to be of benefit only in ≈ 16% (may be more effective with the addition of gentle manipulation of the coccyx *without* general anesthesia[92])
4. caudal epidural steroid injection
5. blockade or neurolysis (with chemicals or by cryoablation[93]) of the ganglion impar (AKA ganglion of Walther, the lowest ganglion of the paired paravertebral sympathetic chain, located just anterior to the sacrococcygeal junction): some success has been described with this technique (traditionally used for intractable sympathetic perineal pain of neoplastic etiology[94])
6. neurolytic techniques directed to S4, S5 and coccygeal nerves
7. coccygectomy (surgical removal of the mobile portion of the coccyx, followed by smoothening of the residual bony prominence on the sacrum): was required in ≈ 20% of patients in one series,[87] with a reported success rate of 90%. However, many practitioners do not view this as a highly effective treatment and feel that great restraint should be used in considering this form of therapy

68.16.5 Recurrence

Occurs in ≈ 20% of conservatively treated cases, usually within the first year. Repeat therapy was often successful in providing permanent relief. More aggressive treatment may be considered for refractory cases.

68.17 Failed back surgery syndrome

68.17.1 General information

Definition: failure to satisfactorily improve low back pain or radiculopathy following back surgery. These patients often require analgesics and are unable to return to work. The failure rate for lumbar discectomy to provide satisfactory long-term pain relief is ≈ 8–25%.[95] Pending legal or worker's compensation claims were the most frequent deterrents to a good outcome.[96]

68.17.2 Etiologies

Factors that may cause or contribute to the failed back syndrome:
1. incorrect initial diagnosis
   a) inadequate pre-op imaging
   b) clinical findings not correlated with abnormality demonstrated on imaging
   c) other causes of symptoms (sometimes in the presence of what was considered to be an appropriate lesion on imaging studies which may have been asymptomatic): e.g. trochanteric bursitis, diabetic amyotrophy...
2. continued nerve root or cauda equina compression caused by:
   a) residual compression (retained disc material, osteophytes...)
   b) recurrent pathology at same level: disc reherniation at the same level, usually have pain-free interval > 6 mos post-op (p. 1061); or restenosis (over many years[97] – was more common with midline fusions)
   c) adjacent level pathology: disc herniation or stenosis[97]
   d) compression of nerve root by peridural scar (granulation) tissue (see below)
   e) pseudomeningocele
   f) epidural hematoma
   g) conjoined nerve roots with compression at another level or in atypical location
   h) segmental instability: 3 patterns,[98] 1) lateral rotational instability, 2) post-op spondylolisthesis, 3) post-op scoliosis

68

3. permanent nerve root injury from the original disc herniation or from surgery, includes deafferentation pain which is usually constant and burning or ice cold
4. adhesive arachnoiditis: responsible for 6–16% of persistent symptoms in post-op patients[99] (see below)
5. discitis (p. 356): usually produces exquisite back pain 2–4 weeks post-op
6. spondylosis
7. other causes of back pain unrelated to the original condition: paraspinal muscle spasm, myofascial syndrome... Look for trigger points, evidence of spasm
8. post-op reflex sympathetic dystrophy, RSD (p. 1054)
9. "non-anatomic factors": poor patient motivation, secondary gains, drug addiction, psychological problems (p. 1053)...

68.17.3 Arachnoiditis (AKA adhesive arachnoiditis)

General information

Inflammatory condition of the lumbar nerve roots. Actually a misnomer, since adhesive arachnoiditis is really an inflammatory process or fibrosis that involves all three meningeal layers (pia, arachnoid, and dura).

Etiologies/risk factors

Many putative "risk factors" have been described for the development of arachnoiditis, including[100]:
1. spinal anesthesia: either due to the anesthetic agents or to detergent contaminants on the syringes used for same
2. spinal meningitis: pyogenic, syphilitic, tuberculous
3. neoplasms
4. myelographic contrast agents: less common with currently available nonionic water soluble contrast agents
5. trauma
   a) post-surgical: especially after multiple operations
   b) external trauma
6. hemorrhage
7. idiopathic

Radiographic findings in arachnoiditis

NB: Radiographic evidence of arachnoiditis may also be found in *asymptomatic* patients.[100] Arachnoiditis must be differentiated from tumor: the central adhesive type (see below) may resemble CSF seeding of tumor, and myelographic block may mimic intrathecal tumor.

Table 68.8 Myelographic classification of arachnoiditis

Type	Description
1	unilateral focal filling defect centered on the nerve root sleeve adjacent to disc space
2	circumferential constriction around thecal sac
3	complete obstruction with "stalactites" or "candle guttering", "candle-dripping", or "paint-brush" filling defects
4	infundibular cul-de-sac with loss of radicular striations

MRI

3 patterns on MRI[101,102]:

1. central adhesion of the nerve roots into 1 or 2 central "cords"
2. "empty thecal sac" pattern: roots adhere to meninges around periphery, only CSF signal is visible intrathecally
3. thecal sac filled with inflammatory tissue, no CSF signal. Corresponds with myelographic block and *candle-dripping* appearance

Enhancement: acute arachnoiditis may enhance. Chronic arachnoiditis usually does not enhance with gadolinium as much as e.g. tumor.

68

Myelogram

May demonstrate complete block, or clumping of nerve roots. One of many myelographic classification systems[103] for arachnoiditis is shown in ▶ Table 68.8.

68.17.4 Peridural scar

General information

Although peridural scar tissue is frequently blamed for causing recurrent symptoms,[104,105] there has been no proof of correlation between the two.[106] Peridural fibrosis is an inevitable sequelae to lumbar disc surgery just as post-op fibrosis is a consequence of any surgical procedure. Even patients who are relieved of their pain following discectomy develop some scar tissue post-op.[107] Although it has been shown that if a patient has recurrent radicular pain following a lumbar discectomy there is a 70% chance that extensive peridural scar will be found on MRI,[106] this study also showed that on post-op MRIs at 6 months, 43% of patients will have extensive scar, but 84% of the time this will be *asymptomatic*.[108] Thus, one must use clinical grounds to determine if a patient with extensive scar on MRI is in the 16% minority of patients with radicular symptoms attributable to scar.[108]

See a discussion of measures to reduce peridural scarring (p. 1053).

Radiologic evaluation

General information

Patients with only persistent low back or hip pain without a strong radicular component, with a neurologic exam that is normal or unchanged from pre-op, should be treated symptomatically. Patients with signs or symptoms of recurrent radiculopathy (positive SLR is a sensitive test for nerve root compression), especially if these follow a period of apparent recovery, should undergo further evaluation.

It is critical to differentiate residual/recurrent disc herniation from scar tissue and adhesive arachnoiditis as surgical treatment has generally poor results with the latter two (below).

MRI without and with IV gadolinium

Diagnostic *test of choice*. The best exam for detecting residual or recurrent disc herniation, and to reliably differentiate disc from scar tissue. Pre-contrast studies with T1WI and T2WI yields an accuracy of ≈ 83%, comparable to IV enhanced CT.[109,110] With the addition of gadolinium, using the protocol below yields 100% sensitivity, 71% specificity, and 89% accuracy.[111] May also detect adhesive arachnoiditis (see above). As scar becomes more fibrotic and calcified with time, the differential enhancement with respect to disc material attenuates and may become undetectable at some point, ≈ 1–2 years post-op[110] (some scar continues to enhance for > 20 yrs).

Recommended MRI protocol

See reference.[111]

Get pre-contrast T1WI and T2WI. Give 0.1 mmol/kg gadolinium IV. Obtain T1WI images within 10 minutes (early post-contrast). No benefit from post-contrast T2WI.

Findings on unenhanced MRI

Signal from a HLD becomes more intense as the sequence is varied from T1WI → T2WI, whereas scar tissue becomes less intense with this transition. Indirect signs (also applicable to CT):

1. mass effect: a nerve root is displaced away from disc material, whereas it may be retracted toward scar tissue by adherence to it
2. location: disc material tends to be in contiguity with the disc interspace (best seen on sagittal MRI)

Findings on enhanced MRI

On early (≤ 10 mins post-contrast) T1WI images: scar enhances inhomogeneously, whereas disc does not enhance at all. A nonenhancing central area surrounded by irregular enhancing material probably represents disc wrapped in scar. Venous plexus also enhances, and may be more pronounced when it is distorted by disc material, but the morphology is easily differentiated from scar tissue in these cases.

On late (> 30 mins post-contrast) T1WI: scar enhances homogeneously, disc had variable or no enhancement. Normal nerve roots do not enhance even on late images.

CT scan without and with IV (iodinated) contrast

Unenhanced CT scan density measurements are unreliable in the postoperative back.[112] Enhanced CT is only fairly good in differentiating scar (enhancing) from disc (unenhancing with possible rim enhancement). Accuracy is about equal to *unenhanced* MRI.

Myelography, with post-myelographic CT

Postoperative myelographic criteria alone are unreliable for distinguishing disc material from scar.[100,113] With the addition of CT scan, neural compression is clearly demonstrated, but scar still cannot be reliably distinguished from disc.

Myelography (especially with post-myelographic CT) is very capable of demonstrating arachnoiditis[113] (see above).

Plain LS x-rays

Generally helpful only in cases of instability, malalignment, or spondylosis.[113] Flexion/extension views are most helpful when trying to demonstrate instability.

68.17.5 Treatment of failed back surgery syndrome

Post-operative discitis

For treatment of intervertebral disc-space infection, see Discitis (p. 356).

Symptomatic treatment

Recommended for patients who do not have radicular signs and symptoms, or for most patients demonstrated to have scar tissue or adhesive arachnoiditis on imaging. As in other cases of non-specific LBP treatment includes: short-term bed rest, analgesics (non-narcotic in most cases), anti-inflammatory medication (non-steroidal, and occasionally a short course of steroids), and physical therapy.

Surgery

Generally reserved for those with recurrent or residual disc herniation, segmental instability, or patients with a pseudomeningocele. Patients with post-op spinal instability should be considered for spinal fusion (p. 1037).[98]

In most series with sufficient follow-up, success rates after reoperation are lower in patients with only epidural scar (as low as 1%) compared to those patients with disc and scar (still only ≈ 37%).[95]

An overall success rate (> 50% pain relief for > 2 yrs) of ≈ 34% was seen in one series,[105] with better results in patients that were young, female, with good results following previous surgery, a small number of previous operations, employment prior to surgery, predominantly radicular (cf axial) pain, and absence of scar requiring lysis.

In addition to the absence of disc material, factors associated with poor outcome were: sensory loss involving more than one dermatome, and patients with past or pending compensation claims.[95,114]

Arachnoiditis:

Surgery for carefully selected patients with arachnoiditis (those with mild radiographic involvement (Types 1 & 2 in ▶ Table 68.8), and < 3 previous back operations)[103] has met with moderate success (although in this series, no patient returned to work). Approximate success rate in other series[115,116]: 50% failure, 20% able to work but with symptoms, 10–19% with no symptoms. Surgery consists of removal of extradural scar enveloping the thecal sac, removing any herniated disc fragments, and performing foraminotomies when indicated. Intradural lysis of adhesions is *not* indicated since no means for preventing reformation of scar has been identified.[116]

References

[1] Bigos S, Bowyer O, Braen G, et al. Acute Low Back Problems in Adults. Clinical Practice Guideline No.14. AHCPR Publication No. 95-0642. Rockville, MD: Agency for Health Care Policy and Research, Public Health Service, U.S. Department of Health and Human Services; 1994

[2] Cypress BK. Characteristics of Physician Visits for Back Symptoms: A National Perspective. Am J Public Health. 1983; 73:389–395

[3] Cunningham LS, Kelsey JL. Epidemiology of Musculoskeletal Impairments and Associated Disability. Am J Public Health. 1984; 74:574–579

[4] Frymoyer JW. Back Pain and Sciatica. N Engl J Med. 1988; 318:291–300

[5] Fardon DF, Milette PC. Nomenclature and classification of lumbar disc pathology. Recommendations of the Combined task Forces of the North American Spine Society, American Society of Spine Radiology, and American Society of Neuroradiology. Spine. 2001; 26:E93–E113

[6] Fardon DF, Williams AL, Dohring EJ, Murtagh FR, Gabriel Rothman SL, Sze GK. Lumbar disc nomenclature: version 2.0: Recommendations of the combined task forces of the North American Spine Society, the American Society of Spine Radiology and the American Society of Neuroradiology. Spine J. 2014. DOI: 10.1016/j.spinee.2014.04.022

[7] McCarron RF, Wimpee MW, Hudkins PG, Laros GS. The Inflammatory Effect of Nucleus Pulposus: A Possible Element in the Pathogenesis of Low-Back Pain. Spine. 1987; 12:760–764

[8] Modic MT. In: Degenerative disorders of the spine. Magnetic Resonance Imaging of the Spine. New York: Yearbook Medical; 1989:83–95

[9] Fairbank JC, Couper J, Davies JB, O'Brien JP. The Oswestry low back pain disability questionnaire. Physiotherapy. 1980; 66:271–273

[10] Fairbank JC, Pynsent PB. The Oswestry Disability Index. Spine. 2000; 25:2940–52; discussion 2952

[11] Baker D, Pynsent P, Fairbank J, Roland M, Jenner J. In: The Oswestry Disability Index revisited. Back pain: New approaches to rehabilitation and education. Manchester: Manchester University Press; 1989:174–186

[12] Roland M, Morris R. A study of the natural history of back pain. Part I: development of a reliable and sensitive measure of disability in low-back pain. Spine (Phila Pa 1976). 1983; 8:141–144

[13] Grevitt M, Khazim R, Webb J, Mulholland R, Shepperd J. The short form-36 health survey questionnaire in spine surgery. J Bone Joint Surg Br. 1997; 79:48–52

[14] Kelsey JL, White AA, Gordon SL. Idiopathic Low Back Pain: Magnitude of the Problem. 1982

[15] Deyo RA, Bigos SJ, Maravilla KR. Diagnostic Imaging Procedures for the Lumbar Spine. Ann Intern Med. 1989; 111:865–867

[16] Hitselberger WE, Witten RM. Abnormal Myelograms in Asymptomatic Patients. J Neurosurg. 1968; 28:204–206

[17] Wiesel SW, Tsourmas N, Feffer HL, Citrin CM, Patronas N. A Study of Computer-Assisted Tomography. I. The Incidence of Positive CAT Scans in an Asymptomatic Group of Patients. Spine. 1984; 9:549–551

[18] Jensen MC, Brant-Zawadzki MN, Obuchowski N, et al. Magnetic Resonance Imaging of the Lumbar Spine in People Without Back Pain. N Engl J Med. 1994; 331:69–73

[19] Boden SD, Davis DO, Dina TS, Patronas NJ, Wiesel SW. Abnormal Magnetic-Resonance Scans of the Lumbar Spine in Asymptomatic Subjects. J Bone Joint Surg. 1990; 72A:403–408

[20] Spitzer WO, LeBlanc FE, Dupuis M, et al. Scientific Approach to the Assessment and Management of Activity-Related Spinal Disorders: A Monograph for Clinicians: Report of the Quebec Task Force on Spinal Disorders. Chapter 3: Diagnosis of the Problem (The Problem of Diagnosis). Spine. 1987; 12: S16–S21

[21] Resnick DK, Choudhri TF, Dailey AT, Groff MW, Khoo L, Matz PG, Mummaneni P, Watters WC, Wang J, Walters BC, Hadley MN. Part 6: Magnetic resonance imaging and discography for patient selection for lumbar fusion. J Neurosurg Spine. 2005; 2:662–669

[22] Holt EP. The Question of Lumbar Discography. J Bone Joint Surg. 1968; 50A:720–726

[23] Carragee EJ, Tanner CM, Khurana S, Hayward C, Welsh J, Date E, Truong T, Rossi M, Hagle C. The rates of false-positive lumbar discography in select patients without low back symptoms. Spine. 2000; 25:1373–80; discussion 1381

[24] Carragee EJ, Paragioudakis SJ, Khurana S. 2000 Volvo Award winner in clinical studies: Lumbar high-intensity zone and discography in subjects without low back problems. Spine. 2000; 25:2987–2992

[25] Nachemson AL. The Lumbar Spine: An Orthopedic Challenge. Spine. 1976; 1:59–71

[26] World Health Organization. A Rational Approach to Radiodiagnostic Investigations. 1983

[27] Scavone JG, Latschaw RF, Rohrer GV. Use of Lumbar Spine Films: Statistical Evaluation of a University Teaching Hospital. JAMA. 1981; 246:1105–1108

[28] Modic MT, Masaryk T, Boumphrey F, et al. Lumbar Herniated Disk Disease and Canal Stenosis: Prospective Evaluation by Surface Coil MR, CT, and Myelography. AJR. 1986; 147:757–765

[29] Jackson RP, Cain JE, Jacobs RR, Cooper BR, McManus GE. The Neuroradiologic Diagnosis of Lumbar Herniated Nucleus Pulposus: II. A Comparison of Computed Tomography (CT), Myelography, CT-

Myelography, and Magnetic Resonance Imaging. Spine. 1989; 14:1362–1367
[30] Modic MT, Pavlicek W, Weinstein MA, Hardy R, et al. Magnetic Resonance Imaging of Intervertebral Disk Disease. Radiology. 1984; 152:103–111
[31] Bosacco SJ, Berman AT, Garbarino JL, et al. A Comparison of CT Scanning and Myelography in the Diagnosis of Lumbar Disc Herniation. Clin Orthop. 1984; 190:124–128
[32] Moufarrij NA, Hardy RW, Weinstein MA. Computed Tomographic, Myelographic, and Operative Findings in Patients with Suspected Herniated Lumbar Discs. Neurosurgery. 1983; 12:184–188
[33] Aejmelaeus R, Hiltunen H, Härkönen M, et al. Myelographic Versus Clinical Diagnostics in Lumbar Disc Disease. Arch Orthop Trauma Surg. 1984; 103:18–25
[34] Herron LD, Turner J. Patient Selection for Lumbar Laminectomy and Discectomy with a Revised Objective Rating System. Clin Orthop. 1985; 199:145–152
[35] Kortelainen P, Puranen J, Koivisto E, Lähde S. Symptoms and Signs of Sciatica and their Relation to the Localization of the Lumbar Disc Herniation. Spine. 1985; 10:88–92
[36] Hirsch C, Nachemson A. The Reliability of Lumbar Disk Surgery. Clin Orthop. 1963; 29
[37] Slebus FG, Braakman R, Schipper J, et al. Non-Corresponding Radiological and Surgical Diagnoses in Patients Operated for Sciatica. Acta Neurochir. 1988; 94:137–143
[38] Walsh TR, Weinstein JN, Spratt KF, et al. Lumbar Discography in Normal Patients. A Controlled, Prospective Study. J Bone Joint Surg. 1990; 72A:1081–1088
[39] Spengler DM, Ouellette EA, Battié M, Zeh J. Elective Discectomy for Herniation of a Lumbar Disc. Additional Experience with an Objective Method. J Bone Joint Surg. 1990; 72A:230–237
[40] Braddom RL, Johnson EW. Standardization of H Reflex and Diagnostic Use in S1 Radiculopathy. Arch Phys Med Rehabil. 1974; 55:161–166
[41] Schütte HE, Park WM. The Diagnostic Value of Bone Scintigraphy in Patients with Low Back Pain. Skeletal Radiol. 1983; 10:1–4
[42] Whalen JL, Brown ML, McLeod R, Fitzgerald RH. Limitations of Indium Leukocyte Imaging for the Diagnosis of Spine Infections. Spine. 1991; 16:193–197
[43] Mills GH, Davies GK, Getty CJM, Conway J. The Evaluation of Liquid Crystal Thermography in the Investigation of Nerve Root Compression due to Lumbosacral Lateral Spinal Stenosis. Spine. 1986; 11:427–432
[44] Harper CM, Low PA, Fealy RD, et al. Utility of Thermography in the Diagnosis of Lumbosacral Radiculopathy. Neurology. 1991; 41:1010–1014
[45] Waddell G, McCulloch JA, Kummel E, Vernner RM. Nonorganic Physical Signs in Low Back Pain. Spine. 1980; 5:117–125
[46] McCombe PF, Fairbank JCT, Cockersole BC, Pynsent PB. Reproducibility of Physical Signs in Low-Back Pain. Spine. 1989; 14:908–918
[47] Nachemson AL. Newest Knowledge of Low Back Pain. A Critical Look. Clin Orthop. 1992; 279:8–20
[48] Deyo RA, Diehl AK, Rosenthal M. How Many Days of Bed Rest for Acute Low Back Pain? A Randomized Clinical Trial. N Engl J Med. 1986; 315:1064–1070
[49] Vroomen PCAJ, de Krom MCTFM, Wilmink JT, et al. Lack of Effectiveness of Bed Rest for Sciatica. N Engl J Med. 1999; 340:418–423
[50] Allen C, Glasziou P, Del Mar C. Bed Rest: A Potentially Harmful Treatment Needing More Careful Evaluation. Lancet. 1999; 354:1229–1233
[51] Lindström I, Ohlund C, Eek C, Wallin L, Peterson L, Fordyce WE, Nachemson AL. The Effect of Graded Activity on Patients with Subacute Low Back Pain: A Randomized Prospective Clinical Study with an Operant-Conditioning Behavioral Approach. Phys Ther. 1992; 72:279–293
[52] Hancock MJ, Maher CG, Latimer J, McLachlan AJ, Cooper CW, Day RO, Spindler MF, McAuley JH. Assessment of diclofenac or spinal manipulative therapy, or both, in addition to recommended first-line treatment for acute low back pain: a randomised controlled trial. Lancet. 2007; 370:1638–1643
[53] Chlorzoxazone Hepatotoxicity. Med Letter. 1996; 38
[54] Deyo RA, Diehl AK. Patient Satisfaction with Medical Care for Low-Back Pain. Spine. 1986; 11:28–30
[55] Thomas KB. General Practice Consultations: Is There Any Point in Being Positive? Br Med J. 1987; 294:1200–1202
[56] Keijsers JFEM, Bouter LM, Meertens RM. Validity and Comparability of Studies on the Effects of Back Schools. Physiother Theory Pract. 1991; 7:177–184
[57] Bergquist-Ullman M, Larsson U. Acute Low Back Pain in Industry. A Controlled Prospective Study with Special Reference to Therapy and Confounding Factors. Acta Orthop Scand. 1977; 170:1–117
[58] Di Fabio RP. Manipulation of the cervical spine: risks and benefits. Phys Ther. 1999; 79:50–65
[59] Ernst E. Life-threatening complications of spinal manipulation. Stroke. 2001; 32:809–810
[60] Stevinson C, Honan W, Cooke B, Ernst E. Neurological complications of cervical spine manipulation. J R Soc Med. 2001; 94:107–110
[61] Cuckler JM, Bernini PA, Wiesel SW, et al. The Use of Epidural Steroids in the Treatment of Lumbar Radicular Pain. A Prospective, Randomized, Double-Blind Study. J Bone Joint Surg. 1985; 67A:63–66
[62] Spaccarelli KC. Lumbar and Caudal Epidural Corticosteroid Injections. Mayo Clin Proc. 1996; 71:169–178
[63] Carette S, Leclaire R, Marcoux S, et al. Epidural Corticosteroid Injections for Sciatica due to Herniated Nucleus Pulposus. N Engl J Med. 1997; 336:1634–1640
[64] Haimovic IC, Beresford HR. Dexamethasone is Not Superior to Placebo for Treating Lumbosacral Radicular Pain. Neurology. 1986; 36:1593–1594
[65] Meek JB, Giudice VW, McFadden JW, Key JD. Colchicine Confirmed as Highly Effective in Disk Disorders. Final Results of a Double-Blind Study. J Neuro & Orthop Med & Surg. 1985; 6:211–218
[66] Schnebel BE, Simmons JW. The Use of Oral Colchicine for Low-Back Pain. A Double-Blind Study. Spine. 1988; 13:354–357
[67] Goodkin K, Gullion CM, Agras WS. A Randomized, Double-Blind, Placebo-Controlled Trial of Trazodone Hydrochloride in Chronic Low Back Pain Syndrome. J Clin Psychopharmacol. 1990; 10:269–278
[68] Deyo RA, Walsh NE, Martin DC, et al. A Controlled Trial of Transcutaneous Electrical Stimulation (TENS) and Exercise for Chronic Low Back Pain. N Engl J Med. 1990; 322:1627–1634
[69] Mathews JA, Hickling J. Lumbar Traction: A Double-Blind Controlled Study for Sciatica. Rheumatol Rehabil. 1975; 14:222–225
[70] van Poppel NNM, Koes BW, van der Ploeg T, et al. Lumbar Supports and Education for the Prevention of Low Back Pain in Industry: A Randomized Controlled Study. JAMA. 1998; 279:1789–1794
[71] Bush C, Ditto B, Feuerstein M. A Controlled Evaluation of Paraspinal EMG Biofeedback in the Treatment of Chronic Low Back Pain. Health Psychol. 1985; 4:307–321
[72] Frost FA, Jessen B, Siggaard-Andersen J. A Control, Double-Blind Comparison of Mepivicaine Injection Versus Saline Injection for Myofascial Pain. Lancet. 1980; 1:499–501
[73] Carette S, Marcoux S, Truchon R, et al. A Controlled Trial of Corticosteroid Injections into Facet Joints for Chronic Low Back Pain. N Engl J Med. 1991; 325:1002–1007
[74] Jackson RP. The Facet Syndrome. Myth or Reality? Clin Orthop Rel Res. 1992; 279:110–121
[75] Manheimer E, White A, Berman B, Forys K, Ernst E. Meta-analysis: acupuncture for low back pain. Ann Intern Med. 2005; 142:651–663
[76] Resnick DK, Choudhri TF, Dailey AT, Groff MW, Khoo L, Matz PG, Mummaneni P, Watters WC,

Wang J, Walters BC, Hadley MN. Part 13: Injection therapies, low-back pain, and lumbar fusion. J Neurosurg: Spine. 2005; 2:707–715

[77] Resnick DK, Choudhri TF, Dailey AT, Groff MW, Khoo L, Matz PG, Mummaneni P, Watters WC, Wang J, Walters BC, Hadley MN. Part 7: Intractable low-back pain without stenosis or spondylolisthesis. J Neurosurg Spine. 2005; 2:670–672

[78] Fritzell P, Hagg O, Wessberg P, Nordwall A. 2001 Volvo Award Winner in Clinical Studies: Lumbar fusion versus nonsurgical treatment for chronic low back pain: a multicenter randomized controlled trial from the Swedish Lumbar Spine Study Group. Spine. 2001; 26:2521–32; discussion 2532-4

[79] Ivar Brox J, Sorensen R, Friis A, Nygaard O, Indahl A, Keller A, Ingebrigtsen T, Eriksen HR, Holm I, Koller AK, Riise R, Reikeras O. Randomized clinical trial of lumbar instrumented fusion and cognitive intervention and exercises in patients with chronic low back pain and disc degeneration. Spine. 2003; 28:1913–1921

[80] Resnick DK, Choudhri TF, Dailey AT, Groff MW, Khoo L, Matz PG, Mummaneni P, Watters WC, Wang J, Walters BC, Hadley MN. Part 11: Interbody techniques for lumbar fusion. J Neurosurg Spine. 2005; 2:692–699

[81] Turner JA, Ersek M, Herron L, et al. Patient Outcomes After Lumbar Spinal Fusions. JAMA. 1992; 268:907–911

[82] Resnick DK, Choudhri TF, Dailey AT, Groff MW, Khoo L, Matz PG, Mummaneni P, Watters WC, Wang J, Walters BC, Hadley MN. Part 8: Lumbar fusion for disc herniation and radiculopathy. J Neurosurg Spine. 2005; 2:673–678

[83] Resnick DK, Choudhri TF, Dailey AT, Groff MW, Khoo L, Matz PG, Mummaneni P, Watters WC, Wang J, Walters BC, Hadley MN. Part 12: Pedicle screw fixation as an adjunct to posterolateral fusion for low-back pain. J Neurosurg Spine. 2005; 2:700–706

[84] Lorenz M, Zindrick M, Schwaegler P, et al. A Comparison of Single-Level Fusions With and Without Hardware. Spine. 1991; 16:S455–S458

[85] Gatchel RJ, Mayer TG, Capra P, et al. Quantification of Lumbar Function, VI: The Use of Psychological Measures in Guiding Physical Functional Restoration. Spine. 1986; 11:36–42

[86] Morley S, Pallin V. Scaling the Affective Domain of Pain: A Study of the Dimensionality of Verbal Descriptors. Pain. 1995; 62:39–49

[87] Wray CC, Easom S, Hoskinson J. Coccydynia. Etiology and Treatment. J Bone Joint Surg. 1991; 73B:335–338

[88] Lath R, Rajshekhar V, Chacko G. Sacral Hemangioma as a Cause of Coccydynia. Neuroradiology. 1998; 40:524–526

[89] Thiele GH. Coccydynia: Cause and Treatment. Dis Colon Rectum. 1963; 6:422–435

[90] Lourie J, Young S. Avascular Necrosis of the Coccyx: A Cause of Coccydynia? Case Report and Histological Findings in Sixteen Patients. Br J Clin Pract. 1985; 39:247–248

[91] Raj PP, Raj PP. In: Miscelleneous Pain Disorders. Pain Medicine: A Comprehensive Review. St. Louis: C V Mosby; 1996:492–501

[92] Boeglin ER. Coccydynia. J Bone Joint Surg. 1991; 73B

[93] Loev MA, Varklet VL, Wilsey BL, Ferrante FM. Cryoablation: A Novel Approach to Neurolysis of the Ganglion Impar. Anesthesiology. 1998; 88:1391–1393

[94] Plancarte R, Amescua C, Patt RB, Aldrette JA. Superior Hypogastric Plexus Block for Pelvic Cancer Pain. Anesthesiology. 1990; 73:236–239

[95] Law JD, Lehman RAW, Kirsch WM, et al. Reoperation After Lumbar Intervertebral Disc Surgery. J Neurosurg. 1978; 48:259–263

[96] Davis RA. A Long-Term Outcome Analysis of 984 Surgically Treated Herniated Lumbar Discs. J Neurosurg. 1994; 80:415–421

[97] Caputy AJ, Luessenhop AJ. Long-Term Evaluation of Decompressive Surgery for Degenerative Lumbar Stenosis. J Neurosurg. 1992; 77:669–676

[98] Markwalder TM, Battaglia M. Failed Back Surgery Syndrome. Part 1: Analysis of the Clinical Presentation and Results of Testing Procedures for Instability of the Lumbar Spine in 171 Patients. Acta Neurochir. 1993; 123:46–51

[99] Burton CV, Kirkaldy-Willis WH, Yong-Hing K, Heithoff KB. Causes of Failure of Surgery on the Lumbar Spine. Clin Orthop. 1981; 157:191–199

[100] Quencer RM, Tenner M, Rothman L. The Postoperative Myelogram: Radiographic Evaluation of Arachnoiditis and Dural/Arachnoidal Tears. Radiology. 1977; 123:667–669

[101] Ross JS, Masaryk TJ, Modic MT, et al. MR Imaging of Lumbar Arachnoiditis. AJNR. 1987; 8:885–892

[102] Delamarter RB, Ross JS, Masaryk TJ, Modic MT, Bohlman HH. Diagnosis of Lumbar Arachnoiditis by Magnetic Resonance Imaging. Spine. 1990; 15:304–310

[103] Roca J, Moreta D, Ubierna MT, et al. The Results of Surgical Treatment of Lumbar Arachnoiditis. Int Orthop. 1993; 17:77–81

[104] Martin-Ferrer S. Failure of Autologous Fat Grafts to Prevent Post Operative Epidural Fibrosis in Surgery of the Lumbar Spine. Neurosurgery. 1989; 24:718–721

[105] North RB, Campbell JN, James CS, et al. Failed Back Surgery Syndrome: 5-Year Follow-Up in 102 Patients Undergoing Repeated Operations. Neurosurgery. 1991; 28:685–691

[106] Ross JS, Robertson JT, Frederickson RCA, et al. Association Between Peridural Scar and Recurrent Radicular Pain After Lumbar Discectomy: Magnetic Resonance Evaluation. Neurosurgery. 1996; 38:855–863

[107] Cooper PR. Comment on Ross JS, et al. Association Between Peridural Scar and Recurrent Radicular Pain After Lumbar Discectomy. Neurosurgery. 1996; 38

[108] Sonntag VKH. Comment on Ross JS, et al. Association Between Peridural Scar and Recurrent Radicular Pain After Lumbar Discectomy. Neurosurgery. 1996; 38

[109] Bundschuh CV, Modic MT, Ross JS, Masaryk TJ, et al. Epidural Fibrosis and Recurrent Disc Herniation in the Lumbar Spine: Assessment with Magnetic Resonance. AJNR. 1988; 9:169–178

[110] Sotiropoulos S, Chafetz NE, Lang P, Winkler M, et al. Differentiation Between Postoperative Scar and Recurrent Disk Herniation: Prospective Comparison of MR, CT, and Contrast-Enhanced CT. AJNR. 1989; 10:639–643

[111] Hueftle MG, Modic MT, Ross JS, Masaryk TJ, et al. Lumbar Spine: Postoperative MR Imaging with Gd-DPTA. Radiology. 1988; 167:817–824

[112] Braun IF, Hoffman JC, Davis PC, Tindall GT, et al. Contrast Enhancement in CT Differentiation between Recurrent Disk Herniation and Postoperative Scar: Prospective Study. AJR. 1985; 145:785–790

[113] Byrd SE, Cohn ML, Biggers SL, Huntington CT, et al. The Radiologic Evaluation of the Symptomatic Postoperative Lumbar Spine Patient. Spine. 1985; 10:652–661

[114] Greenwood J, McGuire TH, Kimbell F. A Study of the Causes of Failure in the Herniated Intervertebral Disc Operation. An Analysis of Sixty-Seven Reoperated Cases. J Neurosurg. 1952; 9:15–20

[115] Jorgensen J, Hansen PH, Steenskov V, Ovesen N. A Clinical and Radiological Study of Chronic Lower Spinal Arachnoiditis. Neuroradiology. 1975; 9:139–144

[116] Johnston JDH, Matheny JB. Microscopic Lysis of Lumbar Adhesive Arachnoiditis. Spine. 1978; 3:36–39

69 Lumbar and Thoracic Intervertebral Disk Herniation / Radiculopathy

69.1 Lumbar disc herniation and lumbar radiculopathy

69.1.1 General information

Key concepts

- Radiculopathy: pain and/or subjective sensory changes (numbness, tingling…) in the distribution of a nerve root dermatome, possibly accompanied by weakness and reflex changes of muscles innervated by that nerve root
- typical disc herniation → radiculopathy in the nerve exiting at the level below
- massive disc herniations can → cauda equina syndrome (a medical emergency). Typical symptoms: saddle anesthesia, urinary retention, LE weakness (p. 1050).
- most patients do as well with conservative treatment as with surgery,∴ initial nonsurgical (conservative) treatment should be attempted for the vast majority
- surgery indications: cauda equina syndrome, progressive symptoms or neurologic deficits despite conservative treatment, or severe radicular pain > ≈ 6 weeks

69

69.1.2 Pathophysiology

Intervertebral discs may undergo degenerative changes (p. 1096); see ▶ Table 68.1 for description: this includes desiccation and fibrosis which further leads to fissuring and tearing which in turn increases the risk of herniation of disc material outside the normal confines of the disc space (see same table for definitions).

Disc herniations may compress one or more nerve roots, producing lumbar radiculopathy or less frequently cauda equina syndrome.

69.1.3 Herniation zones

Central and paramedial disc herniations

The posterior longitudinal ligament is strongest in the midline, and the posterolateral annulus may bear a disproportionate portion of the load exerted by the weight from above. This may explain why most herniated lumbar discs (HLD) occur posteriorly, slightly off to one side within the central canal zone or in the subarticular zone as illustrated in ▶ Fig. 69.1. In the lumbar spine this characteristically compresses the nerve root en passage (that is, the nerve entering the lateral recess just before it exits through the neural foramen of the level *below*).

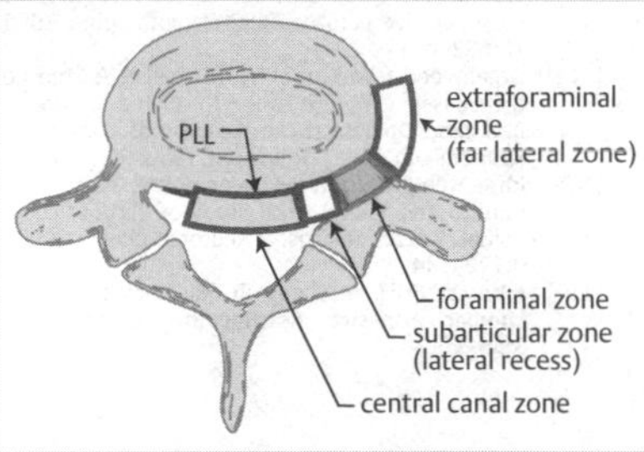

Fig. 69.1 Zones of lumbar disc herniation

Extreme lateral disc herniation

Disc herniations may also occur in the foraminal zone, which typically involves the nerve root exiting at that level.

Disc herniations in the extraforaminal zone occasionally involve the nerve root exiting at that level, however disc herniation here and those herniating anterior to the spine may not result in any nerve root involvement.

69.1.4 Other disc herniation variants

1. intravertebral disc herniation: AKA Schmorl's node. See Herniation through the endplate into the vertebral body (p. 1060)
2. intradural disc herniation (p. 1060)
3. limbus fracture: traumatic separation of a segment of bone from the edge of the vertebral ring apophysis at the site of anular attachment. May accompany HLD

69.1.5 Characteristic findings on the history

- symptoms may start off with back pain, which after days or weeks gradually or sometimes suddenly yields to radicular pain often with reduction of the back pain
- precipitating factors: various factors are often blamed, but are rarely identified[1] with certainty
- pain relief upon flexing the knee and thigh (e.g. lying supine with a pillow under the knees)
- patients generally avoid excessive movements, however, remaining in any one position (sitting, standing, or lying) too long may also exacerbate the pain, sometimes necessitating position changes at intervals that range from every few minutes to 10–20 minutes. This is distinct from constant writhing in pain e.g. with ureteral obstruction
- "cough effect": ↑ pain with coughing, sneezing, or straining at the stool. Occurred in 87% of patients with HLD in one series[2]
- bladder symptoms: the incidence of voiding dysfunction is 1–18%.[3(p 966)] Most common: difficulty voiding, straining, or urinary retention. Reduced bladder sensation may be the earliest finding. The possible causes of this are sensory loss, or incomplete interruption of the preganglionic parasympathetic fibers. Later it is not unusual to see "irritative" symptoms including urinary urgency, frequency (including nocturia), increased post-void residual. Less common: enuresis, and dribbling incontinence[4]; NB: frank urinary retention may indicate cauda equina syndrome (p. 1050). Occasionally a HLD may present only with bladder symptoms which may improve after surgery.[5] Discectomy may improve bladder function, but this cannot be assured

Back pain per se is usually a minor component (only 1% of patients with acute low back pain have sciatica[6]), and when it is the only presenting symptom, other causes should be sought; see Low back pain (p. 1024). Sciatica has such a high sensitivity for disc herniation, that the likelihood of a clinically significant disc herniation[7] in the absence of sciatica is ≈ 1 in 1000. Exceptions include a central disc herniation which may cause symptoms of lumbar stenosis (i.e. neurogenic claudication) or a cauda equina syndrome.

69.1.6 Physical findings in radiculopathy

General information

Nerve root impingement gives rise to a set of signs and symptoms present to variable degrees. Characteristic syndromes are described for the most common nerve roots involved; see Nerve root syndromes (p. 1049).

In a series of patients referred to neurosurgical outpatient clinics for radiating leg pain, 28% had motor loss (yet only 12% listed motor weakness as a presenting complaint), 45% had sensory disturbance, and 51% had reflex changes.[8]

Findings suggestive of nerve root impingement include the following. ▶ Table 69.1 shows the sensitivity and specificity of some findings on the exam among patients with sciatica.

1. signs/symptoms of radiculopathy (▶ Table 69.1)
   a) pain radiating down LE
   b) motor weakness
   c) dermatomal sensory changes
   d) reflex changes: mental factors may influence symmetry[9]
2. positive nerve root tension sign(s): including Lasègue's sign (see below)
3. tenderness over the sciatic notch

69

Table 69.1 Sensitivity and specificity of physical findings for HLD in patients with sciatica[10]

Test	Comment	Sensitivity	Specificity
ipsilateral SLR	positive result: pain at < 60° elevation	0.80	0.40
crossed SLR	reproduction of contralateral pain	0.25	0.90
↓ ankle jerk	HLD usually at L5-S1 (total absence increases specificity)	0.50	0.60
sensory loss	area of loss is poor in localizing level of HLD	0.50	0.50
↓ patellar reflex	suggests upper HLD	0.50	NA
Weakness			
knee extension (quadriceps)	HLD usually at L3–4	< 0.01	0.99
ankle dorsiflexion (anterior tibialis)	HLD usually at L4–5	0.35	0.70
ankle plantarflexion (gastrocs)	HLD usually at L5-S1	0.06	0.95
great toe extension (EHL)	HLD at L5-S1 in 60%, at L4–5 in 30%	0.50	0.70

69

Nerve root tension signs

Includes[11]:

1. Lasègue's sign: AKA straight leg raising (SLR) test. Helps differentiate sciatica from pain due to hip pathology. Test: with patient supine, raise afflicted limb by the ankle until pain is elicited[12] (should occur at < 60°, tension in nerve increases little above this angle). A positive test consists of leg pain or paresthesias in the distribution of pain (back pain alone does not qualify). The patient may also extend the hip (by lifting it off table) to reduce the angle. Although not part of Lasègue's sign, ankle dorsiflexion with SLR usually augments pain due to nerve root compression. SLR primarily tenses L5 and S1, L4 less so, and more proximal roots very little. Nerve-root compression produces a positive Lasègue's sign in ≈ 83% of cases[2] (more likely to be positive in patients < 30 yrs age with HLD[13]). May be positive in lumbosacral plexopathy (p. 544). Note: flexing both thighs with the knees extended ("long-sitting" or sitting knee extension) may be tolerated further than flexing the single symptomatic side alone
2. Cram test: with patient supine, raise the symptomatic leg with the knee slightly flexed. Then, extend the knee. Results similar to SLR
3. crossed straight leg-raising test AKA Fajersztajn's sign: SLR on the painless leg causes contralateral limb pain (a greater degree of elevation is usually required than the painful side). More specific but less sensitive than SLR (97% of patients undergoing surgery with this sign have confirmed HLD[14]). May correlate with a more *central* disc herniation
4. femoral stretch test,[15] AKA reverse straight leg raising: patient prone, examiner's palm at popliteal fossa, knee is maximally dorsiflexed. Often positive with L2, L3, or L4 nerve root compression (e.g. in upper lumbar disc herniation), or with extreme lateral lumbar disc herniation (may also be positive in diabetic femoral neuropathy or psoas hematoma); in these situations SLR (Lasègue's sign) is frequently negative (since L5 & S1 not involved)
5. "bowstring sign": once pain occurs with SLR, lower the foot to the bed by flexing knee, keeping the hip flexed. Sciatic pain ceases with this maneuver, but hip pain persists
6. sitting knee extension test: with patient seated and both hips and knees flexed 90°, slowly extend one knee. Stretches nerve roots as much as a moderate degree of SLR

Other signs useful in evaluation for lumbar radiculopathy

1. FABER: an acronym for Flexion ABduction External-Rotation, AKA FABERE test (the trailing "e" is for extension), AKA Patrick's-test (after Hugh Talbot Patrick). A test of hip motion. Method: the hip and knee are flexed and the lateral malleolus is placed on the contralateral knee. The ipsilateral knee is gently displaced downward towards the exam table. This stresses the hip joint and does not usually exacerbate true nerve-root compression. Often markedly positive in the presence of hip joint disease – e.g. trochanteric bursitis (p. 1101) – sacroiliitis or mechanical low-back pain

2. Trendelenburg sign: examiner observes pelvis from behind while patient raises one leg while standing. Normally the pelvis remains horizontal. A positive sign occurs when the pelvis tilts down toward the side of the lifted leg indicating weakness of the contralateral thigh adductors (primarily L5 innervated)
3. crossed adductors: in eliciting patellar reflex (knee jerk (KJ)), the contralateral thigh adductors contract. In the presence of a hyperactive ipsilateral KJ it may indicate an upper motor neuron lesion, in the presence of a hypoactive ipsilateral KJ it may be a form of pathological spread, indicating nerve root irritability
4. Hoover sign[16]: to distinguish unilateral functional weakness of iliopsoas from organic weakness using synergistic contraction of the contralateral gluteus medius. The supine patient is asked to lift one leg off the bed against resistance from the examiner's hand. The examiner simultaneously places the palm of his/her other hand under the heel of the unlifted leg and gently lifts. Test 1: when the patient lifts the normal leg, if the paretic leg pushes down with more force than was exhibited on manual testing of the limb beforehand, the weakness is judged functional, if the force is equally weak the weakness is judged organic. Test 1 cannot be used if the hip extensor was normal beforehand. Test 2: (the better known test) the patient is asked to lift the weak leg. If the heel on the normal side lifts passively by the examiner, it suggests the weakness is functional (i.e. the patient is not trying). Not totally reliable[17,18]
5. abductor sign: an alternative to the Hoover test, to differentiate functional from organic weakness in the thigh abductors using synergistic contraction of the contralateral thigh abductors.[18] With the patient supine, the examiner places a hand on the lateral aspect of both legs. The patient is asked to abduct one leg, and then the other while the examiner applies resistance with his/her hand. The examiner mentally notes the response of the non-abducting LE. The results are as noted in ▶ Table 69.2

69

Nerve root syndromes

Due to the facts listed below, a herniated lumbar disc (HLD) usually spares the nerve root exiting at that interspace, and impinges on the nerve exiting from the neural foramen one level *below* (e.g. a L5-S1 HLD usually causes S1 radiculopathy). This gives rise to the characteristic lumbar nerve root syndromes shown in ▶ Table 69.3.

Important applied anatomy in lumbar disc disease:

1. in the lumbar region, the nerve root exits *below* and in close proximity to the pedicle of its like-numbered vertebra
2. the intervertebral disc space is located well below the pedicle
3. not all patients have 5 lumbar vertebrae; see Localizing levels in spine surgery (p. 1436)

69.1.7 Radiographic evaluation

See Radiographic evaluation under Low back pain (p. 1416). 70% of herniated discs that migrate do so *inferiorly*.

69.1.8 Nonsurgical treatment

See nonsurgical treatment measures (p. 1033).

69.1.9 Surgical treatment

Indications for surgery

No predictive factors have been identified that can determine which patients are likely to improve on their own and which would be better served with surgery.

Table 69.2 Abductor sign

Abducting LE	Contralateral (nonabducting) LE	
	Organic weakness	Functional weakness
weak LE	maintains position	hyperadducts
normal LE	hyperadducts	maintains position

Table 69.3 Lumbar disc syndromes

Syndrome	Level of herniated lumbar disc		
	L3–4	L4–5	L5-S1
root usually compressed	L4	L5	S1
% of lumbar discs	3–10% (5% average)	40–45%	45–50%
reflex diminished	knee jerk[a] (Westphal's sign)	medial hamstring[b]	Achilles[a] (ankle jerk)
motor weakness	quadriceps femoris (knee extension)	tibialis anterior (foot drop) & EHL[c]	gastrocnemius (plantarflexion), ± EHL[c]
decreased sensation[d]	medial malleolus & medial foot	large toe web & dorsum of foot	lateral malleolus & lateral foot
pain distribution	anterior thigh	posterior LE	posterior LE, often to ankle

[a] **Jendrassik maneuver** may reinforce (see ▶ Table 29.2)
[b]medial hamstring reflex is unreliable (not always pure L5), may also stimulate adductors when eliciting
[c]see WEAKNESS in ▶ Table 69.1 for breakdown
[d]sensory impairment is most common in the distal extremes of the dermatome[19]

Surgical indications in patients with a radiographically identified herniated disc that correlates with findings on the history and physical exam:

1. failure of non-surgical management to control pain after 5–8 weeks: over 85% of patients with acute disc herniation will improve *without* surgical intervention in an average of 6 weeks[20] (70% within 4 weeks[21]). Most clinicians advocate waiting somewhere between 5–8 weeks from the onset of radiculopathy before considering surgery (assuming none of the items listed below applies)
2. " EMERGENT SURGERY": (i.e. before the 5–8 weeks of symptoms have lapsed). Indications:
   a) cauda equina syndrome (CES): (see below)
   b) *progressive* motor deficit (e.g. foot drop). NB: paresis of unknown duration is a doubtful indication for surgery[1,22,23] (no study has documented that there is less motor deficit in surgically treated patients with this finding[24]). However, the acute development or progression of motor weakness is considered an indication for rapid surgical decompression
   c) "urgent" surgery may be indicated for patients whose pain remains intolerable in spite of adequate narcotic pain medication
3. ± patients who do not want to invest the time in a trial of non-surgical treatment if it is possible that they will still require surgery at the end of the trial

Cauda equina syndrome

The clinical condition arising from dysfunction of multiple lumbar and sacral nerve roots within the lumbar spinal canal. Usually due to compression of the cauda equina (the bundle of nerve roots below the conus medullaris arising from the lumbar enlargement and conus). See ▶ Table 53.2 for features to help differentiate CES from a conus lesion.

Possible findings in CES:

1. sphincter disturbance:
   a) urinary retention: the most consistent finding. Sensitivity ≈ 90% (at some point in time during course).[25,26] To evaluate acutely: have patient empty bladder and check post-void residual (by catheterization or with bladder ultrasound). In a patient without retention, only 1 in 1000 will have a CES. Cystometrogram (when done) shows a hypotonic bladder with decreased sensation and increased capacity
   b) urinary and/or fecal incontinence[27]: some patients with urinary retention will present with overflow incontinence
   c) anal sphincter tone: diminished in 60–80%
2. "saddle anesthesia": the most common sensory deficit. Distribution: region of the anus, lower genitals, perineum, over the buttocks, posterior-superior thighs. Sensitivity ≈ 75%. Once total perineal anesthesia develops, patients tend to have permanent bladder paralysis[28]

3. significant motor weakness: usually involves more than a single nerve root (if untreated, may progress to paraplegia)
4. low back pain and/or sciatica (sciatica is usually bilateral, but may be unilateral or entirely absent, prognosis may be worse when absent or bilateral[26])
5. bilateral absence of Achilles reflex has been noted[29]
6. sexual dysfunction (usually not detected until a later time)

Etiologies of CES includes:
1. compression of cauda equina
   a) massive herniated lumbar disc: see below
   b) tumor
      • from compression: e.g. with metastatic disease to the spine with epidural extension
      • intravascular lymphomatosis (B-cell lymphoma) (p. 711): a circulating lymphoma without solid mass. Often presents with CNS findings: dementia, enhancing meninges on MRI, lymphoma cells in CSF, and CES
   c) free fat graft following discectomy[30]
   d) trauma: fracture fragments compressing cauda equina
   e) spinal epidural hematoma
2. infection: may cause neurologic deficit from
   a) compression: typically from spinal epidural abscess complicating discitis or vertebral osteomyelitis
   b) a significant number of cases of CES from infection may be due to vascular compromise resulting from local *septic thrombophlebitis*. This may carry a worse prognosis as surgical decompression cannot correct this mechanism
3. neuropathy:
   a) ischemic
   b) inflammatory
4. ankylosing spondylitis: etiology is often obscure (p. 1123)

69

CES from HLD: May be due to massive herniated disc, usually midline, most common at L4–5, often superimposed on a preexisting condition (spinal stenosis, tethered cord…).[27]

Prevalence of CES
1. 0.0004 in all patients with LBP[7]
2. only ≈ 1–2% of HLD that come to surgery[7]

Time course: CES tends to develop either acutely, or (less typically) slowly (prognosis is worse in the acute onset group, especially for return of bladder function, which occurred in only ≈ 50%).[25] 3 patterns[31]:
• Group I – sudden onset of CES symptoms with no previous low back symptoms
• Group II – previous history of recurrent backache and sciatica, the latest episode combined with CES
• Group III – presentation with backache & bilateral sciatica that later develop CES

Surgical issues: some advise a bilateral laminectomy[27] (but this is not mandatory). Occasionally, when it is difficult to remove a very tense midline disc, transdural removal may be helpful.[29]

Timing of discectomy in CES: controversial, and the point of contention in numerous lawsuits. In spite of early reports emphasizing rapid decompression,[29] other reports found no correlation between the time to surgery after presentation and the return of function.[25,26] Some evidence supports the goal of performing surgery within 48 hours (although performing surgery within 24 hours is desirable if possible, there is no statistically significant proof that delaying up to 48 hrs is detrimental).[32,33]

Booking the case: Lumbar discectomy

Also see defaults & disclaimers (p. 27).
1. position: prone
2. equipment: microscope (if used), minimally invasive retractors (if used)
3. consent (in lay terms for the patient – not all-inclusive):
   a) procedure: through the back to go between the bones and remove the piece of disc that is pressing on the nerve(s)

b) alternatives: nonsurgical management
c) complications: usual spine surgery complications (p. 1018) plus the disc can herniate again in the same place in ≈ 6% of cases, it is possible that a fragment of disc can be missed at the time of surgery, there might not be the amount of pain relief desired (back pain does not respond as well to surgery as nerve-root pain)

Surgical options for lumbar radiculopathy

Once it is decided to treat surgically, options include:

1. trans-canal approaches
   a) standard open lumbar laminectomy and discectomy: 65–85% reported no sciatica one year post-op compared to 36% for conservative treatment.[34] Long-term results (> 1 year) were similar. 10% of patients underwent further back surgery during the first year[34]
   b) "microdiscectomy"[35,36]: similar to standard procedure, however smaller incision is utilized. Advantages may be cosmetic, shortened hospital stay, lower blood loss. May be more difficult to retrieve some fragments.[37 (p 1319),38] Overall efficacy is similar to standard discectomy[39]
   c) sequestrectomy: removal of only the herniated portion of the disc without entering the disc space to remove disc material from there
2. intradiscal procedures (see below): a number of procedures have been devised over the years to percutaneously treat HLD by creating a cavity within the disc. Some have been abandoned for various reasons, not the least of which is controversy regarding the validity of the underlying premise that this can work
   a) chemonucleolysis: using chymopapain to enzymatically dissolve the disc (no longer used)
   b) automated percutaneous lumbar discectomy: utilizes a nucleotome
   c) percutaneous endoscopic intradiscal discectomy: see below
   d) intradiscal endothermal therapy (IDET or IDTA): see below
   e) laser disc decompression

69

Intradiscal surgical procedures (ISP)

ISPs (see below for specific procedures) are among the most controversial procedures for lumbar spine surgery. The theoretical advantage is that epidural scarring is avoided, and that a smaller incision or even just a puncture site is used. This is also purported to reduce postoperative pain and hospital stay (often performed as an outpatient procedure). The conceptual problem with ISPs is that they are directed at removing disc material from the center of the disc space (which is not producing symptoms) and rely on the reduced intradiscal pressure to decompress the herniated portion of the disc from the nerve root. Only ≈ 10–15% of patients considered for surgical treatment of disc disease are candidates for an ISP. ISPs are usually done under local anesthetic in order to permit the patient to report nerve root pain to identify impingement on a nerve root by the surgical instrument or needle. Overall, ISPs are not recommended until rigorous controlled trials prove the efficacy.[10]

Indications utilized by proponents of intradiscal procedures:

1. type of disc herniation: appropriate only for "contained" disc herniation (i.e. outer margin of anulus fibrosus intact)
2. appropriate level: best for L4–5 HLD. May also be used at L3–4. Difficult but often workable (utilizing angled instruments or other techniques) at L5-S1 because of the angle required and interference by iliac crest
3. not recommended in presence of severe neurologic deficit[40]

Results:

"Success" rate (≈ pain free and return to work when appropriate) reported ranges from 37–75%.[41,42,43]

Automated percutaneous lumbar discectomy: AKA nucleoplasty. Utilizes a nucleotome[44] to remove disc material from the center of the intervertebral disc space. 1 year success rate of 37%. Complications include cauda equina syndrome from improper nucleotome placement.[45] In another study, nucleoplasty (with or without IDET (see below)) for HLD showed only modest reduction in pain at 9 months.[46]

Laser disc decompression: Insertion of a needle into the disc, and introduction of a laser fiberoptic cable through the needle to allow a laser to burn a hole in the center of the disc[47,48] (with or without endoscopic visualization).

The 2104 North American Spine Society Coverage Committee[49] position statement:

"**Laser spine surgery** in the **cervical** or **lumbar** spine is NOT indicated at this time. Due to lack of high quality clinical trials concerning laser spine surgery with the cervical or lumbar spine, it cannot be endorsed as an adjunct to open, minimally invasive, or percutaneous surgical techniques."

Percutaneous endoscopic lumbar discectomy (PELD) : This term refers to an essentially intradiscal procedure indicated primarily for contained disc herniations, although some small "noncontained" fragments may be treatable.[50] No large randomized study has been done to compare the technique to the accepted standard, open discectomy (with or without microscope). In one report[51] of 326 patients with L4–5 HLD, only 8 (2.4%) met study criteria (no previous operation, failure of conservative treatment, imaging study proving disc protrusion followed by discography to R/O "disc perforation") for PELD. Of these 8, only 3 were reported as having a good result. This study is not adequate for evaluating the technique.

Intradiscal endothermal therapy (IDET): AKA intradiscal (electro)thermal anuloplasty (IDTA). Efficacy: 23–60% at 1 year for treating "internal disc disruption"[52] (radial fissures in the nucleus pulposus extending into the anulus fibrosus) which is purported to account for 40% of patients with chronic low back pain of unknown etiology.[53]

Adjunctive treatment in lumbar laminectomy

Epidural steroids following discectomy

Perioperative epidural steroids after routine surgery for lumbar degenerative disease may result in a small reduction of post-op pain, length of stay, and the risk of not returning to work at 1 year, but most of the evidence originates from studies not using validated outcome assessment that favor positive results, and further study is recommended (various agents, dosages, co-administered drugs, and delivery methods were reported).[54] However, the combination of systemic steroids at the start of the case (Depo-Medrol® 160 mg IM and methylprednisolone sodium succinate (Solu-Medrol®) 250 mg IV) combined with infiltration of 30 ml of 0.25% bupivacaine (Marcaine®) into the paraspinal muscles at incision and closure, may reduce hospital stay and post-op narcotic requirements.[55]

69

Methods to reduce scar formation

Epidural free fat graft

The use of an autogenous free fat graft in the epidural space has been employed in an attempt to reduce post-op epidural scar formation. Opinion varies widely as to the effectiveness, some feel it is helpful, others feel it actually exacerbates scarring.[56] In some patients, no evidence of the graft will be found on reoperation years later. The fat graft can very rarely be a cause of nerve root compression[57] or cauda equina syndrome[30] within the first few days post-op, and there is a case report of compression 6 years following surgery.[58]

Other measures

Other measures include the placement of barrier films or gels. There are numerous products available, none has been shown to have reproducible benefit.

Risks of lumbar laminectomy

General information

Overall risk of mortality in large series[59,60]: 6 per 10,000 (i.e. 0.06%), most often due to septicemia, MI, or PE. Complication rates are very difficult to determine accurately,[34] but the following is included as a guideline.

Common complications

1. infection:
   a) superficial wound infection: 0.9–5%[61] (risk is increased with age, long term steroids, obesity, ? DM): most are caused by S. aureus; see Laminectomy wound infection (p. 345) for management
   b) deep infection: < 1% (see below under Uncommon complications)
2. increased motor deficit: 1–8% (some transient)
3. unintended "incidental" durotomy (the term "unintended durotomy" has been recommended in preference to "dural tear", see below): incidence is 0.3–13% (risk increases to ≈ 18% in re-do operations).[62] Possible sequelae include those listed in ▶ Table 69.4

Table 69.4 Possible sequelae of dural opening

Well documented
1. CSF leak a) contained: pseudomeningocele b) external: CSF fistula 2. herniation of nerve roots thorough opening 3. associated nerve root contusion, laceration or injury to the cauda equina 4. CSF leak collapses the thecal sac and may increase blood loss from epidural bleeding
Less well documented
1. arachnoiditis 2. chronic pain 3. bladder, bowel and/or sexual dysfunction

a) CSF fistula (external CSF leak): the risk of a CSF fistula requiring operative repair is ≈ 10 per 10,000[59]
b) pseudomeningocele: 0.7–2%[62] (may appear similar radiographically to spinal epidural abscess (SEA), but post-op SEA often enhances, is more irregular, and is associated with muscle edema)

4. recurrent herniated lumbar disc (same level either side) (p. 1061): 4% (with 10 year follow-up)[63]
5. Post-operative urinary retention (POUR): usually temporary, but may delay hospital discharge

69

Uncommon complications

1. direct injury to neural structures. For large disc herniations, consider a bilateral exposure to reduce risk
2. injury to structures anterior to the vertebral bodies (VB): injured by breaching the anterior longitudinal ligament (ALL) through the disc space, e.g. with pituitary rongeur. The depth of disc space penetration with instruments should be kept ≤ 3 cm, since 5% of lumbar discs had diameters as small as 3.3 cm.[64] Asymptomatic perforations of the ALL occur in up to 12% of discectomies. Breach of the ALL risks potential injuries to:
   a) great vessels[65]: risks include potentially fatal hemorrhage, and arteriovenous fistula which may present years later. Most such injuries occur with L4–5 discectomies. Only ≈ 50% bleed into the disc space intraoperatively, the rest bleed into the retroperitoneum. Emergent laparotomy or endovascular treatment[66] is indicated, preferably by a surgeon with vascular surgical experience, if available. Mortality rate is 37–67%
      - aorta: the aortic bifurcation is on the left side of the lower part of the L4 VB, and so the aorta may be injured above this level
      - below L4, the common iliac arteries may be injured
      - veins (more common than arterial injuries): vena cava at and above L4, common iliac veins below L4
   b) ureters
   c) bowel: at L5-S1 the ileum is the most likely viscus to be injured
   d) sympathetic trunk
3. wrong site surgery: incidence in self-reporting survey was 4.5 occurrences per 10,000 lumbar spine operations.[67] Factors identified as potential contributors to the error: unusual patient anatomy, not performing localizing radiograph. 32% of responding neurosurgeons indicated that they removed disc material from the wrong level at some time in their career
4. rare infections:
   a) meningitis
   b) deep infection: < 1%. Including:
      - discitis (p. 356): 0.5%
      - spinal epidural abscess (SEA) (p. 349): 0.67%
5. cauda equina syndrome: may be caused by post-op spinal epidural hematoma (see below). Incidence was 0.21% in one series of 2842 lumbar discectomies[68] and 0.14% in a series of 12,000 spine operations.[69] Red flags: urinary retention, anesthesia that may be saddle or *bilateral* LE
6. postoperative visual loss (POVL)[70]: (see below)
7. complications of positioning:
   a) compression neuropathies: ulnar, peroneal nerves. Use padding over elbows and avoid pressure on posterior popliteal fossa

b) anterior tibial compartment syndrome: due to pressure on anterior compartment of leg (reported with Andrew's frame). An orthopedic emergency that may require emergent fasciotomy
c) pressure on the eye: corneal abrasions, damage to the anterior chamber
d) cervical spine injuries during positioning due to relaxed muscles under anesthesia

8. post-op arachnoiditis (p. 1040): risk factors include epidural hematoma, patients who tend to develop hypertrophic scar, post-op discitis, and intrathecal injection anesthetic agents or steroids. Surgical treatment for this is disappointing. Intrathecal depo-medrol may provide short-term relief (in spite of the fact that steroids are a risk factor for the development of arachnoiditis).
9. thrombophlebitis and deep-vein thrombosis with risk of pulmonary embolism (PE)[59]: 0.1%; see Thromboembolism in neurosurgery (p. 167)
10. complex regional pain syndrome AKA reflex sympathetic dystrophy (RSD) (p. 497): reported in up to 1.2% of cases, usually after posterior decompression with fusion, often following reoperations[71] with onset 4 days to 20 weeks post-op. See also critique of RSD (p. 497). Treatment includes some or all of: PT, sympathetic blocks, oral methylprednisolone, removal of hardware if any
11. very rare: Ogilvie's syndrome (pseudo-obstruction ("ileus") of the colon). Usually seen in hospitalized/debilitated patients. May be related to narcotics, electrolyte deficiencies, possibly from chronic constipation. Also reported following spinal surgery/trauma, spinal/epidural anesthesia, spinal metastases, & myelography[72]

Unintended durotomy

Unintentional opening of the dura during spinal surgery has an incidence of 0–14%.[73]

69

Terminology: The terms "unintended durotomy", "incidental durotomy",[73] or even just "dural opening", have been recommended in preference to "dural tear" which may imply carelessness[62] when none was present. Dural openings have been associated with one or more alleged complications or sequelae in medical malpractice suits involving surgery on the lumbar spine.

The injury: By itself, opening the dura intentionally or otherwise is not expected to have a deleterious effect on the patient.[62,74] In fact, dural opening is often a standard part of the operation for intradural disc herniation,[75] tumors, etc. Although not frequent, (for incidence, see above) unintended durotomy is not an unusual occurrence, and alone, is not considered an act of malpractice. However, it may result from an event or events that produce more serious injuries. These events and injuries should be dealt with on their own merits.

In the SPORT study, there was a 9% incidence of unintended durotomy in patients undergoing first-time open laminectomy.[76] There were no long-term differences in nerve root injuries, mortality, additional operations, or outcome measures. Short-term differences included longer inpatient stay, increased blood loss, and duration of surgery.[76]

Possible sequelae include those listed in ▸ Table 69.4. A CSF leak may produce "spinal headache" (p. 1508) with its associated symptoms and if it breaches the skin it may be a risk factor for meningitis. Pain or sensory/motor deficits may be associated with injuries to nerve roots or delayed herniation of nerve roots through the dural opening.

Etiologies: Potential causes are many, and include[62]: unanticipated anatomic variations, adhesion of the dura to removed bone, slippage of an instrument, an obscured fold of dura caught in a rongeur or curette, thinning of the dura in cases of longstanding stenosis, and the possibility of a delayed CSF leak caused by perforation of the dura when it expands onto a surgically created spicule of bone.[77] The risk may be increased with anterior decompression for OPLL, with revision surgery, and with the use of high-speed drills.[73]

Treatment: If the opening is recognized at the time of surgery, watertight primary closure (with or without patch graft) should be attempted with nonabsorbable suture if at all possible to prevent pseudomeningocele and/or CSF fistula. A cottonoid placed over the opening prevents aspiration of nerve roots.[78] Care must be taken to avoid incorporating a nerve root into the closure. Most repairs will be accomplished with no complication or sequelae to the patient. When the opening is in the far (anterior) side of the dura, consideration may be given to intradural repair accessed through a posterior durotomy which is subsequently closed (this may risk additional injury to the nerve roots). Biocompatible fixatives (e.g. fibrin glue[73]) may be used to supplement primary closure.

Primary repair may be impossible in some situations (e.g. when the opening cannot be found or accessed, as is sometimes the case when it occurs on the nerve root sleeve) and alternatives here include placement of a fat or muscle graft over the suspected leak site, use of a the patient's own blood for a "blood patch" (one technique is to have the anesthesiologist draw ≈ 5–10 ml of the patient's blood from an arm vein, keeping it in the syringe for several minutes until it starts to coagulate, and then to have the anesthesiologist inject the blood onto the dura), use of gelfoam, fibrin glue... Some recommend that the wound not be drained post-op, with a water-tight closure of fascia, fat, and skin to add to the barrier. Others use a subcutaneous drain or epidural catheter. CSF diversionary procedures (e.g. through a drain inserted 1 or more levels away) may also be used.

Although bed rest × 4–7 days is often advocated to reduce symptoms and facilitate healing, when watertight closure has been achieved, normal post-op mobilization is not associated with a high failure rate (bed rest is recommended if symptoms develop).[73]

In one report of 8 patients with leaks that appeared post-op, re-operation was avoided when treated by resuturing the skin under local anesthesia, followed by bed rest in slight Trendelenburg position (to reduce pressure on the leakage site), broad spectrum antibiotics and antibiotic ointment over the skin incision, and daily puncture and drainage of the subcutaneous collection.[79]

See other treatment measures for H/A associated with CSF leak (p. 1049).

Postoperative visual loss

1. ischemic optic neuropathy[80]: the most common cause of the very uncommon post-operative loss of vision. Often bilateral. Usually associated with significant blood loss (median: 2 L), and/or prolonged operative time (≥ 6 hrs). All cases had anesthetic time > 5 hrs or blood loss > 1 L. Blood loss can cause hypotension (may cause release of endogenous vasoconstrictors in addition to reduced blood flow due to low hemodynamic pressure) and increased platelet aggregation. Is not due to direct pressure on the globe in most cases, and can occur at any age and even in otherwise healthy patients. No association with age, HTN, atherosclerosis, smoking or DM.
   The blindness can be extensive and is often permanent. Prevention is critical since there is no known effective treatment.[81]
   a) posterior ischemic optic neuropathy (PION)[80]: may follow surgery (surgical PION). Risk factors as above, plus:
      - surgery in the *prone* position (can cause periorbital edema, and rarely, direct pressure on the orbit)
      - lack of tight glycemic control
      - use of Trendelenburg position
      - hemodilution or overuse of crystalloid vs. colloid (blood) fluid replacement
      - prolonged hypotension
      - cellular hypoxia
      - decreased renal perfusion
   b) 6 independent risk factors for POVL[81]
      - male gender: odds ratio (OR) = 2.53
      - obesity: by clinical assessment or BMI ≥ 30 OR = 2.83
      - use of Wilson frame: OR = 4.30
      - length of anesthesia: OR = 1.39 per hour
      - EBL: OR = 1.34 per Liter
      - use of colloid as a percentage of nonblood replacement: less certain (small difference). OR = 0.67 per 5% colloid
   c) anterior ischemic optic neuropathy (AION): divided into arteritic (as with GCA) and nonarteritic (common with DM)
2. central retinal artery occlusion
3. cortical blindness: from occipital lobe infarction possibly due to embolis

69

Post-op care

Post-op orders

The following are guidelines for post-operative orders for a lumbar laminectomy without intra-operative complications; variations between surgeons and institutions must be taken into consideration:

1. admit post-anesthesia care unit (PACU)
2. vital signs on the nursing unit: q 2° × 4 hrs, q 4° × 24°, then q 8°
3. activity: up with assist, advance as tolerated
4. nursing care
   - I's & O's
   - intermittent catheterization q 4–6° PRN no void
   - optional: TED hose (may reduce risk of DVT) or PCB
   - optional (if drain used): empty drain q 8° and PRN
5. diet: clear liquids, advance as tolerated
6. IV: D5 1/2 NS + 20 mEq KCl/l @ 75 ml/hr, D/C when tolerating PO well (after antibiotics D/C'd if prophylactic antibiotics are used)

7. meds
   - laxative of choice (LOC) PRN
   - sodium docusate (e.g. Colace®) 100 mg PO BID when tolerating PO (stool softener, does not substitute for LOC)
   - optional: prophylactic antibiotics if used at your institution
   - acetaminophen (Tylenol®) 325 mg 1–2 PO or PR q 6° PRN
   - narcotic analgesic
   - optional: steroids are used by some surgeons to reduce nerve-root irritation from surgical manipulation
8. labs
   - optional (if significant blood loss during surgery): CBC

Post-op check

In addition to routine, the following should be checked:

1. strength of lower extremities, especially muscles relevant to nerve root, e.g. gastrocnemius for L5-S1 surgery, EHL for L4–5 surgery…
2. appearance of dressing: look for signs of excessive bleeding, CSF leak…
3. signs of cauda equina syndrome (p. 1050), e.g. by post-op spinal epidural hematoma
   a) loss of perineal sensation ("saddle anesthesia")
   b) inability to void: may not be not unusual after lumbar laminectomy, more concerning if accompanied by loss of perineal sensation
   c) pain out of the ordinary for the post-op period
   d) weakness of multiple muscle groups

69

Any new neurologic deficit should prompt rapid evaluation for spinal epidural hematoma[69] (EDH). Delayed deficits may be due to EDH or epidural abscess. Post-op films in the recovery room can rule out graft or hardware malposition for fusions or instrumentation procedures, or changes in alignment. The diagnostic test of choice is MRI. If contraindicated or not available, CT/myelography may be indicated. An extradural defect immediately post-op suggests EDH.

Outcome of surgical treatment

In a series of 100 patients undergoing discectomy, at 1 year post-op 73% had complete relief of leg pain and 63% had complete relief of back pain; at 5–10 years the numbers were 62% for each category.[2] At 5–10 years post-op, only 14% felt that the pain was the same or worse than pre-op (i.e. 86% felt improved), and 5% qualified as having a failed back surgery syndrome (a heterogeneous not-precisely defined term, here meaning not returned to work, requiring analgesics, receiving worker's compensation, see Failed back surgery syndrome (p. 1039)).

Attempts to measure relative merits of conservative treatment vs. surgery have failed. The recent SPORT study[82,83] suffered from significant selection bias since patients were allowed to crossover to the other arm of the study and thus more nearly approximated the current methodology of surgical selection than an actual RCT.[84] Earlier attempts at randomized trials also suffered from methodological flaws.[1] Conclusions that can be drawn from these studies[84]: most patients with manageable or improving pain and less disability typically choose conservative treatment and most have improvement in symptoms, whereas patients with severe, persistent or worsening pain and/or neurologic deficit are more likely to choose surgery with a resultant excellent outcome.

In patients with a diminished knee-jerk or ankle-jerk pre-op, 35% and 43% (respectively) still had reduced reflexes 1 year post-op[8]; reflexes were lost post-op in 3% and 10% respectively. The same study found that motor loss was improved in 80%, aggravated in 3%, and was newly present in 5% post-op; and that sensory loss was improved in 69% and was worsened in 15% post-op.

Foot drop: severe or complete paralysis of ankle dorsiflexion occurs in 5–10% of HLD, and about 50% of cases recover with or without treatment. Discectomy does not improve the outcome, especially in cases of painless foot drop.[24]

See Recurrent disc herniation (p. 1061).

69.1.10 Herniated upper lumbar discs (levels L1–2, L2–3, and L3–4)

General information

L4–5 & L5-S1 herniated lumbar discs (HLD) account for most cases of HLD (realistically ≈ 90%, possibly as high as 98%[7]). 24% of patients with HLD at L3–4 have a past history of a HLD at L4–5 or L5-S1, suggesting a generalized tendency towards disc herniation. In a series of 1,395 HLDs, there were 4 at L1–2 (0.28% incidence), 18 at L2–3 (1.3%), and 51 at L3–4 (3.6%).[85]

Presentation

Typically presents with LBP, onset following trauma or strain in 51%. With progression, paresthesias and pain in the anterior thigh occur, with complaints of leg weakness (especially on ascending stairs).

Signs

Quadriceps femoris was the most common muscle involved, demonstrating weakness and sometimes atrophy.

Straight leg raising was positive in only 40%. Psoas stretch test was positive in 27%. Femoral stretch test may be positive (p. 1048).

50% had reduced or absent knee jerk; 18% had ankle jerk abnormalities; reflex changes were more common with L3–4 HLD (81%) than L1–2 (none) or L2–3 (44%).

69.1.11 Extreme lateral lumbar disc herniations

General information

Definition: herniation of a disc at (foraminal disc herniation) or distal to (extraforaminal disc herniation) the facet (some authors do not consider foraminal disc herniation to be "extreme lateral"). See ▶ Fig. 69.1.

Incidence (▶ Table 69.5): 3–10% of herniated lumbar discs (HLD) (series with higher numbers[86] include some HLD that are not truly extreme lateral).

69

Occurs most commonly at *L4–5* and next at L3–4 (see ▶ Table 69.5), thus L4 is the most common nerve involved and L3 is next. With a clinical picture of an upper lumbar nerve root compression (i.e. radiculopathy with negative SLR), chances are ≈ 3 to 1 that it is an extremely lateral HLD rather than an upper lumbar disc herniation.

Differs from the more common central and subarticular HLD in that:

- the nerve root involved is usually the one exiting *at* that level (c.f. the root exiting at the level below)
- straight leg raising (SLR) (p. 1048) is negative in 85–90% of cases ≥ 1 week after onset (excluding double herniations; ≈ 65% will be negative if double herniations are included); may have positive femoral stretch test
- pain is reproduced by lateral bending to the side of herniation in 75%
- higher incidence of extruded fragments (60%)
- higher incidence of double herniations on the same side at the same level (15%)
- pain tends to be more severe (may be due to fact that the dorsal root ganglion may be compressed directly) and often has more of a burning dysesthetic quality

Presentation

Quadriceps weakness, reduction of patellar reflex, and diminished sensation in the L3 or L4 dermatome are the most common findings.

Differential diagnosis

1. lateral recess stenosis or superior articular facet hypertrophy
2. retroperitoneal hematoma or tumor

Table 69.5 Incidence of extreme lateral HLD by level[a]

Disc level	No.	%
L1–2	1	1%
L2–3	11	8%
L3–4	35	24%
L4–5	82	60%
L5-S1	9	7%

[a]series of 138 cases[86]

3. diabetic neuropathy (amyotrophy) (p.545)
4. spinal tumor
   a) benign (schwannoma or neurofibroma)
   b) malignant tumors
   c) lymphoma
5. infection
   a) localized (spinal epidural abscess)
   b) psoas muscle abscess
   c) granulomatous disease
6. spondylolisthesis (with pars defect)
7. compression of conjoined nerve root
8. on MRI, enlarged foraminal veins may mimic extreme lateral disc herniation

Radiographic diagnosis

NB: if actively sought, many *asymptomatic* far-lateral disc herniations may be demonstrated on MRI or CT. Careful clinical correlation is usually required.

MRI: diagnostic test of choice. Sagittal views through the neural foramen may help demonstrate the disc herniation.[87] MRI may have ≈ 8% false positive rate due to presence of enlarged foraminal veins that mimic extreme lateral HLD.[88]

Myelography: myelography alone is rarely diagnostic (usually requires post myelo CT.[89,90] Fails to disclose the pathology in 87% of cases due to the fact that the nerve root compression occurs distal to the nerve root sleeve (and therefore beyond the reach of the dye).[91]

CT scan[90]: reveals a mass displacing epidural fat and encroaching on the intervertebral foramen or lateral recess, compromising the emerging root. Or, may be lateral to foramen. Sensitivity is ≈ 50% and is similar with post-myelographic CT.[91] Post-discography CT[91,92] has also been able to demonstrate.

69

Surgical treatment

NB: compression of the dorsal root ganglion may result in a slower recovery from discectomy and overall less satisfying outcome than with the more commonplace paramedian disc herniation.

Foraminal discs

Usually requires mesial facetectomy to gain access to the region lateral to the dural sac without undue retraction on nerve root or cauda equina. Caution: total facetectomy combined with discectomy may result in a high incidence of instability (total facetectomy alone causes ≈ 10% rate of slippage), although other series found this risk to be lower (≈ 1 in 33[93,94]). An alternative technique is to remove just the lateral portion of the superior articular facet below.[95] Endoscopic techniques may be well suited for herniated discs in this location.[96]

Discs herniated beyond (lateral to) the foramen

Numerous approaches are used, including:

1. traditional midline hemilaminectomy: the ipsilateral facet must be partially or completely removed. The safest way to find the exiting nerve root is take the laminectomy of the inferior portion of the upper vertebral level (e.g. L4 for a L4–5 HLD) high enough to expose the nerve root axilla, and then follow the nerve laterally through the neural foramen by removing facet until the HLD is identified
2. lateral approach (i.e. extra-canal) through a paramedian incision.[97] Advantages: the facet joint is preserved (facet removal combined with discectomy may lead to instability), muscle retraction is easier. Disadvantages: unfamiliar approach for most surgeons and the nerve cannot be followed medial to lateral. A localizing x-ray is taken with a spinal needle. A 4–5 cm vertical skin incision is made 3–4 cm lateral to the midline on the side of the disc herniation. The incision is taken down to the thoracolumbar fascia and the subcutaneous tissue is dissected off the fascia. Above L4, one may palpate the groove between multifidus (medial) and longissimus (lateral), where the fascia is incised. The facet joint is palpated, and blunt dissection is used to gain access to the lateral facet joint and transverse processes above and below the level of the disc herniation. The correct level is confirmed on x-ray using a probe as a marker. The intertransversarius muscle and fascia are divided. Care must be taken to avoid mechanical and electrocautery injury to the nerve and dorsal root ganglion (which lies immediately beneath the intertransverse ligament). The radicular artery, vein, and nerve root are located just beneath the transverse processes, usually slightly

medial to this position. The nerve root hugs the pedicle of the level above as it exits the neural foramen (palpating this e.g. with a dental dissector helps locate it), and it may be splayed over the herniated disc fragment. If more medial exposure is necessary, the lateral facet joint may be resected. The HLD is removed. Additional removal of disc material from the disc space may be performed with down-biting pituitary rongeurs. Extracanal approach to L5-S1 requires removal of part of the sacral ala in order to access the space caudal to the L5 transverse process

69.1.12 Lumbar disc herniations in pediatrics

Less than one percent of surgery for herniated lumbar disc is performed on patients between the ages of 10 and 20 yrs (one series at Mayo found 0.4% of operated HLD in patients < 17 yrs age[98]). These patients often have few neurologic findings except for a consistently positive straight leg raising test.[99] Herniated disc material in youths tends to be firm, fibrous and strongly attached to the cartilaginous end-plate unlike the degenerated material usually extruded in adult disc herniation. Plain radiographs disclosed an unusually high frequency of congenital spine anomalies (transitional vertebra, hyperlordosis, spondylolisthesis, spina bifida…). 78% did well after their first operation.[98]

69.1.13 Intradural disc herniation

Herniation of a fragment of disc into the thecal sac, or into the nerve root sleeve (the latter sometimes referred to as "intraradicular" disc herniation) has been recognized with a reported incidence of 0.04–1.1% of disc herniations.[75,100] Although it may be suspected on the basis of pre-op MRI or myelography, the diagnosis is rarely made preoperatively.[100] Intraoperatively, it may be suggested by the appreciation of a tense firm mass within the nerve root sleeve or by the negative exploration of a level with obvious clinical signs and clear cut radiographic abnormalities (after verifying that the correct level is exposed).

69

Surgical treatment:

Although a surgical dural opening may be utilized,[75] others have found this to be necessary in a minority of cases.[101]

69.1.14 Intravertebral disc herniation

General information

AKA Schmorl's node or nodule. Named for German pathologist Christian Georg Schmorl (1861–1932) the term was first used in 1971.[102] AKA Schmor's (no "l") nodule AKA Geipel hernia.[103] Disc herniation through the cartilaginous end plate into the cancellous bone of the vertebral body (VB) (AKA intraspongious disc herniation). Often an incidental finding on x-ray or MRI. Clinical significance is controversial. May produce low back pain initially that lasts ≈ 3–4 months after onset. Diffuse displacement (as may be seen in osteoporosis) is sometimes referred to as a balloon disc.[104]

Clinical findings

During the acute (symptomatic) phase, patients may exhibit LBP that is aggravated by weight bearing and movement. There may be tenderness to percussion or manual compression over the involved segment.

Radiographic findings

MRI: the extrusion of disc material into the VB is easily appreciated on sagittal images. It has been suggested[105] that acute (symptomatic) lesions may appear differentiated from chronic (asymptomatic) lesions by the presence of MRI findings of inflammation in the bone marrow immediately surrounding the node as outlined in ▶ Table 69.6.

CT: demonstrates defect in endplate and vertebral body since disc material has a significantly lower density than bone.

Plain x-ray: ≤ 33% may be seen on plain x-rays.[106] They may not be detectable acutely until sclerotic osseous bone casting develops.

Treatment

Conservative treatment is indicated, usually consisting of non-steroidal anti-inflammatory drugs (NSAIDs). Occasionally stronger pain medication and/or lumbar bracing may be required. Surgery is rarely indicated.

Table 69.6 MRI signal intensity in Schmorl's nodes[a]

Lesion	T1WI	T2WI
symptomatic (acute)	low	high
asymptomatic (chronic)	high[b]	low[b]

[a]signal intensity in surrounding marrow
[b]the same as normal marrow

Outcome

With conservative treatment, symptoms generally resolve within 3–4 months of onset (as with most vertebral body fractures).

69.1.15 Recurrent herniated lumbar disc

General information

Rates quoted in the literature range from 3–19% with the higher rates usually in series with longer follow-up.[107] In an individual series with 10 year mean F/U, the rate of recurrent disc herniation was 4% (same level, either side), one third of which occurred during the 1st year post-op (mean: 4.3 yrs).[63] A *second* recurrence at the same site occurred in 1% in another series[107] with mean F/U of 4.5 yrs. In this series,[107] patients presenting for a second time with disc herniation had a recurrence at the same level in 74%, but 26% had a HLD at another level. Recurrent HLD occurred at L4–5 more than twice as often as L5-S1.[107]

It is often possible for a smaller amount of recurrent herniated disc to cause symptoms than in a "virgin back", due to the fact that the nerve root is often fixated by scar tissue and has little ability to deviate away from the fragment.[56]

Treatment

Initial recommended treatment is as with a first time HLD. Nonsurgical treatment should be utilized in the absence of progressive neurologic deficit, cauda equina syndrome (CES) or intractable pain.

69.1.16 Surgical treatment

Disagreement occurs regarding optimal treatment. See **Practice guideline: Lumbar fusion for disc herniation** (p. 1037).

Surgical outcome:

As with first time HLD, the outcome from surgical treatment is worse in worker's compensation cases and in patients undertaking litigation, only ≈ 40% of these patients benefit.[107,108] A worse prognosis is also associated with: patients with < 6 mos relief after their first operation, cases where fibrosis without recurrent HLD is found at operation.

69.1.17 Spinal cord stimulation

One study actually showed a better response rate to spinal cord stimulation than to reoperation.[109] Since surgery for recurrent HLD carries a higher risk of dural and nerve root injury, and a lower success rate than first time operations, this may be a viable option for some patients.

69.2 Thoracic disc herniation

69.2.1 General information

Key concepts

- comprise only 0.25% of herniated discs, and < 4% of operations for herniated disc
- usually occur at or below T8 (the more mobile portion of the thoracic spine)
- frequently calcified ∴ get CT through disc (may affect choice of surgical approach)

69

- primary indications for surgery: refractory pain, progressive myelopathy
- surgical treatment: laminectomy is usually not appropriate

Account for 0.25–0.75% of all protruded discs.[110] 80% occur between the 3rd and 5th decades. 75% are below T8 (the more mobile portion of the thoracic spine), with a peak of 26% at T11–12. 94% were centrolateral and 6% were lateral.[111] A history of trauma may be elicited in 25% of cases.

Most common symptoms: pain (60%), sensory changes (23%), motor changes (18%). With thoracic radiculopathy, pain and sensory disturbance is in a band-like distribution radiating anteriorly and inferiorly along the involved root's dermatome. Motor involvement is difficult to document.

69.2.2 Evaluation

MRI is the mainstay of diagnosis. However, it is almost mandatory to also obtain a CT scan to determine if the disc is soft or calcified ("hard disc") which can have a profound effect on the approach. The CT is also useful to demonstrate bony detail if instrumentation is needed.

69.2.3 Indications for surgery

Herniated thoracic discs requiring surgery are rare.[111] Indications: refractory pain (usually radicular, bandlike) or progressive myelopathy. Uncommon: symptomatic syringomyelia originating at level of disc herniation.

69

69.2.4 Surgical approaches

Surgery for thoracic disc disease is problematic because of: the difficulty of anterior approaches, the proportionately tighter space between cord and canal compared to the cervical and lumbar regions, and the watershed blood supply which creates a significant risk of cord injury with attempts to manipulate the cord when trying to work anteriorly to it from a posterior approach. Herniated thoracic discs are calcified in 65% of patients considered for surgery[111] (more difficult to remove from a posterior or lateral approach than non-calcified discs).

Open surgical approaches[111,112]:

1. posterior (midline laminectomy): primary indication is for decompression of posteriorly situated intracanalicular pathology (e.g. metastatic tumor) especially over multiple levels. There is a high failure and complication rate when used for single-level anterior pathology (e.g. midline disc herniation)
2. posterolateral
   a) lateral gutter: laminectomy plus removal of pedicle.
   b) transpedicular approach[113]
   c) costotransversectomy (see below)
   d) transfacet pedicle sparing
3. anterolateral (transthoracic): usually through the pleural space
4. lateral extracavitary (retrocolic)[114] staying external to the pleural space

Thoracoscopic surgery is an alternative to open surgery.

69.2.5 Choosing the approach

General information

See anterior approaches to the thoracic spine (p. 1489).

Intraoperative SSEPs and MEPs may be helpful for patients with myelopathy.

For a laterally herniated thoracic disc without myelopathy: posterolateral approach with medial facetectomy is technically simple, and has generally good results. For a central disc herniation, or when myelopathy is present: transthoracic approach has the lowest incidence of cord injury with the best operative results (▶ Table 69.7). For anterior access, unless pathology is predominantly left-sided, a right-sided thoracotomy is preferred because the heart does not impede access.

Costotransversectomy

Indications: in the past this was often used to drain tuberculous spine abscess. It may be used for lateral disc herniation, biopsy of VB or pedicle, limited unilateral decompression of spinal cord from

Table 69.7 Results with various approaches for thoracic spine pathology[115]

Approach	Indication	Total no.	Outcome			
			Normal	Improved	Same	Worse
laminectomy	posteriorly located tumor	129	15%	42%	11%	32%
posterolateral (transpedicular)	radicular pain with lateral disc herniation; biopsy of tumor	27	37%	45%	11%	7%
lateral (costotransversectomy)	fair for midline disc; good ipsilateral access, poor access to opposite side	43	35%	53%	12%	0
transthoracic	best for midline lesions, especially for reaching both sides of cord	12	67%	33%	0	0

tumor or bone fragments, or sympathectomy. Can be used at ≈ any T-spine level. Limitations: difficult to visualize anterior canal to access midline anterior pathology. Better for soft disc than for calcified central disc.

Involves resection of the transverse process and at least ≈ 4–5 cm of the posterior rib. A serious risk of this approach is interruption of a significant radicular artery which may compromise spinal cord blood supply; see Spinal cord vasculature (p. 87). There is also a risk of pneumothorax which is less grave.

69

Booking the case: Costotransversectomy

Also see defaults & disclaimers (p. 27).

1. position: prone, usually on chest rolls
2. equipment:
   a) microscope (not used for all cases)
   b) C-arm
3. implants: if post-op instability is anticipated, thoracic pedicle screws and possibly a cage (e.g. for fracture or tumor, not typically for disc herniation)
4. neuromonitoring: SSEP/MEP
5. blood availability: type and cross 2 U PRBC
6. consent (in lay terms for the patient – not all-inclusive):
   a) procedure: surgery through the back of the chest to remove a small piece of rib to permit removal of the herniated/calcified disc
   b) alternatives: nonsurgical management, surgery from the side through the chest
   c) complications: spinal cord injury with paralysis, lung complications including pneumothorax or hemothorax (blood or air outside lungs), possible seizures with MEPs

69.2.6 Surgical technique

The approach can be somewhat difficult due to the infrequent encounter with the anatomy by most neurosurgeons. Be prepared for a "deep, red hole, where everything initially looks the same and the bony anatomy is not easy to define." With patience and persistence and the help of an anatomic model in the O.R., the surgeon can get his/her bearings. One of the most helpful landmarks is following the NVB (or just the nerve root) medially to the neural foramen.

In the O.R., before the prep and skin incision, localizing x-rays are obtained; a spinal needle inserted between 2 spinous processes may be used as a marker.

Patient position: the approach is from the side of the pathology/symptoms; for central disc herniations a right-sided approach reduces risk of injury to artery of Adamkiewicz (located on the left in 80% (p. 87)). Options:

1. lateral oblique, ≈ 30° elevated from straight prone, a "bean-bag" is good for stabilization. For a thin patient, the surgeon may stand in *front* of the patient (gives more horizontal angle of view – does not work as well with heavier patients due to mass of skin/muscle in the way laterally)

2. prone on chest rolls: the chest roll on the side of the pathology should be more medial to allow the shoulder and scapula to fall forward out of the way

Skin incision options:
1. curved paramedian skin incision: apex oriented away from the midline along the slight depression demarcating the junction of the lateral border of the paraspinal muscles with the ribs (≈ 6–7 cm lateral to midline) centered over the interspace of interest extending ≈ 3 vertebral bodies (VB) above and below. The incision is carried through the skin, subcutaneous fat, trapezius, and (for lower 6 thoracic levels, where most thoracic disc herniations occur) the latissimus dorsi, down to the ribs, and this musculocutaneous flap can be reflected medially as a unit
2. midline incision: need to extend 3–4 levels above and below the level of pathology to get an angle low enough to visualize posterior to the facet in order to access the posterior vertebral body. The inferior aspect can be curved laterally towards the side of pathology. Advantage: a laminectomy can more easily be performed if needed (if the angle does not provide adequate visualization, as a "bail-out" contingency, a facetectomy may be performed, and pedicle may even be removed to access inferior to the disc space. This usually permits easy decompression of the entire thecal sac. In the thoracic spine, stabilization is optional, and if chosen, unilateral pedicle screws and fusion are usually adequate)

Rib removal and thoracic exposure: for a simple biopsy or drainage of a small abscess, removal of only 1 rib may suffice. ✱ The rib to be removed is from the level *inferior* to the disc space to be accessed[116] (e.g. remove the T5 rib to access T4–5 disc space). For most other pathologies, 2 or 3 ribs are often removed.[117] To access a VB, the like-numbered rib *and* the rib below are removed.

69

There are a number of ligaments attached to the rib: the intercostal neurovascular bundle (NVB) courses medial to the superior costotransverse ligament which extends from the superior aspect of the rib to the transverse process of the level above. This ligament and the lateral costotransverse ligament are divided and the transverse process is rongeured off (the base of which lies on the lamina directly posterior to the pedicle). This exposes the rib anterior to the transverse process. The periosteum is incised on the rib from the angle of the rib to the costovertebral articulation, and by subperiosteal dissection around its circumference the pleura is dissected off the anterior surface of the rib. The NVB is dissected from the deep-inferior surface along with the periosteum. The rib is then transected laterally at the angle (≈ 5 cm lateral to the rib head) with rib shears, it is gripped with a clamp, and is rotated while the ligaments (including the radiate ligaments which attach the rib to the both the VB above and the VB below the disc space at the superior and inferior costal facet, respectively, except T1, 11 & 12 which only articulate with their like-numbered VB) are *sharply* dissected off the rib which is then removed. The removed rib material may be used for fusion substrate except in cases of tumor or infection. The pleura is then dissected from the deep surface of the adjacent ribs and VB (taking care not to injure the segmental vessels and to dissect the sympathetic trunk off the VB with the pleura). The pleura is then retracted laterally with a malleable ribbon or Deaver retractor.

The intervertebral foramen of interest may be located by following the NVB of the rib *above* proximally, the intercostal nerve (the ventral ramus of the nerve root at that level) enters between the two pedicles. The dura may then be exposed by enlarging the neural foramen by removing part of the pedicles with a high-speed drill and Kerrison rongeurs.

Instrumentation/fusion are rarely required for simple discectomy. Instability due to fracture, tumor, or extensive resection (e.g. with total facet takedown) necessitates surgical stabilization, typically with pedicle screws/rods extending 2 levels above and 2 levels below. Prior to closure, check for air leak by filling the opening with saline and having the anesthesiologist apply a valsalva maneuver. If an air leak is identified, a Cook catheter may be placed into the pleural space through the surgical exposure, or alternatively a chest tube is placed through a separate intercostal incision after the laminectomy wound is closed. A post-op CXR is obtained regardless of whether an air leak is identified.

Transpedicular approach

Drilling down the pedicle and removing a small amount of bone from the vertebral body, then pushing material from the epidural space into the defect created and removing it. Requires removal of just the rib head. Advantages: minimal risk of pneumothorax, more familiar anatomy. Disadvantages: requires instrumentation especially if done bilaterally, the angle is not very obliques so visualization of epidural space is minimal, may need to be done bilaterally if there are extensive bilateral components to the pathology.

Booking the case: Transpedicular approach

Same as for costotransversectomy (p. 1062).

Transthoracic approach

Indications: thoracic disc disease with central fragment or calcified disc, burst fractures of the thoracic spine, etc.

Advantages[118]:

- excellent anterior exposure (especially advantageous for multiple levels)
- little compromise of stability (due to supporting effect of rib cage)
- low risk of mechanical cord injury

Disadvantages:

- requires thoracic surgeon (or familiarity with thoracic surgery)
- some risk of vascular cord injury (due to sacrifice of intercostal arteries)
- definitive diagnosis may not be possible if it is uncertain prior to procedure

Possible complications:

- pulmonary complications: pleural effusion, atelectasis, pneumonia, empyema, hypoventilation
- CSF-pleural fistula

69

Booking the case: Transthoracic spine surgery

Also see defaults & disclaimers (p. 27).

1. position: typically on the side, often on a beanbag
2. equipment:
   a) microscope (not used for all cases)
   b) C-arm
3. anesthesia: double lumen tube
4. implants: if post-op instability is anticipated, thoracic pedicle screws and possibly a cage (e.g. for fracture or tumor, not typically for disc herniation)
5. neuromonitoring: SSEP/MEP
6. blood availability: type and cross 2 U PRBC
7. some surgeons use chest surgeon for the approach, closure and for follow-up
8. consent (in lay terms for the patient – not all-inclusive):
   a) procedure: surgery through the chest with removal of a small piece of rib to permit removal of the herniated/calcified disc
   b) alternatives: nonsurgical management, surgery from the side or through the back
   c) complications: spinal cord injury with paralysis, pneumothorax, possible seizures with MEPs

Key technical points

1. the services of an experienced thoracic surgeon are usually engaged
2. position: true lateral (facilitates intra-op localizing x-rays); approached from the more involved side. For the upper thoracic *midline* region, some prefer right-side-up to eliminate thoracic aorta from obstructing exposure and to reduce the possibility of encountering the artery of Adamkiewicz,[119] others prefer left-side-up to use the aorta as a landmark[118] (for levels below the cardiophrenic angle, a left-sided approach is preferred because the inferior vena cava is difficult to mobilize)
3. usually one rib is resected; most often the rib of the vertebra immediately *above* the disc space desired (facilitates exposure). Multiple ribs may be resected to increase exposure
4. when removing the vertebral body (VB) (corpectomy, e.g. for osteomyelitis, especially Pott's disease or for kyphoscoliosis)

a) the posterior cortex of the VB must be pulled anteriorly (e.g. with angled curettes) to avoid mechanical cord trauma
b) anterior fusion may be performed using the removed rib. If inadequate, fibula or iliac crest may be used

5. sizeable radicular arteries are spared. The intercostal nerve is used as a guide to the intervertebral foramen (nerve enters foramen superiorly and posteriorly)
6. the disc space is situated off the caudal aspect of the intervertebral foramen for most thoracic levels
7. one or two intervertebral arteries and veins usually have to be sacrificed; to minimize the risk of ischemic cord injury, cut them as close to the midline of the spine as possible (collaterals tend to lie on the lateral aspect of the spine)
8. the sympathetic chain is dissected off the VBs and is pushed posteriorly

Lateral (retrocolic) approach

See reference.[114]

The same instrumentation used for lateral lumbar interbody fusion (p. 1498) may be used to access the lateral thoracic bodies for thoracic disc herniation.

Check the pre-op MRI for the location of the aorta and to rule-out aortic aneurysm. Above T11, enter on the right side. The access retractor is "reversed" so that the center blade is positioned *anteriorly* and the shim is place so that as the retractor is expanded in the AP direction, the lateral blades move posteriorly, giving more access to the posterior disc space. In general, do not penetrate the contralateral anulus because of proximity of aorta. At or just below L12-L1, the diaphragm attaches to the VB. A dual lumen endotracheal tube is *not* required. A chest tube is mandatory if there is an air leak, otherwise it is optional (a pigtail catheter may suffice).

69

References

[1] Weber H. Lumbar Disc Herniation. A Controlled, Prospective Study with Ten Years of Observation. Spine. 1983; 8:131–140
[2] Lewis PJ, Weir BKA, Broad R, et al. Long-Term Prospective Study of Lumbosacral Discectomy. J Neurosurg. 1987; 67:49–53
[3] Wein AJ, Walsh PC, Retik AB, Vaughan ED, Wein AJ. In: Neuromuscular Dysfunction of the Lower Urinary Tract and Its Treatment. Campbell's Urology. 7th ed. Philadelphia: W.B. Saunders; 1998:953–1006
[4] Jones DL, Moore T. The Types of Neuropathic Bladder Dysfunction Associated with Prolapsed Lumbar Intervertebral Discs. Br J Urol. 1973; 45:39–43
[5] Ross JC, Jameson RM. Vesical Dysfunction Due to Prolapsed Disc. Br Med J. 1971; 3:752–754
[6] Frymoyer JW. Back Pain and Sciatica. N Engl J Med. 1988; 318:291–300
[7] Deyo RA, Rainville J, Kent DL. What Can the History and Physical Examination Tell Us About Low Back Pain? JAMA. 1992; 268:760–765
[8] Blaauw G, Braakman R, Gelpke GJ, Singh R, et al. Changes in Radicular Function Following Low-Back Surgery. J Neurosurg. 1988; 69:649–652
[9] Stam J, Speelman HD, van Crevel H. Tendon Reflex Asymmetry by Voluntary Mental Effort in Healthy Subjects. Arch Neurol. 1989; 46:70–73
[10] Bigos S, Bowyer O, Braen G, et al. Acute Low Back Problems in Adults. Clinical Practice Guideline No.14. AHCPR Publication No. 95-0642. Rockville, MD: Agency for Health Care Policy and Research, Public Health Service, U.S. Department of Health and Human Services; 1994
[11] Scham SM, Taylor TKF. Tension Signs in Lumbar Disc Prolapse. Clin Orthop. 1971; 75:195–204
[12] Dyck P. Lumbar Nerve Root: The Enigmatic Eponyms. Spine. 1984; 9:3–6
[13] Spangfort EV. The Lumbar Disc Herniation. A Computer-Aided Analysis of 2,504 Operations. Acta Orthop Scand. 1972; 142:1–93
[14] Rothman RH, Simeone FA. The Spine. Philadelphia 1992
[15] Estridge MN, Rouhe SA, Johnson NG. The Femoral Stretch Test: A Valuable Sign in Diagnosing Upper Lumbar Disc Herniations. J Neurosurg. 1982; 57:813–817
[16] Hoover CF. A new sign for the detection of malingering and functional paresis of the lower extremities. JAMA. 1908; 51:746–747
[17] Archibald KC, Wiechec F. A reappraisal of Hoover's test. Arch Phys Med Rehabil. 1970; 51:234–238
[18] Sonoo M. Abductor sign: A reliable new sign to detect unilateral non-organic paresis of the lower limb. J Neurol Neurosurg Psychiatry. 2004; 75:121–125
[19] Keegan JJ. Dermatome Hypalgesia Associated with Herniation of Intervertebral Disk. Arch Neurol Psychiatry. 1943; 50:67–83
[20] Fager CA. Observations on Spontaneous Recovery from Intervertebral Disc Herniation. Surg Neurol. 1994; 42:282–286
[21] Weber H, Holme I, Amlie E. The Natural Course of Acute Sciatica, with Nerve Root Symptoms in a Double Blind Placebo Controlled Trial Evaluating the Effect of Piroxicam (NSAID). Spine. 1993; 18:1433–1438
[22] Weber H. The Effect of Delayed Disc Surgery on Muscular Paresis. Acta Orthop Scand. 1975; 46:631–642
[23] Saal JA, Saal JS. Nonoperative Treatment of Herniated Lumbar Intervertebral Disc with Radiculopathy: An Outcome Study. Spine. 1989; 14:431–437
[24] Marshall RW. The functional relevance of neurological recovery 20 years or more after lumbar discectomy. J Bone Joint Surg Br. 2008; 90:554–555
[25] Kostuik JP, Harrington I, Alexander D, Rand W, et al. Cauda Equina Syndrome and Lumbar Disc Herniation. J Bone Joint Surg. 1986; 68A:386–391
[26] O'Laoire SA, Crockard HA, Thomas DG. Prognosis for Sphincter Recovery After Operation for Cauda Equina Compression Owing to Lumbar Disc Prolapse. Br Med J. 1981; 282:1852–1854
[27] Shapiro S. Cauda Equina Syndrome Secondary to Lumbar Disc Herniation. Neurosurgery. 1993; 32:743–747
[28] Scott PJ. Bladder Paralysis in Cauda Equina Lesions from Disc Prolapse. J Bone Joint Surg. 1965; 47B:224–235
[29] Tay ECK, Chacha PB. Midline Prolapse of a Lumbar Intervertebral Disc with Compression of the Cauda Equina. J Bone Joint Surg. 1979; 61B:43–46

[30] Prusick VD, Lint DS, Bruder J. Cauda Equina Syndrome as a Complication of Free Epidural Fat-Grafting. J Bone Joint Surg. 1988; 70A:1256–1258
[31] Tandon PN, Sankaran B. Cauda Equina Syndrome due to Lumbar Disc Prolapse. Indian J Orthopedics. 1967; 1:112–119
[32] Shapiro S. Medical Realities of Cauda Equina Syndrome Secondary to Lumbar Disc Herniation. Spine. 2000; 25:348–351
[33] Kostuik JP. Point of View: Comment on Shapiro, S: Medical Realities of Cauda Equina Syndrome Secondary to Lumbar Disc Herniation. Spine. 2000; 25
[34] Hoffman RM, Wheeler KJ, Deyo RA. Surgery for herniated lumbar discs: a literature synthesis. J Gen Intern Med. 1993; 8:487–496
[35] Williams RW. Microlumbar Discectomy: A Conservative Surgical Approach to the Virgin Herniated Lumbar Disc. Spine. 1978; 3:175–182
[36] Caspar W, Campbell B, Barbier DD, et al. The Caspar Microsurgical Discectomy and Comparison with a Conventional Lumbar Disc Procedure. Neurosurgery. 1991; 28:78–87
[37] Schmidek HH, Sweet WH. Operative Neurosurgical Techniques. New York 1982
[38] Fager CA. Lumbar Discectomy: A Contrary Opinion. Clin Neurosurg. 1986; 33:419–456
[39] Tulberg T, Isacson J, Weidenhielm L. Does Microscopic Removal of Lumbar Disc Herniation Lead to Better Results than the Standard Procedure? Results of a One-Year Randomized Study. J Neurosurg. 1993; 70:869–875
[40] Hoppenfield S. Percutaneous Removal of Herniated Lumbar Discs. 50 Cases with Ten-Year Follow-Up Periods. Clin Orthop. 1989; 238:92–97
[41] Kahanovitz N, Viola K, Goldstein T, et al. A Multicenter Analysis of Percutaneous Discectomy. Spine. 1990; 15:713–715
[42] Davis GW, Onik G. Clinical Experience with Automated Percutaneous Lumbar Discectomy. Clin Orthop. 1989; 238:98–103
[43] Revel M, Payan C, Vallee C, et al. Automated Percutaneous Lumbar Discectomy Versus Chemonucleolysis in the Treatment of Sciatica. Spine. 1993; 18:1–7
[44] Maroon JC, Onik G, Sternau L. Percutaneous automated discectomy. A new method for lumbar disc removal. Technical note. J Neurosurg. 1987; 66:143–146
[45] Onik G, Maroon JC, Jackson R. Cauda Equina Syndrome Secondary to an Improperly Placed Nucleotome Probe. Neurosurgery. 1992; 30:412–415
[46] Cohen SP, Williams S, Kurihara C, Griffith S, Larkin TM. Nucleoplasty with or without intradiscal electrothermal therapy (IDET) as a treatment for lumbar herniated disc. J Spinal Disord Tech. 2005; 18 Suppl:S119–S124
[47] Yonezawa T, Onomura T, Kosaka R, et al. The System and Procedures of Percutaneous Intradiscal Laser Nucleotomy. Spine. 1990; 15:1175–1185
[48] Choy DSJ, Ascher PW, Saddekni S, et al. Percutaneous laser disc decompression: A new therapeutic modality. Spine. 1992; 17:949–956
[49] North American Spine Society Coverage Committee. Laser Spine Surgery. Burr Ridge, IL 2014
[50] Mayer HM, Brock M. Percutaneous Endoscopic Discectomy: Surgical Technique and Preliminary Results Compared to Microsurgical Discectomy. J Neurosurg. 1993; 78:216–225
[51] Kleinpeter G, Markowitsch MM, Bock F. Percutaneous Endoscopic Lumbar Discectomy: Minimally Invasive, But Perhaps Only Minimally Useful? Surg Neurol. 1995; 43:534–541
[52] Karasek M, Bogduk N. Twelve-month follow-up of a controlled trial of intradiscal thermal anuloplasty for back pain due to internal disc disruption. Spine. 2000; 25:2601–2607
[53] Schwarzer AC, Aprill CN, Derby R, Fortin J, Kine G, Bogduk N. The prevalence and clinical features of internal disc disruption in patients with chronic low back pain. Spine. 1995; 20:1878–1883
[54] Ranguis SC, Li D, Webster AC. Perioperative epidural steroids for lumbar spine surgery in degenerative spinal disease. J Neurosurg Spine. 2010; 13:745–757
[55] Glasser RS, Knego RS, Delashaw JB, Fessler RG. The Perioperative Use of Corticosteroids and Bipuvicaine in the Management of Lumbar Disc Disease. J Neurosurg. 1993; 78:383–387
[56] Dunsker SB. Comment on Cobanoglu S, et al.: Complication of Epidural Fat Graft in Lumbar Spine Disc Surgery: Case Report. Surg Neurol. 1995; 44:481–482
[57] Cabezudo JM, Lopez A, Bacci F. Symptomatic Root Compression by a Free Fat Transplant After Hemilaminectomy: Case Report. J Neurosurg. 1985; 63:633–635
[58] Cobanoglu S, Imer M, Ozylmaz F, Memis M. Complication of Epidural Fat Graft in Lumbar Spine Disc Surgery: Case Report. Surg Neurol. 1995; 44:479–482
[59] Ramirez LF, Thisted R. Complications and Demographic Characteristics of Patients Undergoing Lumbar Discectomy in Community Hospitals. Neurosurgery. 1989; 25:226–231
[60] Deyo RA, Cherkin DC, Loeser JD, Bigos SJ, et al. Morbidity and mortality in association with operations on the lumbar spine. The influence of age, diagnosis, and procedure. J Bone Joint Surg. 1992; 74A:536–543
[61] Shektman A, Granick MS, Solomon MP, et al. Management of Infected Laminectomy Wounds. Neurosurgery. 1994; 35:307–309
[62] Goodkin R, Laska LL. Unintended 'Incidental' Durotomy During Surgery of the Lumbar Spine: Medicolegal Implications. Surg Neurol. 1995; 43:4–14
[63] Davis RA. A Long-Term Outcome Analysis of 984 Surgically Treated Herniated Lumbar Discs. J Neurosurg. 1994; 80:415–421
[64] Bilsky MH, Shields CB. Complications of Lumbar Disc Surgery. Contemp Neurosurg. 1995; 17:1–6
[65] DeSaussure RL. Vascular Injuries Coincident to Disc Surgery. J Neurosurg. 1959; 16:222–239
[66] Nam TK, Park SW, Shim HJ, Hwang SN. Endovascular treatment for common iliac artery injury complicating lumbar disc surgery: limited usefulness of temporary balloon occlusion. J Korean Neurosurg Soc. 2009; 46:261–264
[67] Jhawar BS, Mitsis D, Duggal N. Wrong-sided and wrong-level neurosurgery: a national survey. J Neurosurg Spine. 2007; 7:467–472
[68] Mclaren AC, Bailey SI. Cauda Equina Syndrome: A Complication of Lumbar Discectomy. Clin Orthop. 1986; 204:143–149
[69] Porter RW, Detwiler PW, Lawton MT, Sonntag VKH, Dickman CA. Postoperative Spinal Epidural Hematomas: Longitudinal Review of 12,000 Spinal Operations. BNI Quarterly. 2000; 16:10–17
[70] Lee LA, Roth S, Posner KL, Cheney FW, Caplan RA, et al. The American Society of Anesthesiologists Postoperative Visual Loss Registry: analysis of 93 spine surgery cases with postoperative visual loss. Anesthesiology. 2006; 105:652–659
[71] Sachs BL, Zindrick MR, Beasley RD. Reflex Sympathetic Dystrophy After Operative Procedures on the Lumbar Spine. J Bone Joint Surg. 1993; 75A:721–725
[72] Feldman RA, Karl RC. Diagnosis and Treatment of Ogilvie's Syndrome After Lumbar Spinal Surgery. J Neurosurg. 1992; 76:1012–1016
[73] Hodges SD, Humphreys C, Eck JC, Covington LA. Management of Incidental Durotomy Without Mandatory Bed Rest. Spine. 1999; 24:2062–2064
[74] Fink LH. Unintended 'incidental' durotomy. Surg Neurol. 1996; 45
[75] Ciappetta P, Delfini R, Cantore GP. Intradural Lumbar Disc Hernia: Description of Three Cases. Neurosurgery. 1981; 8:104–107
[76] Desai A, Ball PA, Bekelis K, Lurie J, Mirza SK, Tosteson TD, Weinstein JN. SPORT: Does incidental durotomy affect longterm outcomes in cases of spinal stenosis? Neurosurgery. 2015; 76 Suppl 1:S57–63; discussion S63
[77] Horwitz NH, Rizzoli HV, Horwitz NH, Rizzoli HV. In: Herniated Intervertebral Discs and Spinal Stenosis. Postoperative Complications of

Extracranial Neurological Surgery. Baltimore: Williams and Wilkins; 1987:1–72
[78] Eismont FL, Wiesel SW, Rothman RH. Treatment of Dural Tears Associated with Spinal Surgery. J Bone Joint Surg. 1981; 63A:1132–1136
[79] Waisman M, Schweppe Y. Postoperative Cerebrospinal Fluid Leakage After Lumbar Spine Operations. Conservative Treatment. Spine. 1991; 15:52–53
[80] Hayreh SS. Ischemic optic neuropathy. Prog Retin Eye Res. 2009; 28:34–62
[81] Postoperative Visual Loss Study Group. Risk factors associated with ischemic optic neuropathy after spinal fusion surgery. Anesthesiology. 2012; 116:15–24
[82] Weinstein JN, Tosteson TD, Lurie JD, Tosteson AN, Hanscom B, Skinner JS, Abdu WA, Hilibrand AS, Boden SD, Deyo RA. Surgical vs nonoperative treatment for lumbar disk herniation: the Spine Patient Outcomes Research Trial (SPORT): a randomized trial. JAMA. 2006; 296:2441–2450
[83] Weinstein JN, Lurie JD, Tosteson TD, Skinner JS, Hanscom B, Tosteson AN, Herkowitz H, Fischgrund J, Cammisa FP, Albert T, Deyo RA. Surgical vs nonoperative treatment for lumbar disk herniation: the Spine Patient Outcomes Research Trial (SPORT) observational cohort. JAMA. 2006; 296:2451–2459
[84] McCormick PC. The Spine Patient Outcomes Research Trial results for lumbar disc herniation: a critical review. J Neurosurg Spine. 2007; 6:513–520
[85] Aronson HA, Dunsmore RH. Herniated Upper Lumbar Discs. J Bone Joint Surg. 1963; 45:311–317
[86] Abdullah AF, Wolber PGH, Warfield JR, et al. Surgical Management of Extreme Lateral Lumbar Disc Herniations: Review of 138 Cases. Neurosurgery. 1988; 22:648–653
[87] Osborn AG, Hood RS, Sherry RG, et al. CT/MR Spectrum of Far Lateral and Anterior Lumbosacral Disk Herniations. AJNR. 1988; 9:775–778
[88] Grenier N, Greselle J-F, Douws C, et al. MR Imaging of Foraminal and Extraforaminal Lumbar Disk Herniations. J Comput Assist Tomogr. 1990; 14:243–249
[89] Godersky JC, Erickson DL, Seljeskog EL. Extreme Lateral Disc Herniation: Diagnosis by CT Scanning. Neurosurgery. 1984; 14:549–552
[90] Osborne DR, Heinz ER, Bullard D, et al. Role of CT in the Radiological Evaluation of Painful Radiculopathy After Negative Myelography. Neurosurgery. 1984; 14:147–153
[91] Jackson RP, Glah JJ. Foraminal and Extraforaminal Lumbar Disc Herniation: Diagnosis and Treatment. Spine. 1987; 12:577–585
[92] Angtuaco EJC, Holder JC, Boop WC, Binet EF. Computed Tomographic Discography in the Evaluation of Extreme Lateral Disc Herniation. Neurosurgery. 1984; 14:350–352
[93] Garrido E, Connaughton PN. Unilateral Facetectomy Approach for Lateral Lumbar Disc Herniation. J Neurosurg. 1991; 74:754–756
[94] Epstein NE, Epstein JA, Carras R, et al. Far Lateral Lumbar Disc Herniations and Associated Structural Abnormalities. An Evaluation in 60 Patients of the Comparative Value of CT, MRI, and Myelo-CT in Diagnosis and Management. Spine. 1990; 15:534–539
[95] Jane JA, Haworth CS, Broaddus WC, Lee JH, Malik J. A Neurosurgical Approach to Far-Lateral Disc Herniation. J Neurosurg. 1990; 72:143–144
[96] Ditsworth DA. Endoscopic Transforaminal Lumbar Discectomy and Reconfiguration: A Posterolateral Approach into the Spinal Canal. Surg Neurol. 1998; 49:588–598
[97] Maroon JC, Kopitnik TA, Schulhof LA, et al. Diagnosis and Microsurgical Approach to Far-Lateral Disc Herniation in the Lumbar Spine. J Neurosurg. 1990; 72:378–382
[98] Ebersold MJ, Quast LM, Bianco AJ. Results of Lumbar Discectomy in the Pediatric Patient. J Neurosurg. 1987; 67:643–647
[99] Epstein JA, Epstein NE, Marc J, Rosenthal AD, et al. Lumbar Intervertebral Disk Herniation in Teenage Children: Recognition and Management of Associated Anomalies. Spine. 1984; 9:427–432
[100] Kataoka O, Nishibayashi Y, Sho T. Intradural Lumbar Disc Herniation: Report of Three Cases with a Review of the Literature. Spine. 1989:529–533
[101] Schisano G, Franco A, Nina P. Intraradicular and Intradural Lumbar Disc Herniation: Experience with Nine Cases. Surg Neurol. 1995; 44:536–543
[102] Schmorl G, Junghanns H. The Human Spine in Health and Disease. New York: Grune & Stratton; 1971
[103] Deeg HJ. Schmorl's nodule. N Engl J Med. 1978; 298
[104] Fardon DF, Milette PC. Nomenclature and classification of lumbar disc pathology. Recommendations of the Combined task Forces of the North American Spine Society, American Society of Spine Radiology, and American Society of Neuroradiology. Spine. 2001; 26:E93–E113
[105] Takahashi K, Miyazaki T, Ohnari H, Takino T, Tomita K. Schmorl's nodes and low-back pain. Analysis of magnetic resonance imaging findings in symptomatic and asymptomatic individuals. Eur Spine J. 1995; 4:56–59
[106] Hamanishi C, Kawabata T, Yosii T, Tanaka S. Schmorl's nodes on magnetic resonance imaging. Spine. 1994; 19:450–453
[107] Herron L. Recurrent Lumbar Disc Herniation: Results of Repeat Laminectomy and Discectomy. J Spinal Disord. 1994; 7:161–166
[108] Waddell G, Crummel EG, Solts WN, Graham JD, Hall H, McCulloch JA. Failed Lumbar Disc Surgery and Repeat Surgery Following Industrial Injuries. J Bone Joint Surg. 1979; 61A:201–207
[109] Bell GK, Kidd D, North RB. Cost-effectiveness analysis of spinal cord stimulation in treatment of failed back surgery syndrome. J Pain Symptom Manage. 1997; 13:286–295
[110] El-Kalliny M, Tew JM, van Loveren H, Dunsker S. Surgical approaches to thoracic disk herniations. Acta Neurochir. 1991; 111:22–32
[111] Stillerman CB, Chen TC, Couldwell WT, Zhang W, Weiss MH. Experience in the surgical management of 82 symptomatic herniated thoracic discs and review of the literature. J Neurosurg. 1998; 88:623–633
[112] Dohn DF. Thoracic Spinal Cord Decompression: Alternative Surgical Approaches and Basis of Choice. Clin Neurosurg. 1980; 27:611–623
[113] Le Roux PD, Haglund MM, Harris AB. Thoracic Disc Disease: Experience with the Transpedicular Approach in Twenty Consecutive Patients. Neurosurgery. 1993; 33:58–66
[114] Uribe JS, Smith WD, Pimenta L, Hartl R, Dakwar E, Modhia UM, Pollock GA, Nagineni V, Smith R, Christian G, Oliveira L, Marchi L, Deviren V. Minimally invasive lateral approach for symptomatic thoracic disc herniation: initial multicenter clinical experience. J Neurosurg Spine. 2012; 16:264–279
[115] Arce AC, Dohrmann GJ. Thoracic Disc Herniation. Surg Neurol. 1985; 23:356–361
[116] Ahlgren BD, Herkowitz HN. A modified posterolateral approach to the thoracic spine. J Spinal Disord. 1195; 8:69–75
[117] O'Leary ST, Ganju A, Rauzzino MJ, et al. Fessler RG, Sekhar L. In: Costotransversectomy. Atlas of Neurosurgical Techniques. New York: Thieme Medical Publishers, Inc.; 2006:441–447
[118] Chou SN, Seljeskog EL. Alternative Surgical Approaches to the Thoracic Spine. Clin Neurosurg. 1972; 20:306–321
[119] Perot PL, Munro DD. Transthoracic Removal of Midline Thoracic Disc Protrusions Causing Spinal Cord Compression. J Neurosurg. 1969; 31:452–461

70 Cervical Disc Herniation

70.1 General information

Important applied anatomy in herniated cervical disc (HCD):

1. in the cervical region, the nerve root exits *above* the pedicle of its like-numbered vertebra (opposite to the situation in the lumbar spine, due to the fact that there are 8 cervical nerve roots and only 7 cervical vertebrae)
2. each root exits passes through its neural foramen in close relation to the undersurface of the pedicle
3. the intervertebral disc space is located close to the inferior portion of the pedicle (unlike the lumbar region)

70.2 Cervical nerve root syndromes (cervical radiculopathy)

70.2.1 General information

Due to the facts listed above, a HCD usually impinges on the nerve exiting from the neural foramen *at* the level of the herniation (e.g. a C6–7 HCD usually causes C7 radiculopathy). This gives rise to the characteristic cervical nerve root syndromes shown in ▶ Table 70.1.

70.2.2 Miscellaneous clinical facts

C4 radiculopathy is not common, and may produce nonradiating axial neck pain.

Left C6 radiculopathy (e.g. from C5–6 HCD) occasionally presents with pain simulating an MI (pseudo-angina).

C8 and T1 nerve root involvement may produce a partial Horner's syndrome.

The most common scenario for patients with herniated cervical disc is that the symptoms were present upon awakening in the morning, without identifiable trauma or stress.[1]

70

70.3 Cervical myelopathy and SCI due to cervical disc herniation

Acute cord compression presenting with myelopathy or spinal cord injury (SCI) (including complete SCI and incomplete syndromes, especially **central cord syndrome** (p.944) and sometimes Brown-Sequard syndrome (p.947) [2] is well described in association with traumatic cervical disc herniation.[3] Less commonly, these findings may occur in non-traumatic cervical disc herniation.

Table 70.1 Cervical disc syndromes

Syndrome	Cervical disc syndromes			
	C4–5	C5–6	C6–7	C7-T1
% of cervical discs	2%	19%	69%	10%
compressed root	C5	C6	C7	C8
reflex diminished	deltoid & pectoralis	biceps & brachioradialis	triceps	finger-jerk[a]
motor weakness	deltoid	forearm flexion	forearm ext (wrist drop)	hand intrinsics
paresthesia & hypesthesia	shoulder	upper arm, thumb, radial forearm	fingers 2 & 3, all fingertips	fingers 4 & 5

[a]not everyone has a finger flexor reflex. Description: gently lift the fingertips of the patient's pronated hand and tap the underside of the fingers with a reflex hammer. When present, fingers flex in response

70.4 Differential diagnosis

See Differential diagnosis (p. 1420).

70.5 Physical exam for cervical disc herniation

70.5.1 Overview

1. evaluation for radiculopathy
   a) lower motor neuron findings
      - weakness usually in one myotome group on one side
      - muscle bulk and tone: atrophy and fasciculations, may be present
   b) sensation: with nerve root compression, sensory loss will follow a dermatomal pattern and will be in the same nerve root distribution as the weakness
   c) muscle stretch reflexes
   d) mechanical signs: reproduction of radicular symptoms with axial loading of the head
2. evidence of spinal cord involvement (myelopathy)
   a) upper motor neuron findings, usually in the lower extremities
      - weakness may occur without atrophy or fasciculations
      - spasticity: poor control of the Legs when walking, scissoring of the legs
   b) sensation: any loss below the level of involvement will follow spinal cord patterns
      - complete loss
      - Brown-Sequard pattern: unilateral loss of pinprick with contralateral vibratory and position sense loss
      - Central cord syndrome: suspended sensory loss in upper extremities, less impaired below
      - Pathologic reflexes: Hoffmann's reflex, Babinski sign, ankle clonus

70

70.5.2 Signs useful in evaluating cervical radiculopathy

General information

Almost all herniated cervical discs cause painful limitation of neck motion. Neck *extension* usually aggravates pain when cervical disc disease is present (a minority of patients instead exhibit pain with flexion). Some patients find relief in elevating the arm and cupping the back or the top of the head with the hand (abduction relief sign, see below for shoulder abduction test). Lhermitte's sign (electrical shock-like sensation radiating down the spine) may be present; see DDx (p. 1421).

Miscellaneous

The following tests were found to be specific, but not particularly sensitive in detecting cervical root compression[4]:

1. Spurling's sign[5]: radicular pain reproduced when the examiner exerts downward pressure on vertex while tilting head towards symptomatic side (sometimes adding neck *extension*). Causes narrowing of the intervertebral foramen and possibly increases disc bulge. Used as a "mechanical sign" analogous to SLR for lumbar disc herniation
2. axial manual traction: 10–15 kg of axial traction is applied to a supine patient with radicular symptoms (pull up on patient's mandible and occiput). The reduction or disappearance of radicular symptoms is a positive finding
3. shoulder abduction test[6]: a sitting patient with radicular symptoms lifts their hand above their head. The reduction or disappearance of radicular symptoms is a positive finding. Moderately sensitive, fairly specific[7]

70.6 Radiologic evaluation

70.6.1 MRI

The study of choice for initial evaluation for herniated cervical disc (HCD). Accuracy is less than water soluble contrast myelogram/CT (≈ 85–90% accuracy for MRI because of only fair to good imaging of neural foramen), but is non-invasive. For *myelopathy*, MRI is > 95% effective in diagnosing.

Protocol:

1. sagittal T1WI
2. multiple echo cardiac gated sagittal images (Tr = 1560, Te = 25, 4th echo)

3. GRASS image: axial partial flip-angle fast scan (Tr = 25, Te = 13, angle = 8°). Dark material adjacent to disc space is bone, disc is higher signal, CSF and flowing blood are high signal.

70.6.2 CT and myelogram/CT

Indications: when MRI cannot be done or when more bony detail than what MRI provides is required. Evaluates for ossification of the posterior longitudinal ligament (OPLL) when suspected.

Plain CT: is usually good at C5–6, is variable at C6–7 (due to artifact from patient's shoulders, depending on body habitus), and is usually poor at C7-T1.

Myelogram/CT (water soluble intrathecal contrast): invasive, on rare occasions requires overnight hospitalization. Accuracy is ≈ 98% for cervical disc disease.

70.6.3 Electrodiagnostics (EMG and NCV)

Compression may occur at the level of the dorsal (pre-ganglionic) sensory root (which, if occurs alone, produces a sensory-only radiculopathy) and/or at the ventral (motor) root. When motor exam is normal, EMG is unlikely to show abnormality. The AANEM practice parameter for cervical radiculopathy[8,9,10] reports sensitivity of 50-71% for the needle EMG examination and correlation between positive needle EMG and radiologic findings of 65-85%.

EMG can also be normal in sensory only radiculopathy, which occasionally occurs in cervical spine, but not in lumbar spine. Since most muscles have at least dual innervation this poses a particular challenge for proximal cervical radiculopathies in which many muscles have the same shared innervation, e.g. biceps, deltoid, brachioradialis, infraspinatus and supraspinatus are all innervated by C5-C6.

For both cervical and lumbosacral radiculopathy, screening 6 muscles representing all root levels to include paraspinal muscles yield consistently high identification rates.[11]

For muscles to demonstrate fibrillations and positive waves there must be axonal loss in the motor nerve axons which innervates a muscle. Muscle demonstrates fibs and positive waves within 1 to 2 weeks following loss of innervation depending on the distance from the nerve to the muscle.

NCV is helpful to assess for peripheral neuropathies which may have symptoms similar to radiculopathy (e.g. carpal tunnel syndrome vs. C6 radiculopathy; ulnar neuropathy vs. C8 radiculopathy). A good physical exam can differentiate these entities in most cases.

70

Practice guideline: EDX guidelines for cervical radiculopathy

See reference.[10]

1. Guideline: EMG needle examination:
   a) needle examination of at least 1 muscle innervated by C5, C6, C7, C8 and T1 spinal roots in a symptomatic limb
   b) cervical paraspinal muscles at 1 or more levels (except in patients with prior posterior approach cervical surgery
   c) if abnormalities are identified, perform studies of 1 or 2 additional muscles innervated by the suspected root and different peripheral nerve
2. Guideline: At least 1 motor and 1 sensory nerve conduction study (NCS) in the clinically involved limb to determine if there is concomitant polyneuropathy or nerve entrapment. Motor and sensory NCS of median and ulnar nerves if symptoms and signs suggest CTS or ulnar neuropathy. If 1 or more NCS are abnormal or if clinical features suggest polyneuropathy, further evaluation may include NCS of other nerves in the ipsilateral and contralateral limb

70.7 Treatment

70.7.1 General information

Over 90% of patients with acute cervical radiculopathy due to cervical disc herniation can improve without surgery,[12] and regression of an extruded cervical disc has been demonstrated radiographically by CT and MRI.[13,14,15] The recovery period may be made more tolerable by adequate pain medication, anti-inflammatory medication (NSAIDs or short-course tapering steroids) and intermittent cervical traction (e.g. gradually escalating up to 10–15 lbs for 10–15 minutes, 2–3 × daily).

Surgery is indicated for those that fail to improve or those with progressive neurologic deficit while undergoing non-surgical management.

Management of myelopathy/central cord syndrome associated with acute cervical disc herniation is controversial, since the natural history is favorable in most cases. However, some patients have poor recovery and experience permanent deficits even with emergency surgery.[16]

70.7.2 Conservative management

Modalities include:

1. physical therapy, which may also include cervical traction.
2. Interventional pain management
   a) Trigger point injections
   b) Facet blocks
   c) Epidural steroid injection: not used as often and with lumbar spine

70.7.3 Surgery

Surgical options

1. anterior cervical discectomy: see below
   a) without any prosthesis or fusion: rarely used today
   b) combined with interbody fusion: the most common approach
      - without anterior cervical plating
      - with anterior cervical plating or with zero profile
   c) with artificial disc AKA cervical disc arthroplasty
2. posterior approaches
   a) cervical laminectomy: not typically used for a herniated cervical disc, more common for cervical spinal stenosis, OPLL
      - without posterior fusion
      - with lateral mass fusion
   b) keyhole laminotomy: sometimes permits removal of disc fragment

For practice guidelines regarding intra-op electrophysiologic, see monitoring for surgery for cervical radiculopathy (p. 1090).

Anterior cervical discectomy with fusion (ACDF)

Without special modifications, a routine anterior approach is usually able to access levels C3–7. In patients with short thick necks, access may be even more limited. In some cases, with long thin necks, up to C2–3 or as low as C7-T1 can be approached anteriorly.

Advantages over posterior (nonfused) approach:

1. safe removal of anterior osteophytes
2. fusion of disc space affords immobility (up to 10% incidence of subluxation with extensive posterior approach)
3. only viable means of directly dealing with centrally herniated disc

Disadvantages over posterior approach: immobility at fused level may increase stress on adjacent disc spaces. If a fusion is performed, some surgeons prescribe a rigid collar (e.g. Philadelphia collar) for 6–12 weeks. Multiple level ACDF can devascularize the vertebral body (or bodies) between discectomies.

Booking the case: ACDF

Also see defaults & disclaimers (p. 27).

1. position: supine, some use halter traction with this
2. equipment:
   a) microscope (not used by all surgeons)
   b) C-arm
3. implants: graft (e.g. PEEK, cadaver bone, titanium cage...) and anterior cervical plate (optional, especially on single level ACDF)

4. neuromonitoring: (optional) some surgeons used SSEP/MEP
5. consent (in lay terms for the patient – not all-inclusive):
   a) procedure: surgery through the front of the neck to remove the degenerated disc and bone spurs, and to place a graft where the disc was, and possibly place a metal plate on the front of the spine. Some surgeons take bone from the hip to replace the removed disc
   b) alternatives: nonsurgical management, surgery from the back of the neck, artificial disc (in some cases)
   c) complications: swallowing difficulties are common but usually resolve, hoarseness of the voice (<4% chance of it being permanent), injury to: foodpipe (esophagus), windpipe (trachea), arteries to the brain (carotid), spinal cord with paralysis, nerve root with paralysis, possible seizures with MEPs

Technique

A summary of the steps involved is included here. For C5–6, the skin incision is made at level of cricoid cartilage, for other levels, appropriate adjustments up or down may be made, sometimes with the assistance of fluoroscopy. The incision is approximately 4–5 cm horizontally, centered on the SCM. Many right handed surgeons prefer operating from the right side of the neck, although the risk to the recurrent laryngeal nerve (RLN) is lower with a left sided approach (the RLN lies in a groove between the esophagus and trachea). The skin may be undermined off the platysma to permit a vertical incision in the platysma in the same orientation as its muscle fibers. Alternatively, some incise the platysma horizontally with scissors horizontally.

Dissect in tissue plane medial to SCM. For the C5–6 interspace, angle slightly cranially during dissection. For the C6–7 disc, proceed almost straight down to spine. Sweep omohyoid medially (to stay out of it and to protect the RLN). The trachea + esophagus are retracted medially. The carotid sheath + SCM are retracted laterally.

After verification of level with lateral C-spine x-ray with spinal needle in the interspace, bipolar the prevertebral fascia and medial edges of the longus coli muscles longitudinally in the midline. Self-retaining retractor blades are inserted underneath the fascia to retract the longus coli muscles laterally. The anesthesiologist is asked to deflate the cuff on the endotracheal tube and then to re-inflate it using minimal leak technique to reduce the risk of compression injury from the retractor. The disc space is incised with a 15 scalpel blade. The discectomy is performed with curettes and pituitary rongeurs; a vertebral body spreader aids the exposure. The posterior longitudinal ligament is incised, one technique is to elevate it with a sharp nerve hook and then incise it with a #11 scalpel. The subligamentous space is probed with a blunt nerve hook. The posterior lip of the VB above and below are removed with a Kerrison rongeur with a small foot-plate. Decompression of the roots is verified with the blunt nerve hook. Fusion is performed at this time if desired by placing the graft in the interspace.

For redo operations (same or different levels): approach is usually from the same side as previous operation(s) since many patients have swallowing issues post-op, and some may be due to partial recurrent laryngeal nerve injury (which can be subclinical) and which could result in a permanent need for a feeding tube if a contralateral injury occurs. If for some reason it is desired to go to the opposite side, an evaluation by an ENT physician is recommended, and should include scoping the patient to rule-out subclinical problems that could turn into major difficulties if bilateral.

Choice of graft material

Autologous bone (usually from iliac crest), non-autologous bone (cadaveric), bone substitutes (e.g. hydroxylapatite[17]) or synthetics (e.g. PEEK or titanium cage) filled with osteogenic material. Substitutes for autologous bone eliminate problems with the donor site (p. 1075), but may have a higher rate of absorption. There were also cases of HIV transmission from cadaveric bone grafts in 1985, however, as a result of the heightened awareness of AIDS since that time together with significant improvements in antibody testing and careful screening of donors, no further cases have been reported.

Anterior cervical plating

Recommendations for plating following ACDF are shown in **Practice guideline: Anterior cervical plating** (p. 1074).

Practice guideline: Anterior cervical plating

1 level ADCF: The addition of an anterior plate to an ACDF is recommended to reduce the pseudarthrosis rate and graft problems (Level D Class III) and to maintain lordosis (Level C Class II) but it does not improve clinical outcome alone (Level B Class II)[18]

2 level ADCF: Plating is recommended to improve arm pain. Plating does not improve other outcome parameters (Level C Class II)[18]

Use of bone morphogenic proteins (BMP)

Practice guideline: Use of BMP in cervical interbody grafting

Current evidence does not support the routine use of rhBMP-2 for cervical arthrodesis (Level C Class II)[19] (**note**: italics added. Use with precautions (see text) may be indicated in cases with high risk of nonunion).

Use of BMP in anterior cervical discectomies is not FDA approved, but has been used off-label. Complication rates as high as 23–27% have been reported (including post-op swallowing or respiratory difficulties as a result of edema which is usually temporary) compared to 3% without BMP.[19] If used, it is recommended that a smaller dose be employed than in the lumbar spine (25% has been advocated) and to avoid contact of BMP with soft tissues in the neck.

70

Post-op check

In addition to routine, the following should be checked

1. evidence of airway obstruction – post-op wound hematoma: should be first consideration. Wound may need to be emergently opened at bedside (before getting to the OR) if airway is compromised, see **Carotid endarterectomy,** disruption of arteriotomy closure, management (p. 1294). Also consider swelling from IJV thrombosis (rare) in differential diagnosis (see below)
   a) respiratory distress
   b) extreme difficulty swallowing: alternatively may indicate anterior extrusion of bone graft impinging upon esophagus (check lateral C-spine x-ray)
   c) tracheal deviation: may be visible or may be seen on AP C-spine x-ray
2. weakness of nerve root of level operated: e.g. biceps for C5–6, triceps for C6–7
3. long tract signs (Babinski sign…) which may indicate cord compression by spinal epidural hematoma
4. hoarseness: may indicate vocal cord paresis from recurrent laryngeal nerve injury: hold oral feeding until this can be further assessed

ACDF complications

General information

Common ones listed below, see references[20,21]for more details. The most common complication following ACDFs: swallowing difficulties (may be multifactorial).

1. exposure injuries
   a) perforation of viscus: minimize risk by blunt retraction until longus colli is separated from its attachment to vertebrae
      - pharynx
      - esophagus: difficult to manage, and require multidisciplinary effort including ENT involvement.[22] The incidence may be higher with use of anterior cervical plate, and injury may not manifest until years after the fusion (may be due to repetitive motion of esophagus over the plate). Treatment of esophageal perforation is usually facilitated by plate removal
      - trachea
   b) vocal cord paresis: due to injury of the recurrent laryngeal nerve (RLN) or vagus. Incidence: 11% temporary, 4% permanent paresis. Symptoms include: hoarseness, breathiness, cough, aspiration, mass sensation, dysphagia, and vocal cord fatigue.[23] Avoid sharp dissection in paratracheal muscles. Some cases may be due to prolonged retraction against trachea and not to nerve division; to reduce this risk, after the self-retaining retractor is placed, have the

anesthesiologist deflate the cuff on the ET tube and then inflate it to minimal leak pressure. More common with right sided approaches, primarily in the lower cervical spine (C5–6 and below) where the RLN is more vulnerable[23]
   c) vertebral artery injury: thrombosis or laceration. 0.3% incidence.[21] Treatment alternatives include: packing, direct repair by temporary clipping with aneurysms clips and repair with 8–0 prolene[24] and endovascular trapping. Risks of treating hemorrhagic complications with packing include: recurrent bleeding, AV fistula, pseudoaneurysm, arterial thrombosis,[21] distal embolic stroke (primarily in cerebellum)
   d) carotid injury: thrombosis, occlusion, or laceration (usually by retraction)
   e) CSF fistula: usually difficult to repair directly. Place fascial graft beneath bone plug. Keep HOB elevated post-op. Consider: dural sealant (fibrin glue, DuraSeal®…), lumbar drain
   f) Horner's syndrome: sympathetic plexus lies within longus coli, thus do not extend dissection far laterally into these muscles
   g) thoracic duct injury: in exposing lower cervical spine, primarily on left
   h) thrombosis of internal jugular vein[25]: rare. Carries 2–3% risk of PE.[26] Treatment options: anticoagulation (oral or IV) may lower the mortality,[27] SVC filter if anticoagulation is contraindicated,[28] percutaneous thrombectomy[29]
2. spinal cord or nerve root injuries
   a) spinal cord injury: especially risky in myelopathy due to narrowed canal. Minimize risk by penetrating the osteophyte at the lateral margin of interspace (however, this increases risk to nerve root)
   b) avoid hyperextension during intubation: anesthesiologist may need to determine patient's tolerance pre-op. Consider fiberoptic guided or awake nasotracheal intubation in extreme stenosis
   c) bone graft must be shorter than interspace depth. Exercise caution in tapping graft into position
   d) sleep induced apnea: rare but serious complications of C3–4 level operations.[30] May be associated with bradycardia & cardiorespiratory instability. Possibly due to disruption of the afferent component of the central respiratory control mechanism
3. bone fusion problems
   a) failure of fusion (pseudarthrosis): see below
   b) anterior (kyphotic) angulation deformity: may be as high as 60% with Cloward technique (may be reduced by collar immobilization). May develop in Hirsch technique with excessive bone removal
   c) graft extrusion: 2% incidence (rarely requires re-operation unless compression of cord posteriorly, or esophagus or trachea anteriorly occurs)
   d) donor site complications: hematoma/seroma, infection, fracture of ilium, injury to lateral femoral cutaneous nerve, persistent pain due to scar, bowel perforation
4. miscellaneous
   a) wound infection: incidence < 1%
   b) post-op hematoma: *see above.* Placing cervical collar in O.R. may delay recognition
   c) dysphagia and hoarseness: common. Usually transient (*see below*)
   d) adjacent level degeneration: controversial whether this represents a sequelae to altered biomechanics from surgery, or a predisposition to cervical spondylosis.[31] Many (≈ 70%) are asymptomatic[32]
   e) postoperative discomfort:
      - globus: the sensation of a lump in throat (see below)
      - nagging discomfort in neck, shoulder, and very commonly in interscapular regions (may last several months). May correlate with amount of distraction of the disc space
   f) complex regional pain syndrome (CRPS) AKA reflex sympathetic dystrophy (**RSD**): rarely described in the literature,[33] possibly due to stellate ganglion injury; see discussion of RSD (p.497)
   g) angioedema: massive edema of the tongue and neck.[34] A dramatic hypersensitivity reaction (not really a direct complication of ACDF, but superficially can mimic some findings of post-op hematoma). If limited to the tongue, the airway is not compromised. See treatment (p.222)
   h) pneumothorax or hemothorax[35]: accessing C7-T1 or lower may expose the pleural apex

70

Dysphagia following ACDF

Symptoms: Include: difficulty swallowing (solids, liquids including saliva), pain with swallowing (odynophagia), globus (sensation of a lump in throat) and compromise of ability to protect against aspiration. Food may stick in the throat (or feel as if it is) and there may be coughing or choking.

Incidence: Early dysphagia is common. Incidence: 60%[36] in retrospective survey after noninstrumented fusion (dysphagia occurred in 23% in a control group undergoing unrelated lumbar spine surgery[36]), 50% in prospective study.[37] At 6 months, only ≈ 5% reported moderate or severe dysphagia.[37] Surgery at multiple levels increased the risk at 1 & 2 months.[37] Decreases significantly in most cases by 6 months.[37]

Etiologies: Etiologies of post-op dysphagia include:

1. post-op hematoma. If severe, may cause tracheal obstruction (see above)
2. post-op edema, due in part to retraction of esophagus
3. effects of general anesthesia: e.g. irritation from ET tube. Accounts for up to 23% of early symptoms (dysphagia occurred in 23% in a control group undergoing unrelated lumbar spine surgery[36]). Usually subsides within ≈ 24–72 hours
4. recurrent laryngeal nerve dysfunction:
   a) temporary: usually due to traction on the nerve
   b) permanent: 1.3% at 12 months[37]
5. esophageal injury
   a) at time of surgery
   b) delayed: possibly from repetitive abrasion on surgical site/hardware or from unrecognized esophageal injury at time of surgery[22]
6. cervical collar
   a) prevents patient from lowering jaw during swallow phase, which compromises effective glottic closure of airway
   b) may be too tight thereby directly squeezing the throat
7. protrusion of graft/hardware anterior to the vertebral bodies
   a) some protrusion is present with most anterior hardware. This may be minimized with "zero profile" instrumentation
   b) hardware failure (screw-pullout/backout/breakage, plate pullout)
   c) interbody graft migration: without anterior plate, or in conjunction with anterior plate displacement
8. excessive adhesions[38]
9. denervation of the pharyngeal plexus[38]
10. rare conditions: swelling from IJV thrombosis, angioedema

70

Management:

1. initial management: rule-out emergent/serious conditions (severe edema, hematoma with airway compromise, risk of aspiration)
   a) if there is significant stridor or dysphonia, especially if tracheal deviation is obvious, someone must stay with the patient as efforts are made to emergently take the patient to the O.R. for wound exploration evacuation. Consider opening the wound at the bedside if delays occur or if symptoms are severe; see Carotid endarterectomy, disruption of arteriotomy closure, management (p. 1294). Emergent anesthesia consultation for airway protection – alert them to the likelihood of deviated trachea which challenges even the most expert at intubating
2. once emergent conditions are ruled out, early management is geared towards amelioration of symptoms
   a) advise patient to eat softer foods (temporarily avoiding steak or bread), to chew food well, to wash down dry foods with a drink. Reassure patient that most cases largely resolve with 6 months[37]
   b) if significant symptoms persist > 2 weeks
      - refer patient to ENT for laryngoscopy to rule out vocal cord paralysis (from RLN injury) or other etiologies. For RLN, see below
      - modified barium swallow
3. persistent symptoms may be amenable to surgical intervention, including hardware removal and lysing of adhesions,[38] management of esophageal perforation usually requires consultation with ENT

Management of esophageal perforation:

There is no consensus on optimal management. A multidisciplinary approach with head and neck surgeons together with the spine surgeon is suggested with the following[22]:

- Closure with a sternocleidomastoid muscle flap, or possibly a pedicle flap
- Removal of all anterior hardware. If there is evidence that the fusion is not solid, posterior instrumentation may be necessary

Recurrent laryngeal nerve paralysis

Heralded by breathy voice, hoarseness, or aspiration. Refer to ENT to have patient scoped to determine if cord is paralyzed and its position. 4 possible positions: 1) median, 2) paramedian, 3) intermediate, 4) lateral (cadaveric). Many patients can compensate for median or paramedian position. Patients requiring intervention usually are treated with medialization technique, either 1) injection, or 2) medialization thyroplasty using an implant. For injections, different materials may be selected for desired duration of effect (Teflon used to be the only available agent, and was essentially permanent) and so early intervention may be employed with temporary materials (instead of waiting 1 year, which was the previous paradigm).

Pseudarthrosis (or pseudoarthrosis) following ACDF

Pseudarthrosis may occur with or without supplemental anterior cervical plating.

Practice guideline: Assessment of subaxial fusion

> 2 mm movement between spinous processes on dynamic (flexion-extension) cervical spine x-rays is recommended as a criteria for pseudarthrosis (Level B Class II), this measurement is unreliable when performed by the treating surgeon (Level C Class II).[39]

Visualization of bone trabeculation across the fusion on static films is a less reliable marker for fusion (Level D Class III) (2D reformatted CT increases the accuracy (Level D Class III))[39]

Incidence: Difficult to assess because of lack of validated criteria. Estimate: 2–20%. Higher with dowel technique (Cloward) than with keystone technique of Bailey & Badgley or with interbody method of Smith-Robinson (10%) or with non-fusion advocated by Hirsch. One criteria: motion > 2 mm between the tips of the spinous processes on lateral flexion/extension x-rays.[40,41] Other criteria: lucencies around the screws of an anterior plate, toggling of the screws on flexion/extension x-rays. 70

Presentation: Not uniformly associated with symptoms or problems.[40,42] Some patients may have chronic or recurrent neck pain, some may present with radicular symptoms. (NB: when DePalma's data is analyzed with patients reclassified as failures if neck and/or arm symptoms persist, the success rate of surgery is lower with pseudarthrosis[43]).

Management: Guidelines are shown in **Practice guideline: Management of anterior cervical pseudarthrosis** (p. 1077). No treatment is required for *asymptomatic* pseudarthrosis. Options for symptomatic patients include re-resection of the bone graft with repeat fusion[44] (some recommend using autologous bone if allograft was used, a plate may be considered if one was not used previously), cervical corpectomy with fusion,[44] or posterior cervical fusion.

Practice guideline: Management of anterior cervical pseudarthrosis

Revision of symptomatic pseudarthrosis should be considered (Level D Class III).[45] Posterior approaches may be associated with higher fusion rates on revision than anterior approaches (Level D Class III)[45]

Cervical disc arthroplasty

An alternative to fusion. Uses an artificial disc to preserve motion at the level of the discectomy. Some of the available cervical disc replacement (CDR) models are shown in ► Table 70.2.[46]

Contraindications described by the FDA have included: isolated axial neck pain, ankylosing spondylitis or pregnancy, rheumatoid arthritis, autoimmune disease, diffuse idiopathic skeletal hyperostosis, severe spondylosis with bridging osteophytes or ossification of the posterior longitudinal ligament, disc height loss > 50%, spinal infection, metal allergy to components of the prosthesis, severe osteoporosis/osteopenia, active malignancy, metabolic bone disease, trauma, segmental instability, 3 or more levels requiring treatment, insulin dependent diabetes mellitus, human immunodeficiency virus, hepatitis B/C, morbid obesity, absence of motion (< 2 degrees), and posterior facet arthrosis.

Table 70.2 Artificial cervical discs

Trade name	Manufacturer	Material	IAR[a]	Comment
Prestige®	Medtronic	MOM[a] (chrome cobalt stainless steel)	variable ball in trough	1st FDA approved CDR; lots of MRI artifact
Bryan®	Medtronic	lubricated elastic nucleus sealed in a flexible membrane	variable in center of disc space	
Advent®	Blackstone (Orthofix)	flexible elastomer core		withdrawn from market
ProDisc-C	Synthes	metal-on-polyethylene	posterior part of inferior VB	midline keel inserts into VB; lots of MRI artifact
Mobi-C®	LDR Spine	metal-on-polyethylene	variable in center of disc space	approved for 1 or 2 levels
PCM®	Cervitech	metal-on-polyethylene	gliding motion	contoured to endplates

[a]Abbreviations: IAR = instantaneous axis of rotation, MOM = metal-on-metal, PCM = Porous-coated Motion

70

Practice guideline: Cervical disc arthroplasty

Cervical arthroplasty is a recommended alternative to ACDF in selected patients for control of arm and neck pain (Level B Class II)[18]

Booking the case: Cervical disc arthroplasty

Also see defaults & disclaimers and/or more significant (p. 27).

1. position: supine, some use halter traction with this
2. equipment:
   a) microscope (not used by all surgeons)
   b) C-arm
3. implants: schedule vendor to provide desired artificial disc
4. neuromonitoring: (optional) some surgeons used SSEP/MEP
5. consent (in lay terms for the patient – not all-inclusive):
   a) procedure: surgery through the front of the neck to remove the degenerated disc and bone spurs, and to place an artificial disc
   b) alternatives: nonsurgical management, surgical fusion (from the front or the back of the neck)
   c) complications: swallowing difficulties are common but usually resolve, hoarseness of the voice (< 4% chance of it being permanent), injury to: foodpipe (esophagus), windpipe (trachea), arteries to the brain (carotid) with stroke, spinal cord with paralysis, nerve root with paralysis, possible seizures with MEPs (if used). The disc may eventually wear out and further surgery may be needed

Post-op orders:

1. no cervical collar (the goal is to preserve motion at the operated level)
2. NSAIDs around the clock for ≈ 2 weeks (this inhibits bone growth which theoretically helps avoid undesirable fusion at the operated level)

Posterior cervical decompression (cervical laminectomy)

Not necessary for unilateral radiculopathy (use either ACD or keyhole laminotomy). Consists of removal of cervical lamina (laminectomy) and spinous processes in order to convert the spinal canal from a "tube" to a "trough."

Usually reserved for the following conditions:

1. multiple cervical discs or osteophytes (anterior cervical discectomy (ACD) is usually used to treat only 2, or possibly 3, levels without) with myelopathy
2. where the anterior pathology is superimposed on cervical stenosis, and the latter is more diffuse and/or more significant (p. 1083)
3. in professional speakers or singers where the 4% risk of permanent voice change due to recurrent laryngeal nerve injury with ACD may be unacceptable

Booking the case: Cervical laminectomy

Also see defaults & disclaimers (p. 27).

1. position: prone, some use pin headholder
2. equipment:
   a) C-arm
   b) high-speed drill
3. implants: cervical lateral mass screws and rods if fusion is being done
4. neuromonitoring: some surgeons used SSEP/MEP
5. consent (in lay terms for the patient – not all-inclusive):
   a) procedure: surgery through the back of the neck to remove the bone over the compressed spinal cord and nerves and possibly to place screws and rods to fuse the boned together
   b) alternatives: nonsurgical management, surgery from the front of the neck, posterior surgery without fusion, laminoplasty
   c) complications: nerve root injury (C5 nerve root is the most common), may not relieve symptoms necessitating further surgery, possible seizures with MEPs. If fusion is not done, risk of progressive bone slippage which would require further surgery

70

Posterior keyhole laminotomy

AKA "keyhole foraminotomy." First described in 1951.[47] A technique to decompress only individual nerve roots (but not the spinal cord) by creating a small "keyhole" in the lamina to access the nerve root.

Practice guideline: Cervical laminoforaminotomy

Cervical laminoforaminotomy is recommended as a surgical treatment option for symptomatic cervical radiculopathy caused by disc herniation or lateral recess narrowing (Level D Class III)[48]

Indications for keyhole approach (as opposed to anterior discectomy):

1. monoradiculopathy with posterolateral *soft* disc sequestration (small *lateral* osteophytic spurs may also be addressed). This approach does *not* provide adequate decompression with central or broad-based disc herniation or with stenosis of the spinal canal
2. radiculopathy in patients who are professional speakers or singers where the risk of recurrent laryngeal nerve injury is untenable (see above)
3. for lower (e.g. C7, C8 or T1) or upper (e.g. C3 or C4) cervical nerve root compression, especially in a patient with a short thick neck, making an anterior approach more difficult
4. in patients with a herniated disc when it is desired to avoid a fusion (as would be done with an anterior approach)

Booking the case: Cervical keyhole laminectomy

Also see defaults & disclaimers (p. 27).

1. position: prone, some use pin headholder
2. equipment:
   a) microscope (not used by all surgeons)
   b) C-arm

3. instrumentation: some surgeons use a tube retractor system
4. neuromonitoring: some surgeons used SSEP/MEP
5. consent (in lay terms for the patient – not all-inclusive):
   a) procedure: surgery through the back of the neck to remove the bone over the compressed nerve root and possibly remove fragment of herniated disc
   b) alternatives: nonsurgical management, surgery from the front of the neck, posterior surgery with fusion
   c) complications: nerve root injury, may not relieve symptoms necessitating further surgery, possible seizures with MEPs

Technique

See references.[49,50,51]

Position:

a) prone, on chest rolls. Adhesive tape is used to retract shoulders down for any level below about C4–5. The head is stabilized on a horse-shoe headrest or in a Mayfield head holder.
b) sitting position: generally abandoned. However, may be used with proper precautions (p. 1445)

"Open" keyhole foraminotomy

The desired level is localized with intra-op fluoroscopy before making the skin incision, a 2–3 cm midline incision is adequate. A unilateral exposure suffices. Periosteal elevators are used to dissect muscles off the lamina and facet joint in the sub-periosteal plane. A Kocher clamp may be placed on the spinous process to permit confirmation of the correct level on intra-operative x-ray. A Scoville retractor or equivalent is employed.

A high-speed drill (e.g. with diamond burr) is used to make an opening in the medial one-third to one-half of the inferior facet of the vertebra above the desired disc space, extending slightly medially into the junction with the lamina. Once the inferior facet is penetrated, the superior facet of the inferior vertebral level will be visualized. This is also thinned with the drill (it is critical to remove the bone of the superior facet of the level below caudally to where it meets the pedicle). A small Kerrison rongeur may be used to slightly enlarge the laminectomy. An opening is made in the ligamentum flavum overlying the lateral aspect of the spinal cord dura. The nerve root can be identified as it exits from the thecal sac, and can be followed as it travels between the pedicles of the vertebrae above and below. Soft tissues (including ligamentum flavum) form fibrous bands across the dorsum of the nerve, and are removed to further expose the dura of the nerve root. The venous plexus around the nerve root is coagulated with bipolar cautery and then divided to mobilize the nerve. The nerve may then be gently moved a few millimeters rostrally using a micro nerve hook. The dura overlying the spinal cord should not be manipulated, and the disc space need not be entered. Inspection for free disc fragments should begin in the nerve root axilla using a probe (e.g. blunt nerve hook). Next, the space anterior to the root (the region of the disc) may be palpated. Any disc fragments that are dislodged are removed with a small pituitary rongeur. If the disc fragment is contained anterior to the posterior longitudinal ligament (PLL), the PLL may be incised in the region of the nerve root axilla with a #11 scalpel blade in a motion that is directed downward and laterally, away from the nerve root and spinal cord. The foraminotomy may be extended slightly laterally if the foramen still feels tight when probed. Small osteophytes can potentially be reduced using a small reversed-angled curette, although some surgeons believe that the need for this is obviated by the decompression provided by the keyhole opening. In some cases, simple posterior decompression of the nerve root (without removing a disc fragment) may be adequate to relieve compression. Spinal stability is usually preserved if less than half the facet joint is removed.

MIS keyhole foraminotomy

Positioning as described above.

1. skin incision
   a) use fluoro to locate the correct level for the incision
   b) incision 1 cm off midline on the side of the pathology at the level of the disc space
   c) remove adhesive plastic barrier (e.g. Ioban®) from around the opening to prevent pieces from being dragged into the incision

2. avoid using a guidewire to reduce the risk of penetrating the interlaminar space. STAY LATERAL and insert the thinnest dilator. Dock the dilator on the lateral mass and insert progressively sized dilators
3. use Bovie to expose lateral lamina and medial facet joint. Start laterally where bone is more easily felt and there is little danger of penetrating the interlaminar space and injuring the spinal cord
4. use a straight curette to expose the inferior edge of the superior lateral lamina and the medial facet joint
5. drill off the medial inferior facet, to expose the superior facet of the level below
6. drill the medial superior facet until you are flush with the superior aspect of the pedicle below
7. this completes the bony work, the soft tissue work proceeds as above under open keyhole foraminotomy

Outcome

A number of large series have reported good or excellent outcome in the range of 90–96%.[50]

References

[1] Mayfield FH. Cervical Spondylosis: A Comparison of the Anterior and Posterior Approaches. Clin Neurosurg. 1966; 13:181–188
[2] Kobayashi N, Asamoto S, Doi H, Sugiyama H. Brown-Sequard syndrome produced by cervical disc herniation: report of two cases and review of the literature. Spine J. 2003; 3:530–533
[3] Dai Liyang, Jia Lianshun. Central Cord Injury Complicating Acute Cervical Disc Herniation in Trauma. Spine. 2000; 25:331–336
[4] Viikari-Juntura E, Porras M, Laasonen EM. Validity of Clinical Tests in the Diagnosis of Root Compression in Cervical Disc Disease. Spine. 1989; 14:253–257
[5] Spurling RG, Scoville WB. Lateral Rupture of the Cervical Intervertebral Discs: A Common Cause of Shoulder and Arm Pain. Surg Gynecol Obstet. 1944; 78:350–358
[6] Davidson RI, Dunn EJ, Metzmaker JN. The shoulder abduction test in the diagnosis of radicular pain in cervical extradural compressive miniradiculopathies. Spine. 1981; 6:441–446
[7] Rubinstein SM, Pool JJ, van Tulder MW, Riphagen II, de Vet HC. A systematic review of the diagnostic accuracy of provocative tests of the neck for diagnosing cervical radiculopathy. Eur Spine J. 2006; 16:307–319
[8] Jablecki CK, Andary MT, Floeter MK, Miller RG, Quartly CA, Vennix MJ, Wilson JR, American Association of Electrodiagnostic Medicine, American Academy of Neurology, American Academy of Physical Medicine, Rehabilitation. Practice parameter: Electrodiagnostic studies in carpal tunnel syndrome. Report of the American Association of Electrodiagnostic Medicine, American Academy of Neurology, and the American Academy of Physical Medicine and Rehabilitation. Neurology. 2002; 58:1589–1592
[9] Campbell WW. Guidelines in electrodiagnostic medicine. Practice parameter for electrodiagnostic studies in ulnar neuropathy at the elbow. Muscle Nerve Suppl. 1999; 8:S171–S205
[10] American Association of Electrodiagnostic Medicine. Chapter 9: Practice parameter for needle electromyographic evaluation of patients with suspected cervical radiculopathy: Summary statement. Muscle Nerve. 1999; 22:S209–S211
[11] Dillingham TR. Evaluating the patient with suspected radiculopathy. PM R. 2013; 5:S41–S49
[12] Saal J, Saal Y, Yurth E. Nonoperative Management of Herniated Cervical Intervertebral Disc with Radiculopathy. Spine. 1996; 21:1877–1883
[13] Maigne JY, Deligne L. Computed tomographic follow-up study of 21 cases of nonoperatively treated cervical intervertebral soft disc herniation. Spine (Phila Pa 1976). 1994; 19:189–191
[14] Mochida K, Komori H, Okawa A, Muneta T, Haro H, Shinomiya K. Regression of cervical disc herniation observed on magnetic resonance images. Spine (Phila Pa 1976). 1998; 23:990–5; discussion 996-7
[15] Bush K, Chaudhuri R, Hillier S, Penny J. The pathomorphologic changes that accompany the resolution of cervical radiculopathy. A prospective study with repeat magnetic resonance imaging. Spine (Phila Pa 1976). 1997; 22:183–6; discussion 187
[16] Joanes V. Cervical disc herniation presenting with acue myelopathy. Surg Neurol. 2000; 54
[17] Senter HJ, Kortyna R, Kemp WR. Anterior Cervical Discectomy with Hydroxylapatite Fusion. Neurosurgery. 1989; 25:39–43
[18] Matz PG, Ryken TC, Groff MW, Vresilovic EJ, Anderson PA, Heary RF, Holly LT, Kaiser MG, Mummaneni PV, Choudhri TF, Resnick DK. Techniques for anterior cervical decompression for radiculopathy. J Neurosurg: Spine. 2009; 11:183–197
[19] Ryken TC, Heary RF, Matz PG, Anderson PA, Groff MW, Holly LT, Kaiser MG, Mummaneni PV, Choudhri TF, Vresilovic EJ, Resnick DK. Techniques for cervical interbody grafting. J Neurosurg: Spine. 2009; 11:203–220
[20] Tew JM, Mayfield FH. Complications of Surgery of the Anterior Cervical Spine. Clin Neurosurg. 1976; 23:424–434
[21] Taylor BA, Vaccaro AR, Albert TJ. Complications of Anterior and Posterior Surgical Approaches in the Treatment of Cervical Degenerative Disc Disease. Semin Spine Surg. 1999; 11:337–346
[22] Dakwar E, Uribe JS, Padhya TA, Vale FL. Management of delayed esophageal perforations after anterior cervical spinal surgery. J Neurosurg Spine. 2009; 11:320–325
[23] Netterville JL, Koriwchak MJ, Winkle M, et al. Vocal Fold Paralysis Following the Anterior Approach to the Cervical Spine. Ann Otol Rhinol Laryngol. 1996; 105:85–91
[24] Pfeifer BA, Freidberg SR, Jewell ER. Repair of Injured Vertebral Artery in Anterior Cervical Procedures. Spine. 1994; 19:1471–1474
[25] Karim A, Knapp J, Nanda A. Internal jugular venous thrombosis as a complication after an elective anterior cervical discectomy: case report. Neurosurgery. 2006; 59
[26] Ascher E, Salles-Cunha S, Hingorani A. Morbidity and mortality associated with internal jugular vein thromboses. Vasc Endovascular Surg. 2005; 39:335–339
[27] Sheikh MA, Topoulos AP, Deitcher SR. Isolated internal jugular vein thrombosis: risk factors and natural history. Vasc Med. 2002; 7:177–179
[28] Ascher E, Hingorani A, Mazzariol F, Jacob T, Yorkovich W, Gade P. Clinical experience with superior vena caval Greenfield filters. J Endovasc Surg. 1999; 6:365–369
[29] Tajima H, Murata S, Kumazaki T, Ichikawa K, Tajiri T, Yamamoto Y. Successful interventional treatment of acute internal jugular vein thrombosis. AJR Am J Roentgenol. 2004; 182:467–469

[30] Krieger AJ, Rosomoff HL. Sleep-Induced Apnea. Part 2: Respiratory Failure After Anterior Spinal Surgery. J Neurosurg. 1974; 39:181–185
[31] Truumees E, Herkowitz HN. Adjacent Segment Degeneration in the Cervical Spine: Incidence and Management. Semin Spine Surg. 1999; 11:373–383
[32] Gore DR, Sepic SB. Anterior Cervical Fusion for Degenerated or Protruded Discs. A Review of One Hundred and Fifty-Six Patients. Spine. 1984; 9:667–671
[33] Hawkins RJ, Bilco T, Bonutti P. Cervical Spine and Shoulder Pain. Clin Orthop Rel Res. 1990; 258:142–146
[34] Krnacik MJ, Heggeness MH. Severe angioedema causing airway obstruction after anterior cervical surgery. Spine. 1997; 22:2188–2190
[35] Harhangi BS, Menovsky T, Wurzer HA. Hemothorax as a complication after anterior cervical discectomy: case report. Neurosurgery. 2005; 56
[36] Winslow CP, Winslow TJ, Wax MK. Dysphonia and dysphagia following the anterior approach to the cervical spine. Arch Otolaryngol Head Neck Surg. 2001; 127:51–55
[37] Bazaz R, Lee MJ, Yoo JU. Incidence of dysphagia after anterior cervical spine surgery: a prospective study. Spine. 2002; 27:2453–2458
[38] Fogel GR, McDonnell MF. Surgical treatment of dysphagia after anterior cervical interbody fusion. Spine J. 2005; 5:140–144
[39] Kaiser MG, Mummaneni PV, Matz PG, Anderson PA, Groff MW, Heary RF, Holly LT, Ryken TC, Choudhri TF, Vresilovic EJ, Resnick DK. Radiographic assessment of cervical subaxial fusion. J Neurosurg: Spine. 2009; 11:221–227
[40] Phillips FM, Carlson G, Emery SE, et al. Anterior Cervical Pseudarthrosis: Natural History and Treatment. Spine. 1997; 22:1585–1589
[41] Cannada LK, Scherping SC, Yoo JU, Jones PK, Emery SE. Pseudoarthrosis of the cervical spine: a comparison of radiographic diagnostic measures. Spine (Phila Pa 1976). 2003; 28:46–51
[42] DePalma AF, Cooke AJ. Results of Anterior Interbody Fusion of The Cervical Spine. Clin Orthop. 1968; 60:169–185
[43] Puschak TJ, Anderson PA. Pseudarthrosis After Anterior Fusion: Treatment Options and Results. Semin Spine Surg. 1999; 11:312–321
[44] Zdeblick TA, Hughes SS, Riew KD, Bohlman HH. Failed anterior cervical discectomy and arthrodesis. Analysis and treatment of thirty-five patients. J Bone Joint Surg. 1997; 79:523–532
[45] Kaiser MG, Mummaneni PV, Matz PG, Anderson PA, Groff MW, Heary RF, Holly LT, Ryken TC, Choudhri TF, Vresilovic EJ, Resnick DK. Management of anterior cervical pseudarthrosis. J Neurosurg: Spine. 2009; 11:228–237
[46] Yi S, Lee DY, Kim DH, Ahn PG, et al. Cervical artificial disc replacement. Part 1: History, design, and overview of the cervical artificial disc. Neurosurg Q. 2008; 18
[47] Scoville WB, Whitcomb BB, McLaurin RL. The Cervical Ruptured Disc: Report of 115 Operative Cases. Trans Am Neurol Assoc. 1951; 76:222–224
[48] Heary RF, Ryken TC, Matz PG, Anderson PA, Groff MW, Holly LT, Kaiser MG, Mummaneni PV, Choudhri TF, Vresilovic EJ, Resnick DK. Cervical laminoforaminotomy for the treatment of cervical degenerative radiculopathy. J Neurosurg: Spine. 2009; 11:198–202
[49] Aldrich F. Posterolateral Microdiscectomy for Cervical Monoradiculopathy Caused by Posterolateral Soft Cervical Disc Sequestration. J Neurosurg. 1990; 72:370–377
[50] Zeidman SM, Ducker TB. Posterior Cervical Laminoforaminotomy for Radiculopathy: Review of 172 Cases. Neurosurgery. 1993; 33:356–362
[51] Collias JC, Roberts MP, Schmidek HH, Sweet WH. In: Posterior Surgical Approaches for Cervical Disc Herniation and Spondylotic Myelopathy. Operative Neurosurgical Techniques. 3rd ed. Philadelphia: W. B. Saunders; 1995:1805–1816

71 Degenerative Cervical Disc Disease and Cervical Myelopathy

71.1 General information

Cervical degenerative disc disease is generally discussed in terms of "cervical spondylosis", a term which is sometimes used synonymously with "cervical spinal stenosis." Spondylosis usually implies a more widespread age-related degenerative condition of the cervical spine including various combinations of the following:

1. congenital spinal stenosis (the "shallow cervical canal"[1])
2. degeneration of the intervertebral disc producing a focal stenosis due to a "cervical bar" which is usually a combination of:
   a) osteophytic spurs ("hard disc" in neurosurgical jargon)
   b) and/or protrusion of intervertebral disc material ("soft disc")
3. hypertrophy of any of the following (which also contributes to canal stenosis):
   a) lamina
   b) dura
   c) articular facets
   d) ligaments, including
      - increased stenosis in extension is more common than with flexion (based on MRI studies[2] and cadaver studies), largely due to posterior inbuckling of ligamentum flavum[3]
      - posterior longitudinal ligament: may include ossification of the posterior longitudinal ligament (OPLL) (p. 1127).[4] May be segmental or diffuse. Often adherent to dura
      - ossification of the ligamentum flavum[5] (yellow ligament)
4. subluxation: due to disc and facet joint degeneration
5. altered mobility: severely spondylotic levels may be fused and are usually stable, however there is often hypermobility at adjacent or other segments
6. telescoping of the spine due to loss of height of VBs → "shingling" of laminae
7. alteration of the normal lordotic curvature[6] (NB: the amount of abnormal curvature did not correlate with the degree of myelopathy)
   a) reduction of lordosis: including
      - straightening
      - reversal of the curvature (kyphosis): may cause "bowstringing" of the spinal cord across osteophytes
   b) exaggerated lordosis (hyperlordosis): the least common variant (may also cause bowstringing)

Although the majority of individuals > 50 yrs old have radiologic evidence of significant degenerative disease of the cervical spine, only a small percentage will experience neurologic symptoms.[7]

71.2 Pathophysiology

Pathogenesis is controversial. Theories include the following alone or in combination:

1. direct cord compression between osteophytic bars and hypertrophy or infolding of the ligamentum flavum, especially if superimposed on congenital narrowing or cervical subluxations
2. ischemia due to compression of vascular structures[8] (arterial deprivation[9] and/or venous stasis[10])
3. repeated local cord trauma by normal movements in the presence of protruded discs and/or osteophytic (spondylotic) bars (cord and root injuries[11])
   a) cephalad/caudad movement with flexion extension[12]
   b) anterior/posterior traction on the cord by dentate ligaments[13] & nerve roots
   c) diameter of spinal canal varies during flexion and extension
      - increased stenosis is more common in extension (see above)
      - unstable segments may sublux (so-called pincer mechanism)[14]

Histologically,[15] there is degeneration of the central grey matter at the level of compression, degeneration of the posterior columns above the lesion (particularly in the anteromedial portion), and demyelination in the lateral columns (especially the corticospinal tracts) below the lesion. Anterior spinal tracts are relatively spared. There may be atrophic changes in the ventral and dorsal roots and neurophagia of anterior horn cells.

71

71.3 Clinical

71.3.1 General information

Cervical spondylosis condition may produce several types of clinical problems[16]:

1. Myeloradiculopathy: some combination of
   a) Radiculopathy: nerve root compression may cause nerve-root (radicular) complaints
   b) spinal cord compression may cause myelopathy. Some stereotypical syndromes are presented below (see Cervical spondylotic myelopathy (CSM) below)
2. pain and paresthesias in the head, neck and shoulders with little or no suggestion of radiculopathy nor abnormal physical findings. This group is the most difficult to diagnose and treat, and often requires a good physician-patient relationship to decide if surgical treatment should be undertaken in an attempt to provide relief

Cervical spondylosis is the most common cause of myelopathy in patients > 55 yrs of age.[17] CSM is rare in patients < 40 years of age.

Cervical spondylotic myelopathy (CSM) develops in almost all patients with ≥ 30% narrowing of the cross-sectional area of the cervical spinal canal[18] (although some patients with more severe cord compression do not have myelopathy[19,20]).

Gait disturbance, often with LE weakness or stiffness, is a common early finding in CSM.[21] Ataxia may result from spinocerebellar tract compression. Early on, patients may experience difficulty running. Cervical pain and mechanical signs are uncommon in cases of pure myelopathy. See ▶ Table 71.1 for the frequency of symptoms in CSM in one series. In most cases the disability is mild, and the prognosis for these is good.

71.3.2 Motor

Findings can be due to cord (UMN) and/or root (LMN) compression. The earliest motor findings are typically weakness in the triceps and hand intrinsics.[23] There may be wasting of the hand muscles.[24] Slow, stiff opening and closing of the fists may occur.[25] Clumsiness with fine motor skills (writing, buttoning buttons…) is common.

There is often *proximal* weakness of the lower extremities (mild to moderate iliopsoas weakness occurs in 54%) and spasticity of the LEs.

71.3.3 Sensory

Sensory disturbance may be minimal, and when present are often not radicular in distribution. There may be a glove-distribution sensory loss in the hands.[26] A sensory level may occur a number of levels below the area of cord compression.

LEs often exhibit loss of vibratory sense (in as many as 82%), and occasionally have reduced pinprick sensation (9%) (almost always restricted to below the ankle). Compression of the spinocerebellar tract may cause difficulty running. Lhermitte's sign was present in only 2 of 37 cases. Some patients may present with a prominence of posterior column dysfunction (impaired joint position sense and 2 point discrimination).[27]

71.3.4 Reflexes

In 72–87%, reflexes are hyperactive at a varying distance below the level of stenosis. Clonus, Babinski's sign (p.90) or Hoffman's sign (p.90) may also be present. Dynamic Hoffman's sign[28] may be more sensitive: test for Hoffman's sign during multiple cervical flexion and extension movements as tolerated by the patient. 94% of asymptomatic individuals with Hoffman's reflex will have significant spinal cord compression on MRI.[29] Inverted radial reflex: flexion of the fingers in response to eliciting the brachioradialis reflex, said to be pathognomonic of CSM.[30]

A hyperactive jaw jerk indicates upper motor neuron lesion *above* the midpons, and distinguishes long tract findings due to pathology above the foramen magnum from those below (e.g. cervical myelopathy): not helpful if absent (a normal variant). Primitive reflexes (grasp, snout, rooting) are not reliable localizing signs (except perhaps the grasp reflex) of frontal lobe pathology.

71.3.5 Sphincter

Urinary urgency and frequency are common in CSM, however these complaints are also protean in the aging population. Urinary incontinence is rare. Anal sphincter disturbances are uncommon.

Table 71.1 Frequency of symptoms in CSM (37 cases[22])

Finding	%
pure myelopathy	**59%**
myelopathy + radiculopathy	**41%**
reflexes	
• hyperreflexia	87%
• Babinski	54%
• Hoffman	13%
sensory deficits	
• sensory level	41%
• posterior column	39%
• dermatomal arm	33%
• paresthesias	21%
• positive Romberg	15%
motor deficits	
• arm weakness	31%
• paraparesis	21%
• hemiparesis	18%
• quadriparesis	10%
• Brown-Séquard	10%
• muscle atrophy	13%
• fasciculations	13%
pain	
• radicular arm	41%
• radicular leg	13%
• cervical	8%
spasticity	**54%**
sphincter disturbance	**49%**
cervical mechanical signs	**26%**

71

71.3.6 Syndromes

Clustering of CSM into these 5 clinical syndromes has been described[25]:

1. transverse lesion syndrome: involvement of corticospinal and spinothalamic tracts and posterior columns, with anterior horn cells *segmentally* involved. Most frequent syndrome, possibly an "end-stage" of the disease process
2. motor system syndrome: primarily corticospinal tract and anterior horn involvement with minimal or no sensory deficit. This creates a mixture of lower motor neuron findings in the upper extremities and upper motor neuron findings (myelopathy) in the lower extremities which can mimic ALS (see below). Reflexes may be hyperactive below the area of maximal stenosis (including the upper extremities), occasionally beginning several levels below the stenosis
3. central cord syndrome: motor and sensory deficit affecting the UEs more than the LEs. This syndrome is characterized by dysfunction of the watershed areas located centrally within the cord,

which may be responsible for prominence of hand symptoms[31] (results in "numb-clumsy hands"[32]). Lhermitte's sign may be more common in this group
4. Brown-Séquard syndrome: often with asymmetric narrowing of the canal with the side of greater narrowing producing ipsilateral corticospinal tract (upper motor neuron weakness) and posterior column dysfunction with contralateral loss of pain and temperature sensation
5. brachialgia and cord syndrome: radicular UE pain with lower motor neuron weakness, and some associated long tract involvement (motor and/or sensory)

71.3.7 Grading

1. the modified Japanese Orthopaedic Association scale (mJOA) (▶ Table 71.2) is a valid and reliable grading system, although it is non-specific
2. Neck Disability Index[33]: a 10 question survey similar to the Oswestry Disability Index for the lumbar spine (see ▶ Table 68.3). Mild disability is defined as a score of 10–28%, moderate = 30–48%, severe = 50–68%, complete ≥ 72%
3. other commonly used scales (not tested for validity or reliability):
   a) Nurick[34] (see ▶ Table 74.2)
   b) Harsh

71.3.8 Natural history

The time course of symptoms is highly variable and unpredictable. In ≈ 75% of cases of CSM, there is progression either in a stepwise fashion (in one-third) or gradually progressive (two-thirds).[35] In some series, the most common pattern was that of an initial phase of deterioration followed by a stabilization that typically lasts for years and may not change thereafter.[36,37] In these cases, the degree of disability may be established early in the course of CSM. Others disagree with such a "benign" outlook and cite that over 50% of cases continue to deteriorate with conservative treatment.[7] Sustained spontaneous improvement is probably rare.[17]

71

In patients < 75 years age and mJOA score > 12 (mild myelopathy), the clinical condition remained stable in 3-years of follow-up (Class I)[38] (however, these patients can still have significant disability that can respond to surgery). Patients with stenosis without myelopathy who have electrodiagnostic abnormalities or clinical radiculopathy are at risk of developing myelopathy (Class I).[38] Longstanding severe stenosis over many years may cause irreversible deficit due to necrosis in gray and white matter (Class III).[38]

71.4 Differential diagnosis

71.4.1 General information

See Myelopathy (p. 1407) for other possible causes. Some of these (e.g. spinal cord tumor, OPLL) may be demonstrated radiographically. Asymptomatic cervical spondylosis is very common, and ≈ 12% of cases of cervical myelopathy attributed to spondylosis are later found to be due to another disease process including:
1. ALS: see below
2. multiple sclerosis (MS): spinal cord demyelination may mimic CSM. With MS, remissions and exacerbations are common, and patients tend to be younger
3. herniated cervical disc (soft disc): patients tend to be younger than with CSM. Course is more rapid
4. subacute combined system disease: abnormal vitamin B12 level and possibly macrocytic anemia (p. 1409)
5. hereditary spastic paraplegia: family history is key. Diagnosis of exclusion[39]
6. (spontaneous) intracranial hypotension (p. 178)

71.4.2 Amyotrophic lateral sclerosis (ALS)

AKA (anterior horn) motor neuron disease; also see Amyotrophic lateral sclerosis (p. 183). Can mimic the motor system syndrome of CSM (see above), and spinal cord compression may be seen on MRI in > 60% of patients with ALS.[40]

"*Triad*" of ALS:
1. atrophic weakness of hands and forearms (early) – LMN finding
2. mild LE spasticity – UMN finding
3. diffuse hyperreflexia – UMN finding

Table 71.2 Modified JOA score for cervical myelopathy[23a]

Score	Description	
	Upper extremity (UE) motor dysfunction	
0	unable to feed self	
1	unable to use knife & fork; can eat with spoon	
2	can use knife & fork with much difficulty	
3	can use knife & fork with slight difficulty	
4	none (normal)	
	Lower extremity (LE) motor dysfunction	
0	unable to walk	
1	can walk on flat surface with walking aid	
2	can walk up and/or down stairs with handrail	
3	lack of smooth and stable gait	
4	none (normal)	
	Sensory deficit	
0	UE	severe sensory loss or pain
1		mild sensory loss
2		none (normal)
0	LE	severe sensory loss or pain
1		mild sensory loss
2		none (normal)
0	trunk	severe sensory loss or pain
1		mild sensory loss
2		none (normal)
	Sphincter dysfunction	
0	unable to void	
1	marked voiding difficulty (retention)	
2	some voiding difficulty (urgency or hesitation)	
3	none (normal)	
[a]total score ranges from 0 to 17 (normal)		

Inevitably, some cases of demyelinating disease will be misdiagnosed initially as CSM until some features suggestive of ALS occur (in one series of 1500 ALS patients, 4% underwent spine surgery (56% cervical, 42% lumbar, 2% thoracic)[40] before ALS was correctly diagnosed).

Features that may help differentiate ALS from CSM:

1. ALS: sensory changes are conspicuously *absent*
2. ALS: bulbar symptoms (dysarthria, hyperactive jaw-jerk…)[41]

71

3. ALS: extensive weakness/muscle atrophy of hands, usually with fasciculations[42]
4. ALS: lower-motor neuron (LMN) findings in the tongue (visible fasciculations, or positive sharp waves on EMG) or in the LEs (e.g. fasciculations and atrophy) favors the diagnosis of ALS over CSM (however, LMN findings in the LEs may occur in CSM if there is coincidental lumbar radiculopathy)
5. CSM or herniated cervical disc: usually includes neck and shoulder pain, limitation of neck movement, sensory changes, and LMN findings restricted to 1 or 2 spinal cord segments

71.5 Evaluation

71.5.1 Plain x-rays

General information

Minimum evaluation consists of AP, lateral (neutral position), and open-mouth odontoid views. If desired, flexion-extension views and/or oblique views may be obtained but requires specific orders.

When MRI is available, the additional information provided by plain cervical spine x-rays in patients with CSM is limited. In this setting, x-rays may be best for:
1. Demonstrating dynamic instability with flexion-extension views (see below)
2. Sagittal balance measured on standing lateral cervical spine x-rays may provide prognostic information[43]
3. X-rays may be able to compensate for the following MRI deficiencies, but cervical CT is much better
   a) Differentiating calcified discs or bone spurs from "soft discs"
   b) Differentiating OPLL form a thickened posterior longitudinal ligament
   c) Bone abnormalities: fractures, bony lytic lesions

Cervical spinal stenosis

71

Cervical spinal stenosis can be inferred from plain x-rays. ✱ NB: Canal diameters measured on x-rays are actually surrogate markers for the entity of interest: viz. spinal canal narrowing sufficient to produce spinal cord compression and thereby spinal cord symptoms. This can be directly demonstrated on MRI or CT/myelo, and MRI can also detect intrinsic spinal cord signal abnormalities.

See Canal diameter (p. 214) for normal dimensions and measurement techniques. Patients with CSM have an average minimal AP canal diameter of 11.8 mm,[44] and values ≤ 10 mm were likely to be associated with myelopathy.[45] Patients with an AP diameter < 14 mm may be at increased risk,[46] and CSM is rare in patients with a diameter > 16 mm, even with significant spurs.[17]

Cervical spinal stenosis is also suggested on plain films when the spinolaminar line is close to the posterior margin of the lateral masses.

Pavlov ratio (AKA Torg ratio[47,48]): the ratio of the AP diameter of the spinal canal at the mid VB level to the VB at the same location. A ratio < 0.8 is sensitive for transient neuropraxia, but has been shown to have poor positive predictive value for CSM.

Oblique views

Oblique views can delineate foraminal compromise caused by osteophytic spurs.

Flexion-extension views

Lateral flexion/extension x-rays may provide valuable information by detecting dynamic instability (abnormalities that manifest with movement) that cannot be appreciated on (static) CT or MRI, including widening of the atlanto-dental interval on flexion (p. 213).

71.5.2 MRI

MRI provides information about the spinal canal, and can also show intrinsic cord abnormalities (demyelination, syringomyelia, spinal cord atrophy, edema…). MRI also rules out other diagnostic possibilities (Chiari malformation, spinal cord tumor…).

Bony structures and calcified ligaments are poorly imaged. These shortcoming and the difficulties in differentiating osteophytes from herniated discs on MRI are overcome with the addition of plain cervical spine films[49] or to better advantage with thin-section CT bone windows.

Findings that correlate with poor outcome (Class III)[50]:
1. *multilevel* T2WI hyperintensity within the spinal cord parenchyma

2. *single* level T2WI hyperintensity with corresponding T1WI hypointensity (single level T2WI hyperintensity without T1WI changes are of uncertain prognostic significance)
3. spinal cord atrophy (transverse area < 45 mm^2)

Other MRI findings seen with CSM:
1. reduced transverse area of the spinal cord (TASC) at the level of maximum compression. A "banana" shaped cord on axial images has a high correlation with the presence of CSM.[46] There is conflicting evidence whether the degree of canal stenosis predicts outcome.[50] Sagittal T2WIs tend to exaggerate the magnitude of spinal cord compression by osteophytes and/or discs, and therefore axial images and T1WIs also need to be considered in the evaluation. Narrowing is not specific for CSM: ≈ 26% of *asymptomatic* individuals > 64 years of age have spinal cord compression on MRI[51]
2. "snake eyes" (AKA "owl's eyes") within the spinal cord on axial T2WI (▶ Fig. 71.1) may be related to cystic necrosis of the cord[52] and may correlate with poor outcome (Class III)[50]

71.5.3 CT and CT/myelogram

Plain CT scans may demonstrate a narrow canal, but do not provide adequate information regarding soft tissues (discs, ligaments, spinal cord and nerve roots). However, bony detail may prove invaluable in the surgical treatment of CSM.

Cervical myelography followed by high-resolution CT scanning provides sagittal and axial information (including spinal cord atrophy), and delineates bony detail better than MRI.[49] Unlike MRI, CT/myelogram is invasive (requires LP) and involves ionizing radiation and does not provide information about changes within the spinal cord parenchyma.

71.5.4 EMG

Not routinely useful in CSM. EMG has poor sensitivity in cervical radiculopathy and is not reliable in predicting outcome from surgery for CSM (Class III).[50] EMG is most helpful in suspicious cases to eliminate etiologies such as peripheral neuropathy or ALS.

71.5.5 Sensory evoked potentials (SEPs)

SSEPs are of limited usefulness, although a normal pre-op SEP or normalization of SEPs in the early post-op period are associated with better outcome.[53]

Practice guideline: Pre-op SEPs in CSM

Pre-op SEPs should be considered if the additional prognostic information would help treatment decisions (Level B Class II)[53]

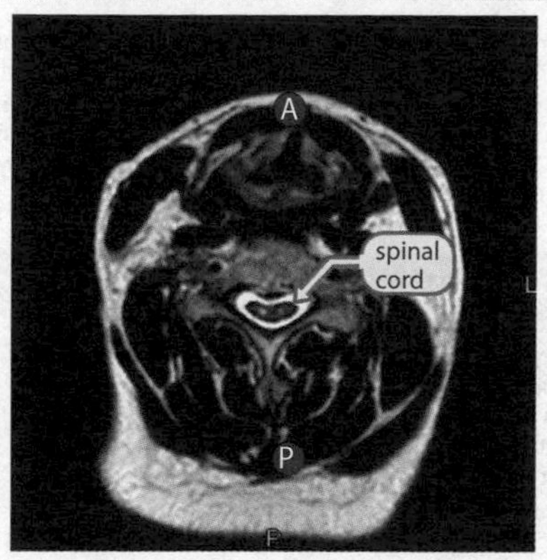

Fig. 71.1 Snake eyes (two foci of high signal) within a slightly flattened and mildly atrophic spinal cord on axial T2WI MRI

71.6 Treatment

71.6.1 Nonoperative management

Measures include: prolonged immobilization with rigid cervical bracing in an attempt to reduce motion and hence the cumulative effects of trauma on the spinal cord, modified activity to eliminate "high-risk" activities or bed rest, and anti-inflammatory medications.[54]

71.6.2 Surgical treatment

Indications for surgery

See **Practice guideline: Surgical vs. nonsurgical management** (p. 1090).

Practice guideline: Surgical vs. nonsurgical management

Mild myelopathy (mJOA score > 12): in the short-term (3 years) patients may be offered the option of surgical decompression or nonoperative management (prolonged immobilization in a rigid cervical collar, anti-inflammatory medications, and "low-risk" activities or bed rest (Level C Class II)).[55] **Note:** patients with mJOA scores > 12 (see ▶ Table 71.2) may not always be mildly impaired, they may derive significant improvement from surgery, and deterioration from this point may be ominous.

More severe myelopathy: should be treated with surgical decompression with benefits maintained at 5 and 15 years post-op (Level D Class III)[55]

Level B Class I[56] Degenerative cervical *radiculopathy*: patients do better with anterior decompression ± fusion (compared to conservative management) for

- rapid relief (within 3–4 months) of arm & neck pain and sensory loss
- relief of longer term (≥ 12 months) symptoms of weakness of wrist extension, elbow extension, shoulder abduction and internal rotation

71

Intraoperative electrophysiologic monitoring

Practice guideline: Intra-operative electrophysiologic monitoring during surgery for CSM or radiculopathy

Use of intra-op EP monitoring during routine surgery for CSM or cervical radiculopathy is not recommended as an indication to alter the surgical plan or administer steroids since this paradigm has not been observed to reduce the incidence of neurologic injury (Level D Class III)[57]

Choice of approach

General information

The debate between anterior approaches (anterior cervical discectomy or corpectomy) and posterior approaches (decompressive cervical laminectomy or laminoplasty) dates back to the time that both became widely practiced.[16] General sentiment is to treat anterior disease at the disc level (e.g. osteophytic bar, herniated disc...) usually limited to ≤ 3 levels (or occasionally 4) with an anterior approach, and to use a posterior approach as the initial procedure in the situations outlined below. Considerations of spinal curvature may need to enter into the decision process.

Practice guideline: Choice of surgical approach for CSM

There was not enough evidence to recommend any of the following techniques over the other (in terms of short-term success in treating CSM): ACDF, anterior corpectomy and fusion, laminectomy (with or without fusion) and laminoplasty (**Level D Class III**)[58]

Laminectomy without fusion, however, is associated with a higher incidence of late kyphotic deformity (**Level D Class III**; incidence 14–47%, not all cases are symptomatic, not all cases need treatment: see text)[58]

Posterior approach

Options include:

1. laminectomy alone laminectomy/arthrodesis (i.e. laminectomy + lateral mass fusion): **Class III** (this procedure was found to be effective, the class shows the strength of the evidence)[59])
2. laminoplasty (**Class III**; this procedure was found to be effective, the class shows the strength of the evidence[60]): methods include unilateral ("open door") and midline enlargement ("French door")
3. multilevel foraminotomies: usually not adequate for central canal stenosis

Situations where a posterior approach would generally be the initial approach:

1. congenital cervical stenosis where removing osteophytes will still not provide at least ≈ 12 mm of AP canal diameter
2. disease over ≥ 3 levels (although up to 4 may occasionally be dealt with anteriorly)
3. primary posterior pathology (e.g. infolding of ligamentum flavum)
4. some cases of OPLL (anterior approach has higher risk of dural tear)

Disadvantages of the posterior approach:

1. laminectomy *without* fusion
   a) degeneration and osteophytes continue to progress following surgery
   b) risk of subsequent subluxation or progressive kyphotic angulation ("swan neck" deformity) (facetiously dubbed "spina bifida neurosurgica")
      - quoted incidence: 14–47%[61,62,63] (risk may be minimized by careful preservation of facet joints)
      - not all cases need to be treated: in one series, 31% (18/58) developed post-op kyphosis, and 16% of these (3/18) required surgical stabilization[64]
      - the development of kyphotic deformity does not appear to diminish the clinical outcome[63] and does not correlate with neurologic deterioration when deterioration occurs[65]
2. more painful initially post-op and sometimes more prolonged rehabilitation
3. long-term complaints of a heaviness of the head possibly associated with atrophy of the paraspinal muscles
4. ✖ contraindicated with pre-existing swan neck deformity, and not recommended in the presence of reversal of the normal cervical lordosis (i.e. kyphotic curve)[66] where the spinal cord won't tend to move away from the anterior compression or in the presence of ≥ 3.5 mm subluxation or > 20° rotation in the sagittal plane[46] and caution must be exercised in hyperlordosis (see below)

Anterior approach

Also shown to be effective (Class III[55]).

Instrumentation options: in terms of *fusion rates* for 2-level anterior operations (i.e. 2 disc spaces) (Class III)[58]:

2-level ACDF with anterior plate = 1-level corpectomy with plate > 1-level corpectomy without plate* > 2-level ACDF without plate

* however, the graft extrusion rate is higher for corpectomy than ACDF

Worsening of myelopathy has been reported in 2–5% of patients after anterior decompression[67,68] (intraoperative SSEP monitoring may reduce this rate[68]) and C5 radiculopathy may occur (see below).

Anterior cervical plating

Many systems are available, with more similarities than differences. All include some method of preventing screw back out. Some general pointers:

1. for single level fusion, typical plate length is 22–24 mm
2. screw length: rule of thumb is 12 mm for females, 14 mm for males
3. do not completely tighten a single screw (to avoid kicking up plate) until the diagonally opposite screws are placed and loosely tightened
4. most systems have fixed and variable angle screws. Variable angle screws allow for load sharing with the graft (here is where a derivative of Wolff's law is often invoked: the weight sharing helps stimulate fusion). Avoid over-angling screws which may prevent the locking mechanism from properly engaging

5. optimal plate placement allows for contact of the plate with the VB at the screw locations. This may require
   a) contouring of plate to follow the lordosis of the c-spine
   b) reduction of anterior osteophytes

Posterior approach

For decompression, some recommend cervical laminectomy extending one or *two* levels beyond the stenosis above and below.[69,70] A C3–6 laminectomy is often considered a "standard" laminectomy. An "extended laminectomy" includes C7 and/or C2.

Curvature considerations: extending the laminectomy to include C2 and sometimes C1 has been recommended for patients with straightening of the cervical curvature.[6] In cases of ***hyperlordosis***, posterior migration of the spinal cord following an extensive laminectomy may put increased tension on the nerve roots and blood vessels (with possible neurologic worsening), and a limited laminectomy just where the cord is compressed is often recommended (below).

"Keyhole foraminotomies" or medial facetectomy with undercutting of the facets may be performed at levels involved with radiculopathy.

Position: choices are primarily: prone, lateral oblique, or sitting. The prone position has a major disadvantage of difficulty elevating the head above the heart, resulting in venous engorgement with significant operative bleeding. The sitting position has a number of inherent risks (p. 1445), including cord hypoperfusion[68] and air embolism. The lateral oblique position may introduce some distortion to the anatomy due to asymmetrical positioning.

The reported rate of post-op spinal deformity is 25–42%. Neurologic worsening has been reported in 2% in some series, higher in others. C5 radiculopathy may occur (see below).

To avoid significant destabilization of the cervical spine:

1. during the dissection, do not remove soft tissue overlying the facet joints (to preserve their blood supply)
2. take the laminectomy only as far lateral as the extent of the spinal canal, carefully preserving the facet joints[7] (use keyhole laminotomies where necessary)
3. avoid removing a total of one facet at any given level

Outcome

General information

Even excluding cases that are later proven to have demyelinating disease, the outcome from surgery for CSM is often disappointing. Once CSM is clinically apparent, complete remission almost never occurs. The prognosis with surgery is worse with increasing severity of involvement at the time of presentation[69] and with longer duration of symptoms (48% showed clinical improvement or cure if operated within 1 yr of onset, whereas only 16% responded after 1 yr[7]). The success of surgery is also lower in patients with other degenerative diseases of the CNS (ALS, MS…).

Progression of myelopathy may be arrested by surgical decompression. This is not always borne out, and some early series[34,37] showed similar results with conservative treatment as with laminectomy which yielded improvement in 56%, no change in 25%, and worsening in 19%. Also as discussed earlier some cases of CSM develop most of the deficit early and then stabilize (p. 1086).

Some series show good results, with ≈ 64–75% patients having improvement in CSM post-op.[22] However, other authors remain less enthusiastic. Utilizing a questionnaire in 32 post-op patients operated anteriorly, 66% had relief from radicular pain, while only 33% had improvement in sensory or motor complaints.[22] In one series, half the patients had improvement in fine motor function of the hands, but the other half worsened postoperatively.[71] Spinal cord atrophy as a result of continued pressure or ischemia may be partly responsible for poor recovery. Bedridden patients with severe myelopathy rarely recover useful function.

Post-op C5 palsy

Criteria: weakness of deltoid and/or biceps with no worsening of myelopathy. Follows ≈ 3–5% of extensive anterior or posterior decompression (including laminoplasty).[67,72] 50% have motor involvement only (deltoid > biceps), 50% also have C5 dermatomal sensory loss and/or C5 dermatomal pain (shoulder). Most occur < 1 week post-op.[72] 92% are unilateral.[72] No pre-op risk factors have been identified.[73] Etiology: unproven, may be related to traction on the nerve root from posterior migration of the cord after decompression or to bone graft displacement. Prognosis for spontaneous recovery is generally good; more severe deficits take longer to recover.[72]

Late developments

Some patients who show early improvement will develop late deterioration (7–12 yrs after reaching a plateau),[46] with no radiographically apparent explanation in up to 20% of these cases.[74] In others, degeneration at levels adjacent to the operated segments may be demonstrated.

Adjacent segment disease (ASD): degeneration that develops at a motion segment adjacent to a previous fusion. Findings include: disc degeneration, stenosis, facet hypertrophy, scoliosis, listhesis and instability. After ACDF, ASD occurred at a rate of 2.9% per year over 10 years observation.[75] Estimate: 25% of patients will develop symptomatic adjacent level changes within 10 years of surgery.[75] This rate was higher with single level fusion at C5–6 or C6–7 than it was with multilevel fusion, and natural progression of the disease was felt to be a significant contributor[75] (i.e. it was not all attributable to the fusion). Most cases of ASD observed radiographically are asymptomatic.

71.7 Coincident cervical and lumbar spinal stenosis

In 5%, lumbar and cervical stenoses are symptomatic simultaneously.[76]

Coincident symptomatic lumbar and cervical spinal stenosis is usually managed by first decompressing the cervical region, and later operating on the lumbar region (unless severe neurogenic claudication dominates the picture). It is also possible, in selected cases, to operate on both in a single sitting.[76,77]

References

[1] Miller CA. Shallow Cervical Canal: Recognition, Clinical Symptoms, and Treatment. Contemp Neurosurg. 1985; 7:1–5

[2] Muhle C, Weinert D, Falliner A, et al. Dynamic changes of the spinal canal in patients with cervical spondyolosis at flexion and extension using mangnetic resonance imaging. Invest Radiol. 1998; 33:444–449

[3] Shedid D, Benzel EC, Benzel EC, Stewart TJ. Cervical spondylosis anatomy: pathophysiology and biomechanics. Neurosurgery. 2007; 60:S1-1-11

[4] Nagashima C. Cervical Myelopathy due to Ossification of the Posterior Longitudinal Ligament. J Neurosurg. 1972; 37:653–660

[5] Miyazawa N, Akiyama I. Ossification of the ligamentum flavum of the cervical spine. J Neurosurg Sci. 2007; 51:139–144

[6] Batzdorf U, Batzdorf A. Analysis of Cervical Spine Curvature in Patients with Cervical Spondylosis. Neurosurgery. 1988; 22:827–836

[7] Cusick JF. Pathophysiology and Treatment of Cervical Spondylotic Myelopathy. Clin Neurosurg. 1989; 37:661–681

[8] Taylor AR. Vascular Factors in the Myelopathy Associated with Cervical Spondylosis. Neurology. 1964; 14:62–68

[9] Bohlman HH, Emery JL. The pathophysiology of cervical spondylosis and myelopathy. Spine. 1988; 13:843–846

[10] Kim RC, Nelson JS, Parisi JE, Schochet SS. In: Spinal cord pathology. Principals and Practice of Neuropathology. St. Louis: C V Mosby; 1993:398–435

[11] Jeffreys RV. The Surgical Treatment of Cervical Myelopathy Due to Spondylosis and Disc Degeneration. J Neurol Neurosurg Psychiatry. 1986; 49:353–361

[12] Adams CBT, Logue V. Studies in Cervical Spondylotic Myelopathy: I. Movement of the Cervical Roots, Dura and Cord, and their Relation to the Course of the Extrathecal Roots. Brain. 1971; 94:557–568

[13] Levine DN. Pathogenesis of Cervical Spondylotic Myelopathy. J Neurol Neurosurg Psychiatry. 1997; 62:334–340

[14] Benzel EC. Biomechanics of Spine Stabilization. Rolling Meadows, IL: American Association of Neurological Surgeons Publications; 2001

[15] Ogino H, Tada K, Okada K, et al. Canal Diameter, Anteroposterior Compression Ratio, and Spondylotic Myelopathy of the Cervical Spine. Spine. 1983; 8:1–15

[16] Mayfield FH. Cervical Spondylosis: A Comparison of the Anterior and Posterior Approaches. Clin Neurosurg. 1966; 13:181–188

[17] Cooper PR. Cervical Spondylotic Myelopathy. Contemp Neurosurg. 1997; 19:1–7

[18] Yu YL, du Boulay GH, Stevens JM, Kendall BE. Computed Tomography in Cervical Spondylotic Myelopathy and Radiculopathy: Visualization of Structures, Myelographic Comparison, Cord Measurements and Clinical Utility. Neuroradiology. 1986; 28:221–236

[19] Epstein JA, Marc JA, Hyman RA, Khan A, et al. Total Myelography in the Evaluation of Lumbar Disks. Spine. 1979; 4:121–128

[20] Houser OW, Onofrio BM, Miller GM, et al. Cervical Spondylotic Stenosis and Myelopathy: Evaluation with Computed Tomographic Myelography. Mayo Clin Proc. 1994; 69:557–563

[21] Emery SE. Cervical spondylotic myelopathy: diagnosis and treatment. J Am Acad Orthop Surg. 2001; 9:376–388

[22] Lunsford LD, Bissonette DJ, Zorub DS. Anterior Surgery for Cervical Disc Disease. Part 2: Treatment of Cervical Spondylotic Myelopathy in 32 Cases. J Neurosurg. 1980; 53:12–19

[23] Chiles BW, III, Leonard MA, Choudhri HF, Cooper PR. Cervical spondylotic myelopathy: Patterns of neurological deficit and recovery after anterior cervical decompression. Neurosurgery. 1999; 44:762–769

[24] Ebara S, Yonenobu K, Fujiwara K, Yamashita K, Ono K. Myelopathy hand characterized by muscle wasting: A different type of myelopathy hand in patients with cervical spondylosis. Spine. 1988; 13:785–791

[25] Crandall PH, Batzdorf U. Cervical Spondylotic Myelopathy. J Neurosurg. 1966; 25:57–66

[26] Voskuhl RR, Hinton RC. Sensory Impairment in the Hands Secondary to Spondylotic Compression of the Cervical Spinal Cord. Arch Neurol. 1990; 47:309–311

[27] MacFadyen DJ. Posterior Column Dysfunction in Cervical Spondylotic Myelopathy. Can J Neurol Sci. 1984; 11:365–370

[28] Denno JJ, Meadows GR. Early diagnosis of cervical spondylotic myelopathy. A useful clinical sign. Spine. 1991; 16:1353–1355

[29] Sung RD, Wang JC. Correlation between a positive Hoffmann's reflex and cervical pathology in asymptomatic individuals. Spine. 2001; 26:67–70

[30] Wiggins GC, Shaffrey CI. Laminectomy in the Cervical Spine: Indications, Surgical Technniques, and Avoidance of Complications. Contemp Neurosurg. 1999; 21:1–10

[31] England JD, Hsu CY, Vera CL, et al. Spondylotic High Cervical Spinal Cord Compression Presenting with Hand Complaints. Surg Neurol. 1986; 25:299–303
[32] Good DC, Couch JR, Wacasser L. "Numb, Clumsy Hands" and High Cervical Spondylosis. Surg Neurol. 1984; 22:285–291
[33] Vernon H, Mior S. The Neck Disability Index: a study of reliability and validity. J Manipulative Physiol Ther. 1991; 14:409–415
[34] Nurick S. The Pathogenesis of the Spinal Cord Disorder Associated with Cervical Spondylosis. Brain. 1972; 95:87–100
[35] Clarke E, Robinson PK. Cervical Myelopathy: A Complication of Cervical Spondylosis. Brain. 1956; 79:483–485
[36] Lees F, Aldren Turner JS. Natural History and Prognosis of Cervical Spondylosis. Br Med J. 1963; 2:1607–1610
[37] Nurick S. The Natural History and the Results of Surgical Treatment of the Spinal Cord Disorder Associated with Cervical Spondylosis. Brain. 1972; 95:101–108
[38] Matz PG, Anderson PA, Holly LT, Groff MW, Heary RF, Kaiser MG, Mummaneni PV, Ryken TC, Choudhri TF, Vresilovic EJ, Resnick DK. The natural history of cervical spondylotic myelopathy. J Neurosurg: Spine. 2009; 11:104–111
[39] Ungar-Sargon JY, Lovelace RE, Brust JC. Spastic paraplegia-paraparesis: A Reappraisal. J Neurol Sci. 1980; 46:1–12
[40] Yoshor D, Klugh A, III, Appel SH, Haverkamp LJ. Incidence and characteristics of spinal decompression surgery after the onset of symptoms of amyotrophic lateral sclerosis. Neurosurgery. 2005; 57:984-9; discussion 984-9
[41] Campbell AMG, Phillips DG. Cervical Disk Lesions with Neurological Disorder. Differential Diagnosis, Treatment, and Prognosis. Br Med J. 1960; 2:481–485
[42] Rowland LP. Diagnosis of amyotrophic lateral sclerosis. J Neurol Sci. 1998; 160:S6–24
[43] Roguski M, Benzel EC, Curran JN, Magge SN, Bisson EF, Krishnaney AA, Steinmetz MP, Butler WE, Heary RF, Ghogawala Z. Postoperative cervical sagittal imbalance negatively affects outcomes after surgery for cervical spondylotic myelopathy. Spine (Phila Pa 1976). 2014; 39:2070–2077
[44] Adams CBT, Logue V. Studies in Cervical Spondylotic Myelopathy: II. The Movement and Contour of the Spine in Relation to the Neural Complications of Cervical Spondylosis. Brain. 1971; 94:569–586
[45] Wolf BS, Khilnani M, Malis L. The Sagittal Diameter of the Bony Cervical Spinal Canal and its Significance in Cervical Spondylosis. J of Mount Sinai Hospital. 1956; 23:283–292
[46] Krauss WE, Ebersold MJ, Quast LM. Cervical Spondylotic Myelopathy: Surgical Indications and Technique. Contemp Neurosurg. 1998; 20:1–6
[47] Pavlov H, Torg JS, Robie B, Jahre C. Cervical Spinal Stenosis: Determination with Vertebral Body Ratio Method. Radiology. 1987; 164:771–775
[48] Torg JS, Naranja RJ, Pavlov H, et al. The Relationship of Developmental Narrowing of the Cervical Spinal Canal to Reversible and Irreversible Injury of the Cervical Spinal Cord in Football Players. J Bone Joint Surg. 1996; 78A:1308–1314
[49] Brown BM, Schwartz RH, Frank E, Blank NK. Preoperative Evaluation of Cervical Radiculopathy and Myelopathy by Surface-Coil MR Imaging. AJNR. 1988; 9:859–866
[50] Mummaneni PV, Kaiser MG, Matz PG, Anderson PA, Groff M, Heary R, Holly L, Ryken T, Choudhri T, Vresilovic E, Resnick D. Preoperative patient selection with magnetic resonance imaging, computed tomography, and electroencephalography: does the test predict outcome after cervical surgery? J Neurosurg: Spine. 2009; 11:119–129
[51] Teresi LM, Lufkin RB, Reicher MA, Moffitt BJ, et al. Asymptomatic degenerative disk disease and spondylosis of the cervical spine: MR imaging. Radiology. 1987; 164:83–88
[52] Mizuno J, Nakagawa H, Inoue T, Hashizume Y. Clinicopathological study of "snake-eye appearance" in compressive myelopathy of the cervical spinal cord. J Neurosurg. 2003; 99:162–168
[53] Holly LT, Matz PG, Anderson PA, Groff MW, Heary RF, Kaiser MG, Mummaneni PV, Ryken TC, Choudhri TF, Vresilovic EJ, Resnick DK. Clinical prognostic indicators of surgical outcome in cervical spondylotic myelopathy. J Neurosurg: Spine. 2009; 11:112–118
[54] Kadanka Z, Bednarik J, Vohanka S, et al. Conservative tratment versus surgery in spondylotic cervical myelopathy treated conservatively or surgically. Eur Spine J. 2000; 9:538–544
[55] Matz PG, Holly LT, Mummaneni PV, Anderson PA, Groff MW, Heary RF, Kaiser MG, Ryken TC, Choudhri TF, Vresilovic EJ, Resnick DK. Anterior cervical surgery for the treatment of cervical degenerative myelopathy. J Neurosurg: Spine. 2009; 11:170–173
[56] Matz PG, Holly LT, Groff MW, Vresilovic EJ, Anderson PA, Heary RF, Kaiser MG, Mummaneni PV, Ryken TC, Choudhri TF, Resnick DK. Indications for anterior cervical decompression for the treatment of cervical degenerative radiculopathy. J Neurosurg: Spine. 2009; 11:174–182
[57] Resnick DK, Anderson PA, Kaiser MG, Groff MW, Heary RF, Holly LT, Mummaneni PV, Ryken TC, Choudhri TF, Vresilovic EJ, Matz PG. Electrophysiological monitoring during surgery for cervical degenerative myelopathy and radiculopathy. J Neurosurg: Spine. 2009; 11:245–252
[58] Mummaneni PV, Kaiser MG, Matz PG, Anderson PA, Groff MW, Heary RF, Holly LT, Ryken TC, Choudhri TF, Vresilovic EJ, Resnick DK. Cervical surgical techniques for the treatment of cervical spondylotic myelopathy. J Neurosurg: Spine. 2009; 11:130–141
[59] Anderson PA, Matz PG, Groff MW, Heary RF, Holly LT, Kaiser MG, Mummaneni PV, Ryken TC, Choudhri TF, Vresilovic EJ, Resnick DK. Laminectomy and fusion for the treatment of cervical degenerative myelopathy. J Neurosurg: Spine. 2009; 11:150–156
[60] Matz PG, Anderson PA, Groff MW, Heary RF, Holly LT, Kaiser MG, Mummaneni PV, Ryken TC, Choudhri TF, Vresilovic EJ, Resnick DK. Cervical laminoplasty for the treatment of cervical degenerative myelopathy. J Neurosurg: Spine. 2009; 11:157–169
[61] Hamanishi C, Tanaka S. Bilateral multilevel laminectomy with or without posterolateral fusion for cervical spondylotic myelopathy: relationship to type of onset and time until operation. J Neurosurg. 1996; 85:447–451
[62] Matsunaga S, Sakou T, Nakanisi K. Analysis of the cervical spine alignment following laminoplasty and laminectomy. Spinal Cord. 1999; 37:20–24
[63] Ryken TC, Heary RF, Matz PG, Anderson PA, Groff MW, Holly LT, Kaiser MG, Mummaneni PV, Choudhri TF, Vresilovic EJ, Resnick DK. Cervical laminectomy for the treatment of cervical degenerative myelopathy. J Neurosurg: Spine. 2009; 11:142–149
[64] Guigui P, Benoist M, Deburge A. Spinal deformity and instability after multilevel cervical laminectomy for spondylotic myelopathy. Spine. 1998; 23:440–447
[65] Kaptain GJ, Simmons NE, Replogle RE, Pobereskin L. Incidence and outcome of kyphotic deformity following laminectomy for cervical spondylotic myelopathy. J Neurosurg. 2000; 93:199–204
[66] Benzel EC, Lancon J, Kesterson L, Hadden T. Cervical laminectomy and dentate ligament section for cervical spondylotic myelopathy. J Spinal Disord. 1991; 4:286 295
[67] Yonenobu K, Hosono N, Iwasaki M, et el.. Neurologic Complications of Surgery for Cervical Compression Myelopathy. Spine. 1991; 16:1277–1282
[68] Epstein NE, Danto J, Nardi D. Evaluation of Intraoperative Somatosensory-Evoked Potential Monitoring During 100 Cervical Operations. Spine. 1993; 18:737–747
[69] Epstein J, Janin Y, Carras R, Lavine LS. A Comparative Study of the Treatment of Cervical Spondylotic Myeloradiculopathy: Experience with 50 Cases Treated by Means of Extensive Laminectomy, Foraminotomy, and Excision of Osteophytes During the Past 10 Years. Acta Neurochir. 1982; 61

[70] Epstein NE, Epstein JA, The Cervical Spine Research Society Editorial Committee. In: Operative Management of Cervical Spondylotic Myelopathy: Technique and Result of Laminectomy. The Cervical Spine. 3rd ed. Philadelphia: Lippincott-Raven; 1998:839–848
[71] Gregorius FK, Estrin T, Crandall PH. Cervical Spondylotic Radiculopathy and Myelopathy. A Long-Term Follow-Up Study. Arch Neurol. 1976; 33:618–625
[72] Sakaura H, Hosono N, Mukai Y, Ishii T, Yoshikawa H. C5 palsy after decompression surgery for cervical myelopathy: review of the literature. Spine. 2003; 28:2447–2451
[73] Komagata M, Nishiyama M, Endo K, Ikegami H, Tanaka S, Imakiire A. Prophylaxis of C5 palsy after cervical expansive laminoplasty by bilateral partial foraminotomy. Spine J. 2004; 4:650–655
[74] Ebersold MJ, Pare MC, Quast LM. Surgical Treatment for Cervical Spondylitic Myelopathy. J Neurosurg. 1995; 82:745–751
[75] Hilibrand AS, Carlson GD, Palumbo MA, Jones PK, Bohlman HH. Radiculopathy and myelopathy at segments adjacent to the site of a previous anterior cervical arthrodesis. J Bone Joint Surg Am. 1999; 81:519–528
[76] Epstein NE, Epstein JA, Carras R, et al. Coexisting Cervical and Lumbar Spinal Stenosis: Diagnosis and Management. Neurosurgery. 1984; 15:489–496
[77] Dagi TF, Tarkington MA, Leech JJ. Tandem Lumbar and Cervical Spinal Stenosis. J Neurosurg. 1987; 66:842–849

72 Thoracic and Lumbar Degenerative Disc Disease

72.1 General information about degenerative disc disease (DDD)

Since structures outside of the disc are usually also involved, the term degenerative spine disease (DSD) may be preferable to degenerative disc disease. Spondylosis is a non-specific term which may include degenerative spine disease. "Cervical spondylosis" is occasionally used synonymously with cervical stenosis (p. 1083).

Symptomatic spinal stenosis in the thoracic region is rare,[1] and is generally seen in the setting of a calcified disc. The majority of this chapter deals with lumbar DSD. For the cervical region, see that chapter (p. 1083).

72.2 Anatomic substrate

72.2.1 General information

DSD is a progressive deterioration of the structures of the spine including:

1. disc abnormalities:
   a) the proteoglycan content of the disc nucleus decreases with age
   b) disc desiccation (loss of hydration) occurs
   c) tears develop in the disc annulus and progress to internal disruption of the lamellar architecture. Herniation of the nucleus may occur from increased nuclear pressure under mechanical loads
   d) mucoid degeneration and ingrowth of fibrous tissue ensues (disc fibrosis)
   e) subsequently disc resorption occurs
   f) there is a loss of disc space height and increased susceptibility to injury
2. facet joint abnormalities: hypertrophy and capsular laxity
3. osteophytes often form on the edges of the VB bordering the degenerated disc
4. spondylolisthesis: subluxation of one VB on another (see Spondylolisthesis below)
5. hypertrophy of the ligamentum flavum

Neurologic involvement in lumbar spinal stenosis may occur in one or more of the following 3 sites:

1. central canal stenosis: narrowing of the AP dimension of the spinal canal below a critical value. The reduction in canal size may cause local neural compression and/or compromise of the blood supply to the spinal cord (cervical) or the cauda equina (lumbar)
   a) Congenital (as in the *achondroplastic dwarf*)
   b) Acquired: as with hypertrophy of facets and ligamentum flavum
   c) Most commonly – acquired superimposed on congenital narrowing.
2. foraminal stenosis: narrowing of the neural foramen. May be the result of any combination of: foraminal disc protrusion, spondylolisthesis, facet hypertrophy, disc space collapse, hypertrophy of uncovertebral joints (cervical), synovial cyst
3. lateral recess stenosis; lumbar spine only (p. 1097)

72.2.2 Lumbar spinal stenosis

Key concepts

- caused by hypertrophy of facets and ligamentum flavum, may be exacerbated by disc bulging or spondylolisthesis, may be superimposed on congenital narrowing
- most common at L4–5 and then at L3–4
- symptomatic stenosis produces gradually progressive back and leg pain with standing and walking that is relieved by sitting or lying (neurogenic claudication)
- symptoms differentiated from vascular claudication which is usually relieved at rest regardless of position
- usually responds to decompressive surgery (sometimes with fusion) or interspinous spacer

Symptomatic lumbar stenosis is most common at L4–5, then L3–4, L2–3 and lastly L5-S1.[2] It is rare at L1–2. Generally occurs in patients with congenitally shallow lumbar canal – see Normal LS spine measurements (p. 1102) – with superimposed acquired degeneration in the form of some combination of facet hypertrophy, hypertrophy of the ligamentum flavum, protruding (and often calcified) intervertebral discs, and spondylolisthesis. First recognized as a distinct clinical entity producing characteristic symptoms in the 1950's and 60's.[3,4]

May be classified as[5]:

1. stable form of lumbar spinal stenosis: hypertrophy of facets and ligamentum flavum accompanied by disc degeneration and collapse
2. unstable: have the above with superimposed
   a) degenerative spondylolisthesis (p. 1098), the unisegmental form
   b) degenerative scoliosis: the multisegmental form

72.2.3 Central canal stenosis

The central canal may be narrowed by a combination of any of the following:

- Hypertrophy of the ligamentum flavum
- Hypertrophy of the facet joints
- Congenitally shot pedicles
- Bulging intervertebral discs
- Osteophytes arising from the posterior VB
- Juxtafacet cysts
- Spondylolisthesis

72.2.4 Lateral recess syndrome

The lateral recess is the "gutter" alongside the pedicle which the nerve root enters just proximal to its exit through the neural foramen (▶ Fig. 72.1). It is bordered anteriorly by the vertebral body, laterally by the pedicle, and posteriorly by the superior articular facet of the inferior vertebral body. Hypertrophy of this superior articular facet compresses the nerve root. Narrowing of the lateral recess is present in essentially all cases of central canal stenosis, but it can be symptomatic by itself.[6] L4–5 is the most commonly involved facet.

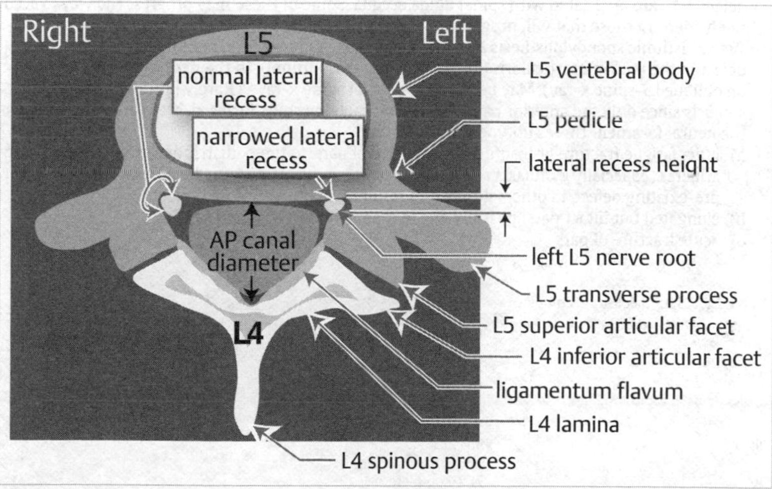

Fig. 72.1 Schematic axial CT through the L4-5 facet joint showing the lateral recesses (normal on patient's right, stenotic on left)

72

72.2.5 Spondylolisthesis

General information

Anterior subluxation of one vertebral body (VB) on another, most commonly the upper VB is anterior to the inferior one. Usually L5 on S1, the next most common is L4 on L5.

Disc herniation and nerve root compression with spondylolisthesis: It is rare for a herniated lumbar disc to occur at the level of the listhesis, however the disc may "roll" out as it is uncovered and produce findings on MRI that may resemble a herniated disc which has been termed a "pseudodisc." It is more common to see a herniated disc at the level *above* the listhesis.

If the listhesis does cause nerve root compression, it tends to involve the nerve exiting below the pedicle of the anteriorly subluxed upper vertebra (e.g. if an L4–5 spondylolisthesis causes nerve root compression, it will generally involve the *L4* root). The compression is usually due to upward displacement of the superior articular facet of the level below together with disc material, and symptoms typically resemble neurogenic claudication, although true radiculopathy may sometimes occur. There also may be a contribution from a fibrous/inflammatory mass from the nonunion.

Isthmic spondylolisthesis rarely produces central canal stenosis since only the anterior part of the vertebral body shifts forward. May present with radiculopathy or neurogenic claudication from compression in the neural foramen, with the nerve exiting under the pedicle at that level being the most vulnerable. May also present with low back pain. Many cases are asymptomatic.

Adolescent spondylolisthesis

In adolescents and teens, spondylolisthesis usually occurs in athletes subject to repetitive hyperextension of the lumbar spine. In girls, this is frequently encountered in gymnasts and softball pitching. In boys, football is common.

In these youngsters, cessation of sports for several months usually produces resolution.

Surgery is sometimes performed for patients who are unwilling to discontinue athletics.

Grading spondylolisthesis

The Meyerding[7,8] grading of subluxation in the sagittal plane is shown in ▶ Table 72.1.

72

Types of spondylolisthesis

1. Type 1: dysplastic: congenital. Upper sacrum or arch of L5 permits the spondylolisthesis. No pars defect. 94% are associated with spinal bifida occulta. Some of these may progress (no way to accurately identify those that will progress)
2. Type 2: isthmic spondylolisthesis AKA spondylolysis: a failure of the neural arch as a result of a defect in the pars interarticularis (identifiable as a discontinuity in the neck of the "Scotty dog" on oblique LS-spine x-ray). May be seen in 5–20% of spine x-rays.[9] Rarely produces central canal stenosis since only the anterior part of the vertebral body shifts forward. May cause narrowing of the neural foramen. Three subtypes:
   a) lytic: fatigue fracture or insufficiency fracture of pars. In the pediatric age group may occur in athletes (especially gymnasts or football players); in some this may be an exacerbation of a pre-existing defect, in others it may be a result of repetitive trauma
   b) elongated but intact pars: possibly due to repetitive fractures and healing
   c) acute fracture of pars

Table 72.1 Spondylolisthesis grading

Grade	% subluxation[a]
I	<25%
II	25–50%
III	50–75%
IV	75%-complete
spondyloptosis	>100%

[a]% of the AP diameter of the VB

3. Type 3: degenerative: due to long-standing intersegmental instability. Usually at L4–5. No break in the pars. Found in 5.8% of men and 9.1% of women (many of whom are asymptomatic)[9]
4. Type 4: traumatic: due to fractures usually in areas other than the pars
5. Type 5: pathologic: generalized or local bone disease, e.g. osteogenesis imperfecta

Natural history

Progression of spondylolisthesis may occur without surgical intervention, but is more common following surgery.[10]

72.2.6 Degenerative scoliosis

One of the main differentiating features from juvenile scoliosis is that in degenerative scoliosis, the disc spaces are asymmetrically narrowed in the coronal plane and the vertebral bodies tend to maintain a more normal configuration.

72.3 Risk factors

1. The risk of developing DSD is multifactorial and includes:
2. * The most powerful determinant in developing DSD in a study of twins was genetic influence, and possibly other unidentified factors.[11] Environmental factors studied (including sedentary vs. active lifestyles, occupation, cigarette smoking…) exerted only a modest influence, which may explain why conflicting findings for these have been reported
3. cumulative effects of microtrauma and macrotrauma to the spine
4. osteoporosis
5. cigarette smoking: several epidemiologic studies have shown that the incidence of back pain, sciatica and spinal degenerative disease is higher among cigarette smokers than among nonsmokers[12,13]
6. in the lumbar spine:
   a) stresses on the spine including effects of excess body weight
   b) loss of muscle tone (primarily abdominals and paraspinals) resulting in increased dependence on the bony spine for structural support

72.4 Associated conditions

1. congenital:
   a) achondroplasia
   b) congenitally narrowed canal
2. acquired:
   a) spondylolisthesis
   b) acromegaly
   c) post-traumatic
   d) Paget's disease (p. 1120)
   e) ankylosing spondylitis (p. 1123)
   f) ossification of the ligamentum flavum: more common in East Asians, rare in Caucasians.[14] Often, but not always, associated with OPLL[15]

72.5 Clinical presentation

72.5.1 General information

1. the degenerative abnormalities may produce spinal stenosis which can lead to neural compromise producing the following symptoms
   a) radicular symptoms (more common in cervical spine than lumbar)
   b) neurogenic claudication (lumbar) or spinal myelopathy (cervical)
2. Sagittal imbalance and scoliosis as a result of degenerative changes can place focal stress on specific spine structures which may be painful. Also, muscles used to compensate for the imbalance can cause pain from overuse fatigue
3. discogenic pain (controversial) may be less prevalent in the late stages of DSD. May contribute to "musculoskeletal low back pain" but the actual pain generators here are not definitively identified

72

4. Many cases of DSD (including spinal stenosis and spondylolisthesis) are asymptomatic, and the degenerative changes are discovered incidentally

72.5.2 Neurogenic claudication

Lumbar spinal stenosis often presents as neurogenic claudication (NC), (claudicate: from Latin, claudico, to limp) AKA pseudoclaudication. To be differentiated from vascular claudication (AKA intermittent claudication) which results from ischemia of exercising muscles (see ▶ Table 72.2 *for distinguishing characteristics*).

NC characteristics: unilateral or bilateral buttock, hip, thigh or leg discomfort that is precipitated by standing or walking and characteristically relieved by a change in posture (usually sitting with the waist flexed, squatting, or lying in the fetal position). Painful burning paresthesias of the lower extremities are also described. Valsalva maneuvers usually do not exacerbate the pain. Many patients report increased pain first thing in the morning that improves once they have been out of bed for varying periods (usually an hour more or less).

The time course is usually gradually progressive over many months to years. As the condition progresses, the ability to get relief from position changes tends to decrease. However, presenting with acute, unrelenting pain is not characteristic and other causes should be sought.

In comparison, a HLD usually causes increased pain on sitting, has a more abrupt onset, has pain on straight leg raising, and is worsened by Valsalva maneuvers.

NC is thought to arise from ischemia of lumbosacral nerve roots, as a result of increased metabolic demand from exercise together with vascular compromise of the nerve root due to pressure from surrounding structures. NC is only moderately sensitive (≈ 60%) but is highly specific for spinal stenosis.[17] Pain may not be the major complaint, instead, some patients may develop paresthesias or LE weakness with walking. Some may complain of muscle cramping, especially in the calves.

Relief from symptoms: occurs with positions that decrease the lumbar lordosis which increases the diameter of the central canal (by reducing inward buckling of the ligamentum flavum) and distracts the facet joints (which enlarges the neural foramina. Favored positions include sitting, squatting and recumbency. Patients may develop "anthropoid posture" (exaggerated waist flexion). "Shopping cart sign" patients often can walk farther if they can lean forward e.g. as on a grocery cart. Riding a bicycle is also often well tolerated.

72

Table 72.2 Clinical features distinguishing neurogenic from vascular claudication[16]

Feature	Neurogenic claudication	Vascular claudication
distribution of pain	in distribution of nerve (dermatomal)	in distribution of muscle group with common vascular supply (sclerotomal)
sensory loss	dermatomal distribution	stocking distribution
inciting factors	variable amounts of exercise, also with prolonged maintenance of a given posture (65% have pain on standing at rest); coughing produces pain in 38%	reliably reproduced with fixed amount of exercise (e.g. distance ambulated) that decreases as disease progresses; rare at rest (27% have pain on standing at rest)
relief with rest	slow (often > 30 min), variable, usually positional (stooped posture or sitting often required, ✱ *standing and resting is usually not sufficient)*	almost immediate; *not* dependent on posture (relief of walking induced symptoms with standing is a key differentiating feature)
claudicating distance	variable day-to-day in 62%	constant day-to-day in 88%
discomfort on lifting or bending	common (67%)	infrequent (15%)
foot pallor on elevation	none	marked
peripheral pulses	normal; or if ↓ usually reduced only unilaterally	↓ or absent; femoral bruits are common
skin temp of feet	normal	decreased

72.5.3 Neurologic exam

The neurologic exam is normal in ≈ 18% of cases (including normal muscle stretch reflexes and negative straight leg raising). Weakness in the anterior tibialis and/or extensor hallicus longus may occur in some cases of central canal stenosis at L4–5, or with foraminal stenosis of L5-S1. Absent or reduced ankle jerks and diminished knee jerks are common,[17] however this is also prevalent in the aged population. Pain may be reproduced by lumbar *extension.*

72.6 Differential diagnosis

72.6.1 General considerations

1. vascular insufficiency: (AKA vascular or intermittent claudication) see above
2. hip disease: trochanteric bursitis (see below), degenerative joint disease
3. disc herniation (lumbar or thoracic)
4. facet joint pain (controversial): may respond to medial branch block (therapeutic & diagnostic)
5. Baastrup's syndrome[18]: AKA arthrosis interspinosa. Radiographically: contact of adjacent spinous processes ("kissing spines") with enlargement, flattening and reactive sclerosis of apposing interspinous surfaces. Produces localized midline lumbar pain & tenderness on back extension relieved by flexion, local anesthetic injection or partial excision of the involved spinous processes
6. juxtafacet cyst: (p. 1143)
7. arachnoiditis
8. intraspinal tumor
9. Type I spinal AVM (spinal dural AVM) (p. 1140)
10. diabetic neuritis: with this, the sole of the foot is usually very tender to pressure from the examiner's thumb
11. delayed onset muscle soreness (DOMS): onset usually 12–48 hours *after* beginning a new activity or changing activities (NC occurs during the activity). Symptoms typically peak within 2 days and subside over several days
12. inguinal hernia: typically produces groin pain
13. functional etiologies

Degenerative hip disease

Trochanteric bursitis (TBS) and degenerative arthritis of the hip are also included in the differential diagnosis of NC.[19,20] Although TBS may be primary, it can also be secondary to other conditions including lumbar stenosis, degenerative arthritis of the lumbar spine or knee, and leg length discrepancy. TBS produces intermittent aching pain over the lateral aspect of the hip. Although usually chronic, it occasionally may have acute or subacute onset. Pain radiates to lateral aspect of thigh in 20–40% (so called "pseudoradiculopathy"), but rarely extends to the posterior thigh or as far distally as the knee. There may be numbness and paresthesia-like symptoms in the upper thigh which are usually not dermatomal in distribution. Like NC, the pain may be triggered by prolonged standing, walking and climbing, but unlike NC it is also painful to lie on the affected side. Localized tenderness over the greater trochanter can be elicited in virtually all patients, with maximal tenderness at the junction of the upper thigh and greater trochanter. Pain increases with weight bearing (and is often present from the very first step, unlike NC) and with certain hip movements, especially external rotation (over half the patients have a positive Patrick-FABERE test (p. 1048), and rarely with hip flexion/extension. Treatment includes NSAIDs, local injection of glucocorticoid (usually with local anesthetic), physical therapy (with stretching and muscle strengthening exercises) and local application of ice. No controlled studies have compared these modalities.

72.7 Diagnostic evaluation

72.7.1 Radiographic evaluation

Comparison of modalities

MRI: demonstrates impingement on neural structures and loss of CSF signal on T2WI due to central canal stenosis, lateral recess stenosis, foraminal stenosis as well as juxtafacet cysts. Increased fluid in the facet joint and vacuum disc MRI is poor for visualizing bone which contributes significantly to the pathology. Asymptomatic abnormalities are demonstrated in up to 33% of patients 50–70 years old without back-related symptoms.[2]

Lumbosacral spine x-rays: may disclose spondylolisthesis. AP diameter of canal is usually narrowed (congenitally or acquired) (below) whereas the interpediculate distance (IPD) may be normal.[16] Oblique films may demonstrate pars defects. Adding flexion/extension views can assess "dynamic" instability.

Standing scoliosis x-rays: provide information about scoliosis and sagittal balance. See Adult degenerative scoliosis for technique and measurements.

CT scan (either routine, or following water-soluble myelography): classically shows "trefoil" canal (cloverleaf shaped, with 3 leaflets). CT also demonstrates AP canal diameter, hypertrophied ligaments, facet arthropathy, pars fractures and occasionally may show bulging annulus or herniated disc

Myelogram: lateral films often show "washboard pattern" (multiple anterior defects), AP films often show "wasp-waisting" (narrowing of dye column), may also show partial or complete (especially in prone position) block. May be difficult to perform LP if stenosis is severe (poor CSF flow and difficulty avoiding nerve roots the LP needle).

Normal LS spine measurements

Normal dimensions of the lumbar spine are shown in ▶ Table 72.3 for plain film and ▶ Table 72.4 for CT.

72.7.2 Adjuncts to radiographic evaluation

"Bicycle test": patients with NC can usually tolerate longer periods of exercise on a bicycle than patients with intermittent (vascular) claudication because the position in bicycling flexes the waist.

Noninvasive studies to rule-out vascular insufficiency: Ratio of ankle to brachial blood pressure (A:B ratio): > 1.0 is normal; mean of 0.59 in patients with intermittent claudication; 0.26 in patients with rest pain; < 0.05 indicates impending gangrene.

EMG with NCV may show multiple nerve-root abnormalities bilaterally.

72

Table 72.3 Normal AP diameter of lumbar spinal canal on lateral *plain film* (from spinolaminar line to posterior vertebral body)[21]

average (normal)	22–25 mm
lower limits of normal	15 mm
severe lumbar stenosis	< 11 mm

Table 72.4 Normal lumbar spine measurements on CT[22]

AP diameter	≥ 11.5 mm
interpediculate distance (IPD)	≥ 16 mm
canal cross-sectional area	≥ $1.45\ cm^2$
ligamentum flavum thickness[23]	≤ 4–5 mm
height of lateral recess (see below)	≥ 3 mm

Table 72.5 Dimensions of lateral recess on CT (bone windows)

Lateral recess height	Degree of lateral recess stenosis
3–4 mm	borderline (symptomatic if other lesion co-exists, e.g. disc bulging)
< 3 mm	suggestive of lateral recess syndrome
< 2 mm	diagnostic of lateral recess syndrome

72.8 Treatment

72.8.1 General information

In one study of 27 unoperated patients, 19 remain unchanged, 4 improved, and 4 worsened (mean follow-up: 49 months; range: 10–103 months).[24]

NSAIDs (acetaminophen may be as effective) and physical therapy are usually the initial measures of nonsurgical management. Unlike the cervical spine, traction is not usually helpful.

Brace therapy, e.g. with an LSO may be attempted. Guidelines are shown below.

Practice guideline: Brace therapy

Level II[25]:

- short-term use (1–3 weeks) of a rigid lumbar support is recommended for treatment of LBP of relatively short duration (< 6 months)
- bracing in patients with LBP > 6 months duration is *not* recommended because it has not been shown to have long-term benefit

Level III[25]:

- lumbar braces may reduce the number of sick days due to LBP among workers with a previous lumbar injury. Braces are *not* recommended for LBP in the general working population
- the use of pre-op bracing or transpedicular external fixation as tools to predict outcome for lumbar fusion is *not* recommended

Interventional pain management s an option for persistent pain. Epidural steroids may provide temporary relief (usually days to weeks at most). Facet blocks and, if helpful, rhizotomies (for longer relief), may be employed.

72.8.2 Management of isthmic spondylolisthesis

72

See reference.[9]

Some special management considerations for isthmic spondylolisthesis as a subset of spinal stenosis.

1. lesions with sclerotic borders are usually well established with little chance of healing.
2. Surgery is reserved for patients with neurologic deficit or incapacitating symptoms or progression of spondylolisthesis
3. lesions without sclerosis that show increased uptake on bone scan (indicating active lesion with potential for healing) or MRI high signal changes on T2WI[26] or STIR may heal in a rigid orthosis such as the **Boston brace** for ≥ 3 months
4. management of symptoms:
   a) LBP only: treat with NSAIDs, PT
   b) LBP with myelopathy, radiculopathy, or neurogenic claudication: surgical treatment[27] (see ▶ Table 72.6 for surgical options)

Table 72.6 Surgical recommendations for spondylolisthesis

Nature of spondylolisthesis	Nature of problem	Type of procedure needed
degenerative	nerve root compression within confines of spinal canal	decompression (preserving facets)
	spinal stenosis at the level of spondylolisthesis	decompression; some advocate with intertransverse-process fusion[29]
	nerve root compression far lateral, outside confines of spinal canal	radical decompression (Gill procedure, see below) plus fusion
traumatic	(does not matter)	decompression plus fusion

5. in pediatrics: may be managed with TLSO and long course of PT (e.g. 6–9 months) for symptoms. Resumption of sports may be considered when symptoms subside, but recurrence should prompt elimination of athletics or consideration of surgery

72.8.3 Indications for surgery

Surgical intervention is undertaken when symptoms become severe in spite of conservative management. The goals of surgery are pain relief, halting progression of symptoms, and possibly reversal of some existing neurologic deficit. Most authors do not consider surgery unless the symptoms have been present > 3 months, and most patients who have surgery for this have symptoms of > 1 year duration.

72.8.4 Surgery

Surgical options

1. laminectomy: posterior (*direct*) decompression of central canal and neural foramina without or with fusion. Fusion options:
   a) posterolateral fusion ± pedicle screw/rod fixation
   b) interbody fusion: generally not done as a "stand-alone" (i.e. usually requires additional stabilization, options here include: pedicle screws, facet screws, facet dowels, spinous process clamp…)
      - posterior lumbar interbody fusion (PLIF) (p. 1497): usually bilateral graft placement
      - transforaminal lumbar interbody fusion (TLIF) (p. 1497): unilateral graft placement though a facet take-down on that side
2. procedures to increase disc space height and thereby *indirectly* decompress neural foramina without direct decompression
   a) anterior lumbar interbody fusion (ALIF) (p. 1493): through laparotomy
   b) lateral lumbar interbody fusion (p. 1498): some techniques trademarked as extreme lateral interbody fusion (XLIF™) or direct-lateral (DLIF™)
   c) axial lumbar interbody fusion (Ax-LIF): L5-S1 only
3. limitation of extension by interspinous spacer: e.g. X-Stop® (see below)

72

Choosing which procedure to use

Items that factor into consideration when choosing which procedure to use include:

1. consider indirect decompression (lateral interbody fusion (e.g. XLIF® or DLIF®), ALIF, interspinous decompression (e.g. X-Stop):
   a) when foraminal stenosis appears to be the dominant problem (e.g. with loss of disc space height, facet hypertrophy, on the concave side of a scoliotic curve)
   b) previous spine surgery that might make exposure of the nerves more difficult or risky
   c) when the disc space is compressed (more difficult to distract an already tall disc space with normal disc)
2. consider direct decompression (e.g. laminectomy)
   a) "pinpoint" central canal stenosis especially when disc height and neural foramina are well preserved
   b) where a significant contributor to the compression is a focal, correctable lesion, e.g. herniated disc, synovial cyst, intraspinal tumor
   c) to avoid a fusion (in select cases)
3. consider motion-preservation surgery when a fusion is undertaken at a level and the adjacent level is already starting to show some degenerative changes that have not yet reached a surgical magnitude. Motion preservation at this adjacent segment theoretically shields it from some of the transmitted stresses from the fused level
4. situations where a fusion should be considered in addition to direct or indirect decompression of the nerves:
   a) spondylolisthesis (especially > Grade I)
   b) symptomatic sagittal imbalance or degenerative scoliosis
   c) dynamic instability on flexion/extension lateral lumbar spine x-rays
   d) expectation that the decompression will destabilize the spine (e.g. facet takedown for a TLIF)
   e) multiply recurrent herniated disc (when this is the third or more operation for the same disc)
   f) controversial: "black disc" on MRI with positive concordant discogram at this level: fusion without decompression has been advocated when there is no neural compression

When spondylolisthesis is present

May occur without decompression, but is more common following surgery.[10] However, lumbar instability following decompressive laminectomy is rare (only ≈ 1% of all laminectomies for stenosis will develop progressive subluxation). Fusion is rarely required to prevent progression of subluxation with degenerative stenosis.[28]

For Grade I and low Grade II spondylolisthesis, laminectomy without fusion may be considered. Stability (without need for instrumentation) is thought to be maintained if > 50–66% of the facets are preserved during surgery and the disc space is not violated (maintains integrity of anterior and middle column). Younger or more active patients are at higher risk of subluxing. Patients with a tall (normal) disc space are at higher risk of subluxing than those with collapsed disc space.

One approach is to obtain flexion/extension x-rays pre-op, and follow patients after decompression. Those who develop symptomatic slippage post-op are treated by fusion, possibly in conjunction with spinal instrumentation.

When surgery is indicated, ▶ Table 72.6 serves as a guide to the type of procedure.

Laminectomy/laminotomy – surgical technique

Posterior approach with removal of the spines and lamina of affected levels (surgical "unroofing"), along with the associated ligamentum flavum. Individual nerve roots are palpated for compression within their neural foramen, with foraminotomies performed at appropriate levels. Doing a total L4 laminectomy for stenosis allows access to the L4–5 foramen, and the upper part of the L5-S1 foramen. If, in addition, the lower part of L3 is also removed, access is gained to the inferior pedicle of L3 and thus the L3–4 neural foramen. Undercutting the superior articular facet is often necessary to decompress the nerves in the lateral recess and neural foramen (p.1097). Treatment of moderate stenosis at adjacent levels appears warranted as these levels have been shown to have a significant likelihood of becoming symptomatic later.[30]

Alternatively, laminotomies (as opposed to laminectomies) may be performed in cases where the central canal has a normal AP diameter, but the lateral canal gutter is stenotic.[31,32] Multilevel subarticular fenestrations are another slight variation on this theme.[33]

Position: either of the following is acceptable

1. prone: on a frame or chest rolls or knee chest position to decompress the abdomen to decrease venous pressure and thus reduce bleeding
2. lateral decubitus position: if there is no laterality to symptoms, right lateral decubitus (left-side-up) is easier for most right-handed surgeons to use angled Kerrison rongeur parallel to nerve roots

72

Booking the case: Lumbar laminectomy

Also see defaults & disclaimers (p.27).

1. position: prone
2. implants: for fusions, schedule with the vendor for the desired implants and associated instrumentation
3. consent (in lay terms for the patient – not all-inclusive):
   a) procedure: through the back to remove bone, ligament and any other tissue that is pressing on the nerve(s). If a fusion is to be done, then typically this will be accomplished using screws, rods and small cages, as required
   b) alternatives: nonsurgical management
   c) complications: usual spine surgery complications (p.28), plus there might not be the amount of pain relief desired (back pain does not respond as well to surgery as nerve-root pain. The surgery slightly weaken the spine, and as a result, about 15% people will need a fusion at a later date

Minimally invasive spine surgery (MISS) decompression

Usually using ≈ 1" incisions and expandable retractors.

1. options include bilateral laminotomies (see above)
2. bilateral decompression through a unilateral laminotomy
   a) entry site: 3.5–4 cm off the midline to permit the needed angle

b) when using a retractor with an "open side" orient the retractor with the open side facing laterally (e.g. with the Nuvasive Maxcess® place the handles medially) to permit the angle needed for contralateral decompression
c) the laminectomy and facet takedown (usually for a TLIF) are done
d) open the ligamentum flavum on the side you're working on, to visualize the posterior extent of the spinal canal, to permit finding the plane between the posterior part of the ligamentum flavum and the undersurface of the bone
e) the ligamentum flavum is left in place on the contralateral side to protect the dura during drilling
f) complete the decompression and disc removal on the side you're working on
g) the undersurface of the bone (spinous process and contralateral lamina) are then drilled to decompress the contralateral side
h) once the undersurface of the contralateral posterior canal has been drilled, the ligamentum flavum is removed with pituitary rongeurs. It is possible to even do a contralateral foraminotomy at this point (curved Kerrison rongeurs are very helpful for this)
i) pedicle screws are placed through the open side, and then percutaneously through the contralateral side
j) this is generally followed by a transforaminal lumber interbody fusion (TLIF)

Interspinous process decompression/stabilization/fusion

Interspinous spacers (e.g. X-Stop™ (Medtronic)) limit extension at 1 or 2 levels (without fusion), preventing narrowing of the associated neural foramen, and may also off-load the facet joints and even the disc. "Success rate": 63% at 2 years. This device may be used as a standalone.

Interspinous plates (e.g. Aspen® (Lanx), Affix™ (Nuvasive), Spire® (Medtronic)) clamp across two spinous processes to fixate them (unlike X-Stop™ which just limits extension). The Aspen® clamps have a space for a graft which may optionally be used to promote fusion between the spinous processes. Interspinous plates may be used to augment other constructs e.g. lateral interbody fusion,[34] but are *not* intended for standalone use. Biomechanical stability is reported to be similar to bilateral pedicle screws in flexion, and unilateral pedicle screws in lateral bending.[35]

Contraindications (includes exclusionary criteria from the IDE study):

72

1. instability at level considered for procedure: spondylolisthesis > Grade 1 or scoliosis with Cobb angle ≥ 25°
2. cauda equina syndrome
3. acute fracture of the spinous process
4. bilateral pars defects (disconnects spinous process from the anterior elements)
5. osteoporosis. Contraindications per the IDE: DEXA scan (p. 1009) with spine or hip T-score < –2.5 (i.e. more than 2.5 SD below the mean for normal adults) in the presence of ≥ 1 fragility fractures. Concerns: spinous process fracture at the time of insertion, or late subsidence due to microfractures. However, Kondrashov[36] interprets a T-score < –2.5 anywhere as indicative of osteoporosis (even without fragility fractures). Options here include:
   a) augmenting the spinous processes by injecting ≈ 0.5–1 cc of PMMA into each spinous process (SP) with a 13 Ga needle inserted ≈ halfway into the SP on lateral fluoro[36] prior to dilating the interspace or placing the X-Stop. Verify central position within SP on AP fluoro, and monitor injection on fluoro
   b) X-Stop^{PK}® made of titanium and PEEK (the modulus of elasticity of PEEK is closer to bone than titanium is)
6. ankylosed level (i.e. already fused)
7. L5-S1 level: the spinous process of S1 is usually too small (not usually an issue since symptomatic stenosis at L5-S1 is rare)
8. age < 50 years: not studied in IDE investigation

Surgical pointers:

1. it is critical that the spacer sit in the anterior third of the spinous process
2. results may be better with the patient awake, under local anesthesia, lying on their side in a position that they feel is relieving their pain (thus opening up the critical levels). This may reduce the risk of undersizing the prosthesis

Post-op (based on manufacturer's recommendations):
1. to avoid spinous process stress fracture: build-up physical activity gradually
2. 1st 6 weeks post-op: no spine hyperextension, no heavy lifting. Minimize stair climbing
3. initially, walking (for < 1 hour) is recommended as long as it is comfortable
4. at 2 weeks post-op: cycling (stationary or bicycle) may be added
5. 6 months post-op: may add sports such as swimming, golf, racquetball, tennis, running or jogging

Gill procedure

This procedure, and its modifications,[37] consist of radical decompression of nerve roots including removal of the loose posterior elements and total facetectomy. This is most usually followed by fusion (posterolateral or interbody). Fusion rate may be enhanced with the use of internal fixation (e.g. transpedicular screw-rod fixation).[38]

Reduction of spondylolisthesis

Reduction of spondylolistheseis can be accomplished with instrumentation, and requires a fusion.

The risk of nerve root injury with reduction of grade I or II spondylolisthesis is low.

Reduction of high-grade (grade III or IV) spondylolisthesis carries a risk of radiculopathy (e.g. L5 radiculopathy in cases of L5-S1 spondylolisthesis) in 50% of cases (some permanent) and may produce a cauda equina syndrome, probably from stretching nerve roots by distraction. Some have recommended intraoperative stimulation of nerve while performing EMG recording as the listhesis is gradually reduced, and stopping if the current required for stimulation increases 50% above baseline.

Isthmic spondylolisthesis (spondylolysis) – pars interarticularis defect

Instrumentation and/or fusion

72

Practice guideline: Fusion in patients with lumbar stenosis without spondylolisthesis

Level III[39]:
- in situ posterolateral fusion is *not* recommended following decompression in patients with lumbar stenosis in whom there is no evidence of preexisting spinal instability or likely iatrogenic instability due to facetectomy
- in situ posterolateral fusion is recommended in patients with lumbar stenosis in whom there is evidence of spinal instability
- the addition of pedicle-screw instrumentation is *not* recommended in conjunction with posterolateral fusion following decompression

Practice guideline: Fusion in patients with lumbar stenosis and spondylolisthesis

Level II[40]: posterolateral fusion is recommended for patients with stenosis and associated degenerative spondylolisthesis who require decompression

Level III[40]: pedicle screw fixation as an adjunct to posterolateral fusion should be considered in patients with stenosis and spondylolisthesis in cases where there is pre-op evidence of spinal instability or kyphosis at the level of the spondylolisthesis or when iatrogenic instability is anticipated (**note:** the definition of "instability" and "kyphosis" varies, and has not been standardized).

Fusion may accelerate degenerative changes at adjacent levels. Some surgeons recommend fusion at levels of spondylolisthetic stenosis.[5,30] Patients with combined degenerative spondylolisthesis, stenosis, and radiculopathy may be reasonable candidates for fusion.[41]

Booking the case: Lumbar lami ± fusion for stenosis

Also see defaults & disclaimers (p. 27).

1. position: prone
2. implants: for fusions, schedule with the vendor for the desired implants and associated instrumentation
3. consent (in lay terms for the patient – not all-inclusive):
   a) procedure: through the back to remove bone, ligament and any other tissue that is pressing on the nerve(s). If a fusion is to be done, then typically this will be accomplished using screws, rods and small cages, as required
   b) alternatives: nonsurgical management
   c) complications: usual spine surgery complications (p. 28), plus there might not be the amount of pain relief desired (back pain does not respond as well to surgery as nerve-root pain). There can be problems with the implants, including breakage, migration (slippage), or undesirable positioning which may require further surgery.

72.9 Outcome

72.9.1 Morbidity/mortality

Risk of in-hospital mortality is 0.32%.[17] Other risks include: unintended durotomy (p. 1055) (0.32%[17] to ≈ 13%[28,42]), deep infection (5.9%), superficial infection (2.3%), and DVT (2.8%); see also Risks of lumbar laminectomy (p. 1053).

72.9.2 Nonunion

72 Risk factors for nonunion in fusion operations (does not necessarily correlate with success of operation):

1. cigarette smoking delays bone healing and increases the risk of pseudoarthrosis following spinal fusion procedures, especially in the lumbar spine[12]
2. number of levels: in lumbar fusions, fusing 2 levels resulted in increased nonunion rates compared to fusing 1 level[43]
3. NSAIDs: controversial
   a) short-term (≤ 5 days) post-op use: high-dose ketorolac (120–240 mg/d) was associated with increased risk of nonunion, but low-dose ketorolac (≤ 110 mg/d), and celecoxib (200–600 mg/d) or rofecoxib (50 mg/d) were not[43].
   b) some feel that long-term NSAID use does lower fusion rate[44]

72.9.3 Success of operation

General information

Patients with a postural component to their pain had much better results (96% good result) than those without a postural component (50% good results), and the relief of leg pain was much more successful than relief of back pain.[45] Surgery is most likely to reduce LE pain and improve walking tolerance.[41]

Outcome studies

SPORT study

There have been many attempts to ascertain the benefit of surgery, including the $13.5 million SPORT study. Shortcomings of the study include: patients were allowed to decline randomization and were then entered into an observational cohort which may introduce bias into the groups, crossovers were allowed between patients randomized to surgery and those randomized to nonsurgical treatment (degrading the "intention to treat" analysis), no standardized surgical or nonsurgical technique, relatively low long-term follow-up (52% at 8 years), change in paradigm from analyzing intention-to-treat to an as-treated analysis.

Results indicated a strong benefit of surgery at 4-years follow-up[46] that appeared to diminish by 8-years in the randomized cohort but persisted in the observational cohort.[47]

Other long-term outcome studies

Literature review[17] with long-term follow-up found good or excellent outcome after surgery with a mean of 64% (range: 26–100%). A patient satisfaction survey indicated that 37% were much improved and 29% somewhat improved (total: 66%) post-op.[48] A prospective study found a success rate of 78–88% at 6 wks and 6 months, which dropped to ≈ 70% at 1 year and 5 yrs.[49] Success rates were slightly lower for lateral recess syndrome.

Reasons for surgical failure

Surgical failure may be divided into two groups:

1. patients with initial improvement who develop recurrent difficulties. Although short-term improvement after surgery is common,[46] many patients progressively deteriorate over time.[47,50] One study found a 27% recurrence of symptoms after 5 years follow-up[30] (30% due to restenosis at the operated level, 30% due to stenosis at a new level ("adjacent segment failure"); 75% of these patients respond to further surgery). Other etiologies include: development of herniated lumbar disc, development of late instability including kyphosis ("proximal junction kyphosis" – PJK), coexisting medical conditions
2. patients who fail to have any post-op pain relief (early treatment failures). In one series of 45 such patients[51]:
   a) the most common finding was a lack of solid clinical and radiographic indications for surgery (e.g. non-radicular LBP coupled with modest stenosis)
   b) technical factors of surgery had less influence on outcome, with the most common finding being failure to decompress the lateral recess (which, in non-fusion cases, requires judicious medial facet resection or undercutting the superior articular facet)
   c) other diagnoses (e.g. arachnoiditis), missed diagnosis (e.g. spinal AVM)

References

[1] Yamamoto I, Matsumae M, Ikeda A, et al. Thoracic Spinal Stenosis: Experience with Seven Cases. J Neurosurg. 1988; 68:37–40
[2] Epstein NE. Symptomatic Lumbar Spinal Stenosis. Surg Neurol. 1998; 50:3–10
[3] Verbiest H. A Radicular Syndrome from Developmental Narrowing of the Lumbar Canal. J Bone Joint Surg. 1954; 36B:230–237
[4] Epstein JA, Epstein BS, Lavine L. Nerve Root Compression Associated with Narrowing of the Lumbar Spinal Canal. J Neurol Neurosurg Psychiatry. 1962; 52:165–176
[5] Duggal N, Sonntag VKH, Dickman CA. Fusion options and indications in the lumbosacral spine. Contemp Neurosurg. 2001; 23:1–8
[6] Ciric I, Mikhael MA, Tarkington JA, et al. The Lateral Recess Syndrome. J Neurosurg. 1980; 53:433–443
[7] Meyerding HW. Spondylolisthesis. Surg Gynecol Obstet. 1932; 54:371–377
[8] Rothman RH, Simeone FA. The Spine. Philadelphia 1982
[9] Frymoyer JW. Back Pain and Sciatica. N Engl J Med. 1988; 318:291–300
[10] Tuite GF, Doran SE, Stern JD, et al. Outcome After Laminectomy for Lumbar Spinal Stenosis. Part II: Radiographic Changes and Clinical Correlations. J Neurosurg. 1994; 81:707–715
[11] Battie MC, Videman T, Gibbons LE, Fisher LD, Manninen H, Gill K. 1995 Volvo Award in clinical sciences: determinants of lumbar disc degeneration. A study relating lifetime exposures and magnetic resonance imaging findings in identical twins. Spine. 1995; 20:2601–2612
[12] Hadley MN, Reddy SV. Smoking and the Human Vertebral Column: A Review of the Impact of Cigarette Use on Vertebral Bone Metabolism and Spinal Fusion. Neurosurgery. 1997; 41:116–124
[13] Fogelholm RR, Alho AV. Smoking and intervertebral disc degeneration. Med Hypotheses. 2001; 56:537–539
[14] Xu R, Sciubba DM, Gokaslan ZL, Bydon A. Ossification of the ligamentum flavum in a Caucasian man. J Neurosurg Spine. 2008; 9:427–437
[15] Miyazawa N, Akiyama I. Ossification of the ligamentum flavum of the cervical spine. J Neurosurg Sci. 2007; 51:139–144
[16] Hawkes CH, Roberts GM. Neurogenic and Vascular Claudication. J Neurol Sci. 1978; 38:337–345
[17] Turner JA, Ersek M, Herron L, Deyo R. Surgery for Lumbar Spinal Stenosis: Attempted Meta-Analysis of the Literature. Spine. 1992; 17:1–8
[18] Kota GK, Kumar NKS, Thomas R. Baastrups Disease An Unusual Cause Of Backpain : A Case Report. 2005
[19] Shbeeb MI, Matteson EL. Trochanteric Bursitis (Greater Trochanter Pain Syndrome). Mayo Clin Proc. 1996; 71:565–569
[20] Deen HG. Diagnosis and Management of Lumbar Disk Disease. Mayo Clin Proc. 1996; 71:283–287
[21] Ehni G. Significance of the Small Lumbar Spinal Canal. J Neurosurg. 1969; 31:490–494
[22] Ullrich CG, Binet EF, Sanecki MG, et al. Quantitative Assessment of the Lumbar Spinal Canal by CT. Radiology. 1980; 134:137–143
[23] Post MJD. Computed Tomography of the Spine. Baltimore 1984
[24] Johnsson KE, Rosén I, Udén A. The Natural Course of Lumbar Spinal Stenosis. Acta Orthop Scand. 1990; 61
[25] Resnick DK, Choudhri TF, Dailey AT, Groff MW, Khoo L, Matz PG, Mummaneni P, Watters WC, Wang J, Walters BC, Hadley MN. Part 14: Brace therapy as an adjunct to or substitute for lumbar fusion. J Neurosurg: Spine. 2005; 2:716–724
[26] Sairyo K, Katoh S, Takata Y, Terai T, Yasui N, Goel VK, Masuda A, Vadapalli S, Biyani A, Ebraheim N. MRI signal changes of the pedicle as an indicator for early diagnosis of spondylolysis in children and adolescents: a clinical and biomechanical study. Spine. 2006; 31:206–211
[27] Weinstein JN, Lurie JD, Tosteson TD, Hanscom B, Tosteson AN, Blood EA, Birkmeyer NJ, Hilibrand AS, Herkowitz H, Cammisa FP, Albert TJ, Emery SE, Lenke LG, Abdu WA, Longley M, Errico TJ, Hu SS. Surgical versus nonsurgical treatment for lumbar degenerative spondylolisthesis. N Engl J Med. 2007; 356:2257–2270

[28] Silvers HR, Lewis PJ, . Decompressive Lumbar Laminectomy for Spinal Stenosis. J Neurosurg. 1993; 78:695–701
[29] Herkowitz HN, Kurz LT. Degenerative Lumbar Spondylolisthesis with Spinal Stenosis: A Prospective Study Comparing Decompression with Decompression and Intertransverse Process Arthrodesis. J Bone Joint Surg. 1991; 73A:802–808
[30] Caputy AJ, Luessenhop AJ. Long-Term Evaluation of Decompressive Surgery for Degenerative Lumbar Stenosis. J Neurosurg. 1992; 77:669–676
[31] Aryanpur J, Ducker T. Multilevel Lumbar Laminotomies for Focal Spinal Stenosis: Case Report. Neurosurgery. 1988; 23:111–115
[32] Aryanpur J, Ducker T. Multilevel Lumbar Laminotomies: An Alternative to Laminectomy in the Treatment of Lumbar Stenosis. Neurosurgery. 1990; 26:429–433
[33] Young S, Veeraoen R, O'Laoire SA. Relief of Lumbar Canal Stenosis Using Multilevel Subarticular Fenestrations as an Alternative to Wide Laminectomy: Preliminary Report. Neurosurgery. 1988; 23:628–633
[34] Wang JC, Haid RW, Jr, Miller JS, Robinson JC. Comparison of CD HORIZON SPIRE spinous process plate stabilization and pedicle screw fixation after anterior lumbar interbody fusion. J Neurosurg Spine. 2006; 4:132–136
[35] Wang JC, Spenciner D, Robinson JC. SPIRE spinous process stabilization plate: biomechanical evaluation of a novel technology. J Neurosurg Spine. 2006; 4:160–164
[36] Kondrashov Dimitriy. 2007
[37] Rombold C. Teatment of Spondylolisthesis by Posterolateral Fusion, Resection of the Pars Interarticularis, and Prompt Mobilization of the Patient: An End-Result Study of Seventy-Three Patients. J Bone Joint Surg. 1966; 48A:1282–1300
[38] Dickman CA, Fessler RG, MacMillan M, Haid RW. Transpedicular Screw-Rod Fixation of the Lumbar Spine: Operative Technique and Outcome in 104 Cases. J Neurosurg. 1992; 77:860–870
[39] Resnick DK, Choudhri TF, Dailey AT, Groff MW, Khoo L, Matz PG, Mummaneni P, Watters WC, Wang J, Walters BC, Hadley MN. Part 10: Fusion following decompression in patients with stenosis without spondylolisthesis. J Neurosurg Spine. 2005; 2:686–691
[40] Resnick DK, Choudhri TF, Dailey AT, Groff MW, Khoo L, Matz PG, Mummaneni P, Watters WC, Wang J, Walters BC, Hadley MN. Part 9: Fusion in patients with stenosis and spondylolisthesis. J Neurosurg Spine. 2005; 2:679–685
[41] Bigos S, Bowyer O, Braen G, et al. Acute Low Back Problems in Adults. Clinical Practice Guideline No.14. AHCPR Publication No. 95-0642. Rockville, MD: Agency for Health Care Policy and Research, Public Health Service, U.S. Department of Health and Human Services; 1994
[42] Deburge A, Lassale B, Benoist M, et al. Le Traitment Chirurgical des Stenosis Lombaires et ses Resultats a Propos d'Une Serie de 163 Cas Operes. Rev Rheum Mal Osteoartic. 1983; 50:47–54
[43] Reuben SS, Ablett D, Kaye R. High dose nonsteroidal anti-inflammatory drugs compromise spinal fusion. Can J Anaesth. 2005; 52:506–512
[44] Thaller J, Walker M, Kline AJ, Anderson DG. The effect of nonsteroidal anti-inflammatory agents on spinal fusion. Orthopedics. 2005; 28:299–303; quiz 304-5
[45] Ganz JC. Lumbar Spinal Stenosis: Postoperative Results in Terms of Preoperative Posture-Related Pain. J Neurosurg. 1990; 72:71–74
[46] Weinstein JN, Tosteson TD, Lurie JD, Tosteson A, Blood E, Herkowitz H, Cammisa F, Albert T, Boden SD, Hilibrand A, Goldberg H, Berven S, An H. Surgical versus nonoperative treatment for lumbar spinal stenosis four-year results of the Spine Patient Outcomes Research Trial. Spine (Phila Pa 1976). 2010; 35:1329–1338
[47] Lurie JD, Tosteson TD, Tosteson A, Abdu WA, Zhao W, Morgan TS, Weinstein JN. Long-term outcomes of lumbar spinal stenosis: eight-year results of the Spine Patient Outcomes Research Trial (SPORT). Spine (Phila Pa 1976). 2015; 40:63–76
[48] Tuite GF, Stern JD, Doran SE, et al. Outcome After Laminectomy for Lumbar Spinal Stenosis. Part I: Clinical Correlations. J Neurosurg. 1994; 81:699–706
[49] Javid MJ, Hadar EJ. Long-Term Follow-Up Review of Patients Who Underwent Laminectomy for Lumbar Stenosis: A Prospective Study. J Neurosurg. 1998; 89:1–7
[50] Katz JN, Lipson SJ, Larson MG, et al. The Outcome of Decompressive Laminectomy for Degenerative Lumbar Stenosis. J Bone Joint Surg. 1991; 73A:809–816
[51] Deen HG, Zimmerman RS, Lyons MK, et al. Analysis of Early Failures After Lumbar Decompressive Laminectomy for Spinal Stenosis. Mayo Clin Proc. 1995; 70:33–36

73 Adult Spinal Deformity and Degenerative Scoliosis

73.1 General information

Key concepts

- Adult spinal deformity (ASD) encompasses scoliosis and sagittal imbalance
- Sagittal balance correlates with quality of life measures
- Basic spine measurements needed: LL, PI, PT, ± SVA
- Major alignment objectives: LL = PI ± 9°, PT < 20°, SVA < 5 cm

Adult spinal deformity (ASD) is a broad term that refers to a wide spectrum of structural abnormalities of a mature spine. ASD encompass abnormalities in the coronal plane (scoliosis) as well as abnormalities in the sagittal plane.

The term "adult degenerative scoliosis" (**ADS**) (as distinguished from idiopathic juvenile scoliosis (IJS)) is often used interchangeably with ASD. Definition of adult degenerative scoliosis: spinal deformity with Cobb angle[1] > 10° in a skeletally mature individual.[2] ADS may be the result of childhood idiopathic scoliosis persisting into adulthood, or may be de novo.

Deformity in ASD can be primarily due to asymmetric disc degeneration or secondary to hip pathology, osteoporosis and asymmetric loads.[3] It subsequently involves posterior elements (including facet joints) and thereafter axial rotation, lateral olisthesis and ligamentous laxity.[2,4] Progressive facet and discogenic degeneration may lead to segmental instability and subsequent central/foraminal stenosis secondary to ligamentum flavum hypertrophy and osteophyte formation[5] and well as spondylolisthesis.

While treatment goals include reduction of pain, symptomatic neural compression and disability due to deformity, the methodology and biomechanics of ADS treatment differ greatly from treating IJS in the adolescent.

ADS tends to progress at an average rate of 3° per year (range: 1–6°).[4] Factors associated with higher rates of progression: Cobb angle > 30°, apical rotation > Grade II (on the Nash-Moe system,[6] which is falling into disuse), lateral listhesis > 6 mm, and an intercrest line through L5.[4] Factors *not* correlated with rate of progression: age and gender. Controversial associations: osteopenia.

73

73.2 Epidemiology

ASD is more prevalent in patients age > 60 years, however true prevalence is not well defined. > 50% of adults hospitalized with spinal deformity are > 65 years.[7] Incidence of asymptomatic scoliosis ranges from 1.4%-32% and up to 68% in patients > 60.[8]

73.3 Clinical evaluation

Location, time and duration pain (leg vs. axial back) are important factors in evaluation of a patient with ASD. These patients may also have symptoms of spinal stenosis (central or radicular), which may require concomitant decompression. The patient's ability to perform activities of daily living and medical co-morbidities (e.g. cardiac, osteoporosis etc.) need be taken into consideration for treatment planning.

Some patients present with obvious spinal deformity (scoliosis, forward flexion at the waist, walking with knees bent).

As with neurogenic claudication, patients tend to be more symptomatic when up on their feet. A significant amount of pain may be generated by attempting to correct for spinal imbalance by using paraspinal muscles as well as retroverting the pelvis (rotating it backward at the hips) and not fully extending the knees. All this extra muscle activity is fatiguing and begins to produce muscle pain in the back and thighs. Patients with ASD tends to be better in the morning when they are rested.

Unlike lumbar spinal stenosis in the absence of scoliosis, symptoms may not relieved by flexion.[2] There may be some relief when supporting the trunk with the arms.

73.4 Diagnostic testing

▸ **CT / MRI.** Both are recommended for the evaluation of symptomatic spondylosis and ASD to determine extent of neural compression.

► **DEXA (dual-energy x-ray absorptiometry).** Patients should be evaluated for osteopenia/osteoporosis prior to surgical planning. Medical treatment may be beneficial in the peri-operative period.

Some surgeons use Forteo for 3 months (off-label use – controversial) in an effort to try and quickly increase osteoporotic bone strength for surgery.

► **Standing scoliosis x-rays.** Recommended for the evaluation of global and regional spinal balance. Pre and postoperative plain films help confirm that alignment objectives are achieved.

Measurements related to sagittal balance are taken from standing scoliosis x-rays (CT & MRI are obtained supine and are not equivalent). Technical requirements for the lateral image:

- x-ray must image from C7 down to the femoral heads
- the patient needs to try to keep the knees straight (extended)
- arms should be folded in front of the chest (and they should not lean or hold on to anything)

Dynamic scoliosis x-rays ("lateral bending films") help determine the degree of curve rigidity preoperatively.

73.5 Pertinent spine measurements

73.5.1 General information

Quantification of severity of spinal deformity and classification helps guide appropriate treatment paradigms.[9,10]

73.5.2 Scoliosis nomenclature

Scoliosis is measured using Cobb angles. On an AP x-ray, the "end vertebrae" are identified at the top and bottom of the scoliotic curve and are defined as the vertebrae with the greatest angle relative to the horizontal plane. One horizontal line is drawn through the superior endplate of the superior "end vertebra", and a second is drawn through the inferior endplate of the inferior "end vertebra." The Cobb angle is the angle between these 2 lines. Curves are named for the convex side (dextroscoliosis = convex to right, levoscoliosis = convex to left).

A non-structural curve can correct on side bending. A structural curve is not flexible.

The major curve is the largest structural curve. A fractional curveis the curve below the major curve.

73

73.5.3 Spino-pelvic parameters

Measurement methodology and pertinent information are shown in ► Table 73.1 and illustrated in ► Fig. 73.1 and ► Fig. 73.2. Basic measurements that can be correlated with pain reduction and quality of life measures:

- LL (lumbar lordosis)
- PI (pelvic incidence)
- PT (pelvic tilt)
- ± SVA (sagittal vertical alignment): while this can be helpful at times, it also appears to be subject to variability depending on how much pain the patient has with standing up straight

With the exception of CSVL, the measurements shown in ► Table 73.1 are all taken from a lateral standing x-ray (► Fig. 73.1 and ► Fig. 73.2).

73.6 SRS-Schwab classification of adult spinal deformity

Adult scoliosis has been classified by the Scoliosis Research Society (**SRS**)[16] based on its regional/global radiographic features (a modification of previously established adolescent King/Moe and Lenke classifications) and most recently by spino-pelvic parameters as it relates to health-related quality of life[17,18,19] is shown here.

- Coronal Curve types
  - T: Thoracic only (with lumbar curve < 30°)
  - L: Thoracolumbar/Lumbar only (with thoracic curve < 30°)
  - D: Double curve (both T and T/L curves > 30°)
  - N: No major coronal deformity (all coronal curves < 30°)
- Sagittal Modifiers
  - Pelvic harmony (PI minus LL)
    - 0: non pathologic (PI–LL < 10°)
    - +: moderate deformity (10° < PI–LL < 20°)
    - ++: marked deformity (PI–LL > 20°)

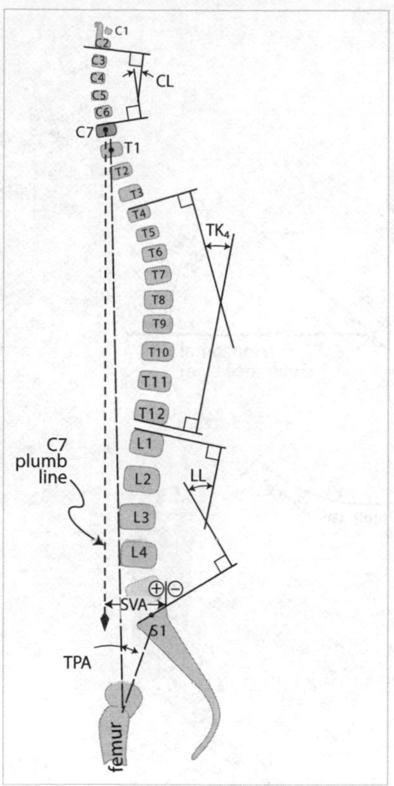

Fig. 73.1 Schematic lateral spine diagram showing method for measuring CL, TK, LL SVA and TPA.

- Global alignment (SVA)
  - 0: non pathologic (SVA < 4 cm)
  - +: moderate deformity (4 cm < SVA < 9.5 cm)
  - ++: marked deformity (SVA > 9.5 cm)
- Pelvic Tilt (PT)
  - 0: non pathologic (PT < 20°)
  - +: moderate deformity (20° < PT < 30°)
  - ++: marked deformity (PT > 30°)

73.7 Treatment/management

73.7.1 Options

1. observation
2. focal decompression
3. surgical correction of deformity
   a) MIS (minimally invasive (spine) surgery)
   b) Hybrid (MIS + open)
   c) Traditional open surgery (transforaminal lumbar interbody fusion (TLIF), posterior lumbar interbody fusion (PLIF)…)

Treatment options are based on clinical symptoms (axial back pain ± radiculopathy vs. radiculopathy alone) and degree of abnormalities in sagittal (balance need for open osteotomies or anterior column release ACR). Neuropathic symptoms most often originate from foraminal compromised on the

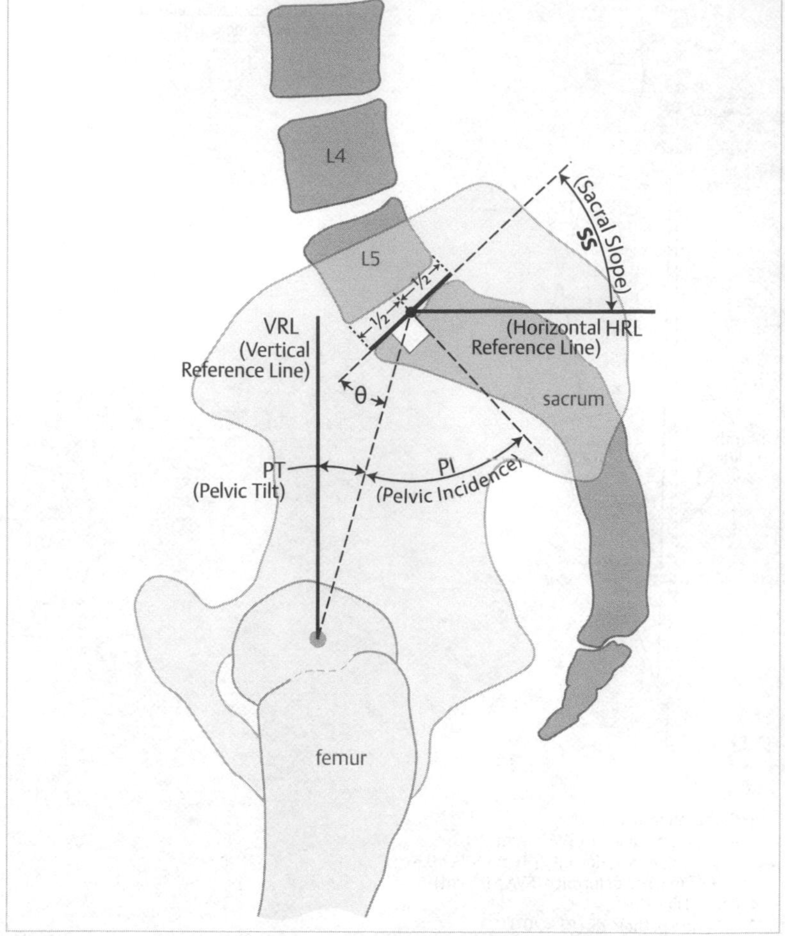

Fig. 73.2 Schematic lateral spine diagram showing method for measuring PT, PI and SS.

concavity of the curve, but can be seen on the convexity in the setting of facet hypertrophy and may improve with indirect decompression and correction in the coronal plane. Significant central stenosis (neurogenic claudication) may require concomitant direct decompression in addition of deformity correction.

Goal of surgery: to improve quality of life measures, neuropathic and axial pain. A surgeon's armamentarium includes traditional open, MIS and hybrid procedures, which is patient and deformity specific. More recently, the surgical decision making paradigms have included MIS techniques to limit approach related morbidity. MIS techniques include lateral interbody fusion, ALLR, MIS-TLIF and percutaneous pedicle screw fixation, which can be used with posterior osteotomies to enhance corrective power.

Table 73.1 Spino-pelvic parameters: Measurement methodology and pertinent information

Parameter	Description	Normal	Alignment objective	Comment
sagittal vertical alignment (SVA) or (C7-SVA)	horizontal distance from the posterior edge of the S1 endplate to a plumb line dropped from the mid-C7 VB	< 5 cm	< 5 cm	numbers are positive if plumb line is anterior. May be susceptible to error depending on patient's stance, resting arms on equipment...
pelvic tilt (PT)	angle between the vertical reference line (VRL) and a line drawn from the midpoint of the femoral head[a] to the midpoint of the S1 endplate	10–25° [11]	< 20°	PT above ≈ 20° indicates the patient is trying to compensate for spinal imbalance (some authors consider up to 25° as normal)
pelvic incidence (PI)	angle between a perpendicular to the S1 endplate and a line drawn from the midpoint of the femoral head[a] to the midpoint of the S1 endplate	≈ 50°	(see lumbar lordosis)	PI is fixed once skeletal maturity is reached[b]. For ease of measurement, PI = 90° – θ[12]
sacral slope (SS)	angle between the horizontal reference line (HRL) and the S1 endplate	36–42°		SS = PI – PT
lumbar lordosis (LL)	angle between the top of S1 and the top of L1	20–40°[13]	LL = PI ± 9°	LL should be within 9° of PI for "pelvic harmony"
Thoracic kyphosis (TK)	angle between the top of T4 and the bottom of T12	41° ± 12°[14]		since T1 is often difficult to visualize, convention is to measure top of T4 to bottom of T12. Sometimes denoted as TK4
TPA (T1Pelvic Angle)	angle between line drawn from center of T1 to center of femoral head and line from femoral head[a] to center of S1 endplate	20°[15]		may be less susceptible to influences than SVA from patient posture during x-ray
central sacral vertical line (CSVL)	(on AP standing scoliosis x-ray) vertically oriented line which bisects the sacrum perpendicular to a tangent drawn across the iliac crests	for coronal balance, a plumb line from the middle of C7 VB should be < 4 cm from CSVL	plumb line from the middle of C7 V B < 4 cm from CSVL	positive numbers are to the right, negative to left

[a] For measurements involving the femoral head (PT, PI & TPA) if the two femoral heads are not superimposed, measure to a point that is midway between the centers of the two femoral heads.
[b] PI is unaffected by posture or degenerative changes (i.e. patients cannot compensate by changing this). A high PI correlates with a higher risk of progression of spondylolisthesis, a low PI correlates with a lower risk.

73

73.7.2 Correction of global spinal balance

Indications for surgery

- Axial back pain ± neuropathic symptoms (deleterious to ADLs)
  - Abnormal SVA
  - ± CSVL (central sacral vertical line) abnormality
  - or derangement of spino-pelvic parameters.
- Patient age and co-morbidities must be taken in to consideration (osteopenia, anesthetic risk and medical co-morbidities can limit correction goal and amount of surgery that is safe)

Summary of spino-pelvic objectives

- LL = PI ± 9°
- PT < 20°
- SVA < 5 cm

In most instances, correction of sagittal imbalance is due to a shortfall of lumbar lordosis (LL) relative to the pelvic incidence (PI) – which can be considered flat back syndrome. That is, LL is usually more than 9° below PI.

Pelvic tilt > 20° suggests the patient is trying to compensate by retroverting the pelvis (some authors accept up to 25° as normal).

The minimum amount of correction that the surgeon tries to achieve is therefore that amount that LL needs to increase to bring it within 9° of PI, and typically also adds in the amount that the patient is compensating (i.e. the amount that PT is greater than 20°) which yields the following approximation (applies when LL is more than 9° lower than PI, and PT is greater than 20°); see Eq (73.1):

$$\text{Increase in LL needed} \approx (\text{PI} - \text{LL} - 9^\circ) + (\text{PT} - 20^\circ) \qquad (73.1)$$

► **Coronal balance.** Measured on AP standing scoliosis x-ray. A plumb line is dropped from the center of the C7 VB. If it falls > 4 cm from the midline of the sacrum (where the CSVL is located), there is coronal imbalance (if the plumb line falls to the right of the CSVL it is positive, to the left it is negative).

73.7.3 Surgical options for increasing lumbar lordosis

Various surgical techniques may be used to increase the lumbar lordosis to bring it within the desired specifications. If necessary, these techniques can be combined with procedures to decompress the neural elements (e.g. laminectomy). A comparison of the approximate amount of lordosis than can be achieved with different techniques is shown in ► Table 73.2.

► **Transforaminal lumbar interbody fusion (TLIF) and posterior lumbar interbody fusion (PLIF).** Traditional operation. May be done open or MIS.

► **Lateral lumbar interbody fusion (LLIF).** E.g. XLIF™, DLIF™, OLIF™. Approach through psoas muscle (XLIF, DLIF) or anterior to psoas muscle (OLIF) through a lateral or anterolateral approach. Can distract the vertebral bodies by increasing the height of the disc space and thereby indirectly decompressing the neural elements. If bone quality is good, and there is no instability nor spondylolisthesis > Grade I, a standalone procedure (i.e. without screw instrumentation) may be an option if cage width of at least 22 mm (or preferably 26 mm) in the AP dimension is used.

Table 73.2 Comparison of the amount of lumbar lordosis that can be obtained from various surgical techniques.

Technique	TLIF/PLIF	LLIF	ALIF	SPO + ACR	PSO
Degrees of lumbar lordosis	< 0 (i.e. kyphosis) up to 2°[20]	1°[21]	6°[20]	16°[22]	30–40°[22,23]

Abbreviations: TLIF = transforaminal lumbar interbody fusion; PLIF = posterior lumbar interbody fusion; LLIF = lateral lumbar interbody fusion; ALIF = anterior lumbar interbody fusion; SPO = Smith-Petersen osteotomy; ACR = anterior column release; PSO = pedicle subtraction osteotomy

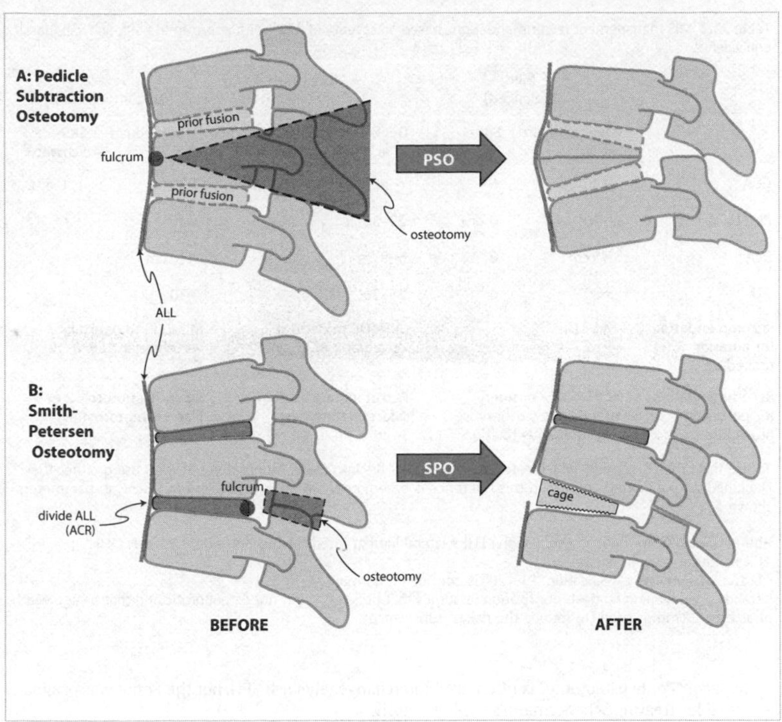

Fig. 73.3 Comparison of A: Pedicle subtraction osteotomy and B: Smith Petersen osteotomy plus ACR. Abbreviations: ALL = anterior longitudinal ligament, ACR = anterior column release.

► **Anterior column release (ACR).** Involves division of the anterior longitudinal ligament (ALL release (ALLR)) typically with placement of a "hyperlordotic" cage (20–30° lordosis) from an anterior approach (e.g. lateral interbody technique). This is followed by posterior fixation, often with a Smith-Petersen osteotomy (especially for 30° cages) and compression. It can increase LL up to 12° per ACR level and improvement of SVA up to 3 cm (depending on the level at which it is performed).[22,24]

Risk of injury to great vessels, either directly (when cutting the ALL) or indirectly by elongating the anterior column. It is critical to evaluate the great vessels on axial MRI or CT or on angiogram and to not do the procedure if the vessels appear tightly approximated to the bodies or to osteophytes, at that level.

► **Smith-Petersen osteotomy (SPO).** AKA "chevron or extension osteotomy" can increase lordosis up to 10° per level. Approximately one degree for each millimeter of bone resected.[25,26] Involves removal of bilateral superior and inferior facets along with the ligamentum flavum and portion of the lamina above and below. The created gap is then closed with compression of the posterior elements to give lordosis (resecting posterior elements and using the middle column as a fulcrum to elongate the anterior column, ► Fig. 73.3 A).[26,27] LL is increased approximately 1° for every 1 mm of bone removed.

Table 73.3 MIS management recommendations based on severity of ASD[9] with approximate SRS-Schwab Class[17] equivalence.

	Mild (balanced)		Moderate (compensated)		Severe (uncompensated)	
	Deukmedjian at al.[9]	SRS-Schwab[17]	Deukmedjian at al.[9]	SRS-Schwab[17]	Deukmedjian et al.[9]	SRS-Schwab[17]
CCA	<30°	N	>30°	T, L or D	>30°	T, L or D
PI – LL	<20°	0 or +	20–30°	++	>30°	++
SVA	<5 cm	0	5–9 cm	+	>10 cm	++
PT[a]	<25°	0	25–30°	+	>30°	++
Recommendations for anterior procedure	**MIS LLIF**		**MIS-LLIF to neutral vertebrae + ACR**		**MIS-LLIF to neutral vertebrae ± ACR**	
Recommendations for posterior procedure	**If PT < 20° consider standalone[b], otherwise percutaneous fixation**		**Percutaneous fixation to S1 ± facetectomy(ies)**		**Open fixation to S2 or iliac + osteotomy(ies)**	

To use this table, determine which category the patient fits into (Mild, Moderate or Severe) using either the Deukmedjian parameters (on which this reference is based) or the roughly equivalent SRS-Schwab parameters shown

Abbreviations: CCA = Cobb coronal angle; LLIF = lateral lumbar interbody fusion (e.g. XLIF, DLIF, OLIF...); ACR = anterior column release
[a] in the SRS-Schwab classification, PT < 20° is considered normal
[b] standalone meaning no posterior fixation, assumes that bone quality is not osteoporotic and that a cage width of at least 22 mm is used (to reduce the risk of subsidence)

The term "Ponte osteotomy" is often used interchangeably with SPO, but the Ponte was originally described for treating Scheuermann's kyphoscoliosis.

73

► **Pedicle subtraction osteotomy (PSO).** Involves removal of the posterior elements including the ligmanetum flavum, lamina and facets widely, followed by isolation and resection of pedicles bilaterally and wedge shaped removal of the vertebral body just barely up to the ventral cortex. The created gap is then closed by compression of the posterior elements and subsequent greenstick fracture of the isolated ventral cortex (► Fig. 73.3 B).[23] Can increase LL by 30°- 40° per level, improvement of SVA 5.5 – 13 cm per level.[22,23]

This procedure is technically challenging and is associated with high blood loss (3 L in 1 series[28]) and increased risk of complications (including proximal junctional kyphosis (**PJK**) in 23%[28]) compared to SPO. Generally reserved for spines that have previously been fused where it is not possible to get the amount of lordosis needed from the unfused levels. The PSO is a spine "shortening" procedure.

Uses the anterior column as a fulcrum. Usually limited to levels below the conus medullaris (i.e. L1–2) due to inward buckling of the dura (L3 is the most common level). Intraoperative electrophysiologic monitoring is required. Relative contraindication: poor bone quality.

► **Anterior lumbar interbody fusion (ALIF).** Best for L5-S1 (where the great vessels tend not to interfere with the access, and where every degree of correction produces a more significant amount of improvement in SVA than at other levels as a result of being at the lowest point in the spine).

73.7.4 Guidelines for MIS treatment for ASD

A simple algorithm for MIS management of sagittal imbalance based on spino-pelvic parameters and the approximate SRS-Schwab class is shown in ► Table 73.3.[9] See references[10,29] for a more detailed protocol.

Currently under investigation by the SRS: when, and to what degree, does improvement in sagittal balance occur with simple decompression (possibly with a minimal fusion) as a result of pain relief permitting the patient to stand up straighter with less pain.

References

[1] Cobb JR. Outline for study of scoliosis. Am Acad Orthop Surg. 1948; 5:261–275

[2] Silva FE, Lenke LG. Adult degenerative scoliosis: evaluation and management. Neurosurg Focus. 2010; 28. DOI: 10.3171/2010.1.FOCUS09271

[3] Wiet RJ, Wiet RJ, Glasscock ME, Shambaugh GE. In: Dissection Manual. Surgical Anatomy of the Temporal Bone Through Dissection. Philadelphia: W.B. Saunders; 1980:677–725

[4] Pritchett JW, Bortel DT. Degenerative symptomatic lumbar scoliosis. Spine (Phila Pa 1976). 1993; 18:700–703

[5] Faldini C, Di Martino A, De Fine M, Miscione MT, Calamelli C, Mazzotti A, Perna F. Current classification systems for adult degenerative scoliosis. Musculoskelet Surg. 2013; 97:1–8

[6] Nash CL, Jr, Moe JH. A study of vertebral rotation. J Bone Joint Surg. 1969; 51:223–229

[7] Drazin D, Shirzadi A, Rosner J, Eboli P, Safee M, Baron EM, Liu JC, Acosta FLJr. Complications and outcomes after spinal deformity surgery in the elderly: review of the existing literature and future directions. Neurosurg Focus. 2011; 31. DOI: 10.3171/2011.7.FOCUS11145

[8] Schwab F, Dubey A, Gamez L, El Fegoun AB, Hwang K, Pagala M, Farcy JP. Adult scoliosis: prevalence, SF-36, and nutritional parameters in an elderly volunteer population. Spine (Phila Pa 1976). 2005; 30:1082–1085

[9] Deukmedjian AR, Ahmadian A, Bach K, Zouzias A, Uribe JS. Minimally invasive lateral approach for adult degenerative scoliosis: lessons learned. Neurosurg Focus. 2013; 35. DOI: 1 0. 3 17 1/2 01 3. 5. FOCUS13173

[10] Haque RM, Mundis GM, Jr, Ahmed Y, El Ahmadieh TY, Wang MY, Mummaneni PV, Uribe JS, Okonkwo DO, Eastlack RK, Anand N, Kanter AS, La Marca F, Akbarnia BA, Park P, Lafage V, Terran JS, Shaffrey CI, Klineberg E, Deviren V, Fessler RG. Comparison of radiographic results after minimally invasive, hybrid, and open surgery for adult spinal deformity: a multicenter study of 184 patients. Neurosurg Focus. 2014; 36. DOI: 10.3171/2014.3.FOCUS1424

[11] Lafage V, Schwab F, Patel A, Hawkinson N, Farcy JP. Pelvic tilt and truncal inclination: two key radiographic parameters in the setting of adults with spinal deformity. Spine (Phila Pa 1976). 2009; 34: E599–E606

[12] Ryan MD. Geometry for Dummies. 2nd ed. Indianapolis, Indiana: Wiley Publishing, Inc.; 2008

[13] Tuzun C, Yorulmaz I, Cindas A, Vatan S. Low back pain and posture. Clin Rheumatol. 1999; 18:308–312

[14] Schwab F, Lafage V, Boyce R, Skalli W, Farcy JP. Gravity line analysis in adult volunteers: age-related correlation with spinal parameters, pelvic parameters, and foot position. Spine (Phila Pa 1976). 2006; 31:E959–E967

[15] Protopsaltis TS, Schwab FJ, Smith JS, et al. The T1 Pelvic Angle (TPA), a Novel Radiographic Parameter of Sagittal Deformity, Correlates Strongly with Clinical Measures of Disability. The Spine Journal. 2013; 13

[16] Lowe T, Berven SH, Schwab FJ, Bridwell KH. The SRS classification for adult spinal deformity: building on the King/Moe and Lenke classification systems. Spine (Phila Pa 1976). 2006; 31:S119–S125

[17] Schwab F, Ungar B, Blondel B, Buchowski J, Coe J, Deinlein D, DeWald C, Mehdian H, Shaffrey C, Tribus C, Lafage V. Scoliosis Research Society-Schwab adult spinal deformity classification: a validation study. Spine (Phila Pa 1976). 2012; 37:1077–1082

[18] Liu Y, Liu Z, Zhu F, Qian BP, Zhu Z, Xu L, Ding Y, Qiu Y. Validation and reliability analysis of the new SRS-Schwab classification for adult spinal deformity. Spine (Phila Pa 1976). 2013; 38:902–908

[19] Ames CP, Smith JS, Scheer JK, Bess S, Bederman SS, Deviren V, Lafage V, Schwab F, Shaffrey CI. Impact of spinopelvic alignment on decision making in deformity surgery in adults: A review. J Neurosurg Spine. 2012; 16:547–564

[20] Hsieh PC, Koski TR, O'Shaughnessy BA, Sugrue P, Salehi S, Ondra S, Liu JC. Anterior lumbar interbody fusion in comparison with transforaminal lumbar interbody fusion: implications for the restoration of foraminal height, local disc angle, lumbar lordosis, and sagittal balance. J Neurosurg Spine. 2007; 7:379–386

[21] Le TV, Vivas AC, Dakwar E, Baaj AA, Uribe JS. The effect of the retroperitoneal transpsoas minimally invasive lateral interbody fusion on segmental and regional lumbar lordosis. ScientificWorldJournal. 2012; 2012. DOI: 10.1100/2012/516706

[22] Manwaring JC, Bach K, Ahmadian AA, Deukmedjian AR, Smith DA, Uribe JS. Management of sagittal balance in adult spinal deformity with minimally invasive anterolateral lumbar interbody fusion: a preliminary radiographic study. J Neurosurg Spine. 2014; 20:515–522

[23] Mummaneni PV, Dhall SS, Ondra SL, Mummaneni VP, Berven S. Pedicle subtraction osteotomy. Neurosurgery. 2008; 63:171–176

[24] Deukmedjian AR, Dakwar E, Ahmadian A, Smith DA, Uribe JS. Early outcomes of minimally invasive anterior longitudinal ligament release for correction of sagittal imbalance in patients with adult spinal deformity. ScientificWorldJournal. 2012; 2012. DOI: 10.1100/2012/789698

[25] Smith-Petersen MN, Larson CB, Aufranc OE. Osteotomy of the spine for correction of flexion deformity in rheumatoid arthritis. Clin Orthop Relat Res. 1969; 66:6–9

[26] Cho KJ, Bridwell KH, Lenke LG, Berra A, Baldus C. Comparison of Smith-Petersen versus pedicle subtraction osteotomy for the correction of fixed sagittal imbalance. Spine (Phila Pa 1976). 2005; 30:2030–7; discussion 2038

[27] La Marca F, Brumblay H. Smith-Petersen osteotomy in thoracolumbar deformity surgery. Neurosurgery. 2008; 63:163–170

[28] Hyun SJ, Rhim SC. Clinical outcomes and complications after pedicle subtraction osteotomy for fixed sagittal imbalance patients : a long-term follow-up data. J Korean Neurosurg Soc. 2010; 47:95–101

[29] Mummaneni PV, Shaffrey CI, Lenke LG, Park P, Wang MY, La Marca F, Smith JS, Mundis GMJr, Okonkwo DO, Moal B, Fessler RG, Anand N, Uribe JS, Kanter AS, Akbarnia B, Fu KM. The minimally invasive spinal deformity surgery algorithm: a reproducible rational framework for decision making in minimally invasive spinal deformity surgery. Neurosurg Focus. 2014; 36. DOI: 10.3171/2014.3.FOCUS1413

74 Special Conditions Affecting the Spine

74.1 Paget's disease of the spine

74.1.1 Pathophysiology

Paget's disease (PD) (AKA osteitis deformans) is a disorder of osteoclasts (possibly virally induced) causing increased rate of bone resorption with reactive osteoblastic overproduction of new, weaker, woven bone, producing characteristic "mosaic pattern."

Initially there is a "hot" phase with elevated osteoclastic activity and increased intraosseous vascularity. Osteoblasts lay down a soft, nonlamellar bone. Later a "cool" phase occurs with disappearance of the vascular stroma and osteoblastic activity leaving sclerotic, radiodense, brittle bone[1] ("ivory bone").

74.1.2 Malignant degeneration

A misnomer, since the malignant changes actually occur in the reactive osteoblastic cells. About 1% (reported range: 1–14%) degenerate into sarcoma (osteogenic sarcoma, fibrous sarcoma, or chondrosarcoma),[2(p 2642)] with the possibility of systemic (e.g. pulmonary) metastases. Malignant degeneration is much less common in the spine than in the skull or femur.

74.1.3 Epidemiology

Prevalence: ≈ 3% of population > 55 years old in the U.S. and Europe, much lower in Asia.[3] Slight male predominance. Family history of Paget's disease is found in 15–30% of cases (accuracy is poor since most are asymptomatic).

74.1.4 Common sites of involvement

Affinity for axial skeleton, long bones and skull. In approximate descending order of frequency: pelvis, thoracic and lumbar spine, skull, femur, tibia, fibula, and clavicles.

74.1.5 Neurosurgical involvement

74

PD may present to the neurosurgeon as a result of:
1. back pain: usually not as a direct result of vertebral bone involvement (see below)
2. spinal cord and/or nerve root symptoms
   a) compression of the spinal cord or cauda equina (relatively rare)
   b) spinal nerve-root compression
   c) vascular steal due to reactive vasodilatation adjacent to involved areas
3. with skull involvement:
   a) compression of cranial nerves as they exit through bony foramina: 8th nerve is most common, producing deafness or ataxia (p.1400)
   b) skull base involvement → basilar invagination
4. to ascertain diagnosis in unclear bone lesions of the spine or skull

74.1.6 Presentation

General information

Only ≈ 30% of pagetic sites are symptomatic,[4] the rest are discovered incidentally. The overproduction of weak bone may produce bone pain (the most common symptom), predilection for fractures and compressive syndromes: cranial nerve (p.1400), spinal nerve root… Painless bowing of a long bone may be the first manifestation. A number of patients present due to pain from joint dysfunction related to PD.

The overwhelming majority of pagetic lesions are asymptomatic[5(p 1413)] with lesions detected on radiographs or bone scan obtained for other reasons or as part of a work-up for an elevated alkaline phosphatase. Although the most common complaint in patients with Paget's disease is of back pain, this is attributable to pagetic involvement alone in only ≈ 12%,[6] in the remainder it is secondary to other factors, some of which are described below.

Symptoms that may be related to the Paget's disease itself

Symptoms from the following are slowly progressive (usually present for > 12 months; rarely < 6 mos):

1. neural compression
   a) causes of compression
      - due to expansion of woven bone
      - due to osteoid tissue
      - pagetic extension into ligamentum flavum and epidural fat[7]
   b) sites of compression
      - spinal cord (see below)
      - nerve root in neural foramen
2. osteoarthritis of facet joints (Paget's disease may precipitate osteoarthritis[6])

Symptoms from the following tend to progress more rapidly:

1. malignant (sarcomatous) change of involved bone (rare, see above)
2. pathologic fracture (pain usually sudden in onset)
3. neurovascular (compromise of vascular supply to nerves or spinal cord) by
   a) compression of blood vessels (arterial or venous)
   b) pagetic vascular steal (see below)

Spinal cord symptoms

Myelopathy or cauda equina syndrome may be due to spinal cord compression or from vascular effects (occlusion, or "steal" due to reactive vasodilatation of nearby blood vessels[5(p 1415)]). Only ≈ 100 cases had been described as of 1981.[8] Characteristically, 3–5 adjacent vertebrae are involved,[9(p 2307)] whereas monostotic involvement is usually asymptomatic.[10] In case reports in the literature, progressive quadri- or paraparesis was the most common presentation.[11] Sensory changes are usually the first manifestation, progressing to weakness and sphincter disturbance. Pain was the only symptom in a neurologically intact patient in only 5.5%.

A rapid course (averaging 6 wks) with a sudden increase in pain is more suggestive of malignant degeneration.

74.1.7 Evaluation

1. lab work (serum markers may be normal in monostotic involvement):
   a) serum alkaline phosphatase: usually elevated (this enzyme is involved in bone synthesis and so may *not* be elevated in purely lytic Paget's disease[5(p 1416)]); mean 380 ± 318 IU/L (normal range: 9–44).[6] Bone-specific alkaline phosphatase may be more sensitive and may be useful in monostotic involvement[3]
   b) calcium: usually normal (if elevated, one should R/O hyperparathyroidism)
   c) urinary hydroxyproline: hydroxyproline is found almost exclusively in cartilage. Due to the high turnover of bone, urinary hydroxyproline is often increased in PD with a mean of 280 ± 262 mg/24 hrs (normal range 18–38)[6]
2. bone scan: lights up in areas of involvement in most, but not all[6] cases
3. plain x-rays:
   a) localized enlargement of bone: a finding unique to PD (not seen in other osteoclastic diseases, such as prostatic bone mets)
   b) cortical thickening
   c) sclerotic changes
   d) osteolytic areas (in skull → osteoporosis circumscripta; in long bones → "V" shaped lesions)
   e) spinal Paget's disease often involves *several contiguous levels.* Pedicles and lamina are thickened, vertebral bodies are usually dense and compressed with increased width. Intervening discs are replaced by bone
4. CT: hypertrophic changes at the facet joints with coarse trabeculations

74.1.8 Treatment

Medical treatment for Paget's disease

General information

There is no cure for Paget's disease. Medical treatment is indicated for cases that are not rapidly progressive where the diagnosis is certain, for patients who are poor surgical candidates, and pre-op if

74

excessive bleeding cannot be tolerated. Medical therapy reverses some neurologic deficit in 50% of cases,[12] but generally requires prolonged treatment (≈ 6–8 months) before improvement occurs, and may need to be continued indefinitely due to propensity for relapses. Medications used include the following.

Calcitonin derivatives

Parenteral salmon calcitonin (Calcimar®)[12]: reduces osteoclastic activity directly, osteoblastic hyperactivity subsides secondarily. Relapse may occur even while on calcitonin. Side effects include nausea, facial flushing, and the development of antibodies to salmon calcitonin (these patients may benefit from a more expensive synthetic human preparation (Cibacalcin®) starting at 0.5 mg SQ q d[13]).

℞ 50–100 IU (medical research council units) SQ q d × 1 month, then 3 injections per week for several months.[3] If used pre-op to help decrease bony vascularity, ≈ 6 months of treatment is ideal. Doses as low as ≈ 50 IU units 3 × per week may be used indefinitely post-op or as a sole treatment (alkaline phosphatase and urinary hydroxyproline decline by 30–50% in > half of patients in 3–6 months, but they rarely normalize).

Bisphosphonates

These drugs are pyrophosphate analogues that bind to hydroxyapatite crystals and inhibit reabsorption. They also alter osteoclastic metabolism, inhibit their activity, and reduce their numbers. They are retained in bone until it is resorbed. Oral absorption of all is poor (especially in the presence of food). Bone formed during treatment is lamellar rather than woven.

Etidronate (Didronel®) (AKA EHDP): reduces normal bone mineralization (especially at doses ≥ 20 mg/kg/d) producing mineralization defects (osteomalacia) which may increase the risk of fracture but which tend to heal between courses.[14] Contraindicated in patients with renal failure, osteomalacia, or severe lytic lesions of a LE. ℞ 5–10 mg/kg PO daily (average dose: 400 mg/d, or 200–300 mg/d in frail elderly patients) for 6 months, may be repeated after a 3–6 month hiatus if biochemical markers indicate relapse.

Tiludronate (Skelid®): unlike etidronate, does not appear to interfere with bone mineralization at recommended doses. Side effects: abdominal pain, diarrhea, N/V. ℞ 400 mg PO qd with 6–8 ounces of plain water > 2 hrs before or after eating × 3 months. Available: 200 mg tablets.

Pamidronate (Aredia®): much more potent than etidronate. May cause a transient acute flu-like syndrome. Oral dosing is hindered by GI intolerance, and IV forms may be required. Mineralization defects do not occur in doses < 180 mg/course. ℞ 90 mg/d IV × 3 days, or as weekly or monthly infusions.

Alendronate (Fosamax®): does not produce mineralization defects (p. 1010).

74

Clodronate (Ostac®, Bonefos®): ℞ 400–1600 mg/d PO × 3–6 months. 300 mg/d IV × 5 days (may be available outside the U.S.).

Risedronate (Actonel®): does not interfere with bone mineralization in recommended doses.[15] ℞: 30 mg PO q d with 6–8 oz. of water at least 30 minutes before the first meal of the day.

Surgical treatment

General information

In general, conservative treatment of fractures in PD are associated with a high rate of delayed union.

Surgical indications for spinal Paget's disease

1. rapid progression: indicating possible malignant change or spinal instability
2. spinal instability: severe kyphosis or compromise of canal by bone fragments from pathologic fracture. Although the collapse is usually gradual, sudden compression may occur
3. uncertain diagnosis: especially to R/O metastatic disease (osteoblastic lesions)
4. failure to improve with medications

Surgical considerations

1. profuse bleeding is common: if significant bleeding would present an unusual problem, treat for as long as feasible pre-op with a bisphosphonate or calcitonin (see above)
   a) use bone wax to help control bleeding
   b) hemostasis may be difficult

2. to treat resultant spinal stenosis: decompressive laminectomy is the standard procedure in the thoracic region.[11] However, if most of the pathology is anterior, consideration should be given to anterior approach
3. bone is often thickened, and may be fused with obliteration of interspace landmarks. A high-speed drill is usually helpful
4. post-op medical treatment may be necessary to prevent recurrences[12]
5. osteogenic sarcoma
   a) surgery and chemotherapy are used, cure is less likely than in primary osteosarcoma of non-pagetic origin
   b) biopsy proven of the scalp requires en-bloc excision of scalp and tumor

Surgical outcome

See reference.[11]

In 65 patients treated with decompressive laminectomy, 55 (85%) had definite but variable degrees of improvement. Patients who had only minimal improvement were often ones with malignant changes. One patient was worse after surgery, and the operative mortality was 7 patients (10%). Survival with malignant degeneration is < 5.5 mos after admission.

74.2 Ankylosing spondylitis

74.2.1 General information

Key concepts

- Prototypical spondyloarthritidy, now referred to as radiographic axial spondyloarthritis
- Seronegative (absence of rheumatoid factor), associated with HLA-B27
- Begins in SI joints (sine qua non of involvement) progressing rostrally
- Clinical: morning back stiffness, kyphotic deformity limits chest expansion
- X-ray findings: "bamboo spine", Andersson lesions, progressive thoracic kyphosis
- Fragile rigid spine highly susceptible to fracture and SCI even after low energy trauma
- Severe deformity, neurologic involvement or unstable fracture warrants surgical intervention

Historically known as Marie-Strümpell disease, Ankylosing spondylitis (AS) is an HLA-B27 associated inflammatory disease and the prototype of a group of diseases known as the spondyloarthritides (SpA). Common features are inflammatory back pain, negative serology for rheumatoid factor and absence of rheumatoid nodules, and asymmetric oligoarthritis predominantly of lower extremities. Currently referred to in the literature as Radiographic axial Spondyloarthritis (RaxSpA), AS is believed to be the late stage of a single disease entity, axial Spondyloarthritis (axSpA) distinguished by definitive evidence of sacroilitis on plain radiographs. Other conditions under this rubric include: psoriatic arthropathy, Reiter's disease, juvenile spondyloarthropathy… AS has in the past also been known as rheumatoid spondylitis, or rheumatoid arthritis of the spine, but use of these terms is discouraged because of the lack of rheumatoid factor. The spine is the primary skeletal site involved, usually starting in the sacroiliac joints and lumbar spine and progressing rostrally.

Enthesopathy: nongranulomatous inflammatory changes at the entheses (attachment points of ligaments, tendons or capsules on bones; the locus of involvement in AS) stimulates re-placement of ligaments by bone ultimately resulting in osteoporotic VBs, calcified intervertebral discs (sparing the nucleus pulposus), and ossified ligaments, producing square appearing VBs with bridging syndesmophytes, the so-called "bamboo spine" or "poker spine". Extra-articular manifestations (EAMs) include: anterior uveitis, inflammatory bowel disease (IBD) and psoriasis.

Neurosurgical involvement usually results from the following:

1. cauda equina syndrome (**CES-AS**) : the etiology of CES in AS is frequently unclear, but is usually *not* due to stenosis or compressive lesion. Onset is slow and insidious and there is a high incidence of dural ectasia.[16] Any patient with AS and neurologic deficit should be assumed to have CES until proven otherwise. Without treatment most patients' neurological status continues to deteriorate[16]
2. rotatory subluxation: at occipitoatlantal and atlantoaxial joints. May occur as these are typically the last mobile segments of the spine. Incidence is much less than with rheumatoid arthritis. Lesions that might be stable in otherwise normal spines are often not stable in AS
3. myelopathy secondary to bow-stringing of the cord: laminectomy may aggravate

74

4. acute spinal cord injury (**SCI**): risk of SCI or CES due to fracture is increased in AS, and may occur following minimal trauma. Injuries are more common in the lower cervical spine. The akylosed spine of AS when fractured creates long lever arms, limiting the ability to absorb impact and rendering even minor fractures very unstable.[17] Delayed deterioration may be due to spinal epidural hematoma.[18]
5. Andersson lesion: discovertebral lesion that results from inflammation or fracture, mechanical stresses prevent lesion from fusion resulting in pseudarthrosis.[19]
6. spinal deformity
7. spinal stenosis: rare
8. basilar impression

74.2.2 Epidemiology

Incidence in the general population is ≈ 0.44-7.3 cases per 100,000.[20] Traditionally reported male: female ratio 3:1, however, likely stems from underdiagnosis in women, and more rapid progression of spinal ankylosis in men.[20] Peak incidence: 17-35 yrs age. > 90% of patients with AS are HLA-B27 positive (only 8% of people without AS have this antigen), but only 2% of people with HLA-B27 develop clinical AS. Although AS is not hereditary, first degree relatives are at increased risk.

74.2.3 Clinical

► **Symptoms.** Typical initial presentation is with nonradiating low back pain, morning back stiffness, hip pain and swelling (due to large joint arthritis), exacerbated by inactivity and improved with exercise.[21]

► **Signs.** **Patrick's test** (p. 1048) usually positive. Compressing the pelvis with the patient in the lateral decubitus position produces pain.

Schober test (measure distraction between skin marks on the back before and after forward flexion to detect reduced mobility of the spine due to fusion). Is not specific for inflammatory spondylopathies[22] but may be helpful for monitoring ongoing physical therapy.

74.2.4 Diagnosis

Diagnosis by experienced rheumatologist is closest thing to a gold standard.[23] The Assessment of SpondyloArthritis international Society (ASAS) recently presented its recommendations for a modified Berlin Algorithm[23] as a potentially useful tool for rheumatologists in diagnosing AS. SI joint involvement is the sine qua non for definite diagnosis. Diagnosis is very involved, and includes: chronic low back pain, buttock pain, sacroiliitis, family history, psoriasis, an inflammatory bowel disease or an arthritis followed in ≤ 1 month with urethritis, cervicitis or acute diarrhea, an enthesopathy, and a family history, and positive x-rays. The (obsolete) New York Criteria (► Table 74.1) are shown here to provide a small insight into early attempts to establish diagnostic criteria, but should no longer be used for definitive diagnosis.

74

74.2.5 Radiographic evaluation

► **Plain x-rays.** Vital for diagnosis and follow-up. Sacroiliac (SI) joint involvement (on AP pelvic x-rays or on oblique views through the plane of the SI joints) is one of the earliest findings, and the often symmetric osteoporosis followed by sclerosis is characteristic. "Bamboo spine" (see above) is also classic. X-ray of the entire spine is recommended since multiple, non-contiguous (and often unsuspected) fractures are not unusual. See ► Fig. 74.1.

► **CT.** Useful for diagnosis of cervical fracture not apparent on plain radiographs, and in preoperative assessment of bony anatomy.

► **MRI.** Can rule out spinal epidural hematoma and the occasional herniated disc. May demonstrate dural ectasia in cases of CES-AS syndrome. Andersson lesions: pathologic changes at ligament insertion sites (MRI signal abnormalities at front and back of the endplates) are characteristic. Erosive changes due to pseudarthrosis at the disc space can mimic discitis (high signal on T1WI & T2WI with enhancement).

► **Bone scan.** Ratio of uptake of SI joint to sacrum > 1.3:1 is suggestive of AS.

Table 74.1 Modified New York Criteria for AS[24] – not to be used for diagnosis (obsolete)
Diagnosis (see criteria below)
Definite AS: radiologic criterion + ≥ 1 clinical criteria
Probable AS: radiological criterion without clinical criteria, or 3 clinical criteria without radiological criterion
Clinical criteria
low back pain > 3 months, improved by exercise, not relieved by rest
limitation of lumbar spine motion in both sagittal and frontal planes
limitation of chest expansion relative to normal values for age and sex
Radiological criterion
sacroiliitis

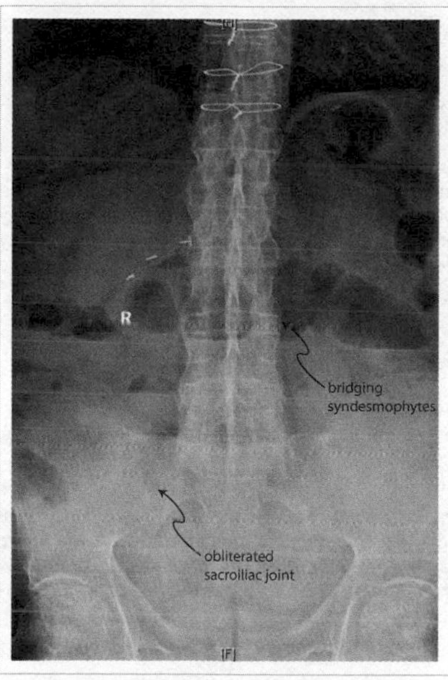

Fig. 74.1 AP lumbar/pelvic x-ray demonstrating "Bamboo spine" and sclerosis of sacroiliac joints

74

74.2.6 Differential diagnosis

1. early on, AS may resemble rheumatoid arthritis. However, in AS nodules do not form in joints, and rheumatoid factor is absent in the serum
2. metastatic prostate Ca in elderly male patients with sacroiliac pain and blastic changes compatible with sacroiliitis
3. Forestier's disease (p. 1130) and DISH (p. 1129): these overlapping conditions produce exuberant bony overgrowth anterior and lateral to the disc without degeneration and ossification of the disc as in AS. Both spare the facets and SI joints, do not produce flexion deformity, and tend to occur in men > 50 yrs old (older than typical AS)[25]
4. Psoriasis, Reactive Arthritis (Reiter's syndrome), Enteropathic (IBD-related) Arthritis: the spondylitis with these tends to be milder and less uniform, and SI joint involvement is *asymmetrical.* Cutaneous findings (erythema nodosum, and pyoderma gangrenosum) are absent in AS.[26]

74.2.7 Natural history

Progression is slow, and patients usually remain functionally active. Thoracic kyphosis with compensatory increase in cervical and lumbar lordosis is common. The shift in center of gravity together with spine stiffness and fragility predisposes to frequent falls and further spine injuries. Eventually can progress to involvement of costovertebral joints resulting in restrictive lung disease pattern. AS patients are also predisposed to development of fibrotic lung disease in late stages.

74.2.8 Treatment

General information

Combined ASAS/EULAR recommendations for management of AS are the most comprehensive currently available (copy available at ASAS website). Multidisciplinary, coordinated by a rheumatologist.[27] Goal of treatment is long term quality of life through symptomatic control and prevention of progressive structural damage. NSAIDs are first line pharmacological management.[27] Management of the disease itself may involve TNF inhibitors in patients with persistently high disease activity.[27]

Surgical treatment

General information

The most common surgical intervention is orthopedic total hip arthroplasty.[27]

Cervical fracture

The cervical spine is the most frequent fracture site in AS patients.[28] Patients often cannot distinguish acute fracture pain from chronic inflammatory pain; therefore there should be a low threshold to obtain imaging. It is imperative to determine pre-injury alignment as application of C-collar may cause hyperextension injury.[29] Gentle, low-weight traction with the force vector directed anteriorly and superiorly may be used for initial stabilization.[30,31] Halo vest or surgery for unstable fracture pattern.

Surgical indications:

- irreducible deformity
- deteriorating neurological status in the presence of epidural hematoma or other source of compression[32]
- unstable fracture (e.g. most 3-column fractures which are very unstable as a result of long lever arms of fused segments above and below): halo-vest immobilization is becoming a less frequently employed option for this

74

Procedures: Decompressive laminectomy if evidence of spinal cord compression.[32] Given poor bone quality and extended lever arms, good fusion bed and a construct extending multiple levels above and below the fracture are critical.[33] Proximally, lateral mass screws up to C3, possible pedicle screw in C2, and pedicle screws in thoracic spine for distal fixation.[33] 360° fusion may provide optimal stabilization in some cases (where feasible).

Thoracolumbar fracture

The majority occur at thoracolumbar junction.[33] Can be divided into 3 types[34]:

1. shearing injury: typically acute. Resembles chance fracture, highly unstable 3 column injury[34]
2. wedge compression: typically chronic
3. pseudarthrosis: typically subacute previously missed fracture

Wedge compression or pseudarthrosis; rule out posterior element involvement to determine if fracture is unstable.[33] Stable fracture can be treated with external orthosis. Unstable fractures, consider thicker rods or more rigid rod material to account for increased forces across fracture, and PMMA augmentation to prevent screw pullout.

Kyphotic deformity

ASAS/EULAR recommendations include corrective osteotomy for severe disabling deformity.[27] Can be accomplished via open wedge osteotomy, polysegmental wedge oseotomy, or closed wedge osteotomy (lowest complication rate).[35] Cervical deformity is most commonly addressed with wedge osteotomy at C7 and T1 given absence of vertebral artery in foramen transversarium at these levels. Current trend in literature is to address deformity simultaneously with acute fracture fixation.[31,32]

Cauda equina syndrome

Although evidence is limited, in the absence of demonstrable neural compression, a lumbo-peritnoneal (LP) shunt may provide the best chance of improving neurologic dysfunction or halting progression of neurologic deficit.[36]

Surgical considerations

- Anesthesia team should be aware of Kyphotic deformity and fracture location: nasotracheal or fiberoptic intubation to prevent hyperextension of the neck and exacerbation of neurologic injury.[33]
- Extensive pre-op evaluation: fracture pattern, posterior ligamentous restraint, neurologic compression and function, preexisting bone quality.[33]
- Surgical positioning modified to account for preexisting deformity; support in all regions to prevent hyperextension and exacerbation of neurologic injury.[33]
- ICBG is gold standard; however, often a significant pain source potentially limiting mobilization and increasing likelihood of stasis sequelae (e.g. DVT), consider allograft.[32]
- Extensive knowledge of lateral mass and pedicle anatomy to ensure adequate hardware placement despite distorted bony anatomy and obscuring of typical landmarks.[32]
- Post-op immobilization via halo-vest or TLSO.[33]
- Expedited mobilization out-of-bed as AS patients are predisposed to pulmonary complications.[33]
- Plastic surgery to help manage skin necrosis and wound closure.[33]

74.3 Ossification of the posterior longitudinal ligament (OPLL)

74.3.1 General information

Key concepts

- fibrosis followed by calcification and then ossification of the posterior longitudinal ligament. The process may involve the dura
- more common in Asian population
- most patients have only mild subjective complaints
- 50% of patients have impaired glucose tolerance, respiratory compromise may result from ossification of the costotransverse and costovertebral ligaments
- surgery is best for moderate neuro involvement (Nurick grade 3 & 4)

The age of patients with OPLL ranges from 32–81 years (mean = 53), with a slight male predominance. The prevalence increases with age. Duration of symptoms averages ~ 13 months. It is more prevalent in the Japanese population (2–3.5%).[37,38]

74.3.2 Pathophysiology

The pathologic basis of OPLL is unknown, but there is an increased incidence of ankylosing hyperostosis which suggests a hereditary basis.

OPLL begins with hypervascular fibrosis in the PLL which is followed by focal areas of calcification, proliferation of periosteal cartilaginous cells and finally ossification.[39] The process frequently extends *into* the dura. Eventually active bone marrow production may occur. The process progresses at varying rates among patients, with an average annual growth rate of 0.67 mm in the AP direction and 4.1 mm longitudinally.[40]

When hypertrophied or ossified, the posterior longitudinal ligament may cause myelopathy (due to direct spinal cord compression, or ischemia) and/or radiculopathy (by nerve root compression or stretching).

Changes within the spinal cord involve the postero-lateral gray matter more than white matter, suggesting an ischemic basis for the neurologic involvement.

74.3.3 Distribution

Average involvement: 2.7–4 levels. Frequency of involvement:
1. cervical: 70–75% of cases of OPLL. Typically begins at C3–4 and proceeds distally, often involving C4–5 and C5–6 but usually sparing C6–7
2. thoracic: 15–20% (usually upper, ≈ T4–6)
3. lumbar: 10–15% (also usually upper, ≈ L1–3)

74.3.4 Pathologic classification

See reference.[41]
1. segmental: confined to space behind vertebral bodies, does not cross disc spaces
2. continuous: extends from VB to VB, spanning disc space(s)
3. mixed: combines elements of both of the above with skip areas
4. other variants: includes a rare type of OPLL that is contiguous with the endplates and is confined to the disc space (involves focal hypertrophy of the PLL with punctate calcification)

74.3.5 Clinical

Most patients are asymptomatic, or have only mild subjective complaints. This is probably explained by the protective effect of the fusion resulting from OPLL and the very gradual compression.

Natural history: 17% of patients without myelopathy developed myelopathy in one study[42] over 1.6 years mean follow-up. Statistically, the myelopathy-free rate in patients without initially presenting with myelopathy was 71% after 30 years.[42]

74.3.6 Evaluation

Plain x-rays

Often fail to demonstrate OPLL. Flexion/extension views may be helpful in assessing stability.

MRI

OPLL appears as a hypointense area and is difficult to appreciate until it reaches ≈ 5 mm thickness. On T1WI it blends in with the hypointensity of the ventral subarachnoid space; on T2WI it remains hypointense while the CSF becomes bright. Sagittal images may be very helpful in providing an overview of the extent of involvement, and T2WI may demonstrate intrinsic spinal cord abnormalities which may be associated with a worse outcome.

Myelography/CT

Myelography with post-myelographic CT (especially with 3D reconstructions) is probably best at demonstrating and accurately diagnosing OPLL.

74.3.7 Treatment

Treatment decisions

Based on clinical grade[41] as follows:
1. Class I: radiographic evidence without clinical signs or symptoms. Most patients with OPLL are asymptomatic.[38] Conservative management unless severe
2. Class II: patients with myelopathy or radiculopathy. Minimal or stable deficit may be followed expectantly. Significant deficit or evidence of progression warrants surgical intervention
3. Class IIIA: moderate to severe myelopathy. Usually requires surgical intervention
4. Class IIIB: severe to complete quadriplegia. Surgery is considered for incomplete quadriplegics showing progressive slow worsening. Rapid deterioration or complete quadriplegia, advanced age or poor medical condition are all associated with worse outcome

In moderate grade patients (Nurick grades 3 & 4,[43] (see ▶ Table 74.2), surgery provided a statistically significant reduction in deterioration. There was no difference between surgery and conservative treatment in mild grade (Nurick 1 or 2), and surgery was ineffective in severe grade (Nurick 5).[42]

Table 74.2 Nurick grade of disability from cervical spondylosis[43]

Grade	Description
0	signs or symptoms of root involvement without myelopathy
1	myelopathy, but no difficulty in walking
2	slight difficulty in walking, able to work
3	difficulty in walking but not needing assistance, unable to work full-time
4	able to walk only with assistance or walker
5	chairbound or bedridden

Pre-op assessment

Appropriate cardiorespiratory assessment should be made knowing that:

1. respiratory compromise may result from ossification of the costotransverse and costovertebral ligaments
2. 50% of patients have impaired glucose tolerance with the attendant risks associated with diabetes

Technical considerations for surgery

Severe OPLL increases the risk of spinal cord injury during neck positioning for intubation, and strong consideration should be given to awake nasotracheal intubation.

An anterior approach is generally favored, although laminectomy may be acceptable. SSEP monitoring has been recommended by some.[39] Distraction should be avoided until the spinal cord has been decompressed from the OPLL.

Some authors advocate complete removal of bone from the dura, while others feel it is permissible to leave a thin rim of bone adherent to the dura. Care must be taken in removing bone because it tends to blend imperceptibly with dura and the next thing one may see is bare spinal cord.

Depending on the distance of vertical involvement, vertebral corpectomy with strut grafting may be required. Internal plate fixation is often used as an adjunct. Post-operative immobilization for at least 3 months is employed with rigid collars for single level ACDF or 1–2 level corpectomies, or halo-vest traction for corpectomies > 2 levels.

74.3.8 Results with surgery

The incidence of pseudarthrosis after vertebral corpectomy and strut graft ranges from 5–10% and increases with the number of levels fused.

In one series there was a 10% incidence of transient worsening of neurologic function following anterior surgery[40] which may have been related to distraction.

The risk of dural tear with CSF leak following an anterior approach depends on the aggressiveness with which bone is removed from the dura, and ranges ≈ 16–25%.

Other risks of anterior approaches, e.g. esophageal injury (p. 1074), also pertain.

74.4 Ossification of the anterior longitudinal ligament (OALL)

OALL of the cervical spine and/or hypertrophic anterior cervical osteophytes may produce dramatic radiographic findings and minimal clinical symptoms. Distinct from Forestier's disease (see below). Cervical involvement may produce dysphagia.[44]

74.5 Diffuse idiopathic skeletal hyperostosis (DISH)

Key concepts

- usually asymptomatic, but may present with globus
- W/U: ✓ speech therapy consult for dysphagia evaluation (usually includes ✓ modified barium swallow), ✓ CT of cervical spine, ± ✓ digital video esophagoscopy

AKA "DISH", AKA spondylitis ossificans ligamentosa, AKA ankylosing hyperostosis, among others. A condition characterized by flowing osteophytic formation of the spine in the absence of degenerative, traumatic, or post-infectious changes. Affects Caucasians and males more commonly, and usually seen in patients in their mid-60s.

97% of cases occur in the thoracic spine, also in the lumbar spine in 90%, cervical spine in 78%, and all three segments in 70%. Sacroiliac joints are *spared*, unlike ankylosing spondylitis (AS) (p. 1123). As with AS, unfused levels may be very unstable.

Risk factors for DISH include: elevated body mass index,[45] elevated serum uric acid,[45] diabetes mellitus,[45] elevated growth hormone or insulin levels.[46]

Usually does not produce clinical symptoms. Patients may have early morning stiffness and mild limitations of activities. Cervical involvement may present with dysphagia or globus pharyngis (the subjective sensation of a lump in the throat, not to be confused with globus hystericus which refers to the sensation of a lump in the throat where there is no identifiable pathology) due to compression of the esophagus between the osteophytes and the rigid laryngeal structures[47] (part of Forestier's disease[48]).

Plain x-rays and CT scan demonstrate the pathology. In cases of dysphagia, evaluation should include speech therapy consult for dysphagia evaluation, barium swallow to help localize the site of obstruction, and DVE (digital video esophagoscopy) to rule-out intrinsic esophageal disease.

In cases of dysphagia, evaluation should include speech therapy consult for dysphagia evaluation, barium swallow to help localize the site of obstruction, and DVE (digital video esophagoscopy) to rule-out intrinsic esophageal disease. Plain x-rays and CT scan helps demonstrate the pathology. Cases that do not respond satisfactorily to dietary modifications in patients who are losing weight or are having recurrent episodes of choking or pneumonia should be considered for surgery. An anterior cervical approach, and utilization of a high-speed drill with careful protection of soft-tissue structures (esophagus, carotid sheath) without need for discectomy nor spine stabilization has been recommended.[47] Patients need to be made aware that post-op they are likely to be *worse* initially (from manipulation of esophagus and possibly disruption of some of the autonomic innervation of the esophagus) and will probably need a gastrostomy feeding tube. By 1 year post-op there may be some improvement.

74.6 Scheuermann's kyphosis

74.6.1 General information

AKA Scheuermann juvenile kyphosis AKA Scheuermann disease AKA juvenile osteochondrosis of the spine.

Definition: anterior wedging of at least 5° of ≥ 3 adjacent thoracic vertebral bodies.

Other findings include: Schmorl nodes (p. 1060) and endplate narrowing.

74

74.6.2 Presentation

Adolescents: often present as a result of the cosmetic deformity associated with progressive kyphosis which may be mistaken for "slouching."

Adults: often present with pain.

74.6.3 Evaluation

Patients require standing scoliosis x-rays and a careful neurologic exam.

The role of MRI is controversial, and not all practitioners obtain this.

74.6.4 Radiographic findings

Anterior wedge deformities at multiple levels. End plate irregularities and Schmorl's nodes.

74.6.5 Treatment

Bracing may be used in adolescents, unless the patient meets surgical criteria listed below.

Adults presenting with pain often respond to nonsurgical treatment including: physical therapy and NSAIDs.

Surgery is generally indicated for:
1. Curves exceeding 70–75°
2. Unacceptable cosmetic appearance
3. Refractory pain
4. Progressive kyphosis
5. Neurologic deficit

74.7 Spinal epidural hematoma

74.7.1 General information

Rare. Over 200 cases of varying etiology have been reported,[49] although one-third of recent cases have been associated with anticoagulation therapy.[50] NSAIDs may also be a risk factor.[51] Etiologies include:
1. traumatic: including following LP or epidural anesthesia,[49,52,53,54] fracture (see below), spinal surgery[55] or chiropractic manipulation.[56] Occurs predominantly in patient who is: anticoagulated,[57] thrombocytopenic, or has bleeding diathesis or a vascular lesion
2. spontaneous[58]: rare. Etiologies: hemorrhage from spinal cord AVM (p. 1140), from vertebral hemangioma (p. 794) or tumor

May occur at any level of the spine, however, thoracic is most common. Most often located posterior to spinal cord (except for hematomas following anterior cervical procedures), facilitating removal via laminectomy.[50]

74.7.2 Traumatic spinal epidural hematoma (TSEH) associated with spine fracture

In one series,[59] among 74 trauma patients who underwent emergent spinal MRI, ≈ half of the patients with spine fractures also had TSEH. Treatment was based solely on the fracture, and the outcome in patients with neurologic deficits was no worse in the group with TSEH than in the group without.

74.7.3 Presentation

The clinical picture of *spontaneous* spinal epidural hematoma is fairly consistent but nonspecific. Usually starts with severe back pain with radicular component. It may occasionally follow minor straining, and is less commonly preceded by major straining or back trauma. Spinal neurologic deficits follow, usually progressing over hours, occasionally over days. Motor weakness may go unnoticed when patients are bedridden with pain.

74.7.4 Treatment

Recovery of neurologic deficit without surgery is rare (only a handful of case reports in the literature[51]), therefore optimal treatment is immediate decompressive laminectomy in those patients who can tolerate surgery.[50] In one series, most patients who recovered underwent decompression within 72 hrs of onset of symptoms.[60] In another, decompression within 6 hours was associated with better outcome.[55]

High-risk patients: for medically high-risk patients (e.g. acute MI) on anticoagulation, surgical mortality and morbidity is extremely high, and this must be considered when making the decision of whether or not to operate. In patients not operated, anticoagulants should be stopped, and reversed if possible; see Correction of coagulopathies or reversal of anticoagulants (p. 166). Consider use of high dose methylprednisolone to minimize cord injury; see Methylprednisolone under spinal cord injury (p. 951). Percutaneous needle aspiration may be a consideration in high-risk patients.

74.8 Spinal subdural hematoma

Rare. May be posttraumatic (including iatrogenic causes) or may occur spontaneously. Spinal subdural hematomas (SSH) that occur spontaneously or following lumbar puncture usually occur in patients with coagulopathies (primary or iatrogenic).[61]

Conservative treatment is possible in nontraumatic SSHs with minimal neurologic impairment.[61]

References

[1] Walpin LA, Singer FR. Paget's Disease: Reversal of Severe Paraparesis Using Calcitonin. Spine. 1979; 4:213–219

[2] Youmans JR. Neurological Surgery. Philadelphia 1990

[3] Delmas PD, Meunier PJ. The Management of Paget's Disease of Bone. N Engl J Med. 1997; 336:558–566

[4] Meunier PJ, Salson C, Mathieu L, et al. Skeletal Distribution and Biochemical Parameters of Paget's Disease. Clin Orthop. 1987; 217:37–44

[5] Rothman RH, Simeone FA. The Spine. Philadelphia 1992

[6] Altman RD, Brown M, Gargano F. Low Back Pain in Paget's Disease of Bone. Clin Orthop. 1987; 217:152–161

[7] Hadjipavlou A, Shaffer N, Lander P, et al. Pagetic Spinal Stenosis with Extradural Pagetoid Ossification. Spine. 1988; 13:128–130

[8] Douglas DL, Duckworth T, Kanis JA, et al. Spinal Cord Dysfunction in Paget's Disease of Bone: Has Medical Treatment a Vascular Basis? J Bone Joint Surg. 1981; 63B:495–503

[9] Wilkins RH, Rengachary SS. Neurosurgery. New York 1985

[10] Dinneen SF, Buckley TF. Spinal Nerve Root Compression due to Monostotic Paget's Disease of a Lumbar Vertebra. Spine. 1987; 12:948–950

[11] Sadar ES, Walton RJ, Gossman HH. Neurological Dysfunction in Paget's Disease of the Vertebral Column. J Neurosurg. 1972; 37:661–665

[12] Chen J-R, Rhee RSC, Wallach S, et al. Neurologic Disturbances in Paget Disease of Bone: Response to Calcitonin. Neurology. 1979; 29:448–457

[13] Human Calcitonin for Paget's Disease. Med Letter. 1987; 29:47–48

[14] Tiludronate for Paget's Disease of Bone. Med Letter. 1997; 39:65–66

[15] Risedronate for Paget's Disease of Bone. Med Letter. 1998; 40:87–88

[16] Ahn NU, Ahn UM, Nallamshetty L, Springer BD, Buchowski JM, Funches L, Garrett ES, Kostuik JP, Kebaish KM, Sponseller PD. Cauda equina syndrome in ankylosing spondylitis (the CES-AS syndrome): meta-analysis of outcomes after medical and surgical treatments. J Spinal Disord. 2001; 14:427–433

[17] Caron T, Bransford R, Nguyen Q, Agel J, Chapman J, Bellabarba C. Spine fractures in patients with ankylosing spinal disorders. Spine (Phila Pa 1976). 2010; 35:E458–E464

[18] Farhat SM, Schneider RC, Gray JM. Traumatic Spinal Epidural Hematoma Associated with Cervical Fractures in Rheumatoid Spondylitis. J Trauma. 1973; 13:591–599

[19] Bron JL, de Vries MK, Snieders MN, van der Horst-Bruinsma IE, van Royen BJ. Discovertebral (Andersson) lesions of the spine in ankylosing spondylitis revisited. Clin Rheumatol. 2009; 28:883–892

[20] Stolwijk C, Boonen A, van Tubergen A, Reveille JD. Epidemiology of spondyloarthritis. Rheum Dis Clin North Am. 2012; 38:441–476

[21] Calin A. Early diagnosis of ankylosing spondylitis. Lancet. 1977; 2

[22] Rae PS, Waddell G, Venner RM. A Simple Technique for Measuring Lumbar Spinal Flexion. J R Coll Surg Edin. 1984; 29:281–284

[23] van den Berg R, de Hooge M, Rudwaleit M, Sieper J, van Gaalen F, Reijnierse M, Landewe R, Huizinga T, van der Heijde D. ASAS modification of the Berlin algorithm for diagnosing axial spondyloarthritis: results from the SPondyloArthritis Caught Early (SPACE)-cohort and from the Assessment of SpondyloArthritis international Society (ASAS)-cohort. Ann Rheum Dis. 2013; 72:1646–1653

[24] van der Linden S, Valkenburg HA, Cats A. Evaluation of diagnostic criteria for ankylosing spondylitis. A proposal for modification of the New York criteria. Arthritis Rheum. 1984; 27:361–368

[25] Bennett GJ. Ankylosing Spondylitis. Clin Neurosurg. 1991; 37:622–635

[26] Qubti MA, Flynn JA, Imboden JB, Hellmann DB, Stone JH. In: Ankylosing spondylitis & the arthritis of inflammatory bowel disease. Current rheumatology diagnosis & treatment. 1st ed. New York: McGraw-Hill; 2004

[27] Braun J, van den Berg R, Baraliakos X, Boehm H, Burgos-Vargas R, Collantes-Estevez E, Dagfinrud H, Dijkmans B, Dougados M, Emery P, Geher P, Hammoudeh M, Inman RD, Jongkees M, Khan MA, Kiltz U, Kvien T, Leirisalo-Repo M, Maksymowych WP, Olivieri I, Pavelka K, Sieper J, Stanislawska-Biernat E, Wendling D, Ozgocmen S, van Drogen C, van Royen B, van der Heijde D. 2010 update of the ASAS/EULAR recommendations for the management of ankylosing spondylitis. Ann Rheum Dis. 2011; 70:896–904

[28] Westerveld LA, Verlaan JJ, Oner FC. Spinal fractures in patients with ankylosing spinal disorders: a systematic review of the literature on treatment, neurological status and complications. Eur Spine J. 2009; 18:145–156

[29] Clarke A, James S, Ahuja S. Ankylosing spondylitis: inadvertent application of a rigid collar after cervical fracture, leading to neurological complications and death. Acta Orthop Belg. 2010; 76:413–415

[30] Detwiler KN, Loftus CM, Godersky JC. Management of Cervical Spine Injuries in Patients with Ankylosing Spondylitis. J Neurosurg. 1990; 72:210–215

[31] Schneider PS, Bouchard J, Moghadam K, Swamy G. Acute cervical fractures in ankylosing spondylitis: an opportunity to correct preexisting deformity. Spine (Phila Pa 1976). 2010; 35:E248–E252

[32] Kanter AS, Wang MY, Mummaneni PV. A treatment algorithm for the management of cervical spine fractures and deformity in patients with ankylosing spondylitis. Neurosurg Focus. 2008; 24. DOI: 10.3171/FOC/2008/24/1/E11

[33] Chaudhary SB, Hullinger H, Vives MJ. Management of acute spinal fractures in ankylosing spondylitis. ISRN Rheumatol. 2011; 2011. DOI: 10.5402/2011/150484

[34] Trent G, Armstrong GW, O'Neil J. Thoracolumbar fractures in ankylosing spondylitis. High-risk injuries. Clin Orthop Relat Res. 1988; 227:61–66

[35] Van Royen BJ, De Gast A. Lumbar osteotomy for correction of thoracolumbar kyphotic deformity in ankylosing spondylitis. A structured review of three methods of treatment. Ann Rheum Dis. 1999; 58:399–406

[36] Dinichert A, Cornelius JF, Lot G. Lumboperitoneal shunt for treatment of dural ectasia in ankylosing spondylitis. J Clin Neurosci. 2008; 15:1179–1182

[37] Tsuyama N. Ossification of the Posterior Longitudinal Ligament of the Spine. Clin Orthop. 1984; 184:71–84

[38] Nakanishi T, Mannen T, Toyokura Y. Asymptomatic Ossification of the Posterior Longitudinal Ligament of the Cervical Spine. J Neurol Sci. 1973; 19:375–381

[39] Epstein N. Diagnosis and Surgical Management of Ossification of the Posterior Longitudinal Ligament. Contemp Neurosurg. 1992; 14:1–6

[40] Harsh GR, Sypert GW, Weinstein PR, et al. Cervical Spine Stenosis Secondary to Ossification of the Posterior Longitudinal Ligament. J Neurosurg. 1987; 67:349–357

[41] Hirabayashi K, Watanabe K, Wakano K, et al. Expansive Cervical Laminoplasty for Cervical Spinal Stenotic Myelopathy. Spine. 1983; 8:693–693

[42] Matsunaga S, Sakou T, Taketomi E, Komiya S. Clinical course of patients with ossification of the posterior longitudinal ligament: a minimum 10-year cohort study. J Neurosurg. 2004; 100:245–248

[43] Nurick S. The Pathogenesis of the Spinal Cord Disorder Associated with Cervical Spondylosis. Brain. 1972; 95:87–100

[44] Epstein NE, Hollingsworth R. Ossification of the Cervical Anterior Longitudinal Ligament Contributing to Dysphagia: Case Report. J Neurosurg. 1999; 90 (Spine 2):261–263

[45] Kiss C, Szilagyi M, Paksy A, Poor G. Risk factors for diffuse idiopathic skeletal hyperostosis: a case-control study. Rheumatology (Oxford). 2002; 41:27–30

[46] Denko CW, Boja B, Moskowitz RW. Growth promoting peptides in osteoarthritis and diffuse idiopathic skeletal hyperostosis–insulin, insulin-like growth factor-I, growth hormone. J Rheumatol. 1994; 21:1725–1730
[47] Burkus JK. Esophageal Obstruction Secondary to Diffuse Idiopathic Skeletal Hyperostosis. Orthopedics. 1988; 11:717–720
[48] McCafferty RR, Harrison MJ, Tamas LB, Larkins MV. Ossification of the Anterior Longitudinal Ligament and Forestier's Disease: An Analysis of Seven Cases. J Neurosurg. 1995; 83:13–17
[49] Tekkok IH, Cataltepe K, Tahta K, Bertan V. Extradural Hematoma After Continuous Extradural Anesthesia. Brit J Anaesth. 1991; 67:112–115
[50] Harik SI, Raichle ME, Reis DJ. Spontaneous Remitting Spinal Epidural Hematoma in a Patient on Anticoagulants. N Engl J Med. 1971; 284:1355–1357
[51] Silber SH. Complete Nonsurgical Resolution of a Spontaneous Spinal Epidural Hematoma. Am J Emergency Med. 1996; 14:391–393
[52] Shnider SM, Levinson G. In: Neurologic Complications of Regional Anesthesia. Anesthesia for Obstetrics. 2nd ed. Baltimore: Williams and Wilkins; 1987:319–320
[53] Sage DJ. Epidurals, Spinals and Bleeding Disorders in Pregnancy: A Review. Anaesth Intens Care. 1990; 18:319–326
[54] Gustafsson H, Rutberg H, Bengtsson M. Spinal Hematoma Following Epidural Analgesia: Report of a Patient with Ankylosing Spondylitis and a Bleeding Diathesis. Anaesthesia. 1988; 43:220–222
[55] Porter RW, Detwiler PW, Lawton MT, Sonntag VKH, Dickman CA. Postoperative Spinal Epidural Hematomas: Longitudinal Review of 12,000 Spinal Operations. BNI Quarterly. 2000; 16:10–17
[56] Domenicucci M, Ramieri A, Salvati M, Brogna C, Raco A. Cervicothoracic epidural hematoma after chiropractic spinal manipulation therapy. Case report and review of the literature. J Neurosurg Spine. 2007; 7:571–574
[57] Dickman CA, Shedd SA, Spetzler RF, Sonntag VKH, et al. Spinal Epidural Hematoma Associated with Epidural Anesthesia: Complications of Systemic Heparinization in Patients Receiving Peripheral Vascular Thrombolytic Therapy. 1990; 72
[58] Packer NP, Cummins BH. Spontaneous Epidural Hemorrhage: A Surgical Emergency. Lancet. 1978; 1:356–358
[59] Bennett DL, George MJ, Ohashi K, El-Khoury GY, Lucas JJ, Peterson MC. Acute traumatic spinal epidural hematoma: imaging and neurologic outcome. Emerg Radiol. 2005; 11:136–144
[60] Rebello MD, Dastur HM. Spinal Epidural Hemorrhage: A Review of Case Reports. Neurol India. 1966; 14:135–145
[61] Domenicucci M, Ramieri A, Ciappetta P, Delfini R. Nontraumatic Acute Spinal Subdural Hematoma. J Neurosurg. 1999; (Spine 1) 91:65–73

75 Other Non-Spine Conditions with Spine Implications

75.1 Rheumatoid arthritis

75.1.1 General information

More than 85% of patients with moderate or severe rheumatoid arthritis (RA) have radiographic evidence of C-spine involvement.[1]

The grading system of Ranawat et al.[1] for myelopathy is shown in ▶ Table 75.1 is used in RA as well as some other etiologies of myelopathy.

75.1.2 Cervical spine involvement in RA

Common involvement

1. upper cervical spine: involved in 44–88% of RA cases[2] (often found together):
   a) anterior atlantoaxial subluxation: the most common manifestation of RA in the cervical spine, found in up to 25% of patients with RA (see below)
   b) basilar impression (BI): upward translocation of the odontoid process, found in ≈ 8% of patients with RA (p. 1138)
   c) pannus of granulation tissue: forms around the odontoid
2. subaxial C-spine (i.e. below C2) subluxation (p. 1138)

Less common involvement of the cervical spine in RA

1. posterior subluxation of the atlantoaxial joint: must have either associated fracture of or near total arthritic erosion of odontoid
2. vertebral artery insufficiency secondary to changes at the cranio-cervical junction[3]

75.1.3 Atlantoaxial subluxation (AAS) in RA

General information

Inflammatory involvement of the atlantoaxial synovial joints causes erosive changes in the odontoid process (anteriorly at the synovial joint with the C1 arch, and posteriorly at the synovial joint with the transverse ligament) and decalcification and loosening of the insertion of the transverse ligament on the atlas. These changes lead to instability allowing a scissoring effect with anterior subluxation of C1 on C2. AAS occurs in ≈ 25% of patients with RA.[3] Mean time between onset of RA symptoms to the diagnosis of AAS in 15 patients: 14 years.[4]

75

Clinical

Signs and symptoms of AAS are shown in ▶ Table 75.2.

AAS is usually slowly progressive. Mean age at onset of AAS symptoms: 57 years.

Pain is experienced locally (upper cervical and suboccipital regions, often from compression of C2 nerve root) or is referred (to mastoid, occipital, temporal, or frontal regions).

VBI may occur from VA involvement (p. 1305).

Table 75.1 Ranawat classification of myelopathy

Class	Description
I	no neural deficit
II	subjective weakness + hyperreflexia + dysesthesia
III	objective weakness + long tract signs III A = ambulatory III B = quadriparetic & non ambulatory

Table 75.2 Signs and symptoms of AAS[a] (15 patients with AAS[4])

Finding	%
pain	
• local	67%
• referred	27%
hyperreflexia	67%
spasticity	27%
paresis	27%
sensory disturbance	20%
[a]other possible findings not reported in this series: clumsiness, neurogenic bladder, Babinski sign	

Radiographic evaluation

General information

The magnitude of AAS is usually increased with neck flexion.

Lateral C-spine x-ray

Both the ADI and PADI below are surrogate markers for instability and for spinal cord compression. With the availability of MRI, the ability to directly assess spinal cord compression has diminished the usefulness of these measures, especially for that aspect.

Anterior atlantodental interval (ADI)

The ADI (p. 213) only gives information about the stability of the C1–2 joint. The normal ADI in adults is < 3–4 mm.[5,6] Widening of the ADI suggests possible incompetence of the transverse ligament. However, the ADI *does not correlate* with the risk of neurologic injury[7,8] and is not predictive of progression from asymptomatic AAS to symptomatic AAS.

Posterior atlantodental interval (PADI)

The amount of room available for the spinal cord can vary for any given ADI depending on the AP diameter of the spinal canal and the thickness of any pannus. The PADI (p. 213) and the AP diameter of the subaxial canal measured on a lateral C-spine x-ray correlates with the presence and severity of paralysis.[7]

The PADI also predicts neurologic recovery following surgery. Patients with paralysis from AAS showed no recovery if the pre-op PADI was < 10 mm.[7] 75

PADI ≤ 14 mm has been proposed as an indication for surgical stabilization.

MRI

The optimal test to evaluate the source and magnitude of upper cord or medulla compression. Demonstrates location of odontoid process, extent of pannus, and effects of subluxation (may need to be performed with head flexed to evaluate this).

Treatment

General information

Requires knowledge of the following information:

1. natural history: AAS in most patients progresses, with a small percentage either stabilizing or fusing spontaneously. In one series[9] with 4.5 years mean follow-up, 45% of patients with 3.5–5 mm subluxation progressed to 5–8 mm, and 10% of these progressed to > 8 mm
2. once myelopathy occurs, it may be irreversible
3. the worse the myelopathy, the higher the risk for sudden death
4. the chances of finding myelopathy are significantly increased once the subluxation reaches ≥ 9 mm[10]

5. associated cranial settling further decreases the tolerance for AAS
6. the life expectancy of patients with RA is 10 years less than the general population[9]
7. the morbidity and mortality of surgical treatment (see below)
8. pannus may regress some after medical treatment

When to treat?

1. symptomatic patients with AAS: almost all require surgical treatment (C1–2 fusion in most cases). For management, see below. Some surgeons do not operate if the maximal dens-C1 distance is < 6 mm
2. asymptomatic patients: controversial
   a) some authors feel surgical fusion is not necessary in asymptomatic patient if the dens-C1 distance is below a certain cutoff. Recommendations for this cutoff have ranged from 6 to 10 mm,[11] with 8 mm commonly cited (an unvalidated delineation)
   b) these patients are often placed in a rigid cervical collar, e.g. while outside the home, even though it is generally acknowledged that a collar probably does not provide significant support or protection
   c) NB: some cases of sudden death in previously asymptomatic RA patients may be due to AAS and may then be erroneously attributed to cardiac arrhythmias, etc.[12]

Surgical management

It is necessary to either reduce the subluxation or to decompress the upper cord before doing a C1-C2 or occipital-C1-C2 fusion.

Menezes assesses all subluxed patients for reducibility using MRI compatible Halo cervical traction as follows: start with 5 lbs, and gradually increase over a period of a week. Most cases reduce within 2–3 days. If not reduced after 7 days then it is probably not reducible. Only ≈ 20% of cases are not reducible (most of these have odontoid > 15 mm above foramen magnum).

Most require stabilization via posterior wiring and fusion, either of C1 to C2, or of occiput to C2. The latter is used when fusion is combined with decompression (posterior laminectomy of C1 with posterior enlargement of the foramen magnum). See Atlantoaxial fusion (C1–2 arthrodesis) (p. 1479).

Posterior fusion alone does not provide adequate relief if the subluxation is irreducible, or if pannus causes significant compression (however, there may be some reduction of pannus after fusion). In these cases, transoral odontoidectomy may be indicated. Performing the posterior stabilization and decompression first allows some patients to avoid a second operation, and permits the remainder to undergo the anterior approach without becoming destabilized. Still, some surgeons do the odontoidectomy first[11] (requires the patient to remain in traction until the fusion).

Reminder: the patient must be able to open the mouth greater than ≈ 25 mm in order to perform transoral odontoidectomy without splitting the mandible.

Posterior fusion

See Atlantoaxial fusion (C1–2 arthrodesis) (p. 1479) for technique. In RA, erosion and osteoporosis weakens the C1 arch, and extra care is needed to avoid fracturing it.

75.1.4 Surgical morbidity and mortality

Because of the frequency of simultaneous involvement of other systems in RA including pulmonary, cardiac, and endocrine, operative mortality ranges from 5–15%.[11]

The non-fusion rate for C1–2 wiring and fusion has been reported as high as 50%,[13] typical rates are lower (with 18% of patients in one series developing a fibrous union[11]). The most common site of failure of osseous fusion is the interface between the bone graft and the posterior arch of C1.[14]

75.1.5 Post-operative care

The patient is usually mobilized almost immediately post-op in halo vest traction (some use an optional period of maintained traction before mobilization). Impaired healing in RA dictates that the Halo be worn until fusion is well established, as seen on x-ray (usually 8–12 weeks). Sonntag evaluates the patient with flexion-extension lateral C-spine x-rays by disconnecting the halo ring from the vest.

75.1.6 Basilar impression in rheumatoid arthritis

General information

AKA atlantoaxial impaction. Erosive changes in the lateral masses of C1 → telescoping of the atlas onto the body of C2 causing ventral migration of C1 with resultant ↓ in AP diameter of the spinal canal. There is concomitant upward displacement of the dens. The posterior arch of C1 often protrudes superiorly through the foramen magnum. All of these factors lead to compression of the pons and medulla. Rheumatoid granulation tissue behind the odontoid also contributes to the brainstem compression. Vertebral artery and/or anterior spinal artery compression may also cause neurologic dysfunction.

The degree of erosion of C1 correlates with the extent of odontoid invagination.

Clinical

See ▶ Table 75.3 for signs & symptoms.

Pain may occur as a result of compression of the C1 and/or C2 nerve roots. Compression of the medulla can cause cranial nerve dysfunction.

Motor exam usually difficult because of severe polyarticular degeneration and associated pain. Sensory findings (all non-localizing): diminished vibratory, position, and light touch.

Radiographic evaluation

See Basilar invagination & basilar impression (BI) (p.217) for radiographic criteria of BI. Erosion of the tip of the odontoid, commonly seen in RA, obviates use of any measurement that is based on the location of the tip of the odontoid.[15] For this reason, other measures have been developed, including the Clark station,[14] Redlund-Johnell criteria,[16] and Ranawat criteria.[1] Since even these methods will miss up to 6% of cases of BI in RA,[15] it is recommended that suspicious cases be investigated further (e.g. with CT and/or MRI).

MRI: optimal for demonstrating brain stem impingement, poor for showing bone. Cervicomedullary angle: the angle between a line drawn through the long axis of the medulla on a sagittal MRI

Table 75.3 Symptoms and signs of BI (45 patients with RA[2])

Finding	%
headache	100%
progressive difficulty ambulating	80%
hyperreflexia + Babinski	80%
limb paresthesias	71%
neurogenic bladder	31%
cranial nerve dysfunction	22%
• trigeminal nerve anesthesia	20%
• glossopharyngeal	
• vagus	
• hypoglossal	
miscellaneous findings	
• internuclear ophthalmoplegia	
• vertigo	
• diplopia	
• downbeat nystagmus	
• sleep apnea	
• spastic quadriparesis	

75

and a line drawn through the cervical spinal cord. The normal CMA is 135–170°. A CMA < 135° correlates with signs of cervicomedullary compression, myelopathy or C2 radiculopathy.[17]

CT: primarily done to assess bony anatomy (erosion, fractures...).

CTA should be performed when surgery is contemplated, to show detail of VA anatomy.

Myelography (water soluble) with *CT*: also good for delineating bony pathology.

Treatment

See also Craniocervical junction and upper cervical spine abnormalities (p. 1151).

Cervical traction

May attempt with Gardner-Wells tongs. Begin with ≈ 7 lbs, and slowly increase up to 15 lbs. Some may require several weeks of traction to reduce.

Surgery

Reducible cases: posterior occipitocervical fusion ± C1 decompressive laminectomy.

Irreducible cases: requires transoral resection of odontoid. May perform before posterior fusion (but then must be kept in traction while waiting for posterior fusion).

75.1.7 Subaxial subluxation in rheumatoid arthritis

The direct effects of RA on the subaxial spine involves the facet joints posteriorly. Degenerative disc disease, which is generally a late manifestation in RA, is not the result of synovitis.[18] Involvement is most common at C2–3 and C3–4.

75.2 Down syndrome

75.2.1 General information

Down syndrome is associated with ligamentous laxity of the spine. This has implications whenever a fusion is contemplated, as adjacent segment failure with kyphosis is very common. Ligamentous laxity may also result in atlantoaxial subluxation (**AAS**).

75.2.2 Atlantoaxial subluxation (AAS) in Down syndrome

General information

Not all cases of AAS are unstable (an unstable spine, by definition, needs treatment).

75 Incidence of AAS in Down syndrome (DS) is 20%,[19] but only 1–2% of DS patients have *symptomatic* AAS.[20] AAS in DS appears to be due to laxity of the transverse atlantal ligament (TAL). This laxity may decrease with age as the TAL stiffens.

Management

Controversial. There have been position statements[21] and rebuttals.[20,22]

Recommendations (modified[23]); ADI = atlantodental interval (p. 213), PADI = posterior atlantodental interval (p. 213):

1. children who have been screened and do not have AAS: no further screening after age 10 years (since AAS does not develop later; the cutoff age is controversial)
2. os odontoideum: surgical fusion
3. symptomatic AAS
   a) symptoms may include: gait difficulties, neck pain, limited neck motion, torticollis, clumsiness, sensory deficits, and other symptoms of myelopathy
   b) for ADI > 4.5 mm or PADI < 14 mm or spinal cord damage on cervical MRI: surgical fusion
4. asymptomatic AAS seen on lateral C-spine x-ray:
   a) for ADI ≤ 4.5 mm *and* PADI ≥ 14 mm: no need for further testing
   b) for ADI > 4.5 mm or PADI < 14 mm: cervical MRI
      - if the MRI shows spinal cord damage: surgical fusion
      - if MRI shows no spinal cord damage: surgical fusion is optional. If fusion is not done, prohibit high-risk activities and restudy in 1 year

75.3 Morbid obesity

Morbid obesity, defined as a body mass index (BMI) > 40. Approximately doubles risks (13.6% vs. 6.9%) of complications of all types (cardiac, renal, pulmonary, wound complications…)[24] with spine surgery. Mortality is tripled (but is still low, 0.41 in morbid obese vs. 0.13).[24] Hospital costs and length of stay is also longer.

References

[1] Ranawat CS, O'Leary P, Pellicci P, et al. Cervical Spine Fusion in Rheumatoid Arthritis. J Bone Joint Surg. 1979; 61A:1003–1010

[2] Menezes AH, VanGilder JC, Clark CR, et al. Odontoid Upward Migration in Rheumatoid Arthritis. J Neurosurg. 1985; 63:500–509

[3] Rana NA, Hancock DO, Taylor AR. Atlanto-Axial Subluxation in Rheumatoid Arthritis. J Bone Joint Surg. 1973; 55B:458–470

[4] Hildebrandt G, Agnoli AL, Zierski J. Atlanto-Axial Dislocation in Rheumatoid Arthritis: Diagnostic and Therapeutic Aspects. Acta Neurochir. 1987; 84:110–117

[5] Hinck VC, Hopkins CE. Measurement of the Atlanto-Dental Interval in the Adult. Am J Roentgenol Radium Ther Nucl Med. 1960; 84:945–951

[6] Meijers KAE, van Beusekom GT, Luyendijk W, et al. Dislocation of the Cervical Spine with Cord Compression in Rheumatoid Arthritis. J Bone Joint Surg. 1974; 56B:668–680

[7] Boden SD, Dodge LD, Bohlman HH, Rechtine GR. Rheumatoid arthritis of the cervical spine. A long-term analysis with predictors of paralysis and recovery. J Bone Joint Surg. 1993; 75:1282–1297

[8] Collins DN, Barnes CL, FitzRandolph RL. Cervical spine instability in rheumatoid patients having total hip or knee arthroplasty. Clin Orthop Relat Res. 1991:127–135

[9] Smith PH, Benn RT, Sharp J. Natural History of Rheumatoid Cervical Luxations. Ann Rheum Dis. 1972; 31:431–439

[10] Weissman BNW, Aliabadi P, Weinfeld MS, et al. Prognostic Features of Atlantoaxial Subluxation in Rheumatoid Arthritis Patients. Radiology. 1982; 144:745–751

[11] Papadopoulos SM, Dickman CA, Sonntag VKH. Atlantoaxial Stabilization in Rheumatoid Arthritis. J Neurosurg. 1991; 74:1–7

[12] Mikulowski P, Wollheim FA, Rotmil P, Olsen I. Sudden death in rheumatoid arthritis with atlanto-axial dislocation. Acta Med Scand. 1975; 198:445–451

[13] Kourtopoulos H, von EssenC. Stabilization of the Unstable Upper Cervical Spine in Rheumatoid Arthritis. Acta Neurochir. 1988; 91:113–115

[14] Clark CR, Goetz DD, Menezes AH. Arthrodesis of the Cervical Spine in Rheumatoid Arthritis. J Bone Joint Surg. 1989; 71A:381–392

[15] Riew KD, Hilibrand AS, Palumbo MA, Sethi N, Bohlman HH. Diagnosing basilar invagination in the rheumatoid patient. The reliability of radiographic criteria. J Bone Joint Surg. 2001; 83-A:194–200

[16] Redlund-Johnell I, Pettersson H. Radiographic measurements of the cranio-vertebral region. Designed for evaluation of abnormalities in rheumatoid arthritis. Acta Radiol Diagn (Stockh). 1984; 25:23–28

[17] Bundschuh C, Modic MT, Kearney F, Morris R, Deal C. Rheumatoid arthritis of the cervical spine: surface-coil MR imaging. AJR Am J Roentgenol. 1988; 151:181–187

[18] Kim DH, Hilibrand AS. Rheumatoid arthritis in the cervical spine. J Am Acad Orthop Surg. 2005; 13:463–474

[19] Martel W, Tishler JM. Observations on the spine in mongoloidism. Am J Roentgenol Radium Ther Nucl Med. 1966; 97:630–638

[20] Pueschel SM. Should children with Down syndrome be screened for atlantoaxial instability? Arch Pediatr Adolesc Med. 1998; 152:123–125

[21] American Academy of Pediatrics Committee on Sports Medicine and Fitness. Atlantoaxial instability in Down syndrome: subject review. Pediatrics. 1995; 96:151–154

[22] Cohen WI. Atlantoaxial instability. What's next? Arch Pediatr Adolesc Med. 1998; 152:119–122

[23] Brockmeyer D. Down syndrome and craniovertebral instability. Topic review and treatment recommendations. Pediatr Neurosurg. 1999; 31:71–77

[24] Kalanithi PA, Arrigo R, Boakye M. Morbid obesity increases cost and complication rates in spinal arthrodesis. Spine (Phila Pa 1976). 2012; 37:982–988

76 Special Conditions Affecting the Spinal Cord

76.1 Spinal vascular malformations

76.1.1 General information

Often also referred to by the term spinal AVMs which technically refers to a subset of spinal vascular malformations (SVMs). Incidence of SVM is about 4% of primary intraspinal masses. 80% occur between age 20 and 60 years.[1 (p 1850–3)]

76.1.2 Classification

For a review of the history of classification systems, see the excellent review by Black[2]).

There are three current era classification systems.

The "American/English/French Connection" classification

References for classification: include[2,3,4,5,6,7,8,9,10]

1. Type I: dural AVM AKA AV-fistula (AVF). The most common type (80%) of SVM in the adult.[11] Fed by radicular artery which forms an AV shunt (fistula) at the dural root sleeve (located in the intervertebral foramen),[8] drains into an engorged spinal vein on *posterior* cord. Usually in lumbar or lower thoracic spine. Slow flow. High pressure in draining vein may cause venous congestion of the cord. Cord involvement may be distant to the fistula. Symptoms: LBP and progressive myeloradiculopathy or cauda equina syndrome (due to venous congestion) with urinary retention usually in middle-aged patients, 90% males. Up to 35% have pain. 15–20% are associated with other AVMs (cutaneous or other). Rarely bleed
   a) Type IA: single arterial feeder
   b) Type IB: two or more arterial feeders
2. intradural AVMs (high flow): 75% present with acute onset of symptoms, usually from hemorrhage (SAH or intramedullary)
   a) Type II: AKA spinal glomus AVM. Intramedullary. True AVM of the spinal cord. 15–20% of all SVMs. Compact nidus fed by medullary arteries with the AV shunt contained at least partially within the spinal cord or pia. May be associated with feeding artery aneurysms. Worse prognosis than dural AVM.[8] Fed by 1, or at most 2–3 feeders 80% of the time
   b) Type III: AKA juvenile spinal AVM. Essentially an enlarged glomus AVM which occupies the entire cross-section of the cord and invades the vertebral body which may cause scoliosis
   c) Type IV[7]: intradural perimedullary AVM (also called arteriovenous fistulae (AVF)). Direct fistula between artery supplying spinal cord (usually anterior spinal artery, often artery of Adamkiewicz) and draining veins. Typically occur in younger patients than Type I, and may present catastrophically with hemorrhage into the subarachnoid space.[12] ▶ Table 76.1 shows the 3 subtypes.[9]
3. miscellaneous spinal vascular lesions:
   a) spinal cord cavernomas
   b) spinal cord venous angiomas: extremely rare. Difficult to visualize angiographically
   c) vertebral body hemangiomas (p.794)

76

Hôpital Bicêtre classification

See reference.[13]

Table 76.1 Merland's subclassification of *Type IV* (perimedullary) AV fistulas[a]

Subtype	Arterial supply	AVF	Venous drainage
I	single (thin ASA)	single, small	slowly ascending perimedullary venous system
II	multiple (dilated ASA & PSA)	multiple, medium	
III		single, giant	giant venous ectasia, rapid metameric venous drainage

[a]AVF = arteriovenous fistula; ASA = anterior spinal artery; PSA = posterior spinal artery

1. AVMs
2. fistulae: micro- or macrofistulae
3. genetic classification of spinal cord

AV shunts
a) genetic hereditary lesions: macrofistulae and hereditary hemorrhagic telangiectasias
b) genetic nonhereditary lesions: multiple lesions with metameric or myelomeric associations
c) single lesions: incomplete associations of categories a or b

Spetzler et al. classification

See reference.[14]

This system reincorporated vascular spinal neoplasms.

1. Neoplastic vascular lesions
   a) hemangioblastoma
   b) cavernous malformation
2. spinal aneurysms (rare)
3. arteriovenous lesions
   a) AVFs
      - extradural
      - intradural: dorsal or ventral
   b) AVMs
      - extradural-intradural
      - intradural
      - intramedullary
      - intramedullary-extramedullary
      - conus medullaris

76.1.3 Presentation

85% present as progressive neuro deficit (back pain associated with progressive sensory loss and LE weakness over months to years). Yet, SVMs account for < 5% of lesions presenting as spinal cord "tumors." 10–20% of SVMs present as sudden onset of myelopathy usually in patients < 30 yrs age,[15,16] secondary to hemorrhage (causing SAH, hematomyelia, epidural hematoma, or watershed infarction). Coup de poignard of Michon = sudden excruciating back pain with SAH (clinical evidence of SVM).

Foix-Alajouanine syndrome (subacute necrotic myelopathy): acute or subacute neurologic deterioration in a patient with a SVM without evidence of hemorrhage. Presents as spastic → flaccid paraplegia, with ascending sensory level and loss of sphincter control. Initially thought to be due to spontaneous thrombosis of the AVM causing subacute necrotizing myelopathy[17] which would be irreversible. However, more recent evidence suggests that the myelopathy may be due to venous hypertension with secondary ischemia, and there may be improvement with treatment.[18]

▶ **Clinical.** Auscultation over spine reveals a bruit in 2–3% of cases. Cutaneous angioma over back is present in 3–25%; valsalva maneuver may enhance the redness of the angioma.[16]

76

76.1.4 Evaluation

Spinal angiography: necessary for treatment planning. Best performed at centers that do this study regularly. For Type I dural AVMs, angiography must encompass all dural feeders of the neuraxis, which includes:

1. ICAs: because of the artery of Bernasconi & Cassinari (p.79)
2. every radicular artery including the artery of Adamkiewicz (p.87)
3. internal iliac arteries: for sacral feeders

MRI: detects some SVMs with greater sensitivity and safety than angiography,[19] but is inadequate for treatment planning. 82% show extramedullary flow voids. Variable degree of cord enhancement (from venous congestion or venous infarction). Negative MRI does not rule out diagnosis.

Myelography: classically shows serpiginous intradural filling defects. Generally superseded by MRI. If done, patient should be imaged prone *and* supine (to avoid missing a dorsal AVM) ✖ Risk of bleeding from puncture of a dilated artery/vein with myelography needle.

76.1.5 Treatment

Type I (dural AVMs): usually require treatment. Usually amenable to endovascular techniques using glue, in which case the proximal vein must be taken as well. If you don't completely eliminate a dural fistula (spinal or intracranial) it will come back!

Type II (spinal glomus AVMs): may be amenable to interventional neuroradiologic procedures including embolization,[20] especially type IIA (single feeder). However recurrence may be higher with endovascular treatment than surgery, and surgery is often preferred for Type IIB (≥ 2 feeders). Surgical strategy: similar to intracranial AVMs except that the parenchyma cannot be retracted, bleeding is rarely life threatening, and arteries of passage must be preserved to avoid devastating deficits. Intraoperative ICG angio is often helpful. The nidus is compact, and the hemosiderin ring around the nidus on MRI often represents a plane that can be exploited.

Type III (juvenile spinal AVMS): the natural history is probably better than the prognosis with any type of treatment.

Type IV (perimedullary fistulae): suggested management[10] is shown in ▶ Table 76.2.

76.2 Spinal meningeal cysts

76.2.1 General information

Spinal meningeal cysts (SMC): diverticula of the meningeal sac, nerve root sheath or arachnoid. May have familial tendency.

Terminology in literature is confusing. One classification system is shown in ▶ Table 76.3. Previously AKA Tarlov's perineural cysts, spinal arachnoid cysts, and extradural diverticula, pouches or cysts. Only congenital lesions are considered here.

1. Type I SMCs above the sacrum usually have a pedicle adjacent to entrance of dorsal nerve root
2. Type II SMCs: formerly called Tarlov's cysts and were differentiated from nerve root diverticula because the former were defined as communicating with subarachnoid space, and the latter not. However, intrathecal contrast CT (ICCT) shows both communicate. Often multiple, occur on dorsal roots anywhere, but are most prominent and symptomatic in sacrum
3. Type III SMCs: may also be multiple and asymptomatic. More common along posterior subarachnoid space. Attributed to proliferation of arachnoid trabeculae

Table 76.2 Suggested management for Type IV arteriovenous fistulae[10]

Subtype	Diagnosis	Embolization	Surgery
Subtype I	difficult; ? reliability of MRI[a]; tomomyelography; angiotomomyelography	difficult	easy on filum terminale; difficult on conus medullaris
Subtype II	easy: MRI or myelography	incomplete occlusion	on posterolateral AVFs
Subtype III		effective	difficult, dangerous

[a]due to inaccuracy, do not delay angiogram to get MRA, etc.

Table 76.3 Types of spinal meningeal cysts[21]

Type	Description
Type I	extradural meningeal cysts without spinal nerve root fibers
IA	"extradural meningeal/arachnoid cyst"
IB	(occult) "sacral meningocele"
Type II	extradural meningeal cysts with spinal nerve root fibers ("Tarlov's perineural cyst", "spinal nerve root diverticulum")
Type III	spinal intradural meningeal cysts ("intradural arachnoid cyst")

76.2.2 Presentation

May be asymptomatic (i.e. incidental finding). May cause radiculopathy by pressure on adjacent nerve root (may or may not cause symptoms of nerve root from which it actually arises). Symptom complex depends on size of SMC, and proximity to spinal cord and nerve roots.

1. Type I SMCs: in thoracic and cervical region, may present with acute myelopathy (spasticity and sensory level); lumbar region → LBP and radiculopathy; sacral region → sphincter disturbance
2. Type II SMCs: often asymptomatic, but sacral lesions may → sciatica and/or sphincter disturbance
3. Type III SMCs: may also be multiple and asymptomatic; more common along posterior subarachnoid space

76.2.3 Evaluation

MRI to identify the mass, then water-soluble ICCT scan to evaluate communication of cyst with subarachnoid space.

1. Type II SMCs: all 18 cases had bony erosion (demonstrated by canal widening, pedicle erosion, foraminal enlargement, or vertebral body scalloping)
2. Type III SMCs: may also cause bony erosion; appear on myelogram as intradural defect, may not appear on ICCT if they communicate with subarachnoid space which causes them to blend with adjacent subarachnoid space

76.2.4 Treatment

1. Type I SMCs: close ostium between cyst and subarachnoid space. Above sacrum, can usually be dissected from dura; occasionally fibrous adhesions prevent this
2. Type II SMCs: no pedicle, thus either partially resect and oversew cyst wall, or excise cyst and involved nerve root. Simple aspiration is not recommended
3. Type III SMCs: excise completely unless dense fibrous adhesions prevent this, in which case marsupialize cyst. Tend to recur if incompletely excised

76.3 Juxtafacet cysts of the lumbar spine

76.3.1 General information

The term juxtafacet cyst (JFC) was originated by Kao et al.[22] in 1974 and includes both synovial cysts (those having a synovial lining membrane) and ganglion cysts (those lacking synovial lining) adjacent to a spinal facet joint or arising from the ligamentum flavum. Distinction between these two types of cysts may be difficult without histology (see below) and is clinically unimportant.[23]

JFC occur primarily in the lumbar spine (although cysts in the cervical[24,25,26] and thoracic[27] spine have been described). They were first reported in 1880 by von Gruker during an autopsy,[28] and were first diagnosed clinically in 1968.[29] The etiology is unknown (possibilities include: synovial fluid extrusion from the joint capsule, latent growth of a developmental rest, myxoid degeneration and cyst formation in collagenous connective tissue…), increased motion seems to have a role in many cysts, and the role of trauma in the pathogenesis is debated[25,30] but probably plays a role in a small number (≈ 14%).[31] JFC are relatively rare, only 3 cases were identified in a series of 1,500 spinal CT exams,[32] but the frequency of diagnosis may be on the rise due to the widespread use of MRI and an increasing awareness of the condition.

76.3.2 Pathology

Cyst walls are composed of fibrous connective tissue of varying thickness and cellularity. There is usually no signs of infection or inflammation. There may be a synovial lining[33] (synovial cyst) or it may be absent[34] (ganglion cyst). The distinction between the two may be difficult,[23] possibly owing in part to the fact that fibroblasts in ganglion cysts may form an incomplete synovial-like lining.[35] Proliferation of small venules is seen in the connective tissue. Hemosiderin staining may be present, and may or may not be associated with a history of trauma.[31]

76.3.3 Clinical

The average age was 63 years in one series[31] and 58 years in a review of 54 cases in the literature[33] (range: 33–87) with a slight female preponderance in both series. Most occur in patients with severe spondylosis and facet joint degeneration,[34] 25% had degenerative spondylolisthesis.[31] L4–5 is the most common level.[31,36] They may be bilateral. Pain is the most common symptom, and is usually radicular. Some JFC may contribute to canal stenosis and can produce neurogenic claudication (p. 1100) [37] or on occasion a cauda equina syndrome. Symptoms may be more intermittent in nature than with firm compressive lesions, such as HLD. A sudden exacerbation in pain may be due to hemorrhage within the cyst. Some JFC may be asymptomatic.[38]

76.3.4 Differential diagnosis

Also see **Differential diagnosis, Sciatica** (p. 1410). Differentiating JFC from other masses relies largely on the appearance and location. Other distinguishing features include:

1. neurofibroma: unlikely to be calcified
2. free fragment of HLD: not cystic in appearance
3. epidural or nerve root metastases: not cystic
4. dural subarachnoid root sleeve dilatation (p. 1142)
5. arachnoid cyst (from arachnoid herniation through a dural defect): not associated with facet joint, margins thinner than JFC[39]
6. perineurial cysts (Tarlov's cyst): arise in space between perineurium and endoneurium, usually on sacral roots,[40] occasionally show delayed filling on myelography. Usually associated with remodelling of adjacent bone

76.3.5 Evaluation

Identifying a JFC pre-op helps the surgeon, as the approach differs slightly from that for HLD, and the cyst might otherwise be missed or unknowingly deflated and unnecessary time wasted afterwards trying to find a compressive lesion. Or, the unwitting surgeon may misinterpret the cyst as a "transdural disc extrusion" and needlessly open the dura. Pre-op diagnoses were incorrect in 30% of operated cases of JFC.[31]

Myelography: posterolateral filling defect (whereas most discs are situated anteriorly, an occasional fragment may migrate posterolaterally, whereas a JFC will always be posterolateral), often with a round extradural appearance.

CT scan: shows a low density epidural cystic lesion typically with a posterolateral juxtaarticular location. Some have calcified rim,[38] and some may have gas within.[41] Erosion of bony lamina is occasionally seen.[36,42]

MRI: variable findings (may be due to differing composition of cyst fluid: serous vs. proteinaceous[43]). Unenhanced signal characteristics of non-hemorrhagic JFC are very similar to CSF. Hemorrhagic JFC are hyperintense. MRI usually misses bony erosion.

76.3.6 Treatment

Optimal treatment is not known. There is one case report of a cyst that resolved spontaneously.[32] If symptoms persist with conservative treatment, some promote cyst aspiration or facet injection with steroids,[44] while most advocate surgical excision of the cyst.

Surgical treatment considerations: The cyst may be adherent to the dura. The cyst may also collapse during the surgical approach and may be missed. A JFC may serve as a marker for possible instability and should prompt an evaluation for the same. Some argue for performing a fusion since JFC may arise from instability, however, it appears that fusion is not required for a good result in many cases.[44] Therefore it is suggested that consideration for fusion be made on the basis of any instability and not merely on the basis of the presence of a JFC.

Minimally invasive spine surgery (MISS) has also been used for removal,[45] long-term follow-up is lacking. A 15 mm entry incision is made 1.5 cm lateral to midline.

Following surgical treatment, symptomatic JFCs may recur or may develop on the contralateral side.[31]

76

76.4 Syringomyelia

76.4.1 General information

Key concepts

- AKA syrinx. Cystic cavitation of the spinal cord
- 70% are associated with Chiari I malformation, 10% with basilar invagination. May also be posttraumatic or associated with tumor, infection...

- symptoms: progressive neurologic deterioration over months to years, usually affecting UE first
- diameter > 5 mm + associated edema predict a more rapid deterioration
- preferred treatment is directed at correcting the causative pathophysiology

AKA syrinx. Cystic cavitation of the spinal cord. Other terms not precisely defined include: hydrosyringomyelia, communicating or noncommunicating syringomyelia.

Syringobulbia: Rostral extension into brainstem (usually medulla). May present with (bilateral) peri-oral tingling and numbness, due to compression of the spinal trigeminal tracts as the fibers decussate.

76.4.2 Etiologies

Primary syringomyelia

This term is used differently by different authors.[46] Herein, refers to syrinx in the absence of identifiable cause

Secondary syringomyelia

Most cases are thought to be secondary to partial obstruction of the spinal subarachnoid space.[46] Unanswered question: Why then do patients with varying degrees of degenerative cervical spinal stenosis generally not get syringomyelia? Etiologies include:

1. Chiari I malformation: the most common cause ofsyrinx (p.277)
2. postinflammatory
   a) postinfectious
      - granulomatous meningitides (TB and fungal)
      - postoperative meningitis, especially after intradural procedure
   b) chemical or other sterile inflammations
      - rarely after SAH
      - after myelography: especially with older oil-based agents no longer in use
3. posttraumatic: also see below
   a) with severe posttraumatic kyphotic deformity: e.g. with retropulsed bone, scarring…
   b) arachnoid scarring without recognized trauma
   c) severe injury to spinal cord and/or its coverings. Blood may be a contributing factor

✖ the older concept of syrinx developing as a coalescence of foci of traumatic hematomyelia has not been borne out

1. postsurgical: has been identified many years after uncomplicated intradural neoplasm removal (e.g. neurofibromas)
2. basilar arachnoiditis:
   a) idiopathic
   b) postinfectious: see above
3. basilar impression, with constriction of the foramen magnum (p.217)
4. associated with spinal tumors: this is distinct from a tumor cyst
5. associated with disc protrusion:
6. cerebellar ectopia
7. Dandy Walker syndrome

76.4.3 Epidemiology

See reference.[47]

Prevalence of non-posttraumatic syringomyelia: 8.4 cases/100,000 population. Usually presents between ages 20–50.

Associated clinical syndromes are shown in ▶ Table 76.4.

76.4.4 Pathophysiology

Major theories of formation of the cyst:

1. hydrodynamic ("water-hammer") theory of Gardner: systolic pulsations are transmitted with each heartbeat from the intracranial cavity to the central canal. Has been essentially disproven using MRI[48]

Table 76.4 Conditions associated with syringomyelia

Condition	%[a]
Chiari type 1 malformation	70
basilar invagination	10
intramedullary spinal cord tumors	4
[a]percent of cases of syringomyelia	

2. Williams' ("craniospinal dissociation") theory: maneuvers that raise CSF pressure (valsalva, coughing...) cause "hydrodissection" through the spinal cord tissue. May be more common in noncommunicating syringomyelia
3. Heiss-Oldfield theory: occlusion at the foramen magnum causes CSF pulsations during cardiac systole to be transmitted through the Virchow-Robin spaces which increases the extracellular fluid which coalesce to form a syrinx[47] (i.e. through the cord parenchyma)

76.4.5 Clinical

Presentation: highly variable. Usually progresses over months to years, with a more rapid deterioration early that gradually slows.[47] Initially, pain, weakness, atrophy and loss of pain & temperature sensation in the upper extremities (with cervical syrinx) is common. Myelopathy that progresses slowly over years ensues.

76.4.6 Characteristic syndrome

(nonspecific for intramedullary spinal cord pathology):
1. sensory loss (similar to central cord syndrome) with a suspended ("cape") dissociated sensory loss (loss of pain and temperature sensation with preserved touch and joint position sense → painless ulcerations from unperceived injuries and/or burns)
2. pain: commonly cervical and occipital. Dysesthetic pain often occurs in the distribution of the sensory loss[47]
3. weakness: lower motor neuron weakness of the hand and arm
4. painless (neurogenic) arthropathies (Charcot's joints) especially in the shoulder & neck due to loss of pain & temperature sensation: seen in < 5%

76.4.7 Evaluation

76

Prior to the CT/MRI era, diagnosis relied on myelography or on autopsy.

MRI: defines anatomy in sagittal as well as axial plane. Test of choice. Cervical & thoracic spine and brain MRI (without & with contrast, to include craniocervical junction) should be obtained. Syringomyelic cavities may be complex, with noncommunicating channels (more common with posttraumatic syrinx).

CT: low attenuation area within cord seen on either plain CT or myelogram/CT (with water soluble contrast).

Myelogram: rarely used alone (usually performed in conjunction with CT). When used alone: often normal (false negative), some → complete block at level of syrinx; iodine contrast studies may show fusiform widening of spinal cord, whereas air contrast studies may show collapse of the cord.[49] Dye may slowly leach into the cyst.

EMG: no characteristic findings, but may be useful to R/O other conditions that may be responsible for symptoms (e.g. peripheral neuropathy causing paresthesias).

76.4.8 Distinguishing from similar entities

1. tumor cyst:
   a) especially with intramedullary spinal cord gliomas. Tumors may secrete fluid, or may cause microcysts that eventually coalesce. Most (but not all) intramedullary tumors will enhance with IV contrast on MRI
   b) tumor cyst fluid is usually highly proteinaceous, syrinx fluid usually has the same MRI characteristics as CSF (NB: true syrinx can occur with tumor)

2. central spinal canal:
   a) residual central spinal canal: the central canal is present within the spinal cord at birth and normally gradually involutes with age.[50] Persistence of the canal is a normal variant. Characteristic imaging features:
      - linear or fusiform on sagittal MRI
      - ≤ 2–4 mm in maximal width
      - may be singular, or there may be several discontinuous regions in the rostral-caudal direction
      - perfectly round in cross-section and centrally located on axial MRI
      - if IV contrast is given, there should be no enhancement
   b) simple dilatation of the central canal with ependymal cell lining has sometimes been called hydromyelia, but this usage is ambiguous

76.4.9 Management

General information

For an incidentally discovered syrinx (i.e. asymptomatic and no neurologic deficit) with no identified etiology, if the size remains stable over 2–3 years of observation, F/U studies at 2–3 year intervals can be done if there are no changes in symptoms.

Surgical treatment

Intervention is considered for symptomatic lesions (not all are symptomatic). If an underlying cause cannot be determined, it may be very difficult to treat a very small syrinx directly (however, these are unlikely to be causing reversible symptoms).

Options include:

1. current philosophy is to treat the underlying pathophysiology (and to use syrinx draining procedures as second choice when this is not feasible)
   a) posterior decompression: procedure of choice when posterior anomalies (e.g. Chiari malformation) are present
   b) decompression if a different site of compression is identified
2. shunts:
   a) disadvantages:
      - complication rate: 16%
      - clinical stabilization rate: 54% at 10 yrs
      - may produce traction on spinal cord with potential for further injury
      - prone to obstruction: 50% at 4 years
      - does not correct underlying pathophysiology and so syrinx may recur
   b) indications: cases of diffuse arachnoiditis (e.g. following tuberculous or chemical meningitis) where the obstruction extends over many levels, and syrinx diameter > 3–4 mm
   c) K or T tube drainage. Choice of distal sites includes:
      - peritoneum[51] (difficult in cervical region): e.g. Edwards-Barbaro syringoperitoneal shunt (distributed by Integra)
      - pleural cavity
      - subarachnoid space (e.g. Heyer-Schulte-Pudenz system): requires normal CSF flow in subarachnoid space, therefore cannot use in arachnoiditis
3. percutaneous aspiration of the cyst[52] (may be used repeatedly)
4. ✖ no longer recommended:
   a) plugging the obex with muscle, teflon or other material
   b) opening the subarachnoid space & removing inferior tonsils
   c) syringostomy: usually fails to remain patent, therefore using a stent or a shunt (syringosubarachnoid or syringoperitoneal) is recommended

Technical considerations:

1. intraoperative ultrasound is often helpful for:
   a) localizing the cyst
   b) assessing for septations (to avoid shunting only part of cyst)
2. if Chiari malformation is not present, consider syringosubarachnoid shunt as the initial procedure. If this fails, then syringoperitoneal shunt may be inserted
3. Rhoton suggests performing the myelotomy in the dorsal root entry zone (DREZ), between the lateral and posterior columns (instead of the midline as with a tumor) because this is consistently

76

the thinnest part and there is usually already an upper extremity proprioceptive deficit from the syrinx.[53(p 1317)] There is ≈ 10% incidence of posterior column dysfunction with shunting
4. with syringosubarachnoid shunts, be sure the distal shunt tip is subarachnoid (and not just subdural) or else it will not function
5. with syringopleural shunt, the pleural opening can be made *posteriorly*, adjacent to one of the ribs as described for ventriculopleural shunt (p. 1515)
6. for peritoneal terminus of shunt: the proximal shunt may be placed in the syrinx with the patient in the prone position, and the peritoneal end of the catheter may be tunneled to an intermediate position in the flank in the midaxillary line where it can be coiled into a small subcutaneous pouch which can be temporarily closed with staples and dressed with Tegaderm. After the spinal incision is closed, the patient can be undraped and rotated to the supine position, the Tegaderm is removed, and the abdomen and the flank incision are prepped, the staples are removed and the catheter is retrieved from the sub-Q pocket and tunneled to the peritoneal opening that is made at this time. A small bump (rolled sheet...) to elevate the flank may be employed in both parts of the operation to facilitate access to the pouch

76.4.10 Outcome

Assessing treatment results is difficult due to rarity of the condition, variability of natural history (which may arrest spontaneously), and too short follow-up.[54] Enthusiasm for direct treatment (shunts, fenestration...) is low among neurosurgeons because of the perceived poor response and risk of iatrogenic neurologic worsening. However, this may remain as the only option for a deteriorating patient and positive outcomes do occur.[55]

76.5 Posttraumatic syringomyelia

76.5.1 General information

Posttraumatic syringomyelia (PTSx) may follow significant spinal trauma (with or without clinical spinal cord injury). Includes penetrating injury or non-penetrating "violent" trauma to the spinal cord (injuries such as post-spinal anesthesia or following thoracic disc herniation are not included).

76.5.2 Epidemiology

Often a late presentation following spinal cord injury, therefore incidence is higher in series with longer follow-up. Incidence increasing with increasing survival following spinal cord injury and with increasing use of MRI. Range: ≈ 0.3–3% of cord injured patients (see ▶ Table 76.5).

In a large number of patients followed via multicenter cooperative data bank, there were fewer cases of syrinx following cervical injuries than following thoracic injuries[57] (may be artifactual since patients with lower lesions may be more aware of ascending levels).

Latency following spinal cord injury:
1. latency to symptoms: 3 mos to 34 yrs (mean 9 yrs) (earlier in complete cord lesions than incomplete: mean 7.5 vs. 9.9 yrs)
2. latency to diagnosis: up to 12 yrs (mean 2.8 yrs) after onset of new symptoms

Table 76.5 Incidence of posttraumatic syringomyelia

Type of injury	No./risk[a]	Incidence
all spinal cord injury patients	30/951	3.2%
complete quadriplegics	14/177	7.9%
incomplete quadriplegics	4/181	4.5%
complete paraplegics	4/282	1.7%
incomplete paraplegics	4/181	2.2%

[a]number occurring over number at risk in 951 patients followed for 11 years[56]

Table 76.6 Presentation (in 30 SCI patients with syrinx[56])

Symptom	Initial	At time of diagnosis
pain[a]	57%	70%
numbness	27%	40%
increased motor deficit	23%	40%
increased spasticity	10%	23%
increased sweating (hyperhidrosis)	3%	13%
autonomic dysreflexia	3%	3%
no symptoms	7%	7%
Signs	**Frequency**	
ascending sensory level	93%	
depressed tendon reflexes	77%	
increased motor deficits	40%	

[a]pain is often quite severe, and unrelieved with analgesics[59]

76.5.3 Clinical

The presentation of patients with PTSx is shown in ▶ Table 76.6. The late appearance of *upper* extremity symptoms in a paraplegic patient should raise a high index of suspicion of posttraumatic syringomyelia.[58]

Hyperhidrosis may be the only feature of *descending* syringomyelia in patients with complete cord lesions.[60] For the differential diagnosis, see Delayed deterioration following spinal cord injuries (p. 1019).

76.5.4 Evaluation

One end of the cavity is often found at a site of spinal column fracture or abnormal angulation.

76.5.5 Management

General information

Many authors advocate early surgical drainage of cyst as a means of reducing increased delayed deficit.[61] Some authors feel that aside from disturbing sensory symptoms, that motor loss was infrequent and therefore conservative management is indicated in most cases.[62]

76

Medical

Managed non-surgically: 31% remained stable, 68% progressed over yrs (longer F/U in latter).

Surgical

There is probably no benefit in operating on a patient with a small syrinx.[56]

Surgical options

Same as in Communicating syringomyelia, with the following differences:

1. cord transection (cordectomy)[63]: an option in *complete* injuries only
2. plugging the obex is probably *not* indicated (controversial in congenital syrinx)

Outcome

In 9 PTSx patients treated with syringosubarachnoid shunt[56]: pain relieved in all 9 (1 only slightly), motor recovery in 5/8, improved tendon reflex in 1/10. Some post-op complications in 9 patients included: 1 incomplete lesion became complete, 1 sensorimotor deterioration, transient pain in 3.

Most results are good for radicular symptoms, with dubious efficacy for autonomic symptoms or spasticity.

76.6 Spinal cord herniation (idiopathic)

76.6.1 General information

Rare. Spinal cord herniates though a defect in the dura usually located anteriorly or anterolaterally between T2–8.[64] Bone erosion anterior to the dural defect may occasionally be seen. Frequently associated with a calcified disc fragment which theoretically may have gradually eroded through the dura.

76.6.2 Differential diagnosis

Main DDx is with dorsal arachnoid cyst (p.1407). Both result in increased subarachnoid space posterior to the cord, and a ventral kinking of the spinal cord. Contiguous CSF pulsation artifact on MRI can be seen with cord herniation, whereas an arachnoid cyst tends to interrupt this.

76.6.3 Presentation

Commonly presents as an incomplete Brown-Séquard syndrome (with relative sparing of posterior columns). Symptoms may be due to distortion of the spinal cord, but vascular injury may also play a role.

76.6.4 Surgery

Requires a lateral or anterolateral approach to minimize spinal cord manipulation (p.1061). The dural defect is widened which usually results in reduction of the spinal cord herniation. A sling of dural substitute can then be slid anterior to the cord to prevent reherniation.

76.7 Spinal epidural lipomatosis (SEL)

76.7.1 General information

Hypertrophy of epidural fat. Most commonly seen with prolonged exogenous steroid therapy (in 75% of cases[65]) usually moderate to high dosage for years,[66] but may also be associated with: Cushing's disease, Cushing's syndrome, obesity,[67] hypothyroidism or may be idiopathic.[68] Male: female = 3:1.[66]

Back pain usually precedes all other symptoms. Progressive LE weakness and sensory changes are common. Sphincter disturbance occurs but is rare. SEL is most common in the thoracic spine (≈ 60% of cases), the rest are in the lumbar spine (no cases reported in cervical spine).

76 It is often very difficult to differentiate the patient with increased epidural fat (even to the point that CSF may be obliterated at the levels of involvement) that is not causing symptoms, from those cases where the exuberant fat is responsible for the findings.

76.7.2 Evaluation

CT: density of adipose tissue is extremely low (-80 to -120 Hounsfield units)[69] which distinguishes SEL from most other lesions (except lipoma).

MRI: signal follows fat (high signal on T1WI, intermediate on T2WI). Suggested diagnostic criteria: epidural adipose should be > 7 mm thick to be considered SEL.[67,70]

76.7.3 Treatment

In those patients who can be weaned off steroids and lose weight, surgery may be avoided in some cases.[71] If SEL is related to obesity, weight loss alone can be successful.

Surgery is indicated for symptomatic patients in whom the above interventions are unsuccessful or not feasible. An effort to normalize cortisol levels in those with endogenous hypercortisolism (Cushing's disease...) should be made before laminectomy is performed. Due to potential complications and slow growth of the tissue, the decision to operate should be made with caution.

Surgery usually consists of laminectomy with removal of adipose tissue. Occasionally repeat surgery is needed for reaccumulation of adipose tissue.

76.7.4 Outcome

Surgery usually results in significant improvement.[70] Idiopathic cases may fare better than those due to steroid excess. Cauda equina compression responds better than thoracic myelopathy.

Complications rates may be higher than expected in part due to medical comorbidities. Fessler et al.[72] reported 22% 1-year mortality.

76.8 Craniocervical junction and upper cervical spine abnormalities

76.8.1 Associated conditions

Also see Axis (C2) vertebra lesions (p. 1391).

Abnormalities in this region are seen in a number of conditions including:

1. rheumatoid arthritis (p. 1134)
2. traumatic & post-traumatic: including fractures of odontoid, occipital condyles…
3. ankylosing spondylitis (p. 1123): may result in fusion of the entire spine which spares the occipitoatlantal and/or atlantoaxial joints which can lead to instability there
4. congenital conditions:
   a) Chiari malformations (p. 277)
   b) Klippel-Feil syndrome (p. 271)
   c) Down syndrome
   d) atlantoaxial dislocation (AAD)
   e) occipitalization of the atlas: seen in 40% of congenital AAD[73]
   f) Morquio syndrome (a mucopolysaccharidosis): atlantoaxial subluxation occurs due to hypoplasia of the odontoid process and joint laxity
5. neoplasms: metastatic (p. 815) or primary
6. infection
7. following surgical procedures of the skull base or cervical spine: e.g. transoral resection of the odontoid

76.8.2 Types of abnormalities

Abnormalities include:

1. basilar impression/invagination: as with Paget's disease
2. atlanto-occipital dislocation
3. atlantoaxial dislocation
4. occipitalization of the atlas, or thin or deficient posterior arch of atlas[74]

76.8.3 Treatment

Fractures of the occipital condyles, atlas or axis are usually adequately treated with external immobilization; also see Occipital condyle fractures (p. 966). Because traumatic occipitocervical dislocations are usually fatal, optimal treatment is not well defined. Occipitalization of the atlas may be treated by creating an "artificial atlas" from the base of the occiput and wiring to that.[74]

Indications and techniques are outlined in Atlantoaxial fusion (C1–2 arthrodesis) (p. 1479).

References

[1] Youmans JR. Neurological Surgery. Philadelphia 1982
[2] Black P. Spinal vascular malformations: an historical perspective. Neurosurg Focus. 2006; 21
[3] Di Chiro G, Doppman J, Ommaya AK. Selective arteriography of arteriovenous aneurysms of spinal cord. Radiology. 1967; 88:1065–1077
[4] Djindjian R. Embolization of angiomas of the spinal cord. Surg Neurol. 1975; 4:411–420
[5] Kendall BE, Logue V. Spinal epidural angiomatous malformations draining into intrathecal veins. Neuroradiology. 1977; 13:181–189
[6] Oldfield EH, Di Chiro G, Quindlen EA, Rieth KG, Doppman JL. Successful treatment of a group of spinal cord arteriovenous malformations by interruption of dural fistula. J Neurosurg. 1983; 59:1019–1030
[7] Heros RC, Debrun GM, Ojemann RG, Lasjaunias PL, Naessens PJ. Direct spinal arteriovenous fistula: a new type of spinal AVM. Case report. J Neurosurg. 1986; 64:134–139
[8] Rosenblum B, Oldfield EH, Doppman JL, Di Chiro G. Spinal Arteriovenous Malformations: A Comparison of Dural Arteriovenous Fistulas and Intradural

76

AVM's in 81 Patients. J Neurosurg. 1987; 67:795–802
[9] Gueguen B, Merland JJ, Riche MC, Rey A. Vascular Malformations of the Spinal Cord: Intrathecal Perimedullary Arteriovanous Fistulas Fed by Medullary Arteries. Neurology. 1987; 37:969–979
[10] Mourier KL, Gobin YP, George B, et al. Intradural Perimedullary Arteriovenous Fistulae: Results of Surgical and Endovascular Treatment in a Series of 35 Cases. Neurosurgery. 1993; 32:885–891
[11] Strugar J, Chyatte D. In Situ Photocoagulation of Spinal Dural Arteriovenous Malformations Using the Nd:YAG Laser. J Neurosurg. 1992; 77:571–574
[12] Bederson JB, Spetzler RF. Pathophysiology of Type I Spinal Dural Arteriovenous Malformations. BNI Quarterly. 1996; 12:23–32
[13] Rodesch G, Hurth M, Alvarez H, Tadie M, Lasjaunias P. Classification of spinal cord arteriovenous shunts: proposal for a reappraisal–the Bicetre experience with 155 consecutive patients treated between 1981 and 1999. Neurosurgery. 2002; 51:374–9; discussion 379-80
[14] Spetzler RF, Detwiler PW, Riina HA, Porter RW. Modified classification of spinal cord vascular lesions. J Neurosurg. 2002; 96:145–156
[15] Aminoff MJ, Logue V. The Prognosis of Patients with Spinal Vascular Malformations. Brain. 1974; 97:211–218
[16] Tobin WD, Layton DD. The Diagnosis and Natural History of Spinal Cord Arteriovenous Malformations. Mayo Clin Proc. 1976; 51:637–646
[17] Wirth FP, Post KD, Di Chiro G, et al. Foix-Alajouanine Disease. Spontaneous Thrombosis of a Spinal Cord Arteriovenous Malformation: A Case Report. Neurology. 1970; 20:1114–1118
[18] Criscuolo GR, Oldfield EH, Doppman JL. Reversible Acute and Subacute Myelopathy in Patients with Dural Arteriovenous Fistulas: Foix-Alajouanine Syndrome Reconsidered. J Neurosurg. 1989; 70:354–359
[19] Barnwell SL, Dowd CF, Davis RL, Wilson CB, et al. Cryptic Vascular Malformations of the Spinal Cord: Diagnosis by Magnetic Resonance Imaging and Outcome of Surgery. J Neurosurg. 1990; 72:403–407
[20] Anson JA, Spetzler RF. Interventional Neuroradiology for Spinal Pathology. Clin Neurosurg. 1991; 39:388–417
[21] Nabors MW, Pait TG, Byrd EB, et al. Updated Assessment and Current Classification of Spinal Meningeal Cysts. J Neurosurg. 1988; 68:366–377
[22] Kao CC, Winkler SS, Turner JH. Synovial Cyst of Spinal Facet. Case Report. J Neurosurg. 1974; 41:372–376
[23] Freidberg SR, Fellows T, Thomas CB, Mancall AC. Experience with Symptomatic Epidural Cysts. Neurosurgery. 1994; 34:989–993
[24] Cartwright MJ, Nehls DG, Carrion CA, Spetzler RF. Synovial Cyst of a Cervical Facet Joint: Case Report. Neurosurgery. 1985; 16:850–852
[25] Onofrio BM, Mih AD. Synovial Cysts of the Spine. Neurosurgery. 1988; 22:642–647
[26] Goffin J, Wilms G, Plets C, et al. Synovial Cyst at the C1-C2 Junction. Neurosurgery. 1992; 30:914–916
[27] Lopes NMM, Aesse FF, Lopes DK. Compression of Thoracic Nerve Root by a Facet Joint Synovial Cyst: Case Report. Surg Neurol. 1992; 38:338–340
[28] Heary RF, Stellar S, Fobben ES. Preoperative Diagnosis of an Extradural Cyst Arising from a Spinal Facet Joint: Case Report. Neurosurgery. 1992; 30:415–418
[29] Kao CC, Uihlein A, Bickel WH, et al. Lumbar Intraspinal Extradural Ganglion Cyst. J Neurosurg. 1968; 29:168–172
[30] Franck JI, King RB, Petro GR, Kanzer MD. A Posttraumatic Lumbar Spinal Synovial Cyst. Case Report. J Neurosurg. 1987; 66:293–296
[31] Sabo RA, Tracy PT, Weinger JM. A Series of 60 Juxtafacet Cysts: Clinical Presentation, the Role of Spinal Instability, and Treatment. J Neurosurg. 1996; 85:560–565
[32] Mercader J, Gomez JM, Cardenal C. Intraspinal Synovial Cyst: Diagnosis by CT. Follow-Up and Spontaneous Remission. Neuroradiology. 1985; 27:346–348
[33] Liu SS, Williams KD, Drayer BP, Spetzler RF, Sonntag VKH. Synovial Cysts of the Lumbosacral Spine: Diagnosis by MR Imaging. AJNR. 1989; 10:1239–1242
[34] Silbergleit R, Gebarski SS, Brunberg JA, McGillicuddy J, Blaivas M. Lumbar Synovial Cysts: Correlation of Myelographic, CT, MR, and Pathologic Findings. AJNR. 1990; 11:777–779
[35] Soren A. Pathogenesis and Treatment of Ganglion. Clin Orthop. 1966; 48:173–179
[36] Gorey MT, Hyman RA, Black KS, et al. Lumbar Synovial Cysts Eroding Bone. AJNR. 1992; 13:161–163
[37] Conrad M, Pitkethly D. Bilateral Synovial Cysts Creating Spinal Stenosis. J Comput Assist Tomogr. 1987; 11:196–197
[38] Hemminghytt S, Daniels DL, Williams ML, et al. Intraspinal Synovial Cysts: Natural History and Diagnosis by CT. Radiology. 1982; 145:375–376
[39] Budris DM. Intraspinal Lumbar Synovial Cyst. Orthopedics. 1991; 14:618–620
[40] Tarlov IM. Spinal Perineurial and Meningeal Cysts. J Neurol Neurosurg Psychiatry. 1970; 33:833–843
[41] Schulz EE, West WL, Hinshaw DB, Johnson DR. Gas in a Lumbar Extradural Juxtaarticular Cyst: Sign of Synovial Origin. Am J Radiol. 1984; 143:875–876
[42] Munz M, Tampieri D, Robitaille Y, Bertrand G. Spinal Synovial Cyst: Case Report Using Magnetic Resonance Imaging. Surg Neurol. 1990; 34:431–434
[43] Martin D, Awwad E, Sundaram M. Lumbar Ganglion Cyst Causing Radiculopathy. Orthopedics. 1990; 13:1182–1183
[44] Kurz LT, Garfin SR, Unger AS, et al. Intraspinal Synovial Cyst Causing Sciatica. J Bone Joint Surg. 1985; 67A:865–871
[45] Sehati N, Khoo LT, Holly LT. Treatment of lumbar synovial cysts using minimally invasive surgical techniques. Neurosurg Focus. 2006; 20:E2–E6
[46] Batzdorf U. Primary spinal syringomyelia. Invited submission from the joint section meeting on disorders of the spine and peripheral nerves, March 2005. J Neurosurg Spine. 2005; 3:429–435
[47] Heiss JD, Oldfield EH. Pathophysiology and treatment of syringomyelia. Contemp Neurosurg. 2003; 25:1–8
[48] Oldfield EH, Muraszko K, Shawker TH, Patronas NJ. Pathophysiology of Syringomyelia Associated with Chiari I Malformation of the Cerebellar Tonsils. J Neurosurg. 1994; 80:3–15
[49] Williams B, Terry AF, Jones F, et al. Syringomyelia as a Sequel to Traumatic Paraplegia. Paraplegia. 1981; 19:67–80
[50] Yasui K, Hashizume Y, Yoshida M, Kameyama T, Sobue G. Age-related morphologic changes of the central canal of the human spinal cord. Acta Neuropathol (Berl). 1999; 97:253–259
[51] Suzuki M, Davis C, Symon L, et al. Syringoperitoneal Shunt for Treatment of Cord Cavitation. J Neurol Neurosurg Psychiatry. 1985; 48:620–627
[52] Booth AE, Kendall BE. Percutaneous Aspiration of Cystic Lesions of the Spinal Cord. J Neurosurg. 1970; 33:140–144
[53] Schmidek HH, Sweet WH. Operative Neurosurgical Techniques. New York 1982
[54] Logue V, Edwards MR. Syringomyelia and its Surgical Treatment. J Neurol Neurosurg Psychiatry. 1981; 44:273–284
[55] Phillips TW, Kindt GW. Syringoperitoneal shunt for syringomyelia: a preliminary report. Surg Neurol. 1981; 16:462–466
[56] Rossier AB, Foo D, Shillito J, et al. Posttraumatic Cervical Syringomyelia. Brain. 1985; 108:439–461
[57] Vernon JD, Chir B, Silver JR, et al. Posttraumatic Syringomyelia. Paraplegia. 1982; 20:339–364
[58] Griffiths ER, McCormick CC. Posttraumatic Syringomyelia (Cystic Myelopathy). Paraplegia. 1981; 19:81–88
[59] Shannon N, Symon L, Logue V, et al. Clinical Features, Investigation and Treatment of Posttraumatic Syringomyelia. J Neurol Neurosurg Psychiatry. 1981; 44:35–42

[60] Stanworth PA. The Significance of Hyperhidrosis in Patients with Posttraumatic Syringomyelia. Paraplegia. 1982; 20:282–287
[61] Dworkin GE, Staas WE. Posttraumatic Syringomyelia. Arch Phys Med Rehabil. 1985; 66:329–331
[62] Watson N. Ascending Cystic Degeneration of the Cord After Spinal Cord Injury. Paraplegia. 1981; 19:89–95
[63] Durward QJ, Rice GP, Ball MJ, et al. Selective Spinal Cordectomy: Clinicopathological Correlation. J Neurosurg. 1982; 56:359–367
[64] Darbar A, Krishnamurthy S, Holsapple JW, Hodge CJ.Jr. Ventral thoracic spinal cord herniation: frequently misdiagnosed entity. Spine. 2006; 31: E600–E605
[65] George WE, Wilmot M, Greenhouse A, et al. Medical Management of Steroid-Induced Epidural Lipomatosis. N Engl J Med. 1983; 308:316–319
[66] Fassett DR, Schmidt MH. Spinal epidural lipomatosis: a review of its causes and recommendations for treatment. Neurosurg Focus. 2004; 16
[67] Kumar K, Nath RK, Nair CPV, Tchang SP. Symptomatic Epidural Lipomatosis Secondary to Obesity: Case Report. J Neurosurg. 1996; 85:348–350
[68] Haddad SF, Hitchon PW, Godersky. Idiopathic and Glucocorticoid-Induced Spinal Epidural Lipomatosis. J Neurosurg. 1991; 74:38–42
[69] Roy-Camille R, Mazel C, Husson JL, et al. Symptomatic spinal epidural lipomatosis induced by a long-term steroid treatment. Review of the iterature and report of two additional cases. Spine. 1991; 16:1365–1371
[70] Robertson SC, Traynelis VC, Follett KA, et al. Idiopathic spinal epidural lipomatosis. Neurosurgery. 1997; 41:68–75
[71] Beges C, Rousselin B, Chevrot A, Godefroy D, Vallee C, Berenbaum F, Deshays C, Amor B. Epidural lipomatosis. Interest of magnetic resonance imaging in a weight-reduction treated case. Spine. 1994; 19:251–254
[72] Fessler RD, Johnson DL, Brown FD, et al. Epidural lipomatosis in steroid-treated patients. Spine. 1992; 17:183–188
[73] Sinh G. Congenital Atlanto-Axial Dislocation. Neurosurg Rev. 1983; 6:211–220
[74] Jain VK, Mittal P, Banerji D, et al. Posterior Occipitoaxial Fusion for Atlantoaxial Dislocation Associated with Occipitalized Axis. J Neurosurg. 1996; 84:559–564

Part XVII

SAH and Aneurysms

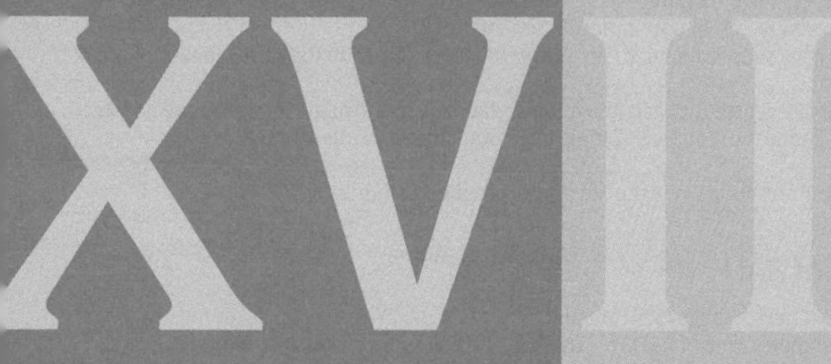

77 Introduction and General Information, Grading, Medical Management, Special Conditions

77.1 Introduction and overview

77.1.1 Definition

Blood in the subarachnoid space, i.e. between the arachnoid membrane and the pia mater.

77.1.2 Miscellaneous facts about SAH

1. May be post-traumatic or spontaneous. Trauma is the most common cause
2. Most cases of spontaneous SAH are due to aneurysmal rupture
3. peak age for aneurysmal SAH is 55–60 years, ≈ 20% of cases occur between ages 15–45 yrs[1]
4. 30% of aneurysmal SAHs occurs during sleep
5. sentinel headaches that precede the SAH-associated ictus have been reported by 10-50% of patients and most commonly occur within 2-8 weeks before overt SAH.[2,3,4]
6. headache is lateralized in 30%, most to the side of the aneurysm
7. SAH is complicated by intracerebral hemorrhage in 20–40%, by intraventricular hemorrhage in 13–28% (p. 1192) and by subdural blood in 2–5%; usually due to p-comm aneurysm when over convexity, or distal anterior intracerebral artery (DACA) aneurysm with interhemispheric subdural (p. 1211)
8. soft evidence suggests that rupture incidence is higher in spring and autumn
9. patients ≥ 70 yrs age have a higher proportion with a severe neurologic grade[5]
10. seizures may occur in up to 20% of patients after SAH, most commonly in the first 24 hours and are associated with ICH, HTN and aneurysm location (MCA & acomm)[6,7]

77.1.3 Outcome of aneurysmal SAH

1. 10–15% of patients die before reaching medical care
2. mortality is 10% within first few days
3. 30-day mortality rate was 46% in one series,[8] and in others over half the patients died within 2 weeks of their SAH[9]
4. median mortality rate in epidemiologicval studies from U.S. has been 32% vs. 44% in Europe and 27% in Japan (may be an underestimate based on underreported prehospital death)[10]
5. causes of mortality
   a) 25% die as a result of medical complications of SAH[11]
      - neurogenic pulmonary edema (p. 1178)
      - neurogenic stunned myocardium (p. 1177)
   b) about 8% die from progressive deterioration from the initial hemorrhage[12 (p 27)]
6. among patients surviving the initial hemorrhage treated without surgery, rebleeding is the major cause of morbidity and mortality (p. 1167), the risk is ~ 15–20% within 2 weeks. The goal of early surgery is to reduce this risk (p. 1200)
7. of those reaching neurosurgical care, vasospasm (p. 1178) kills 7%, and causes severe deficit in another 7%[13]
8. about ≈ 30% of survivors have moderate to severe disability,[14] with rates of persistent dependence estimated between 8-20% in population based studies[10]
9. ≈ 66% of those who have successful aneurysm clipping never return to the same quality of life as before the SAH[14,15]
10. patients ≥ 70 yrs age fare worse for each neurologic grade.[5] A multivariate analysis revealed age and WFNS grade to be most predictive of long-term outcome, regardless of treatment modality[16]
11. the severity of clinical presentation is the strongest prognostic indicator

77.2 Etiologies of SAH

Etiologies of subarachnoid hemorrhage (SAH) include[17]:

1. trauma: the most common cause of SAH.[18,19] In all of the following discussion, only non-traumatic (i.e. "spontaneous") SAH will be considered

2. "spontaneous SAH"
   a) ruptured intracranial aneurysms: **75–80%** of spontaneous SAHs (p. 1191)
   b) cerebral arteriovenous malformation (AVM): 4–5% of cases; AVMs more commonly cause ICH & IVH than SAH (p. 1239)
   c) certain vasculitides that involve the CNS, see Vasculitis and vasculopathy (p. 195)
   d) rarely due to tumor (many case reports[20,21,22,23,24,25,26,27,28,29,30,31])
   e) cerebral artery dissection (may also be post-traumatic)
      - carotid artery (p. 1324)
      - vertebral artery: may cause intraventricular blood (especially 4th and third ventricle) (p. 1325)
   f) rupture of a small superficial artery
   g) rupture of an infundibulum (p. 1161)
   h) coagulation disorders:
      - iatrogenic or bleeding dyscrasias
      - thrombocytopenia
   i) dural sinus thrombosis
   j) spinal AVM: usually cervical or upper thoracic (p. 1140)
   k) cortical subarachnoid hemorrhage
   l) pretruncal nonaneurysmal SAH (p. 1231)
   m) rarely reported with some drugs: e.g. cocaine (p. 207)
   n) sickle cell anemia
   o) pituitary apoplexy (p. 720)
   p) no cause can be determined in 14–22% (p. 1230)

77.3 Incidence

Estimated annual rate of aneurysmal SAH in the United States: 9.7-14.5 per 100,000 population.[32,33] Reported rates are lower in South and Central America,[34] and higher in Japan and Finland.[35] Incident of SAH increases with age (avg. age of onset > 50[33,36,37,38]; tends to be higher in women (1.24 times higher than men),[34] and appears to be higher in African Americans and Hispanics (compared to Caucasians).[32,39,40]

77.4 Risk factors for SAH

See references.[17,41]

1. behavioral
   - hypertension
   - cigarette smoking[42]
   - alcohol abuse
   - sympathomimetic drugs (p. 207)
2. gender and race (see above)
3. history of cerebral aneurysm
   - ruptured aneurysm
   - unruptured aneurysm (esp. those that are symptomatic, larger in size and located in posterior circulation)
   - morphology: bottleneck shape[43] and increased ratio of size of aneurysm to parent vessel have been associated with increased risk of rupture[44,45]
4. family history of aneurysms (at least 1 first-degree family member and especially if ≥ 2 are affected)
5. genetic syndromes
   - autosomal dominant polycystic kidney disease
   - type IV Ehlers-Danlos syndrome
6. pregnancy – there does not appear to be an increased risk of aneurysmal SAH in pregnancy, delivery, and puerperium[46,47]

77.5 Clinical features

77.5.1 Symptoms of SAH

Sudden onset of severe H/A (see below), usually with vomiting, syncope (apoplexy), neck pain (meningismus), and photophobia. If there is LOC, patient may subsequently recover consciousness.[48] Focal cranial nerve deficits may occur (e.g. third nerve palsy from aneurysmal compression of the third cranial nerve, causing diplopia and/or ptosis). Low back pain may develop due to irritation of lumbar nerve roots by dependent blood.

77.5.2 Headache

The most common symptom, present in up to 97% of cases. Usually severe (classic description: "the worst headache of my life") and sudden in onset (paroxysmal). The H/A may clear and the patient may not seek medical attention (referred to as a sentinel hemorrhage or headache, or warning headache; they occur in 30–60% of patients presenting with SAH). If severe or accompanied by reduced level of consciousness, most patients present for medical evaluation. Patients with H/A due to minor hemorrhages will have blood on CT or LP. However, warning headaches may also occur without SAH and may be due to aneurysmal enlargement or to hemorrhage confined within the aneurysmal wall.[49] Warning H/A are usually sudden in onset, milder than that associated with a major rupture, and may last a few days.

Differential diagnosis of severe, acute, paroxysmal headache (25% will have SAH[50]):

1. subarachnoid hemorrhage, AKA "warning headache" or sentinel H/A (see above)
2. benign "thunderclap headaches" (BTH) or crash migraine.[51] Severe global headaches of abrupt onset that reach maximal intensity in < 1 minute, accompanied by vomiting in ≈ 50%. They may recur, and are presumably a form of vascular headache. Some may have transient focal symptoms. There are no clinical criteria that can reliably differentiate these from SAH[52] (although seizures and diplopia, when they occurred, were always associated with SAH). There is no subarachnoid blood on CT and LP, which should probably be performed on at least the first presentation to R/O SAH. Earlier recommendations to angiogram these individuals[53] have since been tempered by experience[54,55]
3. reversible cerebral vasoconstrictive syndrome (RCVS)[56] (AKA benign cerebral angiopathy or vasculitis[57]): severe H/A with paroxysmal onset, ± neurologic deficit, and string of beads appearance on angiography of cerebral vessels that usually clears in 1–3 months. > 50% report prior use of vasoconstrictive substances (cocaine, marijuana, nasal decongestants, ergot derivatives, SSRIs, interferon, nicotine patches) sometimes combined with binge drinking. May also occur post-partum. Complications occurred in 24% including:
   a) usually during the 1st week: SAH, ICH, seizures, RPLS
   b) usually during the 2nd week: ischemic events (TIA, stroke)
4. benign orgasmic cephalgia: a severe, throbbing, sometimes "explosive" H/A with onset just before or at the time of orgasm (distinct from pre-orgasmic headaches which intensify with sexual arousal[58]). In a series of 21 patients[59] neurologic exam was normal in all, and angiography done in 9 was normal. 9 had a history of migraine in the patient or a family member. No other symptoms developed in 18 patients followed for 2–7 yrs. Recommendations for evaluation are similar to that for thunderclap headaches above

77.5.3 Signs

Meningismus (see below), hypertension, focal neurologic deficit (e.g. oculomotor palsy, hemiparesis), obtundation or coma (see below), ocular hemorrhage (see below).

Meningismus

Nuchal rigidity (especially to flexion) often ensues in 6 to 24 hrs. Patients may have a positive Kernig sign (flex thigh to 90° with knee bent, then straighten knee, positive sign if this causes pain in hamstrings) or Brudzinski sign (flex the supine patient's neck, involuntary hip flexion is a positive sign).

Coma following SAH

Coma may follow SAH because of any one or a combination of the following[60]:

1. increased ICP
2. damage to brain tissue from intraparenchymal hemorrhage (may also contribute to increased ICP)
3. hydrocephalus
4. diffuse ischemia (may be secondary to increased ICP)
5. seizure
6. low blood flow (reduced CBF) due to reduced cardiac output (p. 1177)

Ocular hemorrhage

Three types of ocular hemorrhage (OH) may be associated with SAH. They occur alone or in various combinations in 20–40% of patients with SAH.[61]

1. subhyaloid (preretinal) hemorrhage: seen funduscopically in 11–33% of cases as bright red blood near the optic disc that obscures the underlying retinal vessels. May be associated with a higher mortality rate[62]
2. (intra)retinal hemorrhage: may surround the fovea
3. hemorrhage within the vitreous humor (Terson syndrome). First described by the French ophthalmologist Albert Terson. Occurs in 4–27% of cases of aneurysmal SAH,[63,64,65] usually bilateral. May occur with other causes of increased ICP including ruptured AVMs. Funduscopy reveals vitreous opacity. The location of the origin of the vitreous hemorrhage differs in various reports (subhyaloid, epiretinal, subinternal limiting membrane).[66] May be more common with anterior circulation aneurysms (especially ACoA), although 1 study found no correlation with location.[64] Also rarely reported with SDH and traumatic SAH. Often missed on initial examination. When sought, usually present on initial exam, however it may develop as late as 12 days post SAH, and may be associated with rebleeding.[64] The mortality rate may be higher in SAH patients with vitreous hemorrhage than in those without. Patients should be followed for complications of OH (elevated intraocular pressure, retinal membrane formation → retinal detachment, retinal folds[67]). Most cases clear spontaneously in 6–12 mos. Vitrectomy should be considered in patients whose vision fails to improve[65] or if more rapid improvement is desired.[68] The long-term prognosis for vision is good in ≈ 80% of cases with or without vitrectomy[68]

The pathomechanics of OH are controversial. OH was originally attributed to extension of the blood from the subarachnoid space into the vitreous, but no communication exists between these two spaces. In actuality may be due to compression of the central retinal vein and the retinochoroidal anastomoses by elevated CSF pressure[65] causing venous hypertension and disruption of retinal veins.

77.6 Work-up of suspected SAH

77.6.1 Overview

1. tests to diagnose SAH
   a) non-contrast high-resolution CT scan: see below
   b) if CT is negative: LP in suspicious cases (for findings, see below)
2. test to identify *source* of SAH. Options: CTA, MRA, or catheter angiography. The choice needs to take into account the patient's age, renal function, and even best guess of where an aneurysm might be located
   a) MRA: no radiation, and 2D-TOF MRA does not use contrast (p.232). Poor sensitivity for aneurysm detection early after SAH (see below)
   b) CTA vs. angiogram: one needs to balance the risk of the procedure and ease of obtaining it against the information expected to be obtained
      - total iodine load in a healthy adult should be < 90 gm in 24 hours. In older patients and/or possible compromised renal function, this volume should be less. CTA typically uses 65–75 cc of contrast with ≈ 300 mg iodine/ml, or ≈ 21 gm iodine. The amount of contrast with a cerebral arteriogram varies. However if an angiogram is needed after a CTA, in most cases you do not have to wait 24 hours
      - if there is concern about renal function (e.g. serum creatinine > 100 mcmol/L) hydrate the patient and optionally give Mucomyst® (p.221)
      - catheter angiography may be necessary after a positive CTA to better delineate the anatomy, or to determine dominant filling and cross flow, or in highly suspicious cases with a negative CTA (see below). While CTA permits reliable assessment of feasibility of endovascular treatment in most cases,[69] DSA is still necessary in some
3. if CTA/angiogram is negative: see SAH of unknown etiology (p.1230)

77.6.2 Laboratory/radiographic findings

CT scan

A good quality (e.g. no motion artifact) non-contrast high-resolution CT will detect SAH in ≥ 95% of cases if scanned within 48 hrs of SAH. Blood appears as high density (white) within subarachnoid

spaces. For subtle SAH, look in the occipital horns of the lateral ventricles and the dependent portions of the sylvian fissures. CT also assesses:
1. ventricular size: hydrocephalus occurs acutely in 21% of aneurysmal ruptures (p. 1170) [70]
2. hematoma: intracerebral hemorrhage or large amount of subdural blood with mass effect may need emergent evacuation
3. infarct: not sensitive in first 24 hours after infarct (p. 1280)
4. amount of blood in cisterns and fissures: important prognosticator for vasospasm (p. 1180) and can identify pretruncal nonaneurysmal hemorrhage (p. 1231)
5. CT can predict aneurysm location based on the pattern of blood in ≈ 78% of cases (but mostly for MCA and A-comm aneurysms)[71]
   a) blood predominantly in anterior interhemispheric fissure (± blood in lateral ventricles) or within the gyrus rectus suggests a-comm aneurysm
   b) blood predominantly in 1 sylvian fissure is compatible with p-comm or MCA aneurysm on that side
   c) blood predominantly in the prepontine or peduncular cistern suggests a basilar apex or SCA aneurysm
   d) blood predominantly within ventricles (p. 1192)
      - blood primarily in 4th and third ventricle: suggests lower posterior fossa source, such as PICA aneurysm or VA dissection
      - blood primarily in the 3rd ventricle suggests a basilar apex aneurysm
6. with multiple aneurysms, CT may help identify which one bled by the location of blood (see above). See also other "clues" (p. 1226)

Differential diagnosis of SAH on CT

Things that can mimic the appearance of SAH on CT include:
1. pus
2. following contrast administration: sometimes IV, and especially intrathecal
3. occasionally the pachymeningeal thickening seen in spontaneous intracranial hypotension (p. 389)

Lumbar puncture

The most sensitive test for SAH. However, false positives – e.g. with traumatic taps; see Differentiating SAH from traumatic tap (p. 1506) – occur with enough frequency that this test is falling out of favor for diagnosis of SAH.

✖ Caution: lowering the CSF pressure may possibly precipitate rebleeding by increasing the transmural pressure (p. 1170). Therefore remove only a small amount of CSF (several ml) and use a small (≤ 20 Ga) spinal needle.

Findings (also, see ▶ Table 23.4):
1. opening pressure: elevated
2. appearance:
   a) non-clotting bloody fluid that does not clear with sequential tubes
   b) xanthochromia: yellow coloration of CSF supernatant (specimen must be centrifuged in the lab) due to heme pigments released by the breakdown of RBCs. The most reliable means of differentiating traumatic tap from SAH. In patients with a negative head CT, the minimal amount of time required for bilirubin to become detectable in the CSF, as well as the minimal amount of blood the needs to enter the CSF to give a positive xanthochromia remains unknown. However, xanthochromia is usually not apparent until 2–4 hours after the SAH. Is present in almost 100% by 12 hours after the bleed, and remains in 70% at 3 weeks, and is still detectable in 40% at 4 weeks. Spectrophotometry is more sensitive than visual inspection, but may lack sufficient specificity to warrant widespread use.[72,73] False positives: xanthochromia may occur with jaundice or high protein levels in the CSF
3. cell count: RBC count usually > 100,000 RBCs/mm^3. Compare RBC count in first to last tube (should not drop significantly)
4. protein: elevated due to blood breakdown products
5. glucose: normal, or reduced (RBCs may metabolize some glucose with time)

MRI

Not sensitive for SAH acutely within the first 24–48 hrs[74] (too little met-Hb) especially with thin layers of blood. Better after ≈ 4–7 days (excellent for subacute to remote SAH, > 10–20 days). FLAIR

MRI is the most sensitive imaging study for detecting blood in the subarachnoid space. May be helpful in determining which of multiple aneurysms bled (p. 1226).[75]

Magnetic resonance angiography (MRA)

Based on a systematic review, sensitivity is 87% and specificity is 92% for detecting intracranial aneurysms (IAs) (compared to catheter DSA) with significantly poorer sensitivity for aneurysms < 3 mm diameter.[76,77,78]

MRA's ability to detect IAs depends on aneurysm size, rate and direction of blood flow in the aneurysm relative to the magnetic field, and aneurysmal thrombosis and calcification. MRA may be most useful as a screening test in high-risk patients including patient's with two first degree relatives with IAs, especially those who are also smokers or hypertensive themselves.[79]

CT angiography (CTA)

Many centers have shown good results with CTA (p. 227), with a prospective study detecting 97% of aneurysms and demonstrating CTA as safe and effective when used as the initial and sole imaging study for ruptured and unruptured cerebral aneurysms.[80] CTA shows a 3-dimensional image (as can modern catheter angiography) which can help differentiate adherent vessels from those arising from the aneurysm. CTA also demonstrates the relation to nearby bony structures which can be important in surgical planning. CTA use is increasing for evaluation of vasospasm.[81]

Catheter angiogram

General information

Injection of radio-opaque (iodinated) contrast ("dye") into selective vessels using a catheter typically inserted into the femoral artery at the upper thigh, while taking serial x-rays to obtain a "video-like" representation of the vasculature.

The gold standard for evaluation of cerebral aneurysms. Current state of the art uses digital subtraction angiography (DSA). Demonstrates source (usually aneurysm) in ≈ 80–85%; remainder are so-called "SAH of unknown etiology" (p. 1230). Shows if radiographic vasospasm is present – **clinical** vasospasm almost never occurs < 3 days following SAH (p. 1178) – and assesses primary feeding arteries, collateral flow in case of a need for arterial sacrifice.

General principles:

1. study the vessel of highest suspicion first (in case patient's condition should change, necessitating discontinuation of procedure)
2. continue to do complete 4 vessel angiogram (even if aneurysm(s) have been demonstrated) to rule out additional aneurysms and assess collateral circulation
3. if there is an aneurysm or suspicion of one, obtain additional views to help delineate the neck and orientation of the aneurysm (see index for specific aneurysm)
4. ✱ if no aneurysm is seen, before an arteriogram can be considered negative, must:
   a) visualize *both PICA origins*: 1–2% of aneurysms occur at PICA origin. Both PICAs can usually be visualized with one VA injection if there is enough flow to reflux down the contralateral VA. Occasionally it is necessary to see more of the contralateral VA than what refluxes to PICA and selective catheterization may be required
   b) *flow contrast through the ACoA*: if both ACAs fill from one side, this is usually satisfactory. It may be necessary to perform a cross compression AP study with carotid injection (first, rule-out plaque in the carotid to be compressed), or use a higher injection rate to facilitate flow through the ACoA
   c) if an infundibulum (see below) colocalizes to the SAH, it may be unwise to label the case as angiogram-negative and exploration is recommended by some[82]

77

Infundibulum

A funnel shaped initial segment of an artery, to be distinguished from an aneurysm. Found in 7–13% of otherwise normal arteriograms,[83,84] with a higher incidence in cases of multiple or familial aneurysms. Bilateral in 25%.[84] Most commonly found at the origin of the p-comms, but they rarely occur at other sites. Criteria for differentiating infindibula from aneurysms are shown in ▶ Table 77.1. Infundibula may represent incomplete remnants of previous fetal vessels[85 (p 272)]

Although they may bleed,[82,87,88,89] there is less risk of rupture than with a saccular aneurysm (no infundibulum < 3 mm in size bled[90] in the cooperative study). However, infundibula have been documented to progress to an aneurysm (i.e. they are preaneurysmal) which may bleed (13 case reports in the literature as of 2009). Recommended treatment: at the time of surgery for another reason,

Table 77.1 Criteria of an infundibulum
1. triangular in shape 2. mouth (widest portion) < 3 mm[a] [86] 3. vessel at apex
[a]a widely accepted but probably arbitrary dimension

Table 77.2 Hunt and Hess classification[a] of SAH[94]

Grade	Description
1	asymptomatic, or mild H/A and slight nuchal rigidity
2	Cr. N. palsy (e.g. III, VI), moderate to severe H/A, nuchal rigidity
3	mild focal deficit, lethargy, or confusion
4	stupor, moderate to severe hemiparesis, early decerebrate rigidity
5	deep coma, decerebrate rigidity, moribund appearance
Add one grade for serious systemic disease (e.g. HTN, DM, severe atherosclerosis, COPD) or severe vasospasm on arteriography.	
[a]original paper did not consider patient's age, site of aneurysm, or time since bleed; patients were graded on admission and pre-op	

consider treating an infundibulum with wrapping, or placing in an encircling clip, or sacrificing the artery if it can be done safely (infundibula lack a true neck).

Angiographic findings

1. general features to take note of when analyzing an aneurysm on angiogram (special considerations for specific aneurysms are covered in designated sections)
   a) size of aneurysm dome:
      - MRI or CT helps with this since the aneurysm may be partially thrombosed and the portion that is patent and fills with contrast and is therefore visualized on angiogram may be much smaller than the actual size
      - large aneurysms (≥ 15 mm dia.) are associated with lower rates of complete occlusion by endovascular coiling[91,92]
   b) neck size
      - narrow necks < 5 mm are ideal for coiling[93]
      - broad necks ≥ 5 mm are associated with increased risk of incomplete occlusion and recanalization with coiling[92]
      - stent or balloon-assisted coiling may be needed for wide necked aneurysms. Stents should be avoided if possible (p. 1586).
   c) dome:neck ratio ≥ 2 is associated with higher rate of successful coil occlusion[93]
2. for basilar bifurcation aneurysms (p. 1218)

77.7 Grading SAH

77.7.1 General Information

Four grading scales are in common use. The 2 most widely quoted grading scales are presented here.

77.7.2 Hunt and Hess grade

See ► Table 77.2 and ► Table 77.3 for grading system. Grades 1 and 2 were operated upon as soon as an aneurysm was diagnosed. Grade ≥ 3 managed until the condition improved to Grade 2 or 1. Exception: life threatening hematoma or multiple bleeds (which were operated on regardless of grade).

Analysis of data from the International Cooperative Aneurysm Study revealed that with normal consciousness, Hunt and Hess (H&H) grades 1 and 2 had identical outcome, and that hemiparesis and/or aphasia had no effect on mortality.

Table 77.3 Modified classification[95] adds the following

Grade	Description
0	unruptured aneurysm
1 a	no acute meningeal/brain reaction, but with fixed neuro deficit

Table 77.4 WFNS SAH grade[96]

WFNS grade	GCS score[a]	Major focal deficit[b]
0[c]		
1	15	–
2	13–14	–
3	13–14	+
4	7–12	+ or –
5	3–6	+ or –

[a]GCS = Glasgow Coma Scale, see ▶ Table 18.1
[b]aphasia, hemiparesis or hemiplegia (+ = present, – = absent)
[c]intact aneurysm

Mortality:
Admission Hunt and Hess Grade 1 or 2: 20%.
Patients taken to O.R. (for any procedure) at H&H Grade 1 or 2: 14%.
Major cause of death in Grade 1 or 2 is rebleed.
Signs of meningeal irritation increases surgical risk.

77.7.3 World Federation of Neurosurgical Societies / World Federation of Neurological Surgeons (WFNS) grading of SAH

Due to lack of data on the significance of features such as headache, nuchal rigidity, and major focal neurologic deficit, the WFNS Committee on a Universal SAH Grading Scale[96,97] developed a grading system which is shown in ▶ Table 77.4. It uses the Glasgow Coma Scale (GCS) (see ▶ Table 18.1) to evaluate level of consciousness, and uses the presence or absence of major focal neurologic deficit to distinguish grade 2 from grade 3.

77.8 Initial management of SAH

77.8.1 General information

Practice guideline

Practice guideline: Initial management of aneurysmal SAH

Level I[41]:

- administer oral nimodipine to all patients with aneurysmal SAH. The value of other calcium channel blockers is uncertain
- maintain euvolemia and normal circulating blood volume

Level II[41]:

- control of HTN: the ideal BP to reduce the risk of rebleeding has not been established. A reasonable target is to maintain SBP < 160 mm Hg

77

Initial management concerns

1. rebleeding: the major concern during the initial stabilization
2. hydrocephalus: precipitous development acute hydrocephalus may be obstructive (due to blockage of CSF flow by blood clot), but presence of ventriculomegaly early after SAH as well as at later stages is often due to communicating hydrocephalus (p. 1170) (due to toxic effect of blood breakdown products on arachnoid granulations)
3. delayed ischemic neurologic deficit (DIND), usually attributed to vasospasm. Begins to be of concern several days following the SAH
4. hyponatremia with hypovolemia (p. 1166)
5. DVT and pulmonary embolism (p. 167)
6. seizures (p. 1167)
7. determining source of bleeding: should be investigated early with CTA or catheter angiography. The timing and choice of study takes into consideration the patient's condition (unstable or premorbid patients are not candidates), the feasibility of early treatment (ideal), and the likelihood of endovascular therapy (based on patient's age and predicted aneurysm location as well as availability)

Goals of medical management related to neurologic injury

In addition to prevention of hyponatremia, hypovolemia, seizures, etc. (see above), the goals of initial medical management include:

1. augmenting CBF: the main device for accomplishing this is hyperdynamic therapy (p. 1186). Goals are:
   a) increasing cerebral perfusion pressure (CPP)
   b) improving blood rheology: RBC aggregability increases after SAH[98]
   c) maintaining *euvolemia*: the majority of patients become hypovolemic in the first 24 hrs after SAH. Also, avoid prophylactic hypervolemia
   d) maintaining normal ICP
2. neuroprotection: there are currently no medications shown to be effective or approved for use as neuroprotective agents for this or any other type of brain injury. Animal studies have shown time and again that the concept may someday be translated into clinical practice[99]

77.8.2 Monitors/tubes

Also see below.

1. arterial line: for patients who are hemodynamically unstable, stuporous or comatose, those with difficult to control hypertension, or those requiring frequent labs (e.g. ventilator patients)
2. intubate patients who are comatose or unable to protect airway (e.g. stridorous)
3. pulmonary-artery catheter (PA-catheter, AKA Swann-Ganz catheter): the safety and efficacy of this device has been debated in the critical care literature for over a decade now, with some calling for a moratorium on PA catheter use.[100] It is possible that newer technologies may supplant the need for this invasive procedure while allowing close hemodynamic monitoring.[101] Nevertheless, a PA catheter can be considered for:
   a) Hunt and Hess (H&H) grade ≥ 3 (except good grade 3 patients)
   b) patients with possible CSW or SIADH
   c) hemodynamically unstable patients
4. cardiac rhythm monitor: arrhythmias may occur following SAH (p. 1177)
5. intraventricular catheter (IVC) AKA ventriculostomy. Possible indications:
   a) patients developing acute hydrocephalus following SAH or in those with significant intraventricular blood (allows measurement of ICP as well as drainage of blood laden CSF). IVC causes symptomatic improvement in almost two-thirds.[70] May increase the risk of rebleeding (p. 1170), however, the risk of untreated hydrocephalus is probably higher[102]
   b) H&H grade ≥ 3 (except good grade 3 patients). If a high grade patient improves with an IVC, the prognosis may be more favorable. If ICP is elevated, management includes the use of mannitol; see Treatment measures for elevated ICP (p. 866).

77.8.3 Admitting orders

1. admit to ICU (monitored bed)
2. VS with neuro checks q 1 hr

3. activity: BR with HOB at 30°. SAH precautions (i.e. low level of external stimulation, restricted visitation, no loud noises)
4. nursing
   a) strict I's & O's
   b) daily weights
   c) knee high TED hose and pneumatic compression boots (PCB)
   d) indwelling Foley catheter if patient lethargic, incontinent, or unable to void in urinal or bedpan. Consider temperature sensing catheter for strict fever control
5. diet: NPO (in preparation for surgery or endovascular intervention)
6. IV fluids: early aggressive fluid therapy to head off cerebral salt wasting
   a) NS + 20 mEq KCl/L at ≈ 2 ml/kg/hr (typically 140–150 ml/hr) (below)
   b) if Hct < 40%,[103] give 500 ml of 5% albumin over 4 hrs upon admission
7. medications (avoid IM medications to reduce pain)
   a) prophylactic anticonvulsants: see post-SAH seizures below
   b) sedation (not oversedation): e.g. with propofol
   c) analgesics: fentanyl (unlike morphine, does not cause histamine release. Lowers ICP) 25–100 mcg (0.5–2 ml) IVP, q 1–2 hrs PRN (avoid Demerol® because it may lower seizure threshold)
   d) dexamethasone (Decadron®): may help with H/A and neck pain. Effect on edema controversial. Usually given pre-op prior to craniotomy
   e) stool softener in patients able to take PO (docussate 100 mg PO BID)
   f) anti-emetics: avoid phenothiazines (especially in patients who seize) which may lower seizure threshold. Use e.g. Zofran® (ondansetron) 4 mg IV over 2–5 minutes, may repeat in 4 & 8 hours, and then q 8 hours for 1–2 days
   g) calcium channel blockers (p. 1183): nimodipine (Nimotop®) 60 mg PO/NG q 4 hrs initiated within 96 hrs of SAH (some use 30 mg q 2 hrs to avoid periodic dips in BP). IV administration is equally as effective[104] where available. Oral nimodipine should be administered to all patients with aSAH.
   h) H2 blockers (e.g. ranitidine) or proton pump inhibitors (e.g. Prevacid® (lansoprazole) 30 mg p.o. or IV q d): to reduce risk of stress ulceration
   i) ✖ these agents impair coagulation and are *used with caution*: ASA, dextran,[105] heparin, and repeated administration of hetastarch (Hespan®)[106,107] over a period of days
   j) statins: several clinical trials have investigated the utility of statins, with variable results. More recently, a meta-analysis reported no evidence for clinical benefit.[108] In addition, a multicenter randomized phase 3 trial did not detect any short- or long-term benefit with the use of simvastatin[109]
8. oxygenation
   a) in non-intubated patient: O_2 2 L per NC PRN (based on ABG) and if tolerated
   b) in ventilated patient: strive for normocarbia and $pO_2 > 100$ mm Hg
9. temperature (normothermia): medications (Tylenol) and cooling measures (e.g. ice packs, Arctic Sun external cooling device) to reduce and prevent fever are encouraged, as fever has been shown to be independently associated with worse cognitive and functional outcome in survivors of aSAH[110,111,112]
10. HTN: SBP 120–160 mm Hg by cuff is a guideline with unclipped aneurysm (below)
11. labs
    a) ABG, electrolytes, CBC, PT/PTT on admission
    b) ABG, electrolytes, CBC q day (ABG q 6 hrs if patient unstable, electrolytes q 12 hrs if hyponatremia develops, see Hyponatremia following SAH below)
    c) serum and urine osmolality if urine output high or low; see Syndrome of inappropriate antidiuretic hormone secretion (SIADH) (p. 112)
    d) hemoglobin and hematocrit: some studies suggest that higher hemoglobin values are associated with improved outcomes after aSAH.[113,114] However, liberal RBC transfusion has been associated with worse outcomes in aSAH.[115,116] The optimal hemoglobin goal after aSAH in not yet known, and may depend on the presence or absence of vasospasm
    e) serum glucose: effective glucose control after aSAH can significantly reduce the risk of poor outcome[117]
    f) CXR daily until stable: patients undergoing triple-H therapy can develop dangerous pulmonary edema as they "fall off" the Starling curve with volume expansion. Patients with SAH are also rarely at risk for neurogenic pulmonary edema (p. 1178) [118]
    g) if available, transcranial doppler to monitor MCA, ACA, ICA, VA and BA velocities and Lindegaard ratio (p. 1182) q Mon, Weds & Fri

77.8.4 Blood pressure and volume management

General information

With an unsecured (unclipped or uncoiled) aneurysm, gentle volume expansion with slight hemodilution and mild elevation of blood pressure may help prevent or minimize the effects of vasospasm[119] and cerebral salt wasting. However, extreme hypertension must be avoided (to reduce risk of re-bleeding). Hypervolemia is to be avoided since it does not mitigate vasospasm and increases complications.[120]

Initial blood pressure

Ideal blood pressure is controversial, and must take patient's baseline into consideration. The magnitude of blood pressure control to reduce the risk of rebleeding has not been established, but a decrease in systolic blood pressure to < 160 mmHg is reasonable.

If blood pressure is labile, labetalol or nicardipine should be used in conjunction with an arterial-line. Avoid hypotension as it may exacerbate ischemia.

Long acting drugs (e.g. ACE inhibitors should be started in patients requiring continued therapy. In patients who were normotensive prior to SAH with easily controlled hypertension, ACE inhibitors may be used PRN in conjunction with a beta blocker, e.g. labetalol (p. 126).

77.8.5 Hyponatremia following SAH

Background

Hypovolemia and hyponatremia frequently follow SAH as a result of natriuresis and diuresis. The reported incidence of hyponatremia in aSAH ranges from 10-30%.[41] Although hyponatremia had been attributed to a rise in ADH[121] (thought to produce SIADH with hypervolemia), the ADH increment is usually transient, lasting only ≈ 4 days and hypervolemia did not occur. Another theory is based on the fact that there is often a delayed peak in atrial natriuretic factor (ANF) (a 28-amino acid polypeptide) after an initial smaller rise[122] that was frequently followed by urinary loss of sodium (cerebral salt wasting (CSW) (p. 118) that mimics SIADH, and volume depletion. Although CSW has clearly been shown to be the cause of hyponatremia in the majority of these patients,[123] there are still doubts that ANF is the operative natriuretic factor in SAH.[124] A rise in ANP and brain natriuretic peptide (BNP) after SAH is associated with the development of a negative fluid balance.[125]

Routine labs are identical in SIADH and CSW,[126] but the extracellular fluid volume (which is more difficult to measure) is low in CSW and is normal or elevated in SIADH (see ▶ Table 5.5 or a comparison of the two conditions). The neurologic effects of hyponatremia (p. 112) may mimic delayed ischemic neurologic deficit from vasospasm, and hyponatremic patients have about 3 times the incidence of delayed cerebral infarction after SAH than normonatremic patients.[127] Hyponatremia has been chronologically associated with the onset of sonographic and clinical vasospasm[128,129]

Factors that may increase the risk of hyponatremia after SAH include: history of diabetes, CHF, cirrhosis, adrenal insufficiency, or the use of any of the following drugs: NSAIDs, acetaminophen, narcotics, thiazide diuretics.[130]

Treatment

77

✖ Caution! Restricting fluids which is the treatment for SIADH may be hazardous in the case of CSW (which is more likely to occur after SAH than is SIADH) since dehydration increases blood viscosity which exacerbates ischemia from vasospasm.[127]

- reat hypovolemia aggressively with infusions of crystalloid (e.g. NS), PRBCs, or colloids
- hypertonic saline (3%) has been shown to be effective in correcting hyponatremia[131] and appears to increase regional cerebral blood flow, brain tissue oxygen, and pH in patients with high-grade aSAH[132]
- fludrocortisone has been shown to help correct hyponatremia, with a reduced need for fluids.[133,134] Similarly hydrocortisone administration has been associated with reduced natriuresis and a lower rate of hyponatremia[135]

77.8.6 Post-SAH seizures

General information

No RCT has been performed to help guide decisions on prophylaxis or treatment of seizures. There is also conflicting evidence on whether onset seizures are predictive of late seizures or post-SAH epilepsy.[136,137] As such, there is no consensus amongst practitioners regarding the need for AEDs, the best AED to use, which patients should receive prophylactic AEDs, nor the optimal dose or duration of treatment.

Epidemiology

▶ **Incidence.** The incidence of seizure-like episodes varies widely between observational studies. One literature review[138] reported 4-26% of SAH patients had onset seizures, 1-28% had early seizures (w/in first 2 weeks), and 1-35% had late seizures (after 2 weeks).[139] Additionally, non-convulsive status epilepticus has been reported in 3-18% of SAH patients, and should be suspected in patients with a poor neurological exam or in the setting of neurological deterioration.[140,141]

▶ **Risk factors for post-SAH seizures.** [6,41,138,139,140,142,143,144]
- increasing age
- MCA aneurysm
- volume of subarachnoid blood/thickness of clot
- associated intracerebral or subdural hematoma
- poor neurological grade
- Rebleeding
- cerebral infarction
- vasospasm
- hyponatremia
- hydrocephalus
- hypertension
- treatment modality, see coiling vs. clipping (p. 1195)

Outcome

The association between seizures and functional outcome remain unclear. One study[140] showed that an in-hospital seizure was independently predictive of one year mortality (65% with seizures vs. 23% without seizures), but others have shown no association with a poorer prognosis.[138,143,145] Two large, retrospective, single-institution studies of patients with aSAH found that nonconvulsive status epilepticus is a very strong predictor of poor outcome.[41,141,146]

AEDs

Studies have assessed neurological outcome following short- and long-term phenytoin use, with higher doses and longer duration associated with poorer outcomes.[147,148] When Keppra is compared to phenytoin, keppra is associated with a higher rate of short-term seizure recurrence,[149] but improved long-term outcomes and fewer side effects.[139,150] Although use of prophylactic AED for aSAH is controversial, a generalized seizure may be devastating in the presence of a tenuous aneurysm. As such, AEDs are given by many authorities in the acute setting, at least until the aneurysm is secured. One paradigm: Keppra® (levetiracetam) 1 g IV q 12 hours until the aneurysm is secured.

Practice guideline: Post-SAH seizures

- Level II[41]: prophylactic anticonvulsants may be considered in the immediate posthemorrhagic period
- Level III[41]: the routine long-term use of anticonvulsants is not recommended
- Level II[41]: long-term anticonvulsants may be considered with known risk factors for delayed seizure disorder (e.g. prior seizure, intracerebral hematoma, intractable hypertension, infarction, or MCA aneurysm)

77.9 Rebleeding

77.9.1 General information

Approximately 3000 North Americans die each year from rebleeding of ruptured cerebral aneurysms.[151] For untreated ruptured aneurysms, the maximal frequency of rebleeding is in the 1st day (between 4% and 13.6%),[152,153,154,155] with more than 1/3 of rebleeds occurring within 3 hours and 1/2 within 6 hours of symptoms onset.[156] After the first day, the subsequent risk is 1.5% daily for 13 d. Overall, 15–20% rebleed within 14 d, 50% will rebleed within 6 months, thereafter the risk is ≈ 3%/yr with a mortality rate of 2%/yr.[157] (**Note:** to understand the calculation of long-term *cumulative* risk for aneurysmal rupture, see Annual and lifetime risk of hemorrhage and recurrent hemorrhage (p. 1240); that discussion is related to AVMs but the same concepts pertain to aneurysms). 50% of deaths occur in the 1st month.

There is a risk of rebleeding during any period that the aneurysm is untreated. As such, early treatment of the ruptured aneurysm can reduce risk of rebleeding[158] (see Timing of aneurysm intervention). In addition, higher Hunt and Hess grades,[159] larger aneurysm size, and poorly controlled blood pressure (> 160 mmHg) have also been associated with an increased risk of rebleeding.[154,155,160]

Pre-operative ventriculostomy – e.g. for acute post-SAH hydrocephalus (p. 1170) – and possibly lumbar spinal drainage (p. 1202) increase the risk of rebleeding.

The risk of rebleeding in SAH of unknown etiology and with AVMs, as well as the risk of bleeding with incidental multiple unruptured aneurysms, are all similar at ≈ 1%/yr; may actually be less in SAH of unknown etiology (p. 1230).[161]

77.9.2 Prevention of rebleeding

The optimal method of preventing rebleeding is early coiling or surgical clipping. Bed rest and hyperdynamic therapy do *not* prevent rebleeding.[162]

77.9.3 Antifibrinolytic therapy

The role of clot lysis in early rebleeding is uncertain.

Practice guideline: Antifibrinolytic therapy

Level II[41]: for patients with aneurysmal SAH where there is an unavoidable delay in treatment of the aneurysm, in whom there is a significant risk of rebleeding and no compelling medical contraindications, up to 72 hours of therapy with tranexamic acid or aminocaproic acid is reasonable

Drug info: Tranexamic Acid (Cyklokapron®)

Reduces the risk of early rebleeding.[153]

℞: 1 gm IV as soon as diagnosis of SAH is verified (if patient is to be transported to another facility for definitive care, the dose is given before the patient is transported), followed by 1 gm q 6 hours until the aneurysm is occluded; this treatment did not exceed 72 hours.

77

Drug info: Epsilon-aminocaproic acid (Amicar®)

Epsilon-aminocaproic acid (EACA) an antifibrinolytic agent, competitively inhibits activation of plasminogen to plasmin. Existing plasmin is neutralized by endogenous antiplasmins. EACA does reduce the risk of rebleeding. However, the incidence of hydrocephalus and delayed ischemic deficits (vasospasm) have been shown to be higher with prolonged use[163] with prolonged use. There may also be a lag of 24–48 hrs before effectiveness occurs.[164]

Because of the increased rate of cerebral infarction, EACA was found not to reduce early mortality, and its use was discouraged.

Reevaluation in a non-randomized study[165] excluding grade IV and V patients, suggests that the problems with EACA may be minimized by use of an IV loading dose (to eliminate the lag-period to effectiveness) and by limiting the length of time of use to that time until the patient can undergo early surgery. A more recent investigation[166] showed a significant decrease in rebleeding in EACA-treated patients versus non-EACA patients (2.7 vs. 11.4%). There was a 76% reduction in mortality attributable to rebleeding, a 13% increase in favorable outcome in good-grade (Hunt Hess I-III) EACA treated patients, and a 6.8% increase in poor grade patients (Hunt Hess IV/V), but these results did not reach statistical significance. Although there was an 8-fold increase in DVT in the EACA group, there was no increase in pulmonary embolism. Additionally, there was no difference in ischemic complications between groups.

℞ [166]: EACA 4 g IV loading dose, followed by 1 g/h with cessation of infusion 4 hours before angiography for a maximum duration of 72 hours after SAH.

77.10 Pregnancy and intracranial hemorrhage

77.10.1 General information

Intracranial hemorrhage (subarachnoid or intraparenchymal) is a rare occurrence during pregnancy (estimated range of incidence: 0.01–0.05% of all pregnancies[167]) and yet is responsible for 5–12% of maternal deaths during pregnancy.

Intracranial hemorrhage of pregnancy (ICHOP) commonly occurs in the setting of eclampsia, and is more commonly intraparenchymal[168] and may be associated with loss of cerebrovascular autoregulation PRES (p. 194).[169] Symptoms of eclampsia with or without ICHOP include H/A, mental status changes, and seizures.

A literature review of 154 reported cases of ICHOP-related SAH revealed 77% were aneurysmal and 23% were from ruptured AVM (other series show the percentage of AVMs range from 21–48%). Mortality is ≈ 35% for aneurysmal and ≈ 28% for AVM hemorrhage (the latter being higher than in non-gravid patients). There is an increasing tendency for bleeding with advancing gestational age for both aneurysms and AVMs (earlier it had been asserted that this held true for aneurysms only[170]).

Patients with ICHOP having AVMs tend to be younger than those with aneurysm, paralleling the occurrence in the general population. One major oft-quoted study showed an increased risk of hemorrhage from AVMs during pregnancy[171] (citing an 87% hemorrhage rate), however another investigation disputes this assertion,[172] and found the risk of hemorrhage to be 3.5% during the pregnancy in patients with no history of hemorrhage, or 5.8% in those with previous hemorrhage. Another study evaluated risk of aneurysm rupture during pregnancy and delivery form the Nationwide Inpatient data and calculated the rupture risk during pregnancy and delivery to be 1.4% and 0.05%, respectively.[173] Literature review[167] found a risk of recurrent hemorrhage following ICHOP from aneurysm or AVM during the remainder of the pregnancy was 33–50%.

77.10.2 Management modifications for pregnant patients

Modifications of evaluation and treatment techniques may be necessary for the pregnant patient.

1. neuroradiologic studies
   a) CAT scan: with shielding of the fetus, CAT scanning of the brain produces minimal radiation exposure to the child
   b) MRI:
      • generally felt to have low potential for complications, however, many centers will not do MRI during first trimester.
      • gadolinium based contrast agents (GBCAs) are teratogenic in animals in high repeated doses. It has not been studied in human pregnancy. A cohort of 26 women who received GBCAs during the first trimester showed no evidence of teratogenicity or mutagenicity.[174] There have also been no reported issues related to nephrogenic systemic fibrosis. GBCAs are FDA Class C drugs – not recommended for use during pregnancy, but may be used if benefits outweigh potential risks.
   c) angiography: with shielding of the fetus, radiation exposure is minimal. Iodinated contrast agents pose little risk to the fetus, The mother should be well hydrated during and after the study[167]
2. antiepileptic drugs: see Pregnancy and antiepileptic drugs (p. 458)
3. diuretics: the use of mannitol in pregnancy should be avoided to prevent fetal dehydration and maternal hypovolemia with uterine hypoperfusion
4. antihypertensives: nitroprusside should not be used in pregnancy
5. nimodipine is potentially teratogenic in animals, the effect on humans is unknown. It should be used only when the potential benefit justifies the risk

77

77.10.3 Neurosurgical management

The currently recommended treatment of a ruptured aneurysm in the pregnant patient is immediate surgical treatment to avoid rebleeding and ischemic complications due to vasospasm. A meta-analysis has demonstrated that mother and fetus both benefit from surgical treatment – with maternal mortality decreasing from 63% to 11% and fetal mortality decreasing from 27% to 5%.[167,175] Successful endovascular treatment for aSAH has been reported, but fetal exposure to radiation is a concern. The absorbed fetal dose has been estimated to range from 0.17 to 2.8 mGy, corresponding to a fetal risk of a hereditary disease at birth and a cumulative risk for a fatal cancer by age 15 which are both substantially lower than that which naturally occur.[176] Because endovascular treatment requires heparin for systemic anticoagulation, it carries the risk of hemorrhagic implications when labor spontaneously begins during or around the time of embolization.

77.10.4 Obstetric management following ICHOP

Several reports have indicated that the fetal and maternal outcome is no different for vaginal delivery vs. C-section, and is probably more dependent on whether the offending lesion has been treated. However, there are no formal studies to help guide the optimal treatment of pregnant women with aSAH. One strategy[175] is to perform an emergent c-section, followed by aneurysm treatment, if the fetus is mature enough for survival outside the uterus. If the fetus is < 24 weeks, treat the aneurysm and maintain the pregnancy. If the fetus is between 24-28 weeks, a strategy should be tailored according to the maternal and fetal status. C-section may be used for fetal salvage for a moribund mother in the third trimester. During vaginal delivery, the risk of rebleeding may be reduced by the use of caudal or epidural anesthesia, shortening the 2nd stage of labor, and low forceps delivery if necessary.

77.11 Hydrocephalus after SAH

77.11.1 Hydrocephalus after traumatic SAH

See also posttraumatic hydrocephalus (p.920).

77.11.2 Acute hydrocephalus

General information

The frequency of hydrocephalus (HCP) on the initial CT after SAH depends on the defining criteria used, with a reported range of 9–67%.[177] A realistic range is ≈15–20% of SAH patients, with 30–60% of these showing no impairment of consciousness.[177,178] 3% of those *without* HCP on initial CT develop HCP within 1 week.[177]

Factors felt to contribute to acute HCP include: blood interfering with CSF flow through the Sylvian aqueduct, fourth ventricle outlet, or subarachnoid space, and/or with reabsorption at the arachnoid granulations.

Findings associated with acute HCP include[178]:

77

1. increasing age
2. admission CT findings: intraventricular blood, diffuse subarachnoid blood, and thick focal accumulation of subarachnoid blood (intraparenchymal blood did *not* correlate with chronic HCP, and patients with a normal CT had a low incidence)
3. hypertension: on admission, prior to admission (by history), or post-op
4. by location:
   a) posterior circulation aneurysms have a higher incidence of HCP
   b) MCA aneurysms correlate with low incidence of HCP
5. miscellaneous: hyponatremia, patients who were not alert on admission, use of preoperative antifibrinolytic agents, and low Glasgow outcome score

Treatment

About half the patients with acute HCP and impaired consciousness improved spontaneously.[177] Patients in poor grade (H&H IV-V) with large ventricles may be symptomatic from the HCP and consideration should be given to ventriculostomy which caused improvement in ≈ 80% of patients in whom it was used.[177] There may be an increased risk of aneurysmal rebleeding in patients undergoing ventriculostomy shortly after SAH[177,179,180] especially if performed early and if ICP is lowered precipitously. The risk of aneurysm rebleeding with EVD has been studied in retrospective case series with mixed results.[181,182,183] The mechanism is controversial, but may be due to an increase in the transmural pressure (the pressure across the aneurysm wall which equals the difference between arterial pressure and ICP).

When a ventriculostomy is used, it is recommended to keep ICP in the range of 15–25 mm Hg[184] and to avoid rapid pressure reduction (unless absolutely necessary) to decrease the risk of IVC induced aneurysmal rebleeding. One paradigm is to keep the EVD open with the drip chamber nozzle 15-20 cm above the tragus.

Practice guideline: Acute hydrocephalus associated with aSAH

Level B[41]: CSF diversion (EVD or lumbar drain) for acute symptomatic hydrocephalus associated with aSAH.

77.11.3 Chronic HCP

Practice guideline: Chronic hydrocephalus associated with aSAH

- Level B[41]: permanent CSF diversion (shunt) for symptomatic chronic hydrocephalus following aSAH.
- Level C[41]: Weaning an EVD over > 24 hours does not appear to reduce the need for permanent CSF diversion.
- Level C[41]: Routine fenestration of the lamina terminalis is not recommended as it does not reduce the need for permanent CSF diversion.

Chronic HCP is due to pia-arachnoid adhesions or permanent impairment of the arachnoid granulations. Acute HCP does not inevitably lead to chronic HCP. 8–45% (reported range in literature[185]) of all ruptured aneurysm patients, and ≈ 50% of those with acute HCP following SAH need permanent CSF diversion. A number of studies have attempted to identify factors predictive of aSAH-associated shunt dependent chronic hydrocephalus. Intraventricular blood increases this risk.[185] There is controversy as to whether the use of ventriculostomy for acute HCP increases[186] or possibly even decreases[185] the incidence of shunt dependency. There may be a positive association between Fisher grade and likelihood of requiring CSF diversion for chronic hydrocephalus.[187] In addition, Hoh et al.[188] found age (2% increase/ year), comorbidity score (presence of DM, HTN, or alcohol abuse), admission type, insurance type (increased with medicaid and private payer) and hospital aneurysm volume (high > low) to be predictive of shunt placement in ruptured aneurysm patients. Treatment type (clip versus coil) has also been studied with no clear advantage for one modality over the other (p. 1195).

The method of determining which patients require shunt placement has also been studied in a single center RCT.[189] There was no difference in the rate of shunt placement between those who underwent rapid weaning (< 24 hrs) versus gradual weaning (96 hrs) of the EVD (63.4% rapid versus 62.5% gradual).

77

References

[1] Biller J, Toffol GJ, Kassell NF, et al. Spontaneous Subarachnoid Hemorrhage in Young Adults. Neurosurgery. 1987; 21:664–667

[2] Okawara SH. Warning Signs Prior to Rupture of an Intracranial Aneurysm. J Neurosurg. 1973; 38:575–580

[3] de Falco FA. Sentinel headache. Neurol Sci. 2004; 25 Suppl 3:S215–S217

[4] Polmear A. Sentinel headaches in aneurysmal subarachnoid haemorrhage: what is the true incidence? A systematic review. Cephalalgia. 2003; 23:935–941

[5] Yamashita K, Kashiwagi S, Kato S, et al. Cerebral Aneurysms in the Elderly in Yamaguchi, Japan. Analysis of the Yamaguchi Data Bank of Cerebral Aneurysm From 1985 to 1995. Stroke. 1997; 28:1926–1931

[6] Ohman J. Hypertension as a risk factor for epilepsy after aneurysmal subarachnoid hemorrhage and surgery. Neurosurgery. 1990; 27:578–581

[7] Sundaram MB, Chow F. Seizures associated with spontaneous subarachnoid hemorrhage. Can J Neurol Sci. 1986; 13:229–231

[8] Broderick JP, Brott TG, Tomsick T, et al. Intracerebral Hemorrhage More Than Twice as Common as Subarachnoid Hemorrhage. J Neurosurg. 1993; 78:188–191

[9] Sarti C, Tuomilehto J, Salomaa V, et al. Epidemiology of Subarachnoid Hemorrhage in Finland from 1983 to 1985. Stroke. 1991; 22:848–853

[10] Nieuwkamp DJ, Setz LE, Algra A, Linn FH, de Rooij NK, Rinkel GJ. Changes in case fatality of aneurysmal subarachnoid haemorrhage over time, according to age, sex, and region: a meta-analysis. Lancet Neurol. 2009; 8:635–642

[11] Solenski NJ, Haley EC, Kassell NF, et al. Medical complications of aneurysmal subarachnoid hemorrhage: a report of the multicenter, cooperative aneurysm study. Participants of the Multicenter Cooperative Aneurysm Study. Crit Care Med. 1995; 23:1007–1017

[12] Sahs AL, Nibbelink DW, Torner JC. Aneurysmal Subarachnoid Hemorrhage: Report of the Cooperative Study. Baltimore-Munich 1981

[13] Kassell NF, Sasaki T, Colohan ART, et al. Cerebral Vasospasm Following Aneurysmal Subarachnoid Hemorrhage. Stroke. 1985; 16:562–572

[14] Hop JW, Rinkel GJ, Algra A, ven Gijn J. Case-Fatality Rates and Functional Outcome After Subarachnoid Hemorhage: A Systematic Review. Stroke. 1997; 28:660–664

[15] Drake CG. Management of Cerebral Aneurysm. Stroke. 1981; 12:273 283

[16] Park J, Woo H, Kang DH, Kim Y. Critical age affecting 1-year functional outcome in elderly patients aged > /= 70 years with aneurysmal subarachnoid hemorrhage. Acta Neurochir (Wien). 2014; 156:1655–1661

[17] Wirth FP. Surgical Treatment of Incidental Intracranial Aneurysms. Clin Neurosurg. 1986; 33:125–135

[18] Greene KA, Marciano FF, Johnson BA, Jacobowitz R, Spetzler RF, Harrington TR. Impact of Traumatic Subarachnoid Hemorrhage on Outcome in Nonpenetrating Head Injury. J Neurosurg. 1995; 83:445–452

[19] Taneda M, Kataoka K, Akai F, et al. Traumatic Subarachnoid Hemorrhage as a Predictable Indicator of Delayed Ischemic Symptoms. J Neurosurg. 1996; 84:762–768

[20] Dagi TF, Maccabe JJ. Metastatic Trophoblastic Disease Presenting as a Subarachnoid Hemorrhage. Surg Neurol. 1980; 14:175–184

[21] Memon MY, Neal A, Imami R, et al. Low Grade Glioma Presenting as Subarachnoid Hemorrhage. Neurosurgery. 1984; 14:574–577

[22] Miller RH. Spontaneous Subarachnoid Hemorrhage: A Presenting Symptom of a Tumor of the Third Ventricle. Surg Clin N Amer. 1961; 41:1043–1048

[23] Glass B, Abbott KH. Subarachnoid Hemorrhage Consequent to Intracranial Tumors. Arch Neurol Psych. 1955; 73:369–379

[24] Gleeson RK, Butzer JF, Grin OD. Acoustic Neurinoma Presenting as Subarachnoid Hemorrhage. J Neurosurg. 1978; 49:602–604

[25] Yasargil MG, So SC. Cerebellopontine Angle Meningioma Presenting as Subarachnoid Hemorrhage. Surg Neurol. 1976; 6:3–6

[26] Smith VR, Stein PS, MacCarty CS. Subarachnoid Hemorrhage Due to Lateral Ventricular Meningiomas. Surg Neurol. 1975; 4:241 243

[27] Ernsting J. Choroid Plexus Papilloma Causing Spontaneous Subarachnoid Hemorrhage. J Neurol Neurosurg Psychiatry. 1955; 18:134–136

[28] Simonsen J. Fatal Subarachnoid Hemorrhage Originating in an Intracranial Chordoma. Acta Pathol Microbiol Scand. 1963; 59:13–20

[29] Latchaw JP, Dohn DF, Hahn JF, et al. Subarachnoid Hemorrhage from an Intracranial Meningioma. Neurosurgery. 1981; 9:433–435

[30] Fortuna A, Palma L, Ferrante L, et al. Repeated Subarachnoid Hemorrhage with Vasospasm Secondary to Tuberculum Sella Meningioma. J Neurosurg Sci. 1977; 21:251–256

[31] Ellenbogen RG, Winston KR, Kupsky WJ. Tumors of the Choroid Plexus in Children. Neurosurgery. 1989; 25:327–335

[32] Labovitz DL, Halim AX, Brent B, Boden-Albala B, Hauser WA, Sacco RL. Subarachnoid hemorrhage incidence among Whites, Blacks and Caribbean Hispanics: the Northern Manhattan Study. Neuroepidemiology. 2006; 26:147–150

[33] Shea AM, Reed SD, Curtis LH, Alexander MJ, Villani JJ, Schulman KA. Characteristics of nontraumatic subarachnoid hemorrhage in the United States in 2003. Neurosurgery. 2007; 61:1131–7; discussion 1137-8

[34] de Rooij NK, Linn FH, van der Plas JA, Algra A, Rinkel GJ. Incidence of subarachnoid haemorrhage: a systematic review with emphasis on region, age, gender and time trends. J Neurol Neurosurg Psychiatry. 2007; 78:1365–1372

[35] Bederson JB, Awad IA, Wiebers DO, Piepgras D, et al. Recommendations for the management of patients with unruptured intracranial aneurysms. A statement for healthcare professionals from the Stroke Council of the American Heart Association. Circulation. 2000; 102:2300–2308

[36] Ingall T, Asplund K, Mahonen M, Bonita R. A multinational comparison of subarachnoid hemorrhage epidemiology in the WHO MONICA stroke study. Stroke. 2000; 31:1054–1061

[37] Mahindu A, Koivisto T, Ronkainen A, Rinne J, Assaad N, Morgan MK. Similarities and differences in aneurysmal subarachnoid haemorrhage between eastern Finland and northern Sydney. J Clin Neurosci. 2008; 15:617–621

[38] Vadikolias K, Tsivgoulis G, Heliopoulos I, Papaioakim M, Aggelopoulou C, Serdari A, Birbilis T, Piperidou C. Incidence and case fatality of subarachnoid haemorrhage in Northern Greece: the Evros Registry of Subarachnoid Haemorrhage. Int J Stroke. 2009; 4:322–327

[39] Broderick JP, Brott T, Tomsick T, Huster G, Miller R. The risk of subarachnoid and intracerebral hemorrhages in blacks as compared with whites. N Engl J Med. 1992; 326:733–736

[40] Eden SV, Heisler M, Green C, Morgenstern LB. Racial and ethnic disparities in the treatment of cerebrovascular diseases: importance to the practicing neurosurgeon. Neurocrit Care. 2008; 9:55–73

[41] Connolly ES, Jr, Rabinstein AA, Carhuapoma JR, Derdeyn CP, Dion J, Higashida RT, Hoh BL, Kirkness CJ, Naidech AM, Ogilvy CS, Patel AB, Thompson BG, Vespa P, American Heart Association Stroke Council, Council on Cardiovascular Radiology, Intervention, Council on Cardiovascular Nursing, Council on Cardiovascular Surgery, Anesthesia, Council on Clinical Cardiology. Guidelines for the management of aneurysmal subarachnoid hemorrhage: a guideline for healthcare professionals from the American Heart Association/american Stroke Association. Stroke. 2012; 43:1711–1737

[42] Bonita R. Cigarette Smoking, Hypertension and the Risk of Subarachnoid Hemorrhage: A Population-Based Case-Control Study. Stroke. 1986; 17:831–835

[43] Hoh BL, Sistrom CL, Firment CS, Fautheree GL, Velat GJ, Whiting JH, Reavey-Cantwell JF, Lewis SB. Bottleneck factor and height-width ratio: association with ruptured aneurysms in patients with multiple cerebral aneurysms. Neurosurgery. 2007; 61:716–22; discussion 722-3

[44] Dhar S, Tremmel M, Mocco J, Kim M, Yamamoto J, Siddiqui AH, Hopkins LN, Meng H. Morphology parameters for intracranial aneurysm rupture risk assessment. Neurosurgery. 2008; 63:185–96; discussion 196-7

[45] Rahman M, Smietana J, Hauck E, Hoh B, Hopkins N, Siddiqui A, Levy EI, Meng H, Mocco J. Size ratio correlates with intracranial aneurysm rupture status: a prospective study. Stroke. 2010; 41:916–920

[46] Hirsch KG, Froehler MT, Huang J, Ziai WC. Occurrence of perimesencephalic subarachnoid hemorrhage during pregnancy. Neurocrit Care. 2009; 10:339–343

[47] Tiel Groenestege AT, Rinkel GJ, van der Bom JG, Algra A, Klijn CJ. The risk of aneurysmal subarachnoid hemorrhage during pregnancy, delivery, and the puerperium in the Utrecht population: case-crossover study and standardized incidence ratio estimation. Stroke. 2009; 40:1148–1151
[48] Mohr JP, Caplan LR, Melski JW, et al. The Harvard cooperative stroke registry: A prospective study. Neurology. 1978; 28:754–762
[49] Verweij RD, Wijdicks EFM, van Gijn J. Warning Headache in Aneurysmal Subarachnoid Hemorrhage: A Case-Control Study. Arch Neurol. 1988; 45:1019–1020
[50] Linn FHH, Wijdicks EFM, van der Graaf Y, et al. Prospective Study of Sentinel Headache in Aneurysmal Subarachnoid Hemorhage. Lancet. 1994; 344:590–593
[51] Fisher CM. Painful States: A Neurological Commentary. Clin Neurosurg. 1984; 31:32–35
[52] Linn FHH, Rinkel GJE, van Gijn J. Headache Characteristics in Subarachnoid Hemorhage and Benign Thunderclap Headache. J Neurol Neurosurg Psychiatry. 1998; 65:791–793
[53] Day JW, Raskin NH. Thunderclap Headache: Symptom of Unruptured Cerebral Aneurysm. Lancet. 1986; 2:1247–1248
[54] Wijdicks EFM, Kerkhoff H, van Gijn J. Long-Term Follow-Up of 71 Patients with Thunderclap Headache Mimicking Subarachnoid Hemorrhage. Lancet. 1988; 2:68–70
[55] Markus HS. A Prospective Follow-Up of Thunderclap Headache Mimicking Subarachnoid Hemorrhage. J Neurol Neurosurg Psychiatry. 1991; 54:1117–1118
[56] Ducros A, Boukobza M, Porcher R, Sarov M, Valade D, Bousser MG. The clinical and radiological spectrum of reversible cerebral vasoconstriction syndrome. A prospective series of 67 patients. Brain. 2007; 130:3091–3101
[57] Snyder BD, McClelland RR. Isolated benign cerebral vasculitis. Arch Neurol. 1978; 35:612–614
[58] Frese A, Eikermann A, Frese K, Schwaag S, Husstedt IW, Evers S. Headache associated with sexual activity: demography, clinical features, and comorbidity. Neurology. 2003; 61:796–800
[59] Lance JW. Headaches Related to Sexual Activity. J Neurol Neurosurg Psychiatry. 1976; 39:1226–1230
[60] Ogilvy CS, Rordorf G, Bederson JB. In: Mechanisms and Treatment of Coma After Subarachnoid Hemorrhage. Subarachnoid Hemorrhage: Pathophysiology and Management. Park Ridge, IL: American Association of Neurological Surgeons; 1997:157–171
[61] Manschot WA. Subarachnoid Hemorrhage. Intraocular Symptoms and Their Pathogenesis. Am J Ophthalmol. 1954; 38:501–505
[62] Tsementzis SA, Williams A. Ophthalmological Signs and Prognosis in Patients with a Subarachnoid Hemorrhage. Neurochirurgia. 1984; 27:133–135
[63] Vanderlinden RG, Chisholm LD. Vitreous Hemorrhages and Sudden Increased Intracranial Pressure. J Neurosurg. 1974; 41:167–176
[64] Pfausler B, Belcl R, Metzler R, et al. Terson's Syndrome in Spontaneous Subarachnoid Hemorrhage: A Prospective Study in 60 Consecutive Patients. J Neurosurg. 1996; 85:392–394
[65] Garfinkle AM, Danys IR, Nicolle DA, Colohan ART, et al. Terson's Syndrome: A Reversible Cause of Blindness Following Subarachnoid Hemorrhage. J Neurosurg. 1992; 76:766–771
[66] Friedman SM, Margo CE. Bilateral Subinternal Limiting Membrane Hemorrhage with Terson Syndrome. Am J Ophthalmol. 1997; 124:850–851
[67] Keithahn MAZ, Bennett SR, Cameron D, Mieler WF. Retinal Folds in Terson Syndrome. Ophthalmology. 1993; 100:1187–1190
[68] Schultz PN, Sobol WM, Weingeist TA. Long-Term Visual Outcome in Terson Syndrome. Ophthalmology. 1991; 98:1814–1819
[69] van der Jagt M, Flach HZ, Tanghe HL, Bakker SL, Hunink MG, Koudstaal PJ, van der Lugt A. Assessment of feasibility of endovascular treatment of ruptured intracranial aneurysms with 16-detector row CT angiography. Cerebrovasc Dis. 2008; 26:482–488
[70] Milhorat TH. Acute Hydrocephalus After Aneurysmal Subarachnoid Hemorrhage. Neurosurgery. 1987; 20:15–20
[71] Karttunen AI, Jartti PH, Ukkola VA, Sajanti J, Haapea M. Value of the quantity and distribution of subarachnoid haemorrhage on CT in the localization of a ruptured cerebral aneurysm. Acta Neurochir (Wien). 2003; 145:655–61; discussion 661
[72] Perry JJ, Sivilotti ML, Stiell IG, Wells GA, Raymond J, Mortensen M, Symington C. Should spectrophotometry be used to identify xanthochromia in the cerebrospinal fluid of alert patients suspected of having subarachnoid hemorrhage? Stroke. 2006; 37:2467–2472
[73] Gangloff A, Nadeau L, Perry JJ, Baril P, Emond M. Ruptured aneurysmal subarachnoid hemorrhage in the emergency department: Clinical outcome of patients having a lumbar puncture for red blood cell count, visual and spectrophotometric xanthochromia after a negative computed tomography. Clin Biochem. 2015; 48:634–639
[74] Consensus Conference. Magnetic Resonance Imaging. JAMA. 1988; 259:2132–2138
[75] Hackney DB, Lesnick JE, Zimmerman RA, et al. MR Identification of Bleeding Site in Subarachnoid Hemorrhage with Multiple Intracranial Aneurysms. J Comput Assist Tomogr. 1986; 10:878–880
[76] Ross JS, Masaryk TJ, Modic MT, et al. Intracranial Aneurysms: Evaluation by MR Angiography. AJNR. 1990; 11:449–456
[77] Ronkainen A, Hernesniemi J, Puranen M, Niemitukia L, Vanninen R, Ryynanen M, Kuivaniemi H, Tromp G. Familial Intracranial Aneurysms. Lancet. 1997; 349:380–384
[78] White PM, Wardlaw JM, Easton V. Can noninvasive imaging accurately depict intracranial aneurysms? A systematic review. Radiology. 2000; 217:361–370
[79] Broderick JP, Brown RD, Jr, Sauerbeck L, Hornung R, Huston J, III, Woo D, Anderson C, Rouleau G, Kleindorfer D, Flaherty ML, Meissner I, Foroud T, Moomaw EC, Connolly ES. Greater rupture risk for familial as compared to sporadic unruptured intracranial aneurysms. Stroke. 2009; 40:1952–1957
[80] Hoh BL, Cheung AC, Rabinov JD, Pryor JC, Carter BS, Ogilvy CS. Results of a prospective protocol of computed tomographic angiography in place of catheter angiography as the only diagnostic and pretreatment planning study for cerebral aneurysms by a combined neurovascular team. Neurosurgery. 2004; 54:1329–40; discussion 1340-2
[81] Chaudhary SR, Ko N, Dillon WP, Yu MB, Liu S, Criqui GI, Higashida RT, Smith WS, Wintermark M. Prospective evaluation of multidetector-row CT angiography for the diagnosis of vasospasm following subarachnoid hemorrhage: a comparison with digital subtraction angiography. Cerebrovasc Dis. 2008; 25:144–150
[82] Coupe NJ, Athwal RK, Marshman LA, Brydon HL. Subarachnoid hemorrhage emanating from a ruptured infundibulum: case report and literature review. Surg Neurol. 2007; 67:204–206
[83] Saltzman GF. Infundibular Widening of the Posterior Communicating Artery Studied by Carotid Angiography. Acta Radiol. 1959; 51:415–421
[84] Wollschlaeger G, Wollschlaeger PB, Lucas FV, Lopez VF. Experience and Results with Post-Mortem Cerebral Angiography Performed as Routine Procedure of the Autopsy. Am J Roentgenol Radium Ther Nucl Med. 1967; 101:68–87
[85] Osborn AG. Diagnostic Cerebral Angiography. Philadelphia: Lippincott, Williams and Wilkins; 1999
[86] Yoshimoto T, Suzuki J. Surgical Treatment of an Aneurysm on the Funnel-Shaped Bulge of the Posterior Communicating Artery. J Neurosurg. 1974; 41:377–379
[87] Archer CR, Silbert S. Infundibula May Be Clinically Significant. Neuroradiology. 1978; 152:247–251

[88] Trasi S, Vincent LM, Zingesser LH. Development of Aneurysm from Infundibulum of Posterior Communicating Artery with Documentation of Prior Hemorrhage. AJNR. 1981; 2:368–370
[89] Leblanc R, Worsley KJ, Melanson D, Tampieri D. Angiographic Screening and Elective Surgery of Familial Cerebral Aneurysms. Neurosurgery. 1994; 35:9–18
[90] Locksley HB. Report on the Cooperative Study of Intracranial Aneurysms and Subarachnoid Hemorrhage: Section V - Part II: Natural History of Subarachnoid Hemorrhage, Intracranial Aneurysms, and Arteriovenous Malformations - Based on 6368 Cases in the Cooperative Study. J Neurosurg. 1966; 25:321–368
[91] Henkes H, Fischer S, Weber W, Miloslavski E, Felber S, Brew S, Kuehne D. Endovascular coil occlusion of 1811 intracranial aneurysms: early angiographic and clinical results. Neurosurgery. 2004; 54:268–80; discussion 280-5
[92] Henkes H, Fischer S, Mariushi W, Weber W, Liebig T, Miloslavski E, Brew S, Kuhne D. Angiographic and clinical results in 316 coil-treated basilar artery bifurcation aneurysms. J Neurosurg. 2005; 103:990–999
[93] Debrun GM, Aletich VA, Kehrli P, Misra M, Ausman JI, Charbel F. Selection of cerebral aneurysms for treatment using Guglielmi detachable coils: the preliminary University of Illinois at Chicago experience. Neurosurgery. 1998; 43:1281–95; discussion 1296-7
[94] Hunt WE, Hess RM. Surgical Risk as Related to Time of Intervention in the Repair of Intracranial Aneurysms. J Neurosurg. 1968; 28:14–20
[95] Hunt WE, Kosnik EJ. Timing and Perioperative Care in Intracranial Aneurysm Surgery. Clin Neurosurg. 1974; 21:79–89
[96] Drake CG. Report of World Federation of Neurological Surgeons Committee on a Universal Subarachnoid Hemorrhage Grading Scale. J Neurosurg. 1988; 68:985–986
[97] Teasdale GM, Drake CG, Hunt W, Kassell N, Sano K, Pertuiset B, De Villiers JC. A universal subarachnoid hemorrhage scale: report of a committee of the World Federation of Neurosurgical Societies. J Neurol Neurosurg Psychiatry. 1988; 51
[98] Mori K, Arai H, Nakajima K, Tajima A, Maeda M. Hemorheological and Hemodynamic Analysis of Hypervolemic Hemodilution Therapy for Cerebral Vasospasm After Aneurysmal Subarachnoid Hemorrhage. Stroke. 1996; 26:1620–1626
[99] Dirnagl U, Becker K, Meisel A. Preconditioning and tolerance against cerebral ischaemia: from experimental strategies to clinical use. Lancet Neurol. 2009; 8:398–412
[100] Dalen JE, Bone RC. Is it time to pull the pulmonary artery catheter? JAMA. 1996; 276:916–918
[101] Mutoh T, Kazumata K, Ishikawa T, Terasaka S. Performance of bedside transpulmonary thermodilution monitoring for goal-directed hemodynamic management after subarachnoid hemorrhage. Stroke. 2009; 40:2368–2374

77

[102] Redekop G, Ferguson G, Carter LP, Spetzler RF, Hamilton MG. In: Intracranial Aneurysms. Neurovascular Surgery. New York: McGraw-Hill; 1995:625–648
[103] Vermeulen LC, Ratko TA, Erstad BL, et al. The University Hospital Consortium Guidelines for the Use of Albumin, Nonprotein Colloid, and Crystalloid Solutions. Arch Intern Med. 1995; 155:373–379
[104] Kronvall E, Undren P, Romner B, Saveland H, Cronqvist M, Nilsson OG. Nimodipine in aneurysmal subarachnoid hemorrhage: a randomized study of intravenous or peroral administration. J Neurosurg. 2009; 110:58–63
[105] Nearman HS, Herman ML. Toxic Effects of Colloids in the Intensive Care Unit. Crit Care Med. 1991; 7:713–723
[106] Bianchine JR. Intracranial Bleeding During Treatment with Hydroxyethyl Starch - Letter in Reply. New Engl J Med. 1987; 317
[107] Trumble ER, Muizelaar JP, Myseros JS. Coagulopathy with the Use of Hetastarch in the Treatment of Vasospasm. J Neurosurg. 1995; 82:44–47
[108] Vergouwen MD, de Haan RJ, Vermeulen M, Roos YB. Effect of statin treatment on vasospasm, delayed cerebral ischemia, and functional outcome in patients with aneurysmal subarachnoid hemorrhage: a systematic review and meta-analysis update. Stroke. 2010; 41:e47–e52
[109] Kirkpatrick PJ, Turner CL, Smith C, Hutchinson PJ, Murray GD. Simvastatin in aneurysmal subarachnoid haemorrhage (STASH): a multicentre randomised phase 3 trial. Lancet Neurol. 2014; 13:666–675
[110] Fernandez A, Schmidt JM, Claassen J, Pavlicova M, Huddleston D, Kreiter KT, Ostapkovich ND, Kowalski RG, Parra A, Connolly ES, Mayer SA. Fever after subarachnoid hemorrhage: risk factors and impact on outcome. Neurology. 2007; 68:1013–1019
[111] Zhang G, Zhang JH, Qin X. Fever increased in-hospital mortality after subarachnoid hemorrhage. Acta Neurochir Suppl. 2011; 110:239–243
[112] Badjatia N, Fernandez L, Schmidt JM, Lee K, Claassen J, Connolly ES, Mayer SA. Impact of induced normothermia on outcome after subarachnoid hemorrhage: a case-control study. Neurosurgery. 2010; 66:696–700; discussion 700-1
[113] Naidech AM, Drescher J, Ault ML, Shaibani A, Batjer HH, Alberts MJ. Higher hemoglobin is associated with less cerebral infarction, poor outcome, and death after subarachnoid hemorrhage. Neurosurgery. 2006; 59:775–9; discussion 779-80
[114] Naidech AM, Jovanovic B, Wartenberg KE, Parra A, Ostapkovich N, Connolly ES, Mayer SA, Commichau C. Higher hemoglobin is associated with improved outcome after subarachnoid hemorrhage. Crit Care Med. 2007; 35:2383–2389
[115] Kramer AH, Gurka MJ, Nathan B, Dumont AS, Kassell NF, Bleck TP. Complications associated with anemia and blood transfusion in patients with aneurysmal subarachnoid hemorrhage. Crit Care Med. 2008; 36:2070–2075
[116] Smith MJ, Le Roux PD, Elliott JP, Winn HR. Blood transfusion and increased risk for vasospasm and poor outcome after subarachnoid hemorrhage. J Neurosurg. 2004; 101:1–7
[117] Schlenk F, Vajkoczy P, Sarrafzadeh A. Inpatient hyperglycemia following aneurysmal subarachnoid hemorrhage: relation to cerebral metabolism and outcome. Neurocrit Care. 2009; 11:56–63
[118] Ciongoli AK, Poser CM. Pulmonary Edema Secondary to Subarachnoid Hemorrhage. Neurology (NY). 1972; 22:867–870
[119] Solomon RA, Fink ME, Lennihan L. Prophylactic Volume Expansion Therapy for the Prevention of Delayed Cerebral Ischemia After Early Aneurysm Surgery. Arch Neurol. 1988; 45:325–332
[120] Egge A, Waterloo K, Sjoholm H, Solberg T, Ingebrigtsen T, Romner B. Prophylactic hyperdynamic postoperative fluid therapy after aneurysmal subarachnoid hemorrhage: a clinical, prospective, randomized, controlled study. Neurosurgery. 2001; 49:593–605; discussion 605-6
[121] Wise BL. SIADH After Spontaneous Subarachnoid Hemorrhage: A Reversible Cause of Clinical Deterioration. Neurosurgery. 1978; 3:412–414
[122] Wijdicks EFM, Ropper AH, Hunnicutt EJ, Richardson GS, et al. Atrial Natriuretic Factor and Salt Wasting After Aneurysmal Subarachnoid Hemorrhage. Stroke. 1991; 22:1519–1524
[123] Harrigan MR. Cerebral Salt Wasting Syndrome: A Review. Neurosurgery. 1996; 38:152–160
[124] Kröll M, Juhler M, Lindholm J. Hyponatremia in Acute Brain Disease. J Int Med. 1992; 232:291–297
[125] Wijdicks EFM, Schievink WI, Burnett JC. Natriuretic Peptide System and Endothelin in Aneurysmal Subarachnoid Hemorrhage. J Neurosurg. 1997; 87:275–280
[126] Nelson PB, Seif SM, Maroon JC, et al. Hyponatremia in Intracranial Disease. Perhaps Not the Syndrome of Inappropriate Secretion of Antidiuretic Hormone (SIADH). J Neurosurg. 1981; 55:938–941

[127] Wijdicks EFM, Vermeulen M, Hijdra A, et al. Hyponatremia and Cerebral Infarction in Patients with Ruptured Intracranial Aneurysms: Is Fluid Restriction Harmful? Ann Neurol. 1985; 17:137–140
[128] Chandy D, Sy R, Aronow WS, Lee WN, Maguire G, Murali R. Hyponatremia and cerebrovascular spasm in aneurysmal subarachnoid hemorrhage. Neurol India. 2006; 54:273–275
[129] Nakagawa I, Kurokawa S, Takayama K, Wada T, Nakase H. [Increased urinary sodium excretion in the early phase of aneurysmal subarachnoid hemorrhage as a predictor of cerebral salt wasting syndrome]. Brain Nerve. 2009; 61:1419–1423
[130] Harbaugh RE. Aneurysmal Subarachnoid Hemorrhage and Hyponatremia. Contemp Neurosurg. 1993; 15:1–5
[131] Suarez JI, Qureshi AI, Parekh PD, Razumovsky A, Tamargo RJ, Bhardwaj A, Ulatowski JA. Administration of hypertonic (3%) sodium chloride/acetate in hyponatremic patients with symptomatic vasospasm following subarachnoid hemorrhage. J Neurosurg Anesthesiol. 1999; 11:178–184
[132] Al-Rawi PG, Tseng MY, Richards HK, Nortje J, Timofeev I, Matta BF, Hutchinson PJ, Kirkpatrick PJ. Hypertonic saline in patients with poor-grade subarachnoid hemorrhage improves cerebral blood flow, brain tissue oxygen, and pH. Stroke. 2010; 41:122–128
[133] Hasan D, Lindsay KW, Wijdicks EFM, et al. Effect of Fludrocortisone Acetate in Patients with Subarachnoid Hemorrhage. Stroke. 1989; 20:1156–1161
[134] Mori T, Katayama Y, Kawamata T, Hirayama T. Improved efficiency of hypervolemic therapy with inhibition of natriuresis by fludrocortisone in patients with aneurysmal subarachnoid hemorrhage. J Neurosurg. 1999; 91:947–952
[135] Katayama Y, Haraoka J, Hirabayashi H, Kawamata T, Kawamoto K, Kitahara T, Kojima J, Kuroiwa T, Mori T, Moro N, Nagata I, Ogawa A, Ohno K, Seiki Y, Shiokawa Y, Teramoto A, Tominaga T, Yoshimine T. A randomized controlled trial of hydrocortisone against hyponatremia in patients with aneurysmal subarachnoid hemorrhage. Stroke. 2007; 38:2373–2375
[136] Butzkueven H, Evans AH, Pitman A, Leopold C, Jolley DJ, Kaye AH, Kilpatrick CJ, Davis SM. Onset seizures independently predict poor outcome after subarachnoid hemorrhage. Neurology. 2000; 55:1315–1320
[137] Byrne JV, Boardman P, Ioannidis I, Adcock J, Traill Z. Seizures after aneurysmal subarachnoid hemorrhage treated with coil embolization. Neurosurgery. 2003; 52:545–52; discussion 550-2
[138] Lin CL, Dumont AS, Lieu AS, Yen CP, Hwang SL, Kwan AL, Kassell NF, Howng SL. Characterization of perioperative seizures and epilepsy following aneurysmal subarachnoid hemorrhage. J Neurosurg. 2003; 99:978–985
[139] Marigold R, Gunther A, Tiwari D, Kwan J. Antiepileptic drugs for the primary and secondary prevention of seizures after subarachnoid haemorrhage. Cochrane Database Syst Rev. 2013; 6. DOI: 10.1002/14651858.CD008710.pub2
[140] Claassen J, Mayer SA, Kowalski RG, Emerson RG, Hirsch LJ. Detection of electrographic seizures with continuous EEG monitoring in critically ill patients. Neurology. 2004; 62:1743–1748
[141] Dennis LJ, Claassen J, Hirsch LJ, Emerson RG, Connolly ES, Mayer SA. Nonconvulsive status epilepticus after subarachnoid hemorrhage. Neurosurgery. 2002; 51:1136–43; discussion 1144
[142] Ukkola V, Heikkinen ER. Epilepsy after operative treatment of ruptured cerebral aneurysms. Acta Neurochir (Wien). 1990; 106:115–118
[143] Choi KS, Chun HJ, Yi HJ, Ko Y, Kim YS, Kim JM. Seizures and Epilepsy following Aneurysmal Subarachnoid Hemorrhage : Incidence and Risk Factors. J Korean Neurosurg Soc. 2009; 46:93–98
[144] Kotila M, Waltimo O. Epilepsy after stroke. Epilepsia. 1992; 33:495–498
[145] Rhoney DH, Tipps LB, Murry KR, Basham MC, Michael DB, Coplin WM. Anticonvulsant prophylaxis and timing of seizures after aneurysmal subarachnoid hemorrhage. Neurology. 2000; 55:258–265
[146] Little AS, Kerrigan JF, McDougall CG, Zabramski JM, Albuquerque FC, Nakaji P, Spetzler RF. Nonconvulsive status epilepticus in patients suffering spontaneous subarachnoid hemorrhage. J Neurosurg. 2007; 106:805–811
[147] Chumnanvej S, Dunn IF, Kim DH. Three-day phenytoin prophylaxis is adequate after subarachnoid hemorrhage. Neurosurgery. 2007; 60:99–102; discussion 102-3
[148] Naidech AM, Kreiter KT, Janjua N, Ostapkovich N, Parra A, Commichau C, Connolly ES, Mayer SA, Fitzsimmons BF. Phenytoin exposure is associated with functional and cognitive disability after subarachnoid hemorrhage. Stroke. 2005; 36:583–587
[149] Murphy-Human T, Welch E, Zipfel G, Diringer MN, Dhar R. Comparison of short-duration levetiracetam with extended-course phenytoin for seizure prophylaxis after subarachnoid hemorrhage. World Neurosurg. 2011; 75:269–274
[150] Szaflarski JP, Sangha KS, Lindsell CJ, Shutter LA. Prospective, randomized, single-blinded comparative trial of intravenous levetiracetam versus phenytoin for seizure prophylaxis. Neurocrit Care. 2010; 12:165–172
[151] Kassell NF, Drake CG. Review of the Management of Saccular Aneurysms. Neurol Clin. 1983; 1:73–86
[152] Kassell NF, Torner JC. Aneurysmal rebleeding: a preliminary report from the Cooperative Aneurysm Study. Neurosurgery. 1983; 13:479–481
[153] Hillman J, Fridriksson S, Nilsson O, Yu Z, Saveland H, Jakobsson KE. Immediate administration of tranexamic acid and reduced incidence of early rebleeding after aneurysmal subarachnoid hemorrhage: a prospective randomized study. J Neurosurg. 2002; 97:771–778
[154] Naidech AM, Janjua N, Kreiter KT, Ostapkovich ND, Fitzsimmons BF, Parra A, Commichau C, Connolly ES, Mayer SA. Predictors and impact of aneurysm rebleeding after subarachnoid hemorrhage. Arch Neurol. 2005; 62:410–416
[155] Ohkuma H, Tsurutani H, Suzuki S. Incidence and significance of early aneurysmal rebleeding before neurosurgical or neurological management. Stroke. 2001; 32:1176–1180
[156] Tanno Y, Homma M, Oinuma M, Kodama N, Ymamoto T. Rebleeding from ruptured intracranial aneurysms in North Eastern Province of Japan. A cooperative study. J Neurol Sci. 2007; 258:11–16
[157] Winn HR, Richardson AE, Jane JA. The Long-Term Prognosis in Untreated Cerebral Aneurysms. I. The Incidence of Late Hemorrhage in Cerebral Aneurysm: A 10-Year Evaluation of 364 Patients. Ann Neurol. 1977; 1:358–370
[158] Kassell NF, Torner JC, Haley EC, Jr, Jane JA, Adams HP, Kongable GL. The International Cooperative Study on the Timing of Aneurysm Surgery. Part 1: Overall Management Results. J Neurosurg. 1990; 73:18–36
[159] Inagawa T, Kamiya K, Ogasawara H, et al. Rebleeding of Ruptured Intracranial Aneurysms in the Actue Stage. Surg Neurol. 1987; 28:93–99
[160] Matsuda M, Watanabe K, Saito A, Matsumura K, Ichikawa M. Circumstances, activities, and events precipitating aneurysmal subarachnoid hemorrhage. J Stroke Cerebrovasc Dis. 2007; 16:25–29
[161] Jane JA, Kassell NF, Torner JC, et al. The Natural History of Aneurysms and AVMs. J Neurosurg. 1985; 62:321–323
[162] Biller J, Godersky JC, Adams HP. Management of Aneurysmal Subarachnoid Hemorrhage. Stroke. 1988; 19:1300–1305
[163] Kassell NF, Torner JC, Adams HP. Antifibrinolytic Therapy in the Acute Period Following Aneurysmal Subarachnoid Hemorrhage: Preliminary Observations from the Cooperative Aneurysm Study. J Neurosurg. 1984; 61:225–230
[164] Glick R, Green D, Ts'ao C-H, Witt WA, Yu ATW, Raimondi AJ. High Dose e-Aminocaproic Acid Prolongs the Bleeding Time and Increases Rebleeding and Intraoperative Hemorrhage in Patients with

Subarachnoid Hemorrhage. Neurosurgery. 1981; 9:398–401

[165] Leipzig TJ, Redelman K, Horner TG. Reducing the Risk of Rebleeding Before Early Aneurysm Surgery: A Possible Role for Antifibrinolytic Therapy. J Neurosurg. 1997; 86:220–225

[166] Starke RM, Kim GH, Fernandez A, Komotar RJ, Hickman ZL, Otten ML, Ducruet AF, Kellner CP, Hahn DK, Chwajol M, Mayer SA, Connolly ES,Jr. Impact of a protocol for acute antifibrinolytic therapy on aneurysm rebleeding after subarachnoid hemorrhage. Stroke. 2008; 39:2617–2621

[167] Dias MS, Sekhar LN. Intracranial Hemorrhage from Aneurysms and Arteriovenous Malformations during Pregnancy and the Puerperium. Neurosurgery. 1990; 27:855–866

[168] Crawford S, Varner MW, Digre KB, Servais G, et al. Cranial Magnetic Resonance Imaging in Eclampsia. Obstet Gynecol. 1987; 70:474–477

[169] Postma IR, Slager S, Kremer HP, de Groot JC, Zeeman GG. Long-term consequences of the posterior reversible encephalopathy syndrome in eclampsia and preeclampsia: a review of the obstetric and nonobstetric literature. Obstet Gynecol Surv. 2014; 69:287–300

[170] Robinson JL, Hall CJ, Sedzimir CB. Subarachnoid Hemorrhage in Pregnancy. J Neurosurg. 1972; 36:27–33

[171] Robinson JL, Hall CS, Sedzimir CB. Arteriovenous Malformations, Aneurysms, and Pregnancy. J Neurosurg. 1974; 41:63–70

[172] Horton JC, Chambers WA, Lyons SL, Adams RD, et al. Pregnancy and the Risk of Hemorrhage from Cerebral Arteriovenous Malformations. Neurosurgery. 1990; 27:867–872

[173] Kim YW, Neal D, Hoh BL. Cerebral aneurysms in pregnancy and delivery: pregnancy and delivery do not increase the risk of aneurysm rupture. Neurosurgery. 2013; 72:143–9; discussion 150

[174] De Santis M, Straface G, Cavaliere AF, Carducci B, Caruso A. Gadolinium periconceptional exposure: pregnancy and neonatal outcome. Acta Obstet Gynecol Scand. 2007; 86:99–101

[175] Kataoka H, Miyoshi T, Neki R, Yoshimatsu J, Ishibashi-Ueda H, Iihara K. Subarachnoid hemorrhage from intracranial aneurysms during pregnancy and the puerperium. Neurol Med Chir (Tokyo). 2013; 53:549–554

[176] Marshman LA, Rai MS, Aspoas AR. Comment to "Endovascular treatment of ruptured intracranial aneurysms during pregnancy: report of three cases". Arch Gynecol Obstet. 2005; 272. DOI: 10.1007/s00404-004-0707-x

[177] Hasan D, Vermeulen M, Wijdicks EFM, Hijdra A, van Gijn J. Management Problems in Acute Hydrocephalus After Subarchnoid Hemorrhage. Stroke. 1989; 20:747–753

[178] Graff-Radford N, Torner J, Adams HP, Kassell NF, et al. Factors Associated With Hydrocephalus After Subarachnoid Hemorrhage. Arch Neurol. 1989; 46:744–752

[179] Kusske JA, Turner PT, Ojemann GA, Harris AB. Ventriculostomy for the Treatment of Acute Hydrocephalus Following Subarachnoid Hemorrhage. J Neurosurg. 1973; 38:591–595

[180] van Gijn J, Hijdra A, Wijdicks EFM, Vermeulen M, van Crevel H. Acute Hydrocephalus After Aneurysmal Subarachnoid Hemorrhage. J Neurosurg. 1985; 63:355–362

[181] Hellingman CA, van den Bergh WM, Beijer IS, van Dijk GW, Algra A, van Gijn J, Rinkel GJ. Risk of rebleeding after treatment of acute hydrocephalus in patients with aneurysmal subarachnoid hemorrhage. Stroke. 2007; 38:96–99

[182] Pare L, Delfino R, Leblanc R. The relationship of ventricular drainage to aneurysmal rebleeding. J Neurosurg. 1992; 76:422–427

[183] McIver JI, Friedman JA, Wijdicks EF, Piepgras DG, Pichelmann MA, Toussaint LG, III, McClelland RL, Nichols DA, Atkinson JL. Preoperative ventriculostomy and rebleeding after aneurysmal subarachnoid hemorrhage. J Neurosurg. 2002; 97:1042–1044

[184] Voldby B, Enevoldsen EM. Intracranial Pressure Changes Following Aneurysm Rupture. 3. Recurrent Hemorrhage. J Neurosurg. 1982; 56:784–789

[185] Auer LM, Mokry M. Disturbed Cerebrospinal Fluid Circulation After Subarachnoid Hemorrhage and Acute Aneurysm Surgery. Neurosurgery. 1990; 26:804–809

[186] Connolly ES, Kader AA, Frazzini VI, Winfree CJ, Solomon RA. The Safety of Intraoperative Lumbar Subarachnoid Drainage for Acutely Ruptured Intracranial Aneurysm: Technical Note. Surg Neurol. 1997; 48:338–344

[187] Koh KM, Ng Z, Low SY, Chua HZ, Chou N, Low SW, Yeo TT. Management of ruptured intracranial aneurysms in the post-ISAT era: outcome of surgical clipping versus endovascular coiling in a Singapore tertiary institution. Singapore Med J. 2013; 54:332–338

[188] Hoh BL, Kleinhenz DT, Chi YY, Mocco J, Barker FG, II. Incidence of ventricular shunt placement for hydrocephalus with clipping versus coiling for ruptured and unruptured cerebral aneurysms in the Nationwide Inpatient Sample database: 2002 to 2007. World Neurosurg. 2011; 76:548–554

[189] Klopfenstein JD, Kim LJ, Feiz-Erfan I, Hott JS, Goslar P, Zabramski JM, Spetzler RF. Comparison of rapid and gradual weaning from external ventricular drainage in patients with aneurysmal subarachnoid hemorrhage: a prospective randomized trial. J Neurosurg. 2004; 100:225–229

78 Critical Care of Aneurysm Patients

78.1 Neurogenic stress cardiomyopathy (NSC)

78.1.1 General information

Key concepts

- impaired cardiac function (reduced ejection fraction) not attributable to underlying coronary artery disease or myocardial abnormalities. May be reversible
- cardiac enzymes (troponin) tend to be lower than expected for the degree of myocardial impairment, distinguishes NSC from acute MI
- putative mechanism: catecholamine surge (possibly in myocardial sympathetic nerves) as a result of hypothalamic stimulation or injury from the SAH
- possible sequalae: hypotension, CHF, arrhythmias... all of which may further exacerbate cerebral ischemia
- peak incidence: 2 days to 2 weeks post SAH
- risk factors: higher Hunt and Hess grade
- treatment: may include dobutamine (for SBP < 90 and low SVR) and/or milrinone (for SBP > 90 and increased SVR)

Older terms: reversible postischemic myocardial dysfunction,[1] neurogenic stunned myocardium. Classically seen in patients following cardiac surgery, and attributed to a defect in troponin-I (TnI).[2] Some patients may develop myocardial hypokinesis following SAH.[3] May appear compatible with an MI on echocardiography, yet, troponin levels are typically lower (often < 2.8 ng/ml) than would be predicted given the level of myocardial impairment.[4] Peak incidence: 2 days to 2 weeks post SAH. The condition reverses completely in most cases within about 5 days as normal myocardial cells replace those with defective TnI. However, ≈ 10% of patients may progress on to an actual MI.

Stroke volume and cardiac output are reduced. Risk factors include higher Hunt Hess grade (> 3),[5,6,7,8] female gender,[8,9] smoking status and age.[5] Hypotension does not always occur since the reduced cardiac output (CO) may be offset by an increase in SVR. However, the reduced CO may impair the ability to tolerate barbiturates administered for cerebral protection during early surgery due to their myocardial suppressant effect. Intraoperative TEE monitoring may be a useful guide for titrating pressors. The reduced CO may also impede the use of hyperdynamic therapy for vasospasm.

78.1.2 Arrhythmias and EKG changes

EKG changes in over 50% of cases of SAH and include: broad or inverted T-waves, Q-T prolongation, S-T segment elevation or depression, U-waves, premature atrial or ventricular contraction, SVT, V-flutter or V-fib,[10] bradycardia. In some cases EKG abnormalities may be indistinguishable from an acute MI.[11,12]

78.1.3 Possible mechanism

Elevation of intracranial pressure secondary to aSAH is thought to cause sympathetic activation resulting in hypercontraction of cardiac myocytes and subsequent myocardial injury.[5] A related theory invokes hypothalamic ischemia resulting in increased sympathetic tone, whereby the hypothalamic ischemia results in increased sympathetic tone and the resultant catecholamine surge may produce subendocardial ischemia[13] or coronary artery vasospasm.[3] The catecholamine surge appears to be more focal (i.e. in the heart) than systemic.

78.1.4 Treatment

Interventions that have been studied for increasing cardiac output in NSC[14,15]:

1. milrinone: used when SBP > 90 mmHg and normal SVR, or when the patient is on chronic beta blockers
2. dobutamine: more effective with hypotension (SBP < 90 mmHg) and low SVR
3. other options: stellate ganglion block, magnesium

78.2 Neurogenic pulmonary edema

78.2.1 General information

A rare condition associated with a variety of intracranial pathologies, including:
- subarachnoid hemorrhage
- generalized seizures
- and head injury

78.2.2 Pathophysiology

Two possibly synergistic mechanisms. Sudden increased ICP or hypothalamic injury may produce a salvo of sympathetic discharge causing redistribution of blood to the pulmonary circulation, resulting in elevation of pulmonary capillary wedge pressures (PCWP) and increased permeability. Secondly, the associated surge of catecholamines directly disrupts the capillary endothelium which increases alveolar permeability.

78.2.3 Treatment

Supportive, using measures such as positive pressure ventilation with low levels of PEEP (p. 871) and treatment to normalize ICP.

A PA-catheter is usually helpful.

There may be some efficacy in using a dobutamine infusion[16] supplemented with furosemide as needed. The theoretical advantage of dobutamine over previously attempted alpha- and beta-blockers is that dobutamine does not reduce cerebral perfusion.

78.3 Vasospasm

78.3.1 General information

Key concepts

- delayed cerebral ischemic symptoms and/or cerebral arterial narrowing on angiography that follows some cases of SAH (usually), trauma, or other insults
- time course: almost never before day 3 post SAH, peak incidence 6–8 days post SAH, rarely starts after day 17. Main time of risk: 3–14 days post SAH
- risk factors: higher SAH grade, more blood on CT
- results in pathologic changes within the vessel walls (not just vasoconstriction)
- diagnosis: may be clinical, angiographic, or with transcranial Doppler
- treatment: none are curative. Mainstays of treatment:
  - euvolemia and hemodynamic augmentation (formerly "triple H" therapy)
  - neuroendovascular intervention: angioplasty or intraarterial verapamil

78

Cerebral vasospasm is a condition that is most commonly seen following some cases of aneurysmal subarachnoid hemorrhage (SAH), but may also follow other intracranial hemorrhages (e.g. intraventricular hemorrhage from AVM,[17] and SAH of unknown etiology), head trauma (with or without SAH),[18] brain surgery, lumbar puncture, hypothalamic injury, infection, and may be associated with preeclampsia (p. 194). The concept of vasospasm was originated in 1951 by Ecker.[19] Vasospasm has two not-necessarily reconcilable definitions (below):
1. clinical vasospasm: see below
2. radiographic vasospasm: see below

78.3.2 Definitions

Delayed cerebral ischemia (DCI) and early brain injury (EBI)

There has been a move away from thinking of the deleterious effects of SAH in terms of vasospasm, and the concepts of DCI and EBI are coming to the fore.[20]

DCI: Delayed development of a neurological deficit, decline in Glasgow coma scale of at least 2 points, and/or cerebral infarction unrelated to aneurysm treatment or other causes. DCI is an umbrella term that encompasses a number of clinical entities including symptomatic vasospasm, delayed ischemic neurological deficit (DIND), and asymptomatic delayed cerebral infarction.[21]

EBI: In addition to direct mechanical damage from the SAH, EBI also refers to a number of other factors including the transient increase in ICP, reduction of CBF, apoptosis and edema formation.

Clinical vasospasm

Sometimes referred to as delayed ischemic neurologic deficit (DIND), or symptomatic vasospasm. A *delayed* ischemic neurologic deficit following SAH. Clinically characterized by confusion or decreased level of consciousness sometimes with focal neurologic deficit (speech or motor). The diagnosis is one of exclusion, and sometimes cannot be made with certainty.

See clinical findings (p. 1179).

Radiographic vasospasm (AKA angiographic vasospasm)

Arterial narrowing demonstrated on cerebral angiography, often with slowing of contrast filling. The diagnosis is solidified by previous or subsequent angiograms showing the same vessel(s) with normal caliber. In some cases a DIND corresponds to a region of vasospasm seen angiographically. The incidence of angiographic vasospasm following SAH is around 50% (range: 20-100%).[22]

78.3.3 Characteristics of cerebral vasospasm

Clinical findings

Findings usually develop gradually, and may progress or fluctuate. May include:

1. non-localizing findings
   a) new or increasing H/A
   b) alterations in level of consciousness (lethargy…)
   c) disorientation
   d) meningismus
2. focal neurological signs may occur including cranial nerve palsies[23,24] and focal motor deficits. Also, symptoms may cluster into one of the following "syndromes" (vasospasm incidence is higher in the distribution of the ACA than in that of the MCA)
   a) anterior cerebral artery (ACA) syndrome: frontal lobe findings predominate (abulia, grasp/suck reflex, urinary incontinence, drowsiness, slowness, delayed responses, confusion, whispering). Bilateral anterior cerebral artery distribution infarcts are usually due to vasospasm following an AComm aneurysm rupture
   b) middle cerebral artery (MCA) syndrome: hemiparesis, monoparesis, aphasia (or apractagnosia of non-dominant hemisphere – inability to use objects or perform skilled motor activities, due to lesions in the lower occipital or parietal lobes; subtypes: ideomotor apraxia and sensory apraxia)

Incidence

1. Radiographic cerebral vasospasm (CVS) is identified in 20–100% of arteriograms performed around the 7th day following SAH, whereas clinical vasospasm associated with radiographic CVS occurs in only ≈ 30% of patients with SAH[25]
2. radiographic CVS may occur in the absence of clinical deficit, and vice-versa

Severity

1. CVS is a significant cause of morbidity and mortality in patients surviving SAH long enough to reach medical care, exceeded only by the direct effects of aneurysmal rupture as well as re-bleeding[26,27]
2. CVS ranges in severity from mild reversible dysfunction, to severe permanent deficits secondary to ischemic infarction in up to 60% of SAH patients,[28] extensive enough to be fatal in 7% of SAHs[25,28]
3. earlier onset of CVS is associated with greater deficit

Time course of vasospasm

1. onset: almost never before day 3 post-SAH[29]
2. maximal frequency of onset during days 6–8 post-SAH (however, rarely can occur as late as day 17). Typical at-risk period is quoted as days 3–14[30]
3. clinical CVS is almost always resolved by day 12 post-SAH. Once radiographic CVS is demonstrated, it usually resolves slowly over 3–4 weeks
4. onset is usually insidious, but ≈ 10% have an abrupt and severe deterioration

Correlated findings

1. Risk is higher in conditions where arterial blood at high pressure contacts the vessels at the base of the brain. CVS rarely occurs in the setting of intraparenchymal or pure intraventricular hemorrhage (e.g. from AVM) or in SAH with distribution limited to the cerebral convexity
2. blood clots are especially spasmogenic when in direct contact with the proximal 9 cm of the ACA and the MCA
3. not all patients with SAH develop CVS, and CVS can follow other insults besides SAH, such as mass resection,[31] meningitis,[32] amygdalohippocampectomy.[33] Can even be associated with sexual intercourse[34]and over-consumption of black licorice[35]
4. the Hunt and Hess grade on admission correlates with the risk of CVS (▶ Table 78.1)
5. the amount of blood on CT correlates with the severity of CVS[36,37] (▶ Table 78.2; also holds true for traumatic SAH[38])
6. higher incidence with increasing age of patient
7. a history of active cigarette smoking is an independent risk factor[39]
8. history of preexisting hypertension
9. there is good but not perfect correlation between the site of major blood clots on CT, the focality of delayed ischemic neurological deficits, and the visualization of angiographic CVS in corresponding arteries
10. pial enhancement on CT ≈ 3 days after SAH (with IV contrast administration) may correlate with higher risk of CVS (indicates increased permeability of BBB),[40] but this is controversial[41]

Table 78.1 Correlation of DIND with Hunt and Hess grade

Hunt and Hess grade	% DIND (clinical vasospasm)
1	22%
2	33%
3	52%
4	53%
5	74%

Table 78.2 Modified[43] grading system of Fisher[36] (correlation between the amount of blood on CT and the risk of vasospasm)

Modified Fisher scale group	Blood on CT[a]	Symptomatic vasospasm
	No SAH or IVH	
1	focal or diffuse thin SAH, no IVH	24%
2	focal or diffuse thin SAH, with IVH	33%
3	focal or diffuse thick SAH, no IVH	33%
4	focal or diffuse thick SAH, with IVH	40%

[a]measurements made in the greatest longitudinal & transverse dimension on a printed EMI CT scan (no scaling to actual thickness) performed within 5 d of SAH in 47 patients; falx never contributed more than 1 mm thickness to interhemispheric blood

11. for patients undergoing early surgery, if there is little SAH left on a CT done 24 hours post-op, there is little risk of vasospasm
12. antifibrinolytic therapy reduces *rebleeding*, but increases the risk of hydrocephalus and vasospasm (p. 1168) [42]
13. angiographic dye can exacerbate CVS
14. hypovolemia

78.3.4 Pathogenesis

Pathogenesis is still poorly understood.

In humans, CVS is a chronic condition with definite long-term changes in the morphology of the involved vessels. Much of CVS is poorly understood because of lack of a good animal model (humans show a mild acute phase, and most animal studies fail to demonstrate a chronic phase).

Pathological changes observed within the vessel wall are outlined in ▶ Table 78.3.

▶ **Direct mediators.** Vasospasm is caused by smooth muscle contraction, due to either impaired vasodilatory mediators, overactive vasoconstrictive mediators, or more likely, both.

- The formed components of blood have each been shown to contribute to vasospasm
  - Oxyhemoglobin in pure form can cause contraction of cerebral arteries when contacting the abluminal surface of the vessel
  - Hemoglobin scavenges Nitric Oxide, a powerful vasorelaxant[46]
  - Platelet-derived growth factor induces vascular proliferation → vascular stiffening and impaired ability to dilate[47]
- Endothelial dysfunction: theories include decreased production of Nitrous Oxide and prostacyclins, and overproduction of Endothelin-1
- Vessel innervation by the sympathetic nervous system. Interruption of sympathetic innervation prevents vasospasm in rats[48]

▶ **Proposed mechanisms of vasospasm include**

- contraction of the smooth muscle in the media of the vessel wall, as a result of:
  - vasoconstrictors within the hemorrhagic arterial blood[49] (see below)
  - vasoactive substances released into the CSF[50,51]
  - neuronal mechanisms via nervi vasorum (nerves in the vessel wall)
    - increased vasoconstrictor tone (possibly due to denervation supersensitivity)
    - loss of vasodilator tone
    - time dependent relative imbalance favoring vasoconstrictor over vasodilator innervation[52]
    - sympathetic hyperactivity: e.g. due to hypothalamic injury from elevated ICP[53]
  - impairment of endothelial derived relaxant factor (EDRF): vascular endothelium plays an obligatory role in vasodilatation caused by several pharmacologic agents by releasing a relaxant substance called EDRF[54]
- proliferative vasculopathy
- immunoreactive process
- inflammatory process
- mechanical phenomenon
  - stretching of arachnoid fibers
  - direct compression by blood clot
  - platelet aggregation[49]

Table 78.3 Pathological changes in vasospasm

Time	Vessel layer	Pathologic change
day 1–8	adventitia	↑ inflammatory cells (lymphocytes, plasma cells, mast cells) and connective tissue
	media	muscle necrosis and corrugation of elastica
	intima	thickening with endothelial swelling and vacuolization, opening of interendothelial tight junctions[44,45]
day 9–60	intima	proliferation of smooth muscle cells → progressive intimal thickening

78.3.5 Diagnosis of cerebral vasospasm

General information

Diagnosis requires appropriate clinical criteria, and ruling-out other conditions that can produce delayed neurologic deterioration, as shown in ▶ Table 78.4.

Ancillary tests for vasospasm

In addition to angiographically demonstrating vasospasm:
- transcranial doppler (TCD): see below
- alterations in intracranial pulse wave[56]
- CTA: specific for vasospasm, but may overestimate the degree of stenosis[57]
- MRA: may be useful for management of vasospasm (not a practical alternative to conventional angiography)[58]
- continuous quantitatively analyzed EEG monitoring in the ICU:
  - a decline of the percent of alpha activity (defined here as 6–14 Hz) called "relative alpha" (RA) from a mean of 0.45 to 0.17 predicted the onset of vasospasm earlier than TCD or angiographic changes[59]
  - a decline of total EEG power (amplitude) was 91% sensitive for predicting vasospasm[60]
- alterations in cerebral blood flow (CBF):
  - MRI: DWI and PWI may detect early ischemia (p. 232)
  - CT perfusion study (p. 227)
  - Xenon CT: may detect large global changes in CBF, but too insensitive to detect focal blood flow changes[61,62] and does not correlate with increase TCD velocities positron emission tomography (PET)[63] or SPECT scans (nonquantitative, and takes longer than xenon studies)

Transcranial doppler (TCD)

A noninvasive method of semiquantitatively measuring velocity of blood flow in a specific artery through the skull (in regions of thinner bone – insonation windows) utilizing ultrasound phase shift.

Narrowing of the arterial lumen as occurs in vasospasm elevates the blood flow velocity which may be detected with TCD.[64,65,66] Detectable changes may precede clinical symptoms by up to 24–48 hrs. Findings are often more helpful when baseline studies performed before vasospasm is likely to have begun are available.

Typical values are shown for the MCA in ▶ Table 78.5. Also, daily increases of > 50 cm/sec may suggest vasospasm. There is less correlation between velocities and vasospasm in the anterior cerebral

Table 78.4 Diagnosis of clinical vasospasm[55]

- delayed onset or persisting neuro deficit
- onset 4–20 days post-SAH
- deficit appropriate to involved arteries
- rule-out other causes of deterioration
  - rebleeding
  - hydrocephalus
  - cerebral edema
  - seizure
  - metabolic disturbances: hyponatremia...
  - hypoxia
  - sepsis
- ancillary tests (see text)
  - transcranial Doppler
  - CBF studies

78

Table 78.5 Interpretation of transcranial doppler for vasospasm

Mean MCA velocity (cm/sec)	MCA:ICA (Lindegaard) ratio	Interpretation
< 120	< 3	normal
120–200[a]	3–6	mild vasospasm[a]
> 200	> 6	severe vasospasm

[a]velocities in this range are specific for vasospasm but are only ≈ 60% sensitive

arteries (ACA). Distinguishing vasospasm from hyperemia (which increases blood flow velocities in both the MCA and the ICA) is facilitated by using the ratio of these velocities (the so-called Lindegaard ratio) also shown in ▶ Table 78.5.

Once values become elevated, it often takes several weeks to go back down.

Comparison of diagnostic modalities

Determining the sensitivities and specificities for the tests shown in ▶ Table 78.6 have allowed calculation of the positive predictive value (PPV) and negative predictive values (NPV) as listed[21]

78.3.6 Treatment for vasospasm

General information

See management protocol (p. 1185).

Numerous treatments for cerebral arterial vasospasm (CVS) have been evaluated.[67,68] Vasospasm in humans does not respond to the large variety of drugs that reverse experimental vasospasm in animal models.

Prevention of vasospasm

To date, there is no effective prophylactic intervention for CVS.[69] Vasospasm can often be mitigated by preventing post-SAH hypovolemia and anemia by employing hydration and blood transfusion. Although *early* aneurysm treatment (clipping or coiling) does not prevent CVS (in fact, manipulation of vessels may increase the risk), it facilitates treatment of CVS by eliminating the risk of rebleeding (permitting safe use of hypertension as needed) and surgical removal of clot (see below) may reduce the incidence of CVS; see Timing of aneurysm surgery (p. 1200) for discussion of early surgery. *Prophylactic* (i.e. before vasospasm has been diagnosed) hyperdynamic therapy – triple H therapy (p. 1186) – is not indicated (it may cause complications and does not provide any benefit).[70]

Vasospasm treatment options

Treatment options fall into the following categories:

1. direct pharmacological arterial dilatation
   a) smooth muscle relaxants:
      - calcium channel blockers (generally accepted for standard usage): nimodipine does not counteract vasospasm, but does improve neurologic outcomes (p. 1186)
      - endothelin receptor antagonists (experimental or research technique with potential for future application): ET_A antagonists (clazosentan) and $ET_{A/B}$ antagonists[71,72]
      - Ryanodine receptor blocker: Dantrolene. Mediates intracellular calcium release from the sarcoplasmic reticulum. One of the few drugs shown to both prevent and reverse vasospasm[73,74]
      - Magnesium: MASH-2 study showed no improvement in clinical outcome[75]
   b) sympatholytics (technique that is accepted for use but not necessarily standard or available at all centers)

Table 78.6 PPV & NPV of various tests for cerebral vasospasm

Test		PPV (%)	NPV (%)
TCD	MCA	83-100	29-98
	ACA	41-100	37-80
	ICA	73	56
	PCA	37	78
	BA	63	88
	VA	54	82
CTA		43-100	37-100
CTP		71-100	27-99

  c) intra-arterial papaverine[76,77]: short-lived (see below)
  d) αICAM-1 inhibition (antibody to intracellular adhesion molecule; technique that is accepted for use but not necessarily standard or available at all centers)
2. direct mechanical arterial dilatation: balloon angioplasty (see below)
3. indirect arterial dilatation: utilizing hyperdynamic therapy (generally accepted for standard usage; see below)
4. surgical treatment to dilate arteries: cervical sympathectomy (technique *not* generally used or no longer accepted)[78]
5. removal of potential vasospasmogenic agents
  a) removal of blood clot: does not completely prevent vasospasm
    - mechanical removal at the time of aneurysm surgery[79,80]
    - subarachnoid irrigation with thrombolytic agents at the time of surgery or post-op through cisternal catheters[81,82,83,84] (must be initiated within ≈ 48 hrs of clipping) or intrathecally.[85] Hazardous with incompletely clipped aneurysm[84]
  b) CSF drainage: via serial lumbar punctures, continuous ventricular drainage, or postoperative cisternal drainage[86]
6. protection of the CNS from ischemic injury: calcium channel blockers (p. 1183) – generally accepted for standard usage
7. improvement of the rheologic properties of intravascular blood to enhance perfusion of ischemic zones; also an endpoint of hyperdynamic therapy (p. 1185); generally accepted for standard usage
  a) includes: plasma, albumin, low molecular weight dextran (technique *not* generally used or no longer accepted), perfluorocarbons (experimental or research technique with potential for future application), mannitol (p. 1202)
  b) the optimal hematocrit is controversial, but ≈ 30–35% is a good compromise between lowered viscosity without overly reducing O_2 carrying capacity (hemodilution is used to lower Hct; phlebotomy is not used)
8. statins: no benefit was detected with simvastatin[87]
9. extracranial-intracranial bypass around zone of vasospasm (technique *not* generally used or no longer accepted)[88,89]

Vasodilatation by angioplasty

Catheter directed balloon angioplasty of vessels demonstrated to be in vasospasm[90,91]: available only in centers with interventional neuroradiologists. Risks of the procedure: arterial occlusion, arterial rupture, displacement of aneurysm clip,[92,93] arterial dissection. Only feasible in large cerebral vessels (distal arteries not accessible). Clinical improvement occurs in ≈ 60–80%. Improvements in vessel diameter and neuro deficits have been observed in most studies.[94]

Prophylactic TBA: phase II prospective trial failed to show primary end point benefit (Glasgow Outcome Score), but fewer patients developed vasospasm.[95]

Criteria for transluminal balloon angioplasty (TBA):
1. failure of hyperdynamic therapy
2. ruptured aneurysm is repaired
3. optimal results when performed within 12 hours of onset of symptoms
4. may be done immediately post-clipping for vasospasm that was observed pre-op
5. controversial: asymptomatic vasospasm seen on the contralateral side during angioplasty for ipsilateral vasospasm. Some would balloon the asymptomatic side, but others cite the complication rate and would observe
6. ✖recent cerebral infarction (stroke): a contraindication to TBA. Prior to TBA, perform CT or MRI to rule-out

78

Vasodilatation by intra-arterial drug injection

Vasodilatation by intra-arterial drug (IAD) injection produces effects that are shorter-lived and less profound at their peak than with angioplasty. While IAD can be repeated, this requires multiple arterial catheterizations. IAD is also of value to help open up vessels to allow placement of the angioplasty balloon, and for vessels inaccessible to angioplasty balloons.

Agents currently used for chemical spasmolysis (p. 1587):
1. verapamil: the primary drug employed
2. nicardipine: a dihydropiridine calcium channel blocker which acts preferentially on vascular smooth muscle more than cardiac smooth muscle. Restores vessels to at least 60% of normal diameter. 70% of those treated had no stroke on CT. May cause a drop in SBP, but not > 30%.[96] ℞ intra-arterial therapy: 10–40 mg per procedure. Three retrospective case series have reported vessel dilation and transient improvement in neuro deficits.[94]

3. papaverine
4. nitroglycerine

78.3.7 Vasospasm management

Pertinent guidelines

Practice guideline: Management of cerebral vasospasm/DCI after aneurysmal SAH

- Level I[69]: maintain euvolemia and normal circulating blood volume
- Level I[69]:Induce hypertension unless BP is elevated at base-line or if precluded by cardiac stents
- Level II[69]: Endovascular angioplasty and/or selective intra-arterial vasodilator therapy is reasonable for patients not responding rapidly to or candidates for hypertensive therapy

Specific measures for Vasospasm/DCI after aSAH

Patients with clinical suspicion of vasospasm (DIND), or with transcranial doppler (TCD) *increases* of > 50 cm/sec or with absolute velocities > 200:

1. general care measures
   a) serial neuro exams: while important, sensitivity for CVS/DCI is limited in poor grade patients[69]
   b) activity: bed rest, HOB elevated to ≈ 30°
   c) TED hose and/or sequential compression boots
   d) strict I & O measurements
2. diagnostic measures (primarily to rule-out other causes of deficit)
   a) STAT non-contrast CT to rule-out hydrocephalus, edema, infarct or rebleed
   b) option: perfusion CT or MRI (if available)
   c) STAT bloodwork
      - electrolytes to rule-out hyponatremia[97]
      - CBC to assess rheology and rule-out sepsis or anemia
      - ABG to rule out hypoxemia
   d) repeat TCD if available to detect changes indicative of vasospasm
3. monitors
   a) A-line to monitor BP
   b) PA catheter to monitor PCWP and cardiac output when possible (central line to monitor CVP when PA catheter cannot be placed)
   c) insert ICP monitor if ICP felt to be problematic, treat elevated ICP with mannitol or CSF drainage before institution hemodynamic augmentation (caution: the diuresis from mannitol in treating ICP may produce hypovolemia; also, exercise caution in lowering ICP with unsecured aneurysm)
4. treatment measures
   a) continue nimodipine therapy. Give via NG tube if pt unable to swallow
   b) administer O_2 to keep $pO_2 > 70$ mm Hg
5. ensure euvolemia: patients with SAH often develop hypovolemia early in their course.[98,99,100]
   a) primary IV fluid is crystalloid, usually isotonic (e.g. NS)
   b) blood (whole or PRBC) when Hct drops < 40%
   c) colloid: plasma fraction or 5% albumin (at 100 ml/hr) to maintain 40% Hct (if Hct is > 40%, use crystalloids[101])
   d) mannitol 20% at 0.25 gm/kg/hr as a drip may improve rheologic properties of blood in the microcirculation (avoid hypovolemia from resultant diuresis)
   e) replace urinary output (U.O.) with crystalloid (if Hct < 40%, then use 5% albumin, usually @ ≈ 20-25 ml/hr)
   f) avoid hetastarch (Hespan®) (p. 1165) and dextran which impair coagulation
6. monitoring labs
   a) ABG and H/H daily
   b) serum and urine electrolytes and osmolalities q 12 hr (creatinine elevations may indicate peripheral ischemia from vasopressors)

   c) CXR daily
   d) frequent EKG
7. initiate hyperdynamic (triple-H) therapy (see below) unless BP is elevated at baseline or cardiac stents preclude it) for 6 hours
8. if no response to 6 hrs of triple-H therapy, or if doppler or perfusion CT or MRI suggests vasospasm, patient is taken to angiography to confirm presence of vasospasm and for interventional neuroradiologic treatment (intraarterial verapamil, angioplasty...)
1. move patient to the ICU and placed on triple-H therapy for 6 hours if this is not already instituted
2. option: perfusion CT or MRI (if available)
3. if no response to 6 hrs of triple-H therapy, or if perfusion CT suggests vasospasm, patient is taken to angiography to confirm presence of vasospasm and for interventional neuroradiologic treatment (intraarterial verapamil, angioplasty...)

► **Hemodynamic augmentation (formerly "TRIPLE-H" therapy).** Many older treatment schemes for CVS included so-called "triple-H" therapy (for: Hypervolemia, Hypertension and Hemodilution).[102] This has given way to "hemodynamic augmentation" consisting of maintenance of euvolemia and induced arterial hypertension.[103] While potentially confusing, this has now sometimes been referred to as triple-H therapy.[69]

Inducing HTN may be risky with an unclipped ruptured aneurysm. Once the aneurysm is treated, initiating therapy before CVS is apparent may minimize morbidity from CVS.[104,105]

Use fluids to maintain euvolemia.

Administer pressors to increase SBP in 15% increments until neurologically improved or SBP of 220 mm Hg is reached. Agents include:
- dopamine (p. 128)
  - start at 2.5 mcg/kg/min (renal dose)
  - titrate up to 15-20 mcg/kg/min
- levophed
  - start at 1-2 mcg/min
  - titrate every 2-5 minutes: double the rate up to 64 mcg/min, then increase by 10mcg/min
- neosynephrine (phenylephrine): does not exacerbate tachycardia
  - start at 5 mcg/min
  - titrate every 2-5 minutes: double the rate up to 64 mcg/min, then increase by 10mcg/min up to a max of 10 mcg/kg
- dobutamine: positive inotrope
  - start at 5 mcg/kg/min
  - increase dose by 2.5 mcg/kg/min up to a maximum of 20 mcg/kg/min

Complications of hemodynamic augmentation:
- intracranial complications[106]
  - may exacerbate cerebral edema and increase ICP
  - may produce hemorrhagic infarction in an area of previous ischemia
- extracranial complications
  - pulmonary edema in 17%
  - 3 rebleeds (1 fatal)
  - MI in 2%
  - complications of PA catheter[107]:
    - catheter related sepsis: 13%
    - subclavian vein thrombosis: 1.3%
    - pneumothorax: 1%
    - hemothorax: may be promoted by coagulopathy from dextran[106]

78.4 Post-op orders for aneurysm clipping

- admit PACU, transfer to ICU (neuro unit if available) when stable
- VS: q 15 min × 4 hrs, then q 1 hr. Temperature q 4 hrs × 3 d, then q 8 hrs. Neuro check q 1 hr
- activity: bed rest (BR) with HOB elevated 20–30°
- knee high TED hose and pneumatic compression boots
- I & O q 1 hr (if no Foley: straight cath q 4 hrs PRN bladder distension)
- incentive spirometry q 2 hrs while awake (*do not use following transsphenoidal surgery*)
- IVF: NS + 20 mEq KCl/L @ 90 ml/hr

For extubated patients:
- diet: NPO except minimal ice chips and meds as ordered
- O_2: 2 L per NC

For intubated patients:
- diet: NPO. NG tube to intermittent suction. May clamp for 1 hour after meds given
- ventilator orders

For all patients:
- meds:
  a) H2 antagonist, e.g. ranitidine 50 mg IVPB q 8 hrs
  b) Keppra® (levetiracetam): 500 mg PO or IV q 12 hours. Maintain therapeutic AED levels for 2–3 months post-op for most supratentorial craniotomies
  c) Cardene® drip: titrate to keep SBP < 160 mm Hg and/or DBP < 100 mm Hg (use cuff pressures, may use A-line pressures if they correlate with cuff pressures)
  d) analgesics: fentanyl (unlike morphine, does not cause histamine release. Lowers ICP) 25–100 mcg (0.5–2 ml) IVP, q 1–2 hrs PRN
  e) acetaminophen (Tylenol®) 650 mg PO/PR q 4 hrs PRN temperature T > 100.5° F (38 C)
  f) mini-dose heparin or enoxaparin (for DVT prophylaxis; no difference in heparin-induced thrombocytopenia with these 2 agents[108])
  g) calcium channel blockers; see admitting orders (p. 1165): nimodipine (Nimotop®) 60 mg PO/NG q 4 hrs or 30 mg q 2 hrs to avoid dips in BP. May be given IV where available
  h) continue prophylactic antibiotics if used: (e.g. cefazolin (Kefzol®) 500–1000 mg IVPB q 6 hrs x 24 hrs, then D/C)
- if available, transcranial doppler (p. 1182) to monitor MCA, ACA, ICA, VA and BA velocities and Lindegaard ratio (typical protocol is 3 × per week)
- labs:
  a) CBC once stabilized in ICU and q d thereafter
  b) renal profile once stabilized in ICU and q 12 hrs thereafter
  c) ABG once stabilized in ICU and q 12 hrs × 2 days, then D/C (also check ABG after any ventilator change if patient on ventilator)
- call M.D. if any deterioration in crani checks, for T > 101° (38.5 C), sudden increase in SBP, SBP < 120, U.O. < 60 ml/2-hrs

References

[1] Braunwald E, Kloner RA. The Stunned Myocardium: Prolonged Postischemic Ventricular Dysfunction. Circulation. 1982; 66:1146–1149

[2] Murphy AM, Kögler H, Georgakopoulos D, et al. Transgenic Mouse Model of Stunned Myocardium. Science. 2000; 389:491–495

[3] Yuki K, Kodama Y, Onda J, et al. Coronary Vasospasm Following Subarachnoid Hemorhage as a Cause of Stunned Myocardium. J Neurosurg. 1991; 75:308–311

[4] Bulsara KR, McGirt MJ, Liao L, et al. Use of the peak troponin value to differentiate myocardial infarction from reversible neurogenic left ventricual dysfunction associated with aneurysmal subarachnoid hemorrhage. J Neurosurg. 2003; 98:524–528

[5] Malik AN, Gross BA, Rosalind Lai PM, Moses ZB, Du R. Neurogenic Stress Cardiomyopathy After Aneurysmal Subarachnoid Hemorrhage. World Neurosurg. 2015; 83:880–885

[6] Hravnak M, Frangiskakis JM, Crago EA, Chang Y, Tanabe M, Gorcsan J,3rd, Horowitz MB. Elevated cardiac troponin I and relationship to persistence of electrocardiographic and echocardiographic abnormalities after aneurysmal subarachnoid hemorrhage. Stroke. 2009; 40:3478–3484

[7] Kilbourn KJ, Levy S, Staff I, Kureshi I, McCullough L. Clinical characteristics and outcomes of neurogenic stress cadiomyopathy in aneurysmal subarachnoid hemorrhage. Clin Neurol Neurosurg. 2013; 115:909–914

[8] Tung P, Kopelnik A, Banki N, et al. Predictors of neurocardiogenic injury after subarachnoid hemorrhage. Stroke. 2004; 35:548–551

[9] Mayer SA, Lin J, Homma S, Solomon RA, Lennihan L, Sherman D, Fink ME, Beckford A, Klebanoff LM. Myocardial injury and left ventricular performance after subarachnoid hemorrhage. Stroke. 1999; 30:780–786

[10] Harries AD. Subarachnoid Hemorhage and the Electrocardiogram: A Review. Postgrad Med J. 1981; 57:294–296

[11] Beard EF, Robertson JW, Robertson RCL. Spontaneous Subarachnoid Hemorhage Simulating Acute Myocardial Infarction. Am Heart J. 1959; 58:755–759

[12] Gascon P, Ley TJ, Toltzis RJ, et al. Spontaneous Subarachnoid Hemorhage Simulating Acute Transmural Myocardial Infarction. Am Heart J. 1983; 105:511–513

[13] Marion DW, Segal R, Thompson ME. Subarachnoid hemorrhage and the heart. Neurosurgery. 1986; 18:101–106

[14] DiDomenico RJ, Park HY, Southworth MR, et al. Guidelines for acute decompensated heart failure treatment. Ann Pharmacother. 2004; 38:649–660

[15] Naidech A, Du Y, Kreiter KT, Parra A, Fitzsimmons BF, Lavine SD, Connolly ES, Mayer SA, Commichau C. Dobutamine versus milrinone after subarachnoid hemorrhage. Neurosurgery. 2005; 56:21–27

[16] Knudsen F, Jensen HP, Petersen PL. Neurogenic Pulmonary Edema: Treatment with Dobutamine. Neurosurgery. 1991; 29:269–270

[17] Maeda K, Kurita H, Nakamura T, et al. Occurrence of Severe Vasospasm Following Intraventricular Hemorrhage from an Arteriovenous Malformation. J Neurosurg. 1997; 87:436–439

[18] Martin NA, Doberstein C, Zane C, et al. Posttraumatic Cerebral Arterial Spasm: Transcranial Doppler Ultrasound, Cerebral Blood Flow, and Angiographic Findings. J Neurosurg. 1992; 77:575–583
[19] Ecker A, Riemenschneider PA. Arteriographic Demonstration of Spasm of the Intracranial Arteries: With Special Reference to Saccular Aneurysms. J Neurosurg. 1951; 8:660–667
[20] Etminan N. Aneurysmal subarachnoid hemorrhage-status quo and perspective. Transl Stroke Res. 2015; 6:167–170
[21] Washington CW, Zipfel GJ. Detection and monitoring of vasospasm and delayed cerebral ischemia: a review and assessment of the literature. Neurocrit Care. 2011; 15:312–317
[22] Dorsch N. A clinical review of cerebral vasospasm and delayed ischaemia following aneurysm rupture. Acta Neurochir Suppl. 2011; 110:5–6
[23] Wedekind C, Hildebrandt G, Klug N. A case of delayed loss of facial nerve function after acoustic neuroma surgery. Zentralbl Neurochir. 1996; 57:163–166
[24] Kudo T. Postoperative oculomotor palsy due to vasospasm in a patient with a ruptured internal carotid artery aneurysm: a case report. Neurosurgery. 1986; 19:274–277
[25] Kassell NF, Sasaki T, Colohan ART, et al. Cerebral Vasospasm Following Aneurysmal Subarachnoid Hemorrhage. Stroke. 1985; 16:562–572
[26] Awad IA, Carter LP, Spetzler RF, Medina M, Williams FC, Jr. Clinical Vasospasm After Subarachnoid Hemorrhage: Response to Hypervolemic Hemodilution and Arterial Hypertension. Stroke. 1987; 18:365–372
[27] Broderick JP, Brott TG, Duldner JE, Tomsick T, Leach A. Initial and recurrent bleeding are the major causes of death following subarachnoid hemorrhage. Stroke. 1994; 25:1342–1347
[28] Alaraj A, Wallace A, Mander N, Aletich V, Charbel FT, Amin-Hanjani S. Outcome following symptomatic cerebral vasospasm on presentation in aneurysmal subarachnoid hemorrhage: coiling vs. clipping. World Neurosurg. 2010; 74:138–142
[29] Weir B, Grace M, Hansen J, et al. Time Course of Vasospasm in Man. J Neurosurg. 1978; 48:173–178
[30] Pasqualin A. Epidemiology and pathophysiology of cerebral vasospasm following subarachnoid hemorrhage. J Neurosurg Sci. 1998; 42:15–21
[31] Bejjani GK, Sekhar LN, Yost AM, Bank WO, Wright DC. Vasospasm after cranial base tumor resection: pathogenesis, diagnosis, and therapy. Surg Neurol. 1999; 52:577–83; discussion 583-4
[32] Popugaev KA, Savin IA, Lubnin AU, Goriachev AS, Kadashev BA, Kalinin PL, Pronin IN, Oshorov AV, Kutin MA. Unusual cause of cerebral vasospasm after pituitary surgery. Neurol Sci. 2011; 32:673–680
[33] Mandonnet E, Chassoux F, Naggara O, Roux FX, Devaux B. Transient symptomatic vasospasm following antero-mesial temporal lobectomy for refractory epilepsy. Acta Neurochir (Wien). 2009; 151:1723–1726
[34] Valenca MM, Valenca LP, Bordini CA, da Silva WF, Leite JP, Antunes-Rodrigues J, Speciali JG. Cerebral vasospasm and headache during sexual intercourse and masturbatory orgasms. Headache. 2004; 44:244–248
[35] Chatterjee N, Domoto-Reilly K, Fecci PE, Schwamm LH, Singhal AB. Licorice-associated reversible cerebral vasoconstriction with PRES. Neurology. 2010; 75:1939–1941
[36] Fisher CM, Kistler JP, Davis JM. Relation of Cerebral Vasospasm to Subarachnoid Hemorrhage Visualized by CT Scanning. Neurosurgery. 1980; 6:1–9
[37] Kistler JP, Crowell RM, Davis KR, et al. The Relation of Cerebral Vasospasm to the Extent and Location of Subarachnoid Blood Visualized by CT. Neurology. 1983; 33:424–426
[38] Taneda M, Kataoka K, Akai F, et al. Traumatic Subarachnoid Hemorrhage as a Predictable Indicator of Delayed Ischemic Symptoms. J Neurosurg. 1996; 84:762–768
[39] Lasner TM, Weil RJ, Riina HA, et al. Cigarette Smoking-Induced Increase in the Risk of Symptomatic Vasospasm After Aneurysmal Subarachnoid Hemorrhage. J Neurosurg. 1997; 87:381–384
[40] Fox JL, Ko JP. Cerebral Vasospasm: A Clinical Observation. Surg Neurol. 1978; 10
[41] Davis JM, Davis KR, Crowell RM. Subarachnoid Hemorrhage Secondary to Ruptured Intracranial Aneurysm: Prognostic Significance of Cranial CT. AJNR. 1980; 1:17–21
[42] Kassell NF, Torner JC, Adams HP. Antifibrinolytic Therapy in the Acute Period Following Aneurysmal Subarachnoid Hemorrhage: Preliminary Observations from the Cooperative Aneurysm Study. J Neurosurg. 1984; 61:225–230
[43] Frontera JA, Claassen J, Schmidt JM, Wartenberg KE, Temes R, Connolly ES,Jr, MacDonald RL, Mayer SA. Prediction of symptomatic vasospasm after subarachnoid hemorrhage: the modified fisher scale. Neurosurgery. 2006; 59:21–7; discussion 21-7
[44] Sasaki T, Kassell NF, Zuccarello M, et al. Barrier Disruption in the Major Cerebral Arteries During the Acute Stage After Experimental Subarachnoid Hemorrhage. Neurosurgery. 1986; 19:177–184
[45] Sasaki T, Kassell NF, Yamashita M, et al. Barrier Disruption in the Major Cerebral Arteries Following Experimental Subarachnoid Hemorrhage. J Neurosurg. 1985; 63:433–440
[46] Pluta RM, Thompson BG, Afshar JK, Boock RJ, Iuliano B, Oldfield EH. Nitric oxide and vasospasm. Acta Neurochir Suppl. 2001; 77:67–72
[47] Borel CO, McKee A, Parra A, Haglund MM, Solan A, Prabhakar V, Sheng H, Warner DS, Niklason L. Possible role for vascular cell proliferation in cerebral vasospasm after subarachnoid hemorrhage. Stroke. 2003; 34:427–433
[48] Svendgaard NA, Brismar J, Delgado TJ, et al. Subarachnoid Hemorrhage in the Rat: Effect on the Development of Vasospasm of Selective Lesions of the Catecholamine Systems in the Lower Brain Stem. Stroke. 1985; 16:602–608
[49] Honma Y, Clower BR, Haining JL, et al. Comparison of Intimal Platelet Accumulation in Cerebral Arteries in Two Experimental Models of Subarachnoid Hemorrhage. Neurosurgery. 1989; 24:487–490
[50] Allen GS, Gross CJ, French LA, et al. Cerebral Arterial Spasm. Part 5: In Vitro Contractile Activity of Vasoactive Agents Including Human CSF on Human Basilar and Anterior Cerebral Artery. J Neurosurg. 1976; 44:596–600
[51] Sasaki T, Asano T, Takakura K, et al. Nature of the Vasoactive Substance in CSF from Patients with Subarachnoid Hemorrhage. J Neurosurg. 1984; 60:1186–1191
[52] Tew J, Tsai S-H, Greenberg M, Shipley M. Disturbance of Cerebrovascular Innervation After Experimental Subarachnoid Hemorrhage. Baltimore 1987
[53] Wilkins RH. Cerebral Vasospasm. Contemp Neurosurg. 1988; 10-4:1–6
[54] Nakagomi T, Kassell NF, Sasaki T, et al. Effect of Subarachnoid Hemorrhage on Endothelium-Dependent Vasodilatation. J Neurosurg. 1987; 66:915–923
[55] Findlay JM. Current Management of Cerebral Vasospasm. Contemp Neurosurg. 1997; 19:1–6
[56] Cardoso ER, Reddy K, Bose D. Effect of Subarachnoid Hemorrhage on Intracranial Pulse Waves in Cats. J Neurosurg. 1988; 69:712–718
[57] Greenberg ED, Gold R, Reichman M, John M, Ivanidze J, Edwards AM, Johnson CE, Comunale JP, Sanelli P. Diagnostic accuracy of CT angiography and CT perfusion for cerebral vasospasm: a meta-analysis. AJNR Am J Neuroradiol. 2010; 31:1853–1860
[58] Tamatani S, Sasaki O, Takeuchi S, Fujii Y, Koike T, Tanaka R. Detection of delayed cerebral vasospasm, after rupture of intracranial aneurysms, by

magnetic resonance angiography. Neurosurgery. 1997; 40:748–53; discussion 753-4
[59] Vespa PM, Nuwer MR, Juhász C, et al. Early Detection of Vasospasm After Acute Subarachnoid Hemorrhage Using Continuous EEG ICU Monitoring. EEG Clin Neurophys. 1997; 103:607–615
[60] Labar DR, Fisch BJ, Pedley TA, Fink ME, Solomon RA. Quantitative EEG Monitoring for Patients with Subarachnoid Hemorrhage. EEG Clin Neurophys. 1991; 78:325–332
[61] Weir B, Menon D, Overton T. Regional Cerebral Blood Flow in Patients with Aneurysms: Estimation by Xenon 133 Inhalation. Can J Neurol Sci. 1978; 5:301–305
[62] Knuckney NW, Fox RA, Surveyor I, et al. Early Cerebral Blood Flow and CT in Predicting Ischemia After Cerebral Aneurysm Rupture. J Neurosurg. 1985; 62:850–855
[63] Powers WJ, Grubb RL, Baker RP, et al. Regional Cerebral Blood Flow and Metabolism in Reversible Ischemia due to Vasospasm: Determination by Positron Emission Tomography. J Neurosurg. 1985; 62:539–546
[64] Seiler RW, Grolimund P, Aaslid R, et al. Cerebral Vasospasm Evaluated by Transcranial Ultrasound Correlated with Clinical Grade and CT-Visualized Subarachnoid Hemorrhage. J Neurosurg. 1986; 64:594–600
[65] Lindegaard KF, Nornes H, Bakke SJ, et al. Cerebral Vasospasm After Subarachnoid Hemorrhage Investigated by Means of Transcranial Doppler Ultrasound. Acta Neurochir. 1988; 42:81–84
[66] Sekhar LN, Wechsler LR, Yonas H, et al. Value of Transcranial Doppler Examination in the Diagnosis of Cerebral Vasospasm After Subarachnoid Hemorrhage. Neurosurgery. 1988; 22:813–821
[67] Wilkins RH. Attempted Prevention or Treatment of Intracranial Arterial Spasm: A Survey. Neurosurgery. 1980; 6:198–210
[68] Wilkins RH. Attempts at Prevention or Treatment of Intracranial Arterial Spasm: An Update. Neurosurgery. 1986; 18:808–825
[69] Connolly ES, Jr, Rabinstein AA, Carhuapoma JR, Derdeyn CP, Dion J, Higashida RT, Hoh BL, Kirkness CJ, Naidech AM, Ogilvy CS, Patel AB, Thompson BG, Vespa P, American Heart Association Stroke Council, Council on Cardiovascular Radiology, Intervention, Council on Cardiovascular Nursing, Council on Cardiovascular Surgery, Anesthesia, Council on Clinical Cardiology. Guidelines for the management of aneurysmal subarachnoid hemorrhage: a guideline for healthcare professionals from the American Heart Association/american Stroke Association. Stroke. 2012; 43:1711–1737
[70] Egge A, Waterloo K, Sjoholm H, Solberg T, Ingebrigtsen T, Romner B. Prophylactic hyperdynamic postoperative fluid therapy after aneurysmal subarachnoid hemorrhage: a clinical, prospective, randomized, controlled study. Neurosurgery. 2001; 49:593–605; discussion 605-6
[71] Foley PL, Caner HH, Kassell NF, Lee KS. Reversal of Subarachnoid Hemorrhage-Induced Vasoconstriction with an Endothelin Receptor Antagonists. Neurosurgery. 1994; 34:108–113
[72] Zuccarello M, Soattin GB, Lewis AI, Breu V, Hallak H, Rapoport RM. Prevention of Subarachnoid Hemorrhage-Induced Cerebral Vasospasm by Oral Administration of Endothelin Receptor Antagonists. J Neurosurg. 1996; 84:503–507
[73] Muehlschlegel S, Rordorf G, Sims J. Effects of a single dose of dantrolene in patients with cerebral vasospasm after subarachnoid hemorrhage: a prospective pilot study. Stroke. 2011; 42:1301–1306
[74] Majidi S, Grigoryan M, Tekle WG, Qureshi AI. Intra-arterial dantrolene for refractory cerebral vasospasm after aneurysmal subarachnoid hemorrhage. Neurocrit Care. 2012; 17:245–249
[75] Mees SMD, Algra A, Vandertop WP, van Kooten F, Kuijsten HAJM, Boiten J, van Oostenbrugge RF, Salman R, Lavados PM, Rinkel GJE, van den Bergh WM. Magnesium for aneurysmal subarachnoid haemorrhage (MASH-2): a randomised placebo-controlled trial. The Lancet. 2012; 380:44–49
[76] Kaku Y, Yonekawa Y, Tsukahara T, Kazekawa K. Superselective Intra-Arterial Infusion of Papaverine for the Treatment of Cerebral Vasospasm After Subarachnoid Hemorrhage. J Neurosurg. 1992; 77:842–847
[77] Kassell NF, Helm G, Simmons N, et al. Treatment of Cerebral Vasospasm with Intra-Arterial Papaverine. J Neurosurg. 1992; 77:848–852
[78] Hori S, Suzuki J. Early Intracranial Operations for Ruptured Aneurysms. Acta Neurochir. 1979; 46:93–104
[79] Mitzukami M, Kawase T, Tazawa T. Prevention of Vasospasm by Early Operation with Removal of Subarachnoid Blood. Neurosurgery. 1982; 10:301–306
[80] Nosko M, Weir BKA, Lunt A, et al. Effect of Clot Removal at 24 Hours on Chronic Vasospasm After Subarachnoid Hemorrhage in the Primate Model. J Neurosurg. 1987; 66:416–422
[81] Findlay JM, Weir BKA, Steinke D, et al. Effect of Intrathecal Thrombolytic Therapy on Subarachnoid Clot and Chronic Vasospasm in a Primate. J Neurosurg. 1988; 69:723–735
[82] Findlay JM, Weir BKA, Kanamaru K, et al. Intrathecal Fibrinolytic Therapy After Subarachnoid Hemorrhage: Dosage Study in a Primate Model and Review of Literature. Can J Neurol Sci. 1989; 16:28–40
[83] Findlay JM, Weir BKA, Gordon P, et al. Safety and Efficacy of Intrathecal Thrombolytic Therapy in a Primate Model of Cerebral Vasospasm. Neurosurgery. 1989; 24:491–498
[84] Findlay JM, Kassell NF, Weir BKA, et al. A Randomized Trial of Intraoperative, Intracisternal Tissue Plasminogen Activator for the Prevention of Vasospasm. Neurosurgery. 1995; 37:168–178
[85] Mizoi K, Yoshimoto T, Fujiwara S, Takahashi A, et al. Prevention of Vasospasm by Clot Removal and Intrathecal Bolus Injection of Tissue-Type Plasminogen Activator: Preliminary Report. Neurosrugery. 1991; 28:807–813
[86] Ito U, Tomita H, Yamazaki S, et al. Enhanced Cisternal Drainage and Cerebral Vasospasm in Early Aneurysm Surgery. Acta Neurochir. 1986; 80:18–23
[87] Kirkpatrick PJ, Turner CL, Smith C, Hutchinson PJ, Murray GD. Simvastatin in aneurysmal subarachnoid haemorrhage (STASH): a multicentre randomised phase 3 trial. Lancet Neurol. 2014; 13:666–675
[88] Benzel EC, Kesterson L. Extracranial-Intracranial Bypass Surgery for the Management of Vasospasm After Subarachnoid Hemorrhage. Surg Neurol. 1988; 30:231–234
[89] Batjer H, Samson D. Use of Extracranial-Intracranial Bypass in the Management of Symptomatic Vasospasm. Neurosurgery. 1986; 19:235–246
[90] Hieshima GB, Higashida RT, Wapenski J, et al. Balloon Embolization of a Large Distal Basilar Artery Aneurysm: Case Report. J Neurosurg. 1986; 65:413–416
[91] Zubkov YN, Nikiforov BM, Shustin VA. Balloon Catheter Technique for Dilatation of Constricted Cerebral After Aneurysmal Subarachnoid Hemorrhage. Acta Neurochir. 1984; 70:65–79
[92] Newell DW, Eskridge JM, Mayberg MR, Grady MS, et al. Angioplasty for the Treatment of Symptomatic Vasospasm Following Subarachnoid Hemorrhage. J Neurosurg. 1989; 71:654–660
[93] Linskey ME, Horton JA, Rao GR, Yonas H. Fatal Rupture of the Intracranial Carotid Artery During Transluminal Angioplasty for Vasospasm Induced by Subarachnoid Hemorrhage. J Neurosurg. 1991; 74:985–990
[94] Kimball MM, Velat GJ, Hoh BL. Critical care guidelines on the endovascular management of cerebral vasospasm. Neurocrit Care. 2011; 15:336–341
[95] Zwienenberg-Lee M, Hartman J, Rudisill N, Madden LK, Smith K, Eskridge J, Newell D, Verweij B, Bullock MR, Baker A, Coplin W, Mericle R, Dai J, Rocke D, Muizelaar JP. Effect of prophylactic transluminal balloon angioplasty on cerebral vasospasm and outcome in patients with Fisher grade

III subarachnoid hemorrhage: results of a phase II multicenter, randomized, clinical trial. Stroke. 2008; 39:1759–1765
[96] Tejada JG, Taylor RA, Ugurel MS, Hayakawa M, Lee SK, Chaloupka JC. Safety and feasibility of intra-arterial nicardipine for the treatment of subarachnoid hemorrhage-associated vasospasm: initial clinical experience with high-dose infusions. AJNR Am J Neuroradiol. 2007; 28:844–848
[97] Wise BL. SIADH After Spontaneous Subarachnoid Hemorrhage: A Reversible Cause of Clinical Deterioration. Neurosurgery. 1978; 3:412–414
[98] Maroon JC, Nelson PB. Hypovolemia in Patients with Subarachnoid Hemorrhage: Therapeutic Implications. Neurosurgery. 1979; 4:223–226
[99] Wijdicks EFM, Vermeulen M, Hijdra A, et al. Hyponatremia and Cerebral Infarction in Patients with Ruptured Intracranial Aneurysms: Is Fluid Restriction Harmful? Ann Neurol. 1985; 17:137–140
[100] Wijdicks EFM, Vermeulen M, ten Haaf JA, et al. Volume Depletion and Natriuresis in Patients with a Ruptured Intracranial Aneurysm. Ann Neurol. 1985; 18:211–216
[101] Vermeulen LC, Ratko TA, Erstad BL, et al. The University Hospital Consortium Guidelines for the Use of Albumin, Nonprotein Colloid, and Crystalloid Solutions. Arch Intern Med. 1995; 155:373–379
[102] Origitano TC, Wascher TM, Reichman OH, Anderson DE. Sustained Increased Cerebral Blood Flow with Prophylactic Hypertensive Hypervolemic Hemodilution ("Triple-H" Therapy) After Subarachnoid Hemorrhage. Neurosurgery. 1990; 27:729–740
[103] Dankbaar JW, Slooter AJ, Rinkel GJ, Schaaf IC. Effect of different components of triple-H therapy on cerebral perfusion in patients with aneurysmal subarachnoid haemorrhage: a systematic review. Crit Care. 2010; 14. DOI: 10.1186/cc8886
[104] Solomon RA, Fink ME, Lennihan L. Prophylactic Volume Expansion Therapy for the Prevention of Delayed Cerebral Ischemia After Early Aneurysm Surgery. Arch Neurol. 1988; 45:325–332
[105] Solomon RA, Fink ME, Lennihan L. Early Aneurysm Surgery and Prophylactic Hypervolemic Hypertensive Therapy for the Treatment of Aneurysmal Subarachnoid Hemorrhage. Neurosurgery. 1988; 23:699–704
[106] Shimoda M, Oda S, Tsugane R, Sato O. Intracranial Complications of Hypervoemic Therapy in Patients with a Delayed Ischemic Deficit Attributed to Vasospasm. J Neurosurg. 1993; 78:423–429
[107] Rosenwasser RH, Jallo JI, Getch CC, Liebman KE. Complications of Swan-Ganz Catheterization for Hemodynamic Monitoring in Patients with Subarachnoid Hemorrhage. Neurosurgery. 1995; 37:872–876
[108] Kim GH, Hahn DK, Kellner CP, Komotar RJ, Starke R, Garrett MC, Yao J, Cleveland J, Mayer SA, Connolly ES. The incidence of heparin-induced throm bocytopenia Type II in patients with subarachnoid hemorrhage treated with heparin versus enoxaparin. J Neurosurg. 2009; 110:50–57

79 SAH from Cerebral Aneurysm Rupture

79.1 Epidemiology of cerebral aneurysms

The incidence of cerebral aneurysms is difficult to estimate. Range of autopsy prevalence of aneurysms: 0.2–7.9% (variability depends on use of dissecting microscope, hospital referral and autopsy pattern, overall interest). Estimated prevalence of incidental aneurysms range from 1-5% of the population,[1,2,3,4,5] and they are becoming increasingly detected in clinical practice as use of CT and MRI is becoming more common.[6] Ratio of ruptured:unruptured (incidental) aneurysm is 5:3 to 5:6 (rough estimate is 1:1, i.e. 50% of these aneurysms rupture).[7] Unruptured intracranial aneurysms are more common in women (≈3:1 ratio)[8,9]and in the elderly,[10] and only 2% of aneurysms present during childhood.[11] When present in children, they tend to occur more frequently in males (2:1) and to a greater degree in the posterior circulation (40-45%).[12,13]

79.2 Etiology of cerebral aneurysms

The exact pathophysiology of the development of aneurysms is still controversial. In contrast to extracranial blood vessels, there is less elastic in the tunica media and adventitia of cerebral blood vessels, the media has less muscle, the adventitia is thinner, and the internal elastic lamina is more prominent.[14,15] This, together with the fact that large cerebral blood vessels lie within the subarachnoid space with little supporting connective tissue[16(p 1644)] may predispose these vessels to the development of saccular aneurysms. Aneurysms tend to arise in areas where there is a curve in the parent artery, in the angle between it and a significant branching artery, and point in the direction that the parent artery would have continued had the curve not been present.[17]

The etiology of aneurysms may be:

1. congenital predisposition (e.g. defect in the muscular layer of the arterial wall, referred to as a medial gap)
2. "atherosclerotic" or hypertensive: presumed etiology of most saccular aneurysms, probably interacts with congenital predisposition described above
3. embolic: as in atrial myxoma
4. infectious – so called "mycotic aneurysms" (p. 1228)
5. traumatic; see Traumatic aneurysms (p. 1227)
6. associated with other conditions (see below)

79.3 Location of cerebral aneurysms

Saccular aneurysms, AKA berry aneurysms are usually located on major named cerebral arteries at the apex of branch points which is the site of maximum hemodynamic stress in a vessel.[18] More peripheral aneurysms do occur, but tend to be associated with infection (mycotic aneurysms) or trauma. Fusiform aneurysms are more common in the vertebrobasilar system. Dissecting aneurysms should be categorized with arterial dissection (p. 1323).

Saccular aneurysms location:

1. 85–95% in carotid system, with the following 3 most common locations:
   a) ACoA (single most common): 30% (ACoA & ACA more common in males)
   b) p-comm: 25%
   c) middle cerebral artery (MCA): 20%
2. 5–15% in posterior circulation (vertebro-basilar)
   a) ≈ 10% on basilar artery: basilar bifurcation, AKA basilar tip, is the most common, followed by BA-SCA, BA-VA junction, AICA
   b) ≈ 5% on vertebral artery: VA-PICA junction is the most common
3. 20–30% of aneurysm patients have multiple aneurysms (p. 1226) [19]

79

79.4 Presentation of cerebral aneurysms

79.4.1 Major rupture

The most frequent presentation

1. most commonly produces SAH (p. 1167), which may be accompanied by:
2. intracerebral hemorrhage: occurs in 20–40% (more common with aneurysms distal to the Circle of Willis, e.g. MCA aneurysms)

3. intraventricular hemorrhage: occurs in 13–28%[20] (see below)
4. subdural blood occurs in 2–5%

79.4.2 Intraventricular hemorrhage

See also other etiologies of intraventricular hemorrhage (IVH) (p. 1386).

IVH occurs in 13–28% of ruptured aneurysms in clinical series (higher in autopsy series)[20] and appears to carry a worse prognosis (64% mortality).[20] The size of the ventricles on admission was the most important prognosticator (large vents being worse). Patterns that may occur:

1. distal PICA aneurysms: may rupture directly into 4th ventricle through the foramen of Luschka[21]
2. a-comm aneurysm: it has been asserted that IVH occurs from rupture through the lamina terminalis into the anterior 3rd or lateral ventricles, however, this is not always borne out at the time of surgery
3. distal basilar artery or carotid terminus aneurysms: may rupture through the floor of the 3rd ventricle (rare)

79.4.3 Presentation other than major rupture

General information

May be thought of as possible "warning signs."

1. mass effect
   a) giant aneurysms: including brain stem compression producing hemiparesis and cranial neuropathies
   b) cranial neuropathy (average latency from symptom to SAH was 110 days; **note:** the average latency quoted for some of these symptoms comes from a retrospective study of patients presenting with SAH who were identified as having a warning symptom[22]). See below:
   c) intra- or suprasellar aneurysm producing endocrine disturbance[23] due to pituitary gland or stalk compression
2. minor hemorrhage: warning or sentinel hemorrhage; see Headache (p. 1158). This group had the shortest latency (10 days) between symptom and SAH (**note:** the average latency quoted for some of these symptoms comes from a retrospective study of patients presenting with SAH who were identified as having a warning symptom[22])
3. small infarcts or transient ischemia due to distal embolization (including amaurosis fugax, homonymous hemianopsia…)[24]: average latency from symptom to SAH was 21 days A
4. seizures: at surgery, an adjacent area of encephalomalacia may be found.[24] The seizures may arise as a result of localized gliosis and do not necessarily represent aneurysmal expansion as there is no data to indicate an increased risk of hemorrhage in this group
5. headache[24] without hemorrhage: abates after treatment in most cases
   a) acute: may be severe and "thunderclap" in nature,[25] some describe as "worst headache of my life." Has been attributed to aneurysmal expansion, thrombosis, or intramural bleeding,[26] all without rupture
   b) present for ≥ 2 weeks: unilateral in about half (often retro-orbital or periorbital), possibly due to irritation of overlying dura. Diffuse or bilateral in the other half, possibly due to mass effect → increased ICP
6. incidentally discovered (i.e. asymptomatic, e.g. those found on angiography, CT or MRI obtained for other reasons)

Cranial neuropathies from aneurysmal compression

79

1. oculomotor (3rd nerve) palsy (ONP): occurs in ≈ 9% of p-comm aneurysms[27] (ruptured and unruptured), less common with basilar apex aneurysm. Symptoms of ONP may include:
   a) extraocular muscle palsy (eye deviates "down and out" → diplopia
   b) Ptosis
   c) dilated unreactive pupil (✱ non-pupil-sparing third nerve palsy is the classic finding of 3rd nerve compression (p. 562))
2. visual loss due to[24]
   a) compressive optic neuropathy with ophthalmic artery aneurysms: characteristically produces nasal quadrantanopsia
   b) chiasmal syndromes due to ophthalmic, a-comm, or basilar apex aneurysms
3. facial pain syndromes in the ophthalmic or maxillary nerve distribution that may mimic trigeminal neuralgia can occur with intracavernous or supraclinoid aneurysms[24,28]

► **Note.** The development of a third nerve palsy in a patient with an unruptured aneurysm is a medical emergency as it probably results from aneurysmal expansion and may portend impending rupture.

79.5 Conditions associated with aneurysms

79.5.1 Overview

1. autosomal dominant polycystic kidney disease: (see below)
2. fibromuscular dysplasia (**FMD**): prevalence of aneurysms in renal FMD is 7%, in aortocranial FMD 21%
3. arteriovenous malformations (AVM) including moyamoya disease; see AVMs and aneurysms (p. 1241)
4. connective tissue disorders[29]:
   a) Ehlers-Danlos, especially type IV (deficient collagen type III) which also has a high rate of arterial dissection including with angiography or coiling
   b) Marfan syndrome (p. 1322)
   c) pseudoxanthoma elasticum
5. multiple other family members with intracranial aneurysms. Familial intracranial aneurysm syndrome (FIA): 2 or more relatives, third degree or closer, harbor radiographically proven intracranial aneurysms. Also, see Familial aneurysms (p. 1226)
6. coarctation of the aorta[30]
7. Osler-Weber-Rendu syndrome
8. atherosclerosis[31]
9. bacterial endocarditis
10. multiple Endocrine Neoplasia type I[32]
11. hereditary hemorrhagic telangiectasia[33]
12. neurofibromatosis type I[34]

79.5.2 Autosomal dominant polycystic kidney disease

General information

Adult polycystic kidney disease is seen in 1 of every 500 autopsies, and approximately 500,000 people in the U.S. carry the mutant gene for autosomal dominant polycystic kidney disease (ADPKD; there is also an autosomal recessive polycystic kidney disease). Renal function is usually normal during the first few decades of life, with progressive chronic renal failure ensuing. HTN is a common sequelae. Transmission is autosomal dominant, with 100% penetrance by 80 yrs of age.[35] Cystic disease of other organs may occur (viz.: liver in ≈ 33%, and occasionally lung, pancreas).[36]

The first association between ADPKD and cerebral aneurysms is attributed to Dunger in 1904. Reported prevalence of intracranial aneurysms with ADPKD: 10–30%,[37] with 15% being a reasonable estimate.[38] Most were located on the MCA, with multiple aneurysms present in 31%.[39] In addition to the increased incidence of aneurysms, there appears to be an increased risk of rupture,[40] with 64% occurring before age 50. As a result, patients with ADPKD carry a 10–20 fold increased risk of SAH compared to the general population.[41] Aneurysms are rarely detectable before age 20 years. The average rate of rupture of incidental aneurysms is ≈ 2%/yr (p. 1167).

Recommendations

Using the above statistics, together with the life expectancy of patients with ADPKD, and other estimations (of operative morbidity and mortality, etc.), results of decision analysis is that arteriography *not* be routinely employed in patients older than 25 yrs.[37] However, patients with symptoms possibly due to unruptured aneurysms, and those with SAH, should undergo angiography and subsequent treatment of any aneurysms discovered (especially those > 1 cm diameter). A decision analysis study[38] determined that screening with *MRA* was beneficial compared to treating patients once they became symptomatic. Repeat MRA screening may be effectively repeated as follows:

1. every ≈ 2-3 years for a young patient with ADPKD with either:
   a) a history of aneurysms, or
   b) a kindred of ADPKD with aneurysms
2. every 5-20 years for a patient with ADPKD in a kindred of ADPKD with no history of aneurysms.[38]

79.6 Treatment options for aneurysms

79.6.1 General information

The optimal treatment for an aneurysm depends on the age and condition of the patient, the anatomy of the aneurysm and associated vasculature, the ability of the surgeon and the availability of endovascular treatment options, and must be weighed against the natural history of the condition. Also, treatment of the aneurysm facilitates treatment of vasospasm, should it occur.

Natural history:
1. risk of bleeding into subarachnoid space
   a) for ruptured aneurysms: this is the risk of rebleeding (p. 1170)
   b) for unruptured aneurysms (p. 1222)
   c) for cavernous carotid artery aneurysms: this risk is low (p. 1225)
2. spontaneous thrombosis of an aneurysm is a rare occurrence[42,43,44] (estimates in autopsy series is 9–13%[44]). However they may reappear,[45,46] and delayed rupture may occur sometimes even years later
3. enlargement of aneurysm to cause mass effect: some aneurysms go on to become giant aneurysms and can cause mass effect with or without rupture

Although still controversial, endovascular treatment should be initially considered in treating amenable ruptured aneurysms. See also unruptured aneurysms (p. 1225).

79.6.2 Therapies that do not directly address the aneurysm

The hope here is that the aneurysm will not bleed and that it will thrombose (see above).
1. continue medical management initiated on admission: i.e. control of HTN, continue calcium-channel blockers, stool softeners, activity restrictions…
2. treatment options generally *not* used
   a) antifibrinolytic therapy (e.g. ε-aminocaproic acid (EACA)): ✖ NB: *NOT USED*. Reduces rebleeding, but increases the incidence of arterial vasospasm and hydrocephalus[47]
   b) serial LPs: an historical treatment,[48] may increase the risk of aneurysmal re-rupture

79.6.3 Endovascular techniques to treat the aneurysm

1. thrombosing the aneurysm:
   a) "coiling" with Guglielmi electrolytically detachable coils (see below)
   b) Onyx HD 500 (p. 1586) has been used for wide-necked or giant ICA aneurysms.[49] Out of 22 patients, there was 1 parent ICA stenosis and 2 ICA occlusions caused by Onyx migration
   c) "flow diversion" with "covered stents" (tightly woven stents) which promotes thrombosis of the aneurysm (p. 1586)
2. trapping: effective treatment requires distal AND proximal arterial interruption, usually by endovascular techniques,[50] occasionally by direct surgical means (ligation or clip occlusion), or some combination. May also incorporate vascular bypass (e.g. EC-IC bypass) to maintain flow distal to trapped segment[51]
3. proximal ligation (so-called hunterian ligation after Hunter ligated the popliteal artery proximal to a peripheral aneurysm in 1784[52]): useful for giant aneurysms.[53,54] For non-giant aneurysms provides little benefit and adds the risk of thromboembolism (which may be reduced by occluding the CCA rather than the ICA[54]). May also elevate the risk of developing aneurysms in the contralateral circulation[55]

79

79.6.4 Surgical treatment options for aneurysms

1. clipping: the *surgical* gold standard. Surgical placement of a clip across the neck of the aneurysm to exclude the aneurysm from the circulation (see below) without occluding normal vessels
2. wrapping or coating the aneurysm: although this should never be the goal of surgery, situations may arise in which there is little else that can be done (e.g. fusiform basilar trunk aneurysms, aneurysms with significant branches arising from the dome, or part of the neck within the cavernous sinus)
   a) with muscle: the first method used to surgically treat an aneurysm[56] (the patient described died from rebleeding)

b) with cotton or muslin: popularized by Gillingham.[57] An analysis of 60 patients showed that 8.5% rebled in ≤ 6 mos, and the annual rebleeding rate was 1.5% thereafter[58] (similar to the natural history)
c) with plastic resin or other polymer: may be slightly better than muscle or gauze.[59] One study with long follow-up found no protection from rebleeding during the first month, but thereafter the risk was slightly lower than the natural history.[59] Other studies show no difference from natural course[60]
d) teflon and fibrin glue[61]

79.6.5 Treatment decisions: coiling vs. clipping

General information

The use of endovascular treatment for aneurysms has increased, with coil embolization being the most common endovascular modality (see above for other options). From 2002-2008, the rate of aneurysm coiling in the U.S. and U.K. increased from 17 and 35% to 58 and 68%, respectively.[62,63] There is considerable controversy and debate as to the best therapeutic approach for aneurysms (ruptured and unruptured). Impediments to resolving the debate include methodological shortcomings of published studies, the fact that endovascular methods are still rapidly evolving which renders many studies obsolete before completion, and the critical need for long-term follow-up of endovascular results.

This section reviews some of the available information comparing surgical treatment to coil embolization.

Ruptured intracranial aneurysms

To date, four randomized controlled trials have been published comparing functional outcome after coil embolization versus surgical clip ligation for ruptured intracranial aneurysms: the "Finnish Study",[64] ISAT 2002,[65] the "Chinese Study",[66] and BRAT 2012.[67] ▸ Table 79.1 summarizes the treatment data from the 4 RCTs.

▸ **ISAT.** The largest trial, the International Subarachnoid Hemorrhage Aneurysm Trial (ISAT), enrolled 2143 patients and ran from 1997 to 2002, and was stopped prematurely because of a significant outcome difference between the 2 groups favoring endovascular coil embolization. Despite the limitations of ISAT (see below), the findings have often been generalized to all patients with aneurysms, resulting in a dramatic change in management.

Table 79.1 Summary of rebleeding, complete occlusion and retreatment rates as a function of treatment modality (clip vs. coil) for the 4 randomized controlled trials.

	Rebleed[a]: Clip	Rebleed[a]: Coil	Complete occlusion: Clip	Complete occlusion: Coil	Retreatment: Clip	Retreatment: Coil
Finnish	0%	0%	73.7%[b]	50%[b]	7%	23.1%
ISAT	1.0%	2.6%	82%	66%	4.2%	15.1%
$ISAT_5$[c]	0.3%*	0.9%*	n/a	n/a	——	——
$ISAT_{10}$[c]	0.4%	1.6%	n/a	n/a	——	——
Chinese	3.3%	3.2%	83.7%*	64.9%*	——	——
BRAT[d]	0.8%[e]	0%	85%	58%	4.5%*	10.6%*
$BRAT_3$[d]	0%	0%	87%	52%	5%*	13%*

* statistically significant difference ($p < 0.05$)
[a] Rebleeding from target aneurysm after first procedure
[b] Result achieved after treatment during first hospitalization
[c] $ISAT_5$ & $ISAT_{10}$ refer to the 5 and 10 year follow-up studies. Rebleeding results for these studies refer to recurrent SAH after the 1st year of follow-up
[d] $BRAT_3$ refers to the 3-year follow-up study. BRAT & $BRAT_3$ are "as-treated" results
[e] Both rebleeding events occurred during the initial hospitalization

Table 79.2 Methodological shortcomings of ISAT

1. only 20% of 9559 patients presenting with SAH were randomized[a]
   a) selection could introduce bias
   b) more nonrandomized patients underwent MS than EDC
   c) guidelines not provided for which patients to consider for EDC
2. most study centers were located in Europe, Australia & Canada
3. the expertise of the surgeons and the interventionalists were not reported and were not necessarily comparable
4. the following features are not entirely representative of SAH patients at large
   a) 80% of patients were in good clinical condition (H&H grade 1 or 2)
   b) 93% of aneurysms were ≤ 10 mm diameter
   c) 97% were in the anterior circulation
5. rebleeding rate: after EDC (2.4%) or MS (1.0%) was high for both groups, and the difference could be more significant beyond the 1 year follow-up provided

[a]most SAH patients were referred specifically for MS or EDC. The only patients that were randomized were those for whom a panel decided it was not clear which procedure would be superior. Outcomes were not provided for non-randomized patients

Results: At 1 year, there was an absolute reduction of risk of having a poor outcome (i.e. Modified Rankin score > 2) by 7% with coiling (24%) compared to open surgery (31%; p=0.0019). Although not statistically significant, rebleeding in the first year after treatment was higher for coiling (2.6%) than clipping (1.0%). As such, the durability of coil embolization and its ability to prevent subsequent rebleeding of the treated aneurysm was questioned. Additionally, ISAT had many important shortcomings, as detailed in ▶ Table 79.2.

Following the initial report, medium-term follow-up results have been published.[68] In the endovascular cohort, there were 10 episodes of rebleeding from the treated aneurysm after 1 year, in 8447 person-years of follow-up. In the surgical cohort, 3 patients rebled from the treated aneurysm after 1 year, in 8177 person-years of follow-up (one of these patients had declined surgery after randomization and underwent coiling instead). There was a non-significant increased risk of rebleeding from the treated aneurysm in the endovascular cohort (p=0.06), by an intention-to-treat analysis, but a significant difference when analysis was by actual treatment (p=0.02). The probability of death at 5 years was significantly lower in the coiled group (11%) than in the clipping group (14%; p=0.03). However, when patients who died before treatment are excluded from this analysis, the statistical difference is no longer present (p=0.1).[69] The probability of independent survival for those patients alive at 5 years was no different between groups (83% coil; 82% clip).

The 10-year results have been reported for the UK cohort from the initial trial.[70] Similar to the 5-year results, the proportion of patients with a good outcome did not differ between the two groups, but the probability of being alive with a good outcome compared with death or dependence was significantly better for the endovascular group. Thirteen patients in the endovascular group rebled from the target aneurysm (1 per 641 patient-years) compared to 4 in the surgical group (1 per 2041 patient-years). Although the risk of rebleeding was higher in the endovascular group, the overall risk was small and the risk of death or dependency from a rebleed did not differ between the groups.

A follow up study, ISAT II (multicenter RCT), is currently being conducted to help elucidate differences in outcomes between treatment modalities.[71]

▶ **Chinese study[66]** . 192 patients with aSAH randomized to coiling or clipping. Surgical clipping increased the risk of symptomatic vasospasm (OR 1.24), and there were significantly more new cerebral infarctions in the clipping group (21.7 vs. 12.8%). Incidence of complete aneurysm occlusion was significantly lower in the coiling group (64.9 vs. 83.7%). Rebleeding rates were similar in both groups (≈3%). At 1year, there was no significant difference in probability of mortality (coiling: 10.6%, clipping: 15.2%). Furthermore, there was no significant difference in probability of a good outcome (coiling: 75%, clipping: 67.9%).

79

▶ **BRAT[67]** . Initiated at Barrow Neurologic Institute in 2002. Designed to reflect "real-world" practices of ruptured aneurysm treatment in North America. Randomly assigned in an alternate fashion every patient with SAH who agreed to participate. A large number of patients allocated to endovascular treatment crossed over to the surgical arm because patients could be enrolled regardless of whether the aneurysm was amenable to both treatment modalities (75 crossed over from coil to surgery; 4 crossed over from surgery to coil). Proportion of patients with a poor outcome (i.e. mRS > 2) was 33.7% in the surgical group versus 23.2% in the endovascular group (p=0.02, intention-to-treat analsysis). An "as-treated" analysis yielded similar results (33.9 vs 20.4%, p=0.01). There were 2 episodes of rebleeding following treatment – one assigned to and treated with clipping and the other assigned to coil, but treated with surgical clipping. Twelve patients (2.9%) required retreatment during the initial hospitalization (9 surgical and 3 coil patients). Overall, during the 1st year, there was a significant increased probability of retreatment in patients actually treated with coiling compared with those actually treated by clipping (10.6% of coil vs. 4.49% of surgical patients, p=0.03).

At 3years,[72] there was no significant difference in poor-outcome between coiling (30%) and clipping (35.8%). Subgroup analysis: there were no differences in mRS scores between treatment groups at any time point among patients with anterior circulation aneurysms (83%). However, among posterior circulation aneurysms (17%), mRS scores were significantly better after endovascular management than after surgical treatment at every time point. Of note, with the exception of basilar tip aneurysms, the randomization of the posterior circulation aneurysms was unexpectedly skewed (large majority of SCA and PICA were clipped, whereas majority of PCA, vertebral and basilar where coiled). The lack of anatomical parity between the treatment groups makes it difficult to draw strong conclusions. In addition, the degree of aneurysm obliteration (87 vs. 52%), rate of aneurysm recurrence and rate of retreatment (5 vs. 13%) were significantly better in the group treated with clipping compared with coiling. However, no rebleeding occurrences were documented in the 2nd or 3rd year of BRAT.

► **Meta-analyses.** Lanzino et al.[73] conducted a meta-analsysis on the 3 prospective controlled studies (Finnish, ISAT, BRAT). Pooled data showed poor outcome at 1 year to be lower in the embolization group; no difference in mortality between groups; and rebleeding rates within the first month were higher in coiled patients. However, the results were largely skewed by ISAT data.

Li et al.[74] conducted a meta-analysis on the 4 RCTs (see above) and 23 observational studies. The result of the RCT analysis with regard to poor outcome at 1 year paralleled that by Lanzino et al. However, there was no difference in poor outcome between groups in the nonrandomized controlled trial analysis. Additional subgroup analysis showed a higher incidence of rebleeding after coiling (≈2-3 vs. 1%), corresponding to a better complete occlusion rate of clipping (84 vs. 66.5%). Procedural complications rates and 1-year mortality did not differ significantly between the groups.

► **Vasospasm.** Whether coiling or clipping has an independent correlation with symptomatic vasospasm is debatable. One meta-analysis[75] suggested a trend toward less symptomatic vasospasm after coiling compared with clipping. However, the analysis had multiple limitations – the two treatment groups were not comparable (age, clinical grade, aneurysm location); there were differences in study design and definitions of vasospasm; and there was a lack of angiographic diagnosis of vasospasm. In the Chinese RCT (above) symptomatic vasospasm and consequent cerebral infarction was more common in the coiling group. Li et al.[74] found vasospasm was more common after clipping (48.8 vs. 43.1%), however, ischemic infarction did not differ significantly. Treatment choice may also alter the spasm pattern: on one study,[76] patients who underwent clipping developed localized vasospasm around the rupture site, whereas those treated with coiling demonstrated progressive distal vasospasm over time (possibly related to treatment-specific effects on CSF circulation).

► **Shunt-dependent hydrocephalus.** One study showed a lower incidence of shunt-dependent hydrocephalus in the surgical treatment group (19.9 vs. 47.1%),[77] however many others have failed to show this relationship.[74,78,79,80,81,82,83,84,85,86] A suggestion that fenestration of the lamina terminalis at the time of surgery may decrease shunt-dependent chronic hydrocephalus was refuted by a meta-analysis[87] of 11 non-randomized studies (hydrocephalus rates of 10% with fenestration compared to 15% without).

► **Seizures.** A literature review[88] of seizures after aSAH reported a rate of ≈2% following either neurosurgical clipping or endovascular coiling. In contrast, ISAT showed endovascular intervention had lower seizure rates (13.3% to 3.3%) compared to surgical clipping (2.2-5.2%) in the first year. As such, there is no consensus as to whether treatment modality independently impacts seizure and/or epilepsy occurrence.

► **Factors to consider (clipping vs. coiling)**
- health care environment / equipment available
- skill set and experience of the neurosurgeon and interventionalist
  - greater annual numbers of aneurysms treated by individual practitioners were significantly related to decrease in morbidity[89]
- anatomy and location of the aneurysm
  - favorable dome/neck ratio versus wide neck aneurysms
  - MCA aneurysms may be difficult to coil because of a branch near the neck
  - Basilar apex: favors coiling
  - associated IPH/SDH: surgery allows both evacuation of hemorrhage and treatment of aneurysm

  - symptoms due to mass effect: clipping[90,91] may be better than coiling. In 13 patients with p-comm aneurysms and oculomotor nerve (3rd nerve) palsy (**ONP**), 6 of 7 patients clipped vs. 2 of 6 with coiling recovered completely.[27] Partial ONP improved with either treatment, but complete ONP recovered in 3 of 4 patients clipped vs. 0 of 3 coiled[27]
- patient age
  - younger age: lower risk of surgery, and lower lifetime risk of recurrence than with coiling
- clinical state / comorbidities
  - good outcome seen in 63% clip vs. 46% coil in poor grade (WFNS IV/V) pts (contrary to findings in practice guidelines[92]) therefore microsurgery and endovascular treatment, when selected primarily according to angiographic features, were equally likely to achieve good outcome[93]
  - patients on anticoagulation (e.g. Plavix) favor endovascular treatment

Practice guideline: Aneurysm treatment decisions

Level C[92]: Treatment decisions should be multidisciplinary (made by experienced cerebrovascular and endovascular specialists) based on characteristics of the patient and aneurysm.

Level C[92]: Microsurgical clipping may receive increased consideration in patients presenting with large (> 50 ml) intraparenchymal hematomas and middle cerebral artery aneurysms.

Level C[92]: Endovascular coiling may receive increased consideration in the elderly (> 70 yo), in those presenting with poor-grade WFNS classification (IV/V) aSAH, and in those with aneurysms of the basilar apex

Level B[92]: For patients with ruptured aneurysms judged to be technically amenable to both endovascular coiling and neurosurgical clipping, endovascular coiling should be considered

Unruptured intracranial aneurysms

As with ruptured aneurysms, there is controversy over the best treatment method for unruptured intracranial aneurysms (IUAs), and additional uncertainty surrounds the question of which IUAs need to be treated (vs. observed). Darsaut et al.[94] found that practitioners do not agree regarding management of IUAs, even when they share a background in the same specialty, similar capabilities in aneurysm management, or years of practice.

There are no prospective randomized studies of treatment interventions vs. conservative management,[95] or comparing treatment options to each other. Most data are either from personal series or are retrospective.

▸ **Surgical clipping.** One summary of 260 patients (including a retrospective multicenter analysis) show no surgical mortality, and morbidity of 0-10.3% (6.5% major and 8% minor morbidity in the multicenter study).[5] Findings from one meta-analysis of 733 patients who underwent surgical clipping showed a mortality rate of 1% and major morbidity rate of 4%.[96] A larger meta-analysis of 2460 patients revealed mortality and morbidity rates of 2.6% and 10.9%, respectively.[97]

The ISUIA investigators found surgical mortality to be 2.3% at 30days, and 3.8% at 1 year.[98] Additionally, they found a combined morbidity and mortality at 1 year of 12.6% for those without previous hemorrhage and 10.1% for those with previous subarachnoid hemorrhage from another aneurysm. For patients treated with surgical clipping, morbidity and mortality was greatest in those with aneurysms that were large or in the posterior circulation, and in patients older than age 50. In comparison, the combined morbidity and mortality for the 451 patients treated with an endovascular procedure was 9.1% at 30 days and 9.5% at 1 year. Predictors of adverse outcome included aneurysm size and posterior circulation aneurysms. Additionally, the presence of calcification (independent of aneurysm size) has been shown to increase the likelihood of poor outcome.[99]

▸ **Comparison of clipping to coil embolization.** Early retrospective studies have shown a lower incidence of in-hospital death and discharge to skilled nursing facilities with endovascular therapy compared to those treated surgically.[100,101] A recent retrospective study conducted at a single center showed early outcome and lower complication rate favoring clipping, but the results did not remain significant long-term.[102] A meta-analysis[103] showed that clipping resulted in significantly higher disability compared with coiling (OR 2.38-2.83). However, subgroup analysis by outcome-measurement time, revealed clipping to be associated with greater risk of disability in the short-term (< 6 months), but not in the long-term (> 6 months). In addition, mortality (in-hospital and overall), hemorrhage, and infarction were no different between groups. Despite inclusion of a large number of studies and patients, it is very challenging to draw any conclusion from the meta-analysis, as all the studies were observational (i.e. low levels of evidence), and the analysis did not stratify outcomes based on size and/or location of aneurysms.

Lawson et al.[104] compared natural history rupture risk to national treatment risk for coiling and clipping (taken from the Nationwide Inpatient Sample from 2002-2008). Overall mortality rate for clipping and coiling was 2.66% and 2.17%, respectively. Poor outcome was significantly greater for clipping (4.75%) versus coiling (2.16%). Data regarding the homogeneity of the two groups regarding aneurysm size or location was not available. Treatment risk curves were generated and compared against natural history actuarial risk curves calculated from four prominent studies.[105,106,9,107] Overall, the analysis demonstrated rationale for clipping small, unruptured aneurysms in patients < 61-70 years, and coiling small unruptured aneurysms in patients < 70-80 years.

Additional studies have focused on the effect of age on outcomes. Mahaney et al.[108] showed that procedural and in-hospital morbidity and mortality increased with age in patients treated with surgery, but remained relatively constant with endovascular treatment. Poor neurological outcome from aneurysm or procedure-related morbidity and mortality did not differ between management groups for patients 65 years old and younger, but was significantly higher in the surgical group for patients older than 65 years. Surgery appeared to show a surgical benefit in patients < 50 years old at 1 year. Others have suggested an overall benefit of endovascular treatment over surgical clipping, which becomes more pronounced with age.[109]

▶ **Cost.** Several studies have compared total hospital costs for treatment of unruptured aneurysms with mixed results. Halkes et al.[110] and Hoh et al.[111] found endovascular treatment to be associated with higher total hospital costs. A later study by Hoh et al.[112] found that on a national level, surgical clipping was associated with higher costs. A long-term outcome study[113] showed that clipping was associated with higher initial costs, but overall costs at 2 and 5 years were similar to coiling (due to higher number of follow-up angiograms and outpatient costs). More recently, total hospital cost was shown to be lower for clipping, despite higher fixed-direct and fixed-indirect costs.[114] This is a function of much higher variable costs (i.e. the cost of coils and devices) overcoming any substantial cost reduction due to shorter length of stay in patients treated endovascularly.

▶ **Miscellaneous.** *Oculomotor nerve palsy:* Complete recovery of oculomotor nerve palsy associated with p-comm aneurysms is more common with surgical clipping than with endovascular treatment (87 % vs. 44%).[115]

Pregnancy: No studies have directly compared clipping versus coiling. Clipping may be preferred by some[116]; see pregnancy and SAH (p. 1169).

79.7 Timing of aneurysm surgery

79.7.1 Background

Historically, there was controversy between so-called "early surgery" (generally, but not precisely defined as ≤ 48–96 hrs post SAH) and "late surgery" (usually ≥ 10–14 days post SAH). The current consensus is that there should be intervention for a ruptured aneurysm (clipping or coiling) as promptly as possible to secure the aneurysm and prevent rebleeding. In a review of all patients with SAH treated by clipping or coiling in the Nationwide Inpatient Sample between 2002-2010, treatment at non-teaching hospitals and older age (> 80) were associated with delays in time to aneurysm clipping, but these associations were not seen when endovascular treatment was performed.[117] Increased time to procedure (> 3 days) was significantly associated with an increased likelihood of moderate to severe neurological deficit. Ultra-early (< 24 h after SAH) coiling of ruptured aneurysms has also been associated with improved clinical outcomes (mRS 0-2) compared to coiling at > 24 hours in poor grade SAH patients (Hunt-Hess IV/V).[118] This does not rule out a selection bias, however. Additionally, the increased morbidity and mortality associated with surgical intervention on patients who present subacutely with evidence of vasospasm on imaging, may be better suited for endovascular intervention. 79

Early surgery advocated for the following reasons:

1. if successful, virtually eliminates the risk of rebleeding which occurs most frequently in the period immediately following SAH (p. 1167)
2. facilitates treatment of vasospasm which peaks in incidence between days 6–8 post SAH (never seen before day 3) by allowing induction of arterial hypertension and volume expansion without danger of aneurysmal rupture
3. allows lavage to remove potentially vasospasmogenic agents from contact with vessels, including use of thrombolytic agents (p. 1183)
4. although operative mortality is higher, overall patient mortality is lower[119]

Arguments against early surgery, in favor of late surgery include:
1. inflammation and brain edema are most severe immediately following SAH
   a) this necessitates more brain retraction
   b) at the same time this softens the brain making retraction more difficult (retractors have more tendency to lacerate the more friable brain)
2. the presence of solid clot that has not had time to lyse impedes surgery
3. the risk of intra-operative rupture is higher with early surgery
4. possible increased incidence of vasospasm following early surgery from mechanotrauma to vessels

Factors that favor choosing early surgery include:
1. good medical condition of patient
2. good neurologic condition of patient (Hunt and Hess (H&H) grade ≤ 3)
3. large amounts of subarachnoid blood, increasing the likelihood and severity of subsequent vasospasm (p. 1186), ► Table 78.2. Having the aneurysm clipped permits use of hyperdynamic therapy for vasospasm
4. conditions that complicate management in face of unclipped aneurysm: e.g. unstable blood pressure; frequent and/or intractable seizures
5. large clot with mass effect associated with SAH
6. early rebleeding, especially multiple rebleeds
7. indications of imminent rebleeding: (see below)

Factors that favor choosing delayed surgery (10–14 days post SAH) include:
1. poor medical condition and/or advanced age of patient (age may not be a separate factor related to outcome, when patients are stratified by H&H grade[120])
2. poor neurologic condition of patient (H&H grade ≥ 4): *controversial.* Some say the risk of rebleeding and its mortality argues for early surgery even in bad grade patients[121] since denying surgery on clinical grounds may result in withholding treatment in some patients who would do well (54% of H&H grade IV and 24% of H&H grade V patients had favorable outcome in one series[120]). Some data show no difference in surgical complications in good and bad grade patients with anterior circulation aneurysms[122]
3. aneurysms difficult to clip because of large size, or difficult location necessitating a lax brain during surgery (e.g. difficult basilar bifurcation or mid-basilar artery aneurysms, giant aneurysms)
4. significant cerebral edema seen on CT
5. the presence of active vasospasm

79.7.2 Conclusions

Practice guideline: Timing of intervention for ruptured aneurysm

Level B[92]: Surgical clipping or endovascular coiling of a ruptured aneursym causing aSAH should be performed as early as feasible in the majority of patients to reduce the risk of rebleeding.

79.7.3 Imminent aneurysm rupture

Findings that may herald impending aneurysm rupture and may therefore increase the need for expedient intervention include:
1. progressing cranial nerve palsy e.g. development of 3rd nerve palsy with p-comm aneurysm; traditionally regarded as an indication for urgent treatment (p. 1192)
2. increase in aneurysm size on repeat angiography
3. beating aneurysm sign[123]: pulsatile changes in aneurysm size between cuts or slices on imaging (may be seen on angiography, MRA, or CTA)

79

79.8 General technical considerations of aneurysm surgery

79.8.1 General information

The goal of aneurysm surgery is to prevent rupture or further enlargement of the aneurysm, while at the same time preserving all normal vessels and minimizing injury to brain tissue and cranial nerves. This is usually accomplished by excluding the aneurysm from the circulation with a clip across its neck. Placing the clip too low on the aneurysm neck may occlude the parent vessel, while too distal placement may leave a so-called "aneurysmal rest" which is not benign since it may enlarge (see below).

See Intraoperative aneurysm rupture (p.1204) for general measures to reduce the risk of this complication during surgery.

79.8.2 Aneurysmal rest

When a portion of the aneurysm neck is not occluded by a surgical clip, it is referred to as an aneurysmal rest. A "dog-ear" occurs when a clip is angled to leave part of the neck at one end, and obliterates the neck at the other. Rests are not innocuous, even if only 1–2 mm, because they may later expand and possibly rupture years later, especially in younger patients.[124] The incidence of rebleeding was 3.7% in one study, with an annual risk of 0.4–0.8% during the observation period of 4–13 yrs.[125] Patients should be followed with serial angiography, and any increase in size should be treated by reoperation or endovascular techniques if possible.

Booking the case: Craniotomy for aneurysm

Also see defaults & disclaimers (p.27).

1. position: (depends on location of aneurysm), radiolucent head-holder
2. intraoperative angiography (optional)
3. equipment: microscope (with ICG capability if used)
4. blood: type and cross 2 U PRBC
5. post-op: ICU
6. consent (in lay terms for the patient – not all-inclusive):
   a) procedure: surgery through the skull to place a permanent clip on the base of the aneurysm to prevent future bleeding, intraoperative angiogram, possible placement of external (ventricular) drain, possible lumbar drain
   b) alternatives: nonsurgical management, endovascular treatment only for aneurysms that are candidates
   c) complications: usual craniotomy complications (p.28) plus (the following are not really complications of surgery but are possible developments) post-op vasospasm, hydrocephalus, formation of new aneurysms

79.8.3 Surgical exposure

General information

To avoid excessive brain retraction, surgical exposure requires sufficient bony removal and adequate brain relaxation (see below).

Brain relaxation

More critical for ACoA and basilar tip than for easier to reach aneurysms such as p-comm or MCA.... Techniques include:

1. hyperventilation
2. CSF drainage: provides brain relaxation and a field dry of CSF, and removes blood & blood breakdown products along with the CSF. ✖ CSF drainage *before* opening the dura is associated with an increased risk of aneurysmal rebleeding (p.1167)
   a) ventriculostomy: risks include seizures, bleeding from catheter insertion, infection (ventriculitis, meningitis), possible increased risk of vasospasm
      - placed pre-op in cases of acute post-SAH hydrocephalus (p.1170)
      - placed intra-op
   b) lumbar spinal drainage (see below)
   c) intra-operative drainage of CSF from cisterns
3. diuretics: mannitol and/or furosemide. Although proof is lacking, lowering ICP by this or any means may theoretically increase the risk of rebleeding[126]

Lumbar spinal drainage

May be inserted with Tuohy needle following induction of anesthesia (to minimize BP elevation), prior to final positioning. CSF is gradually withdrawn by the anesthesiologist *only* after the dura is opened (to minimize chances of intraoperative aneurysmal bleeding), usually a total of 30–50 cc are removed in ≈ 10 cc aliquots.

Risks include[127]: aneurysmal rebleeding (≤0.3%), back pain (10%, may be chronic in 0.6%), catheter malfunction preventing CSF drainage (< 5%), catheter fracture or laceration resulting in retained catheter tip in the spinal subarachnoid space, post-op CSF fistula, spinal H/A (may be difficult to distinguish from post-craniotomy H/A), infection, neuropathy (from nerve root impingement with needle), epidural hematoma (spinal and/or intracranial).

Cerebral protection during surgery

Pathophysiology of cerebral ischemia

The cerebral metabolic rate of oxygen consumption ($CMRO_2$) (p. 1265) arises from neurons utilizing energy for two functions: 1) maintenance of cell integrity (homeostasis) which normally accounts for ≈ 40% of energy consumption, and 2) conduction of electrical impulses. Occlusion of an artery produces a central core of ischemic tissue where the $CMRO_2$ is not met. The oxygen deficiency precludes aerobic glycolysis and oxidative phosphorylation. ATP production declines and cell homeostasis cannot be maintained, and within minutes irreversible cell death occurs; a so-called cerebral infarction. Surrounding this central core is the penumbra, where collateral flow (usually through leptomeningeal vessels) provides marginal oxygenation which may impair cellular function without immediate irreversible damage. Cells in the penumbra may remain viable for hours.

Cerebral protection by increasing the ischemic tolerance of the CNS

1. drugs that mitigate the toxic effects of ischemia without reducing $CMRO_2$
   a) calcium channel blockers: nimodipine, nicardipine, flunarizine
   b) free radical scavengers: superoxide dismutase, dimethylthiourea, lazaroids, barbiturates, Vitamin C
   c) mannitol: although not a cerebral protectant per se, it may help re-establish blood flow to compromised parenchyma by improving the microvascular perfusion by transiently increasing CBV and decreasing blood viscosity
2. reduction of $CMRO_2$
   a) by reducing the electrical activity of neurons: titrating these agents to a isoelectric EEG reduces $CMRO_2$ by up to a maximum of ≈ 50%
      - barbiturates: in addition to reducing $CMRO_2$, they also redistribute blood flow to ischemic cortex, quench free radicals, and stabilize cell membranes. For dosing of thiopental, see below
      - isoflurane (p. 105): shorter acting and less myocardial depression than with barbiturates
   b) by reducing the maintenance energy of neurons: no drugs developed to date can accomplish this, only hypothermia has any effect on this. Below mild hypothermia, extracerebral effects must be monitored (p. 871)
      - mild hypothermia (core temperatures down to 33° C): in a multicenter RCT[128] mild hypothermia was demonstrated to be safe, but did not improve the neurological outcome after craniotomy among good-grade (Hunt Hess I-III) patients with aSAH
      - moderate hypothermia: 32.5–33° C has been used for head injury
      - deep hypothermia to 18° C permits the brain to tolerate up to 1 hour of circulatory arrest
      - profound hypothermia to < 10° C allows several hours of complete ischemia (the clinical usefulness of this has not been substantiated)

Adjunctive cerebral protection techniques used in aneurysm surgery

1. systemic hypotension
   a) usually used during final approach to aneurysm and during manipulation of aneurysm for clip application
   b) theoretical goals
      - to reduce turgor of aneurysm facilitating clip closure, especially with atherosclerotic neck
      - to decrease transmural pressure (p. 1170) to reduce the risk of intraoperative rupture
   c) One retrospective study[129] suggests that a decrease in MAP > 50% is associated with poor outcome. However, after adjustment for age, this association was no longer statistically significant. Because of the potential danger of hypoxic injury to brain and other organs (including areas of impaired autoregulation as well as normal areas), some surgeons avoid this method.

2. "focal" hypotension: using temporary aneurysm clips (specially designed with low closing force to avoid intimal injury) placed on parent vessel (small perforators will not tolerate temporary clips without injury)
   a) used in conjunction with methods of cerebral protection against ischemia
   b) may be combined with systemic hypertension to increase collateral flow
   c) the proximal ICA can tolerate an hour or more of occlusion in some cases, whereas the perforator bearing segments of the MCA and the basilar apex may tolerate clipping for only a few minutes
   d) in addition to the risk of ischemia, there is the risk of intravascular thrombosis and subsequent release of emboli upon removal of the clip
3. circulatory arrest, utilized in conjunction with deep hypothermia
   a) candidates include patients with large aneurysms that contain significant atherosclerosis and/or thrombosis that impedes clip closure and a dome that is adherent to vital neural structures
4. blood glucose: intraoperative hyperglycemia has been associated with long-term decline in cognition and gross neurologic function[130] and should be avoided

Systematic approach to cerebral protection

See reference.[131]

The following factors may mandate the use of temporary clips (and associated techniques of cerebral protection): giant aneurysm, calcified neck, thin/fragile dome, adherence of dome to critical structures, vital arterial branches near the aneurysm neck, intraoperative rupture. Aside from giant aneurysms, most of these factors may be difficult to identify pre-op. Therefore, Solomon provides some degree of cerebral protection to all patients undergoing aneurysm surgery.

1. spontaneous cooling is permitted during surgery, which usually results in a body temperature of 34° C by the time that dissection around the aneurysm begins
2. if temporary clipping is utilized
   a) if a long segment of the ICA is being trapped, administer 5000 U IV heparin to prevent thrombosis and subsequent emboli
   b) < 5 mins temporary clip occlusion: no further intervention
   c) up to 10 or 15 mins occlusion: administer IV brain protection anesthesia (e.g. thiopental, propofol, and/or etomidate) and titrate to burst suppression on EEG
      - administration of IV brain protection anesthesia to burst suppression has been shown to significantly decrease infarction rate with temporary clipping within this time range[132]
      - intermittent reperfusion has been shown to be advantageous in some studies,[132] while in others findings have been contradictory[133,134]
   d) > 20 mins occlusion: not tolerated (except possibly ICA proximal to p-comm), terminate operation if possible and plan repeat operation utilizing
      - deep hypothermic circulatory arrest (see above)
      - endovascular techniques
      - bypass grafting around the segment to be occluded

79.8.4 Postoperative angiography

Due to the fact that unexpected findings (aneurysmal rest, unclipped aneurysm, or major vessel occlusion) were seen on 19% of post-op angiograms (the only predictive factor identified was a new post-op deficit, which signaled major vessel occlusion) the use of routine post-op angiography has been recommended.[135]

79.8.5 Some drugs useful in aneurysm surgery

Drug info: Propofol (Diprivan®)

May be used to achieve burst suppression[136] with shorter duration of action than other barbiturates. Results are preliminary, further investigation is needed to demonstrate the degree of neuroprotection. Has been reported at doses 170 mcg/kg/min for neuroprotection[137] (if tolerated) but this may be risky. May also be used as a continuous drip for sedation (p. 133), and for ICP management (p. 869). Reverses rapidly upon discontinuation (usually within 5–10 minutes).

Side effects: possible anaphylactic reaction with angioneurotic edema (angioedema) of the airways,[138] Propofol Infusion syndrome (p. 133).

79.8.6 Intraoperative aneurysm rupture

Epidemiology

Reported rates of intraoperative aneurysm rupture (IAR) range from ≈ 18% in the cooperative study (1963–1978)[139] to ≈ 36% in a pre-microscope series[140] (NB: this series had an unexplained high IAR rate of 61% with the microscope) and 40% in a more recent series.[141] Although rupture rate may be higher in early surgery than with late surgery,[141] other series found no difference.[142]

Morbidity and mortality for patients experiencing significant IAR is ≈ 30–35% (vs. ≈ 10% in the absence of this complication), although IAR may primarily affects outcome when it occurs during induction of anesthesia or opening of dura.[141]

See aneurysm rupture during coiling (p. 1587).

Prevention of intraoperative rupture

Presented as a list here to be incorporated into general operative techniques.

1. prevent hypertension from catecholamine response to pain:
   a) insure deep anesthesia during headholder pin placement and skin incision
   b) consider local anesthetic (without epinephrine) in headholder pin-sites and along incision line
2. minimize increases in transmural pressure: reduce MAP to slightly below baseline just prior to dural opening
3. reduce shearing forces on aneurysm during dissection by minimizing brain retraction:
   a) radical removal of sphenoid wing for circle of Willis aneurysms
   b) reduce brain volume by a number of mechanisms: diuretics (mannitol, furosemide), CSF drainage through lumbar subarachnoid drain placed pre-operatively and opened by the anesthesiologist at the time of dural incision, hyperventilation
4. reduce risk of large tear in aneurysm fundus or neck:
   a) utilize sharp dissection in exposing aneurysm and in removing clot from around aneurysm
   b) whenever possible, completely mobilize and inspect aneurysm before attempting clip application

Details of intraoperative rupture

Rupture can occur during any of the three following stages of aneurysm surgery[143]:

1. initial exposure (predissection)
   a) rare. Brain can become surprisingly tight even when bleeding seems to be into open subarachnoid space. Usually carries poor prognosis
   b) possible causes:
      - vibration from bone work: dubious
      - increasing transmural pressure upon opening the dura
      - hypertension from catecholamine response to pain (see above)
   c) management tactics:
      - have anesthesiologist radically drop BP
      - control bleeding (with anterior circulation aneurysms) by placing temporary clip across ICA as it exits from cavernous sinus, or if not possible then compress ICA in patient's neck through drapes
      - if necessary to gain control, resect portions of frontal or temporal lobe
2. dissection of the aneurysm: accounts for the majority of IARs, two basic types:
   a) tears caused by blunt dissection
      - tends to be profuse, proximal to the neck, and difficult to control
      - do not attempt definitive clipping unless adequate exposure has been achieved (which is usually not the case with these tears)
      - temporary clipping: this step is often necessary in this situation, after the temporary clip is in place return the MAP to normal and administer neuroprotective agent (e.g. propofol)
      - once the temporary clip is in place, it is better to take a few extra moments to improve the exposure and apply a well placed permanent clip instead of hastily clipping and trying to restore circulation
      - microsutures may need to be placed to close any portion of the tear that extends onto the parent vessel
   b) laceration by sharp dissection
      - tend to be small, often distally on fundus, and usually easily controlled by a single suction
      - may respond to gentle tamponade with a small cottonoid

Table 79.3 Follow-up schedule for treated aneurysms

Perform indicated study at the following times after treatment	
Coiled aneurysms	*Clipped* aneurysms
Study: CTA or gad-MRA[a]	Study: CTA
6 mos	1 year
1.5 years	5 years
3.5 years	every 10 years thereafter
? every 5–10 years (as with clipped aneurysms)	

[a]gad-MRA indicates gadolinium MRA which is more sensitive here than TOF-MRA (p. 232). Use the same modality for each follow-up to facilitate accurate comparison

- may shrink down with repeated low current strokes with the bipolar (avoid the temptation to use continuous high current)

3. clip application: bleeding at this point is usually due to either
   a) inadequate exposure of aneurysm: clip blade may penetrate unseen lobe of aneurysm. Similar to tears caused by blunt dissection (see above). Bleeding worsens as clip blades become approximated
      - prompt opening and removal of clip at the first hint of bleeding may minimize the extent of the tear
      - utilize 2 suckers to determine if definitive clipping can be done, or what is more common, to allow temporary clipping (see above)
   b) poor technical clip application: tends to abate as clip blades become approximated. Inspect the blade tips for the following:
      - to be certain that they span the breadth of the neck. If not, a second longer clip is usually applied parallel to the first, which may then be advanced
      - to verify that they are closely approximated. If not, tandem clips may be necessary, and sometimes multiple clips are needed

79.8.7 Aneurysm recurrence after treatment

Incompletely treated aneurysms may increase in size and/or bleed. This includes aneurysms that are clipped or coiled where there is still aneurysm filling, as well as a persistent aneurysm rest or a neck (p. 1201). While most aneurysm rests appear to be stable, there is a small subset that may enlarge or rupture.[144]

Additionally, even an aneurysm that has been completely obliterated may recur, and therefore one has to consider the durability of treatment. The risk of recurrence of a completely clipped aneurysm is ≈ 1.5% at 4.4 years.[144]

79.8.8 Follow-up after aneurysm treatment

Based on the above, together with the small risk of de novo aneurysm formation,[144] there is a trend to indefinitely follow patients with known aneurysms. One suggested follow-up schedule is shown in ▶ Table 79.3.

References

[1] Jellinger K. Pathology of intracerebral hemorrhage. Zentralbl Neurochir. 1977; 38:29–42

[2] Jakubowski J, Kendall B. Coincidental aneurysms with tumours of pituitary origin. J Neurol Neurosurg Psychiatry. 1978; 41:972–979

[3] Vlak MH, Algra A, Brandenburg R, Rinkel GJ. Prevalence of unruptured intracranial aneurysms, with emphasis on sex, age, comorbidity, country, and time period: a systematic review and meta-analysis. Lancet Neurol. 2011; 10:626–636

[4] Brown RD, Jr, Broderick JP. Unruptured intracranial aneurysms: epidemiology, natural history, management options, and familial screening. Lancet Neurol. 2014; 13:393–404

[5] Wirth FP. Surgical Treatment of Incidental Intracranial Aneurysms. Clin Neurosurg. 1986; 33:125–135

[6] Menghini VV, Brown RD, Jr, Sicks JD, O'Fallon WM, Wiebers DO. Incidence and prevalence of intracranial aneurysms and hemorrhage in Olmsted

79

County, Minnesota, 1965 to 1995. Neurology. 1998; 51:405–411
[7] Fox JL. Intracranial Aneurysms. New York: Springer-Verlag; 1983
[8] Chason JL, Hindman WM. Berry aneurysms of the circle of Willis; results of a planned autopsy study. Neurology. 1958; 8:41–44
[9] Wiebers DO, Whisnant JP, Huston J, III, Meissner I, Brown RD, Jr, Piepgras DG, Forbes GS, Thielen K, Nichols D, O'Fallon WM, Peacock J, Jaeger L, Kassell NF, Kongable-Beckman GL, Torner JC, International Study of Unruptured Intracranial Aneurysms Investigators. Unruptured intracranial aneurysms: natural history, clinical outcome, and risks of surgical and endovascular treatment. Lancet. 2003; 362:103–110
[10] Inagawa T, Hirano A. Autopsy study of unruptured incidental intracranial aneurysms. Surg Neurol. 1990; 34:361–365
[11] Almeida GM, Pindaro J, Plese P, Bianco E, et al. Intracranial Arterial Aneurysms in Infancy and Childhood. Childs Brain. 1977; 3:193–199
[12] Storrs BB, Humphreys RP, Hendrick EB, Hoffman HJ. Intracranial aneurysms in the pediatric age-group. Childs Brain. 1982; 9:358–361
[13] Meyer FB, Sundt TM, Jr, Fode NC, Morgan MK, Forbes GS, Mellinger JF. Cerebral aneurysms in childhood and adolescence. J Neurosurg. 1989; 70:420-425
[14] Fang H, Wright IS, Millikan CH. In: A Comparison of Blood Vessels of the Brain and Peripheral Blood Vessels. Cerebral Vascular Diseases. New York: Grune and Stratton; 1958:17–22
[15] Wilkinson IMS. The Vertebral Artery: Extracranial and Intracranial Structure. Arch Neurol. 1972; 27:392–396
[16] Youmans JR. Neurological Surgery. Philadelphia 1990
[17] Rhoton AL. Anatomy of Saccular Aneurysms. Surg Neurol. 1981; 14:59–66
[18] Ferguson GG. Physical Factors in the Initiation, Growth, and Rupture of Human Intracranial Saccular Aneurysms. J Neurosurg. 1972; 37:666–677
[19] Nehls DG, Flom RA, Carter LP, et al. Multiple Intracranial Aneurysms: Determining the Site of Rupture. J Neurosurg. 1985; 63:342–348
[20] Mohr G, Ferguson G, Khan M, et al. Intraventricular Hemorrhage from Ruptured Aneurysm: Retrospective Analysis of 91 Cases. J Neurosurg. 1983; 58:482–487
[21] Yeh HS, Tomsick TA, Tew JM. Intraventricular Hemorrhage due to Aneurysms of the Distal Posterior Inferior Cerebellar Artery. J Neurosurg. 1985; 62:772–775
[22] Okawara SH. Warning Signs Prior to Rupture of an Intracranial Aneurysm. J Neurosurg. 1973; 38:575–580
[23] White JC, Ballantine HT. Intrasellar Aneurysms Simulating Hypophyseal Tumors. J Neurosurg. 1961; 18:34–50
[24] Raps EC, Galetta SL, Solomon RA, et al. The Clinical Spectrum of Unruptured Intracranial Aneurysms. Arch Neurol. 1993; 50:265–268
[25] Day JW, Raskin NH. Thunderclap Headache: Symptom of Unruptured Cerebral Aneurysm. Lancet. 1986; 2:1247–1248
[26] Verweij RD, Wijdicks EFM, van Gijn J. Warning Headache in Aneurysmal Subarachnoid Hemorrhage: A Case-Control Study. Arch Neurol. 1988; 45:1019–1020
[27] Chen PR, Amin-Hanjani S, Albuquerque FC, McDougall C, Zabramski JM, Spetzler RF. Outcome of oculomotor nerve palsy from posterior communicating artery aneurysms: comparison of clipping and coiling. Neurosurgery. 2006; 58:1040–6; discussion 1040-6
[28] Sano H, Jain VK, Kato Y, et al. Bilateral Giant Intracavernous Aneurysms: Technique of Unilateral Operation. Surg Neurol. 1988; 29:35–38
[29] ter Berg HWM, Bijlsma JB, Viega PiresJA, et al. Familial association of intracranial aneurysms and multiple congenital anomalies. Arch Neurol. 1986; 43:30–33
[30] Bigelow NH. The association of polycystic kidneys with intracranial aneurysms and other related disorders. Am J Med Sci. 1953; 225:485–494
[31] Longstreth WT, Koepsell TD, Yerby MS, van Belle G. Risk Factors for Subarachnoid Hemorrhage. Stroke. 1985; 16:377–385
[32] Schievink WI. Genetics and aneurysm formation. Neurosurg Clin N Am. 1998; 9:485–495
[33] Maher CO, Piepgras DG, Brown RD, Jr, Friedman JA, Pollock BE. Cerebrovascular manifestations in 321 cases of hereditary hemorrhagic telangiectasia. Stroke. 2001; 32:877–882
[34] Schievink WI, Riedinger M, Maya MM. Frequency of incidental intracranial aneurysms in neurofibromatosis type 1. Am J Med Genet A. 2005; 134A:45–48
[35] Beeson PB, McDermott W. Cecil's Textbook of Medicine. Philadelphia 1979
[36] Peebles BrownR. Polycystic Disease of the Kidneys and Intracranial Aneurysms. Glasgow Med J. 1951; 32:333–348
[37] Levey AS, Pauker SG, Kassirer JP. Occult Intracranial Aneurysms in Polycystic Kidney Disease: When is Cerebral Angiography Indicated? N Engl J Med. 1983; 308:986–994
[38] Butler WE, Barker FG, Crowell RM. Patients with Polycystic Kidney Disease Would Benefit from Routine Magnetic Resonance Angiographic Screening for Intracerebral Aneurysms: A Decision Analysis. Neurosurgery. 1996; 38:506–516
[39] Chauveau D, Pirson Y, Verellen-Dumoulin C, et al. Intracranial aneurysms in autosomal dominant polycystic kidney disease. Kidney Int. 1994; 45:1140–1146
[40] Schievink WI, Prendergast V, Zabramski JM. Rupture of a Previously Documented Small Asymptomatic Intracranial Aneurysm in a Patient with Autosomal Dominant Polycystic Kidney Disease. J Neurosurg. 1998; 89:479–482
[41] Schievink WI, Torres VE, Piepgras DG, Wiebers DO. Saccular Intracranial Aneurysms in Autosomal Dominant Polycystic Kidney Disease. J Am Soc Nephrol. 1992; 3:88–95
[42] Davila S, Oliver B, Molet J, Bartumeus F. Spontaneous Thrombosis of an Intracranial Aneurysm. Surg Neurol. 1984; 22:29–32
[43] Kumar S, Rao VRK, Mandalam KR, Phadke RV. Disappearance of a Cerebral Aneurysm: An Unusual Angiographic Event. Clin Neurol Neurosurg. 1991; 93:151–153
[44] Sobel DF, Dalessio D, Copeland B, Schwartz B. Cerebral Aneurysm Thrombosis, Shrinkage, Then Disappearance After Subarachnoid Hemorrhage. Surg Neurol. 1996; 45:133–137
[45] Spetzler RF, Winestock D, Newton HT, Bodrey EB. Disappearance and Reappearance of Cerebral Aneurysm in Serial Arteriograms: Case Report. J Neurosurg. 1974; 41:508–510
[46] Atkinson JLD, Lane JI, Colbassani HJ, Llewellyn DME. Spontaneous Thrombosis of Posterior Cerebral Artery Aneurysm with Angiographic Reappearance. J Neurosurg. 1993; 79:434–437
[47] Kassell NF, Torner JC, Adams HP. Antifibrinolytic Therapy in the Acute Period Following Aneurysmal Subarachnoid Hemorrhage: Preliminary Observations from the Cooperative Aneurysm Study. J Neurosurg. 1984; 61:225–230
[48] Aring CD. Treatment of Aneurysmal Subarachnoid Hemorrhage. Arch Neurol. 1990; 47:450–451
[49] Weber W, Siekmann R, Kis B, Kuehne D. Treatment and follow-up of 22 unruptured wide-necked intracranial aneurysms of the internal carotid artery with Onyx HD 500. AJNR Am J Neuroradiol. 2005; 26:1909–1915
[50] Fox AJ, Vinuela F, Pelz DM, Peerless SJ, et al. Use of Detachable Balloons for Proximal Artery Occlusion in the Treatment of Unclippable Cerebral Aneurysm. J Neurosurg. 1987; 66:40–46
[51] Bey L, Connolly S, Duong H, et al. Treatment of Inoperable Carotid Aneurysms with Endovascular Carotid Occlusion After Extracranial-Intracranial Bypass Surgery. Neurosurgery. 1997; 41:1225–1234

[52] Drake CG. Giant Intracranial Aneurysms: Experience with Surgical Treatment in 174 Patients. Clin Neurosurg. 1979; 26:12–95
[53] Drake CG. Ligation of the Vertebral (Unilateral or Bilateral) or Basilar Artery in the Treatment of Large Intracranial Aneurysms. J Neurosurg. 1975; 43:255–274
[54] Swearingen B, Heros RC. Common Carotid Occlusion for Unclippable Carotid Aneurysms: An Old but Still Effective Operation. Neurosurgery. 1987; 21:288–295
[55] Drapkin AJ, Rose WS. Serial Development of 'de Novo' Aneurysms After Carotid Ligation: Case Report. Surg Neurol. 1992; 38:302–308
[56] Dott NM. Intracranial Aneurysms: Cerebral Arteriography, Surgical Treatment. Trans Med Chir Soc Edin. 1933; 40:219–234
[57] Gillingham FJ. The Management of Ruptured Intracranial Aneurysms. Hunterian Lecture. Ann R Coll Surg Engl. 1958; 23:89–117
[58] Todd NV, Tocher JL, Jones PA, Miller JD. Outcome Following Aneurysm Wrapping: A 10-Year Follow-Up Review of Clipped and Wrapped Aneurysms. J Neurosurg. 1989; 70:841–846
[59] Cossu M, Pau A, Turtas S, Viola C, Viale GL. Subsequent Bleeding from Ruptured Intracranial Aneurysms Treated by Wrapping or Coating: A Review of the Long-Term Results in 47 Cases. Neurosurgery. 1993; 32:344–347
[60] Minakawa T, Koike T, Fujii Y, et al. Long Term Results of Ruptured Aneurysms Treated by Coating. Neurosurgery. 1987; 21:660–663
[61] Pellissou-Guyotat J, Deruty R, Mottolese C, Amat D. The Use of Teflon as Wrapping Material in Aneurysm Surgery. Neurol Res. 1994; 16:224–227
[62] Gnanalingham KK, Apostolopoulos V, Barazi S, O'Neill K. The impact of the international subarachnoid aneurysm trial (ISAT) on the management of aneurysmal subarachnoid haemorrhage in a neurosurgical unit in the UK. Clin Neurol Neurosurg. 2006; 108:117–123
[63] Smith GA, Dagostino P, Maltenfort MG, Dumont AS, Ratliff JK. Geographic variation and regional trends in adoption of endovascular techniques for cerebral aneurysms. J Neurosurg. 2011; 114:1768–1777
[64] Koivisto T, Vanninen R, Hurskainen H, Saari T, Hernesniemi J, Vapalahti M. Outcomes of early endovascular versus surgical treatment of ruptured cerebral aneurysms. A prospective randomized study. Stroke. 2000; 31:2369–2377
[65] Molyneux A, Kerr R, Stratton I, Sandercock P, Clarke M, Shrimpton J, Holman R. International Subarachnoid Aneurysm Trial (ISAT) of neurosurgical clipping versus endovascular coiling in 2143 patients with ruptured intracranial aneurysms: a randomized trial. J Stroke Cerebrovasc Dis. 2002; 11:304–314
[66] Li ZQ, Wang QH, Chen G, Quan Z. Outcomes of endovascular coiling versus surgical clipping in the treatment of ruptured intracranial aneurysms. J Int Med Res. 2012; 40:2145–2151
[67] McDougall CG, Spetzler RF, Zabramski JM, Partovi S, Hills NK, Nakaji P, Albuquerque FC. The Barrow Ruptured Aneurysm Trial. J Neurosurg. 2012; 116:135–144
[68] Molyneux AJ, Kerr RS, Birks J, Ramzi N, Yarnold J, Sneade M, Rischmiller J. Risk of recurrent subarachnoid haemorrhage, death, or dependence and standardised mortality ratios after clipping or coiling of an intracranial aneurysm in the International Subarachnoid Aneurysm Trial (ISAT): long-term follow-up. Lancet Neurol. 2009; 8:427–433
[69] Bakker NA, Metzemaekers JD, Groen RJ, Mooij JJ, Van Dijk JM. International subarachnoid aneurysm trial 2009: endovascular coiling of ruptured intracranial aneurysms has no significant advantage over neurosurgical clipping. Neurosurgery. 2010; 66:961–962
[70] Molyneux AJ, Birks J, Clarke A, Sneade M, Kerr RS. The durability of endovascular coiling versus neurosurgical clipping of ruptured cerebral aneurysms: 18 year follow-up of the UK cohort of the International Subarachnoid Aneurysm Trial (ISAT). Lancet. 2015; 385:691–697
[71] Darsaut TE, Jack AS, Kerr RS, Raymond J. International Subarachnoid Aneurysm Trial - ISAT part II: study protocol for a randomized controlled trial. Trials. 2013; 14. DOI: 10.1186/1745-6215-14-156
[72] Spetzler RF, McDougall CG, Albuquerque FC, Zabramski JM, Hills NK, Partovi S, Nakaji P, Wallace RC. The Barrow Ruptured Aneurysm Trial: 3-year results. J Neurosurg. 2013; 119:146–157
[73] Lanzino G, Murad MH, d'Urso PI, Rabinstein AA. Coil embolization versus clipping for ruptured intracranial aneurysms: a meta-analysis of prospective controlled published studies. AJNR Am J Neuroradiol. 2013; 34:1764–1768
[74] Li H, Pan R, Wang H, Rong X, Yin Z, Milgrom DP, Shi X, Tang Y, Peng Y. Clipping versus coiling for ruptured intracranial aneurysms: a systematic review and meta-analysis. Stroke. 2013; 44:29–37
[75] de Oliveira JG, Beck J, Ulrich C, Rathert J, Raabe A, Seifert V. Comparison between clipping and coiling on the incidence of cerebral vasospasm after aneurysmal subarachnoid hemorrhage: a systematic review and meta-analysis. Neurosurg Rev. 2007; 30:22–30; discussion 30-1
[76] Jones J, Sayre J, Chang R, Tian J, Szeder V, Gonzalez N, Jahan R, Vinuela F, Duckwiler G, Tateshima S. Cerebral vasospasm patterns following aneurysmal subarachnoid hemorrhage: an angiographic study comparing coils with clips. J Neurointerv Surg. 2015; 7:803–807
[77] Dorai Z, Hynan LS, Kopitnik TA, Samson D. Factors related to hydrocephalus after aneurysmal subarachnoid hemorrhage. Neurosurgery. 2003; 52:763–9; discussion 769-71
[78] Gruber A, Reinprecht A, Bavinzski G, Czech T, Richling B. Chronic shunt-dependent hydrocephalus after early surgical and early endovascular treatment of ruptured intracranial aneurysms. Neurosurgery. 1999; 44:503–9; discussion 509-12
[79] Bae IS, Yi HJ, Choi KS, Chun HJ. Comparison of Incidence and Risk Factors for Shunt-dependent Hydrocephalus in Aneurysmal Subarachnoid Hemorrhage Patients. J Cerebrovasc Endovasc Neurosurg. 2014; 16:78–84
[80] de Oliveira JG, Beck J, Setzer M, Gerlach R, Vatter H, Seifert V, Raabe A. Risk of shunt-dependent hydrocephalus after occlusion of ruptured intracranial aneurysms by surgical clipping or endovascular coiling: a single-institution series and meta-analysis. Neurosurgery. 2007; 61:924–33; discussion 933-4
[81] Varelas P, Helms A, Sinson G, Spanaki M, Hacein-Bey L. Clipping or coiling of ruptured cerebral aneurysms and shunt-dependent hydrocephalus. Neurocrit Care. 2006; 4:223–228
[82] Dehdashti AR, Rilliet B, Rufenacht DA, de Tribolet N. Shunt-dependent hydrocephalus after rupture of intracranial aneurysms: a prospective study of the influence of treatment modality. J Neurosurg. 2004; 101:402–407
[83] Mura J, Rojas-Zalazar D, Ruiz A, Vintimilla LC, Marengo JJ. Improved outcome in high-grade aneurysmal subarachnoid hemorrhage by enhancement of endogenous clearance of cisternal blood clots: a prospective study that demonstrates the role of lamina terminalis fenestration combined with modern microsurgical cisternal blood evacuation. Minim Invasive Neurosurg. 2007; 50:355–362
[84] Jartti P, Karttunen A, Isokangas JM, Jartti A, Koskelainen T, Tervonen O. Chronic hydrocephalus after neurosurgical and endovascular treatment of ruptured intracranial aneurysms. Acta Radiol. 2008; 49:680–686
[85] Sethi H, Moore A, Dervin J, Clifton A, MacSweeney JE. Hydrocephalus: comparison of clipping and embolization in aneurysm treatment. J Neurosurg. 2000; 92:991–994
[86] Hoh BL, Kleinhenz DT, Chi YY, Mocco J, Barker FG, II. Incidence of ventricular shunt placement for hydrocephalus with clipping versus coiling for ruptured and unruptured cerebral aneurysms in

the Nationwide Inpatient Sample database: 2002 to 2007. World Neurosurg. 2011; 76:548–554
[87] Komotar RJ, Hahn DK, Kim GH, Starke RM, Garrett MC, Merkow MB, Otten ML, Sciacca RR, Connolly ES,Jr. Efficacy of lamina terminalis fenestration in reducing shunt-dependent hydrocephalus following aneurysmal subarachnoid hemorrhage: a systematic review. Clinical article. J Neurosurg. 2009; 111:147–154
[88] Lanzino G, D'Urso PI, Suarez J. Seizures and anticonvulsants after aneurysmal subarachnoid hemorrhage. Neurocrit Care. 2011; 15:247–256
[89] Brinjikji W, Rabinstein AA, Lanzino G, Kallmes DF, Cloft HJ. Patient outcomes are better for unruptured cerebral aneurysms treated at centers that preferentially treat with endovascular coiling: a study of the national inpatient sample 2001-2007. AJNR Am J Neuroradiol. 2011; 32:1065–1070
[90] Leivo S, Hernesniemi J, Luukkonen M, et al. Early surgery improves the cure of aneurysm-induced oculmotor palsy. Surg Neurol. 1996; 45:430–434
[91] Feely M, Kapoor S. Third nerve palsy due to posterior communicating artery aneurysm: the importance of early surgery. J Neurol Neurosurg Psychiatry. 1987; 50:1051–1052
[92] Connolly ES, Jr, Rabinstein AA, Carhuapoma JR, Derdeyn CP, Dion J, Higashida RT, Hoh BL, Kirkness CJ, Naidech AM, Ogilvy CS, Patel AB, Thompson BG, Vespa P, American Heart Association Stroke Council, Council on Cardiovascular Radiology, Intervention, Council on Cardiovascular Nursing, Council on Cardiovascular Surgery, Anesthesia, Council on Clinical Cardiology. Guidelines for the management of aneurysmal subarachnoid hemorrhage: a guideline for healthcare professionals from the American Heart Association/american Stroke Association. Stroke. 2012; 43:1711–1737
[93] Sandstrom N, Yan B, Dowling R, Laidlaw J, Mitchell P. Comparison of microsurgery and endovascular treatment on clinical outcome following poor-grade subarachnoid hemorrhage. J Clin Neurosci. 2013; 20:1213–1218
[94] Darsaut TE, Estrade L, Jamali S, Bojanowski MW, Chagnon M, Raymond J. Uncertainty and agreement in the management of unruptured intracranial aneurysms. J Neurosurg. 2014; 120:618–623
[95] Bederson JB, Awad IA, Wiebers DO, Piepgras D, et al. Recommendations for the management of patients with unruptured intracranial aneurysms. A statement for healthcare professionals from the Stroke Council of the American Heart Association. Circulation. 2000; 102:2300–2308
[96] King JT, Jr, Berlin JA, Flamm ES. Morbidity and mortality from elective surgery for asymptomatic, unruptured, intracranial aneurysms: a meta-analysis. J Neurosurg. 1994; 81:837–842
[97] Raaymakers TW, Rinkel GJ, Limburg M, Algra A. Mortality and morbidity of surgery for unruptured intracranial aneurysms: a meta-analysis. Stroke. 1998; 29:1531–1538
[98] The International Study Group of Unruptured Intracranial Aneurysms Investigators (ISUIA). Unruptured Intracranial Aneurysms - Risk of Rupture and Risks of Surgical Intervention. N Engl J Med. 1998; 339:1725–1733
[99] Bhatia S, Sekula RF, Quigley MR, Williams R, Ku A. Role of calcification in the outcomes of treated, unruptured, intracerebral aneurysms. Acta Neurochir (Wien). 2011; 153:905–911
[100] Johnston SC, Zhao S, Dudley RA, Berman MF, Gress DR. Treatment of unruptured cerebral aneurysms in California. Stroke. 2001; 32:597–605
[101] Johnston SC, Dudley RA, Gress DR, Ono L. Surgical and Endovascular Treatment of Unruptured Cerebral Aneurysms at University Hospitals. Neurology. 1999; 52:1799–1805
[102] Birski M, Walesa C, Gaca W, Paczkowski D, Birska J, Harat A. Clipping versus coiling for intracranial aneurysms. Neurol Neurochir Pol. 2014; 48:122–129
[103] Hwang JS, Hyun MK, Lee HJ, Choi JE, Kim JH, Lee NR, Kwon JW, Lee E. Endovascular coiling versus neurosurgical clipping in patients with unruptured intracranial aneurysm: a systematic review. BMC Neurol. 2012; 12. DOI: 10.1186/1471-2377-12-99
[104] Lawson MF, Neal DW, Mocco J, Hoh BL. Rationale for treating unruptured intracranial aneurysms: actuarial analysis of natural history risk versus treatment risk for coiling or clipping based on 14,050 patients in the Nationwide Inpatient Sample database. World Neurosurg. 2013; 79:472–478
[105] Juvela S, Porras M, Poussa K. Natural history of unruptured intracranial aneurysms: probability of and risk factors for aneurysm rupture. J Neurosurg. 2000; 93:379–387
[106] Tsutsumi K, Ueki K, Morita A, Kirino T. Risk of rupture from incidental cerebral aneurysms. J Neurosurg. 2000; 93:550–553
[107] Ishibashi T, Murayama Y, Urashima M, Saguchi T, Ebara M, Arakawa H, Irie K, Takao H, Abe T. Unruptured intracranial aneurysms: incidence of rupture and risk factors. Stroke. 2009; 40:313–316
[108] Mahaney KB, Brown RD, Jr, Meissner I, Piepgras DG, Huston J, III, Zhang J, Torner JC. Age-related differences in unruptured intracranial aneurysms: 1-year outcomes. J Neurosurg. 2014; 121:1024–1038
[109] Brinjikji W, Rabinstein AA, Lanzino G, Kallmes DF, Cloft HJ. Effect of age on outcomes of treatment of unruptured cerebral aneurysms: a study of the National Inpatient Sample 2001-2008. Stroke. 2011; 42:1320–1324
[110] Halkes PH, Wermer MJ, Rinkel GJ, Buskens E. Direct costs of surgical clipping and endovascular coiling of unruptured intracranial aneurysms. Cerebrovasc Dis. 2006; 22:40–45
[111] Hoh BL, Chi YY, Dermott MA, Lipori PJ, Lewis SB. The effect of coiling versus clipping of ruptured and unruptured cerebral aneurysms on length of stay, hospital cost, hospital reimbursement, and surgeon reimbursement at the university of Florida. Neurosurgery. 2009; 64:614-9; discussion 619-21
[112] Hoh BL, Chi YY, Lawson MF, Mocco J, Barker FG, II. Length of stay and total hospital charges of clipping versus coiling for ruptured and unruptured adult cerebral aneurysms in the Nationwide Inpatient Sample database 2002 to 2006. Stroke. 2010; 41:337–342
[113] Lad SP, Babu R, Rhee MS, Franklin RL, Ugiliweneza B, Hodes J, Nimjee SM, Zomorodi AR, Smith TP, Friedman AH, Patil CG, Boakye M. Long-term economic impact of coiling vs clipping for unruptured intracranial aneurysms. Neurosurgery. 2013; 72:1000–11; discussion 1011-3
[114] Duan Y, Blackham K, Nelson J, Selman W, Bambakidis N. Analysis of short-term total hospital costs and current primary cost drivers of coiling versus clipping for unruptured intracranial aneurysms. J Neurointerv Surg. 2015; 7:614–618
[115] Khan SA, Agrawal A, Hailey CE, Smith TP, Gokhale S, Alexander MJ, Britz GW, Zomorodi AR, McDonagh DL, James ML. Effect of surgical clipping versus endovascular coiling on recovery from oculomotor nerve palsy in patients with posterior communicating artery aneurysms: A retrospective comparative study and meta-analysis. Asian J Neurosurg. 2013; 8:117–124
[116] Kataoka H, Miyoshi T, Neki R, Yoshimatsu J, Ishibashi-Ueda H, Iihara K. Subarachnoid hemorrhage from intracranial aneurysms during pregnancy and the puerperium. Neurol Med Chir (Tokyo). 2013; 53:549–554
[117] Attenello FJ, Reid P, Wen T, Cen S, Kim-Tenser M, Sanossian N, Russin J, Amar A, Giannotta S, Mack WJ, Tenser M. Evaluation of time to aneurysm treatment following subarachnoid hemorrhage: comparison of patients treated with clipping versus coiling. J Neurointerv Surg. 2015. DOI: 10.1136/neurintsurg-2014-011642
[118] Luo YC, Shen CS, Mao JL, Liang CY, Zhang Q, He ZJ. Ultra-early versus delayed coil treatment for ruptured poor-grade aneurysm. Neuroradiology. 2015; 57:205–210

[119] Milhorat TH, Krautheim M. Results of Early and Delayed Operations for Ruptured Intracranial Aneurysms in Two Series of 100 Consecutive Patients. Surg Neurol. 1986; 26:123–128
[120] Le Roux PD, Elliott JP, Newell DW, Grady MS, Winn HR. Predicting Outcome in Poor-Grade Patients with Subarachnoid Hemorrhage: A Retrospective Review of 159 Aggressively Managed Cases. J Neurosurg. 1996; 85:39–49
[121] Disney L, Weir B, Grace M, et al. Factors Influencing the Outcome of Aneurysm Rupture in Poor Grade Patients: A Prospective Series. Neurosurgery. 1988; 23:1–9
[122] Le Roux PD, Elliot JP, Newell DW, et al. The Incidence of Surgical Complications is Similar in Good and Poor Grade Patients Undergoing Repair of Ruptured Anterior Circulation Aneurysms: A Retrospective Review of 355 Patients. Neurosurgery. 1996; 38:887–897
[123] Malek AM, Halbach VV, Holmes S, Phatouros CC, Meyers PM, Dowd CF, Higashida RT. Beating aneurysm sign: angiographic evidence of ruptured aneurysm tamponade by intracranial hemorrhage. Case illustration. J Neurosurg. 1999; 91
[124] Lin T, Fox AJ, Drake CG. Regrowth of Aneurysm Sacs from Residual Neck Following Aneurysm Clipping. J Neurosurg. 1989; 70:556–560
[125] Feuerberg I, Lindquist M, Steiner L. Natural History of Postoperative Aneurysm Rests. J Neurosurg. 1987; 66:30–34
[126] Rosenorn J, Westergaard L, Hansen PH. Mannitol-Induced Rebleeding from Intracranial Aneurysm: Case Report. J Neurosurg. 1983; 59:529–530
[127] Connolly ES, Kader AA, Frazzini VI, Winfree CJ, Solomon RA. The Safety of Intraoperative Lumbar Subarachnoid Drainage for Acutely Ruptured Intracranial Aneurysm: Technical Note. Surg Neurol. 1997; 48:338–344
[128] Todd MM, Hindman BJ, Clarke WR, Torner JC. Mild intraoperative hypothermia during surgery for intracranial aneurysm. N Engl J Med. 2005; 352:135–145
[129] Hoff RG, Mettes S, Verweij BH, Algra A, Rinkel GJ, Kalkman CJ. Hypotension in anaesthetized patients during aneurysm clipping: not as bad as expected? Acta Anaesthesiol Scand. 2008; 52:1006–1011
[130] Pasternak JJ, McGregor DG, Schroeder DR, Lanier WL, Shi Q, Hindman BJ, Clarke WR, Torner JC, Weeks JB, Todd MM. Hyperglycemia in patients undergoing cerebral aneurysm surgery: its association with long-term gross neurologic and neuropsychological function. Mayo Clin Proc. 2008; 83:406–417
[131] Solomon RA. Methods of Cerebral Protection During Aneurysm Surgery. Contemp Neurosurg. 1995; 16:1–6
[132] Lavine SD, Masri LS, Levy ML, Giannotta SL. Temporary occlusion of the middle cerebral artery in intracranial aneurysm surgery: time limitation and advantage of brain protection. J Neurosurg. 1997; 87:817–824
[133] Ogilvy CS, Carter BS, Kaplan S, Rich C, Crowell RM. Temporary vessel occlusion for aneurysm surgery: risk factors for stroke in patients protected by induced hypothermia and hypertension and intravenous mannitol administration. J Neurosurg. 1996; 84:785–791
[134] Samson D, Batjer HH, Bowman G, Mootz L, Krippner WJJr, Meyer YJ, Allen BC. A clinical study of the parameters and effects of temporary arterial occlusion in the management of intracranial aneurysms. Neurosurgery. 1994; 34:22–8; discussion 28-9
[135] Macdonald RL, Wallace C, Kestle JRW. Role of Angiography Following Aneurysm Surgery. J Neurosurg. 1993; 79:826–832
[136] Ravussin P, de Tribolet N. Total Intravenous Anesthesia with Propofol for Burst Suppression in Cerebral Aneurysm Surgery: Preliminary Report of 42 Patients. Neurosurgery. 1993; 32:236–240
[137] Batjer HH, Samson DS, Bowman M. Comment on Ravussin R and de Tribolet N: Total Intravenous Anesthesia with Propofol for Burst Suppression in Cerebral Aneurysm Surgery: Preliminary Report of 42 Patients. Neurosurgery. 1993; 32
[138] Couldwell WT, Gianotta SL, Zelman V, DeGiorgio CM. Life-Threatening Reactions to Propofol. Neurosurgery. 1993; 33:1116–1117
[139] Graf CJ, Nibbelink DW, Sahs AL, Nibbelink DW. In: Randomized Treatment Study: Intracranial Surgery. Aneurysmal Subarachnoid Hemorrhage - Report of the Cooperative Study. Baltimore: Urban and Schwarzenburg; 1981:145–202
[140] Pertuiset B, Pia HW, Langmaid C. In: Intraoperative Aneurysmal Rupture and Reduction by Coagulation of the Sac. Cerebral Aneurysms - Advances in Diagnosis and Therapy. Berlin: Springer-Verlag; 1979:398–401
[141] Schramm J, Cedzich C. Outcome and Management of Intraoperative Aneurysm Rupture. Surg Neurol. 1993; 40:26–30
[142] Kassell NF, Boarini DJ, Adams HP, Sahs AL, et al. Overall Management of Ruptured Aneurysm: Comparison of Early and Later Operation. Neurosurgery. 1981; 9:120–128
[143] Batjer H, Samson DS. Management of Intraoperative Aneurysm Rupture. Clin Neurosurg. 1988; 36:275–288
[144] David CA, Vishteh AG, Spetzler RF, et al. Late angiographic follow-up review of surgically treated aneurysms. J Neurosurg. 1999; 91:396–401

80 Aneurysm Type by Location

80.1 Anterior communicating artery aneurysms

80.1.1 General information

The single most common site of aneurysms presenting with SAH.[1] May also present with diabetes insipidus (DI) or other hypothalamic dysfunction.

80.1.2 CT scan

SAH in these aneurysms results in blood in the anterior interhemispheric fissure in essentially all cases, and is associated with intracerebral hematoma in 63% of cases.[2] Intraventricular hematoma is seen in 79% of cases, with the blood entering the ventricles from the intracerebral hematoma in about one-third of these. Acute hydrocephalus was present in 25% of patients (late hydrocephalus, a common sequelae of SAH, was not studied).

Frontal lobe infarcts occur in 20%, usually several days following SAH.[2] One of the few causes of the rare finding of bilateral ACA distribution infarcts is vasospasm following hemorrhage from rupture of an ACoA aneurysm. This results in prefrontal lobotomy-like findings of apathy and abulia.

80.1.3 Angiographic considerations

Also see ▸ Table 102.2 in Endovascular section. Essential to evaluate contralateral carotid, to determine if both ACAs fill the aneurysm. If the aneurysm fills with one side only, it is desirable to inject the other side while cross compressing the side that fills the aneurysm to see if collateral flow is present. Also, determine if either carotid fills both ACAs, or if each ACA fills from the ipsilateral carotid injection (may permit trapping, see below).

▸ **If additional views are needed to better demonstrate aneurysm.** Try oblique 25° away from injection side, center beam 3–4 cm above lateral aspect of ipsilateral orbital rim, orient x-ray tube in Towne's view. A submental vertex view may also visualize the area but the image may be degraded by the large amount of interposed bone.

80.1.4 Surgical treatment

Approaches

General information

1. *pterional approach*: the usual approach (see below)
2. subfrontal approach: especially useful for aneurysms pointing superiorly when there is a large amount of frontal blood clot (allows clot removal during approach)
3. anterior interhemispheric approach[3]: ✖ contraindicated for anteriorly pointing aneurysms as the dome is approached first and proximal control cannot be obtained (see below)
4. transcallosal approach

Pterional approach

Side of craniotomy:

A *right* pterional craniotomy is used with the following exceptions (for which a left pterional crani is used):

1. large ACoA aneurysm pointing to right: left crani exposes neck before dome
2. dominant left A1 feeder to aneurysm (with no filling from right A1): left crani provides proximal control
3. additional left sided aneurysm

See Pterional craniotomy (p. 1453) for positioning, etc. (use shoulder roll, rotate head 60° from vertical; see ▸ Fig. 94.5). Craniotomy is as shown in ▸ Fig. 94.7 (slightly more frontal lobe needs to be exposed than, e.g. for a p-comm aneurysm).

Lumbar drain (if IVC not already inserted) assists with brain relaxation.

Microsurgical dissection

Dissect down sylvian fissure with gentle retraction of frontal lobe away from base of skull. Olfactory nerve visualized first, then optic nerve. Open arachnoid over carotid and optic cistern and drain CSF. Elevate temporal tip, coagulate any bridging temporal tip veins that are present, and expose ICA.

Follow the ICA distally, looking for A1 (exposure of this allows temporary clipping in event of rupture). If the A1 take-off is too high, it may be hidden and would require excessive retraction to expose. Options to increase exposure include

1. gyrus rectus resection: a 1 cm long gyrus rectus corticectomy is performed[4] just medial to the olfactory tract. Helps find the ipsilateral A1 and often ACoA and A2. This is also helpful for down-pointing aneurysms because it permits visualization of the contralateral A1 before exposing the dome of the aneurysm (for proximal control). May lead to neuropsychiatric deficits. A subpial resection is performed with preservation of the small arterial branch that is consistently located here
2. fronto-temporal-orbital-zygoma removal
3. splitting the sylvian fissure: about 50% of experts do this routinely
4. ventricular drainage

Once found, A1 is followed until the ipsilateral A2 is identified. Then the contralateral A2 is identified and is followed proximally until the contralateral A1 is exposed. The a-comm is usually encountered in the process.

Critical branches to preserve: recurrent artery of Heubner; small ACoA perforators (may be adherent to aneurysm dome). If the aneurysm cannot be clipped, it may be trapped by clipping both ends of the ACoA *only* if each ACA fills from the carotid on its own side.

Post clipping, some authors recommend fenestrating the lamina terminalis in an effort to reduce the need for post-op shunting.

Anterior interhemispheric approach

See reference.[3]

Involves minimal brain retraction.

More suitable for an aneurysm that points straight up, but even with this proximal control is poor.

Position: supine with the neck extended ≈ 15°. A transverse skin incision is made in a skin crease in the lower forehead. The authors[3] describe using a 1.5 inch trephine craniotomy in the midline just superior to the glabella. Alternatively, better advantage of the dural opening may be possible with a more rectangular opening. The dural flap is hinged on the superior sagittal sinus. The depth of the aneurysm is ≈ 6 cm from the dura. Proximal control of the A1 branch of the ACA is difficult with this approach.

80.2 Distal anterior cerebral artery aneurysms

80.2.1 General information

Aneurysms of the distal anterior cerebral artery (DACA) (i.e. the ACA distal to the ACoA) are usually located at the origin of the frontopolar artery, or at the bifurcation of the pericallosal and callosomarginal arteries at the genu of the corpus callosum. Aneurysms located more distally are usually posttraumatic, infectious (mycotic), or due to tumor embolus.[5] DACA aneurysms are often associated with intracerebral hematoma or interhemispheric subdural hematoma[6] since the subarachnoid space is limited here. Conservative treatment of DACA aneurysms is often associated with poor results. Unruptured DACA aneurysms have a higher incidence of bleeding than unruptured aneurysms in other locations. These aneurysms are fragile and adherent to the brain, which predisposes to frequent premature intraoperative rupture.

On arteriography, if both ACAs fill from a single sided carotid injection, it may be difficult to make the important determination as to which ACA feeds the aneurysm. Multiple aneurysms are commonly associated with DACA aneurysms.

80.2.2 Treatment

Mycotic aneurysms should be treated as outlined (p. 1228).

Aneurysms up to 1 cm from the ACoA may be approached through a standard pterional craniotomy with partial gyrus rectus resection.

Aneurysms > 1 cm distal to the ACoA up to the genu of the corpus callosum, including those of the pericallosal/callosomarginal bifurcation, may be approached surgically by a basal frontal interhemispheric approach[7] via a frontal craniotomy using a bicoronal skin incision. The patient is positioned supine with the neck slightly extended, positioned vertically or just a few degrees to the left. A right sided craniotomy is preferred in most instances (exception: aneurysm dome buried in the right cerebral hemisphere making retraction hazardous), but should cross to the contralateral side by a couple centimeters. It must be taken all the way to the floor of the frontal fossa to permit exposure of the anterior cerebral artery for proximal control. The craniotomy extends ≈ 8 cm above the supraorbital ridge in order to provide leeway in circumnavigating veins bridging to the superior sagittal sinus. The dural flap is based on the superior sagittal sinus. If the sinus needs to be mobilized, it may be divided low anteriorly.

ACA aneurysms distal to the genu of the corpus callosum may also be approached by an interhemispheric approach using a unilateral skin incision. For these, the patient's neck is not extended, and a parasagittal craniotomy is used that doesn't need to be as low on the frontal fossa. The cingulate gyri may be difficult to separate, and care must be taken because excessive retraction may pull the cingulate gyrus off the dome of the aneurysm and produce premature rupture.

Ideally, A2 proximal to the aneurysm should be identified initially for proximal control and then followed distally to the aneurysm. When this is not possible, dissection should follow distal ACA branches proximally, towards the aneurysm, taking care not to disturb the aneurysm. Often, a portion of the cingulate gyrus may need to be removed and sometimes up to 1–2 cm of the anterior corpus callosum may need to be divided.

Surgical complications: Prolonged retraction on the cingulate gyrus may produce akinetic mutism that is usually temporary. The pericallosal arteries are small in caliber and may be atherosclerotic, which together increases the risk of occlusion of the parent artery with the aneurysm clip.

80.3 Posterior communicating artery aneurysms

80.3.1 General information

May occur at either end of p-comm; that is at the junction with the PCA, or more commonly at the junction with carotid (typically points laterally, posteriorly, and inferiorly). May impinge on the third nerve in either case and cause third nerve palsy (ptosis, mydriasis, "down and out" deviation) that, is *not* pupil sparing in 99% of cases. Surgical clipping may be more advantageous than endovascular coiling to treat oculomotor nerve palsies caused by pcomm aneurysms.[8,9]

80.3.2 Angiographic considerations

Also see ▸ Table 102.2 in Endovascular section. Vertebral artery **(VA)** injection is necessary to help evaluate the p-comm artery:

1. if the p-comm is patent: determine if there is a "fetal circulation" where the posterior circulation is fed only through the p-comm
2. determine if the aneurysm fills from VA injection

If additional views are needed to better demonstrate aneurysm

Try paraorbital oblique 55° away from injection side, center beam 1 cm posterior to inferior portion of lateral rim of ipsilateral orbit, orient x-ray tube 12° cephalad.

80.3.3 Surgical treatment

Pterional approach

See Pterional craniotomy (p. 1453) for positioning, etc. For the more common aneurysm at the ICA-p-comm junction, rotate head 15–30° from vertical (▸ Fig. 94.5). Craniotomy is as shown in ▸ Fig. 94.7 (less frontal lobe needs to be exposed than for an ACoA aneurysm).

Microsurgical dissection

Ultimately, the major vector of retraction will be on tip of temporal lobe (less on frontal lobe than in ACoA aneurysm), but the initial approach will be more anterior to reduce risk of intra-operative rupture.

1. dissect down sylvian fissure, retract frontal lobe and come down on optic nerve

2. cautiously elevate temporal tip (aneurysm may be adherent to temporal tip and/or to tentorium), coagulate bridging temporal tip veins if necessary
3. incise arachnoid membrane along the optic nerve from *anterior* to posterior
4. open arachnoid and drain CSF to gain relaxation
5. start to dissect carotid at anterior margin (at junction with optic nerve) and work towards the posterior margin of carotid where the aneurysm is located (isolating the carotid gives proximal control)

The aneurysm dome usually points laterally, posteriorly and inferiorly, and is encountered before and usually blocks visualization of the p-comm. The aneurysm frequently projects behind the tentorial edge which then obscures the dome.

Critical branches to preserve: anterior choroidal artery, posterior communicating artery (p-comm). If necessary, the p-comm may be sacrificed (e.g. included in clip) without deleterious effect in most cases if there is not a fetal circulation.

80.4 Carotid terminus (bifurcation) aneurysms

80.4.1 Angiographic considerations

See ▶ Table 102.2 in Endovascular section.

▶ **If additional views are needed to better demonstrate aneurysm.** Try oblique 25° away from injection side, center beam 3–4 cm above lateral aspect of ipsilateral orbital rim, orient x-ray tube in Towne's view. Also may try submentovertex view.

80.4.2 Surgical considerations

See Pterional craniotomy (p. 1453) for positioning, etc. (rotate head 30° from vertical, see ▶ Fig. 94.5. Craniotomy is as shown in ▶ Fig. 94.7.

80.5 Middle cerebral artery (MCA) aneurysms

80.5.1 General information

The following considers MCA aneurysms of the M1-M2 junction (referred to as "trifurcation" region, although this is not a true trifurcation (p. 76)).

80.5.2 Surgical treatment

Approaches

1. trans-sylvian approach through a *pterional craniotomy*: this is the most commonly used approach
2. superior temporal gyrus approach[10]:
   a) advantages: minimizes brain retraction, possible reduced vasospasm from manipulation of proximal vessels
   b) disadvantages: proximal control difficult, slightly larger bone flap, possible increased risk of seizures

Craniotomy vs. craniectomy

Primary decompressive craniectomy (vs. craniotomy) for poor-grade MCA aneurysm SAH (WFNS IV/V) with associated IPH (> 30cc) has not shown to provide any survival benefit and is not associated with improved outcome.[11]

Pterional approach

See Pterional craniotomy (p. 1453) for positioning, etc. (rotate head 45° from vertical, ▶ Fig. 94.5).

80

Craniotomy

Craniotomy is as shown in ▶ Fig. 94.7. Less frontal lobe needs to be exposed than for, e.g. an ACoA aneurysm (distance "B" in ▶ Fig. 94.7 only needs to be ≈ 1 cm). The height "H" of the bony opening should be ≈ 5–6 cm (larger than for circle of Willis aneurysms).

Microsurgical dissection

Dissect down sylvian fissure with major vector of retraction on tip of temporal lobe (less on frontal lobe than in ACoA aneurysm). Open arachnoid and drain CSF. Elevate temporal tip, coagulate bridging temporal tip veins, and expose the ICA for proximal control in the event of rupture.

Follow the ICA distally by splitting the sylvian fissure to expose the M1 (again, for proximal control). Although exposure for proximal control is helpful to have as a contingency, one may be able to avoid temporary clipping of the MCA in the event of intraoperative rupture by controlling bleeding with a large suction, and subsequent clip placement (since the blood flow through the MCA is not as voluminous as through the ICA, and the surgical access to these aneurysms is usually fairly unrestricted).

Critical branches to preserve: distal MCA branches, recurrent perforators from the origin of the major MCA branches.

80.6 Supraclinoid aneurysms

See reference.[12]

80.6.1 Applied anatomy

The carotid artery exits the cavernous sinus and enters the subarachnoid space at the dural constriction known as the carotid ring (AKA clinoidal ring). The supraclinoid portion of the carotid artery may be divided into the following segments[13]:

1. ophthalmic segment: the largest portion of the supraclinoid ICA. Lies between the take-off of the ophthalmic artery and the posterior communicating artery (PCoA) origin. The proximal portion of this (including the origin of the ophthalmic artery) is often obscured by the anterior clinoid process. Branches include:
   a) ophthalmic artery: usually originates from the supracavernous ICA just after the ICA enters the subarachnoid space; see variants (p. 79). Enters the optic canal positioned inferolateral to the optic nerve
   b) superior hypophyseal artery: the largest of several perforators supplying the dura of the cavernous sinus and the superior pituitary gland and stalk
2. communicating segment: from the PCoA origin to the origin of the anterior choroidal artery (AChA)
3. choroidal segment: from AChA origin to the terminal bifurcation of the ICA

80.6.2 Ophthalmic segment aneurysms (OSAs)

See reference.[14]

General information

Ophthalmic segment aneurysms (**OSAs**) OSAs include (NB: nomenclature varies among authors):

1. ophthalmic artery aneurysms:
2. superior hypophyseal artery aneurysms:
   a) paraclinoid variant: usually does not produce visual symptoms
   b) suprasellar variant: when giant, may mimic pituitary tumor on CT

Presentation (excluding incidental discovery)

Ophthalmic artery aneurysms

Arise from the ICA just distal to the origin of ophthalmic artery. They project dorsally or dorsomedially towards the lateral portion of the optic nerve.

Presentation:

1. ≈ 45% present as SAH
2. ≈ 45% present as visual field defect:
   a) as the aneurysm enlarges it impinges on the lateral portion of the optic nerve → inferior temporal fiber compression → ipsilateral *monocular superior nasal quadrantanopsia*
   b) continued enlargement → upward displacement of the nerve against the falciform ligament (or fold) → superior temporal fiber compression → *monocular inferior nasal quadrantanopsia*
   c) in addition to near-complete loss of vision in the involved eye, compression of the optic nerve near the chiasm may also produce a superior temporal quadrant defect in the *contralateral*

eye (junctional scotoma AKA "pie in the sky" defect) from injury to the anterior knee of Wilbrand (nasal retinal fibers that course anteriorly for a short distance after they decussate in the contralateral optic nerve[15])
3. ≈ 10% present as both

Superior hypophyseal artery aneurysms

Originate in the small subarachnoid pocket medial to the ICA near the lateral aspect of the sella. The direction of enlargement is dictated by the size of this pocket and the height of the lateral sellar wall, resulting in two variants: paraclinoid & suprasellar.

Suprasellar variant may actually grow to a size large enough to compress the pituitary stalk and cause hypopituitarism and "classic" chiasmal visual symptoms (bilateral temporal hemianopsia).

Angiographic considerations

Also see ▶ Table 102.2 in Endovascular section. A notch can often be observed in the in the anterior, superior, medial aspect of giant ophthalmic artery aneurysms due to the optic nerve.[16]

▶ **If additional views are needed to better demonstrate aneurysm.** Try oblique 25° away from injection side, center beam 3–4 cm above lateral aspect of ipsilateral orbital rim, orient x-ray tube in Towne's view. Try submentovertex view.

80.6.3 Surgical treatment

See reference.[12]

Ophthalmic artery aneurysms

If necessary, the ophthalmic artery may be sacrificed without worsening of vision in the vast majority. Clipping a contralateral ophthalmic artery aneurysm is not technically difficult, and is not uncommonly required as OSAs are often multiple.

The aneurysm arises from the superomedial aspect of the ICA just distal to the ophthalmic artery origin, and projects superiorly.

Cutting the falciform fold early decompresses the nerve, and helps minimize worsening of visual deficit from surgical manipulation.

For unruptured aneurysms, drill off anterior clinoid via an extradural approach before opening dura to approach neck; for ruptured aneurysms, this may not be as safe.

In most cases, a side-angled clip can be placed parallel to the parent artery along the neck of the aneurysm.

Superior hypophyseal artery aneurysms

If necessary, the superior hypophyseal artery on one side may be clipped without demonstrable deleterious effect (due to bilateral supply to stalk and pituitary). Clipping a contralateral superior hypophyseal aneurysms is not really feasible.

With a usual pterional approach, the carotid artery is usually encountered first, and with large aneurysms is usually bowed laterally towards the surgeon. Clinoidal removal is usually required. The entire ICA wall may appear to be involved, and it may necessitate temporary ICA clipping (with cerebral protection) to reconstitute the ICA using encircling clips parallel to the parent vessel.

80.7 Posterior circulation aneurysms

80.7.1 General information

See also basilar tip aneurysms (p. 1218). Clinical syndrome of SAH in the posterior fossa is indistinguishable from that due to anterior circulation aneurysms except for possible increased tendency towards respiratory arrest and subsequent neurogenic pulmonary edema (p. 1178).[17] Vasospasm following posterior fossa SAH may be more likely to cause midbrain symptoms than vasospasm due to SAH elsewhere.

80.7.2 Hydrocephalus

In Yamaura's series,[18] 12% of patients required external ventricular drainage (EVD) following posterior fossa SAH to remove bloody CSF causing hydrocephalus, and 20% eventually required permanent ventricular shunt.

80.7.3 Vertebral artery aneurysms

General information

Traumatic vertebral artery aneurysms (VAA) (AKA dissecting aneurysms) are more common than non-traumatic VAAs. The following discussion concerns non-traumatic VAA.

Most VAAs arise at the VA-PICA junction. Other sites: VA-AICA, VA-BA.

Angiographic considerations

Also see ▶ Table 102.2 in Endovascular section. Angiography of VAA should assess the contralateral VA for patency in case of the need to trap the aneurysm. Allcock test (vertebral artery injection with carotid compression) may be used to assess patency of circle of Willis. Test occlusion with a balloon catheter can determine if patient will tolerate occlusion (a double lumen balloon will even allow measurement of distal back pressure).

PICA aneurysms

General information

For PICA anatomy, see ▶ Fig. 2.6. For arteriogram, see ▶ Fig. 2.7.

Comprise ≈ 3% of cerebral aneurysms. 3 common sites:

1. VA at the VA-PICA junction[19]:
   a) saccular aneurysms: most commonly at the distal (superior) angle. An aneurysm in this location should be suspected with a CT showing blood predominantly in the 4th ventricle[20] (aneurysmal dome may adhere to foramen of Luschka; rupture fills the ventricles with little subarachnoid blood visible on CT). The level is as varied as the PICA origin, and ranges from as low as the foramen magnum to as high as the ponto-medullary junction. Most VA-PICA aneurysms lie in the anterolateral portion of the medullary cistern,[21] anterior to the first dentate ligament.[22] However, the PICA origin may sometimes lie in the midline or across it
   b) fusiform aneurysms: usually the result of prior arterial dissection (p. 1325)
2. PICA aneurysms distal to the VA-PICA junction: tend to be fragile and often develop multiple hemorrhages in a relatively short period, ∴ should be treated promptly, even when discovered incidentally
3. fusiform VA aneurysms involving PICA

Angiographic considerations

See ▶ Table 102.2 in Endovascular section.

Treatment

Options:

1. direct aneurysmal clipping is the preferred treatment
2. endovascular coil embolization: not as effective as clipping for relief of symptoms due to brainstem or cranial nerve compression
3. choices for unclippable and uncoilable aneurysms (e.g. fusiform, giant, or dissecting aneurysms) include:
   a) proximal (hunterian) VA ligation[23] which must be *distal* to the PICA origin to prevent severe morbidity or mortality[24]
   b) occlusion of the VA distal to the PICA origin (usually done endovascularly)
   c) midcervical VA occlusion (allows collateral flow through suboccipital muscular branches) e.g. endovascular Amplatzer plug

Surgical clipping of VA-PICA junction saccular aneurysms

80

One approach to the VA-PICA junction is via a low extreme-lateral p-fossa approach. However, if the aneurysm is too far anterior to the brain stem, it may be totally out of vision or reach. Also, since these aneurysms usually project posteriorly and superiorly, the critical PICA will be directly in harms' way. Direct lateral approach more directly exposes the aneurysm[25] through a lateral suboccipital transcondylar approach.

Position: options include sitting position – less frequently used, see Sitting position (p. 1445) – or lateral oblique ("park bench").

Lateral oblique position

Position: side of involved PICA is up, thorax elevated ≈ 15°. Head in-line with the thorax, neck slightly flexed, and slightly rotated 20° toward the floor (away from the side of the aneurysm). Upper shoulder depressed with adhesive tape. Lumbar spinal subarachnoid catheter placed, allows CSF drainage once dura is opened.

Options for skin incision:

Avoid opening too far laterally, otherwise the muscle mass impedes surgeon's vision.[26(p 1747)]

1. From just above superior nuchal line to C2 vertebra[21]
   a) paramedian vertical incision
   b) midline vertical incision (hockey stick)
2. "sigmoid" incision starting 2 cm medial to mastoid notch, and curving to midline at level of C1 arch[27]

Craniectomy: lateral exposure of bone to the base of the mastoid, medially crossing the midline. Need not be quite as high as the transverse sinus. The foramen magnum is removed to its lateral margin. Removing the posterior arch of C1 from midline to the sulcus arteriosus (under VA) may help with proximal VA exposure[27] but is not usually necessary.[28]

Dural opening: K-shaped dural opening with a linear incision across the band at the foramen magnum (some patients have a sinus known as the arcuate sinus here that may require vascular clips).

Approach: first, gain proximal control of the VA where it first becomes intradural (in case of aneurysmal rupture). Retract cerebellum superiorly (caution: aneurysm dome may be adherent). Follow VA up from point where it enters dura; PICA origin then encountered usually just at neck of aneurysm (PICA origin may be confused for continuation of VA). Dissection must spare branches of pharyngeal filaments of spinal accessory nerve and lower filaments of vagus. May place temporary clip on VA proximal to PICA. Permanent clip usually placed between the fibers of IX & X above and XI below. It is better to leave a small residual aneurysm than to risk compromising PICA.[28]

Postoperative care: when neuropraxia of the lower cranial nerves is likely (in cases of difficult dissection or traction applied during clipping) the patient is kept intubated overnight. Patients who do not tolerate extubation at this point are immediately reintubated and elective tracheostomy is scheduled. Tracheostomy is maintained until the neuropraxia resolves.

Surgical clipping of distal PICA aneurysms

Aneurysms distal to the lateral medullary segment are approached through a craniectomy that extends across the midline.

80.7.4 Vertebrobasilar junction aneurysms

General information

Saccular aneurysms located where the two vertebral arteries join often form at the location of a basilar artery fenestration (basilar fenestration aneurysm).

Angiographic considerations

See ▸ Table 102.2 in Endovascular section.

CT-angiogram may be helpful as an adjunct because it can opacify both vertebral arteries simultaneously (not generally feasible with catheter angiogram).

Surgical approaches

1. suboccipital approach: for most; performed in lateral oblique position
2. subtemporal-transtentorial approach if the vertebrobasilar junction is high; performed in supine position

Suboccipital approach in lateral oblique position

NB: the side of approach must be chosen based on angiogram, as the extreme tortuosity of the VAs may cause the aneurysm of one VA to lie on the contralateral side of the brain stem.

Position: thorax elevated ≈ 15°. Head in-line with the thorax, neck slightly flexed, and slightly rotated away from side of aneurysm. Upper shoulder depressed with adhesive tape. Spinal subarachnoid catheter placed for CSF drainage, opened only once dura is opened.

80.7.5 AICA aneurysms

Angiographic considerations

See ▶ Table 102.2 in Endovascular section.

80.7.6 Basilar bifurcation aneurysms

General information

AKA basilar tip aneurysms. The most common posterior circulation aneurysm. Comprise ≈ 5% of intracranial aneurysms. Considered inoperable until Drake reported 4 cases in 1961,[29] with larger series reported later.[30]

Presentation

Most present with SAH indistinguishable from SAH due to anterior circulation aneurysmal rupture. Enlargement of the aneurysm prior to rupture may rarely compress the optic chiasm → bitemporal field cut (mimicking pituitary tumor), or occasionally may compress the third nerve as it exits from the interpeduncular fossa → oculomotor nerve palsy.[17]

CT/MRI scan

May occasionally be seen on CT or MRI as round mass in region of suprasellar cistern. With SAH, tend to see blood in interpeduncular cistern with some reflux into 4th (and to a lesser extent, third and lateral) ventricle. Occasionally may mimic pretruncal nonaneurysmal SAH (p. 1231).

Angiography

Also see ▶ Table 102.2 in Endovascular section. Dome usually points superiorly. Should evaluate flow through posterior communicating arteries (may require Allcock test) in case trapping is required. Need to assess the height of the basilar bifurcation in relation to the dorsum sella (below).

Critical angiographic features to assess: On angiogram or CTA:

1. general features (p. 1162)
2. orientation: determines whether surgery is an option. Posteriorly pointing aneurysms obscure perforators which may be adherent to the aneurysm, making surgery more difficult
3. patency of PCAs & SCAs
4. patency and size of p-comms
   a) diameter of p-comm > 1 mm is needed to support collateral flow (expert opinion)
   b) to determine if the P1's can be sacrificed
   c) P-comm patency and size is important for endovascular treatment as a potential route for deployment of horizontally oriented stent extending from P1 to contralateral P1[31,32]
   d) which can facilitate temporary clipping, or sacrifice, or placement of stents.
5. height of the aneurysm relative to the posterior clinoid process which will affect the selection of surgical approach[33,34] (the range of height of the posterior clinoid is 4–14 mm[34])
   a) supraclinoidal: aneurysm neck > 5 mm superior to posterior clinoid process
   b) clinoidal: aneurysm neck within 5 mm of posterior clinoid process
   c) infraclinoidal: aneurysm neck > 5 mm inferior to posterior clinoid process

Surgical treatment

Timing

Initial experience tended to favor allowing basilar tip aneurysms to "cool-down" for ≈ 10–14 days after SAH before attempting surgery to permit cerebral edema to subside. More recently, early surgery for these aneurysms has been advocated as for anterior circulation aneurysms (p. 1199).[35] However, some surgeons still recommend waiting ≈ 1 week,[36] and most would agree that if there are obvious technical difficulties because of size, configuration or location of the aneurysm, that early surgery may not be appropriate. Also, if during the craniotomy it becomes apparent that cerebral edema is impairing the exposure, the operation should be aborted and attempted again at a later date.

Approaches

1. right subtemporal craniotomy (classical approach of Drake): approached through the incisura or division of the tentorium. Most basilar tip aneurysms are probably best approached via pterional approach (see below) except for posteriorly pointing aneurysms

a) advantage:
   - less distance to basilar tip
   - may be better than pterional approach for aneurysms projecting posteriorly or posteroinferiorly[36]

b) disadvantages:
   - requires temporal lobe retraction (minimized with lumbar drainage, mannitol, and possibly zygomatic arch section[37])
   - poor visualization of contralateral P1 segment and thalamoperforators

2. pterional approach (described by Yasargil): trans-Sylvian (see below)
   a) advantages:
      - little or no retraction on temporal lobe (unlike subtemporal approach)
      - better visualization of both P1 segments and thalamoperforators
      - other aneurysms, e.g. of the anterior circulation, can be dealt with at the same sitting
   b) disadvantages:
      - increases reach to aneurysm by ≈ 1 cm compared to subtemporal
      - requires wide splitting of the sylvian fissure
      - operating field is narrower than subtemporal approach
      - perforators arising from the posterior aspect of P1 may not be visible
3. modified pterional craniotomy: may allow trans-sylvian or subtemporal approach.[36] The craniotomy is taken further posteriorly than a standard pterional craniotomy
4. orbitozygomatic approach: allows access to portions of the basilar artery below the bifurcation. May be augmented by removal of the top of the clivus

Optional resection of the temporal tip will increase exposure of either approach. Unlike most anterior circulation aneurysms, securing proximal control is very difficult.

If the basilar bifurcation is high above the dorsum sella, then more retraction is required on a subtemporal approach than for a normal bifurcation height (near the dorsum sella). A high bifurcation is dealt with on a trans-sylvian approach by opening the sylvian fissure more widely, or by a subfrontal approach through the third ventricle via the lamina terminalis.[38] A low bifurcation may require splitting the tentorium behind the 4th nerve.

Pterional approach

See reference.[39]

Risks include: oculomotor palsy in ≈ 30% (most are minimal and temporary).

Approach is from the *right* unless:

1. additional left sided aneurysm (e.g. p-comm aneurysm) which could be treated simultaneously by a left sided approach
2. aneurysm points to the right
3. aneurysm is located to the left of midline (the operation is more difficult when the aneurysm is even just 2–3 mm contralateral to the craniotomy)[36]
4. patient has right hemiparesis or left oculomotor palsy

See Pterional craniotomy (p. 1453) for general information. Rotate the head ≈ 30° off the vertical so that the malar eminence points directly upward (▶ Fig. 94.5). Slight neck flexion is used for low-lying aneurysms, slight extension for high ones. Craniotomy is as shown in ▶ Fig. 94.7, with aggressive removal of the sphenoid wing. The sphenoid wing and the orbital roof may be reduced with a drill. The posterior clinoid can be removed to improve exposure.

Approach

The sylvian fissure is split until the take-off of the proximal M1 from the carotid terminus is identified. The approach is medial to the ICA (between the ICA and optic nerve) when this space is ≥ 5–10 mm. If the ICA is close to the optic nerve, an approach lateral to the ICA may be used, aided by medial retraction of the ICA/M1 segment (▶ Fig. 94.8). Here, the exposure is limited by the height of the M1 branch above the skull base, and if the basilar tip height above the skull base greatly exceeds this, clipping via this approach is not feasible.[18]

The 3rd nerve is identified. Also the p-comm and the anterior choroidal artery (AChA) are located as they arise from the posterior surface of the ICA (to differentiate between them: the p-comm origin is proximal to that of the AChA, p-comm courses perpendicular to Liliequist's membrane whereas AChA courses obliquely into the crural cistern). The p-comm is followed posteriorly through Liliequist's membrane which is opened revealing the prepontine cistern. The p-comm is followed until it joins the PCA at the P1/P2 junction. If p-comm is absent, follow the third nerve back to find where it emerges between PCA and SCA. P1 is followed proximally to the basilar bifurcation region where the contralateral P1 and both SCAs are identified. Caudal dissection of Liliequist's membrane exposes the interpeduncular cistern with proximal BA (this exposure is critical for proximal control of BA in the event of aneurysmal rupture).

Thalamoperforating arteries (ThPAs) arise from the distal p-comm and proximal PCA, and often compromise the access. Early poor results with clipping of basilar tip aneurysms has been attributed to sacrificing these vessels, which produces lacunar infarcts in the thalamus, midbrain, subthalamic, and pretectal regions. If hypoplastic, the p-comm may be divided between clips to improve exposure (preserving the ThPAs which will then arise from the stumps). Similarly, a hypoplastic P1 may be divided if the PCA fills from the p-comm. If the ThPAs make it impossible to clip the aneurysm, some may have to be sacrificed, which is best done at their origin. Fortunately, there are some anastamoses[40] and thus they are not entirely end-arteries as originally thought.

Outcome

If the aneurysm cannot be treated with endovascular technique, then the surgical option can be considered. Overall mortality is 5%, and morbidity is 12% (mostly due to injury to perforating vessels).[41]

80.7.7 Basilar trunk aneurysms

Most aneurysms of the basilar trunk are fusiform in morphology. Surgical access for these is extremely difficult.

References

[1] Locksley HB. Report on the Cooperative Study of Intracranial Aneurysms and Subarachnoid Hemorrhage: Section V. J Neurosurg. 1966; 25:219–239

[2] Yock DH, Larson DA. CT of Hemorrhage from Anterior Communicating Artery Aneurysms, with Angiographic Correlation. Radiology. 1980; 134:399–407

[3] Yeh H, Tew JM. Anterior Interhemispheric Approach to Aneurysms of the Anterior Communicating Artery. Surg Neurol. 1985; 23:98–100

[4] VanderArk GD, Kempe LG, Smith DR. Anterior Communicating Aneurysms: The Gyrus Rectus Approach. Clin Neurosurg. 1974; 21:120–133

[5] Olmsted WW, McGee TP. The Pathogenesis of Peripheral Aneurysms of the Central Nervous System: A Subject Review from the AFIP. Radiology. 1977; 123:661–666

[6] Fein JM, Rovit RL. Interhemispheric subdural hematoma secondary to hemorrhage from a calloso-marginal artery aneurysm. Neuroradiology. 1970; 1:183–186

[7] Becker DH, Newton TH. Distal Anterior Cerebral Artery Aneurysm. Neurosurgery. 1979; 4:495–503

[8] Tan H, Huang G, Zhang T, Liu J, Li Z, Wang Z. A retrospective comparison of the influence of surgical clipping and endovascular embolization on recovery of oculomotor nerve palsy in patients with posterior communicating artery aneurysms. Neurosurgery. 2015; 76:687–94; discussion 694

[9] Khan SA, Agrawal A, Hailey CE, Smith TP, Gokhale S, Alexander MJ, Britz GW, Zomorodi AR, McDonagh DL, James ML. Effect of surgical clipping versus endovascular coiling on recovery from oculomotor nerve palsy in patients with posterior communicating artery aneurysms: A retrospective comparative study and meta-analysis. Asian J Neurosurg. 2013; 8:117–124

[10] Heros RC, Ojemann RG, Crowell RM. Superior Temporal Gyrus Approach to Middle Cerebral Artery Aneurysms: Technique and Results. Neurosurgery. 1982; 10:308–313

[11] Zhao B, Zhao Y, Tan X, Cao Y, Wu J, Zhong M, Wang S. Primary decompressive craniectomy for poorgrade middle cerebral artery aneurysms with associated intracerebral hemorrhage. Clin Neurol Neurosurg. 2015; 133:1–5

[12] Day AL. Clinicoanatomic Features of Supraclinoid Aneurysms. Clin Neurosurg. 1988; 36:256–274

[13] Gibo H, Lenkey C, Rhoton AL. Microsurgical Anatomy of the Supraclinoid Portion of the Internal Carotid Artery. J Neurosurg. 1981; 55:560–574

[14] Day AL. Aneurysms of the Ophthalmic Segment: A Clinical and Anatomical Analysis. J Neurosurg. 1990; 72:677–691

[15] Berson EL, Freeman MI, Gay AJ. Visual Field Defects in Giant Suprasellar Aneurysms of Internal Carotid. Arch Ophthalmol. 1966; 76:52–58

[16] Heros RC, Nelson PB, Ojemann RG, et al. Large and Giant Paraclinoid Aneurysms: Surgical Techniques, Complications, and Results. Neurosurgery. 1983; 12:153–163

[17] Drake CG. The Treatment of Aneurysms of the Posterior Circulation. Clin Neurosurg. 1979; 26:96–144

[18] Yamaura A. Surgical Management of Posterior Circulation Aneurysms - Part I. Contemporary Neurosurg. 1985; 7:1–6

[19] Fox JL. Intracranial Aneurysms. New York: Springer-Verlag; 1983

[20] Yeh HS, Tomsick TA, Tew JM. Intraventricular Hemorrhage due to Aneurysms of the Distal Posterior Inferior Cerebellar Artery. J Neurosurg. 1985; 62:772–775

[21] Hammon WM, Kempe LG. The Posterior Fossa Approach to Aneurysms of the Vertebral and Basilar Arteries. J Neurosurg. 1972; 37:339–347

[22] Drake CG. The Surgical Treatment of Vertebral-Basilar Aneurysms. Clin Neurosurg. 1969; 16:114–169

[23] Friedman AH, Drake CG. Subarachnoid hemorrhage from intracraniai dissecting aneurysm. J Neurosurg. 1984; 60:325–334

[24] Yamada K, Hayakawa T, Ushio Y, et al. Therapeutic Occlusion of the Vertebral Artery for Unclippable Vertebral Aneurysm. Neurosurgery. 1984; 15:834–838

[25] Sen CN, Sekhar LN. An Extreme Lateral Approach to Intradural Lesions of the Cervical Spine and Foramen Magnum. Neurosurgery. 1990; 27:197–204

[26] Youmans JR. Neurological Surgery. Philadelphia 1982

[27] Heros RC. Lateral Suboccipital Approach for Vertebral and Vertebrobasilar Artery Aneurysms. J Neurosurg. 1986; 64:559–562

[28] Getch CC, O'Shaughnessy BA, Bendok BR, Parkinson RJ, Batjer HH. Surgical management of intracranial aneurysms involving the posterior inferior cerebellar artery. Contemp Neurosurg. 2004; 26:1–7

[29] Drake CG. Bleeding Aneurysms of the Basilar Artery: Direct Surgical Management in Four Cases. J Neurosurg. 1961; 18:230–238
[30] Drake CG. Further Experience with Surgical Treatment of Aneurysms of the Basilar Artery. J Neurosurg. 1968; 29:372–392
[31] Cross DT, III, Moran CJ, Derdeyn CP, Mazumdar A, Rivet D, Chicoine MM. Neuroform stent deployment for treatment of a basilar tip aneurysm via a posterior communicating artery route. AJNR Am J Neuroradiol. 2005; 26:2578–2581
[32] Wanke I, Gizewski E, Forsting M. Horizontal stent placement plus coiling in a broad-based basilar-tip aneurysm: an alternative to the Y-stent technique. Neuroradiology. 2006; 48:817–820
[33] Friedman RA, Pensak ML, Tauber M, Tew JM, Jr, van Loveren HR. Anterior petrosectomy approach to infraclinoidal basilar artery aneurysms: the emerging role of the neuro-otologist in multidisciplinary management of basilar artery aneurysms. Laryngoscope. 1997; 107:977–983
[34] Aziz KM, van Loveren HR, Tew JM, Jr, Chicoine MR. The Kawase approach to retrosellar and upper clival basilar aneurysms. Neurosurgery. 1999; 44:1225–34; discussion 1234-6
[35] Peerless SJ, Hernesniemi JA, Gutman FB, Drake CG. Early Surgery for Ruptured Vertebrobasilar Aneurysms. J Neurosurg. 1994; 80:643–649
[36] Chyatte D, Philips M. Surgical Approaches for Basilar Artery Aneurysms. Contemp Neurosurg. 1991; 13:1–6
[37] Pitelli SD, Almeida GGM, Nakagawa EJ, et al. Basilar Aneurysm Surgery: The Subtemporal Approach with Section of the Zygomatic Arch. Neurosurgery. 1986; 18:125–128
[38] Canbolt A, Önal Ç, Kiris T. A High-Position Basilar Top Aneurysm Apprached via Third Ventricle: Case Report. Surg Neurol. 1993; 39:196–199
[39] Yasargil MG, Antic J, Laciga R, et al. Microsurgical Pterional Approach to Aneurysms of the Basilar Bifurcation. Surg Neurol. 1976; 6
[40] Marinkovic SV, Milisavljevic MM, Kovacevic MS. Anastamoses Among the Thalamoperforating Branches of the Posterior Cerebral Artery. Arch Neurol. 1986; 43:811–814
[41] Drake CG. Management of Cerebral Aneurysm. Stroke. 1981; 12:273–283

81 Special Aneurysms and Non-Aneurysmal SAH

81.1 Unruptured aneurysms

81.1.1 General information

Unruptured intracranial aneurysms (UIA) includes incidental aneurysms (those that do not produce any symptoms and are discovered incidentally) and aneurysms that produce symptoms other than those due to hemorrhage (e.g. pupillary dilatation due to third nerve compression). UIA merit consideration for treatment since the outcome from SAH with or without surgery is poor even under the best of circumstances. About 65% of patients die from the first SAH,[1] and even in patients with no neurologic deficit after aneurysm rupture, only 46% fully recover, and only 44% return to their former jobs.[2] However, the risk of aneurysmal rupture without intervention should be weighed against the risks of surgical clipping or endovascular treatment. Estimated prevalence of incidental aneurysms is 5–10% of the population.[2]

81.1.2 Presentation

See items other than those listed under "rupture" in Presentation of aneurysms (p. 1191).

81.1.3 Natural history

Risk of bleeding from UIA differs from aneurysms that have ruptured. True risk is not known with certainty. Early studies found annual bleeding rate of 6.25%, whereas later reports estimate lifetime risk for a 20-year-old with an UIA to be 16%, which drops off to 5% for a 60-year-old.[2] A more recent study[3] estimates the annual rupture rate to be ≈ 1%. The International Study of Unruptured aneurysms (ISUIA)[4] was the first large-scale, prospective study evaluating the natural history of unruptured aneurysms as well as the risks of treatment of unruptured aneurysms. The authors concluded that rupture rate was related to size and location of the aneurysm, and that risk is increased with previous aSAH from a separate aneurysm (see below). However, there were important limitations of ISUIA (see ▶ Table 81.1).

> **Σ**
>
> There appears to be 2 distinct types of aneurysms: those that rupture, and those that tend to remain stable. Most UIAs seen in the clinic fall into the latter group

Spontaneous thrombosis of unruptured aneurysms may occur rarely (p. 1194).

Additional retrospective and prospective studies have been conducted to assess the natural history of unruptured aneurysms. Overall, several variables have been identified as risk factors for rupture:

1. patient factors
   a) history of previous aSAH from a separate aneurysm[4,5]
   b) multiple aneurysms[6,7]
   c) age: there is conflicting evidence, as some studies have found an inverse relationship between age and rupture risk,[7,8] while others have found an increased risk of rupture for those aged 40 or older,[9] or no effect of age on rupture risk[10]
   d) medical conditions:
      - hypertension,[7]
      - smoking[8]
   e) geographic location: North America/Europe < Japan < Finland[11]

Table 81.1 Main methodological limitations of ISUIA study

- Patients were not randomized to surgery (vs. no surgery), and there were substantial differences between treated and untreated groups
- Follow-up was < 5 years in of 50% of patients
- Selection bias: low recruitment numbers from each center

f) gender?: Risk of rupture was greater amongst women compared to men in one study, but only approached statistical significance[9]
g) family history?: In the Familial Intracranial Aneurysm study[12] rupture rate in patients with unruptured aneurysm and first-degree relative with intracranial aneurysm was 17x higher than that for patients with unruptured intracranial aneurysm in ISUIA (after matching for aneurysm size and location) – although conclusions are limited secondary to small number of ruptures in the study. Other studies have failed to demonstrate an increased risk in this subgroup

2. aneurysm characteristics
   a) size: risk of rupture appears critically dependent on aneurysm diameter. ISUIA estimated the annual risk of rupture of aneurysms < 10 mm to be 0.05%/year, however a number of other studies have demonstrated a rupture risk closer to ≈1%/year for aneurysms < 10 mm.[5,8,13,14,15] Furthermore, the Small Unruptured Intracranial Aneurysm Verification Study[7] demonstrated that the rupture risk of smaller aneurysms (< 5 mm) is not trivial, and estimated to be ≈0.5%/ year. A more recent retrospective review demonstrated the majority (62%) of ruptured aneurysms to be < 7 mm, with the majority of these being anterior communicating aneurysms.[16] Some speculate that this may be due to a shrinkage of aneurysms following rupture. Larger aneurysms (10-25 mm) are estimated to have ≈ 3-18%/year risk, while giant aneurysms (≥ 25 mm) have a risk of ≈8-50%/year
   b) location: ISUIA showed an increase rupture risk for pcomm and posterior circulation aneurysms.[16] Ishibashi et al.[5] also demonstrated increased risk amongst posterior circulation aneurysms. Conversely, some studies found an increased risk of rupture with anterior communicating aneurysms[8,16,17]
   c) morphology: presence of a daughter sac,[15] bottleneck shape[18] and increased ratio of size of aneurysm to parent vessel have all been associated with increased risk of rupture[19,20]

Estimation of absolute risk of aneurysm rupture in a patient based on a combination of risk factors is complex. Recently, a scoring system (PHASES) was developed by pooling patient data from six prospective studies,[5,7,8,15,21,22] to help estimate 5-year rupture risk by risk factor status.[11] The predictors comprising the PHASES aneurysm rupture risk score and the predicted 5-year cumulative risk of aneurysm rupture based on score is summarized below (▶ Table 81.2). Further studies are needed however to externally validate the score.

81.1.4 Management

Cumulative rupture risk

To understand the calculation of cumulative risk for aneurysmal rupture, see discussion of this issue related to AVMs which is also relevant to aneurysms (p. 1240).

Decision analysis

Decision analysis is a means of mathematically modeling outcomes of various decision options using probabilities and assigning "desirability factors" to the outcomes. This analysis requires data about the natural history (see above), *life expectancy*, and morbidity and mortality of SAH and aneurysm surgery. Although it is only a model, it does yield some insights in some complicated decisions.

In one such study,[23] using the values shown in ▶ Table 81.3, the result obtained was that a life expectancy of 12 more years is the break-even point, i.e. if the patient is not expected to live for 12 more years, then non-surgical management is a better choice than surgery (this result involves numerous assumptions and estimations; e.g. 5% "risk aversiveness" (intermediate) relates to patient's fears of immediate surgical risk vs. risk of rupture spread over many years). Another analysis of various scenarios for a 50 year old female found that treatment was cost effective for UIAs that were symptomatic, ≥ 10 mm diameter, or with a previous history of SAH.[24]

Management recommendations

Decisions are based on natural history data compared with morbidity and mortality of intervention (surgery/endovascular), with recommendations being based mainly on expert opinion as high level evidence is lacking. Size, patient age and location appear to be the most important factors in determining whether to treat and by which means to treat an unruptured aneurysm (in a patient without prior SAH). In addition, treatment should be recommended for patients with a history of aSAH, strong family history, symptomatic aneurysms, and for enlargement or change in configuration of

81

Table 81.2 Predictors comprising the PHASES aneurysm rupture risk score; predicted 5-year cumulative risk of aneurysm rupture based on score[11]

Predictor	Points
(P) Population	
North American, European (other than Finnish)	0
Japanes	3
Finnish	5
(H) Hypertension	
No	0
Yes	1
(A) Age	
< 70 years	0
≥ 70 years	1
(S) Size	
< 7 mm	0
7–9 mm	3
10–19.9 mm	6
20 mm	10
(E) Earlier rupture from another aneurysm	
No	0
Yes	1
PHASES risk score	**5-year risk of aneurysm rupture**
2	0.4%
3	0.7%
4	0.9%
5	1.3%
6	1.7%
7	2.4%
8	3.2%
9	4.3%
10	5.3%
11	7.2%
12	17.8%

the aneurysm.[25] Numerous recommendations have been made for a critical size above which an unruptured aneurysm should be considered for surgery, and have included 3 mm,[26] 5 mm,[27] 7 mm,[28] and 9 mm.[29] The most recent American Heart Association guidelines did not advocate for repair of small incidental aneurysms (< 10 mm) in patients with no history of subarachnoid hemorrhage,[25] but this report was prior to more recent prospective trials. In addition, the patient's expected longevity must also be taken into account, and therefore special consideration for treatment should be

Table 81.3 Data used in decision analysis of management of unruptured aneurysms[23]

	Typical value	Range
annual risk of rupture[a]	1%	0.5–2%
3 month mortality of SAH	55%	50–60%
serious morbidity after SAH	15%	10–20%
surgical morbidity & mortality	2% & 6%	4–10%

[a]this is an intermediate risk for aneurysms 6–10 mm diameter (NB: size may change; small aneurysms may grow)

given to young patients in this group. In all treatment decisions, coexisting medical conditions must also be taken into account.

One recent proposed strategy[30] in management is summarized here:

1. Large and/or symptomatic aneurysms (esp. in young pts) → intervention
2. Patients < 60 years old:
   a) < 7 mm
      - anterior circulation, NO risk factors → medical management or intervention
      - pcomm/posterior circulation, symptomatic aneurysm, strong family hx → intervention
   b) > 7 mm → intervention (surgery or endovascular based on size, location)
3. Patients > 60 years old:
   a) < 7 mm
      - no family hx and asymptomatic → medical management
      - + risk factors → intervention
   b) 7-12 mm
      - anterior circulation → medical management or intervention
      - pcomm/posterior circulation → intervention
   c) > 12 mm → Intervention

Recommended follow-up for UIAs treated conservatively

Σ

Annual follow-up with MRA/CTA is recommended for most incidental aneurysms that are not treated. Intervention is indicated for *any* documented growth. If no growth, may consider repeat imaging at a reduced frequency.

Background: The morbidity from catheter arteriograms is probably too high to recommend them for this purpose. CTA is more accurate than MRA, but involves iodine contrast and radiation. A TOF-MRA (not gadolinium-MRA) has no known risks and does not involve radiation, but has lower spatial resolution.

Unfortunately, most aneurysms rupture without demonstrable enlargement on follow-up. Aneurysms do not grow at a constant rate, and it may take several years to appreciate a millimeter of increased size on MRA.

Studies have identified risk factors for growth, including size,[31,32,33,34] location (MCA, basilar bifurcation),[33,34] *> 1 aneurysm,*[32,33] *family history of SAH*[33] and *smoking.*[31]

Risk of rupture in setting of growth is hard to estimate, given most aneurysms that increase in size are subsequently treated. In one study, the rupture rate was 2.4%/year for aneurysms showing growth (vs. 0.2%/year in those without growth).[31] In another study of 18 Japanese patients, rupture risk after growth was 18.5%/year.[35]

Unruptured cavernous carotid artery aneurysms (CCAAs)

Cavernous carotid artery aneurysms (CCAAs) have a unique risk profile among intracranial aneurysms. Most develop on the horizontal segment of the artery.

Presentation:

1. CCAAs may be discovered incidentally
   a) on arteriography for other reason

b) on MRI
c) occasionally on CT
2. when symptomatic:
a) usually present with:
- headache
- cavernous sinus syndrome (p. 1401): primarily produces diplopia (due to ophthalmoplegia). Classically the third nerve palsy from enlarging CCAA will *not* produce a dilated pupil because the sympathetics which dilate the pupil are also paralyzed[36(p 1492)]
- those that expand through the carotid ring into the subarachnoid space may cause monocular blindness from strangulation of the optic nerve[37]

b) rarely, pain (retro-orbital or pain mimicking trigeminal neuralgia[38,39]) or a carotid-cavernous fistula (**CCF**) are the sole manifestation
c) when CCAAs rupture, they usually produce a CCF
d) life threatening complications are rare, but may be more common with *giant* intracavernous aneurysms.[40] Manifestations include:
- SAH[40,41]: primarily with CCAAs that straddle the carotid ring (subarachnoid extension of CCAAs may be indicated by "waisting" of the aneurysm on angiography[42])
- arterial epistaxis from rupture into sphenoid sinus; usually with traumatic aneurysms (p. 1227); subarachnoid extension of CCAAs may be indicated by "waisting" of the aneurysm on angiography[42]
- emboli

Indications for treatment:
1. unruptured CCAAs: the natural history is not precisely known
a) symptomatic: patients with intolerable pain or visual problems[43]
b) giant aneurysms: especially those that straddle the clinoidal ring (subarachnoid extension of CCAAs may be indicated by "waisting" of the aneurysm on angiography[42])
c) aneurysms that enlarge on serial imaging
d) controversial: incidental aneurysms in the distribution of a stenotic carotid artery for which carotid endarterectomy is indicated. There has been no evidence that doing the endarterectomy increases the risk of rupture, and, as indicated above, most ruptures are not life threatening and so the carotid disease should be treated according to its own merits
2. ruptured CCAAs:
a) emergent treatment for cases with epistaxis or SAH
b) urgent treatment for CCFs with severe eye pain or threat to vision

Treatment options for CCAAs:

Treatment of small incidental intracavernous CCAAs is not generally indicated.[25]

For other unruptured CCAAs, options include detachable coils in an attempt to thrombose the aneurysm (p. 1194). This results in reduction of mass effect in ≈ 50%. Open surgical treatment is rarely appropriate. Aneurysms that rupture and produce a carotid-cavernous fistula may be treated by endovascular occlusion (p. 1256).

81.2 Multiple aneurysms

Multiple aneurysms are present in 15–33.5% of cases of SAH.[2] In one study of multiple factors, hypertension was found to be the most important one associated with multiplicity.[44]

When a patient presents with SAH and is found to have multiple aneurysms, the following may be clues as to which aneurysm has bled:
1. epicenter (center of greatest concentration) of blood on CT or MRI[45,46]
2. area of focal vasospasm on angiogram
3. irregularities in the shape of the aneurysm (so-called "Murphy's teat")
4. if none of the above help, then suspect the largest aneurysm
5. NB: in one series, the most common cause of post-op bleeding in 93 patients with multiple aneurysms was felt to be from rebleeding of the original aneurysm that ruptured that was actually *missed* on initial angiogram[47]

81.3 Familial aneurysms

81.3.1 General information

The role of inheritance in the development of intracranial aneurysms (IA) is well established for disorders such as polycystic kidney disease, and connective tissue disorders such as Ehlers-Danlos type IV, Marfan syndrome, and pseudoxanthoma elasticum (p. 1193). Overall, it is not uncommon for patients with aSAH to have a family history. In one study of patients with subarachnoid hemorrhage,[48] 9.4% had a first-degree relative with aSAH or intracranial aneurysm and 14% had a second-degree relative with these diagnosis In families with two or more affected members, the age-adjusted prevalence of intracranial aneurysm among first-degree relatives was 9.2% in those aged 30 years or older.[49,50]

Additional cases of IAs in identical twins[51,52] as well as familial aggregations of IAs without a recognized inherited disorder have also been reported but are felt to be rare (it has been estimated that < 2% of IAs are familial[53]). Most reported cases consist of only 2 family members with IAs, and these are most commonly siblings.[54] In fact, siblings of an affected aSAH patient have a higher risk of aneurysm, than do children of an affected patient.[30] Analysis of case reports reveals that when IAs occur in siblings they tend to occur at identical or mirror image sites, and in comparison to sporadic IAs, familial IAs tend to rupture at a smaller size and at a younger age, and that the incidence of anterior communicating artery aneurysms is lower.[55] It has been postulated that IAs occurring in siblings may represent a distinct population of IAs.[56]

81.3.2 Screening recommendations

The indications and best method for investigation of asymptomatic relatives of a patient found to harbor an intracranial aneurysm are controversial. Negative studies do not guarantee that at a later date an aneurysm will not be discovered that either subsequently developed or expanded, or was simply not detected on the initial study.[57,58,59] Cerebral angiography is the most sensitive study, however, the risk and expense may not justify its use as a screening test in many cases. Furthermore, there is some evidence that aneurysms that rupture tend to do so shortly after their formation[29] which would reduce the value of screening.

81.3.3 Genetics

A large meta-analysis identified 19 single nucleotide polymorphisms associated with sporadic intracranial aneurysms.[60] The strongest associations were found on chromosomes 9 (CDKN2B; antisense inhibitor gene), 8 (SOX17; transcription regulator gene), and 4 (EDNRA gene).

Screening with either MRA or CTA is typically recommended for first-degree relatives (especially siblings) of affected family members *when two or more* members of the family have an intracranial aneurysm or aSAH.[30] The overall need for screening second-degree relatives is less clear. Screening of first-degree relatives is not typically recommended if only one family member is affected.[25,58] In patients with coarctation of the aorta, screening is typically recommended. Finally, patients with ADPKD who have a family history of intracranial aneurysm or aSAH should be screened. Findings suspicious for intracranial aneurysms should be followed-up with four vessel arteriography to confirm suspected lesions (MRA has a high false-positive rate of ≈ 16%[49]) and to rule-out additional aneurysms.

81.4 Traumatic aneurysms

81.4.1 General information

Traumatic aneurysms **(TAs)** comprise < 1% of intracranial aneurysms.[61,62] Most are actually false aneurysms, AKA pseudoaneurysms (a rupture of all the vessel wall layers with the "wall" of the aneurysm being formed by surrounding cerebral structures[63]). They may occur rarely in childhood. The mechanism of injury usually falls into one of the following groups[64]:

► **Those arising from penetrating trauma.** Usually from gunshot wounds, although penetration with a sharp object (which is less common) may be more prone to cause traumatic aneurysms.[65]

► **Those arising from closed head injury.** More common. Theories of pathogenesis include traction injury to the vessel wall or entrapment within a fracture. Tend to occur either:

1. peripherally
   a) distal anterior cerebral artery aneurysms: secondary to impact against the falcine edge
   b) distal cortical artery aneurysms: often associated with an overlying skull fracture, sometimes a growing skull fracture
2. at the skull base, usually involving the ICA in one of the following sites:
   a) petrous portion (virtually always associated with basal skull fractures):
   b) cavernous carotid artery (virtually always associated with basal skull fractures):

- aneurysm enlargement may cause a progressive cavernous sinus syndrome
- rupture may lead to a posttraumatic carotid-cavernous fistula (p. 1256) or to massive epistaxis in the presence of a sphenoid sinus fracture[66,67,68]

c) supraclinoid carotid artery

▶ **Iatrogenic.** Following surgery in or around the skull base, the sinuses, or orbits (including following transsphenoidal surgery[69]). The first such case was described in 1950

81.4.2 Presentation

1. delayed intracranial hemorrhage (subdural, subarachnoid, intraventricular, or intraparenchymal): the most common presentation. TAs tend to have a high rate of rupture
2. recurrent epistaxis
3. progressive cranial nerve palsy
4. enlarging skull fracture
5. may be incidental finding on CT scan
6. severe headache

81.4.3 Treatment

Although there are case reports of spontaneous resolution, treatment is usually recommended. ICA aneurysms at the skull base should undergo trapping or endovascular embolization. Peripheral lesions should be treated surgically with clipping of aneurysm neck, excision of the aneurysm, coiling, or wrapping if no other method is feasible.

81.5 Mycotic aneurysms

81.5.1 General information

The name *"mycotic"* originated with Osler in whose time the term referred to any infectious process[70] rather than the current usage which infers a fungal etiology. Currently accepted terminology favors infectious aneurysm (or bacterial aneurysm). Infectious aneurysms can, however, also occur with fungal infections.[71] Tend to form in distal (often unnamed) vessels.

81.5.2 Epidemiology and pathophysiology

1. comprise ≈ 4% of intracranial aneurysms
2. occurs in 3–15% of patients with subacute bacterial endocarditis (SBE)
3. most common location: distal MCA branches (75–80%)
4. at least 20% have or develop multiple aneurysms
5. increased frequency in immunocompromised patients (e.g. AIDS) and drug users
6. most probably start in the adventitia (outer layer) and spread inward

81.5.3 Evaluation

Blood cultures and LP may identify the infectious organism. ▶ Table 81.4 shows typical pathogens recovered. Patients with suspected infectious aneurysm(s) should undergo echo-cardiography to look for signs of endocarditis.

81.5.4 Treatment

These aneurysms usually have fusiform morphology and are usually very friable, therefore surgical treatment is difficult and/or risky. Most cases are treated acutely with antibiotics which are continued 4–6 weeks. Serial angiography (at 7–10 days and 1.5, 3, 6 and 12 months, even if aneurysms seem to be getting smaller, they may subsequently increase[73] and new ones may form) helps document effectiveness of medical therapy (serial MRA may be a viable alternative in some cases). Aneurysms may continue to shrink following completion of antibiotic therapy.[74] Delayed clipping may be more feasible; indications include:

1. patients with SAH
2. increasing size of aneurysm while on antibiotics[75] (controversial, some say not mandatory[74])
3. failure of aneurysm to reduce in size after 4–6 weeks of antibiotics[75]

Table 81.4 Pathogens implicated in mycotic aneurysms[72 (p 933–40)]

Organism	%	Comment
streptococcus	44%	*S. viridans* (classic cause of SBE)
staphylococcus	18%	*S. aureus* (cause of acute bacterial endocarditis)
miscellaneous	6%	(pseudomonas, enterococcus, corynebacteria...)
multiple	5%	
no growth	12%	
no info	14%	
total	99%	

Patients with SBE requiring valve replacement should have bioprosthetic (i.e. tissue) valves instead of mechanical valves to eliminate the need for risky anticoagulation.

81.6 Giant aneurysms

81.6.1 General information

Definition: > 2.5 cm (≈ 1 inch) diameter. Two types: saccular (probably an enlarged "berry" aneurysm) and fusiform. Comprise 3 5% of intracranial aneurysms; peak age of presentation 30–60 years; female:male ratio = 3:1.

Drake's series of 174 giant aneurysms[76]: 35% presented as hemorrhage, with 10% showing some evidence of remote bleeding. The bleeding rate is unknown, but is probably less than the ≈ 2%/year for non-giant aneurysms.

May also present as TIAs (by reducing flow or by emboli) or as a mass. About one third have a neck amenable to clipping.

81.6.2 Evaluation

General information

Drake contended that even after thorough radiographic evaluation, actual operative visualization is the only way to definitively assess the aneurysm and its branches. 3D-CTA can add substantial information that rivals and may exceed direct visualization.

Angiogram

Often underestimates the size of the lesion secondary to thrombosed regions of the aneurysm that do not fill with contrast. CT or MRI is required to visualize the thrombosed portion.

CT scan

Frequently have a significant amount of edema surrounding the aneurysm. May see contrast enhancement of the brain surrounding the aneurysm; probably due to increased vascularity secondary to inflammatory reaction to the aneurysm.

MRI scan

Turbulence within → complicated signal on T1WI. Pulsation artifact (linear distortion radiation through aneurysm) on MRI helps differentiate giant aneurysms from solid or cystic lesions.

81.6.3 Treatment

Options include:

1. direct surgical clipping: usually possible in only ≈ 50% of cases
2. vascular bypass of aneurysm with subsequent clipping

3. trapping
4. proximal arterial ligation (hunterian ligation)
   a) for vertebral-basilar aneurysms[77]: results in improvement of cranial nerve deficit in ≈ 95% of patients. A reasonable alternative in the presence of an adequately sized contralateral VA that unites with the VA to be ligated
5. wrapping (p. 1194)
6. endovascular treatment

81.7 Cortical subarachnoid hemorrhage

Cortical SAH (cSAH) appears as SAH over the convexity. Trauma is the most common cause. Nontraumatic etiologies are shown below.

Etiologies of nontraumatic cSAH[78]:

- pial AVMs
- dural AV fistulas
- cerebrovascular arterial dissection
- dural or cortical venous thrombosis
- vasculitis
- Reversible cerebral vasoconstriction syndrome (RCVS), AKA Call-Fleming syndrome,[79] a group of disorders sharing the cardinal clinical and angiographic features of reversible segmental multifocal cerebral vasoconstriction with severe headaches, focal ischemia, and/or seizures. May present as a hemorrhage restricted to a cortical sulcus
- PRES
- Cerebral amyloid angiopathy (CAA)
- Coagulopathies
- Brain tumors (primary or metastatic)

81.8 SAH of unknown etiology

81.8.1 General information

Incidence: traditionally quoted as 20–28% of all SAH, but this includes data from older series (some did not perform true pan-angiography, and/or CT was not available to R/O intracerebral hemorrhage). Recent estimates of incidence: 7–10%. This is a heterogeneous category, and a better term might be "angiogram-negative SAH"; see requirements to be met before considering an arteriogram to be negative (p. 1161). The quantity of blood on CT may predict the chances of an arteriogram disclosing a cerebral aneurysm.[80,81,82,83]

Patients with angiogram-negative SAH tend to be younger, less hypertensive, and more commonly male than those with positive angiography.[81]

Possible causes of SAH with a negative angiogram include:

► **Aneurysm that fails to be demonstrated in initial angiogram:**

1. inadequate angiography, causes include:
   a) incomplete angio: (p. 1161)
      - must see both PICA origins (1–2% of aneurysms occur here)
      - need to cross-fill through the ACoA (p. 1161)
   b) degradation of images due to
      - poor patient cooperation (e.g. from agitation). Either sedate patient (use caution in non-intubated patients) or repeat the study at a later time when patient more cooperative
      - poor quality equipment providing substandard images
2. obliteration of aneurysm by the hemorrhage
3. thrombosis of the aneurysm after SAH (p. 1194)
4. aneurysm too small to be visualized[84]: although "microaneurysms" may be a source of SAH, their natural history and optimal treatment are unknown
5. lack of filling of aneurysm due to vasospasm (of parent artery or of aneurysmal orifice)

► **Nonaneurysmal SAH from source that fails to show up on angiography.** See for etiologies of SAH other than aneurysm (p. 1156) (many of which may not be demonstrated on angiography), including:

1. angiographically occult (or cryptic) vascular malformation (p. 1246)
2. pretruncal nonaneurysmal SAH: see below

81.8.2 Risk of rebleeding

Overall rebleed rate is 0.5%/yr, which is lower than with aneurysmal SAH or rebleeding from AVMs. There is also a smaller risk of delayed cerebral ischemia (vasospasm). Neurological outcome is likewise better.

81.8.3 Management

General measures

These patients are still at risk for the same complications of SAH as with aneurysmal SAH: vasospasm, hydrocephalus, hyponatremia, rebleeding, etc. (p.1164) and (should be managed as any SAH (p.1163). Some subgroups may be at lower risk for complications and may be managed accordingly (e.g. below).

Repeat angiography

Yield of positive second angiogram after technically adequate negative study: 1.8–9.8%)[85] in early (pre-CT) studies, 2–24% quoted more recently.[84,86,87] CT scan findings are helpful in the decision to repeat angiography.[88] 70% of cases with diffuse SAH and thick layering of blood in the anterior interhemispheric fissure were associated with an ACoA aneurysm that showed up on repeat angiography.[82] The absence of blood on CT (performed within 4 days of SAH), or thick blood in the perimesencephalic cisterns alone (see below) were unlikely to be associated with a missed aneurysm.

Recommendations regarding repeat angio:

1. repeat angio after ≈ 10–14 days (allows vasospasm & some clot to resolve; **note**: between 5–10 days there is decreased chance of seeing an aneurysm because of vasospasm; angiography at ≈ day 10 permits surgery to be done if needed ≈ at day 14 which is about the earliest time after the "no-op" window of day 3–12)
   a) technically adequate 4 vessel angiogram is negative, and evidence for SAH is strong
   b) original angio was incomplete or if there are suspicious findings
2. if CT localizes blood clot to particular area, place special attention to this area on repeat angio
3. do not repeat angio for classic pretruncal SAH (see below) or if no blood on CT
4. patients are usually kept in the hospital 10–14 days while waiting for repeat angio (to watch for and manage complication of SAH or rebleeding)

Third arteriogram:

If the 1st 2 arteriograms are negative, and the history is suggestive of aneurysmal SAH, a 3rd arteriogram 3–6 months after SAH has ≈ 1% chance of showing a source of bleeding.

Other studies

1. imaging studies of the brain: MRI (with MRA if available) or CT (with angio-CT if available). This may visualize an aneurysm that fails to show up on angiography, and may identify other sources of SAH such as angiographically occult vascular malformation (p.1246), tumor…
2. tests to rule-out spinal AVM: a rare cause of intracerebral SAH (p.1140)
   a) spinal MRI: cervical, thoracic and lumbar
   b) spinal angiography: too difficult and risky to be justified in most cases of angio negative SAH. Consider in cases with high suspicion of spinal source

Surgical exploration

Advocated by some for cases of SAH with CT findings compatible with an aneurysmal source in which a suspicious area is demonstrated angiographically[84] with careful explanation to the patient and family of the possibility of negative operative findings.

81.9 Pretruncal nonaneurysmal SAH (PNSAH)

81.9.1 General information

Née perimesencephalic nonaneurysmal SAH.[89] The suggestion to change the name to pretruncal nonaneurysmal SAH was proposed because neuroimaging has shown the true anatomic localization of the blood to be in front of the brain stem (truncus cerebri) centered in front of the pons rather than perimesencephalic.[90] The existing literature on PNSAH is somewhat limited by the lack of a rigorous anatomic definition, with criteria of blood pattern differing amongst studies. Blood often extends into the interpeduncular or premedullary cisterns. It has also sometimes been referred to as the "Dutch disease" due to the initial profusion of information in that literature.

A distinct entity considered to be a benign condition with good outcome and less risk of rebleeding and vasospasm than other patients with SAH of unknown etiology[91] (no rebleeding occurred in 37 patients with PNSAH and 45 months mean follow-up,[92] nor in 169 patients with 8–51 months follow-up[87]; vasospasm has been reported in only 3 patients and may have been related to cerebral angiography rather than the PNSAH, and although it is low, the incidence of angiographic vasospasm may be higher than originally thought[93]).

The actual etiology has yet to be determined (there are 3 case reports of patients explored surgically with no abnormal findings[87] and one case where a pontine abnormality resembling a capillary telangiectasia was demonstrated on MRI[94]), but it may be secondary to rupture of a small perimesencephalic vein or capillary.[93] Studies have shown an association with abnormal venous anatomy, including primitive variants of the basal vein of Rosenthal,[95,96] which some authors have hypothesized results in hemorrhage secondary to central cerebral venous hypertension.[97,98] Other proposed etiologies include a ruptured perforating artery, cavernous malformation, intraluminal basilar dissection, and capillary telangiectasia.[99]

81.9.2 Presentation

Patients may present with severe paroxysmal H/A, meningismus, photophobia, and nausea. Loss of consciousness is rare. These patients are usually not critically ill (all were grade 1 or 2 (H&H or WFNS grading scale)), however, complications such as hyponatremia or cardiac abnormalities may still occur. Preretinal hemorrhages and sentinel H/A have not occurred. CT and/or MRI demonstrate characteristic findings (see below) although it may initially be missed on CT,[93] and LP may yield bloody CSF. By definition, all have negative angiography.

81.9.3 Epidemiology

PNSAH has been reported to comprise 20–68% of cases of angiogram-negative SAH[91,100] (depending on the timing of CT, adequacy of angiography, and the definition of PNSAH). However, the true incidence is probably more in the range of 50–75%.[87]

The reported age range is 3–70 years (mean: 50 yrs),[87] 52–59% are male, and pre-existing HTN was present in 3–20% of patients.

81.9.4 Relevant anatomy

Posterior fossa cisterns:

The perimesencephalic cisterns include: interpeduncular, crural, ambient and quadrigeminal cisterns. The prepontine cistern lies immediately anterior to the pons.

Liliequist's membrane (LM)[101]:

Basically considered to separate the interpeduncular cistern from the chiasmatic cistern[102] (forming a competent barrier in only 10–30% of the population). In further detail, the superior leaflet of LM (diencephalic membrane) separates the interpeduncular cistern from the chiasmatic cistern medially and from the carotid cisterns laterally.[103,104] The inferior leaflet (the mesencephalic membrane) separates the interpeduncular from the prepontine cistern.

The diencephalic membrane is thicker and is more often competent, effectively isolating the chiasmatic cistern. However, the carotid cisterns often communicate with the crural cisterns and in turn with the interpeduncular cistern.[104]

Thus, blood in the carotid or prepontine cistern is compatible with a low-pressure pretruncal source of bleeding, however, blood in the chiasmatic cistern should raise concern about aneurysmal rupture.

81.9.5 Diagnostic criteria

Without knowledge of the actual substrate of PNSAH, the following suggested diagnostic criteria must be viewed as empiric (adapted[87]):

1. CT or MRI scan performed ≤ 2 days from ictus meeting the criteria shown in ▶ Table 81.5 (later scans render the diagnosis unreliable, e.g. washout could cause an aneurysmal SAH to fit the criteria). This criteria implies that blood should be contained inferior to Liliequist's membrane (LM) (i.e. perimesencephalic and/or prepontine cisterns). Extension into the suprasellar cistern is

Table 81.5 CT or MRI criteria for PNSAH[93,107]

1. epicenter of hemorrhage immediately anterior to brain stem (interpeduncular or prepontine cistern) 2. there may be extension into anterior part of ambient cistern or basal part of the sylvian fissure 3. absence of complete filling of anterior interhemispheric fissure 4. no more than minute amounts of blood in lateral portion of sylvian fissure 5. absence of frank intraventricular hemorrhage (small amounts of blood sedimenting in the occipital horns of the lateral ventricles is permissible)

Table 81.6 Alternative anatomic CT criteria for PNSAH[108]

• epicenter of bleeding located immediately anterior to and in contact with the brainstem in the prepontine, interpeduncular, or posterior suprasellar cistern • blood limited to the prepontine, interpeduncular, suprasellar, crural, ambient, and/or quadrigeminal cisterns and/or cisterna magna • NO extension of blood into the Sylvian or interhemisheric fissures • intraventricular blood limited to incomplete filling of the fourth ventricle and occipital horns of the lateral ventricles • no intraparenchymal blood

common. Significant amounts of blood penetrating LM to the chiasmatic, sylvian, or interhemispheric cisterns should be viewed with suspicion
2. a negative high-quality 4-vessel cerebral angiogram[105] (radiographic vasospasm is common, and does not preclude the diagnosis nor does it mandate repeat angiography). NB: ≈ 3% of patients with a ruptured basilar bifurcation aneurysm meet the criteria of ▶ Table 81.5,[106] therefore an *initial* arteriogram is mandatory
3. appropriate clinical picture: no loss of consciousness, no sentinel H/A, SAH grade 1 or 2 (Hunt and Hess or WFNS grading scale) (p. 1162), and absence of drug use. Variance from this should raise suspicion of alternate pathogenesis

Recently, a more stringent set of anatomic criteria (see ▶ Table 81.6) was tested and found to result in excellent inter-observer agreement (97.2%) in PNSAH. Additionally, no aneurysms were identified on formal angiography when the anatomical criteria were met.[108]

81.9.6 Repeat angiography

Controversial. Angiography carries ≈ 0.2–0.5% risk of permanent neurologic deficit in this population.[87] Most experts agree that repeat angiography is not indicated in patients meeting the criteria of PNSAH[86,105] (although others recommend repeat angiography in all surgical candidates[84,109]). One should probably repeat the study if any uncertainty exists or if there is a history of a condition associated with increased risk of cerebral aneurysms.[93]

81.9.7 Treatment

Optimal treatment is not known with certainty. The low risk of rebleeding and delayed ischemia suggests that extreme measures are not indicated. The following recommendations are made[87,93] (period not specified):
1. symptomatic treatment
2. cardiac monitoring
3. electrolyte monitoring for hyponatremia
4. follow patient clinically (and if appropriate, with repeat imaging studies) to rule-out hydrocephalus (transient ventricular enlargement is common, however, hydrocephalus requiring shunting is rare (only ≈ 1%)[87])
5. ✖ *not* recommended
   a) hyperdynamic therapy
   b) calcium channel blockers: use has not been investigated in PNSAH, but is probably not warranted due to low incidence of vasospasm and should be discontinued when normal angiographic findings are documented[93]
   c) activity restrictions (except in cases of increasing H/A with mobilization)
   d) anticonvulsants
   e) reduction of blood pressure below normal
   f) surgical exploration

References

[1] Tew JM, Thompson RA, Green JR. In: Guidelines for Management and Surgical Treatment of Intracranial Aneurysms. Controversies in Neurology. New York: Raven Press; 1983:139–154

[2] Wirth FP. Surgical Treatment of Incidental Intracranial Aneurysms. Clin Neurosurg. 1986; 33:125–135

[3] Jane JA, Kassell NF, Torner JC, et al. The Natural History of Aneurysms and AVMs. J Neurosurg. 1985; 62:321–323

[4] The International Study Group of Unruptured Intracranial Aneurysms Investigators (ISUIA). Unruptured Intracranial Aneurysms - Risk of Rupture and Risks of Surgical Intervention. N Engl J Med. 1998; 339:1725–1733

[5] Ishibashi T, Murayama Y, Urashima M, Saguchi T, Ebara M, Arakawa H, Irie K, Takao H, Abe T. Unruptured intracranial aneurysms: incidence of rupture and risk factors. Stroke. 2009; 40:313–316

[6] Yasui N, Suzuki A, Nishimura H, et al. Long-Term Follow-Up Study of Unruptured Intracranial Aneurysms. Neurosurgery. 1997; 40:1155–1160

[7] Sonobe M, Yamazaki T, Yonekura M, Kikuchi H. Small unruptured intracranial aneurysm verification study: SUAVe study, Japan. Stroke. 2010; 41:1969–1977

[8] Juvela S, Poussa K, Lehto H, Porras M. Natural history of unruptured intracranial aneurysms: a long-term follow-up study. Stroke. 2013; 44:2414–2421

[9] Lee EJ, Lee HJ, Hyun MK, Choi JE, Kim JH, Lee NR, Hwang JS, Kwon JW. Rupture rate for patients with untreated unruptured intracranial aneurysms in South Korea during 2006-2009. J Neurosurg. 2012; 117:53–59

[10] Mahaney KB, Brown RD, Jr, Meissner I, Piepgras DG, Huston J,3rd, Zhang J, Torner JC. Age-related differences in unruptured intracranial aneurysms: 1-year outcomes. J Neurosurg. 2014; 121:1024–1038

[11] Greving JP, Wermer MJ, Brown RD, Jr, Morita A, Juvela S, Yonekura M, Ishibashi T, Torner JC, Nakayama T, Rinkel GJ, Algra A. Development of the PHASES score for prediction of risk of rupture of intracranial aneurysms: a pooled analysis of six prospective cohort studies. Lancet Neurol. 2014; 13:59–66

[12] Broderick JP, Brown RD, Jr, Sauerbeck L, Hornung R, Huston J, III, Woo D, Anderson C, Rouleau G, Kleindorfer D, Flaherty ML, Meissner I, Foroud T, Moomaw EC, Connolly ES. Greater rupture risk for familial as compared to sporadic unruptured intracranial aneurysms. Stroke. 2009; 40:1952–1957

[13] Juvela S, Porras M, Poussa K. Natural history of unruptured intracranial aneurysms: probability of and risk factors for aneurysm rupture. J Neurosurg. 2000; 93:379–387

[14] Tsutsumi K, Ueki K, Morita A, Kirino T. Risk of rupture from incidental cerebral aneurysms. J Neurosurg. 2000; 93:550–553

[15] Morita A, Kirino T, Hashi K, Aoki N, Fukuhara S, Hashimoto N, Nakayama T, Sakai M, Teramoto A, Tominari S, Yoshimoto T. The natural course of unruptured cerebral aneurysms in a Japanese cohort. N Engl J Med. 2012; 366:2474–2482

[16] Orz Y, AlYamany M. The impact of size and location on rupture of intracranial aneurysms. Asian J Neurosurg. 2015; 10:26–31

[17] Joo SW, Lee SI, Noh SJ, Jeong YG, Kim MS, Jeong YT. What Is the Significance of a Large Number of Ruptured Aneurysms Smaller than 7 mm in Diameter? J Korean Neurosurg Soc. 2009; 45:85–89

[18] Hoh BL, Sistrom CL, Firment CS, Fautheree GL, Velat GJ, Whiting JH, Reavey-Cantwell JF, Lewis SB. Bottleneck factor and height-width ratio: association with ruptured aneurysms in patients with multiple cerebral aneurysms. Neurosurgery. 2007; 61:716–22; discussion 722-3

[19] Dhar S, Tremmel M, Mocco J, Kim M, Yamamoto J, Siddiqui AH, Hopkins LN, Meng H. Morphology parameters for intracranial aneurysm rupture risk assessment. Neurosurgery. 2008; 63:185–96; discussion 196-7

[20] Rahman M, Smietana J, Hauck E, Hoh B, Hopkins N, Siddiqui A, Levy EI, Meng H, Mocco J. Size ratio correlates with intracranial aneurysm rupture status: a prospective study. Stroke. 2010; 41:916–920

[21] Wiebers DO, Whisnant JP, Huston J, III, Meissner I, Brown RD, Jr, Piepgras DG, Forbes GS, Thielen K, Nichols D, O'Fallon WM, Peacock J, Jaeger L, Kassell NF, Kongable-Beckman GL, Torner JC, International Study of Unruptured Intracranial Aneurysms Investigators. Unruptured intracranial aneurysms: natural history, clinical outcome, and risks of surgical and endovascular treatment. Lancet. 2003; 362:103–110

[22] Wermer MJ, van der Schaaf IC, Velthuis BK, Majoie CB, Albrecht KW, Rinkel GJ. Yield of short-term follow-up CT/MR angiography for small aneurysms detected at screening. Stroke. 2006; 37:414–418

[23] van Crevel H, Habbema JDF, Braakman R. Decision Analysis of the Management of Incidental Intracranial Saccular Aneurysms. Neurology. 1986; 36:1335–1339

[24] Johnston SC, Gress DR, Kahn JG. Which Unruptured Cerebral Aneurysms Should be Treated? A Cost-Utility Analysis. Neurology. 1999; 52:1806–1815

[25] Bederson JB, Awad IA, Wiebers DO, Piepgras D, et al. Recommendations for the management of patients with unruptured intracranial aneurysms. A statement for healthcare professionals from the Stroke Council of the American Heart Association. Circulation. 2000; 102:2300–2308

[26] Solomon RA, Correll JW. Rupture of a Previously Documented Asymptomatic Aneurysm Enhances the Argument for Prophylactic Surgical Intervention. Surg Neurol. 1988; 30:321–323

[27] Ausman JI, Diaz FG, Malik GM, Andrews BT, et al. Management of Cerebral Aneurysms: Further Facts and Additional Myths. Surg Neurol. 1989; 32:21–35

[28] Ojemann RG. Management of the Unruptured Intracranial Aneurysm. N Engl J Med. 1981; 304:725–726

[29] Wiebers DO, Whisnant JP, Sundt TM, et al. The Significance of Unruptured Intracranial Saccular Aneurysms. J Neurosurg. 1987; 66:23–29

[30] Brown RD, Jr, Broderick JP. Unruptured intracranial aneurysms: epidemiology, natural history, management options, and familial screening. Lancet Neurol. 2014; 13:393–404

[31] Villablanca JP, Duckwiler GR, Jahan R, Tateshima S, Martin NA, Frazee J, Gonzalez NR, Sayre J, Vinuela FV. Natural history of asymptomatic unruptured cerebral aneurysms evaluated at CT angiography: growth and rupture incidence and correlation with epidemiologic risk factors. Radiology. 2013; 269:258–265

[32] Burns JD, Huston J, III, Layton KF, Piepgras DG, Brown RD, Jr. Intracranial aneurysm enlargement on serial magnetic resonance angiography: frequency and risk factors. Stroke. 2009; 40:406–411

[33] Miyazawa N, Akiyama I, Yamagata Z. Risk factors for growth of unruptured intracranial aneurysms: follow-up study by serial 0.5-T magnetic resonance angiography. Neurosurgery. 2006; 58:1047–53; discussion 1047-53

[34] Matsubara S, Hadeishi H, Suzuki A, Yasui N, Nishimura H. Incidence and risk factors for the growth of unruptured cerebral aneurysms: observation using serial computerized tomography angiography. J Neurosurg. 2004; 101:908–914

[35] Inoue T, Shimizu H, Fujimura M, Saito A, Tominaga T. Annual rupture risk of growing unruptured cerebral aneurysms detected by magnetic resonance angiography. J Neurosurg. 2012; 117:20–25

[36] Wilkins RH, Rengachary SS. Neurosurgery. New York 1985

[37] Day AL. Clinicoanatomic Features of Supraclinoid Aneurysms. Clin Neurosurg. 1988; 36:256–274

[38] Raps EC, Galetta SL, Solomon RA, et al. The Clinical Spectrum of Unruptured Intracranial Aneurysms. Arch Neurol. 1993; 50:265–268
[39] Sano H, Jain VK, Kato Y, et al. Bilateral Giant Intracavernous Aneurysms: Technique of Unilateral Operation. Surg Neurol. 1988; 29:35–38
[40] Hamada H, Endo S, Fukuda O, et al. Giant Aneurysm in the Cavernous Sinus Causing Subarachnoid Hemorrhage 13 Years After Detection: A Case Report. Surg Neurol. 1996; 45:143–146
[41] Lee AG, Mawad ME, Baskin DS. Fatal Subarachnoid Hemorrhage from the Rupture of a Totally Intracavernous Carotid Artery Aneurysm: Case Report. Neurosurgery. 1996; 38:596–599
[42] White JA, Horowitz MB, Samson D. Dural Waisting as a Sign of Subarachnoid Extension of Cavernous Carotid Aneurysms: A Follow-Up Case Report. Surg Neurol. 1999; 52:607–610
[43] Kupersmith MJ, Hurst R, Berenstein A, Choi IS, Jafar J, Ransohoff J. The Benign Course of Cavernous Carotid Artery Aneurysms. J Neurosurg. 1992; 77:690–693
[44] Ostergaard JR, Hog E. Incidence of Multiple Intracranial Aneurysms. J Neurosurg. 1985; 63:49–55
[45] Hackney DB, Lesnick JE, Zimmerman RA, et al. MR Identification of Bleeding Site in Subarachnoid Hemorrhage with Multiple Intracranial Aneurysms. J Comput Assist Tomogr. 1986; 10:878–880
[46] Karttunen AI, Jartti PH, Ukkola VA, Sajanti J, Haapea M. Value of the quantity and distribution of subarachnoid haemorrhage on CT in the localization of a ruptured cerebral aneurysm. Acta Neurochir (Wien). 2003; 145:655–61; discussion 661
[47] Hino A, Fujimoto M, Iwamoto Y, Yamaki T, Katsumori T. False localization of rupture site in patients with multiple cerebral aneurysms and subarachnoid hemorrhage. Neurosurgery. 2000; 46:825–830
[48] Kissela BM, Sauerbeck L, Woo D, Khoury J, Carrozzella J, Pancioli A, Jauch E, Moomaw CJ, Shukla R, Gebel J, Fontaine R, Broderick J. Subarachnoid hemorrhage: a preventable disease with a heritable component. Stroke. 2002; 33:1321–1326
[49] Ronkainen A, Hernesniemi J, Puranen M, Niemitukia L, Vanninen R, Ryynanen M, Kuivaniemi H, Tromp G. Familial Intracranial Aneurysms. Lancet. 1997; 349:380–384
[50] Ronkainen A, Miettinen H, Karkola K, Papinaho S, Vanninen R, Puranen M, Hernesniemi J. Risk of harboring an unruptured intracranial aneurysm. Stroke. 1998; 29:359–362
[51] Fairburn B. "Twin" Intracranial Aneurysms Causing Subarachnoid Hemorrhage in Identical Twins. Br Med J. 1973; 1:210–211
[52] Schon F, Marshall J. Subarachnoid Hemorrhage in Identical Twins. J Neurol Neurosurg Psychiatry. 1984; 47:81–83
[53] Toglia IU, Samii AR. Familial Intracranial Aneurysms. Dis Nerv Syst. 1972; 33:611–613
[54] Norrgard O, Angquist K-A, Fodstad H, Forsell A, et al. Intracranial Aneurysms and Heredity. Neurosurgery. 1987; 20:236–239
[55] Lozano AM, Leblanc R. Familial Intracranial Aneurysms. J Neurosurg. 1987; 66:522–528
[56] Andrews RJ. Intracranial Aneurysms: Characteristics of Aneurysms in Siblings. N Engl J Med. 1977; 279
[57] Brisman R, Abbassioun K. Familial Intracranial Aneurysms. J Neurosurg. 1971; 34:678–682
[58] Schievink WI, Limburg M, Dreisen JJR, ter Berg HWM, et al. Screening for Unruptured Familial Intracranial Aneurysms: Subarachnoid Hemorrhage 2 Years After Angiography Negative for Aneurysms. Neurosurgery. 1991; 29:434–438
[59] Vanninen RL, Hernesnieni JA, Puranen MI, Tonkainen A. Magnetic Resonance Angiographic Screening for Asymptomatic Intracranial Aneurysms: The Problem of False Negatives: Technical Case Report. Neurosurgery. 1996; 38:838–841
[60] Alg VS, Sofat R, Houlden H, Werring DJ. Genetic risk factors for intracranial aneurysms: a meta-analysis in more than 116,000 individuals. Neurology. 2013; 80:2154–2165
[61] Benoit BG, Wortzman G. Traumatic Cerebral Aneurysms: Clinical Features and Natural History. J Neurol Neurosurg Psychiatry. 1973; 36:127–138
[62] Parkinson D, West M. Traumatic Intracranial Aneurysms. J Neurosurg. 1980; 52:11–20
[63] Morard M, de Tribolet N. Traumatic Aneurysm of the Posterior Inferior Cerebellar Artery: Case Report. Neurosurgery. 1991; 29:438–441
[64] Buckingham MJ, Crone KR, Ball WS, Tomsick TA, Berger TS, Tew JM. Traumatic Intracranial Aneurysms in Childhood: Two Cases and a Review of the Literature. Neurosurgery. 1988; 22:398–408
[65] Kieck CF, de Villiers JC. Vascular Lesions due to Transcranial Stab Wounds. J Neurosurg. 1984; 60:42–46
[66] Handa J, Handa H. Severe Epistaxis caused by Traumatic Aneurysm of Cavernous Carotid Artery. Surg Neurol. 1976; 5:241–243
[67] Maurer JJ, Mills M, German WJ. Triad of Unilateral Blindness, Orbital Fractures and Massive Epistaxis After Head Injury. J Neurosurg. 1961; 18:937–949
[68] Ding MX. Traumatic Aneurysm of the Intracavernous Part of the Internal Carotid Artery Presenting with Epistaxis. Case Report. Surg Neurol. 1988; 30:65–67
[69] Ahuja A, Guterkman LR, Hopkins LN. Carotid Cavernouc Fistula and False Aneurysm of the Cavernous Carotid Artery: Complications of Transsphenoidal Surgery. Neurosurgery. 1992; 31:774–779
[70] Bohmfalk GL, Story JL, Wissinger JP, et al. Bacterial Intracranial Aneurysm. J Neurosurg. 1978; 48:369–382
[71] Horten BC, Abbott GF, Porro RS. Fungal Aneurysms of Intracranial Vessels. Arch Neurol. 1976; 33:577–579
[72] Schmidek HH, Sweet WH. Operative Neurosurgical Techniques. New York 1982
[73] Pootrakul A, Carter LP. Bacterial Intracranial Aneurysm: Importance of Sequential Angiography. Surg Neurol. 1982; 17:429–431
[74] Morawetz RB, Karp RB. Evolution and Resolution of Intracranial Bacterial (Mycotic) Aneurysms. Neurosurgery. 1984; 15:43–49
[75] Bingham WF. Treatment of Mycotic Intracranial Aneurysms. J Neurosurg. 1977; 46:428–437
[76] Drake CG. Giant Intracranial Aneurysms: Experience with Surgical Treatment in 174 Patients. Clin Neurosurg. 1979; 26:12–95
[77] Drake CG. Ligation of the Vertebral (Unilateral or Bilateral) or Basilar Artery in the Treatment of Large Intracranial Aneurysms. J Neurosurg. 1975; 43:255–274
[78] Cuvinciuc V, Viguier A, Calviere L, Raposo N, Larrue V, Cognard C, Bonneville F. Isolated acute nontraumatic cortical subarachnoid hemorrhage. AJNR Am J Neuroradiol. 2010; 31:1355–1362
[79] Call GK, Fleming MC, Sealfon S, Levine H, Kistler JP, Fisher CM. Reversible cerebral segmental vasoconstriction. Stroke. 1988; 19:1159–1170
[80] Hayward RD, O'Reilly GVA. Intracerebral Hemorrhage: Accuracy of Computerized Transverse Axial Scanning in Predicting the Underlying Etiology. Lancet. 1976; 1:1–6
[81] Cioffi F, Pasqualin A, Cavazzani P, et al. Subarachnoid Hemorrhage of Unknown Origin: Clinical and Tomographical Aspects. Acta Neurochir. 1989; 97:31–39
[82] Iwanaga H, Wakai S, Ochiai C, et al. Ruptured Cerebral Aneurysms Missed by Initial Angiographic Study. Neurosurgery. 1990; 27:45–51
[83] Farres MT, Ferraz-Leite H, Schindler E, et al. Spontaneous Subarachnoid Hemorrhage with Negative Angiography: CT Findings. J Comput Assist Tomogr. 1992; 16:534–537
[84] Tatter SB, Crowell RM, Ogilvy CS. Aneurysmal and Microaneurysmal 'Angiogram Negative' Subarachnoid Hemorrhage. Neurosurgery. 1995; 37:48–55
[85] Nishioka H, Torner JC, Graf CJ, et al. Cooperative Study of Intracranial Aneurysms and Subarachnoid Hemorrhage: III. Subarachnoid Hemorrhage of Undetermined Etiology. Arch Neurol. 1984; 41:1147–1151

[86] Kaim A, Proske M, Kirsch E, et al. Value of Repeat-Angiography in Cases of Unexplained Subarachnoid Hemorrhage (SAH). Acta Neurol Scand. 1996; 93:366–373
[87] Schwartz TH, Solomon RA. Perimesencephalic Nonaneurysmal Subarachnoid Hemorrhage: Review of the Literature. Neurosurgery. 1996; 39:433–440
[88] Rinkel GJE, van Gijn J, Wijdicks EFM. Subarachnoid Hemorrhage Without Detectable Aneurysm: A Review of the Causes. Stroke. 1993; 24:1403–1409
[89] van Gijn J, van Dongen KJ, Vermeulen M, Hijdra A. Perimesencephalic Hemorrhage. A Nonaneurysmal and Benign Form of Subarachnoid Hemorrhage. Neurology. 1985; 35:493–497
[90] Schievink WI, Wijdicks EFM. Pretruncal Subarachnoid Hemorrhage: An Anatomically Correct Description of the Perimesencephalic Subarachnoid Hemorhage. Stroke. 1997; 28
[91] van Calenbergh F, Plets C, Goffin J, Velghe L. Nonaneurysmal Subarachnoid Hemorrhage: Prevalence of Perimesencephalic Hemorrhage in a Consecutive Series. Surg Neurol. 1993; 39:320–323
[92] Rinkel GJE, Wijdicks EFM, Vermeulen M, et al. Outcome in Perimesencephalic (Nonaneurysmal) Subarachnoid Hemorrhage: A Follow-Up Study in 37 Patients. Neurology. 1990; 40:1130–1132
[93] Wijdicks EFM, Schievink WI, Miller GM. Pretruncal Nonaneurysmal Subarachnoid Hemorrhage. Mayo Clin Proc. 1998; 73:745–752
[94] Wijdicks EFM, Schievink WI. Perimesencephalic Nonaneurysmal Subarachnoid Hemorhage: First Hint of a Cause? Neurology. 1997; 49:634–636
[95] Buyukkaya R, Yildirim N, Cebeci H, Kocaeli H, Dusak A, Ocakoglu G, Erdogan C, Hakyemez B. The relationship between perimesencephalic subarachnoid hemorrhage and deep venous system drainage pattern and calibrations. Clin Imaging. 2014; 38:226–230
[96] Sabatino G, Della Pepa GM, Scerrati A, Maira G, Rollo M, Albanese A, Marchese E. Anatomical variants of the basal vein of Rosenthal: prevalence in idiopathic subarachnoid hemorrhage. Acta Neurochir (Wien). 2014; 156:45–51
[97] Sangra MS, Teasdale E, Siddiqui MA, Lindsay KW. Perimesencephalic nonaneurysmal subarachnoid hemorrhage caused by jugular venous occlusion: case report. Neurosurgery. 2008; 63:E1202–3; discussion E1203
[98] Mathews MS, Brown D, Brant-Zawadzki M. Perimesencephalic nonaneurysmal hemorrhage associated with vein of Galen stenosis. Neurology. 2008; 70:2410–2411
[99] Lansberg MG. Concurrent presentation of perimesencephalic subarachnoid hemorrhage and ischemic stroke. J Stroke Cerebrovasc Dis. 2008; 17:248–250
[100] Rinkel GJE, Wijdicks EFM, Hasan D, et al. Outcome in Patients with Subarachnoid Hemorrhage and Negative Angiography According to Pattern of Hemorrhage on Computed Tomography. Lancet. 1991; 338:964–968
[101] Liliequist B. The Subarachnoid Cisterns: An Anatomic and Roentgenologic Study. Acta Radiol (Stockh). 1959; 185:1–108
[102] Yasargil MG. Microneurosurgery. New York: Thieme-Stratton Inc.; 1985
[103] Matsuno H, Rhoton AL, Peace D. Microsurgical Anatomy of the Posterior Fossa Cisterns. Neurosurgery. 1988; 23:58–80
[104] Brasil AVB, Schneider FL. Anatomy of Liliequist's Membrane. Neurosurgery. 1993; 32:956–961
[105] Adams HP, Gordon DL. Nonaneurysmal Subarachnoid Hemorrhage. Ann Neurol. 1991; 29:461–462
[106] Pinto AN, Ferro JM, Canhao P, Campos J. How Often is a Perimesencephalic Subarachnoid Hemorrhage CT Pattern Caused by Ruptured Aneurysms? Acta Neurochir. 1993; 124:79–81
[107] Rinkel GJE, Wijdicks EFM, Vermeulen M, Ramos LMP, et al. Nonaneurysmal Perimesencephalic Subarachnoid Hemorrhage: CT and MR Patterns that Differ from Aneurysmal Rupture. AJNR. 1991; 12:829–834
[108] Wallace AN, Vyhmeister R, Dines JN, Chatterjee AR, Kansagra AP, Viets R, Whisenant JT, Moran CJ, Cross DT,3rd, Derdeyn CP. Evaluation of an anatomic definition of non-aneurysmal perimesencephalic subarachnhoid hemorrhage. J Neurointerv Surg. 2015. DOI: 10.1136/neurintsurg-2015-01168 0
[109] Cloft HJ, Kallmes DF, Dion JE. A Second Look at the Second-Look Angiogram in Cases of Subarachnoid Hemorhage. Radiology. 1997; 205:323–324

Part XVIII

Vascular Malformations

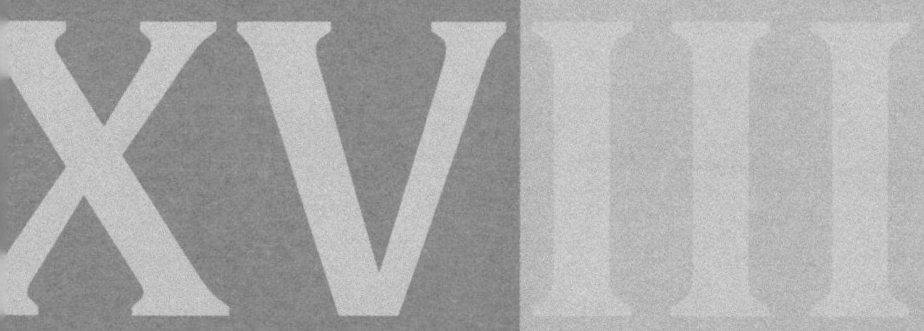

82 Vascular Malformations

82.1 General information and classification

This designation encompasses a number of non-neoplastic vascular lesions of the CNS. The four types originally described by McCormick in 1966 are shown in ▶ Table 82.1.[1]

Possible additional categories:

1. direct fistula AKA arteriovenous fistula (AV- fistula, *not* AVM). Single or multiple dilated arterioles that connect directly to a vein *without* a nidus. These are high-flow, high-pressure. Low incidence of hemorrhage. Usually amenable to interventional neuroradiological procedures. Examples include:
   a) vein of Galen malformation (aneurysm) (p. 1255)
   b) dural AVM (p. 1251)
   c) carotid-cavernous fistula (p. 1256)
2. mixed or unclassified angiomas: 11% of AOVM[2]

82.2 Arteriovenous malformation (AVM)

82.2.1 General information

Key concepts

- dilated arteries and veins with dysplastic vessels. Arterial blood flows directly between them with no capillary bed and no intervening neural parenchyma in nidus
- AVMs are medium-to-high pressure and high-flow
- usually presents with hemorrhage, less often with seizures
- these usually are congenital lesions with a lifelong risk of bleeding of ≈ 2–4% per year
- demonstrable on angiography, MRI, or CT (especially with contrast)
- main treatment options: stereotactic radiosurgery (usually for deep lesions < 3 cm dia) or surgical excision

82.2.2 Description

An abnormal collection of blood vessels wherein arterial blood flows directly into draining veins without the normal interposed capillary beds. There is no brain parenchyma contained within the nidus. AVMs are usually congenital lesions, that tend to enlarge somewhat with age and often progress from low flow juvenile lesions at birth to medium-to-high-flow high-pressure lesions in adulthood. AVMs appear grossly as a "tangle" of vessels, often with a fairly well-circumscribed center (nidus), and draining "red veins" (veins containing oxygenated blood). May be classified as:

1. parenchymal AVMs (discussed below). Subclassified as:
   a) pial
   b) subcortical
   c) paraventricular
   d) combined

Table 82.1 4 classic types of vascular malformation

Type	Prevalence %
Arteriovenous malformation (AVM)[a]	44–60%
Cavernous malformation (p. 1247)	19–31%
Capillary telangiectasia (p. 1247)	4–12%
Developmental venous anomaly (DVA) – formerly venous angioma	9–10%

[a]Sometimes referred to as "pial AVM" to distinguish it e.g. from dural AVM

2. pure dural AVM (p. 1251)
3. mixed parenchymal and dural (rare)

82.2.3 Epidemiology

Prevalence: probably slightly greater than the usually quoted 0.14%.

Slight male preponderance. Congenital (therefore risk of hemorrhage is lifelong).

A few types are known to be hereditary. Other types are part of known hereditary syndromes: 15–20% of patients with Osler-Weber-Rendu syndrome (hereditary hemorrhagic telangiectasia) have cerebral AVMs.

82.2.4 Comparison to aneurysms

See reference.[3]

AVM:aneurysm ratio in U.S. is 1:5.3 (pre-CT era data). The average age of patients diagnosed with AVMs is ≈ 33 yrs, which is ≈ 10 yrs younger than aneurysms.[4] 64% of AVMs are diagnosed before age 40 (c.f. 26% for aneurysms).

82.2.5 Presentation

General information

1. hemorrhage (most common)[5]: 50% (61% quoted elsewhere,[3] compared to 92% for aneurysms) (see below)
2. seizures
3. mass effect: e.g. trigeminal neuralgia due to CPA AVM
4. ischemia: by steal
5. H/A: rare. AVMs may occasionally be associated with migraines. Occipital AVMs may present with visual disturbance (typically hemianopsia or quadrantanopsia) and H/A that are indistinguishable from migraine[6]
6. bruit: especially with dural AVMs (p. 1251)
7. increased ICP
8. findings limited almost exclusively to peds, usually with large midline AVMs that drain into an enlarged vein of Galen ("vein of Galen malformation" (p. 1255)):
   a) hydrocephalus with macrocephaly: due to compression of Sylvian aqueduct by enlarged vein of Galen or to increased venous pressure
   b) congestive heart failure with cardiomegaly
   c) prominence of forehead veins (due to increased venous pressure)

Hemorrhage

General information

Peak age for hemorrhage is between 15–20 yrs.[3] The reported morbidity and mortality from AVM hemorrhage varies widely. An estimate is 10% mortality, 30–50% morbidity[7] (neurological deficit) from each bleed. For a discussion of hemorrhage during pregnancy, also see Pregnancy & intracranial hemorrhage (p. 1169).

Hemorrhage location with AVMs

1. intraparenchymal (CH): 82% (the most common site of bleeding)[8]
2. intraventricular hemorrhage:
   a) usually accompanied by ICH as the result of rupture of the ICH into the ventricle
   b) pure IVH (with no ICH) may indicate an intraventricular AVM
3. subarachnoid: SAH may also be due to rupture of an aneurysm on a feeding artery; common with AVMs (p. 1156)
4. subdural: uncommon. May be the sourced of a spontaneous SDH (p. 904)

Hemorrhage rate related to AVM size

Small AVMs tend to present more often as hemorrhage than do large ones.[9,10] It was postulated that larger AVMs presented as seizure more often simply because their size made them more likely to involve the cortex. However, small AVMs are now thought to have much higher pressure in the feeding arteries[10] (see ▶ Table 82.2). Conclusion: small AVMs are more lethal than larger ones.

Table 82.2 Risk of bleeding by size of AVM[10]

Characteristic	Size of AVM		
	Small (<3 cm)	Medium (3–6 cm)	Large (>6 cm)
number of patients	44	31	17
% that bled	82%	29%	12%
size of hematoma (ave)	4.9 cm	2.7 cm	2.0 cm
feeding artery pressure (mm Hg)	66	47	35

Table 82.3 Annual average hemorrhage rates for various AVM subgroups[12]

Venous drainage	No Prior hemorrhage	Prior hemorrhage	Nidus location
No deep venous drainage	0.9%	4.5%	Not deep
	3.1%	14.8%	Deep
Deep venous drainage	8.0%	34.4%	
	2.4%	11.4%	Not deep

Hemorrhage rate related to Spetzler-Martin grade

Controversial. Some studies show increased risk with Spetzler-Martin (S-M) grade 4–5 AVMs (p. 1242) [11] (high grade), others show the opposite effect as:

S-M grade 1–3: annual risk of hemorrhage is 3.5%.
S-M grade 4–5: annual risk of hemorrhage is 2.5%.

Hemorrhage rate based on nidus depth, venous drainage and prior bleed

Breakdown of the risk of bleeding based on history of prior bleeding, venous drainage pattern, and nidus location using data from Stapf et al. is shown in ▶ Table 82.3.

Annual and lifetime risk of hemorrhage and recurrent hemorrhage

The average risk of hemorrhage from an AVM is ≈ 2–4% per year[13] (reminder: risk varies by AVM size, see above). The risk of bleeding over the remainder of one's life is given by Eq (82.1); this analysis includes a number of assumptions, among them: a constant risk of rebleeding even early after an initial bleed, no change in risk during the lifetime (which may not be true in pregnancy), no difference in risk for various AVM locations or age groups.

$$\text{risk of bleeding (at least once)} = 1 - (\text{annual risk of not bleeding})^{\text{expected years of remaining life}} \quad (82.1)$$

where the annual risk of not bleeding is equal to 1 – the annual risk of bleeding. For example, if a 3% annual risk of bleeding is used as an average, and the remaining life expectancy is 25 years, the result is as illustrated in Eq (82.2).

$$\text{risk of bleeding (at least once in 25 years)}^{*} = 1 - 0.97^{25} = 0.53 - 53\% \quad (82.2)$$

A simple to apply first approximation to Eq (82.1) is shown in Eq (82.3).

$$\text{risk of bleeding (at least once)}^{*} \approx 105 - \text{age in years} \quad (82.3)$$

* Note: Eq (82.3) assumes a 3% per year bleeding rate.

▶ Table 82.4 shows the risk for various ages using Eq (82.1) (longevity is taken from insurance life-tables).

Table 82.4 Lifetime risk of hemorrhage[a]

Age at presentation	Estimated years to live[b]	Lifetime risk of hemorrhage		
		For 1% annual risk[c]	For 2% annual risk	For 3% annual risk
0	76	53%	78%	90%
15	62	46%	71%	85%
25	52	41%	65%	79%
35	43	35%	58%	73%
45	34	29%	50%	64%
55	25	22%	40%	53%
65	18	16%	30%	42%
75	11	10%	20%	28%
85	6	5.8%	11%	17%

[a]modified from reference[13]
[b]based on 1992 Preliminary Life tables prepared by Metropolitan Life Insurance Company
[c]1% annual risk is also presented because it may be appropriate for incidental aneurysms (p. 1222)

A study of 166 *symptomatic* AVMS with long average follow-up (mean: 23.7 yrs)[4] found the risk of major bleeding was constant at 4% per year, and that this was independent of whether the AVM presented with or without hemorrhage. The mean time between presentation and hemorrhage was 7.7 yrs. The mortality rate was 1% per year, and the combined major morbidity and mortality rate was 2.7% per year.

Older studies may suffer from smaller numbers[9] or short follow up (mean: 6.5 yrs).[3,5] These studies suggested a higher risk of (re)bleeding depending on whether the initial presentation was hemorrhage (≈ 3.7% per year) vs. seizure (1–2% per year). Crawford found that none of 8 incidental (*asymptomatic*) AVMs bled in 20 yrs follow-up; all died of unrelated causes.[9]

The hemorrhage risk (but not the rate) may be higher in pediatrics or with posterior-fossa AVMs.[13]

Rebleeding

The literature contains conflicting information. Reported rebleeding rate in the first year after hemorrhage was 6% in one series,[14] 18% in another series[15] which declined to 2% per year after 10 years, and in another large series[4] the annual rate was 4% and did not vary regardless of presentation as discussed above.

Seizures

The younger the patient at the time of diagnosis, the higher the risk of developing convulsions. 20 yr risk: diagnosis at age 10–19 → 44% risk; age 20–29 → 31%; age 30–60 → 6%. Patients presenting with hemorrhage have 22% risk of developing epilepsy in 20 yrs. No AVM found incidentally or presenting with neuro deficit developed seizures.[9]

AVMs and aneurysms

7% of patients with AVMs have aneurysms. 75% of these are located on major feeding artery (probably from increased flow).[9] These aneurysms may be classified into 1 of 5 types shown in ▶ Table 82.5. Aneurysms also may form within the nidus or on draining veins. When treating tandem AVMs and aneurysms, the symptomatic one is usually treated first (when feasible, both may be treated at the same operation).[16] If it is not clear which bled, the odds are that it was the aneurysm. Although a significant number (≈ 66%) of related aneurysms will regress following removal of the AVM, this does not always occur. In one series, none of the 9 associated aneurysms ruptured or enlarged following AVM removal[16]

82

Table 82.5 Categories of aneurysms associated with AVMs[a] [16]

Type	Aneurysm location
I	proximal on ipsilateral major artery feeding AVM
IA	proximal on major artery related but contralateral to AVM
II	distal on superficial feeding artery
III	proximal or distal on deep feeding artery ("bizarre")
IV	on artery unrelated to AVM

[a]excludes intra-nidal and venous aneurysms

82.2.6 Evaluation

CT

Unenhanced brain CT is the best study to rule-out acute hemorrhage. Can also demonstrate calcifications within the lesion. Adding a contrast CT will show enhancement within the vessels, and can delineate the nidus (dense central area of an AVM). See below for CTA.

MRI

Characteristics of AVM on MRI:
1. flow void on T1WI or T2WI within the AVM
2. feeding arteries
3. draining veins
4. increased intensity on partial flip-angle (to differentiate signal dropout on T1WI or T2WI from calcium)
5. significant edema around the lesion may indicate a tumor that has bled rather than an AVM
6. gradient echo sequences (GRASS…) help demonstrate surrounding hemosiderin which suggests a previous significant hemorrhage
7. a complete ring of low density (due to hemosiderin) surrounding the lesion suggests AVM over neoplasm

82.2.7 CT angiography (CTA)

MR angiography (MRA)

Angiography

Characteristics of AVM on angiography:
1. tangle of vessels
2. large feeding artery
3. large draining veins
4. draining veins are visualized in the same images as arteries (arterial phase)

Most, but not all AVMs show up on angiography; see Angiographically occult vascular malformations (p. 1246). Fewer cavernous malformations and venous angiomas do.

Grading

Spetzler-Martin grade of AVMs

Grade = sum of points from ▸ Table 82.6, ranges from 1 to 5. A separate grade 6 is reserved for untreatable lesions (by any means: surgery, SRS…), resection of these would almost unavoidably be associated with disabling deficit or death. This scale has been shown to have good prognostic predictability.[17] May not be applicable to pediatrics (AVMs are immature and change with time; AVMs mature at ≈ age 18 yrs and tend to become more compact).

Outcome based on Spetzler-Martin grade: 100 consecutive cases operated by an expert (Spetzler) had the outcomes shown in ▸ Table 82.7 (no deaths).

✱ Spetzler has since published a 3-tiered management recommendation scheme[19] as follows:
- Class A (S-M Grade I & II): surgical resection

Table 82.6 Spetzler-Martin AVM grading system[18]

Graded feature	Points
Size[a]	
small (<3 cm)	1
medium (3–6 cm)	2
large (>6 cm)	3
Eloquence of adjacent brain	
non-eloquent[b]	0
eloquent[b]	1
Pattern of venous drainage[c]	
superficial only	0
deep	1

[a]largest diameter of nidus on non-magnified angiogram (is related to and therefore implicitly includes other factors relating to difficulty of AVM excision, e.g. number of feeding arteries, degree of steal, etc.)
[b]eloquent brain: sensorimotor, language and visual cortex; hypothalamus and thalamus; internal capsule; brain stem; cerebellar peduncles; deep cerebellar nuclei
[c]considered superficial if all drainage is through cortical venous system; considered deep if any or all is through deep veins (e.g. internal cerebral vein, basal vein, or pre-central cerebellar vein)

Table 82.7 Surgical outcome by Spetzler-Martin grade operated on by Spetzler

Grade	No.	No deficit		Minor deficit[a]		Major deficit[b]	
1	23	23	(100%)	0		0	
2	21	20	(95%)	1	(5%)	0	
3	25	21	(84%)	3	(12%)	1	(4%)
4	15	11	(73%)	3	(20%)	1	(7%)
5	16	11	(69%)	3	(19%)	2	(12%)

[a]minor deficit: mild brainstem deficit, mild aphasia, mild ataxia
[b]major deficit: hemiparesis, increased aphasia, homonymous hemianopsia

- Class B (S-M Grade III): multimodality treatment
- Class C (S-M Grade IV & V): follow clinically and repeat angiogram every 5 years. Treatment only for progressive neurologic deficit, steal-related symptoms, or aneurysms identified on surveillance angiograms

82.2.8 Treatment

General information

Options and some pros and cons of each include:

1. surgery: the treatment of choice for AVMs. When surgical risk is unacceptably high, alternative procedures (e.g. SRS) may be an option
   a) pros: eliminates risk of bleeding almost immediately. Seizure control improves
   b) cons: invasive, risk of surgery, cost (high initial cost of treatment may be offset by effectiveness or may be increased by complications)
2. radiation treatment
   a) conventional radiation: effective in ≈ 20% or less of cases.[20,21] Therefore not considered effective therapy
   b) stereotactic radiosurgery (SRS): accepted for some small (≤ 2.5–3 cm nidus), deep AVMs; see Stereotactic radiosurgery & radiotherapy (p. 1564)

 - pros: done as an outpatient, non-invasive, gradual reduction of AVM flow, no recovery period
 - cons: takes 1–3 years to work (latency period). During that time there is a risk of bleeding, controversial whether it is increased or decreased); limited to lesions with nidus ≤ 3 cm

3. endovascular techniques: e.g. embolization (see below)
   a) pros: facilitates surgery
   b) cons: sometimes inadequate by itself to permanently obliterate AVMs, induces acute hemodynamic changes, may require multiple procedures, embolization prior to SRS reduces the obliteration rate from 70% (without embolization) to 47% (with embolization)[22]
4. combination techniques: e.g. embolization to shrink nidus then stereotactic radiosurgery

Considerations to take into account in managing AVMs:
1. associated aneurysms: on feeding vessels, draining veins or intra-nidal
2. flow: high or low
3. age of patient
4. history of previous hemorrhage
5. size and compactness of nidus
6. availability of interventional neuroradiologist
7. general medical condition of the patient

Embolization

Used as an initial procedure, embolization facilitates surgery[23] and possibly SRS. It is usually inadequate by itself to treat conventional AVMs (may recanalize later). See AVM embolization (p. 1589) in Endovascular neurosurgery section.

Surgical treatment

Pre-op medical management

Before direct surgical treatment, patient should ideally be pre-treated with propranolol 20 mg PO QID for 3 days to minimize post-op normal perfusion pressure breakthrough (postulated cause of postoperative bleeding and edema,[24] see below). Labetalol has also been used perioperatively to keep MAP 70–80 mm Hg.[25]

Booking the case: Craniotomy for AVM

Also see defaults & disclaimers (p. 27).
1. position: (depends on location of AVM), radiolucent headholder
2. pre-op embolization (by neuroendovascular interventionalist): typically 24–48 hours pre-op
3. intraoperative angiography (optional)
4. equipment
   a) microscope (with ICG capability if used)
   b) image-guided navigation: primarily for the bone flap placement
5. blood availability: type and cross 2 U PRBC
6. post-op: ICU
7. consent (in lay terms for the patient – not all-inclusive):
   a) procedure: surgery to open the skull and remove the abnormal tangle of blood vessels in the brain, intraoperative angiography
   b) alternatives: stereotactic radiosurgery, endovascular techniques (not considered definitive treatment for most AVMs, but often used as an adjunct)
   c) complications: usual craniotomy complications (p. 28) plus stroke (the main concern), bleeding intra-op (requiring transfusion) and post-op, neurologic deficit related to the area of AVM location, failure to be able to remove entire AVM, recurrence in future

Basic tenets of AVM surgery

1. wide exposure
2. occlude feeding (terminal) arteries before draining veins (lesions with a single draining vein can become impossible to deal with if premature blockage of the draining vein occurs, e.g. by kinking, coagulation)

3. excision of whole nidus is necessary to protect against rebleeding (occluding feeding arteries is not adequate)
4. identify and spare vessels of passage and adjacent (uninvolved) arteries
5. dissect directly on nidus of AVM, work in sulci and fissures whenever possible
6. in lesions that are high-flow on angiography, consider preoperative embolization
7. lesions with supplies from multiple vascular territories may require staging
8. clip accessible aneurysms on feeding arteries

Delayed postoperative deterioration

May be due to any of the following:

1. normal perfusion pressure breakthrough[24]: characterized by post-op swelling or hemorrhage. Thought to be due to loss of autoregulation, although this theory has been challenged.[26] Risk may be reduced by pre-op medication (see above)
2. occlusive hyperemia[27]: in the immediate post-op period probably due to obstruction of venous outflow from adjacent normal brain, in a delayed presentation may be due to delayed thrombosis of draining vein or dural sinus.[28] Risk may be elevated by keeping the patient "dry" post-op
3. rebleeding from a retained nidus of AVM
4. seizures

82.2.9 Follow-up of treated AVMs

When satisfactory complete angiographic obliteration of an AVM has been accomplished, recommended follow-up is with *catheter angiogram* (not CTA or MRA) at 1 & 5 years post treatment.

82.3 Venous angiomas

82.3.1 General information

Key concepts

- a vascular malformation that is part of the venous drainage of the involved area with intervening brain present. Therefore direct treatment is rarely indicated
- low-flow, low-pressure
- usually demonstrable on angiography as a starburst pattern
- rarely symptomatic: seizures rare, hemorrhage even more uncommon. Venous infarcts may occur (controversial)
- may have an associated cavernous malformation (p. 1247) which is more likely to be symptomatic

AKA venous malformation or (developmental) venous anomaly (DVA). A tuft of medullary veins that converge into an enlarged central trunk that drains either to the deep or superficial venous system. The veins lack large amounts of smooth muscle and elastic. No abnormal arteries are found. There is neural parenchyma between the vessels. Most common in regions supplied by the MCA[29] or in the region of the vein of Galen. They may be associated with a cavernous malformation (p. 1247). Non hereditary. These are low-flow and low-pressure.

Most are clinically silent, but rarely seizures and even less frequently hemorrhage may occur. Venous infarcts have been described, but may be coincidental. If symptoms are present, look for an associated cavernous malformation (GRASS MRI images may reveal some cavernous malformations that might otherwise be occult).

82.3.2 Imaging

MRI

There may be some T2 hyperintensity on FLAIR.

Angiogram

Occasionally may be angiographically occult, however, they classically produce a distinct caput medusae (other descriptive terms include: a hydra, spokes of a wheel, a spider, an umbrella, a mushroom, or a sunburst or starburst).[30(p 1471)] Other angiographic characteristics: appears as a long draining vein (longer than a normal vein) draining an excessive amount of brain tissue (it is theorized that venous restrictive disease occurs because of the length), arterial phase should show no AV shunting (characteristic of AVM).

82.3.3 Treatment

In general, these should not be treated as they are the venous drainage of the brain in that vicinity. If surgery is indicated for associated cavernous malformations, the angioma should be left alone. Surgery for the angioma itself is reserved only for documented bleeding or for intractable seizures that can be definitely attributed to the lesion.

82.4 Angiographically occult vascular malformations

82.4.1 General information

Terminology is controversial. The term "cryptic cerebrovascular malformations" was originally applied to angiographically and clinically silent lesions regardless of size.

Recommendation: use the term " ***angiographically*** occult (or cryptic) vascular malformations" (AOVM) to refer to cerebrovascular malformations that are not demonstrable on technically satisfactory catheter cerebral angiography (i.e. good quality films, with subtraction views, and the following as appropriate: magnification, angiotomography, rapid serial angiograms or delayed films).[31] Many lesions have large patent vessels at surgery in spite of negative angiography.[32] Other imaging modalities (i.e. CT, MRI) may be able to reveal these lesions. Although often used interchangeably, the term "occult malformation" (omitting the word "angiographically") is suggested for use with lesions that also do not appear on these other imaging modalities.

The reasons for a vascular lesion being angiographically cryptic include:

1. lesion that have hemorrhaged
   a) the bleeding may obliterate the lesion: difficult to substantiate[33]
   b) the clot may temporarily compress the lesion[33] which may re-open after weeks to months as clot dissolves
2. sluggish flow
3. small size of the abnormal vessels
4. may require very late angiographic films (i.e. delayed films) to visualize due to late filling

82.4.2 Epidemiology

Incidence of AOVM has been estimated as ≈ 10% of cerebrovascular malformations.[29] AOVMs were found at necropsy in 21 (4.5%) of 461 patients with spontaneous intracranial hemorrhage (**ICH**),[34] but refinements in angiography have occurred since this 1954 report.

The average age at diagnosis in one literature review[31] was 28 yrs.

82.4.3 Presentation

AOVM most often present with seizures or H/A. Less commonly they may present with progressive neurologic symptoms (usually as a result of spontaneous ICH).[35] They may also be discovered incidentally.

The natural history of this group of lesions is not accurately known.

82.5 Osler-Weber-Rendu syndrome

82.5.1 General information

AKA hereditary hemorrhagic telangiectasia (HHT), AKA capillary telangiectasia: slightly enlarged capillaries with low flow. Cannot be imaged on any radiographic study. Usually incidentally found at necropsy without clinical significance (risk of hemorrhage is very low, except possibly in brain stem). Has intervening neural tissue[29] (unlike cavernous malformations). Usually solitary, but may be multiple when seen as a part of a syndrome: Osler-Weber-Rendu (see below), Louis -Barr (ataxia telangiectasia), Myburn-Mason, Sturge-Weber.

Associated cerebrovascular malformations (CVM) include: telangiectasias, AVMs (the most common CVM, seen in 5–13% of HHT patients[36]), venous angiomas and aneurysms. Patients are also prone to pulmonary arteriovenous fistulas with associated risk of paradoxical cerebral embolism which predisposes to embolic stroke and cerebral abscess formation (p.320).

82.5.2 Epidemiology

Rare autosomal dominant genetic disorder of blood vessels affecting ≈ 1 in 5,000 people. 95% have recurrent epistaxis.

82.5.3 Imaging

CT

May show a well demarcated homogeneous or mottled high density[35] (high density due to hematoma, calcification, thrombosis, hemosiderin deposition, alterations in BBB, and/or increased blood volume[31]) with some form of contrast enhancement (around or within lesion) in 17 of 24 patients.[35] Surrounding edema or mass effect is rare (except in cases that have recently hemorrhaged).

MRI

May demonstrate previous hemorrhage(s),[37] (may be important when the presence of multiple occurrences affects therapeutic choices). T2WI finding: reticulated core of increased and decreased intensity, a prominent surrounding rim of reduced intensity may be present (due to hemosiderin laden macrophages from previous hemorrhages). GRASS image demonstrates flow related enhancement in ≈ 60% of cases, which allows signal dropout from flowing blood on other sequences to be differentiated from that due to calcium (and thus, bone) or air (limitations: hemosiderin causes signal dropout, and slow in-plane flow does not enhance).[38]

82.5.4 Treatment

Surgery is indicated mainly for evacuation of hematoma or diagnosis, especially when favorably located. Also consider surgery for recurrent hemorrhages (rupture has been reported even after normal angiography) or medically intractable seizures. Stereotactic radiosurgery has not had a satisfactorily high enough benefit to risk ratio to justify its use.[39]

82.6 Cavernous malformation

82.6.1 General information

Key concepts

- usually angiographically occult. May show up on MRI (open channels → flow void on T2WI, previous hemorrhage → "popcorn" pattern especially on T2* gradient echo) or contrast CT
- low-flow. No intervening neural parenchyma, no arteries. Associated with venous anomaly (represents venous outflow and should be preserved)
- XRT is a risk factor for developing cavernous malformation
- presentation: usually seizures. Hemorrhage: rare, risk is difficult to predict
- treatment:
  a) ♦ surgery is the treatment of choice for symptomatic accessible lesions
  b) ✖ radiosurgery should not be considered as a treatment option

AKA: cavernous hemangioma, cavernoma, cavernous angioma, angioma, and in medical jargon "cavmal." A well-circumscribed, benign vascular hamartoma consisting of irregular thick and thin walled sinusoidal vascular channels located within the brain but *lacking intervening neural parenchyma*,[29] large feeding arteries, or large draining veins. Usually 1–5 cm in size. May hemorrhage, calcify, or thrombose. Occur rarely in the spinal cord.[40] Caverns are filled with blood in various stages of thrombus formation/organization/dissolution. Frequently associated with venous angiomas (p.1245). Capillary telangiectasias may be found adjacent to lesions and may represent a precursor. Stain positive for angiogenesis factor.[41] Lesions may arise de novo,[42] and may grow (although slower than hemangioblastomas), shrink, or remain unchanged with time.[43]

82.6.2 Pathology

Gross appearance resembles a mulberry (facetiously dubbed a "hemorrhoid of the brain"). Light microscopy: stains for von Willebrand's factor. Smooth muscle layer is absent (except for some tiny portions). EM: shows abnormal gapping of the tight junctions between endothelial cells[44] (may permit leakage of blood) and sparse or poorly characterized subendothelial smooth muscle cells.[44]

82.6.3 Epidemiology

Cerebral cavernous malformations (CM) comprise 5–13% of CNS vascular malformations, and develop in 0.02–0.13% of the population (based on large autopsy[45] and MRI[46] series). 48–86% are supratentorial, 4–35% brainstem, 5–10% basal ganglia.[47] Multiple in 23%[48] to 50%[49] of cases, and multiplicity may be more common in hereditary cases.[50]

Spinal CMs: CMs rarely may occur in spinal cord. XRT appears to be a risk factor,[51] (e.g. following craniospinal XRT[52] for medulloblastoma) especially for spinal CMs. 42% of patients with spinal CMs also harbor ≥ 1 intracranial CM.[53]

82.6.4 Genetics

Two types: sporadic and hereditary. The latter may be inherited in a Mendelian autosomal dominant pattern with variable expressivity.[54] There appears to be at least 3 gene loci (see ▸ Table 82.8.

Multiple lesions are more common in the familial form.[46]

82.6.5 Presentation/natural history

See references.[55,56,57]

General information

Seizures (60%), progressive neurologic deficit (50%), hemorrhage (20%, usually intraparenchymal; **note:** here, hemorrhage is defined as symptomatic, radiologically proven extralesional bleeding), hydrocephalus, or as in incidental finding (over 50% in one series).

Hemorrhage

Risk is not well delineated. Even the definition of hemorrhage is controversial since, by definition, all CMs have surrounding hemosiderin indicative of small leaks. The Angioma Alliance[58] definition of hemorrhage: acute or subacute symptoms (any of: headache, seizure, impaired consciousness, or new/worsened focal neurological deficit referable to the anatomic location of the CM) accompanied by radiological, pathological, surgical, or rarely only cerebrospinal fluid evidence of recent extra- or intralesional hemorrhage. This definition does not include either an increase in CM diameter without other evidence of recent hemorrhage, nor the presence of a hemosiderin halo. Risk of significant hemorrhage is much less than with AVMs. CMs are prone to recurrent small hemorrhages that are rarely devastating. Hemorrhage rate tends to be low in cohort studies ≈ 2.6–3.1%/yr; appears higher in females (4.2%/yr) than males (0.9%/yr).[46] Bleeding risk is not related to the size of the CM. Controversial if hemorrhage increases the risk of future bleeding: it did not in one study[46] whereas another study[59] found only a 0.6%/yr risk of bleeding in lesions without prior hemorrhage. Some CMs behave benignly after an initial hemorrhage. Others behave more malignantly with (> 2 hemorrhages) with increasingly more detrimental outcome. Pregnancy and parturition are not known to be risk factors for hemorrhage.[54]

Table 82.8 Subtypes of CCM

	CCM1	CCM2	CCM3
locus	7q11-q22	7p15-13	3q25.2-q27
gene	KRIT1	MGC4607 (malcavernin)	PDCD10
feature	more common in Hispanics		

Σ

The bleeding rate is variable & the criteria for what constitutes "bleeding" has not been uniform. Each patient appears to have their own natural history ∴ it is difficult to assign a risk of hemorrhage for any individual patient.

Seizures

The rate of new-seizure onset is 2.4%/yr.[46]

82.6.6 Evaluation

CT

Not sensitive: CT misses many small lesions, some large ones, and even some that have bled. Not specific: CT findings may overlap with low grade tumors, hemorrhages, granulomas.

MRI

Gradient-echo T2WI MRI is the most sensitive test due to high sensitivity to susceptibility artifact. Findings are similar to AOVM in general (mixed signal core with low signal rim – sometimes described as "popcorn" pattern; see above). The diagnosis is strongly suggested by finding multiple lesions with these characteristics and a positive family history.[19] A venous malformation may be seen adjacent to a solitary CM, but not with multiple CMs.[60] Diffusion tensor imaging/white matter tractography[61] and pre-op 3D-constructive interference in steady-state (CISS) MRI[62] may improve localization, approach, and post-op outcomes.

Angiography

Does not demonstrate lesion. MRI appearance is nearly pathognomonic, and angiography is not necessary in classically appearing cases. Angiography may be needed to R/O other diagnoses in questionable cases.

Familial considerations

First degree relatives of patients with more than one family member having a cavernous malformation should have MRI screening and appropriate genetic counselling.

82.6.7 Treatment/management

Overview

Options:

1. observe
2. surgical excision
3. XRT or stereotactic radiosurgery.[63,64,65,66] Controversial: results appear comparable to natural history

No randomized prospective study has been done. Determining treatment response is difficult since no imaging study can prove elimination of the lesion. Therefore it has been suggested that recurrent hemorrhage rate be followed as an endpoint.

Recommendations

Incidental lesions

Asymptomatic, incidentally discovered CMs should be managed expectantly with serial imaging studies for about 2–3 years (to rule-out frequent subclinical bleeds); additional studies thereafter based on clinical grounds. However, some experts recommend removal for single, easily accessible incidental CMs in non-eloquent brain.[67]

✖ Since the radiographic appearance is almost pathognomonic, biopsy or excision solely to verify the diagnosis is rarely appropriate.

82

Brainstem CMs

Surgery is almost never indicated for brainstem CMs that have not bled. With a bleed rate of 2–6%, Gross et. al[68] suggest operative management for a history of > 2 prior hemorrhages and "pial/ependymal representation" on T1WI MRI.

Bleeds that do not come to the surface cannot be removed without creating neurologic deficit (worsening of neurologic outcome was 9% vs. 29% in superficial vs. deep brainstem CM resections, respectively[69]). The approach is chosen to expose the site where the bleed comes closest to the surface. Spetzler says brainstem CMs are almost always associated with a venous angioma (p. 1245) (which, again, must be preserved since it provides the venous outflow). Outcome was worse with surgery through the floor of the 4th ventricle than with a lateral approach. Significant short-term neurologic deficit is expected with brainstem CM resection.[68]

Spinal cord CMs

Managed essentially the same as brainstem CMs.

Cranial nerve CMs

Many case reports and reviews document CMs of cranial nerves (rarely extra-axial) with various presentations.[70,71,72] Case reports suggest patients may benefit from early surgical decompression from hemorrhagic chiasmal cavernomas since they are at risk for recurrent micro-hemorrhages.[73]

Surgery

General information

Indications for surgery for intracranial CMs:

1. accessible lesions with
   a) focal deficit
   b) or symptomatic hemorrhage
   c) or seizures:
      - **new onset** seizures (p. 461): there is a suggestion that removing CMs before "kindling" occurs may have a better chance of preventing future seizures
      - difficult to manage seizures
2. less accessible lesions that repeatedly bleed with progressive neurologic deterioration may be considered for excision, even in delicate regions such as the brain stem[74,75,76] or spinal cord

Surgical technique

Goal of surgery: complete removal of the malformation. Since CMs are not particularly bloody, piecemeal excision is an option; especially important in brainstem lesions.

Stereotactic localization or intraoperative ultrasound may be particularly helpful in localizing. When operating on CMs that have bled, one usually encounters a cavity containing the CM and blood degradation products.[77] Initial dissection is directed at separating the lesion from the adjacent brain. Although bleeding is usually not a problem, it occasionally may be brisk if the CM is entered before the dissection and devascularization is complete. Once the dissection is complete, the contents of the CM capsule may be removed piecemeal to minimize the parenchymal opening (especially important in the brainstem). For supratentorial CMs presenting with seizures, it is desirable to also remove the hemosiderin-stained brain immediately surrounding the CM.

Keep in mind the relatively common association of CMs with venous angiomas (p. 1245), which if encountered should not be removed as they represent the venous drainage of the area.

Brainstem CMs

The use of retractors is to be avoided; cottonoids and exploitation of hematoma cavity may be used to gain access. Brainstem CMs may be extremely adherent to brain parenchyma[76] unlike supratentorial CMs. Bipolar cautery: use on low power with constant irrigation to reduce thermal injury. Unlike supratentorial CMs with seizures (where you want to remove adjacent hemosiderin-stained brain), just remove the CM itself.

Post-op follow-up

Follow-up MRI ≈ 3 months post-op is recommended. It never looks "normal" but can determine if removal was complete.

Stereotactic radiosurgery (SRS)

Some non-controlled studies have shown a possible reduction in recurrent hemorrhage rate following a 2 year latency period after SRS,[66] however, radiation induced morbidity was significant.[78,79] Other series have failed to show reduction.[80] Findings may reflect the natural history of CMs with temporal clustering of hemorrhagic events with decrease in hemorrhage rates after 28 months.[81]

Σ

SRS is not an alternative to surgery and should not be considered for the treatment of CMs.

82.6.8 Prognosis

When CMs can be completely removed, the risk of further growth or hemorrhage is essentially permanently eliminated[77] (however, recurrence of symptoms has been reported after partial and even seemingly-complete removal[76,82]).

For CMs treated surgically, patients need to be aware that post-op neurologic worsening is very common, especially with brainstem CMs.[83] Worsening may be transient,[84] but may take months to resolve.

82.7 Dural arteriovenous fistulae (DAVF)

82.7.1 General information

AKA dural AVMs (DAVM). Vascular abnormality in which an arteriovenous shunt is contained within the leaflets of the dura mater, exclusively supplied by branches of the internal/external carotid or vertebral arteries.[85] Because they are considered acquired rather than congenital lesions, the term fistula is preferred over malformation, although the latter term has also been used in the literature. Multiple fistulas may be found in up to 8% of cases.

Usually found adjacent to dural venous sinuses. Common locations:

1. transverse/sigmoid: the most common[86] (63% of cases) with a slight left-sided predominance,[87] with the epicenter of these almost invariably at the junction of the transverse and sigmoid sinuses
2. tentorial/petrosal
3. anterior fossa/ethmoidal
4. middle fossa/Sylvian
5. cavernous sinus (carotid-cavernous fistula – CCF)
6. superior sagittal sinus
7. foramen magnum

82.7.2 Etiology

Evidence suggests that most DAVFs are acquired, idiopathic lesions, and they have a well-recognized association with venous sinus thrombosis, although their exact pathogenesis is not fully understood. Theories include:

1. venous sinus occlusion awakens dormant embryonic dural arteriovenous channels[86]
2. venous hypertension/thrombosis promotes local angiogenesis and the de novo formation of DAVF[88]
3. the DAVF may arise first and itself result in venous sinus thrombosis[89]

82.7.3 Epidemiology

DAVFs comprise 10–15% of all intracranial AVMs.[87] 61–66% occur in females, and patients are usually in their 40 s or 50 s. They occur rarely in children, and when they do they tend to be complex, bilateral dural sinus malformations.[90]

82.7.4 Presentation

Common findings are listed in ► Table 82.9. Pulsatile tinnitus is the most common presenting symptom of a DAVF. Cortical venous drainage with resultant venous hypertension can produce IC-HTN,

Table 82.9 Clinical findings in 27 patients with dural AVMs[91]

Sign/symptom	No. (%)
pulsatile tinnitus	25 (92%)
occipital bruit	24 (89%)
headache	11 (41%)
visual impairment	9 (33%)
papilledema	7 (26%)

Table 82.10 Borden classification

Type	Features
I	DAVF drainage into a dural venous sinus or meningeal veins, with normal anterograde flow. Usually clinically benign.
II	DAVF draining anterograde into dural venous sinus, but with retrograde flow into cortical veins.
III	DAVF with direct retrograde flow from fistula into cortical veins causing venous hypertension.
Above further subclassified into a: with single hole and b: multiple holes	

and this is the most common cause of morbidity and mortality and thus the strongest indication for DAVF treatment. DAVFs may also cause global cerebral edema or hydrocephalus due to poor cerebral venous drainage or by impairing the function of the arachnoid granulations, respectively. Other DAVF symptoms/signs include headaches, seizures, cranial nerve palsies, and orbital venous congestion. a.

82.7.5 Evaluation

General information

Brain CT or MRI without contrast are often normal. CTA may reveal dilated tortuous vessels corresponding to enlarged arterial feeders or ectatic draining veins. MRA may reveal dilated pial vessels, early prominent venous sinus filling, sinus enlargement or occlusion, and white matter edema related to venous hypertension. Full 6 vessel cerebral angiography (bilateral ICAs, bilateral ECAs, bilateral vertebral arteries) is required to establish the diagnosis and to plan treatment.

Angiographic classification

Several classification systems have been described to characterize DAVFs. The Borden[92] (▶ Table 82.10) and the Cognard[93] (▶ Table 82.11) systems have emerged as the most commonly utilized contemporary grading schemes. See Tables. Cortical venous drainage is the defining angiographic feature that distinguishes benign (low-grade) from aggressive (high-grade) fistulas. (Borden I, Cognard I, and Cognard IIa are low-grade, all others are high-grade.)

Borden classification system

The Borden classification[92] is shown in ▶ Table 82.10.

Cognard angiographic classification

The Cognard system[93] is shown in ▶ Table 82.11. This system is generally most applicable to DAVFs involving the transverse sinus.

Cognard found 54% had no cortical venous reflux (Types I and IIa) and usually exhibit benign behavior.

* Key determinant: in the Cognard system, the pattern of venous drainage is the most critical factor. As a general rule, lesions with retrograde flow in the cortical veins (IIb, IIa+b, III & IV – red frames in ▶ Table 82.11) are high risk (for bleeding or intracranial hypertension…).

82.7.6 Natural history

The concept of benign vs aggressive DAVF behavior based on the absence or presence, respectively, of cortical venous drainage was validated by data reported by University of Toronto group. Over a 3 year period, 98% of benign lesions (no cortical venous drainage) remained benign.[94] On the other hand, over a 4 year period, annual rates of hemorrhage, non-hemorrhagic neurologic deficit, and mortality were 8.1%, 6.9%, and 10.4% for aggressive lesions (with cortical venous drainage).[95]

In a meta-analysis of 377 cases,[96] three DAVF locations were associated with particularly aggressive behavior (aggressive:benign ratio) – tentorial (31:1), middle fossa/sylvian (2.5:1), anterior fossa/ethmoidal 2.1:1).

82.7.7 Management

General information

Lesions with cortical venous drainage should generally be treated. Lesions without cortical venous drainage should be followed radiographically and clinically (2% may evolve to develop cortical venous drainage). A change in a bruit (either worsening, or disappearance) should prompt restudy.

Indications for intervention:

1. presence of cortical venous drainage
2. neurologic dysfunction
3. hemorrhage
4. orbital venous congestion
5. refractory symptoms (headache, pulsatile tinnitus)

Manual carotid self compression

Advocated by some, the thrombosis rate of ≈ 22% and clinical improvement rate of 33%[97] may mimic the natural course. Patients are advised to compress with the hand that would be affected by ischemia if it were to occur (e.g. with a left-sided DAVF, the right hand should be used to compress the left carotid artery). That way, the hand would fall away if ischemia develops. Recommendations vary, one option: start with 10 minutes once a day, gradually increase frequency and duration.

Endovascular embolization

May be performed transarterial or transvenous. Before the availability of liquid embolic agents (Onyx and NBCA), treatment was directed at the *venous* drainage (unlike pial AVMs) which had higher success, because the coils could be deployed to sacrifice the venous drainage very close to point of arteriovenous shunting, resulting in thrombosis of the fistula. It is more difficult to deploy coils across the point of arteriovenous shunting from the arterial side, whereas the liquid embolic agents, particularly Onyx, can be injected at somewhat of a distance and pushed forward across the fistulous point. Whether a transarterial, transvenous, or combined approach is utilized depends on the unique angioarchitecture of the fistula.

Surgery

While endovascular approaches have emerged as the primary treatment for most DAVFs, certain fistula types are still best dealt with via open surgery as the first line strategy.[98] Furthermore, surgery has been used to successfully treat DAVFs after previous partial, incomplete, or failed endovascular treatment. Finally, surgery can be used adjunctively in a combined approach to provide direct access for embolization of DAVFs that are inaccessible by a purely endovascular route.

Preoperative embolization may facilitate surgical treatment[99] by lessening the risk of catastrophic hemorrhage, which may occur simply during the performance of the craniotomy.[91] The use of the crainiotome is discouraged, as a sinus or venous laceration could produce a fatal hemorrhage. Contingencies for the rapid administration of blood products must be made (large bore central lines). The scalp incision, craniotomy flap, and dural incision should be planned in a strategic manner to control and sequentially eliminate the blood supply to the lesion at each step, while maximizing the exposure as needed. Surgical options for the treatment of DAVFs include the following techniques[98]:

1. radical fistula excision
2. sinus skeletonization

Table 82.11 Angiographic classification of dural AVMS[93a]

<table>
<tr><th colspan="2">Venous drainage: sinus</th></tr>
<tr><td>Type I
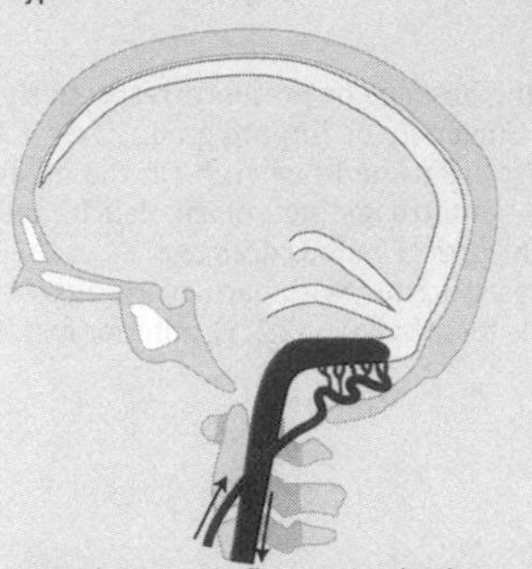
Normal antegrade flow into a dural venous sinus
Course: benign[b]</td><td>Type IIa
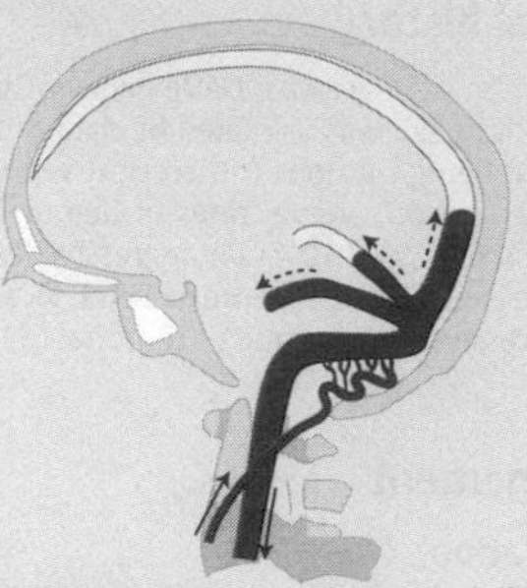
Drainage into a sinus with retrograde flow within the sinus[c]
Course: sinus reflux caused IC-HTN in 20%</td></tr>
<tr><td>Type IIb
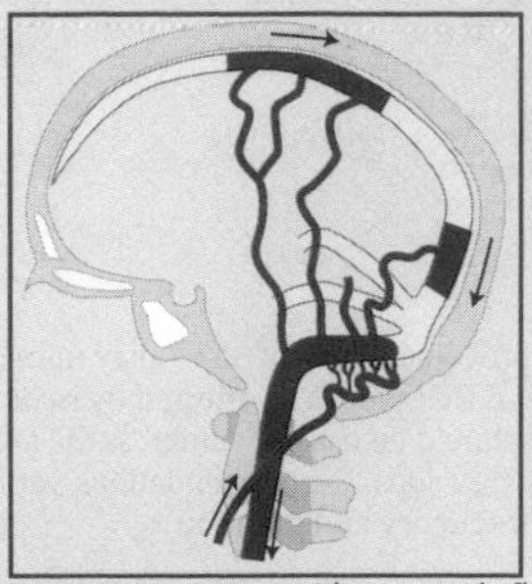
Drainage into a sinus with retrograde flow into cortical vein(s)
Course: reflux into veins induced hemorrhage in 10%</td><td>Type IIa + b
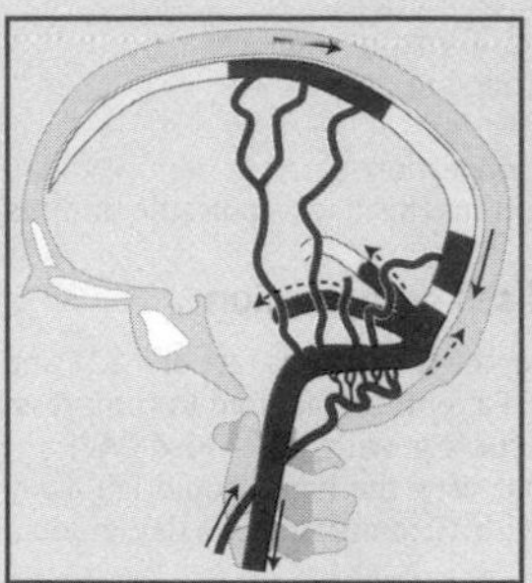
Drainage into a sinus with retrograde flow within the sinus[c] and cortical vein(s)
Course: aggressive in 66% with bleeding and/or IC-HTN</td></tr>
<tr><th colspan="2">Venous drainage: directly into cortical veins</th></tr>
<tr><td>Type III
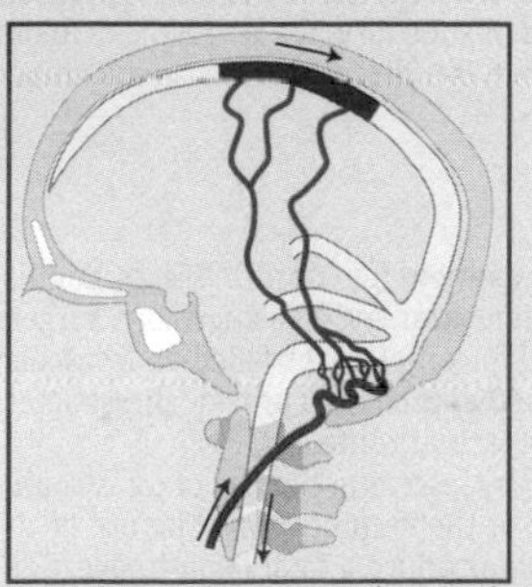
Direct drainage into a cortical vein without venous ectasia Description: direct cortical venous drainage without venous ectasia
Course: hemorrhage occurs in 40%</td><td>Type IV
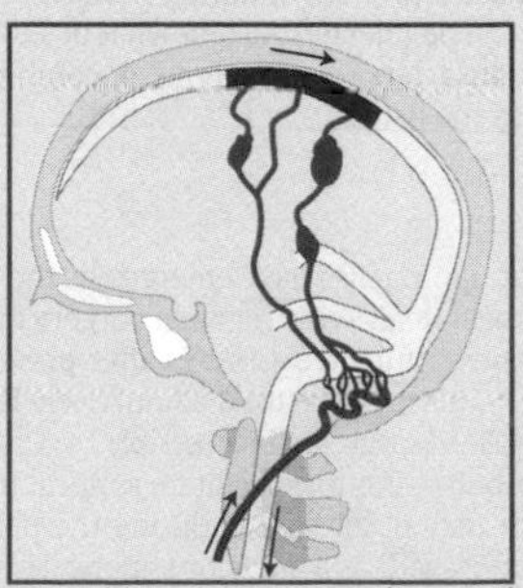
Direct drainage into a cortical vein with venous ectasia
Course: hemorrhage occurs in 65%</td></tr>
</table>

Venous drainage: spinal in addition to all of the above
Type V 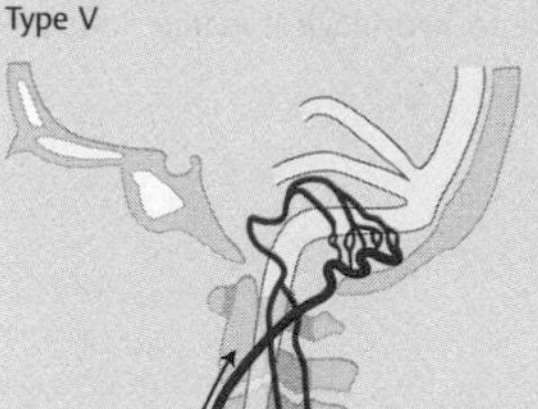 Direct drainage into spinal perimedullary veins in addition to all of the above Course: progressive myelopathy in 50%
[a]those in red boxes are high risk for bleeding or intracranial hypertension [b]despite a usually good prognosis, ≈ 2% will progress and therefore follow-up studies may be warranted [c]dashed arrows signify retrograde flow

3. disconnection of cortical venous drainage
4. ligation of the fistulous point and/or outflow vein
5. sinus packing
6. coagulation of arterial feeders to the lesion

While surgery vs. endovascular treatment can be considered for all DAVF locations, two locations generally remain more favorable for surgery:
1. anterior fossa/ethmoidal
2. tentorial DAVFs

The endovascular approach to these fistulas is difficult whereas the surgical approach is often straightforward. Surgically-assisted embolization, whereby a craniotomy is performed followed by direct puncture for embolization of the target vessel, may be utilized in select cases.

Stereotactic radiosurgery

May be used post-embolization.[100] Pan et al[101] reported a complete obliteration rate of 58% of transverse/sigmoid fistulae treated with only radiosurgery (1650–1900 cGy) or with radiosurgery after surgery/embolization had failed to produce complete obliteration. 71% of the patients were cured of their symptoms.

With the continued improvement of endovascular technology over the past two decades, the role of radiosurgery for DAVF treatment has steadily decreased; however, it remains an option for those difficult lesions in which endovascular/surgical options have been exhausted.

82.8 Vein of Galen malformation

82.8.1 General information

Enlargement of the great cerebral vein of Galen (VOG) may occur in "vein of Galen malformations" (VOGM) (some refer to these as vein of Galen aneurysms). Congenital, develop before the 3-month embryo stage, and probably consists not of the vein of Galen but rather of the medial vein of the prosencephalon) or secondarily to high flow from adjacent deep parenchymatous AVMs or pial fistulae. Parenchymatous AVMs can be distinguished from true VOG malformations by retrograde filling of the of the internal cerebral vein in the former.[102]

True VOG malformations are predictably fed from the medial and lateral choroidal, circumferential, mesencephalic, anterior choroidal, pericallosal and meningeal arteries.[102,103] Agenesis of the straight sinus may be an associated finding.

82.8.2 Presentation

Newborns tend to present with congestive heart failure in first few weeks of life (due to high blood flow)[104] and a cranial bruit. Hydrocephalus may result from obstruction of the sylvian aqueduct by the enlarged VOG, or it may be caused by the increased venous pressure (which can also produce prominence of the scalp veins[105]).

Parenchymatous AVMs are usually diagnosed later in life due to neurological manifestations[106] including focal neurologic deficit and hemorrhage.

82.8.3 Classification

Classified based on the location of the fistula[107,108]:

1. pure internal fistulae: single or multiple
2. fistulae between thalamoperforators and the VOG
3. mixed form: the most common
4. plexiform AVMs

82.8.4 Natural history

Untreated VOG malformations have a poor prognosis, with neonates having nearly 100% mortality, and 1–12 month olds having ≈ 60% mortality, 7% major morbidity, and 21% being normal.[109]

Parenchymatous AVMs behave similar to other AVMs.

82.8.5 Treatment

Hydrocephalus

Hydrocephalus associated with VOGM is obstructive, due to the varix. Although admonitions about shunting were common due to fear of precipitating a hemorrhage, when hydrocephalus is present the patient needs a shunt.

Vein of Galen malformations

Pediatric patients are often in poor medical condition, limiting the efficacy of operative treatment. Treatment options for these include embolization of the main feeding arteries. Prognosis is poor. Those presenting with hydrocephalus from aqueductal obstruction often do so at the end of the first year of life. Neurosurgical excision may be considered here, and the prognosis is better.

Repeated embolization while monitoring the venous drainage is employed.

Parenchymal AVM with enlarged VOG

The AVM is treated by the same methods as other AVMs (embolization, resection or radiosurgery).

82.9 Carotid-cavernous fistula

82.9.1 General information

Key concepts

- direct (high flow, from ICA) or indirect (low flow, from meningeal branches)
- classic triad (more common with direct CCF): chemosis, pulsatile proptosis, ocular bruit
- risk of SAH is low. Major risk is to vision
- natural history of low flow CCF is up to 50% spontaneous thrombosis

See also anatomy and venous inflow and outflow of the cavernous sinus (p. 86).

Carotid-cavernous fistula (CCF): divided into direct (Type A) and indirect (Types B-D)[110]:

1. Type A: direct high-flow shunts between the *internal* carotid artery and cavernous sinus:
   a) traumatic (including iatrogenic): occur in 0.2% of patients with craniocerebral trauma. Iatrogenic: may follow percutaneous trigeminal rhizotomy,[111] endovascular procedures…
   b) spontaneous: usually due to ruptured cavernous sinus ICA aneurysm. May also occur in patients with connective tissue disorders
2. indirect (dural): most are shunts: from dural arteries that are branches of the *external* carotid (not from ICA) (exception: Type B) – low flow

a) Type B: from meningeal branches of the internal carotid artery (ICA)
b) Type C: from meningeal branches of the external carotid artery (ECA)
c) Type D: from meningeal branches of both the ICA and ECA

82.9.2 Presentation

1. orbital and/or retro-orbital pain
2. chemosis (arteriolization of conjunctiva)
3. pulsatile proptosis
4. ocular and/or cranial bruit
5. deterioration of visual acuity: may be due to hypoxic retinopathy as a result of reduced arterial pressure and increased venous pressure and increased intraocular pressure
6. diplopia: abducens (VI) palsy is the most common
7. pupillary dilatation
8. ophthalmoplegia (usually unilateral, but may present initially as bilateral or may progress to bilateral)
9. increased intraocular pressure
10. neo-vascularization of the iris or retina
11. rarely: SAH

Indirect CCFs generally have a more gradual onset and milder presentation than direct.

82.9.3 Evaluation

CT or MRI: usually demonstrates proptosis. Serpiginous and engorged intraocular vessels including the superior ophthalmic vein (best seen on T2WI coronals – helps to differentiate from rectus muscles) and convexity of lateral wall of cavernous sinus.

Angiography: shunting of blood from ICA into cavernous sinus. Rapid opacification of petrosal sinus and/or ophthalmic vein may be seen.

1. Huber maneuver: lateral view, inject VA and manually compress affected carotid. Helps identify upper extent of fistula, multiple fistulous openings, and complete transection of ICA
2. Mehringer-Hieshima maneuver: inject contrast at a rate of 2 3 ml/s into affected carotid while compressing the carotid in the neck (below the catheter tip) to control flow to help demonstrate the fistula

82.9.4 Treatment

General information

20–50% of *low flow* CCF spontaneously thrombose, therefore one may observe these as long as visual acuity is stable and intra-ocular pressure is <≈ 25. Symptomatic (e.g. progressive visual deterioration) high-flow CCFs rarely resolve spontaneously, and urgent treatment is usually indicated. Treatment is usually in the form of embolization by an interventional neuroradiologist or trapping between surgically placed clips.

Even if normal ocular motility cannot be achieved in affected eye, preservation of vision is desirable because:

1. for some oclar motility abnormalities, surgical treatment may reduce diplopia
2. patient may be provided with frosted eyeglass lens which will eliminate diplopia but will maintain peripheral vision
3. in the rare event of injury to contralateral eye (trauma, central retinal artery occlusion…) there would be "reserve" vision in the eye with reduced motility (with loss of the other eye, there would not be diplopia)

Indications for treatment

1. proptosis
2. visual loss
3. cranial nerve VI palsy
4. intractable bruit
5. severely elevated intraocular pressure
6. increased filling of cortical veins on angiography

Endovascular treatment

Options include:
1. Electrolytically detachable coils
2. Amplatzer vascular plug

Routes available include:
1. transarterial through internal carotid. If this fails (e.g. wide aneurysm neck), the carotid artery may be occluded on either side of fistula to trap it (sacrifices carotid artery, therefore test occlusion must be done first to determine if patient can tolerate this; however **note**: test occlusion with an open fistula may give false positive result because steal through the fistula may reduce CBF and cause neurologic symptoms not related to the occlusion acting alone). The distal occlusion needs to be proximal to the ophthalmic artery
2. transarterial through external carotid: useful only for dural fistulas
3. transvenous:
   a) traversing heart to enter jugular vein, then through petrosal sinus to cavernous sinus. Lower success rate (≈ 20%) than transarterial route
   b) via superior ophthalmic vein: entered where supra-optic vein enters orbit to become superior ophthalmic vein. If possible, it is best to wait for the vein to become arterialized by the high flow pressure. Reports of "disasters" due to injury to the fragile vein performed before arteriolization took place may have been due to more primitive balloon catheters that were standard before current commercially produced versions were available (which are softer than original). Must avoid lacerating the vein inside the orbit, and avoid distal ligation of the vein without proximal occlusion (shunts even more blood into eye)

Choice of technique

With indirect fistulas, it is mandatory to place coils on the venous side (otherwise new feeders will be recruited).

Coils or clips may be used to occlude direct fistulas.

82.10 Sigmoid sinus diverticulum

Sigmoid sinus diverticulum (SSD, see ▶ Fig. 82.1) or sigmoid sinus dehiscence is found in 1.2% of asymptomatic patients.[112] However, these abnormalities may be found ipsilaterally in up to 23% of patients with pulsatile tinnitus, presumably due to turbulent flow which may occur in these abnormalities.[113] SSD are more common in women.

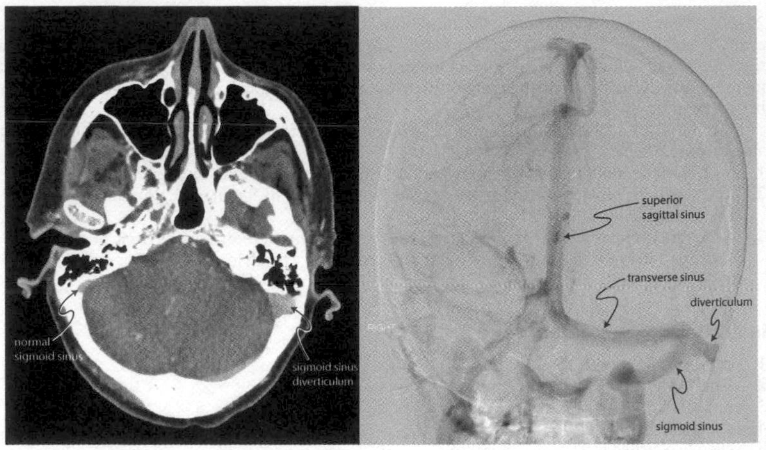

Fig. 82.1 Axial contrast head CT (left) and AP venous phase angiogram (right) showing sigmoid sinus diverticulum on the patient's left side.

When treatments such as masking noise generators fail, surgical intervention can be considered. Surgical treatment options include:

- Endovascular coiling/stenting
- Transmastoid "resurfacing" (see below)
- Craniectomy with clip reconstruction

Transmastoid "resurfacing" consists of partial mastoidectomy, and subtotal obliteration of the area of the diverticulum (so-called sinus wall resurfacing[[113]Otto, 2007 #7186][114]) with e.g. bone chips, fibrin glue, or muscle.

References

[1] McCormick WF. The Pathology of Vascular ('Arteriovenous') Malformations. J Neurosurg. 1966; 24:807–816

[2] Lobato RD, Perez C, Rivas JJ, Cordobes F. Clinical, Radiological, and Pathological Spectrum of Angiographically Occult Intracrtanial Vascular Malformations. J Neurosurg. 1988; 68:518–531

[3] Perret G, Nishioka H. Report on the Cooperative Study of Intracranial Aneurysms and Subarachnoid Hemorrhage: Arteriovenous Malformations. J Neurosurg. 1966; 25:467–490

[4] Ondra SL, Troupp H, George ED, Schwab K. The Natural History of Symptomatic Arteriovenous Malformations of the Brain: A 24-Year Follow-Up Assessment. J Neurosurg. 1990; 73:387–391

[5] Drake CG. Cerebral AVMs: Considerations for and Experience with Surgical Treatment in 166 Cases. Clin Neurosurg. 1979; 26:145–208

[6] Kupersmith MJ, Vargas ME, Yashar A, Madrid M, Nelson K, Seton A, Berenstein A. Occipital arteriovenous malformations: visual disturbances and presentation. Neurology. 1996; 46:953–957

[7] Hartmann A, Mast H, Mohr JP, et al. Morbidity of Intracranial Hemorrhage in Patients with Cerebral Arteriovenous Malformation. Stroke. 1998; 29:931–934

[8] Morgan M, Sekhon L, Rahman Z, Dandie G. Morbidity of Intracranial Hemorrhage in Patients with Cerebral Arteriovenous Malformation. Stroke. 1998; 29

[9] Crawford PM, West CR, Chadwick DW, Shaw MDM. Arteriovenous Malformations of the Brain: Natural History in Unoperated Patients. J Neurol Neurosurg Psychiatry. 1986; 49:1–10

[10] Spetzler RF, Hargraves RW, McCormick PW, Zabramski JM, et al. Relationship of Perfusion Pressure and Size to Risk of Hemorrhage from Arteriovenous Malformations. J Neurosurg. 1992; 76:918–923

[11] Jayaraman MV, Marcellus ML, Do HM, Chang SD, Rosenberg JK, Steinberg GK, Marks MP. Hemorrhage rate in patients with Spetzler-Martin grades IV and V arteriovenous malformations: is treatment justified? Stroke. 2007; 38:325–329

[12] Stapf C, Mast H, Sciacca RR, Choi JH, Khaw AV, Connolly ES, Pile-Spellman J, Mohr JP. Predictors of hemorrhage in patients with untreated brain arteriovenous malformation. Neurology. 2006; 66:1350–1355

[13] Kondziolka D, McLaughlin MR, Kestle JRW. Simple Risk Predictions for Arteriovenous Malformation Hemorrhage. Neurosurgery. 1995; 37:851–855

[14] Graf CJ, Perret GE, Torner JC. Bleeding from Cerebral Arteriovenous Malformations as Part of Their Natural History. J Neurosurg. 1983; 58:331–337

[15] Fults D, Kelly DL. Natural History of Arteriovenous Malformations of the Brain: A Clinical Study. Neurosurgery. 1984; 15:658–662

[16] Cunha MJ, Stein BM, Solomon RA, McCormick PC. The Treatment of Associated Intracranial Aneurysms and Arteriovenous Malformations. J Neurosurg. 1992; 77:853–859

[17] Hamilton MG, Spetzler RF. The Prospective Application of a Grading System for Arteriovenous Malformations. Neurosurgery. 1994; 34:2–7

[18] Spetzler RF, Martin NA. A Proposed Grading System for Arteriovenous Malformations. J Neurosurg. 1986; 65:476–483

[19] Spetzler RF, Ponce FA. A 3-tier classification of cerebral arteriovenous malformations. Clinical article. J Neurosurg. 2011; 114:842–849

[20] Laing RW, Childs J, Brada M. Failure of Conventionally Fractionated Radiotherapy to Decrease the Risk of Hemorrhage in Inoperable Arteriovenous Malformations. Neurosurgery. 1992; 30:872–876

[21] Redekop GJ, Elisevich KV, Gaspar LE, Wiese KP, Drake CG. Conventional Radiation Therapy of Intracranial Arteriovenous Malformations: Long-Term Results. J Neurosurg. 1993; 78:413–422

[22] Andrade-Souza YM, Ramani M, Scora D, Tsao MN, terBrugge K, Schwartz ML. Embolization before radiosurgery reduces the obliteration rate of arteriovenous malformations. Neurosurgery. 2007; 60:443–51; discussion 451-2

[23] Jafar JJ, Davis AJ, Berenstein A, et al. The Effect of Embolization with N-Butyl Cyanoacrylate Prior to Surgical Resection of Cerebral Arteriovenous Malformations. J Neurosurg. 1993; 78:60–69

[24] Spetzler RF, Wilson CB, Weinstein P, et al. Normal Perfusion Pressure Breakthrough Theory. Clin Neurosurg. 1978; 25:651–672

[25] Orlowski JP, Shiesley D, Vidt DG, Barnett GH, et al. Labetalol to Control Blood Pressure After Cerebrovascular Surgery. Crit Care Med. 1988; 16:765–768

[26] Young WL, Kader A, Prohovnik I, et al. Pressure Autoregulation Is Intact After Arteriovenous Malformation Resection. Neurosurgery. 1993; 32:491–497

[27] al-Rodhan NRF, Sundt TM, Piepgras DG, et al. Occlusive Hyperemia: A Theory for the Hemodynamic Complications Following Resection of Intracerebral Arteriovenous Malformations. J Neurosurg. 1993; 78:167–175

[28] Wilson CB, Hieshima G. Occlusive hyperemia: A new way to think about an old problem. J Neurosurg. 1993; 78:165–166

[29] Steiger HJ, Tew JM. Hemorrhage and Epilepsy in Cryptic Cerebrovascular Malformations. Arch Neurol. 1984; 41:722–724

[30] Wilkins RH, Rengachary SS. Neurosurgery. New York 1985

[31] Cohen HCM, Tucker WS, Humphreys RP, et al. Angiographically Cryptic Histologically Verified Cerebrovascular Malformations. Neurosurgery. 1982; 10:704–714

[32] Shuey HM, Day AL, Quisling RG, et al. Angiographically Cryptic Cerebrovascular Malformations. Neurosurgery. 1979; 5:476–479

[33] Ropper AH, Davis KR. Lobar Cerebral Hemorrhages: Acute Clinical Syndromes in 26 Cases. Ann Neurol. 1980; 8:141–147

[34] Russell DS. The Pathology of Spontaneous Intracranial Hemorrhage. Proc R Soc Med. 1954; 47:689–693

[35] Bitoh S, Hasegawa H, Fujiwara M, et al. Angiographically Occult Vascular Malformations Causing Intracranial Hemorrhage. Surg Neurol. 1982; 17:35–42

[36] Willemse RB, Mager JJ, Westermann CJ, Overtoom TT, Mauser H, Wolbers JG. Bleeding risk of cerebrovascular malformations in hereditary hemorrhagic telangiectasia. J Neurosurg. 2000; 92:779–784

[37] Lemme-Plaghos L, Kucharczyk W, Brant-Zawalski M, et al. MRI of Angiographically Occult Vascular Malformations. AJNR. 1986; 7:217–222

[38] Needell WM, Maravilla KR. MR Flow Imaging in Vascular Malformations Using Gradient Recalled Acquisition. AJNR. 1988; 9:637–642

[39] Lindquist C, Guo W-Y, Kerlsson B, Steiner L. Radiosurgery for Venous Angiomas. J Neurosurg. 1993; 78:531–536

[40] Cosgrove GR, Bertrand G, Fontaine S, et al. Cavernous Angiomas of the Spinal Cord. J Neurosurg. 1988; 68:31–36

[41] Uranishi R, Baev NI, Ng PY, Kim JH, Awad IA. Expression of endothelial cell angiogenesis receptors in human cerebrovascular malformations. Neurosurgery. 2001; 48:359–67; discussion 367-8

[42] Detwiler PW, Porter RW, Zabramski JM, Spetzler RF. De novo formation of a central nervous system cavernous malformation: implications for predicting risk of hemorrhage. Case report and review of the literature. J Neurosurg. 1997; 87:629–632

[43] Clatterbuck RE, Moriarity JL, Elmaci I, Lee RR, Breiter SN, Rigamonti D. Dynamic nature of cavernous malformations: a prospective magnetic resonance imaging study with volumetric analysis. J Neurosurg. 2000; 93:981–986

[44] Wong JH, Awad IA, Kim JH. Ultrastructural pathological features of cerebrovascular malformations: a preliminary report. Neurosurgery. 2000; 46:1454–1459

[45] Simard JM, Garcia-Bengochea, Ballinger WE, et al. Cavernous angioma: A review of 126 collected and 12 new clinical cases. Neurosurgery. 1986; 18:162–172

[46] Moriarity JL, Wetzel M, Clatterbuck RE, et al. The natural history of cavernous malformations: a prospective study of 68 patients. Neurosurgery. 1999; 44:1166–1173

[47] Gross BA, Batjer HH, Awad IA, Bendok BR. Cavernous malformations of the basal ganglia and thalamus. Neurosurgery. 2009; 65:7–18; discussion 18-9

[48] Moran NF, Fish DR, Kitchen N, Shorvon S, Kendall BE, Stevens JM. Supratentorial cavernous haemangiomas and epilepsy: a review of the literature and case series. J Neurol Neurosurg Psychiatry. 1999; 66:561–568

[49] Rigamonti D, Drayer BP, Johnson PC, Hadley MN, Zabramski J, Spetzler RF. The MRI Appearance of Cavernous Malformations (Angiomas). J Neurosurg. 1987; 67:518–524

[50] Perlemuter G, Bejanin H, Fritsch J, Prat F, Gaudric M, Chaussade S, Buffet C. Biliary obstruction caused by portal cavernoma: a study of 8 cases. J Hepatol. 1996; 25:58–63

[51] Detwiler PW, Porter RW, Zabramski JM, Spetzler RF. Radiation-induced cavernous malformation. J Neurosurg. 1998; 89:167–169

[52] Maraire JN, Abdulrauf SI, Berger S, Knisely J, Awad IA. De novo development of a cavernous malformation of the spinal cord following spinal axis radiation. Case report. J Neurosurg. 1999; 90:234–238

[53] Cohen-Gadol AA, Jacob JT, Edwards DA, Krauss WE. Coexistence of intracranial and spinal cavernous malformations: a study of prevalence and natural history. J Neurosurg. 2006; 104:376–381

[54] Hayman LA, Evans RA, Ferrell RE, et al. Familial Cavernous Angiomas: Natural History and Genetic Study Over a 5-Year Period. Am J Med Genet. 1982; 11:147–160

[55] Robinson JR, Awad IA, Little JR. Natural history of the cavernous angioma. J Neurosurg. 1991; 75:709–714

[56] Del Curling OJr, Kelly DL, Jr, Elster AD, Craven TE. An analysis of the natural history of cavernous angiomas. J Neurosurg. 1991; 75:702–708

[57] Kim DS, Park YG, Choi JU, Chung SS, Lee KC. An analysis of the natural history of cavernous malformations. Surg Neurol. 1997; 48:9–17; discussion 17-8

[58] Al-Shahi Salman R, Berg MJ, Morrison L, Awad IA. Hemorrhage from cavernous malformations of the brain: definition and reporting standards. Angioma Alliance Scientific Advisory Board. Stroke. 2008; 39:3222–3230

[59] Kondziolka D, Lunsford LD, Kestle JRW. The natural history of cerebral cavernous malformations. J Neurosurg. 1995; 83:820–824

[60] Abdulrauf SI, Kaynar MY, Awad IA. A comparison of the clinical profile of cavernous malformations with and without associated venous malformations. Neurosurgery. 1999; 44:41–6; discussion 46-7

[61] Chen X, Weigel D, Ganslandt O, Buchfelder M, Nimsky C. Diffusion tensor imaging and white matter tractography in patients with brainstem lesions. Acta Neurochir (Wien). 2007; 149:1117–31; discussion 1131

[62] Zausinger S, Yousry I, Brueckmann H, Schmid-Elsaesser R, Tonn JC. Cavernous malformations of the brainstem: three-dimensional-constructive interference in steady-state magnetic resonance imaging for improvement of surgical approach and clinical results. Neurosurgery. 2006; 58:322–30; discussion 322-30

[63] Kondziolka D, Lunsford LD, Flickinger JC, Kestle JR. Reduction of hemorrhage risk after stereotactic radiosurgery for cavernous malformations. J Neurosurg. 1995; 83:825–831

[64] Porter RW, Detwiler PW, Han PP, Spetzler RF. Stereotactic radiosurgery for cavernous malformations: Kjellberg's experience with proton beam therapy in 98 cases at the Harvard Cyclotron. Neurosurgery. 1999; 44:424–425

[65] Zhang N, Pan L, Wang BJ, et al. Gamma knife radiosurgery for cavernous hemangiomas. J Neurosurg. 2000; 93:74–77

[66] Pollock BE, Garces YI, Stafford SL, Foote RL, Schomberg PJ, Link MJ. Stereotactic radiosurgery for cavernous malformations. J Neurosurg. 2000; 93:987–991

[67] Scott. Orlando, FL 2008

[68] Gross BA, Batjer HH, Awad IA, Bendok BR. Brainstem cavernous malformations. Neurosurgery. 2009; 64:E805–18; discussion E818

[69] Ferroli P, Sinisi M, Franzini A, Giombini S, Solero CL, Broggi G. Brainstem cavernomas: long-term results of microsurgical resection in 52 patients. Neurosurgery. 2005; 56:1203–12; discussion 1212-4

[70] Deshmukh VR, Albuquerque FC, Zabramski JM, Spetzler RF. Surgical management of cavernous malformations involving the cranial nerves. Neurosurgery. 2003; 53:352–7; discussion 357

[71] Albanese A, Sturiale CL, D'Alessandris QG, Capone G, Maira G. Calcified extra-axial cavernoma involving lower cranial nerves: technical case report. Neurosurgery. 2009; 64:135–6; discussion 136

[72] Itshayek E, Perez-Sanchez X, Cohen JE, Umansky F, Spektor S. Cavernous hemangioma of the third cranial nerve: case report. Neurosurgery. 2007; 61. DOI: 10.1227/01.NEU.0000290916.63094.8E

[73] Crocker M, Desouza R, King A, Connor S, Thomas N. Cavernous hemangioma of the optic chiasm: a surgical review. Skull Base. 2008; 18:201–212

[74] Bicknell JM. Familial Cavernous Angioma of the Brain Stem Dominantly Inherited in Hispanics. Neurosurgery. 1989; 24:102–105

[75] Ondra SL, Doty JR, Mahla ME, et al. Surgical Excision of a Cavernous Hemangioma of the Rostral Brain Stem: Case Report. Neurosurgery. 1988; 23:490–493

[76] Zimmerman RS, Spetzler RF, Lee KS, Zabramski JM, et al. Cavernous Malformations of the Brain Stem. J Neurosurg. 1991; 75:32–39

[77] Wascher TM, Spetzler RF, Carter LP, Spetzler RF, Hamilton MG. In: Cavernous malformations of the brain stem. Neurovascular Surgery. New York: McGraw-Hill; 1995:541–555

[78] Hasegawa T, McInerney J, Kondziolka D, Lee JY, Flickinger JC, Lunsford LD. Long-term results after stereotactic radiosurgery for patients with cavernous malformations. Neurosurgery. 2002; 50:1190–7; discussion 1197-8

[79] Liu KD, Chung WY, Wu HM, Shiau CY, Wang LW, Guo WY, Pan DH. Gamma knife surgery for cavernous hemangiomas: an analysis of 125 patients. J Neurosurg. 2005; 102 Suppl:81–86

[80] Karlsson B, Kihlstrom L, Lindquist C, Ericson K, Steiner L. Radiosurgery for cavernous malformations. J Neurosurg. 1998; 88:293–297
[81] Barker FG, II, Amin-Hanjani S, Butler WE, Lyons S, Ojemann RG, Chapman PH, Ogilvy CS. Temporal clustering of hemorrhages from untreated cavernous malformations of the central nervous system. Neurosurgery. 2001; 49:15–24; discussion 24-5
[82] Bertalanffy H, Gilsbach JM, Eggert HR, et al. Microsurgery of deep-seated cavernous angiomas: report of 26 cases. Acta Neurochir. 1991; 108:91–99
[83] Weil SM, Tew JM,Jr. Surgical management of brain stem vascular malformations. Acta Neurochir (Wien). 1990; 105:14–23
[84] Bartolomei J, Wecht DA, Chaloupka J, Fayad P, Awad IA. Occipital lobe vascular malformations: prevalence of visual field deficits and prognosis after therapeutic intervention. Neurosurgery. 1998; 43:415–21; discussion 421-3
[85] Malik GM, Pearce JE, Ausman JI. Dural Arteriovenous Malformations and Intracranial Hemorrhage. Neurosurgery. 1984; 15:332–339
[86] Graeb DA, Dolman CL. Radiological and Pathological Aspects of Dural Arteriovenous Fistulas. J Neurosurg. 1986; 64:962–967
[87] Arnautovic KI, Krisht AF. Transverse-Sigmoid Sinus Dural Arteriovenous Malformations. Contemp Neurosurg. 2000; 21:1–6
[88] Houser OW, Campbell JK, Campbell RJ, Sundt TM, Jr. Arteriovenous malformation affecting the transverse dural venous sinus–an acquired lesion. Mayo Clin Proc. 1979; 54:651–661
[89] Aminoff MJ. Vascular anomalies in the intracranial dura mater. Brain. 1973; 96:601–612
[90] Ashour R, Aziz-Sultan MA, Soltanolkotabi M, Schoeneman SE, Alden TD, Hurley MC, Dipatri AJ, Tomita T, Elhammady MS, Shaibani A. Safety and efficacy of onyx embolization for pediatric cranial and spinal vascular lesions and tumors. Neurosurgery. 2012; 71:773–784
[91] Sundt TM, Piepgras DG. The Surgical Approach to Arteriovenous Malformations of the Lateral and Sigmoid Dural Sinuses. J Neurosurg. 1983; 59:32–39
[92] Borden JA, Wu JK, Shucart WA. A proposed classification for spinal and cranial dural arteriovenous fistulous malformations and implications for treatment. J Neurosurg. 1995; 82:166–179
[93] Cognard C, Gobin YP, Pierot L, Bailly AL, Houdart E, Casasco A, Chiras J, Merland JJ. Cerebral dural arteriovenous fistulas: clinical and angiographic correlation with a revised classification of venous drainage. Radiology. 1995; 194:671–680
[94] Davies MA, Saleh J, Ter Brugge K, Willinsky R, Wallace MC. The natural history and management of intracranial dural arteriovenous fistulae. Part 1: benign lesions. Interv Neuroradiol. 1997; 3:295–302
[95] van Dijk JM, terBrugge KG, Willinsky RA, Wallace MC. Clinical course of cranial dural arteriovenous fistulas with long-term persistent cortical venous reflux. Stroke. 2002; 33:1233–1236
[96] Awad IA, Little JR, Akarawi WP, Ahl J. Intracranial dural arteriovenous malformations: factors predisposing to an aggressive neurological course. J Neurosurg. 1990; 72:839–850
[97] Halbach V, Higashida R, Hieshima G, Goto K, Norman D, Newton T. Dural fistulas involving the transverse and sigmoid sinuses: results of the treatment in 28 patients. Radiology. 1987; 163:443–447
[98] Ashour R, Morcos JJ, Spetzler RF, Kondziolka DS. In: Surgical Management of Cerebral Dural Arteriovenous Fistulae. Comprehensive Management of Arteriovenous Malformations of the Brain and Spine. Cambridge: Cambridge University Press; 2015:144–170
[99] Barnwell SL, Halbach VV, Higashida RT, Wilson CB, et al. Complex Dural Arteriovenous Fistulas: Results of Combined Endovascular and Neurosurgical Treatment in 16 Patients. J Neurosurg. 1989; 71:352–358
[100] Lewis AI, Tomsick TA, Tew JM. Management of Tentorial Dural Arteriovenous Malformations: Transarterial Embolization Combined with Stereotactic Radiation or Surgery. J Neurosurg. 1994; 81:851–859
[101] Pan DH, Chung WY, Guo WY, Wu HM, Liu KD, Shiau CY, Wang LW. Stereotactic radiosurgery for the treatment of dural arteriovenous fistulas involving the transverse-sigmoid sinus. J Neurosurg. 2002; 96:823–829
[102] Khayata MH, Casaco A, Wakhloo AK, Rekate HL, Carter LP, Spetzler RF, Hamilton MG. In: Vein of Galen malformations: intravascular techniques. Neurovascular Surgery. New York: McGraw-Hill; 1995:1029–1039
[103] Lasjaunias P, Rodesch G, Pruvost P, et al. Treatment of vein of Galen aneurysmal malformation. J Neurosurg. 1989; 70:746–750
[104] Cummings GR. Circulation in neonates with intracranial arteriovenous fistula and cardiac failure. Am J Cardiol. 1980; 45:1019–1024
[105] Strassburg HM. Macrocephaly is Not Always Due to Hydrocephalus. J Child Neurol. 1989; 4:S32–S40
[106] Clarisse J, Dobbelaere P, Rey C, et al. Aneurysms of the great vein of Galen. Radiological-anatomical study of 22 cases. J Neuroradiol. 1978; 5:91–102
[107] Yasargil MG. In: AVM of the brain, clinical considerations, general and specific operative techniques, surgical results, nonoperated cases, cavernous and venous angiomas, neuroanesthesia. Microneurosurgery. Stuttgart: Georg Thieme; 1988:317–396
[108] Litvak J, Yahr MD, Ransohoff J. Aneurysms of the great vein of Galen and mid-line cerebral arteriovenous anomalies. J Neurosurg. 1960; 17:945–954
[109] Johnston IH, Whittle IR, Besser M, Morgan MK. Vein of Galen malformation: diagnosis and management. Neurosurgery. 1987; 20:747–758
[110] Barrow DL, Spector RH, Braun IF, Tindall GT, et al. Classification and Treatment of Spontaneous Carotid-Cavernous Fistulas. J Neurosurg. 1985; 62:248–256
[111] Kuether TA, O'Neill OR, Nesbit GM, Barnwell SL. Direct Carotid Cavernous Fistula After Trigeminal Balloon Microcompression Gangliolysis: Case Report. Neurosurgery. 1996; 39:853–856
[112] Schoeff S, Nicholas B, Mukherjee S, Kesser BW. Imaging prevalence of sigmoid sinus dehiscence among patients with and without pulsatile tinnitus. Otolaryngol Head Neck Surg. 2014; 150:841–846
[113] Song JJ, Kim YJ, Kim SY, An YS, Kim K, Lee SY, Koo JW. Sinus Wall Resurfacing for Patients With Temporal Bone Venous Sinus Diverticulum and Ipsilateral Pulsatile Tinnitus. Neurosurgery. 2015; 77:709–717
[114] Santa Maria PL. Sigmoid sinus dehiscence resurfacing as treatment for pulsatile tinnitus. J Laryngol Otol. 2013; 127 Suppl 2:S57–S59

Part XIX

Stroke and Occlusive Cerebrovascular Disease

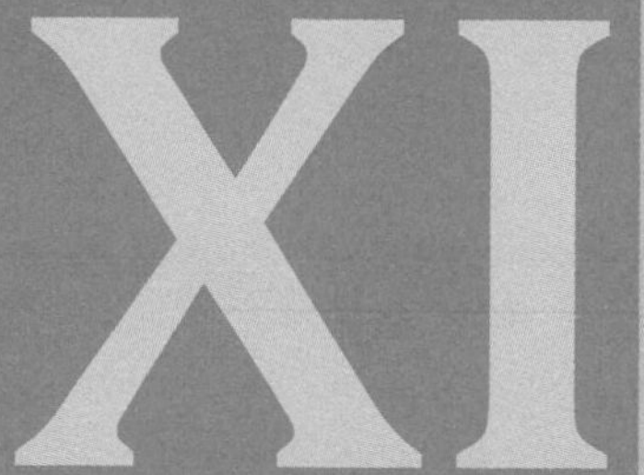

83 General Information and Stroke Physiology

83.1 Definitions

83

Stroke AKA cerebral infarction. Obsolete term: cerebrovascular accident (CVA).

► **TIA.** (Transient ischemic attack): transient neuronal dysfunction secondary to focal ischemia (of brain, spinal cord, or retina) without (permanent) acute infarction[1] (**note:** obsolete operational definitions used an arbitrary 24 hour cutoff for duration of symptoms).

10–15% of patients with TIA have a stroke within 3 months, 50% of which occur within 48 hours.

► **Stroke.** Permanent (i.e. irreversible) death of neurons caused by inadequate perfusion of a region of brain or brain stem.

► **Watershed infarct.** Ischemic infarction in a territory located at the periphery of two bordering arterial distributions due to a disturbance in flow in one or both of the arteries.

83.2 Cerebrovascular hemodynamics

83.2.1 Cerebral blood flow (CBF) and oxygen utilization

► Table 83.1 shows typical CBF values and the corresponding neurophysiologic state. CBF < 20 is generally associated with ischemia and if prolonged will produce cell death.[2] However, this assumes normal metabolic rate and may be more applicable to global cerebral hypoperfusion.[3] There is a higher CBF threshold for loss of electrical excitability than that for cell death – this has led to the concept of the ischemic penumbra – nonfunctioning cells that are still viable.[2]

CBF is related to blood pressure as shown in Eq (83.1).

$$CBF = \frac{CPP}{CVR} = \frac{MAP - ICP}{CVR} \quad (83.1)$$

where CPP = cerebral perfusion pressure (p.856), CVR = cerebrovascular resistance (see below), and MAP = mean arterial pressure.

83.2.2 Cerebrovascular resistance (CVR)

CVR is affected by the $PaCO_2$ such that there is a linear increase in CBF with increasing $PaCO_2$ within the range of 20–80 mm Hg.

CVR is also affected by changes in CPP which produce changes in blood vessel tone via a myogenic mechanism. In the range of CPP = 50–150 mm Hg the CVR of normal brain tissue varies linearly to

Table 83.1 Correlates of CBF

CBF (ml per 100 gm tissue/min)	Condition
> 60 (approx)	hyperemia (CBF > tissue demand)
45–60	normal brain at rest
75–80	gray matter
20–30	white matter
< 20: Ischemia	
16–18	EEG becomes flatline
15	physiologic paralysis
12	brainstem auditory evoked response (BAER) changes
10	alterations in cell membrane transport (cell death; stroke)

maintain an almost constant CBF. This phenomenon is called (cerebral) autoregulation, which is altered in pathologic states.

83.2.3 Cerebral metabolic rate of oxygen consumption ($CMRO_2$)

$CMRO_2$ averages 3.0–3.8 ml/100 gm tissue/min. The ratio of CBF to $CMRO_2$ (the coupling ratio[4]) in the quiescent brain is 14–18. With focal cortical activity, local CBF increases ≈ 30% while $CMRO_2$ increases ≈ 5%.[5] $CMRO_2$ can be manipulated to some degree.

83.2.4 Cerebrovascular reserve and reactivity

May be evaluated with xenon-enhanced CT, CTP (p.228), TCD, SPECT, or MRI.[6,7,8,9] Response of CBF to a vasodilator challenge with 1000 mg of IV acetazolamide (ACZ) (Diamox®) is classified as[8,9]:

Type I: normal baseline CBF with 30–60% increase following ACZ challenge

Type II: decreased baseline CBF with blunted response of < 10% increase or < 10 ml/100 g/min absolute increase after ACZ challenge

Type III: decreased baseline CBF with paradoxical decrease of regional CBF following ACZ challenge, suggesting a steal phenomenon in regions with maximally dilated vasculature at baseline

83.3 Collateral circulation

83.3.1 Collateral circulation for ICA stenosis/occlusion

The effects of ICA stenosis/occlusion may be ameliorated by collateral blood flow. Potential alternate routes for blood to reach brain tissue include:

1. flow through the circle of Willis
   a) from contralateral ICA through anterior communicating a.
   b) from forward flow through the ipsilateral posterior communicating a.
2. retrograde flow through *ophthalmic a.* parasitizing blood from *both* ECAs via:
   a) facial a. → angular a. → dorsal nasal a. & medial palpebral a.
   b) maxillary a.
      - middle meningeal a. → lacrimal a.
      - vidian a. (a. of the pterygoid canal)
   c) transverse facial a. → lateral palpebral a.
   d) superficial temporal a. → supraorbital a.
3. proximal maxillary a. → anterior tympanic a. → caroticotympanic branch of ICA
4. cortical-cortical anastomoses
5. dural-leptomeningeal anastomoses

83.3.2 Collateral circulation for vertebrobasilar stenosis/occlusion

Available collaterals depend on the site of occlusion.

Basilar artery occlusion. Collateral flow via:

1. posterior communicating aa.
2. anastomoses between SCA and PICA

Proximal vertebral artery (VA) occlusion. Collateral flow via:

1. ECA → occipital a. → muscular branches of VA → VA
2. thyrocervical trunk → ascending cervical a. → direct connection or spinal radicular aa.→ VA
3. contralateral VA and/or ascending cervical a. via spinal radicular branches and anterior spinal artery

83.4 "Occlusion" syndromes

83.4.1 Occlusion of major vessels organized by vascular territories

See ► Fig. 2.1 for the distribution territories of the major cerebral arteries. To indicate lateralization of findings, {CL} = contralateral, {IL} = ipsilateral.

83

Internal carotid artery and its branches

Risk and extent of stroke is influenced by suddenness of occlusion, location of occlusion, and collateral circulation (see above)

1. statistics:
   a) acute ICA occlusion (all comers): 26–49% risk of stroke[10] (not all of these strokes are severe)
   b) annual stroke risk in 1261 patients with symptomatic ICA occlusion: 7% overall, 5.9% ipsilateral to the occlusion (mean follow-up = 45.5 mos) (even with anticoagulation or antiplatelets drugs) (12 prospective studies[11])
   c) St. Louis Carotid Occlusion Study[12]: 2-year ipsilateral ischemic stroke rate in patients with symptomatic ICA occlusion = 5% in patients with normal O_2 extraction fraction (OEF) by PET scan, and 26% in patients with increased OEF
   d) stroke risk is less when one includes asymptomatic ICA occlusions (i.e. there are people walking around with ICA occlusion and no symptoms)
   e) in patients presenting with ICA territory stroke or TIA, complete ICA occlusion is found in 10–15%[12]
2. worst-case scenario of total ICA occlusion with no a-comm or p-comm flow and no collateral rescue: stroke in ACA and MCA territories (▶ Table 83.2)
3. anterior cerebral artery: {CL} weakness of LE > UE
4. posterior cerebral artery
   a) unilateral occipital lobe infarction → homonymous hemianopsia with macular sparing (visual cortex of the macula receives dual blood supply from MCA and PCA)
   b) Balint syndrome
   c) cortical blindness (Anton syndrome)
   d) Weber syndrome
   e) alexia without agraphia
   f) thalamic pain syndrome (Dejerine-Roussy syndrome)
5. artery of Percheron (p. 83): bilateral thalamic and mesencephalic infarctions[13]

Posterior circulation

1. vertebral artery
   a) medial medullary syndrome (Dejerine syndrome)
   b) lateral medullary syndrome (Wallenberg syndrome): see below
2. basilar artery
3. AICA: lateral pontine syndrome (Marie-Foix syndrome)

Table 83.2 Total ICA occlusion

Deficit[a]	complete (M1 occlusion)	superior division	inferior division
[CL] weakness of UE > LE	X	X	
[CL] weakness of lower face	X	X	
[CL] hemisensory loss (UE & LE)	X	X	
[CL] hemisensory loss face (all modalities)	X	X	
[CL] neglect[b]	X	X	
[IL] gaze preference	X		
[CL] homonymous hemianopsia	X		X[c]
receptive aphasia[d] (Wernicke's area)	X		X
expressive aphasia[d] (Broca's area)	X	X	
Gerstmann syndrome (p. 98): with dominant parietal lobe infarct			

[a][CL] = contralateral, [IL] = ipsilateral. An "X" indicates that the deficit is present
[b]with involvement on side of nondominant hemisphere
[c]plus [CL] upper quadrantanopsia
[d]with involvement on the side of the dominant hemisphere

4. PICA: sometimes lateral medullary (Wallenberg) syndrome: see below
5. SCA: infarction of superior cerebellar vermis and superior cerebellum
6. anterior spinal artery
7. recurrent medial striate artery (of Heubner): expressive aphasia + mild hemiparesis (UE > LE, proximal muscles weaker than distal)
8. anterior choroidal artery (AChA) syndrome: first described by Foix et al. in 1925. The complete triad consists of {CL} hemiplegia, hemihypesthesia and homonymous hemianopsia (mnemonic: 3 H's), however, incomplete forms are more common.[14] Occlusion is usually due to small vessel disease and CT or MRI usually shows infarct in posterior limb of IC (just above temporal horn of lateral vent)[15] and white matter posterior and lateral to it. Occlusion is usually tolerated fairly well, and ligation of this artery was actually utilized in treatment of Parkinsonism sometimes without ill effect[16(p 540)] – see Surgical treatment of Parkinson's disease (p. 1524) – but internal capsule infarct occurred in ≈ 15%.

Lateral medullary syndrome (LMS)

AKA Wallenberg's syndrome, AKA PICA syndrome. Classically attributed to PICA occlusion, but in 80–85% of cases the *vertebral artery* is also involved.[17] No cases have been reported arising from brainstem hemorrhage. Onset is usually acute. The findings are listed in ▶ Table 83.3(NB: *absence of pyramidal tract findings*, and *no change in sensorium*). The location of the lesion and medullary structures are shown in ▶ Fig. 83.1.

▶ **Note.** This is essentially the only location where a lesion will produce sensory loss on one side of the face (ipsilateral to the lesion) and contralateral sensory loss in the body. All in the absence of pyramidal tract findings (i.e. overt weakness).

These patients sometimes develop severe cerebellar swelling that responds to neurosurgical decompression (the tissue aspirates easily).

In a patient presenting with LMS, one needs to rule-out vertebral dissection (p. 1325) since this would be treated with heparin. MRI including fat-suppressed T1WI and MRA would detect dissection in most cases.

Prognosis: 12% of 43 patients died during the acute phase from respiratory and cardiovascular complications and 2 new posterior-fossa strokes occurred.[18] Recurrent vertebrobasilar territory stroke rate was 1.9% per year.[18]

83.4.2 Lacunar strokes

General information

Small infarcts in deep noncortical cerebrum or brainstem (▶ Table 83.4) resulting from occlusion of penetrating branches of cerebral arteries. Size of infarcts ranges from 3–20 mm (CT detects larger ones; better sensitivity in white matter).

Table 83.3 Findings in lateral medullary syndrome[16(p 547)]

GENERALIZED symptoms	Responsible lesion
• vertigo, N/V, nystagmus, diplopia, oscillopsia	vestibular nuclei & connections
• hiccups	?
IPSILATERAL to lesion	**Responsible lesion**
• facial pain, paresthesias, & impaired sensation	descending tract and nucleus V over half of face
• ataxia of limbs	(restiform body?)
• Horner's syndrome	descending sympathetic tract
• dysphagia, diminished gag, hoarseness	exiting fibers of IX & X
• numbness of arm, trunk, or leg	cuneate & gracile nuclei
CONTRALATERAL to lesion	**Responsible lesion**
• impaired pain & temp sense over half of body	spinothalamic tract

83

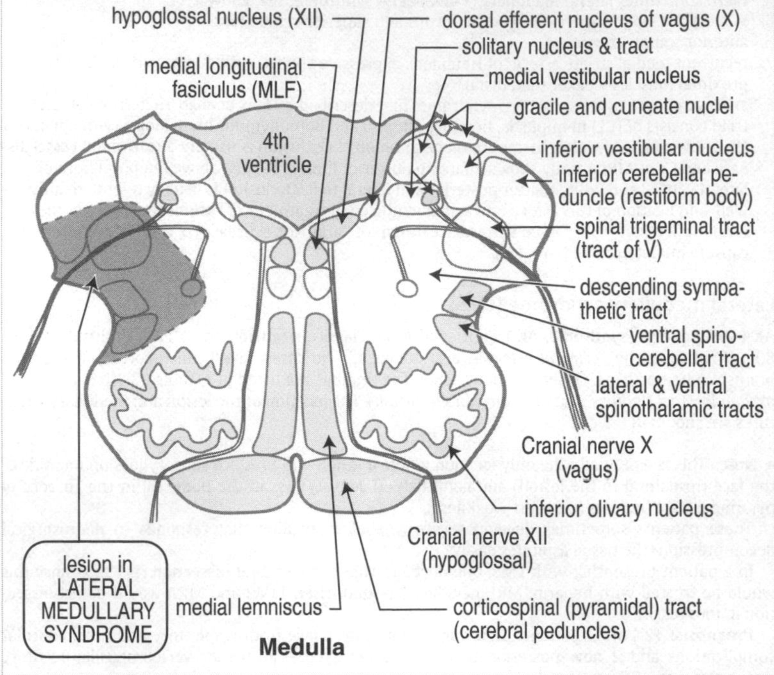

Fig. 83.1 Typical lesion in lateral medullary syndrome (indicated as shaded area)

Table 83.4 Typical locations for lacunar strokes *(in descending frequency)*

- putamen
- caudate
- thalamus
- pons
- internal capsule (IC)
- convolutional white matter

Small (3–7 mm) lacunes may be due to lipohyalinosis (vasculopathy due to HTN) of arteries < 200 microns (may also be cause of many ICHs); this vasculopathy is indicative of small vessel disease, unlikely to be prevented by carotid endarterectomy.

Clinically, diagnosis virtually *excluded* by: aphasia, apractagnosia, sensorimotor stroke, monoplegia, homonymous hemianopsia (**HH**), severe isolated memory impairment, stupor, coma, LOC, or seizures.

L'etat lacunaire: multiple lacunes → chronic progressive neuro decline with one or more episodes of hemiparesis; results in invalidism, dysarthria, small-step gait (marche á petits pas), imbalance, incontinence, pseudobulbar signs, dementia. Many signs and symptoms are possibly due to NPH (unrecognized originally).

Lacunar syndromes

Major syndromes (see reference[19] for others):

1. pure sensory stroke or TIA: (the most common lacunar manifestation) usually isolated unilateral numbness of face, arm, and leg. Only 10% of TIA go on to stroke. Lacune in sensory (posteroventral) thalamus → CT detection is poor. Dejerine-Roussy = rare thalamic pain syndrome that may develop late

2. pure motor hemiparesis (PMH): (2nd most common lacunar manifestation) pure unilateral motor deficit of face, arm and leg without sensory deficit, HH, etc. Lacune in posterior limb of IC, or in lower basis pontis where corticospinal (CS) tracts coalesce, or rarely in mid-cerebral peduncle
3. ataxic hemiparesis: contralateral PMH + cerebellar ataxia of affected limbs (if they can move). Lacune in basis pontis at junction of upper third and lower two-thirds → dysarthria, nystagmus and unidirectional toppling possible. Differential severity in face, arm and leg possible because CS fibers dispersed by nuclei pontis (unlike compact pyramids and peduncle)
   a) variant: dysarthria-clumsy hand syndrome: lesion in same location or genu of IC. May be mimicked by a cortical infarct, but latter will have numb lips
4. PMH sparing the face: lacune in medullary pyramid; at onset, there may be vertigo and nystagmus (approaching lateral medullary syndrome)
   a) variant: thalamic dementia: central region of one thalamus + adjacent subthalamus → abulia, memory impairment + partial Horner's (miosis + anhydrosis)
5. mesencephalothalamic syndrome: "top o' the basilar syndrome." Usually caused by embolus. Infarct typically butterfly shaped & bilateral involving rostral brainstem and cerebral hemisphere regions fed by the distal basilar artery. Clinical: III palsy, Parinaud's syndrome & abulia, may have amnesia, hallucinations and somnolence, usually without significant motor dysfunction
6. Weber's syndrome: Cr. N. III palsy with contralateral PMH (no sensory loss). Usually due to occlusion of interpeduncular branches of basilar artery → central midbrain infarction, disrupting cerebral peduncle and issuing fibers of III. May also be due to aneurysm of basilar bifurcation or BA-SCA junction
7. PMH with crossed VI palsy: lacune in paramedian inferior pons
8. cerebellar ataxia with crossed III palsy (*Claude* syndrome): lacune in dentatorubral tract (superior cerebellar peduncle)
9. hemiballism: classically, infarct or hemorrhage in subthalamic semilunar nucleus of Luys
10. lateral medullary syndrome: see below
11. locked-in syndrome: bilateral PMH from infarct at IC, pons, pyramid or (rarely) cerebral peduncles

83.5 Stroke in young adults

83.5.1 General information

Only 3% of ischemic strokes occur in patients < 40 yrs age.[20] Over 10% of ischemic strokes occur in patients ≤ 55 yrs.[21] Incidence: 10 per 100,000 persons age 35–44 yrs,[22] 73 per 100,000 for age < 55 yrs.[21]

83.5.2 Etiologies

The differential diagnosis is lengthy,[20] with *trauma* being the most common cause of strokes (22%) in patients under 45 yrs.[23] Most of the rest are covered by the small number of etiologies listed below (excludes: trauma, post-op stroke, SAH, and intracerebral hemorrhage).

1. atherosclerosis: 20% – less common than in older population (all 18 patients in one series had either ID-DM, or were males > 35 yrs with ≥ 1 risk factors (see below), most had TIAs earlier)
2. embolism with recognized source: 20%
   a) cardiac origin is the most common (above), most have previously known cardiac disease:
      - rheumatic heart disease
      - prosthetic valve
      - endocarditis
      - mitral valve prolapse (MVP): present in 5–10% of young adults, in 20–40% of young adults with stroke (although one series found MVP in only 2% of stroke in young adults[22])
      - A-fib
      - left-atrial myxoma
   b) fat embolism syndrome: neurologic manifestation is usually global neurologic dysfunction; see Fat embolism syndrome (p. 835)
   c) paradoxical embolism: e.g. ASD, pulmonary AVM including Osler-Weber-Rendu syndrome, patent foramen ovale (above)
   d) amniotic fluid embolism: may occur typically in the post-partum period
3. vasculopathy: 10%
   a) inflammatory
      - Takayasu's
      - infective: TB, syphilis, ophthalmic zoster

- amphetamine abuse
- herpes zoster ophthalmicus (HZO): usually presents with delayed contralateral hemiplegia with a mean of ≈ 8 weeks following HZO[24]
- mucormycosis: a nasal and orbital fungal infection primarily in diabetics and immunocompromised patients that causes an arteritis which may thrombose the orbital veins and ICA or ACA. Produces proptosis, ocular palsy, and hemiplegia
- associated with systemic disease such as: SLE (lupus), (also see below under Coagulopathy); arteritis (especially periarteritis nodosa (p. 199)) when confined to CNS is usually multifocal and progressive, but may mimic stroke early; multiple sclerosis (MS); cancer; rheumatoid arthritis

b) non-inflammatory
- fibromuscular dysplasia (p. 200)
- carotid or vertebral artery dissections (including posttraumatic)
- moyamoya disease (p. 1313)
- homocystinuria: a genetic defect in methionine metabolism that produces intimal thickening and fibrosis in almost all vessels with associated thromboembolic events (arterial and venous, including dural venous sinuses). Estimated risk of stroke is 10–16%. Patients have a Marfan syndrome-like physical appearance, malar blotches, mental retardation, and elevated levels of urinary homocysteine
- pseudoxanthoma elasticum

4. coagulopathy: 10%. The following are associated with hypercoagulable states
   a) SLE: lupus anticoagulant → prolonged PTT incompletely corrects with 50/50 mix. Collagen vascular disease only rarely presents initially with stroke
   b) polycythemia or thrombocytosis
   c) sickle cell disease
   d) TTP (thrombotic thrombocytopenic purpura)
   e) antithrombin III deficiency (controversial – not seen in large series of young adults with stroke)
   f) protein C or protein S deficiency (familial): protein C attenuates hemostatic reactions, homozygous deficiency is fatal in the neonatal period. Heterozygous deficiency is associated with *thrombotic* strokes. A rare complication during initial therapy with warfarin is a drop in protein C before other coagulation factors resulting in a hypercoagulable state
   g) antiphospholipid-antibody syndrome (APLAS)[25,26]: causes venous and/or arterial thrombosis. The two best known antiphospholipid-antibodies are anticardiolipin antibodies (ACLA), and lupus anticoagulant (LAC). Once they become symptomatic, treatment is high-intensity warfarin therapy to an INR ≥ 3.[27] There is a dramatic increase in thrombotic events after discontinuing warfarin. Aspirin is useless
   h) following use of the drug 3,4-methylenedioxymethamphetamine (MDMA, known on the street as ecstasy),[28] possibly independent of the hypercoagulable state that occurs with hyperthermia when insufficient fluids are consumed in conjunction with use of the drug
5. peripartum: 5% (usually within 2 wks of parturition)
6. miscellaneous causes: 35%
   a) uncertain etiology
   b) oral contraceptives (BCP): associated with ninefold increased risk for stroke, many with prior migraine history
   c) venous thrombosis (including dural sinus thrombosis): incidence may be increased with use of BCP
   d) migraine[29]: widely accepted, but difficult to assess objectively (incidence of stroke in these patients may be same as general population). *Rare*. Usually occurs in women, with a benign long-term course; recurs in < 3%. Possible mechanisms include: vasospasm, platelet dysfunction and arteriopathy.[30] strokes often occur during a migrainous attack[31] or shortly thereafter
   e) cocaine abuse[32]: stroke may result from vasoconstriction, or from HTN in the presence of aneurysms or AVMs (frank vasculitis occurs[33] but is rare with cocaine, unlike amphetamines); strokes with alkaloidal cocaine ("crack") are ≈ equally divided between ischemic and hemorrhagic
   f) posterior reversible encephalopathy syndrome (PRES) (p. 194)

83.5.3 Risk factors

In a retrospective "neighborhood control" study of 201 Australian patients aged 15–55 (mean = 45.5) with first-time strokes, the following risk factors were identified[21]:

1. diabetes: odds ratio = 12
2. HTN: odds ratio = 6.8

3. current cigarette smoking: odds ratio = 2.5
4. long-term heavy alcohol consumption: odds ratio = 15 (heavy alcohol ingestion within 24 hrs preceding the stroke was *not* a risk factor)

83.5.4 Evaluation

1. history & physical exam directed at uncovering systemic disease (see above) and modifiable risk factors (see above)
2. cardiology work-up including EKG and echocardiogram
3. bloodwork (include as appropriate):
   a) routine: electrolytes, CBC, platelet count and/or function, ESR (elevation may suggest SLE, arteritis, atrial myxoma… but a normal ESR does not rule-out vasculitis), PT/PTT, VDRL (should be obtained in all young adults with stroke), fasting lipid profile
   b) for unexplained stroke: ANA, antithrombin III, protein C, protein S, homocysteine, factor V Leiden, PPD, sickle-cell screen, toxicology screen (blood and urine, to R/O drugs such as cocaine), SPEP, lupus anticoagulant, serum amino acid, tissue plasminogen-activator and -inhibitor
4. miscellaneous tests: U/A, CXR, CSF exam when indicated
5. cerebral angiography: not always necessary for patients with obvious systemic disease or strong evidence for cardiac embolism; may occasionally diagnose cerebral embolism if performed within 48 hrs of ictus

83.6 Atherosclerotic carotid artery disease

83.6.1 General information

Atherosclerotic plaques begin to form in the carotid artery at 20 yrs of age. In the extracranial cerebral circulation, plaques typically start on the back wall of the common carotid artery (CCA). As they enlarge, they encroach on the lumen of the ICA. Calcified hard plaques may not change with time. The risk of stroke correlates with the degree of stenosis and with certain types of plaque morphology, and is also increased in hypercoagulable states and with increased blood viscosity.

Plaque morphology

"Vulnerable" plaques are atherosclerotic plaques likely to cause thrombotic complications, or those that tend to progress rapidly. Criteria for vulnerable plaques include: intimal thickening, plaque fissure, lipid/necrotic core with thin fibrous cap, calcification, thrombus, intraplaque hemorrhage, and outward remodeling. Some of these features can be identified with high-resolution MRI.[34,35,36,37]

83.6.2 Presentation

General information

Carotid artery lesions are considered symptomatic if there is one or more lateralizing ischemic episodes appropriate to the distribution of the lesion. A lesion is considered to be *asymptomatic* if the patient only has non-specific visual complaints, dizziness, or syncope not associated with TIA or stroke.[38] The majority (80%) of carotid atherothrombotic strokes occur without warning symptoms.[39]

Asymptomatic carotid stenosis

Usually discovered as a carotid bruit. Asymptomatic bruit: prevalence increases with age (2.3% in ages 45–54 yrs, 8.2% at ≥ 75).[40] Accuracy of a bruit in predicting ICA stenosis: 50–83% (depending on cohort, criteria for stenosis…). Sensitivity is as low as 24%.[41]

Symptomatic carotid disease

May present as a TIA, RIND or stroke with any of the following findings; see also ICA occlusion syndromes (p. 1265):

1. retinal insufficiency or infarction (central retinal artery is a branch of the ophthalmic artery): ipsilateral monocular blindness
   a) may be temporary: amaurosis fugax, AKA transient monocular blindness (TMB). Four types:

Type I: embolic. Described "like a black curtain coming down" in *one eye*. Complete loss of vision, usually lasts 1–2 minutes

Type II: flow related. Retinal hypoperfusion → desaturation of color, usually described as a graying of vision

Type III: vasospastic. May occur with migraines

Type IV: miscellaneous. May occur with anticardiolipin antibodies

a) blindness may be permanent

1. middle cerebral artery symptoms:
   a) contralateral motor or sensory TIA (arm and face worse than leg) with hyperreflexia and upgoing toe
   b) language deficits if dominant hemisphere involved

83.6.3 Evaluation of the extent of carotid disease

Overview

Symptomatic patients will usually be assessed as part of a stroke/TIA protocol.

Check CBC with platelet count, fibrinogen, PT/PTT/INR (to R/O hypercoagulable state).

Funduscopic exam may show Hollenhorst plaques (cholesterol crystal emboli) in the retina.

Classification of patients based on the hemodynamics and also the embolic propensity of carotid lesions has thus far been too complex to be utilized in large studies. The tests described below place a great deal of emphasis on the greatest degree of stenosis which is probably an oversimplification. Plaque composition and morphology is probably important.

Recommendations for screening for carotid stenosis

1. the U.S. Preventive Services Task Force (USPSTF) currently recommends against screening for carotid stenosis in the adult general population (grade D recommendation: moderate or high certainty that the service has no net benefit or that the harm outweighs the benefit)[42]
2. the AHA Primary Prevention of Stroke Guidelines does not recommend screening for asymptomatic carotid stenosis[43]
3. the American Society of Neuroimaging advised that screening should be considered only for age ≥ 65 years with 3 or more cardiovascular risk factors[44]
4. the Society of Vascular Surgery recommends ultrasonography screening for age ≥ 55 years with cardiovascular risk factors, such as a HTN, diabetes, smoking, hypercholesterolemia, or known cardiovascular disease[45]

Assessment options

See also recommendations for which tests to use (p. 1274).

Angiography

The "gold standard" test is a catheter arteriogram. It cannot be justified as a *screening* test because it is invasive, and too costly and risky (recent data show < 1% risk of transient or permanent deficit (risk is 2–3 times higher in symptomatic patients than in asymptomatic)[46,47,48] in good hands). Also, unlike duplex doppler and MRA, it does not provide any information about the thickness of the plaque. Different definitions of the degree of stenosis are employed, ▶ Table 83.5 compares the definitions used by the NASCET study[49] to that of the ECST.[50] For both, N is the linear diameter of the carotid artery at the site of greatest narrowing. The studies differ in the denominator, NASCET uses D (the diameter of the normal artery *distal* to the carotid bulb – taken at the first point at which the arterial walls become parallel), whereas the ECST uses B (the estimated carotid bulb diameter).

For example, using the NASCET definition, the degree of stenosis is shown in Eq (83.2).

$$\% \text{ stenosis (NASCET)} = \left(1 - \frac{N}{D}\right) \times 100 \qquad (83.2)$$

The relationship between the degree of narrowing based on the NASCET definition vs. that of the ECST has also been estimated by equation[51] as shown in Eq (83.3).

Table 83.5 Comparison of NASCET and ECST measurements of ICA stenosis[a]

NASCET	ECST
$1 - \frac{N}{D}$	$1 - \frac{N}{B}$
Approximate equivalent degrees of ICA stenosis based on direct comparison (%)	
30[b]	65[b]
40[b]	70
50	75
60	80
70	85
80	91
90	97

[a]adapted from Donnan G A, Davis S M, Chambers B R, et al.: Surgery for the Prevention of Stroke. Lancet 351: 1372, 1998, with permission
[b]indicates degrees of stenosis for which surgery was NOT of clear benefit for symptomatic stenosis (p. 1290)

$$\% \text{ stenosis (by ECST)} = 0.6 \times \% \text{ stenosis (by NASCET)} + 40\% \qquad (83.3)$$

Angiography also affords the opportunity to perform endovascular intervention if indicated.

Duplex doppler ultrasound

B-mode image evaluates the artery in cross-sectional plane, and spectrum analysis shows blood flow. Performs poorly with a “string sign.” Cannot scan above the angle of the mandible. Lower frequencies give greater depth of penetration, but signal definition is sacrificed (used in transcranial doppler). Sensitivity: 88%, specificity: 76%.[52]

Magnetic resonance angiography (MRA)

May obviate the need for angiography in some cases of carotid stenosis, specifically in symptomatic patients with a focal “gap” of signal intensity loss with distal reappearance of signal.[53,54] Sometimes overestimates the degree of stenosis.[55] Sensitivity: 91%, specificity: 88% for extracranial carotid disease.[56] 2D TOF-MRA is adequate (contrast-MRA shows more, but is not necessary for surgical lesions[57]).

Can be performed at the time as MRI with stroke protocol in TIA/stroke patients, and also detects thrombus or dissection. As with Doppler, has difficulties distinguishing very severe stenosis from occlusion. Less operator dependent than Doppler, but is more expensive and time-consuming. MRA is more difficult to perform if the patient is critically ill, unable to lie supine, or has claustrophobia, a pacemaker or ferromagnetic implants. High-resolution MRI may also detect vulnerable plaques (p. 1271).

Computed tomography angiography (CTA)

CTA involves ionizing radiation (x-rays) and IV iodinated contrast, limiting its use in patients with dye allergies and renal dysfunction. Results are comparable to MRA and Doppler. CTA can be performed within a few seconds and yields high-resolution images of all vessels from the aortic arch through the intracranial/extracranial vessels as well as the surrounding soft tissues. In a metaana lysis, sensitivity and specificity for detection of a 70% to 99% stenosis were 85% and 93%, respectively.[58] CTA is still evolving and may help detect vulnerable plaques (p. 1271). Another potential advantage: ability to obtain CT-perfusion (p. 228) studies at the same time.

Choice of imaging test/management decisions

Despite a great deal of research on the subject, there are no data to support a particular testing algorithm.[1] Doppler, CTA, or MRA are acceptable initial screening tests. In patients with an abnormal screening test, a common strategy is to obtain a second confirmatory noninvasive test to evaluate the carotid bifurcation before intervention. The combination of carotid ultrasound and MRA has proved cost effective with good interobserver reliability.[59] If 2 noninvasive tests are discordant, catheter angiography should be considered before intervention.

83.6.4 Treatment

Treatment alternatives are primarily between the following.
1. "best medical management": see below
2. carotid endarterectomy (p. 1290)
3. endovascular techniques: combined angioplasty and stenting (± distal embolus protection)

Medical treatment

General information

What constitutes "best medical management" has not been precisely determined, and recommendations are constantly changing. Some or all of the following are utilized:
1. antiplatelet therapy (p. 164):
   a) usually aspirin (ASA) (see below)
   b) clopidogrel, either alone or in combination with ASA (see below)
   c) combination of extended release dipyridamole and ASA (Aggrenox®) (no benefit from dipyridamole (Persantine®) alone)
2. antihypertensive therapy as appropriate
3. good control of diabetes if present
4. patients with asymptomatic A-fib should be treated with anticoagulation; see Cardiogenic brain embolism (p. 1304)
5. antilipid therapy if needed – Statins
6. intervention to help patients to quit smoking

Antiplatelet therapy

Drug info: Aspirin

Irreversibly inhibits cyclooxygenase preventing synthesis of vascular prostacyclin (a vasodilator and platelet inhibitor) and platelet thromboxane A2 (a vasoconstrictor and platelet activator). Platelets, lacking cellular organelles, cannot resynthesize cyclooxygenase whereas the vascular tissues do so rapidly.[60] NB: < 1000 mg ASA per day probably does not help with high grade stenosis where there is perfusion failure or flow failure. Some (but not all) studies show less effectiveness in women,[61] and no large study has shown that ASA prevents a second stroke in patients that have already had one.

℞: For angina, a bolus dose of 160–325 mg PO is followed by maintenance doses of 80–160 mg/d (lower doses appear to be as effective as higher doses).[62] Optimal dose for cerebrovascular ischemia continues to be debated. 325 mg PO qd reduces risk of stroke following TIA by 25–30%. Daily doses of 81 or 325 mg when compared to higher doses were associated with a lower rate of stroke, MI and death (6.2% vs. 8.4%) following carotid endarterectomy.[63]

Drug info: Aspirin/ER-Dipyridamole (Aggrenox®)

Combination of extended release dipyridamole and ASA (Aggrenox) is more effective than ASA alone for prevention of TIA, stroke, and myocardial infarction.[64,65,66] Aggrenox was not superior to clopidogrel, with increased hemorrhage with Aggrenox.[67] **Side effects:** H/A with initial therapy.

℞: 1 capsule PO BID. **Supplied:** fixed dose capsules of aspirin 25 mg/extended-release with dipyridamole 200 mg.

Drug info: Clopidogrel (Plavix®)

A thienopyridine. Incidence of severe neutropenia (0.04%) is close to that of ASA (≈ 0.02%).[68] Interferes with platelet membrane function by inhibiting ADP-induced platelet fibrinogen binding and release of platelet granule contents, as well as subsequent platelet-platelet interactions. Produces a time and dose dependent irreversible inhibition of platelet aggregation and prolongation of bleeding time. May replace ASA if intolerance or resistance. Used in combination with ASA for some endovascular procedures. Although clopidogrel plus aspirin is recommended over aspirin for acute coronary syndromes, the MATCH[69] results do not suggest a similar benefit for stroke and TIA. Combination therapy significantly increased risk of hemorrhage.[69]

Pharmacokinetics: Dosed once daily. Requires several days to reach maximal effect (∴ a loading dose may used, e.g. after an *acute* event such as an MI, or before stenting). Takes ≈ 5 days off the drug for platelet inhibition to reverse.

℞: 75 mg PO qd. Loading dose: 225 mg (3 pills) the first day of therapy. **Supplied:** 75 mg film-coated tablet.

Choice of antiplatelet agents

Individualization is recommend for antiplatelet agents for secondary stroke prevention. ASA is effective, and its low cost may help compliance. A small reduction of vascular events with Aggrenox may justify its expense from a broader healthcare perspective. Clopidogrel is appropriate for those intolerant or resistant to ASA. Clopidogrel plus ASA may be indicated in patients with recent cardiac ischemia or vascular stenting.[70]

Asymptomatic carotid artery stenosis

Key concepts

- natural history: reveals low stroke rate (2%/yr) half of which are not disabling
- large randomized trials have revealed moderate surgical benefit versus medical management for: asymptomatic stenosis > 60%
- treatment selection criteria depend on patient's age, gender and comorbidities (and therefore life expectancy), and on perioperative complication rate

Practice guideline: Asymptomatic carotid stenosis

- Level I[71]: CEA is reasonable in asymptomatic patients with > 70% ICA stenosis if risk of perioperative stroke, MI and death is low
- Level II[71]: It is reasonable to choose CEA over CAS when revascularization is indicated in older patients especially when the anatomy is unfavorable for endovascular intervention
- Level II[71]: It is reasonable to choose CAS over CEA when revascularization is indicated in patients with anatomy unfavorable for surgery
- Level II[71]: prophylactic CAS may be considered in highly selected patients with asymptomatic ICA stenosis (≥ 60% by angiography, > 70% by validated Doppler ultrasound), but the effectiveness compared to medical therapy alone is not well established

- Level II[71]: In patients with high risk of complications by either CEA or CAS (includes: age > 80 years, NYHA heart failure class II or IV, LVEF < 30%, class III or OV angina pectoris, left main or multivessel CAD, need for cardiac surgery within 30 days, MI within 4 weeks, and severe chronic lung disease), the effectiveness of revascularization over medical therapy alone is not well established

Abbreviations: CEA = carotid endarterectomy, CAS = carotid artery stenting

Natural history

Prevalence of carotid stenosis > 50% in men and women > 65 years of age is 5–10%, with 1% having stenosis > 80%.[72,73,74]

Natural history studies reflect an annual stroke risk of 1–3.4% with asymptomatic carotid artery stenosis of 50–99% at 2–3 years.[75,76,77,78,79,80] A cohort study found similar cumulative rates of ipsilateral stroke over 10 years (9.3%, or 0.9%/year) and 15 years (16.6%, or 1.1%/year).[81]

Attempts to identify subgroups of patients with asymptomatic carotid stenosis at elevated stroke risk suggest that the rate of unheralded stroke ipsilateral to a hemodynamically significant extracranial carotid artery stenosis is 1–2% annually, with some data suggesting that the stroke rate may be higher with progressing stenosis or with more severe stenosis. Asymptomatic carotid stenosis is an important marker of concomitant ischemic cardiac disease.[75,76,77,80,81] In the REACH Study,[82] patients with asymptomatic carotid stenosis (n = 3164) had statistically significantly higher age- and sex-adjusted 1-year rates of transient ischemic attack, non-fatal stroke, fatal stroke, and cardiovascular death compared with patients without asymptomatic carotid stenosis (n = 30 329).

Surgery vs. medical management: the studies

ACST

See reference.[83]

Σ

The largest multicenter randomized trial to date[83] revealed a moderate benefit for immediate CEA vs. medical management in patients age < 75 with asymptomatic stenosis ≥ 60%.

Details: 3,120 patients with ≥ 60% stenosis by duplex ultrasound were randomized to immediate CEA (50% had CEA within 1 month, 88% within 1 year) or medical therapy at the discretion of the treating physician. Mean follow-up: 3.4 years. Exclusion criteria included: poor surgical risk, prior ipsilateral CEA, and probable cardiac emboli. Surgeons were required to have a perioperative morbidity and mortality rate of < 6%.

Net five-year risk for all stroke or perioperative stroke or death: 6.4% in the CEA group, vs. 11.8% in the medical group ($p < 0.0001$). Fatal or disabling stroke: 3.5 vs. 6.1%. Fatal stroke alone: 2.1 vs. 4.2%. Although men and women benefited, men benefited more. CEA did not demonstrate a statistically significant benefit for patients over the age of 75. Statistical benefit was not seen in the immediate CEA group until nearly two years after surgery, despite a relatively low perioperative morbidity and mortality rate of 3.1%, (in contrast to patients with symptomatic stenosis (NASCET[84]) where benefit was seen much earlier).

ACAS

See reference.[85]

Σ

Large trial that randomized patients in good health with asymptomatic stenosis (calculated in the same manner as the NASCET study) ≥ 60% to CEA plus aspirin, or aspirin alone[85] found a reduced 5-year risk of ipsilateral stroke if CEA was performed with < 3% perioperative morbidity and mortality and is added to aggressive management of modifiable risk factors.

83

Details: CEA reduced 5-year stroke risk 66% in males, 17% in females (not statistically significant), and 53% overall (males & females lumped together). CEA did *not* significantly protect against major stroke or death (P = 0.16) (half of the strokes were not disabling), and was somewhat protective against any stroke or death (P = 0.08). The study group was 95% caucasian, and 66% were male. Excluded patients (age > 79 yrs, unstable CAD, uncontrolled HTN) may have been higher risk. Surgeons were carefully selected and the surgical morbidity (1.5%) and mortality (0.1%) was very low. Surprisingly, ≈ half of the total morbidity (1.2%) was related to angiography. The implication is that for a generally healthy white male with ACAS > 60%, management with CEA (when performed by a surgeon with a low complication rate, as described) reduces his annual risk of all strokes from 0.5% to 0.17% (the reduction of risk for severe stroke is less). The benefit from CEA is realized within less than one year after the CEA. This is in contrast to the ACST trial (see above) and is most likely due to the lower perioperative event rate. The risk from mortality from other causes (including MI) is ≈ 3.9% per year. Combined stroke and death rates in community hospitals[86] while improved over the last 20 yrs, remains higher at ≈ 6.3% than at centers used in this study.

Veteran's Administration Cooperative Study (VACS)

See reference.[84]

CEA reduces ipsilateral neurologic events, but did not reduce the rate of ipsilateral strokes nor death (most deaths were secondary to MI). This trial did not include women and was not powered to detect differences in outcome subgroups.

CASANOVA Study

See reference.[87]

No difference in outcome between CEA vs. aspirin (new stroke or death), but an unusual protocol lessened its statistical validity.[88]

Mayo Clinic Asymptomatic Carotid Endarterectomy (MACE) Study

See reference.[89]

There were no major strokes or deaths in either the medical or the endarterectomy group. Surgically treated patients were not given aspirin, and 26% had an MI compared to 9% in the aspirin-treated medical arm, reflecting the high incidence of concomitant CAD in patients with an asymptomatic carotid artery stenosis.

References

[1] Easton JD, Saver JL, Albers GW, Alberts MJ, Chaturvedi S, Feldmann E, Hatsukami TS, Higashida RT, Johnston SC, Kidwell CS, Lutsep HL, Miller E, Sacco RL. Definition and evaluation of transient ischemic attack. Stroke. 2009; 40:2276–2293

[2] Astrup J, Siesjö BK, Symon L. Thresholds in Cerebral Ischemia - The Ischemic Penumbra. Stroke. 1981; 12:723–725

[3] Powers WJ, Grubb RL, Darriet D, et al. Cerebral Blood Flow and Cerebral Metabolic Rate of Oxygen Requirements for Cerebral Function and Viability in Humans. J Cereb Blood Flow Metab. 1985; 5:600–608

[4] Raichle ME, Grubb RL, Gado MH, et al. Correlation Between Regional Cerebral Blood Flow and Oxidative Metabolism. In Vivo Studies in Man. Arch Neurol. 1976; 33:523–526

[5] Henegar MM, Silbergeld DL. Pharmacology for Neurosurgeons. Part II: Anesthetic Agents, ICP Management, Corticosteroids, Cerebral Protectants. Contemp Neurosurg. 1996; 18:1–6

[6] Chimowitz MI, Furlan AJ, Jones SC, Sila CA, Lorig RL, Paranandi L, Beck GJ. Transcranial Doppler assessment of cerebral perfusion reserve in patients with carotid occlusive disease and no evidence of cerebral infarction. Neurology. 1993; 43:353–357

[7] Guckel FJ, Brix G, Schmiedek P, Piepgras Z, Becker G, Kopke J, Gross H, Georgi M. Cerebrovascular reserve capacity in patients with occlusive cerebrovascular disease: assessment with dynamic susceptibility contrast-enhanced MR imaging and the acetazolamide stimulation test. Radiology. 1996; 201:405–412

[8] Rogg J, Rutigliano M, Yonas H, Johnson DW, Pentheny S, Latchaw RE. The acetazolamide challenge: imaging techniques designed to evaluate cerebral blood flow reserve. AJR Am J Roentgenol. 1989; 153:605–612

[9] Vagal AS, Leach JL, Fernandez-Ulloa M, Zuccarello M. The acetazolamide challenge: techniques and applications in the evaluation of chronic cerebral ischemia. AJNR Am J Neuroradiol. 2009; 30:876–884

[10] Allen JW. Proximal internal carotid artery branches: prevalence and importance for balloon occlusion test. J Neurosurg. 2005; 102:45–52

[11] Hankey GJ, Warlow CP. Prognosis of symptomatic carotid artery occlusion: an overview. Cerebrovasc Dis. 1991; 1:245–256

[12] Grubb RL, Jr, Powers WJ, Derdeyn CP, Adams HP,Jr, Clarke WR. The Carotid Occlusion Surgery Study. Neurosurg Focus. 2003; 14

[13] Matheus MG, Castillo M. Imaging of acute bilateral paramedian thalamic and mesencephalic infarcts. AJNR Am J Neuroradiol. 2003; 24:2005–2008

[14] Derex L, Ostrowsky K, Nighoghossian N, Trouillas P. Severe Pathological Crying After Left Anterior Choroidal Artery Infarction: Reversibility with Paroxetine Treatment. Stroke. 1997; 28:1464–1466

[15] Helgason C, Caplan LR, Goodwin J, Hedges T. Anterior Choroidal Artery-Territory Infarction: Report of Cases and Review. Arch Neurol. 1986; 43:681–686

[16] Adams RD, Victor M. Principles of Neurology. 2nd ed. New York: McGraw-Hill; 1981

[17] Fisher CM, Karnes WE, Kubik CS. Lateral Medullary Infarction: The Pattern of Vascular Occlusion. J Neuropath Exp Neurol. 1961; 29:323–379

[18] Norrving B, Cronqvist S. Lateral medullary infarction: prognosis in an unselected series. Neurology. 1991; 41:244–248
[19] Fisher CM. Lacunar Strokes and Infarcts: A Review. Neurology (NY). 1982; 32:871–876
[20] Hart RG, Miller VT. Cerebral Infarction in Young Adults: A Practical Approach. Stroke. 1983; 14:110–114
[21] You RX, McNeil JJ, O'Malley HM, et al. Risk factors for stroke due to cerebral infarction in young adults. Stroke. 1997; 28:1913–1918
[22] Adams HP, Butler MJ, Biller J, et al. Nonhemorrhagic Cerebral Infarction in Young Adults. Arch Neurol. 1986; 43:793–796
[23] Hilton-Jones D, Warlow CP. The causes of stroke in the young. J Neurol. 1985; 232:137–143
[24] Verghese A, Sugar AM. Herpes zoster ophthalmicus and granulomatous angiitis: An ill-appreciated cause of stroke. J Am Geriatr Soc. 1986; 34:309–312
[25] Toschi V, Motta A, Castelli C, et al. High Prevalence of Antiphosphatidylinositol Antibodies in Young Patients with Cerebral Ischemia of Undetermined Cause. Stroke. 1998; 29:1759–1764
[26] Tanne D, Triplett DA, Levine SR. Antiphospholipid-protein antibodies and ischemic stroke: Not just cardiolipin anymore. Stroke. 1998; 29:1755–1758
[27] Khamashta MA, Cuadrado MJ, Mujic F, et al. The Management of Thrombosis in the Antiphospholipid-Antibody Syndrome. N Engl J Med. 1995; 332:993–997
[28] Milroy CM, Clark JC, Forrest AR. Pathology of Deaths Associated with "Ecstasy" and "Eve" Misuse. J Clin Pathol. 1996; 49:149–153
[29] Welch KMA, Levine SR. Migraine-related stroke in the context of the International Headache Society Classification of head pain. Arch Neurol. 1990; 47:458–462
[30] Rothrock JF, Walicke P, Swenson MR, et al. Migrainous stroke. Arch Neurol. 1988; 45:63–67
[31] Spaccavento LJ, Solomon GD. Migraine as an etiology of stroke in young adults. Headache. 1984; 24:19–22
[32] Levine SR, Brust JCM, Futrell N, Ho KL, et al. Cerebrovascular Complications of the Use of the 'Crack' Form of Alkaloidal Cocaine. N Engl J Med. 1990; 323:699–704
[33] Kaye BR, Fainstat M. Cerebral Vasculitis Associated with Cocaine Abuse. JAMA. 1987; 258:2104–2106
[34] Cai JM, Hatsukami TS, Ferguson MS, Small R, Polissar NL, Yuan C. Classification of human carotid atherosclerotic lesions with in vivo multicontrast magnetic resonance imaging. Circulation. 2002; 106:1368–1373
[35] Saam T, Cai J, Ma L, Cai YQ, Ferguson MS, Polissar NL, Hatsukami TS, Yuan C. Comparison of symptomatic and asymptomatic atherosclerotic carotid plaque features with in vivo MR imaging. Radiology. 2006; 240:464–472
[36] Saam T, Hatsukami TS, Takaya N, Chu B, Underhill H, Kerwin WS, Cai J, Ferguson MS, Yuan C. The vulnerable, or high-risk, atherosclerotic plaque: noninvasive MR imaging for characterization and assessment. Radiology. 2007; 244:64–77
[37] Nighoghossian N, Derex L, Douek P. The vulnerable carotid artery plaque: current imaging methods and new perspectives. Stroke. 2005; 36:2764–2772
[38] Moneta GL, Taylor DC, Nicholls SC, et al. Operative Versus Nonoperative Management of Asymptomatic High-Grade Internal Carotid Artery Stenosis. Stroke. 1987; 18:1005–1010
[39] Kistler JP, Furie KL. Carotid Endarterectomy Revisited. N Engl J Med. 2000; 342:1743–1745
[40] Heyman A, Wilkinson WE, Heyden S, Helms MJ, Bartel AG, Karp HR, Tyroler HA, Hames CG. Risk of stroke in asymptomatic persons with cervical arterial bruits: a population study in Evans County, Georgia. N Engl J Med. 1980; 302:838–841
[41] Sonecha TN, Delis KT, Henein MY. Predictive value of asymptomatic cervical bruit for carotid artery disease in coronary artery surgery revisited. Int J Cardiol. 2006; 107:225–229
[42] U.S. Preventive Services Task Force. Screening for carotid artery stenosis: U.S. Preventive Services Task Force recommendation statement. Ann Intern Med. 2007; 147:854–859
[43] Goldstein LB, Adams R, Alberts MJ, Appel LJ, Brass LM, Bushnell CD, Culebras A, Degraba TJ, Gorelick PB, Guyton JR, Hart RG, Howard G, Kelly-Hayes M, Nixon JV, Sacco RL. Primary prevention of ischemic stroke. Stroke. 2006; 37:1583–1633
[44] Qureshi AI, Alexandrov AV, Tegeler CH, Hobson RW,2nd, Dennis Baker J, Hopkins LN. Guidelines for screening of extracranial carotid artery disease. J Neuroimaging. 2007; 17:19–47
[45] Society for Vascular Surgery. SVS Position Statement on Vascular Screenings, 2007. 2007
[46] Connors JJ, III, Sacks D, Furlan AJ, Selman WR, Russell EJ, Stieg PE, Hadley MN, Wojak JC, Koroshetz WJ, Heros RC, Strother CM, Duckwiler GR, Durham JD, Tomsick TO, Rosenwasser RH, McDougall CG, Haughton VM, Derdeyn CP, Wechsler LR, Hudgins PA, Alberts MJ, Raabe RD, Gomez CR, Cawley CM, III, Krol KL, Futrell N, Hauser RA, Frank JI. Training, competency, and credentialing standards for diagnostic cervicocerebral angiography, carotid stenting, and cerebrovascular intervention: a joint statement from the American Academy of Neurology, the American Association of Neurological Surgeons, the American Society of Interventional and Therapeutic Neuroradiology, the American Society of Neuroradiology, the Congress of Neurological Surgeons, the AANS/CNS Cerebrovascular Section, and the Society of Interventional Radiology. Neurology. 2005; 64:190–198
[47] Willinsky RA, Taylor SM, TerBrugge K, Farb RI, Tomlinson G, Montanera W. Neurologic complications of cerebral angiography: prospective analysis of 2,899 procedures and review of the literature. Radiology. 2003; 227:522–528
[48] Kaufmann TJ, Huston J, III, Mandrekar JN, Schleck CD, Thielen KR, Kallmes DF. Complications of diagnostic cerebral angiography: evaluation of 19,826 consecutive patients. Radiology. 2007; 243:812–819
[49] The North American Symptomatic Carotid Endarterectomy Trial. Beneficial Effect of Carotid Endarterectomy in Symptomatic Patients with High-Grade Carotid Stenosis. N Engl J Med. 1991; 325:445–453
[50] The European Carotid Surgery Trialists' Collaborative Group. Randomized Trial of Endartectomy for Recently Symptomatic Carotid Stenosis: Final Results of the MRC European Carotid Surgery Trial (ECST). Lancet. 1998; 351:1379–1387
[51] Rothwell PM, Gibson RJ, Slattery J, et al. Equivalence of Measurements of Carotid Stenosis: A Comparison of Three Methods on 1001 Angiograms. Stroke. 1994; 25:2435–2439
[52] Buskens E, Nederkoorn PJ, Buijs-Van Der Woude T, Mali WP, Kappelle LJ, Eikelboom BC, Van Der Graaf Y, Hunink MG. Imaging of carotid arteries in symptomatic patients: cost-effectiveness of diagnostic strategies. Radiology. 2004; 233:101–112
[53] Anson JA, Heiserman JE, Drayer BP, Spetzler RF. Surgical Decisions on the Basis of Magnetic Resonance Angiography of the Carotid Arteries. Neurosurgery. 1993; 32:335–343
[54] Heiserman JE, Zabramski JM, Drayer BP, Keller PJ. Clinical Significance of the Flow Gap in Carotid Magnetic Resonance Angiography. J Neurosurg. 1996; 85:384–387
[55] Anderson CM, Saloner D, Lee RE, et al. Assessment of Carotid Artery Stenosis by MR Angiography: Comparison with X-Ray Angiography and Color-Coded Doppler Ultrasound. AJNR. 1992; 13:989–1003
[56] Debrey SM, Yu H, Lynch JK, Lovblad KO, Wright VL, Janket SJ, Baird AE. Diagnostic accuracy of magnetic resonance angiography for internal carotid artery disease: a systematic review and meta-analysis. Stroke. 2008; 39:2237–2248
[57] Babiarz LS, Romero JM, Murphy EK, Brobeck B, Schaefer PW, Gonzalez RG, Lev MH. Contrast-enhanced MR angiography is not more accurate than unenhanced 2D time-of-flight MR angiography for determining > or = 70% internal carotid

artery stenosis. AJNR Am J Neuroradiol. 2009; 30:761–768

[58] Koelemay MJ, Nederkoorn PJ, Reitsma JB, Majoie CB. Systematic review of computed tomographic angiography for assessment of carotid artery disease. Stroke. 2004; 35:2306–2312

[59] Kent KC, Kuntz KM, Patel MR, Kim D, Klufas RA, Whittemore AD, Polak JF, Skillman JJ, Edelman RR. Perioperative imaging strategies for carotid endarterectomy. An analysis of morbidity and cost-effectiveness in symptomatic patients. JAMA. 1995; 274:888–893

[60] Weksler BB, Pett SB, Alonso D, et al. Differential Inhibition by Aspirin of Vascular and Platelet Prostaglandin Synthesis in Atherosclerotic Patients. N Engl J Med. 1983; 308:800–805

[61] Grotta JC. Current Medical and Surgical Therapy for Cerebrovascular Disease. N Engl J Med. 1987; 317:1505–1516

[62] Théroux P, Fuster V. Acute Coronary Syndromes: Unstable Angina and Non-Q-Wave Myocardial Infarction. Circulation. 1998; 97:1195–1206

[63] Taylor DW, Barnett HJM, Haynes RB, et al. Low-Dose and High-Dose Acetylsalicylic Acid for Patients Undergoing Carotid Endarterectomy: A Randomized Controlled Trial. Lancet. 1999; 353:2179–2184

[64] Halkes PH, van Gijn J, Kappelle LJ, Koudstaal PJ, Algra A. Aspirin plus dipyridamole versus aspirin alone after cerebral ischaemia of arterial origin (ESPRIT): randomised controlled trial. Lancet. 2006; 367:1665–1673

[65] Diener HC, Cunha L, Forbes C, Sivenius J, Smets P, Lowenthal A. European Stroke Prevention Study. 2. Dipyridamole and acetylsalicylic acid in the secondary prevention of stroke. J Neurol Sci. 1996; 143:1–13

[66] Verro P, Gorelick PB, Nguyen D. Aspirin plus dipyridamole versus aspirin for prevention of vascular events after stroke or TIA: a meta-analysis. Stroke. 2008; 39:1358–1363

[67] Sacco RL, Diener HC, Yusuf S, Cotton D, Ounpuu S, Lawton WA, Palesch Y, Martin RH, Albers GW, Bath P, Bornstein N, Chan BP, Chen ST, Cunha L, Dahlof B, De Keyser J, Donnan GA, Estol C, Gorelick P, Gu V, Hermansson K, Hilbrich L, Kaste M, Lu C, Machnig T, Pais P, Roberts R, Skvortsova V, Teal P, Toni D, Vandermaelen C, Voigt T, Weber M, Yoon BW, . Aspirin and extended-release dipyridamole versus clopidogrel for recurrent stroke. N Engl J Med. 2008; 359:1238–1251

[68] Clopidogrel for Reduction of Atherosclerotic Events. Med Letter. 1998; 40:59–60

[69] Diener HC, Bogousslavsky J, Brass LM, Cimminiello C, Csiba L, Kaste M, Leys D, Matias-Guiu J, Rupprecht HJ. Aspirin and clopidogrel compared with clopidogrel alone after recent ischaemic stroke or transient ischaemic attack in high-risk patients (MATCH): randomised, double-blind, placebo-controlled trial. Lancet. 2004; 364:331–337

[70] Sacco RL, Adams R, Albers G, Alberts MJ, Benavente O, Furie K, Goldstein LB, Gorelick P, Halperin J, Harbaugh R, Johnston SC, Katzan I, Kelly-Hayes M, Kenton EJ, Marks M, Schwamm LH, Tomsick T. Guidelines for prevention of stroke in patients with ischemic stroke or transient ischemic attack: a statement for healthcare professionals. Stroke. 2006; 37:577–617

[71] Brott TG, Halperin JL, Abbara S, Bacharach JM, Barr JD, Bush RL, Cates CU, Creager MA, Fowler SB, Friday G, Hertzberg VS, McIff EB, Moore WS, Panagos PD, Riles TS, Rosenwasser RH, Taylor AJ. 2011 ASA/ACCF/AHA/AANN/AANS/ACR/ASNR/CNS/SAIP/SCAI/SIR/SNIS/SVM/SVS guideline on the management of patients with extracranial carotid and vertebral artery disease. Stroke. 2011; 42:e464–e540

[72] O'Leary DH, Polak JF, Kronmal RA, Kittner SJ, Bond MG, Wolfson SKJr, Bommer W, Price TR, Gardin JM, Savage PJ. Distribution and correlates of sonographically detected carotid artery disease in the Cardiovascular Health Study. The CHS Collaborative Research Group. Stroke. 1992; 23:1752–1760

[73] Fine-Edelstein JS, Wolf PA, O'Leary DH, Poehlman H, Belanger AJ, Kase CS, D'Agostino RB. Precursors of extracranial carotid atherosclerosis in the Framingham Study. Neurology. 1994; 44:1046–1050

[74] Hillen T, Nieczaj R, Munzberg H, Schaub R, Borchelt M, Steinhagen-Thiessen E. Carotid atherosclerosis, vascular risk profile and mortality in a population-based sample of functionally healthy elderly subjects: the Berlin ageing study. J Intern Med. 2000; 247:679–688

[75] Autret A, Pourcelot L, Saudeau D, Marchal C, Bertrand P, de Boisvilliers S. Stroke risk in patients with carotid stenosis. Lancet. 1987; 1:888–890

[76] Bogousslavsky J, Despland P-A, Regli F. Asymptomatic Tight Stenosis of the Internal Carotid Artery. Neurology. 1986; 36:861–863

[77] Chambers BR, Norris JW. Outcome in patients with asymptomatic neck bruits. N Engl J Med. 1986; 315:860–865

[78] Hennerici M, Hulsbomer HB, Hefter H, Lammerts D, Rautenberg W. Natural history of asymptomatic extracranial arterial disease. Results of a long-term prospective study. Brain. 1987; 110 (Pt 3):777–791

[79] Mackey AE, Abrahamowicz M, Langlois Y, Battista R, Simard D, Bourque F, Leclerc J, Cote R. Outcome of asymptomatic patients with carotid disease. Asymptomatic Cervical Bruit Study Group. Neurology. 1997; 48:896–903

[80] Meissner I, Wiebers DO, Whisnant JP, O'Fallon WM. The natural history of asymptomatic carotid artery occlusive lesions. JAMA. 1987; 258:2704–2707

[81] Nadareishvili ZG, Rothwell PM, Beletsky V, Pagniello A, Norris JW. Long-term risk of stroke and other vascular events in patients with asymptomatic carotid artery stenosis. Arch Neurol. 2002; 59:1162–1166

[82] Aichner FT, Topakian R, Alberts MJ, Bhatt DL, Haring HP, Hill MD, Montalescot G, Goto S, Touze E, Mas JL, Steg PG, Rother J. High cardiovascular event rates in patients with asymptomatic carotid stenosis: the REACH registry. Eur J Neurol. 2009. DOI: 10.1111/j.1468-1331.2009.02614.x

[83] Halliday A, Mansfield A, Marro J, Peto C, Peto R, Potter J, Thomas D. Prevention of disabling and fatal strokes by successful carotid endarterectomy in patients without recent neurological symptoms: randomised controlled trial. Lancet. 2004; 363:1491–1502

[84] Hobson RW, Weiss DG, Fields WS, et al. Efficacy of Carotid Endarterectomy for Asymptomatic Carotid Stenosis. N Engl J Med. 1993; 328:221–227

[85] The Executive Committee for the Asymptomatic Carotid Atherosclerosis Study. Endarterectomy for Asymptomatic Carotid Artery Stenosis. JAMA. 1995; 273:1421–1428

[86] Mattos MA, Modi JR, Mansour MA, et al. Evolution of Carotid Endarterectomy in Two Community Hospitals: Springfield Revisited - Seventeen Years and 2243 Operations Later. J Vasc Surg. 1995; 21:719–728

[87] CASANOVA Study Group. Carotid Surgery Versus Medical Therapy in Asymptomatic Carotid Stenosis. Stroke. 1991; 22:1229–1235

[88] Mayberg MR, Winn HR. Endarterectomy for Asymptomatic Carotid Artery Stenosis. Resolving the Controversy. JAMA. 1995; 273:1459–1461

[89] Mayo Asymptomatic Carotid Endarterectomy Study Group. Results of a randomized controlled trial of carotid endarterectomy for asymptomatic carotid stenosis. Mayo Clin Proc. 1992; 67:513–518

84 Evaluation and Treatment for Stroke

84.1 Rationale for acute stroke treatment

84.1.1 General information

In the complete absence of blood flow, neuronal death occurs within 2–3 minutes from exhaustion of energy stores. However, in most strokes, there is a salvageable penumbra (tissue at risk) that retains viability for a period of time through suboptimal perfusion from collaterals. Progression of local cerebral edema from the injury results in compromise of these collaterals and progression of ischemic penumbra to infarction if flow is not restored and maintained. Prevention of this secondary neuronal injury drives the treatment of stroke and has led to the creation of designated Primary Stroke Centers that offer appropriate and timely triage and treatment of all potential stroke patients.

Current standard of care requires the administration of IV tPA to all eligible patients. Documentation is necessary to justify deviation from this standard of care in the current medico-legal environment.

In centers with advanced capabilities (Comprehensive Stroke Centers), other treatment modalities are also offered.

84.2 Evaluation

84.2.1 History – key components

1. time last seen normal (stroke on awakening being increasingly evaluated by perfusion studies to ensure the presence of viable tissue)
2. current deficit and clinical presentation
3. NIH Stroke Scale score (p. 1282) should be assessed and recorded
4. reasons for not administering IV tPA (if any) should be documented

84.2.2 CAT scan (emergent)

General information

Upon presentation with symptoms of a potential stroke, a noncontrast brain CT scan should be done immediately to rule-out hemorrhage (intraparenchymal or SAH), hematoma, early signs of ischemia, old infarcts or injuries, and other lesions (e.g. tumor).

CAT scan findings with ischemic stroke ("pale" infarcts)

General information

NB: These principles do *not* apply to small lacunar infarcts, nor to hemorrhagic strokes. NB: CT is normal in 8–69% of MCA strokes in the first 24 hours.[1]

Findings at various times after ischemic stroke

► **Hyperacute (< 6 hours after stroke).** Early signs of infarction involving large areas of the MCA territory correlate with poor outcome.[2] Early findings may include[3]:

1. hyperdense artery sign (see below): low sensitivity, but helpful if present
2. focal low attenuation within the gray matter*
3. loss of the gray-white interface*
4. attenuation of the lentiform nucleus
5. mass effect*
   a) early: effacement of the cerebral sulci (often subtle)[4]
   b) late: midline shift in large territory infarction
6. loss of the insular ribbon (hypodensity involving the insular region)
7. enhancement with IV contrast: occurs in only 33%. Stroke becomes isodense (called "masking" effect) or hyperdense with normal brain, and, rarely, may be the only indication of infarction[4]

* These findings are probably due to increased water content resulting from the following: cellular edema arising from altered cell permeability which produces a shift of sodium and water from the extracellular to the intracellular compartment, which also increases the extracellular osmotic pressure causing transudation of water from capillaries into the interstitium.[5]

► **24 hrs.** Most strokes can be identified as a low density by this time.

► **1–2 wks.** Strokes are sharply demarcated. In 5–10% there may be a short window (at around day 7–10) where the stroke becomes isodense, called “fogging effect.” IV contrast will usually demonstrate these.

► **3 wks.** Stroke approaches CSF density.

► **Mass effect.** Common between day 1 to 25. Then atrophy is usually seen by ≈ 5 wks (2 wks at the earliest). Serial CT scans have shown that midline shift increases after ischemic stroke and reaches a maximum 2–4 days after the insult.

► **Calcifications.** Over a long period of time (months to years) approximately 1–2% of strokes calcify (in adults, it is probably a much smaller fraction than this; and in peds it is a higher percentage than this). Therefore, in an adult, calcifications almost rule-out a stroke (consider AVM, low grade tumor…).

Hyperdense artery sign

First described in the MCA in 1983.[6] The cerebral vessel (usually the MCA) appears as a high density on unenhanced CT, indicating intra-arterial clot (thrombus or embolus).[7] Seen in 12% of 50 patients scanned within 24 hrs of stroke, and in 34% of 23 *very* early CTs done to R/O hemorrhage. Sensitivity for MCA occlusion is low, but specificity is high (although it may also be seen with carotid dissection, or (usually bilaterally) with calcific atherosclerosis or high hematocrit[7]). Does *not* have independent prognostic significance.[8]

Enhancement

CT enhancement with IV contrast in stroke:

1. many enhance by day 6, most by day 10, some will enhance up to 5 wks
2. rule of 2’s: 2% enhance at 2 days, 2% enhance at 2 mos
3. gyral enhancement: AKA called “ribbon” enhancement. Common. Usually seen by 1 week (grey matter enhances > white). DDx includes inflammatory infiltrating lesions such as lymphoma, neurosarcoidosis… (due to breakdown of BBB)
4. rule of thumb: there should not be enhancement at the same time there is mass effect

84.2.3 CT angio (CTA)

CTA (p. 227) is useful for assessing the location and extent of vascular occlusion in acute ischemic stroke,[9] and may identify the bleeding source in subarachnoid hemorrhage. Findings can direct treatment towards endovascular options when a proximal or significant large vessel occlusion is seen.

84.2.4 CT perfusion

Theoretically identifies salvageable penumbra as a region of mismatch between CBF and CBV. Assumption: the infarcted core (with no salvageable tissue) has decreased CBF within a region of decreased CBV (CBF/CBV match). A mismatched area (decreased CBV *without* a decrease in CBF) represents potentially salvageable penumbra.[10] Implication: thrombolytics and interventional treatment modalities without mismatch will likely increase morbidity and mortality without clinical benefit.

84.2.5 MRI

With newer, faster acquisition times, and with gradient echo sequences that are highly sensitive to hemorrhage, MRI is increasingly being utilized in the hyperacute setting and is at times replacing CT as the initial evaluation. More sensitive than CT (especially DWI-MRI (p. 232) – and particularly in the 1st 24 hrs after stroke), and especially with brainstem or cerebellar infarction. More contraindications (p. 230) than CT.

Contrast MRI: not often used. 4 enhancement patterns[11]:

1. intravascular enhancement: occurs in ≈ 75% of 1–3 day-old cortical infarcts, and is probably due to sluggish flow and vasodilatation (thus, it is not seen with complete occlusion). May indicate areas of brain at risk of infarction
2. meningeal enhancement: especially involving the dura. Seen in 35% of cortical strokes 1–3 days old (not seen in deep cerebral or brainstem strokes). No angiographic nor CT equivalent

3. transitional enhancement: above two types of enhancement coexist with early evidence of BBB breakdown; usually seen on days 3–6
4. parenchymal enhancement: classically appears as a cortical or subcortical gyral ribbon enhancement. May not be apparent for the first 1–2 days, and gradually approaches 100% by 1 week. Enhancement may eliminate "fogging effect" (as on CT) which may obscure some strokes at ≈ 2 weeks on unenhanced T2WI

84.2.6 MRI perfusion

Similar to CT perfusion (p. 228), areas of matched DWI and PWI abnormality are thought to represent infarcted tissue. PWI abnormalities that do not have a DWI correlate are thought to represent potentially salvageable penumbra.[12]

84.2.7 Emergency cerebral catheter angiography

Indications:
1. early stroke in carotid distribution + history of amaurosis fugax or bruit or retinal emboli, etc. suggesting increasing carotid stenosis, thrombogenic ulcerated plaque, or carotid dissection
2. if diagnosis still questionable (e.g. aneurysm, vasculitis)
3. with rapid recovery, suggesting carotid TIA in face of increasing stenosis
4. *AVOID* angio if unstable or if severe disabling neuro deficit

Findings:
1. cutoff sign: vessel ends abruptly at the point of obstruction
2. string sign: narrow strand of contrast in a vessel with high grade stenosis
3. "luxury perfusion": reactive hyperemia is a recognized response of cerebral tissue to injury (trauma, infarction, epileptogenic focus…). Luxury perfusion is blood flow in excess of demand due to abolition of CBF autoregulation due to acidosis.[13] The exact nature of the perfusion is not known (i.e. if it is capillary, arteriole…). On angiography it shows up as accelerated circulation adjacent to the infarct with a stain or blush and early venous drainage

84.2.8 NIH stroke scale (NIHSS)

Administer in order shown (▶ Table 84.1). Record initial performance only (do not go back).

84.3 Management of TIA or stroke

84.3.1 Treatment options timeline

See ▶ Fig. 84.1.

Σ

1. within 4.5 hours of onset of symptoms:
   a) patients may be candidates for IV tPA (p. 1286)
   b) failures to respond to IV tPA who are in good clinical grade)NIHSS (p. 1282) > 8–10) may be candidates for
      • intraarterial tPA (IA tPA) or
      • mechanical embolectomy/clot disruption
2. 4.5–6 hours after onset:
   a) intraarterial tPA (IA tPA) or
   b) mechanical embolectomy/clot disruption
3. 6–8 hours, check perfusion with CTP or MRI-DWI before mechanical embolectomy (studied up to 8 hours after onset). ✖ Embolectomy contraindicated if stroke > 1/3 of MCA distribution (risk of ICH with reperfusion)

These times are more applicable to anterior circulation strokes. Posterior circulation occlusions may be treated more aggressively, e.g. IA tPA has been used up to 12 hrs.

Table 84.1 NIH Stroke scale[a]

Scale	Finding
1a. Level of consciousness (LOC)	
0	alert; keenly responsive
1	not alert, but arousable by minor stimulation to obey, answer or respond
2	not alert, requires repeated stimulation to attend, or is obtunded and requires strong painful stimulation to make movements (not stereotyped)
3	comatose: responds only with reflex motor (posturing) or autonomic effects, or totally unresponsive, flaccid and areflexic
1b. Level of consciousness questions	
Patient is asked the month and their age.	
0	answers both questions correctly: must be correct (no credit for being close)
1	answers one question correctly, or cannot answer because of: ET tube, orotracheal trauma, severe dysarthria, language barrier, or any other problem not secondary to aphasia.
2	answers neither question correctly, or is: aphasic, stuporous, or does not comprehend the questions
1c. Level of consciousness commands	
Patient is asked to open and close the eyes, and then to grip and release the non-paretic hand. Substitute another 1-step command if both hands cannot be used. Credit is given for an unequivocal attempt even if it cannot be completed due to weakness. If there is no response to commands, demonstrate (pantomime) the task. Record only first attempt.	
0	performs both tasks correctly
1	performs one task correctly
2	performs neither task correctly
2. Best gaze	
Test only horizontal eye movement. Use motion to attract attention of aphasic patients.	
0	normal
1	partial gaze palsy (gaze abnormal in one or both eyes, but forced deviation or total gaze paresis are not present) or patient has an isolated cranial nerve III, IV or VI paresis
2	forced deviation or total gaze paresis not overcome by oculocephalic (Doll's eyes) maneuver (do not do caloric testing)
3. Visual	
Visual fields (upper and lower quadrants) are tested by confrontation. May be scored as normal if patient looks at side of finger movement. Use ocular threat where consciousness or comprehension limits testing. Then test with double sided simultaneous stimulation (DSSS).	
0	no visual loss
1	partial hemianopia (clear cut asymmetry), or extinction to DSSS
2	complete hemianopia
3	bilateral hemianopia (blind, including cortical blindness)
4. Facial palsy	
Ask patient (or pantomime) to show their teeth, or raise eyebrows and close eyes. Use painful stimulus and grade grimace response in poorly responsive or non-comprehending patients.	
0	normal symmetrical movement
1	minor paralysis (flattened nasolabial fold, asymmetry on smiling)

Table 84.1 continued

Scale	Finding
2	partial paralysis (total or near total paralysis of lower face)
3	complete paralysis of one or both sides (absent facial movement in upper and lower face)
5. Motor Arm (5a = left, 5b = right)	
Instruct patient to hold the arms outstretched, palms down (at 90° if sitting, or 45° if supine). If consciousness or comprehension impaired, cue patient by actively lifting arms into position while verbally instructing patient to maintain position.	
0	no drift (holds arm at 90° or 45° for full 10 seconds)
1	drift (holds limbs at 90° or 45° position, but drifts before full 10 seconds but does not hit bed or other support)
2	some effort against gravity (cannot get to or hold initial position, drifts down to bed)
3	no effort against gravity, limb falls
4	no movement
9	amputation or joint fusion: explain
6. Motor leg (6a = left, 6b = right)	
While supine, instruct patient to maintain the non-paretic leg at 30°. If consciousness or comprehension impaired, cue patient by actively lifting leg into position while verbally instructing patient to maintain position. Then repeat in paretic leg.	
0	no drift (holds leg at 30° full 5 seconds)
1	drift (leg falls before 5 seconds, but does not hit bed)
2	some effort against gravity (leg falls to bed by 5 seconds)
3	no effort against gravity (leg falls to bed immediately)
4	no movement
9	amputation or joint fusion: explain
7. Limb ataxia	
Looking for unilateral cerebellar lesion). Finger-nose-finger and heel-knee-shin tests are performed on both sides. Ataxia is scored only if clearly out of proportion to weakness. Ataxia is absent in the patient who cannot comprehend or is paralyzed.	
0	absent
1	present in one limb
2	present in two limbs
9	amputation or joint fusion: explain
8. Sensory	
Test with pin. When consciousness or comprehension impaired, score sensation normal unless deficit clearly recognized (e. g. clear-cut asymmetry of grimace or withdrawal). Only hemisensory losses attributed to stroke are counted as abnormal.	
0	normal, no sensory loss
1	mild to moderate sensory loss (pinprick dull or less sharp on the affected side, or loss of superficial pain to pinprick but patient aware of being touched)
2	severe to total (patient unaware of being touched in the face, arm and leg)
9. Best language	
In addition to judging comprehension of commands in the preceding neurologic exam, the patient is asked to describe a standard picture, to name common items, and to read and interpret the standard text in the box below. The intubated patient should be asked to write:	

Table 84.1 continued

Scale	Finding
• You know how. • Down to earth. • I got home from work. • Near the table in the dining room. • They heard him speak on the radio last night.	
0	normal, no aphasia
1	mild to moderate aphasia (some loss of fluency, word finding errors, naming errors, paraphasias and/or impairment of communication by either comprehension or expression disability)
2	severe aphasia (great need for inference, questioning and guessing by listener; limited range of information can be exchanged)
3	mute or global aphasia (no usable speech or auditory comprehension) or patient in coma (item 1a = 3)
10. Dysarthria	
Patient may be graded based on information already gleaned during evaluation. If patient is thought to be normal, have them read (or repeat) the standard text shown in this box. • MAMA • TIP-TOP • FIFTY-FIFTY • THANKS • HUCKLEBERRY • BASEBALL PLAYER • CATERPILLAR	
0	normal speech
1	mild to moderate (slurs some words, can be understood with some difficulty)
2	severe (unintelligible slurred speech in the absence of, or out of proportion to any dysphasia, or is mute/anarthric)
9	intubated or other physical barrier
11. Extinction and inattention (formerly neglect)	
Sufficient information to identify neglect may already be gleaned during evaluation. If the patient has severe visual loss preventing visual DSSS, and the cutaneous stimuli are normal, the score is normal. Scored as abnormal only if present.	
0	normal, no sensory loss
1	visual, tactile, auditory, spatial or personal inattention or extinction to DSSS in one of the sensory modalities
2	profound hemi-inattention or hemi-inattention to more than one modality. Does not recognize own hand or orients to only one side of space.
A. Distal motor function (not part of NIHSS) (a = left arm, b = right)	
Patients hand is held up at the forearm by the examiner, and is asked to extend the fingers as much as possible. If patient cannot do so, the examiner does it for them. Do not repeat the command.	
0	normal (no finger flexion after 5 seconds)
1	at least some extension after 5 seconds (any finger movement is scored)
2	no voluntary extension after 5 seconds
Higher NIHSS scores correlate with more proximal vascular lesions (larger vessel occlusion causes more widespread deficit).	
[a]Revised 1/24/91. Based on Cincinnati stroke scale.[14] Contact the Public Health Service, National Institutes of Health, National Institute of Neurologic Disorders and Stroke, Bethesda, Maryland, U.S.A. for copies of a grading form (which has more details on some aspects of grading) and for training information.[15]	

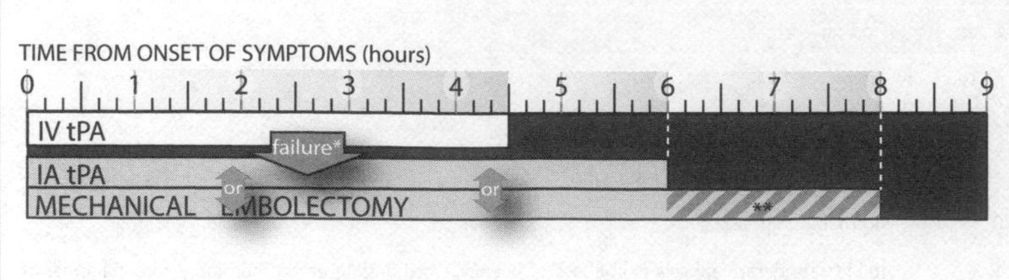

Fig. 84.1 Treatment options timeline.
* option for failures with NIHSS > 8-10
** from 6-8 hrs, check perfusion before mechanical embolectomy

84.3.2 Thrombolytic therapy

General information

Plasminogen activators catalyze the conversion of plasminogen to the fibrinolytic compound plasmin. The primary agent used is alteplase (recombinant tissue plasminogen activator (rtPA, or just tPA)) (Activase®) which is FDA approved for the IV treatment of acute ischemic stroke (see below).

Tissue plasminogen activator

IV tPA

For *intraarterial* tPA see endovascular therapy.

A randomized double-blind NINDS study of 624 patients with an ischemic stroke having a clearly defined time of onset and a CT scan prior to drug administration, found improved neurologic outcome at 3 months in patients who received alteplase (these patients were 30% more likely to have minimal or no disability)[16] which persisted at 6 and 12 mos[17] in all subgroups of ischemic stroke. The recurrent stroke rate in control and tPA patients was similar (5%). In contrast, statistical benefit at 90 days could not be confirmed in the second European Cooperative Acute Stroke Study (ECASS II).[18]

Early data indicated tPA had to be given ≤ 3 hrs after the onset of symptoms, however, this window was extended to 4.5 hours after the ECASS-3[19] looked at 821 stroke patients randomized between placebo or tPA in the 3- to 4.5-hour time-window. Compared to placebo, tPA-treated patients experienced a 7.2% absolute increase in the rate of excellent recovery at 90-day follow-up (P=0.04). Although tPA therapy was associated with an increased rate of symptomatic intracerebral hemorrhage (7.9% for tPA versus 3.5% for placebo, P < 0.001), it was not associated with an increased rate of death (7.7% for tPA versus 8.4% for placebo, P=0.68). For every 100 acute ischemic stroke patients given tPA in accordance with the NINDS protocols, 32 will benefit and 3 will be harmed.[20]

Guidelines for the administration of IV tPA

Eligibility:

1. age ≥ 18 years (although use in childhood stroke is increasing[21]
2. time since last seen normal < 3 hrs prior to administration (ECASS III extends window to 4.5 hours in select patients[22]; ECASS III did not include: patients ≥ 80 years of age, patients with baseline NIHSS (p. 1282) scores > 25, and prior stroke in diabetics. These patients are not excluded from treatment with IV tPA in the 0–3-hour window by the regulatory authorities in the United States and Canada.)
3. "wake-up" stroke (seen in 25% of ischemic stroke patients) may also be safe to treat in select circumstances[23]

Contraindications (see reference[16]):

1. intracerebral hemorrhage (ICH): on admitting CT, or history of prior ICH
2. clinical presentation of SAH (even with negative CT)
3. known intracranial aneurysm or AVM
4. active internal bleeding
5. known bleeding diathesis, including but not limited to:
   a) patients on anticoagulants, or those who received heparin in past 48 hrs
   b) platelet count < 100,000/mm³

6. serious head trauma, serious stroke, or intracranial surgery within past 3 months
7. SBP > 185 mm Hg, or DBP > 110 mm Hg that cannot be controlled despite use of nicardipine infusion or IV labetalol

✖ Cautions:
1. seizure witnessed at the time of onset of stroke symptoms
2. major surgery within the last 14 days
3. arterial puncture at non-compressible site within past 7 days
4. recent lumbar puncture
5. rapidly improving or minor symptoms
6. blood glucose > 400 mg/dl or < 50 mg/dl
7. history of GI or urinary tract hemorrhage within past 21 days
8. post myocardial infarction pericarditis

Treatment protocol: Also, see Contraindications (p. 1286).

℞ alteplase (Activase®): initiate < 4.5 hrs from onset of deficit. NINDS protocol: 0.09 mg/kg IV bolus over 1 min, followed by 0.81 mg/kg constant infusion over 60 minutes (up to a maximum of 90 mg total, including the bolus).[16]

HTN is aggressively controlled.

Anticoagulants and antiplatelet drugs are held for 24 hrs after treatment. If there is an indication for anticoagulation, obtain a non-contrast CT 24 hours prior to starting anticoagulation since there is a risk of subclinical intracerebral hemorrhage.

ICH following IV tPA

There is an increased risk of symptomatic intracerebral hemorrhage (ICH) with the use of tPA (NINDS study: 6.4% vs. 0.6% with placebo; ECASS II: 8.8% vs. 3.4%). In spite of this, the NINDS study found that mortality in the tPA group was similar to controls at 3 mos (17% vs. 21%). The following factors were associated with an increased risk of symptomatic ICH (with only a 57% efficiency rate of predicting ICH): severity of NIHSS score, or pre-treatment CT showing brain edema or mass effect. In one study, ICH did not influence outcome except in the rare instance when a massive hematoma occurred.[24] Outcomes were still better in the treated group, and the conclusion is that these patients are still reasonable candidates for tPA.[25] Since then, multicenter analyses have demonstrated that size of infarction and elevated blood sugar are independent risk factors for symptomatic ICH.[26]

Management of post-tPA ICH:
1. discontinue tPA infusion of and obtain STAT head CT
2. send labs: PT, aPTT, platelet count, fibrinogen, and type & cross
3. prepare to administer 6–8 units cryoprecipitate containing Factor VIII
4. prepare to administer 6–8 units of platelets
5. if emergent EVD placement or other interventional procedure is needed, consider the use of recombinant Factor VIIa (40–80 mg/kg) immediately beforehand (NB: this is only a temporizing measure and cryoprecipitate needs to still be given)

84.3.3 Endovascular therapy for stroke

Recent trials favor rapid endovascular intervention in acute ischemic stroke with proximal vessel occlusion, small infarct core and moderate to good collateral circulation.[27,28,29,30] Techniques include intraarterial tPA, mechanical clot retrieval. See Endovascular neurosurgery section (p. 1595) for details.

84.3.4 Management of patients not undergoing therapy directed at thrombus

Admitting orders

These guidelines are for TIA or stroke, but not SAH (p. 1163) nor intracerebral hemorrhage (ICH) (p. 1339). See reference[31] for rationale for these recommendations. The following guidelines for initial management should be maintained 48 hrs after last neuro deterioration.
1. frequent VS with crani checks (q 1 hr × 12 hrs, then q 2 hrs)
2. activity: bed rest

3. labs:
   a) routine: CBC + platelet count, electrolytes, PT/PTT, U/A, EKG, CXR, ABG
   b) "special" (when appropriate): RPR (to rule-out neurosyphilis), ESR (to rule-out giant cell arteritis), hepatic profile, cardiac profile
   c) at 24 hrs: CBC, platelet count, cardiac profile, lipid profile, EKG
4. O_2 at 2 L per NC; repeat ABG on 2 L O_2
5. monitor cardiac rhythm × 24 hrs (literature quotes 5–10% prevalence of EKG changes, and 2–3% acute MIs in patients with stroke)
6. diet: NPO

7. nursing care
   a) indwelling Foley (urinary) catheter if consciousness impaired or if unable to use urinal or bedpan; intermittent catheterization q 4–6 hrs PRN no void if Foley not used
   b) accurate I's & O's; notify M.D. for urine output < 20 cc/hr × 2 hrs by Foley, or < 160 cc in 8 hrs if no Foley
8. IV fluids: NS or 1/2 NS at 75–125 cc/hr for most patients (to eliminate dehydration if present)
   a) *avoid glucose*: hyperglycemia may extend ischemic zone (penumbra).[32] Although hyperglycemia may be a stress response and may not be neurotoxic,[33] recommendations are to strive for normoglycemia[34]
   b) avoid overhydration in cases of ICH, CHF, or SBP > 180. It had been suggested that an optimal Hct for compromise between O_2 delivery and decreased viscosity was ≈ 33% and that fluid management should strive for this, however the early promise of this theory has not been borne out
9. treat CHF and arrhythmias (check CXR & EKG). MI or myocardial ischemia may present with neuro deficit, these patients should be admitted to CCU
10. avoid diuretics unless volume overloaded
11. blood pressure (BP) management:
    a) for patients presenting with HTN: management must take baseline BP into account: see Hypertension in stroke patients below for management
    b) for patients presenting with hypotension (SBP < 110 or DBP < 70):
       - unless contraindicated (viz.: ICH, cerebellar infarct, or decreased cardiac output) give 250 cc NS over 1 hr, then 500 cc over 4 hrs, then 500 cc over 8 hrs
       - if fluid ineffective or contraindicated: consider pressors
12. medications
    a) ASA 325 mg PO q d (unless hemorrhagic stroke proven or suspected)
    b) stool softener
13. see following sections for discussion of anticoagulation (p. 1289), steroids (p. 1289), and mannitol (p. 1290)

Hypertension in stroke patients

General information

HTN may actually be needed to maintain CBF in the face of elevated ICP, and it usually resolves spontaneously. Therefore treat HTN cautiously and slowly to avoid rapid reduction and overshooting the target. Avoid treating mild HTN. Indications to treat HTN emergently include:

1. acute LV failure (rare)
2. acute aortic dissection (rare)
3. acute hypertensive renal failure (rare)
4. neurologic complications of HTN
   a) hypertensive encephalopathy
   b) converting a massive pale (ischemic) infarct into a hemorrhagic infarct
   c) patients with ICH; some HTN is needed to maintain CBF, see Initial management of ICH (p. 1339)

Hypertension treatment algorithm (modified)

See reference.[31]

Recommended lower limits for treatment endpoints are shown in ▶ Table 84.2.

1. If DBP > 140 (malignant hypertension): ≈ 20–30% reduction is desirable. Cardene infusion or IV labetalol are agents of choice; arterial-line monitor recommended; sympatholytics (e.g. trimethaphan) contraindicated (they reduce CBF)
2. SBP > 230 or DBP 120–140 × 20 mins: **labetalol** (p. 126) (unless contraindicated): start at 10 mg slow IVP over 2 mins, then double q 10 min (20, 40, 80, then 160 mg slow IVP) until controlled or

Table 84.2 Guidelines for lower limits of treatment endpoints for HTN in strokes

	No prior history of HTN	Prior history of HTN
do not lower SBP below	160–170 mm Hg	180–185 mm Hg
do not lower DBP below	95–105 mm Hg	105–110 mm Hg

total of 300 mg given. Maintenance: effective dose (from above) q 6–8 hrs PRN SBP > 180 or DBP > 110

3. SBP 180–230 or DBP 105–120: defer emergency treatment unless there is evidence of LV failure or if readings persist × 60 mins
   a) oral **labetalol** (p. 126) (unless contraindicated) dosed as follows:
      - for SBP > 210 or DBP > 110: 300 mg PO BID
      - for SBP 180–210 or DBP 100–110: 200 mg PO BID
   b) if labetalol contraindicated:
      nicardipine (p. 126)

Anticoagulants

Heparin

A prospective trial[35] administering continuous IV infusion of unfractionated heparin titrated to keep APTT 1.5–2.5 × control found no significant improvement in outcome.[36] The recurrent stroke rate in the 7 days following a stroke was only 0.6–2.2% per week.[35,37] Effectiveness is unproven in strokes and TIAs except with cardiogenic brain embolism (p. 1304). Anticoagulation may also be hazardous,[38] however the complication rate has not been assessed prospectively (small, nonrandomized studies have found symptomatic ICH in 1–8%, and other bleeding complications in 3–12%[35]). Conversion rate of pale → hemorrhagic stroke is 2–5% (dog studies suggest the risk is increased only when HTN not well controlled). Conclusion: the risk of heparin therapy for acute focal cerebral ischemia exceeds any proven benefit,[35] and is *not* justified in most cases (especially when used just to placate the frustrated clinician).[39,40] The American Heart Association has recommended: "Until more data are available, the use of heparin remains a matter of preference of the treating physician".[35] A small but significant reduction in recurrent stroke has been shown with ASA.

Warfarin

High-intensity warfarin therapy has proven helpful for the antiphospholipid antibody syndrome (APLAS) (p. 1270).

For the rare indication for anticoagulation therapy:

1. first, R/O hemorrhage by CT before beginning therapy
2. ASA 325 mg PO q d in all patients with non-hemorrhagic stroke where anticoagulants or surgery not indicated (NB: angiography may be slightly more difficult in patients on ASA)
3. anticoagulants (heparin/warfarin):
   a) indications (*rare*)
      - probably effective for cardiogenic emboli (below)
      - shown *ineffective* for stroke in evolution (neuro deficit that begins, recurs, fluctuates, or worsens while patient in hospital), crescendo TIA or completed stroke. **Note:** in 74 patients with recent TIAs, elevating PTT 1.5–2.5 x normal with heparin did not reduce recurrent TIAs nor strokes. Bleeding occurred in 9 (12.2%). Additional risk: hemorrhage from heparin induced thrombocytopenia.[41]
      - unproven, but generally used for carotid dissection
   b) contraindicated with large cardiac embolism, large stroke (risk of hemorrhagic conversion), peptic-ulcer disease that has bled in past 6 mos, uncontrolled severe HTN
   c) start IV heparin and simultaneous warfarin (Coumadin®). Maintain heparin during first ≈ 3 days of warfarin because of initial *hypercoagulability*, see Anticoagulation (p. 156) for target APTT and INR
   d) stop warfarin after 6 months (benefits decline, risks rise)

Steroids (including Dexamethasone (Decadron®))

Indications:

1. steroid responsive vasculitis, e.g. giant cell arteritis (temporal arteritis)
2. cerebellar infarct/bleed with mass effect

Mannitol

1. indicated for cerebellar infarct/bleed, prior to surgery, or if mass effect
2. contraindicated in hypotension
3. initial dose: 50 to 100 gm IV over 20 minutes

Emergency surgery

Possible indications:

1. herniation from subdural hematoma
2. suboccipital craniectomy for progressive neurologic deterioration due to brainstem compression from cerebellar hemorrhage/infarction (see below)
3. decompressive craniectomy for malignant MCA territory stroke (see below)
4. carotid endarterectomy for high grade carotid stenosis ipsilateral to *fluctuating* neuro deficit; see Emergency carotid endarterectomy (p. 1295)

84.4 Carotid endarterectomy

84.4.1 Indications

Trials and results

▶ Table 84.3 shows the status of current studies for the surgical treatment of carotid stenosis (NB: some of the results may be contradictory).

The North American Symptomatic Carotid Endarterectomy Trial[43] (NASCET) found that for patients with a hemispheric or retinal TIA or a mild (non-disabling) stroke within 120 days and *ipsilateral high-grade* stenosis (> 70%), that carotid endarterectomy (CEA) reduced the rate of fatal and non-fatal strokes (by 17% at 18 months) and death from any cause (by 7% at 18 months) when compared to best medical management (when surgery was performed with perioperative risk of stroke

Table 84.3 Summary of study findings for carotid endarterectomy (CEA)[a] (modified[42])

Stenosis	Relevant study	Recommendation	Risk reduction[b]
	Symptomatic Narrowing		
70–99%	NASCET[43]	CEA	16.5 @ 2 yrs
> 60%	ECST[44]	CEA	11.6 @ 3 yrs
50–69%	NASCET[45]	CEA[c]	10.1 @ 5 yrs
< 30%	NASCET[45]	BMM	0.8 @ 5 yrs
< 40%	ECST[46]	BMM	CEA worse @ 3 yrs
	Asymptomatic Narrowing (p. 1275)		
> 60%	ACST[47]	CEA if age < 75 yrs	5.4% @ 5 yrs
> 60%	ACAS,[48] ACST[d]	CEA[d]	6.3 @ 5 yrs
> 50%	VACS	± CEA[e]	
< 90%	CASANOVA	BMM[e]	

[a]abbreviations: NASCET = North American Symptomatic Carotid Endarterectomy Trial; ECST = European Carotid Surgery Trial; CASANOVA = Carotid Artery Stenosis with Asymptomatic Narrowing Operation Versus Aspirin; ACAS = Asymptomatic Carotid Atherosclerosis Study; ACST = Asymptomatic Carotid Atherosclerosis Study; VACS = Veteran's Administration Cooperative Study; CEA = carotid endarterectomy; BMM = best medical management
[b]reduction in risk of all nonfatal strokes and death from any cause with CEA vs. BMM (e.g. with an absolute risk reduction of 16.5 at 2 yrs, for every 100 patients treated, 16.5 nonfatal strokes or deaths were prevented over a 2 year period)
[c]surgery moderately beneficial (requires low complication rate)
[d]the overall health of the patient is critical
[e]results equivocal

or death of 5.8%). Results were twice as good for patients with stenosis from 90–99% than for those with 70–79%. Furthermore, with CEA the frequency of major functional impairment was reduced at 2 years.[49] NB: see differences in techniques for measuring stenosis between NASCET and ECST ▸ Table 83.5.

See also **asymptomatic** patients (p. 1275).

Unresolved controversies

Include:

1. progressive STROKE ("stroke in evolution"): see Emergency carotid endarterectomy (p. 1295)
2. abrupt occlusion: see Emergency endarterectomy (p. 1295)
3. tandem lesions (e.g. carotid siphon and bifurcation stenosis): although this topic remains controversial, CEA in patients with tandem lesions has not been associated with increased postoperative stroke rates.[50,51] Recent case series also report success with endovascular treatment
4. progressive retinal ischemia

84.4.2 Timing with respect to acute stroke

For patients with small fixed deficits or small infarcts on CT or MRI, the risk of early CEA is not increased.[50,52] In the pooled analysis of the three symptomatic CEA studies, patients randomized in the trials within 2 weeks of the last symptomatic event had greater benefit from CEA.[53] Data from Sundt (see below) indicates that a stroke is a risk factor for a complication only if it occurred within 7 days pre-op.

Since the introduction of tPA for the treatment of acute ischemic stroke, there have been reports on the successful treatment of residual critical ICA stenosis following tPA recanalization as early as 24 hours after administration of tPA in patients with small fixed deficit or small ischemic areas on MRI.[53,54]

84.4.3 Pre-op risk factors for CEA

Σ

The characteristics of patients who are high risk for complications from CEA has not been well defined, despite the perception that this group exists.

Identifying patients at high risk for complications after CEA has proven challenging. Typically, the exclusion criteria from studies is cited, but in most cases these are simply patients that were not included in the study because it was the investigators perception these patients might be "high risk." Therefore these risk factors are not validated. They are included here for completeness.

NASCET and ACAS: age > 80 years, prior ipsilateral CEA, prior contralateral CEA within 4 months, prior neck XRT, tandem lesion larger than target lesion, other conditions that could cause symptoms (atrial fibrillation, prior stroke with persistent major deficit, valvular heart disease), major organ failure, uncontrolled hypertension or diabetes mellitus, and significant coronary artery disease[55,56]).

The SAPPHIRE Trial (Stenting and Angioplasty with Protection in Patients at High-Risk for Endarterectomy): patients with clinically significant cardiac disease (CHF, abnormal stress test, or need for open-heart surgery), severe pulmonary disease, contralateral carotid occlusion, contralateral laryngeal-nerve palsy, previous radical neck surgery or neck XRT, recurrent stenosis after endarterectomy, and age > 80 years.[57] The ARCHeR Trial (ACCULINK for Revascularization of Carotids in High-Risk patients) also included patients with tracheostomy, spinal immobility, and dialysis-dependant renal failure.[58]

84.4.4 Carotid endarterectomy – surgical considerations

Perioperative management

Pre-op management (carotid endarterectomy)

1. ASA 325 mg TID for at least 2 days, preferably 5 days pre-op[59] (NB: patients should be kept on their ASA for surgery, and if not on ASA they should be started, in order to reduce risks of MI and TIA[60])

Post-op management (carotid endarterectomy)

1. patient monitored in ICU with A-line
2. keep patient well hydrated (run IVF ≥ 100 cc/hr for most adults)
3. SBP ideally 110 – 150 mm Hg (higher pressures are permitted in patients with chronic severe HTN)
   a) BP frequently labile in 1st 24 hrs post-op, may be due to "new" pressure in carotid bulb; to prevent rebound hyper- or hypo-tension, avoid long acting agents
   b) hypotension
      - check EKG – R/O cardiogenic shock
      - if mild, start with fluids (crystalloid or colloid)
      - phenylephrine (Neo-Synephrine®) for resistant hypotension
   c) hypertension: nicardipine (Cardene®) (p. 126) is the agent of choice. Avoid rebound hypotension
4. avoid antiplatelet drugs for 24–48 hrs post-op (causes oozing); may start these 24–72 hrs post-op (note: ASA 325 mg + dipyridamole 75 mg TID have been shown *not* to reduce the rate of restenosis after endarterectomy[61])
5. optional: reverse half of heparin with protamine 10 minutes after closing arteriotomy

Post-op check (carotid endarterectomy)

In addition to routine, the following should be checked:

1. change in neurologic status due to cerebral dysfunction, including:
   a) pronator drift (R/O new hemiparesis)
   b) signs of dysphasia (especially for left sided surgery)
   c) mimetic muscle symmetry (assesses facial nerve function)
2. pupil diameter and reaction (R/O stroke, Horner's syndrome)
3. severe H/A (especially unilateral) > may indicate hyperperfusion syndrome
4. STA pulses (R/O external carotid occlusion)
5. tongue deviation (R/O hypoglossal nerve injury)
6. symmetry of lips (R/O weakness of lower lip depressors due to retraction of marginal mandibular branch of facial nerve against mandible, usually resolves in 6–12 wks, must differentiate from central VII palsy due to stroke)
7. check for hoarseness (R/O recurrent laryngeal nerve injury)
8. assess for hematoma in operative site: note any tracheal deviation, dysphagia

Post-op complications (carotid endarterectomy)

To justify CEA, the absolute upper limit of (significant) complication rate should be ≤ 3%.

1. overall in-hospital mortality: 1%[62]
2. disruption of arteriotomy closure: rare, but emergent (see below)
   a) evidenced by:
      - swelling of neck: rupture may produce a pseudoaneurysm
      - tracheal deviation (visible, palpable, or on CXR)
      - symptoms: dysphagia, air hunger or worsening hoarseness, difficulty swallowing
   b) dangers:
      - asphyxiation: most immediate danger
      - stroke
      - exsanguination (unlikely, unless skin closure is also disrupted)
   c) late (often delayed weeks to months): false aneurysm.[63] Risk = 0.33%. Presents as neck mass. Risk is increased with wound infection and possibly with patch graft as compared to endarterectomy alone[63,64,65]
3. stroke (cerebral infarction) intra-op or post-op rate[66]: 5%
   a) embolic (the most common cause of *minor* post-op neurologic deficit): source may be denuded media of endarterectomy
   b) intracerebral hemorrhagic (ICH) (breakthrough bleeding): occurs in < 0.6%.[67] Related to cerebral hyperperfusion in most[68,69] (see below). Usually occurs within first 2 weeks, often in basal ganglion 3–4 days post-op with hypertensive episode. Patients at greatest risk are those with severe stenosis and limited hemispheric collateral flow
   c) post-op ICA occlusion
      - most common cause of *major* post-op stroke, but may be asymptomatic
      - risk is reduced by attention to technical details at surgery[70 (p 249)]
      - some may be due to hypercoagulable state induced by heparin (predictable in patients whose platelet count drops while on heparin. No known therapy for this condition[70 (p 249–50)])

- the endarterectomized surface is highly thrombogenic for 4 hrs following endarterectomy (Sundt recommends not reversing heparin)
- in Sundt's series using patch graft[70(p 229)]: 0.8% incidence, associated with major stroke in 33% and minor stroke in 20%
- occlusion rate with primary closure: 4% in Sundt's experience, 2–5% in literature[70(p 249)]

4. post-op TIAs: most due to ICA occlusion. Some may be due to microemboli. Hyperperfusion syndrome produces a 1% incidence of post-op TIAs[70(p 229)]
5. seizures[71]: usually focal in onset with possible generalization, most occur late (post-op day 5–13) with an incidence of ≈ 0.4%[67] to 1%.[72] May be due to cerebral hyperperfusion,[67] emboli,[73] and/or intracerebral hemorrhage. Usually difficult to control initially, lorazepam and phenytoin are recommended (p.205)
6. late restenosis: identifiable restenosis occurs in ≈ 25% by 1 yr, and half of these reduce luminal diameters by > 50%.[74] Restenosis within 2 yrs is usually due to fibrous hyperplasia, after 2 yrs it is typically due to atherosclerosis[75]
7. cerebral hyperperfusion syndrome (AKA normal pressure hyperperfusion breakthrough): classically thought to result from return of blood flow to an area that has lost autoregulation due to chronic cerebral ischemia typically from high-grade stenosis. Controversial.[69] Usually presents as ipsilateral vascular H/A or eye pain that subsides within several days[76] or with seizures (± PLEDs on EEG, more common with Halothane®, due to petechial hemorrhages[67]). May cause ICH.[77] Most complications occur several days post-op
8. hoarseness: the most common cause is laryngeal edema and *not* superior nor recurrent laryngeal nerve injury
9. cranial nerve injury: the most common complication after CEA with an incidence of up to 8–10%[78]
   a) hypoglossal nerve → tongue deviation towards the side of injury: incidence ≈ 1% (with mobilizing XII to allow displacement). Unilateral injury may cause speaking, chewing and swallowing difficulties. Bilateral injuries can cause upper airway obstruction.[79] The presence of a unilateral palsy is a contraindication to doing contralateral endarterectomy until the first side recovers. May last as long as four months
   b) vagus or recurrent laryngeal nerve → unilateral vocal cord paralysis: 1% risk
   c) mandibular branch of facial nerve → loss of ipsilateral lip depressor
10. headache[67]
11. hypertension[80,81]: may develop 5–7 days post-op. Longstanding HTN may occur as a result of the loss of the carotid sinus baroreceptor reflex

Complication management

1. post-op TIAs
   a) if TIA occurs in recovery room, emergency CT (to R/O hemorrhage) and then angiogram recommended to assess for ICA or CCA occlusion (vs. emboli)
   b) if TIA occurs later, consider emergent OPG; if abnormal → emergent surgery (if neurologically intact, pre-op angiogram is appropriate)[70]
2. fixed post-op deficit in distribution of endarterectomized carotid
   a) if deficit occurs immediately post-op (i.e. in PACU), recommend immediate re-exploration without delay for CT or angiogram[82] (case reports of no deficit when flow re-established in ≤ 45 mins). For later onset, workup is indicated. Technical considerations for emergency re-operation[70(p 255)]:
      - isolate the 3 arteries (CCA, ECA, & ICA)
      - occlude CCA 1st, then ECA, and ICA last (to minimize emboli)
      - open arteriotomy, check backflow; if none, pass a No. 4 Fogarty catheter into ICA, gently inflate and withdraw (avoid intimal tears)
      - if good backflow established, close with patch graft
      - remove tortuous vessel loops and kinks before closing
   b) immediate management (unless ICH or SDH are likely) includes
      - fluids (e.g. Plasmanate®) to improve rheology and to elevate BP
      - pressors (e.g. phenylephrine) to elevate SBP to ≈ 180 mm Hg
      - oxygen
      - heparinization (may be controversial)
   c) theoretical benefits of radiographic evaluation include:
      - CT: identifies ICH or SDH that might require treatment other than re-exploration of the surgical site, elevating BP, etc.

84

- angiogram: identifies whether ICA is occluded, or if deficit is from another cause (e.g. emboli from endarterectomy site) that would not benefit from re-exploration or possibly endovascular treatment

3. disruption of arteriotomy closure, management
   a) OPEN WOUND – if there is any stridor, it is critical to do this before trying to intubate (although ideally performed in O.R., the delay may be decisive). Evacuate clot (start with a sterile gloved finger) and stop bleeding, preferably without traumatizing the artery, a DeBakey clamp is optimal
   b) INTUBATION – high priority, may be difficult or impossible if trachea is deviated (open wound immediately). Preferably done by anesthesiologist in controlled setting (i.e. O.R.) unless there is acute airway obstruction
   c) call O.R. and have them prepare set-up for endarterectomy, and take patient to O.R.

84.4.5 Operative technique

Anesthesia and monitoring

Most (but not all) surgeons monitor some parameter of neurologic function during carotid endarterectomy, and will alter technique (e.g. insert a vascular shunt) if there is evidence of hemodynamic intolerance of carotid clamping (only occurs in ≈ 1–4%).

1. local/regional anesthesia: permits "clinical" monitoring of patient's neurologic function.[83,84] Disadvantages: patient movement during procedure (often exacerbated by sedation and alterations in CBF), lack of cerebral protection from anesthetic and adjunctive agents. The only prospective randomized study found no difference between local and general anesthesia.[85] The multicenter, randomized controlled General Anesthesia versus Local Anesthesia (GALA) Trial[86] found no significant differences in the prevention of stroke, MI, or death for either anesthetic technique. Subgroup analysis showed trends (not statistically significant) favoring local anesthesia for perioperative death, event-free survival at 1 year, and patients with contralateral occlusion. Local anesthesia was associated with a significant reduction of shunt insertion.[86] A Cochrane Database Review found no evidence from randomized trials to favor either anesthetic technique[87]
2. general anesthesia, possibly including barbiturates (thiopental boluses of 125–250 mg until 15–30 second burst suppression on EEG, followed by small bolus injections or constant infusion to maintain burst suppression[59])
   a) EEG monitoring
   b) SSEP monitoring
   c) measurement of distal stump pressure after CCA occlusion (unreliable), e.g. using a shunt if stump pressure < 25 mm Hg
   d) transcranial Doppler
   e) near-infrared spectroscopy

Position and incision

1. supine, neck slightly extended and rotated slightly (≈ 30°) away from the operative side
2. the incision curves gently and follows the anterior border of the sternocleidomastoid muscle, and curves posteriorly at the rostral end
3. keep the horizontal portion of the incision ≈ 1 cm away from the mandible to avoid injury to marginal mandibular branch of facial nerve (which lies in the inferior parotid gland and supplies lip depressor) due to retraction against mandible
4. retractors should not be placed deeper than the platysma to avoid injury to recurrent laryngeal nerve which runs between the esophagus and trachea. Blunt retractors are used to avoid internal jugular vein injury

Dissection

1. the common facial vein (CFV) usually crosses the field over the carotid bifurcation, it is doubly ligated and divided. It leads to the internal jugular vein (IJV)
2. identifying the IJV is key, dissection is carried down between the carotid artery and the IJV
3. the *ansa hypoglossi* runs superficial to the ICA and serves as a useful guide to the *hypoglossal nerve* (XII) which should be identified since it is at greater risk when it is not seen. XII can arise anywhere from the carotid bifurcation to the angle of the mandible, although it is usually in the vicinity of the CFV. Mobilization can be facilitated by dividing the small artery (sternocleidomastoid branch of the ECA) and vein that cross over it[79]

4. the ansa hypoglossi can usually be spared, and if mobilized, allows medial retraction of the hypoglossal nerve out of harm's way. If it is necessary to divide the ansa it is done close to the hypoglossal nerve to be certain it is not a branch of the vagus and to minimize neurologic deficit (the ansa has an anterior cervical limb from the cervical plexus)
5. the superior thyroid artery is the first branch of the ECA, and helps differentiate ECA from the ICA (the ICA is located posterior to the ECA)
6. the carotid bulb may be anesthetized with ≈ 2–3 ml of 1% plain lidocaine using a 27 Ga needle. This may be done routinely, or, as some prefer only if hypotension and/or bradycardia occur during dissection (indicating IX nerve stimulation)
7. the ICA must be exposed beyond the extent of the plaque which can be determined by gentle palpation with a moistened finger and by visualization as the area where the artery turns from yellowish to its normal pinker color

Occlusion and arteriotomy

1. a vessel loop is placed around the ECA at least 2 cm above the bifurcation
2. a vessel loop is also placed around the ICA but is looped only once
3. umbilical tape with a choke is placed around the CCA 2–3 cm below the bifurcation
4. IV heparin (usually 5,000 IU) is given 1 minute prior to cross clamping
5. a temporary aneurysm clip is placed on the superior thyroid artery
6. the order of *occlusion* of the vessels is as follows (mnemonic: "ICE"):
   a) ICA (e.g. with temporary aneurysm clip)
   b) CCA (e.g. with a small DeBakey clamp)
   c) ECA (e.g. with temporary aneurysm clip)
7. during ICA clamping, mild hypertension is maintained by the anesthesiologist
8. shunt: some surgeons use some form of monitoring (EEG, BSAER, etc.) to determine if a shunt is needed – see Anesthesia and monitoring (p. 1294) -, yet others routinely use a shunt whenever possible without assessing the need
9. the arteriotomy is begun in the CCA with a #11 scalpel, and once the lumen is entered, a Potts' scissors carries the incision through to the ICA beyond the plaque. Stay in the midline to facilitate arteriotomy closure

Plaque removal

1. the plaque usually cannot be completely removed from the CCA, and thus it is usually transected with a Potts' scissors taking care not to inadvertently incise the artery wall and to leave as smooth an edge as possible
2. in the ICA, great care must be made to avoid leaving an intimal flap which could become a nidus for an arterial dissection. If necessary the intima may be tacked down by suturing from the lumen out on both ends (using double armed suture) and tying the knot outside the vessel

Arteriotomy closure and vessel release

1. arteriotomy may be performed with a running Prolene suture using either
   a) primary closure
   b) or with a patch graft to increase the caliber of the vessel and reduce the risk of re-stenosis
   c) limited evidence suggests that carotid patch angioplasty may reduce the risk of perioperative arterial occlusion and re-stenosis. Synthetic patches (Dacron, PTFE) are preferred to autologous vein (risk of aneurysmal dilatation, thrombogenic surface)[88,89]
2. the order of releasing the vessels (reverse that of the clamping order):
   a) ECA
   b) CCA (allows air and debris to be washed into the ECA)
   c) ICA

84.4.6 Emergency carotid endarterectomy

General information

Emergency CEA indications include crescendo TIAs and stroke in evolution. The treatment paradigm of these conditions has shifted towards the use of interventional methods, such as thrombolysis and stenting, although there are no randomized controlled trial data to support that approach. A recent meta-analysis of emergent CEA has shown that the pooled stroke and stroke/death rates after CEA for crescendo TIA in 176 patients were 6.5% and 9.0%, respectively. For those with stroke in evolution, the overall stroke and stroke/death rates in 114 patients were 16.9% and 20.0%, respectively.[90]

After retrospective analysis of 64 emergency endarterectomies[91] the guidelines given below were suggested. However, the efficacy of immediate surgical removal of obstruction is controversial and unproven. In one early study, over 50% of patients suffered fatal intracranial hemorrhage within 72 hours of emergency carotid endarterectomy.

Initial management of patient presenting with acute neuro deficit

1. obtain history directed at determining presence of previous stroke and other serious medical illness, and to try to differentiate from seizure
2. baseline neurological assessment including evaluation of STA pulses and carotid bruits
3. during evaluation: close control of BP. O_2 per NC. Labs + EKG; see Management of TIA or stroke (p. 1282). Consider hemodilution with LMD
4. CT to R/O ICH or infarction (early stroke will not be visible)
5. when carotid disease is suspected, and CT is negative for ICH or acute infarct, emergency angiography, MRI/MRA or CTA is performed

Indications for emergency carotid endarterectomy

General information

In patients with acute neurological deficits, the need for rapid decision making often does not allow differentiating between TIA, stroke in evolution and acute stroke, nor in assessing the stability or fluctuating nature of the deficit.

Indications

1. stroke in evolution
2. crescendo TIAs: TIAs that abruptly increase in frequency to ≥ several per day
3. following intra-arterial thrombolysis, emergent/urgent CEA is indicated for residual critical carotid stenosis[54,92]

Contraindications

See also more details (p. 1286). Patients with depressed levels of consciousness or acute fixed deficits.

Surgical management

Again, most cases would now be managed initially with endovascular thrombolysis and stenting. Surgery would considered if this is not an option.

1. for emergency surgery, it is essential that blood pressure be stable
2. in patients with complete occlusion, ICA is not occluded intra-op (to avoid breaking up thrombus, if present)
3. if thrombus present
   a) attempt spontaneous extrusion using back pressure
   b) if this fails, attempt to remove with smoothened suction catheter
   c) if this fails, pass balloon embolectomy catheter as far as base of skull (caution: avoid injury to distal ICA that could cause CCF)
   d) obtain intra-op angiogram unless thrombus emerges and backflow is excellent
   e) plicate ICA (avoid creating a blind pouch at origin) if there is good backflow or if satisfactory angiography cannot be obtained

Surgical results

Highest correlation was with presenting neurologic status (▶ Table 84.4).

Table 84.4 Surgical results

Presenting deficit	Same or improved	Deaths
intact or mild	92%	0
moderate	80%	1 (7%)
severe	77%	3 (13%)

84.5 Carotid angioplasty/stenting

84.5.1 General information

Σ

There are no well-designed studies that convincingly show superiority of angioplasty/stenting over CEA in *average risk* symptomatic patients, and the recommendation in these patients is to continue with the time-tested technique of CEA.

There is a paucity of randomized control trials[57,58,93,94,95,96] comparing carotid angioplasty/stenting with CEA, and many nonrandomized registries.[58,97,98,99,100,101,102,103,104,105]

However, data from multicenter randomized trials showing that carotid angioplasty/stenting is as safe over the short term or as efficacious over the long term as CEA in average-risk symptomatic patients are lacking. Published trials are heterogeneous (clinically and methodologically), too small to provide robust and convincing data, and limited in long-term follow-up. Only the SAPPHIRE study[57] comparing CEA with stenting (using a distal embolic protection device) for moderate to severe carotid stenosis with comorbidities that might increase the risk of CEA (high-risk patients), found that angioplasty/stenting was not inferior (risk within 3%, P = 0.004) to CEA (based on a composite primary end point of stroke, death, or MI within 30 days, or death from neurologic causes or ipsilateral stroke between 31 days and 1 year).[57] However, the study methodology has been criticized.[106,107,108]

A 2007 Cochrane review concluded that available data on carotid angioplasty/stenting are difficult to interpret and does not support a change in clinical practice away from recommending CEA as the treatment of choice for suitable carotid artery stenosis.[109]

84.5.2 Indications for angioplasty/stenting

Carotid stenting performed with adequate procedural quality levels, should be considered instead of CEA in the presence of[110]:

1. severe vascular and cardiac comorbidities:
   a) congestive heart failure (New York Heart Association class III/IV) and/or known severe left ventricular dysfunction
   b) open heart surgery needed within 6 weeks
   c) recent myocardial infarction (< 24 hours and > 4 weeks)
   d) unstable angina (Canadian Cardiovascular Society class III/IV)
   e) contralateral carotid occlusion
2. specific conditions:
   a) contralateral laryngeal nerve palsy
   b) radiation therapy to the neck
   c) previous CEA with recurrent restenosis
   d) high cervical internal carotid/below the clavicle common carotid lesions
   e) severe tandem lesions
   f) age > 80 years
   g) severe pulmonary disease

The 2009 European Society for Vascular Surgery (ESVS) Guidelines state that carotid angioplasty/stenting is indicated in cases of: contralateral laryngeal nerve palsy, previous radical neck dissection or cervical XRT, prior CEA (re-stenosis), high bifurcation or intracranial extension of a carotid lesion, provided that the peri-interventional stroke or death rate is not higher than that accepted for CEA (Class C recommendation).[88]

AHA Guidelines state that angioplasty/stenting might be a reasonable alternative to CEA in ***asymptomatic high risk*** patients. However, they stress that it remains uncertain whether this group of patients should have either procedure.[111]

References

[1] Moulin T, Cattin F, Crépin-Leblond T, et al. Early CT Signs in Acute Middle Cerebral Artery Infarction: Predictive Value for Subsequent Infarct Locations and Outcome. Neurology. 1996; 47:366–375

[2] Marks MP, Holmgren EB, Fox AJ, Patel S, von Kummer R, Froehlich J. Evaluation of early computed tomographic findings in acute ischemic stroke. Stroke. 1999; 30:389–392

[3] Tomandl BF, Klotz E, Handschu R, Stemper B, Reinhardt F, Huk WJ, Eberhardt KE, Fateh-Moghadam S. Comprehensive imaging of ischemic stroke with multisection CT. Radiographics. 2003; 23:565–592
[4] Wall SD, Brant-Zawadzki M, Jeffrey RB, Barnes B. High Frequency CT Findings Within 24 Hours After Cerebral Infarction. AJR. 1982; 138:307–311
[5] Aarabi B, Long DM. Dynamics of Cerebral Edema. J Neurosurg. 1979; 51:779–784
[6] Gacs G, Fox AJ, Barnett HJM, Vinuela F. CT Visualization of Intracranial Thromboembolism. Stroke. 1983; 14:756–762
[7] Tomsick TA, Brott TG, Olinger CP, Adams H, et al. Hyperdense Middle Cerebral Artery: Incidence and Quantitative Significance. Neuroradiology. 1989; 31:312–315
[8] Manelfe C, Larrue V, von Kummer R, et al. Association of Hyperdense Middle Cerebral Artery Sign With Clinical Outcome in Patients Treated With Plasminogen Activator. Stroke. 1999; 30:769–772
[9] Sims JR, Rordorf G, Smith EE, Koroshetz WJ, Lev MH, Buonanno F, Schwamm LH. Arterial occlusion revealed by CT angiography predicts NIH stroke score and acute outcomes after IV tPA treatment. AJNR Am J Neuroradiol. 2005; 26:246–251
[10] Nabavi DG, Cenic A, Craen RA, Gelb AW, Bennett JD, Kozak R, Lee TY. CT assessment of cerebral perfusion: experimental validation and initial clinical experience. Radiology. 1999; 213:141–149
[11] Elster AD, Moody DM. Early Cerebral Infarction: Gadopentetate Dimeglumine Enhancement. Radiology. 1990; 177:627–632
[12] Barber PA, Darby DG, Desmond PM, Yang Q, Gerraty RP, Jolley D, Donnan GA, Tress BM, Davis SM. Prediction of stroke outcome with echoplanar perfusion- and diffusion-weighted MRI. Neurology. 1998; 51:418–426
[13] Lassen NA. Control of Cerebral Circulation in Health and Disease. Circ Res. 1974; 34:749–760
[14] Brott T, Adams HP, Ollinger CP, et al. Measurements of Acute Cerebral Infarction: A Clinical Examination Scale. Stroke. 1991; 20:864–870
[15] Lyden P, Brott T, Tilley B, et al. Improved reliability of the NIH stroke scale using video training. Stroke. 1994; 25:2220–2226
[16] The National Institute of Neurological Disorders and Stroke rt-PA Stroke Study Group. Tissue plasminogen activator for acute ischemic stroke. N Engl J Med. 1995; 333:1581–1587
[17] Kwiatkowski TG, Libman RB, Frankel M, et al. Effects of plasminogen activator for acute ischemic stroke at one year. N Engl J Med. 1999; 340:1781–1787
[18] Hacke W, Kaste M, Fieschi C, et al. Randomized double-blind placebo-controlled trial of thrombolytic therapy with intravenous alteplase in acute ischemic stroke (ECASS II). Lancet. 1998; 352:1245–1251
[19] Lansberg MG, Bluhmki E, Thijs VN. Efficacy and safety of tissue plasminogen activator 3 to 4.5 hours after acute ischemic stroke: a metaanalysis. Stroke. 2009; 40:2438–2441
[20] Saver JL. Hemorrhage after thrombolytic therapy for stroke: the clinically relevant number needed to harm. Stroke. 2007; 38:2279–2283
[21] Benedict SL, Ni OK, Schloesser P, White KS, Bale JF, Jr. Intra-arterial thrombolysis in a 2-year-old with cardioembolic stroke. J Child Neurol. 2007; 22:225–227
[22] Fisher M, Hachinski V. European Cooperative Acute Stroke Study III: support for and questions about a truly emerging therapy. Stroke. 2009; 40:2262–2263
[23] Barreto AD, Martin-Schild S, Hallevi H, Morales MM, Abraham AT, Gonzales NR, Illoh K, Grotta JC, Savitz SI. Thrombolytic therapy for patients who wake-up with stroke. Stroke. 2009; 40:827–832
[24] Toni D, Fiorelli M, Bastianello S, et al. Hemorrhagic transformation of brain infarct: Predictability in the first 5 hours from stroke onset and influence on clinical outcome. Neurology. 1996; 46:341–345
[25] The National Institute of Neurological Disorders and Stroke rt-PA Stroke Study Group. Intracerebral hemorrhage after intravenous t-PA therapy for ischemic stroke. Stroke. 1997; 28:2109–2118
[26] Paciaroni M, Agnelli G, Corea F, Ageno W, Alberti A, Lanari A, Caso V, Micheli S, Bertolani L, Venti M, Palmerini F, Biagini S, Comi G, Previdi P, Silvestrelli G. Early hemorrhagic transformation of brain infarction: rate, predictive factors, and influence on clinical outcome: results of a prospective multicenter study. Stroke. 2008; 39:2249–2256
[27] Campbell BC, Mitchell PJ, Kleinig TJ, Dewey HM, Churilov L, Yassi N, Yan B, Dowling RJ, Parsons MW, Oxley TJ, Wu TY, Brooks M, Simpson MA, Miteff F, Levi CR, Krause M, Harrington TJ, Faulder KC, Steinfort BS, Priglinger M, Ang T, Scroop R, Barber PA, McGuinness B, Wijeratne T, Phan TG, Chong W, Chandra RV, Bladin CF, Badve M, Rice H, de Villiers L, Ma H, Desmond PM, Donnan GA, Davis SM. Endovascular therapy for ischemic stroke with perfusion-imaging selection. N Engl J Med. 2015; 372:1009–1018
[28] Goyal M, Demchuk AM, Menon BK, Eesa M, Rempel JL, Thornton J, Roy D, Jovin TG, Willinsky RA, Sapkota BL, Dowlatshahi D, Frei DF, Kamal NR, Montanera WJ, Poppe AY, Ryckborst KJ, Silver FL, Shuaib A, Tampieri D, Williams D, Bang OY, Baxter BW, Burns PA, Choe H, Heo JH, Holmstedt CA, Jankowitz B, Kelly M, Linares G, Mandzia JL, Shankar J, Sohn SI, Swartz RH, Barber PA, Coutts SB, Smith EE, Morrish WF, Weill A, Subramaniam S, Mitha AP, Wong JH, Lowerison MW, Sajobi TT, Hill MD. Randomized assessment of rapid endovascular treatment of ischemic stroke. N Engl J Med. 2015; 372:1019–1030
[29] Berkhemer OA, Fransen PS, Beumer D, van den Berg LA, Lingsma HF, Yoo AJ, Schonewille WJ, Vos JA, Nederkoorn PJ, Wermer MJ, van Walderveen MA, Staals J, Hofmeijer J, van Oostayen JA, Lycklama a Nijeholt GJ, Boiten J, Brouwer PA, Emmer BJ, de Bruijn SF, van Dijk LC, Kappelle LJ, Lo RH, van Dijk EJ, de Vries J, de Kort PL, van Rooij WJ, van den Berg JS, van Hasselt BA, Aerden LA, Dallinga RJ, Visser MC, Bot JC, Vroomen PC, Eshghi O, Schreuder TH, Heijboer RJ, Keizer K, Tielbeek AV, den Hertog HM, Gerrits DG, van den Berg-Vos RM, Karas GB, Steyerberg EW, Flach HZ, Marquering HA, Sprengers ME, Jenniskens SF, Beenen LF, van den Berg R, Koudstaal PJ, van Zwam WH, Roos YB, van der Lugt A, van Oostenbrugge RJ, Majoie CB, Dippel DW. A randomized trial of intraarterial treatment for acute ischemic stroke. N Engl J Med. 2015; 372:11–20
[30] Fransen PS, Beumer D, Berkhemer OA, van den Berg LA, Lingsma H, van der Lugt A, van Zwam WH, van Oostenbrugge RJ, Roos YB, Majoie CB, Dippel DW. MR CLEAN, a multicenter randomized clinical trial of endovascular treatment for acute ischemic stroke in the Netherlands: study protocol for a randomized controlled trial. Trials. 2014; 15. DOI: 10.1186/1745-6215-15-343
[31] Brott T, Reed RL. Intensive care for acute stroke in the community hospital setting: The first 24 hours. Stroke. 1989; 20:694–697
[32] Pulsinelli WA, Levy DE, Sigsbee B, Scherer B, et al. Increased damage after ischemic stroke in patients with hyperglycemia with or without established diabetes mellitus. Am J Med. 1983; 74:540–544
[33] Tracey F, Crawford VLS, Lawson JT, Buchanan KD, Stour RW. Hyperglycemia and mortality from acute stroke. Quart J Med. 1993; 86:439–446
[34] Wass CT, Lanier WL. Glucose Modulation of Ischemic Brain Injury: Review and Clinical Recommendations. Mayo Clin Proc. 1996; 71:801–812
[35] Swanson RA. Intravenous heparin for acute stroke. What can we learn from the megatrials? Neurology. 1999; 52:1746–1750
[36] Duke RJ, Bloch RF, Turpie AG, et al. Intravenous heparin for the prevention of stroke progression in acute partial stable stroke. Ann Intern Med. 1986; 105:825–828
[37] Barer D. Interpretation of IST and CAST stroke trials. Lancet. 1997; 350

[38] Genton E, Barnett HJM, Fields WS, et al. Cerebral Ischemia: The Role of Thrombosis and of Antithrombotic Therapy. Stroke. 1977; 8:150–175
[39] Scheinberg P. Heparin Anticoagulation. Stroke. 1989; 20:173–174
[40] Phillips SJ. An Alternative View of Heparin Anticoagulation in Acute Focal Brain Ischemia. Stroke. 1989; 20:295–298
[41] Ramirez-Lassepas M, Quiñones MR, Nino HH. Treatment of acute ischemic stroke: Open trial with continuous intravenous heparinization. Arch Neurol. 1986; 43:386–390
[42] Chassin MR. Appropriate Use of Carotid Endarterectomy. N Engl J Med. 1998; 339:1468–1471
[43] The North American Symptomatic Carotid Endarterectomy Trial. Beneficial Effect of Carotid Endarterectomy in Symptomatic Patients with High-Grade Carotid Stenosis. N Engl J Med. 1991; 325:445–453
[44] The European Carotid Surgery Trialists' Collaborative Group. Randomized Trial of Endartectomy for Recently Symptomatic Carotid Stenosis: Final Results of the MRC European Carotid Surgery Trial (ECST). Lancet. 1998; 351:1379–1387
[45] Barnett HJM, Taylor W, Eliasziw M, et al. Benefit of Carotid Endarterectomy in Patients with Symptomatic Moderate or Severe Stenosis. N Engl J Med. 1998; 339:1415–1425
[46] The European Carotid Surgery Trialists' Collaborative Group. Endartectomy for Moderate Symptomatic Carotid Stenosis: Interim Results of the MRC European Carotid Surgery Trial. Lancet. 1996; 347:1591–1593
[47] Halliday A, Mansfield A, Marro J, Peto C, Peto R, Potter J, Thomas D. Prevention of disabling and fatal strokes by successful carotid endarterectomy in patients without recent neurological symptoms: randomised controlled trial. Lancet. 2004; 363:1491–1502
[48] The Executive Committee for the Asymptomatic Carotid Atherosclerosis Study. Endarterectomy for Asymptomatic Carotid Artery Stenosis. JAMA. 1995; 273:1421–1428
[49] Haynes RB, Taylor DW, Sackett DL, et al. Prevention of Functional Impairment by Endarterectomy for Symptomatic High-Grade Stenosis. Lancet. 1994; 351:1379–1387
[50] Faries PL, Chaer RA, Patel S, Lin SC, DeRubertis B, Kent KC. Current management of extracranial carotid artery disease. Vasc Endovascular Surg. 2006; 40:165–175
[51] Rouleau PA, Huston J, III, Gilbertson J, Brown RD,Jr, Meyer FB, Bower TC. Carotid artery tandem lesions: frequency of angiographic detection and consequences for endarterectomy. AJNR Am J Neuroradiol. 1999; 20:621–625
[52] Bond R, Rerkasem K, Rothwell PM. Systematic review of the risks of carotid endarterectomy in relation to the clinical indication for and timing of surgery. Stroke. 2003; 34:2290–2301
[53] Rothwell PM, Eliasziw M, Gutnikov SA, Warlow CP, Barnett HJ. Endarterectomy for symptomatic carotid stenosis in relation to clinical subgroups and timing of surgery. Lancet. 2004; 363:915–924
[54] Bartoli MA, Squarcioni C, Nicoli F, Magnan PE, Malikov S, Berger L, Lerussi GB, Branchereau A. Early carotid endarterectomy after intravenous thrombolysis for acute ischaemic stroke. Eur J Vasc Endovasc Surg. 2009; 37:512–518
[55] Nguyen LL, Conte MS, Reed AB, Belkin M. Carotid endarterectomy: who is the high-risk patient? Semin Vasc Surg. 2004; 17:219–223
[56] Kang JL, Chung TK, Lancaster RT, Lamuraglia GM, Conrad MF, Cambria RP. Outcomes after carotid endarterectomy: is there a high-risk population? A National Surgical Quality Improvement Program report. J Vasc Surg. 2009; 49:331–8, 339 e1; discussion 338-9
[57] Yadav JS, Wholey MH, Kuntz RE, Fayad P, Katzen BT, Mishkel GJ, Bajwa TK, Whitlow P, Strickman NE, Jaff MR, Popma JJ, Snead DB, Cutlip DE, Firth BG, Ouriel K. Protected carotid-artery stenting versus endarterectomy in high-risk patients. N Engl J Med. 2004; 351:1493–1501
[58] Gray WA, Hopkins LN, Yadav S, Davis T, Wholey M, Atkinson R, Cremonesi A, Fairman R, Walker G, Verta P, Popma J, Virmani R, Cohen DJ. Protected carotid stenting in high-surgical-risk patients: the ARCHeR results. J Vasc Surg. 2006; 44:258–268
[59] Spetzler RF, Martin N, Hadley MN, et al. Microsurgical Endarterectomy Under Barbiturate Protection: A Prospective Study. J Neurosurg. 1986; 65:63–73
[60] Mayo Asymptomatic Carotid Endarterectomy Study Group. Results of a Randomized Controlled Trial of Carotid Endarterectomy for Asymptomatic Carotid Stenosis. Mayo Clin Proc. 1992; 67:513–518
[61] Harker LA, Bernstein EF, Dilley RB, Scala TE, et al. Failure of Aspirin plus Dipyridamole to Prevent Restenosis After Carotid Endarterectomy. Ann Int Med. 1992; 116:731–736
[62] McPhee JT, Hill JS, Ciocca RG, Messina LM, Eslami MH. Carotid endarterectomy was performed with lower stroke and death rates than carotid artery stenting in the United States in 2003 and 2004. J Vasc Surg. 2007; 46:1112–1118
[63] Branch CL, Davis CH. False Aneurysm Complicating Carotid Endarterectomy. Neurosurgery. 1986; 19:421–425
[64] McCollum CH, Wheeler WG, Noon GP, et al. Aneurysms of the Extracranial Carotid Artery. Am J Surg. 1979; 137:196–200
[65] Welling RE, Taha A, Goel T, et al. Extracranial Carotid Artery Aneurysms. Surgery. 1983; 93:319–323
[66] Brott TG, Labutta RJ, Kempczinski RF. Changing Patterns in the Practice of Carotid Endarterectomy in a Large Metropolitan Area. JAMA. 1986; 255:2609–2612
[67] Reigel MM, Hollier LH, Sundt TM, et al. Cerebral Hyperperfusion Syndrome: A Cause of Neurologic Dysfunction After Carotid Endarterectomy. J Vasc Surg. 1987; 5:628–634
[68] Piepgras DG, Morgan MK, Sundt TM, et al. Intracerebral Hemorrhage After Carotid Endarterectomy. J Neurosurg. 1988; 68:532–536
[69] Ascher E, Markevich N, Schutzer RW, Kallakuri S, Jacob T, Hingorani AP. Cerebral hyperperfusion syndrome after carotid endarterectomy: predictive factors and hemodynamic changes. J Vasc Surg. 2003; 37:769–777
[70] Sundt TM. Occlusive Cerebrovascular Disease. Philadelphia: W. B. Saunders; 1987
[71] Kieburtz K, Ricotta JJ, Moxley RT. Seizures Following Carotid Endarterectomy. Arch Neurol. 1990; 47:568–570
[72] Sundt TM, Sharbrough FW, Piepgras DG, et al. Correlation of Cerebral Blood Flow and Electroencephalographic Changes During Carotid Endarterectomy. Mayo Clin Proc. 1981; 56:533–543
[73] Wilkinson JT, Adams HP, Wright CB. Convulsions After Carotid Endarterectomy. JAMA. 1980; 244:1827–1828
[74] Bernstein EF, Humber PB, Collins GM, et al. Life expectancy and late stroke following carotid enderterectomy. Ann Surg. 1983; 198:80–86
[75] Callow AD. Recurrent Stenosis After Carotid Endarterectomy. Arch Surg. 1982; 117:1082–1085
[76] Dolan JG, Mushlin AI. Hypertension, Vascular Headaches, and Seizures After Carotid Endarterectomy. Arch Intern Med. 1984; 144:1489–1491
[77] Caplan LR, Skillman J, Ojemann R, Fields W. Intracerebral Hemorrhage Following Carotid Endarterectomy: A Hypertensive Complication. Stroke. 1979; 9:457–460
[78] Sajid MS, Vijaynagar B, Singh P, Hamilton G. Literature review of cranial nerve injuries during carotid endarterectomy. Acta Chir Belg. 2007; 107:25–28
[79] Imparato AM, Bracco A, Kim GE, Bergmann L. The Hypoglossal Nerve in Carotid Arterial Reconstructions. Stroke. 1972; 3:576–578
[80] Skydell JL, Machleder HI, Baker JD, et al. Incidence and Mechanism of Postcarotid Endarterectomy Hypertension. Arch Surg. 1987; 122:1153–1155

[81] Lehv MS, Salzman EW, Silen W. Hypertension Complicating Carotid Endarterectomy. Stroke. 1970; 1:307–313
[82] Baker WH, Bergan JJ, Yao JST. In: Management of stroke during and after carotid surgery. Cerebrovascular Insufficiency. New York: Grune and Stratton; 1983:481–495
[83] Zuccarello M, Yeh H-S, Tew JM. Morbidity and Mortality of Carotid Endarterectomy under Local Anesthesia: A Retrospective Study. Neurosurgery. 1988; 23:445–450
[84] Lee KS, Courtland CH, McWhorter JM. Low Morbidity and Mortality of Carotid Endarterectomy Performed with Regional Anesthesia. J Neurosurg. 1988; 69:483–487
[85] Forssell C, Takolander R, Bergqvist D, et al. Local Versus General Anesthesia in Carotid Surgery. A Prospective Randomized Study. Eur J Vasc Surg. 1989; 3:503–509
[86] Lewis SC, Warlow CP, Bodenham AR, Colam B, Rothwell PM, Torgerson D, Dellagrammaticas D, Horrocks M, Liapis C, Banning AP, Gough M, Gough MJ. General anaesthesia versus local anaesthesia for carotid surgery (GALA): a multicentre, randomised controlled trial. Lancet. 2008; 372:2132–2142
[87] Rerkasem K, Rothwell PM. Local versus general anaesthesia for carotid endarterectomy. Cochrane Database Syst Rev. 2008. DOI: 10.1002/14651858.CD000126.pub3
[88] Liapis CD, Bell PR, Mikhailidis D, Sivenius J, Nicolaides A, Fernandes e Fernandes J, Biasi G, Norgren L. ESVS guidelines. Invasive treatment for carotid stenosis: indications, techniques. Eur J Vasc Endovasc Surg. 2009; 37:1–19
[89] Bond R, Rerkasem K, AbuRahma AF, Naylor AR, Rothwell PM. Patch angioplasty versus primary closure for carotid endarterectomy. Cochrane Database Syst Rev. 2004. DOI: 10.1002/14651858.CD000160.pub2
[90] Karkos CD, Hernandez-Lahoz I, Naylor AR. Urgent carotid surgery in patients with crescendo transient ischaemic attacks and stroke-in-evolution: a systematic review. Eur J Vasc Endovasc Surg. 2009; 37:279–288
[91] Walters BB, Ojemann RG, Heros RC. Emergency Carotid Endarterectomy. J Neurosurg. 1987; 66:817–823
[92] Mayo Asymptomatic Carotid Endarterectomy Study Group. Results of a randomized controlled trial of carotid endarterectomy for asymptomatic carotid stenosis. Mayo Clin Proc. 1992; 67:513–518
[93] CAVATAS Investigators. Endovascular versus surgical treatment in patients with carotid stenosis in the Carotid and Vertebral Artery Transluminal Angioplasty Study (CAVATAS): a randomised trial. Lancet. 2001; 357:1729–1737
[94] Alberts MJ. Results of a multicenter prospective randomized trial of carotid artery stenting vs. carotid endarterectomy. Stroke. 2001; 32
[95] Mas JL, Chatellier G, Beyssen B, Branchereau A, Moulin T, Becquemin JP, Larrue V, Lievre M, Leys D, Bonneville JF, Watelet J, Pruvo JP, Albucher JF, Viguier A, Piquet P, Garnier P, Viader F, Touze E, Giroud M, Hosseini H, Pillet JC, Favrole P, Neau JP, Ducrocq X. Endarterectomy versus stenting in patients with symptomatic severe carotid stenosis. N Engl J Med. 2006; 355:1660–1671
[96] Ringleb PA, Allenberg J, Bruckmann H, Eckstein HH, Fraedrich G, Hartmann M, Hennerici M, Jansen O, Klein G, Kunze A, Marx P, Niederkorn K, Schmiedt W, Solymosi L, Stingele R, Zeumer H, Hacke W. 30 day results from the SPACE trial of stent-protected angioplasty versus carotid endarterectomy in symptomatic patients: a randomised non-inferiority trial. Lancet. 2006; 368:1239–1247
[97] CaRESS Steering Committee. Carotid Revascularization Using Endarterectomy or Stenting Systems (CaRESS) phase I clinical trial: 1-year results. J Vasc Surg. 2005; 42:213–219
[98] White CJ, Iyer SS, Hopkins LN, Katzen BT, Russell ME. Carotid stenting with distal protection in high surgical risk patients: the BEACH trial 30 day results. Catheter Cardiovasc Interv. 2006; 67:503–512
[99] Safian RD, Bresnahan JF, Jaff MR, Foster M, Bacharach JM, Maini B, Turco M, Myla S, Eles G, Ansel GM. Protected carotid stenting in high-risk patients with severe carotid artery stenosis. J Am Coll Cardiol. 2006; 47:2384–2389
[100] Hill MD, Morrish W, Soulez G, Nevelsteen A, Maleux G, Rogers C, Hauptmann KE, Bonafe A, Beyar R, Gruberg L, Schofer J. Multicenter evaluation of a self-expanding carotid stent system with distal protection in the treatment of carotid stenosis. AJNR Am J Neuroradiol. 2006; 27:759–765
[101] Fairman R, Gray WA, Scicli AP, Wilburn O, Verta P, Atkinson R, Yadav JS, Wholey M, Hopkins LN, Raabe R, Barnwell S, Green R. The CAPTURE registry: analysis of strokes resulting from carotid artery stenting in the post approval setting: timing, location, severity, and type. Ann Surg. 2007; 246:551-6; discussion 556-8
[102] Iyer SS, White CJ, Hopkins LN, Katzen BT, Safian R, Wholey MH, Gray WA, Ciocca R, Bachinsky WB, Ansel G, Joye JD, Russell ME. Carotid artery revascularization in high-surgical-risk patients using the Carotid WALLSTENT and FilterWire EX/EZ: 1-year outcomes in the BEACH Pivotal Group. J Am Coll Cardiol. 2008; 51:427–434
[103] Bosiers M, Peeters P, Deloose K, Verbist J, Sievert H, Sugita J, Castriota F, Cremonesi A. Does carotid artery stenting work on the long run: 5-year results in high-volume centers (ELOCAS Registry). J Cardiovasc Surg (Torino). 2005; 46:241–247
[104] Theiss W, Hermanek P, Mathias K, Ahmadi R, Heuser L, Hoffmann FJ, Kerner R, Leisch F, Sievert H, von Sommoggy S. Pro-CAS: a prospective registry of carotid angioplasty and stenting. Stroke. 2004; 35:2134–2139
[105] Zahn R, Roth E, Ischinger T, Mark B, Hochadel M, Zeymer U, Haerten K, Hauptmann KE, von Leitner ER, Schramm A, Kasper W, Senges J. Carotid artery stenting in clinical practice results from the Carotid Artery Stenting (CAS)-registry of the Arbeitsgemeinschaft Leitende Kardiologische Krankenhausarzte (ALKK). Z Kardiol. 2005; 94:163–172
[106] Goldstein LB. New data about stenting versus endarterectomy for symptomatic carotid artery stenosis. Curr Treat Options Cardiovasc Med. 2009; 11:232–240
[107] Fayad P. Endarterectomy and stenting for asymptomatic carotid stenosis: a race at breakneck speed. Stroke. 2007; 38:707–714
[108] Naylor AR, Bell PR. Treatment of asymptomatic carotid disease with stenting: con. Semin Vasc Surg. 2008; 21:100–107
[109] Ederle J, Featherstone RL, Brown MM. Percutaneous transluminal angioplasty and stenting for carotid artery stenosis. Cochrane Database Syst Rev. 2007. DOI: 10.1002/14651858.CD000515.pub3
[110] Cremonesi A, Setacci C, Bignamini A, Bolognese L, Briganti F, Di Sciascio G, Inzitari D, Lanza G, Lupattelli L, Mangiafico S, Pratesi C, Reimers B, Ricci S, de Donato G, Ugolotti U, Zaninelli A, Gensini GF. Carotid artery stenting: first consensus document of the ICCS-SPREAD Joint Committee. Stroke. 2006; 37:2400–2409
[111] Goldstein LB, Adams R, Alberts MJ, Appel LJ, Brass LM, Bushnell CD, Culebras A, Degraba TJ, Gorelick PB, Guyton JR, Hart RG, Howard G, Kelly-Hayes M, Nixon JV, Sacco RL. Primary prevention of ischemic stroke. Stroke. 2006; 37:1583–1633

85 Special Conditions

85.1 Totally occluded internal carotid artery

85.1.1 General information

10–15% of patients presenting with carotid territory stroke or transient ischemic attacks (TIA) are found to have carotid occlusion. This amounts to an estimated 61,000 first ever strokes and 19,000 TIAs per year in the United States. Prevention of subsequent stroke in symptomatic patients with carotid artery occlusion remains a difficult challenge. The overall rate of subsequent stroke is 7% per year for all stroke and 5.9% per year for ischemic stroke ipsilateral to the occluded carotid artery.[1] These risks persist even despite treatment with antiaggregants and anticoagulants.[2] The prevalence of asymptomatic carotid occlusion is not known, and the incidence of ipsilateral stroke in never-symptomatic carotid occlusion is negligible.[3]

85

85.1.2 Presentation

3 patterns of stroke with acute carotid artery occlusion:

1. stump emboli: produces cortical infarcts. Emboli usually go up the external carotid (higher flow, and reverse flow that may occur through ICA initially prevents emboli from ICA). Later, ICA emboli may occur.
2. whole hemisphere stroke
3. watershed infarct

In symptomatic patients[4]: hemiparetic TIA 53%, dysphasic TIA 34%, fixed neuro deficit 21%, crescendo TIAs 21%, amaurosis fugax 17%, acute hemiplegia 6%. One series had 27% asymptomatic.[5] Patients may have the so-called "slow carotid stroke" of carotid occlusion which is a stuttering progressive stroke.

85.1.3 Natural history

See reference.[6]

Patients with mild deficit and angiographically proven ICA occlusion have a stroke rate (in two series) of 3 or 5% per year (2 or 3.3% related to occluded side). In patients with acute ICA occlusion and profound neurological deficit, 2–12% make good recovery, 40–69% will have profound deficit, and 16–55% will have died by the time of follow-up.

85.1.4 Endovascular thrombolysis and stenting for acute carotid occlusion

Case reports and series of endovascular treatment of internal carotid artery occlusion have confirmed the feasibility of this technique. Intra-arterial thrombolysis within 6 hours of stroke onset may increase recanalization rates to 37%-100% and clinical improvement to 53%-94% without significant increase in hemorrhagic transformation when compared with intravenous thrombolytic therapy alone.[7,8,9,10,11,12] Although results appear promising, randomized controlled trials on cervical carotid thrombolysis and/or stenting are lacking.

85.1.5 Surgery

Options include: endarterectomy, Fogarty balloon catheter embolectomy (utilizing a No. 2 French catheter with 0.2 ml balloon gently passed 10–12 cm up ICA from small arteriotomy made distal to atheromatous plaque[13]), extracranial-intracranial bypass. Restored patency rate is inversely related to suspected duration of occlusion. Chronically occluded ICA has poor patency rate and little gain from re-opening.

Determining the exact time of occlusion is frequently impossible. One must often rely on clinical grounds, therefore an occasional chronic occlusion will be included.

Retrograde filling of ICA to petrous or cavernous segment from ECA (e.g. via ophthalmic) or from contralateral ICA is a good sign of operability.[4]

Surgical results[4]

32% (15/47 cases) immediate surgical failures (no or minimal back bleeding), at least 3 deaths. Among immediate successes no strokes and no TIAs. If operated < 2 days reported patency rate 70–100%, from 3–7 days 50–100%, 8–14 days 27–58%, 15–30 days 4–61%, over 1 month (2 series) 20–50%.

85.1.6 Guidelines

Emergency operations for acute neuro deficit associated with total occlusion should not be performed after about 2 hrs. Extremely poor neuro status (lethargy/coma) is a contraindication to surgery. Patients without persistent neuro deficit: operate ASAP. If the patient has recurrent TIAs (despite maximal medical therapy) following recent carotid occlusion, and no definite infarct on MRI, consider by-pass surgery.

85.2 Cerebellar infarction

85.2.1 General information

Relatively rare (seen on only 0.6% of all CTs obtained for any reason[14]). Cerebellar infarcts may be classified as involving the PICA distribution (cerebellar tonsil and/or inferior vermis), superior cerebellar artery distribution (superior hemisphere or superior vermis), or other indeterminate patterns.[15] 80% of patients developing signs of brainstem compression will die, usually within hours to days.

85.2.2 Early clinical findings

In most cases the onset is sudden, without premonitory symptoms.[16] The first 12 hrs after onset were characterized by lack of progression. Early findings are due to the *intrinsic* cerebellar lesion (ischemic infarction or hemorrhage):

1. symptoms
   a) dizziness or vertigo
   b) nausea/vomiting
   c) loss of balance, often with a fall and inability to get up
   d) headache (infrequent in one series[16])
2. signs
   a) truncal and appendicular ataxia
   b) nystagmus
   c) dysarthria

85.2.3 Later clinical findings

Patients with cerebellar infarction may subsequently develop increased pressure within the posterior fossa (due to cerebellar edema or mass effect from clot), with brainstem compression (particularly posterior pons). Clinical findings generally increase between 12–96 hrs following onset. Compression the sylvian aqueduct can cause acute hydrocephalus with attendant increased ICP.

85.2.4 Imaging studies

CT scan: may be normal very early in these patients. There may be subtle findings of a tight posterior fossa: compression or obliteration of basal cisterns or 4th ventricle or hydrocephalus.

MRI: (including DWI) more sensitive for ischemia, especially in the posterior fossa.

85.2.5 Surgical indications

Surgical decompression (see below) should probably be done as soon as any of the following signs develop if there is no response to medical therapy.[17] It is important to recognize a lateral medullary syndrome (LMS) (p. 1267) which may often accompany a cerebellar infarct. With LMS, the signs are usually present from the onset (dysphagia, dysarthria, Horner's syndrome, ipsilateral facial numbness, crossed sensory loss…), and are not accompanied by a change in sensorium. There is no place for surgical decompression in LMS since it represents primary brainstem ischemia and not compression.

Findings proceed in the approximate following sequence if there is no intervention:

1. abducens (VI) nerve palsy
2. loss of ipsilateral gaze (compression of VI nucleus and lateral gaze center)
3. peripheral facial nerve paresis (compression of facial colliculus)
4. confusion and somnolence (may be partly due to developing hydrocephalus)
5. Babinski sign
6. hemiparesis
7. lethargy
8. small but reactive pupils
9. coma
10. posturing → flaccidity
11. ataxic respirations

85.2.6 Suboccipital craniectomy for cerebellar infarction

Unlike the situation with supratentorial masses causing herniation, there are several reports of patients in deep coma from direct brainstem compression who were operated upon quickly who made useful recovery.[17,18,19] See also Guidelines for patients with cerebellar hemorrhage (p. 1344).

The operation of choice is a suboccipital decompression to include enlargement of the foramen magnum. The dura is then opened and the infarcted cerebellar tissue usually exudes "like toothpaste" and is easily aspirated. Avoid using ventricular drainage alone as this may cause upward cerebellar herniation (p. 303) and does not relieve the direct brainstem compression.

85.3 Malignant middle cerebral artery territory infarction

85.3.1 General information

A distinct syndrome that occurs in up to 10% of stroke patients,[20,21] which carries a mortality of up to 80% (mostly due to severe postischemic cerebral edema → increased ICP → herniation).[21]

Patients usually present with findings of severe hemispheric stroke (hemiplegia, forced eye and head deviation) often with CT findings of major infarct within the first 12 hours. Most develop drowsiness shortly after admission. There is progressive deterioration during the first 2 days, and subsequent transtentorial herniation usually within 2–4 days of stroke. Fatalities are often associated with: severe drowsiness, dense hemiplegia, age > 45–50 yrs,[22] early parenchymal hypodensity involving > 50% of the MCA distribution on CT scan,[23] midline shift > 8–10 mm, early sulci effacement and hyperdense artery sign (p. 1281) [22] in MCA.

Neurosurgeons may become involved in caring for these patients because aggressive therapies in these patients may reduce morbidity and mortality. Options include:

1. conventional measures to control ICP (with or without ICP monitor): mortality is still high in this group, and elevated ICP is not a common cause of initial neurologic deterioration in large hemispheric stroke
2. hemicraniectomy (decompressive craniectomy): see below
3. ✖ to date, the following treatments have not improved outcome: agents to lyse clot, hyperventilation, mannitol, or barbiturate coma

85.3.2 Hemicraniectomy for malignant MCA territory infarction

May reduce mortality to as low as 32% in nondominant hemisphere strokes[24] (37% in all comers[25]) with surprising reduction of hemiplegia, and in dominant hemisphere strokes, with only mild-moderate aphasia (better results occur with early surgery, especially if surgery is performed *before* any changes associated with herniation occur). Meta-analysis[26] of 3 randomized controlled trials found that hemicraniectomy within 48 hours after stroke onset resulted in decreased mortality and increased the number of patients with a favorable functional outcome.

Indications: No firm indications. Guidelines:

1. age < 70 years
2. more strongly considered in nondominant hemisphere (usually right)
3. clinical & CT evidence of acute, complete ICA or MCA infarcts and direct signs of impending or complete severe hemispheric brain swelling (severe post-admission neurologic deterioration is the usual event that triggers surgical intervention)

See also **Technique** (p. 1467).

85.4 Cardiogenic brain embolism

85.4.1 General information

About one stroke in six is cardioembolic. Emboli may be composed of fibrin-rich thrombi (e.g. mural thrombi due to segmental myocardial hypokinesis following MI or ventricular aneurysm), platelets (e.g. nonbacterial thrombotic endocarditis), calcified material (e.g. in aortic stenosis), or tumor particles (e.g. atrial myxoma).

85.4.2 Following acute myocardial infarction (AMI)

2.5% of patients will have a stroke within 1–2 weeks of an AMI (the period when most emboli occur). The risk is higher with anterior wall MI (≈ 6%) vs. inferior wall MI (≈ 1%).

85.4.3 Atrial fibrillation (A-fib)

Nonrheumatic patients with a-fib have a 3–5 fold increased risk of stroke,[27] with a 4.5% rate of stroke per year without treatment.[28] The incidence of a-fib in the U.S. is 2.2 million. About 75% of strokes in patients with A-fib are due to left atrial thrombi.[29] Independent risk factors for stroke in patients with A-fib are: advanced age, prior embolism (stroke or TIA), HTN, DM, and echocardiographic evidence of left atrial enlargement or left ventricular dysfunction.[27]

The CHADS2 scoring system for patients with a-fib has been widely validated[30] and is shown in ▶ Table 85.1. The points are totaled and risk assessment is shown in ▶ Table 85.2. For patients with a CHADS2 score ≥ 2, warfarin therapy was significantly protective for out-of-hospital death or hospitalization for stroke, MI or hemorrhage (CI = 0.61–0.91).[31]

85.4.4 Prosthetic heart valves

Patients with mechanical prosthetic heart valves on long-term anticoagulation have an embolism rate of 3%/year for mitral and 1.5%/year for aortic valves. With bioprosthetic heart valves and no anticoagulation the risk is 2–4%/year.

Table 85.1 CHADS2 scoring items

Item	Points
CHF (any history)	1
HTN (prior history)	1
Age > 75 yrs	1
Diabetes mellitus	1
Secondary prevention: in patients with prior ischemic stroke or TIA; most also include systemic embolic events	2

Table 85.2 Risk based on CHADS2 score

CHADS 2 score	Annual stroke risk (%/year)
0	1.9
1	2.8
2	4
3	5.9
4	8.5
5	12.5
6	18.2

85.4.5 Paradoxical embolism

Paradoxical embolism can occur with a patent foramen ovale which is present in 10–18% of the general population, but in up to 56% of young adults with unexplained stroke.[32]

85.4.6 Endocarditis

Diagnosis

Blood cultures and TEE help evaluate.

No specific neurologic features can distinguish these patients. The diagnosis is suggested in imaging studies showing multiple intracranial ischemic strokes in different arterial distributions, the differential diagnosis includes: vasculitis, intracranial atherosclerosis (focal plaques, more common in Asian populations that consume Western diets), and intravascular lymphomatosis.

The diagnosis of cardiogenic brain embolism (CBE) as a cause of a stroke relies on demonstrating a potential cardiac source, the absence of cerebrovascular disease, and non-lacunar stroke.

Large areas of hemorrhagic transformation within an ischemic infarct may be more indicative of CBE due to thrombolysis of the clot and reperfusion of infarcted brain with subsequent hemorrhagic conversion. Hemorrhagic transformation most often occurs within 48 hrs of a CBE stroke, and is more common with larger strokes.

Detection of cardiac source

Most centers rely on echocardiography (without transesophageal ability). Using restricted criteria (i. e. excluding mitral valve prolapse), about 10% of patients with ischemic stroke will have potential cardiac source detected by echo, and most of these patients have other manifestations of cardiac disease. In stroke patients without clinical heart disease, only 1.5% will have a positive echo; the yield is higher in younger patients without cerebrovascular disease.[33]

EKG may detect atrial fibrillation which may be seen in 6–24% of ischemic strokes, and may be associated with a 5-fold increased risk of stroke (see below).

Treatment

CBE is essentially the only condition for which anticoagulation has been shown to significantly reduce the rate of further strokes.

One must balance the risk of recurrent emboli (12% of patients with a cardioembolic stroke will have a second embolic stroke within 2 weeks) against that of converting a pale infarct into a hemorrhagic one. No study has shown a clear benefit of *early* anticoagulation.

Recommendations for anticoagulation:

1. if anticoagulation is to be used, it should not be instituted within the first 48 hrs of a probable CBE stroke
2. CT should be obtained after 48 hrs following a CBE stroke and before starting anticoagulation (to R/O hemorrhage)
3. anticoagulation should not be used in the face of large infarcts
4. start heparin and warfarin simultaneously. Continue heparin for 3 days into warfarin therapy, see Anticoagulation (p. 156)
5. optimal range of oral anticoagulation to minimize subsequent embolism and/or hemorrhage has not been determined, but pending further data, an INR of 2–3 appears satisfactory
6. patients with asymptomatic A-fib have 66–86% reduction in stroke risk with warfarin (Coumadin®).[27,34] ASA is only about half as effective, but may be sufficient for those without associated risk factors (p. 1304) [27]

85.5 Vertebrobasilar insufficiency

85.5.1 General information

Signs and symptoms resulting from inadequate blood flow through the posterior cerebral circulation (vertabral arteries, basilar artery and their branches).

85.5.2 Symptoms

▶ Table 85.3 shows a mnemonic of the symptoms of vertebrobasilar insufficiency (VBI). Predicting the site of the lesion based only on clinical evaluation is very unreliable.

Diagnostic criteria for VBI are shown in ▶ Table 85.3.

VBI may also be suspected in a patient with transient episodes of "dizziness" (vertigo that is otherwise unexplained, e.g. absence of orthostatic hypotension or benign positional vertigo) that is initiated by positional changes. VBI may sometimes be due to compression of the VA at the C1-C2 level with:

1. head turning (below)
2. os odontoideum (p. 981)
3. anterior atlantoaxial subluxation: e.g. in rheumatoid arthritis (p. 1134)
4. with rotatory atlantoaxial subluxation (p. 968)

85.5.3 Pathophysiology

Atheromatous and stenotic lesions of the posterior circulation occur most frequently at the VA origin.

VBI symptoms may be due to:

1. hemodynamic insufficiency (may be the most common etiology), including:
   a) subclavian steal: reversed flow in VA due to proximal stenosis of subclavian artery
   b) stenosis of both VAs or of one VA where the other is hypofunctional (e.g. hypoplastic, occluded, or terminates in PICA) causing reduced distal flow in face of inadequate collaterals (below)
2. embolism from ulcerations
3. atherosclerotic occlusion of brainstem perforators
4. Vertebrobasilar hypoplasia: reported as a possible etiology for cerebellar stroke.

85.5.4 Natural history

No clinical study accurately defines the natural history. The estimated stroke rate is 22–35% over 5 years, or 4.5–7% per year[35] (one study estimating 35% stroke rate in 5 years did not use angiography).

Risk of stroke after first VBI-TIA has been estimated as 22% for first year.[36]

85.5.5 Evaluation

Adequate investigation usually requires selective four-vessel angiography,[37] sometimes with provocative maneuvers (see e.g. Bow Hunter's Syndreome below). CTA may also be useful.

85.5.6 Treatment

Anticoagulation is the mainstay of medical management. Alternatives include anti-platelet drugs such as ASA (efficacy of either remains unproven[35,37]).

Table 85.3 Mnemonic: "The 5 D's of VBI"

- "drop attack"
- diplopia
- dysarthria
- defect (visual field)
- dizziness

Table 85.4 Criteria for clinical diagnosis of VBI

Clinical diagnosis requires 2 or more of the following
- motor or sensory symptoms or both, occurring bilaterally in the same event
- diplopia: ischemia of upper brainstem (midbrain) near ocular nuclei
- dysarthria: ischemia of lower brainstem
- homonymous hemianopsia: ischemia of occipital cortex (NB: this is *binocular*, in contrast to amaurosis fugax which is monocular)

Surgical treatment includes:

1. vertebral endarterectomy
2. transposition of VA to ICA (with or without carotid endarterectomy, with or without saphenous vein patch graft) or to thyrocervical trunk or to subclavian artery[38]
3. bypass grafting (e.g. occipital artery to PICA)
4. C1–2 posterior arthrodesis (p. 1479) may prevent potentially life-threatening stroke in cases of os odontoideum (p. 982)

85.6 Bow hunter's stroke

85.6.1 General information

A special subset of VBI. The term was coined in 1978 by Sorensen.[39] Bow hunter's stroke (BHS): hemodynamic VBI induced by intermittent VA occlusion resulting from head rotation[40] (ischemic sequelae range from TIA (bow hunter's sign) to completed stroke). May occur with forced (e.g. with chiropractic neck manipulation[41]) or voluntary[42] head rotation.

Occlusion usually involves the VA *contralateral* to the direction of rotation, and usually occurs at the C1-C2 junction (due to the immobility of the VA at this location).[43] However, other sites have also been reported.[44,45]

VA occlusion does not produce symptoms in most individuals due to collateral flow through the contralateral VA and/or the circle of Willis. Symptomatic occlusion usually involves the dominant VA,[46] however, may also occur with non-dominant VA[42]). Most cases of BHS occur in patients with an isolated posterior circulation (incompetent posterior communicating arteries).

BHS has also been postulated as one possible cause of SIDS.[47]

85.6.2 Contributing factors

1. external VA compression[45]
   a) spondylotic bone spurs: particularly in the foramen transversarium[48]
   b) tumors
   c) fibrous bands (e.g. proximal to entrance of VA into C6 foramen transversarium[44])
   d) infectious processes
   e) trauma
2. tethering of the VA
   a) at the transverse foramina of C1 & C2
   b) along the sulcus arteriosus proximal to where the VA enters the dura
3. defect in odontoid process[49]
4. atherosclerotic vascular disease

85.6.3 Diagnosis

General information

BHS should be suspected in patient with symptoms of VBI precipitated by head movement. This may be very difficult to differentiate from vertigo and nausea due to vestibular dysfunction (which can also be induced by head movement) – (rotation of the body keeping the head motionless should not cause symptoms from vestibular symptoms and might help distinguish these conditions[50]).

Dynamic cerebral angiography (DCA)

✖ NB: significant consequences can be precipitated during DCA in patients with BHS.[43] The involved VA shows loss of flow as the head is rotated from the neutral position to the contralateral side. Carotid injections demonstrate patency of P-comms and the presence of any persistent fetal anastomoses.

CT angiogram (CTA)

Same precautions as with DCA (see above). Probably not the initial diagnostic study of choice. If the DCA is negative, CTA is not needed. If DCA is positive, CTA may be helpful to demonstrate the arterial relationship to the bony anatomy.

85.6.4 Treatment

Options include:
1. anticoagulation[50]
2. cervical collar: to remind patient not to turn their head
3. for VA compression at C1–2 (see ► Table 85.5 for a comparison):
   a) C1–2 fusion (p. 1481)
   b) VA decompression: C1 "hemilaminectomy" via a posterior approach[51]
4. for compression at other sites: elimination of the source of compression where possible (e.g. sectioning of offending fibrous band,[44] removal of osteophytic spurs[48]...)

85

Management recommendations: For compression at C1–2, it is suggested that VA decompression be performed as the initial treatment. This should be followed by DCA to verify maintenance of patency with head turning. Patients who fail clinically or on DCA should undergo C1–2 fusion.[43] Patients need to know pros and cons of each option.

85.7 Cerebrovascular venous thrombosis

85.7.1 General information

There are 3 types of cerebrovascular venous thrombosis (CVVT) (any of which may produce venous infarctions):
1. dural sinus thrombosis (DST)
2. cortical venous thrombosis
3. deep venous thrombosis

85.7.2 Etiologies

Partial list of etiologies

Many conditions have been incriminated with CVVT. Some common ones are listed here[53 (p 1301)]:
1. infection
   a) usually local, e.g. otitis media[54,55] (leading to the now obsolete term otitic hydrocephalus), sinusitis, peritonsillar abscess, paranasal sinusitis[56]: in the pre-antibiotic era, CVVT was most commonly associated with chronic suppurative infection
   b) meningitis
2. pregnancy & puerperium: see below
3. birth control pills (BCP) (oral contraceptives)[57]
4. dehydration and cachexia (marantic thrombosis): includes burns and cachexia of neoplastic disease
5. cardiac disease (including CHF)
6. ulcerative colitis (UC): 1% of UC patients have some thrombotic complication (not necessarily all intracranial), and this is the cause of ≈ 33% of deaths (usually pulmonary embolism, PE)
7. periarteritis nodosa
8. sickle cell trait
9. trauma: including closed head injury (see below)
10. iatrogenic: e.g. S/P radical neck surgery,[58] transvenous pacemaker placement, post-craniotomy
11. malignancy: including myeloproliferative disorders
12. hypercoagulable state (AKA thrombophilia)
    a) protein C deficiency or resistance to activated protein C: hereditary factor V Leiden mutation may produce resistance to activated protein C.[59] Apparent protein C deficiency may be an artifact of dehydration in some cases
    b) antithrombin III deficiency
    c) protein S deficiency

Table 85.5 Comparison of surgical treatment for positional VA occlusion at C1–2

Procedure	Advantages	Disadvantages
C1–2 fusion	high success rate in eliminating symptoms	loss of 50–70% of neck rotation with possible discomfort
VA decompression	no loss of motion	33% continue to have symptoms[52]

d) antiphospholipid antibodies: associated with a variety of clinical syndromes including ischemic stroke, DVTs, thrombocytopenia, systemic lupus erythematosus SLE. The best known antibodies include
   - anticardiolipin antibodies
   - lupus anticoagulant

e) paroxysmal nocturnal hemoglobinuria (PNH)
f) plasminogen deficiency
g) systemic lupus erythematosus[60]
h) factor VIII elevation[61]: may explain some cases of CVVT in pregnancy (see below)

13. diabetes mellitus: especially with ketoacidosis
14. homocystinuria (p. 200)
15. Behçet's syndrome (p. 200) [62]
16. rarely associated with lumbar puncture, associated with hereditary activated protein C resistance due to the factor V R506Q mutation (FV Leiden) in one report[63]

* In the absence of factors such as BCP use, CVVT is highly suggestive of myeloproliferative disorder.

Pregnancy/puerperium

Highest risk is in first 2 wks post-partum. One series[64] found no case of CVVT occurred later than 16 days post-partum. Incidence ≈ 1/10,000 births. Etiology may be related to elevation of clotting factors (VII, X and especially factor VIII[65]).

Trauma

A rare sequelae of closed head injury.[66] CVVT occurs in ≈ 10% of combat injuries involving the brain. May occur in absence of skull fracture. CVVT should be suspected in patients with fractures or missiles crossing sinus.

85.7.3 Relative frequency of involvement

The relative frequency of involvement of dural sinuses and other veins with thrombotic issues

1. sinuses
   a) superior sagittal sinus (**SSS**) and left transverse sinus (**TS**) (70% each)
   b) multiple sinuses in 71%
   c) isolated inferior sagittal sinus: rare, first case report in 1997[67]
   d) straight sinus[68]
2. superficial cortical veins
3. deep venous system (e.g. internal cerebral vein)
4. cavernous sinus[69,70]: rare. Thrombophlebitis of the cavernous sinus may be caused by sphenoid sinusitis. MRI may show enlargement and abnormal enhancement of the cavernous sinus, increased signal of the petrous apex and clivus on T2WI, and narrowing of the cavernous portion of the ICA[70]

85.7.4 Pathophysiology

Venous thrombosis reduces venous outflow from the brain and diminishes effective blood flow to the involved area. This venous engorgement causes white matter edema. The increased venous pressure may also lead to infarction and/or hemorrhage. These processes may all elevate ICP. Thus, clinical findings may be due to elevated ICP, and focal findings may be due to edema and/or hemorrhage. Cerebral infarction due to venous stasis is called venous infarction.

85.7.5 Clinical

Clinical presentations of DST are shown in ▶ Table 85.6. There are no pathognomonic findings. Many signs and symptoms are due to elevated ICP. May present as a syndrome clinically indistinguishable from idiopathic intracranial hypertension; see pseudotumor cerebri (p. 768).

There is a high association of concurrent thromboembolic disease in other organs.

The anterior 1/3 of the SSS may occlude often without sequelae. Posterior to this, venous infarction is more likely to develop. Midportion SSS occlusion usually → increased muscle tone ranging from spastic hemi- or quadri-paresis to decerebration. Posterior SSS thrombosis → field cuts or cortical blindness, or massive stroke with cerebral edema and death. Occlusion of the TS may occur

85

Table 85.6 Presentation of dural sinus thrombosis

Sign/symptom	Series A[a]	Series B[a]
H/A	100%	74%
N/V	75%	–
seizures	70%	29%
hemiparesis	70%	34%
papilledema	70%	45%
blurred vision	60%	–
altered consciousness	35%	26%

[a]series A: 20 young females[64]; series B: 38 cases from France[72]

without deficit unless the contralateral TS is hypoplastic, in which cases presentation is similar to posterior SSS occlusion.

SSS occlusion alone will not cause cranial nerve findings except perhaps for visual obscuration and abducens (VI) nerve palsy from elevated of ICP. Thrombosis in the jugular bulb may compress the nerves in the jugular foramen pars nervosa causing hoarseness, aphonia, difficulty swallowing and breathlessness; see Vernet's syndrome (p. 100).[71]

85.7.6 Diagnosis of DST

General information

Catheter angiography is better at demonstrating the presence of residual flow, and can identify areas of reversal of flow, and can sometimes demonstrate clot as a filling defect. However, CT (especially CTA) & MRI are better for identifying areas of clot. Angiography is often used as a complementary test[73] when the diagnosis is suggested by CT or MRI.

CT scan

Non-contrast CT

May be normal in 10–20% of cases of DST. Findings include:
1. hyperdense sinuses and veins (high density clots in cortical veins has been dubbed the cord sign which is pathognomonic for cerebral venous thrombosis; seen in only 2/30 patients)
2. petechial "flame" hemorrhages (intraparenchymal): seen in 20% (suspect sinus thrombosis with intracerebral hemorrhages in unusual locations for aneurysm or "hypertensive" hemorrhage)
3. small ventricles: seen in 50%
4. thrombosis of superior sagittal sinus may produce a triangular-shaped high density within the sinus posteriorly near the Torcular herophili on axial CT images (some refer to this as the delta sign, but this causes confusion with the "empty delta sign", see below) (there is also confusion when an apparent "empty delta sign" is seen *without* contrast, this may occur when there is blood surrounding the SSS, e.g. following subarachnoid hemorrhage, this has been called a "false delta sign" or pseudodelta sign[74]). Recommendation: avoid the confusion of the variations on "delta signs" and describe the findings
5. white matter edema
6. above changes occurring *bilaterally*

IV contrast CT

Findings of DST include:
1. with *contrast*, the dura around the sinus may enhance and become denser than clot in 35% of cases.[75] Near the Torcular herophili this produces what has been called the empty delta sign,[76] but sometimes this, too, is called the delta sign
2. gyral enhancement occurs in 32%
3. dense deep (white matter) veins (collateral flow)
4. intense tentorial enhancement (common)

MRI

MRI excels for diagnosis and follow-up. Shows absence of flow and clot burden, also demonstrates parenchymal changes. Can differentiate occluded sinus from congenital absence. Shows cerebral edema and non-acute hemorrhagic changes to better advantage than CT. Also may help estimate age of clots (▶ Table 85.7). MR-angiography may increase the utility. MR-venography (MRV) tends to overestimate the degree of occlusion.

Angiography for DST

Accuracy is close to MRI, and some still consider it to be the standard of diagnosis. MRI has some advantages over angiography (e.g. on angiography a hypoplastic transverse sinus may not visualize, or non-opacified blood entering a sinus may mimic a filling defect).

Findings include:

1. non-filling of segments of sinuses, or filling defects in segments that are visualized
2. prolonged circulation time: present in 50% of cases (may need delayed films to see veins)
3. stumps and abnormal collateral pathways

LP

OP usually increased. CSF may be bloody or xanthochromic.

Bloodwork

To detect predisposing conditions when the etiology is unknown. Some tests that may be useful include evaluation for thrombophilia (protein C and S levels, antiphospholipid antibodies = anticardiolipin antibodies and lupus anticoagulant) as well as tests for specific predisposing conditions (CBC, Factor II level, serum homocysteine level, paroxysmal nocturnal hemoglobinuria (PNH) panel, leukocyte alkaline phosphatase).

Ultrasound for DST

May be used in diagnosis of superior sagittal sinus thrombosis in the neonate.[77]

Evaluation for underlying disorder

At the time of presentation, work-up is difficult because the acute process will cause numerous abnormalities in the clotting system. The best time to work these patients up is ≈ 3 months after they recover from the acute phase.

85.7.7 Treatment

General information

Driving principle: treat the underlying abnormality (if possible).

Should be aggressive because recoverability of brain is probably greater than with arterial occlusive stroke. Management is complicated because measures that counteract thrombosis (e.g. anticoagulation) tend to increase the risk of hemorrhagic infarct (the risk of which is already increased), and measures that lower ICP tend to increase blood viscosity → increased coagulability.

Table 85.7 MRI appearance of thrombosed sinuses at various stages

Age of clot in sinus	Appearance of clotted sinus	
	T1WI	T2WI
acute	iso-intense	decreased (black): can mimic flow void
subacute	increased (1st)	increased (2nd)
late (> 10 d, recanalized)	black (flow void)	black (flow void)

85

Specific measures

1. correct underlying abnormality when possible (e.g. antibiotics for infection)
2. heparin (systemic): see dosing information (p. 164) especially if patient is in DIC. Several studies show a lower mortality rate with heparin than without.[78,79,80] It remains the best treatment even when there is evidence of intracerebral hemorrhage ICH with the attendant risk of increasing the size of the hemorrhage.[73] There is no consensus on duration of treatment or if warfarin should be used afterwards. Success rate may be higher if administered before patient becomes moribund
3. avoid steroids (reduces fibrinolysis, increases coagulation)
4. control HTN
5. anticonvulsants to control seizures
6. monitor ICP if patient continues to deteriorate: ventriculostomy preferred, but caution must be used if patient is on heparin
   a) hydrate aggressively as ICP tolerates
   b) measures to lower ICP: in general, order is almost reverse of that for traumatic intracranial hypertension because diuretics → hypertonicity → ↑ viscosity → ↑ coagulation:
      - elevate HOB
      - hyperventilate
      - drain CSF
      - pentobarbital coma
      - reserve hyperosmotic and/or loop diuretics for last (replace fluid loss with isotonic IV fluids to prevent dehydration; i.e. goal is hypertonic euvolemia)
7. thrombolytic therapy: either systemically or infused directly into clotted sinus,[73,81] may be followed with heparin. Many reports, but no controlled trials have been published
   a) urokinase[68,81] or streptokinase
   b) intravenous tissue plasminogen activator (tPA): promising animal evidence,[82] not yet reported in humans
8. when above measures fail, either
   a) decompressive craniectomy (± decompressive lobectomy): this decreases ICP, but may not improve outcome
   b) OR direct "attack" on clotted sinus: direct surgical treatment when deficit progresses in spite of above measures, or ICP not manageable (i.e. failure of medical therapy) (see below)
9. interventional neuroradiology: effectiveness is much reduced with chronic clot
   a) Penumbra® system: sucks out clot, only takes out a small amount of clot
   b) AngioJet®: not FDA approved for this. Not used for arterial clots because of injury to cerebral tissue, but may have some efficacy with venous clot
10. visual loss with papilledema may be treated with optic nerve sheath fenestration/decompression[83]
11. long-term treatment after resolution of acute phase with heparin and/or warfarin × 3–6 months

Direct surgical treatment for DST

Rarely indicated. Thrombectomy and sinus reconstruction are technically possible, but rethrombosis is common. Surgery may be indicated for abscess requiring excision.

Surgical technique for direct treatment of SSS thrombosis

Have available: blood for massive transfusion, large bore IV access, sinus shunt (pre-fabricated, or improvise with high-vacuum silicone grease inside & outside pediatric anode endotracheal tube with cuff on both ends, gas sterilize, prepared pre-op), tissue for sinus reconstruction (e.g. 20 cm of saphenous vein (arteries have a high rate of fibrosis, and there is no published experience with synthetics grafts). Vein grafts are dilated with heparinized saline and should be oriented correctly in case of valves).

Expose a wide portion of the sinus.

Consider ligation when lesion in non-critical location (SSS anterior to rolandic vein, non-dominant transverse or sigmoid, minor sinuses on skull base).

Hemorrhage is controlled by digital pressure, Fogarty catheter (insert directly, or insert a no. 7 Fogarty thru tiny sinotomy proximal to bleeding which allows repair of bleeding site), and/or insertion of shunt.

85.7.8 Prognosis

Mortality: approximately 30% (range: 5–70%) (10% in French series[72]).

Poor prognosticators:

1. clinical status:
   a) coma[84];
   b) rapid neurologic deterioration,[84] focal signs.
2. demographics
   a) age: extremes of age (infancy or elderly)[84] and age > 37 years
   b) male gender
3. radiographic findings:
   a) hemorrhages, especially larger hemorrhages
   b) venous infarcts
4. deep venous involvement

85.8 Moyamoya disease

85.8.1 General information

Key concepts

- progressive bilateral spontaneous occlusion of ICAs with compensatory capillary collaterals that look like a "puff of smoke" (Japanese: moyamoya) on angio
- typical presentation: juvenile form → ischemic infarcts/TIAs (suspect diagnosis in any child presenting with TIAs). Adult form → hemorrhage
- pathology: intimal thickening w/o inflammation, may also involve heart, kidneys. Associated aneurysms may be source of bleeding
- evaluation: cerebral angiography is necessary to delineate degree of stenosis as well as to evaluate potential extracranial donor vessels for revascularization. Also identifies aneurysms
- treatment:
  a) medical treatment (antiplatelet drugs, anticoagulation, vasodilators...): not shown to be effective although antiplatelet/anticoagulation is often used
  b) surgical revascularization: reduces the incidence of strokes and TIAs, but benefit on reducing the rate of hemorrhage is unproven

Progressive spontaneous occlusion of one or usually both ICAs (usually at the level of the carotid siphon) and their major branches, with secondary formation of an anastomotic collateral capillary network at the base of the brain which has been termed "moyamoya", the Japanese word for something hazy like a "puff of cigarette smoke"[85] (which it fancifully resembles on angiography) (first described in 1957,[86] and named in 1969[85]). With progression, involvement includes the proximal MCAs and ACAs and on rare occasion the vertebrobasilar system. Associated aneurysms (see below) and rarely AVMs[87,88] may be observed.

Eventually the dilated capillary (moyamoya) vessels disappear with the development of collaterals from the ECA (meningeal collaterals are called "rete mirabile").

85.8.2 Pathophysiology

Primary moyamoya disease

The most common pathology is stenosis of the proximal anterior and middle cerebral arteries that is neither atherosclerotic nor inflammatory in origin. Exact etiology is unknown but some studies show elevated basic fibroblast growth factor in the dura and scalp arteries in patients with moyamoya.[89] The internal elastic lamina of affected vessels may be thinned or duplicated. Similar vascular changes may also occur in the heart, kidney and other organs, suggesting it may be a systemic vascular disease.

Secondary moyamoya disease

AKA "quasi-moyamoya disease" or "moyamoya syndrome".[90] Angiographic findings of moyamoya associated with e.g.:

1. Graves' disease/thyrotoxicosis
2. history of cerebral inflammatory disease, including meningitis (especially tubercular (TB) meningitis and leptospirosis)

3. retinitis pigmentosa
4. vascular disorders: atherosclerosis, fibromuscular dysplasia, pseudoxanthoma elasticum
5. congenital disorders: Down syndrome, Marfan syndrome, Turner syndrome, neurofibromatosis type 1, tuberous sclerosis, Apert syndrome
6. hematologic disorders: Fanconi anemia, sickle cell anemia (in the U.S. one of the more common associations) and sickle cell trait
7. following radiation therapy for skull base glioma in children[91]
8. head trauma
9. systemic lupus erythematosus (SLE)

Associated aneurysms

85

Intracranial *aneurysms* are frequently associated with moyamoya disease (MMD). This may be a result of the increased flow through dilated collaterals, or it may be that patients with moyamoya may also have a congenital defect in the arterial wall that predisposes them to aneurysms. 3 types: 1) usual sites of aneurysms in the Circle of Willis, 2) in peripheral portions of cerebral arteries, e.g. posterior/anterior choroidal, Heubner's, and 3) within moyamoya vessels. The frequency of aneurysms in the vertebrobasilar system is ≈ 62% which is much higher than in the general population.[92] Aneurysmal SAH may be the actual cause of some hemorrhages that were erroneously attributed to moyamoya vessels.

85.8.3 Epidemiology

Risk factors

A history of inflammation in the head & neck region has been implicated.

Demographics

Incidence in Japan is higher (0.35/100,000/yr) than in North America. Two peaks (may not be same disease): juvenile (highest peak), age < 10 yrs (mean 3); adult, 3rd & 4th decade. Slight female predominance (1.8:1). Some evidence for familial tendency (some Asian families have an incidence as high as 7%), genetics appears autosomal dominant with low penetrance. Associated with some HLA antigens (B40 in juvenile form; B54(20) in adult) and anti-double-stranded DNA antibody.

85.8.4 Presentation

Juvenile form

Moyamoya is associated with 6% of childhood strokes.[89] Ischemic presentation more common (81%); includes TIAs (41%) which may alternate sides (alternating hemiplegia is a suggestive clinical finding), RINDs, or infarct (40%). Neurologic events are often provoked by straining or by hyperventilation (e.g. during crying or blowing a wind instrument) which is thought to produce hypocapnea with reactive vasoconstriction.

Headache is the most common presenting symptom, but seizures, focal neurologic deficits, choreoathetotic movements and hemorrhages can also be presenting symptoms. The risk of hemorrhage is increased in stages 5 & 6 of MMD.

Adult form

Hemorrhage has been described as being more common (60%), but in a Stanford series[93] 89% presented with ischemia. Rupture of the fragile moyamoya vessels produces bleeding in the basal ganglia (BG), thalamus or ventricles (from the ventricular wall) in 70–80% of hemorrhages. SAH may occur, usually due to rupture of associated aneurysms (see above). In the pre-CT era, the most common form of hemorrhage was thought to be SAH from the rupture of moyamoya vessels, but most cases were probably intraventricular blood or SAH from associated aneurysms.[94]

85.8.5 Natural history

Incidence of disease progression in one study was 20% in adult patients with MMD.[95] Female patients had a higher risk of disease progression than males.

Prognosis of untreated MMD is poor, with 73% rate of major deficit or death within 2 years of diagnosis in children, and similarly poor outlook in adults.[93]

85.8.6 Evaluation and diagnosis

Diagnostic criteria

Diagnosis of moyamoya requires bilateral symmetrical stenosis or occlusion of the terminal portion of the ICAs as well as the presence of dilated collateral vessels at the base of the brain.[89] (If unilateral, the diagnosis is considered questionable,[96] and these cases may progress to bilateral involvement).

Other characteristic findings include:

1. stenosis/occlusion starting at termination of ICA and at origins of ACA and MCA
2. abnormal vascular network in region of BG (intraparenchymal anastamosis)
3. transdural anastomosis (rete mirabile), AKA "vault moyamoya." Contributing arteries: anterior falcial, middle meningeal, ethmoidal, occipital, tentorial, STA
4. moyamoya collaterals may also form from internal maxillary artery via ethmoid sinus to forebrain in frontobasal region

CT

Work-up in suspected cases typically begins with a non-enhanced head CT. Up to 40% of ischemic cases have normal CT. Low density areas (LDAs) may be seen, usually confined to cortical and subcortical areas (unlike atherosclerotic disease or acute infantile hemiplegia which tend to have LDAs in basal ganglia as well). LDAs tend to be multiple and bilateral, especially in the PCA distribution (poor collaterals), and are more common in children.

MRI and MRA

MRA usually discloses the stenosis or occlusion of the ICA. Moyamoya vessels appear as flow voids on MRI (especially in basal ganglia) and a fine network of vessels on MRA, and are demonstrated better in children than adults. Parenchymal ischemic changes are commonly shown, usually in watershed areas.

Angiography

In addition to helping to establish the diagnosis, angiography also identifies suitable vessels for revascularization procedures and unearths associated aneurysms. The angiography-related complication rate is higher than with atherosclerotic occlusive disease. Avoid dehydration prior to and hypotension during the procedure. Six angiographic stages of MMD are described in ▶ Table 85.8 [85] that tend to progress up until adolescence and stabilize by age 20.

EEG

Non-specific in the adult. Juvenile cases: high-voltage slow waves may be seen at rest, predominantly in the occipital and frontal lobes. Hyperventilation produces a normal buildup of monophasic slow waves (delta-bursts) that return to normal 20–60 seconds after hyperventilation. In > 50% of cases, after or sometimes continuous with buildup is a second phase of slow waves (this characteristic finding is called "rebuildup") which are more irregular and slower than the earlier waves, and usually normalize in ≤ 10 minutes.[97]

Table 85.8 Six angiographic stages of MMD[85]

Stage	Finding
1	stenosis of suprasellar ICA, usually bilateral
2	development of moyamoya vessels at base of brain; ACA MCA & PCA dilated
3	increasing ICA stenosis & prominence of moya-moya vessels (most cases diagnosed at this stage); maximal basal moyamoya
4	entire circle of Willis and PCAs occluded, extracranial collaterals start to appear, moyamoya vessels begin to diminish
5	further progression of stage 4
6	complete absence of moyamoya vessels and major cerebral arteries

Cerebral blood flow (CBF) studies

CBF is decreased in children with MMD, but relatively normal in adults. There is a shift of CBF from the frontal to the occipital lobes[98] probably reflecting the increasing dependency of CBF on the posterior circulation. Children with MMD have impaired autoregulation of CBF to blood pressure and CO_2 (with more impairment of vasodilatation in response to hypercapnia or hypotension than vasoconstriction in response to hypocapnia or hypertension).[99]

Xenon (Xe-133) CT can identify areas of low perfusion. Repeating the study after an acetazolamide challenge (which causes vasodilatation) evaluates reserve capacity of CBF and can identify areas of "steal" which are at high risk of future infarction.

85.8.7 Treatment

General information

No medical or surgical treatment has been proven effective in reducing the rate of hemorrhage in the adult with MMD. However, multiple large case series have supported the efficacy of cerebral revascularization for reducing the incidence of ischemic strokes and TIA's.[90]

Asymptomatic moyamoya disease

Guidelines for management of asymptomatic moyamoya disease have not yet been established. A multi-center, nation-wide survey in Japan focusing on asymptomatic moyamoya disease provided the following findings[100]: subtle findings of cerebral infarction and disturbed cerebral hemodynamics were detected in 20% and 40% of the involved hemispheres, respectively. Angiographic stage was more advanced in elderly patients. Of 34 medically-treated patients, 7 experienced TIA, ischemic stroke or hemorrhage during a mean follow-up period of 43.7 months. Cerebral infarction or hemorrhage did not occur in the 6 patients who underwent surgical revascularization.

Medical treatment

Medical treatment with platelet inhibitors, anticoagulants, calcium channel blockers,[93] steroids, mannitol, low-molecular-weight dextran and antibiotics have not proven to be of benefit. Steroids may be considered for involuntary movements and acutely during recurrent TIAs.

Surgical treatment

General information

Patients with mass effect from clot may be candidates for urgent decompression. Revascularization procedures, however, should be performed when the patient is stable under nonemergent conditions.

Perioperative management

During any surgical procedure:

1. avoid hyperventilation: due to increased sensitivity of collaterals, keep $PaCO_2$ 40–50 mm Hg to avoid ischemic infarction
2. avoid hypotension: maintain BP at normotensive levels
3. avoid alpha-adrenergic agents because of vasoconstrictive effects
4. cerebral protection: mild hypothermia (32–43° C) and barbiturates are routinely used
5. papaverine helps prevent vascular spasm

Postoperatively following STA-MAC bypass procedures:

1. avoid hypertension: may cause bleeding at anastomotic site and in areas of increased perfusion within the brain
2. avoid hypotension: may result in graft occlusion
3. aspirin is started on the post-op day #1
4. watch for evidence of CSF leak
5. monitor coag studies and correct abnormalities
6. cerebral arteriogram is recommended 2–6 months post-op

Suggested criteria for revascularization procedures

See reference.[90]

1. patients presenting with infarction or hemorrhage but are in good neurologic condition

2. infarction < 2 cm maximal diameter on CT, and all previous hemorrhages have completely resolved
3. angiographic stage is II-IV (see ▶ Table 85.8)
4. timing of operation: ≥ 2 months after most recent attack

Surgical revascularization options

Various methods to revascularize the ischemic brain, used primarily in children, include:

1. direct revascularization procedures:
   a) results are superior to indirect revascularization procedures[101,102] if a donor and recipient vessel of sufficient caliber (≥ 1 mm outer dia) can be identified (may be difficult in the pediatric age group who are the most likely to benefit[103]). Otherwise, indirect revascularization procedures (see below) are options.
   b) Among direct revascularization procedures, STA-MCA bypass[104] is the procedure of choice
2. indirect revascularization procedures: usually reserved for younger patients (suggested cutoff age ≈ 15 years). May be combined with STA-MCA bypass. Includes:
   a) encephalomyosynangiosis (**EMS**): laying the temporalis muscle on the surface of the brain (may cause problems with muscle contractions during talking and chewing, and neural impulses on surface of brain)
   b) encephaloduroarteriosynangiosis (**EDAS**)[105,106]: suturing the STA with a galeal cuff to a linear defect created in the dura. Variations on this technique include splitting the dura[107]
   c) omental transposition[108]: either as a pedicle graft or as a vascularized free flap. Felt to have higher potential to revascularize ischemic tissue than above procedures, but there is greater risk of mass effect from the thickness of the omentum
3. the above indirect revascularization procedures improve blood flow in the MCA distribution, but not ACA circulation. This may be rectified by:
   a) simple placement of frontal burr holes with opening of the underlying dura and arachnoid[109]
   b) "ribbon EDAS" where a pedicle of galea is inserted into the interhemispheric fissure on both sides[110]
4. stellate ganglionectomy and perivascular sympathectomy: unproven that this increases CBF permanently

Outcome with surgical treatment

Neurologic status at time of treatment generally predicts long-term outcome.[89] The mortality rate in adults (≈ 10%) is higher than for juveniles (≈ 4.3%).[96] The cause of death was bleeding in 56% of 9 children and 63% of 30 adults. With treatment the prognosis is good in 58%.[94]

85.9 Extracranial-intracranial (EC/IC) bypass

85.9.1 EC/IC bypass for atherosclerotic occlusive disease

The EC/IC bypass study

The EC/IC bypass, pioneered by Donaghy and Yasargil in 1967,[111] plummeted in popularity[112] after publication of the international cooperative EC/IC bypass study[113] in 1985. The EC/IC trial randomized 1377 patients with symptomatic ICA or MCA stenosis to either STA-MCA bypass or medical therapy with ASA. Despite a graft patency rate of 96%, surgical patients suffered more and earlier fatal and nonfatal strokes. Patients with severe MCA stenosis and those with persistent symptoms following ICA occlusion fared especially worse with bypass. During the 55.8 months mean follow-up, the percentage of patients experiencing 1 or more strokes in the medical group compared to the surgical group was 29% vs. 31%.

Critics highlight the failure of the study's inclusion criteria to distinguish between hemodynamic vs. thromboembolic causes of stroke[2,114,115] (ischemia secondary to thromboembolic events would not be expected to improve with flow augmentation, and inclusion of such patients in the surgical arm could therefore artificially lower the apparent efficacy of the procedure).

Current state of affairs

Imaging technologies introduced since the EC/IC trial can identify flow-dependent ischemia. Xenon-CT, TCD, SPECT, and MRI may be used in combination with acetazolamide challenge to evaluate cerebrovascular reserve and reactivity (p. 1265).

As cerebral perfusion pressure decreases in severe atherosclerotic occlusive disease, cerebral autoregulation is unable to maintain adequate CBF to meet metabolic demands. In this state of "misery perfusion", oxygen extraction fraction (OEF) of available blood flow will increase.[116,117] Abnormal OEF, as quantified by PET, is an independent predicator of subsequent stroke.[2] Patients with abnormal response to acetazolamide challenge (p.228) and/or with elevated OEF are therefore potential candidates for cerebral revascularization.[2,115,118,119,120]

Indications for EC/IC bypass

1. Patients with misery perfusion (see above)
2. aneurysms: certain aneurysms are not amendable to either direct microsurgical clipping or endovascular coiling due to extreme size, location, calcification or atherosclerosis, dissection, or the incorporation of perforators or major arteries. EC/IC bypass remains a highly viable adjunctive measure in patients requiring Hunterian occlusion of parent vessel or prolonged temporary occlusion for definite treatment.[121,122,123,124,125] Cerebrovascular reserve and need for bypass can be assessed preoperatively using balloon test occlusion (BTO) with hypotensive challenge
3. tumors encasing or invading major arteries
4. moyamoya disease (p.1313)

Bypass types

The type of graft used depends on preoperative determination of amount of flow augmentation necessary, the size of the recipient graft and the availability of donor vessel[126]:

1. pedicled arterial grafts: STA, occipital artery
   a) low-flow (15 – 25 ml/min)
   b) only one anastomosis required
   c) 95% graft patency in superficial temporal artery-middle cerebral artery (STA-MCA) bypasses
2. radial artery graft
   a) moderate to high flow (40 – 70 ml/min)
   b) advantages: physiological conduit for arterial blood; constant location makes it easy to harvest; lumen size closely approximates that of M2 or P1 and reduces flow mismatch with subsequent flow turbulence and graft thrombosis
   c) disadvantages: risk of vasospasm (reduced with pressure distension technique)
   d) > 90% graft patency at 5 years
3. saphenous vein graft
   a) high flow (70 – 140 ml/min)
   b) advantages: easy accessibility; longer length
   c) disadvantages: risk of thrombosis at distal anastomosis due to flow mismatch and turbulence; lower graft patency rates
   d) 82% graft patency at 5 years

References

[1] Hankey GJ, Warlow CP. Prognosis of symptomatic carotid artery occlusion: an overview. Cerebrovasc Dis. 1991; 1:245–256

[2] Grubb RLJr, Derdeyn CP, Fritsch SM, Carpenter DA, Yundt KD, Videen TO, Spitznagel EL, Powers WJ. Importance of hemodynamic factors in the prognosis of symptomatic carotid occlusion. JAMA. 1998; 280:1055–1060

[3] Powers WJ, Derdeyn CP, Fritsch SM, Carpenter DA, Yundt KD, Videen TO, Grubb RLJr. Benign prognosis of never-symptomatic carotid occlusion. Neurology. 2000; 54:878–882

[4] Hafner CD, Tew JM. Surgical Management of the Totally Occluded Internal Carotid Artery. Surgery. 1981; 89:710–717

[5] Satiani B, Burns J, Vasko JS. Surgical and Nonsurgical Treatment of Total Carotid Artery Occlusion. Am J Surg. 1985; 149:362–367

[6] Walters BB, Ojemann RG, Heros RC. Emergency Carotid Endarterectomy. J Neurosurg. 1987; 66:817–823

[7] Sugg RM, Malkoff MD, Noser EA, Shaltoni HM, Weir R, Cacayorin ED, Grotta JC. Endovascular recanalization of internal carotid artery occlusion in acute ischemic stroke. AJNR Am J Neuroradiol. 2005; 26:2591–2594

[8] Nesbit GM, Clark WM, O'Neill OR, Barnwell SL. Intracranial intraarterial thrombolysis facilitated by microcatheter navigation through an occluded cervical internal carotid artery. J Neurosurg. 1996; 84:387–392

[9] Endo S, Kuwayama N, Hirashima Y, Akai T, Nishijima M, Takaku A. Results of urgent thrombolysis in patients with major stroke and atherothrombotic occlusion of the cervical internal carotid artery. AJNR Am J Neuroradiol. 1998; 19:1169–1175

[10] Srinivasan A, Goyal M, Stys P, Sharma M, Lum C. Microcatheter navigation and thrombolysis in acute symptomatic cervical internal carotid occlusion. AJNR Am J Neuroradiol. 2006; 27:774–779

[11] Imai K, Mori T, Izumoto H, Watanabe M, Majima K. Emergency carotid artery stent placement in patients with acute ischemic stroke. AJNR Am J Neuroradiol. 2005; 26:1249–1258

[12] Jovin TG, Gupta R, Uchino K, Jungreis CA, Wechsler LR, Hammer MD, Tayal A, Horowitz MB. Emergent stenting of extracranial internal carotid artery occlusion in acute stroke has a high revascularization rate. Stroke. 2005; 36:2426–2430

[13] McCormick PW, Spetzler RF, Bailes JE, Zabramski JM, Frey JL. Thromboendarterectomy of the

Symptomatic Occluded Internal Carotid Artery. J Neurosurg. 1992; 76:752–758
[14] Tomaszek DE, Rosner MJ. Cerebellar Infarction: Analysis of Twenty-One Cases. Surg Neurol. 1985; 24:223–226
[15] Hinshaw D, Thompson J, Haso A, Casselman E. Infarctions of the Brain Stem and Cerebellum: A Correlation of Computer Tomography and Angiography. Radiology. 1980; 137:105–112
[16] Sypert GW, Alvord EC. Cerebellar Infarction: A Clinicopathological Study. Arch Neurol. 1975; 32:357–363
[17] Heros RC. Surgical Treatment of Cerebellar Infarction. Stroke. 1992; 23:937–938
[18] Heros RC. Cerebellar Hemorrhage and Infarction. Stroke. 1982; 13:106–109
[19] Chen H-J, Lee T-C, Wei C-P. Treatment of Cerebellar Infarction by Decompressive Suboccipital Craniectomy. Stroke. 1992; 23:957–961
[20] Moulin DE, Lo R, Chiang J, Barnett HJM. Prognosis in Middle Cerebral Artery Occlusion. Stroke. 1985; 16:282–284
[21] Hacke W, Schwab S, Horn M, et al. Malignant Middle Cerebral Artery Territory Infarction: Clinical Course and Prognostic Signs. Arch Neurol. 1996; 53:309–315
[22] Wijdicks EFM, Diringer MN. Middle Cerebral Artery Territory Infarction and Early Brain Swelling: Progression and Effect of Age on Outcome. Mayo Clin Proc. 1998; 73:829–836
[23] von Kummer R, Meyding-Lamadé U, Forsting M, Rosin L, Rieke K, Hacke W, et al. Sensitivity and Prognostic Value of Early CT in Occlusion of the Middle Cerebral Artery Trunk. AJNR. 1994; 15:9–15
[24] Carter BS, Ogilvy CS, Candia GJ, et al. One-Year Outcome After Decompressive Surgery for Massive Nondominant Hemispheric Infarction. Neurosurgery. 1997; 40:1168–1176
[25] Schwab S, Steiner T, Aschoff A, et al. Early Hemicraniectomy in Patients With Complete Middle Cerebral Artery Infarction. Stroke. 1998; 29:1888–1893
[26] Vahedi K, Hofmeijer J, Juettler E, Vicaut E, George B, Algra A, Amelink GJ, Schmiedeck P, Schwab S, Rothwell PM, Bousser MG, van der Worp HB, Hacke W, Decimal Destiny, . Early decompressive surgery in malignant infarction of the middle cerebral artery: a pooled analysis of three randomised controlled trials. Lancet Neurol. 2007; 6:215–222
[27] Blackshear JL, Kopecky SL, Litin SC, et al. Management of Atrial Fibrillation in Adults: Prevention of Thromboembolism and Symptomatic Treatment. Mayo Clin Proc. 1996; 71:150–160
[28] Atrial Fibrillation Investigators. Risk factors for stroke and efficacy of antithrombotic therapy in atrial fibrillation: Analysis of pooled data from five randomized controlled trials. Arch Intern Med. 1994; 154:1449–1457
[29] Hart RG, Helperin JL. Atrial fibrillation and stroke: Revisiting the dilemmas. Stroke. 1994; 25:1337–1341
[30] Gage BF, Waterman AD, Shannon W, Boechler M, Rich MW, Radford MJ. Validation of clinical classification schemes for predicting stroke: results from the National Registry of Atrial Fibrillation. JAMA. 2001; 285:2864–2870
[31] Gage BF, Birman-Deych E, Kerzner R, Radford MJ, Nilasena DS, Rich MW. Incidence of intracranial hemorrhage in patients with atrial fibrillation who are prone to fall. Am J Med. 2005; 118:612–617
[32] Lechat P, Mas JL, Lascault G, et al. Prevalence of patent foramen ovale in patients with stroke. N Engl J Med. 1988; 318:1148–1152
[33] Cerebral Embolism Task Force. Cardiogenic Brain Embolism. Arch Neurol. 1989; 46:727–743
[34] Stroke Prevention in Atrial Fibrillation Study Group. Preliminary report of the stroke prevention in atrial fibrillation study. N Engl J Med. 1990; 322:863–868
[35] Hopkins LN, Martin NA, Hadley MN, et al. Vertebrobasilar Insufficiency, Part 2: Microsurgical Treatment of Intracranial Vertebrobasilar Disease. J Neurosurg. 1987; 66:662–674
[36] Robertson JT. Current Management of Vertebral Basilar Occlusive Disease. Clin Neurosurg. 1983; 31:165–187
[37] Ausman JI, Shrontz CE, Pearce JE, et al. Vertebrobasilar Insufficiency: A Review. Arch Neurol. 1985; 42:803–808
[38] Diaz FG, Ausman JI, de los Reyes RA, et al. Surgical Reconstruction of the Proximal Vertebral Artery. J Neurosurg. 1984; 61:874–881
[39] Sorensen BF. Bow hunter's stroke. Neurosurgery. 1978; 2:259–261
[40] Fox MW, Piepgras DG, Bartleson JD. Anterolateral decompression of the atlantoaxial vertebral artery for symptomatic positional occlusion of the vertebral artery. J Neurosurg. 1995; 83:737–740
[41] Pratt-Thomas HR, Berger KE. Cerebellar and spinal injuries after chiropractic manipulation. JAMA. 1947; 133:600–603
[42] Matsuyama T, Morimoto T, Sakaki T. Bow hunter's stroke caused by a nondominant vertebral artery occlusion: Case report. Neurosurgery. 1997; 41:1393–1395
[43] Lemole GM, Henn JS, Spetzler RF, Zabramski JM. Bow hunter's stroke. BNI Quarterly. 2001; 17:4–10
[44] Mapstone T, Spetzler RF. Vertebrobasilar insufficiency secondary to vertebral artery occlusion from a fibrous band. Case report. J Neurosurg. 1982; 56:581–583
[45] George B, Laurian C. Impairment of vertebral artery flow caused by extrinsic lesions. Neurosurgery. 1989; 24:206–214
[46] Kuether TA, Nesbit GM, Clark WM, et al. Rotational Vertebral Artery Occlusion: A Mechanism of Vertebrobasilar Insufficiency. Neurosurgery. 1997; 41:427–433
[47] Pamphlett R, Raisanen J, Kum-Jew S. Vertebral artery compression resulting from head movement: a possible cause of the sudden infant death syndrome. Pediatrics. 1999; 103:460–468
[48] Okawara S, Nibbelink D. Vertebral artery occlusion following hyperextension and rotation of the head. Stroke. 1974; 5:640–642
[49] Ford FR. Syncope, vertigo and disturbances of vision resulting from intermittent obstruction of vertebral arteries due to defect in odontoid process and excessive mobility of second cervical vertebra. Bull Johns Hopkins Hosp. 1952; 91:168–173
[50] Tatlow WFT, Bammer HG. Syndrome of vertebral artery compression. Neurology. 1957; 7:331–340
[51] Shimizu T, Waga S, Kojima T, Niwa S. Decompression of the vertebral artery for bow-hunter's stroke. Case report. J Neurosurg. 1988; 69:127–131
[52] Matsuyama T, Morimoto T, Sakaki T. Comparison of C1-2 posterior fusion and decompression of the vertebral artery in the treatment of bow hunter's stroke. J Neurosurg. 1997; 86:619–623
[53] Wilkins RH, Rengachary SS. Neurosurgery. New York 1985
[54] Symonds CP. Otitic Hydrocephalus. Brain. 1931; 54:55–71
[55] Garcia RDJ, Baker AS, Cunningham MJ, Weber AL. Lateral Sinus Thrombosis Associated with Otitis Media and Mastoiditis in Children. Pediatr Infect Dis J. 1995; 14:617–623
[56] Dolan RW, Chowdry K. Diagnosis and Treatment of Intracranial Complications of Paranasal Sinus Infections. J Oral Maxillofac Surg. 1995; 53:1080–1087
[57] Shende MC, Lourie H. Sagittal Sinus Thrombosis Related to Oral Contraceptives: Case Report. J Neurosurg. 1970; 33:714–717
[58] Mahasin ZZ, Saleem M, Gangopadhyay K. Transverse Sinus Thrombosis and Venous Infarction of the Brain Following Unilateral Radical Neck Dissection. J Laryngol Otol. 1998; 112:88–91
[59] Martinelli I, Landi G, Merati G, et al. Factor V Gene Mutation is a Risk Factor for Cerebral Venous Thrombosis. Thromb Maemost. 1996; 75:393–394
[60] Flusser D, Abu-Shakra M, Baumgarten-Kleiner A, et al. Superior Sagittal Sinus Thrombosis in a

Patient with Systemic Lupus Erythematosus. Lupus. 1996; 5:334–336

[61] Bugnicourt JM, Roussel B, Tramier B, Lamy C, Godefroy O. Cerebral venous thrombosis and plasma concentrations of factor VIII and von Willebrand factor: a case control study. J Neurol Neurosurg Psychiatry. 2007; 78:699–701

[62] Bousser MG. Cerebral Vein Thrombosis in Bechet's Syndrome. Arch Neurol. 1982; 39

[63] Wilder-Smith E, Kothbauer-Margreiter I, Lämmle B, et al. Dural Puncture and Activated protein C Resistance: Risk Factors for Cerebral Venous Sinus Thrombosis. J Neurol Neurosurg Psychiatry. 1997; 63:351–356

[64] Estanol B, Rodriguez A, Conte G, et al. Intracranial Venous Thrombosis in Young Women. Stroke. 1979; 10:680–684

[65] Brenner B. Haemostatic changes in pregnancy. Thromb Res. 2004; 114:409–414

[66] Ferrera PC, Pauze DR, Chan L. Sagittal Sinus Thrombosis After Closed Head Injury. Am J Emerg Med. 1998; 16:382–385

[67] Elsherbiny SM, Grunewald RA, Powell T. Isolated Inferior Sagittal Sinus Thrombosis: A Case Report. Neuroradiology. 1997; 39:411–413

[68] Gerszten PC, Welch WC, Spearman MP, et al. Isolated Deep Cerebral Venous Thrombosis Treated by Direct Endovascular Thrombolysis. Surg Neurol. 1997; 48:261–266

[69] Sofferman RA. Cavernous Sinus Thrombosis Secondary to Sphenoid Sinusitis. Laryngoscope. 1983; 93:797–800

[70] Kriss TC, Kriss VM, Warf BC. Cavernous Sinus Thrombophlebitis: Case Report. Neurosurgery. 1996; 39:385–389

[71] Kalbag RM, Kapp JP, Schmidek HH. In: Cerebral Venous Thrombosis. The Cerebral Venous System and its Disorders. Orlando: Grune and Stratton; 1984:505–536

[72] Bousser MG, Chiras J, Bories J, et al. Cerebral Venous Thrombosis - A Review of 38 Cases. Stroke. 1985; 16:199–213

[73] Perkin GD. Cerebral Venous Thrombosis: Developments in Imaging and Treatment. J Neurol Neurosurg Psychiatry. 1995; 59:1–3

[74] Yeakley JW, Mayer JS, Patchell LL, et al. The Pseudodelta Sign in Acute Head Trauma. J Neurosurg. 1988; 69:867–868

[75] Rao KCVG, Knipp HC, Wagner EJ. CT Findings in Cerebral Sinus and Venous Thrombosis. Radiology. 1981; 140:391–398

[76] Virapongse C, Cazenave C, Quisling R, et al. The empty delta sign: Frequency and significance in 76 cases of dural sinus thrombosis. Radiology. 1987; 162:779–785

[77] Lam AH. Doppler Imaging of Superior Sagittal Sinus Thrombosis. J Ultrasound Med. 1995; 14:41–46

[78] Levine SR, Twyman RE, Gilman S. The Role of Anticoagulation in Cavernous Sinus Thrombosis. Neurology. 1988; 38:517–522

[79] Villringer A, Garner C, Meister W, er al.. High-Dose Heparin Treatment in Cerebral Sinus Thrombosis. Stroke. 1988; 19

[80] Einhäupl KM, Villringer A, Meister W, et al. Heparin Treatment in Sinus Venous Thrombosis. Lancet. 1991; 338:597–600

[81] Horowitz M, Purdy P, Unwin H, et al. Treatment of Dural Sinus Thrombosis Using Selective Catheterization and Urokinase. Ann Neurol. 1995; 38:58–67

[82] Alexander LF, Tamamoto Y, Ayoubi S, Al-Mefty O, et al. Efficacy of Tissue Plasminogen Activator in the Lysis of Thrombosis of the Cerebral Venous Sinus. Neurosurgery. 1990; 26:559–564

[83] Horton JC, Seiff SR, Pitts LH, Weinstein PR, Rosenblum ML, Hoyt WF. Decompression of the Optic Nerve Sheath for Vision-Threatening Papilledema Caused by Dural Sinus Occlusion. Neurosurgery. 1992; 31:203–212

[84] Stam J, Majoie CB, van Delden OM, van Lienden KP, Reekers JA. Endovascular thrombectomy and thrombolysis for severe cerebral sinus thrombosis: a prospective study. Stroke. 2008; 39:1487–1490

[85] Suzuki J, Takaku A. Cerebrovascular "Moyamoya" Disease: Disease Showing Abnormal Net-Like Vessels in Base of Brain. Arch Neurol. 1969; 20:288–299

[86] Takeuchi K, Shimuzi K. Hypogenesis of Bilateral Interanl Carotid Arteries. No To Shinkei. 1957; 9:37–37

[87] Kayama T, Suzuki S, Sakurai Y, et al. A Case of Moyamoya Disease Accompanied by an Arteriovenous Malformation. Neurosurgery. 1986; 18:465–468

[88] Lichtor T, Mullan S. Arteriovenous Malformation in Moyamoya Syndrome: Report of Three Cases. J Neurosurg. 1987; 67:603–608

[89] Smith ER, Scott RM. Surgical management of moyamoya syndrome. Skull Base. 2005; 15:15–26

[90] Zipfel GJ, Fox DJ,Jr, Rivet DJ. Moyamoya disease in adults: the role of cerebral revascularization. Skull Base. 2005; 15:27–41

[91] Rajakulasingam K, Cerullo LJ, Raimondi AJ. Childhood Moyamoya Syndrome: Postradiation Pathogenesis. Childs Brain. 1979; 5:467–475

[92] Kwak R, Ito S, Yamamoto N, Kadoya S. Significance of Intracranial Aneurysms Associated with Moyamoya Disease (Part I): Differences Between Intracranial Aneurysms Associated with Moyamoya Disease and Usual Saccular Aneurysms - Review of the Literature. Neurol Med Chir. 1984; 24:97–103

[93] Chang SD, Steinberg GK. Surgical Management of Moyamoya Disease. Contemp Neurosurg. 2000; 22:1–9

[94] Ueki K, Meyer FB, Mellinger JF. Moyamoya Disease: The Disorder and Surgical Treatment. Mayo Clin Proc. 1994; 69:749–757

[95] Kuroda S, Ishikawa T, Houkin K, Nanba R, Hokari M, Iwasaki Y. Incidence and clinical features of disease progression in adult moyamoya disease. Stroke. 2005; 36:2148–2153

[96] Nishimoto A. Moyamoya Disease. Neurol Med Chir. 1979; 19:221–228

[97] Kodama N, Aoki Y, Hiraga H, et al. Electroencephalographic Findings in Children with Moyamoya Disease. Arch Neurol. 1979; 36:16–19

[98] Ogawa A, Yoshimoto T, Suzuki J, Sakurai J. Cerebral Blood Flow in Moyamoya Disease. Part 1. Correlation with Age and Regional Distribution. Acta Neurochir. 1990; 105:30–34

[99] Ogawa A, Nakamura N, Yoshimoto T, Suzuki J. Cerebral Blood Flow in Moyamoya Disease. Part 2. Autoregulation and CO2 Response. Acta Neurochir. 1990; 105:107–111

[100] Kuroda S, Hashimoto N, Yoshimoto T, Iwasaki Y. Radiological findings, clinical course, and outcome in asymptomatic moyamoya disease: results of multicenter survey in Japan. Stroke. 2007; 38:1430–1435

[101] Matsushima Y, Inoue T, Suzuki SO, et al. Surgical Treatment of Moyamoya Disease in Pediatric Patients - Comparison between the Results of Indirect and Direct Vascularization. Neurosurgery. 1992; 31:401–405

[102] Ishikawa T, Houkin K, Kamiyama H, Abe H. Effects of Surgical Revascularization on Outcome of Patients with Pediatric Moyamoya Disease. Stroke. 1997; 28:1170–1173

[103] Fabi AY, Meyer FB. Moyamoya Disease. Contemp Neurosurg. 1997; 19:1–6

[104] Karasawa J, Kikuchi H, Furuse S, et al. Treatment of Moyamoya Disease with STA-MCA Anastamosis. J Neurosurg. 1978; 49:679–688

[105] Matsushima Y, Fukai N, Tanaka K, et al. A new surgical treatment of moyamoya disease in children: A preliminary report. Surg Neurol. 1980; 15:313–320

[106] Matsushima Y, Inaba Y. Moyamoya Disease in Children and Its Surgical Treatment. Childs Brain. 1984; 11:155–170

[107] Kashiwagi S, Kato S, Yasuhara S, et al. Use of Split Dura for Revascularization if Ischemic Hemispheres in Moyamoya Disease. J Neurosurg. 1996; 85:380–383

[108] Karasawa J, Kikuchi H, Kawamura J, et al. Intracranial Transplantation of the Omentum for Cerebrovascular Moyamoya Disease: A Two-Year Follow-Up Study. Surg Neurol. 1980; 14:444–449
[109] Endo M, Kawano N, Miyasaka Y, et al. Cranial Burr Hole for Revascularization in Moyamoya Disease. J Neurosurg. 1989; 71:180–185
[110] Kinugasa K, Mandai S, Tokunaga K, et al. Ribbon Encephalo-Duro-Arterio-Myo-Synangiosis for Moyamoya Disease. Surg Neurol. 1994; 41:455–461
[111] Crowley RW, Medel R, Dumont AS. Evolution of cerebral revascularization techniques. Neurosurg Focus. 2008; 24. DOI: 10.3171/FOC/2008/24/2/E3
[112] Amin-Hanjani S, Butler WE, Ogilvy CS, Carter BS, Barker FG, II. Extracranial-intracranial bypass in the treatment of occlusive cerebrovascular disease and intracranial aneurysms in the United States between 1992 and 2001: a population-based study. J Neurosurg. 2005; 103:794–804
[113] EC/IC Study Group. Failure of EC-IC arterial bypass to reduce the risk of ischemic stroke. N Engl J Med. 1985; 313:1191–1200
[114] Garrett MC, Komotar RJ, Merkow MB, Starke RM, Otten ML, Connolly ES. The extracranial-intracranial bypass trial: implications for future investigations. Neurosurg Focus. 2008; 24. DOI: 10.3171/FOC/2008/24/2/E4
[115] Garrett MC, Komotar RJ, Starke RM, Merkow MB, Otten ML, Sciacca RR, Connolly ES. The efficacy of direct extracranial-intracranial bypass in the treatment of symptomatic hemodynamic failure secondary to athero-occlusive disease: a systematic review. Clin Neurol Neurosurg. 2009; 111:319–326
[116] Baron JC, Bousser MG, Rey A, Guillard A, Comar D, Castaigne P. Reversal of focal "misery-perfusion syndrome" by extra-intracranial arterial bypass in hemodynamic cerebral ischemia. A case study with 15O positron emission tomography. Stroke. 1981; 12:454–459
[117] Powers WJ, Press GA, Grubb RL, Jr, Gado M, Raichle ME. The effect of hemodynamically significant carotid artery disease on the hemodynamic status of the cerebral circulation. Ann Intern Med. 1987; 106:27–34
[118] Grubb RL,Jr, Powers WJ, Derdeyn CP, Adams HP,Jr, Clarke WR. The Carotid Occlusion Surgery Study. Neurosurg Focus. 2003; 14
[119] Kappelle LJ, Klijn CJ, Tulleken CA. Management of patients with symptomatic carotid artery occlusion. Clin Exp Hypertens. 2002; 24:631–637
[120] Kuroda S, Houkin K, Kamiyama H, Mitsumori K, Iwasaki Y, Abe H. Long-term prognosis of medically treated patients with internal carotid or middle cerebral artery occlusion: can acetazolamide test predict it? Stroke. 2001; 32:2110–2116
[121] Cantore G, Santoro A, Guidetti G, Delfinis CP, Colonnese C, Passacantilli E. Surgical treatment of giant intracranial aneurysms: current viewpoint. Neurosurgery. 2008; 63:279–89; discussion 289-90
[122] Mohit AA, Sekhar LN, Natarajan SK, Britz GW, Ghodke B. High-flow bypass grafts in the management of complex intracranial aneurysms. Neurosurgery. 2007; 60:ONS105–22; discussion ONS122-3
[123] O'Shaughnessy BA, Salehi SA, Mindea SA, Batjer HH. Selective cerebral revascularization as an adjunct in the treatment of giant anterior circulation aneurysms. Neurosurg Focus. 2003; 14
[124] Schaller B. Extracranial-intracranial bypass to reduce the risk of ischemic stroke in intracranial aneurysms of the anterior cerebral circulation: a systematic review. J Stroke Cerebrovasc Dis. 2008; 17:287–298
[125] Sekhar LN, Bucur SD, Bank WO, Wright DC. Venous and arterial bypass grafts for difficult tumors, aneurysms, and occlusive vascular lesions: evolution of surgical treatment and improved graft results. Neurosurgery. 1999; 44:1207–23; discussion 1223-4
[126] Liu JK, Kan P, Karwande SV, Couldwell WT. Conduits for cerebrovascular bypass and lessons learned from the cardiovascular experience. Neurosurg Focus. 2003; 14

86 Cerebral Arterial Dissections

86.1 General information

Key concepts

- hemorrhage into the tunica media of an artery
- may be spontaneous, post-traumatic, or iatrogenic [e.g. angiography-related], may be intracranial or extracranial
- may present with pain (usually ipsilateral H/A or carotidynia), Horner's syndrome
- (in carotid dissections), TIA/stroke, or SAH
- extracranial dissections are usually treated medically (anticoagulation), intracranial dissections with SAH are treated surgically

This section primarily discusses "spontaneous" dissections. ICA dissection following blunt cervical trauma is much more common (p.851).

86.2 Nomenclature

Some confusion has arisen because of inconsistent terminology in the literature. Although by no means standard, Yamaura[1] has suggested the following:

► **Dissection.** Extravasation of blood between the intima and media, creating luminal narrowing or occlusion.

► **Dissecting aneurysm.** Dissection of blood between the media and adventitia, or at the media, causing aneurysmal dilatation, which may rupture into the subarachnoid space.

► **Pseudoaneurysm.** Rupture of artery with subsequent encapsulation of the extravascular hematoma, may or may not produce luminal narrowing.

86.3 Pathophysiology

The lesion common to all dissections is hemorrhage outside of the vascular lumen due to pathological trans-intimal extravasation of blood from the true lumen into the vessel wall. The hematoma may either dissect the internal elastic membrane from the intima[2] causing narrowing of the true lumen, or it may dissect into the subadventitial plane producing an adventitial outpouching from the vessel wall (pseudoaneurysm). Rupture through the vessel wall producing SAH occurs occasionally.

Subintimal dissection is more common with intracranial dissections, whereas extracranial vessels (including the aorta) usually dissect at the media or between media and adventitia.

"Spontaneous" dissections have been associated with a large number of conditions, oftentimes the association is unproven. These conditions include:

- fibromuscular dysplasia (FMD): found in ≈ 15% of cases[3]
- cystic medial necrosis (or degeneration): originally thought to be a common finding, now thought to perhaps be linked to a higher likelihood of *fatal* dissection
- saccular aneurysm
- Marfan syndrome: autosomal dominant inherited disorder of connective tissue. Phenotypic manifestations are due to production of abnormal fibrillin, the main component of extracellular microfibrils, a component in the media of certain blood vessels, encoded by the FBN1 gene on chromosome 15q21
- Ehlers-Danlos syndrome
- atherosclerosis: only rarely implicated as an etiology. More likely to be a factor with subintimal dissection of *extra*cranial arteries
- Takayasu's disease
- medial degeneration
- syphilitic arteritis (more common in the past, associated with 60% of dissections before 1950)

- autosomal dominant polycystic kidney disease (p. 1193): associated with a higher incidence of cerebral aneurysms
- variant periarteritis nodosa
- allergic arteritis
- homocystinuria
- moyamoya disease (p. 1313)[4]
- strenuous physical activity

86.4 Epidemiology

Occurs primarily in middle aged patients, with a mean age of ≈ 45 yrs (average age of traumatic dissections is slightly younger). More frequent in men.[1,3] Incidence is unknown, since often times the condition produces mild, transient symptoms. Increased awareness of the condition has resulted in an increased rate of diagnosis. ICA dissection accounts for 1-2.5% of first strokes.[5] However, in middle aged and young adults it comprises 10-25% of strokes.[6]

86.5 Sites of dissection

A review of 260 cases[1] (literature review + new cases) found the incidence by location shown in ▶ Table 86.1. The vertebral artery was the most common intracranial site. Previously, it was believed that the ICA was the most common site. This change may be due to the recent increased recognition of arterial dissections as a source of SAH (and vertebral dissections most often present as SAH). Multiple dissections occur in ≈ 10% (the most common: bilateral vertebrobasilar lesions).

86.6 Clinical

Cerebral arterial dissections may cause symptoms by:

1. embolization secondary to:
   a) platelet aggregation stimulated by the exposed surfaces
   b) dislodged thrombus (formation of which is enhanced by reduced flow)
2. reduced distal flow secondary to:
   a) thrombosis due to reduced flow
   b) occlusion of the true lumen by the expansion of the mural hematoma
3. subarachnoid hemorrhage (atypical presentation, may be more common with posterior circulation dissection than with anterior circulation)[7]

The most common presentation in patients < 30 yrs of age was due to internal carotid dissection without SAH. In patients > 30 yrs, vertebrobasilar artery (VBA) dissection with SAH was the most common.[1]

Headache, usually severe, often predates neurologic deficit by days or weeks (p. 1228). See sections ICA (p. 1324) and vertebrobasilar (p. 1325) for specifics.

Table 86.1 Spontaneous intracranial dissections by site

Location	Left	Right	Total
vertebral	122	82	204
basilar	35		35
internal carotid	17	13	30
middle cerebral	16	10	26
anterior cerebral	10	3	13
posterior cerebral	7	9	16
PICA	4	10	14
Total	**176**	**127**	**338**

86.7 Evaluation

► **CT.** More useful for evaluating brain for infarction. Dissection can sometimes be visualized directly.[8]

► **CT angiogram (CTA).** Often obviates the need for cerebral angiography since CTA scanners with ≥ 16 detectors are equal in predictive value and have an accuracy near 99%.[9]

► **Angiography.** The definitive diagnostic study. However, diagnosis may be delayed if the dissection is misinterpreted as:
1. an unusual saccular aneurysm (the most common error)
2. atherosclerotic lesions: with dissections, the location is unusual, the lesion may be isolated, the age is usually younger, and the stenosis is smooth. Cervical ICA dissection typically spares the carotid bulb whereas cervical ICA atherosclerosis tends to involve the bulb.
3. vasospasm following SAH: however, the narrowing with vasospasm is delayed in onset vs. the changes with dissection which are present from the beginning

Angiographic findings may include:
1. luminal stenosis: irregular stenosis over long segments of the artery often with focal areas of near total stenosis ("string sign")
2. fusiform dilation with proximal or distal narrowing (string and pearl sign)
3. occlusion: artery usually tapers to a point
4. intimal flap: when seen, usually found at proximal end of dissection
5. may see proximal beading ("string of beads" configuration, indicative of FMD)
6. "double lumen sign": true vessel lumen and an intramural false lumen with an intimal flap. Usually with retention of contrast within the false lumen well into the venous phase. The only pathognomonic sign
7. wavy "ripple" appearance
8. severe kinking (frequently bilateral). With VBA lesions: dolichoectasia

A characteristic of arterial dissections is that they often change configuration on repeat angiography[10] (some resolve, and some worsen). NB: forceful intra-arterial contrast injection during the performance of angiography carries a potential for worsening the dissection.

► **MRI.** Probably not as accurate as CTA or angiography. Optimal MRI study is source *T1WI axial images with fat suppression* ("fat sat"), look for loss of visualization over several slices, with good visualization above and below. May visualize intimal flap and distinguish a dissection from a fusiform aneurysm.

Crescent sign: bright signal in wall of ICA on T2WI axial images (hematoma in vessel wall).

86.8 Overall outcome

An early review of the literature found an 83% mortality within a few weeks of presentation with vertebrobasilar artery (VBA) dissection.[11] A later report tempered that grim prognosis.[12]

Based on a review of 260 cases,[1] an overall mortality of 26% was found. 70% had a favorable outcome (assessed using Glasgow Outcome scale), 5% poor. Mortality was higher in ICA lesions (49%) than VBA lesions (22%). Mortality was 24% in the SAH group, and 29% in non-SAH cases.

86.9 Vessel specific information

86.9.1 Internal carotid dissection

See above for general information. Posttraumatic ICA dissection (p. 1323) is much more common than spontaneous.

Some cases considered "spontaneous" may actually be due to trivial trauma, including violent coughing, nose blowing, and simple neck turning. Usually seen in young women.

In spontaneous dissection, the most common initial symptom is ipsilateral headache. Most of these (60%) are orbital or periorbital, but they may also be auricular or mastoid (39%), frontal (36%), temporal (27%). May also produce sudden onset of severe pain over carotid artery (carotidynia).[13]

Incomplete Horner's syndrome (oculosympathetic palsy): ptosis and miosis without anhidrosis (due to involvement of plexus around the ICA, sparing the ECA plexus which innervates facial sweat glands) may occur. Bruits may be heard by the examiner or by the patient. These and other clinical features are shown in ▶ Table 86.2.

May be a cause of some cases of infantile and childhood hemiplegia and hemiparesis.[14]

86.9.2 Vertebrobasilar system artery dissection

Vertebral artery dissections

General information

See general information on cerebral arterial dissections (p. 1322). See also posttraumatic vertebrobasilar dissection (p. 852).

Less common than carotid. Extracranial lesions outnumber intracranial.

Traumatic dissections tend to occur where the VA crosses bony prominences, e.g. at the C1–2 junction or where it enters the foramen transversarium (usually at C6). Spontaneous dissections tend to be intracranial and commonly occur on the *dominant* VA. Unlike cervical ICA dissections, which tend not to propagate intracranially through the carotid canal, high cervical VA dissections can readily propagate intracranially through the foramen magnum.

Spontaneous VA dissections have been associated with FMD, migraine, and oral contraceptives.[15] Unrecognized or forgotten trauma or sudden head motion may have occurred in some cases reported as spontaneous. Commonly occurs in young adults (mean age: 48 yrs). With spontaneous dissections, 36% of patients have dissections at other sites, 21% of cases have bilateral VA dissections.[16]

Dissecting aneurysms of the VA (possibly a distinct entity) are also described.[17,18,19] They tend to be fusiform, and may be amenable to clipping, and were associated with vertebral dissections in 5 of 7 cases reported in one series.[20] As of 1984, only ≈ 50 cases of dissecting aneurysms were published.[20]

Presentation

In spontaneous extradural dissections, neck pain is a prominent early finding in most patients, and is commonly located over the occiput and posterior cervical region. Generalized severe headache is also common. TIAs or stroke (usually lateral medullary syndrome (p. 1267) [21] or cerebellar infarction, especially in patients with occlusion of the third or fourth portion of the VA[22]). None of 5 patients developed new neurologic symptoms after the original stroke in an average of 21 months follow-up.[22] In 3 of these 5, VA dissection was bilateral.

Dissecting aneurysms may present with altered consciousness, and may cause SAH (seen in 6 of 30 cases of vertebrobasilar complex dissections).[20] Rebleeding occurs in 24–30% of those cases presenting with SAH,[16] making these lesions treacherous, with a very high mortality.[23,24]

Traumatic extradural dissections or pseudoaneurysms may have a similar presentation, but can also produce massive external hemorrhage or neck hematomas.[16]

Evaluation

See section under Cerebral arterial dissections, Evaluation (p. 1324).

Table 86.2 Clinical features of spontaneous ICA dissection[3]

Feature	%
focal cerebral ischemia	76%
headache	59%
oculosympathetic palsy	30%
bruit	25%
amaurosis fugax	10%
neck pain	9%
syncope	4%
scalp tenderness	2%
neck swelling	2%

► **Angiography.** Diagnosis by angiography may be difficult in many cases (the most common misdiagnosis is ruptured saccular aneurysm of unusual shape[25]).

In post-traumatic dissections, the most common finding is irregular stenosis of horizontal loops of distal extracranial VAs as they pass behind C1, often bilateral.

In 14 of 15 post-traumatic VA dissections, the lesion was located posterior to the atlas (distal extracranial 3rd segment), the single exception being a patient with direct trauma causing proximal VA involvement. This predilection is possibly explained by the fact that the first and third portions of the VA are movable, whereas the second and fourth are relatively immobilized by bone.

Treatment

Except for cases presenting with hemorrhage or large ischemic stroke, medical therapy should be started emergently. Classically consists of anticoagulation, with heparin acutely, followed by oral agents (e.g. Coumadin) probably for a total of 6 months. Recent preliminary study showed antiplatelet therapy was equally as effective.[26]

As with traumatic dissections, endovascular techniques are now assuming more prominent role in management.

► **Indications for intervention.** Surgery or endovascular techniques (mostly stents, but also occlusion, angioplasty[16]) are required for dissections presenting with SAH (due to their propensity to rebleed) and is recommended for most intradural dissections. For extradural lesions it is indicated for dissections that progress (angiographically) or for persistent symptoms in spite of adequate medical therapy. Some less malignant lesions may be amenable to endovascular stenting.

► **Endovascular treatment.** Balloon-mounted, self-expandable, or covered stents have been used relatively infrequently to treat dissections of the internal carotid or vertebral arteries, with good technical results and low procedure-related complication rates[27] 2011]. Given the small number of patients treated and the fact that medical therapy is generally effective, the role of stenting for dissection remains to be defined. It should be reserved for patients in whom medical therapy is ineffective or contra-indicated or when the dissection causes symptomatic flow-limiting stenosis.

► **Surgical treatment.** At the time of surgery, the site of dissection may be recognized by fusiform or tubular enlargement of the artery with discoloration due to blood within the arterial wall (the discoloration has been described as black, bluish, purple, purple red, or brown[25]).

Surgical treatment of intradural dissection when endovascular techniques are not an option includes the following alternatives:

1. non-clippable aneurysms may be candidates for Hunterian occlusion of the VA proximal to the BA (either by microsurgical technique, or by endovascular techniques which may not be as precise). Some may not tolerate clipping the dominant VA, especially if the contralateral VA is hypoplastic. Conversely, some may tolerate bilateral VA occlusion.[28] Balloon test occlusion[16] is recommended
   a) if the dissection involves the PICA origin, then clip proximal to dissection. PICA then fills from retrograde flow, and the reversal of flow across the site of dissection should push the intima back against the wall
   b) if the dissection is proximal to PICA and doesn't involve PICA, then trap the aneurysm between clips. PICA fills by retrograde flow
   c) if the aneurysm begins distal to the PICA origin, occlude the VA[7] *distal* to the PICA takeoff[29]
2. combining VA clipping (non-clippable aneurysms may be candidates for Hunterian occlusion of the VA proximal to the aneurysm) with vascular bypass, options:
   a) side-to-side PICA-PICA anastomosis
   b) transplantation of the PICA origin to the VA outside the aneurysm
   c) occipital artery-to-PICA bypass
3. resection accompanied by autogenous interposition vein graft
4. non occlusive surgical techniques
   a) clipping with specially designed clips for fusiform aneurysms (e.g. Sundt-Kees clip)
   b) wrapping: of dubious benefit

86.9.3 Vertebrobasilar system dissections excluding the VA

Basilar artery dissections tend to present with brain stem infarction and more rarely with SAH.[24] The prognosis is generally regarded as poor. Endovascular techniques may be able to treat some.

References

[1] Yamaura A. Nontraumatic Intracranial Arterial Dissection: Natural History, Diagnosis, and Treatment. Contemp Neurosurg. 1994; 16:1–6

[2] Goldstein SJ. Dissecting Hematoma of the Cervical Vertebral Artery: Case Report. J Neurosurg. 1982; 56:451–454

[3] Anson J, Crowell RM. Cervicocranial Arterial Dissection. Neurosurgery. 1991; 29:89–96

[4] Yamashita M, Tanaka K, Matsuo T, et al. Cerebral dissecting aneurysms in patients with moyamoya disease. J Neurosurg. 1983; 58:120–125

[5] Bogousslavsky J, Despland PA, Regli F. Spontaneous carotid dissection with acute stroke. Arch Neurol. 1987; 44:137–140

[6] Debette S, Leys D. Cervical-artery dissections: predisposing factors, diagnosis, and outcome. Lancet Neurol. 2009; 8:668–678

[7] Friedman AH, Drake CG. Subarachnoid hemorrhage from intracraniai dissecting aneurysm. J Neurosurg. 1984; 60:325–334

[8] Hodge C, Leeson M, Cacayorin E, et al. Computed Tomographic Evaluation of Extracranial Carotid Artery Disease. Neurosurgery. 1987; 21:167–176

[9] Eastman AL, Chason DP, Perez CL, McAnulty AL, Minei JP. Computed tomographic angiography for the diagnosis of blunt cervical vascular injury: is it ready for primetime? J Trauma. 2006; 60:925–9; discussion 929

[10] Kitanaka C, Tanaki J-I, Kuwahara M, et al. Nonsurgical Treatment of Unruptured Intracranial Vertebral Artery Dissection with Serial Follow-Up Angiography. J Neurosurg. 1994; 80:667–674

[11] Berger MS, Wilson CB. Intracranial dissecting aneurysms of the posterior circulation. Report of six cases and review of the literature. J Neurosurg. 1984; 61:882–894

[12] Pozzati E, Padovani R, Fabrizi A, et al. Benign Arterial Dissection of the Posterior Circulation. J Neurosurg. 1991; 75:69–72

[13] Welling RE, Taha A, Goel T, et al. Extracranial Carotid Artery Aneurysms. Surgery. 1983; 93:319–323

[14] Chang V, Newcastle NB, Harwood-Nash DCF, Norman MG. Bilateral dissecting aneurysms of the intracranial internal carotid arteries in an 8-year-old boy. Neurology. 1975; 25:573–579

[15] Leys D, Lesoin F, Pruvo JP, et al. Bilateral Spontaneous Dissection of Extracranial Vertebral Arteries. J Neurol. 1987; 234:237–240

[16] Halbach VV, Higashida RT, Dowd CF, Fraser KW, Smith TP, Teitelmaum GP, Wilson CB, Hieshima GB. Endovascular Treatment of Vertebral Artery Dissections and Pseudoaneurysms. J Neurosurg. 1993; 79:183–191

[17] Miyazaki S, Yamaura A, Kamata K, et al. A dissecting aneurysm of the vertebral artery. Surg Neurol. 1984; 21:171–174

[18] Hugenholtz H, Pokrupa R, Montpetit VJA, et al. Spontaneous dissecting aneurysm of the extracranial vertebral artery. Neurosurgery. 1982; 10:96–100

[19] Senter HJ, Sarwar M. Nontraumatic dissecting aneurysm of the vertebral artery. J Neurosurg. 1982; 56:128–130

[20] Shimoji T, Bando K, Nakajima K, et al. Dissecting Aneurysm of the Vertebral Artery. J Neurosurg. 1984; 61:1038–1046

[21] Okuchi K, Watabe Y, Hiramatsu K, et al. [Dissecting Aneurysm of the Vertebral Artery as a Cause of Wallenberg's Syndrome]. No Shinkei Geka. 1990; 18:721–727

[22] Caplan LR, Zarins CK, Hemmati M. Spontaneous Dissection of the Extracranial Vertebral Arteries. Stroke. 1985; 16:1030–1038

[23] Aoki N, Sakai T. Rebleeding from intracranial dissecting aneurysm in the vertebral artery. Stroke. 1990; 21:1628–1631

[24] Pozzati E, Andreoli A, Limoni P, Casmiro M. Dissecting Aneurysms of the Vertebrobasilar System: Study of 16 Cases. Surg Neurol. 1994; 41:119–124

[25] Yamaura A, Watanabe Y, Saeki N. Dissecting Aneurysms of the Intracranial Vertebral Artery. J Neurosurg. 1990; 72:183–188

[26] Markus HS, Hayter E, Levi C, Feldman A, Venables G, Norris J. Antiplatelet treatment compared with anticoagulation treatment for cervical artery dissection (CADISS): a randomised trial. Lancet Neurol. 2015; 14:361–367

[27] Pham MH, Rahme RJ, Arnaout O, Hurley MC, Bernstein RA, Batjer HH, Bendok BR. Endovascular stenting of extracranial carotid and vertebral artery dissections: a systematic review of the literature. Neurosurgery. 2011; 68:856–66; discussion 866

[28] Six EG, Stringer WL, Cowley AR, et al. Posttraumatic Bilateral Vertebral Artery Occlusion. Case Report. J Neurosurg. 1981; 54:814–817

[29] Yamada K, Hayakawa T, Ushio Y, et al. Therapeutic Occlusion of the Vertebral Artery for Unclippable Vertebral Aneurysm. Neurosurgery. 1984; 15:834–838

Part XX

Intracerebral Hemorrhage

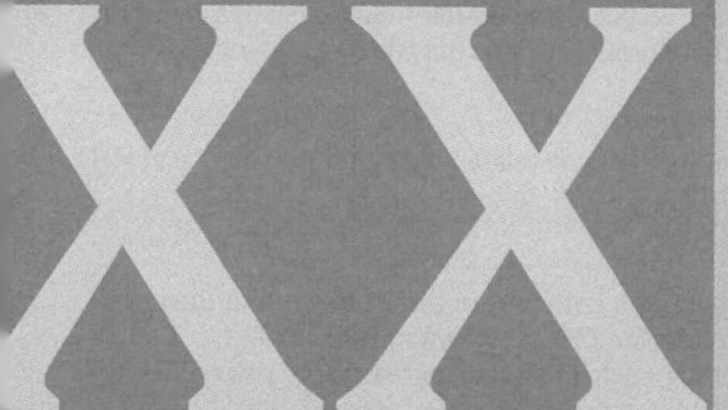

87 Intracerebral Hemorrhage

87.1 General Information

Intracerebral hemorrhage (ICH) is a hemorrhage within the brain parenchyma. Formerly commonly referred to as "hypertensive hemorrhage", but hypertension is a debatable etiology in many cases; see *Hypertension as a cause?* (p. 1334).

87.2 Intracerebral hemorrhage in adults

Key concepts

- the second most common form of stroke (15–30% of strokes), but the most deadly
- unlike ischemic infarct: smooth progressive onset over minutes to hours, often with severe headache, vomiting and alterations in level of consciousness
- unenhanced CT scan of the brain is the initial diagnostic study of choice
- the volume of the hematoma correlates highly with morbidity and mortality
- the clot enlarges in at least 33% of cases within the first 3 hours of onset
- angiography is recommended (as long as it doesn't delay emergent treatment) except for patients > 45 yrs of age with preexisting hypertension and ICH in thalamus, putamen or posterior fossa
- treatment
  a) still controversial. The initial promise of rFVIIa has not been actualized
  b) the usefulness of surgery is still controversial, but seems limited to some cerebellar hemorrhages and select supratentorial hemorrhages that come within 1 cm of the cortical surface

87

87.3 Epidemiology

87.3.1 Incidence

The second most common form of stroke (≈ 15–30% of all strokes) (earlier estimates: 10%[1]), and the most deadly. Approximately 12–15 cases per 100,000/yr. Early studies estimated an incidence equal to SAH, but more recent studies in the CT era show approximately twice the incidence as SAH[2] (pre-CT studies may have misclassified some ICH as ischemic stroke, and some cases of ICH that rupture into the subarachnoid space (occurs in ≈ 7%) may have been misclassified as SAH). After a decline in the 1970's, the incidence increased in the 1980s for those age ≥ 65 years.[3] Onset is usually during activity (rarely during sleep), which may be related to elevation of BP or increased CBF; see Etiologies (p. 1332).

87.3.2 Risk factors

The following are epidemiologic risk factors; see also others (p. 1332).

1. age: the incidence increases significantly after age 55 years and doubles with each decade of age until age > 80 yrs where incidence is 25 times that during previous decade. Relative risk for age > 70 yrs is 7
2. gender: more common in men
3. race: in the U.S., ICH affects blacks more than whites. May be related to higher prevalence of HTN in blacks. Incidence may also be higher in Asians[4]
4. previous stroke (any type) increases risk to 23:1
5. alcohol consumption[4,5]:
   a) recent use: moderate or heavy alcohol consumption both within the 24 hours and the week preceding the ICH were independent risk factors for ICH[6] as shown in ▶ Table 87.1
   b) chronic use: one study suggests that consuming > 3 drinks a day increases the risk of ICH by ≈ 7 times[7(p 15)]
   c) ICH in patients with high ethanol consumption were more commonly lobar than the typical "hypertensive hemorrhages" in the basal ganglia[8]

Table 87.1 Relative risk of ICH with EtOH consumption

Period prior to ICH	Amount[a] (g EtOH)	Relative risk
24 hours	41–120	4.6
	>120	11.3
1 week	1–150	2.0
	151–300	4.3
	>300	6.5

[a]1 standard drink = 12 g EtOH

Table 87.2 Common sites for ICH (modified[13])

%	Location
50%	striate body (basal ganglia); putamen most common; also includes: lenticular nucleus, internal capsule, globus pallidus
15%	thalamus
10–15%	pons (≈ 90% of these are genuinely hypertensive)
10%	cerebellum
10–20%	cerebral white matter
1–6%	brain stem

6. cigarette smoking: increases the risk of SAH and ischemic infarction but probably does *not* increase the risk of ICH,[9,10] further clarification is needed
7. street drugs: cocaine, amphetamines, phencyclidine[11]
8. liver dysfunction: hemostasis may be impaired on the basis of thrombocytopenia, reduced coagulation factors, and hyperfibrinolysis[12] (may be responsible for the increased risk of ICH with chronic EtOH consumption)

87.4 Locations of hemorrhage within the brain

87.4.1 General information

Common sites of ICH are shown in ▶ Table 87.2. Common arterial feeders of ICHs:

1. lenticulostriates: the source of putaminal hemorrhages (possibly secondary to microaneurysms of Charcot-Bouchard, see below)
2. thalamoperforators
3. paramedian branches of BA

87.4.2 Lobar hemorrhage

This term was popularized in 1980 after a report delineating 4 clinical syndromes associated with hemorrhage in each of the cerebral lobes.[14] It incorporates primary hemorrhages into the occipital, temporal, frontal and parietal lobes (including ICH arising from cortex and subcortical white matter), as opposed to hemorrhage of deep structures (e.g. basal ganglion, thalamus, and infratentorial structures).[14] Accounts for 10–32% of nontraumatic ICHs.[14] With large hemorrhages, it may be difficult to make a distinction between lobar and deep ICH.

Lobar hemorrhages are more likely to be associated with structural abnormalities than deep hemorrhages (see below). They may also be more common in patients with high alcohol consumption (see above). Lobar hemorrhages may also have a more benign outcome than ganglionic-thalamic hemorrhages.[14]

Etiologies of lobar hemorrhage: Although many causes of ICH can produce lobar hemorrhages (see below for a detailed list), those that are more likely to produce lobar hemorrhages include:
1. extension of a deep hemorrhage
2. cerebral amyloid angiopathy (p. 1334): the most common cause of lobar ICH in elderly normotensive patients
3. trauma
4. hemorrhagic transformation of an ischemic infarct: see below
5. hemorrhagic tumor (p. 1335). Multiple lobar hemorrhages may occur with metastases
6. cerebrovascular malformation (especially AVM) (p. 1246)
7. rupture of an aneurysm: see below for circumstances likely to produce this
8. idiopathic

87.4.3 Internal capsule hemorrhages

There may be prognostic significance with regard to contralateral motor function if the hemorrhage is medial to and/or extending through the internal capsule (IC), or lateral to the IC and merely compressing it, making the clot more accessible to surgical treatment without damaging the IC.

87.5 Etiologies

87.5.1 History check list

Based on information in this chapter, the following check-list is presented to assist in the gathering of historical information important in evaluating the adult with ICH:
1. hypertension
2. drugs:
   a) sympathomimetics:
      - amphetamines, cocaine
      - appetite suppressants or nasal decongestants (phenylpropanolamine, pseudoephedrine)
   b) dietary supplements: especially ephedra alkaloids (ma huang)
   c) anticoagulants: warfarin in particular
   d) antiplatelet drugs: aspirin (patients often forget taking low dose 81 mg), Plavix, NSAIDS
   e) oral contraceptive (birth control pills): questionable association
3. history of alcohol abuse
4. coagulopathies
5. leukemia
6. previous stroke
7. history of known vascular abnormalities (AVM, venous angioma…)
8. tumor: known history of cancer, especially those that tend to go to brain (lung, breast, GI, renal, melanoma…)
9. recent surgery: especially carotid endarterectomy, procedures requiring heparin…
10. recent childbirth and/or eclampsia or preeclampsia
11. history of recent trauma

87.5.2 Etiology list

1. "hypertension" (debatable as a cause or effect, see below) but is a risk factor
   a) acute hypertension (HTN): as may occur in eclampsia (see below) or with use of certain drugs, e.g. cocaine, phenylpropanolamine… (p. 1334)
   b) chronic HTN: possibly causes degenerative changes within blood vessels
2. possibly associated with acutely increased CBF (globally or focally),[15] especially to areas previously rendered ischemic:
   a) following carotid endarterectomy[16,17]
   b) following repair of congenital heart defects in children[18]
   c) previous stroke (embolic[19] or otherwise): hemorrhagic transformation may occur in up to 43% of strokes during the first month.[20] May follow dislodgment or recanalization of an arterial occlusion, although it has been demonstrated with persistent occlusion.[21] May occur as early as ≤ 24 hrs after a stroke in patients with a negative CT done within 6 hours.[22] Two types[20,23]:
      - type 1: diffuse or multifocal. Heterogeneous or mottled appearance within the boundaries of the stroke. Less hyperdense than primary ICH

- type 2: extensive hematoma. Probably unifocal source. As hyperdense as primary ICH and may extend outside the original stroke boundaries. Unlike type 1, classically associated with anticoagulation therapy, and tends to occur in initial few days after stroke and is often associated with clinical worsening. May be difficult to distinguish from primary ICH, and may be frequently misdiagnosed as such[22]
- migraine: during[24] or following[25] a migraine attack (probably an exceedingly rare event)

a) following surgery to remove an AVM: " normal perfusion pressure breakthrough." Some cases may be due to incomplete AVM excision
b) physical factors: following strenuous physical exertion,[26] exposure to cold[27]...

3. vascular anomalies
   a) AVM: rupture; see Arteriovenous malformation (p. 1239)
   b) aneurysm rupture
      - saccular ("berry") aneurysms: (i) **aneurysms of the circle of Willis (COW)**: aneurysms that have become adherent to brain surface by fibrosis as a result of inflammation or previous hemorrhage may produce ICH when they rupture instead of the usual SAH; (ii) **aneurysms distal to the COW** (e.g. MCA aneurysms)
      - microaneurysms of Charcot-Bouchard (p. 1334)
4. venous angioma rupture: significant ICH from these common lesions is a very rare event
   a) "arteriopathies"
      - amyloid angiopathy: usually → repeated lobar hemorrhages (see below)
      - fibrinoid necrosis[1,28] (sometimes seen in cases of amyloid angiopathy)
      - lipohyalinosis: subintimal lipid-rich hyaline material[29]
      - cerebral arteritis (including necrotizing angiitis)
5. brain tumor (primary or met): below
6. coagulation or clotting disorders
   a) leukemia
   b) thrombocytopenia:
      - thrombotic thrombocytopenic purpura
      - aplastic anemia
   c) patients receiving anticoagulation therapy (p. 1336)
   d) patients receiving thrombolytic therapy:
      - for acute ischemic stroke: incidence of *symptomatic* ICH within 36 hrs of treatment with rtPA is 6.4% (vs. 0.6% in the placebo treated group)[30]
      - for acute MI or other thrombosis: incidence is ≈ 0.36–2%.[31,32,33] Risk is increased with higher doses than the recommended 100 mg of alteplase (Activase®, recombinant tissue plasminogen activator (rt-PA)),[34] in older patients, in those with anterior MI or higher Killip class, and with bolus administration (vs. infusion).[35] When heparin was used adjunctively, higher doses were associated with higher risk of ICH.[36] ICH is thought to occur in those patients with some preexisting underlying vascular abnormality.[37] Immediate coronary angioplasty is safer than rt-PA when available[33]
   e) aspirin therapy:
      - one ASA qod was associated with increased risk of ICH,[38] with a rate of 0.2–0.8% per year[39]
      - ASA 100 mg/d did not increase the risk of significant ICH in patients > 60 yrs with mild to moderate head injury (GCS ≥ 9)[40]
      - Vitamin E supplements[41]: associated with reduction of 1 ischemic stroke in 476 individuals, and increase of 1 ICH in 1250 patients taking vitamin E
7. CNS infection:
   a) especially fungal, which attack blood vessels
   b) granulomas
   c) herpes simplex encephalitis: may initially produce low density lesions that progress to hemorrhagic ones
8. venous or dural sinus thrombosis (p. 1308)
9. drug related
   a) substance abuse
      - alcohol: consumption of > 3 drinks/day increases the risk of ICH ≈ 7-fold (p. 1330)
      - drug abuse: especially sympathomimetics (cocaine,[42,43] amphetamine[44])
   b) drugs that raise BP:
      - alpha-adrenergic agonists (sympathomimetics): phenylpropanolamine[45,46] (may also cause ischemic stroke (p. 1287)) which was removed on the order of the FDA from OTC nasal decongestants and appetite suppressants, but other OTC alpha agonists (including phenylephrine, ephedrine,[47] and pseudoephedrine[48]) are also problematic[49]
      - ephedra alkaloids: sold as a dietary supplement (ma huang) to suppress appetite and increase energy. Associated in case reports with HTN, SAH, ICH, seizures and death[50]

10. post-traumatic: often in a delayed fashion[51,52]; see **Hemorrhagic contusion** (p. 891)
11. pregnancy related: the risk of ICH in pregnancy and puerperium (up to 6 weeks post partum) is ≈ 1 in 9,500 births[53]
    a) most commonly associated with eclampsia or preeclampsia: the mortality of eclampsia is ≈ 6% with ICH being the most frequent direct cause[54]; also see Pregnancy & intracranial hemorrhage (p. 1169)
    b) postpartum ICH (median 8 days, range 3–35 days) in the absence of eclampsia has been reported[55]; when associated with vasculopathy the term **postpartum cerebral angiopathy** has been used
    c) vascular findings:
        - some cases associated with isolated cerebral vasculopathy in the absence of systemic vasculitis[56]
        - some cases demonstrate vasospasm
        - some cases show findings (e.g. patchy enhancement in occipital lobes) suggestive of cerebrovascular dysautoregulation (p. 1264)
        - some cases show no vascular-related abnormalities
12. post-operative:
    a) following carotid endarterectomy (see above)
    b) following craniotomy:
        - at site of craniotomy[57]: risk factors identified: within residual astrocytoma after subtotal resection, following craniotomy for AVM (see above)
        - at site remote from craniotomy. In a series of 37 patients, unlike hematomas at craniotomy site, the following were identified as *not* being related to risk of hemorrhage: HTN, coagulopathy, CSF drainage, underlying occult lesion,
        following drainage of chronic SDH (p. 899)
        cerebellar hemorrhage following pterional craniotomy[58] (this author incriminated possibly rapid overdrainage of CSF), or following temporal lobectomy[59]
13. idiopathic[14]

87

87.5.3 Cerebellar hemorrhage etiologies

Etiologies are similar to ICH of any location, however, some nuances:
1. HTN is a factor in up to two-thirds of cerebellar hemorrhages
2. AVM is a consideration, aneurysm is very rare (possibly AICA aneurysm, but usually only in association with other high-flow lesion, e.g. AVM[60])
3. may be related to recent previous spinal or supratentorial surgery

87.5.4 Hypertension as a cause?

Hypertension (HTN) is controversial as cause of ICH since the incidence of both ICH and HTN increases with age (66% of patients > 65 yrs have HTN). The relative risk for ICH with HTN is 3.9–5.4, depending on the definition of HTN used.[61] Many patients with ICH are dramatically hypertensive on presentation, however, acute elevations of ICP from the hemorrhage may actually precipitate HTN (part of Cushing's triad, see ▸ Table 56.2). HTN is probably a risk factor primarily for pontine/cerebellar ICH and is probably not a factor in at least 35% of basal ganglion hemorrhages.

87.5.5 Microaneurysms of Charcot-Bouchard

AKA miliary aneurysms.[62] Occur primarily at bifurcation of small (< 300 mcm) perforating branches of lateral lenticulostriate arteries in basal ganglia (found in 46% of hypertensive patients over age 66, but only in 7% of controls[63]). Possibly the origin of some "hypertensive" ganglionic (putaminal) hemorrhages,[64] but this is controversial.

87.5.6 (Cerebral) amyloid angiopathy

Cerebral amyloid angiopathy (CAA) AKA congophilic angiopathy. Pathologic deposition of beta amyloid protein (appears as birefringent "apple-green" under polarized light when stained with congo red) within the media of small meningeal and cortical vessels (especially those in white matter) without evidence of systemic amyloidosis.[65] Some vessels may show fibrinoid necrosis of vessel wall.[66,67]

CAA should be suspected in patients with *recurrent* hemorrhages (uncommon with "hypertensive hemorrhages" (p. 1330) [68]) that are *lobar* in location. Gradient-echo MRI may identify petechial hemorrhages or hemosiderin deposits from small cortical hemorrhages which may be associated with CAA.[69] Less likely in the case of basal ganglion or brain stem hemorrhages.[14]

Incidence increases with age: CAA is present in ≈ 50% of those over 70 years of age,[70] however, most do not hemorrhage. CAA is probably responsible for ≈ 10% of cases of ICH. May be associated with genetic factors (including the apolipoprotein E ε4 allele[71]), and may be more prevalent in patients with Down syndrome. Although they are distinct diseases, there is some overlap between CAA and Alzheimer's disease; the amyloid in CAA is identical to that found in senile plaques of Alzheimer's disease. CAA may increase the risk of ICH by potentiating plasminogen[72] (may be of special relevance to patients receiving tissue plasminogen activator (t-PA) to treat MI or stroke).

Patients with CAA may present with a TIA-like prodrome (see below).

Among patients with lobar hemorrhage, those with the apoE ε4 allele typically have their first hemorrhage > 5 yrs earlier than noncarriers (73 ± 8 yrs vs./ 79 ± 7 yrs).[71]

Diagnostic tests are useful mainly to rule-out other conditions. The definitive diagnosis of CAA requires pathologic evaluation of brain tissue. Criteria for the diagnosis of CAA are shown in ▶ Table 87.3.[73]

87.5.7 Hemorrhagic brain tumors

Although any brain tumor can hemorrhage, tumoral ICH is usually associated with malignancies. Tumors on occasion can also produce SAH or subdural hematomas.

Malignant tumors most commonly associated with ICH:

1. glioblastoma
2. lymphoma
3. metastatic tumors
   a) melanoma[74,75]: ≈ 40% hemorrhage
   b) choriocarcinoma[74,76,77]: ≈ 60% hemorrhage
   c) renal cell carcinoma
   d) bronchogenic carcinoma: although only ≈ 9% hemorrhage, this tumor is such a frequent source of cerebral mets that it therefore is a more common source of tumoral ICH

Malignant tumors that hemorrhage less commonly include:

1. medulloblastoma[78,79,80,81] (most commonly in children)
2. gliomas[82,83]

Some *benign* brain tumors that have been associated with ICH include:

1. meningiomas have been associated with intratumoral, subdural, and nearby parenchymal hemorrhage.[84,85,86,87] Tendency to bleed is similar for angioblastic variety as for other highly vascular meningiomas

Table 87.3 Criteria for the diagnosis of cerebral amyloid angiopathy (CAA)[73]

Diagnosis	Criteria
Definite CAA	Full postmortem exam showing all 3 of the following: a) lobar, cortical, or corticosubcortical hemorrhage b) severe CAA c) absence of another diagnostic lesion
Probable CAA with supporting pathological evidence	Clinical data & pathological tissue showing all 3 of the following: a) lobar, cortical, or corticosubcortical hemorrhage b) some degree of vascular amyloid deposition in specimen c) absence of another diagnostic lesion
Probable CAA	Clinical data and MRI findings showing all 3 of the following: a) age ≥ 60 yrs b) multiple hemorrhages restricted to the lobar, cortical, or corticosubcortical region c) absence of another cause of hemorrhage[a]
Possible CAA	Clinical data and MRI findings: a) age ≥ 60 yrs b) single lobar, cortical, or corticosubcortical hemorrhage without another cause[a], or multiple hemorrhages with a possible but not a definite cause[a] or with some hemorrhages in an atypical location (e.g. brain stem)
[a]e.g. excessive anticoagulation (INR > 3.0), head trauma, ischemic stroke, CNS tumor, cerebrovascular malformation, vasculitis or blood dyscrasia	

87

2. pituitary adenoma, see Pituitary apoplexy (p. 720)
3. oligodendroglioma (relatively benign): rarely presents with hemorrhage,[88] classically after years of causing seizures
4. hemangioblastoma[89]
5. vestibular schwannoma[90,91,92]
6. cerebellar astrocytoma[93]

87.5.8 Anticoagulation preceding ICH

10% of patients on warfarin (Coumadin®) develop a significant bleeding complication per year (not all are intracranial), including ICH (65% mortality in this group). The risk of ICH in patients treated with warfarin for A-fib varies between 0–0.3% per year[39] (historically, this was as high as ≈ 1.8% in older studies[94] from the 1960s and 1970s), but when an elderly subgroup (mean age 80 yrs) was analyzed, this rate was 1.8% per year.[39] ICH was the only cause of fatal bleeding complications of warfarin therapy in one series where the cumulative risk of a fatal hemorrhage was 1% at 1 year and 2% at 3 yrs.[95]

The risk of hemorrhagic complications was increased with the length and also the variability of the PT, and during the first three months of anticoagulation.[95] Patients with cerebral amyloid angiopathy (CAA) (see above) are also at increased risk of ICH following administration of antiplatelet drugs or anticoagulants.[73]

87

87.6 Clinical

87.6.1 General information

In general, the neurologic deficit with ICH is characterized by a smooth progressive onset over minutes to hours, unlike embolic/ischemic stroke where deficit is maximal at onset. With ICH, severe headache, vomiting and alterations in level of consciousness may be more common (H/A may not be more prevalent than in embolic stroke, but it is often a first and prominent symptom[14]).

87.6.2 Prodrome

TIA-like symptoms may precede lobar hemorrhages[96,97] in patients with CAA, and may occur in up to ≈ 50% of patients for whom a complete history is obtainable. Unlike typical TIAs, these usually consist of numbness, tingling or weakness (corresponding to the area where the hemorrhage will subsequently occur) that gradually spreads in a manner reminiscent of a Jacksonian-march and may spill-over vascular territories (probably an electrical phenomenon rather than an ischemic event). This is suggestive of but not pathognomonic for the subsequent development of lobar ICH.

87.6.3 Concomitants of specific lesions in ICH

Putaminal hemorrhage

The most common site for ICH. Smooth gradual deterioration in 62% (maximal deficit at onset in 30%); never fluctuating. Contralateral hemiparesis, may progress to hemiplegia or even coma or death. H/A in 14% at onset. No H/A at any time in 72%. Papilledema and subhyaloid preretinal hemorrhage are rare.

Thalamic hemorrhage

Classically, contralateral hemisensory loss. Also hemiparesis when the internal capsule is involved. Extension into upper brain stem → vertical gaze palsy, retraction nystagmus, skew deviation, loss of convergence, ptosis, miosis, anisocoria, ± unreactive pupils. H/A in 20–40%. Motor deficit similar to putaminal hemorrhage, but contralateral sensory deficit widespread and striking. Hydrocephalus may occur from compression of CSF pathways.

In 41 patients, when hemorrhage > 3.3 cm on CT, all died. Smaller hematomas usually caused permanent disability.

Cerebellar hemorrhage

May include any combination of the following:
1. symptoms of increased ICP (lethargy, N/V, HTN with bradycardia…) due to hydrocephalus which may occur as a result of:
   a) compression of the 4th ventricle → obstruction of CSF
   b) extension of the hemorrhage into the ventricular system
2. direct compression of brain stem may produce:
   a) facial palsy: due to pressure on the facial colliculus
   b) these patients classically become comatose without first having hemiparesis, unlike many supratentorial etiologies

Lobar hemorrhage

Syndromes associated with hemorrhage in the 4 cerebral lobes[14] (≈ 50% have H/A as a first and prominent symptom):
1. frontal lobe (the most distinctive of the syndromes): frontal H/A with contralateral hemiparesis, usually in the arm with mild leg and facial weakness
2. parietal lobe: contralateral hemisensory deficit and mild hemiparesis
3. occipital lobe: ipsilateral eye pain and contralateral homonymous hemianopsia, some may spare superior quadrant
4. temporal lobe: on dominant side, produces fluent dysphasia with poor auditory comprehension but relatively good repetition

87

87.6.4 Delayed deterioration

General information

Deterioration after the initial hemorrhage is usually due to any combination of the following:
1. rebleeding: see below
2. edema: see below
3. hydrocephalus: higher risk with intraventricular extension or posterior fossa ICH
4. seizures

Rebleeding or extension of bleed

Early rebleeding: Rebleeding (more so in basal ganglion hemorrhages than in lobar hemorrhages) has been documented during the first hour by "ultra-early" scanning and repeating CT scans. Rebleeding is usually accompanied by clinical deterioration.[98] The incidence of hematoma enlargement decreases with time, 33–38% in 1–3 hours,[99] 16% in 3–6 hrs, and 14% between 24 hrs of onset and a second CT within 24 hrs of the first.[100] Patients with enlarging hematomas were more likely to have larger hematomas and/or coagulopathy, and had a worse outcome.[100] Rebleeding may still occur following surgical evacuation of clot even with satisfactory intraoperative hemostasis. Hemostatic agents (e.g. NovoSeven®) may reduce this risk (p. 1339). The "spot sign"[101] on CTA (small enhancing foci within acute ICH) correlated with increased risk of hematoma expansion.

Late rebleeding: Quoted rates for late rebleeding from ICH range from 1.8–5.3% (depending on length of follow-up).[102] Diastolic BP was significantly higher in the group with recurrent hemorrhage, with a 10%/yr risk for DBP > 90 mm Hg vs. < 1.5% for DBP ≤ 90 (mean F/U of 67 months).[102] Other risk factors include diabetes and tobacco and alcohol abuse.[103] Recurrent hemorrhages may indicate underlying vascular malformations or amyloid angiopathy (lobar rebleeding is likely to be due to amyloid angiopathy[103]).

Edema

Edema and ischemic necrosis around the hemorrhage may cause delayed deterioration.[1] Although necrosis from mass effect of the clot contributes a small part to the edema, experiments indicate that by itself, the mass effect is insufficient to account for the amount of edema that occurs. It is believed that an edemogenic toxin is released from the clot. Experiments with various components of blood clots has disclosed that thrombinin concentrations that could be released from the clot causes increased permeability of the blood-brain-barrier, and is also a potent vasoconstrictor. This is the leading suspect as the major cause of delayed edema and deterioration. Also see Cerebral edema (p. 90).

87.7 Evaluation

87.7.1 CT scan

CT scan is rapid, and easily demonstrates blood as high density within the brain parenchyma immediately after hemorrhage. Although mass effect is common, the tendency for the hemorrhage to dissect through brain tissue often results in less mass effect than would be anticipated from the size of the clot.

Clot volume carries prognostic significance (p. 1343). It can be measured volumetrically using computer algorithms available on some CT scanners, or it can very simply be approximated by the ellipsoid method[104] (originally developed for AVMs, based on the principal that the volume of an ellipsoid is approximately half of that of a parallelepiped into which it is placed)[105] and is simpler than other slightly more accurate estimation methods[106] as shown in Eq (87.1), where AP, LAT and HT are the *diameters* of the clot in each of the 3 dimensions (antero-posterior, lateral, and height). To estimate height of a lesion when only axial images are available (as on most initial CTs), count the number of images on which the lesion is seen, and multiply by the slice thickness of the CT cuts[104,106,107](this information is usually printed on the CT), or, subtract the table position of the highest cut that shows the clot from the table position of the lowest cut showing clot.

$$\text{ellipsoid volume} \approx \frac{\text{AP} \times \text{LAT} \times \text{HT}}{2} \tag{87.1}$$

On the average, the size of the clot decreases ≈ 0.75 mm/day, and the density decreases by ≈ 2 CT units/day, with little change for 1st 2 wks.

87.7.2 MRI

Usually *not* the procedure of choice for initial study. Does not show blood well within the first few hours. Difficult to ventilate or access patient during the study. Slower and more expensive than CT. May be useful later, e.g. to help diagnose cerebral amyloid angiopathy (CAA) (p. 1334).

The appearance of ICH on MRI is very complicated. It is highly dependent on the age of the clot[108] with 5 stages identified (▶ Table 87.4).

87.7.3 Cerebral angiography

For making the diagnosis of the ICH itself, angiography cannot reliably differentiate the mass effect from an ICH from that due to an ischemic infarct or tumor.[109] May demonstrate AVMs and aneurysms when they are associated with the ICH. The yield may be increased by delaying the study.[14]

Table 87.4 Variation of MRI appearance of ICH with time since hemorrhage[a] [108]

Stage	Age	Condition of hemoglobin	T1WI	T2WI
hyperacute	< 24 hrs	oxy-Hgb (intracellular)	iso	sl. ↑
acute	1–3 d	deoxy-Hgb (intracellular)	sl. ↓	very ↓
subacute				
• early	> 3 d	met-Hgb (intracellular)	very ↑	very ↓
• late	> 7 d	met-Hgb (extracellular[b])	very ↑	very ↑
chronic				
• center	> 14 d	hemichromes[c] (extracellular)	iso	sl. ↑
• rim		hemosiderin (intracellular)	sl. ↓	very ↓

[a]Abbreviations: oxy-Hgb = oxyhemoglobin, deoxy-Hgb = deoxyhemoglobin, met-Hgb =methemoglobin, iso = isointense to brain, ↓ = hypo-intense, ↑ = hyperintense, sl = slightly
[b]when the RBCs lyse, the Hgb becomes extracellular
[c]diamagnetic (non-paramagnetic) heme derivatives

May demonstrate vascular blush in some cases of tumor. Normal arteriography cannot eliminate cerebral amyloid angiopathy as the etiology of ICH in the elderly.[110]

For indications for cerebral angiography in ICH, see below.

87.7.4 ICH score

The system of Hemphill et al.[111] assigns points based on 5 features as indicated in ▶ Table 87.5. The points are then summed for the "ICH score." The associated 30 day mortality is tabulated in ▶ Table 87.6.

87.8 Initial management of ICH

87.8.1 Outline

(The following assumes the diagnosis has already been made, usually on CT scan.) There is not uniform agreement on almost all aspects of the management of ICH from the optimal BP to the indications for surgery. The following is offered as a guide.

Most aspects of management are controversial. The following is offered as a guide.

1. patients should be managed in an ICU
2. HTN: controversial. Issues: HTN may contribute to further bleeding, especially within the first hour.[98] However, some HTN may be needed to maintain perfusion. Some say reduce MAP to pre-morbid level if known, or by ≈ 20% if unknown. **Note:** A study of 8 ICHs showed autoregulation was maintained, but with an elevated lower limit. However, CBF fell when MAP was lowered pharmacologically below the usual MAP, which averaged 80% of the admission MAP (admission HTN followed the ICH).[112]
3. intubate if stuporous or comatose
4. maintain euglycemia
5. maintain normothermia
6. anticonvulsants
   a) seizures are treated with appropriate AEDs
   b) prophylactic AEDs: optional. May decrease risk of early seizures in patients with lobar hemorrhages
   c) AED options
      - Keppra has a very favorable therapeutic/toxic profile. Dose 500 mg BID
      - OR phenytoin: load with 17 mg/kg slow IV over 1 hour, follow with 100 mg q 8 hrs; see phenytoin (PHT, Dilantin®) (p. 446)

Table 87.5 ICH Score[111]

Feature	Finding	Points
GCS score (▶ Table 18.1)	3–4	2
	5–12	1
	13–15	0
Age[a]	≥ 80 years	1
	< 80	0
Location	infratentorial	1
	supratentorial	0
ICH volume see (87.1)	≥ 30 cc	1
	< 30 cc	0
Intraventricular blood	yes	1
	no	0
"ICH Score" = Total Points		0–6

[a]possible bias since treatment decisions in elderly patients may have differed from younger patients

Table 87.6 Mortality based on ICH Score

ICH Score[a]	30 day mortality	
0	0%	(26 pts)
1	13%	(32 pts)
2	26%	(27 pts)
3	72%	(32 pts)
4	97%	(29 pts)
5	100%	(6 pts)
6	? 100%[b]	(0 pts)

[a]from ▶ Table 87.5
[b]no pt. in the study had a score of 6, but "it is expected this would be associated with high rate of mortality"

7. hemostatic issues:
   a) check INR (or PT), PTT & platelet count (PC), platelet function assay (PFA)
      - correct coagulopathies, see Correction of coagulopathies or reversal of anticoagulants (p. 166)
      - platelets: correct thrombocytopenia or platelet inhibiting drugs as discussed below
   b) bleeding time: not generally helpful
   c) ✱ hemostatic agents: NovoSeven® (recombinant activated coagulation factor VII (rFVIIa)) given IV within 4 hours of onset,[113] see below
8. steroids: controversial. No benefit from dexamethasone in ICH, with significantly more complications (primarily infectious, GI bleeding and diabetogenic).[114] Consider use if significant perihemorrhage edema on imaging (suggested dosage[115]: 4 mg dexamethasone IV q 6 hrs, tapered over 7–14 days)
9. treat intracranial hypertension presumptively: mannitol and/or furosemide as tolerated, also helps with HTN; for more, see Treatment measures for elevated ICP (p. 866). If significant problems from suspected increased ICP, consider ICP monitor
10. external ventricular drain (EVD): for hydrocephalus, some cases of intraventricular blood, or to manage ICP (see below). ✖ R/O coagulopathy before placing
11. follow electrolytes and osmolarity
    a) aggressively treat hyperglycemia (insulin drip if problematic)
    b) watch for SIADH (p. 114)
12. angiography: primarily to R/O underlying vascular malformation, but also to R/O aneurysm (a less common cause of ICH), and tumor (which is usually better diagnosed on contrast CT or MRI)
    a) if urgent surgery is indicated (e.g. for herniation), the delay in obtaining an angiogram may be detrimental and it may be best deferred to post-op
    b) ✱ indications: angiography is recommended *except* for patients > 45 yrs of age with preexisting hypertension *and* ICH in thalamus, putamen or posterior fossa because there was a 0% yield out of 29 patients in this group[116] and low yield in all patients with isolated deep ICH[117]
       - patients > 45 yrs with a history of HTN and a *lobar* ICH: angiography had a 10% yield,[116] with the ratio of AVM:aneurysm ≈ 4.3:1
       - patients with intraventricular hemorrhage (without parenchymal hematoma): the yield of angiography was ≈ 65%,[116] primarily AVM
    c) an underlying lesion may be obliterated by ICH, especially acutely. If initial angio is negative, repeat after CT shows resorption of clot (≈ in 2–3 mos). If still negative, follow CT or MRI q 4–6 mos for ≈ 1 year to R/O tumor.[1] Delaying the initial angiogram for several weeks may increase the yield and is also an option[14]
    d) the literature indicates that MRI/MRA has only ≈ 90% sensitivity for detecting structural abnormalities in this setting, and so a negative study cannot completely exclude this possibility[116]
    e) the yield of angiography in ICH would be expected to be lower in patients at increased risk of ICH: patients on warfarin (Coumadin®), chronic alcoholics, patients with amyloid angiopathy…

Σ

Treat HTN. Suggested target BP ≈ 140/90. Avoid overcorrection (relative or absolute hypotension)

87.8.2 Thrombocytopenia or platelet inhibiting drugs

1. thrombocytopenia: although platelet transfusions are generally recommended only for PC < 50K, ICH is so serious that a suggestion is ideally to keep PC > 100K (if this is difficult to attain, aim for platelet count > 75K)
2. patients on platelet inhibiting drugs (e.g. aspirin or Plavix®) should receive platelets
3. when needed: start with 6 units of platelets; see Platelets (p. 154)

87.8.3 NovoSeven® (recombinant activated coagulation factor VII (rFVIIa))

At the site of a tissue factor (TF) bearing cell, rFVIIa forms a complex with TF resulting in thrombin production. It also converts factor X to its active form, Xa on the surface of activated platelets resulting in a "thrombin burst" at the site of damage.[118] Half life: 2.6 hrs. Expensive (≈ $10,000 per dose).

FDA approved for various bleeding diatheses (including hemophiliacs with antibodies to factor VIII or IX). Phase II "off label" Factor Seven for Acute Hemorrhagic Stroke (FAST) study for ICH[113] appeared promising, however, preliminary results of the phase 3 trial showed no difference in death or major disability at 90 days.

℞ for ICH. Doses studied: 40, 80 & 160 mcg/kg IV over 1–2 minutes given IV within 4 hours of symptom onset reduces 90 day morbidity & mortality, with a dose-related reduction in mean increase of ICH volume at 24 hrs, and a small increase in thrombotic complications (studied in patients with GCS > 5, with no plan for surgical evacuation within 24 hours and no history of thrombotic or vaso-occlusive disease). **Side effects:** thrombotic events (MI, stroke…) primarily with higher doses (≥ 120 mcg/kg),[119] risk may be increased in presence of DIC, predisposing coagulopathy, advanced atherosclerotic disease, crush injury, septicemia, or concomitant treatment with activated or nonactivated prothrombin complex concentrates (aPCC/PCCs) due to increased levels of circulating TF.

87.8.4 Anticoagulation following ICH

Patients with ICH who subsequently require anticoagulation (e.g. for embolic ischemic stroke or for mechanical heart valve) pose a management dilemma. In the case of embolic disease, the fear of converting an ischemic infarct to a hematoma or increasing the size a small ICH with continued anticoagulation has traditionally outweighed the possible benefit of protection from further embolization. However, an anecdotal (retrospective uncontrolled) report of 12 such patients found no incidence of increased intracranial bleeding with either continued anticoagulation (6 patients) or resumption of anticoagulation after an hiatus (several days in 4 patients, 5 days in 1, and 14 days in 1).[120] In another study[121] none of 35 patients who had resumption of warfarin had recurrent intracranial hemorrhage (ICH, SAH or subdural hematoma). While this does not prove that anticoagulation is safe after ICH, it does demonstrate that if there is a strong indication for anticoagulation, and if there is not an acceptable alternative (e.g. Greenfield filter for DVT (p. 170)), that anticoagulation in this setting is not always met with disastrous results.

The probability of having an ischemic stroke at 30 days following cessation of warfarin for a median of 10 days using Kaplan-Meier survival estimates are approximately 2.9% for patients who had originally been treated with warfarin for prosthetic heart valves, 2.6% for those treated for atrial fibrillation, and 4.8% for those treated for cardioembolic stroke.[121] These numbers may be gross underestimates as many patients died within 2 weeks, and follow-up imaging was scant[122]; another study[123] showed a much higher rate of 20%; see Cardiogenic brain embolism (p. 1304) for more details.

Antiplatelet therapy after ICH is not associated with a substantially increased risk of recurrent ICH[124] (prospective cohort study).

Recommendations

A-fib: long-term anticoagulation should be *avoided* after ICH.[125]

Mechanical heart valves: 1–2 weeks off anticoagulation (to observe ICH, or to evacuate a SDH or clip an aneurysm).[121,126] Patients with deep hemispheric ICH at high-risk for thromboembolic stroke may benefit from resumption of long-term anticoagulation).[125]

Patients requiring hemodialysis after ICH: heparin-free dialysis may be used.

87.8.5 Ventriculostomy (IVC) AKA external ventricular drainage (EVD)

Indications:

1. intraventricular extension of blood causing acute obstruction of the third ventricular outlet. In these cases, the IVC is usually placed in the lateral ventricle *contralateral* to the hemorrhage (to avoid putting the catheter directly in clot, which may obstruct the inlets). The prognosis for patients with a significant volume of intraventricular blood is poor. It may be difficult to maintain the patency of the catheter due to occlusion by clot, tissue plasminogen activator may help (see below)
2. acute hydrocephalus
3. ↑ICP management

87.9 Surgical treatment

87.9.1 General information

The first successful evacuation of an intracerebral hematoma was reported by MacEwan in 1888.[127] The patient recovered completely from an upper extremity monoplegia.

Booking the case: Craniotomy for ICH

Also see defaults & disclaimers (p. 27).

1. position: (depends on location of bleed)
2. equipment:
   a) microscope (not used for all cases)
   b) image guided navigation (not typically used)
3. post-op: ICU
4. consent (in lay terms for the patient – not all-inclusive):
   a) procedure: surgery through the skull to remove blood clot, stop any bleeding identified, possible placement of external (ventricular) drain
   b) alternatives: nonsurgical management
   c) complications: usual craniotomy complications (p. 28) plus further bleeding which may cause problems (especially in patients taking blood thinners, antiplatelet drugs including aspirin, or those with coagulation abnormalities or previous bleeds) and may require further surgery, areas of the brain that have already been damaged by the bleeding are not likely to recover, hydrocephalus

87.9.2 Indications for surgery

General information

Amazingly, after repeated attempts to resolve this dilemma, considerable controversy persists regarding indications for surgery. Surgery may lower morbidity from rebleeding (especially if an aneurysm or AVM is identified as the cause of the ICH), edema, or necrosis from mass effect of hematoma (unproven), but rarely causes neurologic improvement. Meta-analyses[128,129] yield inconclusive or conflicting results and could not identify whether there was a favorable effect of surgery, the types of ICH and patients that are likely to benefit, and the relative effectiveness of the various available surgical options.

Randomized prospective studies (RPS) in the current CT/surgical era

One RPS[130] found lower mortality for patients with GCS 7–10 treated surgically (**note**: only 20% of these patients were operated on < 8 hrs from the bleed, and the mean time for all patients to operation was 14.5 hours (range: 6–48 hrs), which may be long). However, survivors in this group were all severely disabled (none were independent).

Another[115] found no benefit from surgery for *putaminal* hemorrhages, also with poor outcomes in all patients.

International STICH[131]: enrolled 1,033 patient. Study shortcomings: possible selection bias (the responsible neurosurgeon had to be uncertain of the benefits of medical vs. surgical treatment), "early surgery" had a somewhat long median time to treatment of 30 hours, and 26% of medically treated patients crossed over and had surgery at a mean of 60 hours (late). Given these limitations, the conclusion was that for supratentorial ICH there was no benefit of early surgery (although there may have been some benefit in the subgroup with a hematoma within 1 cm of the cortical surface). This trial may be more accurately considered to be a comparison of early vs. delayed surgery in patients subjectively judged to need surgery by the investigator.

Conclusion

The decision to operate therefore must be individualized based on patient's neurologic condition, size and location of hematoma, patient's age, and the patient's expressed preferences (e.g. by a "living will") and the family's wishes concerning "heroic" measures in the face of catastrophic illness.

87

Guidelines for considering surgery vs. medical management

(for separate indications for surgery for *cerebellar* hemorrhage, see below)

1. NON-SURGICAL: factors that favor medical management
   a) minimally symptomatic lesions: e.g. alert patient with subtle hemiparesis (especially patients with GCS > 10[130])
   b) situations with little chance of good outcome
      - high ICH score (p. 1339), which overlaps with the following
      - massive hemorrhage with significant neuronal destruction (see below)
      - large hemorrhage in dominant hemisphere
      - poor neurologic condition: e.g. comatose with posturing (i.e. GCS ≤ 5), loss of brain stem function (fixed pupils, posturing…)
      - ≈ age > 75 yrs: do not do well with surgery for this
   c) severe coagulopathy or other significant underlying medical disorder(s): in the event of herniation, rapid decompression surgery may be considered in spite of the risks
   d) basal ganglion (putaminal) or thalamic hemorrhage: surgery is no better than medical management, and both have little to offer[115,132] (see below)
2. SURGICAL: factors that favor rapid surgical removal of the blood clot
   a) lesions with marked mass effect, edema, or midline shift on imaging (removal is considered due to the potential for herniation)
   b) lesions where the symptoms (e.g. hemiparesis/plegia, aphasia, or sometimes just confusion or agitation…) appear to be due to increased ICP or to mass effect (i.e. compression) from the clot or surrounding edema. Symptoms attributable directly to brain injury from the hemorrhage are unlikely to be reversed by surgical evacuation
   c) volume: surgery for *moderate volume* hematomas (i.e. ≈ 10–30 cc, Eq (87.1)) may be more appropriate than with:
      - ✖ small clot (< 10 cc): mass effect from clot + edema is usually not significant enough to require surgery
      - ✖ large clot: > 30 cc: associated with poor outcome (only 1 of 71 patients could function independently at 30 days[133])
      - ✖ massive hemorrhage > 60 cc with GCS ≤ 8: 91% 30-day mortality[133]
      - ✖ massive hemorrhage > 85 cc (the volume of a sphere with a diameter of 5.5 cm): no patient survived, regardless of treatment in one series[134]
   d) persistent elevated ICP in spite of therapy (failure of medical management). Evacuating clot definitely lowers ICP, but the effect on outcome is uncertain
   e) rapid deterioration (especially with signs of brain stem compression) regardless of location in a patient considered to be salvageable
   f) favorable location, for example:
      - lobar (as opposed to deep hemispheric): in spite of optimistic results in a non-randomized study done in 1983 indicating good outcomes in patients with deep hemorrhages treated with early surgery,[64] a later randomized study failed to confirm this benefit[115]
      - cerebellar: see below

- external capsule
- non-dominant hemisphere

g) young patient (especially age ≤ 50 yrs): they tolerate surgery better than elderly patients, and, unlike elderly patients with brain atrophy, they also have less room in the head to accommodate the mass effect of clot + edema
h) early intervention following hemorrhage: surgery after 24 hrs from onset of symptoms or deterioration may be of less benefit[130]

Management of cerebellar hemorrhage

Recommendations[135]:

1. patients with a Glasgow Coma Scale (GCS) score ≥ 14 and hematoma < 4 cm diameter: treat conservatively
2. patients with GCS ≤ 13 or with a hematoma ≥ 4 cm: surgical evacuation
3. patients with absent brain stem reflexes and flaccid quadriplegia: intensive therapy is not indicated. **Note:** some authors contend that the loss of brain stem reflexes from direct compression may not be irreversible,[136] and that cerebellar hemorrhage represents a surgical emergency (and that the above criteria would thus deny potentially helpful surgery to some, see discussion of cerebellar infarction and decompression (p. 1302)).
4. patients with hydrocephalus: ventricular catheter (if no coagulopathy). Caution: do not overdrain to avoid upward cerebellar herniation (p. 303). Most cases with hydrocephalus also require evacuation of the clot

87

87.9.3 Surgical considerations

General recommendations

1. send specimens (hematoma, abnormal looking tangle of blood vessels if present, and possibly biopsy walls of hematoma cavity) to pathology for analysis[137] (to rule-out tumor, AVM, amyloid angiopathy…)
2. surgical options:
   a) "standard approach": craniotomy with evacuation of the clot under direct vision (with or without microscope)
   b) stereotactic aspiration with thrombolytic agents has also been used; see **Stereotactic surgery** (p. 1441), evacuation of intracerebral hemorrhage
   c) endoscopic surgery[138]

Surgical techniques for cerebellar hemorrhage

1. position: lateral oblique (p. 1446) with the involved side up
2. if rapidity is crucial, a midline skin incision is preferred because it can be taken down quickly with little fear of encountering a vertebral artery
3. craniectomy (without bone replacement) is preferred over craniotomy to accommodate post-op swelling
4. a prophylactic Frazier burr hole is recommended to allow rapid treatment if post-op hydrocephalus develops – see placement (p. 1450) and use (p. 1452) -, or a ventricular catheter may be placed to monitor ICP and allow CSF drainage post-op
5. in cases where there has been rupture into the ventricular system, the surgical microscope should be used to follow the clot to the fourth ventricle which is then cleared of clot

Intraventricular tissue plasminogen activator (rt-PA)

Intraventricular rt-PA may help lyse clot and maintain catheter patency or reopen a clotted catheter. No well-designed randomized study has been done; but anecdotal evidence suggests it is relatively safe. ✖ In cases of suspected aneurysm, AVM or other vascular malformation, it cannot be used until the source of bleeding has been corrected.[139,140]

℞: 2–5 mg of rt-PA[139,141,142] in NS is administered through an intraventricular catheter (IVC). The IVC is closed for 2 hours after injection.[142] In the low dose CLEAR-IVH (Clot Lysis: Evaluating Accelerated Resolution of Intraventricular Hemorrhage) trial (a phase II trial with 52 patients), 1 mg tPA intrathecally via a ventricular catheter every 8 hours up to a maximum of 4 days, was associated with a 30 d mortality of 15% (compared to an expected 80–85%).[143] Hemorrhagic complication rate was 6%. A phase III trialhttp://clinicaltrials.gov/ct2/show/NCT00784134?term=clear+III+stroke&rank=1 is underway to confirm this.

87.10 Outcome

Thalamic hemorrhages that tend to destroy the internal capsule (IC) are more likely to produce hemiplegia than hemorrhages lateral to the IC that compress but do not disrupt the IC.

Mortality: The chief cause of death (in a series testing the effects of dexamethasone) is cerebral herniation,[114] occurring mainly during the first week and mostly in patients with initial Glasgow Coma Scale scores ≤ 7. The in-hospital death rate decreased overall during the 1980s but increased for patients ≥ 65 years of age.[3]

Quoted mortality rates vary widely, and depend on size and location of clot, age and medical condition of the patient, and etiology of the hemorrhage. Overall, the 30-day mortality rate is ≈ 44% for ICH,[2] which is similar to that for SAH (≈ 46%). Patients with lobar hemorrhages (p. 1336) tend to fare better than deep ICH (basal ganglion, thalamus…) with only ≈ 11% mortality in 26 patients.[14]

87.11 ICH in young adults

87.11.1 General information

In a review of 72 patients age 15–45 yrs suffering nontraumatic ICH,[144] a presumed cause was found in 76% (▶ Table 87.7). 3 patients had labor or post-partum hemorrhages (p. 1334); see also Pregnancy & intracranial hemorrhage (p. 1169).

AVM: lobar hemorrhages in this age group are highly suggestive of AVM. Of 40 lobar hemorrhages, 37.5% were determined to be from AVMs.[144]

Herpes simplex encephalitis: may produce hemorrhagic changes on CT, especially in the temporal lobes; see Herpes simplex encephalitis (p. 364).

Drug abuse: especially with sympathomimetics such as cocaine (p. 1333) should also be considered in young adults.

Leukemia: ICH may the initial presentation of leukemia in a young adult (may be due to metastases (chloroma) or to thrombocytopenia).

87.11.2 Outcome

Overall in-hospital survival (including those treated medically) was 87.5%.

Table 87.7 Causes of spontaneous ICH in young adults[144]

Etiology	%
ruptured AVM	29.1%
arterial hypertension	15.3%
ruptured saccular aneurysm	9.7%
sympathomimetic drug abuse	6.9%
tumor[a]	4.2%
acute EtOH intoxication	2.8%
pre-eclampsia/eclampsia	2.8%
superior sagittal sinus thrombosis	1.4%
moyamoya	1.4%
cryoglobulinemia	1.4%
undetermined	23.6%

[a]hemangioma, ependymoma, metastatic choriocarcinoma...see Hemorrhagic brain tumors (p. 1335)

87.12 Intracerebral hemorrhage in the newborn

87.12.1 General information

Occurs primarily in premature infants. Alternate terms: subependymal hemorrhage (SEH), germinal matrix hemorrhage (GMH), periventricular-intraventricular hemorrhage (PIVH). Intraventricular hemorrhage (IVH) arises from extension of SEH through ependymal lining of ventricle and occurs in 80% of cases of SEH.[145]

87.12.2 Etiology

87

The highly vascular germinal matrix is part of the primordial tissue of the developing brain and is the source of future neurons and glial cells. It is located just beneath the ependymal lining of the lateral ventricles, and undergoes progressive involution until 36 weeks gestational age (GA). Thus, the matrix may persist out of utero in premature infants. A disproportionate amount of the total CBF perfuses the periventricular circulation through these capillaries which are immature and fragile and have impaired autoregulation.[146,147] The site of hemorrhage is age dependent. Between 24–28 weeks GA they occur over the body of the caudate nucleus and at 29 weeks GA or greater they arise over the head of the caudate nucleus.[148]

87.12.3 Pathogenesis of PIVH in the pre-term infant

The metabolically active GM is susceptible to hypotension and hypoperfusion which can lead to infarction. The GM is a vulnerable watershed zone supplied by Heubner's artery (from the anterior cerebral artery), terminal branches of the lateral striate arteries (off the middle cerebral artery) and the anterior choroidal artery (off the internal carotid or middle cerebral artery).

1. postnatal hypoxia due to respiratory distress syndrome related to hyaline membrane disease, pneumothorax and/or anemia can deprive the metabolically active GM of oxygen. This ischemia to the endothelial cells lining the capillaries makes them vulnerable to infarction and then disruption
2. hypercapnia maximally dilates the thin walled vessels of the GM. If this is followed by sudden increases in perfusion the result can be rupture of the vessels
3. increased venous pressure from any cause (labor and delivery, positive pressure ventilation, stimulation, endotracheal suctioning, myocardial failure from ischemia) can result in increased venous pressure in the GM leading to hemorrhage
4. dehydration followed by rapid resuscitation with hyperosmolar solutions increases the intravascular volume by osmotically encouraging the movement of fluid from tissues into the intravascular space. With associated increases in systemic blood pressure the GM capillaries are at increased risk of rupture

87.12.4 Risk factors for PIVH

Increased cerebral perfusion pressure (CPP) with the associated increased cerebral blood flow (CBF) and hypoxia are the common denominators for most risk factors for PIVH. The elevated pressure may cause the hemorrhage by rupturing the fragile vessels of the germinal matrix, possibly already damaged by previous insults of high or fluctuating CBF and hypoxia.

Risk factors for PIVH include[149]:

1. those associated primarily with increased CBF or CPP:
   a) asphyxia: including hypercapnia (see above)
   b) rapid volume expansion
   c) seizures
   d) pneumothorax
   e) cyanotic heart disease (including PDA)
   f) infants being mechanically ventilated having RDS and fluctuating CBF velocity documented by Doppler flow meter[150]
   g) anemia
   h) decreased blood glucose
   i) arterial catheterization
   j) blood pressure fluctuations
2. younger gestational age (GA)
3. low birth weight
4. acute amnionitis

5. failure to give antenatal steroids (p. 1347) during the 48 hours prior to pre-term delivery[151] (i.e. to women at risk of delivering low birth-weight infants):
6. APGAR's < 4 at 1 minute and < 8 at 5 minutes
7. acidosis
8. coagulopathies
9. general anesthesia for C-section
10. extracorporeal membrane oxygenation (ECMO): due to heparinization in addition to increased CPP
11. maternal cocaine abuse[152]
12. maternal aspirin use

87.12.5 Epidemiology

Incidence

Depends on the method used for detection (many PIVHs are asymptomatic) and the population being evaluated. 540,000 pre-term infants are born in the United States annually. 85,000 are very pre-term (< 32 weeks GA) and 385,000 are late pre-term (34–36 weeks GA). 63,000 very low birth weight (< 1500 grams) infants are born each year. Of the preemies weighing < 1500 gm birth weight, 20–25% will suffer from a PIVH.[153,154]

87

In a 1978 study, PIVH was found by CT in 43% (20/46) of preemies with birth-weight < 1500 gm.[155] Mortality in infants with PIVH was 55%, compared to 23% in those without PIVH.[155] Ultrasound (U/S) detected PIVH in 90% of 113 preemies < 34 weeks gestation[156] (49% were grade III or IV, see ▶ Table 87.8 for grading).

Timing

The timing of PIVH has a bimodal distribution. A substantial number occur within 6 hours of birth with 50% occurring within 12 hours of birth.[157,158] At postnatal days 3–4, a second peak occurs. Only 5% of bleeds will develop after postnatal day 4. Progression of hemorrhage has been documented in 10–20% of infants.[158] Early onset PIVH is more likely to progress and has a higher mortality.[159]

87.12.6 Prevention

Numerous studies have been conducted to find a method of directly reducing the incidence of PIVH among premature infants. Many are controversial. Optimal resuscitation and neonatal care, with an emphasis on measures which minimize cerebral blood flow fluctuations are key.

1. good prenatal care and avoiding pre-term labor
2. antenatal corticosteroids: administration of one course of antenatal corticosteroids to women at risk of having premature birth infants reduces neonatal mortality, respiratory distress syndrome and PIVH.[160] Multiple courses of antenatal corticosteroids did not improve outcomes and were associated with decreased head circumference, weight and length at birth[161]
3. indomethacin: results in cerebral vasoconstriction and reduces the responsiveness of CBF to changes in CO_2, lowers CBF and increases arterial oxygenation reducing patent ductus arteriosus (PDA). However, use is possibly associated with increased risk of intestinal perforation
4. antenatal vitamin K given IM > 4 hrs prior to delivery decreases PIVH from 33% to 5%
5. sluicing umbilical cord blood and delaying umbilical cord clamping by 30–120 seconds in *premature* babies increased hematocrit and decreased PIVH in 5 of 7 studies[162]
6. using surfactant to reduce RDS
7. minimizing external stimulation (some centers use fentanyl drips)
8. steroids to stabilize the GM vessels

Table 87.8 Grading subependymal hemorrhage[155]

Grade	Description
I	subependymal
II	IVH without ventricular dilatation
III	IVH with ventricular dilatation
IV	IVH with parenchymal hemorrhage

87.12.7 Clinical

Grading

The most commonly used grading system of Papile et al. based on CT or U/S findings is shown in ▶ Table 87.8. PIVH may present acutely, subacutely. Most commonly, it is discovered incidentally on surveillance U/S.

There is a direct correlation between younger gestational age (GA) and the severity of PIVH. In infants 24–26 weeks GA, 32% will have a Grade III PIVH and 19% will have a Grade IV PIVH compared with infants 31–32 weeks GA, 11% will have a Grade III PIVH and 5% will have a Grade IV PIVH.[163]

Presentation

Asymptomatic PIVH

Most PIVHs will be clinically unsuspected, usually with smaller hemorrhages. Retrospectively, these PIVHs may have been suggested by a fall in Hct or delays in neurologic development. These have a 78% 6-month survival, vs. 20% for PIVH showing signs.

Subacute presentation

Usually smaller or more slowly developing hemorrhages. Clinically may present as irritability, reduced motor activity, or abnormal eye movements.

Acute presentation

1. changes in muscle tone or activity: usually decerebrate or decorticate posturing, sometimes flaccid paralysis
2. seizures: often subclinical
3. tense fontanelle
4. hypotension
5. respiratory and cardiac irregularities: apnea & bradycardia ("A's and B's")
6. unreactive pupils and/or loss of extraocular muscle movements
7. Hct drop > 10%

Hydrocephalus

General information

20–50% of infants with PIVH will develop either transient or progressive hydrocephalus (HCP). Grades III and IV are more often associated with progressive ventricular dilatation than are lower grades (however, HCP may develop even after low grade PIVH[164]). Younger gestational age infants may be at *lower* risk.

Post PIVH hydrocephalus usually occurs 1–3 weeks after the hemorrhage. Probably caused by cellular debris and/or the toxic effects of blood breakdown products on the arachnoid granulations (communicating HCP), or by an adhesive arachnoiditis in the posterior fossa or rarely by compression or blockage of critical pathways, e.g. at the sylvian aqueduct (obstructive HCP). In a case of HCP following intra-uterine PIVH, aqueductal gliosis was found at autopsy.[165]

Differential diagnosis of ventriculomegaly in PIVH

When ventriculomegaly is detected, it needs to be differentiated from the following:

1. transient ventriculomegaly: occurs in the first few days after PIVH. This may not cause elevated ICP. As implied, it is self limited
2. progressive ventriculomegaly: occurs in 20–50% of cases (true hydrocephalus)
3. "hydrocephalus ex vacuo": due to loss of brain tissue or maldevelopment. Is not progressive on serial U/S. OFCs may fall below normal due to lack of growing brain as stimulus for head growth

Possible presentations

Abnormally increasing OFC (crossing percentile curves faster than body weight), lethargy, apnea and bradycardia, vomiting. There is progressive dilatation of the ventricular system on serial U/S or CT or MRI evaluations.

87.12.8 Pathophysiologic effects of PIVH

Deleterious effects of PIVH on the brain are due to[166]:
1. destruction of the germinal matrix and glial precursors
2. direct injury to neural tissue from hematoma: once hemorrhage resorbs may leave patient with porencephaly or cystic lesions
3. pressure of hematoma on nearby brain tissue reducing CBF even to parts of the same hemisphere distant from the hemorrhage[167]
4. diffuse decreased CBF following the hemorrhage[168] due to elevated ICP
5. injury from the same hypoxic event that precipitated the PIVH
6. decreased CPP leads to periventricular leukomalacia (PVL) and cerebral infarction
7. periventricular hemorrhagic infarction
8. hydrocephalus (see above): numerous deleterious effects on the CNS
9. seizures: repeated or prolonged seizures may be deleterious to neuronal function

87.12.9 Diagnosis

Ultrasound (U/S)

Performed through the open fontanelles.[156] Accuracy ≈ 88% (91% sensitivity, 85% specificity).[169] U/S is invaluable because:
1. it demonstrates the size of the ventricles, the location and size of the hematoma, and the thickness of the cortical mantle
2. it may be brought to the infant's bedside (obviating transportation)
3. it is non-invasive
4. it is not adversely affected by occasional infant movements (eliminating the need for sedation)
5. there is no exposure to ionizing radiation (radiation from diagnostic imaging in children has long-term risks for cancer[170] and damage to the lens)
6. it may be followed serially with relative ease

CT scan

Sometimes necessary when U/S is not readily available, or in complicated cases where anatomy is difficult to deduce from U/S images. Many ICUs have portable CT scans available which obviates need for patient transport.

Rapid sequence MRI

Pros: Eliminates the risk of ionizing radiation associated with CT scan.

Cons: Requires moving the infant from the neonatal ICU to the radiology suite.

87.12.10 Treatment

General measures

General measures are directed at optimizing CPP without further excessive elevation of CBF by carefully maintaining normal MAP and normalizing pCO_2, and by treating active hydrocephalus as needed (see above).

While daily LPs can control the deleterious effects of posthemorrhagic HCP, they do not reduce the frequency of long-term HCP (requiring permanent shunting). Ventricular size must be monitored with serial U/S.

Medical treatment

1. not very effective. Treated patients fared worse in several studies
2. osmotic agents: isosorbide, glycerol. Effects are short-lived
3. ✖ diuretic therapy: has been used, but a large study showed increased nephrocalcinosis and biochemical abnormalities, resulting in a borderline increase in the risk for motor impairment at one year.[171] The results were so compelling, the data-monitoring committee terminated the study prematurely. Furosemide and acetazolamide therapy was deemed neither safe nor effective in treating post-hemorrhagic ventricular dilatation and cannot therefore be recommended[172]

Surgical/interventional treatment for the clot

Due to poor operative results, surgical evacuation of an intracerebral hemorrhage in the newborn is not indicated with the possible exception of a posterior fossa hemorrhage causing brain stem compression that does not respond to medical treatment.[173] Supportive measures are usually in order.

Intervention for intraventricular blood

General information

34% of infants < 1500 g require shunt/reservoir drainage after failed medical management. Grade III and IV PIVH: > 70% of cases develop progressive ventricular dilatation, and 32–47% of this subset will ultimately require shunting.[174]

Indications for intervention

Intervention for intraventricular blood is indicated in the setting of progressive ventriculomegaly with the OFC crossing percentile curves and clinical evidence of increased ICP (split sutures, tense fontanelle…).

87

Serial lumbar punctures

Used at many facilities for hemorrhages with intraventricular extension and communicating hydrocephalus (the usual type of HCP that occurs with PIVH).[175]

This should be undertaken with the knowledge that meta-analysis[176] showed sequential lumbar or ventricular taps of ≈ 10 ml/kg/tap for prophylaxis or treatment of progressive hydrocephalus offers no clear benefit over conservative treatment, and had an infection rate of 5–9%. In rare cases, LPs may succeed in temporizing progressive HCP for a few weeks until the infant is large enough for shunt placement.

Infants < 800 gm may not tolerate LPs because of desaturation when lying on their side, or the LP itself may be difficult. In these patients, consider 1–2 ventricular taps to at least obtain fluid for analysis (in some cases nothing further needs to be done).

Serial ventricular taps

May be a viable short-term option for those infants who cannot tolerate LPs or in whom there is obstruction to CSF flow in the lumbar subarachnoid space (e.g. due to spinal subdural hematoma from previous LP). However it is not desirable for long-term use because of repeated trauma to brain (risk of porencephaly) and risk of intracerebral, intraventricular, or subdural hemorrhage.

If continued taps are likely (i.e. large hemorrhage, or rapid recurrence of intracranial hypertension as determined by palpation of fullness of anterior fontanelle (AF) following several taps) the acceptable options include:

1. continuing serial LPs (see below)
2. percutaneous ventricular taps: not recommended for more than a few treatments as it causes porencephaly
3. placement of a temporary ventricular access device (TVAD) – a *ventricular catheter* connected to a subgaleal *reservoir* (either a Rickham reservoir, or a low profile McComb reservoir[177]). These can be inserted safely at the bedside, obviating the need for transport to the O.R.[178]
   a) temporary ventricular access: the reservoir can be used for serial percutaneous taps. Usually tapped QD or QOD (see below). Use a 27 Ga butterfly needle, clean with at least 3 betadine stick swabs, withdraw ≈ 10 ml and send for culture. Reported infection rate: 8–12%[179]
   b) ventricular-subgaleal shunt: the side-port of the reservoir is left uncapped. A subgaleal pocket must be created at the time of surgery. Fluid is reabsorbed from this potential space. First performed in 1893 by Mikulicz-Radecki (1850–1905). Use has been reported up to 35 days.[180] Infection rate: ≈ 6%
   c) the reservoir may be converted to VP shunt if and when appropriate. Not recommended in infants < 1100 gms due to very high infection rate
4. external ventricular drainage (EVD): similar to reservoir placement, but with possibility of inadvertent dislodgment (13%) and comparable infection rate (6%)
5. early VP shunting: high infection rate, peritoneal cavity not suitable in many cases, e.g. due to necrotizing enterocolitis (NEC), paucity of subcutaneous tissue through which to pass shunt tube… Not recommended for infants < 2000 gms

Temporary ventricular access device (TVAD)

Advantages of TVAD

1. avoids shunt in unhealthy children at risk of infection, skin breakdown or other operative/anesthetic complications
2. clears protein and cellular debris (more favorable for subsequent shunting)
3. avoids repeated penetration of brain with risk of porencephaly
4. provides port for infusion of medication (e.g. antibiotics) PRN
5. avoids cumbersome, easily dislodged EVD with infection risk 6% on average of 13 days of EVD
6. up to 25% of patients will recover and avoid permanent shunt placement[181,182]

Disadvantages of TVAD

1. requires services of a neurosurgeon (not always available)
2. increases risk of infection of subsequent permanent shunt from 5% to 13%([183]
3. inherent risks of surgery including hemorrhage, infection, ventriculitis, meningitis, CSF leak
4. risks of overdrainage including subdural hematoma, impaired skull growth

Technical considerations for serial taps (via ventricular reservoir or LP)

8–20 cc of fluid are removed initially, and this is repeated daily (or more often if AF become very tense before 24 hours elapse) for several days, and then usually varies from 5–20 cc qod to 15 cc TID depending on response. The frequency and volume of the taps are modified based on:

1. fullness of AF: attempt to keep AF from becoming tense
2. appearance of ventricles on serial U/S: strive to prevent progressive enlargement, reduction in size can usually be achieved
3. follow OFC: should not cross percentile curves (need to differentiate from the so-called "catch-up phase" of brain growth which may occur once the infant overcomes their overall medical problems and is able to adequately utilize nutrition[184,185]; serial U/S will show rapid brain growth without progressive ventriculomegaly in cases of catch-up brain growth)
4. CSF protein concentration: controversial. Diminishes with serial taps. Some feel that as long as it is ≥ 100 mg/dl it is unlikely that significant spontaneous resorption will occur and continued serial taps will probably be needed
5. NB: removal of this volume of fluid may cause electrolyte disturbances, primarily hyponatremia; ∴ follow serum electrolytes on regular basis

Follow with serial U/S on day 3–5, and then weekly for several weeks, and then bi-weekly. A baseline CT scan is often obtained prior to placement of a permanent shunt.

Insertion of VP shunt or conversion of sub-Q reservoir to VP shunt

Indications and requirements:

1. symptomatic hydrocephalus (p. 1348) and/or progressive ventriculomegaly
2. infant is extubated (and thus off ventilator)
3. infant weighs ≥ 2000 grams (some prefer ≥ 2500 grams)
4. no evidence of NEC (might create problems with peritoneal end of catheter)
5. CSF proteinideally < 100 mg/dl (because of concerns about plugging of the shunt, or causing ileus or malabsorption of the fluid – which was not seen with high protein fluid shunted from the subdural space[186] – and also to see if patient will start reabsorbing CSF on their own)

Technical recommendations:

1. do not tap reservoir for at least 24 hrs before inserting a new ventricular catheter (allows ventricles to expand to facilitate catheterization)
2. obtain U/S the day prior to conversion
3. use a low or very-low pressure system (if CSF protein is high, consider a valveless system), upgrade later in infancy if necessary
4. avoid placing shunt hardware in areas on which these debilitated infants tend to lay (to prevent skin breakdown with hardware exposure)

87.12.11 Outcome

Short-term

Preemies with PIVH have higher mortality than matched preemies without PIVH.

The incidence of mortality and progression of hemorrhage is higher the earlier the hemorrhage occurs. The more severe the hemorrhage, the higher the mortality and the higher the risk of HCP (▶ Table 87.9).

87

Table 87.9 Short-term outcome of PIVH (≈ 250 cases[145])

Severity of hemorrhage	Deaths (%)	Progressive hydrocephalus (%)
mild	0	0–10
moderate	5–15	15–25
severe	50–65	65–100

Long-term

The effect of low grade PIVH on long-term neurodevelopment has not been studied well. Most investigators feel that higher grades of PIVH are associated with greater degrees of handicaps than matched controls.

In one study of 12 infants with Grade II PIVH treated with serial LPs and in the 7 with progressive ventriculomegaly with VP shunt followed for a mean of 4.5 years found all were ambulatory and 75% had IQ within normal range.[187]

87

A recent study of very low birth weight infants showed that children 18–22 months of age with severe PIVH and shunts had significantly lower scores on the Bayley Scales of Infant Development IIR compared with children with no PIVH and children with equal grades of PIVH who did not require a shunt.[188]

87.13 Other causes of intracerebral hemorrhage in the newborn

1. birth trauma may result in subdural hemorrhage, tentorial hemorrhage, parenchymal hemorrhage and/or subarachnoid blood. This is usually detected by imaging (U/S or CT) when an infant develops seizures, apnea, bradycardia or rarely focal neurological deficits. It rarely requires surgical intervention
2. choroid plexus hemorrhage can result in IVH. In some cases HCP can develop and require shunt placement
3. hemorrhagic stroke has been identified in 6.2 per 100,000 live births.[189] The usual presentation was with encephalopathy (100%) and seizures (65%). 75% of the strokes were idiopathic. Other identified etiologies were thrombocytopenia and a single case of a cavernous malformation. Risk factors for perinatal hemorrhagic stroke include: male gender, fetal distress, emergent c-section, prematurity and post-maturity
4. tumors in the neonate can present with hemorrhage
5. vascular malformations of any form can present in the neonate with hemorrhage, although this is uncommon. Vein of Galen malformations are diagnosed in the neonate in about 40% of cases.[190] Most of these infants present with fulminant congestive heart failure and 50% have ventriculomegaly

References

[1] Ojemann RG, Heros RC. Spontaneous Brain Hemorrhage. Stroke. 1983; 14:468–475
[2] Broderick JP, Brott TG, Tomsick T, et al. Intracerebral Hemorrhage More Than Twice as Common as Subarachnoid Hemorrhage. J Neurosurg. 1993; 78:188–191
[3] Chyatte D, Easley K, Brass LM. Increasing Hospital Admission Rates for Intracerebral Hemorrhage During the Last Decade. J Stroke Cerebrovasc Dis. 1997; 6:354–360
[4] Gorelick PB, Kelly MA, Feldman E. In: Ethanol. Intracerebral Hemorrhage. Armonk, New York: Futura Publishing Co.; 1994:195–208
[5] Camargo CA. Moderate alcohol consumption and stroke: The epidemiological evidence. Stroke. 1989; 20:1611–1626
[6] Juvela S, Hillbom M, Palomäki H. Risk Factors for Spontaneous Intracerebral Hemorrhage. Stroke. 1995; 26:1558–1564
[7] Feldman E. Intracerebral Hemorrhage. Armonk, NY 1994
[8] Monforte R, Estruch R, Graus F, et al. High Ethanol Consumption as Risk Factor for Intracerebral Hemorrhage in Young and Middle-Aged People. Stroke. 1990; 21:1529–1532
[9] Shinton R, Beevers G. Meta-analysis of relation between cigarette smoking and stroke. Br Med J. 1989; 298:789–794
[10] Fogelholm R, Murros K. Cigarette Smoking and Risk of Primary Intracerebral Hemorrhage: A Population-Based Case-Control Study. Acta Neurol Scand. 1993; 87:367–370
[11] Gorelick PB. Stroke from alcohol and drug abuse. A current social peril. Postgrad Med. 1990; 88:171–178
[12] Niizuma H, Shimizu Y, Nakasato N, et al. Influence of Liver Dysfunction on Volume of Putaminal Hemorrhage. Stroke. 1988; 19:987–990
[13] Schmidek HH, Sweet WH. Operative Neurosurgical Techniques. New York 1982
[14] Ropper AH, Davis KR. Lobar Cerebral Hemorrhages: Acute Clinical Syndromes in 26 Cases. Ann Neurol. 1980; 8:141–147
[15] Caplan L. Intracerebral Hemorrhage Revisited. Neurology. 1988; 38:624–627

[16] Caplan LR, Skillman J, Ojemann R, Fields W. Intracerebral Hemorrhage Following Carotid Endarterectomy: A Hypertensive Complication. Stroke. 1979; 9:457–460
[17] Bernstein M, Fleming JFR, Deck JHN. Cerebral Hyperperfusion After Carotid Endarterectomy: A Cause of Cerebral Hemorrhage. Neurosurgery. 1984; 15:50–56
[18] Humphreys RP, Hoffman HJ, Mustard WT, et al. Cerebral hemorrhage following heart surgery. J Neurosurg. 1975; 43:671–675
[19] Fisher CM, Adams RD. Observations on Brain Embolism with Special Reference to the Mechanism of Hemorrhagic Infarction. J Neuropathol Exp Neurol. 1951; 10:92–93
[20] Hornig CR, Dorndorf W, Agnoli AL. Hemorrhagic Cerebral Infarction: A Prospective Study. Stroke. 1986; 17:179–185
[21] Okada Y, Yamaguchi T, Minematsu K, et al. Hemorrhagic Transformation in Cerebral Embolism. Stroke. 1989; 20:598–603
[22] Bogousslavsky J, Regli F, Uske A, Maeder P. Early Spontaneous Hematoma in Cerebral Infarct: Is Primary Cerebral Hemorrhage Overdiagnosed? Neurology. 1991; 41:837–840
[23] Cerebral Embolism Study Group. Cardioembolic stroke, early anticoagulation, and brain hemorrhage. Arch Intern Med. 1987; 147:626–630
[24] Raabe A, Krug U. Migraine associated bilateral intracerebral hemorrhages. Clin Neurol Neurosurg. 1999; 101:193–195
[25] Cole A, Aube M. Late-Onset Migraine with Intracerebral Hemorrhage: A Recognizable Syndrome. Neurology. 1987; 37S1
[26] Lee K-C, Clough C. Intracerebral Hemorrhage After Break Dancing. N Engl J Med. 1990; 323:615–616
[27] Caplan LR, Neely S, Gorelick P. Cold-Related Intracerebral Hemorrhage. Arch Neurol. 1984; 41
[28] Rosenblum WI. Miliary Aneurysms and 'Fibrinoid' Degeneration of Cerebral Blood Vessels. Hum Pathol. 1977; 8:133–139
[29] Fisher CM. Pathological Observations in Hypertensive Cerebral Hemorrhage. J Neuropathol Exp Neurol. 1971; 30:536–550
[30] The National Institute of Neurological Disorders and Stroke rt-PA Stroke Study Group. Tissue plasminogen activator for acute ischemic stroke. N Engl J Med. 1995; 333:1581–1587
[31] Aldrich MS, Sherman SA, Greenberg HS. Cerebro vascular Complications of Streptokinase Infusion. JAMA. 1985; 253:1777–1779
[32] Maggioni AP, Franzosi MG, Santoro E, et al. The risk of stroke in patients with acute myocardial infarction after thrombolytic and antithrombotic treatment. N Engl J Med. 1992; 327:1–6
[33] Grines CL, Browne KF, Marco J, et al. A Comparison of Immediate Angioplasty with Thrombolytic Therapy for Acute Myocardial Infarction. N Engl J Med. 1993; 328:673–679
[34] Public Health Service. Approval of Thrombolytic Agents. FDA Drug Bull. 1988; 18:6–7
[35] Mehta SR, Eikelboom JW, Yusuf S. Risk of intracranial hemorrhage with bolus versus infusion thrombolytic therapy: a meta-analysis. Lancet. 2000; 356:449–454
[36] Tenecteplase (TNKase) for thrombolysis. Med Letter. 2000; 42:106–108
[37] DaSilva VF, Bormanis J. Intracerebral Hemorrhage After Combined Anticoagulant-Thrombolytic Therapy for Myocardial Infarction: Two Case Reports and a Short Review. Neurosurgery. 1992; 30:943–945
[38] The Steering Committee of the Physician's Health Study Group. Preliminary Report: Findings from the Aspirin Component of the Ongoing Physician's Health Study. N Engl J Med. 1988; 318:262–264
[39] Blackshear JL, Kopecky SL, Litin SC, et al. Management of Atrial Fibrillation in Adults: Prevention of Thromboembolism and Symptomatic Treatment. Mayo Clin Proc. 1996; 71:150–160
[40] Spektor S, Agus S, Merkin V, Constantini S. Low-dose aspirin prophylaxis and risk of intracranial hemorrhage in patients older than 60 years of age with mild or moderate head injury: a prospective study. J Neurosurg. 2003; 99:661–665
[41] Schurks M, Glynn RJ, Rist PM, Tzourio C, Kurth T. Effects of vitamin E on stroke subtypes: meta-analysis of randomised controlled trials. BMJ. 2010; 341
[42] Lowenstein DH, Collins SD, Massa SM, McKinney HE, et al. The Neurologic Complications of Cocaine Abuse. Neurology. 1987; 37S1
[43] Levine S. Cocaine and stroke. Current concepts of cerebrovascular disease. Stroke. 1987; 22:25–29
[44] Harrington H, Heller A, Dawson D, Caplan L, et al. Intracerebral Hemorrhage and Oral Amphetamines. Arch Neurol. 1983; 40:503–507
[45] Kase CS, Foster TE, Reed JE, Spatz EL, et al. Intracerebral Hemorrhage and Phenylpropanolamine Use. Neurology. 1987; 37:399–404
[46] Kernan WN, Viscoli CM, Brass LM, Broderick JP, Brott T, et al. Phenylpropanolamine and the risk of hemorrhagic stroke. N Engl J Med. 2000; 343:1826–1832
[47] Bruno A, Nolte KB, Chapin J. Stroke associated with ephedrine use. Neurology. 1993; 43:1313–1316
[48] Stoessl AJ, Young GB, Feasby TE. Intracerebral hemorrhage and angiographic beading following ingestion of catechoaminergics. Stroke. 1985; 16:734–736
[49] Phenylpropanolamine and other OTC alpha-adrenergic agonists. Med Letter. 2000; 42
[50] Haller CA, Benowitz NL. Adverse cardiovascular and central nervous system events associated with dietary supplements containing ephedra alkaloids. N Engl J Med. 2000; 343:1833–1838
[51] Gudeman SK, Kishore PR, Miller JD, Girevendulis AK. The Genesis and Significance of Delayed Traumatic Intracerebral Hematoma. Neurosurgery. 1979; 5:309–313
[52] Young HA, Gleave JRW, Schmidek HH, Gregory S. Delayed Traumatic Intracerebral Hematoma: Report of 15 Cases Operatively Treated. Neurosurgery. 1984; 14:22–25
[53] Wang KC, Chen CP, Yang YC, Wang KG, Hung FY, Su TH. Stroke complicating pregnancy and the puerperium. Zhonghua Yi Xue Za Zhi (Taipei). 1999; 62:13–19
[54] Salerni A, Wald S, Flannagan M. Relationships Among Cortical Ischemia, Infarction, and Hemorrhage in Eclampsia. Neurosurgery. 1988; 22:408–410
[55] Witlin AG, Mattar F, Sibai BM. Postpartum stroke: a twenty-year experience. Am J Obstet Gynecol. 2000; 183:83–88
[56] Geocadin RG, Razumovsky AY, Wityk RJ, Bhardwaj A, Ulatowski JA. Intracerebral hemorrhage and postpartum cerebral vasculopathy. J Neurol Sci. 2002; 205:29–34
[57] Kalfas IH, Little JR. Postoperative Hemorrhage: A Survey of 4992 Intracranial Procedures. Neurosurgery. 1988; 23:343–347
[58] Papanastassiou V, Kerr R, Adams C. Contralateral Cerebellar Hemorrhagic Infarction After Pterional Craniotomy: Report of Five Cases and Review of the Literature. Neurosurgery. 1996; 39:841–852
[59] Toczek MT, Morrell MJ, Silverberg GA, Lowe GM. Cerebellar Hemorrhage Complicating Temporal Lobectomy: Report of Four Cases. J Neurosurg. 1996; 85:718–722
[60] Menovsky T, Andre Grotenhuis J, Bartels RH. Aneurysm of the anterior inferior cerebellar artery (AICA) associated with high-flow lesion: report of two cases and review of literature. J Clin Neurosci. 2002; 9:207–211
[61] Brott T, Thalinger K, Hertzberg V. Hypertension as a Risk Factor for Spontaneous Intracerebral Hemorrhage. Stroke. 1986; 17:1078–1083
[62] Wakai S, Nagai M. Histological Verification of Microaneurysms as a Cause of Cerebral Hemorrhage in Surgical Specimens. J Neurol Neurosurg Psychiatry. 1989; 52:595–599
[63] Newton TH, Potts DG. Radiology of the Skull and Brain. Saint Louis 1971
[64] Kaneko M, Tanaka K, Shimada T, Sato K, et al. Long-Term Evaluation of Ultra-Early Operation for

Hypertensive Intracerebral Hemorrhage in 100 Cases. J Neurosurg. 1983; 58:838–842
[65] Gilles C, Brucher JM, Khoubesserian P, et al. Cerebral Amyloid Angiopathy as a Cause of Multiple Intracerebral Hemorrhages. Neurology. 1984; 34:730–735
[66] Mandybur TI. Cerebral Amyloid Angiopathy: The Vascular Pathology and Complications. J Neuropathol Exp Neurol. 1986; 45:79–90
[67] Vonsattel JP, Myers RH, Hedley-White ET, Ropper AH, et al. Cerebral Amyloid Angiopathy Without and With Cerebral Hemorrhages: A Comparative Histological Study. Ann Neurol. 1991; 30:637–649
[68] Kase CS, Kase CS, Caplan LR. In: Cerebral Amyloid Angiopathy. Intracerebral Hemorrhage. Boston: Butterworth-Heinemann; 1994:179–200
[69] Greenberg SM, Briggs ME, Hyman BT, et al. Apolipoprotein E e4 Is Associated With the Presence and Earlier Onset of Hemorrhage in Cerebral Amyloid Angiopathy. Stroke. 1996; 27:1333–1337
[70] Vinters HV, Gilbert JJ. Amyloid Angiopathy: Its Incidence and Complications in the Aging Brain. Stroke. 1981; 12
[71] Greenberg SM, Rebeck GW, Vonsattel JPV, et al. Apolipoprotein E e4 and Cerebral Hemorrhage Associated with Amyloid Angiopathy. Ann Neurol. 1995; 38:254–259
[72] Kingston IB, Castro MJ, Anderson S. In Vitro Stimulation of Tissue-Type Plasminogen Activator by Alzheimer Amyloid Beta-Peptide Analogues. Nature Med. 1995; 1:138–142
[73] Greenberg SM, Edgar MA. Cerebral Hemorrhage in a 69-Year Old Woman Receiving Warfarin. Case Records of the Massachusetts General Hospital. Case 22-1996. N Engl J Med. 1996; 335:189–186
[74] Scott M. Spontaneous Intracerebral Hematoma caused by Cerebral Neoplasms. J Neurosurg. 1975; 42:338–342
[75] Dublin AB, Norman D. Fluid-Fluid Level in Cystic Cerebral Metastatic Melanoma. J Comput Assist Tomogr. 1979; 3:650–652
[76] Acosta-Sison H. Extensive Cerebral Hemorrhage Caused by the Rupture of a Cerebral Blood Vessel due to a Chorionepithelioma Embolus. Am J Ob Gyn. 1956; 71
[77] Weir B, MacDonald N, Mielke B. Intracranial Vascular Complications of Choriocarcinoma. Neurosurgery. 1978; 2
[78] Weinstein ZR, Downey EF. Spontaneous Hemorrhage in Medulloblastomas. AJNR. 1983; 4:986–988
[79] McCormick WF, Ugajin K. Fatal Hemorrhage into a Medulloblastoma. J Neurosurg. 1967; 26:78–81
[80] Chugani HT, Rosemblat AM, Lavenstein BL, et al. Childhood Medulloblastoma Presenting with Hemorrhage. Childs Brain. 1984; 11:135–140
[81] Zee CS, Segall HD, Miller C, et al. Less Common CT Features of Medulloblastoma. Radiology. 1982; 144:97–102
[82] Oldberg E. Hemorrhage into Gliomas. Arch Neurol Psych. 1933; 30:1061–1073
[83] Richardson RR, Siqueira EB, Cerullo LJ. Malignant Glioma: Its Initial Presentation as Intracranial Hemorrhage. Acta Neurochir. 1979; 46:77–84
[84] Nakao S, Sato S, Ban S, et al. Massive Intracerebral Hemorrhage Caused by Angioblastic Meningioma. Surg Neurol. 1977; 7:245–247
[85] Modesti LM, Binet EF, Collins GH. Meningiomas causing Spontaneous Intracranial Hematomas. J Neurosurg. 1976; 45:437–441
[86] Goran A, Ciminello VJ, Fisher RG. Hemorrhage into Meningiomas. Arch Neurol. 1965; 13:65–69
[87] Cabezudo-Artero, Areito-Cebrecos, Vaquero-Crespo J. Hemorrhage Associated with Meningioma. J Neurol Neurosurg Psych. 1981; 44
[88] Little JR, Dial B, Belanger G, et al. Brain Hemorrhage from Intracranial Tumor. Stroke. 1979; 10:283–288
[89] Wakai S, Inoh S, Ueda Y, et al. Hemangioblastoma Presenting with Intraparenchymatous Hemorrhage. J Neurosurg. 1984; 61:956–960
[90] McCoyd K, Barron KD, Cassidy RJ. Acoustic Neurinoma Presenting as Subarachnoid Hemorrhage. J Neurosurg. 1974; 41:391–393
[91] Gleeson RK, Butzer JF, Grin OD. Acoustic Neurinoma Presenting as Subarachnoid Hemorrhage. J Neurosurg. 1978; 49:602–604
[92] Yonemitsu T, Niizuna H, Kodama N, et al. Acoustic Neurinoma Presenting as Subarachnoid Hemorrhage. Surg Neurol. 1983; 20:125–130
[93] Vincent FM, Bartone JR, Jones MZ. Cerebellar Astrocytoma Presenting as a Cerebellar Hemorrhage in a Child. Neurology. 1980; 30:91–93
[94] Kawamata T, Takeshita M, Kubo O, et al. Management of Intracranial Hemorrhage Associated with Anticoagulant Therapy. Surg Neurol. 1995; 44:438–443
[95] Fihn SD, McDonell M, Martin D, et al. Risk Factors for Complications of Chronic Anticoagulation: A Multicenter Study. Ann Intern Med. 1993; 118:511–520
[96] Smith DB, Hitchcock M, Philpot PJ. Cerebral Amyloid Angiopathy Presenting as Transient Ischemic Attacks: Case Report. J Neurosurg. 1985; 63:963–964
[97] Greenberg SM, Vonsattel JP, Stakes JW, Gruber M, Finklestein SP. The Clinical Spectrum of Cerebral Amyloid Angiopathy: Presentations without Lobar Hemorrhage. Neurology. 1993; 43:2073–2079
[98] Broderick JP, Brott TG, Tomsick T, et al. Ultra-Early Evaluation of Intracerebral Hemorrhage. J Neurosurg. 1990; 72:195–199
[99] Brott T, Broderick J, Kothari R, Barsan W, Tomsick T, Sauerbeck L, Spilker J, Duldner J, Khoury J. Early hemorrhage growth in patients with intracerebral hemorrhage. Stroke. 1997; 28:1–5
[100] Fujii Y, Tanaka R, Takeuchi S, et al. Hematoma Enlargement in Spontaneous Intracerebral Hemorrhage. J Neurosurg. 1994; 80:51–57
[101] Wada R, Aviv RI, Fox AJ, Sahlas DJ, Gladstone DJ, Tomlinson G, Symons SP. CT angiography "spot sign" predicts hematoma expansion in acute intracerebral hemorrhage. Stroke. 2007; 38:1257–1262
[102] Arakawa S, Saku Y, Ibayashi S, et al. Blood Pressure Control and Recurrence of Hypertensive Brain Hemorrhage. Stroke. 1998; 29:1806–1809
[103] Gonzalez-Duarte A, Cantu C, Ruiz-Sandoval JL, Barinagarrementeria F. Recurrent Primary Cerebral Hemorrhage: Frequency, Mechanisms, and Prognosis. Stroke. 1998; 29:1802–1805
[104] Stocchetti N, Croci M, Spagnoli D, Gilardoni F, Resta F, Colombo A. Mass volume measurement in severe head injury: accuracy and feasibility of two pragmatic methods. J Neurol Neurosurg Psychiatry. 2000; 68:14–17
[105] Pasqualin A, Barone G, Cioffi F, Rosta L, Scienza R, Da Pian R. The relevance of anatomic and hemodynamic factors to a classification of cerebral arteriovenous malformations. Neurosurgery. 1991; 28:370–379
[106] Bullock MR, Chesnut RM, Ghajar J, et al. Appendix I: Post-traumatic mass volume measurements in traumatic brain injury. Neurosurgery. 2006; 58
[107] Kothari RU, Brott T, Broderick JP, Barsan WG, Sauerbeck LR, Zuccarello M, Khoury J. The ABCs of measuring intracerebral hemorrhage volumes. Stroke. 1996; 27:1304–1305
[108] Bradley WG. MR Appearance of Hemorrhage in the Brain. Radiology. 1993; 189:15–26
[109] Taveras JM, Gilson JM, Davis DO, et al. Angiography in Cerebral Infarction. Radiology. 1969; 93:549–558
[110] Toffol GJ, Biller J, Adams HP, Smoker WRK. The Predicted Value of Arteriography in Nontraumatic Intracerebral Hemorrhage. Stroke. 1986; 17:881–883
[111] Hemphill JC,3rd, Bonovich DC, Besmertis L, Manley GT, Johnston SC. The ICH score: a simple, reliable grading scale for intracerebral hemorrhage. Stroke. 2001; 32:891–897
[112] Kaneko T, Sawada T, Niimi T, et al. Lower Limit of Blood Pressure in Treatment of Acute Hypertensive Intracranial Hemorrhage. J Cereb Blood Flow Metab. 1983; 3S1:S51–S52

[113] Mayer SA, Brun NC, Begtrup K, Broderick J, Davis S, Diringer MN, Skolnick BE, Steiner T. Recombinant activated factor VII for acute intracerebral hemorrhage. N Engl J Med. 2005; 352:777–785
[114] Poungvarin N, Bhoopat W, Viriyavejakul A, et al. Effects of Dexamethasone in Primary Supratentorial Intracerebral Hemorrhage. N Engl J Med. 1987; 316:1229–1233
[115] Batjer HH, Reisch JS, Plaizier LJ, Su CJ. Failure of Surgery to Improve Outcome in Hypertensive Putaminal Hemorrhage: A Prospective Randomized Trial. Arch Neurol. 1990; 47:1103–1106
[116] Zhu XL, Chan MSY, Poon WS. Spontaneous Intracranial Hemorrhage: Which Patients Need Diagnostic Cerebral Angiography? A Prospective Study of 206 Cases and Review of the Literature. Stroke. 1997; 28:1406–1409
[117] Laissy JP, Normand G, Monroc M, et al. Spontaneous Intracerebral Hematomas from Vascular Causes: Predictive Value of CT Compared with Angiography. Neuroradiology. 1991; 33:291–295
[118] Hoffman M, Monroe DM, III. A cell-based model of hemostasis. Thromb Haemost. 2001; 85:958–965
[119] Diringer MN, Skolnick BE, Mayer SA, Steiner T, Davis SM, Brun NC, Broderick JP. Risk of thromboembolic events in controlled trials of rFVIIa in spontaneous intracerebral hemorrhage. Stroke. 2008; 39:850–856
[120] Pessin MS, Estol CJ, Lafranchise F, Caplan LR. Safety of Anticoagulation After Hemorrhagic Infarction. Neurology. 1993; 43:1298–1303
[121] Phan TG, Koh M, Wijdicks EF. Safety of discontinuation of anticoagulation in patients with intracranial hemorrhage at high thromboembolic risk. Arch Neurol. 2000; 57:1710 1713
[122] Hacke W. The dilemma of reinstituting anticoagulation for patients with cardioembolic sources and intracranial hemorrhage: how wide is the strait between skylla and karybdis? Arch Neurol. 2000; 57:1682–1684
[123] Bertram M, Bonsanto M, Hacke W, Schwab S. Managing the therapeutic dilemma: patients with spontaneous intracerebral hemorrhage and urgent need for anticoagulation. J Neurol. 2000, 247:209–214
[124] Viswanathan A, Rakich SM, Engel C, Snider R, Rosand J, Greenberg SM, Smith EE. Antiplatelet use after intracerebral hemorrhage. Neurology. 2006; 66:206–209
[125] Eckman MH, Rosand J, Knudsen KA, Singer DE, Greenberg SM. Can patients be anticoagulated after intracerebral hemorrhage? A decision analysis. Stroke. 2003; 34:1710–1716
[126] Wijdicks EF, Schievink WI, Brown RD, Mullany CJ. The dilemma of discontinuation of anticoagulation therapy for patients with intracranial hemorrhage and mechanical heart valves. Neurosurgery. 1998; 42:769–773
[127] MacEwen W. An Address on the Surgery of the Brain and Spinal Cord. Br Med J. 1888; 2:302–309
[128] Hankey GJ, Hon C. Surgery for Primary Intracerebral Hemorrhage: Is It Safe and Effective? A Systematic Review of Case Series and Randomized Trials. Stroke. 1997; 28:2126–2132
[129] Teernstra OP, Evers SM, Kessels AH. Meta analyses in treatment of spontaneous supratentorial intracerebral haematoma. Acta Neurochir (Wien). 2006; 148:521–8; discussion 528
[130] Juvela S, Heiskanen O, Poranen A, et al. The Treatment of Spontaneous Intracerebral Hemorrhage: A Prospective Randomized Trial of Surgical and Conservative Treatment. J Neurosurg. 1989; 70:755–758
[131] Mendelow AD, Gregson BA, Fernandes HM, Murray GD, Teasdale GM, Hope DT, Karimi A, Shaw MD, Barer DH. Early surgery versus initial conservative treatment in patients with spontaneous supratentorial intracerebral haematomas in the International Surgical Trial in Intracerebral Haemorrhage (STICH): a randomised trial. Lancet. 2005; 365:387–397
[132] Waga S, Miyazaki M, Okada M, et al. Hypertensive Putaminal Hemorrhage: Analysis of 182 Patients. Surg Neurol. 1986; 26:159–166
[133] Broderick JP, Brott TG, Duldner JE, Tomsick T, Huster G. Volume of intracerebral hemorrhage. A powerful and easy-to-use predictor of 30-day mortality. Stroke. 1993; 24:987–993
[134] Volpin L, Cervellini P, Colombo F, et al. Spontaneous intracerebral hematomas: A new proposal about the usefulness and limits of surgical treatment. Neurosurgery. 1984; 15:663–666
[135] Kobayashi S, Sato A, Kageyama Y, et al. Treatment of Hypertensive Cerebellar Hemorrhage - Surgical or Conservative Management. Neurosurgery. 1994; 34:246–251
[136] Heros RC. Surgical Treatment of Cerebellar Infarction. Stroke. 1992; 23:937–938
[137] Hinton DR, Dolan E, Sima AF. The Value of Histopathological Examination of Surgically Removed Blood Clot in Determining the Etiology of Spontaneous Intracerebral Hemorrhage. Stroke. 1984; 15:517–520
[138] Auer LM, Deinsberger W, Niederkorn K, et al. Endoscopic Surgery Versus Medical Treatment for Spontaneous Intracerebral Hematoma: A Randomized Study. J Neurosurg. 1989; 70:530–535
[139] Findlay JM, Grace MGA, Weir BKA. Treatment of Intraventricular Hemorrhage with Tissue Plasminogen Activator. Neurosurgery. 1993; 32:941–947
[140] Engelhard HH, Andrews CO, Slavin KV, Charbel FT. Current management of intraventricular hemorrhage. Surg Neurol. 2003; 60:15–21; discussion 21-2
[141] Grabb PA. Traumatic intraventricular hemorrhage treated with intraventricular recombinant-tissue plasminogen activator: technical case report. Neurosurgery. 1998; 43:966–969
[142] Rohde V, Schaller C, Hassler WE. Intraventricular recombinant tissue plasminogen activator for lysis of intraventricular hemorrhage. J Neurol Neurosurg Psychiatry. 1995; 58:447–451
[143] CLEAR result: low-dose tPA safe, effective in treating intraventricular hemorrhage. Nice, France 2008
[144] Toffol GJ, Biller J, Adams HP. Nontraumatic Intracerebral Hemorrhage in Young Adults. Arch Neurol. 1987; 44:483–485
[145] Volpe JJ. Neonatal Intraventricular Hemorrhage. N Engl J Med. 1981; 304:886–891
[146] Lou HC, Lassen NA, Friis-Hansen B. Impaired Autoregulation of Cerebral Blood Flow in the Distressed Newborn Infant. J Pediatr. 1979; 94:118–121
[147] Milligan DWA. Failure of Autoregulation and Intraventricular Hemorrhage in Preterm Infants. Lancet. 1980; 1:896–898
[148] Hambleton G, Wigglesworth JS. Origin of intraventricular haemorrhage in the preterm infant. Arch Dis Child. 1976; 51:651–659
[149] Dykes FD, Lazzara A, Ahmann P, Blumenstein B, et al. Intraventricular Hemorrhage: A Prospective Evaluation of Etiopathologies. Pediatrics. 1980; 66:42–49
[150] Perlman JM, McMenamin JB, Volpe JJ. Fluctuating Cerebral Blood-Flow Velocity in Respiratory Distress Syndrome. N Engl J Med. 1983; 309:204–209
[151] Wirtschafter DD, Danielsen BH, Main EK, Korst LM, Gregory KD, Wertz A, Stevenson DK, Gould JB. Promoting antenatal steroid use for fetal maturation: results from the California Perinatal Quality Care Collaborative. J Pediatr. 2006; 148:606–612
[152] Volpe JJ. Effect of Cocaine Use on the Fetus. N Engl J Med. 1992; 327:399–407
[153] Murphy BP, Inder TE, Rooks V, Taylor GA, Anderson NJ, Mogridge N, Horwood LJ, Volpe JJ. Posthaemorrhagic ventricular dilatation in the premature infant: natural history and predictors of outcome. Arch Dis Child Fetal Neonatal Ed. 2002; 87:F37–F41
[154] Sheth RD. Trends in incidence and severity of intraventricular hemorrhage. J Child Neurol. 1998; 13:261–264

[155] Papile LA, Burstein J, Burstein R, et al. Incidence and Evolution of Subependymal and Intraventricular Hemorrhage: A Study of Infants with Birth Weights Less Than 1,500 Gm. J Pediatr. 1978; 92:529–534

[156] Bejar R, Curbelo V, Coen RW, et al. Diagnosis and Follow-Up of Intraventricular and Intracerebral Hemorrhages by Ultrasound Studies of Infant's Brain Through the Fontanelles and Sutures. Pediatrics. 1980; 66:661–673

[157] Tsiantos A, Victorin L, Relier JP, Dyer N, et al. Intracranial Hemorrhage in the Prematurely Born Infant. J Pediatr. 1974; 85:854–859

[158] Perlman JM, Volpe JJ. Cerebral Blood Flow Velocity in Relation to Intraventricular Hemorrhage in the Premature Newborn Infant. J Pediatr. 1982; 100:956–959

[159] Ment LR, Oh W, Philip AG, Ehrenkranz RA, Duncan CC, Allan W, Taylor KJ, Schneider K, Katz KH, Makuch RW. Risk factors for early intraventricular hemorrhage in low birth weight infants. J Pediatr. 1992; 121:776–783

[160] Crowley P, Chalmers I, Keirse MJ. The effects of corticosteroid administration before preterm delivery: an overview of the evidence from controlled trials. Br J Obstet Gynaecol. 1990; 97:11–25

[161] Murphy KE, Hannah ME, Willan AR, Hewson SA, Ohlsson A, Kelly EN, Matthews SG, Saigal S, Asztalos E, Ross S, Delisle MF, Amankwah K, Guselle P, Gafni A, Lee SK, Armson BA. Multiple courses of antenatal corticosteroids for preterm birth (MACS): a randomised controlled trial. Lancet. 2008; 372:2143–2151

[162] Rabe H, Reynolds G, Diaz-Rossello J. Early versus delayed umbilical cord clamping in preterm infants. Cochrane Database Syst Rev. 2004. DOI: 10.1002/14651858.CD003248.pub2

[163] Volpe JJ. Neurology of the Newborn. 4th ed. Philadelphia: W. B. Saunders; 2008

[164] Fishman MA, Dutton RY, Okumura S. Progressive Ventriculomegaly following Minor Intracranial Hemorrhage in Premature Infants. Dev Med Child Neurol. 1984; 26:725–731

[165] Hill A, Rozdilsky B. Congenital Hydrocephalus Secondary to Intra-Uterine Germinal Matrix/Intraventricular Hemorrhage. Dev Med Child Neurol. 1984; 26:509–527

[166] James HE, Bejar R, Merritt A, et al. Management of Hydrocephalus Secondary to Intracranial Hemorrhage in the High Risk Newborn. Neurosurgery. 1984; 14:612–618

[167] Volpe JJ, Herscovitch P, Perlman JM, Raichle ME. Positron Emission Tomography in the Newborn: Extensive Impairment of Regional Cerebral Blood Flow with Intraventricular Hemorrhage and Hemorrhagic Intracerebral Involvement. Pediatrics. 1983

[168] Ment LR, Duncan CC, Ehrenkranz RA, Lange RC, et al. Intraventricular Hemorrhage in the Preterm Neonate: Timing and Cerebral Blood Flow Changes. J Pediatr. 1984; 104:419–425

[169] Trounce JQ, Fagan D, Levene MI. Intraventricular Hemorrhage and Periventricular Leucomalacia: Ultrasound and Autopsy Correlation. Arch Dis Child. 1983; 61:1203–1207

[170] Brenner DJ. Estimating cancer risks from pediatric CT: going from the qualitative to the quantitative. Pediatr Radiol. 2002; 32:228–3; discussion 242-4

[171] International PHVD Drug Trial Group. International randomised controlled trial of acetazolamide and furosemide in posthaemorrhagic ventricular dilatation in infancy. Lancet. 1998; 352:433–440

[172] Whitelaw A, Kennedy CR, Brion LP. Diuretic therapy for newborn infants with posthemorrhagic ventricular dilatation. Cochrane Database Syst Rev. 2001. DOI: 10.1002/14651858.CD002270

[173] Rom S, Serfontein GL, Humphreys RP. Intracerebellar Hematoma in the Neonate. J Pediatr. 1978; 93:486–488

[174] Murphy BP, Inder TE, Rooks V, Taylor GA, Anderson NJ, Mogridge N, Horwood LJ, Volpe JJ. Posthaemorrhagic ventricular dilatation in the premature infant: natural history and predictors of outcome. Arch Dis Child Fetal Neonatal Ed. 2002; 87:F37–F41

[175] Kreusser KL, Tarby TJ, Kovnar E, et al. Serial Lumbar Punctures for at Least Temporary Amelioration of Neonatal Posthemorrhagic Hydrocephalus. Pediatrics. 1985; 75

[176] Whitelaw A. Repeated lumbar or ventricular punctures in newborns with intraventricular hemorrhage. Cochrane Database Syst Rev. 2001

[177] Benzel EC, Reeves JP, Nguyen PK, Hadden TA. The treatment of hydrocephalus in preterm infants with intraventricular haemorrhage. Acta Neurochir (Wien). 1993; 122:200–203

[178] Marlin AE, Rivera S, Gaskill SJ. Treatment of posthemorrhagic ventriculomegaly in the pretern infant: Use of the subcutaneous ventricular reservoir. Concepts in Pediatric Neurosurgery. 1988; 8:15–22

[179] Hudgins RJ, Boydston WR, Gilreath CL. Treatment of posthemorrhagic hydrocephalus in the preterm infant with a ventricular access device. Pediatr Neurosurg. 1998; 29:309–313

[180] Tubbs RS, Smyth MD, Wellons JC,3rd, Blount JP, Grabb PA, Oakes WJ. Alternative uses for the subgaleal shunt in pediatric neurosurgery. Pediatr Neurosurg. 2003; 39:22–24

[181] Fulmer BB, Grabb PA, Oakes WJ, Mapstone TB. Neonatal ventriculosubgaleal shunts. Neurosurgery. 2000; 47:80–3; discussion 83-4

[182] Rahman S, Teo C, Morris W, Lao D, Boop FA. Ventriculosubgaleal shunt: a treatment option for progressive posthemorrhagic hydrocephalus. Childs Nerv Syst. 1995; 11:650–654

[183] Wellons JC, Shannon CN, Kulkarni AV, Simon TD, Riva-Cambrin J, Whitehead WE, Oakes WJ, Drake JM, Luerssen TG, Walker ML, Kestle JR. A multicenter retrospective comparison of conversion from temporary to permanent cerebrospinal fluid diversion in very low birth weight infants with posthemorrhagic hydrocephalus. J Neurosurg Pediatr. 2009; 4:50–55

[184] Bridgers SL, Ment LR. Absence of Hydrocephalus despite Disproportionately Increasing Head Size After the Neonatal Period in Preterm Infants with Known Intraventricular Hemorrhage. Childs Brain. 1981; 8:423–426

[185] Sher PK, Brown SA. A Longitudinal Study of Head Growth in Preterm Infants: II. Differentiation between 'Catch-Up' Head-Growth and Early Infantile Hydrocephalus. Dev Med Child Neurol. 1975; 17:711–718

[186] Aoki N, Miztani H, Masuzawa H. Unilateral Subdural-Peritoneal Shunting for Bilateral Chronic Subdural Hematomas in Infancy. J Neurosurg. 1985; 63:134–137

[187] Krishnamoorthy K, Kuehnle KJ, Todres ID, et al. Neurodevelopmental Outcome of Survivors with Posthemorrhagic Hydrocephalus. Ann Neurol. 1984; 15:201–204

[188] Adams-Chapman I, Hansen NI, Stoll BJ, Higgins R. Neurodevelopmental outcome of extremely low birth weight infants with posthemorrhagic hydrocephalus requiring shunt insertion. Pediatrics. 2008; 121:e1167–e1177

[189] Armstrong-Wells J, Johnston SC, Wu YW, Sidney S, Fullerton HJ. Prevalence and predictors of perinatal hemorrhagic stroke: results from the Kaiser Pediatric Stroke Study. Pediatrics. 2009; 123:823–828

[190] Alexander MJ, Spetzler RF. Pediatric Neurovascular Disease. New York: Thieme Medical Publishers, Inc.; 2006

Part XXI

Outcome Assessment

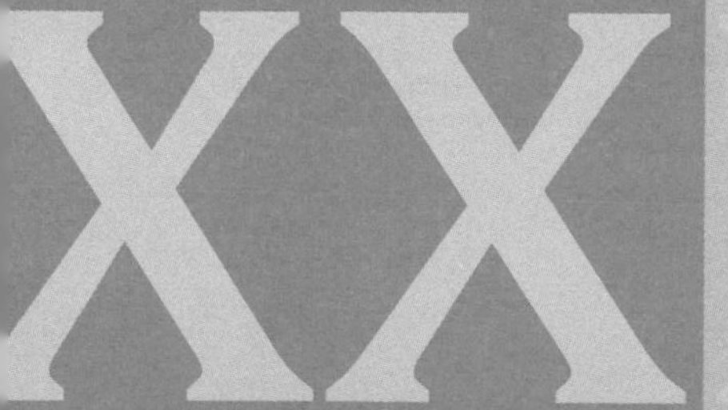

88 Outcome Assessment

88.1 Cancer

► **Karnofsky performance scale (KPS).** ► Table 88.1, (after David A. Karnofsky) often used for grading functional status in patients with cancer. A KPS score < 70 (particularly with brain tumors) often identifies patients with a worse prognosis for any given treatment.

WHO performance score. ► Table 88.2, the WHO Performance score[3] (AKA The Eastern Cooperative Oncology Group (ECOG) score, AKA Zubrod score (after C. Gordon Zubrod), ranges from 0 to 5, with 0 indicating perfect health and 5 death. The advantage over the Karnofsky scale is its simplicity.

88.2 Head injury

The **Ranchos Los Amigos scale** (► Table 88.3) is often used in rating disability following head injury. The Glasgow outcome scale (► Table 88.4) is frequently employed in outcome assessment.

88.3 Cerebrovascular events

88

88.3.1 General information

Several outcome grading scales have come to be favored for use following strokes or SAH. Each emphasizes different aspects of outcome. The Barthel Index (► Table 88.6) places weight on activities of daily living (ADLs), while others, such as the modified Rankin scale[5] (► Table 88.5) assess levels of independence and includes a comparison to previous activity levels and shows fairly good interobserver consistency.[6] While it does measure functional status, the modified Rankin is not sensitive to subtle neurologic deficits such as dysphasia or visual field defects.

Table 88.1 Karnofsky performance status scale (modified[1,2])

Score	Criteria	General category
100	normal: no complaints, no evidence of disease	Able to carry on normal activity and work. No special care is needed
90	able to carry on normal activity: minor signs or symptoms	
80	normal activity with effort: some signs or symptoms	
70	cares for self: unable to carry on normal activity or to do active work	Unable to work. Able to live at home, care for most personal needs. Variable assistance is required
60	requires occasional assistance: cares for most of needs	
50	requires considerable assistance and frequent care	
40	disabled: requires special care and assistance	Unable to care for self. Requires equivalent of institutional or hospital care. Disease may be rapidly progressing
30	severely disabled: hospitalized; death not imminent	
20	very sick: hospitalized; active supportive care needed	
10	moribund: fatal processes are progressing rapidly	
0	dead	

Table 88.2 WHO performance scale

Grade	Description
0	Fully active, no performance restriction as a result of disease.
1	Restricted in physically strenuous activity. Ambulatory. Able to do light work, e.g. light house work, desk work.
2	Unable to perform any work activities. Ambulatory. Up & about > 50% of waking hours.
3	Only able to perform limited self care. Wheelchair confined > 50% of waking hours.
4	Completely disabled. Unable to perform self care. Totally bed or chair confined.
5	Dead

Table 88.3 Ranchos Los Amigos cognitive scale

Level	Meaning
I	No response to pain, touch, sight or sound.
II	Generalized reflex responses to pain.
III	Localized response. Blinks to strong light, turns towards/away from sound, responds to physical discomfort, inconsistent responses to commands.
IV	Confused – Agitated Alert, very active, agitated, aggressive, or bizarre behaviors. Performs motor activities but behavior is non-purposeful, extremely short attention span.
V	Confused – Non agitated Gross attention to environment, easily distracted, requires continual redirection, difficulty learning new tasks, agitated by excess stimulation. May converse socially but with inappropriate verbalizations.
VI	Confused – Appropriate Inconsistent orientation to time and place. Retention span and recent memory impaired. Begins to recall past, consistently follows simple commands, goal directed behavior with assistance.
VII	Automatic – Appropriate Performs daily routine in highly familiar environment in a non-confused but automatic "robot-like" fashion. Skills deteriorate in unfamiliar environment. Lacks realistic planning for future.
VIII	Purposeful – Appropriate

Table 88.4 Glasgow outcome scale[4]

Score	Meaning
5	good recovery – resumption of normal life despite minor deficits ("return to work" not reliable)
4	moderate disability (disabled but independent) – travel by public transportation, can work in sheltered setting (exceeds mere ability to perform "activities of daily living")
3	severe disability (conscious but disabled) – dependent for daily support (may be institutionalized, but this is not a criteria)
2	persistent vegetative state – unresponsive & speechless; after 2–3 weeks, may open eyes & have sleep/wake cycles
1	death – most deaths ascribable to primary head injury occur within 48 hrs

Table 88.5 The modified* Rankin scale

Grade	Description
0	no symptoms at all
1	no significant disability despite symptoms: able to carry out all usual duties & activities
2	slight disability: unable to carry out all previous activities. Able to look after own affairs without assistance
3	moderate disability: requiring some help, but able to walk without assistance
4	moderately severe disability: unable to walk without assistance, and unable to attend to own bodily needs without assistance
5	severe disability: bedridden, incontinent, and requiring constant nursing care and attention

* the original Rankin scale[7]: did not have Grade 0, Grade 1 did not include the words "despite symptoms" and "& activities", and it defined Grade 2 as "unable to carry out some of previous activities..."

Table 88.6 The Barthel index

Item	Original Barthel Index			Modified Barthel Index				
	Unable to perform task	Needs assistance	Fully independent	CODE 1	CODE 2	CODE 3	CODE 4	CODE 5
				Unable to perform task	Attempts task but unsafe	Moderate help required	Minimal help required	Fully independent
Personal hygiene	0	0	5	0	1	3	4	5
Self bathing	0	0	5	0	1	3	4	5
Feeding	0	5	10	0	2	5	8	10
Toilet	0	5	10	0	2	5	8	10
Stair climbing	0	5	10	0	2	5	8	10
Dressing	0	5	10	0	2	5	8	10
Bowel control	0	5	10	0	2	5	8	10
Bladder control	0	5	10	0	2	5	8	10
Ambulation	0	5–10	15	0	3	8	12	15
Wheelchair[a]	0	0	5	0	1	3	4	5
Chair/bed transfers	0	5–10	15	0	3	8	12	15
Total (range)	**0**	→→	**100**	**0**		→→→→		**100**

[a] score only if unable to walk and patient trained in wheelchair management

88.3.2 Scales

▶ **Modified Rankin scale (▶ Table 88.5)**

▶ **Barthel index (▶ Table 88.6).** The original Barthel index[8,9] assigns one of three scores to 10 ratable ADLs, and then the individual scores are summed. The modified Barthel index (MBI) with a 5-step scoring system appears to have greater sensitivity.[10] The total ranges from 0 to 100 (a score of 100 implies functional independence, not necessarily normality).

Table 88.7 The Functional Independence Measure™ (FIM)

Classification	Item
	Motor
Self-care	Eating
	Grooming
	Bathing
	Dressing – upper body
	Dressing – lower body
	Toileting
Sphincter control	Bladder management
	Bowel management
Mobility	Bed, chair, wheelchair
	Toilet
	Tub, shower
Locomotion	Walk or wheelchair
	Stairs
	Cognitive
Communication	Comprehension
	Expression
Social cognition	Social interaction
	Problem solving
	Memory

Table 88.8 The 7 FIM™ rating levels of disability

Degree of dependency	Level of function	Score
No helper	Complete independence	7
	Modified independence	6
Modified dependence on a helper	Supervision	5
	Minimal assist (≥ 75% independent)	4
	Moderate assist (≥ 50% independent)	3
Complete dependence on a helper	Maximal assist (≥ 25% independence)	2
	Total assist (< 25% independence)	1

Of all the factors, independence in bathing was the most difficult. Abilities on the Barthel index tend to return in a fairly consistent order, and so most patients with the same score will have similar patterns of disability.

88.4 Spinal cord injury

► **Functional Independence Measure™ (FIM™)** [11,12,13] **(FIM™)**. Developed to provide uniform evaluation of disability for spinal cord injuries. Rates 18 items shown in ► Table 88.7 (13 motor, 5 cognitive) on the 7 level scale shown in ► Table 88.8.

The FIM™ has high internal consistency and is a good indicator of burden of care.[14,15]

References

[1] Karnofsky DA, Burchenal JH, Macleod CM. Evaluation of Chemotherapy Agents. New York: Columbia University Press; 1949:191–205

[2] Karnofsky D, Burchenal JH, Armistead GC, et al. Triethylene melamine in the treatment of neoplastic disease. Arch Intern Med. 1951; 87:477–516

[3] Oken MM, Creech RH, Tormey DC, Horton J, Davis TE, McFadden ET, Carbone PP. Toxicity and response criteria of the Eastern Cooperative Oncology Group. Am J Clin Oncol. 1982; 5:649–655

[4] Jennett B, Bond M. Assessment of Outcome After Severe Brain Damage: A Practical Scale. Lancet. 1975; i:480–484

[5] UK-TIA Study Group. The UK-TIA Aspirin Trial: Interim Results. Br Med J. 1988; 296:316–320

[6] van Swieten JC, Koudstaal PJ, Visser MC. Interobserver agreement for the assessment of handicap in stroke patients. Stroke. 1988; 19:604–607

[7] Rankin J. Cerebral Vascular Accidents in Patients Over the Age of 60. 2. Prognosis. Scott Med J. 1957; 2:200–215

[8] Mahoney FI, Barthel DW. Functional Evaluation: The Barthel Index. Maryland State Med J. 1965; 14:61–65

[9] Wade DT, Hewer RL. Functional abilities after stroke: Measurement, natural history and prognosis. J Neurol Neurosurg Psychiatry. 1987; 50:177–182

[10] Shah S, Vanclay F, Cooper B. Improving the sensitivity of the Barthel Index for stroke rehabilitation. J Clin Epidemiol. 1989; 42:703–709

[11] Forer S, Granger C, et al. Functional Independence Measure. Buffalo, NY: The Buffalo General Hospital, State University of New York at Buffalo; 1987

[12] Ditunno JF.Jr. New spinal cord injury standards, 1992. Paraplegia. 1992; 30:90–91

[13] Ditunno JF.Jr. Functional assessment measures in CNS trauma. J Neurotrauma. 1992; 9:S301–S305

[14] Dodds TA, Martin DP, Stolov WC, Deyo RA. A validation of the functional independence measurement and its performance among rehabilitation inpatients. Arch Phys Med Rehabil. 1993; 74:531–536

[15] Linacre JM, Heinemann AW, Wright BD, Granger CV, Hamilton BB. The structure and stability of the Functional Independence Measure. Arch Phys Med Rehabil. 1994; 75:127–132

Part XXII

Differential Diagnosis

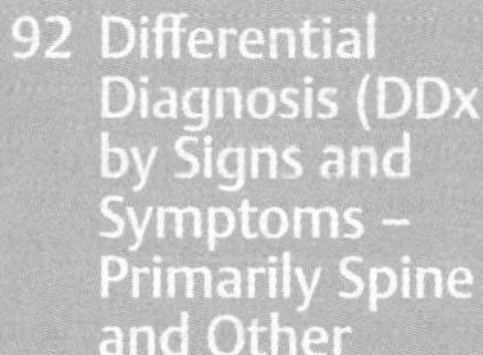

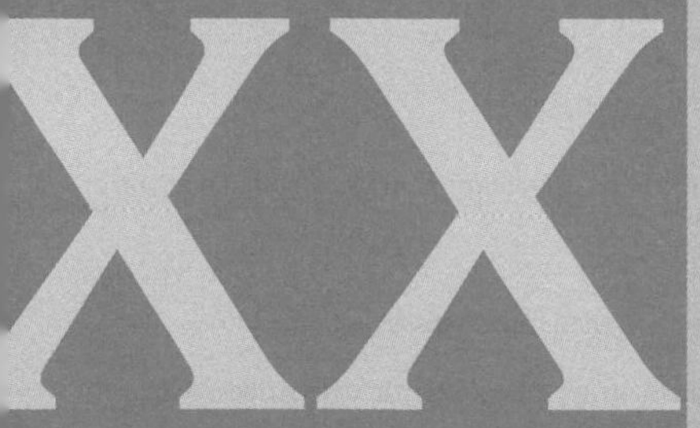

89 Differential Diagnosis by Location or Radiographic Finding – Intracranial

89.1 Diagnoses covered outside this chapter

Table 89.1 Differential diagnoses by location or radiographic finding, intracranial – covered outside this chapter

DDx
chordomas (p. 778)
extra-axial fluid (peds) (p. 903)
gyral enhancement (p. 1281)
hydrocephalus (p. 399)
pineal region tumors (p. 658)
pneumocephalus (p. 887)
schizencephaly (p. 288)

89

89.2 Posterior fossa lesions

89.2.1 Cerebellar lesions

General information

The following addresses *intra*-axial p-fossa abnormalities (for extra-axial lesions, below).

Adult

Single lesion

► **Note.** Rule of thumb: "the differential diagnosis of a solitary intraparenchymal lesion in an adult p-fossa is metastasis, metastasis, metastasis, until proven otherwise."

1. tumors:
   a) metastasis
   b) hemangioblastoma (p. 701): the most common PRIMARY intra-axial p-fossa tumor in adults (7–12% of p-fossa tumors). Very vascular nodule, often has cyst. Almost all p-fossa tumors are relatively avascular on angiography *except* these (look for serpentine signal voids especially in the periphery of the lesion on MRI,[1] much less common in cavernous hemangioma)
   c) cerebellar (pilocytic) astrocytoma (p. 630): may be solid or cystic, tends to occurs in younger adults
   d) brainstem glioma: an isolated glioblastoma in the posterior fossa of an adult is a reportable rarity
   e) choroid plexus tumor: usually infratentorial in adults (p. 1380)
   f) cerebellar liponeurocytoma (p. 646)
2. infectious: abscess
3. vascular
   a) cavernous hemangioma
   b) hemorrhage
   c) infarction: cerebellar stroke may be associated with H/A and/or pain in suboccipital region or upper neck
      - embolic
      - thrombotic/plaque related
      - vertebral artery dissection: much less common than carotid dissection (p. 1325)
      - vertebrobasilar hypoplasia (p. 1306)
4. Lhermitte-Duclos (p. 647): Focal or diffuse. Nonenhancing. Characteristic tiger stripes. Widens folia (c.f. most neoplasms which destroy folial pattern)

Multiple lesions

1. metastases
2. hemangioblastoma (possibly as part of von Hippel-Lindau) (p. 703)
3. abscesses
4. cavernous hemangiomas

Pediatric

Also see Pediatric brain tumors (p. 593).

Early data: 67% of childhood brain tumors occur in p-fossa, and astrocytomas were the most common there. Currently: p-fossa tumors comprise 54–60% of childhood brain tumors (breakdown listed below). 4 types account for ≈ 95% of infratentorial tumors in patients ≤ 18 yrs age.[2] The 3 most common are equal in incidence (expressed as percent of p-fossa tumors pooled from 1350 pediatric brain tumors[3]):

1. PNET, including medulloblastoma (p. 663): 27%
   a) most start in *roof* of 4th ventricle (fastigium), and most are solid
   b) differentiating medulloblastoma (MB) from ependymoma:
      - 4th ventricle drapes around medulloblastoma ("banana sign") from the anterior aspect, c.f. ependymoma which tends to grow into 4th ventricle from floor. Ependymoma may grow through foramen of Luschka and/or Magendie
      - ependymomas tend to be inhomogeneous on T1WI MRI (unlike MB)
      - the exophytic component of ependymomas tends to be high signal on T2WI MRI (with MB this is only mildly hyperintense)
      - calcifications: common in ependymomas, but only in < 10% of MB
2. cerebellar (pilocytic) astrocytoma (p. 630): 27%. Most start in cerebellar hemisphere. Often cystic with enhancing mural nodule
3. brainstem gliomas (p. 633): 28%. Usually present with multiple cranial nerve palsies and long tract findings
4. ependymoma (p. 642): usually arise in *floor* of 4th ventricle
5. choroid plexus papilloma (p. 648): majority of patients are < 2 yrs old
6. atypical teratoid/rhabdoid tumor (AT/RT) (p. 666)
7. metastasis: neuroblastoma, rhabdomyosarcoma, Wilm's tumor…
8. PHACES syndrome: acronym for a group of findings including Posterior fossa malformations, cervicofacial Hemangioma, Arterial anomalies of the head and neck, Coarctation of the aorta and cardiac defects, Eye anomalies and Sternal cleft. Ratio girls:boys = 9:1. Thought to begin during gestation weeks 8–10

89.2.2 Cerebellopontine angle (CPA) lesions

Lesions in general

Vestibular schwannoma, meningioma, and epidermoid account for most. For those lesions that may be cystic, see below.

1. vestibular schwannoma: (80–90% of CPA lesions); see below for differentiating from meningioma (p. 1366)
2. meningioma: (5–10%); see below for differentiating from vestibular schwannoma (p. 1366)
3. ectodermal inclusion tumors (p. 761)
   a) epidermoid (cholesteatoma): 5–7%. High signal on DWMRI (p. 761). Tumor passing from the posterior fossa to the middle fossa though the incisura is highly suggestive of epidermoid
   b) dermoid
4. metastases
5. neuroma from cranial nerves other than VIII (also see below for some differentiating features)
   a) trigeminal neuroma: expands towards Meckel's cave
   b) facial nerve neuroma[4]: may arise in any portion of the VII nerve, with a predilection for the geniculate ganglion.[5] Even in these tumors, hearing loss tends to precede facial paresis. Hearing loss may be sensorineural from VIII nerve compression from tumors arising in the proximal portion of VII (cisternal or internal auditory canal (IAC) segment), or it may be conductive from erosion of the ossicles by tumors arising in the second (tympanic, or horizontal) segment of VII. Facial palsy (peripheral) (p. 576) may also develop, usually late[4]
   c) neurinoma of lowest 4 cranial nerves (IX, X, XI, XII)
6. arachnoid cyst (p. 248)

89

7. neurenteric cyst (p. 290): rare.[6] May secrete mucin
8. cholesterol granuloma (distinct from epidermoid) (p. 761)
9. lipoma
10. aneurysm: PICA, AICA, vertebrobasilar
11. dolichobasilar ectasia
12. cysticercosis
13. extensions of:
    a) brain stem or cerebellar glioma
    b) pituitary adenoma
    c) craniopharyngioma
    d) chordoma & tumors of skull base
    e) fourth ventricle tumors (ependymoma, medulloblastoma)
    f) choroid plexus papilloma: from 4th ventricle through foramen of Luschka
    g) glomus tumor
        - glomus jugulare
        - glomus tympanicum
    h) primary tumors of temporal bone (e.g. sarcoma or carcinoma)

Cystic lesions of the CPA

CPA lesions from the above list that may be cystic or have a cystic component[6]:
1. arachnoid cyst: same intensity as CSF on all MRI sequences, homogeneous
2. epidermoid cyst (p. 270): ✱ high signal on DWMRI differentiates this from arachnoid cyst
3. dermoid cyst: high intensity areas on T1WI similar to fat; usually midline
4. cystic schwannoma
5. cholesterol granuloma: ✱ ≈ only lesion that is high signal on T1WI (due to blood breakdown products; exception: the rare "white" epidermoid). Also high signal on T2WI. Usually extradural, especially near petrous apex. Bone destruction is common
6. neurenteric cyst: nonenhancing. Low intensity on DWMRI
7. choroidal cyst
8. cysticercosis: enhancing nodule (scolex)

89

Differentiating neuromas of V, VII and VIII cranial nerves

All 3 of these tumors may present in the CPA and may cross from posterior fossa to middle fossa, but they tend to do so in different manners. Vestibular schwannomas show "transhiatal" extension by passing through the tentorial hiatus medially. Most trigeminal neuromas show "transapicopetrosal" extension by crossing into the middle fossa via the petrous apex (although some show transhiatal extension). When facial neuromas cross, they tend to spread across the midpetrosal bone, which is characteristic for facial neuromas spread across the midpetrosal bone is characteristic for facial neuromas.[4] When a facial neuroma enlarges the IAC, unlike a vestibular schwannoma, it tends to erode the anterosuperior aspect of the IAC.

Differentiating vestibular schwannoma from CPA meningioma

1. vestibular schwannoma (VS) (AKA acoustic neuroma):
    a) clinical: progressive unilateral hearing loss, usually with tinnitus. Progression results in unsteadiness, with true vertigo being rare. The facial nerve is more resistant to stretching, thus facial nerve signs and symptoms occur late. Trigeminal nerve involvement may occur with tumors > 3 cm (check corneal reflex), with tic douloureux-like symptoms being unusual
    b) imaging: often heterogeneous signal and nonuniform enhancement. Medium size tumors look like ice cream in a cone (IAC is the cone). Rarely calcified. Except for very small tumors, IAC is frequently enlarged. Look for an acute angle between the tumor and the petrous bone (meningiomas usually have an obtuse angle)
2. meningiomas: may mimic VSs with these differences:
    a) clinical: since they often arise from the superior anterior edge of the IAC, early facial nerve involvement is more common, and hearing loss is usually *late*. Trigeminal neuralgia-like pain is more common than with VSs
    b) imaging: homogeneous signal and enhancement. The tumor may enter the IAC but it tends not to enlarge it. IAC often eccentric in tumor. Tumor is flat against petrous bone with an obtuse angle to the bone. *Calcification and bony hypertrophy* may occur (which occasionally *narrows* the IAC).

89.2.3 Petrous apex lesions

1. infection/inflammatory:
   a) osteomyelitis: may produce Gradenigo's syndrome (p. 570)
   b) cholesterol granuloma (bright on T1WI epidermoid cyst are bright on DWI, neither enhance)
2. vascular lesions: aneurysm
3. neoplastic:
   a) squamous cell cancer
   b) glomus tumor
   c) chondrosarcoma: will displace the carotid from medial to lateral (almost every other tumor in this region encases the carotid)

89.2.4 Foramen magnum lesions

Differential diagnosis

See Foramen magnum lesions (p. 1367) for *nonneoplastic* lesions. Most foramen magnum (FM) region tumors are extra-axial. This includes:

1. Extra-axial tumors
   a) meningioma: the anterior lip of the foramen magnum is the second most common site of origin of posterior fossa meningiomas. Meningiomas (p. 698) comprise 38–46% of FM tumors[7,8] and most are intradural
   b) Chordoma (p. 778): a mass behind the dens compressing the spinal cord is a chordoma until proven otherwise
   c) neurilemmoma
   d) epidermoid
   e) chondroma
   f) chondrosarcoma
   g) metastases
2. Exophytic component of a brainstem tumor
3. Non-neoplastic lesions
   a) aneurysms or ectasia of the vertebral artery
   b) odontoid process in cases of basilar invagination (p. 278)
   c) pannus from involvement of the odontoid with rheumatoid arthritis or old nonunion of fracture
   d) synovial cyst of the quadrate ligament of the odontoid[9]

Presentation

In the pre-imaging era (i.e. before CT & MRI) these lesions were often diagnosed relatively late due to the unusual associated clinical syndromes and the rarity of visualizing this region on myelography.

Clinical findings

Symptoms:

1. sensory
   a) craniocervical pain: usually an early symptom, commonly in neck and occiput. Aching in nature. ↑ with head movement
   b) sensory findings: usually occur later. Numbness and tingling of the fingers
2. motor
   a) spastic weakness of the extremities: weakness usually starts in the ipsilateral UE, then the ipsilateral LE, then contralateral LE, and finally contralateral UE ("rotating paralysis")

Signs:

1. sensory
   a) dissociated sensory loss: loss of pain and temperature contralateral to lesion with preservation of tactile sensation
   b) loss of position and vibratory sense, greater in the upper than the lower extremities
2. motor
   a) spastic weakness of the extremities
   b) atrophy of the intrinsic hand muscles: a lower motor nerve finding
   c) cerebellar findings may rarely be present with extensive intracranial extension
3. long tract findings
   a) brisk muscle stretch reflexes (hyperreflexia, spasticity)

89

b) loss of abdominal cutaneous reflexes
c) neurogenic bladder: usually a very late finding
4. ipsilateral Horner's syndrome: due to compression of cervical sympathetics
5. nystagmus: classically downbeat (p. 558) but other types can occur

It had been postulated that long tract findings were due to direct compression at the cervicomedullary junction, and that lower motor nerve findings in the upper extremities were due to central necrosis of the grey matter as a result of compression of arterial blood supply. Anatomic study suggests that it is actually *venous* infarction at lower cervical levels (C8-T1) that is responsible for the lower motor neuron findings.

89.3 Multiple intracranial lesions on CT or MRI

89

1. neoplastic
   a) primary
      - multicentric gliomas; ≈ 6% of gliomas are multicentric, more common in neurofibromatosis, see Multiple gliomas (p. 619)
      - tuberous sclerosis (including giant cell astrocytomas); (usually periventricular)
      - multiple meningiomas
      - lymphoma
      - PNET
      - multiple neuromas (usually in neurofibromatosis, including bilateral vestibular schwannomas)
   b) metastatic: usually cortical or subcortical, surrounded by prominent vasogenic edema (p. 803). More common tumors include:
      - lung
      - breast
      - melanoma: may be higher density than brain on unenhanced CT
      - renal cell
      - gastrointestinal tumors
      - genitourinary tract tumors
      - choriocarcinoma
      - testicular
      - atrial myxoma
      - leukemia
2. infection: mostly abscess or cerebritis. Most commonly due to:
   a) pyogenic bacteria
   b) toxoplasmosis: common in AIDS patients (p. 371)
   c) fungal
      - cryptococcus
      - mycoplasma
      - coccidiomycosis
      - aspergilloisis
      - candidiasis
   d) echinococcus
   e) schistosomiasis
   f) paragonimiasis
   g) herpes simplex encephalitis (HSE): usually temporal lobe (p. 364)
3. inflammatory
   a) demyelinating disease
      - MS: usually in white matter, periventricular, with little mass effect, margins are usually very sharp. Ring enhancing lesions can occur with tumefactive demyelinating lesions (p. 179)
      - progressive multifocal leukoencephalopathy (PML): primarily in white matter. No enhancement. Patients are usually very sick
   b) gummas
   c) granulomas
   d) amyloidosis
   e) sarcoidosis
   f) vasculitis or arteritis
   g) collagen vascular disease, including:
      - periarteritis nodosa (PAN) (p. 199)

- systemic lupus erythematosus (SLE)
- granulomatous arteritis

4. vascular
   a) multiple aneurysms (congenital or atherosclerotic)
   b) multiple hemorrhages, e.g. associated with DIC or other coagulopathies (including anticoagulant therapy)
   c) venous infarctions, especially in dural sinus thrombosis (p. 1308)
   d) moyamoya disease (p. 1313)
   e) subacute hypertension (as in malignant HTN, eclampsia…) → symmetric confluent lesions with mild mass effect and patchy enhancement usually in occipital subcortical white matter
   f) multiple strokes
      - lacunar strokes (l'etat lacunaire)
      - multiple emboli (e.g. in atrial fibrillation, mitral valve prolapse, SBE, air emboli)
      - sickle cell disease
      - vasculitis
      - intravascular lymphomatosis (p. 711)
5. hematomas and contusions
   a) traumatic (multiple hemorrhagic contusions, multiple SDH)
   b) multiple "hypertensive" hemorrhages (amyloid angiopathy, etc.)
6. intracranial calcifications (p. 1380)
7. miscellaneous
   a) radiation necrosis
   b) foreign bodies (e.g. post gunshot wound)
   c) periventricular low densities
      - Binswanger's disease
      - transependymal absorption of CSF (e.g. in active hydrocephalus)

89

► **Evaluation.** Deciding which of the following tests are needed to evaluate a patient with multiple intracranial lesions must be individualized for the appropriate clinical setting.

1. cardiac echo: to R/O SBE that could shed septic emboli
2. "metastatic workup" (p. 806) including:
   a) CT of chest/abdomen/pelvis with and without contrast: has become a relatively standard part of the metastatic workup. It has largely supplanted CXR, lower GI (barium enema) and IVP. Rationale:
      - Chest: R/O primary bronchogenic Ca or pulmonary metastases of another Ca. Can demonstrate mediastinal lymphadenopathy. Also to R/O pulmonary abscess that could shed septic emboli.
      - Assesses for possible primary lesions: e.g. kidneys, GI, prostate
      - Evaluates for metastases to liver, adrenal, and even spine.
   b) mammogram in women
   c) PSA in men

89.4 Ring-enhancing lesions on CT/MRI

89.4.1 Abscess vs. tumor

See ► Fig. 89.1 and ► Fig. 89.2. Tumor: the enhancing ring may be incomplete and irregular. Abscess: ring is usually complete, often thinner and smoother than with tumor. Abscess: usually brighter than tumor on DWI MRI.

MRS should theoretically be ideal for differentiating tumor from abscess (abscess should show reduced NAA, Cr and choline, and "atypical peaks" may be present), but in practice is often not conclusive.

89.4.2 Short list

Multiple lesions: metastases or abscess are much more likely than astrocytoma.

In adults, the main differential (short list) is:

1. High grade glioma (glioblastoma)
2. Metastasis
3. Abscess
4. Lymphoma should also always be tacked on as a possibility

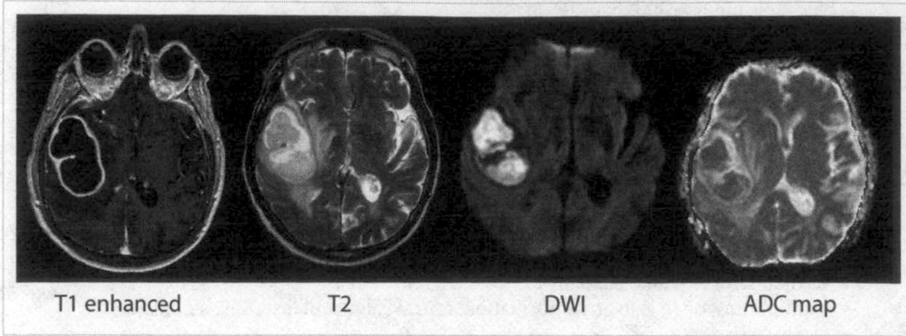

Fig. 89.1 MRI of right hemispheric cerebral *abscess* (bright on DWI)

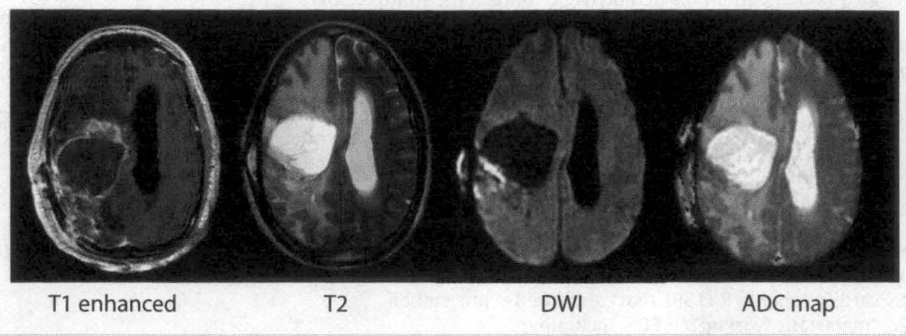

Fig. 89.2 MRI of right hemispheric *glioblastoma* (dark on DWI)

89.4.3 Long list

Mnemonic: "Magic Dr" (metastasis (including lymphoma), abscess, glioma, infarct, contusion, demyelination, radiation).

1. astrocytoma: usually glioblastoma multiforme
2. metastases (p. 800): especially lung
3. abscess (p. 320):
   a) may see visible growth over several days on serial imaging
   b) pyogenic abscesses are often (but not always) associated with fever and rapidly progressing neurologic deficit
   c) Nocardia abscesses (p. 335) are often *multiloculated* and are usually associated with a lung lesion
4. others
   a) lymphoma (primary brain lymphoma or metastatic systemic lymphoma): wall is thicker than abscess.[10] Incidence is increasing (p. 712)
   b) radiation necrosis
   c) resolving intracerebral hematoma: on T1 gradient echo sequence, a continuous ring suggests hematoma, an interrupted ring suggests malignancy
   d) cystic lesions with enhancing wall or mural nodule (see also intracranial cysts):
      - cysticercosis cyst, see Neurocysticercosis (p. 371)
      - hemangioblastoma
      - pilocytic astrocytoma
      - cystic acoustic neuroma
   e) trauma
   f) recent infarct
   g) thrombosed giant aneurysm

89.5 White matter lesions

89.5.1 Leukoencephalopathy

Disease largely confined to the white matter. Demyelinating disease cause most.

Appear as white matter low density on CT or low signal on T1WI MRI, and high-intensity on T2WI. Usually does not enhance. Unlike a stroke, changes tend to spare the cortex. Conditions such as metabolic derangements, leuko-araiosis, etc. tend to produce fairly symmetric findings.

Differential diagnosis:

1. anoxia/ischemia
2. demyelinating disease
   a) MS
   b) ADEM (p. 182)
3. intoxication: cyanide, organic solvents, carbon monoxide
4. vitamin deficiencies: B12 with subacute combined degeneration
5. infectious, especially viral:
   a) progressive multifocal leukoencephalopathy (PML) (p. 331)
   b) herpes varicella-zoster leukoencephalitis (p. 366)
   c) HIV infection (AIDS): perivascular pattern of demyelination
   d) cytomegalovirus infection
   e) Creutzfeldt-Jakob disease: small and perivascular demyelination
6. metabolic derangements: hyponatremia (p. 110), excessively rapid correction of hyponatremia (causing osmotic myelinolysis)
7. hereditary: metachromatic leukodystrophy, adult-onset Schilder's disease
8. leuko-araiosis (p. 1384)
9. multiple myeloma (p. 714)
10. low grade (WHO grade II infiltrating) glioma

89

89.5.2 Corpus callosum lesions

1. lymphoma
2. MS plaque
3. tumefactive demyelinating lesions (p. 181)
4. lipoma
5. diffuse axonal injury from trauma

89.6 Sellar, suprasellar and parasellar lesions

89.6.1 General information

May enlarge, erode or destroy the sella turcica. Considerations in adults (adenoma is the most common enhancing pituitary lesion) are different than for children (adenomas are rare, craniopharyngioma and germinoma are more common). Includes (modified[11]):

89.6.2 Tumors/pseudotumors

Tumors having epicenter within the sella

► **Pituitary tumor:**

1. adenohypophyseal tumors
   a) adenoma
      - microadenoma: < 1 cm diameter (p. 718)
      - macroadenoma: ≥ 1 cm diameter
      - invasive adenoma (p. 721): Includes aggressive tumors of Nelson's syndrome (p. 724)
   b) pituitary carcinoma or carcinosarcoma (p. 718)
2. neurohypophyseal tumors
   a) metastases: the most common tumor found in the posterior pituitary (presumably due to rich blood supply): breast and lung are most common primaries[12]
   b) pituicytoma (p. 728): the most common tumor arising from neurohypophysis/pituitary stalk (i.e. primary)
   c) astrocytoma: arising from stalk or posterior pituitary

► **Pituitary "pseudotumor":**

1. hyperplasia (enlargement)
   a) thyrotroph hyperplasia due to primary hypothyroidism[13] (see ► Table 46.2) causing chronic pituitary stimulation by TRH. Typically: free T4 low or normal, TSH ↑↑, symmetrical sellar mass on MRI
   b) gonadotroph hyperplasia: due to primary hypogonadism
   c) somatotroph hyperplasia: due to ectopic GH-RH secretion
   d) lactotroph hyperplasia: in pregnancy
2. pituitary enlargement may occur in intracranial hypotension (p. 391)
3. the pituitary gland of young women of childbearing potential is normally slightly enlarged

Juxtasellar or suprasellar tumors or masses: any of these lesions may extend into the sella

1. craniopharyngioma (p. 763): in this region, these account for 20% of tumors in adult, 54% in peds
2. Rathke cleft cyst (p. 756)
3. meningioma (parasellar, tuberculum sellae, or diaphragma sellae): to differentiate tuberculum sellae meningioma from pituitary macroadenoma on MRI (► Fig. 89.3), 3 characteristics of meningioma are: 1) bright homogeneous enhancement with gadolinium (c.f. heterogeneous, poor enhancement with macroadenoma), 2) suprasellar epicenter (vs. sellar), 3) tapered extension of intracranial dural base[14] (*dural tail*). Also, the *sella is usually not enlarged*, and even large suprasellar meningiomas rarely produce endocrine disturbances.[15] The pituitary stalk is sometimes seen being pushed posteriorly by a meningioma. Tuberculum sellae meningiomas may be associated with sphenoid pneumosinus dilatans[16] (enlargement of the underlying sphenoid sinus without bone erosion)
4. pituitary tumor (mostly adenomas) with extrasellar extension: tends to push carotids laterally (unlike meningioma which may encase carotid), more symmetric than meningioma
5. germ cell tumors (GCT) (p. 659): choriocarcinoma, germinoma, teratoma, embryonal carcinoma, endodermal sinus tumor. In females, suprasellar GCTs are more common; in males pineal region is more common
   a) *suprasellar* GCT: triad of diabetes insipidus, visual deficit and panhypopituitarism.[17] May also present with obstructive hydrocephalus
   b) simultaneous suprasellar and pineal lesions is diagnostic of GCT (so-called synchronous germ cell tumors (p. 659))
6. glioma
7. hypothalamic glioma
8. optic nerve or chiasm (optic glioma) (p. 631)
9. metastasis
10. chordoma
11. parasitic infections: cysticercosis
12. epidermoid cyst

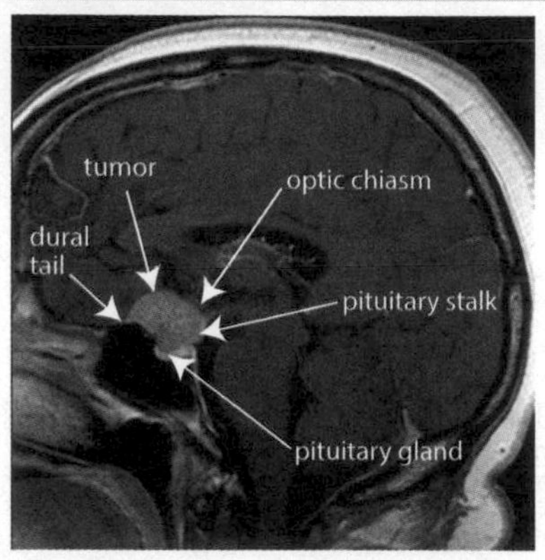

Fig. 89.3 Tuberculum sellae meningioma that could be mistaken for a pituitary adenoma. Contrast enhanced T1WI sagittal MRI

89

13. suprasellar arachnoid cyst: see Arachnoid cysts (p. 265)
14. sarcoidosis (p. 189): hypothalamic involvement is a more likely site as a cause of anterior and/or posterior pituitary insufficiency
15. bone abnormalities
    a) giant cell tumor (p. 794)
    b) chondromyxoid fibroma
    c) brown tumor of hyperparathyroidism
    d) bone spur
    e) extramedullary hematopoiesis[18]

89.6.3 Vascular lesions

a) aneurysm: ACoA, ICA (p. 1334) (cavernous carotid or suprasellar variant of superior hypophyseal artery aneurysm), ophthalmic, basilar bifurcation. Giant aneurysms may produce mass effect
b) carotid cavernous fistula (CCF) (p. 1256)

89.6.4 Inflammatory

a) (autoimmune) hypophysitis (see below):
    - distinguishing imaging characteristics are shown in ▶ Table 89.2
    - the most important clinical feature: pregnancy
    - the most important laboratory feature: diabetes insipidus (if DI is present, it is unlikely to be an adenoma)
b) pituitary granuloma[19]

89

89.6.5 Empty sella syndrome

1. primary (p. 773)
2. secondary: following pituitary tumor resection (p. 773)

89.6.6 Hypophysitis

AKA autoimmune hypophysitis (AH)

Two main forms:

1. lymphocytic (adeno)hypophysitis[20] AKA lymphoid adenohypophysitis: the more commonly encountered form. Inflammation of the pituitary stalk with lymphocytic infiltrate. Well established autoimmune etiology, although the antigens have not been identified. Primarily affects women in late pregnancy or early postpartum period
2. granulomatous hypophysitis: more aggressive. No gender bias. No association with pregnancy. May be autoimmune, but pathogenesis not definitely known

Table 89.2 Imaging characteristics of hypophysitis vs. adenoma[20]

Feature	Hypophysitis	Adenoma
Enlargement	symmetric	asymmetric
Pituitary stalk	thickened, nontapering	not thickened, tapering, deviated
Sellar floor[a]	spared	may be eroded
Enhancement	intense, may be heterogeneous	less intense, usually homogeneous
Mean size at time of presentation	3 cm^3	10 cm^3
Posterior pituitary bright spot[b]	lost	preserved in 97%

[a] on CT scan
[b] the normal hyperintensity of the posterior pituitary on T1WI MRI (p. 737) [21]

Because AH often mimics a nonsecretory pituitary macroadenoma (enhancing sellar mass on imaging, with negative endocrine tests), these lesions often undergo surgical resection instead of what may be more appropriate medical therapy (e.g. steroids,[22] or discontinuing possible offending agents such as ipilimumab[23]).

For distinguishing imaging characteristics, see ▶ Table 89.2.

89.7 Intracranial cysts

89.7.1 In general

Modified[24]:

1. arachnoid cysts (p. 265): Typically lined with meningothelial cells
2. suprasellar cyst from dilated third ventricle
3. interhemispheric cyst from porencephaly
4. neuroectodermal cysts (glioependymal cysts): intraparenchymal, located near ventricles
5. old infarct: if it communicates with ventricle it is called a porencephalic cyst
6. tumor cysts (the solid portion may sometimes be isodense to brain on CT):
   a) ganglioglioma (p. 652): usually solid but may appear cystic on CT
   b) pilocytic astrocytoma (p. 629): usually has enhancing mural nodule
   c) neurilemmomas may be cystic
   d) supratentorial ependymomas are often cystic (p. 643)
7. infectious
   a) abscess
   b) cysticercosis: see Neurocysticercosis (p. 371)
   c) hydatid cyst: see Echinococcosis (p. 375)
8. pineal cysts (p. 658)
9. colloid cyst (p. 756)
10. Rathke's cleft cyst (p. 756)
11. giant aneurysm
12. on CT, a low density non-enhancing tumor can mimic a cyst
13. chronic subdural hematoma or hygroma may mimic a cyst
14. posterior fossa: (for cysts of the CPA) (p. 1366). Includes:
    a) cyst associated with Dandy-Walker malformation (p. 256)
    b) epidermoid (p. 760)
    c) enlarged cisterna magna may mimic a cyst
    d) cerebellar hemangioblastoma: often has an enhancing mural nodule (p. 704)
    e) arachnoid cyst of posterior fossa
    f) neurenteric cyst (p. 290)
    g) pilocytic astrocytoma of the cerebellum (p. 629): usually has an enhancing mural nodule

89

89.7.2 Midline cavities

Three potential supratentorial midline cavities in the center of the brain and differentiating features are shown in ▶ Table 89.3.

Table 89.3 Features of midline brain cavities[25]

Cavity	Anatomy	Frequency	Clinical significance
cavum septum pellucidum (CSP) (see text)	located between leaflets of septum pellucidum	100% of preemies, 97% of newborns, 10% of adults	no known association with pathologic conditions
cavum vergae	directly posterior to, and often communicating with CSP	relatively uncommon	possible association with neurologic abnormalities[a]
cavum velum interpositum	due to separation of crura of fornix between thalami above the 3rd ventricle	present in 60% of children < 1 yr age, and in 30% between 1 and 10 yrs	no known association with pathologic conditions

[a]including developmental delay, macrocephaly, Apert's syndrome, abnormal EE

89.7.3 Cavum septum pellucidum (CSP)

AKA fifth ventricle, among others. A variable slit-like fluid-filled space between the leaflets of the left and right septum pellucidum. The compartment is usually isolated, although some communicate with third ventricle. The CSP is part of normal development, and persists until shortly after birth. Thus, it is present in ≈ all preemies. It is found in ≈ 10% of the adult population, usually representing an asymptomatic developmental anomaly. However, it is also commonly seen in boxers suffering from chronic traumatic encephalopathy (p. 924).

89.8 Orbital lesions

89.8.1 General information

4 compartments of the orbit:

1. ocular (AKA globe, AKA bulbar)
2. optic nerve sheath
3. intraconal
4. extraconal

CT remains a strong imaging modality within the orbit (less susceptible to motion artifact than MRI because of the speed, images bony structures to good advantage).

89.8.2 Orbital lesions in adults

Orbital pseudotumor is the most common.

1. neoplastic
   a) discrete tumors that may occur adjacent to but not envelope the optic nerve sheath
      - cavernous hemangioma: the most common *benign* primary intra-orbital neoplasm. Choroidal hemangioma is seen in Sturge-Weber syndrome
      - fibrohistiocytoma
      - hemangiopericytoma
   b) capillary hemangioma: produces infantile proptosis. Regresses spontaneously
   c) lymphangioma: produces infantile proptosis. Does *not* regress
   d) melanoma: the most common primary ocular malignancy of adulthood
   e) retinoblastoma: congenital, malignant primary retinal tumor. 40% are bilateral, 90% are calcified (often a key differentiating feature; does not portend benignity as with other lesions). CT may show retinal detachment
   f) lymphoma of the orbit: causes painless proptosis. The 3rd most common cause of proptosis
   g) intraorbital meningioma
   h) primary optic nerve tumors
      - optic glioma
      - optic nerve sheath tumor (schwannoma)
2. congenital
   a) Coats disease: telangiectatic vascular malformation of retina which leaks a lipid exudate causing retinal detachment. May mimic retinoblastoma. Vitreous is hyperintense on MRI on both T1WI and T2WI due to lipid
   b) persistent hyperplastic primary vitreous
   c) retinopathy of prematurity (retrolental fibroplasia)
3. infectious
   a) toxocara endophthalmitis
4. inflammatory/collagen vascular disease: usually bilateral
   a) scleritis
   b) pseudotumor of the orbit: the most common intraconal lesion. Usually unilateral (p. 569)
   c) sarcoidosis: usually affects the conjunctiva and lacrimal gland and spares connective tissues and intraorbital muscles
   d) Sjögren's syndrome
5. vascular
   a) enlargement of the superior orbital vein: may occur in thrombosis of cavernous sinus or in carotid-cavernous fistula
   b) dural AVM
6. miscellaneous
   a) drusen: degenerated retinal pigment cells in the posterior globe that may resemble calcified masses on CT

b) thyroid ophthalmopathy: Graves' disease (hyperthyroidism & swelling of EOMs → *painless* proptosis). 80% of cases are bilateral. The ophthalmopathy is independent of the level of thyroid hormone (possibly an autoimmune process). NB: a swollen inferior rectus muscle may resemble an orbital tumor if seen only on lower CT cut through the orbit
c) EOM enlargement can also occur with steroid use or occasionally with obesity
d) fibrous dysplasia

89.8.3 Orbital tumors in pediatrics

1. dermoid cyst: 37%. The most common lesion in children
2. hemangioma: 12%. Most regress spontaneously without surgery
3. rhabdomyosarcoma: 9%. The most common malignant tumor of the orbit
4. optic nerve glioma: 6%
5. lymphangioma: < 7%. Imaging resembles hemangioma. But will not regress spontantously, requires surgery. Proptosis may worsen after a URI. May bleed into itself (chocolate cysts)

89.9 Cavernous sinus lesions

Modified[26]:
1. primary tumors (rare)
   a) meningiomas[27]
   b) neurinomas
2. tumors from adjacent areas that may extend into cavernous sinus (head and neck cancers may track intracranially along cranial nerves, especially V)
   a) meningiomas
   b) neurinomas
   c) chordomas
   d) chondromas
   e) Chondrosarcomas
   f) pituitary tumors[28]
   g) nasopharyngeal carcinomas
   h) esthesioneuroblastomas
   i) nasopharyngeal angiofibromas
   j) metastatic tumors
3. inflammation: e.g. Tolosa-Hunt (p. 569)
4. infection: mucormycosis (phycomycosis) (p. 568). Usually in diabetics
5. vascular
   a) cavernous carotid aneurysm
   b) carotid-cavernous fistula (p. 1256)
   c) cavernous sinus thrombosis

89.10 Skull lesions

89.10.1 General information

The most common *benign* tumors of skull are osteoma and hemangioma. Osteogenic sarcoma is the most common *malignancy*. See also specific skull tumors (p. 775).

Evaluating roentgenographic skull lucencies

There is enough overlap of features to prevent any systematic means of determining the etiology of all or even most radiographic skull lucencies. The following features should be noted for any lucency, some are more helpful than others (modified[29]):
1. multiplicity (single or multiple?): except for multiple venous lakes, the presence of 6 or more defects is usually indicative of a malignancy
2. origin (intradiploic, full thickness, inner or outer table only):
   a) most vault lesions originate intradiploically, so limitation to this space may merely signify early recognition of a lesion
   b) expansion of the diploë with bulging of one or both tables almost always signifies a benign lesion
   c) full thickness lesions affecting both tables congruently usually indicates malignancy, whereas non-congruent erosion is more common with benign lesions

3. edges (smooth or ragged):
   a) smooth edges, whether regular, distinct or indistinct: no predictive value
   b) irregular margins (especially ragged undermined edges): more suggestive of infection (osteomyelitis) or malignancy
   c) sharply demarcated, full thickness punched out defects: suggest myeloma
4. presence of peripheral sclerosis: circumferential bony sclerosis suggests benignity (may indicate slow expansion and longstanding nature). The ring of sclerosis is generally narrow except in fibrous dysplasia
5. presence or absence of peripheral vascular channels: presence is highly suggestive of benign lesions (seen in ≈ 66% of venous lakes and ≈ 50% of hemangiomas)
6. pattern within the lucency:
   a) ✱ hemangiomas classically show *honeycomb* or *trabecular* pattern (seen in ≈ 50% of cases) or *sunburst* pattern (seen in ≈ 11% of cases)
   b) fibrous dysplasia may show well defined islands of bone, or a grossly mottled appearance with randomly arranged cystic and dense areas
7. location on the cranial vault (high vs. low): poor correlation with benign vs. malignant lesions
8. pain: Langerhans cell histiocytosis lesions are often *tender*

NB: keep in mind that skull lesions may have an intracranial component. CT scanning is good for assessing bone (MRI is poor for this), however, CT may miss small intracranial lesions tucked within the convexity of the calvaria due to bone hardening artifact (MRI has better sensitivity in this setting).

Nuclear bone scan may be a helpful adjunctive test (see specific lesion for findings).

Biopsy: indicated for questionable skull lesions. If the bone has not been destroyed by soft tissue, biopsy may be accomplished with a Craig needle, and the specimen may need decalcification by the pathologist before histologic evaluation can be completed.

89

89.10.2 Radiolucent lesion or bone defect in skull (AKA lytic lesions)

1. congenital or developmental
   a) epidermoid (cholesteatoma): *sclerotic* edge
   b) congenital: encephalocele, meningoencephalocele, dermal sinus
   c) fibrous dysplasia (p.779). A benign condition in which normal bone is replaced by fibrous connective tissue. Tends to occur higher in calvaria. 3 types:
      - cystic: widening of the diplöe usually with thinning of the outer table and little involvement of the inner table. Typically involves calvaria
      - sclerotic: usually involves skull base (especially sphenoid bone) and facial bones
      - mixed: appearance is similar to cystic type with patches of increased density within the lucent lesions
   d) hemangioma or AVM of bone or scalp
   e) pacchionian depression: arachnoid granulations (older terms: Pacchioni's granulation (after Italian anatomist Antonio Pacchioni) or pacchionian bodies) resorb CSF into vascular system and occasionally cause a bony lucency, usually near the superior sagittal sinus
   f) Albright's syndrome
   g) congenital foramina: "holes" in skull traversed by emissary veins
   h) parietal thinning: usually a bilateral process
   i) frontal fenestrae
   j) venous lakes
   k) cerebral herniations: AKA occipital pacchionian granulations
2. traumatic
   a) surgical defect: burr hole, craniectomy
   b) fracture
   c) post-traumatic leptomeningeal cyst (p.915)
   d) following trauma in children[30]
3. inflammatory
   a) osteomyelitis: including tuberculosis[31]
   b) sarcoidosis
   c) syphilis
4. neoplastic
   a) hemangioma: fine, honeycombed matrix. Classic x-ray finding: "starburst" appearance due to radiating bone spicules (may occur in as few as ≈ 11% of cases[29])
   b) intracranial tumor with erosion

c) lymphoma, leukemia
d) meningioma
e) metastasis: usually hot on bone scan
f) multiple myeloma, plasmacytoma (p. 714). Usually cool on bone scan
g) sarcoma or fibrosarcoma of bone
h) skin tumor with invasion (rodent ulcer)
i) neuroblastoma
j) lipoma
k) epidermoid (may also be considered congenital, thus also see above)

5. miscellaneous
   a) Langerhans cell histiocytosis (p. 777). Perfectly round *non-sclerotic* punched out lesion, may be single (formerly called eosinophilic granuloma) or multiple, tender
   b) Paget's disease (when seen as a zone of osteolysis without osteoblastic sclerosis on skull films, this is defined as osteoporosis circumscripta). Usually "hot" on bone scan
   c) aneurysmal bone cyst: rare. Arises in diploë and expands both tables which become thin but remain intact
   d) brown tumor of hyperparathyroidism

89.10.3 Diffuse demineralization or destruction of the skull

Includes "salt and pepper skull."

1. common
   a) hyperparathyroidism, primary or secondary
   b) metastatic carcinoma or neuroblastoma
   c) multiple myeloma
   d) osteoporosis
2. uncommon
   a) Paget's disease (osteoporosis circumscripta)

89

89.10.4 "Hair-On-End" appearance in skull

1. common
   a) congenital hemolytic anemia (e.g. thalassemia, sickle cell, hereditary spherocytosis, pyruvate kinase deficiency)
2. uncommon
   a) hemangioma
   b) cyanotic congenital heart disease (with secondary polycythemia)
   c) iron deficiency anemia
   d) metastases: especially neuroblastoma, thyroid carcinoma
   e) multiple myeloma
   f) meningioma
   g) osteosarcoma
   h) polycythemia vera

89.10.5 Diffuse increased density, hyperostosis, or calvarial thickening

1. common
   a) anemia (sickle cell, iron deficiency, thalassemia, hereditary spherocytosis)
   b) fibrous dysplasia
      - leontiasis ossea ("lion-like facies"): a form of polyostotic fibrous dysplasia
   c) hyperostosis interna generalisata
   d) osteoblastic metastases (especially prostate, breast)
   e) Paget's disease (begins with lytic zone and diploic thickening)
   f) treated hydrocephalus
2. uncommon
   a) chronic phenytoin therapy
   b) Engelman's disease (progressive diaphyseal dysplasia)
   c) fluorosis
   d) hypervitaminosis D
   e) hypoparathyroidism, pseudohypoparathyroidism
   f) meningioma

g) osteogenesis imperfecta
h) osteopetrosis (p. 1401)
i) secondary polycythemia
j) syphilitic osteitis
k) tuberous sclerosis

89.10.6 Focal increased density of skull base

1. common
   a) fibrous dysplasia
   b) meningioma
2. uncommon
   a) mastoiditis
   b) nasopharyngeal carcinoma
   c) osteoblastic metastasis
   d) osteoma of the outer table or diploe
   e) chondroma
   f) sarcoma of bone (e.g. osteosarcoma, chondrosarcoma)
   g) sphenoid sinusitis

89.10.7 Generalized increased density of skull base

1. common
   a) fibrous dysplasia
   b) Paget's disease
2. uncommon
   a) severe anemia (e.g. thalassemia, sickle cell)
   b) Engelman's disease (progressive diaphyseal dysplasia)
   c) fluorosis
   d) hyperparathyroidism, primary or secondary (treated)
   e) hypervitaminosis D
   f) idiopathic hypercalcemia
   g) meningioma
   h) osteopetrosis (p. 1401)

89.10.8 Localized increased density or hyperostosis of the calvaria

1. common
   a) anatomic variation (e.g. sutural sclerosis)
   b) fibrous dysplasia
   c) osteoma (p. 775)
   d) meningioma
   e) hyperostosis frontalis interna (p. 779)
   f) osteoblastic metastases (especially: prostate, breast)
   g) Paget's disease (begins with lytic zone and diploic thickening)
   h) cephalhematoma
   i) depressed skull fracture
2. uncommon
   a) osteosarcoma
   b) chronic osteomyelitis, tuberculosis
   c) tuberous sclerosis
   d) osteoid osteomas: radiolucent nidus with surrounding zone of dense sclerosis
   e) osteoblastoma:
   f) ossifying fibromas: predilection for frontotemporal region
   g) radiation necrosis

89.10.9 Pneumocele

Pneumocele: enlargement of an air sinus often with bone erosion. Pneumosinus dilatans (p. 1372) generally denotes enlargement of an air sinus *without* bone erosion, as may occur with tuberculum sellae or planum sphenoidale meningiomas.

Pneumoceles occur primarily in the maxillary antrum. Involvement of frontal sinus. usually involves pneumosinus dilatans. Etiology is unknown, and may involve a trap-valve mechanism, ruptured mucocele, or possibly congenital. May occur with fibrous dysplasia.

Presentation of pneumocele or pneumosinus dilatans:

1. headache
2. neuralgia
3. facial asymmetry
4. frontal bossing (with frontal pneumosinus dilatans)
5. exophthalmous
6. CSF fistula (leak)
7. Treatment for maxillary pneumocele: opening the sinus into the nasal cavity via endoscopic approach. Watch for encephalocele.

89.11 Combined intracranial/extracranial lesions

Lesion causing mass outside skull with intracranial component.

1. intra-axial: rule of thumb – "there is no intra-axial lesion that grows out of skull", however untreated fungating malignant gliomas may do this
2. extra-axial:
   a) meningioma
      - may arise in diploe, grows outward and inward
      - intracranial meningioma can grow through bone by destroying it
      - intracranial meningioma can induce hyperostosis that causes extracranial mass

89

   b) metastatic disease (e.g. GI carcinoma, and especially prostate Ca)
   c) bone (skull) lesion:
      - hemangioma
      - epidermoid
      - fibrous dysplasia (rare)
      - giant cell tumor (rare)
      - Ewing's sarcoma (rare in skull)
      - aneurysmal bone cyst (5% occur in skull, occipital bone most common)

89.12 Intracranial hyperdensities

I.e. Differential diagnosis of an intracranial structure that is hyperdense with respect to brain (i.e. appear "whiter" than brain) on non-contrast CT):

1. acute blood
2. calcium
3. vessels with low flow
4. melanoma: may be slightly hyperdense to brain due to melanin

89.13 Intracranial calcifications

89.13.1 Single intracranial calcifications

1. physiologic
   a) choroid plexus: calcifications usually bilateral (see below)
   b) arachnoid granulation
   c) diaphragma sellae
   d) dural (falcine, tentorial, sagittal sinus)
   e) habenular commissure
   f) petroclinoid or interclinoid ligaments
   g) pineal: 55% of patients > 20 yrs age have a calcified pineal gland visible on plain skull x-ray
2. infection
   a) cysticercosis cyst: single or multiple, see Neurocysticercosis (p. 371)
   b) encephalitis, meningitis, cerebral abscess (acute and healed)
   c) granuloma (torulosis and other fungi)
   d) hydatid cyst
   e) tuberculoma
   f) paragonimiasis
   g) rubella
   h) syphilitic gumma

3. vascular
   a) aneurysm, including:
      - vein of Galen aneurysm
      - giant aneurysm
   b) arteriosclerosis (especially carotid artery in siphon region)
   c) hemangioma, AVM, Sturge-Weber syndrome
4. neoplastic: calcifications usually suggest a more benign process
   a) meningioma (p. 690)
   b) craniopharyngioma
   c) choroid plexus papilloma
   d) ependymoma
   e) glioma (especially oligodendroglioma, also astrocytoma)
   f) ganglioglioma
   g) lipoma of corpus callosum
   h) pinealoma
   i) hamartoma of tuber cinereum
5. miscellaneous
   a) hematoma: ICH, EDH or SDH. Calcifications usually only when chronic
   b) idiopathic
   c) tuberous sclerosis (p. 606)

89.13.2 Multiple intracranial calcifications

1. common
   a) choroid plexus: the most common site for physiologic calcification (in lateral ventricles where it is usually bilateral and symmetric; rare in 3rd & 4th ventricles). Increases in frequency and extent with age (prevalence: 75% by 5th decade). Rare under age 3. Under age 10, consider possible choroid plexus papilloma. Involvement in the temporal horns is often associated with neurofibromatosis
   b) basal ganglia (BG): slight bilateral BG calcifications on CT are common, especially in the elderly. Considered a normal radiographic variant by some. They may be idiopathic, secondary to conditions such as hypoparathyroidism or long-term anticonvulsant use, or part of rare conditions such as Fahr's disease (see below). BG calcifications > 0.5 cm dia are possibly association with cognitive impairment and a high prevalence of psychiatric symptoms (including bipolar and obsessive-compulsive disorders, but no patients had schizophreniform disorders)[32]
2. uncommon
   a) Fahr's disease: progressive idiopathic calcification of medial portions of basal ganglia, sulcal depths of cerebral cortex, and dentate nuclei[33]
   b) hemangioma, AVM, Sturge-Weber syndrome, von Hippel-Lindau disease
   c) basal cell nevus syndrome (falx, tentorium)
   d) Gorlin's syndrome. Associated findings: mandibular cysts, rib and vertebral deformities, short metacarpals. Medulloblastoma seen in several patients
   e) deposition of calcium in the media of medium-sized blood vessels without compromise of the lumen. Usually asymptomatic. May become symptomatic by the time the involvement is significant enough to be visible on plain x-ray in a young person
   f) cytomegalic inclusion disease
   g) encephalitis (e.g. measles, chickenpox, neonatal herpes simplex)
   h) hematomas (SDH or EDH, chronic)
   i) neurofibromatosis (choroid plexi)
   j) toxoplasmosis
   k) tuberculomas; tuberculous meningitis (treated)
   l) tuberous sclerosis
   m) hypoparathyroidism (including post-thyroidectomy cases[34]) and pseudohypoparathyroidism
   n) multiple tumors (e.g. meningiomas, gliomas, metastases)
   o) cysticercosis cyst: may be single or multiple, see Neurocysticercosis (p. 371)

89.14 Intraventricular lesions

89.14.1 General information

Intraventricular tumors represent only ≈ 10% of CNS neoplasms. A clue to differentiating a tumor located within the ventricle from an intraparenchymal tumor invaginating into the ventricle is a "cap" of CSF surrounding an intraventricular tumor on CT or MRI.

89

89.14.2 Differential diagnosis

(Percentages quoted here are from a series of 73 patients with an intraventricular lesion on *CT* seen at UCSF[35]).

1. astrocytoma: (20%) the most common lesion. Hydrocephalus (HCP) is present in 73%. Hyperdense on non-contrast CT (NCCT) in 77%.
   Locations in descending order of frequency:
   a) frontal horn
   b) third ventricle
   c) atrium (AKA trigone)
   d) fourth ventricle
2. colloid cyst: (14%) essentially seen only in anterior third ventricle at foramen of Monro (other sites have been described but are exceedingly rare). 50% are hyperdense on NCCT. MRI appearance is variable, and may occasionally be missed. Little or no enhancement on CT/MRI (p.756). DDx includes xanthogranuloma
3. meningioma: (12%) most in atrium, rarely in frontal horn. All hyperdense with dense uniform enhancement. May be calcified. Most have dense tumor blush on angiogram, most supplied from anterior choroidal artery, posterior choroidal less common. Thought to arise from arachnoidal cells within the choroid plexus
4. ependymoma: (10%) most in 4th ventricle, may occur in body of lateral ventricle. Often hyperdense on CT because of high cellularity
5. craniopharyngioma: (7%) primarily in 3rd ventricle. Most have punctate calcification. Squamous epithelial rests in region of lamina terminalis are felt to give rise to this uncommon variety of craniopharyngioma
6. medulloblastoma: (5%) often fill 4th ventricle. Hyperdense on CT with homogeneous enhancement
7. cysticercosis: (5%) may involve any ventricle or may be panventricular (NB: incidence related to geographic location),
8. choroid plexus papilloma: (5%) most common in lateral ventricle (may be bilateral), but also may be seen in 4th and occasionally in 3rd. Non-obstructive HCP may occur (possible CSF overproduction). Intense blush on angiogram
9. epidermoid: (4%) mostly in 4th ventricle. Hypodense on CT with no enhancement (tend to follow CSF signal). The most common 4th ventricular low density lesion in the U.S.
10. dermoid: (3%) common in 4th ventricle. May see free floating fat in ventricles suggestive of cyst rupture. Tendency to form in midline
11. choroid plexus carcinoma: (3%) common in atrium of lateral ventricle. May extended into adjacent brain parenchyma with edema and shift. Intense blush on angio. NB: very rare lesion
12. subependymoma: (3%) 4th ventricle or frontal horn. Typically isodense on CT with *minimal enhancement*. May have calcification or cystic degeneration (more common in ependymoma). Most commonly in floor of 4th ventricle near obex
13. ependymal cyst: (3%) common in lateral ventricle. Absence of communication demonstrated by water soluble contrast cisternography
14. arachnoid cyst: (1%) lateral ventricle. Absence of communication demonstrated by water soluble contrast cisternography
15. arteriovenous malformation (AVM): (3%)
16. teratoma: (1%) Located in anterior 3rd ventricle. Partially calcified with foci of fat density. Marked enhancement
17. central neurocytoma (p.645)
18. metastases: breast and lung reported[36]
19. chordoid glioma of the 3rd ventricle[37]

89.14.3 Features to help identify type of intraventricular lesions

By location within ventricular system

▸ Table 89.4 shows the breakdown of lesion type by location within the ventricular system.

By location and age within lateral ventricle

See reference.[38]

See ▸ Table 89.5. This study excluded tumors that were clearly arising in the third ventricle or were predominantly parenchymal with intraventricular extension.

Table 89.4 Type of intraventricular lesions by location[35] (numbers are patients out of 73[a])

3rd ventricle		4th ventricle		Lateral ventricle					
				Atrium		Body		Frontal horn	
colloid cyst	10	medulloblast.	4	meningioma	8	ependymoma	3	astrocytoma	7
craniopharyng	5	ependymoma	4	astrocytoma	3	ch. plexus papil.[b]	1	meningioma	1
astrocytoma	4	epidermoid	3	ch. plexus papil.	1	ch. plexus carc.	1	subependym.	1
teratoma	1	cysticercosis	2	ch. plexus carc.	1	ependym. cyst	1	dermoid	1
ch. plexus papil.	1	astrocytoma	1	arachnoid cyst	1	AVM	1		
cysticercosis	1	subependym.	1	ependym. cyst	1				
dermoid	1								
ch. plexus carc.	1								
AVM	1								

[a]1 patient had cysticercosis diffusely throughout ventricles
[b] 1 patient with bilateral lateral ventricle papillomas

Table 89.5 Lateral ventricle tumor type by location & age

Age (yrs)	Location within lateral ventricle[a]		
	Foramen of Monro region	Trigone	Body
0–5	0	8 CPP	2 PNETs 1 teratoma
6–30	5 SEGAs 2 pilocytic astrocytomas 1 CPP 1 meningioma 1 oligodendroglioma	1 ependymoma 1 oligodendroglioma	1 mixed glioma 1 ependymoma 1 pilocytic astrocytoma
> 30	2 metastases	8 meningiomas	2 glioblastomas 1 lymphoma 1 metastasis 6 subependymomas

[a]abbreviations: CPP = choroid plexus papillomas, PNET = primitive neuroectodermal tumor, SEGA = subependymal giant cell astrocytoma

The teratoma and both PNETs occurred in age < 1 year, and all showed calcifications. Only one CPP occurred above age 5 years.

In adults > 30 years age, the only tumors found in the trigone were meningiomas. Subependymomas were the *only* nonenhancing tumor in this age group.

By location within third ventricle

1. anterior third ventricle
   a) colloid cyst
   b) sellar mass

c) sarcoidosis
d) aneurysm
e) hypothalamic glioma
f) histiocytosis
g) meningioma
h) optic glioma
2. posterior third ventricle
a) pinealoma (dysgerminoma)
b) meningioma
c) arachnoid cyst
d) vein of Galen aneurysm

By enhancement

All lesions enhanced except: cysts (ependymal and arachnoid), dermoids and epidermoids. There are differences of opinion of the tendency for subependymomas to enhance, Jelinek et al.[38] found that they did not.

By multiplicity

Multiple lesions are more suggestive of: neurocysticercosis, metastases, or ruptured epidermoid cyst.

89.15 Periventricular lesions

89.15.1 Periventricular solid enhancing lesions (in decreasing frequency)

1. lymphoma; CNS involvement from systemic, or rarely primary brain (p. 710): must be included in differential diagnosis of any solid enhancing periventricular brain tumor. Very radiosensitive.
2. ependymoma (usually invaginates)
3. metastatic Ca: especially malignant melanoma or choriocarcinoma
4. ventriculitis
5. medulloblastoma (in peds), AKA cerebellar sarcoma in adults
6. pineal tumor (dysgerminoma type): usually midline, young patient
7. occasionally, glioblastoma can present like this

89.15.2 Periventricular low density on CT, or high signal on T2WI MRI

1. increased extracellular or intracellular water content (edema)
   a) in hydrocephalus: transependymal CSF absorption (p. 399)
   b) necrosis from infarction
   c) edema from tumor
2. uncommon late variants of adrenoleukodystrophy
3. vascular disorders
   a) subacute arteriosclerotic encephalopathy (Binswanger's disease)[39,40]
   b) cerebral embolism
   c) vasculitis
   d) amyloid angiopathy
   e) low flow states
4. demyelination: including multiple sclerosis
5. leukoaraiosis[41]: a term coined to describe white matter disease with symmetric (or nearly so) periventricular white matter changes on CT or MRI. May be asymptomatic or may present with findings including dementia. May be related to:
   a) Binswanger's encephalopathy
   b) watershed infarction[42]
   c) normal aging[43]: increases each decade after age 60, usually patchy
   d) hypoxia
   e) hypoglycemia[44]
6. heterotopias: islands of grey matter in abnormal locations
7. following radiation therapy (XRT)

89.16 Meningeal thickening/enhancement

89.16.1 Dural enhancement

See reference.[45]

Visible beneath the inner table of the skull. Unlike leptomeningeal enhancement, does not follow the gyral convolutions. May be either focal or diffuse:

1. focal
   a) adjacent to meningioma: so called "dural tail"
   b) pleomorphic xanthoastrocytoma: also can have "dural tail"
2. diffuse dural enhancement[46]: associated with extraaxial neoplastic processes in ≈ 65%. Clinically: H/A, multiple cranial nerve palsies, seizures; may be indistinguishable from leptomeningeal metastases
   a) intracranial hypotension: diffuse pachymeningeal enhancement on cerebral MRI (p. 389)
   b) bacterial meningitis
   c) primary CNS tumors: medulloblastoma, malignant meningioma
   d) sarcoidosis
   e) following craniotomy
   f) metastases (mostly carcinomas):
      - bony mets to skull: present in 10 of 13 patients
      - dural metastases
      - leptomeningeal
   g) following subdural hemorrhage[47]

89

89.16.2 Leptomeningeal enhancement

See reference.[45]

1. thin linear enhancement that closely follows the gyri
2. small nodules attached to the brain

89.17 Ependymal and subependymal enhancement

Some overlap with periventricular enhancement. Ependymal enhancement often heralds a serious condition.[48] Main DDx is tumor vs. infectious process.

1. ventriculitis or ependymitis: ependymal enhancement occurs in 64% of cases of pyogenic ventriculitis.[49]
   a) Infection may occur in the following settings
      - following shunt surgery
      - after intraventricular surgery
      - with indwelling prosthetic devices (e.g. Ommaya reservoir)
      - with use of intrathecal chemotherapy
      - with meningitis
      - with viral ependymitis
      - in some cases of CMV encephalitis in immunocompromised patients
      - granulomatous involvement: esp. in immunocompromised patients; e.g. tuberculosis, mycobacterium, syphilis
   b) Infections may be[48]
      - bacterial (pyogenic) ventriculitis
      - tuberculous ventriculitis
      - cystic lesions suggest cysticercosis
2. carcinomatous meningitis: typically also produces meningeal enhancement (p. 812)
3. multiple sclerosis: usually more *peri*ventricular (in the white matter)
4. tumors
   a) lymphoproliferative disorders
      - CNS lymphoma (p. 710)
      - leukemia
   b) ependymoma
      - with tumor spread
      - transient enhancement reported in a child with ependymoma in the absence of tumor spread[50]
   c) Metastasis
   d) Germ cell tumors

5. tuberous sclerosis: subependymal hamartomas appear as nodules which occasionally enhance (p. 606). These gradually calcify with age
6. in the presence of appropriate constitutional symptoms: rare causes of linear enhancement include: neurosarcoidosis, Whipple's disease, metastatic multiple myeloma (usually nodular)

In immunocompromised patients, the enhancement pattern may help distinguish between the following (which tend to occur in this population[48]):
1. thin linear enhancement: suggests virus (CMV or varicella-zoster)
2. nodular enhancement: suggests CNS lymphoma
3. band enhancement: less specific (may occur with virus, lymphoma, or tuberculosis (TB))

89.18 Intraventricular hemorrhage

Etiologies:
1. most occur as a result of extension of intraparenchymal hemorrhages
   a) in the adult:
      - spontaneous ICH: especially thalamic or putaminal hemorrhages (p. 1336)
      - associated with AVM
   b) in newborns: extension of subependymal hemorrhage (p. 1346)
2. *pure* intraventricular hemorrhage (IVH) is usually the result of a rupture of
   a) aneurysm: accounts for ≈ 25% of IVH in adults, and is second only to extension of intracerebral hemorrhage as the most common cause. IVH occurs in 13–28% of ruptured aneurysms in clinical series.[51] More common with the following aneurysms: a-comm, distal basilar artery or carotid terminus, VA or distal PICA (p. 1192) (for patterns)
   b) vertebral artery dissection (or dissecting aneurysms) (p. 1323)
   c) intraventricular AVM
   d) intraventricular tumor
   e) SAH outside the ventricles refluxing into foramina of Luschka and/or Magendie

89

89.19 Medial temporal lobe lesions

May be responsible for seizures, especially "uncal fits" (temporal lobe seizures).
1. hamartoma
2. mesial temporal sclerosis (p. 441): should see atrophy of the parenchyma in this area with dilatation of the temporal horn of the lateral ventricle
3. glioma: may be low grade. Look for mass effect and possibly enhancement

89.20 Basal ganglion abnormalities

1. generally symmetric abnormalities
   a) calcification (p. 1381)
   b) Wilson's disease (hepatolenticular degeneration): autosomal recessive disease causing accumulation of copper in tissues
   c) Huntington's disease (or chorea): caused by > 40 trinucleotide CAG repeats in the Huntington gene (4p16.3) which leads to the production of the protein huntingtin. Cell loss in caudate nucleus can be seen on CT or MRI
   d) manganese: symmetrical high signal abnormalities on T1WI primarily in the globus pallidus with essentially no findings on T2WI or GRASS (almost pathognomonic) (p. 177)
   e) globus pallidus (low density on CT):
      - severe carbon monoxide intoxication
      - cyanide poisoning
      - hypoxia
   f) putamen
      - hypoglycemia: affects corpus striatum (caudate and putamen)
2. stroke

89.21 Thalamic lesions

Astrocytomas are the most common tumors.

1. Common neoplasms
   a) Adults
      - anaplastic astrocytoma
      - glioblastoma multiforme
      - metastasis
      - primary CNS lymphoma
   b) Pediatrics
      - anaplastic astrocytoma
      - astrocytoma (WHO grade II)
      - glioblastoma multiforme
      - pilocytic astrocytoma
2. Uncommon neoplasms
   a) Adults
      - astrocytoma (WHO grade II)
      - neurocytoma
      - oligodendroglioma
      - pilocytic astrocytoma
      - hamartoma
   b) Pediatrics
      - germinoma
      - oligodendroglioma
      - PNET
      - subependymal giant cell tumor
3. non-neoplastic (pediatric and adult)
   a) cavernous angioma
   b) granuloma
   c) heterotopias
   d) AVM
   e) infarct

89.22 Intranasal/intracranial lesions

Lesions within the nose that may communicate with the intracranial cavity:

1. infectious
   a) tuberculosis
   b) syphilis
   c) Hansen's disease (leprosy)
   d) fungal infections, especially:
      - aspergillosis
      - mucormycosis: seen primarily in diabetics or immunocompromised patients (p. 568)
      - Sporothrix schenckii
      - Coccidioides
   e) Wegener's granulomatosis (p. 199): necrotizing granulomatous vasculitis of the upper and lower respiratory tracts with glomerulonephritis and nasal destruction[52]
   f) lethal midline granuloma (p. 199): a locally destructive lymphomatoid infiltrative disease that may not have true granulomas, and may also cause local nasal destruction. However, renal and tracheal involvement do not occur as in Wegener's granulomatosis
   g) polymorphic reticulosis: may be a nasal lymphoma. Possibly the same disease as lethal midline granuloma (see above)
2. mucocele: a retention cyst of an air sinus that results from an occluded ostium and may cause expansive erosion of the involved sinus. Often enhances with IV contrast (MRI or CT), and may contain mucus or pus
3. neoplasms
   a) carcinoma of the nasal sinus
      - squamous cell
      - glandular
      - nasopharyngeal carcinomas: may be related to Epstein-Barr Virus (EBV) infection
      - sinonasal undifferentiated carcinoma (SNUC)[53]: distinct from lymphoepithelioma (less keratinizing). Rare, aggressive carcinoma (more lethal variant of squamous cell carcinoma) with poor prognosis. Incidence may be higher with prior XRT and in woodworkers and nickel factory workers. May invade adjacent structures, those relevant to neurosurgeons: frontal fossa, and cavernous sinus. No relation to EBV. Treatment: tri-modal therapy (XRT, chemotherapy and salvage surgery)

Table 89.6 Encephalocele vs. nasal glioma

Finding	Encephalocele	Nasal glioma
pulsatile?	frequently (may not be if small)	no
changes with Valsalva maneuver	swells (Furstenberg sign)	no change
presence of hypertelorism	suggests encephalocele	does not correlate
attachment to CNS	stalk	none, or minimal
probe	can be passed lateral	cannot be passed lateral

b) esthesioneuroblastoma[54] or aesthesioneuroblastoma AKA olfactory neuroblastoma: named for the stem cell of the olfactory epithelium (esthesioneuroblast). A malignant tumor arising from crest cells of the nasal vault, often with intracranial invasion. Very rare (≈ 200 reported cases). Presents with epistaxis (76%), nasal obstruction (71%), tearing (14%), pain (11%), diplopia, proptosis, anosmia and endocrinopathies.[55] Treatment: surgical resection followed by XRT, ± chemotherapy
c) metastatic tumors: very rare, possibly with renal cell carcinoma
d) benign tumors
   - frontal meningioma: rarely erodes into nasal cavity
   - rhabdomyoma
   - benign hemangiopericytoma
   - cholesteatoma
   - chordoma

89

4. congenital lesions
   a) **encephalocele** : a nasal polypoid mass in a *newborn* should be considered an encephalocele until proven otherwise. Classifications:
      - cranial vault
      - frontal ethmoidal
      - basal
      - posterior fossa
   b) nasal glioma: non-neoplastic glial tissue located within the nose, often conceptually and diagnostically confused with an encephalocele (▶ Table 89.6). The term "glioma" is a misnomer, and nasal glial heterotopia is preferred. Does not communicate with the subarachnoid space

References

[1] Ho VB, Smirniotopoulos JG, Murphy FM, Rushing EJ. Radiologic-Pathologic Correlation: Hemangioblastoma. AJNR. 1992; 13:1343–1352
[2] Laurent JP, Cheek WR. Brain Tumors in Children. J Pediatr Neurosci. 1985; 1:15–32
[3] Section of Pediatric Neurosurgery of the American Association of Neurological Surgeons. Pediatric Neurosurgery. New York 1982
[4] Inoue Y, Tabuchi T, Hakuba A, et al. Facial Nerve Neuromas: CT Findings. J Comput Assist Tomogr. 1987; 11:942–947
[5] Tew JM, Yeh HS, Miller GW, Shahbabian S. Intratemporal Schwannoma of the Facial Nerve. Neurosurgery. 1983; 13:186–188
[6] Enyon-Lewis NJ, Kitchen N, Scaravilli F, Brookes GB. Neurenteric Cyst of the Cerebellopontine Angle. Neurosurgery. 1998; 42:655–658
[7] George B, Lot G, Boissonnet H. Meningioma of the Foramen Magnum: A Series of 40 Cases. Surg Neurol. 1997; 47:371–379
[8] George B, Lot G, Velut S. Tumors of the Foramen Magnum. Neurochirurgie. 1993; 39:1–89
[9] Onofrio BM, Mih AD. Synovial Cysts of the Spine. Neurosurgery. 1988; 22:642–647
[10] O'Neill BP, Illig JJ. Primary Central Nervous System Lymphoma. Mayo Clin Proc. 1989; 64:1005–1020
[11] Davis DO. Sellar and Parasellar Lesions. Clin Neurosurg. 1970; 17:160–188
[12] Kovacs K. Metastatic cancer of the pituitary gland. Oncology. 1973; 27:533–542
[13] Atchison JA, Lee PA, Albright L. Reversible Suprasellar Pituitary Mass Secondary to Hypothyroidism. JAMA. 1989; 262:3175–3177
[14] Taylor SL, Barakos JA, Harsh GR, Wilson CB. Magnetic Resonance Imaging of Tuberculum Sellae Meningiomas: Preventing Preoperative Misdiagnosis as Pituitary Macroadenoma. Neurosurgery. 1992; 31:621–627
[15] Symon L, Rosenstein J. Surgical Management of Suprasellar Meningioma. J Neurosurg. 1984; 61:633–641
[16] Mai A, Karis J, Sivakumar K. Meningioma with pneumosinus dilatans. Neurology. 2003; 60
[17] Hoffman HJ, Ostubo H, Hendrick EB, et al. Intracranial Germ-Cell Tumors in Children. J Neurosurg. 1991; 74:545–551
[18] Aarabi B, Haghshenas M, Rakeii V. Visual failure caused by suprasellar extramedullary hematopoiesis in beta thalassemia: case report. Neurosurgery. 1998; 42:922–5; discussion 925-6
[19] Daniels DL, Williams AL, Thornton RS, et al. Differential Diagnosis of Intrasellar Tumors by Computed Tomography. Radiology. 1981; 141:697–701
[20] Gutenberg A, Larsen J, Lupi I, Rohde V, Caturegli P. A radiologic score to distinguish autoimmune hypophysitis from nonsecreting pituitary adenoma

preoperatively. AJNR Am J Neuroradiol. 2009; 30:1766–1772
[21] Kucharczyk W, Davis DO, Kelly WM, et al. Pituitary adenomas: high-resolution MR imaging at 1.5 T. Radiology. 1986; 161:761–765
[22] Miyake I, Takeuchi Y, Kuramoto T, et al. Autoimmune hypophysitis treated with intravenous glucocorticoid therapy. Intern Med. 2006; 45:1249–1252
[23] Carpenter KJ, Murtagh RD, Lilienfeld J, Weber J, Murtagh FR. Ipilimumab-induced hypophysitis: MR imaging findings. AJNR. 2009; 30:1751–1753
[24] Harsh GR, Edwards MSB, Wilson CB. Intracranial Arachnoid Cysts in Children. J Neurosurg. 1986; 64:835–842
[25] Miller ME, Kido D, Horner F. Cavum Vergae: Association With Neurologic Abnormality and Diagnosis by Magnetic Resonance Imaging. Arch Neurol. 1986; 43:821–823
[26] Sekhar LN, Moller AR. Operative Management of Tumors Involving the Cavernous Sinus. J Neurosurg. 1986; 64:879–889
[27] Knosp E, Perneczky A, Koos WT, et al. Meningiomas of the Space of the Cavernous Sinus. Neurosurgery. 1996; 38:434–444
[28] Knosp E, Steiner E, Kitz K, Matula C. Pituitary Adenomas with Invasion of the Cavernous Sinus Space: A Magnetic Resonance Imaging Classification Compared with Surgical Findings. Neurosurgery. 1993; 33:610–618
[29] Thomas JE, Baker HL. Assessment of Roentgenographic Lucencies of the Skull: A Systematic Approach. Neurology. 1975; 25:99–106
[30] Horning GW, Beatty RM. Osteolytic Skull Lesions Secondary to Trauma. J Neurosurg. 1990; 72:506–508
[31] Le Roux PD, Griffin GE, Marsh HT, Winn HR. Tuberculosis of the Skull - A Rare Condition: Case Report and Review of the Literature. Neurosurgery. 1990; 26:851–856
[32] Lopez-Villegas D, Kulisevsky J, Deus J, et al. Neuropsychological Alterations in Patients with Computed Tomography-Detected Basal Ganglia Calcification. Arch Neurol. 1996; 53:251–256
[33] Ang LC, Alport EC, Tchang S. Fahr's Disease Associated with Astrocytic Proliferation and Astrocytoma. Surg Neurol. 1993; 39:365–369
[34] Bhimani S, Sarwar M, Virapongse C, Freilich M. Computed Tomography of Cerebrovascular Calcifications in Postsurgical Hypoparathyroidism. J Comput Assist Tomogr. 1985; 9:121–124
[35] Morrison G, Sobel DF, Kelley WM, et al. Intraventricular Mass Lesions. Radiology. 1984; 153:435–442
[36] D'Angelo VA, Galarza M, Catapano D, et al. Lateral ventricle tumors: Surgical strategies according to tumor origin and development - a series of 72 cases. Neurosurgery. 2005; 56:ONS36–ONS45
[37] Brat DJ, Scheithauer BW, Staugaitis SM, Cortez SC, Brecher K, Burger PC. Third ventricular chordoid glioma: a distinct clinicopathologic entity. J Neuropathol Exp Neurol. 1998; 57:283–290
[38] Jelinek J, Smirniotopoulos JG, Parisi JE, et al. Lateral Ventricular Neoplasms of the Brain: Differential Diagnosis Based on Clinical, CT, and MR Findings. AJNR. 1990; 11:567–574
[39] Kinkel WR, Jacobs L, Polachini I, Bates V, et al. Subcortical Arteriosclerotic Encephalopathy (Binswanger's Disease). Arch Neurol. 1985; 42:951–959
[40] Roman GC. Senile Dementia of the Binswanger Type: A Vascular Form of Dementia in the Elderly. JAMA. 1987; 258:1782–1788
[41] Hachinski VC, Potter P, Merskey H. Leuko-Araiosis. Arch Neurol. 1987; 44:21–23
[42] Steingart A, Hachinski VC, Lau C, Fox AJ, et al. Cognitive and Neurologic Findings in Subjects With Diffuse White Matter Lucencies on Computed Tomographic Scan (Leuko-Araiosis). Arch Neurol. 1987; 44:32–35
[43] Zatz LM, Jernigan TL, Ahumada AJ. White Matter Changes in Cerebral Computed Tomography Related to Aging. J Comput Assist Tomogr. 1982; 6:19–23
[44] Janota I, Mirsen TR, Hachinski VC, Lee DH, et al. Neuropathologic Correlates of Leuko-Araiosis. Arch Neurol. 1989; 46:1124–1128
[45] Paakko E, Patronas NJ, Schellinger D. Meningeal Gd-DTPA enhancement in patients with malignancies. J Comput Assist Tomogr. 1990; 14:542–546
[46] River Y, Schwartz A, Gomori JM, Soffer D, Siegal T. Clinical significance of diffuse dural enhancement detected by magnetic resonance imaging. J Neurosurg. 1996; 85:777–783
[47] Sze G, Soletsky S, Bronen R, Krol G. MR Imaging of the Cranial Meninges with Emphasis on Contrast Enhancement and Meningeal Carcinomatosis. AJNR. 1989; 10:965–975
[48] Guerini H, Helie O, Leveque C, Adem C, Hauret L, Cordoliani YS. [Diagnosis of periventricular ependymal enhancement in MRI in adults]. J Neuroradiol. 2003; 30:46–56
[49] Fukui MB, Williams RL, Mudigonda S. CT and MR imaging features of pyogenic ventriculitis. AJNR Am J Neuroradiol. 2001; 22:1510–1516
[50] Butler WE, Khan A, Khan SA. Posterior fossa ependymoma with intense but transient disseminated enhancement but not metastasis. Pediatr Neurosurg. 2002; 37:27–31
[51] Mohr G, Ferguson G, Khan M, et al. Intraventricular Hemorrhage from Ruptured Aneurysm: Retrospective Analysis of 91 Cases. J Neurosurg. 1983; 58:482–487
[52] Brandwein S, Esdaile J, Danoff D, et al. Wegener's Granulomatosis: Clinical Features and Outcome in 13 Patients. Arch Intern Med. 1983; 143:476–479
[53] Jeng YM, Sung MT, Fang CL, Huang HY, Mao TL, Cheng W, Hsiao CH. Sinonasal undifferentiated carcinoma and nasopharyngeal-type undifferentiated carcinoma: two clinically, biologically, and histopathologically distinct entities. Am J Surg Pathol. 2002; 26:371–376
[54] Morita A, Ebersold MJ, Olsen KD, et al. Esthesioneuroblastoma: Prognosis and Management. Neurosurgery. 1993; 32:706–715
[55] Hlavac PJ, Henson SL, Popp AJ. Esthesioneuroblastoma: Advances in Diagnosis and Treatment. Contemp Neurosurg. 1998; 20:1–5

90 Differential Diagnosis by Location or Radiographic Finding – Spine

90.1 Diagnoses covered outside this chapter

Table 90.1 Differential diagnoses by location or radiographic finding, spine – covered outside this chapter

DDx
chordomas (p. 778)
lateral disc herniation (p. 1058)
spinal cord tumors (p. 783)
spinal epidural abscess (p. 350)
spinal stenosis
• lumbar (p. 1101)
synovial cyst (spinal) (p. 1144)
thoracic outlet syndrome (p. 554)

90.2 Atlantoaxial subluxation

1. incompetence of the transverse atlantal ligament (TAL): results in *increased* atlanto-dental interval (ADI) (p. 213)
   a) rheumatoid arthritis: erosion of insertion points of the TAL (p. 1134)
   b) traumatic
      - disruption (tear) of the TAL (rare)
      - avulsion of the insertion points of the TAL (as in comminuted C1 fx)
   c) congenital laxity of the TAL:
      - Down syndrome: 20% incidence (p. 1138) [1]
      - may be associated with neurofibromatosis
   d) retropharyngeal infections: chronic tonsillitis (p. 968), Grisel syndrome
   e) chronic steroid use
2. incompetence of the odontoid process: ADI is *normal*
   a) odontoid fractures (p. 978)
   b) os odontoideum (p. 981)
   c) erosion of the odontoid due to rheumatoid arthritis (RA) (p. 1134)
   d) neoplastic erosion of the odontoid:
      - metastases to the upper cervical spine (p. 815)
      - other tumors of the axis
   e) Morquio syndrome: hypoplasia of the dens (p. 1151)
   f) congenital absence/dysplasia of the odontoid
   g) following transoral odontoidectomy: creates severe ligamentous instability (p. 1472)
   h) local infection

► **Note.** Chronic AAS seen in conditions such as rheumatoid arthritis or Down syndrome may be significant yet asymptomatic. Treatment decisions in this group are difficult. Acute AAS is more commonly symptomatic and may be life threatening.

90.3 Abnormalities in vertebral bodies

See also lesions unique to the craniocervical junction & upper cervical spine (p. 1151).

For abnormalities unique to the axis (C2), see below.

1. neoplasms; see more extensive list (p. 542)
   a) metastases: prostate, breast, lung, renal cell, thyroid, lymphoma & myeloma commonly go to bone. Four patterns (≈ all are *low intensity* on T1WI):
      - focal lytic (most common): T1WI = hypointense, T2WI = hyperintense

- focal sclerotic: hypointense on T1WI and T2WI
- diffuse homogeneous: T1WI = hypointense, T2WI = hyperintense or heterogeneous
- diffuse heterogeneous: mixed signal intensities on T1WI & T2WI

b) primary bone tumors; see more extensive discussion (p. 792)
- vertebral hemangioma
- osteoblastoma

2. infection: osteomyelitis/discitis
3. fatty infiltrate or replacement of bone marrow: with age, hematopoietic red marrow of VBs is gradually replaced by yellow marrow in a splotchy pattern at a slower rate than in many other locations, e.g. distal appendicular bones.[2] T1WI: yellow marrow (MRI characteristics similar to subcutaneous fat) is hyperintense to red marrow (caution: bright areas on T1WI may be fat, or may be a normal area next to a low intensity met). T2WI: yellow marrow is bright
4. degenerative changes (Modic changes), see ▶ Table 68.2
5. metabolic
   a) Paget's disease: plain x-rays → enlargement of VBs with cortical thickening usually involving **several contiguous levels** (p. 1121)
   b) osteoporosis: reduced bone density. Vertebral compression fractures may be seen
   c) ankylosing spondylitis (p. 1123): osteoporotic VBs, calcified intervertebral discs (sparing the nucleus pulposus), and ossified ligaments, → square VBs with bridging syndesmophytes ("bamboo spine"). Starts in sacroiliac joints & lumbar spine

90.4 Axis (C2) vertebra lesions

1. tumors: rare. Possibilities include those that involve the spine at any location. Some factors pertinent to this location[3]:
   a) primary bone
      - chondroma
      - chondrosarcoma: rare in the craniovertebral junction. Lobulated tumors with calcified areas
      - chordoma: slow-growing radioresistant malignancy (p. 778)
      - osteochondroma (chondroma)
      - osteoblastoma (p. 792)
      - osteoid osteoma (p. 792): more common in posterior elements than VB[4]
      - giant-cell tumors of bone: typically arise in adolescence. Lytic with bony collapse[5]
   b) metastatic: including
      - typical metastases that spread hematogenously to bone, including: breast cancer, prostate cancer, malignant melanoma, paraganglioma, renal cell carcinoma
      - extension of regional tumors: nasopharyngeal tumors, craniopharyngioma
   c) miscellaneous
      - plasmacytoma
      - multiple myeloma
      - Langerhans cell histiocytosis: osteolytic defect with progressive vertebral collapse. Occasionally occur in C2[6]
      - Ewing's sarcoma: malignant. Peak incidence during 2nd decade of life
      - aneurysmal bone cyst[7]
2. infection: osteomyelitis of the axis
3. pannus from old nonunion of fracture or from rheumatoid arthritis (**RA**)
4. erosive changes in the odontoid process with RA (p. 1134)

90.5 Pathologic fractures of the spine

90.5.1 General information

Fractures due to metastatic involvement are hypointense on T1WI and hyperintense on T2WI. Benign VB collapse should be isointense to normal VBs on all sequences[8,9] and the VB should look homogeneous. On T2WI or STIR images, the cortex of the VB (which should be dark border around the VB due to low water content of cortical bone) should be intact.

90.5.2 Etiologies

1. osteoporosis
2. neoplasm: short list
   a) metastases: common sources of spine mets: lung, breast, prostate, myeloma

   b) Langerhans cell histiocytosis (p. 777): may cause vertebra plana (see below)
   c) lymphoma
   d) hemangioma (p. 794)
3. infection
4. avascular necrosis of the vertebral body
   a) Calve-Kummel-Verneuil disease (see below)
   b) with steroid use

90.5.3 Vertebra plana

Criteria:

1. uniform collapse of vertebral body into flat thin disc
2. increased density of vertebra
3. spares neural arches
4. normal disc and intervertebral disc space
5. intervertebral vacuum cleft sign (pathognomonic)
6. no kyphosis

Etiologies include:

1. Langerhans cell histiocytosis
2. Calve-Kummel-Verneuil disease: avascular necrosis of the vertebral body. Occurs in 2–15 year olds
3. hemangioma

90.6 Spinal epidural masses

See items marked with a dagger (†) under Myelopathy (p. 1407).

90.7 Destructive lesions of the spine

90.7.1 Etiologies

1. neoplastic; see Differential diagnosis: spine & spinal cord **tumors** (p. 783) for more:
   a) metastatic tumors with a predilection for bone: prostate, breast, renal cell, lymphoma, thyroid, lung…; see Spinal epidural metastases (p. 814)
   b) primary bone tumors: chordomas (p. 778), osteoid osteoma (p. 792), hemangioma (p. 794)
2. infection:
   a) vertebral osteomyelitis: occurs mostly in IV drug abusers, patients with diabetes mellitus, and hemodialysis patients. May have associated spinal epidural abscess. Also see Vertebral osteomyelitis (p. 353)
   b) Discitis (p. 356)
3. chronic renal failure: some patients develop a destructive spondyloarthropathy that resembles infection[10,11]
4. ankylosing spondylitis (p. 1123): bamboo spine (square VBs with bridging syndesmophytes)
5. lesions producing *posterior* scalloping of VB (mnemonic: AMEN)

A acromegaly or achondroplasia
M Marfan syndrome or mucopolysaccharidosis
E Ehlers-Danols
N neurofibromatosis
also: dural ectasia

1. lesions producing *anterior* scalloping of VB
   a) aortic aneurysm
   b) lymphoma
   c) spinal TB

90.7.2 Differentiating factors

Of the many lytic or destructive lesions that involve the vertebra, destruction of the disc space is highly suggestive of *infection* which often involves at least two adjacent vertebral levels. Although tumors may involve adjacent vertebral levels and cause collapse of disc height, the disc space is usually not destroyed[12] (possible exceptions include: some vertebral plasmacytomas, a reported metastatic cervical carcinoma, and there may occasionally be destruction of the disc in ankylosing spondylitis[13]). Unlike pyogenic infections, the disc may be relatively resistant to tuberculous involvement in Pott's disease.[14] Also, since metastatic tumor involvement usually produces widespread bony involvement, it is less likely with involvement of a single bone.

90.8 Vertebral hyperostosis

1. Paget's disease (p. 1120): classic "ivory bone" with cortical thickening ("picture frame" appearance on plain x-rays). Consider Paget's with a *dense* vertebra on x-ray in an older patient, commonly involving several contiguous vertebrae
2. osteoblastic metastases
   a) in men: prostate
   b) in women: breast
   c) lymphoma

90.9 Sacral lesions

Tumors:

1. metastases: the most common sacral neoplasm
2. primary neoplasms of the sacrum are uncommon and include:
   a) giant cell tumor (p. 1412)
   b) chordoma
   c) teratoma:
      - adults: pre-sacral or sacro-coccygeal teratomas may arise from cells sequestered from Hensen's node in the caudal embryo. Rarely cause neurologic involvement (distinguishing this from chordoma). Sacrum may be normal in up to 50% (abnormal in almost all chordomas). Treatment is complete removal usually by general surgeon
      - peds: malignant pre-sacral teratoma is a rare tumor seen primarily in female children

Infection:

Most infections of the sacrum or sacroiliac joint are due to contiguous spread from a suppurative focus

Arthritic disorders:

1. ankylosing spondylitis (p. 1124): involves SI joint almost by definition
2. osteoarthritis

Sacral fractures, may be due to:

1. trauma
2. repetitive stress
3. sacral insufficiency (p. 1415)

Congenital:

sacral agenesis (caudal regression syndrome): rare (prevalence: 0.005–0.01%; higher (0.1–0.2%) in children of diabetic mothers (16–20% of children with sacral agenesis have diabetic mothers)). Increased incidence of associated spinal abnormalities including: syrinx, tethered cord, lipoma, and lipomyelomeningocele.

1. Four types:
   a) Type 1: partial unilateral agenesis, localized to the sacrum or coccyx
   b) Type 2: partial bilaterally symmetric defects in the sacrum. Iliac bones articulate with S1, and distal segments of the sacrum and coccyx fail to develop
   c) Type 3: total sacral agenesis + iliac bones articulate with the lowest segment of the lumbar spine present
   d) Type 4: total sacral agenesis + iliac bones fused posteriorly along the midline
2. in cases of total sacral agenesis (types 3 & 4), MR findings include: absence of the sacrum and coccyx and variable absence of a portion of the lumbar spine, with a characteristic club-shaped configuration of the conus medullaris

Miscellaneous:

osteitis condensans ilii: increased density in ilium, usually asymptomatic (incidental) finding. Occasionally may produce low back pain or tenderness

90

90.10 Enhancing nerve roots

1. tumor
   a) meningeal carcinomatosis
   b) lymphoma
2. infection: especially CMV (often seen in AIDS patients)
3. inflammatory
   a) Guillain-Barre
   b) arachnoiditis
   c) sarcoid

90.11 Nodular enhancing lesions in the spinal canal

1. neurofibromatosis (NFT)
2. tumor
   a) drop mets
   b) neurofibroma
   c) schwannoma

90.12 Intraspinal cysts

1. spinal meningeal cysts (p. 1142)
2. cystic neurofibroma
3. ependymoma: may be cystic. In filum terminale: myxopapillary ependymoma (p. 789)
4. syringomyelia (p. 1144)
5. dilated central canal (p. 1144)

90.13 Diffuse enhancement of nerve roots/cauda equina

(As distinct from nodular enhancement, see above)
1. Guillain-Barre (p. 184)
2. meningitis
3. cytomegalovirus (CMV) (especially in AIDS)
4. lymphoma
5. sarcoid (look for hilar adenopathy)

References

[1] Martel W, Tishler JM. Observations on the spine in mongoloidism. Am J Roentgenol Radium Ther Nucl Med. 1966; 97:630–638

[2] Lakhkar BN, Aggarwal M, Jose J. Pictorial essay: MR appearances of osseous spine tumors. Indian J Radiol Imaging. 2002; 12:383–390

[3] Piper JG, Menezes AH. Management Strategies for Tumors of the Axis Vertebra. J Neurosurg. 1996; 84:543–551

[4] Molloy S, Saifuddin A, Allibone J, Taylor BA. Excision of an osteoid osteoma from the body of the axis through an anterior approach. Eur Spine J. 2002; 11:599–601

[5] Honma G, Murota K, Shiba R, et al. Mandible and Tongue-Splitting Approach for Giant Cell Tumor of Axis. Spine. 1989; 14:1204–1210

[6] Osenbach RK, Youngblood LA, Menezes AH. Atlanto-Axial Instability Secondary to Solitary Eosinophilic Granuloma of C2 in a 12-Year-Old Girl. Case Report. J Spinal Disord. 1990; 3:408–412

[7] Verbiest H, The Cervical Spine Research Society Editorial Committee. In: Benign Cervical Spine Tumors: Clinical Experience. The Cervical Spine. 2nd ed. Philadelphia: J.B. Lippincott; 1989:723–774

[8] Li KC, Poon PY. Sensitivity and specificity of MRI in detecting spinal cord compression and in distinguishing malignant from benign compression fractures of vertebrae. Magn Reson Imaging. 1988; 6:547–556

[9] Yuh WTC, Zachar CK, Barloon TJ, Sato Y, Sickels WJ. Vertebral compression fractures: distinction between benign and malignant causes with MR imaging . Radiology. 1989; 172:215–218

[10] Kuntz D, Naveau B, Bardin T, Druecke T, et al. Destructive spondyloarthropathy in hemodialyzed patients: A new syndrome. Arthritis Rheum. 1984; 27:369–375

[11] Alcalay M, Goupy M-C, Azais I, Bontoux D. Hemodialysis is not Essential for the Development of Destructive Spondyloarthropathy in Patients with Chronic Renal Failure. Arthritis Rheum. 1987; 30:1182–1186

[12] Borges LF. Case Records of the Massachusetts General Hospital: Case 24-1989. N Engl J Med. 1989; 320:1610–1618

[13] Cawley MD, Chalmers TM, Kellgren JH, Ball J. Destructive Lesions of Vertebral Bodies in Ankylosing Spondylitis. Ann Rheum Dis. 1972; 31:345–348

[14] Rothman RH, Simeone FA. The Spine. Philadelphia 1992

91 Differential Diagnosis (DDx) by Signs and Symptoms – Primarily Intracranial

91.1 Diagnoses covered outside this chapter

Table 91.1 Differential diagnoses by signs and symptoms, primarily intracranial – covered outside this chapter

DDx
abducens palsy (p. 567)
anisocoria (p. 561)
chordomas (p. 778)
chronic meningitis (p. 319)
coma (p. 297)
Creutzfeldt-Jakob disease (p. 370)
diabetes insipidus (p. 120)
dizziness (p. 572)
facial nerve palsy (Bell's palsy) (p. 576)
giant cell arteritis (p. 195)
gyral enhancement (p. 1281)
hemiplegia/hemiparesis – see spine section (p. 1414)
internuclear ophthalmoplegia (p. 565)
Menlere's disease (p. 573)
multiple sclerosis (p. 180)
ophthalmoplegia
• painful (p. 568)
• painless (p. 569)
papilledema (p. 558)
Parinaud's syndrome (p. 99)
Parkinson's disease (p. 177)
pneumocephalus (p. 887)
prolactin elevation (► Table 46.4)
pseudotumor cerebri (p. 770)
retinal hemorrhage (p. 916)
sarcoidosis (p. 191)
seizures
• new onset, adult (p. 461)
• new onset, peds (p. 462)
• nonepileptic (p. 464)

91

Table 91.1 continued

DDx
• status epilepticus (p. 470)
schizencephaly (p. 288)
torticollis (p. 1533)
trigeminal neuralgia (p. 481)
vertigo (p. 572)

91.2 Encephalopathy

Many etiologies are similar to that for coma (p. 297). EEG may be helpful in distinguishing some etiologies (p. 238).

1. a rare cause may be (spontaneous) intracranial hypotension (p. 389)
2. hypertensive encephalopathy from malignant hypertension

91.3 Syncope and apoplexy

91.3.1 General information

Syncope may be defined as one or more episodes of brief loss of consciousness (LOC) with prompt recovery (this term is considered by many to signify a vasovagal episode). The uncommonly used term lipothymia may be less likely to imply an etiology. Prevalence may be as high as ≈ 50% (higher in the elderly). Apoplexy is traditionally considered a form of hemorrhage, usually intracerebral. The recovery from apoplexy would therefore usually be slower than for syncope.

91.3.2 Etiologies

Adapted[1,2]). NB: in a large number of cases no cause can be determined.

1. vascular: a few myotonic jerks may be seen in cerebral ischemia
   a) cerebrovascular
      - subarachnoid hemorrhage (most commonly aneurysmal)
      - intracerebral hemorrhage
      - brain stem infarction
      - pituitary apoplexy (p. 720) (rare)
      - vertebrobasilar insufficiency (VBI) (p. 1305)
      - rarely with migraine
   b) cardiovascular
      - Stokes-Adams attacks: disorder of AV-node conduction in the heart resulting in syncope with bradycardia
      - carotid sinus syncope: minimal stimulation (e.g. tight shirt collar, syncope while shaving…) causes reflex bradycardia with hypotension, more common in patients with carotid vascular disease. Bedside carotid massage with ECG and BP monitor may diagnose[2]
      - cardiac standstill: seen rarely in patients with glossopharyngeal neuralgia (p. 492)
      - vasodepressor syncope (the common faint), AKA vasovagal response, and recently AKA neurocardiogenic syncope[3]: the most common cause of transient LOC. Hypotension usually with any of the following autonomic manifestations: pallor, nausea, heavy perspiration, pupillary dilatation, bradycardia, hyperventilation, salivation. Usually benign. Most common in age < 35 yrs
      - orthostatic hypotension: drop in SBP ≥ 25 mm Hg on standing
      - triggered syncope: includes micturition syncope, tussive syncope, weight lifting syncope… (most involve elevation of intrathoracic pressure)
2. infectious
   a) meningitis
   b) encephalitis
3. seizure (p. 443): in general, there are involuntary movements and confusion afterwards, lasts at least several minutes. Todd's paralysis may follow and usually resolves slowly over a period of a few hours. There may be irritative special-sense phenomena (visual, auditory, or olfactory hallucinations)
   a) generalized

b) complex partial
c) akinetic seizure
d) drop attack (loss of posture without LOC): seen in Lennox-Gastaut
4. metabolic: hypoglycemia (may produce seizure, usually generalized)
5. miscellaneous
a) intermittent ventricular obstruction: the classic example is a colloid cyst of the third ventricle (p. 756), but this mechanism is questionable
b) narcoleptic cataplexy: narcolepsy is characterized by somnolence and sudden attacks of weakness (cataplexy) when awake. Easy arousal and lack of post-ictal drowsiness distinguishes cataplexy from a seizure. The somnolence is treated with CNS stimulants (such as amphetamines or modafinil (Provigil®) 200 mg PO q AM), and cataplexy is treated with antidepressants
c) psychogenic
6. intracranial hypotension: usually with CSF shunt when upright (p. 389)
7. unknown: in ≈ 40% of cases no cause can be diagnosed

91.3.3 Practical approach to syncope

Introduction

The core of diagnosis and management are the H&P, orthostatic vital signs, and the ECG, with a combined diagnostic yield of 50%[4] covering:
1. reflex mediated such as vasovagal or valsalva/stress-induced: 36 -62%
2. cardiac valvular etiology or arrhythmia: 10–30%
3. orthostatic due to autonomic dysregulation, dehydration or polypharmacy: 2–24%
4. cerebrovascular due to stroke: ≈ 1%
5. seizure

Evaluation

1. history: includes
a) medication list: look for drugs that may cause orthostatic hypotension, especially blood pressure medication, beta blockers
b) precipitating factors: e.g. change in position, sensitivity to tight collars…
c) premonitory factors: e.g. sweating and tremulousness may signify hypoglycemia, bradycardia is associated with vasovagal events, tonic-clonic movements may occur with a seizure
d) post-ictal emergence: usually rapid after a simple faint, slower after seizure which may also exhibit Todd's paralysis (p. 443)
2. cardiovascular etiologies: Testing is also guided by H&P, vital signs & ECG:
a) cardiac arrhythmia evaluation: 12-lead ECG & 24-hour Holter monitor, and may lead to electrophysiologic (EP) testing/intervention[4,5]
b) abnormal orthostatics warrants a formal tilt-table test
c) history of cardiomyopathy or CAD merits an echocardiogram and formal stress testing. These results determine the need for cardiac catheterization
3. neurologic etiologies: comprise < 1% of cases.[6] In the absence of clinical evidence of a neurologic etiology, neurodiagnostic testing (EEG, CT scan, MRI/MRA, carotid doppler) have a diagnostic yield of 2–6%. ∴ These tests are warranted only when clinically indicated[5] (seizures, altered consciousness, gradually resolving Todd's paralysis, known history of cerebrovascular compromise). Tests include:
a) unenhanced brain CT: rules out most acute neurosurgical etiologies (bleed, hydrocephalus, edema which may be associated with tumor)
b) MRI without and with enhancement in cases with unexplained CT findings, or with a negative CT but high suspicion of a CNS etiology
c) seizure evaluation: when symptoms suggest possible seizure:
• EEG: usually a sleep deprived EEG. Not very sensitive
• 24 hour video EEG monitoring: in cases with high index of suspicion of seizures or nonepileptic seizures

Management

Admission and inpatient management is warranted for patients with diagnosed cardiac or neurologic syncope, either by suggestive history (family history of sudden death, syncope during exertion, witnessed seizure) or diagnostic testing (arrhythmia, severe orthostatic changes, hemodynamic instability).[4,7]

91

91.4 Transient neurologic deficit

For apoplexy, etc., see Syncope and apoplexy (p. 1396).

The first three etiologies listed below cover most cases of transient neurologic deficit:

1. transient ischemic attack (TIA) (p. 1264): temporary neurologic dysfunction as a result of ischemia. Maximum deficit usually at onset. Most resolve in < 20 mins
2. migraine: unlike TIA, tends to progress in a march-like fashion over several minutes. May or may not be followed by headache; see Migraine (p. 175)
3. seizure: may be followed by a Todd's paralysis (p. 443)
4. TIA-like syndrome
   a) "tumor TIA": a transient deficit in a patient with a tumor, may be clinically indistinguishable from an ischemic TIA. Intravascular lymphomatosis may mimic TIAs (p. 711)
   b) TIA-like symptoms may occur as a prodrome (p. 1336) to a lobar intracerebral hemorrhage[8,9] in cases of cerebral amyloid angiopathy (CAA). Unlike typical TIAs, these usually consist of numbness, tingling or weakness that gradually spreads in a manner reminiscent of a Jacksonian-march and may cross-over vascular territories. Caution: antiplatelet drugs and anticoagulation may increase the risk of hemorrhage in patients with CAA (p. 1334)
   c) chronic subdural hematoma: may cause recurrent TIA-like symptoms of the involved hemisphere[10] (including transient aphasia with dominant hemisphere involvement, hemisensory or motor abnormalities). The duration of symptoms tends to be longer than the typical TIA.[10] Postulated mechanisms include:
      - electrical basis: the possibility of epileptic activity due (e.g. due to irritation of the cortex by blood breakdown products) has not been supported in the literature; however, spreading depression of Leao has been considered[11]
      - impairment of venous outflow by compression of surface veins
      - compromised regional cerebral perfusion by indirect shifting of the anterior and posterior cerebral arteries[12]
      - transient ICP elevations → variations in cerebral perfusion pressure

91

91.5 Ataxia/balance difficulties

1. cerebellar origin: usually with involvement of UEs in addition to LEs
   a) cerebellar tumors
   b) cerebellar hemorrhage
   c) acute cerebellar ataxia: usually follows viral infection in a child < 3 years. Usually self-limited with good prognosis for complete recovery
2. spinal cord: usually worse with eyes closed (loss of proprioceptive input)
   a) spinal stenosis
   b) neoplastic cord compression
   c) syringomyelia (may be part of Chiari malformation)
3. degenerative
   a) ataxia-telangiectasia syndrome
   b) ataxia oculomotor apraxia
   c) Friedreich's ataxia
   d) spinocerebellar degeneration
4. metabolic/nutritional
   a) vitamin B12 deficiency
   b) drugs
      - AEDs (especially phenytoin or carbamazepine)
      - alcohol: acutely with intoxication and chronic
      - heavy metal poisoning
5. conditions that may mimic ataxia
   a) weakness
   b) peripheral neuropathy
   c) dizziness: including orthostatic hypotension; see Dizziness and vertigo (p. 572)
6. peripheral neuropathy:
   a) ataxia can occur with Guillain-Barré syndrome (p. 185), especially Miller Fisher variant (p. 186)
   b) balance difficulties are common with chronic immune demyelinating polyradiculoneuropathy (CIDP) (p. 186)

91.6 Diplopia

1. cranial nerve palsy of any one or combination of III, IV (rare), or VI
   a) for multiple cranial nerve palsies, below
   b) VI palsy (p. 567): can occur with increased intracranial pressure, e.g. in idiopathic intracranial hypertension (pseudotumor cerebri) (p. 766), sphenoid sinusitis…; see other causes of abducens palsy (p. 321)
   c) isolated muscle paresis of III suggests nuclear lesion or myasthenia gravis
2. intraorbital mass compressing extraocular muscles
   a) orbital pseudotumor (p. 569)
   b) meningioma
3. Graves' disease: hyperthyroidism + ophthalmopathy (p. 1375)
4. myasthenia gravis
5. giant cell arteritis (p. 196)
6. botulism: due to toxin from Clostridium botulinum (in adults: ingested or in wound). N/V, abdominal cramps, and diarrhea often precede neurologic symptoms. Neurologic involvement is typically symmetric. Dry mouth & cranial nerves palsies (diplopia, ptosis, loss of accommodation and pupillary light reflex) are followed by descending weakness. Bulbar paresis (dysarthria, dysphagia, dysphonia, flaccid facial muscles) follows. Muscles of the trunk/extremities and respiration progressively weaken in a descending fashion. Sensory disturbances are absent. Sensorium usually remains clear
7. following head trauma: includes injury to EOMs, orbital hematoma, VI palsy from increased ICP

91.7 Anosmia

1. abrupt onset of anosmia
   a) severe upper respiratory infection with damage to the neuroepithelium: the most common cause
   b) head trauma: second most common cause. Anosmia occurs in 7–15% of patients with significant head trauma
2. gradual onset of anosmia
   a) allergic rhinitis and sinus disease[13]: third most common cause of anosmia (anosmia in this setting may be intermittent)
   b) intracranial neoplasms: olfactory groove meningioma, see Foster Kennedy syndrome (p. 99), esthesioneuroblastoma (p. 1387)
   c) may also be associated with Alzheimer's disease
   d) olfactory sense diminishes with age: ≈ 50% of patients 65–85 years of age have some loss of sense of smell
   e) metabolic abnormalities: vitamin deficiency
   f) physical blockage of nasal passages: nasal polyps…
   g) endocrine abnormalities: diabetes…
   h) chemical: alcohol abuse, exposure to solvents,[14] cocaine (ischemic infarction of olfactory mucosa from vasoconstriction)
3. congenital anosmia: Kallmann syndrome (anosmia with hypogonadotrophic hypogonadism[15])

91.8 Multiple cranial nerve palsies (cranial neuropathies)

91.8.1 Framework

The differential diagnosis is legion. The following is a framework (modified[16]):

1. congenital
   a) Möbius syndrome: AKA congenital facial diplegia. Facial plegia is complete in ≈ 35% (in rest, affects upper face more than lower face, unlike central or peripheral facial palsy), associated with abducens palsy in 70%, external ophthalmoplegia in 25%, ptosis in 10%, lingual palsy in 18%
   b) congenital facial diplegia may be part of facioscapulohumeral or myotonic muscular dystrophy
2. infectious
   a) chronic meningitis:
      - spirochetal, fungal, mycoplasma, viral (including AIDS)
      - mycobacterial AKA tuberculous (TB) meningitis: 6th nerve involved first and most frequently. CSF shows lymphocytic pleocytosis and hypoglycorrhachia. Smears are usually negative and multiple cultures are needed to diagnose

91

b) stage II Lyme disease (p.576). Facial nerve weakness is common, sometimes bilateral (Lyme disease is the most common cause of facial diplegia in endemic areas). Other cranial nerve involvement is rare
c) neurosyphilis: rare nowadays except with AIDS. Diagnosed by serologic testing
d) fungal infection
 - cryptococcal meningitis (p.376): CSF analysis for cryptococcal antigen and India ink prep can detect
 - aspergillosis: may extend to the orbit from sinuses and involve cranial nerves
 - mucormycosis (phycomycosis) (p.1269): produces cavernous sinus syndrome, usually occurs in diabetics
e) cysticercosis: especially with basal form; see Neurocysticercosis (p.371)
3. traumatic: especially with basal skull fractures. Lower cranial nerve palsies may occur (sometimes delayed in onset) with occipital condyle fractures (p.966) or atlanto-occipital dislocation (p.963)
4. neoplastic (brain stem compression and intrinsic lesions usually also produce long tract findings early). Also see Jugular foramen syndromes (p.100)
a) chordoma (p.778)
b) sphenoid-ridge meningioma
c) neoplasms of the temporal bone (often in conjunction with chronic otitis media and otalgia): adenoid cystic carcinoma, adenocarcinoma, mucoepidermoid carcinoma
d) glomus jugulare tumors: often affects nerves IX, X, and XI. May cause pulsatile tinnitus; see Paraganglioma (p.652)
e) carcinomatous or lymphomatous meningitis (p.811): CSF pleocytosis and elevated protein. Palsies are painless or associated with diffuse headache. Sensory palsies are common, resulting in deafness and blindness
f) invasive pituitary adenomas involving the cavernous sinus (p.720): extraocular cranial neuropathies tend to develop after visual field deficits in these tumors, and are less common when compared to other intracavernous solid tumors[17]
g) primary CNS lymphoma (p.712)
h) multiple myeloma involving the skull base (p.714)
i) intrinsic brain stem tumors: gliomas, ependymoma, metastases…
5. vascular
a) aneurysm: intracranial or cavernous sinus (p.1225)
b) brain stem stroke: usually also produces long tract findings (p.99)
 - Weber's syndrome: Cr N III (usually pupil sparing) + contralateral hemiparesis
 - Millard-Gubler syndrome: Cr N VI + VII + contralateral hemiparesis
c) vasculitis: Wegener's granulomatosis usually affects eighth nerve in addition to others
6. granulomatous
a) sarcoidosis: ≈ 5% have CNS involvement, usually as fluctuating single or multiple cranial neuropathies (facial nerve is most common, and may be indistinguishable from Bell's palsy). CSF pleocytosis (p.200) is common
7. inflammatory
8. neuropathies
a) Guillain-Barré syndrome (GBS) (p.184): cranial nerve involvement includes facial diplegia, oropharyngeal paresis. Peripheral neuropathy usually presents with ascending weakness, proximal muscle weakness > distal, and absent deep tendon reflexes
b) Miller-Fisher variant GBS: ataxia, areflexia & ophthalmoplegia. Serum marker: anti-GQ1b antibodies
c) idiopathic cranial polyneuropathy: subacute onset of constant facial pain, usually retro-orbital. Frequently precedes sudden onset of cranial-nerve palsies usually involving III, IV & VI, less frequently V, VII, and lower nerves (IX through XII). Olfactory and auditory nerves usually spared. Acute and chronic inflammation of unknown etiology similar to Tolosa-Hunt and orbital pseudotumor. Steroids reduce pain and expedite recovery
9. entrapment in abnormal bone
a) hyperostosis cranialis interna: a rare autosomal dominant abnormality of the bone of the base of the skull causing recurrent facial palsy and other cranial nerve palsies[18]
b) osteopetrosis: see below
c) Paget's disease (p.1120) involving the skull: 8th nerve involvement (deafness) is most common. Optic nerve atrophy, and palsies of oculomotor, facial, IX, XI, olfactory nerves and others may also occur[19]
d) fibrous dysplasia (p.779)

91

91.8.2 Specific syndromes

Facial diplegia

Items culled from the above list that have facial diplegia (p. 576) as a prominent finding:
1. congenital: Möbius syndrome, congenital facial diplegia
2. infectious: Lyme disease
3. neuropathies: Guillain-Barré syndrome
4. isolated 4th ventricle (p. 576): compression at the facial colliculus
5. granulomatous: sarcoidosis

Cavernous sinus syndrome

Multiple cranial nerve palsies (involving any of the cavernous sinus cranial nerves: III, IV, V1, V2, VI) which primarily produce diplopia (due to ophthalmoplegia). Classically the third nerve palsy (e.g. from an enlarging cavernous carotid artery aneurysm) will *not* produce a dilated pupil because the sympathetics which dilate the pupil are also paralyzed.[20(p 1492)] Facial pain or altered facial sensation may occur.

See list of lesions that may produce cavernous sinus syndrome (p. 1376).

Osteopetrosis

AKA "marble bone disease" (there is also some confusion with the term osteosclerosis; osteosclerosis fragilis generalisata is the obsolete term for osteopetrosis). A rare group of genetic disorders of defective osteoclastic resorption of bone resulting in increased bone density, may be transmitted either as autosomal dominant or recessive.[21] The dominant form is usually benign and is seen in adults and adolescents. The recessive ("malignant") form is often associated with consanguinity, and is similar to hyperostosis cranialis interna (see above), but in addition to the proclivity for the skull, also involves ribs, clavicles, long bones, and pelvis (long-bone involvement results in destruction of marrow and subsequent anemia). Cranial nerves involved primarily include optic (optic atrophy and blindness are the most common neurologic manifestation), facial, and vestibulo-acoustic (with deafness), trigeminal nerve may also be involved. There may also be extensive intracranial calcifications, hydrocephalus, intracranial hemorrhage and seizures.

Bilateral optic nerve decompression via a supraorbital approach may improve or stabilize vision.[21]

91.9 Binocular blindness

▶ **Bilateral occipital lobe dysfunction:**
1. bilateral posterior cerebral artery flow impairment
   a) top of the basilar syndrome
   b) increased intracranial pressure
      - hydrocephalus with shunt malfunction
      - pseudotumor cerebri (idiopathic intracranial hypertension) (p. 768)
      - cryptococcal meningitis: decreased visual acuity (p. 376)
2. trauma: bilateral occipital lobe injury (e.g. contrecoup injury)

▶ **Seizures.** Epileptic blindness

▶ **Migraine.** Cortical spreading depression

▶ **Posterior ischemic optic neuropathy.** Usually in the setting of shock

▶ **Bilateral vitreous hemorrhage.** E.g. with SAH (Terson's syndrome)

▶ **Functional.** Conversion reaction, hysterical blindness…

91.10 Monocular blindness

Due to a lesion anterior to the optic chiasm.
1. Amaurosis fugax: often described as a "shade coming down" over one eye
   a) TIA: usually due to occlusion of the retinal artery (p. 1271)
   b) giant cell arteritis (GCA) (p. 195): usually due to ischemia of optic nerve or tracts (less commonly due to retinal artery occlusion)[22]

2. trauma: optic nerve injury
3. ruptured carotid cavernous aneurysm: resultant carotid cavernous fistula increases intraocular pressure by impeding venous return
4. intraorbital pathology: tumors
5. injury within the globe: retinal detachment, ocular trauma
6. unilateral vitreous hemorrhage: e.g. with SAH (Terson's syndrome)

91.11 Exophthalmos

91.11.1 General information

Alternate spelling: exophthalmus.

Definition: abnormal protrusion of the eyeball. Some authors reserve the term exophthalmos for cases due to endocrinopathies and use proptosis (of the eye) for other causes, but these terms are widely used interchangeably.

Criteria: different criteria are proposed. Anterior displacement of 18 mm (Hertal exophthalmometry can be used to measure clinically – requires intact lateral orbital bone). CT criteria: for most accurate results, the patient's should have their eyes open and fixated on a point in the primary gaze position. position of equator of the globe (widest part) is distal to a line drawn from lateral orbit to medial canthus, > 2/3 of the globe anterior to this line.

91.11.2 Pulsatile

1. carotid cavernous fistula (CCF) (p. 1256)
2. transmitted intracranial pulsation due to defect in orbital roof
   a) seen unilaterally e.g. in neurofibromatosis type 1 (p. 604)
   b) post-op following procedures that remove orbital roof or wall
3. vascular tumors

91

91.11.3 Non-pulsatile

1. tumor
   a) intraorbital tumor: may be due to mass effect from tumor or to compromised venous drainage from the orbit
      - optic glioma (p. 631)
      - optic sheath neuroma
      - lymphoma
      - optic sheath meningioma[23]
      - orbital involvement with multiple myeloma (p. 714)
      - orbital invasion by invasive pituitary adenoma (p. 771)
      - in peds: metastatic neuroblastoma
      - in peds: Langerhans cell histiocytosis (p. 777) as part of Hand-Schüller-Christian (triad: DI, exophthalmos and lytic bone lesions (particularly of cranium))
   b) due to hyperostosis from a sphenoid ridge meningioma
2. Graves' disease (hyperthyroidism + exophthalmos) (p. 1375): even though the exophthalmos is usually bilateral with this (80%), thyroid disease is still the most common cause of *unilateral* proptosis[24]
3. enlargement of periorbital fat[25]
4. infection: orbital cellulitis (usually has concomitant sinusitis)
5. inflammatory: orbital pseudotumor. Usually unilateral (p. 569)
6. hemorrhage
   a) traumatic
   b) spontaneous
7. 3rd nerve palsy: can cause up to 3 mm proptosis from relaxation of the rectus muscles
8. cavernous sinus occlusion (may affect both eyes)
   a) cavernous sinus thrombosis (p. 1309)
   b) cavernous sinus tumor obstructing venous outflow
9. pseudo-exophthalmos
   a) congenital macrophthalmos (bull's eye)
   b) lid retraction: e.g. in Graves' disease (p. 1403)
   c) coronal craniosynostosis can cause a "relative" proptosis (p. 253)

91.12 Ptosis

AKA blepharoptosis. Drooping of the upper eyelid.

Distinguished from pseudoptosis (lid droop not resulting from weakness of levator palpebrae superioris (LPS)) which can be due to enophthalmos (globe displaced posteriorly, e.g. with orbital floor blow-out fracture), microphthalmia, blepharospasm, Duane syndrome.

Etiologies of ptosis:

1. congenital: most are simple (autosomal dominant inheritance), complicated ptosis is associated with other findings (e.g. ptosis with ophthalmoplegia)
2. traumatic: injury to eyelid, orbital roof fracture…
3. neurogenic:
   a) third nerve palsy (p.565)
      - involvement of main trunk of third nerve: can occur intradurally or within cavernous sinus. Ptosis may be an early sign of pituitary tumor expansion (apoplexy) (p.720)
      - involvement of the superior division of the third nerve within the orbit
   b) Horner's syndrome (p.564): ptosis here is partial (may be a pseudoptosis since weakness is in tarsal muscles, not LPS), and the lower eyelid will higher than the uninvolved contralateral lower eyelid
4. myogenic ptosis
   a) botulinum toxin injection (e.g. Botox®)
   b) myasthenia gravis
5. mechanical ptosis
   a) tumors: neurofibroma, hemangioma, malignant melanoma, mets…
   b) extension of mucocele of frontal sinus
6. pharmacologic (drugs). Partial list:
   a) corticosteroids: including topical
   b) alcohol
   c) opium

91

91.13 Pathologic lid retraction

1. hyperthyroidism (p.1376)
2. psychiatric: schizophrenia…
3. steroids
4. Parinaud's syndrome (p.99)

91.14 Macrocephaly

Macrocephaly means increased size of the head.[26] Although sometimes used synonymously, some contend that the term macrocrania by convention refers to a head circumference > 98th percentile.[27(p 203)] Also, not to be confused with macrencephaly AKA megalencephaly (see below). In a pediatric practice the 3 most common etiologics in decreasing order of frequency: familial (parents have big heads), benign subdural fluid collections of infancy (p.904), and hydrocephalus.

1. with ventricular enlargement
   a) (hydrostatic) hydrocephalus (HCP), see for etiologies (p.394)
      - communicating
      - obstructive
   b) hydranencephaly (p.288)
   c) constitutional ventriculomegaly: ventricular enlargement of no known etiology with normal neurologic function
   d) hydrocephalus ex vacuo: loss of cerebral tissue (more often associated with *micro*cephaly, e.g. with TORCH infections)
   e) vein of Galen aneurysms: see below
2. with normal or mildly enlarged ventricles
   a) "external hydrocephalus": prominent subarachnoid spaces and basal cisterns; see External hydrocephalus (AKA benign external hydrocephalus) (p.400)
   b) subdural fluid
      - hematoma
      - hygroma
      - effusion benign and symptomatic
      - benign subdural collections of infancy (p.904)

c) cerebral edema: some consider this to be a form of pseudotumor cerebri[26]
   - toxic: e.g. lead encephalopathy (from chronic lead poisoning)
   - endocrine: hypoparathyroidism, galactosemia, hypophosphatasia, hypervitaminosis A, adrenal insufficiency…

d) familial (hereditary) macrocrania: parents also have large heads, the brains eventually "catch up"
e) idiopathic
f) megalencephaly (AKA macrencephaly): an enlarged brain (p.289)
g) neurocutaneous syndromes: usually due to increased volume of brain tissue (megalencephaly, see above).[26] Seen especially in neurofibromatosis and congenital hypermelanosis (Ito's syndrome). Less common in tuberous sclerosis and Sturge-Weber. Also seen in the rare hemimegalencephaly syndrome
h) arachnoid cyst (AKA subependymal or subarachnoid cyst)[26]: a duplication of the ependyma or arachnoid layer filled with CSF. Usually reach maximal size by 1 month of age and do not enlarge further. Treatment is required in ≈ 30% due to rapid enlargement or growth beyond first month. Cyst may be shunted or fenestrated. Prognosis with true arachnoid cyst is generally good (unlike porencephalic cyst) if no increased ICP or progressive macrocephaly during 1st year of life
i) arteriovenous malformation: especially vein of Galen "aneurysm" (p.1255). Auscultate for cranial bruit. With vein of Galen aneurysms, macrocephaly may be due to HCP from obstruction of the sylvian aqueduct.[26] With other malformations, macrocrania may be due to increased pressure in venous system without HCP
j) brain tumors without hydrocephalus: brain tumors are rare in infancy, and most cause obstructive HCP. Tumors that occasionally present without HCP includes astrocytomas. May also be seen in the rare diencephalic syndrome, see tumor of anterior hypothalamus (p.632)
k) "gigantism syndromes"
   - Soto's syndrome: associated with advanced bone age on x-ray, and multiple dysplastic features of face, skin and bones
   - exomphalomacroglossia-gigantism (EMG) syndrome: hypoglycemia (from abnormalities in islets of Langerhans), large birth weight, large umbilicus or umbilical hernia and macroglossia

91

l) "craniocerebral disproportion" (p.903) [26]: may be the same as benign extra-axial fluid of infancy
m) achondroplastic dwarf: cranial structures are enlarged but the skull base is small, giving rise to a prominent forehead and an OFC ≥ 97th percentile for age, hypoplasia of midface, and stenosis at foramen magnum. Head growth follows different curve than normal (OFC ≥ 97th percentile for age is not unusual and does not necessitate shunting)
n) Canavan's disease: AKA spongy degeneration of the brain, an autosomal recessive disease of infancy prevalent among Ashkenazi Jews. Produces symmetrical low attenuation of hemispheric white matter on CT[28] and macrocephaly
o) neurometabolic diseases: usually due to deposition of metabolic substances in the brain. Seen in Tay-Sachs gangliosidosis, Krabbe disease…

3. due to thickening of the skull
   a) anemia: e.g. thalassemia
   b) skull dysplasia: e.g. osteopetrosis (p.1401)

91.15 Tinnitus

91.15.1 General information

May be either subjective (heard only by patient) or objective (e.g. cranial bruit, can be heard by examiner as well, usually with a stethoscope place over the cranium, orbit, or carotid arteries in the neck). Objective tinnitus is almost always due to vascular turbulence (from increased flow or partial obstruction).

91.15.2 Pulsatile tinnitus

Most cases are due to vascular lesions.

1. pulse synchronous:
   a) carotid cavernous fistula (p.1256)

b) AVM:
   - cerebral (pial) AVM
   - dural AVM (p. 1251)
c) glomus jugulare tumor (p. 654)
d) cerebral aneurysm: (rare) possibly with turbulent flow in giant aneurysm
e) hypertension
f) hyperthyroidism
g) idiopathic intracranial hypertension (pseudotumor cerebri) (p. 766)
h) transmitted bruit: from heart (e.g. aortic stenosis), carotid artery stenosis (especially external carotid)
i) dehiscent jugular bulb or high riding jugular bulb: normal venous variant
j) rarely with posterior fossa tumors: CP-angle tumors e.g. vestibular schwannoma or meningioma, vascular intraparenchymal tumors e.g. hemangioblastoma (especially in CPA)
k) lesions that can present with a red tympanic membrane
   - aberrant carotid artery in middle ear
   - persistent stapedial artery: rare. Arises from aberrant ICA or from junction of horizontal and vertical petrous ICA. Foramen spinosum is absent on the affected side. Enlargement of anterior tympanic segment of seventh nerve canal
   - glomus tympanicum tumor (p. 654)
l) sigmoid sinus diverticulum

2. non pulse-synchronous: asymmetrical enlargement of sigmoid sinus and jugular vein may produce a low grade hum

Workup for pulsatile tinnitus:
1. MRI without and with enhancement: to look for tumors, e.g. glomus jugulare
2. angiogram: include internal and external carotid injections
3. tests that are usually *not* helpful and should not be ordered routinely
   a) carotid ultrasound: nonspecific, not sensitive
   b) MRI/MRV: may miss small dural fistulas and do not give details needed for treatment for large ones

91.15.3 Non-pulsatile tinnitus

1. occlusion of external ear: cerumen, foreign body
2. middle ear infection (otitis media)
3. otosclerosis
4. stapedial muscle spasms: as occurs in hemifacial spasm
5. CP-angle tumors: including vestibular schwannoma (p. 670)
6. Meniere's disease (p. 573)
7. labyrinthitis
8. endolymphatic sac tumors: e.g. as in von Hippel-Lindau disease (p. 705)
9. drugs
   a) salicylates: aspirin, bismuth subsalicylate (Pepto Bismol®)
   b) quinine
   c) aminoglycoside toxicity: streptomycin, tobramycin (tinnitus precedes hearing loss)

91.16 Facial sensory changes

1. circumoral paresthesias
   a) hypocalcemia
   b) syringobulbia
2. unilateral facial sensory changes
   a) trigeminal nerve neuroma
   b) vestibular schwannoma (VS): to involve Cr. N. V a VS has to be > 2 cm diameter; see symptoms from 5th nerve compression under vestibular schwannoma (p. 671)
   c) compression of the spinal trigeminal tract (large compressive lesions may cause bilateral alteration of facial sensation) that chiefly manifests in diminution of pain and temperature sense with little effect on touch sense.[29] The tract usually extends down into the spinal cord as far as ≈ the C2 vertebral level (although it may occasionally extend down to C4)

91.17 Language disturbance

1. aphasia:
   a) injury to speech areas of brain
      - Wernicke's aphasia (p. 98): classically produces *fluent* aphasia (normal sentence length & intonation, devoid of meaning)
      - Broca's aphasia (p. 98): faltering, dysarthric
      - conduction aphasia (p. 98): fluent spontaneous speech and paraphasias, but patients understand spoken or written words, and are aware of their deficit
   b) transitory aphasia following a seizure; see Todd's paralysis (p. 443)
   c) primary progressive aphasia of adulthood: idiopathic & degenerative
2. akinetic mutism: seen with bilateral frontal lobe dysfunction (e.g. with bilateral ACA distribution infarction due to vasospasm from a-comm aneurysm rupture or with large bilateral frontal lesions; may actually be abulia) or with bilateral cingulate gyrus lesions
3. muteness of cerebellar origin[30,31]
4. following transcallosal surgery: as a result of bilateral cingulate gyrus retraction or thalamic injury together with section of the midportion of the corpus callosum[32]

91

References

[1] Cardoso ER, Peterson EW. Pituitary Apoplexy: A Review. Neurosurgery. 1984; 14:363–373
[2] Kapoor WN. Evaluation and Management of the Patient with Syncope. JAMA. 1992; 268:2553–2560
[3] Barron SA, Rogovski Z, Hemli Y. Vagal Cardiovascular Reflexes in Young Persons with Syncope. Ann Intern Med. 1993; 118:943–946
[4] Miller TH, Kruse JE. Evaluation of syncope. Am Fam Physician. 2005; 72:1492–1500
[5] Linzer M, Yang EH, Estes NA, III, Wang P, Vorperian VR, Kapoor WN. Diagnosing syncope. Part 1: Value of history, physical examination, and electrocardiography. Clinical Efficacy Assessment Project of the American College of Physicians. Ann Intern Med. 1997; 126:989–996
[6] Sarasin FP, Louis-Simonet M, Carballo D, Slama S, Rajeswaran A, Metzger JT, Lovis C, Unger PF, Junod AF. Prospective evaluation of patients with syncope: a population-based study. Am J Med. 2001; 111:177–184
[7] Brignole M, Alboni P, Benditt D, Bergfeldt L, Blanc JJ, Bloch Thomsen PE, van Dijk JG, Fitzpatrick A, Hohnloser S, Janousek J, Kapoor W, Kenny RA, Kulakowski P, Moya A, Raviele A, Sutton R, Theodorakis G, Wieling W. Guidelines on management (diagnosis and treatment) of syncope. Eur Heart J. 2001; 22:1256–1306
[8] Smith DB, Hitchcock M, Philpot PJ. Cerebral Amyloid Angiopathy Presenting as Transient Ischemic Attacks: Case Report. J Neurosurg. 1985; 63:963–964
[9] Greenberg SM, Vonsattel JP, Stakes JW, Gruber M, Finklestein SP. The Clinical Spectrum of Cerebral Amyloid Angiopathy: Presentations without Lobar Hemorrhage. Neurology. 1993; 43:2073–2079
[10] Kaminski HJ, Hlavin ML, Likavec MJ, Schmidley JW. Transient Neurologic Deficit Caused by Chronic Subdural Hematoma. Am J Med. 1992; 92:698–700
[11] Moster M, Johnston D, Reinmuth O. Chronic Subdural Hematoma with Transient Neurologic Deficits: A Review of 15 Cases. Ann Neurol. 1983; 14:539–542
[12] McLaurin R. Contributions of Angiography to the Pathophysiology of Subdural Hematomas. Neurology. 1965; 15:866–873
[13] Apter AJ, Mott AE, Frank ME, Clive JM. Allergic rhinitis and olfactory loss. Ann Allergy Asthma Immunol. 1995; 75:311–316
[14] Emmett EA. Parosmia and hyposmia induced by solvent exposure. Br J Ind Med. 1976; 33:196–196
[15] Lieblich JM, Rogol AD, White BJ, Rosen SW. Syndrome of anosmia with hypogonadotropic hypogonadism (Kallmann syndrome): clinical and laboratory studies in 23 cases. Am J Med. 1982; 73:506–519
[16] Beal MF. Multiple Cranial-Nerve Palsies - A Diagnostic Challenge. N Engl J Med. 1990; 322:461–463
[17] Krisht AF. Giant Invasive Pituitary Adenomas. Contemp Neurosurg. 1999; 21:1–6
[18] Manni JJ, Scaf JJ, Huygen PLM, et al. Hyperostosis cranialis interna: A new hereditary syndrome with cranial-nerve entrapment. N Engl J Med. 1990; 322:450–454
[19] Chen J-R, Rhee RSC, Wallach S, et al. Neurologic Disturbances in Paget Disease of Bone: Response to Calcitonin. Neurology. 1979; 29:448–457
[20] Wilkins RH, Rengachary SS. Neurosurgery. New York 1985
[21] Al-Mefty O, Fox JL, Al-Rodhan N, Dew JH. Optic Nerve Decompression in Osteopetrosis. J Neurosurg. 1988; 68:80–84
[22] Salvarani C, Cantini F, Boiardi L, Hunder GG. Polymyalgia rheumatica and giant-cell arteritis. N Engl J Med. 2002; 347:261–271
[23] Clark WC, Theofilos CS, Fleming JC. Primary Optic Sheath Meningiomas: Report of Nine Cases. J Neurosurg. 1989; 70:37–40
[24] Gibson RD. Measurement of proptosis (exophthalmos) by computerised tomography. Australas Radiol. 1984; 28:9–11
[25] Peyster RG, Ginsberg F, Silber JH, Adler LP. Exophthalmos caused by excessive fat: CT volumetric analysis and differential diagnosis. AJR Am J Roentgenol. 1986; 146:459–464
[26] Strassburg HM. Macrocephaly is Not Always Due to Hydrocephalus. J Child Neurol. 1989; 4:S32–S40
[27] Section of Pediatric Neurosurgery of the American Association of Neurological Surgeons. Pediatric Neurosurgery. New York 1982
[28] Rushton AR, Shaywitz BA, Duncan CC, et al. Computed Tomography in the Diagnosis of Canavan's Disease. Ann Neurol. 1981; 10:57–60
[29] Carpenter MB. Core Text of Neuroanatomy. 2nd ed. Baltimore: Williams and Wilkins; 1978
[30] Rekate H, Grubb R, Aram D, et al. Muteness of Cerebellar Origin. Arch Neurol. 1985; 42:637–638
[31] Ammirati M, Mirzai S, Samii M. Transient Mutism Following Removal of a Cerebellar Tumor: A Case Report and Review of the Literature. Childs Nerv Syst. 1989; 5:12–14
[32] Apuzzo MLJ. Surgery of Masses Affecting the Third Ventricular Chamber: Techniques and Strategies. Clin Neurosurg. 1988; 34:499–522

92 Differential Diagnosis (DDx) by Signs and Symptoms – Primarily Spine and Other

92.1 Diagnoses covered outside this chapter

Table 92.1 Differential diagnoses by signs and symptoms, spine and other – covered outside this chapter

DDx
ankylosing spondylitis (p. 1125)
bladder dysfunction (p. 92)
brachial plexopathy (p. 542)
carpal tunnel syndrome (p. 521)
cervical stenosis (p. 1086)
lateral disc herniation (p. 1059)
meralgia paresthetica (p. 534)
myopathy
spinal cord tumors (p. 783)
spinal epidural abscess (p. 349)
spinal stenosis • lumbar (p. 1101)
synovial cyst (spinal) (p. 1144)
thoracic outlet syndrome (p. 554)
torticollis (p. 1533)
urinary retention (p. 94)

92

92.2 Myelopathy

Items marked with a dagger (†) may present as a *spinal epidural mass.*

► **Congenital:**
1. (Arnold)-Chiari malformation (p. 284): Type I often presents in early adulthood
2. tethered cord: often may not present until after some trauma
3. syringomyelia: may be congenital or post-traumatic in quadriplegics, usually presents with a central cord syndrome – see Syringomyelia (p. 1144) – or progressive myelopathy
4. neurenteric cyst (p. 290)
5. cord compression that occurs with some mucopolysaccharidoses: e.g. Morquio syndrome (due to atlanto-axial subluxation), Hurler syndrome
6. hereditary spastic paraplegia: family history is key. Diagnosis of exclusion[1]

► **Acquired:**
1. cervical or thoracic spinal stenosis: often degenerative disease superimposed on congenitally narrow canal (congenital narrowing is frequent in achondroplastic dwarfs)
2. traumatic: including spinal shock, hematomyelia, spinal epidural hematoma (see vascular below), barotrauma, electrical injuries, compression by bone fracture†. May follow minor trauma in the setting of spinal stenosis
3. herniated intervertebral disc†: myelopathy more common in thoracic region, radiculopathy more common in cervical region (long tract signs are rare with herniated cervical disc)
4. kyphosis

5. extramedullary hematopoiesis† (p. 171): hypertrophy of marrow → cord compression. Primarily in chronic anemias (e.g. thalassemia major)
6. bony compression secondary to incompetence of odontoid process or transverse atlantal ligament†. May be congenital, traumatic (p. 978), neoplastic, or inflammatory (especially rheumatoid arthritis)
7. epidural lipomatosis† (p. 1150): hypertrophy of epidural fat most often due to years of exogenous steroid therapy[2]
8. ossification of the posterior longitudinal ligament (OPLL) (p. 1127)[3]
9. arachnoiditis ossificans: a rare condition (only ≈ 43 case reports as of 1998[4]) involving calcification of the arachnoid membrane. In the T-spine, may occur as ossified plaques or in a cylindrical form surrounding the spinal cord. May be difficult to detect on MRI and myelography. Plain unenhanced CT may be optimal for diagnosis
10. vertebral Paget's disease† (p. 1120)
11. idiopathic spinal cord herniation (p. 1150)[5,6]: rare. Thoracic spinal cord herniates through an anterior dural defect frequently producing a Brown-Séquard syndrome or spastic paraparesis

► **Neoplastic:**
1. spine/spinal cord tumors† (p. 783) (for details)
   a) extradural (55%):
      - primary tumors (rare) include: neurofibromas, chordomas, osteoid osteoma, aneurysmal bone cyst, vertebral hemangioma[7]
      - if age > 40 yrs, suspect extradural lymphoma (primary or secondary) or leukemic deposits (chloroma), especially with pre-existing diagnosis of hematopoietic or lymphatic disorder
      - epidural metastases (p. 814) become increasingly common after age 50 yrs. Occurs in up to 10% of cancer patients. 5–10% of malignancies present initially with cord compression
   b) intradural-extramedullary (40%): meningiomas, neurofibromas
   c) intradural-intramedullary: primary cord tumors (p. 784) (ependymoma, astrocytoma) and rarely intramedullary mets
2. carcinomatous meningitis (p. 811): neurologic deficit usually cannot be localized to a single level
3. paraneoplastic syndrome (p. 542): including effects on spinal cord or on peripheral nerves

92

► **Vascular:**
1. hematoma/hemorrhage
   a) spinal epidural hematoma† (p. 1131): usually associated with anticoagulation therapy[8]
      - traumatic: following LP or epidural anesthesia (p. 1131)
      - spontaneous[9]: rare. Includes hemorrhage from spinal cord AVM (p. 1131) or from vertebral hemangioma (p. 1140)
   b) spinal subarachnoid hemorrhage: as in spinal epidural hematoma (p. 165), this may also be post-traumatic (e.g. following LP[10,11]) or secondary to spinal cord AVM
   c) spinal subdural hematoma
   d) hematomyelia
2. spinal cord infarction: uncommon with the elimination of syphilitic endarteritis. Most often in the territory of the anterior spinal artery, sparing posterior columns. Most commonly ≈ T4 level (watershed zone)
   a) atherosclerosis of radicular artery in elderly patient with hypotension is now the major cause of this rare condition
   b) clamping aorta during surgery (e.g. for abdominal aortic aneurysm)
   c) hypotension (relative or absolute) during surgery in the sitting position in the presence of spinal stenosis.[12] May be improved by avoiding absolute hypotension, using awake fiber-optic intubation and positioning, intraoperative SSEP monitoring and inducing hypertension if changes occur with positioning, avoidance of sitting position, and avoiding hyperflexion, hyperextension and traction
   d) aortic dissection
   e) embolization of spinal arteries
3. spinal cord vascular malformations† (p. 1140): 10–20% present as sudden onset of myelopathy usually in patients < 30 yrs,[13] myelopathy may be secondary to:
   a) mass effect from AVM: spinal AVMs account for < 5% of lesions presenting as cord "tumors"
   b) rupture → SAH, hematomyelia, or epidural hematoma
   c) watershed infarction due to "steal"
   d) spontaneous thrombosis (necrotizing myelopathy of Foix-Alajouanine disease (p. 1141)[14]): presents as spastic → flaccid paraplegia, with ascending sensory level
4. radiation myelopathy: due to microvascular occlusion (p. 1563)

5. secondary to iodinated contrast material used for mesenteric or aortic angiography. Especially when angiogrammed in presence of hypotension, where cardiac output is shunted away from viscera and into spinal radicular arteries. Treatment: place patient sitting, remove ≥ 100 ml of CSF via LP and replace with equal amount of saline over 30 mins[15]

► **Autoimmune:**

1. post-viral (or post-vaccination): may actually be etiology of auto-immune process (i.e. transverse myelitis). Viral prodrome present in ≈ 37% of cases of ATM. Viral infection is usually most damaging to gray matter (e.g. poliomyelitis)

► **Demyelinating:**

1. acute (idiopathic) transverse myelitis (ATM) (p. 187). Peak incidence during first 2 decades of life. Abrupt onset of LE weakness, sensory loss, back pain, and sphincter disturbance indistinguishable from spinal cord compression. Thoracic region most common. CT and myelogram are normal. MRI may demonstrate. CSF → pleocytosis and hyperproteinemia
2. multiple sclerosis (**MS**): diagnosed in only 7% of patients presenting as acute transverse myelopathy. Although more common in young adults, MS can occur at any time in life. Myelopathy of MS is usually insidious, and is usually incomplete (i.e. some sparing). Affects myelin, thus sparing gray matter. Abdominal cutaneous reflexes are almost always absent in MS
3. **Devic syndrome** (neuromyelitis optica (NMO)): a variant of MS characterized by acute bilateral optic neuritis and transverse myelitis (extending ≥ 3 levels,[16] often causing cervical myelopathy). Spinal cord edema may become so severe as to cause complete block on myelography. More common in Asia and India than U.S. or Europe. Compared to classic MS: the myelopathy tends to be more severe (pathology: more necrosis as opposed to incomplete demyelination) and with less chance of recovery. Distinct serum IgG antibodies (NMO-IgG) may help differentiate from MS[17]

► **Metabolic/toxic:**

1. (subacute) combined system disease (CSD) (AKA subacute combined columnal degeneration): due to vitamin B12 (cyanocobalamin) deficiency.
   a) etiologies:
      - dietary deficiency of B12 (B12 is a water soluble vitamin present in meats and animal products)
      - pernicious anemia: intestinal malabsorption of B12 in the distal ileum due to lack of secretion of intrinsic factor (a small polypeptide) by gastric parietal cells[18])
      - other gastric disorders: low gastric pH e.g. in Zollinger-Ellison syndrome can inhibit attachment of intrinsic factor to ileal receptors
2. clinical: onset is gradual and uniform. Begins with symmetrical paresthesias in feet or hands (posterior column involvement) → leg stiffness, weakness, and proprioceptive deficits with unsteadiness that is worse in the dark → spasticity → paraplegia → bowel and bladder dysfunction. Dementia (confusion, memory impairment, irritability…) occurs in advanced cases due to cerebral white matter changes. Visual disturbances with or without optic atrophy may be due to optic nerve demyelination
3. labs:
   a) serum B12: the most sensitive test. However, normal B12 levels do not R/O B12 deficiency. If there are neurologic symptoms then check malonic acid or other markers of B12 deficiency such as methylmalonic acid (also check homocysteine to R/O folate deficiency)
   b) CBC: most (but not all) patients will have a *macrocytic* (megalocytic) anemia (folic acid deficiency also produces megaloblastic anemia. Folic acid corrects the anemia, even with CSD, but *not* the neurologic deficits which may actually worsen)
   c) **Schilling test**: determines the cause of the B12 deficiency even if B12 injections have already been given (radiolabeled cyanocobalamin is given orally, followed by a parenteral flushing dose of nonradioactive vitamin, and the percentage of radioactivity is measured in the urine over 24 hours, performed once without and then once with added intrinsic factor, and then once following antibiotic therapy)
4. imaging: T2WI MRI may demonstrate increased signal within the white matter of the spinal cord, predominantly in the posterior columns but may also be seen in spinothalamic tracts
5. treatment: B12 injections q 1–3 months or large doses of oral preparations[19] (other transport systems independent of intrinsic factor results in absorption of ≈ 1% of orally administered B12, doses of 300–100,000 mcg result in absorption of more than the daily requirement of 1–2.5 mcg)
6. toxins: e.g. local anesthetics used for spinal anesthesia rarely cause myelopathy

92

▶ **Infectious:**
1. (para) spinal abscess, AKA **spinal epidural abscess** or epidural empyema (p. 349) †: often history of staphylococcus infection, usually a skin furuncle. Vertebral osteomyelitis often accompanies.[20] Produces local tenderness, back pain, fever, elevated ESR
2. vertebral osteitis/osteomyelitis (p. 353) †
3. pyogenic discitis†: spontaneous or following procedures (p. 356)
4. HIV or AIDS related myelopathy: similar to B12 deficiency. Spastic weakness & ataxia. Can cause vacuolization of spinal cord. "Tropical (spastic) paraparesis of AIDS" also seen in HTLV-I infection[21]
5. tuberculosis: Pott's disease, see Tuberculous vertebral osteomyelitis (p. 354)
6. spinal meningitis with pachymeningitis
7. viral:
   a) herpes varicella-zoster: rarely causes necrotizing myelopathy
   b) Herpes simplex type 2: may cause ascending myelitis
   c) cytomegalovirus: may cause transverse myelitis
8. syphilitic involvement: may cause tabes dorsalis, syphilitic meningomyelitis, or spinal vascular syphilis. Diagnosed by serum and CSF serology
9. parasitic cysts†
10. some forms of Creutzfeldt-Jakob disease (CJD) with predominant initial muscle wasting may mimic spinal cord disease or ALS (p. 367)

▶ **Peripheral neuromuscular disorder:**
1. Guillain-Barré syndrome (GBS) (p. 184): rapidly ascending weakness (mimics cord compression) with areflexia and near normal sensation
2. chronic dysimmune neuropathies: presumed to be immune mediated[22]
   a) chronic immune demyelinating polyradiculoneuropathy (CIDP) (p. 186): similar to GBS but can progress over a longer period of time
   b) multifocal motor neuropathy (MMN): characterized by asymmetric muscle wasting, cramping & LE twitching. May mimic ALS, but is treatable (with IVIg or immunosuppression)
3. myopathies: including steroid myopathy (usually affects proximal > distal muscles)

▶ **Motor neuron diseases:**
1. amyotrophic lateral sclerosis (ALS) (p. 183): upper and lower motor neuron disease. *Slight* spasticity of LEs (extreme spasticity is rare), atrophic weakness of the hands and forearms, fasciculations in the UEs, absence of sensory changes (including lack of pain), sphincter control usually preserved
2. primary lateral sclerosis: age > 50. No LMN signs. Slower progression than ALS (yrs to decades). Pseudobulbar palsy (p. 178) is common[23]

† items with dagger may also present as a spinal epidural mass

92.3 Sciatica

92.3.1 General information

Definition: pain in the distribution of the sciatic nerve. The sciatic nerve is comprised of components of nerve roots of L4-S3. The nerve passes out of the pelvis through the greater sciatic foramen along the back of the thigh. In the lower third of the thigh it divides into the tibial and common peroneal nerves.

92.3.2 Etiologies

The most common cause of sciatica is *radiculopathy* due to a herniated lumbar disc.[24] The differential diagnosis is similar to that for myelopathy (see above) but also includes:
1. congenital:
   a) meningeal cyst (perineural cyst); see Spinal meningeal cysts (p. 1142)
   b) conjoined nerve root (p. 275): initially dismissed as a possible cause of radiculopathy, but current thinking recognizes that these may be symptomatic possibly by tethering
2. acquired:
   a) spinal stenosis/spondylosis/spondylolysis/spondylolisthesis
   b) juxtafacet cyst: includes synovial cyst and ganglion cyst (p. 1143) [25]: detection is increasing with the use of MRI

c) nerve root sheath cyst: may be congenital or acquired. May arise near axilla of nerve root and cause compression of adjacent roots. Treatment: excise cyst and oversew the ostium
d) arachnoiditis ossificans (p. 1408): rare. In the lumbar region may occur as columnar, cylindrical, or irregularly shaped masses.[26] May produce low back pain, radiculopathy, or cauda equina syndrome
e) heterotopic ossification around the hip[27]
f) injection injuries from misplaced IM injections
g) compartment syndrome of the posterior thigh
h) injury complicating total hip arthroplasty[28]
i) radiation injury following treatment of nearby tumors

3. infectious:
a) discitis (p. 356): usually causes excruciating pain with any movement
b) Lyme disease (p. 334)
c) herpes zoster: a rare cause of radiculopathy.[29] Lumbosacral dermatomes are involved in ≈ 10–15% of zoster cases. Pain is usually independent of position. Typical herpetic skin lesions usually follow onset of pain by 3–5 days. 1–5% develop motor weakness (usually in arms or trunk). Sacral zoster can cause detrusor paralysis, producing urinary retention. 55% of those with motor symptoms have good recovery, 30% have fair to good recovery

4. neoplastic:
a) spine tumors: multiple myeloma (p. 714), metastases (p. 821)
b) bone or soft-tissue tumors along the course of the sciatic nerve: may result in erroneous laminectomy for herniated lumbar disc.[30] Pain is usually *insidious* in onset, and *not positional* (see below)
   - intra-abdominal or pelvic neoplasm
   - tumors of the thigh
   - tumors in the popliteal fossa or calf

5. inflammatory:
a) trochanteric bursitis (p. 1101): may produce pseudoradiculopathy. Rarely extends to the posterior thigh or as far distally as the knee
b) myositis ossificans of the biceps femoris muscle[31]

6. vascular:
a) sciatica may be mimicked by intermittent (i.e. vascular) claudication
b) psoas hematoma: usually in patient on anticoagulant. Sometimes drainage is required

7. referred pain of nonspinal origin: not dermatomal. Nerve root tensions signs (p. 1101) are usually negative. Includes:
a) pyelonephritis
b) renolithiasis including ureteral obstruction
c) cholecystitis
d) appendicitis
e) endometritis/endometriosis
f) posterior perforating duodenal ulcer
g) inguinal hernia, especially if incarcerated
h) aortic dissection (p. 1414)

8. piriformis syndrome (PS): controversial. Piriformis muscle originates on anterior S2–4 VBs, sacrotuberous ligament and passes through the greater sciatic notch to attach to the greater trochanter of the femur. It is innervated by L5-S1. It is the principle *external* rotator of the extended hip. It may irritate or compress the sciatic nerve (AKA pseudosciatica, can mimic symptoms of a herniated disc). The superior gluteal nerve is spared as it has a take-off proximal to the muscle. Conversely, PS may occur secondary to lower lumbar radiculopathy. Produces pain in the sciatic distribution and weakness of external rotation and abduction of the hip. Signs: Freiberg test (pain with forced internal rotation of the hip with thigh extension) or the Pace test (pain on resisted abduction/external rotation of the hip). No well designed studies of treatments. Advocated therapies include: PT, stretching, injection of the muscle localized by digital rectal exam taking care not to inject the sciatic nerve itself & piriformis muscle section. Sometimes long-lasting relief can follow injection with local anesthetic. Use of botulinum toxin (Botox®) injections has been described

9. more peripheral involvement (i.e. neuropathy) that may be confused with radiculopathy. Including:
a) femoral neuropathy mistaken for L4 radiculopathy (see below)
b) proximal sacral plexus lesion mistaken for S1 radiculopathy (see below)
c) diabetic neuropathy (p. 545) including diabetic amyotrophy
d) tumors (see below)

92.3.3 Extraspinal tumors causing sciatica

* Pain characteristics: pain is almost always insidious in onset.[30] It may be intermittent initially, but eventually all patients develop pain that is constant, progressive and unaffected by position or rest.[30] Significant night pain is described in ≈ 80%.

Straight leg raising was positive in most, but in more than half the pain was localized to a specific point along the course of the nerve, distal to the sciatic notch.[30] Conservative treatment brings either no or only temporary relief.

Approximately 20% will have a previous history of tumor (usually neurofibromatosis or previous malignancy). Malignancies include[30]: metastatic lesions, primary bone sarcomas (chondrosarcoma…), soft-tissue sarcomas (liposarcoma…). Benign tumors include: lipoma, neurofibroma, schwannoma, aneurysmal bone cyst of the sacrum, giant cell tumor of the sacrum, tenosynovial giant cell tumor.

In two-thirds of cases, a detailed medical history and physical exam allowed localization and even determining the nature (bone tumor vs. soft-tissue) of the lesion.[30] Radiographs that show the entire pelvis and the proximal femur will demonstrate almost all tumors in these locations.[30,32]

92.3.4 Features differentiating radiculopathy in sciatica

General information

Sciatica may result from nerve root involvement within the spinal canal (e.g. with lumbar disc herniation). Clinically this produces a nerve root syndrome; see Nerve root syndromes (p. 1049). Spinal imaging studies (MRI, myelogram/CT) will usually detect nerve root compression here. More peripheral involvement may be difficult to image.

L4 involvement

Femoral neuropathy is often mistakenly identified as an L4 radiculopathy. Distinguishing features are shown in ▶ Table 92.2.

92

L5 involvement

Peroneal nerve palsy may be mistaken for L5 radiculopathy (p. 1416).

S1 involvement

Outside the spinal canal, S1 can also be involved as it enters the sacral plexus, e.g. by a pelvic tumor. In plexus lesions, EMG will show sparing of the paraspinal muscles (nerves to paraspinal muscles exit in the region of the neural foramen) and the gluteus maximus and medius (superior and inferior gluteal nerves take-off just distal to the paraspinal nerves).

Table 92.2 Distinguishing femoral neuropathy from L4 radiculopathy

Feature	Femoral neuropathy	L4 radiculopathy
	Sensory loss	
distribution (▶ Fig. 1.14)	anterior thigh	dermatome from ≈ knee to medial malleolus, spares anterior thigh
	Muscle weakness	
iliopsoas	weak	normal
thigh adductors	normal (innervated by obturator nerve)	may be weak
quadriceps	weak	weak

92.4 Acute paraplegia or quadriplegia

92.4.1 General information

Entities causing spinal cord compression usually present as: paraplegia or -paresis (or quadriplegia/paresis), urinary retention (may require bladder ultrasound or checking a post-void residual to detect), and impaired sensation below level of compression. May develop over hours or days. Reflexes may be hyper- or hypo-active. There may or may not be a Babinski sign. Excluding trauma, the most common cause is compression by tumor or bone.

92.4.2 Etiologies

Some overlap with myelopathy.

1. in infancy (may produce "floppy infant syndrome")
   a) spinal muscular atrophy (the most severe form is called Werdnig-Hoffmann disease and is usually fatal within months): autosomal recessive congenital disease of childhood with degeneration of anterior horn cells. Only rarely evident at birth (where it presents as a paucity of movement), produces weakness, areflexia, muscle and tongue fasciculations with normal sensation. Severe cases progress over the first year or two to quadriplegia
   b) spinal cord injury during parturition: a rare sequela of breech delivery
   c) congenital myopathies: e.g. infantile acid maltase deficiency (Pompe disease)
   d) infantile botulism: ileus, hypotonia, weakness, mydriasis, Clostridium botulinum bacteria and toxin in feces
2. traumatic spinal cord injury
   a) major trauma: diagnosis is usually evident
   b) minor trauma: may cause cord injury in setting of spinal stenosis, may → central cord syndrome; see Central cord syndrome (p.944)
   c) atlantoaxial dislocation: from major trauma or due to instability from tumor or rheumatoid arthritis
3. congenital
   a) extradural spinal cord compression by bone secondary to cervical hemivertebra (symptoms not present at birth, may develop decades later, occasionally after minor trauma)
   b) cervical stenosis (p.1088) (usually with superimposed spondylosis): quadriplegia or central cord syndrome may follow minor trauma
   c) achondroplastic dwarfism: spinal stenosis (animal model: dachshund)
   d) syringomyelia: usually presents with central cord syndrome
4. metabolic
   a) combined system disease* (p.1409)
   b) thallium poisoning: usually causes sensory and autonomic symptoms, quadriplegia and dysarthria may be seen in severe cases
   c) central pontine myelinolysis (p.115)
5. infectious
   a) epidural spinal infection (abscess or empyema)*
   b) post-viral (or post-vaccination): may be a transverse myelitis*
6. peripheral neuromuscular disorder*
   a) Guillain-Barré syndrome (p.186): classically an *ascending* paralysis, but paraparesis mimicking a spinal cord lesion is an unusual variant[33]
   b) myopathies
7. neoplastic*: spinal cord tumors
8. autoimmune*
9. vascular
   a) acute pontomedullary infarction: age usually > 50 yrs. Patient is quadriplegic, alert, with bulbar palsies (eye movement abnormalities, impaired gag and speech)
   b) spinal cord infarction*: including AVM, radiation myelopathy...
10. miscellaneous compressive*: including epidural hematoma, bony compression, epidural lipomatosis
11. functional: hysteria, malingering
12. bilateral cerebral hemisphere lesion (involving both motor strips): e.g. post-cerebral irradiation or parasagittal lesion. Will not have sensory *level*

* For items with asterisk, see Myelopathy (p.1407) for details.

92

92.5 Hemiparesis or hemiplegia

92.5.1 General information

May be produced by anything that interrupts the corticospinal tract from its origin in the pyramidal cells of Betz in the motor strip down to the cervical spine. This results an upper motor neuron paralysis (see ► Table 29.4) which should also produce long tract findings, including Babinski sign ipsilateral to hemiplegia.

92.5.2 Etiologies

► **Lesions of the cerebral hemisphere in the region of the contralateral motor strip.** Large lesions may also involve sensory cortex producing reduced sensation ipsilateral to the hemiparesis

1. tumor (neoplasm): primary or metastatic
2. traumatic: epidural or subdural hematoma, hemorrhagic contusion of the brain, compression by depressed skull fracture
3. vascular:
   a) infarction
      - ischemic: embolic, low flow (due to atherosclerosis, arterial dissection…)
      - hemorrhagic: intracerebral hemorrhage, aneurysmal SAH…

   b) TIA (p. 1264)
4. infection: cerebritis, abscess

► **Lesions of the contralateral internal capsule.** Produces pure motor hemiplegia without sensory loss. Most common etiology is ischemic lacunar infarct

► **Lesions of the brainstem.** Ischemic infarct, hemorrhage, tumor

► **Lesions of cervicomedullary junction.** Foramen magnum lesions (p. 1367).

► **Unilateral spinal cord lesions.** Above ≈ C5 ipsilateral to the weakness producing a Brown-Séquard syndrome (p. 947) with contralateral sensory loss to pain and temperature. See etiologies (p. 947).

92

► **Hypoglycemia.** Can sometimes be associated with hemiparesis that clears after administration of glucose

► **Note.** In a patient with unexplained hemiparesis/hemiplegia, especially after trauma, consider carotid dissection.

92.6 Low back pain

92.6.1 General information

The following considers primarily low back pain (LBP) *without* radiculopathy or myelopathy, although some overlap occurs. Trauma is usually obvious and is not discussed. See Sciatica (p. 1410) for differential diagnosis of that and also Low back pain and radiculopathy (p. 1414) for evaluation.

92.6.2 Acute low back pain

Similar to list for myelopathy (p. 1407). Most cases are non-specific (e.g. lumbosacral sprain), only 10–20% can be given a precise pathoanatomical diagnosis[34]:

► **Patients writhing in pain.** Should be evaluated for an intraabdominal or vascular condition (e.g. pain of aortic dissection is typically described as a "tearing" pain): patients with neurogenic LBP tend to remain as still as possible, possibly needing to change positions at intervals

► **Unrelenting pain at rest:**

1. spinal tumor (intradural or extradural) (p. 1032)
   a) primary or metastatic spine tumor: suspected in patients with pain duration > 1 month, unrelieved by bed rest, failure to improve with conservative therapy, unexplained weight loss, age > 50 yrs[35]

b) nocturnal back pain relieved by aspirin is suggestive of osteoid osteoma or benign osteoblastoma (p. 792) [36]
2. infection (especially in IV drug abusers, diabetics, post spinal surgery, immunosuppressed patients, or those with pyelonephritis or UTI post-GU surgery). Fever is somewhat insensitive for spinal infections. Spine tenderness to percussion has 86% sensitivity with bacterial infections, but a low specificity of 60%.[35] Types of infections include:
a) discitis
b) spinal epidural abscess: should be considered in patients with back pain, fever, spine tenderness, or skin infection (furuncle)
c) vertebral osteomyelitis
3. inflammatory
4. sacroiliitis: may produce pain and tenderness over one or both SI joints. Pelvic x-rays may show sclerosis of one or both sacroiliac joints.
a) bilateral & symmetric
• ankylosing spondylitis (p. 1123): morning back stiffness, no relief at rest, improvement with exercise.[37] Usually seen in males with symptom onset before age 40 yrs. Positive Patrick's test (p. 1048) and pain on compressing the pelvis with the patient in the lateral decubitus position
• Reiter syndrome (after Hans Reiter, a German bacteriologist): a reactive arthritis (usually 1–3 weeks following certain bacterial infections) with involvement of at least one other non-joint area (urethritis, uveitis/conjunctivitis, skin lesions, mucosal ulcerations…). 75% are HLA-B27 positive
• may occur in Crohn's disease
b) bilateral & asymmetric
• psoriatic arthritis
• rheumatoid arthritis: adult & juvenile forms
c) unilateral
• gout
• osteoarthritis
• infection

► **Evolving neurologic deficit.** (**Cauda equina syndrome**: perineal anesthesia, urinary incontinence or urgency or retention, progressive weakness) all require emergent diagnostic evaluation to rule-out treatable conditions such as:
1. spinal epidural abscess (p. 349)
2. spinal epidural hematoma (p. 1131)
3. spinal tumor (intradural or extradural) (p. 783)
4. massive central disc herniation (p. 1051)

► **Pathologic fracture.** Acute pain in patients at risk for osteoporosis or with known Ca should prompt evaluation for pathologic fractures
1. lumbar compression fracture: see Osteoporotic spine fractures (p. 1008)
2. sacral insufficiency fracture[38]: especially in rheumatoid arthritis patients on chronic steroids, often with no antecedent history of trauma. May cause back pain and/or radiculopathy. Often missed on plain films, best seen on CT, but may also be detected on bone scan

► **Coccydynia** (p. 1038). Pain and tenderness around the coccyx

► **Tears in the anulus fibrosus.** ("Anular tears")[39] (NB: also present in 40% of asymptomatic patients between 50–60 yrs age, and 75% between 60–70 yrs[40])

► **Rarely following subarachnoid hemorrhage.** (SAH) due to irritation of lumbar nerve roots and dura: usually accompanied by other signs of SAH (p. 1156)

► **Myalgia.** May be a side-effect of "statins" (drugs used to lower serum concentration of LDL cholesterol) with or without elevation of serum creatinine phosphokinase, sometimes with accompanying weakness and rarely with severe rhabdomyolysis and myoglobinuria leading to renal failure (risk may be increased with renal or hepatic dysfunction, advanced age, hypothyroidism, or serious infection)[41]

► **Drug induced:**
1. statins: see above under myalgia

92

2. phosphodiesterase type 5 (PDE5) inhibitors used for erectile dysfunction: all may be associated with LBP, but the incidence is higher with tadalafil,[42] etiology unknown. Usually occurs 12–24 hours post-dose and resolves by 48 hours. Most respond to simple analgesics

92.6.3 Subacute low back pain

10% of patients with LBP have symptoms that persists > 6 weeks.

Differential diagnosis includes causes of acute LBP (above) and also:

1. continued pain at rest should prompt evaluation for spinal osteomyelitis (especially with fever and elevated ESR) or neoplasm if not already done
2. plain spine x-rays may show possibly causative conditions, although many or all of the following may also be seen in *asymptomatic* patients
   a) spondylolisthesis (p. 1098)
   b) spinal osteophytes
   c) lumbar stenosis
   d) **Schmorl's node** or **nodule** (p. 1060): disc herniation through cartilaginous end-plate into vertebral body (NB: may also be seen in 19% of asymptomatic patients[43])

Chronic low back pain

After 3 months, only ≈ 5% of patients with LBP will continue to have persistent symptoms. A structural diagnosis is possible in only ≈ 50% of these patients. These patients account for 85% of the cost in lost work and compensation.[34]

Differential diagnosis includes causes of acute and subacute LBP listed above, as well as:

1. degenerative conditions
   a) degenerative spondylolisthesis (p. 1099)
   b) spinal stenosis (affecting the spinal canal)
   c) lateral recess syndrome
2. spondyloarthropathies
   a) ankylosing spondylitis: look for erosive changes adjacent to SI joint and positive test for HLA-B27 antigen
   b) Paget's disease of the spine: vertebral involvement is very common in a patients with Paget's disease
3. osteitis condensans ilii: increased density in ilium, usually asymptomatic (incidental) finding. Occasionally may produce low back pain or tenderness. Usually found in women who have been pregnant
4. psychological overlay: including secondary gain (financial, emotional...)

92.7 Foot drop

92.7.1 General information

Key concepts

- weak anterior tibialis (foot extension) innervated by deep peroneal nerve (L4, 5)
- most common etiologies: L4/L5 radiculopathy, common peroneal nerve palsy
- in a patient with foot drop, check posterior tibialis (foot inversion) and gluteus medius (internal rotation of flexed hip) – both are spared in peroneal nerve palsy and both should be involved with L4/5 radiculopathy
- EMG can assist in localization and prognostication

Definition: weakness of anterior tibialis (primarily L4 and to a lesser extent L5), often accompanied by a weak extensor digitorum longus and extensor hallicus longus (primarily L5 with some S1 contribution), all of which are innervated by the *deep peroneal nerve*.

92.7.2 Underlying substrates of foot drop

The most common dilemma is to distinguish foot drop due to radiculopathy from that due to peroneal nerve palsy (usually common peroneal nerve). With common peroneal nerve (CPN) palsy, there is *sparing* of posterior tibialis (foot inversion, innervated by posterior tibial nerve) and gluteus medius (internal rotation of the thigh with the hip flexed, innervated by superior gluteal nerve, primarily L5 with some L4, the takeoff is shortly after the roots exit from neural foramen). With L4 or L5 root lesions these muscles will also be weak, see ▶ Fig. 92.1.

Flail foot results from paralysis of dorsiflexors *plus* plantarflexors, e.g. in sciatic nerve dysfunction as can occur during surgery for hip fracture/dislocation[44] or injection injuries (IM injections should be give superiorly and laterally to a line drawn between the posterior superior iliac spine and the greater trochanter of the hip). NB: the peroneal division of the sciatic nerve tends to be more vulnerable to injury than the tibial division.

92.7.3 Etiologies of foot drop

Three major categories: 1) muscular, 2) neurologic, 3) anatomic.

1. peripheral nerve palsies (more common). See ▶ Table 92.3 and ▶ Fig. 92.1.
   a) peroneal nerve injury (also, see Common peroneal nerve palsy (p. 535) for details including etiologies). Branches that may be involved:
      - deep peroneal nerve: isolated foot drop with minimal sensory loss (except possibly in great toe web space)
      - superficial peroneal nerve: weakness of peroneus longus and brevis (foot eversion) with *no* foot drop. Sensory loss: lateral aspect of lower half of leg and foot
      - common peroneal nerve: combination of above (i.e. foot drop + weak foot eversion, with sparing of tibialis posterior (foot inversion). Sensory loss: lateral aspect of lower half of leg and foot)
   b) L5 radiculopathy: (or, less commonly, L4). The most common cause is HLD at L4–5, other etiologies include: lumbar spinal stenosis at L4–5, sacral ala fracture (p. 1014)
      - results in pain and/or sensory changes in L5 (or L4) dermatome
      - weakness with radiculopathy tends to be more pronounced in distal muscles (e.g. anterior tibialis) than in proximal (e.g. gluteus maximus)
      - *painless* foot drop is unlikely to be due to radiculopathy; consider peroneal neuropathy, diabetic neuropathy, lesion anywhere along pyramidal tract, motor neuron disease…
   c) lumbar plexus injury
   d) lumbosacral plexus neuropathy (p. 544)
   e) injury to lateral trunk of sciatic nerve

92

Table 92.3 Localization of lesion with foot drop

Lesion	Motor deficit[a]					Sensory changes
	anterior tibialis (L4. 5 ankle dorsiflexion)	peroneus longus/ brevis (L5, S1 foot eversion)	tibialis posterior (L4, 5 foot inversion)	biceps femoris (L5, S1, 2 knee flexion)	gastrocnemius (S1, 2 plantarflexion)	
deep peroneal nerve	x					minimal, or great toe web space
superficial peroneal nerve		x				lateral distal leg and dorsum of foot
common peroneal nerve (CPN)	x	x				all of the above
L4 or L5 radiculopathy	x	x	x			dermatomal (▶ Fig. 1.14)
peroneal division of sciatic nerve[b]	x	x	x	x		as with common peroneal
main trunk of sciatic nerve	x	x	X	x	x	lateral distal leg and entire foot

[a]x denotes that the indicated muscle is involved (i.e. weak)
[b]see footnote (b) under ▶ Fig. 92.1

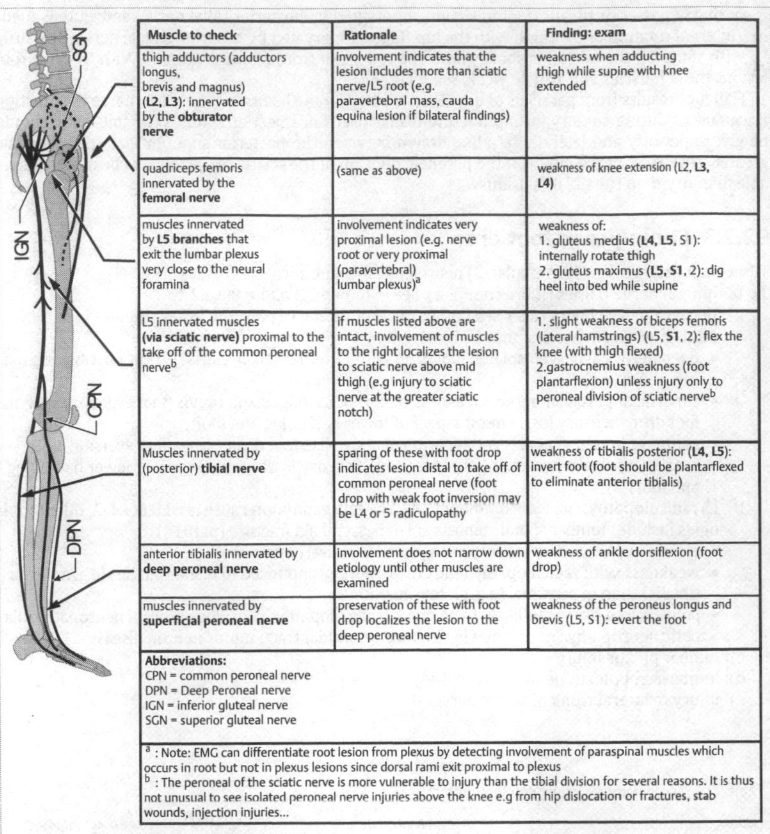

Muscle to check	Rationale	Finding: exam
thigh adductors (adductors longus, brevis and magnus) (**L2, L3**): innervated by the **obturator nerve**	involvement indicates that the lesion includes more than sciatic nerve/L5 root (e.g. paravertebral mass, cauda equina lesion if bilateral findings)	weakness when adducting thigh while supine with knee extended
quadriceps femoris innervated by the **femoral nerve**	(same as above)	weakness of knee extension (L2, **L3, L4**)
muscles innervated by **L5 branches** that exit the lumbar plexus very close to the neural foramina	involvement indicates very proximal lesion (e.g. nerve root or very proximal (paravertebral) lumbar plexus)[a]	weakness of: 1. gluteus medius (**L4, L5**, S1): internally rotate thigh 2. gluteus maximus (**L5, S1**, 2): dig heel into bed while supine
L5 innervated muscles **(via sciatic nerve)** proximal to the take off of the common peroneal nerve[b]	if muscles listed above are intact, involvement of muscles to the right localizes the lesion to sciatic nerve above mid thigh (e.g injury to sciatic nerve at the greater sciatic notch)	1. slight weakness of biceps femoris (lateral hamstrings) (L5, **S1**, 2): flex the knee (with thigh flexed) 2.gastrocnemius weakness (foot plantarflexion) unless injury only to peroneal division of sciatic nerve[b]
Muscles innervated by (posterior) **tibial nerve**	sparing of these with foot drop indicates lesion distal to take off of common peroneal nerve (foot drop with weak foot inversion may be L4 or 5 radiculopathy	weakness of tibialis posterior (**L4, L5**): invert foot (foot should be plantarflexed to eliminate anterior tibialis)
anterior tibialis innervated by **deep peroneal nerve**	involvement does not narrow down etiology until other muscles are examined	weakness of ankle dorsiflexion (foot drop)
muscles innervated by **superficial peroneal nerve**	preservation of these with foot drop localizes the lesion to the deep peroneal nerve	weakness of the peroneus longus and brevis (L5, S1): evert the foot

Abbreviations:
CPN = common peroneal nerve
DPN = Deep Peroneal nerve
IGN = inferior gluteal nerve
SGN = superior gluteal nerve

[a] : Note: EMG can differentiate root lesion from plexus by detecting involvement of paraspinal muscles which occurs in root but not in plexus lesions since dorsal rami exit proximal to plexus
[b] : The peroneal of the sciatic nerve is more vulnerable to injury than the tibial division for several reasons. It is thus not unusual to see isolated peroneal nerve injuries above the knee e.g from hip dislocation or fractures, stab wounds, injection injuries...

Fig. 92.1 Physical exam to localize the lesion in a patient with LE weakness

f) peripheral neuropathy: weakness tends to be greater distally, producing wrist or foot drop. Classic example: Charcot-Marie-Tooth (p. 541), findings tend to be rather dramatic in spite of the fact that it often doesn't seem to bother the patient very much
g) early in the course of motor neuron disease (ALS)
h) heavy metal poisoning

2. central nervous system causes (foot drop here is usually painless)
   a) cortical lesion (UMN): parasagittal lesions in region of motor strip (sensation will be spared if the lesion does not extend posteriorly to the sensory cortex).[45] There may be a Babinski sign or hyperactive Achilles reflex (so-called "spastic foot drop"). Usually painless
   b) spinal cord injury: including cervical spinal myelopathy
3. non-neurogenic causes
   a) muscular dystrophy
   b) lead toxicity: in children may cause foot drop with no sensory loss
   c) anterior compartment syndrome

92.7.4 Clinical

Loss of dorsiflexion causes foot slap with the front of the foot when the heel strikes the ground while walking. Also during the swing phase of gait the front of the foot may snag the ground (especially on uneven surfaces) which may cause tripping; thus patients develop steppage gait (exaggerated thigh & knee flexion) on the affected side. Associated weakness of tibialis posterior, when present (e.g. with L5 radiculopathy) destabilizes the ankle permitting eversion which also predisposes to falls and to ankle fractures. Chronic foot drop may produce achilles tendon contracture with talipes equinus.

Wasting of the extensor digitorum brevis may be seen.

92.7.5 Evaluation

1. bloodwork: glucose, ESR
2. EMG: can help differentiate L5 radiculopathy from peroneal nerve palsy, plexus lesion (▶ Fig. 92.1) or motor neuron disease (p. 182) (for details). EMG is not reliable until symptoms have been present at least ≈ 3 weeks
3. For suspected radiculopathy: MRI (or CT/myelogram if MRI is not possible)

92.8 Weakness/atrophy of the hands/UEs

92.8.1 Hand/UE weakness or atrophy with relatively preserved function in the LEs

1. cervical spondylosis (p. 1083): often causes sensory disturbance
2. cervical radiculopathy (p. 1069)
3. amyotrophic lateral sclerosis (ALS): no sensory involvement. One of the few causes of clinically prominent *fasciculations*. See details of ALS (p. 1410), other distinguishing features (p. 1410), fibrillations (p. 505)
4. spinal cord pathology
   a) central cord syndrome (p. 944): typically causes more involvement (weakness, sensory disturbance) in the UE than the LE
   b) syringomyelia (p. 1144): usually burning dysesthesias of the hands with dissociated sensory loss
5. brachial plexus injury (p. 550)
6. brachial plexus neuropathy (includes Parsonage-Turner syndrome) (p. 542)
7. peripheral nerve problems, including
   a) carpal tunnel syndrome (p. 519)
   b) ulnar neuropathy (p. 526)
   c) other peripheral nerve entrapment syndromes (p. 515)
8. foramen magnum lesions (p. 1367): can cause (Bell's) cruciate paralysis[46] due to compression above the pyramidal decussation which produces bilateral UE weakness and possibly atrophy of the hands with sparing of the LEs[47] (in the differential diagnosis for central cord syndrome). Compression on one side may produce the similarly named but clinically different hemiplegia cruciata (spastic palsy of one UE and the contralateral LE)[47]
9. thoracic outlet syndrome (p. 554)
10. botulism (p. 1399)
11. pharyngeal-cervical-brachial variant of Guillain-Barré syndrome (p. 186)

92.8.2 Atrophy of the first dorsal interosseous muscle

Etiologies: either C8/T1 nerve root or ulnar nerve involvement (either may be focal or diffuse). There are 4 main differential diagnoses:

1. ulnar neuropathy: check median nerve to see if findings extend to a nearby but separate nerve
   a) at the elbow (p. 531)
   b) at Guyon's canal (p. 531)
2. nerve root involvement:
   a) cervical radiculopathy: C8 or T1
   b) nerve root avulsion: weakness + sensory loss with normal SNAP on EMG (p. 243) usually with a history of precipitating trauma
3. lower brachial plexus involvement
   a) thoracic outlet syndrome (p. 554)
   b) Pancoast tumor (p. 542)
4. neurodegenerative disorders

a) amyotrophic lateral sclerosis (ALS) (p.1086)
b) multifocal motor neuropathy (MMN) (p.1410): a chronic dysimmune neuropathy with asymmetric muscle wasting, cramping & LE twitching

92.9 Radiculopathy, upper extremity (cervical)

See Weakness/atrophy of the hands/UEs (p.1420). In addition to those items:

1. primary shoulder pathology: characteristically, pain is aggravated by active and/or passive shoulder movement. In general, shoulder pathology does not produce pain referred to the neck
   a) rotator cuff tear
   b) bicipital tendonitis: tenderness over biceps tendon
   c) subacromial bursitis: there may be tenderness over the AC joint
   d) adhesive capsulitis
   e) impingement syndrome: the "empty can test" is usually positive (each arm held out in front, 30° lateral to straight forward, thumbs pointing down, as in emptying out a soda can. Examiner pushes down on the patient's hands while the patient resists. Test is positive if it reproduces pain)
2. shoulder pain is very common in polymyalgia rheumatica (p.198), typically worsens with movement
3. interscapular pain: a common location for referred pain with cervical radiculopathy, may also occur with cholecystitis or some shoulder pathologies
4. MI: some cases of cervical radiculopathy (especially left C6) may present with symptoms that are suggestive of an acute myocardial infarction
5. complex regional pain syndrome AKA reflex sympathetic dystrophy (p.497): may be difficult to distinguish from cervical radiculopathy. Stellate ganglion blocks may help.[48]

92.10 Neck pain (cervical pain)

This section deals primarily with axial neck-pain without radicular features. For radicular features, see Radiculopathy, upper extremity (cervical) above.

92

1. cervical spondylosis (including facet arthritis)
2. cervical sprain: including whiplash associated disorder
3. fracture of the cervical spine: with upper cervical spine fractures (e.g. odontoid), patients characteristically hold their head in their hands, especially when going from recumbent to upright position
   a) traumatic
   b) pathologic (tumor invasion, rheumatoid arthritis)
4. occipital neuralgia (p.515)
5. herniated cervical disc:
   a) lateral herniated disc: if symptomatic, tends to produce more radicular symptoms in the UE than actual neck pain
   b) central disc herniation: if symptomatic, tends to produce myelopathy, does not produce any neck pain whatsoever in many cases
6. abnormalities of the craniocervical junction:
   a) Chiari 1 malformation (p.277)
   b) atlantoaxial subluxation
7. fibromyalgia: idiopathic chronic pain syndrome characterized by widespread nonarticular musculoskeletal pain, nodularity and stiffness[49,50] without pathologic inflammation. Possible link to neuroendocrine dysfunction.[51] Afflicts 2% of the population,[50] female:male ratio is 7:1. No diagnostic laboratory study. May be associated with psychiatric illness and multiple non-specific somatic complaints including malaise, fatigue, impaired sleep, GI complaints and cognitive impairment
8. Eagle's syndrome: elongation of the styloid process. Surgical resection can ameliorate the pain. Two variants:
   a) typical variant: history of tonsillectomy. Pharyngeal pain, dysphagia and otalgia
   b) second variant: AKA carotid artery-styloid process syndrome. Carotidynia radiating into ipsilateral eye and vertex
9. crystal deposition diseases: gout, pseudogout, hydroxyapatite (HA) or calcium pyrophosphate dihydrate (CPPD) crystal deposition diseases. May appear as a crown-like density encompassing the odontoid process (crowned-dens syndrome)[52] representing calcifications in the transverse ligament, seen best on cervical CT. May be treated with a short course of prednisolone (e.g. 15 mg/d) followed by NSAIDs

92.11 Burning hands/feet

1. spinal cord syndromes:
   a) central cord syndrome (CCS) (p. 944)
   b) burning hands syndrome (p. 937): a possible variant of CCS, described in football-related cervical spine injury
   c) numb-clumsy hand syndrome (p. 1085): seen in cervical myelopathy
2. complex regional pain syndrome (CRPS) AKA reflex sympathetic dystrophy (p. 497)
3. peripheral neuropathy
   a) diabetic amyotrophy AKA Bruns-Garland syndrome (p. 545)
4. erythermalgia AKA erythromelalgia: rare disorder characterized by erythema, edema, increased skin temperature, and burning pain of the hands and/or feet. Usually refractory to medical management, some success reported with epidural bupivacaine,[53] lidocaine patches,[54] or cold soaks
   a) primary erythermalgia: etiology is idiopathic
   b) secondary erythermalgia: associated with autoimmune and rheumatologic factors
5. vascular:
   a) occlusive arterial disease: atherosclerosis, Raynaud's syndrome
   b) venous insufficiency

92.12 Muscle pain/tenderness

1. fibromyalgia: see above
2. myopathy
3. statin induced myopathy: can vary from mild (with symptoms of muscles aches, symptoms usually abate rapidly after discontinuation of the statin although, occasionally up to 2 months may be required) to severe (with rhabdomyolysis which can → nephropathy)
4. diffuse severe sensitivity to light touch is a marker of nonorganic pain[55]

92.13 Lhermitte's sign

92.13.1 General information

Technically, a symptom (not a sign). Electrical shock-like sensation radiating down the spine usually provoked by neck flexion (shocks radiating up the spine are sometimes referred to as reverse Lhermitte's sign). Classically attributed to MS, but may occur in any process involving primarily the posterior columns of the spinal cord.

92.13.2 Etiologies

1. multiple sclerosis (MS) (p. 179)
2. cervical spondylosis
3. subacute combined degeneration (p. 1409): check for vitamin B12 deficiency
4. cervical cord tumor
5. cervical disc herniation
6. radiation myelopathy (p. 1563)
7. Chiari type I malformation (p. 277)
8. central cord syndrome (p. 944)
9. SCIWORA (spinal cord injury without radiographic abnormality) (p. 999)

92.14 Swallowing difficulties

1. mechanical: the term globus describes a sensation of a lump in the throat
   a) ossification of the anterior longitudinal ligament (OALL) (p. 1129)
   b) diffuse idiopathic skeletal hyperostosis (DISH) (AKA Forestier disease) (p. 1129): An enthesopathy
   c) post-op following ACDF
      - it is normal to have a little swelling and fullness early post-op
      - may be increased with multiple levels and with anterior plating
      - as a complication from post-op hematoma
2. neurologic

92

References

[1] Ungar-Sargon JY, Lovelace RE, Brust JC. Spastic paraplegia-paraparesis: A Reappraisal. J Neurol Sci. 1980; 46:1–12
[2] George WE, Wilmot M, Greenhouse A, et al. Medical Management of Steroid-Induced Epidural Lipomatosis. N Engl J Med. 1983; 308:316–319
[3] Nagashima C. Cervical Myelopathy due to Ossification of the Posterior Longitudinal Ligament. J Neurosurg. 1972; 37:653–660
[4] Lucchesi AC, White WL, Heiserman JE, Flom RA. Review of Arachnoiditis Ossificans with a Case Report. BNI Quarterly. 1998; 14:4–9
[5] Marshman LAG, Hardwidge C, Ford-Dunn SZ, Olney JS. Idiopathic Spinal Cord Herniation: Case Report and Review of the Literature. Neurosurgery. 1999; 44:1129–1133
[6] Darbar A, Krishnamurthy S, Holsapple JW, Hodge CJJr. Ventral thoracic spinal cord herniation: frequently misdiagnosed entity. Spine. 2006; 31: E600–E605
[7] Fox MW, Onofrio BM. The Natural History and Management of Symptomatic and Asymptomatic Vertebral Hemangiomas. J Neurosurg. 1993; 78:36–45
[8] Harik SI, Raichle ME, Reis DJ. Spontaneous Remitting Spinal Epidural Hematoma in a Patient on Anticoagulants. N Engl J Med. 1971; 284:1355–1357
[9] Packer NP, Cummins BH. Spontaneous Epidural Hemorrhage: A Surgical Emergency. Lancet. 1978; 1:356–358
[10] Brem SS, Hafler DA, Van Uitert RL, et al. Spinal Subarachnoid Hematoma: A Hazard of Lumbar Puncture Resulting in Reversible Paraplegia. N Engl J Med. 1981; 303:1020–1021
[11] Rengachary SS, Murphy D. Subarachnoid Hematoma Following Lumbar Puncture Causing Compression of the Cauda Equina. J Neurosurg. 1974; 41:252–254
[12] Epstein NE, Danto J, Nardi D. Evaluation of Intraoperative Somatosensory-Evoked Potential Monitoring During 100 Cervical Operations. Spine. 1993; 18:737–747
[13] Tobin WD, Layton DD. The Diagnosis and Natural History of Spinal Cord Arteriovenous Malformations. Mayo Clin Proc. 1976; 51:637–646
[14] Wirth FP, Post KD, Di Chiro G, et al. Foix-Alajouanine Disease. Spontaneous Thrombosis of a Spinal Cord Arteriovenous Malformation: A Case Report. Neurology. 1970; 20:1114–1118
[15] Rothman RH, Simeone FA. The Spine. Philadelphia 1982
[16] Wingerchuk DM, Lennon VA, Pittock SJ, et al. Revised diagnostic criteria for neuromyelitis optica. Neurology. 2006; 66:1485–1489
[17] Lennon VA, Wingerchuk DM, Kryzer TJ. A serum autoantibody marker of neuromyelitis optica: distinction from multiple sclerosis. Lancet. 2004; 364:2106–2112
[18] Pruthi RK, Tefferi A. Pernicious Anemia Revisited. Mayo Clin Proc. 1994; 69:144–150
[19] Elia M. Oral or Parental Therapy for B12 Deficiency. Lancet. 1998; 352:1721–1722
[20] Altrocchi PH. Acute Spinal Epidural Abscess vs Acute Transverse Myelopathy: A Plea for Neurosurgical Caution. Arch Neurol. 1963; 9:17–25
[21] Sheremata WA, Berger JR, Harrington WJ, et al. Human T Lymphotropic Virus Type I-Associated Myelopathy: A Report of 10 Patients Born in the United States. Arch Neurol. 1992; 49:1113–1118
[22] Busby M, Donaghy M. Chronic dysimmune neuropathy. A subclassification based upon the clinical features of 102 patients. J Neurol. 2003; 250:714–724
[23] Rowland LP. Diagnosis of amyotrophic lateral sclerosis. J Neurol Sci. 1998; 160:S6–24
[24] Deen HG. Diagnosis and Management of Lumbar Disk Disease. Mayo Clin Proc. 1996; 71:283–287
[25] Gritza T, Taylor TKF. A Ganglion Arising from a Lumbar Articular Facet Associated with Low Back Pain and Sciatica. J Bone Joint Surg. 1970; 52:528–531
[26] Kitigawa H, Kanamori M, Tatezaki S, et al. Multiple Spinal Ossified Arachnoiditis. A Case Report. Spine. 1990; 15:1236–1238
[27] Thakkar DH, Porter RW. Heterotopic Ossification Enveloping the Sciatic Nerve Following Posterior Fracture-Dislocation of the Hip: A Case Report. Injury. 1981; 13:207–209
[28] Johanson NA, Pellici PM, Tsairis P, Salvati EA. Nerve Injury in Total Hip Arthroplasty. Clin Orthop. 1983; 179:214–222
[29] Burkman KA, Gaines RW, Kashani SR, Smith RD. Herpes Zoster: A Consideration in the Differential Diagnosis of Radiculopathy. Arch Phys Med Rehabil. 1988; 69:132–134
[30] Bickels J, Kahanovitz N, Rupert CK, et al. Extraspinal Bone and Soft-Tissue Tumors as a Cause of Sciatica. Clinical Diagnosis and Recommendations: Analysis of 32 Cases. Spine. 1999; 24:1611–1616
[31] Jones BV, Ward MW. Myositis Ossificans in the Biceps Femoris Muscles Causing Sciatic Nerve Palsy: A Case Report. J Bone Joint Surg. 1980; 62B:506–507
[32] Thompson RC, Berg TL. Primary Bone Tumors of Pelvis Presenting as Spinal Disease. Orthopedics. 1996; 19:1011–1016
[33] Ropper AH. Unusual clinical variants and signs in Guillain-Barre syndrome. Arch Neurol. 1986; 43:1150–1152
[34] Frymoyer JW. Back Pain and Sciatica. N Engl J Med. 1988; 318:291–300
[35] Deyo RA, Rainville J, Kent DL. What Can the History and Physical Examination Tell Us About Low Back Pain? JAMA. 1992; 268:760–765
[36] Janin Y, Epstein JA, Carras R, et al. Osteoid Osteomas and Osteoblastomas of the Spine. Neurosurgery. 1981; 8:31–38
[37] Calin A, Porta J, Fries JF, Schurman DJ. Clinical History as a Screening Test for Ankylosing Spondylitis. JAMA. 1977; 237:2613–2614
[38] Crayton HE, Bell CL, De Smet AA. Sacral Insufficiency Fractures. Sem Arth Rheum. 1991; 20:378–384
[39] McCarron RF, Wimpee MW, Hudkins PG, et al. The Inflammatory Effect of Nucleus Pulposus: A Possible Element in the Pathogenesis of Low-Back Pain. Spine. 1987; 12:760–764
[40] Hirsch C, Schajowicz F. Studies on Structural Changes in the Lumbar Annulus Fibrosus. Acta Orthop Scand. 1952; 22:184–231
[41] Choice of lipid-regulating drugs. Med Letter. 2001; 43:43–48
[42] Seftel AD, Farber J, Fletcher J, Deeley MC, Elion-Mboussa A, Hoover A, Yu A, Fredlund P. A three-part study to investigate the incidence and potential etiologies of tadalafil-associated back pain or myalgia. Int J Impot Res. 2005; 17:455–461
[43] Jensen MC, Brant-Zawadzki MN, Obuchowski N, et al. Magnetic Resonance Imaging of the Lumbar Spine in People Without Back Pain. N Engl J Med. 1994; 331:69–73
[44] Bonney G. Iatrogenic Injuries of Nerves. J Bone Joint Surg. 1986; 68B:9–13
[45] Eskandary H, Hamzel A, Yasamy MT. Foot Drop Following Brain Lesion. Surg Neurol. 1995; 43:89–90
[46] Bell HS. Paralysis of both arms from injury of the upper portion of the pyramidal decussation: "cruciate paralysis". J Neurosurg. 1970; 33:376–380
[47] Yayama T, Uchida K, Kobayashi S, Nakajima H, Kubota C, Sato R, Baba H. Cruciate paralysis and hemiplegia cruciata: report of three cases. Spinal Cord. 2006; 44:393–398
[48] Hawkins RJ, Bilco T, Bonutti P. Cervical Spine and Shoulder Pain. Clin Orthop Rel Res. 1990; 258:142–146

[49] Goldenberg DL. Fibromyalgia Syndrome. JAMA. 1987; 257:2782–2787
[50] Wolfe F, Smythe HA, Yunus MB, et al. The American College of Rheumatology 1990 Criteria for the Classification of Fibromyalgia: Report of the Multicenter Criteria Committee. Arthritis Rheum. 1990; 33:160–172
[51] Adler GK, Kinsley BT, Hurwitz S, et al. Reduced Hypothalamic-Pituitary and Sympathoadrenal Responses to Hypoglycemia in Women with Fibromyalgia Syndrome. Am J Med. 1999; 106:534–543
[52] Goto S, Umehara J, Aizawa T, Kokubun S. Crowned Dens syndrome. J Bone Joint Surg Am. 2007; 89:2732–2736
[53] Stricker LJ, Green CR. Resolution of refractory symptoms of secondary erythermalgia with intermittent epidural bupivacaine. Reg Anesth Pain Med. 2001; 26:488–490
[54] Davis MD, Sandroni P. Lidocaine patch for pain of erythromelalgia. Arch Dermatol. 2002; 138:17–19
[55] Sobel JB, Sollenberger P, Robinson R, Polatin PB, Gatchel RJ. Cervical nonorganic signs: A new clinical tool to assess abnormal illness behavior in neck pain patients. Arch Phys Med Rehabil. 2000; 81:170–175

Part XXIII

Procedures, Interventions, Operations

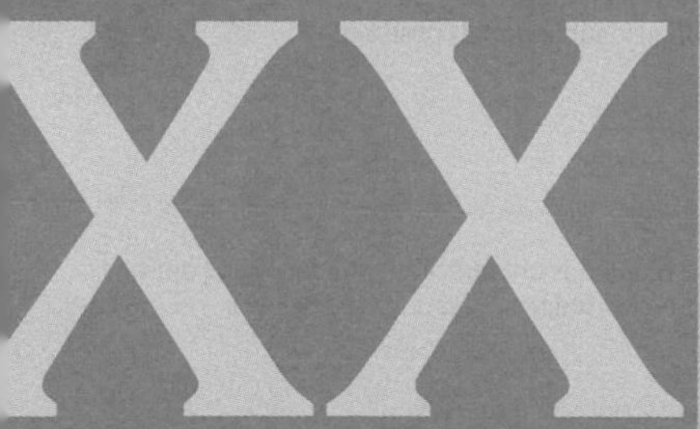

93 General Information

93.1 Introduction

This section provides information useful in the O.R. that apply to a number of different topics. Some items that are pertinent to only one topic will be found in that section instead (e.g. transsphenoidal tumor removal is found in the section on pituitary tumors).

REMEMBER: before performing any invasive procedure, know the patient's coagulation status (history of anticoagulant and/or antiplatelet function medications, and if indicated: PT, PTT, INR, platelet count and platelet function assay, FDP…).

93.2 Intraoperative dyes

This section covers visible dyes that may be useful in the operating room. For radio-opaque dyes, see Contrast agents in neuroradiology (p. 219). There is little information available in the literature regarding the intrathecal (IT) use of the following agents.

Indigo carmine: a blue dye which has been used intrathecally to locate CSF leaks. There are few published reports, and no accounts of adverse effects. In 1933 a report[1] of IT injection of 5 ml of 0.6% indigo carmine solution produced blue-green discoloration of the CSF draining through a fistula into the nose within 15 minutes, lasting for 5 hours, with no indication of toxicity. It is excreted in the urine (and not in mucous membranes). The consensus is that it should be relatively safe for IT use, but the manufacturer did not recommend this application.

✖ Methylene blue: methylene blue is probably *cytotoxic* and appears to become fixed to neural tissue. It should therefore *not* be used as a stain in neurosurgical operations or diagnostic tests. CNS damage (some permanent) occurred in 14 patients given an IT injection of a 1% solution. Symptoms included: paraparesis, quadriplegia, multiple cranial nerve involvement (including anosmia and optic atrophy), dementia and hydrocephalus.[2]

Fluorescein: although intrathecal injection (e.g. to look for CSF leak) has been used by ENT surgeons with apparently acceptable results, there is a risk of seizures. 2.5% fluorescein is diluted 1:10 with CSF or saline and ≈ 6 ml is injected into the spinal subarachnoid space (or 0.5 ml of 5% fluorescein mixed with 5–10 ml of CSF[3]).

93

Fluorescein has also been used *IV* (adult dose: 1 amp IV) to help mark areas of the brain where there is breakdown of the blood brain barrier (BBB), e.g. in tumors (p. 596), however, fluorescein is eventually excreted in mucus, urine, etc., and just about everything turns orange. It has also been used to perform intraoperative "visible angiograms" during the removal of AVMs.

Indigocyanine green (ICG): used for intraoperative angiography (p. 1597).

93.3 Operating room equipment

93.3.1 Operating microscope – observer's eyepiece

For spine cases, the ideal location of the observer eyepiece is usually directly opposite the surgeon. For intracranial work, the observer's (assistant's) eyepiece is placed to *right* of operator's except in the following cases where it is placed to the left:
1. transsphenoidal surgery (when the surgeon stands to the patient's right)
2. *right* posterior fossa craniotomy in the lateral oblique (suboccipital) position

93.3.2 Head stabilization

General information

Options include
1. Non-pin head stabilization: When absolute head fixation is not indicated, the following options avoid some of the complications associated with pin-based head fixation (see below):
   a) Horse-shoe head rest
   b) Doughnut fashioned out of stockinette
   c) Prone-view® for prone position e.g. during posterior spine surgery
2. Pin-based head-fixation: The most common system is the Mayfield head-holder.

Pin-based head-fixation

Indications for pin stabilization:

1. ✖ not recommended for use in age < 3 years, use pediatric pins with care in ages 3–10 years (this age cutoff is not based on scientific evidence, most reported complications occur in age > 3 years)
2. craniotomies:
   a) most intracranial vascular operations: a radiolucent head-holder should be used if intraoperative angiogram is to be performed
   b) often for tumor operations, especially if there is need for a self-retaining retractor system that attaches to the Mayfield head-holder (e.g. Budde halo)
   c) when intraoperative image-guidance (IG) systems are used (an alternative here is to used mask-based or strap-on registration array holders)
3. cervical spine: often used for posterior cervical operations (laminectomies, instrumentation, fusions…)

Application of pin head holder:

1. "skull block" (p. 1434) (blockade of scalp innervation) may be administered prior to pin placement. Critical for awake craniotomies (for the wake-up), and for vascular cases and cases with increased ICP where the block blunts the precipitous increase in blood pressure[4,5] that may otherwise accompany pinning which may → increased ICP. For technique, see Typical sequence of anesthesia (p. 1434).
2. plan pin placement
   a) the manufacturer recommends that the pins be placed within a band-like area similar to a "sweatband" worn just above the orbits and the pinna
   b) avoid placing pins on the thin temporal squamosa, and use with caution over the frontal sinus[6]
   c) the single pin is typically placed anteriorly when the patient is in the supine position (▶ Fig. 94.5), for a posterior fossa approach in the prone position, if the craniotomy is on one side the single pin is placed on that side
   d) the pins in the dual pin "rocker" should be equidistant from the centerline for maximal stability
3. appropriately sized sterile pins are placed in the head-holder:
   a) ✖ children < 3 yrs age A: increased risk of calvarial penetration or depressed skull fractures. A padded cerebellar head rest should be used instead[6,7]
   b) children ≥ 3 yrs age and < 10 yrs age: special pediatric pins should be employed (these pins have a "shoulder" to insure shorter depth of penetration)
4. the pins are often coated with appropriate antibiotic ointment
5. the clamp is squeezed together, allowing the ratchet gears to slide, until the pins are initially seated in the skull
6. the knob housing the tension spring and gauge is tightened (each ring = 20 lbs)
   a) adults: tighten until the third ring (60 lbs) is visible; up to 80 lbs has been described
   b) pediatrics: less pressure should be applied, 30–40 lbs has been suggested.[6] 6 Even with pediatric pins & decreased pressure, complications may occur, consider horseshoe headrest

Complications of pin head-fixation:

1. malposition of pins:
   a) through unintended anatomic structures: pinna, orbit, superficial temporal artery, shunt hardware, prior craniotomy defect
   b) poor fixation by not properly placing pins close to "equator" resulting in movement during surgery (with risk of cervical spine injury, injury to structures being operated on due to the sudden movement, loss of image guided registration) and possible skin laceration
2. skin penetration by pins: can cause injury to intracranial structures, infection including delayed abscess, epidural hematoma[6]…
   a) overtightening of pins
   b) incorrect pin selection: see above
   c) soft skull: in elderly patients, poorly calcified skulls, pediatric patients[6]
3. skin necrosis: especially with pediatric pins due to the "shoulder" of the pins
4. skull fracture: including "ping-pong ball" fractures in young children
5. slippage of any of the joints or connections to the O.R. table
6. clamp breakage[8,9]: inspect the head-holder for cracks prior to each application, store properly and maintain per the manufacturer's specifications

93

7. bleeding from pin site: usually when the head-holder is removed. If bleeding does not stop after a minute or so of pressure, a suture or surgical staple may be used

93.4 Surgical hemostasis

93.4.1 Basic options

1. thermocoagulation
   a) electrical coagulation:
      - monopolar (Bovie) cautery: electric current passes through the patient to a grounding pad. Because of possible transmission through electrically and thermally sensitive neural structures, this modality is not used directly on the brain or in proximity to named nerves (including cranial nerves) & nerve roots
      - bipolar cautery: current passes only between the tips of the cautery device. Used for precise coagulation. When used directly on or near to the brain or nerves, the current setting is typically reduced from that employed for general use

   b) thermal units: e.g. AccuTemp® disposable eye cautery units (particularly useful to coagulate dura when inserting a ventriculostomy in the ICU)
   c) laser: especially neodymium:yttrium-aluminum-garnet (Nd:YAG) laser
2. mechanical
   a) bone wax: originated by Sir Victor Horsely. *Inhibits bone formation*
   b) ligature: less commonly used in neurosurgery than other specialties
   c) "silver clips" (e.g. HemoClips®)
3. chemical hemostasis: see below

93.4.2 Chemical hemostasis

See review[10] for more information. Some key points:

1. gelatin sponge (Gelfoam®): no intrinsic coagulating effect. Absorbs 45 times its weight in blood which causes it to expand and tamponade bleeding. Absorbable. May be combined with thrombin as patties or as powder (e.g. FLOSEAL®, SurgiFlo®)
2. oxidized cellulose (Oxycel®) and oxidized regenerated cellulose (Surgicel®): absorbable. Acidic material that reacts with blood to form a reddish brown "pseudoclot." Bactericidal to over 20 different organisms. May retard bone growth. Oxycel® interferes with epithelialization more than Surgicel®
3. microfibrillar collagen (Avitene®): promotes adhesion and aggregation of platelets. Loses effectiveness in severe thrombocytopenia (< 10,000/ml). May be used on bone bleeding. Remove excess material to reduce risk of infection
4. thrombin (Thrombostat®): does not depend on any intermediate physiological agent. Caution: although thrombin may cause significant edema when placed on brain where the pia has been disrupted, practical experience indicates this is uncommon

93.5 Craniotomy general information

93.5.1 Cranial perforators

Perforators are one means used to create burr holes which enable the surgeon to access the brain for intracranial procedures. Many brands of perforators are designed with a slip clutch that disengages the drill and stops the outer shaft from spinning and entering the skull once the central part of the drill penetrates the inner table. While these clutches are generally reliable and immensely helpful, there is a possibility of malfunction such that the outer shaft continues to rotate and if it penetrates the inner table, the entire drill can plunge into the brain. In 8 months of 2005 the FDA received reports of 200 injuries as a result of the drill failing to disengage.[11] The FDA released a number of recommendations to reduce the risk of injury,[11] excerpts of which are shown here:

- select the appropriate perforator based on the skull thickness (pediatric vs. adult)
- keep the perforator perpendicular to the skull throughout the drilling process
- do not rock, rotate, or change the angle of the device during drilling
- avoid using excessive pressure on the drill. Brace the hand holding the drill on the other hand which should rest on the patient's skull, and thereby prevent plunging if the drill completely penetrates the skull
- use caution when:
  - drilling through areas of irregular bone contour, curvature or variations in thickness

- drilling on skulls of infants/children, the elderly, or any other patient who might have softer bone consistency (including osteogenesis imperfecta...)
- perforating bone in an area where the bone might be diseased or incompetent or have loose fragments

93.5.2 Intraparenchymal cyst aspiration

When a cystic tumor or intracerebral hemorrhage is being operated on, an attempt should be made to insert a ventricular needle into the lesion and aspirate some but not all of the cyst contents. This often produces significant decompression. Avoid evacuating all of the contents otherwise the lesion might be difficult to find. The needle may then be left in place to allow localization of the lesion (or the needle track can be followed, which may occasionally be difficult).

93.5.3 Intra-operative brain swelling

Background

Under certain circumstances during surgery, the brain may start to severely swell out of the craniotomy wound. Etiologies of this emergency situation include:

1. extraparenchymal bleeding: from a vessel or intraoperative aneurysm rupture, remotely situated epidural/subdural hematoma
2. intracerebral hemorrhage
3. venous outflow obstruction
4. vasodilatation induced by hypercarbia
5. severe diffuse cerebral edema following stroke or traumatic brain injury (TBI)

Management

First efforts should be aimed at ruling out and correcting the aforementioned causes as well as some adjunctive measures. Most maneuvers are similar to those used in controlling an ICP crisis. During the process, it is critical to try to avoid having the brain compress itself against the craniotomy bone edges which can lacerate the cortex and can also further compromise cortical veins which impairs venous outflow causing more brain edema and swelling which accelerates the vicious cycle.

1. elevate the head of the patient (e.g. with reverse Trendelenburg of the O.R. table)
2. make sure the jugular veins are not kinked: this may require rotating the head by loosening the pivot that connects the table adapter to the Mayfield head holder and rotating the head to a more neutral position
3. rule-out hypercarbia: make sure the endotracheal tube is not kinked, check the patient's end-tidal pCO_2
4. measures to lower ICP and protect the brain
   a) give Mannitol 1 gm/kg IV bolus
   b) drain CSF if an option: from adjacent cistern or lumbar drain
   c) have anesthesiologist hyperventilate to a PCO_2 of 30–35 mm Hg
   d) have anesthesiologist induce burst suppression
5. emergently intubate patients who are undergoing awake craniotomy
6. consider intraoperative ultrasound if rapidly available to rule-out hematoma (intracerebral, EDH, SDH) which could potentially be immediately evacuated
7. during the above steps, place a moist sponge on the surface of the brain and gently but firmly apply evenly distributed pressure to push the brain back into the wound
8. if all else is failing, the craniotomy flap can be enlarged as much as possible to create a decompressive craniotomy. Enlarging the skin incision to do so is preferable to having too small a bony opening which risks brain compression/laceration against the edges. The skin is closed without the bone flap and without dural closure as in a decompressive craniectomy (p. 1467)
9. a last ditch life-saving measure for continued uncontrollable swelling which is to be taken under advisement with eloquent cortex: use a gloved hand to sweep the herniating brain out of the wound (i.e. remove it from the patient)

93.5.4 Craniotomy pre- and post-op management

Risks

Many risks cannot be generalized for all craniotomies and are specific to various tumors, aneurysms, etc. General information:

1. post-operative hemorrhage
   a) overall risk of post-operative hemorrhage[12,13]: 0.8–1.1%. The most common indication for craniotomy in these series was for meningioma, followed by trauma, aneurysm, and then intrinsic supratentorial tumors. 43–60% of the hematomas were intraparenchymal, 28–33% epidural, 5–7% subdural, 5% intrasellar, 8% mixed, 11% confined to superficial wound. Overall mortality was 32%
   b) hematoma may occur at the surgical site or in remote locations, e.g. intracerebellar hemorrhage after pterional[14] and temporal[15] craniotomies
2. in craniotomy for brain tumor[16]:
   a) risk of anesthetic complications: 0.2%
   b) increased neurologic deficit in 1st 24 hours post-op: ≈ 10%
   c) wound infection: 2%
3. postoperative headache (p. 1431)

Pre-op orders

1. for tumor: if patient on steroids, give ≈ 50% higher dose 6 hrs before and on-call to O.R. (stress doses); if not on steroids give dexamethasone 10 mg PO 6 hrs before and on call to O.R. (in A.M., give with sip water)
2. antiepileptic medication
   a) if there is a history of seizures:
      - if already on antiepileptic drugs (AEDs) continue same doses
      - if not on AEDs, load with Keppra 500 mg or oral PHT (may give 300 mg PO q 4 hrs × 3 doses (total 900 mg) to load orally)
   b) if no history of seizures
      - if surgery does not require a cortical incision (e.g. aneurysm) then AEDs are generally not used
      - if a cortical incision is anticipated, option to load with AEDs as above
3. prophylactic antibiotics: (optional) ideally 30–60 minutes before incision. For most antibiotics, it is given in the O.R. before the skin incision. For antibiotics that take a long time to infuse (e.g. vancomycin) it may help to order it to be given "on call to O.R."
4. DVT prophylaxis: pneumatic compression boots or knee-high TED® hose

Post-op orders

93

Guidelines (individualize as appropriate) for patient to be extubated

1. admit PACU, transfer to ICU (neuro unit if available) when stable
2. VS: q 15 min x 4 hrs, then q 1 hr. Temperature q 4 hrs x 3 d, then q 8 hrs. Neuro check q 1 hr
3. activity: bed rest (BR) with HOB elevated 20–30°
4. knee high TED hose or pneumatic compression boots
5. I & O q 1 hr (if no Foley: straight cath q 4 hrs PRN bladder distension)
6. incentive spirometry q 2 hrs while awake (*do not use following transsphenoidal surgery*)
7. diet: NPO except minimal ice chips and meds as ordered
8. IVF: NS + 20 mEq KCl/L @ 90 ml/hr
9. O_2: 2 L per NC
10. meds:
    a) dexamethasone (Decadron®): if not on chronic steroids, give 4 mg IV q 6 hrs. Otherwise give stress doses based on patients current dose and length of treatment
    b) H2 antagonist, e.g. ranitidine 50 mg IVPB q 8 hrs
    c) Anti-epileptic drug (AED) especially when cerebral cortex is violated: typically Keppra® (levetiracetam): 500 mg PO or IV q 12 hours. If there is no prior history of seizure, typically discontinue after ≈ 1 week
    d) Cardene® drip: titrate to keep SBP < 160 mm Hg and/or DBP < 100 mm Hg (use cuff pressures, may use A-line pressures if they correlate with cuff pressures)
    e) codeine 30–60 mg IM q 3–4 hrs PRN H/A
    f) acetaminophen (Tylenol®) 650 mg PO/PR q 4 hrs PRN temperature > 100.5° F (38 C)
    g) continue prophylactic antibiotics if used: (e.g. cefazolin (Kefzol®) 500–1000 mg IVPB q 6 hrs x 24 hrs, then D/C)
11. labs:
    a) CBC once stabilized in ICU and q d thereafter
    b) renal profile once stabilized in ICU and q 12 hrs thereafter
    c) ABG once stabilized in ICU and q 12 hrs x 2 days, then D/C (also check ABG after any ventilator change if patient on ventilator)

12. call M.D. if any deterioration in crani checks, for T > 101° (38.5 C), sudden increase in SBP, SBP < 120, U.O. < 60 ml/2-hrs
13. post-op CT: non-contrast post-op head CT is performed if the patient does not return to baseline neurologic function within a reasonable amount of time, also, performed routinely at many institutions following all craniotomies

93.5.5 Postoperative deterioration

General information

When the postoperative neurologic status is worse than pre-op, especially in a patient who deteriorates after initially doing well following surgery, emergency evaluation and treatment is indicated.

Possible etiologies:

1. hematoma (p. 1429)
   a) intracerebral hemorrhage (ICH)
   b) epidural hematoma: at or remote from surgical site
   c) subdural hematoma
2. cerebral infarction
   a) arterial
   b) venous infarction: especially with surgery on or around the venous sinuses (p. 1466)
3. postoperative seizure: may be due to inadequate anticonvulsant levels, and may be exacerbated by any of the above (see below for management)
4. acute hydrocephalus
5. pneumocephalus; also see Pneumocephalus (p. 887):
   a) tension pneumocephalus: see Tension pneumocephalus (p. 888)
   b) simple pneumocephalus: the simple presence of air in the cranium can cause neurologic symptoms even if not under tension (as would commonly occur following the now outdated pneumoencephalogram). Symptoms include: lethargy, confusion, severe headache, nausea & vomiting, seizures. Air may be located over the cerebral convexities, in the p-fossa, and/or in the ventricles and usually resorbs with symptomatic improvement in 1–3 days
6. edema: may improve with steroids
   a) worsening of cerebral edema: moderate post-op worsening of cortical function of immediately adjacent brain is not unexpected in many operations, and is usually transient. However, reversible etiologies (such as subdural hematoma (SDH)) must be ruled out
   b) traction or manipulation of cranial nerves may cause dysfunction that may be temporary. Division of cranial nerves can cause permanent dysfunction
7. persistent anesthetic effect (including paralytics): unlikely in a patient who deteriorates after initially doing well post-op. Consider reversing medication given during surgery (caution re hypertension and agitation), e.g. naloxone, flumazenil (p. 298), or reversal of pharmacologic muscle block (p. 136)
8. vasospasm: following SAH or may be due to manipulation of blood vessels

Postoperative seizure management

1. intubate if patient does not rapidly regain consciousness, is not protecting airway, or has labored respirations
2. CT scan: rule out hematoma (intracerebral or extra-axial) or hydrocephalus
3. anticonvulsants:
   a) draw blood for appropriate anticonvulsant level
   b) bolus with additional anticonvulsants: do not wait for levels

93.5.6 Postoperative headache

General information

Persistent headache (H/A) is well described following posterior fossa craniectomy (incidence range: 0–83%[17]). The time course in one series[18] was: 23% at 3 mos, 16% at 1 yr, and 9% at 2 yrs.

Persistent H/A may also be observed following supratentorial craniotomy[19] (prevalence 1 year after anterior temporal lobectomy for seizures: 12%[19]). The "syndrome of the trephined" was first described in the French literature during World War I, and consisted of: headache and sometimes pulsatile pain (usually localized to the area of the skull defect), amnesia, inability to concentrate, insomnia... similar in some ways to postconcussive syndrome (p. 923).

93

These H/A have been attributed to: traction on the dura when the bone is not replaced, tension on the dura due to tight dural closure, temporalis or nuchal muscle dissection, nerve entrapment in the closing sutures or in the healing scar, intradural blood and/or bone dust, CSF leak.[19]

Prevention

No single method or group of methods has been successful in completely eliminating the complaint of post-op H/A.[20,21] Until further research can further advance the understanding of the cause and prevention of these H/A, it seems reasonable to employ the following measures as much as possible in an attempt to minimize these debilitating symptoms: restoring function of the temporalis or suboccipital musculature, rigid fixation of bone flaps, cranioplasty for large craniectomies, meticulous tension-free dural closure (using duraplasty when necessary), and keeping intradural blood clot and bone dust to the minimum possible.[22] Cranioplasty following posterior fossa surgery for vestibular schwannoma reduced the incidence of post-op H/A from 17% to 4%.[23]

Treatment

Initially, symptomatic treatment is indicated. Referral to a H/A specialist may be appropriate when it becomes apparent that the H/A are not resolving spontaneously after ≈ 3 months.[22]

93.6 Intraoperative cortical mapping (brain mapping)

93.6.1 General information

Indications: typically used to locate motor strip, sensory cortex, or speech centers intraoperatively for surgery in and around these eloquent areas. Localization of these areas based on visible anatomy alone is unreliable. These techniques are typically employed in seizure surgery as well as in treating lesions in areas of eloquent brain.

Some techniques require an awake patient, with the surgery being done under local anesthesia with sedation. Motor and sensory cortex can also be localized in anesthetized patients using SSEPs (see below).

93

93.6.2 Phase reversal method for localizing primary sensory and motor cortex

General information

Utilizes intra-operative SSEPs to localize primary sensory and motor cortex in patients under general anesthesia (as opposed to using brain mapping techniques in awake patients).[24,25]

Technique

See anesthesia requirements for intraoperative EP monitoring (p. 107). A strip grid is placed on the surface of the brain perpendicular to the anticipated orientation of the central sulcus. SSEP stimulation is performed while recording through the strip grid. Phase reversal of the N20/P20 peak between a pair of electrodes in the strip grid indicates that those electrodes straddle the central sulcus (► Fig. 93.1) with primary motor cortex located anteriorly, and sensory cortex posteriorly. The grid is then repositioned and the test is run again to verify the findings.

93.6.3 Awake craniotomy

General information

Usually employed for brain mapping, especially for speech areas. Numerous techniques and protocols have been described. Typically, the patient is temporarily anesthetized with short acting agents (inhalational and/or injectable). This is supplemented with local anesthetic. The craniotomy is then performed and the patient is allowed to wake up while the brain is exposed to permit neurophysiologic testing during surgery. If (short-acting) paralytics are used, it is critical to reverse these agents 15–30 minutes prior to applying the electrical stimulation and that a train-of-four muscle twitch can be elicited.

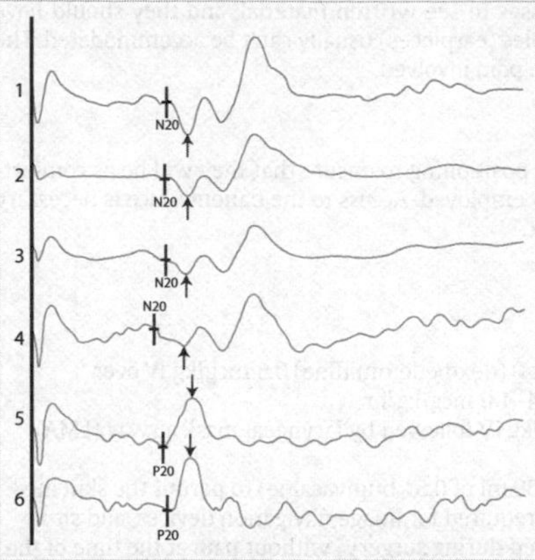

Fig. 93.1 Phase reversal
Intra-op 6-electrode recording strip placed on the brain during SSEP recording. Phase reversal of the negative N20 peak (arrows) to a positive P20 peak between electrodes #4 & 5 indicates that electrodes #4 & 5 straddle the central sulcus.

Booking the case: Awake craniotomy

Also see defaults & disclaimers (p. 27) and pre-op counselling (see below).

1. position: depends on lesion location, with pin headholder (for image guided navigation if used)
2. equipment:
   a) microscope if needed e.g. for tumor dissection
   b) image guided navigation system (if used)
   c) ultrasonic aspirator (for tumors)
3. anesthesia: pre-op consult for "awake craniotomy" & skull block
4. consult neurology or neuropsychology to be available during surgery for intra-op neurologic testing for "awake craniotomy"
5. EEG techs to perform intra-op EEG and provide brain stimulator
6. post-op: ICU
7. consent (in lay terms for the patient – not all-inclusive):
   a) procedure: surgery on the brain to be performed with periods where the patient will be woken up for testing, (plus whatever else is planned, e.g. removal of tumor, removal of seizure source...)
   b) alternatives: the same surgery under general anesthesia, nonsurgical management, (for some diagnoses, e.g. tumor, radiation therapy)
   c) complications: (usual craniotomy complications: stroke, bleeding, coma, death, infection, seizures), difficulty accurately mapping the desired areas of the brain

93

Indications

1. surgery in eloquent brain (near motor strip (Brodmann's area 4 in ▶ Fig. 1.1) or speech/language centers (Wernicke's & Broca's areas)) or thalamus, including tumors and epileptic foci
2. removal of brainstem tumors
3. some seizure surgery to look for seizure focus

Contraindications to awake craniotomy

1. patient unlikely to be able to cooperate: very young or very elderly patients, confused patients, those with significant speech deficits already present or language barrier

Patient counselling pre-op

Patients need to be aware of what the sequence of events will be and what will be expected of them. It may be helpful to have them practice reading some typical material that will be used in the O.R.

Patients over age ≈ 40 usually need reading glasses to see written material, and they should have their own available in the O.R., although the temples (earpieces) usually can't be accommodated. The patient should be advised that there may be some pain involved.

Patient positioning for surgery

Significantly more time must be spent on patient positioning to ensure that they will be as comfortable as possible without moving. Extra padding is employed. Access to the patient's face is necessary for the anesthesiologist and the neurophysiologist.

Typical sequence for anesthesia

See reference.[26]

1. in the pre-op holding area, load with Precedex® (dexmedetomidine) 0.5 mcg/kg IV over 20 minutes followed by intra-op infusion at 0.4–1.0 mcg/kg/hr
2. induction of anesthesia utilizes propofol 3 mg/kg IV followed by laryngeal mask airway (LMA) placement
3. skull block[4]: injection of local anesthetic (e.g. 30 ml of 0.5% bupivacaine) to permit the skin incision and also rigid head fixation with pins (as required for image navigation devices, and situations where no head movement can be tolerated during surgery) without pain at the time of the wake-up. Injection at 4 regions on each side as shown in ▶ Fig. 93.2:

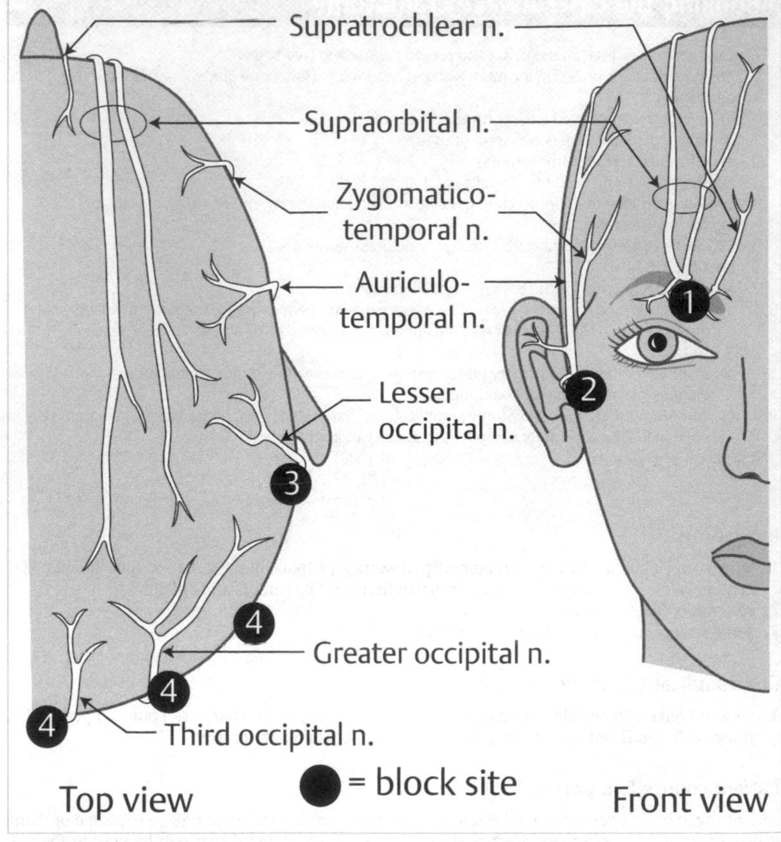

Fig. 93.2 Infiltration sites for skull block

❶ supraorbital & supratrochlear nerves: 2 ml injected 1.5 cm above the supraorbital foramen above the medial third of the orbit. NB: if you are going to use surface matching to register the patient for image guidance (e.g. BrainLab or Stealth), injecting here may deform the skin and affect the registration accuracy. Consider injecting a lower volume of higher concentration agent (e.g. 2% lidocaine)
❷ auriculotemporal nerve: 5 ml injected 1.5 cm anterior to the tragus. ✖ Caution: to avoid anesthetizing the facial nerve, inject just deep to the subcutaneous tissue
❸ postauricular branches of the greater auricular nerve: 2 ml 1.5 cm posterior to the antitragus
❹ greater, lesser & third occipital nerves: inject 5 ml with a 22 gauge spinal needle at the mastoid process and proceed along the nuchal ridge until the midline is reached

4. start inhalational anesthesia with 0.5 MAC desflurane with the patient breathing spontaneously while the scalp incision, craniotomy, and dural opening are performed (the dura is pain sensitive, the brain is not)
5. as the dural opening is begun, the desflurane is turned off and a remifentanil infusion of 0.1–0.2 mcg/kg/min IV is started
6. by the time the dural opening is completed, the desflurane has usually worn off and the LMA can be removed
7. remifentanil is then titrated for pain control
8. neurophysiologic testing can usually be performed at this time (e.g. below)
9. the operation may often be carried to completion with the patient awake, although once the intracranial part of the operation is completed, more pain relief may be desired and general anesthesia may be needed for pain control or agitation (LMA may suffice here)

93.6.4 Speech mapping

General information

Typical settings for a constant current generator using a bipolar electrode are shown in ▶ Table 93.1. If a voltage based unit is used, start at 1 volt and increase.

Techniques for speech mapping

There are numerous methodologies. One protocol:

1. requires awake craniotomy
2. once temporal lobe is exposed, a recording electrode strip is place on the brain surface
3. using a bipolar stimulator, start with a low current (e.g. 2 mA) and begin stimulate an area of cortex for 3–5 seconds, and observe for afterdischarges (akin to a focal seizure) on the recording strip. If no afterdischarges, increase the current in 2 mA increments up to a maximum of ≈ 10 mA. If afterdischarges occur, back off by 1–2 mA and then test that area for speech changes as follows
4. stimulate cortex while patient names objects shown on picture cards (automatic verbalization, such as counting, is robust and may persist). Observe for effects ranging from total speech arrest to paraphasic errors
5. repeat the above steps at the next area (first finding threshold for afterdischarges and then stimulating while testing)

Table 93.1 Settings for constant current generator

Control	Setting[a]
frequency	50–60 Hz
waveform	biphasic square wave
duration	2–4 mS peak-to-peak
mode	repeat
polarity	normal
current	varies between 2–16 mA

[a]not all settings are present on all models

93

93.7 Cranioplasty

93.7.1 Indications

1. cosmetic restoration of external skull symmetry
2. relief of symptoms due to craniotomy defect (p. 1431)
3. protection from trauma (blunt or penetrating) in area of post-craniotomy or posttraumatic skull defect

93.7.2 Timing

In certain cases, no consensus is possible. To avoid the risk of infection, some authors recommend delaying cranioplasty with a "foreign body" (e.g. tantalum mesh) at least 6 months after an open (i.e. contaminated) wound or one that traverses the nasal sinuses. Others perform primary closure at the time of repair of the skull fracture. In "clean" cases (e.g. repair of defect after removing hemangioma of the skull) there is little argument against immediate cranioplasty.

93.7.3 Material

Options for material include:
1. the patient's own bone if it was previously removed in a sterile fashion and saved either in a sterile manner under refrigeration, or in an abdominal pocket at the time of craniectomy
2. materials that can be formed by the surgeon
   a) methylmethacrylate: mixed in the O.R., molded to desired shape, and allowed to set before being attached to the skull usually with plates (alternatively, sutures or wire may be used). Setting is an exothermic reaction and ample irrigation and preferably removal from the operative site during the process avoids undesirable transmission of heat to the brain
   b) mesh: may be made of titanium or tantalum.
3. pre-fabricated custom flaps may be made by a number of commercial vendors using thin-cut CT scans to generate computer models of the defect and, if available, to use the contralateral side as a "mirror image" model for the desired shape
   a) methylmethacrylate
   b) PEEK (poly-ether-ether-ketone)
   c) titanium
4. split thickness calvaria

93

When foreign material is used, some recommend perforating the flap with a dozen or so drill holes to prevent the accumulation of fluid (either underneath the flap, or between the flap and the skull). This cannot be done with tantalum plates.

Localizing levels in spine surgery

Identifying the correct level in spine surgery may be extremely challenging in certain situations. With the proliferation of minimally invasive spine techniques and the associated reduction in the structures that are directly visualized, the reliance on intraoperative imaging to determine the spinal level has increased.

Potential pitfalls which increase the chances of error, including:
1. pre-op, pathology is usually identified on MRI, and there are problems in translating MRI images to imaging available in the O.R.
   a) thoracic lesions: pre-op MRI usually counts from the top (C2) down, and in surgery it is often necessary to count from the bottom up, the count could be off if there are not 5 lumbar vertebra and 12 pairs of ribs
   b) lumbar spine: a well developed S1–2 disc (so-called lumbarized S1) or an L5 vertebra fused to the sacrum (sacralized L5) can confuse the count
2. not all patients have 12 ribs, or 5 "lumbar" vertebrae. In the modal (most common) human spine, there are 24 presacral vertebrae, however some individuals have 23 and others have 25 (variations include: 11 or 13 rib bearing vertebrae, or a lumbosacral transitional vertebrae; the terminology of a "lumbarized S1 vertebrae" or a "sacralized L5 vertebrae" is imprecise and confusing). A HLD at the ultimate disc space (usually L5-S1) most often impinges on the 25th nerve root (however, in the variant cases, it may actually impinge on the 24th or 26th root)[27]

3. patients may have variant or ambiguous anatomy (e.g. a well-developed S1–2 disc space, an enlarged L1 transverse process which mimics a rib)
4. some "landmarks" used for localizing levels are unreliable or changeable
5. plain radiographs (and fluoroscopy) has difficult imaging the upper thoracic and sometimes the lower cervical spine
   a) on lateral imaging, the shoulder often obscure lower cervical/upper thoracic levels
   b) on AP imaging, the pronounced kyphosis of this region requires cranio-caudal angulation of the x-ray beam, which throws off imaging at other levels
6. spinous processes of lumbar and especially thoracic levels are below the corresponding VB
7. changes may occur between the time of the pre-op imaging and the surgery

Aids in determining spinal levels:
1. image guided systems, when available
2. some O.R. suites have intra-op MRI or CT (or CT-like modalities, e.g. O-arm™ by Medtronic or ARCADIS® C-arm by Siemens) or image guided spine technology
3. ✱ pre-op plain x-rays: lumbar (for lumbar pathology) and lumbar + thoracic (for thoracic pathology) to verify there are 12 thoracic vertebrae and 5 lumbar
4. on lateral lumbar spine x-rays, the top of the iliac crests are even with the L4 spinous process or the L4–5 interspinous space
5. on sagittal MRI there are generally no numbering cues, but on axial MRI, the sacral ala are reliably identifiable and this can be used to identify L5-S1 disc space
6. counting methods (if possible, using more than 1 method is highly recommended)
   a) counting up from T12 or L5 on fluoro: be sure there are 12 ribs. You can "bridge" from lumbar or lower thoracic spine to higher thoracic levels using an instrument on the patient as a marker, or you can count up to one level (e.g. T9) and then while a hemostat is placed at this level on the fluoro screen, under real-time fluoro the machine is slowly moved up the spine and the hemostat is moved along with T9 (to count up from L5, verify there are 5 lumbar (i.e. non-rib bearing) presacral vertebrae). Radiation safety: avoid live fluoro as much as possible
   b) AP view: starting at T12 (lowest rib) or from L5
   c) lateral view: starting at the L5 and counting up
   d) counting down from T1 (first rib) on AP fluoro: the fluoro machine may need to be angled caudally from the anterior position because of the thoracic kyphosis. Sometimes counting pedicles helps
   e) by palpation: with thoracotomy, in the upper T-spine you can palpate the ribs from the inside from T1 and count down. The rib inserts at the upper end of the thoracic vertebra near the junction with the VB above (e.g. the T5 rib joins T5 close to the T4–5 disc space)

93.8 Bone graft

93.8.1 Use of bone graft extenders/substitutes as an adjunct to fusion

Practice guideline: Bone graft extenders and substitutes

Level I[28]: autologous bone or recombinant human bone morphogenic protein (rhBMP-2) bone graft substitute is recommended in the setting of an ALIF in conjunction with a threaded titanium cage

Level III[28]:
- rhBMP-2 in conjunction with hydroxyapatite and tricalcium phosphate may be substituted for autograft in some cases of posterolateral fusion
- calcium phosphate is recommended as a bone graft extender, especially when combined with autologous bone

93.8.2 Assessing surgical lumbar fusion

See **Practice guideline: Radiographic assessment of fusion** (p. 1438).

Practice guideline: Radiographic assessment of fusion

Level I[29]: static x-rays alone are *not* recommended

Level II[29]:

- in the *absence* of rigid instrumentation, lack of motion between vertebrae on lateral flexion/extension x-rays is highly suggestive of successful fusion
- ✖ technetium-99 bone scanning is *not* recommended

Level III[29]: radiographic techniques, often in combination, may be used when failed lumbar fusion is suspected, including: static and flexion/extension x-rays, CT scan

Practice guideline: Correlation between fusion and outcome

Level III[30]: the correlation between fusion and clinical outcome is not strong, and in any given situation fusion status may be unrelated to outcome

93.8.3 Bone graft properties

General information

For spine fusions, components of bone graft that are important for fusion:

1. osteoinduction: recruitment of mesenchymal cells and the stimulation of these cells to develop into osteoblasts and osteoclasts
2. osteogenesis: formation of new bone by host or graft mesenchymal stem cells transformed into osteoblasts
3. osteoconduction: the structure of the graft that acts as a scaffold upon which new bone and blood vessels form
4. mechanical stability: the structural anatomical biomechanical support provided, e.g. following discectomy, corpectomy or resection of vertebral tumor

93

▶ Table 93.2 summarizes the properties of various bone graft materials (adapted[31,32,33]). See the sections that follow for more details.

Table 93.2 Characteristics of bone graft materials[a] (see text for details)

Material	Mechanical stability	Osteogenic	Osteo-inductive	Osteo-conductive
Cancellous autograft	±	++++	++	++++
Cortical autograft	+++	+	+	+
Vascularized autograft	+++	+++	++	+++
Allograft	+	–	±	+
Bone marrow aspirate	–	+	±	+
Demineralized bone matrix (DBM)	–	–	+	+
Bone morphogenic protein (BMP)	–	–	++++	–
Collagen	–	–	–	–
Ceramics	+	–	–	+++

[a] – no effect, ± minimal or no effect, + mild, ++ moderate, +++ strong, ++++ very strong effect

Autograft

Common donor sites: iliac crest, rib,[34] fibula, bone removed during decompression. Characteristics:
1. PROS: no histocompatibility or disease transmission issues
2. CONS:
   a) persistent post-op donor site pain: occurs in as many as 34% of patients (the severity of which was graded as "unacceptable" in 3%)[35]
   b) increased surgical risks of:
      - blood loss
      - wound infection
      - fracture
      - cosmetic deformity
      - increased operative time to procure
      - numbness from nerve injury (e.g. cluneal nerves see below)
      - hematoma
3. subtypes
   a) cancellous bone: provides all graft components except mechanical stability
   b) cortical bone:
      - provides superior and immediate mechanical strength
      - has diminished osteoinduction and osteoconduction capacity
   c) corticocancellous bone: e.g. tricortical iliac crest wedge. Contains all bone graft components
   d) vascularized autograft:
      - technically challenging
      - best suited for areas that are scarred, irradiated, or that span long segments
   e) autologous bone marrow:
      - source of osteoprogenitor cells and osteoinductive substrates
      - diminished donor site risks
      - no osteoconductive nor structural properties

Allograft

Acquired through organ procurement agencies. Primarily frozen or freeze dried. Donor sites include: ilium, tibia, fibula, femur, rib.
1. PROS: eliminates risks associated with harvesting autograft
2. CONS:
   a) small but real risk of disease transmission
   b) provide only osteoconduction (lacks osteoinduction and osteogenesis)
   c) availability may vary from time-to-time
3. subtypes
   a) tricortical block, bicortical plug, or unicortical dowel
   b) corticocancellous: matchsticks, crushed
   c) cancellous: cubes, block, crushed, bone powder
4. uses: allografts are acceptable for structural grafts such as in anterior spinal interbody fusion, where compressive forces are applied to the graft. However, for onlay grafts such as for posterior cervical fusion, the lack of osteoinductive and osteogenetic properties is a critical shortcoming

Demineralized bone matrix (DBM)

Prepared by acid extraction, reducing antigenicity, but preserving some osteoconductive and variable osteoinductive properties.
1. available as putty, gel, chips, granules or powder
2. primarily used as an adjunct to other grafting materials
3. CONS:
   a) increased cost
   b) variable efficacy between preparations and batches of the same preparation
   c) no mechanical or structural properties

Bone morphogenic proteins (BMP)

(AKA bone morphogenetic proteins). Biological compounds that induce the transformation of mesenchymal stem cells into osteoblasts (osteoinduction) with the potential to induce ectopic bone formation. There are ≈ 20 different proteins from the transforming growth factor-β family. Produced using recombinant DNA technology.

93

1. a carrier matrix is required to retain the soluble factor at the graft site (i.e. to prevent the BMP from diffusing into adjacent tissues, thereby reducing the desired effect and possibly inducing bone growth at undesired foci)
2. FDA approved in U.S. only for ALIF. Other uses are "off label"
3. available preparations: rhBMP-2 (Infuse® by Medtronic)
4. PROS: increases fusion rates
5. CONS:
   a) expensive
   b) ectopic bone formation, bone resorption (so-called osteolysis) or remodelling at the graft site[36]
   c) in anterior cervical spine surgery: neck swelling with airway compromise, hematoma, painful seroma[36]

Collagen

Used primarily as a carrier for other osteoinductive, osteoconductive, or osteogenetic materials and as a composite with other graft extenders
1. PROS: contributes to vascular ingrowth, mineral deposition, and growth factor binding
2. CONS:
   a) minimal structural support
   b) potential immunogenicity

Ceramics

Includes tricalcium phosphate, calcium carbonate & hydroxyapatite.
1. PROS: no risk of disease transmission
2. CONS: only recommended for use as bone graft extenders (i.e. must be combined with autograft, bone marrow aspirate, BMP…)

93.8.4 Bone graft procurement

Iliac crest

Anterior iliac bone graft

93

Should be obtained at least ≈ 3–4 cm lateral to the anterior superior iliac spine (ASIS) to avoid the lateral femoral cutaneous nerve and to reduce the risk of avulsion fractures of the remaining ilium. When a tricortical graft is taken, keep the dissection in the subperiosteal plane and avoid electrocautery on the medial (inner) surface when detaching the iliacus muscle to avoid injury to the ilioinguinal, iliohypogastric and lateral femoral cutaneous nerves.

Posterior iliac crest bone graft

May be used to obtain corticocancellous strips or plates for onlay bone grafts, or tricortical grafts which may be used as strut grafts or for C1–2 arthrodesis.

Posterior bone grafts (▶ Fig. 93.3) are taken from the medial 6–8 cm of the iliac crest to avoid the superior cluneal nerves (which cross the posterior iliac crest ≈ 8 cm lateral to the posterior superior iliac spine) with resultant buttock numbness or the development of painful neuromas. A vertical incision just medial to the posterior superior iliac spine usually works well.

The spine may sometimes be found on corpulent patients by locating the "dimple of Venus" (fossae lumbales laterales – indentation sometimes visible superior to the gluteal cleft, directly superficial to the sacroiliac joint) and incising slightly lateral to it. Avoid mistaking the sacrum for the iliac spine.

The gluteus maximus is dissected off the lateral surface subperiosteally. To avoid fractures extending into the iliac crest, a wide osteotome should be used to create a "stop cut"; alternatively, a sagittal saw may be used. Avoid penetration through the inner cortical surface of the crest so as not to enter the pelvis and possibly cause an intra-abdominal hematoma. Another potential complication is fracture extension into the greater sciatic notch with possible injury to the gluteal arteries and sciatic nerve among others. Once the graft is removed and cancellous bone is gouged out, the exposed bone surfaces should be waxed and closed system drainage should be used to reduce the risk of local hematoma formation.

Fibula

Autogenous fibular graft provides a high arthrodesis rate,[37] but may be associated with significant morbidity, and so may be best reserved for salvage procedures.[38] Preserve the proximal fibular head

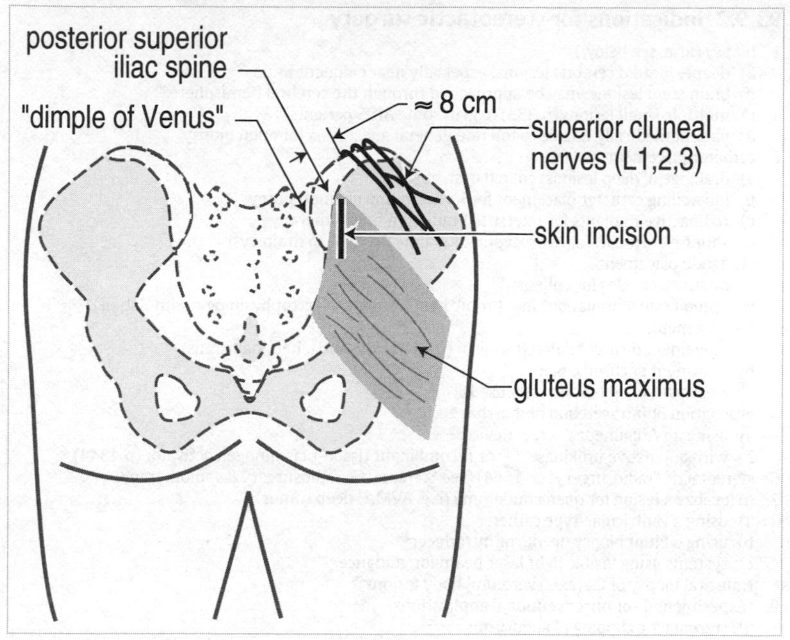

Fig. 93.3 Posterior iliac crest bone donor site

to avoid injury to the peroneal nerve. At least 7 cm of distal fibular should be maintained to preserve ankle stability.[34]

93.9 Stereotactic surgery

93.9.1 General information

The term stereotactic (Greek: stereo = 3-dimensional, tactic = to touch) surgery was initially used in animals, and was based on atlases of three dimensional coordinates compiled from dissections. The term was then used for surgery performed in humans, usually for thalamic lesioning to treat Parkinsonism (see Surgical treatment of Parkinson's disease (p. 1524)), where the target site to be lesioned was located relative to landmarks with intraoperative pneumoencephalography or contrast ventriculography. Use of this procedure fell off dramatically in the late 1960's with the introduction of L-dopa for Parkinsonism.[39]

Current techniques would be more appropriately termed *image-guided* stereotactic surgery. In the first part of the procedure, a CT scan or MRI (or occasionally, angiogram) is performed. For increased precision, some sort of "fiucial" markers or frame is attached to the patient's head during this image acquisition phase. Acceptable accuracy can often be obtained using high resolution thin cut imaging slices (usually with a 0 angle of the gantry) and then surface matching algorithms in the guidance system will match the pre-op CT/MRI to the patient's head.

The second part of the procedure usually takes place in an operating room. The patient is "reiistered" with the pre-op images, and then tracking cameras follow the movement of instruments with appropriate attachments to show in "real-time" the location of the instrument with respect to the pre-op image. An important limitation to be aware of is the fact that the pre-op images are "historical" and are not updated as the surgical procedure alters the anatomy of the patient. For example, even the administration of mannitol can cause brain shifts that may cause the target of the surgery to move away from its pre-op location by several millimeters.

93.9.2 Indications for stereotactic surgery

1. biopsy (also, see below)
   a) deeply located cerebral lesions: especially near eloquent brain
   b) brain stem lesions: may be approached through the cerebral hemisphere[40]
   c) multiple small lesions (p. 333) (e.g. in some AIDS patients)
   d) patient medically unable to tolerate general anesthesia for open biopsy
2. catheter placement
   a) drainage of deep lesions: colloid cyst, abscess
   b) indwelling catheter placement for intratumoral chemotherapy
   c) radioactive implants for interstitial radiation brachytherapy[41]
   d) shunt placement: for hydrocephalus (rarely used) or to drain cyst
3. electrode placement
   a) depth electrodes for epilepsy
   b) "deep brain stimulation" for chronic pain (requires electrophysiologic stimulation)
4. lesion generation
   a) movement disorders: Parkinsonism (p. 1526), dystonia, hemiballismus
   b) treatment of chronic pain
   c) treatment of epilepsy (rarely used)
5. evacuation of intracerebral hemorrhage
   a) using an Archimedes' screw device[42,43]
   b) with adjunctive urokinase[44,45] or recombinant tissue-plasminogen activator (p. 1344) [46]
6. stereotactic "radiosurgery" (p. 1564) (see Stereotactic radiosurgery & radiotherapy)
7. to localize a lesion for open craniotomy (e.g. AVM,[47] deep tumor)
   a) using a ventricular-type catheter
   b) using a blunt biopsy needle or introducer[48]
   c) systems using visible light laser beam for guidance
8. transoral biopsy of C2 (axis) vertebral body lesions[49]
9. "experimental" or unconventional applications
   a) stereotactic clipping of aneurysms[50]
   b) stereotactic laser surgery
   c) CNS transplantation[51]: e.g. for Parkinsonism (p. 1525)
   d) foreign body removal[52]

93

93.9.3 Stereotactic biopsy

This section presents information regarding stereotactic brain biopsy (SBB) in general. For SBB in specific conditions, see the index entry for that condition. Biopsy may be through a small "cookie cutter" craniotomy, or through a smaller burr hole with a needle. Although it may be performed under local or general anesthesia, it is more commonly done under general.

Contraindications

1. coagulation disorders
   a) coagulopathies: bleeding diatheses, iatrogenic (heparin or coumadin)
   b) low platelet count (PC): PC < 50,000/ml is an absolute contraindication, it is desirable to get the PC ≥ 100,000
2. inability to tolerate general anesthesia and to cooperate for local anesthesia

Yield

The yield rate (i.e. the ability to make a diagnosis from a SBB) reported in large series in the literature ranges from 82–99% in nonimmunocompromised (NIC) patients, and is slightly lower in AIDS patients at 56–96%. Higher yield rates in AIDS may result from improved surgical technique and histologic evaluation.[53]

The yield rate is higher for lesions that enhance with contrast on CT or MRI (99% in NIC patients) than with lesions that do not enhance (74%).[54]

Complications

The most frequent complication is hemorrhage, although most are too small to have clinical impact. The risk of a major complication (mostly due to hemorrhage) in NIC patients ranges from 0–3% (with most < 1%), and 0–12% in AIDS.[54] Higher complication rates seen in AIDS patients in some series may be due to reduced platelet count or function, and to vessel fragility in primary CNS lymphoma. In NIC patients, multifocal high grade gliomas had the highest complication rate.

Infection is an infrequent complication with needle biopsy.

References

[1] Fox N. Cure in a Case of Cerebrospinal Rhinorrhea. Arch Otolaryngol. 1933; 17:85–87

[2] Evans JP, Keegan HR. Danger in the Use of Intrathecal Methylene Blue. JAMA. 1960; 174:856–859

[3] Calcaterra TC. Extracranial Repair of Cerebrospinal Rhinorrhea. Ann Otol Rhinol Laryngol. 1980; 89:108–116

[4] Pinosky ML, Fishman RL, Reeves ST, Harvey SC, Patel S, Palesch Y, Dorman BH. The effect of bipuvicaine skull block on the hemodynamic response to craniotomy. Neurosurgical Anesthesia. 1996; 83:1256–1261

[5] el Gohary M, Gamil M, Girgis K, et al. Scalp nerve blocks in children undergoing a supratentorial craniotomy: A randomized controlled study. Asian J Sci Res. 2009; 2:105–112

[6] Vitali AM, Steinbok P. Depressed skull fracture and epidural hematoma from head fixation with pins for craniotomy in children. Childs Nerv Syst. 2008; 24:917–23; discussion 925

[7] Agrawal D, Steinbok P. Simple technique of head fixation for image-guided neurosurgery in infants. Childs Nerv Syst. 2006; 22:1473–1474

[8] Lee TH, Kim SJ, Cho do S. Broken mayfield head clamp. J Korean Neurosurg Soc. 2009; 45:306–308

[9] Taira T, Tanikawa T. Breakage of Mayfield head rest. J Neurosurg. 1992; 77:160–161

[10] Arand AG, Sawaya R. Intraoperative Chemical Hemostasis. Neurosurgery. 1986; 18:223–233

[11] . Cranial Perforators with an Automatic Clutch Mechanism, Failure to Disengage: FDA Safety Communication. 2015

[12] Kalfas IH, Little JR. Postoperative Hemorrhage: A Survey of 4992 Intracranial Procedures. Neurosurgery. 1988; 23:343–347

[13] Palmer JD, Sparrow OC, Iannottl FI. Postoperative Hematoma: A 5-Year Survey and Identification of Avoidable Risk Factors. Neurosurgery. 1994; 35:1061–1065

[14] Papanastassiou V, Kerr R, Adams C. Contralateral Cerebellar Hemorrhagic Infarction After Pterional Craniotomy: Report of Five Cases and Review of the Literature. Neurosurgery. 1996; 39:841–852

[15] Toczek MT, Morrell MJ, Silverberg GA, Lowe GM. Cerebellar Hemorrhage Complicating Temporal Lobectomy: Report of Four Cases. J Neurosurg. 1996; 85:718–722

[16] Mahaley MS, Mettlin C, Natarajan N, Laws ER, et al. National Survey of Patterns of Care for Brain-Tumor Patients. J Neurosurg. 1989; 71:826–836

[17] Driscoll CL, Beatty CW. Pain After Acoustic Neuroma Surgery. Otolaryngol Clin North Am. 1997; 30:893–903

[18] Harner SG, Beatty CW, Ebershold MJ. Headache After Acoustic Neuroma Excision. Am J Otolaryngol. 1993; 14:552–555

[19] Kaur A, Selwa L, Fromes G, Ross DA. Persistent Headache After Supratentorial Craniotomy. Neurosurgery. 2000; 47:633–636

[20] Catalano PJ, Jacobowitz O, Post KD. Prevention of Headache After Retrosigmoid Removal of Acoustic Tumors. Am J Otol. 1996; 17:904–908

[21] Lovely TJ, Lowry DW, Jannetta PJ. Functional Outcome and the Effect of Cranioplasty After Retromastoid Craniectomy for Microvascular Decompression. Surg Neurol. 1999; 51:191–197

[22] Long DM. Comment on Kaur A et al.: Persistent Headache After Supratentorial Craniotomy. Neurosurgery. 2000; 47

[23] Harner SG, Beatty CW, Ebersold MJ. Impact of cranioplasty on headache after acoustic neuroma removal. Neurosurgery. 1995; 36:1097–9; discussion 1099-100

[24] Gregori EM, Goldring S. Localization of Function in the Excision of Lesions from the Sensorimotor Region. J Neurosurg. 1984; 61:1047–1054

[25] Woolsey CN, Erickson TC, Gibson WE. Localization in Somatic Sensory and Motor Areas of Human Cerebral Cortex as Determined by Direct Recording of Evoked Potentials and Electrical Stimulation. J Neurosurg. 1979; 51:476–506

[26] Dreier JD, Williams B, Mangar D, Camporesi EM. Patients selection for awake neurosurgery. HSR Proc. 2009; 1:19–27

[27] Wigh RE. Classification of the Human Vertebral Column: Phylogenic Departures and Junctional Anomalies. Med Radiogr Photogr. 1980; 56:2–11

[28] Resnick DK, Choudhri TF, Dailey AT, Groff MW, Khoo L, Matz PG, Mummaneni P, Watters WC, Wang J, Walters BC, Hadley MN. Part 16: Bone graft extenders and substitutes. J Neurosurg: Spine. 2005; 2:733–736

[29] Resnick DK, Choudhri TF, Dailey AT, Groff MW, Khoo L, Matz PG, Mummaneni P, Watters WC, Wang J, Walters BC, Hadley MN. Part 4: Radiographic assessment of fusion. J Neurosurg Spine. 2005; 2:653–657

[30] Resnick DK, Choudhri TF, Dailey AT, Groff MW, Khoo L, Matz PG, Mummaneni P, Watters WC, Wang J, Walters BC, Hadley MN. Part 5: Correlation between radiographic and functional outcome. J Neurosurg Spine. 2005; 2:658–661

[31] Whang PG, Wang JC. Bone graft substitutes for spinal fusion. Spine J. 2003; 3:155–165

[32] Giannoudis PV, Dinopoulos H, Tsiridis E. Bone substitutes: an update. Injury. 2005; 36 Suppl 3:S20–S27

[33] Shen FH, Samartzis D, An HS. Cell technologies for spinal fusion. Spine J. 2005; 5:231S–239S

[34] Galler RM, Sonntag VKH. Bone graft harvest. BNI Quarterly. 2003; 19:13–19

[35] Heary RF, Schlenk RP, Sacchieri TA, Barone D, Brotea C. Persistent iliac crest donor site pain: independent outcome assessment. Neurosurgery. 2002; 50:510–6; discussion 516-7

[36] Vaidya R, Sethi A, Bartol S, Jacobson M, Coe C, Craig JG. Complications in the use of rhBMP-2 in PEEK cages for interbody spinal fusions. J Spinal Disord Tech. 2008; 21:557–562

[37] Gore DR. The arthrodesis rate in multilevel anterior cervical fusions using autogenous fibula. Spine. 2001; 26:1259–1263

[38] Kim CW, Abrams R, Lee G, et al. Use of vascularized fibular strut grafts as a salvage procedure for previously failed spinal arthrodesis. Spine. 2001; 19:2171–2175

[39] Gildenberg PL. Whatever Happened to Stereotactic Surgery? Neurosurgery. 1987; 20:983–987

[40] Hood TW, Gebarski SS, McKeever PE, Venes JL, et al. Stereotactic Biopsy of Intrinsic Lesions of the Brain Stem. J Neurosurg. 1986; 65:172–176

[41] Coffey RJ, Friedman WA. Interstitial Brachytherapy of Malignant Brain Tumors Using Computed Tomography-guided Stereotaxis and Available Imaging Software: Technical Report. Neurosurgery. 1987; 20:4–7

[42] Backlund E-O, von Holst H. Controlled Subtotal Evacuation of Intracerebral Hematomas by Stereotactic Technique. Surg Neurol. 1978; 9:99–101

[43] Tanikawa T, Amano K, Kawamura H, et al. CT-Guided Stereotactic Surgery for Evacuation of Hypertensive Intracerebral Hematoma. Appl Neurophysiol. 1985; 48:431–439

[44] Niizuma H, Otsuki T, Johkura H, et al. CT-Guided Stereotactic Aspiration of Intracerebral Hematoma - Result of a Hematoma-Lysis Method Using Urokinase. Appl Neurophysiol. 1985; 48:427–430

[45] Niizuma H, Shimizu Y, Yonemitsu T, Nakasato N, et al. Results of Stereotactic Aspiration in 175 Cases of Putaminal Hemorrhage. Neurosurgery. 1989; 24:814–819

[46] Schaller C, Rohde V, Meyer B, Hassler W. Stereotactic Puncture and Lysis of Spontaneous Intracerebral Hemorrhage Using Recombinant Tissue-Plasminogen Activator. Neurosurgery. 1995; 36:328–335

[47] Sisti MB, Solomon RA, Stein BM. Stereotactic Craniotomy in the Resection of Small Arteriovenous Malformations. J Neurosurg. 1991; 75:40–44

[48] Moore MR, Black PM, Ellenbogen R, Gall CM, et al. Stereotactic Craniotomy: Methods and Results Using the Brown-Roberts-Wells Stereotactic Frame. Neurosurgery. 1989; 25:572–578

[49] Patil AA. Transoral Stereotactic Biopsy of the Second Cervical Vertebral Body: Case Report with Technical Note. Neurosurgery. 1989; 25:999–1002

[50] Kandel EI, Peresedov VV. Stereotaxic Clipping of Arterial Aneurysms and Arteriovenous Malformations. J Neurosurg. 1977; 46:12–23

[51] Backlund E-O, Granberg P-O, Hamberger B, Knutson E, et al. Transplantation of Adrenal Medullary Tissue to Striatum in Parkinsonism: First Clinical Trials. J Neurosurg. 1985; 62:169–173

[52] Blacklock JB, Maxwell RE. Stereotactic Removal of a Migrating Ventricular Catheter. Neurosurgery. 1985; 16:230–231

[53] Levy RM, Russell E, Yungbluth M, et al. The efficacy of image-guided stereotactis brain biopsy in neurologically symptomatic acquired immunodeficiency syndrome patients. Neurosurgery. 1992; 30:186–190

[54] Nicolato A, Gerosa M, Piovan E, et al. Computerized Tomography and Magnetic Resonance Guided Stereotactic Brain Biopsy in Nonimmunocompromised and AIDS Patients. Surg Neurol. 1997; 48:267–277

94 Specific Craniotomies

94.1 Posterior fossa (suboccipital) craniectomy

94.1.1 Indications

To gain access to the cerebellum, cerebellopontine angle (CPA), to one vertebral artery, posterior brainstem, fourth ventricle, pineal region, or, using extreme lateral posterior fossa approach to the antero-lateral brain stem. See paramedian (p. 1447) and midline (p. 1450) suboccipital craniectomies for details.

94.1.2 Position

Options

Position options include:
1. sitting position: see below
2. lateral oblique (p. 1446): patient three-quarters oblique (almost prone),
3. semi-sitting
4. supine with shoulder roll, head almost horizontal
5. prone
6. Concorde position: prone, thorax elevated, neck flexed and tilted away from the side on which the surgeon will be standing

Sitting position

Used less frequently than in the past because of associated complications and acceptable alternative positions (except for some specific circumstances). However, some experts feel that the risks of the sitting position have been greatly overstated.[1]

Advantages
1. improved drainage of blood and CSF out of surgical site
2. enhanced venous drainage which helps reduce venous bleeding and also ICP
3. easy ventilation due to unencumbered chest
4. patient's head may be kept exactly midline, aiding operator orientation, and reducing risk of kinking of vertebral arteries

Disadvantages/risks
1. possible air embolism (see below)
2. fatigue of operators hands
3. increased surgical risks from placement of CVP catheter (required to treat possible AE): e.g. pneumothorax with subclavian vein catheterization, thrombosis
4. risk of post-op hematoma at the operative site may be increased since potential venous bleeders may remain occult while the patient is sitting, but may manifest when patient returns to a horizontal position post-op. However, one study found no such increased incidence[2]
5. risk of post-op subdural hematoma: 1.3% of p-fossa cases[3]
6. possible brachial plexus injury: prevent this by not allowing patient's arms to hang at the side. Instead, fold them across abdomen
7. midcervical quadriplegia[4,5]: presumably due to flexion myelopathy.[6,7,8] The combination of the sitting position with hypotension[9] or neck flexion with possible compression of the anterior spinal artery, ± cervical bar, and elevation of the head thus reducing the arterial pressure may all contribute
8. sciatic nerve injury (piriformis syndrome)[10]: prevent this by flexing patient's knees (reduces tension on sciatic nerve)
9. extent of post-op pneumocephalus is more pronounced, and may increase the risk of tension pneumocephalus[11]; see Pneumocephalus (p. 887)
10. venous pooling of blood in the LEs under anesthesia may cause relative hypovolemia and should be counteracted by binding the LEs prior to positioning
11. decreased cerebral blood flow due to lower hemodynamic arterial pressure[12]

Air embolism (AE): A potentially fatal complication of any operation when an opening to air occurs in a non-collapsible vein (e.g. diploic vein or a dural sinus) when there is a negative pressure in the vein (e.g. when the head is elevated above the heart).[13] Air is entrained in the vein and can become trapped in the right atrium of the heart which may impair venous return causing hypotension. May also produce cardiac arrhythmias. Paradoxical air embolism can occur in the presence of a patent foramen ovale[14] or pulmonary AV fistula, and may produce ischemic cerebral infarction.

Greater negative pressures occur in the sitting position due to the extreme elevation of the head, but AE can occur in any operation with the head elevated higher than the heart. Incidence: a wide range has been quoted in the literature, and depends on the monitoring method used: ≈ 7–25% incidence with the sitting position using Doppler monitoring is an estimate.[3]

For operations with a *significant* risk of AE, a right atrial CVP line is recommended (to aspirate air), and monitoring for air embolism; options include: transesophageal echo (the most sensitive), precordial Doppler monitoring. (Although technically the risk of air embolism includes *any* case where the head is higher than the right cardiac atrium, practically it is limited to cases where the head of the bed is ≈ > 30° which is mostly limited to the sitting position for posterior fossa tumors.)

Diagnosis and treatment:

AE should be suspected in any operative case in which the surgical site is higher than the heart when there is any unexplained hypotension or decrease in $EtCO_2$.[16]

- transesophageal echocardiography (TEE). Bubbles can be seen on the 2D echo display
  pros: considered the most sensitive monitoring modality
  cons: significant false positive rate, expensive, invasive, requires experience and vigilance
- precordial doppler U/S: probe may be placed over 2nd to 4th intercostal space either to right or left of sternum, or posteriorly between the scapula and spine. AE is heralded by a change in sonic intensity and character at first by a superimposed irregular high-pitched swishing sound, and then as more air is entrained so called "mill wheel" or machinery sounds dominate
  pros: the most sensitive of the non-invasive techniques
  cons: difficult in morbidly obese patients and in certain patient positions (e.g. prone or lateral), interference from other sounds in the OR, requires vigilance

The earliest indication of AE may be a rise in the end-tidal nitrogen (requires mass-spectrometer on monitor), then a fall in the end tidal pCO_2 occurs. Machinery sounds in the precordial Doppler also suggest AE. Hypotension may develop. Measures shown in ▶ Table 94.1 should be immediately instituted.

Lateral oblique position

AKA "park bench" position.

- Axillary roll for the down side arm (see ▶ Fig. 94.1) (or, position the patient so that the down side arm extends over the edge of the table and is held in place by a sling formed by the Mayfield table attachment with copious padding)
- Upper arm supported on pillows or towels (avoid using a Mayo stand which restricts the ability to laterally tilt the OR table during surgery)
- Adhesive tape to gently pull down on the upper shoulder
- Bring the patient's back as close to the side edge of the table as possible (usually limited by the travel of the head clamp) to bring the patient closer to the surgeon
- Elevate thorax 10-15°
- Tilt the vertex of the head towards the floor (see below)
- Optional spinal drainage (usually for large tumors)
- Pillow between the legs
- Secure patient with adhesive tape over pads so the table can be "airplaned" (rolled) during the operation

94

Table 94.1 Treatment for air embolism

1. find and occlude site of air entry, or else rapidly pack wound with sopping wet sponges/laps and wax bone edges
2. lower patient's head if at all possible (30° or less from horizontal)
3. jugular venous compression (bilateral best; second choice: right only)
4. rotate patient *LEFT* side down (attempt to trap air in right atrium)
5. aspirate air from right atrium via CVP catheter
6. ventilate patient with 100% O_2
7. discontinue nitrous oxide if used (may expand AE)[15]
8. use pressors and volume expanders to maintain BP
9. PEEP is *ineffective* in preventing or treating AE; may increase the risk of paradoxical AE[13]

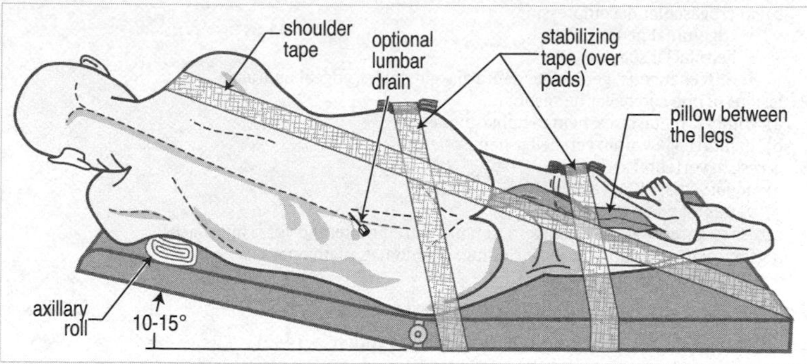

Fig. 94.1 Lateral oblique ("park bench") position

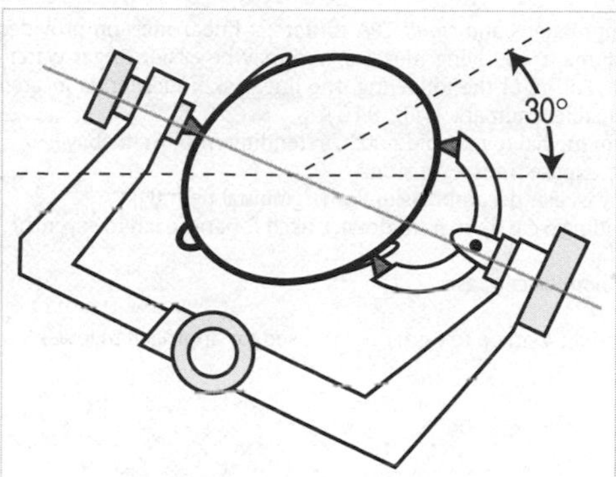

Fig. 94.2 Position of head and headholder for right suboccipital craniectomy (looking down on top of patient's head)

For access to the porus acusticus or more caudally

(e.g. for vestibular schwannomas; not necessary for microvascular decompression for trigeminal neuralgia).

Get the shoulders out of the way by flexing the neck as much as possible while maintaining patent airway (aided by use of non-kinking wire-reinforced ET tube, so-called **"armored tube"**). The upper shoulder is retracted caudally by adhesive tape (avoid excess traction which may injure brachial plexus).

Head positioning

A Mayfield head-clamp is placed with the single pin on the side of the lesion, slightly anterior to a true-lateral on the skull (▶ Fig. 94.2.). The head is then rotated 20–30° face-down from the horizontal.

94.1.3 Paramedian suboccipital craniectomy

Indications

1. access to the cerebellopontine angle (CPA)
   a) CPA tumors, including:
      - vestibular schwannoma
      - CPA meningioma
      - epidermoid

   b) microvascular decompression
      - trigeminal neuralgia
      - hemifacial spasm
      - miscellaneous: geniculate neuralgia, glossopharyngeal neuralgia
2. lesions of one cerebellar hemisphere:
   a) tumors: metastases, hemangioblastomas...
   b) hemorrhage within cerebellar hemisphere
3. access to vertebral artery
   a) aneurysms: PICA, vertebrobasilar junction
   b) vertebral endarterectomy
4. access to antero-lateral brainstem tumors (extreme lateral p-fossa approach)
   a) foramen magnum tumors, including: chordomas, meningiomas

Position, skin incision, craniectomy, approach...

See list of alternatives (p. 1445). See lateral oblique position (p. 1446).

Skin incision

Linear (paramedian) incisions

Access to CPA. For microvascular decompressions and *small* CPA tumors, a linear incision provides adequate exposure and involves less trauma to overlying muscles, and may be easier to get water-tight closure than with midline incision. For all of the following, the linear skin incision is located 5 mm medial to the mastoid notch (a palpable landmark, ▶ Fig. 94.3):

1. "5–6–4" incision (incision placed 5 mm medial to mastoid notch, extending from 6 cm above notch to 4 cm below). High enough to expose transverse sinus:
   a) for approach to fifth nerve: microvascular decompression for trigeminal neuralgia
2. "5–5–5" incision (5 mm medial, extending 5 cm up to 5 cm down), used for approach to seventh/ eighth nerve complex:
   a) microvascular decompression for hemifacial spasm
   b) small vestibular schwannoma
3. "5–4–6" incision (5 mm medial, extending 4 cm up to 6 cm down): used for approach to lower cranial nerves:
   a) glossopharyngeal neuralgia

"Hockey-stick" incision

94 Useful for cerebellar hemispheric lesions as well as for larger CPA lesions where getting the muscles out of the way will facilitate maneuvering instruments about the posterior fossa.

Incision is made in the midline starting at ≈ C2 spinous process, proceeding superiorly to just above the inion, and then laterally to just beyond the mastoid tip (▶ Fig. 94.4). A short optional caudal curve may be made laterally to further remove the muscle from the operative field.

Craniectomy

Landmarks

The location of the inferior margin of the transverse sinus is quite accurately estimated at two finger-breadths above the upper limit of the mastoid notch (usually just above the superior nuchal line). This should be the upper limit of the skull opening.

For microvascular decompression

Craniectomy ≈ 2 cm diameter placed in the angle between transverse and sigmoid sinuses.

For small tumors (< 2.5 cm)

Craniectomy ≈ 4 cm diameter placed in the angle between transverse and sigmoid sinuses.

For large tumors

A larger craniectomy may be needed, the size of which is limited by:

1. transverse sinus superiorly
2. foramen magnum inferiorly (which may be opened as prophylaxis against tonsillar herniation in the event of p-fossa edema post-op)

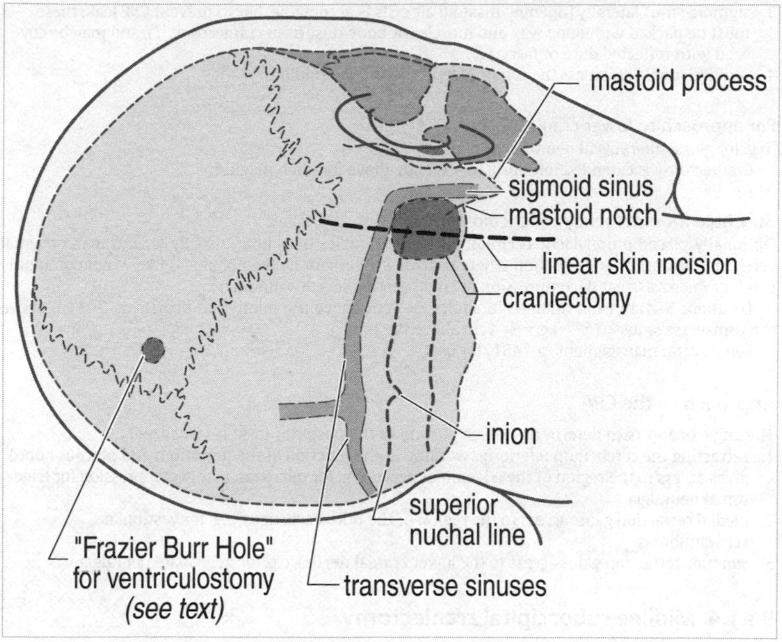

mastoid process
sigmoid sinus
mastoid notch
linear skin incision
craniectomy
inion
superior nuchal line
"Frazier Burr Hole" for ventriculostomy *(see text)*
transverse sinuses

Fig. 94.3 Paramedian suboccipital craniectomy

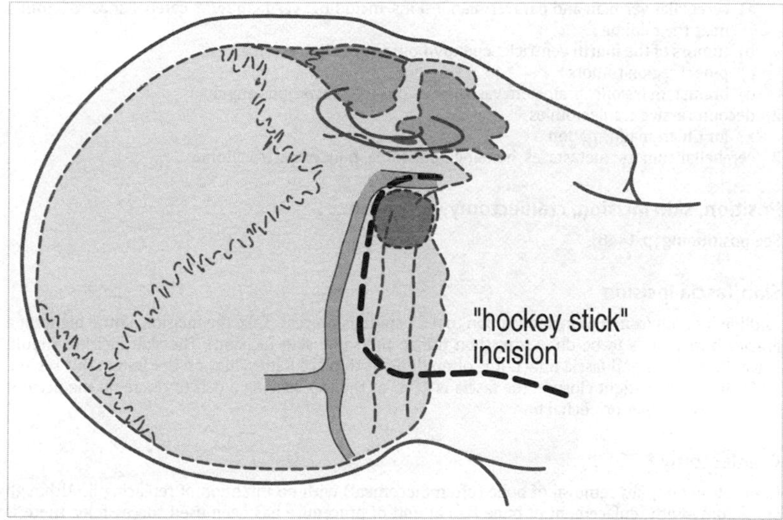

Fig. 94.4 "Hockey-stick" skin incision

3. sigmoid sinus laterally (opening mastoid air cells is acceptable, but to prevent CSF leak, these must be packed with bone wax and muscle (or bone dust from craniectomy[17]), and may be covered with reflected dura or fascia)
4. midline medially (unless the tumor extends across the midline)

For approach to lower cranial nerves

(e.g. for glossopharyngeal neuralgia).

Craniectomy is extended inferiorly to ≈ 1/2 cm above foramen magnum.

Burr hole for emergency ventriculostomy

Optionally placed prophylactic occipital burr hole (**Frazier burr hole**) usually for intraparenchymal cerebellar tumors or any situation where post-op swelling or hydrocephalus is likely (not commonly used for microvascular decompression or small vestibular schwannomas).

Location: 3–4 cm from midline. In adults, 6–7 cm above the inion[18]; in pediatrics, 2–3 cm above the transverse sinus[19(p 429)] (i.e. ≈ 3–4 cm above the inion).

See Post-op management (p. 1451) for use.

Approach to the CPA

The angle of approach determines which portion of the posterior fossa is visualized.

1. retracting the cerebellum *inferiorly* (working in the junction of the tentorium and petrous bone) gives access to the region of the trigeminal nerve, e.g. for microvascular decompression for trigeminal neuralgia
2. *medial* retraction gains access to the region of the porus acusticus, e.g. for vestibular schwannomas
3. *superior* retraction gains access to the lower cranial nerves, e.g. for geniculate neuralgia

94.1.4 Midline suboccipital craniectomy

Indications

Access to the midline or both sides of the posterior fossa

1. midline posterior fossa lesions
   a) cerebellar vermian and paravermian lesions, including: vermian AVM, cerebellar astrocytoma near the midline
   b) tumors of the fourth ventricle: ependymoma, medulloblastoma
   c) pineal region tumors
   d) brainstem lesions: brainstem vascular lesions (e.g. cavernous angioma)
2. decompressive craniectomies
   a) for Chiari malformation
3. cerebellar tumors: metastases, hemangioblastoma, pilocytic astrocytoma…

Position, skin incision, craniectomy, approach…

See positioning (p. 1446).

Skin/fascia incision

Midline incision from ≈ 6 cm above inion to ≈ C2 spinous process. Take the incision a little higher if a Frazier burr hole is to be done (can then utilize the same skin incision). The skin incision should leave the muscles and fascia intact. It is often difficult to place Raney clips on the skin in this region. To facilitate water-tight closure, the fascia is "T'd" at the top, leaving a cuff of tissue on the occiput just above the superior nuchal line.

Craniectomy

Craniectomy implies removal of bone (often piecemeal) with no intention of replacing it. Although craniotomy with replacement of bone flap at end of procedure has been used successfully, there is some concern that if there is post-op swelling, the inelastic bone flap may cause more pressure to be transmitted to the brain stem.

Usually taken down to foramen magnum. For cerebellar hemisphere tumors, many remove the posterior arch of C1 (caution re vertebral arteries on superior aspect of C1).

Approach

A "Y" shaped durotomy is often used. If the lesion has a cystic component, aspiration through a ventricular needle is used to partially decompress it.

94.1.5 Extreme lateral posterior fossa approach

Allows access to antero-lateral region of brain stem. Differs from above in that the skin incision is designed to get the bulk of the skin and muscle flap out of the way.

Key: remove the lip of the foramen magnum as far laterally as possible, best done with a diamond drill.

94.1.6 Cranioplasty for suboccipital craniectomy

Methylmethacrylate cranioplasty as part of the closure following suboccipital crani for vestibular schwannoma reduced the incidence of post-op H/A from 17% to 4%.[20]

94.1.7 Post-op considerations for p-fossa cranis

Post-op check

In addition to routine, the following should be checked:
1. respirations: rate, pattern (see Intubation below)
2. follow closely for hypertension (see below)
3. evidence of CSF leak through wound

Post-op management

Intubation

Post-op intubation for 24–48 hours is sometimes maintained on a precautionary basis: many complications often have respiratory arrest as the initial manifestation (see below), and the patient may deteriorate precipitously from this point. There is a trade-off as the stimulus of the endotracheal tube may exacerbate hypertension and patient agitation, and so sedation is often required, which may obscure the neuro exam and depress respirations. If the patient wakes up extremely well from an uncomplicated p-fossa crani and it is not late at night, most surgeons will extubate.

Hypertension

Hypertension should be avoided at all costs to prevent bleeding from tenuous vessels (e.g. nitroprusside should be prepared prior to termination of the operation, and should be hanging and ready to titrate to keep SBP ≥ 160 mm Hg during the reversal of anesthesia and post-op).

Physician should be called for any sudden changes in BP post-op (may indicate elevated pressure in posterior fossa, see below).

Post-op complications

Posterior fossa edema and/or hematoma

In the posterior fossa, a small amount of mass effect can be rapidly fatal due to the paucity of room and the immediate transmission of pressure directly to the brain stem. It can also occlude CSF circulation through the aqueduct and cause *acute hydrocephalus* with the attendant risk of tonsillar herniation. Increased pressure in the p-fossa is usually heralded by sudden increases in BP or changes in respiratory pattern (pupillary reflexes, level of consciousness and ICP are *not* affected until late). See ▶ Table 94.2 for emergency treatment measures.

Table 94.2 Emergency treatment for p-fossa swelling
✱ Rapid intubation, ventricular tap (through previously placed burr hole, if possible, see below), and reoperation is indicated. The wound should be opened immediately wherever patient is (recovery room, ICU, floor...). CT scanning may cost valuable minutes; it is rarely appropriate to delay treatment for this (must be judged on an individual basis).

94

To expedite ventricular taps, a prophylactic occipital burr hole (Frazier burr hole) is often placed during posterior fossa surgery to permit drainage of CSF from the lateral ventricles in the event of acute hydrocephalus from blockage of the 4th ventricle or aqueduct. If acute hydrocephalus develops (e.g. from a hematoma), an emergent percutaneous ventricular tap with ventricular needle (or, if not available, spinal needle) is performed, passing the needle through the burr hole aiming for the middle of the forehead. In the presence of acute hydrocephalus, CSF should be encountered at a depth of 3–5 cm. NB: this maneuver may provide a few more minutes while preparing for the definitive treatment of re-opening the wound; however, hydrocephalus may not initially be present since it takes some time to develop.

Suboccipital pseudomeningocele

An "internal" CSF fistula. Incidence following suboccipital craniectomy: 8[21]-28%.[22]

May be asymptomatic, but also may be associated with H/A, nausea/vomiting, local pain/tenderness. Some are soft and compressible, others may be tense.

Indications for operation:

1. external leak (CSF fistula, see below)
2. threatening integrity of incision
3. cosmetic deformity
4. causing symptoms

Treatment options (up to 67% require permanent CSF drainage[23]):

1. noninvasive measures: expectant management, fluid restriction, head wrapping, keeping HOB elevated, acetazolamide. Steroids may be used if aseptic meningitis is suspected
2. percutaneous aspiration: "tap and wrap".[19 (p 436),24] Risks introducing bacteria, causing infection
3. direct surgical exploration with multilayer re-closure[19 (p 436)]
4. lumbar drain: effective only if pseudomeningocele communicates with the subarachnoid space. ✖ May produce acute posterior fossa syndrome (H/A, nausea, vomiting, ataxia…)[21] especially if the pseudomeningocele doesn't communicate. Symptoms usually resolve with prompt discontinuation of lumbar drainage.[21,22] Other potential complications: vagal nerve palsy, tonsillar herniation, subdural hematoma, kinking of PCA → stroke. Drainage options:
   a) external drain (temporary)
   b) lumboperitoneal shunt (permanent)
5. ventricular drainage
   a) EVD (temporary)
   b) shunt (permanent)

94

CSF fistula

Occurs in 5–17% of cases. A potential source of meningitis, thus CSF leak must be treated immediately.

Etiologies: controversial. May include:

1. abnormal CSF hydrodynamics (i.e. hydrocephalus). Maneuvers to stem the leak will likely fail until the CSF is shunted or hydrodynamics normalize
2. poor wound closure: probably blamed more often than it is the actual cause
3. subarachnoid scarring

May be associated with meningitis (aseptic or infectious), multiple operations. Formation may be facilitated by coughing/sneezing, postural changes, one-way ball-valve mechanism due to a tissue flap.

An external CSF leak may occur through:

1. the skin incision
2. via the eustachian tube; see possible routes of egress following suboccipital vestibular schwannoma removal (p.683):
   a) through the nose (CSF rhinorrhea)
   b) down the back of the throat
3. the ear (CSF otorrhea) in cases with perforated TM

Treatment:

Initial treatment measures to temporize in the hope that CSF hydrodynamics will normalize and/or that the leak site will scar closed within a few days:

1. elevate the HOB

2. lumbar subarachnoid drainage
3. if the leak occurs through the skin incision:
   a) reinforce the incision with sutures, e.g. running locked 3–0 nylon after preparation of the skin with antimicrobial and local anesthetic
   b) alternatively, the incision may be painted with several coats of collodion

If persistent, a CSF fistula requires surgical correction, see CSF fistula (cranial), for general information (p. 384), see CSF fistula following suboccipital removal of vestibular schwannoma (p. 684).

Fifth or seventh nerve injuries

Causes diminished corneal reflex with potential corneal ulceration; initially managed with isotonic eye drops (e.g. Natural Tears®) q 2–4 hrs & PRN, or with a moisturizing insert (e.g. Lacricert®) q day, and at night with an eye patch or taping eyelid shut.

Miscellaneous

Supratentorial intracerebral hemorrhage has been described, and may result from transient hypertension.[25]

94.2 Pterional craniotomy

94.2.1 Indications

1. aneurysms
   a) all aneurysms of anterior circulation
   b) basilar tip aneurysms
2. direct surgical approach to cavernous sinus
3. suprasellar tumors
   a) pituitary adenoma (when there is a large suprasellar component)
   b) craniopharyngioma

94.2.2 Technique

Position, skin incision, craniectomy, approach...

1. supine, ipsilateral shoulder roll if head turned > 30° (see below)
2. elevate thorax 10–15°: reduces venous distension
3. flex knees
4. Mayfield 3 pin head-holder: applied between true AP and true lateral (so that it is ≈ horizontal when head is rotated to the necessary position, see ► Fig. 94.5)
5. neck extended 15°: allows gravity to retract frontal lobe away from skull base
6. head rotated from vertical as shown in ► Fig. 94.5

Room arrangement

1. microscope: observer tube to operator's *right* for either right or left pterional crani

Skin incision

See ► Fig. 94.6. From zygomatic arch 1 cm in front of tragus (to avoid frontalis branch of facial nerve and frontal branch of superficial temporal artery), curving slightly anteriorly, staying behind hairline to widow's peak, optional additional curve beyond midline to aid in skin retraction. Over temporalis muscle, incise skin down to but not through temporalis fascia.

The temporalis muscle may be incised caudal to the skin incision (i.e. closer to zygomatic arch): this minimizes the muscle mass that needs to be retracted inferiorly and yet keeps the scar behind hairline (note: there is an increased risk of frontalis weakness with this technique than if the temporalis muscle is incised in-line with the skin incision).

Craniotomy

There are numerous ways to cross the pterion (the lesser wing of the sphenoid makes this difficult). One method is outlined here, ► Fig. 94.7.

94

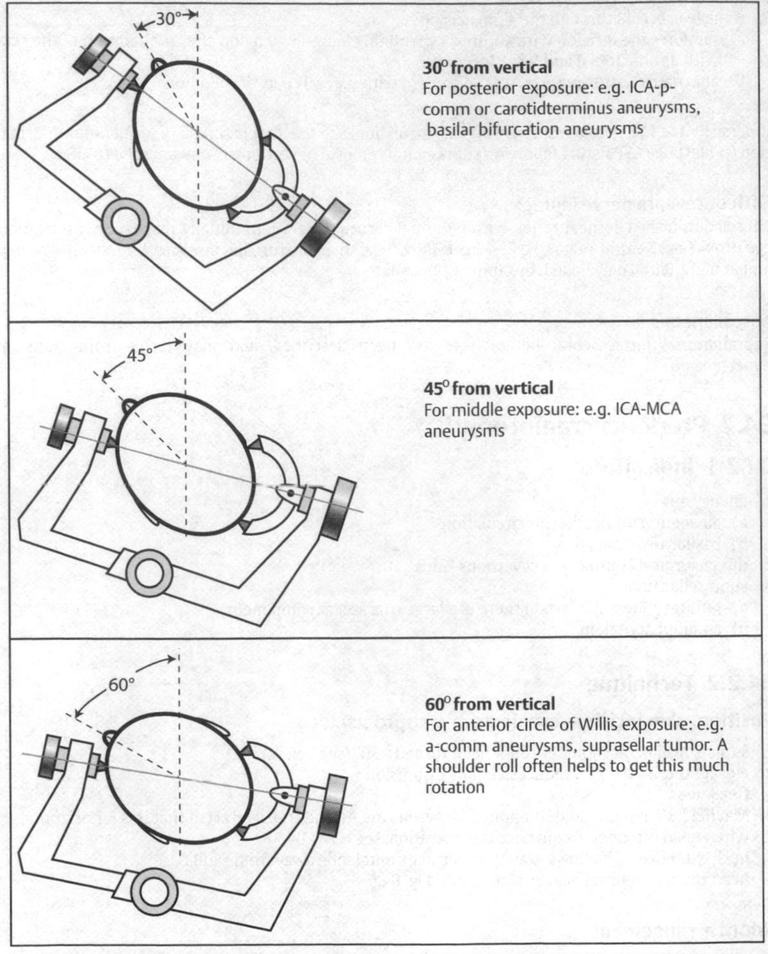

30°
30° from vertical
For posterior exposure: e.g. ICA-p-comm or carotidterminus aneurysms, basilar bifurcation aneurysms
45°
45° from vertical
For middle exposure: e.g. ICA-MCA aneurysms
60°
60° from vertical
For anterior circle of Willis exposure: e.g. a-comm aneurysms, suprasellar tumor. A shoulder roll often helps to get this much rotation

Fig. 94.5 Head position for pterional craniotomy depending on exposure required. The blue line indicates the approximate centerline.

Burr holes

Two burr holes are sufficient; made as far caudally as possible to minimize the amount of bone to be rongeured off to gain access to the floor of the middle cranial fossa. One burr hole is made at the posterior insertion of the zygomatic arch ("A" in ▶ Fig. 94.7); this burr hole may be placed slightly forward when exposure is centered over structures around the ACoA (e.g. suprasellar tumor). The second burr hole ("Z") is made at the intersection of the zygomatic bone (near the frontozygomatic suture), the superior temporal line and the supraorbital ridge. The hole should be as low as possible on the orbit; aim the drill slightly superiorly to avoid actually entering the orbit. The dura is dissected off the inner table with a Penfield #3 dissector.

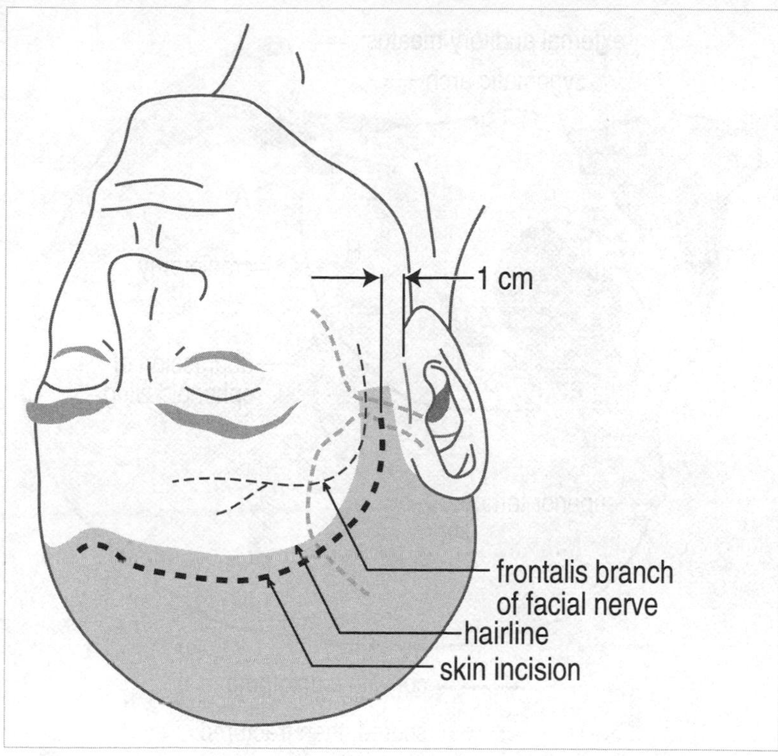

Fig. 94.6 Skin incision for pterional craniotomy

Craniotomy

The resulting bone flap is centered over the depression of the sphenoid ridge. Approximately 33% of the craniotomy is anterior to the anterior margin of temporalis muscle insertion, ≈ 66% is posterior.

With the craniotome, starting at the frontal burr hole the craniotomy is taken anteriorly across the anterior margin of the superior temporal line staying as low as possible on the orbit (to obviate having to rongeur bone, which is unsightly on the forehead). The distance "**B**" from the medial extent of the craniotomy to the frontal burr hole is 3 cm for anterior circulation aneurysms. For the approaches to skull base (e.g. Dolenc approach), distance "B" is larger and takes the opening to ≈ the mid orbit. Then from point "B", a sharp superior turn is made and the opening is taken back to point "A." The height ("**H**") of the craniotomy needs to be only ≈ 3 cm for aneurysms of the Circle of Willis, and slightly larger (≈ 5 cm) for middle cerebral artery aneurysms. Minimal exposure of temporal cortex is necessary for aneurysms of the skull base region. For large flaps (e.g. for tumors), "H" is made larger to expose more temporal lobe.

From the frontal burr hole, the craniotomy is then taken posteriorly towards the depression corresponding to the sphenoid wing until the drill hangs up.

The craniotomy from the posterior burr hole is taken forward towards the depression corresponding to the sphenoid wing until the drill hangs up.

The bone between the two points where the drill hangs up is scored with the craniotome, and then the bone is fractured at this point. A rongeur is used to remove as much sphenoid wing as possible.

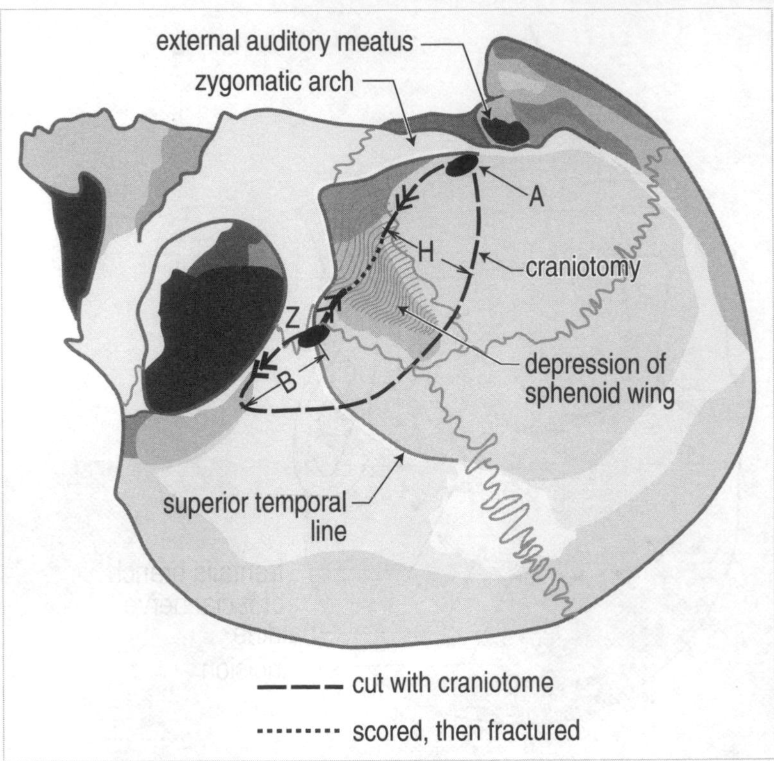

Fig. 94.7 Skull landmarks for right pterional craniotomy

Dural flap

Curvilinear, centered over sphenoid wing, retracted inferiorly with dural stitch.

Dissection

For some anterior circulation aneurysms (e.g. MCA aneurysms) and for the Yasargil approach to basilar tip aneurysms, the sylvian fissure needs to be split. This can be accomplished by working from the lateral aspect of the fissure medially, or, by starting at the point where the carotid artery penetrates the fissure and working laterally. The latter method may be easier when prolific veins overly the junction of the frontal and temporal lobe. There are no arteries that cross the sylvian fissure, and so if the correct plane is maintained, no arteries need to be sacrificed.

▶ Fig. 94.8 shows a theoretical exposure of the circle of Willis possible through a pterional craniotomy. This diagram is semi-schematic, and in reality dissection would be directed either anteriorly (e.g. to expose ACoA) or posteriorly (e.g. for basilar tip aneurysms) but not both.

94.3 Temporal craniotomy

94.3.1 Indications

1. temporal lobe biopsy: herpes simplex encephalitis
2. temporal lobectomy: for resection of seizure focus, decompression post-trauma…

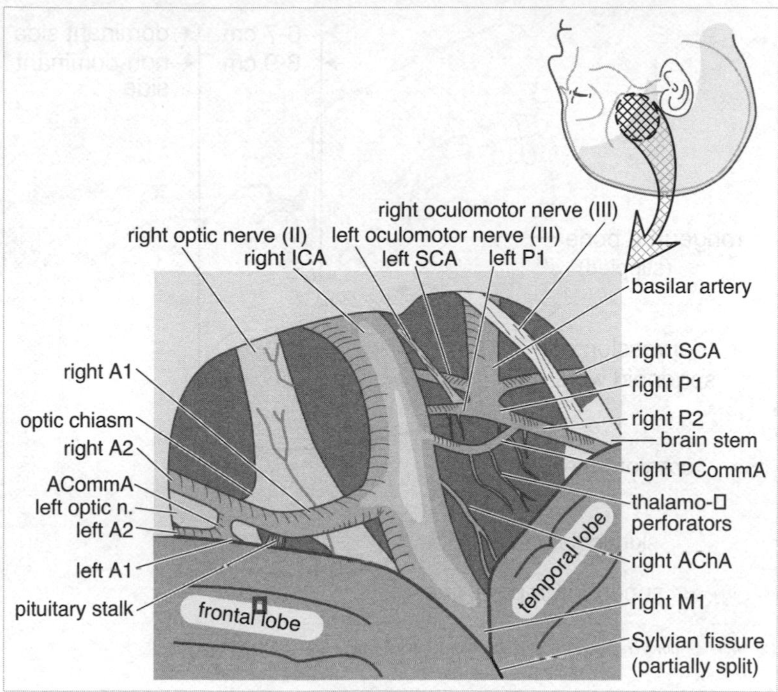

Fig. 94.8 Right sided sylvian fissure dissection, surgical view

3. hematoma (epidural or subdural) overlying temporal lobe
4. tumors of the temporal lobe
5. small, laterally located vestibular schwannomas[26]
6. access to the floor of the middle cranial fossa (including foramen ovale/Meckel's cave, the labyrinthine and upper tympanic portion of the facial nerve)
7. access to medial temporal lobe e.g. for amygdalo-hippocampectomy (p. 1556) or for mesial temporal sclerosis (p. 441)

94.3.2 Technique

See ▶ Fig. 94.9. Two basic methods for temporal craniotomy:

1. small craniotomy or craniectomy through a linear skin incision: good for cortical biopsy or draining chronic subdural hematoma. Also permits access to floor of middle fossa. Simple quick closure
2. question-mark skin incision with standard craniotomy flap: useful for temporal lobe exposure for tumor or acute hematoma

94.3.3 Position, skin incision, craniectomy, approach...

1. patient supine with shoulder roll (to assist in rotating neck to get head almost horizontal)
2. elevate thorax 10–15°: reduces venous distension
3. flex knees slightly
4. Mayfield 3 pin head-holder: true AP with single pin anteriorly
5. head rotated almost horizontal to floor: avoid over-extending to prevent kinking neck veins

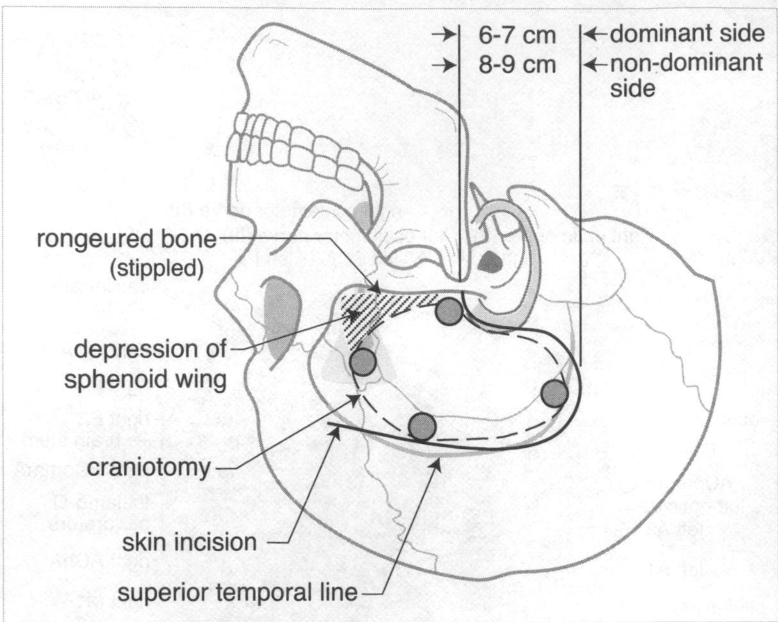

Fig. 94.9 Temporal craniotomy (exposing entire temporal lobe)

94.3.4 Craniotomies

94

Small craniectomy

Linear skin incision completely within the extent of the temporalis muscle. To access the temporal tip: place the incision midway between the lateral canthus and external auditory canal (EAC); extend it from the zygomatic arch upward for ≈ 6 cm. For small, laterally located vestibular schwannomas, the incision is made 0.5 cm anterior to the EAC extending ≈ 7–8 cm above the zygomatic arch.[26] To drain a subdural, place the incision just anterior to the tragus and start it 1–2 cm above the zygomatic arch for ≈ 6 cm (modified based on the location of the epicenter of the subdural). Take the incision down to temporalis fascia with the knife, and incise the fascia and muscle with Bovie cautery. Spread with self-retaining retractors, and make a burr hole. Enlarge with rongeurs and/or Kerrison punches.

Standard craniotomy

Question-mark skin incision

See ▶ Fig. 94.9. Used for access to the temporal lobe including tip (a reverse question mark incision may be used to gain access to the middle and posterior temporal lobe).

1. the pinna is either sutured inferiorly out of the way before draping, or it can be folded under the drapes which may be stapled to the skin
2. the lower limb extends from the zygomatic arch just anterior to the tragus (to avoid the superficial temporal artery)
3. curve as far posteriorly as ≈ 6–7 cm on the non-dominant side, or ≈ 8–9 cm on the dominant side at the level of the top of the pinna (these dimensions allow access to the "safe" area of temporal tip for lobectomy)
4. then superiorly to the level of the superior temporal line
5. then anteriorly towards the forehead, stopping at the hair line

Burr hole placement

1. at the posterior insertion of the zygomatic arch
2. at upper anterior junction of zygomatic arch
3. one or two burr holes along posterior and superior aspect of the skin incision

Craniotomy

Connect the burr holes with the craniotome, keeping as low as possible in the middle fossa to minimize the amount of bone that must be rongeured. The remaining bone is rongeured down to the floor of the middle fossa (cross-hatched area in ▶ Fig. 94.9).

Temporal lobectomy

✖ Danger points:

1. dominant hemisphere: Wernicke's speech area. Although variable (see Temporal lobectomy (p. 1556)), one can usually safely resect up to 4–5 cm from temporal tip without use of mapping techniques to localize speech
2. non-dominant hemisphere: one can resect up to 6–7 cm before running the risk of injuring the optic radiation
3. sylvian fissure (middle cerebral artery): it is best to amputate the temporal lobe backward from the tip for the extent of the desired resection, and then work deep
4. medially, the incisura should be identified to avoid injury to the brain stem which lies just medial to this

94.4 Frontal craniotomy

94.4.1 Indications

1. access to frontal lobe: e.g. for infiltrating tumor
2. approach to third ventricle or to sellar region tumors in some situations, including craniopharyngiomas, planum sphenoidale meningiomas
3. repair of ethmoidal CSF fistula

94.4.2 ✖ Danger points

1. anterior cerebral arteries in the midline (deep)
2. superior sagittal sinus (SSS) in the midline (note: the SSS may be sacrificed in its anterior third without engendering venous infarction in most cases, whereas venous infarction will almost always occur with division of the SSS posterior to that)
3. avoid inadvertently crossing the midline into the contralateral hemisphere through the corpus callosum
4. dominant hemisphere: Broca's (motor speech) area is located in the inferior frontal gyrus

94.4.3 Technique

Craniotomy options

Two basic choices for craniotomy:

1. unilateral craniotomy through a curved skin incision taken anteriorly up to the hairline: used when one does not need to be low in the frontal fossa in the midline (otherwise the skin incision would have to be taken far into forehead) and when there is no need to cross the midline
2. large bifrontal skin incision from "ear-to-ear" (souttar skin incision[27]) allowing low approach to one or both frontal fossa

Unilateral frontal craniotomy

▶ Fig. 94.10. Skin incision starts < 1 cm anterior to the tragus, and does not need to go all the way down to the zygomatic arch. It curves superiorly and slightly posteriorly before being taken to the midline frontally.

Burr holes

1. at the junction of the superior temporal line and the orbital rim

94

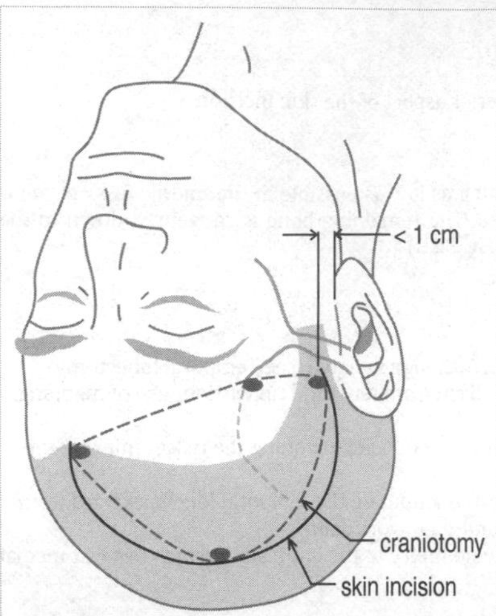

Fig. 94.10 Unilateral frontal craniotomy

2. just posterior to the depression of the sphenoid wing (behind the pterion)
3. anteriorly just behind the hairline to avoid having a burr hole under the forehead (which causes an unsightly depression)
4. superiorly

Bilateral frontal craniotomy

1. "ear-to-ear" or souttar skin incision
   a) just behind hairline with a slight widow's peak at the front
   b) does not need to go all the way to the zygomatic arch, it just needs to be ≈ as low as the orbital roof
   c) unlike pterional craniotomy, usually do not need to incise the temporalis muscle and fascia. Dissect the flap off the muscle/fascia
   d) if a periosteal flap is likely to be needed, it sometimes helps not to incise the periosteum at the same time as the skin incision. Then, the periosteum can be incised behind the skin incision to yield a longer periosteal graft than would have otherwise been obtained
2. burr holes: to avoid burr hole defects on the forehead, the bone flap can be created with two burr holes straddling the superior sagittal sinus (SSS) close to the skin incision, and two burr holes laterally
3. the SSS may be divided low, near the orbital roof, with little risk
4. if the frontal sinus is entered, it is dealt with as outlined under Frontal sinus fractures (p. 886)

94

94.5 Petrosal craniotomy

94.5.1 Indications

1. lesions of the petrous apex (e.g. petroclival meningiomas)
2. lesions of the clivus (e.g. chordomas) with both posterior fossa and supratentorial components

94.5.2 Advantages

Spares sinus and otologic apparatuses. Minimizes cerebellar and temporal lobe retraction.

94.5.3 Technique

See reference.[28]

Position

1. patient supine, ipsilateral shoulder roll
2. elevate thorax 10°: reduces venous distension
3. flex knees
4. Mayfield 3 pin head-holder: close to true AP with single pin on forehead
5. head positioned to place petrous base at highest point of field:
   a) head rotated 40–60° from vertical
   b) head abducted towards contralateral shoulder
   c) neck extended 15°: allows gravity to retract frontal lobe away from skull base

Skin incision

Reverse question mark starting from zygomatic arch 1 cm anterior to tragus, arcing posteriorly over ear, descending to 0.5–1 cm medial to mastoid notch.

Temporalis muscle and periosteum reflected anteriorly and inferiorly.

Craniotomy

Four burr holes are utilized, two on each side of the sinuses (near the junction of the transverse and sigmoid sinuses).

94.6 Approaches to the lateral ventricle

Surgical approaches to the trigone – Contemporary Neurosurgery Vol. 27 No.5[29]

Classic review[18(p 561–74)] summarized:

1. atrium (AKA trigone); numerous approaches include[29]:
   a) middle temporal gyrus: through the dilated temporal horn
   b) lateral temporal parietal
   c) superior parietal occipital
   d) transcallosal (see below)
   e) transtemporal horn: access to temporal horn is via lobectomy of the temporal tip
   f) occipital lobe incision or occipital lobectomy: recommended only if patient has homonymous hemianopsia pre-op
2. frontal horn
   a) middle frontal gyrus
3. midventricular body
   a) transcallosal
   b) middle frontal gyrus: usually prevents access to vascular supply until most of the tumor is removed (especially for tumors supplied primarily by posterior choroidal artery)
4. temporal horn
   a) middle temporal gyrus
   b) transtemporal horn

94

94.7 Approaches to the third ventricle

94.7.1 General information

Classic references review the microsurgical anatomy[30] and surgical approaches,[31] and are briefly summarized below.

Alternative approaches for lesions of the anterior third ventricle[32]:

1. transcortical: approach is through the lateral ventricle and is feasible only in the presence of hydrocephalus; especially useful if the tumor extends from the third ventricle into one of the lateral ventricles. Risk of seizures is 5% (higher then with transcallosal) (p. 1466).
2. transcallosal: may be preferable in the absence of hydrocephalus (see below)
   a) anterior transcallosal: good visualization of both walls of third ventricle; risk of bilateral fornicial damage
   b) posterior transcallosal: allows approach to quadrigeminal plate or pineal region; risk of damage to deep veins
3. subfrontal: allows four different approaches
   a) subchiasmatic: between optic nerve and optic chiasm
   b) optico-carotid: through the triangular space bordered by optic nerve medially, carotid artery laterally, and ACA posteriorly

    c) lamina terminalis: above the optic chiasm[33]
    d) transsphenoidal: requires removal of tuberculum sellae, planum sphenoidale, and anterior wall of the sella turcica
4. transsphenoidal
5. subtemporal
6. stereotactic: may be useful for aspiration of colloid cysts; see Stereotactic drainage of colloid cysts (p. 759)

94.7.2 General principles of tumor removal

Summarized.[31] During the approach, deep veins should be preserved at all costs, even if it means stretching them to the point that they may rupture.

It is helpful to place a suture through the tumor capsule to act as a tether.

The tumor should first be removed from within the capsule; techniques include aspiration, and then opening the capsule and debulking from within. The capsule may then be collapsed and dissected from adherent structures. If the capsule adhesions seem unyielding, the most likely cause is incomplete intracapsular evacuation.

Vessels on the surface of the tumor should be presumed to be supplying normal brain, and should be dissected off the capsule once it is completely emptied.

94.7.3 Transcallosal approach to lateral or third ventricle

General information

Performed through an interhemispheric approach to the corpus callosum (CC) via a parietal craniotomy, usually right sided in a left-hemisphere dominant patient.

Indications

Primarily for tumors or lesions of the lateral or third ventricle, including:
1. colloid cysts
2. craniopharyngiomas
3. cysticercosis cysts
4. thalamic glioma
5. AVM

94

Booking the case: Transcallosal surgery

Also see defaults & disclaimers (p. 27).
1. position: supine with pin headholder
2. equipment:
    a) microscope
    b) image guided navigation system
3. post-op: ICU
4. consent (in lay terms for the patient – not all-inclusive):
    a) procedure: operation between the two halves of the brain to remove lesion
    b) alternatives: non-surgical management, surgery through the surface of the brain (transcortical), radiation therapy for some diagnoses
    c) complications: stroke, "disconnection syndrome" (uncommon) (p. 1556), hydrocephalus with possible need for a shunt, memory deficits

Technique

See references.[30,31,34]

General information

▶ Fig. 94.11. Image-guided navigation is very helpful in ascertaining the correct trajectory which permits minimizing the size of the callosotomy, and helps distinguish the corpus callosum from the cingulate gyri.

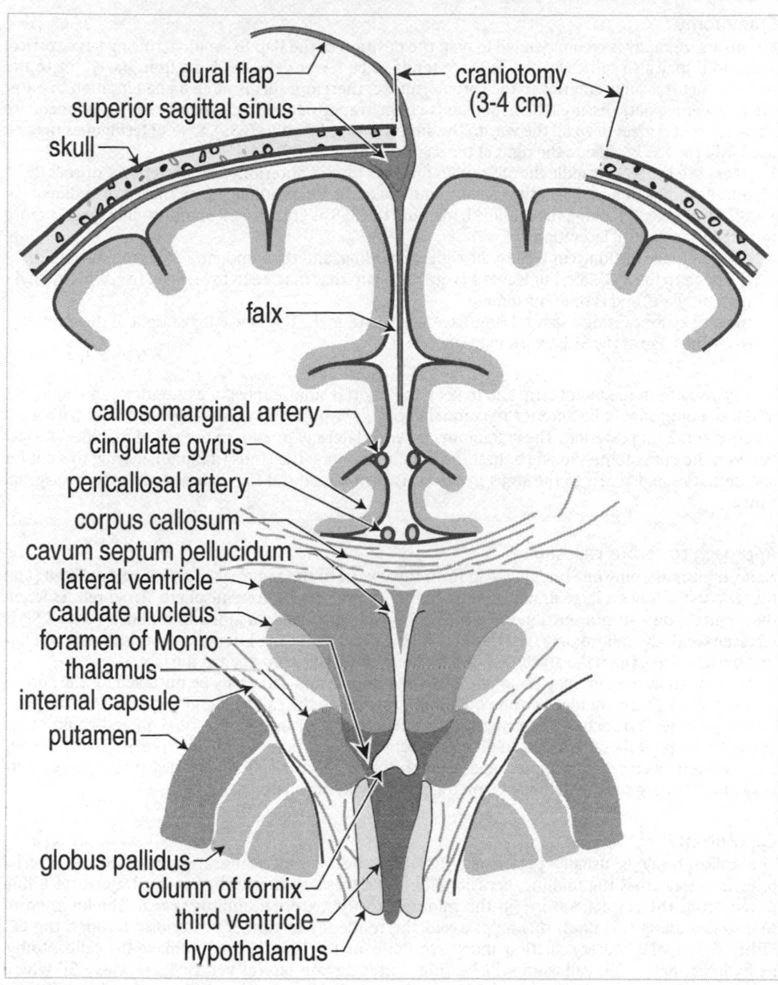

Fig. 94.11 Transcallosal approach to the third ventricle: frontal view

Position

Supine with neck flexed. Thorax elevated 20°. Spinal drain *not* used. Keep the head perfectly vertical to minimize disorientation that can easily occur with this approach. Alternatively, gravity retraction may be employed either by tilting the head slightly to the right (causing the right hemisphere to fall away) or by using the lateral position.

Skin incision

Either of the following may be used:

1. inverted "U" with the top just left of midline, extending from 6 cm anterior to the coronal suture to 2 cm behind the coronal suture, taking the sides for 7–8 cm
2. souttar skin incision

Craniotomy

Pre-op angiography is recommended to plan the position of the flap to avoid sacrificing large cortical veins. MRI may also suffice for this.[35] There tends to be fewer veins bridging from the cortex to the superior sagittal sinus anterior to the coronal suture, therefore this is often a good location to enter the interhemispheric fissure. The bone flap is either trapezoidal or triangular in shape, for adequate exposure it is *critical* to go all the way to the superior sagittal sinus (SSS). Several techniques may be used. NB: the SSS is often to the right of the sagittal suture (p.61).

1. to expose the SSS, straddle the SSS with paired burr holes anteriorly and posteriorly, dissect the dura from the inner table between pairs, and make the longitudinal cut on the *left* of midline. Disadvantage: removing the midline bone puts the SSS at greater risk of injury and makes it more difficult to control lacerations
2. one can make the long cut well to the right of midline, and then under direct vision rongeur off the bone to the SSS. Safe, but leaves a large bone gap that may need to be filled (e.g. with methyl methacrylate) and is time consuming
3. most risky for causing a sagittal sinus laceration is to make the long cut just right of the midline (over the edge of the SSS, which may lacerate it)

To stay away from the motor strip and to keep the sagittal sinus exposure as anterior as possible, 2/3 of the opening should lie anterior to coronal suture, 1/3 posterior (generally: 6 cm total with 4 cm anterior and 2 cm posterior). The craniotomy extends laterally to 3–4 cm to right of midline. The last cut with the craniotome should connect the burr holes along the sinus (midline); leaving this cut for last permits rapid access to the sinus in case it is torn. The dural flap is based towards the sagittal sinus.

Approach to corpus callosum

None, or at most, only one bridging vein from the cortex to the sagittal sinus may be sacrificed (and then, only if it is not a large draining vein). Gently retract the right hemisphere. Avoid retractors on the sagittal sinus to prevent injury to the SSS which may lead to sinus thrombosis (once CSF is released (with the callosotomy) retraction will be easier). Enter the interhemispheric fissure and follow the falx deep. Open the arachnoid membrane beyond the deep edge of the falx.

The two cingulate gyri may be adherent in the midline, and can easily be mistaken for the corpus callosum (CC). This error may be compounded by mistaking the callosomarginal arteries for the pericallosal arteries. Erroneously entering the cingulate gyrus disorients the surgeon and could cause injury to the pericallosal arteries. To differentiate: the CC is a pure white structure, is usually deeper than one anticipates, and is appreciated beneath the paired pericallosal arteries. Image guided surgery or measuring the depth to the CC on the pre-op MRI may help.

Callosotomy

The callosotomy is usually performed between the two pericallosal arteries. Some arterial branches may cross the midline, occasionally it is necessary to sacrifice some. Trajectory: a line drawn from the coronal suture (in the midline) to the external auditory canal (the foramen of Monro lies along this line); this helps avoid the tendency to tunnel posteriorly through the CC. Either the bipolar cautery, suction and sharp knife, or the laser is used to make the callosotomy. In hydrocephalus, the callosum will be thin. Entering the lateral ventricle releases CSF which aids retraction. When the foramen of Monro is occluded (e.g. with colloid cyst), it helps to fenestrate the septum pellucidum to prevent it from bulging into the ventricle in which one is operating (otherwise, as CSF is aspirated from the ipsilateral lateral ventricle, it cannot escape from the other).

Disconnection syndrome (p.1556): more common with posterior callosotomy (near the splenium) where more visual information crosses. The risk is reduced by creating a callosotomy < 2.5 cm in length extending posteriorly from a point 1–2 cm behind the tip of the genu.[36] For an interfornicial approach, the callosotomy must be perfectly midline.

Approach to third ventricle

Usually, the callosotomy will not be exactly midline, and one of the lateral ventricles will be entered. Great care must be taken to correctly identify which lateral ventricle has been entered, another potentially disorienting pitfall. For orientation (▶ Fig. 94.12), the choroid plexus passes forward in the choroidal fissure to the foramen of Monro (which is medial) where it converges with the thalamostriate vein approaching from a more lateral position in the groove between the thalamus and caudate. The septal and caudate veins approach the foramen from anterior. With colloid cysts, the

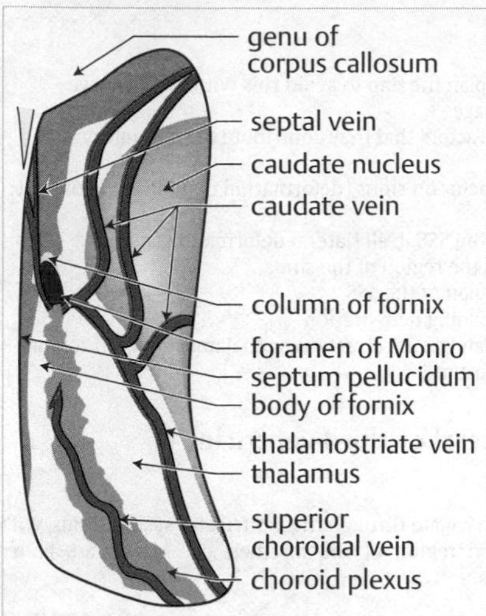

Fig. 94.12 Right foramen of Monro viewed from above through right lateral ventricle[30])

foramen of Monro may be hard to recognize initially as it will be plugged with the cyst which can resemble the ependymal lining of the ventricle, but on close inspection is usually slightly grayer (the choroid plexus enters the posterior aspect of the foramen).

Another possible pitfall upon incising the CC is entering a cavum septum pellucidum (p. 1375). The give-away here is that *no* landmarks will be visible.

Alternative approaches to third ventricle

1. interfornicial[36]: go *above* body of fornix, approaches *roof* of third ventricle. Well suited for lesions of the mid and posterior third ventricle. Callosotomy should be as close to midline as possible
2. from lateral ventricle through the foramen of Monro: with hydrocephalus, the foramen of Monro is usually dilated. If the foramen is too small for adequate access to the third ventricle, one can:
   a) return to the interfornicial approach (see above) or
   b) enlarge the foramen of Monro only if absolutely necessary. Either by:
      - opening the foramen laterally
      - the "subchoroidal" approach, making the incision posteriorly (sacrificing the thalamostriate vein) which is reportedly well tolerated[31,37]
      - last resort: incising the antero-superior margin of the foramen through the column of one fornix.[36] Caution: if the other fornix is non-functional for any reason, this would produce a bilateral forniceal lesion and may (but not definitely[36]) result in loss of short term memory and ability for new learning

Colloid cyst removal

It is critical to debulk and empty a cystic lesion, such as a colloid cyst, before delivering it from the third ventricle through the foramen of Monro. This will minimize the retraction and manipulation of the fornix. Inserting a needle and aspirating may work. The partially emptied cyst is grasped with a micro-pituitary and is delivered into the lateral ventricle through the foramen of Monro. One should only attempt to deliver the empty capsule through the foramen of Monro (p. 1462). There is usually a stalk attaching the lesion to the roof of the third ventricle, this is coagulated with bipolar cautery and divided.

For other tumors, if the tumor is too large to fit through the foramen of Monro, it should be gutted from within.

94

Complications

1. venous infarction, may be due to:
   a) sacrifice of critical cortical draining veins: plan the flap to avoid this with preoperative angiography, or with sagittal T2WI MRI images[38]
   b) superior sagittal sinus (SSS) thrombosis.[39] Factors that may contribute to sinus injury include[35]:
      - injury from retractor: avoid placing retractor on sinus (deformation of midline should not exceed 5 mm)
      - over-retraction of the dural sinus flap or on SSS itself (lateral deformation should be < 2 cm)
      - injury during the opening of the bone in the region of the sinus
      - over-use of bipolar coagulation in the region of the SSS
      - hypercoagulable state of the patient, including dehydration
2. transient mutism as a result of bilateral cingulate gyrus retraction or thalamic injury in conjunction with section of the midportion of the callosum[38]

94.7.4 Transcortical approach to lateral or third ventricle

Indications

In the absence of hydrocephalus, it is difficult to navigate through the ventricular system. Thus, with normal sized ventricles, the third ventricle and region of the foramen of Monro are better approached transcallosally (p. 1462).

1. tumors of the atrium of the lateral ventricle
2. tumors of the roof of the third ventricle
3. third ventricular tumors with significant extension into one lateral ventricle

Approaches

1. posterior parietal
2. middle temporal gyrus: useful when temporal horn of lateral ventricle is dilated due to hydrocephalus caused by the tumor; access is through the temporal horn
3. middle frontal gyrus approach: a 4 cm incision is made parallel to the axis of the middle frontal gyrus, above and anterior to the expressive speech center (Broca's area) and anterior to the motor strip[31]; about the same point as used for frontal ventriculostomy, see Kocher's point (p. 1512)

94.8 Interhemispheric approach

94.8.1 Indications

For lesions abutting on midline, deep to surface, but superficial to corpus callosum (lesions that can "fall away" from midline). Similar to transcallosal approach above, except that the pathology can be placed on the down side, which allows gravity to retract the hemisphere and thus minimizes pressure necrosis injury from mechanical retractors.

94.8.2 Technique

Position

True lateral (prevents getting lost from unusual angles). Head tilted slightly up.

Approach

Similar to transcallosal (p. 1462). Need to be sure that lateral portion of craniotomy extends at least 4 cm from midline to minimize the necessity of retraction of brain against bone.

94.9 Occipital craniotomy

94.9.1 Indications

Occipital lobe tumors including posterior falx meningiomas or tentorial meningiomas with only supratentorial component. Occipital lobe intracerebral hemorrhages.

94.9.2 Positions

Supine

Shoulder roll on affected side; elevate thorax 15°. Mayfield 3 pin headholder with single pin in forehead off to the side of the crani, double pin just over midline on opposite side.

Lateral oblique

1. affected side up, can operate either
   a) from behind patient similar to p-fossa crani for CPA lesion
   OR
   b) from top of table
2. alternative approach: affected side down. Useful in lesions adjacent to the falx; see **Interhemispheric approach** (p. 1466)

94.10 Decompressive craniectomy

94.10.1 Indications

Indications (controversial) include:
1. malignant middle cerebral artery occlusion syndrome (p. 1303) primarily for nondominant hemisphere. Use on dominant side is more controversial
2. traumatic intracranial hypertension
   a) as an adjunct for persistent intracranial hypertension when other ICP control measures fail (p. 914) [40]
   b) early in the management: may be considered for patients undergoing emergent surgery (for fracture, EDH, SDH...)[41]
3. uncontrollable brain swelling during craniotomy (p. 1429)
4. reported in children with refractory nontraumatic intracranial hypertension[42] (e.g. infection, infarction, Reye's syndrome...)

94.10.2 Potential complications

1. bleeding
2. herniation of the brain through the opening, compressing and lacerating the brain on the bone edges (risk may be reduced by making generous craniectomy)
3. post-op injury to the brain from inadvertent external pressure applied to the now relatively less protected brain
4. post-op fluid collections: hygromas or hematomas at the operative site, on the contralateral side, or interhemispheric

94.10.3 Techniques

General considerations

1. it is necessary to open the dura
2. options for the removed bone flap
   a) discard it: this may be the best option when the bone flap has been contaminated as a result of an open traumatic scalp laceration
   b) place it in a separate subcutaneous pouch in the patient's abdomen for later retrieval and reimplantation into the skull. This is especially helpful if the patient's own skull is preferred and the patient does not live in the area where he/she is having the surgery
   c) store it for future implantation: saturate with sterile solution (e.g. RPMI medium 1640 www.invitrogen.com/GIBCO) and then place within sterile storage (e.g. intestinal bags which are then placed in a sterile plastic container) and store in a bone freezer at -80° C
   d) for non-contaminated situations (e.g. stroke): reimplantation can be considered after 6–12 weeks
3. bone openings need to be large (e.g. > 12 cm diameter,[43] often > 15 cm)

Hemicraniectomy

1. some prefer use of a Mayfield headholder placed low (▶ Fig. 94.13) to give greater access[41] (not feasible with severe comminuted skull fractures)

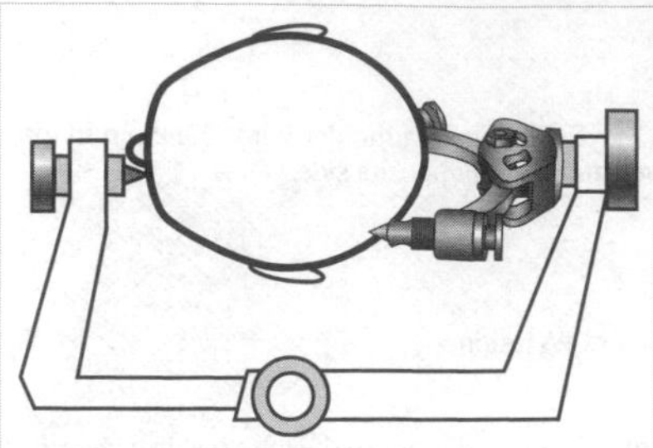

Fig. 94.13 Position of head and headholder for right hemicraniectomy (looking down on top of patient's head)

2. AP axis of head is placed horizontal to floor (unless C-spine not cleared or if neck too immobile – one may compensate for this by rotating table)
3. skin incision: two options
   a) ► Fig. 94.14A starts at widow's peak, similar to trauma flap (p.837), but with increased exposure by taking it posteriorly close to the inion then turning sharply anteriorly and hugging the ear to preserve blood supply
   b) ► Fig. 94.14B "T" incision. Less risk of flap ischemia. The "T" joins the midline incision behind the coronal suture to preserve the STA[41]
   c) burr holes (► Fig. 94.15): a burr hole is made just above the posterior root of the zygomatic arch, a second one may be made just behind the frontal insertion of the zygomatic arch, inferior to the superior temporal line
   d) bone flap: proceed posteriorly from the posterior zygomatic arch using the footplated craniotome. Posteriorly, stay ≈ 1 cm superior to asterion to avoid the transverse sinus. The flap is taken 1 cm beyond the lambdoid suture, and then up towards the sagittal suture, crossing the lambdoid suture again (this leaves a small amount of bone posteriorly on which the head can rest post-op). An anterior turn is made 1 cm short of the sagittal suture to avoid the superior sagittal sinus, and the sagittal suture is paralleled. The coronal suture is crossed and the drill is taken as low as possible in the frontal fossa near the midline. Staying as low as possible, the orbital roof is followed posteriorly towards the second burr hole. The burr holes are then connected
   e) some bone may need to be rongeured to expose the floor of the middle fossa (stippled area in ► Fig. 94.15)
   f) dural opening: based inferiorly, taken to 1 cm short of the craniotomy edge. Dural releasing incisions may be made at intervals up to the bone margin to avoid strangulation of the brain on the dural edge
   g) duraplasty
      - onlay: 2 cm wide strips of dural substitute can then be placed partway under the dural edge around the periphery to isolate the brain from the undersurface of the skin flap where there will be a gap in the dura
      - some authors suture a dural draft in place
   h) the dural flap is then replaced on top of the brain and dural substitute strips, and is not sutured

Bilateral craniectomy

The above procedure can be performed bilaterally, however, it is difficult to position the head to do this. Alternatively, a bifrontal craniectomy can be performed.

1. skin incision: bicoronal, posterior to the coronal suture (► Fig. 94.16)
2. burr holes: may use the same ones as for hemicraniectomy (see above) bilaterally. Addition burr holes to straddle the superior sagittal sinus may be made if a large single bone flap is planned
3. bone flap (► Fig. 94.17): two options, both are taken back to the coronal suture
   a) a single large bone flap[44] extending back to the coronal sutures, or
   b) two frontal flaps leaving a thin strip of bone in the midline overlying the superior sagittal sinus (if this strip is too wide, it can damage the brain)
4. dural opening: bilateral, based against the midline (superior sagittal sinus)

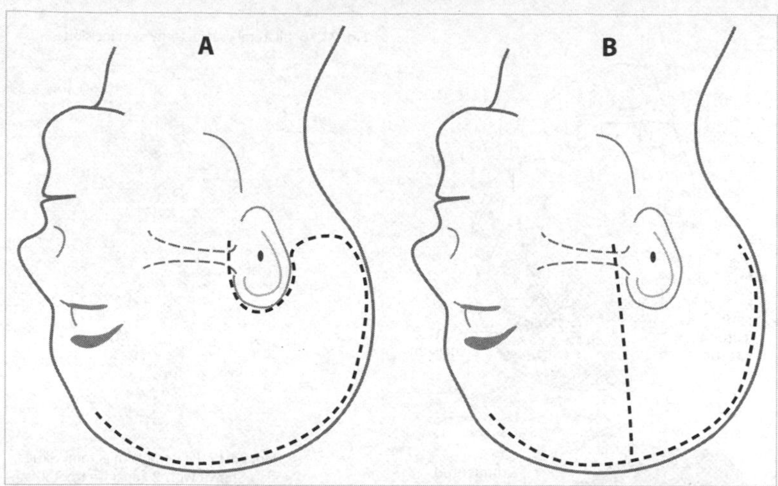

Fig. 94.14 Two options for skin incision for hemicraniectomy (see text)

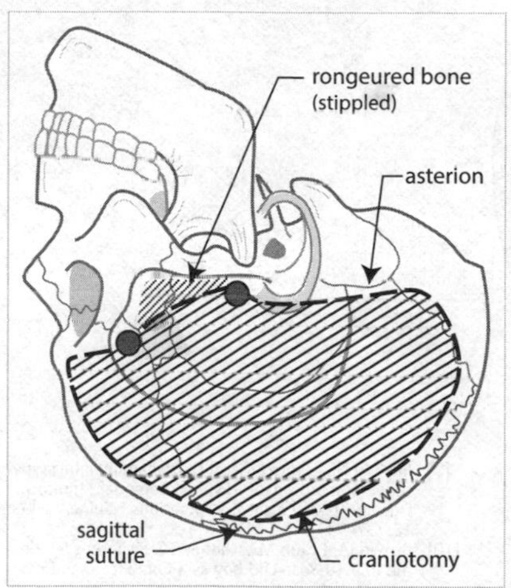

Fig. 94.15 Hemicraniectomy bone flap

Posterior fossa decompressive craniectomy

1. skin incision: midline skin incision from above inion to ≈ C2 spinous process
2. bone opening: laterally to sigmoid sinuses, superiorly to transverse sinus. C1 laminectomy is typically performed as well[42]
3. dural opening: "Y" shaped incision

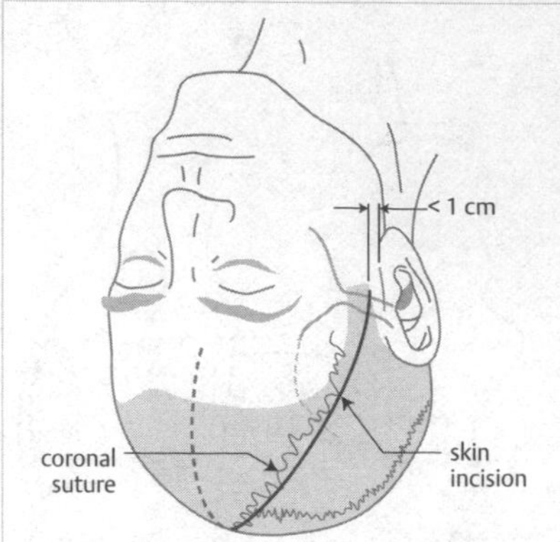

Fig. 94.16 Bilateral craniectomy skin incision

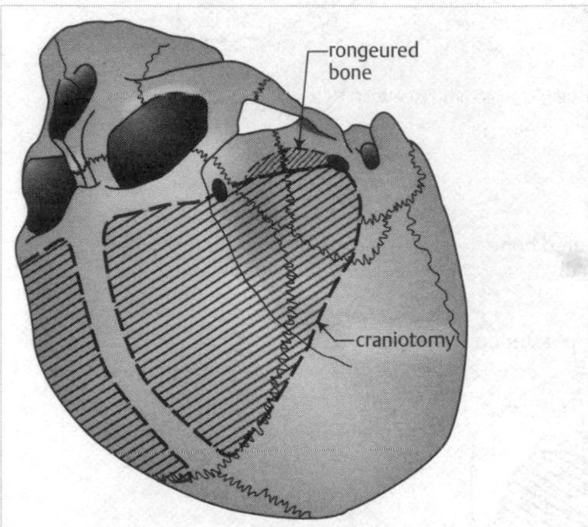

Fig. 94.17 Bilateral craniectomy skull flap Shown with 2 separate frontal flaps (the preserved midline bone strip over the superior sagittal sinus is optional)

References

[1] Fager CA. Comment on Zeidman S M and Ducker T B: Posterior Cervical Laminoforaminotomy for Radiculopathy: Review of 172 Cases. Neurosurgery. 1993; 33

[2] Kalfas IH, Little JR. Postoperative Hemorrhage: A Survey of 4992 Intracranial Procedures. Neurosurgery. 1988; 23:343–347

[3] Standefer MS, Bay JW, Trusso R. The Sitting Position in Neurosurgery. Neurosurgery. 1984; 14:649–658

[4] Kurze T. Microsurgery of the Posterior Fossa. Clin Neurosurg. 1979; 26:463–478

[5] Hitselberger WE, House WF. A Warning Regarding the Sitting Position for Acoustic Tumor Surgery. Arch Otolaryngol. 1980; 106

[6] Wilder BL. Hypothesis: The Etiology of Midcervical Quadriplegia After Operation with the Patient in the Sitting Position. Neurosurgery. 1982; 11:530–531

[7] Iwasaki Y, Tashiro K, Kikuchi S, et al. Cervical Flexion Myelopathy: A "Tight Dural Canal Mechanism". J Neurosurg. 1987; 66:935–937

[8] Haisa T, Kondo T. Midcervical Flexion Myelopathy After Posterior Fossa Surgery in the Sitting Position: Case Report. Neurosurgery. 1996; 38:819–822

[9] Epstein NE, Danto J, Nardi D. Evaluation of Intraoperative Somatosensory-Evoked Potential Monitoring During 100 Cervical Operations. Spine. 1993; 18:737–747

[10] Brown JA, Braun MA, Namey TC. Piriformis Syndrome in a 10-Year-Old Boy as a Complication of Operation with the Patient in the Sitting Position. Neurosurgery. 1988; 23:117–119

[11] Lunsford LD, Maroon JC, Sheptak PE, et al. Subdural Tension Pneumocephalus: Report of Two Cases. J Neurosurg. 1979; 50:525–527

[12] Tindall GT, Craddock A, Greenfield JC. Effects of the Sitting Position on Blood Flow in the Internal Carotid Artery of Man During General Anesthesia. J Neurosurg. 1967; 26:383–389

[13] Grady MS, Bedford RF, Park TS. Changes in Superior Sagittal Sinus Pressure in Children with Head Elevation, Jugular Venous Compression, and PEEP. J Neurosurg. 1986; 65:199–202

[14] Black S, Cucchiara RF, Nishimura RA, et al. Parameters Affecting Occurrence of Paradoxical Air Embolism. Anesthesiology. 1989; 71:235–241

[15] Munson ES, Merrick HC. Effect of Nitrous Oxide on Venous Air Embolism. Anesthesiology. 1966; 27:783–787

[16] Mirski MA, Lele AV, Fitzsimmons L, Toung TJ. Diagnosis and treatment of vascular air embolism. Anesthesiology. 2007; 106:164–177

[17] Symon L, Pell MF. Cerebrospinal Fluid Rhinorrhea Following Acoustic Neurinoma Surgery: Technical Note. J Neurosurg. 1991; 74:152–153

[18] Schmidek HH, Sweet WH. Operative Neurosurgical Techniques. New York 1982

[19] Matson DD. Neurosurgery of Infancy and Childhood. 2nd ed. Springfield: Charles C Thomas; 1969

[20] Harner SG, Beatty CW, Ebersold MJ. Impact of cranioplasty on headache after acoustic neuroma removal. Neurosurgery. 1995; 36:1097–9; discussion 1099-100

[21] Manley GT, Dillon W. Acute posterior fossa syndrome following lumbar drainage for treatment of suboccipital pseudomeningocele. Report of three cases. J Neurosurg. 2000; 92:469–474

[22] Roland PS, Marple BF, Meyerhoff WL, Mickey B. Complications of lumbar spinal fluid drainage. Otolaryngol Head Neck Surg. 1992; 107:564–569

[23] Culley DJ, Berger MS, Shaw D, Geyer R. An Analysis of Factors Determining the Need for Ventriculoperitoneal Shunts After Posterior Fossa Tumor Surgery in Children. Neurosurgery. 1994; 34:402–408

[24] Stein BM, Tenner MS, Fraser RAR. Hydrocephalus Following Removal of Cerebellar Astrocytomas in Children. J Neurosurg. 1972; 36:763–768

[25] Haines SJ, Maroon JC, Jannetta PJ. Supratentorial Intracerebral Hemorrhage following Posterior Fossa Surgery. J Neurosurg. 1978; 49:881–886

[26] Brackmann DE, Sekhar LN, Janecka IP. In: The Middle Fossa Approach. Surgery of Cranial Base Tumors. New York: Raven Press; 1993:367–377

[27] Souttar HS. New methods of surgical access to the brain. Br Med J. 1928; 1:295–300

[28] Al-Mefty O, Fox JL, Smith RR. Petrosal Approach to Petroclival Meningiomas. Neurosurgery. 1988; 22:510–517

[29] Rowe R. Surgical approaches to the trigone. Contemp Neurosurg. 2005; 27:1–5

[30] Yamamoto I, Rhoton AL, Peace DA. Microsurgery of the Third Ventricle: Part 1. Neurosurgery. 1981; 8:334–356

[31] Rhoton AL, Yamamoto I, Peace DA. Microsurgery of the Third Ventricle: Part 2. Operative Approaches. Neurosurgery. 1981; 8:357–373

[32] Carmel PW. Tumors of the Third Ventricle. Acta Neurochir. 1985; 75:136–146

[33] Klein HJ, Rath SA. Removal of Tumors of the III Ventricle Using Lamina Terminalis Approach: Three Cases of Isolated Growth of Craniopharyngiomas in the III Ventricle. Childs Nerv Syst. 1989; 5:144–147

[34] Shucart WA, Stein BM. Transcallosal Approach to the Anterior Ventricular System. Neurosurgery. 1978; 3:339–343

[35] Apuzzo MLJ. Comment on Garrido E, et al.: Cerebral Venous and Sagittal Sinus Thrombosis After Transcallosal Removal of a Colloid Cyst of the Third Ventricle: Case Report. Neurosurgery. 1990; 26

[36] Apuzzo MLJ, Chikovani OK, Gott PS, et al. Transcallosal, Interforniceal Approaches for Lesions Affecting the Third Ventricle: Surgical Considerations and Consequences. Neurosurgery. 1982; 10:547–554

[37] Hirsch JF, Zouaoui A, Renier D, et al. A new surgical approach to the third ventricle with interruption of the striothalamic vein. Acta Neurochir. 1979; 47:135–147

[38] Apuzzo MLJ. Surgery of Masses Affecting the Third Ventricular Chamber: Techniques and Strategies. Clin Neurosurg. 1988; 34:499–522

[39] Garrido E, Fahs GR. Cerebral Venous and Sagittal Sinus Thrombosis After Transcallosal Removal of a Colloid Cyst of the Third Ventricle: Case Report. Neurosurgery. 1990; 26:540–542

[40] Bullock MR, Chesnut RM, Ghajar J, et al. Surgical management of traumatic parenchymal lesions. Neurosurgery. 2006; 58:S25–S46

[41] Holland M, Nakaji P. Craniectomy: Surgical indications and technique. Operative Techniques in Neurosurgery. 2004; 7:10–15

[42] Aghakhani Nozar, Durand Philippe, Chevret Laurent, Parker Fabrice, Devictor Denis, Tardieu Marc, Tadi√© Marc. Decompressive craniectomy in children with nontraumatic refractory high intracranial pressure. Journal of Neurosurgery: Pediatrics. 2009; 3:66–69

[43] Delashaw JB, Broaddus WC, Kassell NF, et al. Treatment of Right Hemispheric Cerebral Infarction by Hemicraniectomy. Stroke. 1990; 21:874–881

[44] Polin RS, Shaffrey ME, Bogaev CA, et al. Decompressive Bifrontal Craniectomy in the Treatment of Severe Refractory Posttraumatic Cerebral Edema. Neurosurgery. 1997; 41:84–94

95 Spine, Cervical

95.1 Anterior approaches to the cervical spine

1. anterior odontoid screw (p. 1476)
2. C1–3 (upper cervical spine):
   a) transoral approach: including odontoidectomy (p. 1472)
   b) extrapharyngeal approaches: use nasotracheal intubation (so that the mandible can be completely closed) through the contralateral nares. The head is slightly extended and is rotated 15° to the contralateral side. Avoid any oral tubes
      - medial extrapharyngeal approach: medial to carotid sheath. Provides a more anterior position than the lateral retropharyngeal approach. Structures encountered: branches of external carotid artery, upper laryngeal nerves, hypoglossal nerve
      - lateral retropharyngeal approach: only the spinal accessory nerve is encountered
3. C3-C7: standard anterior cervical discectomy approach
   a) For 1 or 2 level ACDF or 1 level corpectomy, a horizontal incision is usually employed
   b) For more levels, a vertically oriented incision may be preferred to facilitate access

95.2 Transoral approach to anterior craniocervical junction

95.2.1 General information

Primarily useful for midline *extradural* lesions (approach to intradural lesions has been described,[1] but the use has been extremely limited because of difficulties obtaining watertight closure and increased risk of meningitis). Refinements in techniques and equipment (e.g. flexible reinforced oral endotracheal tube, McGarver or Crockard retractor, operating microscope, and suturing transnasal red-rubber catheters to the uvula to aid in retraction) allows access from as high as the inferior third of the clivus to as low as C3 (and sometimes C4[2]) vertebral body without need for tracheostomy or splitting of the tongue. Additional access can be achieved with use of extended techniques including splitting of the hard & soft palate, tongue splitting, and transmandibular approach.

95.2.2 Transoral odontoidectomy

Indications

Anterior extradural compression of the cervicomedullary junction as with pannus from rheumatoid arthritis, irreducible basilar invagination, tumors of C2, infection.

Stabilization

75% of patients undergoing transoral removal of the odontoid process required posterior fusion afterwards[3] due to ligamentous instability.[4,5] While the stabilization intuitively seems like it should be done first, it is often done following the decompression at the same sitting or at a soon to follow date. Some reasons for decompressing before stabilization:

1. positioning the patient for fusion may cause neurologic compromise if there is cord compression
2. a post-op MRI can be done to determine if enough decompression was achieved from the odontoidectomy. If not, a laminectomy can be done at the same time as the posterior stabilization
3. the amount of destabilization may not be known until after the odontoidectomy – in some cases a C1–2 fusion may suffice[5]

Stabilization usually entails posterior occipitocervical fusion. Occasionally fusion may be limited to C1–2 or C1–3 without the occiput. It is also possible to place an anterior strut between the body of C2 and the clivus, or between C2 and C1. Fibula is recommended. Metal instrumentation should be avoided.

Pre-op preparation

1. make sure that the patient can open the mouth at least 25 mm. If not, then other approaches such as translabiomandibular should be considered

2. for conditions resulting in malalignment or basilar invagination, cervical traction for 1 or more days is sometimes required
3. radiographic evaluation
   a) cervical MRI without and with contrast to define the soft tissue pathology
   b) CT of the craniocervical junction with sagittal and coronal reconstruction
   c) CTA to assess the position and involvement of the vertebral arteries. Measuring the distance between the VAs provides useful information

Booking the case: Transoral approach

Also see defaults & disclaimers (p. 27).
1. position: supine with pin headholder
2. equipment
   a) microscope
   b) high-speed drill with long bits
   c) C-arm
   d) image guided navigation system (if used)
3. instruments
   a) transoral set (usually includes oral retractor such as Crockard, Dingman, Dickman-Sonntag...)
   b) long instruments: microdiscectomy instruments often work
4. anesthesia: awake, fiberoptic endotracheal intubation
5. some surgeons use ENT to perform the approach and closure and for follow-up
6. consent (in lay terms for the patient – not all-inclusive):
   a) procedure: transoral resection of odontoid, placement of halo-vest immobilization, MEP monitoring (MEP should be consented specifically due to risk of seizures). Need for posterior stabilization at the same setting or in the immediate future
   b) alternatives: nonsurgical management, radiation therapy for some diagnoses
   c) complications: CSF leak with possible meningitis, spinal cord injury, wound breakdown, swallowing difficulties (may require PEG tube), breathing problems (may require tracheostomy), seizures with MEP

Technical considerations

For details, see references.[2,3,6] Some key points:

Awake fiberoptic orotracheal intubation is employed. Nasotracheal (NT) is used by some, but at the narrow upper part of the exposure the NT tube tends to get in the way.

SSEP and MEP monitoring are used in appropriate cases.

Positioning: 3-point fixation with a Mayfield headholder is typically used. The patient is supine with no *neck rotation* (distorts the anatomical relationships and may bring one VA closer to the midline). Tilt the whole patient or the table towards the surgeon. 10–15° neck extension improves the exposure. Alternatively, the surgeon can stand above the patient who is kept perfectly supine.

A specialized retractor (e.g. Crockard transoral retractor) or a conventional Dingman retractor is placed. Verify that the tongue is not being compressed against the teeth.

Landmark: the tubercle of the atlas can be palpated through the posterior pharynx to locate the midline and for craniocaudal orientation.

The mucosa of the posterior pharynx is infiltrated with 1% lidocaine with epinephrine. Some authors culture the oropharynx to obtain drug sensitivities of organisms for use in the event of infection. Some advocate liberal topical use of 1% hydrocortisone ointment to the mucosa of the oropharynx and posterior tongue at the beginning and also during the operation to reduce intra-op and post-op swelling. Others feel it has no effect, and IV Decadron is used by some.

A 3 cm long vertical midline incision is made.

To reduce the risk of C1 spreading and allowing basilar invagination, C1 ring-sparing surgery may be attempted by removing only the inferior half to two-thirds of the anterior C1. When C1 ring-sparing is not done, the central 3 cm of the atlas is removed with a high-speed drill.

There is ≈ about 20–25 mm working distance between the two vertebral arteries at their point of closest approximation where they enter the foramen transversarium at the inferior aspect of the lateral mass of C2.

The odontoid is hollowed out "like a canoe") using a high speed drill, checking progress on lateral fluoro at frequent intervals. Once the bone has been reduced to a thin shell, it can be fractured in towards the hollowed out portion using curettes. The superior tip of the odontoid is particularly challenging due to the apical ligament.

Closure: a two layer closure is preferred by some. Others recommend a single layer closure incorporating deep muscle, superficial muscle, and mucosa.[2] If the dura has been violated, a fascial patch is secured with tissue adhesive and a lumbar subarachnoid drain is placed in the O.R. and maintained at low pressure for 3–4 days. An NG tube is placed under direct visualization to avoid injury or penetration of the mucosal closure.

Posterior stabilization

Transoral odontoidectomy produces instability in most cases (sometimes delayed).[4,5]

For basilar invagination or occipitocervical instability, an occipitocervical fusion is recommended (p. 1474).[6]

For C1–2 instability alone, a posterior C1–2 arthrodesis may be performed (p. 1479).[6]

Possible complications

1. dural tear with CSF leak and risk of meningitis
2. vertebral artery injury
3. spinal cord injury

Post-op care

1. NG feeding or IV hyperalimentation is used initially (in anticipation of oropharyngeal swelling (lasts 2–3 days) and to avoid disruption of the mucosal closure)
2. intubation is maintained until the swelling subsides. Initial removal of the endotracheal tube over a tube changer facilitates reintubation if needed; the tube changer can be removed if no problem develops after 1 hour[6]
3. if the NG tube comes out, it should only be replaced under direct vision (usually by ENT physician) to avoid injury/penetration of the mucosal incision
4. halo-vest immobilization is maintained until the posterior fusion is performed
5. for staged procedures when the fusion is being done at a later date, a post-op MRI should be done to assess the degree of decompression. If further decompression is needed, then a laminectomy can be added to the posterior fusion

95.3 Occipitocervical fusion

95

The patient will lose about 30% of neck flexion mobility with an occipital to C1 fusion.

Indications for occipitocervical fusion[7]:

1. traumatic occipitoatlantal dislocation
2. absence of a complete arch of C1. **Note:** Alternatively, C1–2 lateral mass fusion (with or without lateral mass screws) (p. 1479) may be used in cases b and c if only the posterior arch of C1 is compromised
   a) congenital
   b) post-decompression
   c) posttraumatic: "bursting" C1 fracture (bilateral or multiple C1 ring fractures). NB: some feel that this may be satisfactorily treated with halo immobilization until the atlas fracture heals (as they almost all do) followed by C1 to C2 wiring/fusion.[8]
3. congenital anomalies of the occipitocervical joints
4. upward migration of the odontoid into the foramen magnum
5. marked irreducible shifts of C1 or C2

Disadvantages of occipitocervical fusion:

1. loss of movement at the occipitoatlantal junction further reduces the range of motion as follows[9]:
   a) flexion/extension: reduced by ≈ 30% (13° occurs at occiput-C1 junction)
   b) lateral rotation: 10° is lost
   c) lateral bending: 8° is lost
2. non-union rate is higher than with C1–2 fusion alone[10]

Options:
1. keel plate (placed centrally over the thickest portion of the occipital bone) connected via rods to cervical screws (C2 pedicle screws and C3 lateral mass screws): reduced range of motion (ROM) to 17% of normal in a cadaver study[11] (for technique, see below)
2. occipital condyle (OC)-C1 polyaxial screws[12]: see below
3. occipital-C1 (AKA atlantooccipital) transarticular screws (see below)
4. looped rod wired to the occiput via wire cables placed through holes drilled in the occiput. Reduced ROM only to 31% of normal[11]

95.3.1 Keel plate occipital-cervical fusion

Pre-op planning:
1. CT scan through C2
   a) to rule-out aberrant position of foramen transversarium
   b) to measure diameter of pedicles (may be best done on coronal sections due to the fact that the axial images are not usually oriented along path of pedicle) and estimate length of screws to be used
   c) to verify trajectory of screws
2. measure thickness of occipital bone to determine screw-length for occipital screws

Technique:
1. occipital keel screws/plate
   a) a drill, tap and screwdriver with flexible shafts or universal joints are usually needed because of interference from patient's skin
   b) midline holes are preferred since occipital bone is thickest here
   c) drill with drill guide to 8 mm, check depth with probe, if the inner cortex has not been breached, drill to 10 mm, check depth again, keep drilling 2 mm at a time until the inner cortex is breached, use that screw length
   d) SCREWS 4.5 diameter **blunt** screws, 8–12 mm length
2. C2 pedicle screws (p. 1485)
3. C3 lateral mass screws (p. 1485) (if used)

95.3.2 Occipital condyle to C1 polyaxial screw fusion

See references.[12,13]

Utilizes polyaxial screws placed in the occipital condyles that are then connected to screws placed at lower levels (see below) via connecting rods.
1. PROS compared to occipital plate/keel instrumentation:
   a) circumvents problem of poor occipital bone purchase which may occur with keel plates
   b) can be used even following posterior fossa craniectomy
   c) greater surface area for fusion
   d) avoids risk of intracranial injury from occipital screws
2. CONS: due to condylar variability, not all patients are candidates
3. biomechanics: compared to occipital plate, similar stiffness in flexion-extension and axial rotation, increased stiffness to lateral bending[14]
4. clinical: 1 patient, 2 years F/U with solid OC fusion[15]

Pre-op planning: CT scan occiput through C2.

Technique:

✖ Structures to avoid include: hypoglossal nerve in hypoglossal canal (just above the occipital condyles (OC)), carotid and vertebral arteries, jugular bulb. IG may be helpful
1. occipital condyle screws
   a) ENTRY 4–5 mm lateral to the foramen magnum, 1–2 mm rostral to the atlanto-occipital joint (do not need to or want to expose the entire condyle – there is an emissary vein laterally which is best left alone)
   b) TRAJ 12–22° medial (mean: 17°), 5° maximal superior angulation
   c) SCREWS 3.5 mm diameter polyaxial screws; bicortical purchase obtained using 20–24 mm length (mean: 22 mm)
2. condyle screws are connected with 3 mm diameter rods to either:
   a) screws in C1 lateral mass and C2 pedicles (p. 1483), or
   b) C1–2 transarticular screws (p. 1480)

95.3.3 Occipital-C1 (AKA atlantooccipital) transarticular screws

See references.[16,17]

1. PROS: no compromise of C1–2 joint
2. CONS: steep trajectory requires additional incision at level of C-T junction
3. ENTRY midpoint of posterior C1 lateral mass
4. TRAJ 10–20° medially, aiming cranially to TARGET middle of occipital condyle
5. SCREWS 28–32 mm cannulated lag screws
6. biomechanics: ≈ equal to occipital plate-C1 lateral mass fusion[18]
7. clinical data: 2 cases reported, 2 year F/U, co complication

95.3.4 Post-op immobilization/bracing

1. for severe C1 fractures, or those with impaired bone healing capacity (elderly or unreliable patients, smokers…) a halo-vest is recommended × 8–12 weeks
2. otherwise, if C1 is not badly damaged, a collar that limits flexion (e.g. Miami-J collar) suffices × 8–12 weeks

95.4 Anterior odontoid screw fixation

95.4.1 Introduction

50% of axial rotation of the head occurs at the C1-C2 complex. Treatment of odontoid fractures by C1–2 fusion significantly reduces this mobility (although subaxial articulations will compensate to some degree over time). Odontoid screw fixation (OSF) attempts to treat odontoid fractures by restoring the structural integrity of the odontoid process (osteosynthesis) without sacrificing the normal mobility.

Stability of the C1–2 joint depends primarily on the integrity of the odontoid process and the atlantal transverse ligament (p.70) (which is the most important structure holding the odontoid process in position against the anterior arch of C1).

95.4.2 Evaluation

A full set of C-spine x-rays is needed, including an open-mouth odontoid view. MRI is recommended to rule-out disruption of atlantal transverse ligament. Cervical axial CT with coronal and sagittal reconstructions are also recommended to demonstrate the orientation of the fracture path and to verify the integrity of the posterior elements. Complex motion polytomography may be used if the CT findings are unclear.

95

95.4.3 Indications

Reducible odontoid Type II fracture (and Type III fractures where the fracture line is in the cephalad portion of the body of C2 in an elderly patient who may not fuse as well with immobilization as a younger patient[19]). The transverse ligament *must be* intact.

95.4.4 Contraindications

1. fractures of the C2 vertebral *body* (except cephalad Type III fracture)
2. disruption of atlantal transverse ligament: see Transverse atlantal ligament (TAL) injuries (p.1479). May be directly demonstrated on MRI. Indirect evidence: if the sum of the overhang of the lateral masses of C1 on C2 exceeds 7 mm (rule of Spence (p.970))
3. large odontoid fracture gap
4. irreducible fracture
5. age of fracture: controversial. Fusion rates in fracture > 18 months old was 25%.[20] Fracture < 6 months old have ≈ 90% fusion rate[20]
6. patients with short, thick necks and/or barrel chest: makes it difficult to achieve the proper angle. May be circumvented by the instrumentation distributed by Richard-Nephew which utilize a cannulated flexible drill, tap and screwdriver
7. pathologic odontoid fracture
8. fracture line in oblique orientation to frontal plane (shearing forces can cause malalignment during screw tightening)

Booking the case: Odontoid screw fixation

See defaults & disclaimers (p. 27).

1. position: supine head on horseshoe headrest, halter traction
2. anesthesia: awake fiberoptic or nasotracheal intubation. Do NOT use a wire reinforced endotracheal tube
3. equipment: **2** C-arms for biplane fluoro, or O-arm image guidance
4. instrumentation:
   a) ACDF surgical set
   b) tube retractor (e.g. METRx® by Medtronic)
   c) some surgeons use specialized instrumentation (e.g. Apfelbaum set)
5. implants: cannulated screw set
6. consent (in lay terms for the patient – not all-inclusive):
   a) procedure: surgery to place screw(s) from the front of the neck across the fractured odontoid bone. Possible posterior approach in case the anterior approach cannot be completed
   b) alternatives: nonsurgical management in a collar, fusion
   c) complications: screw breakage/pullout, failure to fuse which might require addition surgery (which will reduce neck motion)

95.4.5 Technique summary

Preparation

Various instrumentation systems have been developed to facilitate the procedure. The following describes some of the basic elements that are not specific to any one instrumentation (see reference by Apfelbaum[21] for details of his instrumentation distributed by Aesculap Instrument Corporation, South San Francisco, CA).

Two C-arm fluoroscopy machines are mandatory for bi-plane imaging (simultaneous AP and lateral views). Some surgeons prefer placing 2 screws if there is enough bone to accommodate them, however, this may also reduce the amount of bone surface that can heal and the fusion rate appears to be the same.[22]

Anesthetic considerations

The anesthesiologist is positioned at the *foot* of the table. Awake fiberoptic or nasotracheal intubation is recommended, especially for easily dislocatable fractures. Do NOT use a wire reinforced endotracheal tube since the wire interferes with the AP imaging.

Position

95

Supine. The neck is placed in *extension* (critical to performing the procedure) either with Holter traction and a small shoulder roll with the head on a doughnut (a strip of tape across the forehead stabilizes the head), or a radiolucent head holder may be used. Place the *lateral* fluoro unit first, then the AP unit slides into the "C" of the lateral unit. Lateral fluoroscopy is used to assess reduction of the fracture fragment, and the head is repositioned to try and achieve reduction. If there is retrolisthesis of the odontoid, the neck may need to be slightly less extended. A radiolucent mouth gag is placed to hold the mouth open for AP transoral imaging (a small tape roll works well). Abort the procedure if AP and lateral fluoroscopic views do not adequately image the odontoid.

Approach

A Cloward-type of horizontal skin incision at ≈ C5–6 (the entry site can be localized by placing a guidewire adjacent to the patients neck and taking a lateral fluoro) and approach identical to anterior cervical discectomy is used (all the way to exposing the longus coli muscles (p. 1073)). A Kittner is used to dissect superiorly anterior to the longus coli muscles in the loose areolar tissue up to C2. A self-retaining retractor (e.g. Caspar retractor – not distractor) with a superior retractor blade is attached (or a hand-held retractor, preferably radiolucent, may be used). Alternatively, a retractor tube system[23] (e.g. METRx® by Medtronic) may be used. The bovie is used to remove the soft tissue over the inferior front of C2.

Procedure

Localization: lateral fluoro is used to place the tip of an awl *as far anteriorly as possible* on the inferior endplate of C2 (▶ Fig. 95.1; a common error is to go too far back along the inferior margin of C2, then the guidewire end up towards the back of the dens). AP fluoro is used place the awl in the exact center of the C2 body in the lateral dimension. The awl is used to make a pilot hole at this location.

Guidewire placement, drilling, tapping and ultimately screw placement are performed while monitoring the progress on frequent fluoro images, aiming for the exact middle of the dens on AP fluoro, and aiming towards the apex of the odontoid fracture fragment (skimming just within the anterior part of the C2 vertebral body) on lateral fluoro.

Drilling is performed under fluoro all the way *through* the apical cortex of the dens to avoid cracking the dens with the screw (the area just distal to the apex of the dens is safe).

A titanium partially threaded (lag) screw is placed. If an appropriately sized lag screw is not available, one can overdrill the part of the path through the body of C2 up to the fracture. In this way, a fully threaded screws can be used which will slip through the overdrilled hole and still have a lag effect on the fracture fragment. If a second side-by-side screw is used, it may be fully threaded. In chronic nonunion cases, prior to advancing the screw a bifaced curette may be inserted within the fracture space to freshen the fracture site. The screw(s) should be drawn up tightly to the inferior edge of C2. ▶ Fig. 95.1 shows the final position of an anterior odontoid screw.

At the end of the procedure confirm integrity of the transverse ligament by carefully flexing the neck under lateral fluoro.

95

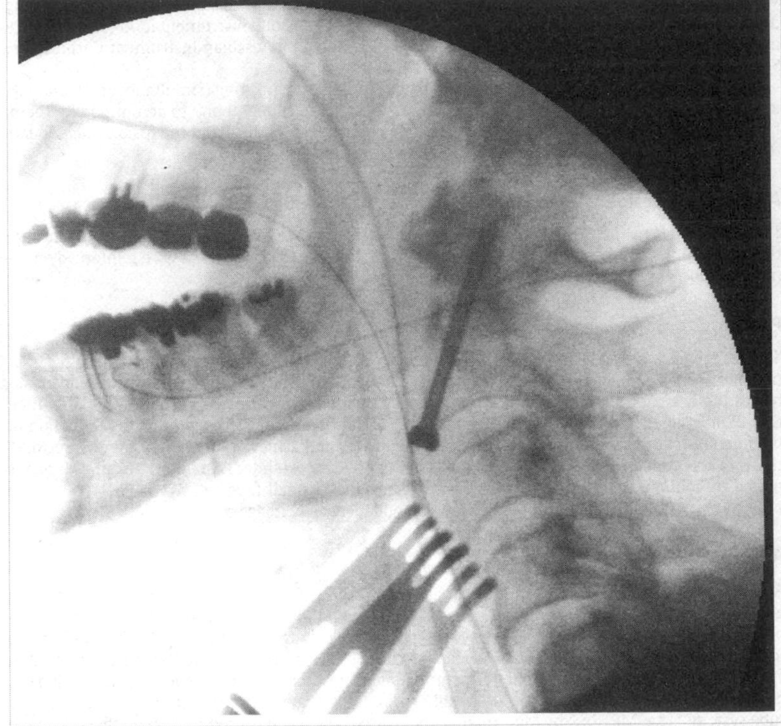

Fig. 95.1 Final position of anterior odontoid screw

Postoperative immobilization

The immediate post-op strength of the odontoid + screw is only ≈ 50% of the normal odontoid. Therefore, a cervical brace is recommended for 6 weeks[19] (although some authors don't use one[21]). If the patient has significant osteoporosis, a halo brace is recommended.

Results

Healing takes ≈ 3 months (or longer with chronic nonunion). With fractures < 6 months old, the union rate was 95%. Chronic nonunions > 6 months old have a significant risk of hardware failure (screw breakage or pull-out), with a bony union rate of 31%, and 38% rate of presumed fibrous union.[21] Thus, in cases of chronic nonunion > 6 months old, C1–2 arthrodesis is probably a better choice unless the need to maintain motion is worth the risk of needing a second operation if this one fails.

The average technical complication rate is ≈ 6% (2% screw malposition, 1.5% screw breakout).

95.5 Atlantoaxial fusion (C1–2 arthrodesis)

95.5.1 Indications

NB: The patient will lose ≈ 50% of head rotation with C1–2 fusion.

▸ **Instability of the C1–2 joints, including:**

1. atlantoaxial dislocation due to incompetence of the transverse atlantal ligament (TAL):
   a) rheumatoid arthritis (p. 1136): symptomatic patients, or asymptomatic patients with subluxation ≥ 8 mm
   b) local infection
   c) trauma
   d) Down syndrome (p. 1138): due to laxity of the TAL
2. incompetence of the odontoid process
   a) odontoid fractures meeting surgical criteria, including
      - Type II fractures with > 6 mm displacement
      - instability at the fracture site in halo-vest traction
      - chronic nonunion of odontoid fractures
      - disruption of the transverse ligament
   b) following transoral odontoidectomy
   c) tumors destroying the odontoid process

▸ **Vertebrobasilar insufficiency with head turning** (p. 1307) **(bow hunter's sign)**

95.5.2 Technical considerations

Come cases require incorporation of the occiput in addition to C1–2.

Surgical options include:

▸ **Rigid instrumentation:**

1. C1-C2 fusion using polyaxial screws connected by rods:
   a) C1: screws placed in lateral masses. May be used in cases where the posterior arch of C1 is compromised
   b) C2 screw options:
      - screws may be placed in pedicles (pars)
      - screws may be placed in lateral masses
      - crossed C2 laminar screws[24]
2. C1–2 posterior transarticular facet screws (TAS)[25,26,27]

▸ **Posterior cervical wiring and fusion.** With the development of rigid fixation, these techniques are used less frequently. While they are poor in limiting rotation, they are effective in limiting flexion. And since the Dickman & Sonntag technique is effective in limiting extension, it has recently been used to offload C1 lateral mass screws which have a tendency to break at the point of entry to the bone of C1

1. interspinous fusion technique of Dickman and Sonntag (p. 1483)
2. not presented here:

95

a) Brooks fusion[28] (the Smith-Robinson technique as modified by Griswold[29]): C1 to C2 sublaminar wires with 2 wedge bone grafts
b) Gallie fusion[30(p 1477–93)] and its modifications: midline wire under the arch of C1 with an "H" bone graft

▶ **Halifax clamps with fusion.**[31] These clamps are effective in minimizing movement in flexion, but are less stable in extension or with rotation

▶ **Odontoid compression screw fixation** (p. 1476). Essentially only for odontoid Type II fractures < 6 months old with intact transverse ligament (p. 1476).[32] Preserves more mobility than C1–2 fusion

▶ **Combined anterolateral and posterior bone grafting.**[32]

▶ **Combining anterior (transoral) decompression with posterior fusion.** Indicated when a significant anterior mass is present causing neural compression and/or making passage of sublaminar wires at C1 unsafe

95.5.3 Techniques of atlantoaxial fusion

Positioning

The patient is placed in a halo ring (with a gap in the back and secured to the table using a Mayfield adapter) or Mayfield pin fixation and is then placed prone on the O.R. table on chest rolls. The table will usually need to be positioned in a maximal reverse-Trendelenburg position to bring up the surgical area. The patient's feet are allowed to rest on a padded footplate on the table to prevent the patient from sliding down. Lateral intraoperative x-rays are taken after patient positioning.

Incision and approach

A midline skin incision is made from just below the inion to the spinous process of C5 or C6.

C1–2 transarticular facet screws (TAS)

May be used as an adjunct to posterior C1–2 wiring and bone graft – e.g. technique of Dickman and Sonntag (p. 1483) – to achieve immediate stabilization without the need for postoperative external orthosis, or in cases where the posterior arch of C1 is fractured or absent. ✖ A major risk of the procedure is vertebral artery (VA) injury. Therefore many practitioners have adopted C1 lateral mass screws (p. 1481).

Selection of candidates

95

May be appropriate in elderly patients or those with rheumatoid arthritis, in whom there may be slow fusion, or for those who have failed a previous attempt at C1–2 wiring/fusion. Also in young individuals who have ligamentous laxity.

All patients must have thin cut CT scans from the occipital condyles through C3 with sagittal reconstruction through the C1–2 facet on both sides to look for the presence of a vertebral artery in the intended path of the screw. Also, risk of VA injury can be reduced using CT scans reconstructed along the planned trajectory of the screw (aiming from a point 4 mm above the inferior C2 facet to a point in the anterior C1 button on CT[33]).

Technique summary

A number of instrumentation sets are available for the procedure, and each has its own nuances. The following is intended to primarily cover the basic procedure common to most or all (see reference by Apfelbaum[21] for details with that system).

Position:

Patient supine, with the head clamped in a Mayfield head-holder with a slight military tuck of the chin. Lateral C-arm fluoroscopy is used for the procedure, and some have advocated biplane fluoro.

Approach:

Utilize a standard midline posterior laminectomy approach from occiput to the C3 spinous process. The lamina of C2 and the posterior arch of C1 are exposed to the lateral aspect of the C2 inferior articular facet. The lateral extent of the spinal canal is defined using a small angled curette. The C1–2 facet is curetted to facilitate arthrodesis and permits observation of the drill as it crosses the joint.

ENTRY 1–2 mm superior to the C2–3 facet on the midline axis of the pars interarticularis. The trajectory is determined fluoroscopically using a K-wire placed on the side of the neck as a guide, aiming it through the C2 inferior articular process, pars interarticularis, superior articular process and across the C1–2 articulation into the lateral mass of C1. This helps establish the appropriate entry site for the drill guide through a separate stab wound, usually around the T1–2 level, 2–3 cm off the midline.

TRAJ A pilot hole is then drilled using visual guidance to maintain a straight parasagittal course (it helps to stand on 1 or 2 footstools to eliminate some of the parallax error) and fluoroscopic guidance to maintain the trajectory towards the C1 lateral mass. An assistant can reduce any atlanto-axial translational malalignment using a towel clip on C1 or C2 just prior to the drill crossing the C1–2 facet joint. To minimize the risk of VA injury, keep the drill as far dorsally as possible within the pars interarticularis. The pilot hole is then tapped and a fully threaded titanium screw is placed. If brisk arterial bleeding (not bone bleeding) occurs after drilling or tapping the first side, the VA may have been injured. The screw may still be placed but the contralateral hole and screw should *not* be placed. A post-op arteriogram is then performed to assess for propagating thrombus or dissection. Barring any contraindications, the procedure is repeated on the contralateral side. After screw placement, then posterior bone fusion – e.g. technique of Dickman and Sonntag (p. 1483) – is performed. External immobilization is usually not employed post-op (the screws are considered to supply adequate internal immobilization).

Results

A fusion rate of up to 99% with no complications has been reported.[25] Injury to the vertebral artery is the main potential complication.

C1–2 lateral mass screws

Placement of polyaxial mini screws in C1 lateral mass and C2 pedicle with rod fixation. Originated by Goel and Laheri[34] in 1994 and promulgated in 2001 by Harms and Melcher.[35]

Advantages over C1–2 transarticular screws (see above):

1. the more superior and medial trajectory should reduce the risk of VA injury[35]
2. may be used in the presence of C1–2 subluxation
3. may be usable in certain cases of aberrant VA course
4. in selected cases, this can be used for temporary fixation without fusion (since joint spaces remain intact) and the hardware may be removed after an appropriate time to reclaim motion in the C1–2 articulation

Booking the case: C1–2 lateral mass fusion

Also see defaults & disclaimers (p. 27) and pre-op assessment (see below).

1. position: prone, pin headholder
2. anesthesia: awake fiberoptic or nasotracheal intubation
3. equipment: C-arm or O-arm image guidance
4. implants:
   a) mini-polyaxial screws (smooth shank screws needed for C1)
   b) cable required for interspinous graft (optional, but recommended)
   c) have rep bring in occipital plates and instrumentation in case of inability to place C1 screws therefore enabling occipital-cervical fusion as a bail-out option
5. consent (in lay terms for the patient – not all-inclusive):
   a) procedure: surgery to place screws & rods from the back of the neck to stabilize, and usually to fuse the top 2 bones of the neck
   b) alternatives: nonsurgical management in a collar, in some cases screws may be temporary and no fusion would be done
   c) complications: screw breakage/pullout, failure to fuse which might require addition surgery, loss of some neck bending motion is expected (≈ 20% is typical)

Surgical technique (excerpted highlights)

See references.[35,36]

NB: if fusion is to accompany screw placement (i.e. permanent screw placement), strong consideration should be given to supplemental interspinous fusion, if not contraindicated (p. 1483) to prevent fatigue breakage of C1 screws.

Applied anatomy: there is no true neural foramen at C1–2, the C2 nerve root lies on the posterior surface of the capsule of the C1–2 articular joint.

Pre-op assessment

It is mandatory to know the position of the VA on both sides (and in particular, the location of both foramina transversarium of C1), and the following bony information (requires thin-cut CT scan):

1. cranio-caudal thickness (height) of the posterior arch of C1 (in case the arch needs to be drilled to facilitate screw placement)
2. to determine screw length: distance from the planned entry point (see below) to the planned exit target (midposition of the anterior part of the superior C1 VB)
3. to estimate medio-lateral angle for screws

Approach

Completely expose the C1–C2 complex. Dissect over the superior surface of the C2 pars interarticularis to expose the C1–C2 joint to accurately locate the entry point for the C1 lateral mass screws. Bleeding is controlled with bipolar cautery and/or Gelfoam-thrombin. Complete exposure of the posterior face of the inferior C1 facet also mobilizes the C2 root from the underlying attachments and facilitates its inferior mobilization.

1. C1 lateral mass screws ENTRY visualization commonly requires caudal retraction of the C2 dorsal root ganglion (occasionally this may not be feasible[36]; sacrificing the C2 root may be required but this can lead to post-op pain and numbness[37]; technique is to divide the *preganglionic* nerve fibers and to close the dural defect[36]). The screw entry point is the midpoint of the inferior part of the C1 lateral mass (for both mediolateral and cranio-caudal directions). An awl or a 1- to 2-mm high-speed drill is used to mark the position to prevent slippage while drilling the hole. Drilling a portion of the inferior arch of C1 is sometimes needed to allow screw placement (caution: the thickness of the arch in the cranio-caudal dimension varies widely, and the horizontal segment of the VA lies immediately above – use pre-op CT for planning)
2. C1 screw TRAJ averages ≈ 17° medially, ≈ 22° rostrally, TARGET the superior aspect of the anterior tubercle of C1 on lateral fluoro (see ▶ Fig. 95.2)
3. C1 SCREWS 3.5 or 4 mm diameter, length is determined from pre-op fine-cut CT to obtain bicortical purchase (✖ CAUTION: the ICA may be as close as 1 mm to the ideal exit site of the screw[38] ∴ some authors use only unicortical purchase). The screw needs to be proud to bring it up to the level of the C2 screw (it may actually be necessary to have the C1 screw protruding 1–2 mm more than the C2 screw in order to allow rod attachment[36]), and it should have an ≈ 8 mm unthreaded superficial portion to minimize irritation of the C2 nerve which could produce occipital neuralgia
4. C2 pedicle (pars) screws, see description of placement (p. 1483)
5. if a fusion is to be performed: the posterior arch of C1 and the C2 lamina are decorticated with a drill. Onlay fusion substrate is then placed, taking care not to compress the dura. Optional adjunct: intra-articular decortication and packing bone within the C1–2 joint

95

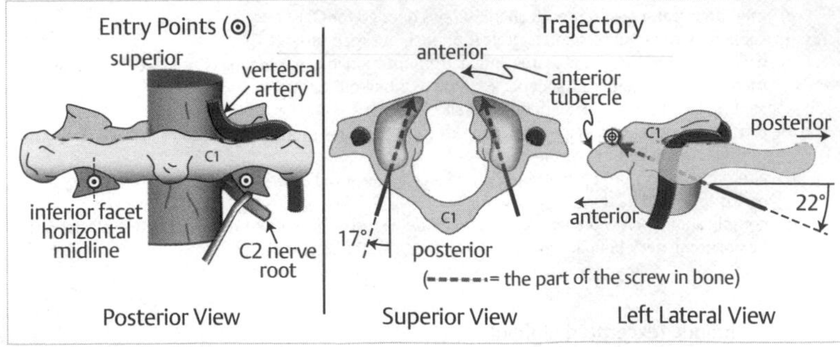

Fig. 95.2 Screw entry point and trajectory for C1 lateral mass screws

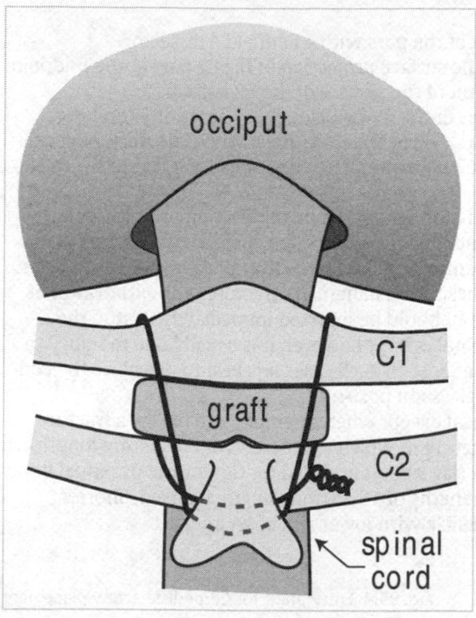

Fig. 95.3 Dickman and Sonntag C1–2 interspinous fusion

Post-op care

A cervical collar (soft or rigid, as preferred) for 4–6 weeks suffices.

Interspinous fusion technique of Dickman and Sonntag

A single bicortical graft is used, with multistranded cable passed sublaminar to C1 only. The bone graft is wedged between C1 and C2 (trapping it between loops of cable),[39,40] see ▶ Fig. 95.3. Currently, this technique is infrequently used as the primary fixation for C1–2 fusion (unless technical difficulties prevent e.g. C1–2 lateral mass fusion). However, it may be most useful for limiting extension to offload C1 lateral mass screws to reduce the risk of screw breakage.[41]

Cannot be used if the posterior ring of C1 or C2 is fractured.

Bone graft

Autologous bone is preferred. Bone is often taken from the posterior iliac crest (p. 1440). A tricortical graft of ≈ 4 cm length and > 1 cm height is obtained. The top edged is removed to create a bicortical graft of ≈ 1 cm height.

95

95.6 C2 screws

95.6.1 Options

1. pedicle screws (pars interarticularis screws): directed medially (see below)
2. lateral mass screws: directed laterally. Length is sized to fall short of foramen transversarium
3. C1–2 transarticular screws (p. 1480): associated with more risk of VA injury
4. translaminar screws[42,43]: 1 year stability appears to be less than C2 pedicle screws when used for subaxial fusions, but was ≈ as effective for axial fusions (C1–2 or C1–3).[44] May be useful as a “bail-out” for subaxial fusions when the C2 pars diameter is too small for pedicle screws[45]

95.6.2 C2 pedicle (pars) screws

Check CT scan or MRI to rule-out aberrant location of vertebral artery or unusual location of foramen transversarium before placing C2 pedicle screws. Some find image guided navigation systems to be helpful.

Technique:

1. ENTRY palpate the medial and superior aspect of the pars with a Penfield 4 dissector (▶ Fig. 95.4). Enter at the estimated center of the surface projection of the C2 pars at the midpoint medio-laterally[35] in the supero-medial quadrant of the surface of the C2 isthmus
2. TRAJ **20–30° medially** (through the central axis of the C2 pedicle),[46] 25° superiorly (on lateral fluoroscopy, place the screw parallel to the pars) (▶ Fig. 95.5). To assist with trajectory, expose the proximal upper and medial border of the C2 pars interarticularis, and use a Penfield 4 to palpate during drilling (▶ Fig. 95.4)
3. drill a shallow entry point, then drill with drill-stop set at 12 mm, monitoring progress at intervals under fluoro and palpating with probe, and if no breakout, then complete drilling by gradually increasing drilling depth by 2 mm increments either up to 15-20 mm to stay in the pedicles, or up to ≈ 30 mm depth to perform osteosynthesis for a hangman's fracture. ✖ If withdrawal of the drill is followed by brisk bleeding, the screw should be inserted immediately to stop the bleeding. This bleeding may be from the vertebral artery; however, it is usually due to injury to the venous plexuses, and will not have any ill effects. In such cases it is best to not place the contralateral screw and to obtain an angiogram very soon post-op
4. SCREWS **3.5 mm dia.** Screw length is not critical except when attempting to bridge a fracture gap (osteosynthesis) e.g. with a hangman's fracture in which case screws of 20–30 mm length are placed to avoid penetrating anterior C2 cortex (lag screws are used for this, or the proximal bone can be overdrilled); for most purposes screw lengths of 15–20 mm length are used. Shorter screws (15-16 mm length) can still grip the pedicle with lower risk of VA injury

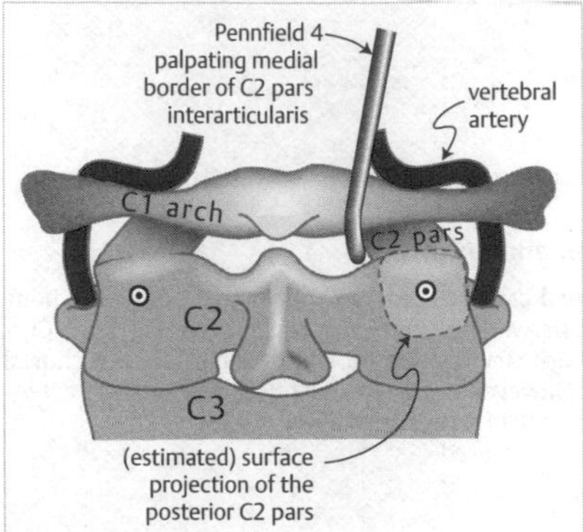

Fig. 95.4 Entry point for C2 pedicle screw placement (posterior view)

95

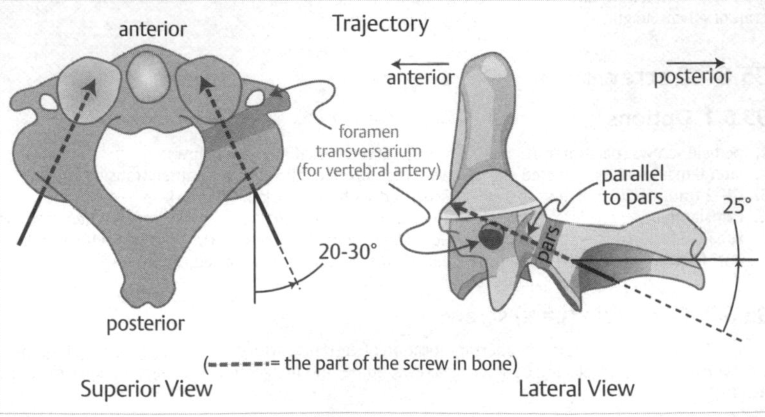

Fig. 95.5 Screw trajectory for C2 pedicle screws

95.6.3 C3–6 fixation

Lateral mass screws

Generally applicable to C3–6. The lateral masses of the thoracic spine are usually too small and not strong enough[47] for these screws. C7 is a transitional level, and lateral mass screws may sometimes be used. Occasionally even T1 may be amenable (see below).

Technique:

A number of methods have been promulgated with various screw entry points and trajectories (some are shown in ▶ Table 95.1). Comparing 3 techniques[48] there was a lower risk of nerve injury with the following (method of An[49]):

1. ENTRY[49] 1 mm medial to the midpoint of the lateral mass (▶ Fig. 95.6). In the cranial-caudal direction, the midpoint is used. A Penfield 4 may be used to palpate the medial wall of the pars to help determine entry point and trajectory
2. TRAJ 30° laterally, 15° cephalad (editor's note: for upper cervical levels more cephalad trajectory is used, for caudal cervical levels 15° or less may be closer) (▶ Fig. 95.6).[49] To get the lateral angulation, the holes are best drilled from the contralateral side of the patient, holding the drill shaft almost up against the spinous processes (if they are still present)
   a) SCREWS 3.5 mm diameter, 14–16 mm length (for C3–6)
   b) rod size: 3.5 mm diameter rods are usually used, and can be placed as far caudally as T3 as long as there is not gross instability (below T3, 5.5 mm diameter rods are used either via transitional rods or with rod connectors, e.g. "domino" connector)

Spinous process wiring may be used with intact spinous processes to help secure the bone graft.[47]

Transarticular screw fixation

An alternative to lateral mass fusion. First described in 1972 by Roy Camille. May be used alone or as an anchor point.

Table 95.1 Comparison of methods for lateral mass screw placement for C3–6

Method	Entry point		Trajectory angle	
	Medio-lateral	Cranio-caudal	Medio-lateral	Cranio-caudal
An	1 mm medial to mid-point	midpoint	30° lateral	15° cephalad
Magerl	2 mm medial to midpoint	2 mm cranial to midpoint	20–25° lateral	parallel to facet joint[a]
Roy-Camille	midpoint	midpoint	0–10° lateral	0°

[a] angle can be determined by inserting probe into the joint

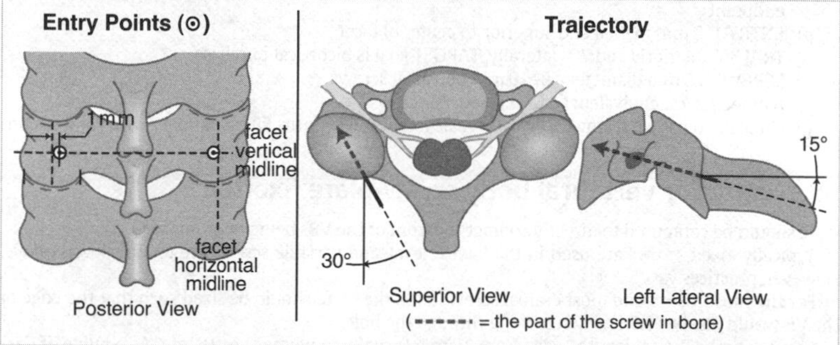

Fig. 95.6 Screw entry point and trajectory for C3–6 lateral mass screws (method of An)

95

1. PROS:
   a) screws cross 4 cortical surfaces for better purchase
   b) compresses across the joint to promote fusion
   c) useful at cervico-thoracic junction where trajectory preserves facet capsule
   d) lower implant profile
2. CONS: cannot correct deformity
3. ENTRY midpoint of lateral mass
4. TRAJ perpendicular to joint, neutral to 5° lateral (to avoid VA and exiting root)
5. biomechanics: stability equivalent to lateral mass screws[50]
6. clinical: 25 patients (81 screws), 71 anchor, 10 fixation, 3.5 years F/U: solid fusion, no complications[51]

Translaminar cervical screw fixation

May be used in cervical or thoracic spine.[52,53]

1. indications: salvage technique when anatomy precludes pedicle screws
2. PROS:
   a) avoids complications related to pedicle screws
   b) no need for fluoroscopy (reduces radiation exposure)
3. CONS: requires intact posterior elements (cannot do with laminectomy)
4. ENTRY contralateral spinolaminar junction (at base of spinous process)
5. TARGET junction of the transverse process and the superior facet contralateral to the entry point
6. SCREWS 3.5–4.5 mm × 26 mm polyaxial screw
7. biomechanics: no data
8. clinical: 7 patients (C-T fixation), 14 months F/U, no hardware complications. Inconsequential ventral penetration in 5%[52]

C7 screws

C7 is a transitional level, and as a result either the lateral masses or the pedicles or both may be relatively small.

Screw fixation options:

1. pedicle screws (p. 1489): recommended especially when the C7 lateral mass is of inadequate size for lateral mass screws.[49] Placement with fluoroscopy may be difficult due to shoulder artifact on lateral fluoro, and direct visualization of the medial wall of the pedicle may be required as in the thoracic spine
2. lateral mass screws[46]:
   a) ENTRY as for C3–6 (see above)
   b) TRAJ compared to C3–6 screws, slightly less lateral at ≈ 15° and a little less cephalad at ≈ 10°
   c) SCREWS 3.5 mm diameter, 14 mm length
   d) biomechanics: lab studies indicate that C7 lateral mass screws are biomechanically equivalent to C7 pedicle screws in constructs extending down to C7[54]
3. C7 transfacet screw[55]:
   a) PROS: reduced risk to spinal cord and nerve roots
   b) CONS: disrupts C7-T1 facet capsule, so T1 must be included in fusion. short screws result in low pullout strength ∴ may be best used as an intermediate anchor point and not an construct endpoint
   c) ENTRY 1–2 mm medial and superior to center of facet
   d) TRAJ 30° inferiorly and 20° laterally, TARGET goal is bicortical purchase
   e) SCREWS 3.5 mm diameter × 8–10 mm polyaxial screws
   f) biomechanics: equivalent to C7-T1 pedicle screws[56]
   g) clinical: 10 patients, long cervico-thoracic fixation, 6 months F/U, 3 patients with solid fusion

95.7 Anterior vertebral body screw-plate fixation

Plate should be contoured to directly contact the front of the VBs being instrumented.

Typically, fixed screws are used in the lowest level, and variable screws are used at levels above. However, practices vary.

For the most rostral and most cranial screw holes, the plate should be sized such that the edge of the VB would just be visible when looking through the hole.

Screw length: Typical lengths vary from 12 mm (usually in women) to 16 mm. As a guide, if Caspar pins are used during the operation, most have 14 mm of threads in the VB, the screw length can be chosen based on how close these Caspar pins come to the posterior VB. The screws in the plate are usually angled, so an additional 1–2 mm can be accommodated beyond this length.

95.8 Zero profile interbody devices

These devices incorporate holders for screw placement into an interbody cage without need for a separate anterior plate. Most often used in cervical spine.

1. PROS:
   a) Are often easier to place adjacent to a previously placed anterior plate (because the plate will often cover too much of the VB to provide enough room for another plate on the same VB)
   b) Avoids plates that are not parallel to the long axis of the spine
   c) Posterior migration of the cage is prevented once the screws are placed
2. CONS: Biomechanical stability is less than that with a plate (4-screw devices are more stable than 3 screw devices)

References

[1] Crockard HA, Sen CN. The Transoral Approach for the Management of Intradural Lesions at the Craniovertebral Junction: Review of 7 Cases. Neurosurgery. 1991; 28:88–98

[2] Hadley MN, Spetzler RF, Sonntag VKH. The Transoral Approach to the Superior Cervical Spine. A Review of 53 Cases of Extradural Cervicomedullary Compression. J Neurosurg. 1989; 71:16–23

[3] Menezes AH, VanGilder JC. Transoral-Transpharyngeal Approach to the Anterior Craniocervical Junction. J Neurosurg. 1988; 69:895–903

[4] Dickman CA, Locantro J, Fessler RG. The Influence of Transoral Odontoid Resection on Stability of the Craniocervical Junction. J Neurosurg. 1992; 77:525–530

[5] Dickman CA, Crawford NR, Brantley AGU, et al. Biomechanical Effects of Transoral Odontoidectomy. Neurosurgery. 1995; 36:1146–1153

[6] Mummaneni PV, Haid RW. Transoral odontoidectomy. Neurosurgery. 2005; 56:1045–50; discussion 1045-50

[7] Fielding JW. The Status of Arthrodesis of the Cervical Spine. J Bone Joint Surg. 1988; 70A:1571–1574

[8] Lipson SJ. Fractures of the Atlas Associated with Fractures of the Odontoid Process and Transverse Ligament Ruptures. J Bone Joint Surg. 1977; 59A:940–943

[9] White A, Panjabi M, White AA. In: Kinematics of the Spine. Clinical Biomechanics of the Spine. 2nd ed. Philadelphia: J B Lippincott; 1990:85–126

[10] Roberts A, Wickstrom J. Prognosis of Odontoid Fractures. J Bone Joint Surg. 1972; 54A

[11] Bambakidis NC, Feiz-Erfan I, Horn EM, Gonzalez LF, Baek S, Yuksel KZ, Brantley AG, Sonntag VK, Crawford NR. Biomechanical comparison of occipitoatlantal screw fixation techniques. J Neurosurg Spine. 2008; 8:143–152

[12] Uribe JS, Ramos E, Vale F. Feasibility of occipital condyle screw placement for occipitocervical fixation: a cadaveric study and description of a novel technique. J Spinal Disord Tech. 2008; 21:540–546

[13] La Marca F, Zubay G, Morrison T, Karahalios D. Cadaveric study for placement of occipital condyle screws: technique and effects on surrounding anatomic structures. J Neurosurg Spine. 2008; 9:347–353

[14] Uribe JS, Ramos E, Youssef AS, Levine N, Johnson WM, Vale F. Craniocervical fixation with occipital condyle screws: biomechanical analysis of a novel technique. Spine. 2010; 35:931–938

[15] Uribe JS, Ramos E, Baaj A, Youssef AS, Vale FL. Occipital cervical stabilization using occipital condyles for cranial fixation: Technical case report. Neurosurgery. 2009; 65:E1216–E1217

[16] Grob D. Transarticular screw fixation for atlanto-occipital dislocation. Spine. 2001; 26:703–707

[17] Feiz-Erfan I, Gonzalez LF, Dickman CA. Atlantooccipital transarticular screw fixation for the treatment of traumatic occipitoatlantal dislocation. Technical note. J Neurosurg Spine. 2005; 2:381–385

[18] Gonzalez LF, Crawford NR, Chamberlain RH, Perez Garza LE, Preul MC, Sonntag VK, Dickman CA. Craniovertebral junction fixation with transarticular screws: biomechanical analysis of a novel technique. J Neurosurg. 2003; 98:202–209

[19] Morone MA, Rodts GR, Erwood S, Haid RW. Anterior Odontoid Screw Fixation: Indications, Complication Avoidance, and Operative Technique. Contemp Neurosurg. 1996; 18:1–6

[20] Rao G, Apfelbaum RI. Odontid screw fixation for fresh and remote fractures. Neurol India. 2005; 53:416–423

[21] Apfelbaum RI. Screw Fixation of the Upper Cervical Spine: Indications and Techniques. Contemp Neurosurg. 1994; 16:1–8

[22] Sasso R, Doherty BJ, Crawford MJ, Heggeness MH. Comparison of the One- and Two-Screw Technique. Spine. 1993; 18:1950–1950

[23] Hott JS, Henn JS, Sonntag VKH. A new table-fixed retractor for anterior odontoid screw fixation: technical note. J Neurosurg. 2003; 98:118–120

[24] Wang MY. C2 crossing laminar screws: cadaveric morphometric analysis. Neurosurgery. 2006; 59: ONS84–8; discussion ONS84-8

[25] Grob D, Jeanneret B, Aeb M, Markwalder T. Atlanto-Axial Fusion with Transarticular Screw Fixation. J Bone Joint Surg. 1991; 73B:972–976

[26] Stillerman CD, Wilson JA. Atlanto-Axial Stabilization with Posterior Transarticular Screw Fixation: Technical Description and Report of 22 Cases. Neurosurgery. 1993; 32:948–955

[27] Marcotte P, Dickman CA, Sonntag VKH, et al. Posterior Atlantoaxial Facet Screw Fixation. J Neurosurg. 1993; 79:234–237

[28] Brooks AL, Jenkins EB. Atlanto-Axial Arthrodesis by the Wedge Compression Method. J Bone Joint Surg. 1978; 60A:279–284

[29] Griswold DM, Albright JA, Schiffman E, et al. Atlanto-Axial Fusion for Instability. J Bone Joint Surg. 1978; 60A:285–292

[30] Schmidek HH, Sweet WH. Operative Neurosurgical Techniques. New York 1982

[31] Aldrich EF, Crow WN, Weber PB, Spagnolia TN. Use of MR Imaging-Compatible Halifax Interlaminar Clamps for Posterior Cervical Fusion. J Neurosurg. 1991; 74:185–189

[32] Bohler J. Anterior Stabilization for Acute Fractures and Non-Unions of the Dens. J Bone Joint Surg. 1982; 64:18–28

[33] Paramore CG, Dickman CA, Sonntag VKH. The Anatomical Suitability of the C1-2 Complex for Transarticular Screw Fixation. J Neurosurg. 1996; 85:221–224

[34] Goel A, Laheri V. Plate and screw fixation for atlanto-axial subluxation. Acta Neurochir (Wien). 1994; 129:47–53

95

[35] Harms J, Melcher RP. Posterior C1-C2 fusion with polyaxial screw and rod fixation. Spine. 2001; 26:2467–2471

[36] Rocha R, Safavi-Abbasi S, Reis C, Theodore N, Bambakidis N, de Oliveira E, Sonntag VKH, Crawford NR. Working area, safety zones, and angles of approach for posterior C-1 lateral mass screw placement: a quantitative anatomical and morphometric evaluation. J Neurosurg Spine. 2007; 6:247–254

[37] McCormick PC, Kaiser MG. Comment on Goel A et al.: Atlantoaxial fixation using plate and screw method: a report of 160 treated patients. Neurosurgery. 2002; 51

[38] Currier BL, Todd LT, Maus TP, Fisher DR, Yaszemski MJ. Anatomic relationship of the internal carotid artery to the C1 vertebra: A case report of cervical reconstruction for chordoma and pilot study to assess the risk of screw fixation of the atlas. Spine. 2003; 28:E461–E467

[39] Papadopoulos SM, Dickman CA, Sonntag VKH. Atlantoaxial Stabilization in Rheumatoid Arthritis. J Neurosurg. 1991; 74:1–7

[40] Dickman CA, Sonntag VKH, Papadopoulos SM, Hadley MN. The Interspinous Method of Posterior Atlantoaxial Arthrodesis. J Neurosurg. 1991; 74:190–198

[41] Hott JS, Lynch JJ, Chamberlain RH, Sonntag VK, Crawford NR. Biomechanical comparison of C1-2 posterior fixation techniques. J Neurosurg Spine. 2005; 2:175–181

[42] Wright NM. Posterior C2 fixation using bilateral, crossing C2 laminar screws: case series and technical note. J Spinal Disord Tech. 2004; 17:158–162

[43] Jea A, Sheth RN, Vanni S, Green BA, Levi AD. Modification of Wright's technique for placement of bilateral crossing C2 translaminar screws: technical note. Spine J. 2008; 8:656–660

[44] Parker SL, McGirt MJ, Garces-Ambrossi GL, Mehta VA, Sciubba DM, Witham TF, Gokaslan ZL, Wolinksy JP. Translaminar versus pedicle screw fixation of C2: comparison of surgical morbidity and accuracy of 313 consecutive screws. Neurosurgery. 2009; 64:343–8; discussion 348-9

[45] Wang MY. Comment on Parker, SL, McGirt, MJ et al., Translaminar versus pedicle screw fixation of C2: comparison of surgical morbidity and accuracy of 313 consecutive screws. Neurosurgery. 2009; 64. DOI: 10.1227/01.NEU.0000338955.36649.4F

[46] Dickman CA, Sonntag VKH, Marcotte PJ. Techniques of Screw Fixation of the Cervical Spine. BNI Quarterly. 1993; 9:27–39

[47] Chapman JR, Anderson PA, Pepin C, Toomey S, et al. Posterior Instrumentation of the Unstable Cervicothoracic Spine. J Neurosurg. 1996; 84:552–558

[48] Xu R, Haman SP, Ebraheim NA, Yeasting RA. The Anatomic Relation of Lateral Mass Screws to the Spinal Nerves. A Comparison of the Magerl, Anderson and An Techniques. Spine. 1999; 24:2057–2061

[49] An HS, Gordin R, Renner K. Anatomic Considerations for Plate-Screw Fixation of the Cervical Spine. Spine. 1991; 16:S548–S551

[50] Miyanji F, Mahar A, Oka R, Newton P. Biomechanical differences between transfacet and lateral mass screw-rod constructs for multilevel posterior cervical spine stabilization. Spine (Phila Pa 1976). 2008; 33:E865–E869

[51] Takayasu M, Hara M, Yamauchi K, Yoshida M, Yoshida J. Transarticular screw fixation in the middle and lower cervical spine. Technical note. J Neurosurg. 2003; 99:132–136

[52] Kretzer RM, Sciubba DM, Bagley CA, Wolinsky JP, Gokaslan ZL, Garonzik IM. Translaminar screw fixation in the upper thoracic spine. J Neurosurg Spine. 2006; 5:527–533

[53] Gardner A, Millner P, Liddington M, Towns G. Translaminar screw fixation of a kyphosis of the cervical and thoracic spine in neurofibromatosis. J Bone Joint Surg Br. 2009; 91:1252–1255

[54] Xu R, McGirt MJ, Sutter EG, Sciubba DM, Wolinsky JP, Witham TF, Gokaslan ZL, Bydon A. Biomechanical comparison between C-7 lateral mass and pedicle screws in subaxial cervical constructs. Presented at the 2009 Joint Spine Meeting. Laboratory investigation. J Neurosurg Spine. 2010; 13:688–694

[55] Horn EM, Theodore N, Crawford NR, Bambakidis NC, Sonntag VK. Transfacet screw placement for posterior fixation of C-7. J Neurosurg Spine. 2008; 9:200–206

[56] Horn EM, Reyes PM, Baek S, Senoglu M, Theodore N, Sonntag VK, Crawford NR. Biomechanics of C-7 transfacet screw fixation. J Neurosurg Spine. 2009; 11:338–343

96 Spine, Thoracic and Lumbar

96.1 Anterior access to the cervico-thoracic junction/upper thoracic spine

96.1.1 Sternal splitting procedure

Permits access down to T3 (occasionally as far as T5) from an anterior midline approach (access to this region with a lateral (transthoracic) approach is poor due to the small volume of the pulmonary apices).

The neck and thorax are prepped down to the umbilicus. A hockey stick incision may be used, the horizontal portion is the usual for an ACDF. The vertical limb is centered over the sternum. In most cases, the services of a CV surgeon are employed to split the sternum and divide the sternocleidomastoid. This approach does not violate the pericardium or pleura, and a chest tube is not required (but is often used as a large bore drain to prevent hemomediastinum, and also as a precaution in case the parietal pleura is cut during the exposure). Because of the depth of the approach, longer instruments than the routine 7 inch length instruments used for an ACDF are required.

The exposed edges of the sternum may also be used to obtain cancellous bone for the graft.

96.2 Anterior access to mid and lower thoracic spine

96.2.1 Transthoracic approach

Position: lateral position on a bean-bag on the O.R. table with the break in the table under the level of pathology (remember to unbreak the table prior to instrumenting). Stabilize the patient using adhesive tape over surgical towels. An axillary roll is placed. A double-lumen endotracheal tube is used to permit deflating the lung on the side of the thoracotomy. If the patient does not tolerate completely deflating one lung, it is often adequate to just *partially* deflate the lung.

To increase the exposure, a rib may be resected. Generally, the level opened and the rib removed are one or two levels above the level of pathology (e.g. for T7 VB tumor, the T6 or T5 rib are removed).

If a compression plate is going to be used, the goal is to be lateral on the VB, to achieve this try to position it as far posterior as possible (rongeur off a little bit of the rib heads to facilitate this).

96.2.2 Anterior access to mid thoracic spine

Laterality of approach: if the pathology does not dictate use of one side over another:

1. advantages of right-sided thoracotomy: the heart, mediastinum and brachiocephalic vein do not impede access
2. advantages of left-sided thoracotomy: aorta is easier to mobilize and retract

Determining the level in the upper T-spine can be quite difficult intraoperatively. Counting up from the sacrum on an AP view using live fluoro sometimes will work when lateral spine x-rays cannot penetrate the lower c-spine due to the shoulders.

96.2.3 Anterior access to lower thoracic spine

Unless pathology is predominantly right-sided, a left-sided thoracotomy is preferred (easier to mobilize aorta than vena cava).

At about T10 and below, the attachment of the diaphragm increases the difficulty of the approach. In this area, a retrocoelmic approach (outside the pleural cavity) can facilitate surgery.

96.3 Thoracic pedicle screws

96.3.1 General information

Preferable to lateral mass screws because the transverse processes (which are analogous to the lateral masses in the cervical spine) of most thoracic vertebrae are not as strong.[1] Thoracic pedicles are usually very narrow in the lateral dimension (the width is a little larger at the cranial end) and are very tall in cranio-rostral direction. Image guidance systems may also be helpful.

Accurate placement of thoracic pedicle screws is generally more challenging than the lumbar spine. There are at least 4 methods to place these screws, and a combination of methods may be used.

1. Intra-operative fluoro: for parts of the thoracic spine, biplane fluoro may be used as in the lumbar spine (see above)
   a) PROS:
      - Allows percutaneous screw placement
      - generally good accuracy in screw placement
   b) CONS:
      - due to the dense bone of the shoulders, the thoracic spine is usually difficult to image from T1 to about T4 on lateral fluoroscopy. For non-percutaneous cases, Steinman pins may be placed at the estimated entry points for the screws, and AP fluoro is used to fine-tune the position so that the screw enters the pedicle at the desired location
      - may increase radiation exposure to surgery team and patient
2. "Free hand" placement based on anatomic landmarks. X-rays are usually still obtained at the end, and any screws with unsatisfactory placement must be revised
   a) PROS:
      - As the number of levels (and therefore, screws) placed in a patient increases, may save time over other methods
      - The small facetectomies that are needed to visualize the facet joint of the level below can facilitate correction of spinal curves and provide a good fusion surface
      - likely reduces radiation to the surgical team and the patient
   b) CONS: Steep learning curve: this method probably takes the most practice to perfect
3. Performing small laminotomies at each level where pedicles are not exposed by a laminecrtomy, and use position of pedicle either by visualization or by palpate of the medial and superior aspect of the pedicles with a dissector to get an approximation of the entry point and pedicle trajectory
   a) PROS: can permit accurate placement at essentially any level with potentially less radiation (depending on how often the surgeon checks screw position)
   b) CONS: takes a little time at each level, but is over all comparable to other methods
4. Image guidance using instruments that are fitted with specialized markers that are tracked real-time by "cameras" that project the drill and/or screw location on a CT or x-ray image viewed in the OR.
   a) PROS:
      - reduces intra-operative radiation to surgical team, and to a lesser extent to the patient
      - Allows percutaneous screw placement
   b) CONS: accuracy may be compromised by movement of spinal segments relative to the registration array, or by technical errors. The surgeon must be vigilant for screw placement that does not look appropriate based on the anatomy

96.3.2 Fluoro and laminotomy thoracic pedicle screw placement technique:

96

1. ENTRY: See Freehand thoracic pedicle screw placement technique (p. 1491) for entry points using landmarks. Alternatives: making a small laminotomy to palpate the medial and cephalad edges of the pedicle with a Penfield #4 dissector, using Steinman pins at estimated entry points and taking AP fluoro to fine tune (see ► Fig. 96.1).
2. TRAJ
   a) below T1: 5–10° *medially* and 10–20° *caudad*[1] (► Fig. 96.2). A thoracic Lenke probe may be used as a pedicle finder.
   b) T1: if a *lateral mass* screw is placed at T1 (instead of a pedicle screw), aim almost straight down at the floor (with patient positioned horizontally, i.e. without Trendelenberg or reverse-Trendelenberg)
3. SCREWS Smaller pedicles (usually T1–4, especially in females) usually require the smallest screw diameter (typically 4.5 mm). Others may accommodate 5.5 mm. Typical length: 20–25 mm
4. **Rod size:** when connecting to a cervical rod, down to ≈ T3 you can use a 3.5 mm diameter cervical rod throughout (here, the stiffer cobalt-chrome rod may be advantageous over titanium) with some systems (e.g. Mountaineer by DePuy using a 4.35 diameter screw). Below T3, ≈ 5.5 mm diameter rods (or 6.35 mm for scoliosis surgery) are usually used either via a transitional rod or using a domino connector to mate the two rods

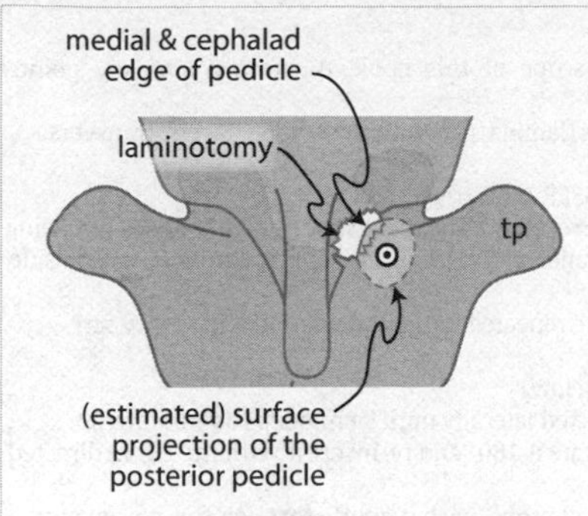

Fig. 96.1 Entry point for thoracic *pedicle* screws (posterior view) tp = transverse process

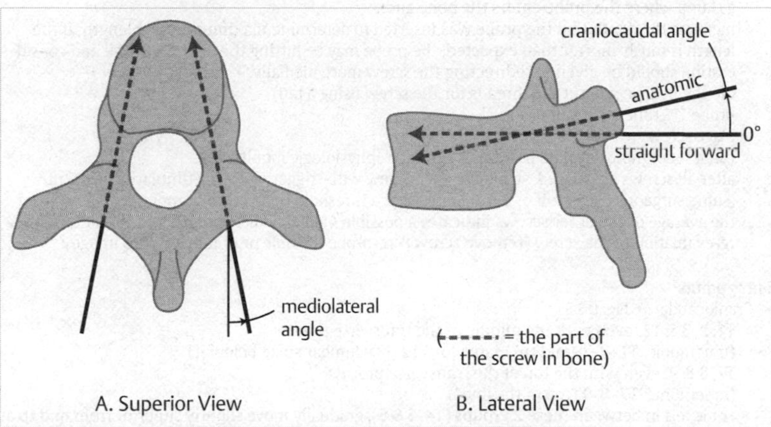

Fig. 96.2 Screw trajectory for thoracic *pedicle* screws

96.3.3 Freehand thoracic pedicle screw placement technique

Advantages and disadvantages

Possible advantages

- May speed up surgery especially when instrumenting a large number of levels
- Reduces the amount of x-rays/fluoroscopy needed during surgery
- Avoids the challenges of getting fluoro aligned for each level in a scoliotic spine especially when a rotational component is present
- Not impeded in areas that are difficult to image on fluoroscopy (typically upper thoracic spine)
- Accuracy as good or better than other techniques
- Obtains bone for use in graft (from facetectomies)
- Exposes bone (of facet joints) to assist in fusion
- Releases joints which facilitates reduction of scoliosis

Possible disadvantages

- Cannot be used if anatomy distorted by previous fusions, congenital anomalies…
- Steep learning curve: requires learning new aspects of anatomy, necessitates performing numerous screw placements, usually with a mentor, to become proficient
- Possible increased blood loss from increased exposure and facetectomies

Procedure

The details of the procedure are beyond the scope of this book. A summary of key points/ information[2]:

- Complete exposure of entire posterior elements (lamina, pars interarticularis, facets, transverse process (tp)…) at every level is mandatory
- Intraoperative electrophysiologic monitoring: SSEP, MEP, triggered EMG
- Facetectomies: performed bilaterally at every level except the most superior (that one is not being fused to the level above). Make 2 cuts: 1st is parallel to canal. Caution: spinal cord is at risk on side of concavity
- It is essential to develop a series of steps that are repeated without deviation with every screw placement:
  - make pilot hole at entry point (as indicated below)
  - insert curved pedicle finder with the tip directed laterally until 2 cm deep (do not force)
  - completely remove the pedicle finder and rotate it 180° and re-insert it with the curve directed medially
  - palpate all 4 walls and the deep end with a ball probe, push it gently through the cancellous bone until the tip strikes the cortical bone of the anterior vertebral body (sound and feel). Place a clamp where the probe enters the bone and…
  - measure the depth that the probe was inserted to determine maximum screw length; if the length is much shorter than expected, the probe may be hitting the lateral VB wall and consideration should be given to redirecting the screw more medially
  - tap the pedicle (i.e. cut the threads for the screw using a tap)
  - probe 2nd time with ball probe
  - place screw
  - run a set of motor evoked potentials on electrophysiologic monitoring
  - after all screws are placed, stimulate each screw with triggered EMG: stimulation at < 6 mA (some surgeons use cutoff of 8 mA instead) or a threshold that is 65% or more decreased from the average of the other screws indicates a possible medial pedicle breach and should prompt a re-evaluation of the screw (remove screw & re-probe the hole or obtain a fluoro image)[2]

Entry points[2]

- Craniocaudal (▶ Fig. 96.3)
  - T1, 2, 3 & 12: even with the middle of the transverse process (mnemonic: T1–2-3 “mid tp”) same for T12 (like lumbar spine below it)
  - T7, 8 & 9: even with the top of the transverse process (mnemonic: T7–8-9 “top of the line”)
  - For levels in between these 2 groups (T4, 5 & 6), gradually move slightly superior from mid tp at T1–2-3 to the top of the tp at T7–8-9
- Mediolateral (▶ Fig. 96.3)
  - T1, 2 & 3: even with the lateral edge of the pars
  - T7, 8 & 9: just lateral to midposition of the base of the superior articular facet (the most medial starting points)
  - T11, 12: at or just medial to lateral edge of pars
  - Levels in between these groups: gradually transition the position

96

Trajectories

- Trajectories using landmarks
  - Practitioners of freehand screw placement use landmarks more than angles. The advantage is that angles are difficult to estimate, and using landmarks allows screws to be placed even in rotated, scoliotic spines.
  - The screw is inserted perpendicular to the surface of the superior articular facet (that is exposed during the facetectomies) while also “aiming” at the contralateral pedicle.
- Trajectories using angles: may be helpful to conceptualize
  - Craniocaudal angle (▶ Fig. 96.2 – B): either of 2 trajectories are used[3]
    - Straightforward screw placement: 0° to horizontal (parallel to the superior endplate – allows fixed-head screws for spine derotation)
    - Anatomic screw placement: 10–15° caudal[4] (parallel to the pedicle – provides a longer path for screw contact with bone but requires a multiaxial screw head)
  - Mediolateral trajectory[4] (▶ Fig. 96.2 – A)
    - the angle gradually becomes more medial as you progress from
    - T12 where the angle is slightly lateral (≈ –5°) to

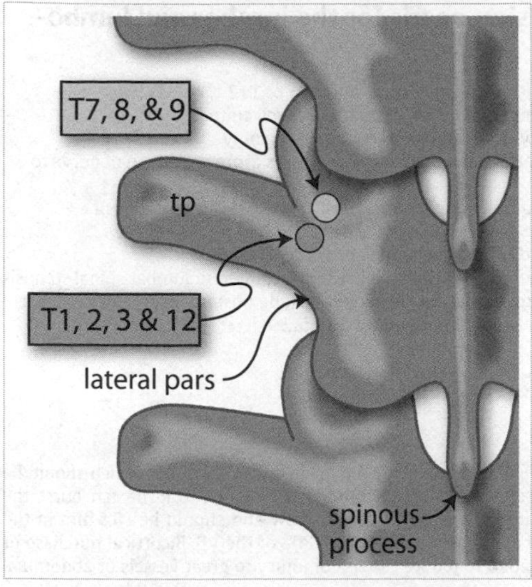

Fig. 96.3 Entry points for freehand thoracic pedicle screw placement on left side. Posterior view, stylized representation of generic thoracic level.

- T1 where the angle is ≈ 27° medial
- (at T11 it is close to 0° and as a rough approximation it increases by 2° per level above this)

Screw size

- Length: the depth to the anterior cortex varies from 40–45 mm when measured along axis of pedicle (or 30–42 mm when measured parallel to sagittal plane).[4] Typical thoracic screw length is 35–40 mm.
- Diameter: the narrowest pedicles in the mediolateral dimension are typically T4–7.[4] Screw diameter should be approximately 80% of the pedicle diameter.

96.4 Anterior access to thoracolumbar junction

96.4.1 Retroperitoneal approach

Unless the pathology is predominantly left-sided, a left-sided approach is preferred because the spleen is easier to retract than the liver, and the aorta is easier to mobilize than the inferior vena cava. It is important to flex the ipsilateral leg to relax the psoas muscle, permitting safer retraction of the ipsilateral lumbosacral plexus.

96

96.5 Anterior access to the lumbar spine

96.5.1 Anterior lumbar interbody fusion (ALIF)

Retroperitoneal usually through a Pfannenstiel's abdominal incision.

Relatively contraindicated in males because of risk of retrograde ejaculation in 1–2% (as high as 45% in some reviews). Other risks: injury to great vessels, especially with calcified arteries, especially at L4–5.

Bowel prep the day before surgery for complex cases.

Position: Trendelenburg position, place the level of the iliac crests over the kidney rest or use a sacral bump to increase lordosis.

As a result of the bifurcation of the great vessels (aorta and inferior vena cava) which ranges from just above to just below the L4–5 disc space, this approach is best suited for access to L5-S1.

At L5-S1, the anterior sacral artery runs down the midline of the VB and has to be sacrificed to do an ALIF.

96.6 Instrumentation/fusion pearls for the lumbar and lumbosacral spine

1. a lumbar fusion that includes L1 should not be terminated at L1 or T12
2. the taller the disc space the less likely that interbody grafts are well suited:
   a) the disc may not be significantly degenerated to require discectomy
   b) tall disc space means larger interbody implants which requires more retraction of nerve to insert (using a PLIF technique)
3. a long fusion should not be terminated at or near a vertebral level that is at the apex of scoliosis[5(p 382)]
4. laminectomy without fusion should be avoided at the apex of scoliosis
5. posterior midline fusion: early experience with midline fusions resulted in lumbar spinal stenosis as a late complication. Therefore, current fusion techniques include postero-lateral fusion, interbody fusion (from anterior or posterior approach), facet fusion…

96.7 Lumbosacral pedicle screws

96.7.1 General information

Pedicle screw pull out strength is determined in part by the major screw diameter which should be 70–80% of pedicle diameter (larger screws can break through the pedicle wall or can burst the pedicle). The minor diameter determines the strength of the screw and should be ≥ 5.5 mm in the adult lumbar spine. The length should allow penetration of 70–80% of the VB. Bicortical purchase or anterior VB penetration should be avoided to reduce the risk of injury to great vessels or abdominal viscera.

96.7.2 Placement techniques

There are at least 4 screw placement techniques
1. Intra-operative fluoro: biplane fluoro facilitates this technique
   a) PROS:
      - allows percutaneous screw placement
      - generally good accuracy in screw placement
   b) CONS:
      - imaging may be difficult in some parts of the lumbar spine, especially in larger patients. In these cases, the Steinman pin method below can be used to supplement
      - may increase radiation exposure to surgery team and patient
2. Steinman pin method: Steinman pins are placed at the estimated entry points for the screws, and AP and lateral fluoro is used to fine-tune the position so that the screw enters the pedicle at the desired location
3. Freehand placement based on anatomic landmarks. Usually with X-ray assistance. Greatly facilitated at levels where a laminectomy has been performed since the medial pedicle is exposed and is easily palpated
   a) PROS: likely reduces radiation to the surgical team and the patient
   b) CONS: requires somewhat more experience than the other methods
4. Image guidance using instruments that are fitted with specialized markers that are tracked real-time by "cameras" that project the drill and/or screw location on a CT or x-ray image viewed in the O.R.
   a) PROS:
      - reduces intra-operative radiation to surgical team, and to a lesser extent to the patient
      - allows percutaneous screw placement
   b) CONS: accuracy may be compromised by movement of spinal segments relative to the registration array, or by technical errors. The surgeon must be vigilant for screw placement that does not look appropriate based on the anatomy

96.7.3 Open lumbar pedicle screw technique (see below for percutaneous placement)

1. ENTRY at the base of the transverse process, at the intersection of the center of the transverse process (in the rostral-caudal direction) and the sagittal plane through the lateral aspect of the

superior facet. If a laminectomy has been performed at that level, the location of the pedicle is then verified by palpation using a probe within the spinal canal, otherwise fluoroscopy is used

2. TRAJ
   a) the approximate mediolateral trajectory is shown in ▶ Table 96.1, and equals the lumbar vertebral number multiplied by 5° for each level from L1 to L5.[6] The angle of the screw in the rostral-caudal direction is determined by fluoroscopy, maintaining a course that is parallel to the vertebral end plate. A frameless stereotactic navigation system may help orient screw trajectory
   b) S2 screws are oriented laterally and superiorly and can be as long as 60 mm
3. SCREWS goal is for screw to cross ≈ 2/3 of the VB (typical screw lengths: 40-55 mm except for S1 which are usually only 35-40 mm long)
4. rod diameter: typically 5–6.5 mm

X-ray verification once pedicle screws are placed: on AP view if the screw tip crosses the midline to the contralateral side, there is likely to be a breach of the medial pedicle (sensitivity 0.87, specificity 0.97, accuracy 0.98),[7] and if the screw does not pass medial to the medial pedicle wall there is likely to be lateral pedicle/VB violation (sensitivity 0.94, specificity 0.90, accuracy 0.96)[7]).

96.7.4 Percutaneous pedicle screws

The principles here are also employed in accessing the pedicles for e.g. vertebroplasty/kyphoplasty, percutaneous biopsy of pathology in the pedicle and/or vertebral body.

Basic principles:

1. requires AP and lateral fluoroscopy, or "O-arm" imaging (essentially an image guided intra-operative CT scan). With fluoroscopy, biplane fluoro (1 C-arm dedicated for AP view, another for lateral) greatly expedites the procedure
2. this method can be employed essentially from T1 through S1 as long as adequate AP & lateral imaging of the involved level is possible. Using fluoro for upper thoracic placement (e.g. above ≈ T5) is challenging (small pedicles, and the shoulders interfere with lateral x-ray)
3. the skin entry site is lateral to the lateral edge of the pedicle. This permits the needle to pass through the pedicle in a medial direction into the VB. The degree of angulation and therefore the distance off the midline for the entry site depends on the vertebral level being accessed (thoracic pedicles are oriented in a more AP direction, lumbar pedicles angulate medially inward) as well as the amount of overlying muscle/fat

Procedure:

1. a needle, typically a Jamshidi needle, is placed such that the tip is just short of entering the pedicle on the lateral fluoro (on left in ▶ Fig. 96.4)
2. at this point, on the AP view the needle tip should be at or just barely lateral to the lateral edge of the pedicle near the equator of the pedicle (on the right side, this would be at the "3:00" position on the left side this would be at the "9:00" position)
3. the needle is advanced to just enter the pedicle on lateral fluoro, at this point it should be just within the pedicle margin at the 3:00 or 9:00 position on the AP view (as shown on the right in ▶ Fig. 96.4)

96

Table 96.1 Medial angles for lumbar pedicle screw

Level	Medial angle
L1	5° medially
L2	10° medially
L3	15° medially
L4	20° medially
L5 & S1[a]	25° medially
S2	40–45° *laterally*

[a]aim for sacral promontory

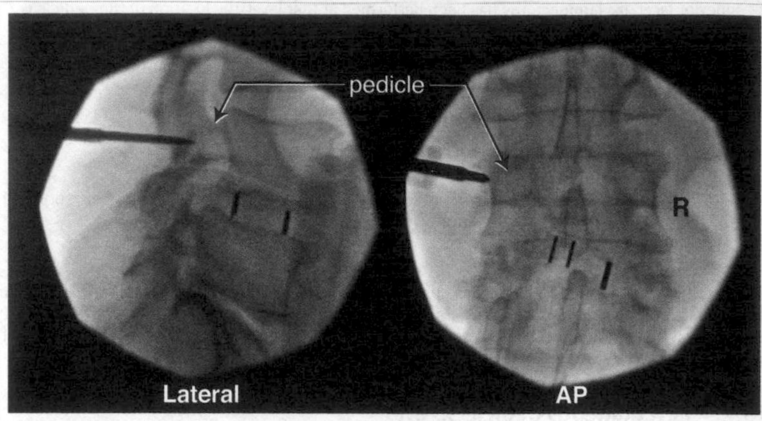

Fig. 96.4 Pedicle cannulation – entering pedicle

4. continue advancing the needle into the pedicle. Intermediate fluoro images can be obtained (e.g. to monitor trajectory on the lateral fluoro), but the next critical landmark is when the needle tip is just traversing the junction of the pedicle and the VB on the lateral fluoro (i.e. just entering the VB, as shown on the left in ▶ Fig. 96.5). it should be close to but never more medial than the medial border of the pedicle on the AP view (as shown on right in ▶ Fig. 96.5). If this criteria is maintained, the needle cannot breech the medial wall of the pedicle where it can threaten neural structures or compromise the purchase of the pedicle screw
5. subsequent steps differ for various procedures and manufacturers

96.7.5 Pedicle-screw rod diameters

Approximate weight guidelines for pedicle-screw *rod* diameters are shown in ▶ Table 96.2.

96.7.6 Lumbar lateral mass screw fixation

Trademarked names for equipment related to this procedure include "Cortical Screws."

These screws enter the bone of the lumbar spine near the infero-medial border, and are directed superiorly and laterally, thereby passing close to 3 cortical margins, which provides a pull-out strength close to (but probably slightly less) than pedicle screws.

96

1. PROS: placement through a midline incision is somewhat easier than trying to get a more laterally situate entry point for a pedicle screw, and the supero-lateral trajecdtory does not require fighting the paraspinal muscles as occurs in trying to get a medial trajectory with pedicle screws
2. CONS:
   a) pull-out strength slightly less than pedicle screws
   b) the bone that has to be left unviolated at the screw entry site may interfere with some of the decompression

96.7.7 Translaminar lumbar screw fixation

1. indications:
   a) short segment lumbar fusion
   b) posterior component in a 360° fixation combined with interbody fusion
2. PROS:
   a) small incision, minimal soft tissue disruption
   b) decreased cost (fewer screws implanted)
   c) decreased blood loss
   d) adjacent facet joint spared

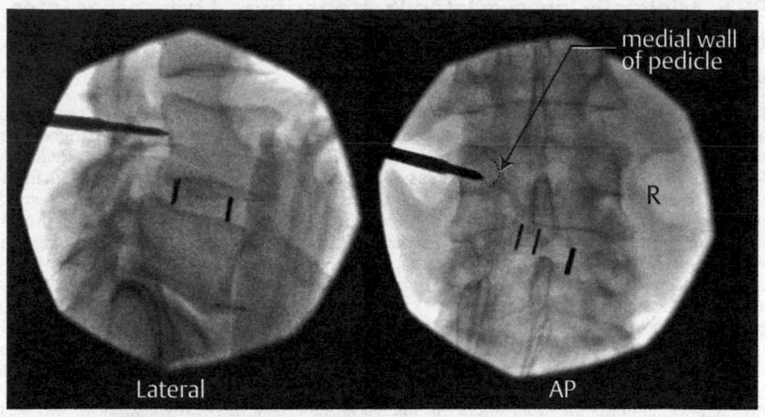

Fig. 96.5 Pedicle cannulation – entering the vertebral body

Table 96.2 Minimum recommended titanium rod diameter for lumbar pedicle-screw fixation

Patient weight		Rod diameter (mm)
(lbs)	(kg)	
30–90	12–40	4.5
90–225	40–100	5.5
> 225	> 100	6.35 (1/4 inch)

3. CONS:
   a) requires intact posterior elements (cannot use with laminectomy)
   b) cannot reduce
4. ENTRY skin incision 5–7 off midline, screw entry into bone in contralateral spinous process. Can be placed bilaterally
5. drill between the tables of the lamina across the center of the facet joint, terminating at the base of the transverse process
6. SCREWS 4.5 mm diameter fully threaded screws (no polyaxial head)
7. biomechanics: equivalent to bilateral pedicle screws.[8] Limited in extension[9]
8. clinical: 476 patients, 10 years mean F/U, 74% good outcomes[9]

96

96.7.8 Posterior lumbar interbody fusion (PLIF and TLIF)

Originally developed by Cloward[10] in 1943. Bilateral laminectomy and aggressive discectomy followed by the placement of bone grafts into the decorticated disc space. It has been advocated to reduce the movement in an abnormal "motion segment" (defined as the area between two vertebra). Relatively contraindicated with well preserved disc-space height.

Many PLIFs when studied ≈ 1 year later show re-collapse of the disc space, which raises the question as to whether the PLIF has any benefit over simple discectomy. Areas of concern include: concerns regarding injury to nerves at the time of surgery or later due to retropulsion of bone graft.

Transforaminal lumbar interbody fusion (TLIF): a variation on a PLIF where the graft is placed from one side (via the "neural foramen) after complete removal of the facet joint on that side. Requires much less nerve root retraction than PLIF, and is often advantageous for re-operations with primarily unilateral pathology where going through the foramen avoids the scar tissue.

Stand-alone PLIFs or TLIFs may be associated with progressive spondylolisthesis at that level and are usually supplemented with pedicle screws/rods.

96.8 Minimally invasive lateral retroperitoneal transpsoas interbody fusion

96.8.1 General information

First introduced by Luiz Pimenta in 2001[11,12] as an adaptation of an endoscopic lateral transpsoas approach to lumbar fusion described by Bergey et al.[13] Trademarked names include "extreme-lateral" (XLIF™, NuVasive, San Diego, CA) or "direct-lateral" lumbar interbody fusion (DLIF™, Medtronic, Memphis, TN); the generic term lateral lumbar interbody fusion (LLIF) will be used here. Variants to the approach include the oblique lumbar interbody fusion (OLIF™, Medtronic, Memphis, TN) which utilizes a pre-psoas approach (at L5-S1 the OLIF is halfway between an ALIF and a LLIF). A retroperitoneal approach. Indirectly decompresses nerves by distracting the disc space and fuses the spine with an interbody cage having a large cross-sectional area. Access is best from L1–5. For L1–2, one can retract the 12th rib, or go between 11th & 12th rib, or excise the 12th rib. Iliac crest prevents access to L5-S1 (axial-LIF may be used here) and occasionally to L4–5 (see below). A similar retropleural approach may be employed in the thoracic spine up to T4. ✖ With *thoracic* lateral interbody fusions, DO NOT penetrate the contralateral anulus. Intra-operative EMG monitoring is critical, so the anesthesiologist needs to use only *short-acting* neuromuscular blockade at beginning of case. In males, implants are typically 55-60 mm in length (oriented along patient's lateral axis) if placed in the midposition of the VB, or 45 mm in the anterior portion (lengths are 10% shorter in females).[14] Potential advantages include less tissue trauma, minimal blood loss, shorter operation time, less wound issues, placement of a larger cage, early patient mobilization,[15,16] no risk of durotomy with CSF leak.

96.8.2 Indications

- central lumbar spinal stenosis (mild to moderate only) with neurogenic claudication
- foraminal stenosis (indirect decompression)
- spondylolisthesis grade 1 or 2
- axial low back pain associated with degenerative disc disease
- total disc replacement
- for correction of sagittal or coronal imbalance
- adjacent segment failure: LLIF is particularly attractive here because it obviates dealing with scar tissue and (often) hardware from previous surgery and which also reduces risk of durotomy
- burst fractures and tumors in the thoracolumbar area (corpectomy)
- to retrieve damaged or malpositioned lumbar disc replacement devices[17]
- adult spinal deformity: can be used to correct scoliosis and to increase lumbar lordosis especially when combined with release of the anterior longitudinal ligament (ALL release)[16]

96.8.3 Contraindications

96

1. cases requiring direct decompression: includes
   a) pathology within the spinal canal e.g. herniated disc, synovial cyst, where simply distracting the disc space is less likely to correct the pathology
   b) somewhat imprecisely defined "pinpoint" central canal stenosis (some cases may still respond)
2. tall disc spaces: disc space height > 12 mm usually implies that further distraction may be difficult to achieve. However, the interbody cage can still prevent compression at these levels when the patient stands up
3. prior retroperitoneal surgery on the planned side of LLIF (can still be done on contralateral side, sometimes may still be feasible on ipsilateral side)
4. pathology at L5-S1: the technique cannot reliably access L5-S1 due to the interference from the ilium of the pelvis
5. may not be able to access L4–5 if the iliac crest extends more than ≈ halfway up the L4 VB. Sometimes it is necessary to position the patient on the O.R. table with the table flexed and a bump under the hip to see if the space will "open up" and permit access. Angled instruments can usually permit acceptable access to the space of the lumbar plexus is not located too far forward on the VB
6. anomalous vascular anatomy interfering with approach: check position of great vessels on pre
7. relative contraindications:
   a) osteoporosis: may also be contraindication to lateral plates
   b) active infection (relatively contraindicated with any fusion technique)

96.8.4 Surgical Technique (MIS retroperitoneal transposas approach)

1. Positon
   a) lateral decubitus position with the top of the iliac crest just superior to the table break
   b) choice of side: If there is no reason not to do so, the left side is usually up. Factors that might influence which side is to be up:
      - right side up if access is needed to L4-5 and the iliac crest is higher on left and would interfere (use AP x-rays, lateral x-rays and/or lumbar CT to evaluate)
      - previous retroperitoneal surgery would cause one to consider placing the contralateral side up
      - if scoliosis is present and the intent is to correct this, the concave side is usually up: this usually provides better access to L4/5 if it is an operative level. Also usually allows access to multiple levels through potentially fewer and smaller incisions because the corridors to each disc space tend to converge
      - if ACR is planned, a posterior location of the great vessels and especially the lack of any soft tissue between the vertebral body/osteophyte and the vessel would speak for using the contralateral side if that is more favorable (if not, ACR may not be advisable)
   c) true orthogonal position: the c-arm fluoroscopy is place horizontal with 0° tilt, the patient position is then find-tuned until the spinous process is exactly in the center between the pedicles on the AP view. If this is not possible due to rotation between levels, a relatively neutral level is chosen to start, and the OR table will need to be rotated slightly for each level as it is being worked on in order to make that level true lateral (centering spinous process). Adhesive tape is applied to maintain the patient in this position
2. lateral fluoroscopy is used to mark the index disc space transversely and the posterior third of the disc space vertically. An exception is at L4/5, where the vertical mark is at the middle of the disc space based on the anatomic safe zones[18]
3. retroperitoneal access through a single lateral skin incision and blunt dissection through abdominal muscles and fascia (external oblique, internal oblique, transversalis)
4. transpsoas approach and retractor placement is achieved using sequential tubular dilators that are placed under the guidance of fluoroscopic imaging (or navigation) and using directional EMG monitoring (Neurovision™, NuVasive, San Diego, CA) allowing the dilator placed anterior to the main lumbar plexus
5. discectomy and preparation of the disc space without violation of the endplates (to reduce the risk of subsidence) are performed. Work straight up-and-down in the ventral-dorsal plane (to avoid injuring the ALL anteriorly or entering the spinal canal posteriorly)
6. interbody spacer is placed usually with the posterior edge in the posterior third of the disc space (as the EMG monitoring allows)
7. for anterior column release (MIS-ACR), additional steps have to be performed after diskectomy, which include dissection/section of the ALL, and placement of hyperlordotic cages (20 or 30 degrees) usually more anteriorly in the disc space than a routine cage. This is a technique for the advanced lateral access surgeon

96.8.5 Instrumented augmentation (pedicle screws or lateral plate)

96

Standalone cage

May be feasible in the following circumstances:

- no osteoporosis
- no instability on pre-op lateral flexion/extension x-rays
- the ALL was not disrupted during LLIF surgery
- a cage width of at least 22 mm (26 mm or larger is optimal) has been placed: the large surface area reduces the risk of subsidence

When these conditions are not met, additional instrumentation should be considered.

Lateral plate and screws

May be applied through the same exposure. May not be optimal in patients with osteoporosis or age > 55 due to increased risk of subsidence from weaker bone. Not as practical for multilevel LLIFs.

Posterior instrumentation

For cases with instability, posterior instrumentation (e.g. pedicle screws, including percutaneously placement) may be superior. Also, may be indicated if laminectomy is needed for direct decompression.

96.8.6 Complications

1. thigh numbness: incidence is ≈ 10-12%.[16,19] Due to injury to the genitofemoral nerve. Risk of direct injury in the quadrant anterior to the midline at L2-3 and in the anterior quadrant at L3-4 and L4-5.[18] A sensory nerve – cannot be monitored with EMG. Usually transient, resolves in ≈ 2 weeks
2. thigh flexion weakness: due to psoas injury. Risk increases if > 2 levels are done. Usually transient, resolves in 1–8 weeks
3. femoral nerve injury with quadriceps weakness: due to nerve root/plexus injury[20] (probably from psoas retraction – shorter operations may have lower risk) or psoas hematoma. Onset may be delayed 1–2 d post-op. Incidence < 1%. May improve slowly over a long time (> 9 months)
4. Lumbar plexus injuries: the risk of direct injury to the lumbar plexus is reduced by staying at or anterior to "safe" working zones defined by Uribe et al.[18] as follows (NB: it is often possible to work posterior to these zones using EMG monitoring to ascertain the proximity of the plexus, and conversely injuries can occur even in these safe zones):
   - L1-2 through L3-4: middle of the posterior quarter of the VB
   - L4-5: midpoint of the VB
5. contralateral femoral nerve injury
6. genitofemoral neuralgia
7. abdominal viscera perforation
8. vascular injury[21] including common iliac artery (at the L4-5 level) or aortic injury (above L4-5), common iliac vein or inferior vena cava
9. kidney-ureter injury
10. graft subsidence
11. unintended rupture of anterior longitudinal ligament
12. psoas/retroperitoneal hematoma ipsilateral/contralateral
13. abdominal wall paresis or hernia[22]
14. rhabdomyolysis
15. retrograde ejaculation (primarily with ACR and pre-psoas approaches)

96.8.7 Postoperative care

- for single-level lumbar LLIF: mobilize the patient in the immediate post-op period without a brace
- hip flexion pain on the approach side is anticipated during the immediate postoperative period
- transient hip flexion weakness related to psoas muscle manipulation is usually self-limited and improves by 8 weeks post-op
- in case of significant leg weakness (femoral nerve injury), a lumbar CT or MRI is indicated to rule out compression by a psoas hematoma, disc extrusion or malposition of cage or screw. If compression is ruled out, patients can be followed by postoperative EMG at 6 weeks to define extent of injury (neuropraxia, axonotomesis, neuronotomesis), again at 3 months to evaluate if the expected interval improvement from neuropraxia has occurred and 5 months to follow up axonal growth[20]

96.8.8 Outcomes

- fusion rates range from 91-100%[23]
- outcomes scales (ODI and VAS leg and back) are significantly improved at follow up[24]

Booking the case: Lateral interbody fusion

Also see defaults & disclaimers (p. 27) and pre-op orders (see below).
1. position: lateral decubitus, typically left-side up unless specified otherwise
2. equipment: C-arm
3. implants:
   a) interbody graft
   b) some stabilizing hardware is usually needed, especially if spondylolisthesis is present. Options:
   - pedicle screws: bilateral, or unilateral
   - interspinous clamps
4. consent (in lay terms for the patient – not all-inclusive):
   a) procedure: surgery through the side to place a spacer between two of the vertebrae (backbones) to make more space for the nerves and to stop painful movement, screws/plates etc. will then need to be placed either from the side through the same opening or sometimes from the back. In case the procdure cannot be done from the side due to the position of the lumbar plexus (uncommon, when it occurs it is usually an issue at L4-5) determine if patient wants to have a posterior procedure (e.g. TLIF) and put that on the consent. Be sure to notify the vendor of this possibility
   b) alternatives: nonsurgical management, open surgery through the back
   c) complications: thigh weakness (usually temporary), knee weakness (uncommon), thigh numbness, graft subsidence/migration, failure to achieve desired relief

96.9 Transfacet pedicle screws

96.9.1 General information

Screws place directly across the lumbar facet joint into the pedicle of the level below. No rod is needed. Immobilizes only, does not provide any decompression, distraction or fusion. Therefore not intended for use as a standalone. Can be placed percutaneously.

96.9.2 Indications

Placement is optimal for L3–4, L4–5 or L5-S1. Difficulty increases in upper lumbar levels.

May be used as adjunct to:
1. ALIF
2. LLIF (when lateral plate not used)
3. contralateral to TLIF (pedicle screws could be used on the side of the TLIF, or a spinous process clamp could be used)
4. axial-LIF (Ax-LIF)

96.9.3 Contraindications

A transfacet pedicle screw cannot be used where the facet has been removed (e.g. for a TLIF) or with a pars defect in the upper of the two levels to be fused.

96.9.4 Technique

1. placed percutaneously or via an open procedure usually in the prone position
2. approximate skin incision site: a single midline ≈ 1.5 cm vertical incision is used
   a) for L5-S1 or L4–5: incision at L3 spinous process
   b) for L3–4: incision at L2 spinous process

3. use AP & lateral fluoro to guide trajectory
   a) AP fluoro: lay a guidewire on the patient's back and orient it to pass through the desired pedicle. Use a skin marker on the patient's back to mark the guidewire's trajectory
   b) lateral fluoro: initial bony target is the midpoint of the inferior facet of the upper level. The tip of the guidewire should contact the bone directly posterior to the inferior endplate of the upper level

96.10 Facet fusion

A bone dowel (e.g. TruFUSE® by MinSURG) is placed into a predrilled opening in the facet joint to promote fusion across the joint. Marketed as a possible standalone.

96.11 S2 screws

May be directed medially (analogous to pedicle screws), or more commonly, directed laterally and superiorly into the ala. In either case, bicortical purchase is necessary.

The main structure to avoid is penetrating the sacroiliac (SI) joint with the screw.

96.12 Iliac screws

Wide exposure is needed. On the initial few cases, the surgeon may be better served by exposing all the way to the posterosuperior aspect of the sciatic notch so that the screw trajectory can be aimed using a palpating finger.

A small amount of bone is removed just below and medial to the posterior superior iliac spine. This prevents the head of the screw from being too superficial which may cause discomfort or skin breakdown. The screw trajectory aims towards the acetabulum to pass approximately 1 cm superior to the sciatic notch on AP fluoro. Avoid penetrating the cortex, especially in the sciatic notch.

An offset adapter is usually required to connect to rods passing through pedicle screws in the levels above.

SCREWS Length 50–70 mm (the screw should end just above midpoint of the sciatic notch, or slightly medial to that). Diameter: 6–8 mm.

96.13 Post-op clinic visits – lumbar and/or thoracic spine fusion

96.13.1 Visit schedule

Patients are seen in the clinic at intervals depending on the preference of the surgeon. A typical follow-up schedule with studies routinely performed is shown in ▶ Table 96.3. For specific problems, additional investigations are usually needed.

96

Table 96.3 Sample post-op lumbar fusion clinic visit schedule[a]

Time post-op	Agenda
7–10 d	wound check, D/C sutures/staples if used
6 wks	AP & lateral LS-spine x-ray in brace
10–12 wks	• AP & lateral LS-spine x-rays with flexion/extension views out of brace • if x-rays look good and patient is doing well, begin weaning brace
6 months	• AP & lateral LS-spine x-rays with flexion/extension views • some surgeons release patients at this time if they are doing well
1 year (optional)	• AP & lateral LS-spine x-rays with flexion/extension views • release patient if they are doing well

[a]the same schedule can be used for thoracic fusions with the difference that standing AP & lateral x-rays are done in place of flexion/extension views

96.13.2 Post-op x-rays

Items to check on post-op x-rays include:

1. alignment
2. position of grafts if used (e.g. interbody grafts)
3. integrity of hardware (look for screw or rod breakage, screw pullout, rod disconnection)
4. lucencies around screws which may indicate motion and implies nonunion
5. any evidence of fusion (may be difficult, e.g. with synthetic interbody cages)
6. on flexion/extension films: look for motion across fused segments (sometimes absence of motion may be the only evidence of fusion on plain x-rays) and the development of abnormal motion at adjacent segments.

References

[1] Chapman JR, Anderson PA, Pepin C, Toomey S, et al. Posterior Instrumentation of the Unstable Cervicothoracic Spine. J Neurosurg. 1996; 84:552–558

[2] Kim YJ, Lenke LG, Bridwell KH, Cho YS, Riew KD. Free hand pedicle screw placement in the thoracic spine: is it safe? Spine (Phila Pa 1976). 2004; 29:333–42; discussion 342

[3] Rosner MK, Polly DW,Jr, Kuklo TR, Ondra SL. Thoracic pedicle screw fixation for spinal deformity. Neurosurg Focus. 2003; 14

[4] Zindrick MR, Wiltse LL, Doornik A, Widell EH, Knight GW, Patwardhan AG, Thomas JC, Rothman SL, Fields BT. Analysis of the morphometric characteristics of the thoracic and lumbar pedicles. Spine (Phila Pa 1976). 1987; 12:160–166

[5] Benzel EC. Biomechanics of Spine Stabilization. Rolling Meadows, IL: American Association of Neurological Surgeons Publications; 2001

[6] Dickman CA, Fessler RG, MacMillan M, Haid RW. Transpedicular Screw-Rod Fixation of the Lumbar Spine: Operative Technique and Outcome in 104 Cases. J Neurosurg. 1992; 77:860–870

[7] Kim YJ, Lenke LG, Cheh G, Riew KD. Evaluation of pedicle screw placement in the deformed spine using intraoperative plain radiographs: A comparison with computerized tomography. Spine. 2005; 30:2084–2088

[8] Ferrara LA, Secor JL, Jin BH, Wakefield A, Inceoglu S, Benzel EC. A biomechanical comparison of facet screw fixation and pedicle screw fixation: effects of short-term and long-term repetitive cycling. Spine. 2003; 28:1226–1234

[9] Aepli M, Mannion AF, Grob D. Translaminar screw fixation of the lumbar spine: long-term outcome. Spine (Phila Pa 1976). 2009; 34:1492–1498

[10] Cloward RB. The Treatment of Ruptured Lumbar Intervertebral Discs by Vertebral Body Fusion. J Neurosurg. 1953; 10:154–168

[11] Pimenta L. Lateral endoscopic transpsoas retroperitoneal approach for lumbar spine surgery. Belo Horizo te, Minas Gerais, Brazil 2001

[12] Ozgur BM, Aryan HE, Pimenta L, Taylor WR. Extreme Lateral Interbody Fusion (XLIF): a novel surgical technique for anterior lumbar interbody fusion. Spine J. 2006; 6:435–443

[13] Bergey DL, Villavicencio AT, Goldstein T, Regan JJ. Endoscopic lateral transpsoas approach to the lumbar spine. Spine (Phila Pa 1976). 2004; 29:1681–1688

[14] Hall LT, Esses SI, Noble PC, Kamaric E. Morphology of the lumbar vertebral endplates. Spine. 1998; 23:1517–22; discussion 1522-3

[15] Rodgers WB, Gerber EJ, Patterson J. Intraoperative and early postoperative complications in extreme lateral interbody fusion: an analysis of 600 cases. Spine (Phila Pa 1976). 2011; 36:26–32

[16] Dakwar E, Cardona RF, Smith DA, Uribe JS. Early outcomes and safety of the minimally invasive, lateral retroperitoneal transpsoas approach for adult degenerative scoliosis. Neurosurg Focus. 2010; 28. DOI: 10.3171/2010.1.FOCUS09282

[17] Pimenta L, Diaz RC, Guerrero LG. Charite lumbar artificial disc retrieval: use of a lateral minimally invasive technique. Technical note. J Neurosurg Spine. 2006; 5:556–561

[18] Uribe JS, Arredondo N, Dakwar E, Vale FL. Defining the safe working zones using the minimally invasive lateral retroperitoneal transpsoas approach: an anatomical study. J Neurosurg Spine. 2010; 13:260–266

[19] Knight RQ, Schwaegler P, Hanscom D, Roh J. Direct lateral lumbar interbody fusion for degenerative conditions: early complication profile. J Spinal Disord Tech. 2009; 22:34–37

[20] Ahmadian A, Deukmedjian AR, Abel N, Dakwar E, Uribe JS. Analysis of lumbar plexopathies and nerve injury after lateral retroperitoneal transpsoas approach: diagnostic standardization. J Neurosurg Spine. 2013; 18:289–297

[21] Assina R, Majmundar NJ, Herschman Y, Heary RF. First report of major vascular injury due to lateral transpsoas approach leading to fatality. J Neurosurg Spine. 2014; 21:794–798

[22] Dakwar E, Vale FL, Uribe JS. Trajectory of the main sensory and motor branches of the lumbar plexus outside the psoas muscle related to the lateral retroperitoneal transpsoas approach. J Neurosurg Spine. 2011; 14:290–295

[23] Youssef JA, McAfee PC, Patty CA, Raley E, DeBauche S, Shucosky E, Chotikul L. Minimally invasive surgery: lateral approach interbody fusion: results and review. Spine (Phila Pa 1976). 2010; 35:S302–S311

[24] Alimi M, Hofstetter CP, Cong GT, Tsiouris AJ, James AR, Paulo D, Elowitz E, Hartl R. Radiological and clinical outcomes following extreme lateral interbody fusion. J Neurosurg Spine. 2014; 20:623–635

97 Miscellaneous Surgical Procedures

97.1 Percutaneous ventricular puncture

97.1.1 Indications

In pediatrics, may be used to remove hemorrhagic ventricular fluid following intraventricular hemorrhage, or to obtain CSF specimen in cases of suspected ventriculitis. May be used emergently in pediatrics or adult as a temporizing measure in patient herniating from obstructive hydrocephalus.

97.1.2 Peds

Shave hair. 5 minute Betadine® prep.

The right side is preferred. Enter through coronal suture just lateral to anterior fontanelle (AF) using a 20–22 Ga. spinal needle. If a CT scan has been done, it may be used to help judge angulation (usually varies between contra- and ipsi-lateral medial canthus and intersection with EAM).

97.1.3 Adult

See reference.[1]

Only used emergently. Takes advantage of thin orbital roof in adult.

Prep conjunctiva and skin with antiseptic (e.g. ophthalmic betadine). Elevate the eyelid and depress the globe. Using a 16–18 Ga. spinal needle, penetrate the anterior third of orbital roof (1–2 cm behind orbital rim) with firm pressure (may need gentle tapping). Aim at coronal suture in the midline. The frontal horn should be about 3–4 cm deep.

97.2 Percutaneous subdural tap

97.2.1 Indications

Utilized in pediatrics. Used to be done for diagnostic purposes, but this has been supplanted by CT, MRI & ultrasound. Currently, this procedure may be used emergently for decompression, to drain subdural collections and to obtain fluid for diagnostic tests, such as culture (repeat taps may be used, but surgery should be considered after ≈ 5–6).

97.2.2 Technique

Shave hair. Prep 5 minutes with povidone iodine (Betadine®). Using a short 20–21 Ga. spinal needle (spinal needle is recommended because the stylet may reduce the risk of implanting epidermal cells into the CNS), penetrate the lateral margin of the anterior fontanelle (AF) or coronal suture at least 2 cm off midline. Remove the stylet and aspirate. With bilateral fluid collections, bilateral taps should be done.

97.3 Lumbar puncture

97.3.1 Contraindications

1. risk of tonsillar herniation (see below)
   a) known or suspected intracranial mass
   b) non-communicating hydrocephalus
2. infection in region desired for puncture: choose another site if possible
3. coagulopathy
   a) platelet count should be > 50,000/mm^3 (p. 154)
   b) patient should not be on anticoagulants because of risk of epidural hematoma (p. 1131) or subarachnoid hemorrhage[2] with secondary cord compression
4. use caution in suspected aneurysmal SAH: excessive lowering of the CSF pressure increases the transmural pressure (pressure across the aneurysm wall) and may precipitate rerupture
5. caution in patients with complete spinal block: 14% will deteriorate after LP[3]

6. relative contraindication: Chiari malformation. There is some evidence that draining CSF may precipitate herniation. This is less of a concern with successfully surgically treated Chiari malformation.

Elevated ICP and/or papilledema by themselves are *NOT* contraindications (e.g. LP is actually used diagnostically and as a treatment in idiopathic intracranial hypertension, see below).

97.3.2 Technique

Background and anatomy

The spinal cord and column are the same length in a 3-month fetus. After that, the spinal column grows faster than the cord. As a result, the conus medullaris is located rostral to the termination of the thecal sac in the adult, situated between the middle thirds of the vertebral bodies of L1 and L2 in 51–68% of adults (the most common location), T12-L1 in ≈ 30%, and L2–3 in ≈ 10% (with 94% of cords terminating within the territory of L1 and L2 vertebral bodies).[4] The thecal sac ends ≈ S2. The tips of the spinous processes as palpated on the surface are located caudal to the corresponding VB. The intercristal line (connecting the superior border of the iliac crests) crosses the spine at the L4 spinous process or between the L4 and L5 spinous processes in most adults.

Procedure

Position: the procedure is usually performed in the lateral decubitus position. As the needle is advanced, it is helpful to have the patient bring the knees up and to flex the neck in order to open up the spaces between the posterior elements of the spine.

For diagnostic LP, a 20 Ga spinal needle is often selected. Larger needles (e.g. 18 Ga) may be used e.g. with pseudotumor cerebri to encourage post-procedure drainage of CSF into the soft tissues of the back.

The back is prepped and draped to create a sterile working area.

Entry point: in an adult, use the L4–5 interspace in most cases (located at or just below the intercristal line) or 1 level higher (L3–4). Peds: L4–5 is preferred over L3–4.

The needle is always advanced with the *stylet in place* at least through the skin and some subcutaneous tissue to avoid introducing epidermal cells which may cause iatrogenic *epidermoid tumors*; see Complications following LP (p. 1507). The needle is aimed slightly cranially (to parallel the spinous processes) and usually a little down towards the bed (aiming towards the umbilicus). If a Quincke LP (standard) needle is used, the bevel is turned parallel to the length of the spinal column to reduce the risk of post-LP H/A (p. 1509). In general, if bone is encountered it is more often due to deviation from a true midline trajectory rather than a failure to aim correctly in the rostral-caudal direction. The needle should be withdrawn to just below the skin surface before attempting a new trajectory.

If during insertion of the needle the patient experiences pain radiating down one LE, this usually indicates that a nerve root has been encountered. The needle should be withdrawn immediately and reinserted aiming more towards the side *contralateral* to the extremity that experienced the pain. The stylet is removed at intervals during the insertion to look for CSF (a distinct pop is sometimes felt as the needle penetrates the dura).

Once CSF flows, the needle is connected to a manometer through a 3-way stopcock, the pressure is measured and recorded (see below), and CSF is drained into sterile tubes (1–2 ml for each tube) for laboratory analysis (see below). The practitioner should also note the color of the fluid (clear, blood tinged, xanthochromic...) and the clarity (clear, cloudy, purulent...).

At the end of the procedure, the stylet should be replaced before the needle is withdrawn (to reduce post-LP H/A, see below).

Opening pressure: The opening pressure (OP) should be measured and recorded for every LP. To be meaningful, the patient should be lying down and as relaxed as possible (should not be in forced fetal position), with the bed flat. The variation of pressure with respirations is usually a good indication of a communicating fluid column (the fluctuation is in-phase with the respiratory pressures in the inferior vena cava, rising with inspiration and falling with expiration[5]). Normal values: in the left lateral decubitus position, average OP = 12.2 ± 3.4 cm H_2O (8.8 ± 0.9 mm Hg).[6] Also, see ▶ Table 23.1 for peds.

Queckenstedt's test: if a subarachnoid block is suspected (e.g. from spinal tumor), compress the jugular vein (JV) first on one side then on both (do not compress carotid arteries). If there is no block, the pressure will rise to 10–20 cm of fluid, and will drop to the original level within 10 seconds of release of the JV.[7(p 11)] Do *not* do JV compression if intracranial disease is suspected.

97

97.3.3 Laboratory analysis

Routinely, three tubes are sent for analysis as shown in ▶ Table 97.1. See ▶ Table 23.4 for interpreting the results of the laboratory analysis.

If the tap is possibly traumatic (i.e. bloody), or if having an accurate cell count is essential (e.g. to R/O SAH) then 4 tubes are collected, and the first and last are sent for cell counts and are compared; see Traumatic tap (p. 1506).

If special cultures are required (e.g. acid fast, fungal, viral) they are also specified on the tube for culture & sensitivity (C & S).

If CSF for cytology is desired (e.g. to R/O carcinomatous meningitis or CNS lymphoma), then at least 10 ml of CSF must be sent in one tube to pathology (where it is spun down, and examined for cells).

97.3.4 Mining useful data with a traumatic tap

General information

A traumatic tap (TT) occurs when the spinal needle damages a blood vessel with the result that (usually venous) blood either alone or admixed with CSF will be obtained.

Estimating true WBC count in CSF with a traumatic tap

When many RBCs and WBCs are present in the CSF due to a traumatic tap (TT), it is difficult to know if there is a true leukocytosis on the CSF. It may help to determine if the WBCs are elevated or if they are present in the same ratio as in the peripheral blood. In non-anemic patients, there should be ≈ 1–2 WBCs for every 1000 RBCs (as a correction[8(p 176)]: subtract 1 WBC for every 700 RBCs[8(p 176)]). In the presence of anemia or ***peripheral*** leukocytosis, use Fishman's formula[8(p 176)] shown in Eq (97.1) to estimate the original WBC count in the CSF *before* the TT,

$$WBC_{CSF\ Original} = WBC_{CSF} - \frac{WBC_{Blood} \times RBC_{CSF}}{RBC_{Blood}} \quad (97.1)$$

where WBCCSF original = WBC count in the CSF before the TT, WBCCSF & RBCCSF = WBC & RBC counts measured in the CSF, and WBCBlood & RBCBlood = WBC & RBC per mm^3 in the peripheral blood.

Estimating true total CSF protein content with a traumatic tap

If the hemogram and peripheral protein are normal, then have the cell count and protein content run on the *same tube*, and the correction is[8(p 176)]:

- subtract 1 mg per 100 ml of protein for every 1000 RBC per mm^3

Differentiating SAH from traumatic tap

97

See typical findings in SAH (p. 1160). Some features helpful in differentiating SAH from TT are shown in ▶ Table 97.2.

Table 97.1 Routine tests for CSF

Test	If there is *no* concern about possible traumatic tap	If there is concern about traumatic tap
cell count		Tube 1
gram stain + C & S (culture & sensitivity)	Tube 1	Tube 2
protein and glucose	Tube 2	Tube 3
cell count	Tube 3	Tube 4

Table 97.2 Features distinguishing traumatic tap from SAH

Feature	Traumatic tap (TT)	SAH
RBC count (and gross appearance of bloodiness)	declines as CSF drains (compare first tube to last tube)	usually > 100,000 RBCs/mm^3, changes little as CSF drains
ratio of WBC:RBC	similar to the ratio in peripheral blood (above)	usually promotes a leukocytosis (elevated WBC count)
supernatant	clear	xanthochromic[a] (rarely in < 2 hrs, present in 70% by 6 hrs, and > 90% by 12 hrs after SAH)
clotting of fluid	usually clots if erythrocyte count > 200,000/mm^3	usually does not clot
protein concentration	fresh bleeding elevates CSF protein from normal by only ≈ 1 mg per 1000 RBC	blood breakdown products elevate this more than TT (measured protein exceeds the sum of normal protein + 1 mg protein/1000 RBC)
repeat LP at higher level	usually clear	remains bloody
opening pressure	usually normal	usually elevated

[a] NB: other conditions can cause xanthochromia

97.3.5 Complications following LP

General information

The overall risk of disabling or persistent symptoms (defined as severe H/A lasting > 7 days, cranial nerve palsies, major exacerbation of pre-existing neurological disease, prolonged back pain, aseptic meningitis, and nerve root or peripheral nerve injuries) has been estimated at 0.1–0.5%.[9] Severe side effects, which include brainstem herniation, infection, subdural hematoma or effusion, and SAH, are rare.[10(p 171–2)]

Possible complications

1. tonsillar herniation
   a) acute herniation in the presence of mass lesion (see below)
   b) chronic tonsillar herniation (acquired Chiari 1 malformation): this has been reported after multiple traumatic LPs with presumed post-LP CSF leak[11]
2. infection (spinal meningitis)
3. "spinal headache": usually positional (diminishes with recumbency) (see below)
4. spinal epidural hematoma (p. 1131): usually seen only with coagulopathy
5. spinal epidural CSF collection: may be fairly common in patients with post-LP H/A. Usually resolves spontaneously
6. epidermoid tumor: risk may be increased by advancing LP needle without stylet (transplanting a core of epidermal tissue)[12,13,14]
7. impinging nerve root with needle: usually causes transient radicular pain, may cause permanent radiculopathy in some
8. *intracranial* subdural hygroma or hematoma[15,16] (rare)
9. vestibulocochlear dysfunction[17]:
   a) subclinical (demonstrated on audiogram) or moderate reduction in hearing may occur, and seems to correlate with post-procedure CSF leakage. Most studies show reduction is at frequencies < 1000 Hz
   b) sudden hearing loss may occur. Perform audiogram to quantify loss. Treat with bedrest for several days, prednisone 60 mg/d tapered over 2–3 weeks
   c) pathogenesis: reduced CSF pressure may reduce perilymph pressure through the cochlear aqueduct (may be especially pronounced with a patent aqueduct),[18] producing endolymphatic hydrops
10. ocular abnormalities
    a) abducens palsy: almost invariably unilateral. Often delayed 5–14 days post-LP, usually recovers after 4–6 wks[19]
11. dural sinus thrombosis[20] (usually with underlying thrombophilia)

Risk of acute tonsillar herniation following lumbar puncture

The question of when to do LP first (to save time) and when to obtain CT scan first to R/O intracranial mass (for safety) before performing an LP is controversial.

Issues

The time delay to initiating antibiotics is the most important variable in the outcome of meningitis. Time may be more crucial in community acquired meningitis, where a virulent organism infects a sometimes immune compromised host (e.g. children or the elderly), than in post-op neurosurgical meningitis (usually a low virulence organism, e.g. Staph. aureus, in an immune intact host where the BBB has been disrupted).

The theoretical risk in performing an LP with an intracranial mass is that the resultant shift in pressure may precipitate tonsillar herniation.

Starting antibiotics without first having a CSF specimen from an LP may prevent cultures from growing in the lab which then risks the difficulties inherent in managing partially treated meningitis, or a suboptimal choice of antibiotic medication.

Clinical evaluation for possible contraindication to LP is unreliable. Papilledema is one possible indication of increased ICP. Papilledema takes a minimum of 6 hrs to develop after the onset of increased ICP, and in most cases it requires up to 24 hrs to develop. Therefore, its absence does not insure normal intracranial pressure. Furthermore, papilledema may be seen in conditions where there is not a contraindication to LP, e.g. idiopathic intracranial hypertension, where LP is one of the accepted treatments (p. 766).

The ready availability of CT scans, often within the emergency department itself, may involve a delay of only a few minutes, if qualified personnel to interpret the study are also immediately available. However, in a busy E/R, there may be delays related to other patients also requiring emergency CT, the need to transmit scans to an off-site radiologist…

Historical information

Herniation following LP was more common prior to ≈ 1950, long before CT scans were available, where the procedure was performed even when some patients had clear evidence of ↑ ICP, large bore spinal needles (12–16 gauge) were more commonly employed, and large quantities of CSF were removed for therapeutic purposes. In a 1969 report of 30 patients who deteriorated after LP,[21] 73% had localizing signs (hemiparesis, anisocoria…) and 30% had papilledema. None of 5 patients with cerebral abscess deteriorated after the first of multiple LPs.

In a series of 129 patients with ↑ ICP,[22] the complication rate reported was 6%; however, some of these complications were probably unrelated to LP, and many of these patients were in extremis. In 7 series totalling 418 patients, a complication rate of 1.2% was calculated.[22]

Σ

97 Herniation as a result of LP is consistently reported only in patients with severe non-infectious processes, often with accompanying signs of mass effect (localizing signs, papilledema…). Thus, in cases of suspected meningitis in the absence of focal findings and papilledema, if a CT scan cannot be performed and interpreted within a few minutes, the benefits of performing an LP with a needle 20 gauge or smaller and removing only a few ml of CSF and starting empiric antibiotics probably outweigh the small risk of herniation. In the unlikely event that there is acute deterioration associated with the withdrawal of a few ml of CSF, the (anecdotal) recommendation is to immediately replace the fluid through the LP needle.

Post LP (myelogram) H/A

General information

AKA "postspinal headache" or "spinal headache." May also follow procedures other than LP/myelogram, such as dural opening (p. 1055). Can also occur with spontaneous intracranial hypotension (p. 389) and following decompressive craniectomy.[23]

Clinical features

Important distinctive characteristic: H/A occurs when patient is erect, and is completely or partially (but significantly) relieved when recumbent. May be associated with nausea, vomiting, dizziness, or visual disturbances.

► **Time course.** Most post-LP headaches (PLPHA) have a delayed onset 24–48 hrs after the LP, and although they may occur weeks post-LP, most also develop within 3 days. The duration of PLPHA varies, with a mean of 4 days,[24] and reports of duration of months[25] and even > 1 year.[26]

Pathophysiology

Thought to be due to continued CSF leakage through the hole in the dura,[27] which reduces the CSF "cushion" of the brain. In the upright position, the pull of gravity on the brain produces traction on the blood vessels and any structures tethering the brain to the pain-sensitive dura. CSF may sometimes be demonstrable in the *epidural* space.

Epidemiology following LP

Reported incidence range is 2–40% (typically ≈ 20%), higher after diagnostic LP than for epidural anesthesia.[24]

See also variables in LP that impact upon the risk of PLPHA (p. 1508) (e.g. incidence is lower with smaller gauge spinal needle).

1. Risk factors for post-LP H/A outside the control of the physician:
   a) age: incidence ↑ in younger patients
   b) sex: incidence ↑ in females
   c) prior headache history (including previous PLPHA)
   d) body size: ↑ with small body mass index = weight/height2[28]
   e) pregnancy
2. Variables that have been shown to influence the incidence of PLPHA:
   a) needle size: larger needles carry increased risk[29]
   b) bevel orientation: orienting the bevel parallel to the longitudinally running fibers of the dura reduces the risk of PLPHA[30]
   c) replacing the stylet prior to needle removal lowers the incidence[28]
   d) the number of dural punctures (may not be totally under the physician's control)
3. Variables that may or may not influence the incidence of PLPHA:needle type
   a) Quincke needle: bevelled edge with cutting tip (the standard LP needle). Incidence of PLPHA with 20 and 22 gauge Quincke needles: 36%[31])
   b) atraumatic needles: a number of types are available (Sprotte, Whitacre…). Most are "pencil pointed" and may produce a hole with a lower incidence of transdural leak.[32] Unproven[28]
4. Factors found *not* to affect the incidence of PLPHA:
   a) the position of the patient after LP (does not seem to prevent PLPHA, but may delay the onset of symptoms[33,34])
   b) volume of fluid removed at the time of LP
   c) hydration following LP[28]

Treatment for H/A following LP

Initial "conservative" measures include:

1. flat in bed for at least 24 hrs
2. hydration (PO or IV)
3. analgesics for H/A
4. tight abdominal binder
5. desoxycortisone acetate 5 mg IM q 8 hrs[24]
6. caffeine sodium benzoate 500 mg in 2 cc IV q 8 hrs up to 3 d max (70% of patients had relief with 1 or 2 injections)[35]
7. high-dose steroids: report of success in a case of intracranial hypotension associated with spontaneous slit ventricles tapering down from a starting dose of dexamethasone 20 mg/day[36]
8. blood patch if refractory

► **Epidural blood patch.** For refractory post-lumbar puncture or post-myelogram H/A. Works in one application in over 90% of cases, may be repeated if ineffective.[25] Theoretical risks: infection, cauda equina compression, failure to relieve H/A.

► **Technique.** Summary: 10 ml of non-heparinized autologous blood injected into *epidural* space.

Accessing epidural space (one of several techniques): proceed as routine LP. When ligaments are traversed, and needle tip is nearing spinal canal, stylet is removed. Then, either place drop of sterile saline in hub (hanging drop technique) and advance while watching for it to be drawn into needle as epidural space is entered, or gently try injecting air with small syringe (preferably glass, lower resistance) while advancing, when the epidural space is entered, resistance to injection disappears, but CSF cannot be aspirated.

A venipuncture site is prepared aseptically. 10 ml of the patient's blood is withdrawn. After verifying CSF cannot be aspirated through the spinal needle, the blood is injected into the epidural space. After 30 minutes supine, patient may ambulate ad lib.

97.4 Lumbar catheter CSF drainage

97.4.1 General information

Insertion of a catheter into the lumbar subarachnoid space for the purpose of draining CSF. Usually connected to a closed drainage system similar to that for an EVD. Generally used for periods of only a few days or so.

97.4.2 Indications

1. to reduce CSF pressure on a site of CSF leak/fistula. Example situations:
   a) dural breach during spine surgery or craniotomy (especially posterior fossa)
   b) for spontaneous CSF fistula (rare) (p.386)
2. to reduce intracranial pressure in cases of *communicating* hydrocephalus: e.g. drain test for NPH, or when an infected shunt has been removed
3. to reduce CSF pressure to attempt to increase perfusion of the spinal cord: e.g. during surgery for abdominal aortic aneurysm, or following spinal cord injury

97.4.3 Contraindications

As with lumbar puncture (see above).

97.4.4 Insertion technique

Positioning, entry site, and trajectory are all similar to lumbar puncture (see above). Instead of a spinal needle, a Tuohy needle is used. The bevel is inserted parallel to the fibers of the dura (rostrocaudal). The needle is then rotated 90° (usually pointing rostrally) and the catheter is threaded into the needle. ✖ If the catheter does not thread, the needle must be withdrawn *together* with the catheter – attempting to withdraw the catheter through the needle will shear off the catheter at the tip of the needle.

97.4.5 Management

The orders for the nursing staff to maintain the catheter include:

1. instructions as to how to regulate the CSF drainage. Most commonly one of:
   a) by pressure: accomplished by specifying a height of the drip chamber, usually at the level of the tragus or shoulder
   b) by withdrawing a specified amount of CSF per hour: usually 10–20 cc. This method reduces the risk of overdrainage if the dip chamber is too low
2. instructions for the exit site: usually treated as an arterial-line

97.4.6 Complications

1. infection
2. overdrainage: usually as a result of the drainage bag being too low when using the pressure drainage method described above (either from falling to the floor, or not being raised when the patient sits or stands up) or from catheter disconnection. Can cause:
   a) subdural hematoma from tearing of bridging veins from downward displacement of the brain
   b) headache
3. pneumocephalus: usually from placing the drain height below the site of a fistula, and air is drawn in through the fistula tract
   a) tension pneumocephalus: usually with a ball-valve effect at the fistula site
4. catheter pull out: frequently occurs simply as a result of patient movement in bed or with patient transfers

97.5 C1–2 puncture and cisternal tap

97.5.1 Indications

Situations where CSF specimen is required but access via LP is difficult or contraindicated (lumbar arachnoiditis, superficial infection, marked obesity, patients who cannot be turned on their sides...), or to instill contrast to demonstrate the rostral extent of a block documented by dye injected via LP. Spinal headache is less common with these procedures than with LP. C1–2 puncture is safer than cisternal tap.

✖ Contraindicated: in patient with Chiari malformation (often present in myelomeningocele) due to low lying cerebellar tonsils and medullary kink.

Normal CSF values for glucose and protein differ only slightly from CSF obtained by lumbar puncture. Opening pressures averaged 18 cm of fluid with lateral puncture.

97.5.2 C1–2 puncture

AKA lateral cervical puncture. Equipment: LP tray (useful for the specimen tubes, extension tube for contrast injection under fluoroscopy, lidocaine, and spinal needle) with a standard 20 Ga spinal needle, contrast if needed (e.g. Iohexol®). It is preferred to perform the procedure under fluoro, however it has also been described without fluoroscopic guidance with a completely cooperative patient.[37]

Patient position: supine in bed without a pillow, with the head straight up. Avoid any head rotation which may bring the vertebral artery (VA) into the needle path.[38] Place head within lateral fluoroscopy unit (since this is rarely available, a C-arm fluoro positioned horizontally may be used).

If iodinated dye is being injected for myelography, the head should be elevated to prevent contrast from running into posterior fossa; in cases with cervical spine injury, one can put the entire bed in reverse Trendelenburg.

Entry point: 1 cm caudal and 1 cm posterior (dorsal) to the tip of the mastoid process. Needle insertion: use a 25 Ga. needle to anesthetize the skin at the entry point. Under fluoro, advance a larger needle (e.g. 21 Ga.) towards the C1–2 interspace while injecting local anesthetic: aim for a target in the middle of the posterior third of the bony spinal canal (or, alternatively, 2–3 mm anterior to the posterior margin of the bony canal) ("X" in ▸ Fig. 97.1). Leave this needle in as a marker. Insert the 20 Ga. spinal needle parallel to the marker needle. Verify the course with fluoro. If fluoro is not used, insert the spinal needle at the entry point, and advance it parallel to the plane of the bed, perpendicular to the neck.[37] If the needle penetrates deeply without encountering bone or CSF, it is most likely that the tip is too par posterior. If bone is encountered, redirect the needle in the rostro-caudal plane.

Several "pops" may be felt, and the stylet should be removed after each to check for CSF return. The subarachnoid space is ≈ 5–6 cm deep to the skin surface in most adults.[39] The needle must be supported more than with a lumbar puncture.

To inject iodinated contrast, use e.g. ≈ 5 ml of 180 mg% Iohexol® for cervical myelogram, watch dye on fluoro (should be able to see it in subarachnoid space).

Risks

Case report of a death from subdural hematoma due to puncture of an anomalous vertebral artery[40] (found in ≈ 0.4% of population). If the VA is penetrated, the needle is withdrawn and local pressure is applied. Penetration of the upper spinal cord/lower medulla (risk of serious neurologic sequelae, even from this, is small). Herniation (as with LP) when there is increased ICP.

97.5.3 Cisternal tap

Suboccipital access to the cisterna magna. Usually done with patient sitting, with neck slightly flexed.[41] Overlying hair should be shaved. Local anesthetic is infiltrated. A 22 gauge spinal needle is inserted exactly in the midline between the inion and the C2 spinous process, directed superiorly towards the glabella until the needle strikes the occiput or enters the cisterna magna. If the occiput is encountered, the needle is withdrawn slightly and reinserted directed slightly inferiorly, the process is repeated ("walking down the occiput") until the cisterna magna is entered (a "pop" will be felt).

The distance from the skin surface to the cisterna magna is 4–6 cm, and from the dura to the medulla is ≈ 2.5 cm. However, due to tenting of the dura, the needle may be very close to the medulla before entering the subarachnoid space.

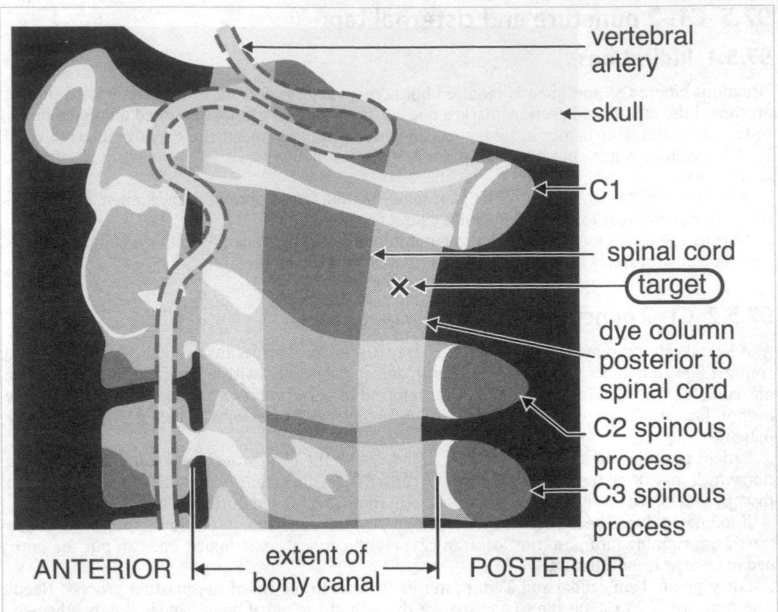

Fig. 97.1 C1–2 puncture target*
* left lateral view through upper C-spine: composite diagram of a myelogram and vertebral arteriogram illustrating the relative location of the spinal cord, CSF space, and VA. Only bony landmarks will be visible with fluoroscopy

Risks

1. hemorrhage in the cisterna magna: may be due to perforation of a large vessel[37]
2. piercing the medulla oblongata: may cause vomiting, respiratory arrest…
3. positioning may compromise blood flow in the vertebral artery in elderly patients

97.6 CSF diversionary procedures

97.6.1 Ventricular catheterization

Most common insertion sites[42(p 151–3)]:

97

1. ✱ Kocher's point (coronal): localizes an entry point into the frontal horn of the lateral ventricle that passes anterior to the motor strip. The right side is usually used. Often employed for ICP monitors, EVDs, shunts, ventriculoscopes…. Originally described as, "about 2 cm from the central line and 3 cm from the precentral fissure.".[43] A number of surface landmarks have been described to locate a point anterior to the motor strip that is in this general vicinity, and the author will often refer to the position as "Kocher's point." Commonly cited landmarks:
   a) entry site: 2–3 cm from midline which is approximately the mid-pupillary line with forward gaze, 1 cm anterior to coronal suture which is approximately 11 cm up from the nasion (to avoid the motor strip)
   b) trajectory: direct catheter perpendicular to surface of brain, which can be approximated by aiming in coronal plane towards medial canthus of ipsilateral eye and in AP plane towards EAM
   c) insertion length: advance catheter with stylet until CSF is obtained (should be < 5–7 cm depth; this may be 3–4 cm with markedly dilated ventricles). Advance catheter without stylet 1 cm deeper. ✖ CAUTION: if CSF is not obtained until very long insertion length (e.g. ≥ 8 cm) the tip is probably in a cistern (e.g. prepontine cistern) which is undesirable

2. ✱ occipital-parietal region: commonly used for CSF shunt
   a) entry site: a number of means have been described, including:
      - Frazier burr hole: placed prophylactically before p-fossa crani for emergency ventriculostomy in event of post-op swelling. Location: 3–4 cm from midline, 6–7 cm above inion[44(p 520)] (caution: an error in locating the inion could put the catheter in an undesirable location if this method alone is used)
      - parietal boss: flat portion of parietal bone
      - follow point from mid-pupillary line parallel to sagittal suture until it intersects line extending posteriorly from the top of the pinna
      - ≈ 3 cm above and ≈ 3 cm posterior to top of pinna
   b) trajectory: insert the catheter parallel to skull base:
      - initially aim for middle of forehead
      - if this fails, aim for ipsilateral medial canthus
   c) insertion length: ideally, the tip should be just anterior to the foramen of Monro in the frontal horn.[45] Ventriculoscopic guidance (if available) increases the accuracy to a significant degree. In the absence of this:
      - intracranial length should be ≈ two-thirds of the length of the skull (this is short enough to prevent penetration of frontal brain parenchyma, but long enough to take tip beyond the foramen of Monro to prevent catheter from ending up in the temporal horn where choroid plexus increases the chance of obstruction)
      - in adults without macrocrania the inserted length is usually ≈ 12 cm when the burr hole is in line with the axis of the lateral ventricle[46] (lengths > 12 cm are rarely required). In hydrocephalic infants usually ≈ 7–8 cm is required
      - use the stylet for the initial ≈ 6 cm of insertion, then remove it and insert the remaining length (keeps the catheter straight during penetration of occipital parenchyma and prevents the tip from dropping into the temporal horn where there is choroid plexus, also the temporal horn may collapse and occlude the catheter when the HCP is resolved)
3. Keen's point (posterior parietal): (placement in trigone) 2.5–3 cm posterior and 2.5–3 cm superior to pinna (was the usual site of occurrence of cerebral abscesses arising from otitis media, and was often used to tap these)
4. Dandy's point: 2 cm from midline, 3 cm above inion (may be more prone to damage visual pathways than above)

97.6.2 Ventriculostomy/ICP monitor

General information

AKA intraventricular catheter (IVC) or external ventricular drainage (EVD).

Elevated INR: for patients with an elevated INR (such as patients on warfarin), it has generally been recommended that placement of intraparenchymal catheters be delayed until the INR be ≤ 1.6 in order to reduce the risk of hemorrhage to an acceptable level.[47] However, intraparenchymal ICP monitors were placed without hemorrhagic or thrombotic complications in 11 patients with grade III/IV hepatic encephalopathy associated with fulminant hepatic failure who had an average INR of 3 when it was performed within 15-120 minutes after receiving 36.7 micrograms/kg IV of recombinant activated factor VII (rFVIIa).[48]

Insertion technique

Unless contraindicated (e.g. right ventricular bleed), the right (non-dominant) side is preferred. Shave entire ipsilateral hemicranium and contralateral frontal portion. Clip the hair around the planned incision site and the exit site for the tunneled catheter (avoid shaving which degrades the skin's barrier function against infection). Prep with any acceptable surgical prep (betadine prep for 5 minutes, Chloroprep, Duraprep…)

Site: approximately Kocher's point (see above). To avoid motor strip, enter *1–2 cm anterior to coronal suture* (estimated position of coronal suture: follow line up midway between lateral canthus and EAM, or measure 11 cm up from the nasion), and to avoid the sagittal sinus, *2–3 cm lateral to midline* (2 fingerbreadths or ≈ 3 cm is commonly employed as an approximation). Incision oriented in sagittal plane (in case it needs to be incorporated in flap); elevate periosteum; place self-retaining retractor; make twist drill hole. Bone-wax edges to stop bone bleeding; cauterize dura with bipolar coagulator; incise dura in cruciate fashion with #11 scalpel blade; cauterize incised dural edges and then pia/arachnoid with bipolar.

For ventriculostomy: insert catheter *perpendicular* to brain surface[49] to a depth of 5–7 cm (most catheters are marked at 5 and 10 cm). With any ventricular enlargement, CSF should flow at least by

3–4 cm depth (with normal ventricles, this may be 4–5 cm). If no CSF is encountered here and the catheter is passed further until CSF is obtained, it is unlikely to be due to catheterization of frontal horn of lateral ventricle (in this case, at ≈ 9–11 cm the tip will often be in the pre-pontine cistern, a subarachnoid space, which is undesirable). If unsuccessful after a maximum of three attempted passes, then place a subarachnoid bolt or intraparenchymal monitor.

For (Richmond) subarachnoid bolt: screw in until tip is flush with inner table.

Removal

Patients receiving anticoagulants need to have normal coagulation and platelet function before discontinuing the catheter to reduce the risk of intracranial hemorrhage. For heparin and LMW heparin, stop the drug 24 hours prior to discontinuing the drain.

"Sump drainage"

The tip of a 25 gauge butterfly may be bent at a 90° angle, and inserted into a subcutaneous reservoir for prolonged ventricular drainage.[50] In one series OF 34 patients, this was used for prolonged periods (up to 44 days) with acceptably low infection rate.[51] The use of a one-way valve, continuous antibiotics (ampicillin and cloxacillin) and meticulous technique was credited for the lack of infection.

97.6.3 Ventricular shunts

Booking the case: Ventricular shunt

Also see defaults & disclaimers (p. 27).

1. position: supine with shoulder roll
2. implants: need to specify shunt manufacturer and valve type (e.g. programmable, low profile...) Uncommon components (e.g. ultra-low pressure, tumor filter) may need special order
3. equipment:
   a) C-arm for ventriculo-atrial shunts
   b) endoscopic display (e.g. if NeuroPen is used)
   c) image guided navigation system (infrequently used)
4. consent (in lay terms for the patient – not all-inclusive):
   a) procedure: surgery to insert a permanent drainage tube from the brain to the abdomen, outside of the lungs, vein near the heart (as appropriate) to drain excess cerebrospinal fluid
   b) alternatives: nonsurgical management (rarely effective for hydrocephalus), third ventriculostomy (for certain cases)
   c) complications: infection, suboptimal position which might require re-operation, failure to relieve hydrocephalus/symptoms, subdural hematoma, bleeding in the brain, shunts are mechanical devices and will eventually fail (break, block up, move...) and need repair/replacement (sometimes sooner rather than later). Abdominal shunts: risk of bowel injury (which could require further surgery)

97

Ventricular catheter

Kocher's point is currently used in most cases for insertion site of ventricular catheter; see Ventricular catheterization (p. 1512) for technique. An alternative is an occipital burr hole aiming toward the frontal horn of the lateral ventricle.

An inverted "J" shaped incision is used to keep hardware from lying directly under the skin incision (minimizes risk of skin breakdown and also creates additional barrier to infection of subjacent hardware). CSF should be sent for culture at the time of insertion since it has been estimated that in ≈ 3% of patients the CSF is already infected. 4 mg of preservative-free gentamicin may instilled into the ventricular catheter by the technique of barbotage, (a technique to administer a drug while reducing the amount of drug lost in the dead space of the catheter: a portion of the antibiotic solution is injected into the CSF, then a lesser amount of CSF is aspirated, a second portion is then injected and the process is repeated until all of the medication is administered).

If you think the catheter is in the ventricle, but you don't get CSF flow, it may be due to low pressure, you can compress the jugular veins or lower the head of the bed to try and induce CSF flow.

Connectors

If a connector must be used near the clavicle, place it rostral to (above) the clavicle. ✖ Avoid placing it caudal to the clavicle which increases the risk of disconnection.

Distal catheter placement options

All things being equal, the general order of preference for distal catheter placement:
1. peritoneal cavity: see below
2. pleural space (p. 416): not for age ≤ 7 years. For technique, see below
3. right atrium or superior vena cava (p. 1516)
4. infrequently used distal shunt sites
   a) gall bladder
   b) internal jugular vein (with the catheter pointing "upstream")
   c) superior sagittal sinus

Ventriculoperitoneal shunt

Peritoneal catheter

For small children, use at least 30 cm length of intraperitoneal tubing to allow for continued growth (120 cm total length of peritoneal tubing was associated with a lower revision rate for growth without significant increase in other complications[52]). A silver clip is placed at the point where the catheter enters the peritoneum so that the amount of residual intraperitoneal catheter can be determined on later films (more important in growing children).

Distal slits on the peritoneal catheter may increase the risk of distal obstruction,[53] and some authors recommend that they be trimmed off. Wire reinforced catheters should not be used because of excessively high rate of viscus perforation, and this tubing was designed to prevent kinking which is not a problem with modern shunts.

Open technique

A vertical incision lateral and superior to the umbilicus is one of several choices. The following layers should be identified as they are traversed to avoid confusing preperitoneal fat with omentum and erroneously placing the tip in the preperitoneal space:
1. subcutaneous fat
2. anterior sheath of the abdominis rectus muscle (anterior rectus sheath)
3. abdominis rectus muscle fibers: should be split longitudinally
4. posterior rectus sheath
5. preperitoneal fat (may be very well developed in a few individuals, but is essentially nonexistent in most)
6. peritoneum (usually closely adherent to the posterior rectus sheath)

Trocar technique

1. place a Foley catheter to decompress the bladder
2. 1 cm skin incision above and lateral to the umbilicus
3. pull abdominal skin anteriorly (away from patient)
4. insert trocar aiming toward the ipsilateral iliac crest
5. feel 2 "pops" of penetration: 1 = anterior rectus sheath, 2 = posterior rectus sheath/peritoneum
6. peritoneal catheter should feed easily through trocar
7. ✖ contraindications: prior abdominal surgery, extremely overweight patients

VP shunt, post-op orders (adult)

1. flat in bed (to avoid overshunting and possible subdural hematoma) with gradual mobilization
2. if peritoneal end is new or revised, do not feed until bowel sounds resume (usually at least 24 hrs, due to ileus from manipulation of peritoneum)
3. shunt series (AP & lateral skull, and chest/abdominal x-ray) as baseline for future comparison (some surgeons obtain these films immediately post-op in case some immediate revision is indicated, e.g. ventricular catheter tip in temporal horn)

Ventriculopleural shunt insertion

See reference.[54]

97

See also more details (p.416). Not for age ≤ 7 years. A 3 cm horizontal incision is made just below the level of the breast either in the midclavicular line or in the anterior axillary line. Divide the subcutaneous tissue, deep fascia, and pectoralis muscle. The external and internal intercostal muscles are divided along the *superior* margin of the inferior of the two ribs exposed (to avoid the neurovascular bundle running along the inferior margin of each rib). A self retaining retractor between the ribs aids the exposure. The parietal pleura is visualized with the visceral pleura sliding underneath with each respiration. The pleura is not opened until the catheter is brought out subcutaneously at this incision. Have the anesthesiologist hold respirations, and nick the parietal pleura (or use a blunt-tip hemostat to pop through) to admit the catheter. Allow the lung to drop away and insert 20–40 cm of tubing into the pleural cavity. If the pleural opening is lax around the catheter, it can be snugged with a 4–0 absorbable suture. Have the anesthesiologist provide a valsalva maneuver before cinching down the pleural suture, and again before closing the deep muscle layer. A chest tube is usually not required. A maneuver that may sometimes be helpful is to place a red-rubber catheter next to the shunt tube at the same time (to permit the escape of air from the pleural space). Begin closing, but prior to placing the last deep suture, have the anesthesiologist perform a valsalva maneuver and allow air to escape through the red-rubber catheter (you can place the end in saline to see the bubbles). Once the bubbles stop, pull the red-rubber catheter and close the last stitch. If the bubbles don't stop, there is an air leak in the visceral pleura and a pigtail catheter or a chest tube connected to a Pleur-evac® should be used.

Ventriculo-atrial shunt insertion

Open method

The common facial vein (CFV) is located by making a diagonal cervical incision across the anterior border of the sternocleidomastoid at or just below the level of the angle of the mandible (the CFV may be as far as ≈ 2 cm below this point). The platysma is divided, and the CFV is located as it joins the internal jugular vein (IJV) at the level of the hyoid bone. The CFV is cannulated with the atrial tubing, and is secured with a snug ligature close to the junction with the IJV. If the CFV is not suitable, a purse string suture is placed directly in the IJV, and the IJV is then opened in the center of the purse string and cannulated.

Percutaneous method

May be utilized in adults (and possibly peds). The IJV is catheterized using the Seldinger technique[55] with a guide-wire and needle through a stab wound at the anterior margin of the SCM. Fluoroscopy is used to place the tip of the wire at the desired location (see below). A No. 13 French peel-away introducer and dilator are then inserted over the wire, which is then bent at the skin edge and withdrawn[56] (for a pediatric case: may use a No. 7 French introducer with a 1.5 mm O.D. *lumboperitoneal* catheter for the distal atrial catheter). The atrial catheter is cut to the length of the wire distal to the bend, and the catheter is then threaded into the introducer. The position of the catheter tip should again be confirmed (e.g. with radio-opaque contrast under fluoroscopy). A short skin incision is then made starting at the point where the catheter penetrates the skin to permit subcutaneous tunneling of the tubing.

Location of distal tip

Placement pointer: if the catheter repeatedly goes down the wrong vessel (e.g. the subclavian vein), a "J" guidewire may help. Also, rotating the head to a more neutral position sometimes works.

97

The ideal location of the distal tip is in the right atrium (unlike the location for central catheters in the superior vena cava (SVC)) so that the turbulent blood flow will reduce the risk of thrombus formation. The tip may enter the right atrium, but must not penetrate the tricuspid valve. A number of methods for optimal placement of the distal shunt tip may be employed, and include:

1. using an intraoperative chest x-ray to locate the tip between the level of T6-T8 vertebra in an adult. In a growing child, initially insert to ≈ T10 level. This method is subject to error due to malalignment of the x-ray beam (parallax error)
2. locating the tip near the level described above, then inject iodinated contrast, e.g. 20 ml of Omnipaque 180 (iohexol) (p.219) under intraoperative fluoroscopy to locate the tip in SVC
3. fill the catheter with normal or 3% saline and use the catheter as an EKG electrode. The P-wave changes from a downward to a biphasic morphology as the tip enters the atrium. A sharp upward deflection occurs as the tricuspid valve is approached.[57] Some recommend advancing the tip to maximal P-wave amplitude and then backing off a centimeter or two
4. fill the catheter with heparinized saline (1–5 U per cc NS) and measure the pressure as the tip is advanced,[58] leave tip just short of where atrial pressure tracing occurs
5. utilizing intraoperative echocardiography[59]

A growing patient is followed with annual CXRs. When the catheter tip is above ≈ T4, the catheter must be lengthened or converted to a VP shunt.

97.6.4 Third ventriculostomy

General information

See also indications and complications (p.415).

Older techniques include a subfrontal approach, opening the chiasmatic and lamina terminalis cisterns, and making a 5–10 mm opening in the lamina terminalis. Stereotactic third ventriculostomy (using contrast ventriculography[60] or CT guided) has also been described. Current technique, endoscopic third ventriculostomy (ETV) often with assistance of image-guidance consists of fenestrating the floor of the third ventricle using a ventriculoscope.

Ventriculoscopic technique

1. equipment: requires a rigid endoscope (does not work well with flexible)
2. image guided stereotactic technology helps immensely with the trajectory, but once you've entered the third ventricle, you must navigate by visual landmarks and cannot rely on image guidance because of the limitations of the accuracy
3. burr hole: 2–3 cm lateral to the midline just anterior to the coronal suture (Kocher's point)
4. pass through the foramen of Monro and fixate the sheath just within the third ventricle
5. the floor of the third ventricle is inspected and must be thin enough and translucent enough to permit visualization of the basilar artery and mammillary bodies. If these structures cannot be visualized then the procedure should be aborted
6. the location of the opening is chosen:
   a) in the midline (avoids p-comm and PCA)
   b) in the region of the tuber cinereum (prominence of the base of the hypothalamus, extending ventrally into the infundibulum and pituitary stalk)
   c) posterior to the infundibular recess
   d) anterior to the mammillary bodies
   e) anterior to the tip of the basilar artery
7. an effective technique consists of "rubbing through" the floor of the third ventricle either with a probe or Decq forceps. Alternatively, hydrodissection or bipolar electrocautery may be used to thin down the lamina. ✖ Do not use laser due to possibility of injury to basilar artery![61]
8. the opening can be enlarged with the Decq forceps, or a 3 french use of a Fogarty balloon or a double balloon (Fogarty or Neuroballoon™ catheter (Integra LifeSciences 7CBD10)). The balloon is inflated distal to the opening in the floor and is then withdrawn through the opening
9. the opening does not need to be large (unlike e.g. fenestrating an arachnoid cyst): ≈ 4–5 mm is usually adequate[62,63]
10. after penetrating through the floor of the third ventricle, make certain that you can see vessels (sometimes the arachnoid is not perforated, or there is a second membrane or webs of membranes that need to be lysed)
11. consider injection of diluted iohexol or other intrathecal contrast agent into the lateral/third ventricle (see ventriculogram) prior to removal of scope. CT head 1 hour after surgery will show diffuse subarachnoid contrast in cisterns and over convexity if ETV successful
12. sagittal T2 weighted, thin-slice sequence will show drop out of T2 signal at stoma of ETV

97.6.5 LP shunt placement

Technique of insertion

See reference.[64]

1. position: lateral decubitus position, both knees flexed (right side up preferred)
2. prep back, flank and abdomen
3. 1 cm skin incision over L4–5 or L5-S1 (in obese patients, use larger skin incision carried down to fascia overlying spinous processes. This may also be superficially incised between spinous processes to aid insertion)
4. tilt table to 30° reverse-Trendelenburg to expand lumbar subarachnoid space
5. insert 14 gauge Tuohy needle into subarachnoid space, with opening directed rostrally (caudal placement also acceptable). Confirm placement by CSF flow
6. remove trocar, insert shunt tubing such that ≤ 8 cm of catheter (for L4–5 insertion) lies within spinal canal (minimizes conus medullaris irritation)
7. needle then withdrawn over catheter

8. make flank incision, pass tunneler from flank to back incision. Feed catheter from back to flank. Withdraw tunneler over catheter
9. abdominal placement:
   a) open: incision made through peritoneum. Catgut (or other absorbable suture) purse-string placed in peritoneal opening
   b) trocar
10. pass tunneler from abdominal incision to flank incision. Feed catheter from flank to abdomen. Withdraw tunneler over catheter
11. verify CSF flow. Place catheter inside peritoneum. For open technique: cinch purse-string snugly, but loose enough to allow catheter to slide with gentle pushing
12. snug fitting retaining sleeve placed around catheter at all three incisions, and secured to subcutaneous tissue with non-absorbable suture

Lumboperitoneal (LP) shunt evaluation

When problems develop, evaluation of function may be more difficult than with VP shunt. Evaluation may include:
1. abdominal x-rays: AP & lateral x-rays can rule out breakage or migration of a shunt component
2. noncontrast brain CT scan: can rule-out complication such as subdural hematoma
3. LP: perform LP just above or below level of lumbar catheter. The pressure may be 0 or negative, and it may be necessary to aspirate CSF to confirm placement
   a) can give indirect evidence of shunt function by measuring the CSF pressure, which should be low if the shunt is working (only helpful in cases where the shunt was placed for elevated CSF pressure, e.g. pseudotumor cerebri; not helpful in NPH).
   b) "shunt-o-gram": inject contrast into subarachnoid space through LP needle
      - radionuclide (p.421): inject radio-isotope via LP and look for subsequent tracer activity in peritoneal cavity
      - with water-soluble contrast[65]: inject 10 ml of iohexol and monitor the flow of contrast fluoroscopically as the patient is brought vertical. Coughing or valsalva maneuver will accelerate the flow of contrast
4. shunt tap: if an antechamber has been installed, it is accessed after cleaning the skin with antiseptic using a 22 Ga. or smaller needle placed perpendicular to the dome to prevent leakage. If there is no access chamber, it is sometimes possible to tap the tubing itself with a 27 gauge butterfly needle

97.7 Ventricular access device

97.7.1 General information

An indwelling ventricular catheter connected to a reservoir that is situated under the scalp for the purpose of chronic access to the intrathecal space (usually the ventricular system), or sometimes other intracranial compartments such as tumor cysts. Sometimes referred to as an Ommaya® reservoir, this is actually a trade name.

97.7.2 Indications

1. administration of intrathecal (IT) antineoplastic chemotherapy:
   a) for CNS neoplasms, including: carcinomatous meningitis, methotrexate for CNS lymphoma or leukemia (p.713)
   b) IT chemotherapy is often used for the following even in the absence of CNS involvement because of the high relapse rate in the CNS: acute lymphoblastic leukemia, lymphoblastic lymphoma, Burkitt's lymphoma
2. administration of intrathecal antibiotic for chronic meningitis
3. chronic removal of CSF from infants with intraventricular hemorrhage
4. for fluid aspiration from a chronic tumor cyst that is resistant to therapy (radiation or surgery)

Booking the case: Ventricular access device

Also see defaults & disclaimers (p. 27).

1. position: supine
2. equipment
   a) endoscopic display (e.g. if NeuroPen is used)
   b) C-arm (optional) to verify position of ventricular catheter
   c) image guided navigation system (infrequently used)
3. implants: need to specify reservoir manufacturer
4. consent (in lay terms for the patient – not all-inclusive):
   a) procedure: surgery to insert a tube into the fluid space within the brain (ventricle) which is connected to a port under the skin so that fluids can be removed or injected (usually medication)
   b) alternatives: sometimes fluid can be removed and medication can be injected using a lumbar puncture (spinal tap). The effectiveness of this may not be the same as the operation being discussed here
   c) complications: infection, suboptimal position which might require re-operation, subdural hematoma, bleeding in the brain, this is a mechanical device and may eventually fail (break, block up...) and need repair/replacement

97.7.3 Technique of insertion

See reference.[66]

Preferably placed in the right frontal region, unless indicated otherwise (e.g. for tumor cyst). Usually placed under endotracheal general anesthesia, although local anesthesia occasionally may be used (e.g. for patients too ill to tolerate general anesthesia).

Patient position: supine, head midline, neck flexed 5°.

Incision: inverted "U", slightly larger than the reservoir (the original Ommaya® reservoir is 3.4 cm diameter), with the center over the coronal suture approximately 3 cm from midline, roughly centered near Kocher's point (p. 1512). A circle of pericranium of diameter equal to that of the reservoir is excised and saved. Alternatively, the pericranium may be flapped separately in the opposite direction (i.e. a right-side-up "U"), and closed over the reservoir to help secure it in position.

Make a burr hole over the coronal suture 3 cm off midline. A cruciate incision in the dura is made large enough to visualize the cortical surface, minimal cortical bipolar coagulation is used, and a pial/cortical incision is made to avoid surface vessels.

One may inject 15–20 cc of filtered air into the ventricles with a ventricular needle prior to the catheter insertion to guide the tip of the catheter with intra-operative lateral skull x-rays (intraoperative pneumoencephalogram). The trajectory is towards a point intersecting a plane 2 cm anterior to the EAM aiming minimally towards the midline (1–2°). Alternatively, one may aim perpendicular to the surface of the skull.[49] A total length of ≈ 7.25 cm of catheter is fixed to the base of the reservoir which allows the catheter to lie on the floor of the anterior horn of the lateral ventricle in most adults. This location can be verified with intraoperative pneumoencephalography[66] or with ventriculoscopic techniques.

The excised pericranium is placed over the dura, and the reservoir is sutured to the pericranium. Note: the dome of the original Ommaya® reservoir has a low resistance, and may be easily collapsed if too much tension is placed on the overlying scalp. If early use of the reservoir is desired (i.e. within 48 hrs post-op), the skin closure should be performed with a running nonabsorbable suture (e.g. nylon) and coated with collodion, and the surgical site can then be left without a gauze dressing for easier access to the reservoir. A skin tattoo can be created over the center of the reservoir (to assist in localizing the reservoir for injection) using India ink and a pricking the skin with a sterile needle.

97.7.4 Reservoir puncture

The scalp is prepped with antimicrobial scrub, and using sterile technique, a 25 gauge or smaller butterfly needle is introduced at an oblique angle, preferably with a non-coring needle. The original (Ommaya®) reservoir has firm plastic bottom surface which can be penetrated if too much force is applied.

97.8 Sural nerve biopsy

97.8.1 General information

Although a number of peripheral nerves may be biopsied, the sural nerve fulfills the criteria of being well studied, expendable with minimal deficit, easily accessible, and often involved in the pathologic process in question.

97.8.2 Indications

Nerve biopsy plays a small role in diagnosing peripheral neuropathies, but may be very accurate for vasculitis, amyloidosis, Hansen's disease, metachromatic and globoid leukodystrophy, neoplastic infiltration of peripheral nerve, and relapsing polyneuritis.[67(p 316)] May help distinguish the two types of Charcot-Marie-Tooth syndrome. May show demyelination in diabetic amyotrophy (p.545). The yield of sural nerve biopsy may be low if it is normal on nerve conduction testing. Disadvantages of the sural nerve is that it will usually be spared in purely motor neuropathies.

97.8.3 Risks of procedure

1. sensory loss in the sural nerve distribution is expected, but often does not persist for more than several weeks (unless the underlying disease process prevents this)
2. problems with wound healing: the ankle is a notorious region for poor circulation and the loss of sensation (from the disease or biopsy) may render the area subject to repeated trauma without the patient being aware. Furthermore, many patients with an undiagnosed systemic disease requiring a sural nerve biopsy will have poor wound healing (a significant number are also diabetic)
3. failure to make a diagnosis: although biopsy may be able to exclude some contingencies, it often does not make a specific diagnosis

97.8.4 Applied anatomy

The sural nerve is formed by the merging of the distal portion of the medial sural cutaneous nerve (one of the terminal branches of the tibial nerve) and the anastomotic ramus of the common peroneal nerve. It is entirely sensory except for some unmyelinated autonomic fibers. It supplies cutaneous sensation to the posterolateral third of the leg, the lateral heel and foot, and the little toe. At the level of the ankle it lies between the Achilles tendon and the lateral malleolus. This location is constant, superficial, and relatively protected from external trauma which might otherwise confuse the analysis.

97.8.5 Technique

Modified technique.[68(p 771–2)] Usually done under local anesthesia with sedation. Side to biopsy: if one leg shows more involvement, that is often the preferred side to biopsy.

Position: patient prone. If patient is not under general anesthesia, use 3/4 oblique (not prone) pillow between the legs. The leg to be biopsied is uppermost and is flexed 90° at the knee to relax tension on the nerve, the ankle is slightly everted. Compressing the calf (can be done using a sterile Penrose drain as a temporary tourniquet during surgery) distends the lesser saphenous vein (LSV) at the lateral malleolus (LM), which (when visible) reliably locates the sural nerve usually deep and anterior to the vein.

97

After prepping, drape the limb with a sterile stockinette or similar drape, infiltrate local anesthetic subcutaneously just posterior to the LM and proximally, paralleling the Achilles tendon for ≈ 10 cm. A 7–10 cm incision is made overlying the course of the LSV beginning usually just posterior to and ≈ 1 cm proximal to the LM. The vein can be seen through the translucent Scarpa's fascia. The fascia is incised over the vein which is gently retracted to reveal the nerve usually deep to the vein. A common pitfall is to go too deep, the nerve is fairly superficial; it is not necessary to go through the thick fascia. If at any time you see tendons to the toes, you have gone too deep.

To differentiate the sural nerve from the LSV (which may resemble the nerve in some cases): the nerve has many branches at acute angles especially proximal to the LM, vs. the vein which has right angle branches. If in doubt, a frozen section may be helpful to verify that the biopsied structure is a nerve in order to avoid potentially embarrassing explanations and the possible need to repeat the procedure.

After exposing at least 3–5 cm of the nerve, anesthetize the proximal portion with 0.5% lidocaine using a 27 Ga. needle and cut it sharply just distal to the infiltration site (note: sometimes a biopsy of only a portion of the nerve's fascicles may suffice: this is accomplished by opening the epineurium for the length of the exposure and teasing out a fascicle with minimal branching). Cut the nerve with slight tension on it to allow the ends to retract deep to the skin incision to prevent the formation of a scar neuroma. Some pathologists request that the proximal end of the nerve be marked, e.g. with a suture.

If it is desired to obtain a biopsy of the sural nerve higher up for comparison, it may be accessed in the mid upper calf between the heads of the gastrocnemius muscle. Here it may be as deep as ≈ 2 cm. Gently tugging on the exposed nerve in the ankle may help in localization.

A dissolvable subcuticular closure may be used. Generous padding should be placed over the incision to protect it from bumps (since many patients are numb from the pathology and/or surgery, there is increased risk of inadvertent surgical wound injuries). An elastic pressure dressing is applied after closure.

97.8.6 Nerve handling

For light microscopy which suffices in most cases, immerse the nerve in formalin. For electron microscopy, glutaraldehyde is used. For biochemical and immunofluorescence studies, use rapid freezing.

97.8.7 Post-op care

Pressure dressing should be worn for protection for two weeks. The patient is allowed to walk but should restrict their activity for 2–3 days. If nonabsorbable sutures are used instead of subcuticular closure, they should be left in place 10–14 days.

97.9 Nerve blocks

Also see Occipital nerve block (p. 516).

97.9.1 Stellate ganglion block

General information

✖ Do not perform stellate ganglion block bilaterally (can cause bilateral laryngeal paralysis → respiratory compromise). Stellate ganglion is actually closer to C7 than C6, but risks at C7 are much higher (closer to pleura → pneumothorax, vertebral artery → arterial injection → seizures and/or hematoma, recurrent laryngeal nerve → unilateral vocal cord paralysis → hoarseness (common), brachial plexus → UE weakness). Other complications: intradural injection → spinal anesthesia, phrenic nerve block.

Technique

Patient supine; interscapular roll; head tilted backward, mouth slightly open to relax strap muscles. Displace SCM and carotid sheath laterally, insert 1.5 inch 22 Ga. needle to contact Chassaignac's tubercle (anterior tubercle of transverse process of C6) AKA carotid tubercle (the most prominent in the C-spine) usually at the level of the cricoid cartilage, approximately 1.5–2 inches above clavicle.

Withdraw needle 1–2 mm and aspirate (do not inject intravascularly). Inject small test dose, then full 10 ml of 0.5% bupivacaine (Marcaine®) or 20 ml of 1% lidocaine. Remove needle and elevate patient's head on pillow to facilitate spread.

Verify block by Horner's syndrome, and anhidrosis and increased warmth of ipsilateral hand.

97.9.2 Lumbar sympathetic block

Technique

Patient prone on fluoro table. Use local anesthetic to allow insertion of 20–22 gauge spinal needles (10 to 12.5 cm long) at L2, L3 and L4 levels. Needle inserted 4.5–5 cm lateral to spinous process until transverse process contacted, then redirected caudally and inserted to a depth 3.5–4 cm deeper than transverse process. Final needle tip position should be just anterolateral to vertebral bodies. At each level, instill ≈ 8 ml of 1% lidocaine local after verifying that nothing can be aspirated.

Keep patient on bed rest for several hours, then ambulate with assist; watch for orthostatic hypotension due to vascular pooling in blocked lower extremity.

97.9.3 Intercostal nerve block

Indications

1. postthoracotomy pain
2. intercostal neuralgia
3. postherpetic neuralgia
4. pain from rib fractures

General principles

In order to obtain good anesthesia, the following should be noted:

1. a good site for injection is in the *posterior axillary line* (PAL) because
   a) this is proximal to the origin of the lateral cutaneous nerve (which originates ≈ in the anterior axillary line)
   b) this avoids the scapula for nerves above ≈ T7
   c) this reduces the risk of pneumothorax from injecting closer to the spine (the latter requires a longer needle path and there is increased difficulty palpating landmarks)
2. due to overlap, at least 3 intercostal nerves usually need to be blocked to achieve at least some area of anesthesia; it is usually necessary to block 1–2 intercostal nerves both above and below the affected dermatome
3. the intercostal nerves lie on the undersurface of the corresponding rib in close proximity to the pleura; the order of structures from top down is: rib, vein, artery, nerve

Technique

1. after raising a skin wheal at the desired level in the PAL, insert a 22 Ga. or smaller needle directly against the rib
2. walk the needle down the rib millimeter by millimeter until the needle just slips under the rib; to avoid pleural puncture, do not advance the needle more than one-eighth inch deep to the anterior surface of the rib
3. aspirate to be certain that there is no air (from lung penetration) or blood (from entering the intercostal artery or vein)
4. if no air or blood returns, inject 3–5 ml of local anesthetic
5. if there is any question about lung penetration, obtain a portable CXR to R/O pneumothorax

References

[1] Navarro IM, Renteria JAG, Peralta VHR, et al. Transorbital Ventricular Puncture for Emergency Ventricular Decompression. J Neurosurg. 1981; 54:273–274
[2] Brem SS, Hafler DA, Van Uitert RL, et al. Spinal Subarachnoid Hematoma: A Hazard of Lumbar Puncture Resulting in Reversible Paraplegia. N Engl J Med. 1981; 303:1020–1021
[3] Hollis PH, Malis LI, Zappulla RA. Neurological Deterioration After Lumbar Puncture Below Complete Spinal Subarachnoid Block. J Neurosurg. 1986; 64:253–256
[4] Reimann AE, Anson BJ. Vertebral Level of Termination of the Spinal Cord with a Report of a Case of Sacral Cord. Anat Rec. 1944; 88
[5] Antoni N. Pressure Curves from the Cerebrospinal Fluid. Acta Med Scand Suppl. 1946; 170:439–462
[6] Bono F, Lupo MR, Serra P, Cantafio C, et al. Obesity does not induce abnormal CSF pressure in subjects with normal cerebral MR venography. Neurology. 2002; 59:1641–1643
[7] Adams RD, Victor M. Principles of Neurology. 2nd ed. New York: McGraw-Hill; 1981
[8] Fishman RA. Cerebrospinal Fluid in Diseases of the Nervous System. Philadelphia: W. B. Saunders; 1980
[9] Wiesel J, Rose DN, Silver AL, et al. Lumbar Puncture in Asymptomatic Late Syphilis. An Analysis of the Benefits and Risks. Arch Intern Med. 1985; 145:465–468
[10] Fishman RA. Cerebrospinal Fluid in Diseases of the Nervous System. Philadelphia: W. B. Saunders; 1992
[11] Sathi S, Stieg PE. "Acquired" Chiari I Malformation After Multiple Lumbar Punctures: Case Report. Neurosurgery. 1993; 32:306–309
[12] Stern WE. Localization and Diagnosis of Spinal Cord Tumors. Clin Neurosurg. 1977; 25:480–494
[13] DeSousa AL, Kalsbeck JE, Mealey J, et al. Intraspinal Tumors in Children. A Review of 81 Cases. J Neurosurg. 1979; 51:437–445
[14] McDonald JV, Klump TE. Intraspinal Epidermoid Tumors Caused by Lumbar Puncture. Arch Neurol. 1986; 43:936–939
[15] Pavlin J, McDonald JS, Child B, Rusch V. Acute Subdural Hematoma: An Unusual Sequela to Lumbar Puncture. Anesthesiology. 1979; 52:338–340
[16] Rudehill A, Gordon E, Rahu T. Subdural Hematoma: A Rare but Life Threatening Complication After Spinal Anesthesia. Acta Anaesthesiol Scand. 1983; 17:376–377
[17] Sundberg A, Wang LP, Fog J. Influence of hearing of 22 G Whitacre and 22 G Quincke needles. Anaesthesia. 1992; 47:981–983
[18] Michel O, Brusis T. Hearing Loss as a Sequel of Lumbar Puncture. Ann Otol Rhinol Laryngol. 1992; 101:390–394
[19] Kestenbaum A. Clinical Methods of Neuroophthalmologic Examination. 2nd ed. New York: Grune and Stratton; 1961
[20] Wilder-Smith E, Kothbauer-Margreiter I, Lämmle B, et al. Dural Puncture and Activated protein C Resistance: Risk Factors for Cerebral Venous Sinus Thrombosis. J Neurol Neurosurg Psychiatry. 1997; 63:351–356

[21] Duffy GP. Lumbar Puncture in the Presence of Raised Intracranial Pressure. Brit Med J. 1969; 1:407–409
[22] Korein J, Cravioto H, Leicach M. Reevaluation of Lumbar Puncture: A Study of 129 Patients with Papilledema or Intracranial Hypertension. Neurology. 1959; 9:290–297
[23] Mokri B. Orthostatic headaches in the syndrome of the trephined: resolution following cranioplasty. Headache. 2010; 50:1206–1211
[24] DiGiovanni AJ, Dunbar BS. Epidural Injections of Autologous Blood for Postlumbar-Puncture Headache. Anesth and Analg. 1970; 49:268–271
[25] Seebacher J, Ribeiro V, Le Guillou JL, et al. Epidural Blood Patch in the Treatment of Post Dural Puncture Headache: A Double Blind Study. Headache. 1989; 29:630–632
[26] Lance JW, Branch GB. Persistent Headache After Lumbar Puncture. Lancet. 1994; 343
[27] Gass H, Goldstein AS, Ruskin R, et al. Chronic Postmyelogram Headache. Arch Neurol. 1971; 25:168–170
[28] Evans RW, Armon MD, Frohman MHS, Goodin DS. Assessment: prevention of post-lumbar puncture headaches: report of the therapeutics and technology assessment subcommittee of the American Academy of Neurology. Neurology. 2000; 55:909–914
[29] Tourtellotte WW, Henderson WG, Tucker RP, et al. A Randomized, Double Blind Clinical Trial Comparing the 22 Versus 26 Gauge Needle in the Production of the Post-Lumbar Puncture Syndrome in Normal Individuals. Headache. 1972; 12:73–78
[30] Mihic DN. Postspinal Headache and Relationship of Needle Bevel to Longitudinal Dural Fibres. Reg Anesth. 1985; 10:76–81
[31] Kuntz KM, Kokmen E, Stevens JC, et al. Post-Lumbar Puncture Headaches: Experience in 501 Consecutive Procedures. Neurology. 1992; 42
[32] Carson D, Serpell M. Choosing the Best Needle for Diagnostic Lumbar Puncture. Neurology. 1996; 47:33–37
[33] Hilton-Jones D, Harrad RA, Gill MW, et al. Failure of Postural Maneuvers to Prevent Lumbar Puncture Headache. J Neurol Neurosurg Psychiatry. 1982; 45:743–746
[34] Carbaat PAT, van Crevel H. Lumbar Puncture Headache: Controlled Study on the Preventive Effect of 24 Hours Bed Rest. Lancet. 1981; 1:1133–1135
[35] Sechzer PH, Abel L. Post-Spinal Anesthesia Headache Treated with Caffeine: Evaluation with Demand Method. Part 1. Cur Ther Res. 1978; 24:307–312
[36] Murros K, Fogelholm R. Spontaneous Intracranial Hypotension with Slit Ventricles. J Neurol Neurosurg Psychiatry. 1983; 46:1149–1151
[37] Zivin JA. Lateral Cervical Puncture: An Alternative to Lumbar Puncture. Neurology. 1978; 28:616–618
[38] Penning L. Normal Movements of the Cervical Spine. AJR. 1978; 130:317–326
[39] Section of Pediatric Neurosurgery of the American Association of Neurological Surgeons. Pediatric Neurosurgery. New York 1982
[40] Rogers LA. Acute Subdural Hematoma and Death Following Lateral Cervical Spinal Puncture. J Neurosurg. 1983; 58:284–286
[41] Ward E, Orrison WW, Watridge CB. Anatomic Evaluation of Cisternal Puncture. Neurosurgery. 1989; 25:412–415
[42] Wilkins RH, Rengachary SS. Neurosurgery. New York 1985
[43] Tillmanns H. Something about puncture of the brain. Sheffield, England 1908
[44] Schmidek HH, Sweet WH. Operative Neurosurgical Techniques. New York 1982
[45] Becker DP, Nulsen FE. Control of Hydrocephalus by Valve-Regulated Venous Shunt: Avoidance of Complications in Prolonged Shunt Maintenance. J Neurosurg. 1968; 28:215–226
[46] Keskil SI, Ceviker N, Baykaner K, Alp H. Index for Optimum Ventricular Catheter Length: Technical Note. J Neurosurg. 1991; 75:152–153
[47] Davis JW, Davis IC, Bennink LD, Hysell SE, Curtis BV, Kaups KL, Bilello JF. Placement of intracranial pressure monitors: are "normal" coagulation parameters necessary? J Trauma. 2004; 57:1173–1177
[48] Le TV, Rumbak MJ, Liu SS, Alsina AE, van Loveren H, Agazzi S. Insertion of intracranial pressure monitors in fulminant hepatic failure patients: early experience using recombinant factor VII. Neurosurgery. 2010; 66:455–8; discussion 458
[49] Ghajar JBG. A Guide for Ventricular Catheter Placement: Technical Note. J Neurosurg. 1985; 63:985–986
[50] Mann KS, Yue CP, Ong GB. Percutaneous Sump Drainage: A Palliation for Oft-Recurring Intracranial Cystic Lesions. Surg Neurol. 1983; 19:86–90
[51] Chan KH, Mann KS. Prolonged Therapeutic External Ventricular Drainage: A Prospective Study. Neurosurgery. 1988; 23:436–438
[52] Couldwell WT, LeMay DR, McComb JG. Experience with Use of Extended Length Peritoneal Shunt Catheters. J Neurosurg. 1996; 85:425–427
[53] Cozzens JW, Chandler JP. Increased Risk of Distal Ventriculoperitoneal Shunt Obstruction Associated With Slit Valves or Distal Slits in the Peritoneal Catheter. J Neurosurg. 1997; 87:682–686
[54] McComb JG, Scott RM. In: Techniques for CSF Diversion. Hydrocephalus. Baltimore: Williams and Wilkins; 1990:47–65
[55] Seldinger SI. Catheter replacement of the needle in percutaneous arteriography. A new technique. Acta Radiol. 1953; 39:368–376
[56] Harrison MJ, Welling BG, DuBois JJ. A new method for inserting the atrial end of a ventriculoatrial shunt. technical note. J Neurosurg. 1996; 84:705–707
[57] Robertson JT, Schick RW, Morgan F, et al. Accurate Placement of Ventriculo-Atrial Shunt for Hydrocephalus under Electrocardiographic Control. J Neurosurg. 1961; 18:255–257
[58] Cantu RC, Mark VH, Austen WG. Accurate Placement of the Distal End of a Ventriculo-Atrial Shunt Catheter Using Vascular Pressure Changes. J Neurosurg. 1967; 27:584–596
[59] Szczerbicki MR, Michalak M. Echocardiograhic Placement of Cardiac Tube in Ventriculoatrial Shunt. Technical Note. J Neurosurg. 1996; 85:723–724
[60] Hoffman HJ. Technical Problems in Shunts. Monogr Neural Sci. 1982; 8:158–169
[61] McLaughlin MR, Wahlig JB, Kaufmann AM, Albright AL. Traumatic Basilar Aneurysm After Endoscopic Third Ventriculostomy: Case Report. Neurosurgery. 1997; 41:1400–1404
[62] Grant JA, McLone DG. Third ventriculostomy; a review. Surg Neurol. 1997; 47:210–212
[63] Jones RF, Stening WA, Brydon M. Endoscopic third ventriculostomy. Neurosurgery. 1990; 26:86–91; discussion 91-2
[64] Spetzler R, Wilson CB, Schulte R. Simplified Percutaneous Lumboperitoneal Shunting. Surg Neurol. 1977; 7:25–29
[65] Ishiwata Y, Yamashita T, Ide K, et al. A new technique for percutanous study of lumboperitoneal shunt patency. J Neurosurg. 1988; 68:152–154
[66] Leavens ME, Aldama-Luebert A. Ommaya Reservoir Placement: Technical Note. Neurosurgery. 1979; 5:264–266
[67] Youmans JR. Neurological Surgery. Philadelphia 1990
[68] Dyck PJ, Thomas PK. Peripheral Neuropathy. 2nd ed. Philadelphia: W. B. Saunders; 1984

98 Functional Neurosurgery

For functional neurosurgery related to pain, see Pain procedures (p. 1541).

98.1 Deep brain stimulation

A variety of conditions may be treated including:

1. movement disorders
   a) Parkinson's disease: STN stimulation may be superior to best medical management[1,2] because of similar efficacy to levodopa with fewer side effects (primarily dyskinesias) (see below)
   b) dystonia (p. 1528)
   c) tremor (p. 1537)
2. epilepsy (p. 1554)
3. pain (p. 1550): response is variable, typically only 25–60% respond
4. potential uses
   a) psychiatric disorders: mainly
      - Tourette syndrome: thalamic & pallidal DBS (case reports[3,4])
      - obsessive compulsive disorders: anterior capsule and STN stimulation[5] and, recently, targets more posterior and rostral[6]
      - depression: subgenual cingulate gyrus[7] and anterior capsule stimulation[8]
   b) obesity[9]
   c) drug addiction[10]
   d) hypertension (case report of lowering BP in a patient who was being treated for pain[11])

98.2 Typical targets used in functional brain surgery

▶ Fig. 98.1 depicts relationships of typical targets to other structures and effects of DBS (or lesioning). This figure is intended for illustrative purposes only, and is not presented for purposes of performing surgical procedures.

98.3 Surgical treatment of Parkinson's disease

98.3.1 Historical background

Prior to the availability of effective medications, surgical procedures were developed to treat Parkinson's disease. An early procedure was ligation of the anterior choroidal artery. Due to variability in distribution, destruction often extended beyond the desired confines of the pallidum and the results were too unpredictable. Anterodorsal pallidotomy became an accepted procedure in the 1950's, but long-term improvement was mainly in rigidity, while tremor and bradykinesia did not improve.[12] The ventrolateral thalamus subsequently became the preferred target. Lesions there were most effective in diminishing tremor. In actuality, the tremor was often not the most debilitating symptom, particularly since it is a resting tremor at first (it may become more pervasive later). Bradykinesia and rigidity were frequently more problematic. Furthermore, the procedure only reduces tremor in the contralateral half of the body, and bilateral thalamotomies were not recommended due to an unacceptably high risk of post-op dysarthria and gait disturbance. Use of thalamotomy fell off dramatically in the late 1960's with the introduction of L-dopa.[13]

98.3.2 Current trends

However, at some point most patients will experience problematic side effects and/or resistance to treatment with antiparkinsonian drugs. This, together with recent refinements in surgical techniques resulting in improved outcomes have produced in a resurgence of interest in the operative treatment of Parkinson's disease. Tissue transplantation (e.g. with adrenal medullary tissue) appears to have only modest benefits (see below). Lesioning or stimulation techniques have therefore gained in popularity with renewed interest in the posteroventral pallidum as the target, which was actually pioneered by Leksell around the time that thalamotomy came into vogue.[12]

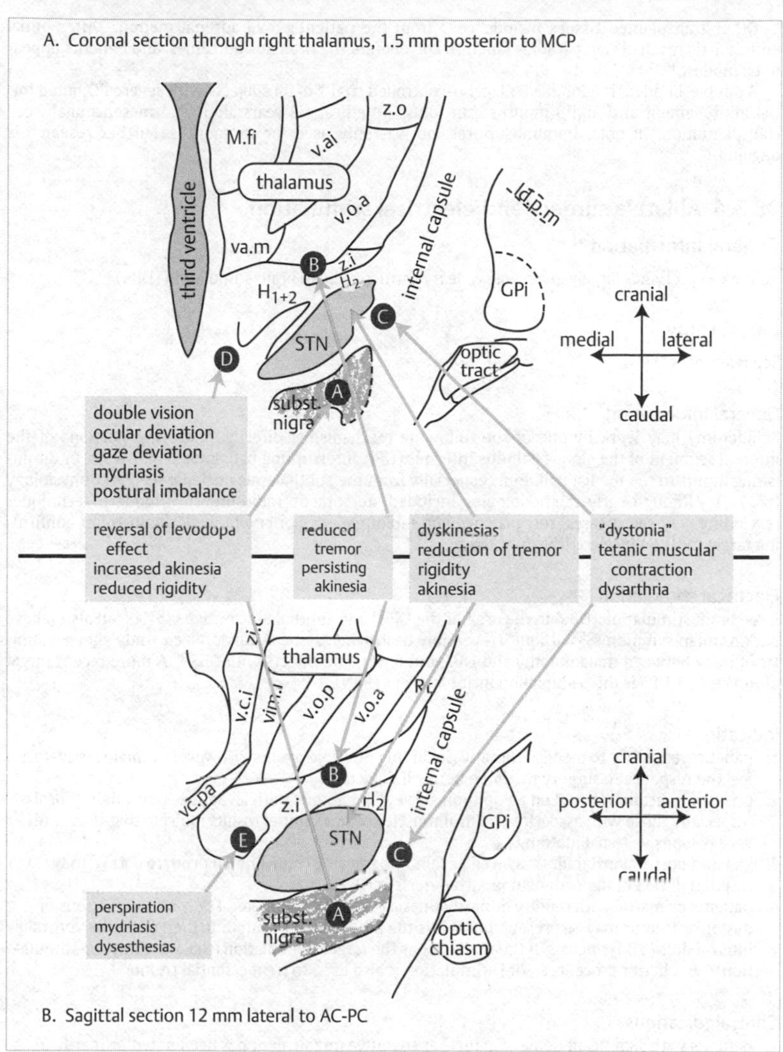

Fig. 98.1 Illustration of some targets for functional brain surgery
Abbreviations: AC = anterior commissure, GPi = globus pallidus interna, H_1 = Forel's H_1 field, MCP = midcommissural point (halfway between AC & PC), PC = posterior commissure, STN = subthalamic nucleus, subst.nigr = substantia nigra, z.i = zona incerta

98.3.3 Tissue transplantation

Tissue transplantation for Parkinson's disease is generally limited to research centers. The present status of implantation of fetal dopaminergic brain cells into Parkinson's disease patients is that it may reduce the severity of the illness and increase the effectiveness of levodopa.[14] For ethical reasons, this procedure is rarely performed in the U.S.

Other transplanted tissues include cells from the patient's own adrenal medulla. After initial enthusiastic results,[15] later studies failed to corroborate the dramatic outcomes, and benefits appear to be modest.[16,17,18]

A double-blinded, randomized, placebo-controlled trial[19] of 34 subjects with severe PD noted initial improvement at 6 and 9 months, but found no efficacy 2 years after fetal mesencephalic cell transplantation. Of note: immunosuppression was only used for six months. Further research is ongoing.[20]

98.3.4 Ablative surgery and electrical stimulation

General information

Ablative surgery has largely given way to less destructive beep brain stimulation (DBS).

Pallidotomy

See references.[21,22]

General information

Pallidotomy may work by one of the following mechanisms: directly destroying portions of the internal segment of the globus pallidus internus (GPi), interrupting pallidofugal pathways, or diminishing inputs to the medial pallidum (especially from the subthalamic nucleus; see Pathophysiology (p. 177)). Although early methodologies included stereotactic radiosurgery,[23] modern techniques (excluding very select cases) rely primarily on radiofrequency or cryoprobe lesioning after confirming target location by electrical stimulation.

Electrical stimulation

Deep brain stimulation (DBS) in the area of the GPi[24] and subthalamic nucleus (STN) can also relieve parkinsonian symptoms[25] without irreversibly destroying tissue. A randomized study showed similar efficacy between thalamotomy and DBS, but fewer side-effects with DBS.[26] A more recent target of interest for DBS is the pedunculopontine nucleus (PPN).

Indications

1. patients refractory to medical therapy (including multiple agents). However, some investigators feel the response to surgery might be better if done early
2. primary indication (based on an opinion survey[27]): patients with levodopa-induced dyskinesias (especially those with associated painful muscle spasms). Initial results indicate that these are very responsive to pallidotomy
3. gait and postural instability[28] as well as falls and freezing (non-human primate data)[29] may respond to DBS of the pedunculopontine nucleus (PPN)
4. patients primarily with rigidity or bradykinesia (unilateral or bilateral), on-off fluctuations or dystonia. Tremor may be present, but if it is the predominant symptom, then using the ventralis intermedius (VIM) nucleus of the thalamus as the target (for ablation (thalamotomy) or stimulation)[30] is a better procedure. VIM stimulation is also used to treat essential tremor[31]

Contraindications

98

1. patients with significant dementia: further cognitive impairment has been noted primarily in patients with cognitive deficits prior to treatment
2. patients with risk of intracerebral hemorrhage: those with coagulopathy, poorly controlled hypertension, those on anti-platelet drugs that cannot be withheld (may consider stereotactic radiosurgery lesions for these rare patients, see below)
3. patients with ipsilateral hemianopsia: due to the risk of post-op contralateral hemianopsia from optic tract injury which would make the patient blind
4. age ≥ 85 yrs
5. patients with secondary Parkinsonism (p. 177) i.e. *not* idiopathic Parkinson's disease: respond poorly, presumably due to different pathophysiology. Look for:
   a) signs of autonomic nervous system dysfunction (suggests Shy-Drager)
   b) EOM abnormalities (may occur in progressive supranuclear palsy (PSNP))
   c) long-tract signs
   d) cerebellar findings (as in olivo-ponto-cerebellar atrophy (OPCA))
   e) failure to improve with levodopa

f) MRI: lacunar infarcts in basal ganglia (as in arteriosclerotic Parkinsonism), or tumor in region of substantia nigra
g) PET scanning (if available): decreased striatal metabolism detected by deoxyglucose PET scan (suggests striato-nigral degeneration (SND))

Technique

General information

Antiparkinsonian medications are withheld the morning of the procedure to bring out symptoms. A stereotactic frame is applied under local anesthetic parallel to the orbitomeatal line (which aligns with the anterior-posterior commissural (AC-PC) line).

Radiologic target localization

May utilize: MRI, CT, and/or ventriculography. MRI is the most common imaging modality, and may best demonstrate the desired anatomy, but is susceptible to geometric distortion. Therefore many centers also utilize CT and/or ventriculography to supplement MRI. T1WI images are commonly employed, however some feel that optimal MRI imaging may be performed with gadolinium-enhanced axial and coronal projections using 1 mm slice intervals and a STIR or spoiled GRASS volume acquisition protocol.

The posterior commissure is the white-matter band at the level of the pineal that crosses at the posterior third ventricle.

The typical initial target[27] is shown in ▶ Table 98.1. Avoid encroachment on internal capsule (medial to GPi) and optic tract (inferior to GPi). Lesions of the subthalamic nucleus are associated with hemiballismus. An entry site is chosen from imaging studies, and is usually just anterior to the coronal suture and 15–20 mm lateral to the midline. A 4 mm twist drill hole is used. The trajectory should avoid midline venous structures, arterioles within sulci (therefore enter through a gyrus), and passage through the lateral ventricle.

Electrophysiologic target localization

Stimulation:

The patient must be awake for the procedure. For patients with dyskinesias that occur only following a dose of medication, their normal dose of medicine is given after imaging to bring out the symptoms for the procedure. Stimulation is required to verify the neurophysiologic target which varies between individuals. Macroelectrode stimulation may be done with the lesioning electrode. Impedance typically drops when a white matter tract is encountered. The impedance of the desired target is usually > 600 Ω. Stimulate with square wave at 1, 5, 50 and 100 Hz with voltage range of 0.5–3 volts (NB: above ≈ 2 V you may be seeing wide-field stimulation). Pallidum stimulation usually increases (but occasionally decreases) contralateral muscle tone. Also look for reduction of tremor or dyskinesia. Contralateral weakness or hypotonia indicates proximity to the internal capsule. Visual scotomata suggests stimulation of the optic tract.

Micro-electrode recording:

About half the institutions surveyed perform microelectrode recording, and half the remaining centers were considering starting it.

Lesioning

Kondziolka et al.[22] use a 1.1 mm diameter probe with a 3 mm exposed tip. A small lesion is made at 45°C for 30 seconds, before making the definitive lesion at 70–80°C for 60 seconds. The probe is withdrawn 3–4 mm and a second lesion is made. Lesions with cryoprobes may be associated with a higher incidence of intracerebral hemorrhage.

For the very rare patient in whom insertion of an electrode is contraindicated (e.g. refractory coagulopathy), lesioning may be done with stereotactic radiosurgery, however, this eliminates the

Table 98.1 Target for pallidotomy

Typical initial target	Median
1–3 mm anterior to the midpoint of the AC-PC line	2 mm
18–23 mm lateral[a]	21 mm
2–6 mm inferior	5 mm
[a]may be decreased in women (start at ≈ 19 mm), or increased when the 3rd ventricle is dilated	

critical ability to verify the site of the planned lesion electrophysiologically before a permanent lesion is made.

Unilateral pallidotomy produces primarily contralateral effects, although some ipsilateral changes occur. Bilateral procedures are usually staged separately with a 3–12 hiatus between sides. Although they can been done in one sitting, bilateral pallidotomies may carry an increased risk of speech difficulties and cognitive decline.

Results

At present, the major focus of therapy has been on improvement of motor symptoms. Although 97% of patients showed at least some improvement (some poor results may derive from inclusion of some patients with secondary Parkinsonism), in 17% the degree of improvement was graded as mild.

Significant reduction of levodopa induced dyskinesias occurred in 90%.Bradykinesia improved in 85%, rigidity in 75%, and tremor in 57%. Other areas of improvement include: speech, gait, posture, and reduction of on-off phenomenon and freezing. Although symptoms may be ameliorated, overall functional improvement may not be remarkable.[32]

Although dosages of antiparkinsonian medication are often reduced, continued medical therapy is usually required, and no change is made for at least 2 months following pallidotomy.

Indications are that beneficial surgical effects can last ≥ 5 years, with early failures possibly due to production of too small of a lesion, and late failures possibly due to progression of the disease.

Ongoing studies are investigating longer term results, microelectrode recording, alternate lesioning targets, the role of early surgery… Until more information is available, one cannot make any statements about the optimal target, localizing method, etc.

Complications

Visual field deficit occurs in 2.5% due to proximity of the optic tract to the globus pallidus. Hemiparesis may occur due to the nearby passage of the internal capsule. Intracerebral hemorrhage may also occur. Dysarthria occurs in ≈ 8%, but is usually temporary. Speech difficulties and also cognitive decline may be more risky when bilateral pallidotomies are performed at the same sitting.

Thalamic lesions

Lesioning the thalamic ventralis intermedius nucleus (VIM) nucleus reduces Parkinsonian tremor in > 85%. It can also be useful in the treatment of rigidity and drug induced dyskinesias by extending the lesioning anteriorly to include the ventral oralis. However thalamotomy does not improve symptoms of akinesia or bradykinesia and can result in worsening of gait symptoms or speech problems.

Subthalamotomy

Lesioning the subthalamic nucleus (STN) is classically associated with intractable hemiballism. There are few studies as a result, but the limited data suggests that selective lesioning in this region provides relief on par with pallidotomy. Postoperative hemichorea is a known complication but is generally transitory and mild.[33] DBS in this region may be a better option (p. 1524).

98.4 Dystonia

98

Pallidal stimulation is the primary surgical treatment for dystonia.[34] Response is better for primary dystonias, e.g. tardive dystonias than for secondary dystonias such as postanoxic, postencephalitic, perinatal and poststroke dystonias[34] (other targets need to be assessed).

For primary dystonias, the globus pallidus internus (GPi) is the most common primary target (► Fig. 98.1). Good results have also been reported with STN DBS.

98.5 Spasticity

98.5.1 General information

Results from lesions in upper motor neuron pathway, causing absence of inhibitory influence on alpha motor-neurons (αMN) (alpha spasticity) as well as on gamma motor neurons (intrafusal fibers) (gamma spasticity). Causes uninhibited reflex arc between αMN and Ia afferents from muscle spindles resulting in a hypertonic state of muscles with clonus, and sometimes with involuntary movements. Etiologies include: injury to cerebrum (e.g. stroke) or spinal cord (spasticity is an expected sequelae of spinal cord injury rostral to the conus medullaris), multiple sclerosis, and congenital abnormalities (e.g. cerebral palsy, spinal dysraphism).

98.5.2 Clinical

General information

Increased resistance to passive movement, hyperactive muscle stretch reflexes, simultaneous activation of antagonistic muscle groups, may occur spontaneously or in response to minimal stimuli. Characteristic postures include scissoring of legs or hyperflexion of thighs. May be painful, or may disrupt patient's ability to sit in wheelchair, lay in bed, drive modified vehicles, sleep, etc. May also promote development of decubitus ulcers. A spastic bladder will have low capacity and will empty spontaneously.

Spasticity is often exacerbated by same type of stimuli that aggravate autonomic hyperreflexia; see Autonomic hyperreflexia (p. 1020).

The onset of spasticity following spinal cord injury may be delayed for several days to months (the latency period is attributed to **"spinal shock"** (p. 931), during which time there is decreased tone and reflexes).[35] Onset of spasticity following spinal shock starts with increasing flexor synergistic activity over 3–6 mos, with more gradual increases of extensor synergy which ultimately predominates in most cases.

Some "beneficial" aspects of mild spasticity:

1. maintains muscle tone and therefore bulk: provides support for patient when sitting in wheelchair, helps prevent decubitus ulcers over bony prominences
2. muscle contractions may help prevent DVTs
3. may be useful in bracing

Grading spasticity

Assessment should be performed with patient supine and relaxed. The Ashworth scale (▶ Table 98.2) is commonly used for the clinical grading of the *severity* of spasticity. Many attempts have been made to quantitate spasticity electrodiagnostically, the most reliable has been H-reflex measurement.

98.5.3 Treatment

General information

Depends on extent of useful function (or potential for same) present in areas at and below the level where spasticity starts (complete spinal cord injuries usually have little function, whereas patients with MS may have significant function).

Medical treatment

1. "prevention": measures to decrease inciting stimuli (physical therapy to prevent joint damage, good skin & bladder care… see Autonomic hyperreflexia (p. 1020))
2. prolonged stretching (more than just range of motion): not only prevents joint and muscle contractures, but modulates spasticity
3. oral medications[37]; (see Surgical treatment (p. 1530) for intrathecal medications: few drugs are effective without significant undesirable side effects

Table 98.2 Ashworth scores[36]

Ashworth score	Degree of muscle tone
1	no increase in tone (normal)
2	slight increase, a "catch" with flexion or extension
3	more marked increase, passive movements easy
4	considerable increase, passive movements difficult
5	affected part rigid in flexion or extension

a) *diazepam* (Valium®): activates GABAA receptors, increases pre-synaptic inhibition of αMN. Most useful in patients with complete spinal cord injuries.
℞ start with 2 mg PO BID-TID, increase by 2 mg per day q 3 days up to a max of 20 mg TID.

Side effects: may cause sedation, weakness, decreased stamina (most of which may be minimized by gradual increases in dosage). Abrupt discontinuation may cause depression, seizures, withdrawal syndrome

a) *baclofen* (Lioresal®): activates presynaptic GABAB receptors of Ia muscle spindle afferents, causes pre-synaptic inhibition of αMN and decreases nociception. May be most useful in patients with spinal cord lesions (complete or incomplete).
℞ start with 5 mg PO BID-TID, increase in 5 mg increments q 3 days up to max of 20 mg QID. **Side effects:** sedation, lowers seizure threshold. Must be tapered to discontinue (abrupt discontinuation may result in seizures, rebound hyper-spasticity or hallucinations).
b) *dantrolene* (Dantrium®): reduces depolarization induced Ca^{++} influx into sarcoplasmic reticulum of skeletal muscle; acts on all skeletal muscle (with no preferential effect on spasmogenic reflex arc).
℞ start with 25 mg PO q d, increase q 4–7 days to BID, TID, then QID, then by 25 mg per day up to max of ≈ 100 mg QID (may take 1 week at new steady state to see effect); **Side effects:** muscle weakness (may make ambulation impossible), sedation, idiosyncratic hepatitis (may be fatal; more common in patients on > 300 mg/d x > 2 mos) that is often preceded by anorexia, abdominal pain, N/V; D/C if no benefit is seen by ≈ 45 days; follow LFTs (SGPT or SGOT)
c) progabide: activates both GABAA and GABAB receptors. Useful for patients with severe flexor spasms
d) theoretical benefits may be derived from other agents, but they have not been used for some practical reason in each case[35] (e.g. phenothiazines reduce gamma spasticity, but only at high PO doses or parenterally; clonidine; tetrahydrocannabinol…)

Surgical treatment

General information

Reserved for spasticity refractory to medical treatment, or where side effects of medications are intolerable. Generally either orthopedic (e.g. tendon release operations (tenotomies) of heel cord or hamstrings, iliopsoas myotomies, etc.) or neurosurgical (e.g. nerve blocks, neurectomies, myelotomy, etc.). Herz et al.[38] recommend percutaneous radiofrequency foraminal rhizotomy, usually with percutaneous radiofrequency sciatic neurectomy as the initial ablative procedure (see below).

1. nonablative procedures
   a) intrathecal (IT) baclofen (see below)
   b) intrathecal morphine (tolerance and dependence may develop)
   c) electrical stimulation via percutaneously placed epidural electrodes[39]
2. ablative procedures, with *preservation* of potential for ambulation
   a) motor point block[35] (intramuscular phenol neurolysis): preserves sensation and existing voluntary function. Especially useful in patients with incomplete myelopathies; time consuming
   b) phenol nerve block: similar to motor point block, but used when spasticity more severe and complete block of muscle desired. Open phenol block used instead of percutaneous when nerve is mixed and sensory preservation is desired (also reduces post-block dysesthesias)[40]
   c) selective neurectomies[35]
      - sciatic neurectomy (may be done with RF lesion)[38]
      - obturator neurectomy: useful if strong hip adductor spasticity that causes scissoring and wasted energy expenditure in ambulating
      - pudendal neurectomy: useful if excessive detrusor dyssynergy interferes with bladder retraining
   d) percutaneous radiofrequency foraminal rhizotomy: small unmyelinated sensory fibers are more sensitive to RF lesions than larger myelinated A-alpha fibers of motor units.
   Technique: start at S1 on one side, and work up to T12, then repeat on other side. At each level: verify needle position by stimulating with 0.1–0.5 V and watch for movement in appropriate myotome (tip should be extradural, avoid subarachnoid placement), ablate with 70–80° C × 2 mins for S1, and 70° C × 2 mins for L5 to T12 (to preserve motor function). If symptoms recur, may repeat with lesions at 90° C × 2 mins
   e) myelotomies[41]
      - Bischof's myelotomy: divides anterior and posterior horns via laterally placed incision, disrupts reflex arc. No effect on α-spasticity

98

- midline "T" myelotomy: interrupts reflex arc from sensory to motor units without disrupting connections from corticospinal tract to anterior motor neurons. Slightly higher risk of losing motor function.
  Technique: laminectomy from T11 to L1. Mobilize midline dorsal longitudinal vein and incise cord in midline from T12 at a depth of 3 mm to S1 at a depth of 4 mm (preserving S2-S4 maintains bladder reflex pathways. Unilateral extension up to conus medullaris reduces bladder spasticity and increases capacity before reflex emptying occurs)

f) selective dorsal rhizotomy[42,43]: uses intraoperative EMG and electrophysiological stimulation to eliminate sensory rootlets involved in "handicapping spasticity" (leaves rootlets subserving "useful spasticity" intact). Interrupts the afferent limb of pathologic reflex arc. May be temporary, but seems to persist at least ≈ 5 yrs. No effect on α-spasticity. Ambulatory children with cerebral palsy have improved gait, nonambulatory children are improved but are still not able to ambulate afterwards

g) stereotactic thalamotomy or dentatotomy: may be useful in cerebral palsy.[44] Useful for unilateral dystonia, but cannot be used for bilateral dystonia as bilateral lesions would be required which jeopardizes speech. Effective only for dystonia *distal* to shoulders or hips, and should not be used if the condition is rapidly progressive

3. ablative procedures, with *sacrifice* of potential for ambulation (in complete cord injuries, nonablative procedures are not indicated because there is no motor function to recover). Used after failure of percutaneous rhizotomy (see above) and "T" myelotomy (see above)
   a) intrathecal injection of 6 ml of 10% phenol (by weight) in glycerin mixed with 4 ml of iohexol (Omnipaque® 300) (p. 219) for a final concentration of 6% phenol and ≈ 120 mg iodine/ml. Administered via LP at L2–3 interspace with patient in lateral decubitus position (most symptomatic side down) under fluoro until T12-S1 nerve root sleeves are filled (sparing S2–4 for bladder function). Patient is maintained in this position × 20–30 mins and then kept sitting upright × 4 hrs[45] (absolute alcohol provides more permanent blocks, but is hypobaric and more difficult to control)
   b) selective anterior rhizotomy: results in flaccid paralysis with denervation atrophy of muscles
   c) neurectomies, often combined with tenotomies[38]
   d) intramuscular neurolysis by phenol injection[38]
   e) cordectomy[46]: most drastic measure, reserved for patients who do not respond to any other measure. Results in total flaccidity with loss of benefits from mild spasticity. Converts bladder from UMN to LMN control. Works well for progressive deficit from syringomyelia and for spasticity, but poor for "phantom" leg pain[47]
   f) cordotomy: rarely used

Intrathecal baclofen

See references.[48,49,50,51]

Selection criteria used in one study[50] are shown in ▶ Table 98.3. Other indications include: stroke,[52] cerebral palsy, TBI, dystonia, stiff-man syndrome.

Test doses: incremental test doses of 50, 75, and then 100 mcg intrathecal baclofen (ITB) via lumbar puncture or temporary catheter were used,[50] randomly alternated with placebo, with dose escalation halted if a response to active drug occurred. The following parameters were evaluated at 0.5, 1, 2, 4, 8 & 24 hrs post injection: pulse and respiratory rate, BP, hypertonia (Ashworth score, ▶ Table 98.2), reflexes, spasm score, voluntary muscle movement, and adverse effects (if any, including seizures). Pump implantation was offered if there was a 2 point reduction in the Ashworth score and muscle spasm score for ≥ 4 hrs after bolus injection of active drug without intolerable side effects. Usual daily dose for ITB is twice the test dose, typically 200 micrograms/d.

98

Table 98.3 Selection criteria for baclofen pump
• age 18–65 yrs (older patients treated on compassionate use basis) • able to give informed consent • severe, chronic spasticity (≥ 12 mos duration) due to spinal cord lesion or MS • spasticity refractory to oral drugs (including baclofen), or unacceptable side effects • no CSF block (e.g. on myelography) • positive response to IT baclofen at test dose ≤ 100 mcg and no response to placebo • no implanted programmable device such as cardiac pacemaker[a] • females of childbearing potential: not pregnant & using adequate contraception • no hypersensitivity (allergy) to baclofen • no history of stroke, impaired renal function, or severe hepatic or GI disease
[a]this study used a programmable IT pump

Alternatively, give 25 mcg IT in the O.R., and if the patient improves, insert subcutaneous pump.[37]

Pump systems: Available programmable systems include N'Vision, manufactured by Medtronic, Inc., Minneapolis, MN.

Insertion technique: IT catheter is typically inserted ≈ L2–3, and is threaded rostrally ≈ 3 levels, but should be no higher than T10 (risk of rostral progression of hypotonia).

Post-op orders: Guidelines for post-operative orders following baclofen pump insertion

1. admit PACU, transfer to:
   a) floor if insertion follows test dosing or if patient has just been transitioned from stable PO dose
   b) ICU if there has been a hiatus in baclofen therapy
2. neuro checks q 2 hrs for 1st 24 hours
3. baclofen:
   a) for patients on oral or IV baclofen: continue baclofen at the previous dose via the same route (oral or IV) until the ITB takes effect (usually 2–4 hrs, full effect is delayed up to 24 hrs). The IV/PO drug is then tapered
   b) if there has been a hiatus in baclofen therapy: baclofen 20 mg PO QID
4. have 2 vials of IV physostigmine available and labeled "FOR EMERGENCY USE ONLY" for possible baclofen overdose

Baclofen overdose:

ABCs (airway/breathing/circulation). Intubate if necessary

1. empty pump reservoir to stop drug flow (record amount withdrawn)
2. administer physostigmine if not contraindicated:
   a) ℞ adult: 0.5–1.0 mg IM or IV @ rate ≤ 1 mg/min (may repeat q 10–30 minutes PRN)
   b) ℞ peds: 0.02 mg/kg IM or IV @ rate ≤ 0.5 mg/min (may repeat q 5–10 min up to 2 mg max)
3. withdraw 30–40 ml CSF either via LP or through catheter access port
4. notify the pump manufacturer

Complications: Device-related complications are shown in ▶ Table 98.4. The frequency of most is ≈ 1%, except catheter-related problems which had a rate of ≈ 30%[50]

Complications related to the drug therapy itself include: overdosage problems (rostral progression of hypotonia, respiratory depression, coma, and seizures.

Intrathecal baclofen withdrawal: Interruption of ITB therapy may occur as a result of: empty pump reservoir, pump battery failure, catheter migration/breakage/kinking/disconnection/occlusion, programming error. Steps in assessing the infusion system are shown in ▶ Table 98.5.

The severity of withdrawal syndrome depends on dose of drug used (increased with higher dose) and duration of therapy (increased with longer therapy).

Syndromes: with abrupt discontinuation of ITB

Table 98.4 ITB pump complications[a]
1. mechanical problems a) pump underinfusion b) catheter problems: occlusion, kink, dislodgment, cut, break or disconnection 2. wound complications a) pocket erosion b) incisional pain c) infection d) seroma (may require aspiration) e) CSF collection
[a]device-related complications requiring a secondary invasive procedure

98

Table 98.5 Assessing ITB infusion systems
• interrogate the pump (with device programmer) • refill reservoir with drug if empty (by experienced ITB practitioner) • obtain AP & lateral x-rays to assess location of catheter tip and to look for breaks, kinks or migration

1. mild withdrawal symptoms: return of spasticity and rigidity, tachycardia, piloerection (goosebumps) & pruritus
2. more significant withdrawal symptoms: seizures & hallucinations
3. severe withdrawal symptoms (estimated incidence: 3–5%)[53]: increased rebound spasticity, rigidity, fever, labile BP, and reduced level of consciousness – resembling but distinct from malignant hyperthermia (p. 108) or neuroleptic malignant syndrome. If untreated, the severe syndrome can progress over 24–72 hours to rhabdomyolysis (with elevated creatine kinase (CK) and transaminase), hepatic and renal failure, DIC, and occasionally death

Management of *abrupt* ITB withdrawal syndrome[53]:

1. ABCs (airway/breathing/circulation). Intubate if necessary
2. primary goal is to reestablish ITB therapy at the same dose as soon as possible
3. assess pump/system as outlined in ▶ Table 98.5
4. early use of high-dose oral/enteral baclofen: ≥ 120 mg/d in 6–8 divided doses if the patient's condition permits (NB: PO baclofen is not reliable as the lone treatment for ITB withdrawal, and safety not established for age < 12 yrs)
5. attempt to restore ITB therapy at or near pre-withdrawal dosage by experienced physician by one of the following:
   a) using a programmed bolus through the pump
   b) via the catheter access port
   c) via LP
   d) via new externalized catheter
6. if restoration of ITB therapy is delayed and if symptoms persist
   a) move pt. to ICU if not already there
   b) parenteral benzodiazepine infusion: diazepam or midazolam. Titrate dose to reduce muscle rigidity, hyperthermia, BP lability, seizures
   c) cyproheptadine[54]: a serotonin antagonist. Start with 4 mg po q 6 hrs
   d) diphenhydramine 50 mg PO or IM, may repeat q 6 hrs for pruritis
   e) dantrolene may *not* be as effective as it is for malignant hyperthermia
   f) rectal baclofen

If it is necessary to electively (or semi-electively) remove a pump system, the optimal scenario is to gradually taper the drug by reprogramming the pump and/or by filling the reservoir with solution of decreased baclofen concentration.

98.6 Torticollis

98.6.1 General information

AKA wry neck. A form of dystonia resulting in a failure to control head position (if shoulders or trunk are also involved, dystonia is a more proper label).

98.6.2 Etiologies

A symptom of diverse causes. Differential diagnosis includes:

1. congenital torticollis (may be the initial presentation of dystonia musculorum deformans)
2. spasmodic torticollis, AKA wry neck: a specific subtype of torticollis that is idiopathic by definition. The shortened sternocleidomastoid (SCM) muscle is usually in spasm
3. extrapyramidal lesions (including degenerative): often alleviated by lying down; EMG shows abnormal grouped activity
4. psychogenic (often mentioned, seldom verified)
5. torticollis from atlantoaxial rotatory subluxation (p. 968): the *elongated* SCM may be in spasm (opposite of that in spasmodic torticollis)
6. neurovascular compression of the 11th nerve (see below)
7. hemorrhage into sternocleidomastoid muscle (with subsequent contracture)
8. infection of the cervical spine
9. cervical adenitis
10. syringomyelia
11. cerebellar tumors in children
12. bulbar palsies

98

13. "pseudotorticollis" may develop as an unconscious correction to reduce diplopia that occurs with imbalance of extraocular eye musculature

98.6.3 Non-surgical treatment of torticollis

Should be attempted first, and includes:
1. relaxation training, including biofeedback
2. thorough neuropsychiatric evaluation
3. trans-epidermal neuro-stimulation (TENS) to the neck

98.6.4 Surgical procedures

Reserved for disabling, refractory cases. Includes:
1. dorsal cord stimulation
2. local injection of botulinum toxin: may work for retrocollis, is poor for lateral torticollis (must inject posterior cervicals and both SCM, and may cause temporary pharyngeal muscle dysfunction resulting in dysphagia), and is totally ineffective for anterocollis
3. selective rhizotomy and spinal accessory nerve section

98.6.5 Other treatments for torticollis

Stereotactic electrocoagulation of Forel's H1 field.

98.6.6 Torticollis of 11th nerve origin

1. usually a horizontal type (manifests as horizontal head movement) which may be exacerbated when supine (unlike extrapyramidal torticollis)
2. contraction of SCM is usually accompanied by activity in contralateral agonist muscles
3. may be treated surgically. Procedures include
   a) sectioning of the anastomotic branches between the 11th nerve and the upper cervical posterior root (C1 anastomotic branch is sensory only)
   b) microvascular decompression of the 11th nerve (most cases caused by vertebral artery, but PICA compression is also described[55]). Relief takes several weeks post-op

98.7 Neurovascular compression syndromes

98.7.1 General information

Syndromes due to compression of cranial nerves at the root entry zone (REZ) (or in the case of motor nerves, root exit zone). The REZ (AKA Obersteiner-Redlich zone) is the point where central myelin (from oligodendroglial cells) changes to peripheral myelin (from Schwann cells).

Syndromes include:
1. trigeminal neuralgia, see Trigeminal neuralgia (p. 479)
2. hemifacial spasm: see below
3. disabling positional vertigo
4. some forms of torticollis of 11th nerve origin (above)

98

98.7.2 Hemifacial spasm

General information

Key concepts

- intermittent unilateral painless contractions of facial muscles
- typically caused by compression of VII nerve by AICA
- along with palatal myoclonus: the only movement disorder that persists in sleep
- responds well to microvascular decompression, but risk of hearing loss is ≈ 20%

Hemifacial spasm (HFS) is a condition of intermittent, painless, involuntary, spasmodic contractions of muscles innervated by the facial nerve in one side of the face only. May be limited to the upper or lower half of the face only, and excess lacrimation may be present. HFS usually begins with rare contractions of the orbicularis oculi, and slowly progresses to involve the entire half of the face and increases in frequency until the ability to see out of the affected eye is impaired.

HFS may be associated with trigeminal neuralgia, geniculate neuralgia; see **Tic convulsif** (p.493), or vestibular and/or cochlear[56] nerve dysfunction.

HFS is more common in women, is seen more often on the left, and usually presents after the teenages. Auditory function testing reveals abnormal acoustic middle ear reflex in almost half of patients, indicating some degree of VIII compromise.[56]

Meige's syndrome: hemifacial spasm with oral movements.

▸ **Note.** HFS and palatal myoclonus are the only involuntary movement disorders that persist during sleep.[57]

Etiologies

1. vascular compression syndrome (see below): the most common etiology (much more common than with trigeminal neuralgia)
2. idiopathic
3. tumor compressing the nerve
4. can follow some cases of Bell's palsy
5. conditions that can mimic HFS
   a) blepharospasm (bilateral spasmodic closure of the orbicularis oculi muscles) which is more common in the elderly, and may be associated with organic brain syndrome. Blepharospasm is notorious for disappearing when the patient presents for medical evaluation (an effect of alerting), but may be elicited by asking patient to gently close the eyes and then rapidly open them, following which a blepharospasm may occur. HFS usually involves more than the ocular muscles
   b) facial myokymia: continuous facial spasm which may be a manifestation of an intrinsic brainstem glioma or of multiple sclerosis. Often associated with other findings

Vascular compression

HFS is usually caused by compression of the facial nerve at the root exit zone (REZ) by a vessel, which is most often an artery (most commonly *AICA*[58] (either pre- or postmeatal[59]), but other vascular possibilities include an elongated PICA, SCA, a tortuous VA, the cochlear artery, a dolichoectatic basilar artery, AICA branches…), aneurysm, a vascular malformation, and rarely, veins have been implicated. In typical HFS (onset in the orbicularis oculi, and progressing downward over the face), the vessel impinges on the antero-caudal aspect of the VII/VIII nerve complex, in atypical HFS (beginning in the buccal muscles and progressing upward over the face) the compression is rostral or posterior to VII.[60]

Vessels contacting the REZ of the vestibular nerve may cause vertigo, whereas tinnitus or hearing loss may result from cochlear nerve REZ compression.

Infrequently, benign tumors or a cyst in the cerebellopontine angle, multiple sclerosis, adhesions, or osseous skull deformities will be the cause of HFS.

Evidence indicates that there is not cross (ephaptic) conduction at the compressed REZ, but that the facial motonucleus is involved secondarily as a result of the REZ compression, via a phenomenon similar to kindling.[61] In addition to the spasm, a 2nd electrophysiological phenomenon associated with HFS is synkinesis, where stimulation of one branch of the facial nerve results in delayed discharges through another branch (average latency: 11 mSec[62]).

Evaluation

In typical cases of HFS, the diagnostic work-up is negative.

Most patients should have MRI of the posterior fossa (CT scan is less sensitive here) to R/O tumors or AVMs.

Vertebral angiography is usually not performed if imaging is normal. The neurovascular compression responsible for HFS usually cannot be identified on angiography.

Treatment

Medical management

HFS is generally a surgical condition. Early, mild cases may be managed expectantly. Carbamazepine and phenytoin are generally ineffective, unlike the situation with the causally similar condition of trigeminal neuralgia. Local injection of botulinum **toxin** (Oculinum®) may be effective in treating HFS and/or blepharospasm.[63,64] Baclofen has been advocated but is not very effective.

Surgical management

General information

Many ablative procedures are effective for HFS (including sectioning of divisions of the facial nerve), however, this leaves the patient with some degree of facial paresis. The current procedure of choice for HFS is microvascular decompression (MVD) wherein the offending vessel is physically moved off of the nerve, and a sponge (e.g. Ivalon®, polyvinyl formyl alcohol foam) is interposed as a cushion. Other cushions may not prove to be as satisfactory (muscle may disappear, and Teflon felt may thin[65]).

Most often, the offending vessel approaches the nerve at a right angle, and causes grooving in the nerve. Compression must occur at the root exit zone; decompression of vessels impinging distal to this area is usually ineffective.

Operative risks: see below.

Post-operatively, there may be episodes of mild HFS, however they usually begin to diminish 2–3 days following MVD. Severe spasm that does not abate suggests failure to achieve adequate decompression, and reoperation should be considered.

Surgical results of MVD depends on the duration of symptoms (shorter duration has better prognosis) as well as on the age of the patient (elderly patients do less well). Complete resolution of HFS occurred in 44 (81%) of 54 patients undergoing MVD, however, 6 of these patients had relapse.[66] 5 patients (9%) had partial improvement, and 5 (9%) had no relief.

Technique of MVD

Intra-operative brainstem auditory evoked potential (BAER),[67] or more applicable, direct VIII nerve monitoring[68] may help prevent hearing loss during MVD for 7th or 8th nerve dysfunction. Furthermore, monitoring for the disappearance of the (delayed) synkinetic response may aid in determining when adequate decompression has been achieved (generally reserved for teaching institutions).[61]

For a diagram of the normal anatomy of the CPA, see ▸ Fig. 1.9. The facial nerve should not be manipulated, and one should avoid dissection around the VII and VIII nerves near the IAC.[69] Vessels must be preserved, especially the cochlear artery and small perforators.

Place gentle medial traction on the cerebellum (< 1 cm is recommended[69]), and incise the arachnoid membrane between the flocculus and the eighth nerve (to avoid tension on nerves that could cause post-op deficit). The IX nerve may be followed medially from the jugular foramen to locate the origin of the VII nerve (the origin of VII is 4 mm cephalad and 2 mm anterior to that of the IX nerve[70]).

Surgical results

Complete resolution of spasm occurs in ≈ 85–93%.[65,71,72,73,74] Spasm is diminished in 9%, and unchanged in 6%.[74] Of 29 patients with complete relief, 25 (86%) had immediate post-op resolution, and the remaining 4 patients took from 3 mos to 3 yrs to attain quiescence.

Recurrence

Return of symptoms after a period of complete resolution of HFS occurs in up to 10% of patients, 86% of recurrences happen within 2 yrs of surgery, and the risk of developing recurrence after 2 yrs of post-op relief is only ≈ 1%.[74]

Surgical complications

1. ipsilateral hearing loss: may occur from traction injury or a vasospasm
   a) total hearing loss occurs in ≈ 13% (range: 1.6–15%) (2.8% in one series,[56] 15% in another series[66])
   b) partial hearing loss: 6%
2. facial weakness
   a) transient: 18%
   b) permanent facial weakness: 6%[72]

3. ataxia in 1–6%
4. other complications that are minor or temporary include:
   a) aseptic meningitis (AKA hemogenic meningitis) in 8.2%
   b) hoarseness or dysphagia in 14%
   c) CSF rhinorrhea in 0.3%
   d) perioral herpes in 3%[69]

98.8 Hyperhidrosis

98.8.1 General information

Either essential (primary, or idiopathic) or secondary (etiologies include: hyperthyroidism, diabetes mellitus, pheochromocytoma, acromegaly, parkinsonism, CNS trauma, syringomyelia, hypothalamic tumors, menopause).[75]

Due to overactivity of eccrine sweat glands (found over entire body, highest concentration in palms and soles of feet). They produce a hypotonic secretion with saline as the primary constituent. These glands are under control of the sympathetic nervous system, however, the neurotransmitter is paradoxically acetylcholine (i.e. they are cholinergic, unlike most sympathetic end organs which are adrenergic). Most eccrine sweat glands serve a thermoregulatory function, however, those on the palms and soles respond primarily to emotional stress.[75]

Essential hyperhidrosis is a generalized condition that usually manifests mostly in the palms. The incidence is unknown, although it was ≈ 1% in an Israeli study (probably high).

98.8.2 Treatment

Mild cases are treated medically with:
1. topical agents: astringents (potassium permanganate, tannic acid…) or antiperspirants (contact dermatitis usually limits use of these agents)
2. or systemically with anticholinergics: including atropine, propantheline bromide… (side effects of dry mouth and blurred vision usually limits use of these)
3. tap water iontophoresis: may produce keratinization of palmar epithelium

Severe cases refractory to medical therapy may be candidates for surgical sympathectomy (see below).

98.9 Tremor

Thalamotomy or thalamic stimulation may be useful for tremors that are refractory to medical treatment, including parkinsonian (p. 1526), essential,[76,77] cerebellar and post-traumatic.[30]

98.10 Sympathectomy

98.10.1 Cardiac sympathectomy

With the advances in percutaneous coronary artery techniques, cardiovascular surgery and drugs, cardiac sympathectomy for angina pectoris has found less application. However, it may still be useful in patients who have no further treatment options. Bilateral sympathectomy from the stellate ganglion through the T7 ganglia is required. Newer thoracoscopic techniques may revive some interest in this.

98.10.2 Upper extremity sympathectomy

Various pathologies that may be indications for upper extremity sympathectomy are shown in ▶ Table 98.6.

Table 98.6 Indications for UE sympathectomy

- essential hyperhidrosis
- primary Raynaud's disease
- shoulder-hand syndrome
- intractable angina
- ± causalgia major (p. 497)

Removal of the only second thoracic ganglion is probably adequate, and avoids a Horner's syndrome in most. Techniques used include: anterior transthoracic, thoracic endoscopic,[78] percutaneous radiofrequency, and supraclavicular. An approach via a midline posterior incision with a T3 costotransversectomy allows bilateral access.[75,79] The risk of significant complications is ≈ 5% and include pneumothorax, intercostal neuralgia, spinal cord injury, and Horner's syndrome.

98.10.3 Upper thoracic sympathectomy

Approaches include:
1. posterior paravertebral approach
2. axillary thoracotomy with transthoracic exposure of the sympathetic chain
3. supraclavicular, retropleural exposure
4. percutaneous radiofrequency technique[80,81]
5. video endoscopic approach[82]

98.10.4 Lumbar sympathectomy

Primary indication is for causalgia major of the lower extremity. Preoperative lumbar sympathetic blocks may be utilized to evaluate patient for response.

Removal of the L2 and L3 sympathetic ganglion is usually adequate to remove sympathetic tone from the lower extremities (occasionally L1 and sometimes T12 are also removed for causalgia of the thigh).

The most common approach is a retroperitoneal approach through a flank incision. The patient is placed in a lateral oblique position, and the skin incision is made from the anterior superior iliac spine to the tip of the 12th rib. The peritoneum is dissected from the muscular wall and is retracted anteriorly. The kidney and ureter are retracted anteriorly; injury to the ureter being a major risk of the operation. The sympathetic chain is identified on the lateral aspect of the vertebral bodies. The vena cava makes a right-sided approach more difficult as the aorta is easier to deal with on left-sided approaches.

References

[1] Deuschl G, Schade-Brittinger C, Krack P, Volkmann J, Schafer H, Botzel K, Daniels C, Deutschlander A, Dillmann U, Eisner W, Gruber D, Hamel W, Herzog J, Hilker R, Klebe S, Kloss M, Koy J, Krause M, Kupsch A, Lorenz D, Lorenzl S, Mehdorn HM, Moringlane JR, Oertel W, Pinsker MO, Reichmann H, Reuss A, Schneider GH, Schnitzler A, Steude U, Sturm V, Timmermann L, Tronnier V, Trottenberg T, Wojtecki L, Wolf E, Poewe W, Voges J. A randomized trial of deep-brain stimulation for Parkinson's disease. N Engl J Med. 2006; 355:896–908

[2] Weaver FM, Follett K, Stern M, Hur K, Harris C, Marks WJ,Jr, Rothlind J, Sagher O, Reda D, Moy CS, Pahwa R, Burchiel K, Hogarth P, Lai EC, Duda JE, Holloway K, Samii A, Horn S, Bronstein J, Stoner G, Heemskerk J, Huang GD. Bilateral deep brain stimulation vs best medical therapy for patients with advanced Parkinson disease: a randomized controlled trial. JAMA. 2009; 301:63–73

[3] Diederich NJ, Kalteis K, Stamenkovic M, Pieri V, Alesch F. Efficient internal pallidal stimulation in Gilles de la Tourette syndrome: a case report. Mov Disord. 2005; 20:1496–1499

[4] Dehning S, Mehrkens JH, Muller N, Botzel K. Therapy-refractory Tourette syndrome: beneficial outcome with globus pallidus internus deep brain stimulation. Mov Disord. 2008; 23:1300–1302

[5] Mallet L, Polosan M, Jaafari N, Baup N, Welter ML, Fontaine D, du Montcel ST, Yelnik J, Chereau I, Arbus C, Raoul S, Aouizerate B, Damier P, Chabardes S, Czernecki V, Ardouin C, Krebs MO, Bardinet E, Chaynes P, Burbaud P, Cornu P, Derost P, Bougerol T, Bataille B, Mattei V, Dormont D, Devaux B, Verin M, Houeto JL, Pollak P, Benabid AL, Agid Y, Krack P, Millet B, Pelissolo A. Subthalamic nucleus stimulation in severe obsessive-compulsive disorder. N Engl J Med. 2008; 359:2121–2134

[6] Greenberg BD, Malone DA, Friehs GM, Rezai AR, Kubu CS, Malloy PF, Salloway SP, Okun MS, Goodman WK, Rasmussen SA. Three-year outcomes in deep brain stimulation for highly resistant obsessive-compulsive disorder. Neuropsychopharmacology. 2006; 31:2384–2393

[7] Lozano AM, Mayberg HS, Giacobbe P, Hamani C, Craddock RC, Kennedy SH. Subcallosal cingulate gyrus deep brain stimulation for treatment-resistant depression. Biol Psychiatry. 2008; 64:461–467

[8] Malone DA, Jr, Dougherty DD, Rezai AR, Carpenter LL, Friehs GM, Eskandar EN, Rauch SL, Rasmussen SA, Machado AG, Kubu CS, Tyrka AR, Price LH, Stypulkowski PH, Giftakis JE, Rise MT, Malloy PF, Salloway SP, Greenberg BD. Deep brain stimulation of the ventral capsule/ventral striatum for treatment-resistant depression. Biol Psychiatry. 2009; 65:267–275

[9] Halpern CH, Wolf JA, Bale TL, Stunkard AJ, Danish SF, Grossman M, Jaggi JL, Grady MS, Baltuch GH. Deep brain stimulation in the treatment of obesity. J Neurosurg. 2008; 109:625–634

[10] Stelten BM, Noblesse LH, Ackermans L, Temel Y, Visser-Vandewalle V. The neurosurgical treatment of addiction. Neurosurg Focus. 2008; 25. DOI: 10.3171/FOC/2008/25/7/E5

[11] Green AL, Wang S, Bittar RG, Owen SL, Paterson DJ, Stein JF, Bain PG, Shlugman D, Aziz TZ. Deep brain stimulation: a new treatment for hypertension? J Clin Neurosci. 2007; 14:592–595

[12] Laitinen LV, Bergenheim AT, Hariz MI. Leksell's Posteroventral Pallidotomy in the Treatment of Parkinson's Disease. J Neurosurg. 1992; 76:53–61

[13] Gildenberg PL. Whatever Happened to Stereotactic Surgery? Neurosurgery. 1987; 20:983–987

[14] Fahn S. Fetal-Tissue Transplantation in Parkinson's Disease. N Engl J Med. 1992; 327:1589–1590

[15] Madrazo I, Drucker-Colin R, Diaz V, et al. Open Microsurgical Autograft of Adrenal Medulla to the Right Caudate Nucleus in Two Patients with Intractable Parkinson's Disease. N Engl J Med. 1987; 316:831–834

[16] Penn RD, Goetz CG, Tanner CM, et al. The Adrenal Medullary Transplant Operation for Parkinson's Disease: Clinical Observation in Five Patients. Neurosurgery. 1988; 22:999–1004
[17] Goetz CG, Stebbins GT, Klawans HL, et al. United Parkinson Foundation Neurotransplantation Registry on Adrenal Medullary Transplants: Presurgical, and 1- and 2-Year Follow-Up. Neurology. 1991; 41:1719–1722
[18] Boyer KL, Bakay RAE. The History, Theory, and Present Status of Brain Transplantation. Neurosurg Clin North Amer. 1995; 6:113–125
[19] Olanow CW, Goetz CG, Kordower JH, Stoessl AJ, Sossi V, Brin MF, Shannon KM, Nauert GM, Perl DP, Godbold J, Freeman TB. A double-blind controlled trial of bilateral fetal nigral transplantation in Parkinson's disease. Ann Neurol. 2003; 54:403–414
[20] Snyder BJ, Olanow CW. Stem cell treatment for Parkinson's disease: an update for 2005. Curr Opin Neurol. 2005; 18:376–385
[21] Iacono RP, Shima F, Lonser RR, et al. The Results, Indications, and Physiology of Posteroventral Pallidotomy for Patients with Parkinson's Disease. Neurosurgery. 1995; 36:1118–1127
[22] Kondziolka D, Bonaroti EA, Lunsford LD. Pallidotomy for Parkinson's Disease. Contemp Neurosurg. 1996; 18:1–6
[23] Leksell L. Stereotactic Radiosurgery. J Neurol Neurosurg Psychiatry. 1983; 46:797–803
[24] Iacono RP, Lonser RR, Mandybur G, Yamada S. Stimulation of the Globus Pallidus in Parkinson's Disease. Br J Neurosurg. 1995; 9:505–510
[25] Limousin P, Pollack P, Benazzouz A, et al. Bilateral Subthalamic Nucleus Stimulation for Severe Parkinson's Disease. Mov Disord. 1995; 10:672–674
[26] Schuurman PR, Bosch DA, Bossuyt PM, Bonsel GJ, van Someren EJ, de Bie RM, Merkus MP, Speelman JD. A comparison of continuous thalamic stimulation and thalamotomy for suppression of severe tremor. N Engl J Med. 2000; 342:461–468
[27] Favre J, Taha JM, Nguyen TT, Gildenberg PL, Burchiel KJ. Pallidotomy: A Survey of Current Practice in North America. Neurosurgery. 1996; 39:883–892
[28] Stefani A, Lozano AM, Peppe A, Stanzione P, Galati S, Tropepi D, Pierantozzi M, Brusa L, Scarnati E, Mazzone P. Bilateral deep brain stimulation of the pedunculopontine and subthalamic nuclei in severe Parkinson's disease. Brain. 2007; 130:1596–1607
[29] Pereira EA, Muthusamy KA, De Pennington N, Joint CA, Aziz TZ. Deep brain stimulation of the pedunculopontine nucleus in Parkinson's disease. Preliminary experience at Oxford. Br J Neurosurg. 2008; 22 Suppl 1:S41–S44
[30] Jankovic J, Cardoso F, Grossman RG, Hamilton WJ. Outcome After Stereotactic Thalamotomy for Parkinsonian, Essential, and Other Types of Tremor. Neurosurgery. 1995; 37:680–687
[31] Pahwa R, Lyons KE, Wilkinson SB, Simpson RK Jr, Ondo WG, Tarsy D, Norregaard T, Hubble JP, Smith DA, Hauser RA, Jankovic J. Long-term evaluation of deep brain stimulation of the thalamus. J Neurosurg. 2006; 104:506–512
[32] Sutton JP, Couldwell W, Lew MF, et al. Ventroposterior Medial Pallidotomy in Patients with Advanced Parkinson's Disease. Neurosurgery. 1995; 36:1112–1117
[33] Walter BL, Vitek JL. Surgical treatment for Parkinson's disease. Lancet Neurol. 2004; 3:719–728
[34] Awan NR, Lozano A, Hamani C. Deep brain stimulation: current and future perspectives. Neurosurg Focus. 2009; 27. DOI: 10.3171/2009.4.FOCUS0982
[35] Merritt JL. Management of Spasticity in Spinal Cord Injury. Mayo Clin Proc. 1981; 56:614–622
[36] Ashworth B. Preliminary Trial of Carisoprodal in Multiple Sclerosis. Practitioner. 1964; 192:540–542
[37] Scott BA, Pulliam MW. Management of Spasticity and Painful Spasms in Paraplegia. Contemp Neurosurg. 1987; 9:1–6
[38] Herz DA, Looman JE, Tiberio A, et al. The Management of Paralytic Spasticity. Neurosurgery. 1990; 26:300–306
[39] Richardson RR, Cerullo LJ, McLone DG, et al. Percutaneous Epidural Neurostimulation in Modulation of Paraplegic Spasticity. Acta Neurochir. 1979; 49:235–243
[40] Garland DE, Lucie RS, Waters RL. Current use of open phenol block for adult acquired spasticity. Clin Ortho Rel Res. 1982; 165:217–222
[41] Padovani R, Tognetti F, Pozzati E, et al. The Treatment of Spasticity by Means of Dorsal Longitudinal Myelotomy and Lozenge-Shaped Griseotomy. Spine. 1982; 7:103–109
[42] Privat JM, Benezech J, Frerebeau P, et al. Sectorial posterior rhizotomy, a new technique of surgical treatment for spasticity. Acta Neurochir. 1976; 35:181–195
[43] Sindou M, Millet MF, Mortamais J, et al. Results of Selective Posterior Rhizotomy in the Treatment of Painful and Spastic Paraplegia Secondary to Multiple Sclerosis. Appl Neurophysiol. 1982; 45:335–340
[44] Gornall P, Hitchcock E, Kirkland IS. Stereotaxic Neurosurgery in the Management of Cerebral Palsy. Dev Med Child Neurol. 1975; 17:279–286
[45] Scott BA, Weinstein Z, Chiteman R, et al. Intrathecal Phenol and Glycerin in Metrizamide for Treatment of Intractable Spasms in Paraplegia. J Neurosurg. 1985; 63:125–127
[46] McCarty CS. The Treatment of Spastic Paraplegia by Selective Spinal Cordectomy. J Neurosurg. 1954; 11:539–545
[47] Durward QJ, Rice GP, Ball MJ, et al. Selective Spinal Cordectomy: Clinicopathological Correlation. J Neurosurg. 1982; 56:359–367
[48] Albright AL, Cervi A, Singletary J. Intrathecal Baclofen for Spasticity in Cerebral Palsy. JAMA. 1991; 265:1418–1422
[49] Penn RD. Intrathecal Baclofen for Spasticity of Spinal Origin: Seven Years of Experience. J Neurosurg. 1992; 77:236–240
[50] Coffey RJ, Cahill D, Steers W, et al. Intrathecal Baclofen for Intractable Spasticity of Spinal Origin: Results of a Long-Term Multicenter Study. J Neurosurg. 1993; 78:226–232
[51] Albright AL, Barron WB, Fasick P, Polinko P, Janosky J. Continuous Intrathecal Baclofen Infusion for Spasticity of Cerebral Origin. JAMA. 1993; 270:2475–2477
[52] Meythaler JM, Guin-Renfroe S, Brunner RC, Johnson A, Hadley MN. Intrathecal baclofen for spastic hypertonia from stroke. Stroke. 2001; 32:2099–2119
[53] Coffey RJ, Edgar TS, Francisco GE, Graziani V, et al. Abrupt withdrawal from intrathecal baclofen: Recognition and management of a potentially life-threatening syndrome. Arch Phys Med Rehabil. 2002; 83:735–741
[54] Meythaler JM, Roper JF, Brunner RC. Cyproheptadine for intrathecal baclofen withdrawal. Arch Phys Med Rehabil. 2003; 84:638–642
[55] Shima F, Fukui M, Kitamura K, et al. Diagnosis and Surgical Treatment of Spasmodic Torticollis of 11th Nerve Origin. Neurosurgery. 1988; 22:358–363
[56] Moller MB, Moller AR. Loss of Auditory Function in Microvascular Decompression for Hemifacial Spasm: Results in 143 Consecutive Cases. J Neurosurg. 1985; 63:17–20
[57] Tew JM, Yeh HS. Hemifacial Spasm. Neurosurgery (Japan). 1983; 2:267–278
[58] Yeh HS, Tew JM, Ramirez RM. Microsurgical Treatment of Intractable Hemifacial Spasm. Neurosurgery. 1981; 9:383–386
[59] Martin RG, Grant JL, Peace D, Rhoton AL, et al. Microsurgical Relationships of the Anterior Inferior Cerebellar Artery and the Facial-vestibulocochlear Nerve Complex. Neurosurgery. 1980; 6:483–507
[60] Wilkins RH, Rengachary SS. Neurosurgery. New York 1985
[61] Moller AR, Jannetta PJ. Microvascular Decompression in Hemifacial Spasm: Intraoperative Electrophysiological Observations. Neurosurgery. 1985; 16:612–618
[62] Moller AR, Jannetta PJ. Hemifacial Spasm: Results of Electrophysiologic Recording During Microvascular Decompression Operations. Neurology. 1985; 35:969–974

[63] Dutton JJ, Buckley EG. Botulinum Toxin in the Management of Blepharospasm. Arch Neurol. 1986; 43:380–382

[64] Kennedy RH, Bartley GB, Flanagan JC, et al. Treatment of Blepharospasm With Botulinum Toxin. Mayo Clin Proc. 1989; 64:1085–1090

[65] Rhoton AL. Comment on Payner T D and Tew J M: Recurrence of Hemifacial Spasm After Microvascular Decompression. Neurosurgery. 1996; 38

[66] Auger RG, Peipgras DG, Laws ER. Hemifacial Spasm: Results of Microvascular Decompression of the Facial Nerve in 54 Patients. Mayo Clin Proc. 1986; 61:640–644

[67] Friedman WA, Kaplan BJ, Gravenstein D, et al. Intraoperative Brain-Stem Auditory Evoked Potentials During Posterior Fossa Microvascular Decompression. J Neurosurg. 1985; 62:552–557

[68] Moller AR, Jannetta PJ. Monitoring Auditory Functions During Cranial Nerve Microvascular Decompression Operations by Direct Recording from the Eighth Nerve. J Neurosurg. 1983; 59:493–499

[69] Fukushima T, Carter LP, Spetzler RF, Hamilton MG. In: Microvascular Decompression for Hemifacial Spasm: Results in 2890 Cases. Neurovascular Surgery. New York: McGraw-Hill; 1995:1133–1145

[70] Rhoton AL. Microsurgical Anatomy of the Brainstem Surface Facing an Acoustic Neuroma. Surg Neurol. 1986; 25:326–339

[71] Jannetta PJ. Neurovascular Compression in Cranial Nerve and Systemic Disease. Ann Surg. 1980; 192:518–525

[72] Loeser JD, Chen J. Hemifacial Spasm: Treatment by Microsurgical Facial Nerve Decompression. Neurosurgery. 1983; 13:141–146

[73] Huang CI, Chen IH, Lee LS. Microvascular Decompression for Hemifacial Spasm: Analyses of Operative Findings and Results in 310 Patients. Neurosurgery. 1992; 30:53–57

[74] Payner TD, Tew JM. Recurrence of Hemifacial Spasm After Microvascular Decompression. Neurosurgery. 1996; 38:686–691

[75] Bay JW. Management of Essential Hyperhidrosis. Contemp Neurosurg. 1988; 10:1–5

[76] Sydow O, Thobois S, Alesch F, Speelman JD. Multicentre European study of thalamic stimulation in essential tremor: a six year follow up. J Neurol Neurosurg Psychiatry. 2003; 74:1387–1391

[77] Schuurman PR, Bosch DA, Merkus MP, Speelman JD. Long-term follow-up of thalamic stimulation versus thalamotomy for tremor suppression. Mov Disord. 2008; 23:1146–1153

[78] Kao M-C. Video Endoscopic Sympathectomy Using a Fiberoptic CO2 Laser to Treat Palmar Hyperhidrosis. Neurosurgery. 1992; 30:131–135

[79] Dohn DF, Sava GM. Sympathectomy for Vascular Syndromes and Hyperhidrosis of the Upper Extremities. Clin Neurosurg. 1978; 25:637–650

[80] Wilkinson HA. Percutaneous radiofrequency upper thoracic sympathectomy: A new technique. Neurosurgery. 1984; 15:811–814

[81] Wilkinson HA. Percutaneous Radiofrequency Upper Thoracic Sympathectomy. Neurosurgery. 1996; 38:715–725

[82] Lee KH, Hwang PYK. Video Endoscopic Sympathectomy for Palmar Hyperhidrosis. J Neurosurg. 1996; 84:484–486

99 Pain Procedures

99.1 General information

Medical therapy must be maximized before a patient is a candidate for a pain procedure. Usually this requires escalating the dose of oral narcotic pain medications until the point that the pain is relieved or the side effects (usually somnolence or hallucinations) are intolerable (e.g. up to 300–400 mg/day of MS Contin may sometimes be necessary).

99.2 Choice of pain procedure

▶ Table 99.1 shows some pain procedures that may be used for various indications (the list is not intended to be all inclusive, but is rather to serve as a starting point for organizing pain procedures). In general, nonablative procedures are exhausted before resorting to ablative procedures.

99.3 Types of pain procedures

See pain procedures particular to trigeminal neuralgia (p. 482).

Techniques for other conditions include:

1. electrical stimulation
   a) deep brain stimulation (p. 1524) [1]: targets include thalamus and periaqueductal or periventricular gray matter
   b) spinal cord stimulation (p. 1547)
2. direct drug administration into the CNS:
   a) different routes: spinal (p. 1545), epidural or intrathecal, intraventricular (p. 1547)
   b) different agents: local anesthetics, narcotics (without motor, sensory, or sympathetic impairment seen with local anesthetics) (p. 1545)
3. intracranial ablative procedures:
   a) cingulotomy: theoretically reduces the unpleasant affect of pain without eliminating the pain. Must be done bilaterally, recently with MRI. Intolerable pain usually recurs after ≈ 3 mos. 10–30% develop flattened affect
   b) medial thalamotomy: no longer used (presented for historical reasons). Controversial. Was used for some for nociceptive cancer pain. Performed stereotactically
   c) **stereotactic mesencephalotomy**[2]: for unilateral head, neck, face and/or UE pain. Use MRI to create lesion 5 mm lateral to sylvian aqueduct at the level of the inferior colliculus. Unlike spinal cordotomy, the lesion is not near any motor tracts. Main complication is diplopia due to interference with vertical eye movement, often transient
4. spinal ablative surgical procedures
   a) cordotomy: see below
      - open
      - percutaneous
   b) cordectomy
   c) commissural myelotomy: for bilateral pain (p. 1544)
   d) punctate midline myelotomy: for relief of visceral cancer pain
   e) dorsal root entry zone lesion (p. 1550)
   f) dorsal rhizotomy: not useful for large areas of involvement

Table 99.1 Choice of pain procedures[a]

Unilateral pain		Bilateral or midline pain	
Head, face, neck, UE	Pain at or below C5 dermatome	Below diaphragm	Above diaphragm
DBS	cordotomy[b]	spinal IT narcotics ↓ commissural myelotomy	intraventricular narcotics
stereotactic mesencephalotomy			

[a] abbreviations: IT = intrathecal, UE or LE = upper or lower extremity
[b] cordotomy (open or percutaneous) if pain is unresponsive to or too high for spinal IT narcotics

99

    g) dorsal root ganglionectomy (an extraspinal procedure)
    h) sacral cordotomy: for patients with pelvic pain who have colostomy and ileostomy. A ligature is tied around the dural sac below S1 nerve roots
5. sympathectomy: possibly for causalgia major; see Sympathectomy (p. 1537) and Complex regional pain syndrome (CRPS) (p. 497)
6. peripheral nerve procedures
    a) nerve block[3]:
        - neurolytic: injection neurodestructive agents (e.g. phenol or absolute alcohol) on or near the target nerve
        - nonneurolytic: using local anesthetics, sometimes in combination with corticosteroids
    b) neurectomy: (e.g. intercostal neurectomy for pain due to infiltration of chest wall by malignancy). Performed open or percutaneously with radiofrequency lesion. May sacrifice motor function with mixed nerves
    c) peripheral nerve stimulators: rarely discussed

99.4 Cordotomy

99.4.1 General information

Interruption of the lateral spinothalamic tract fibers in the spinal cord. Cordotomy is the procedure of choice for *unilateral* pain below the C5 dermatomal level (≈ nipple; occasionally pain as high up as the mandible may be treated), in a terminally ill patient. Better for aching pain, poor for central pain, dysesthesias, causalgia (deafferentation pain) midline visceral pain. May be performed as an open procedure, but is more easily performed percutaneously at the C1–2 interspace (which limits the procedure to the cervical region). If there is any contralateral pain, it will tend to be magnified following the procedure and often leads to dissatisfaction with cordotomy. If there is any bladder dysfunction, it will usually be worse following cordotomy. Bilateral cervical cordotomies carries a risk of the loss of automaticity of breathing[4] (one form of sleep apnea, so-called Ondine's curse[5]). Therefore, if bilateral cordotomies are desired, the second should be staged after normal respiratory function and CO_2 responsiveness are verified following the first procedure, or the second stage may be done as an open procedure in the thoracic region.

Review the cross sectional spinal cord anatomy for relationships of the critical tracts (spinothalamic and corticospinal) to the dentate ligament, the anterior spinal artery, respiratory (▶ Fig. 1.13), and bladder areas (▶ Fig. 3.1).

99.4.2 Pre-op evaluation

Spirometric measurement of minute volume before and after breathing a mixture of 5% CO_2 and 95% O_2 for 5 minutes. If the MV decreases, these patients are at increased risk of having sleep apnea (usually transient), no increased risk if MV increases or stays the same. Also, patients with < 50% of predicted values on PFTs are not candidates.

In patients with pulmonary cancer contralateral to the planned side of cordotomy, check that the contralateral diaphragm is functioning with fluoroscopy, otherwise if the ipsilateral diaphragm is lost due to cordotomy, the patient may be hypopneic.

99.4.3 Percutaneous cordotomy

General information

Indicated for unilateral pain below ≈ C4–5 in a terminally ill patient. Radiofrequency current is used to lesion the lateral spinothalamic tract.

Technique

Patient does not need to be NPO. Usual pain medications should be given. The patient must be awake and cooperative (any movement with the needle in the cord may lacerate the cord), however one may give e.g. hydroxyzine (Vistaril®) 50 mg IM on call to procedure for relaxation.

The procedure is performed in the x-ray department with either fluoroscopic or CT guidance. For fluoroscopy, the head is placed in a Rosomoff headholder with the height adjusted to keep the mastoid process in the same horizontal plane as the acromioclavicular joint. Working on the side *contralateral* to the pain, local anesthetic without epinephrine is infiltrated 1 cm caudal to the mastoid tip. An 18 gauge lumbar puncture needle is inserted perfectly horizontal aiming halfway between the posterior margin of the body of C2 and the anterior portion of the C2 spinous process. Stay rostral to the C2 lamina to avoid the nerve (which is painful).

The dura will be penetrated at about the time that the tip of the needle is approximately even with the midline of the odontoid process on AP fluoro. A few ml of CSF are aspirated and shaken in a syringe together with a few ml of Pantopaque®, and several ml of the mixture are injected into the subarachnoid space under lateral fluoro guidance (**note:** Pantopaque is no longer available, and water soluble agents are less effective). A needle endoscopic technique may be able to localize the spinal cord anterior to the dentate ligaments. Some dye will layer on the anterior cord, some on the dentate ligament, and most in the posterior thecal space. The dye will only stay momentarily on the dentate ligament, thus be ready to immediately advance the needle just barely anterior to this while monitoring the tip impedance which will jump from ≈ 300–500 Ω (ohms) in the CSF to ≈ 1200–1500 Ω as the spinal cord is penetrated.

Stimulation at 100 Hz. should produce contralateral tingling at a threshold of ≤ 1 volt. No motor response should be elicited with 100 Hz. in the spinothalamic tract, and if muscle tetany occurs, lesioning must *not* be performed. If tingling is in the arm, lesioning will usually render from the arm and below analgesic. If tingling is in the lower extremity it will render only that limb analgesic. Stimulation at 2 Hz. should produce ipsilateral twitching of the arm or neck at ≈ 1–3 volts.

Radiofrequency lesioning is performed for 30 seconds while the patient sustains contraction of the *ipsilateral* hand and the voltage is gradually increased from zero. Any twitching of the hand is indication to back down on the voltage. A second lesion is performed in the same region and is usually less painful. The appropriate body area is then checked for analgesia to pinprick.

If the procedure is performed satisfactorily, an ipsilateral Horner's syndrome usually occurs.

Complications

For complications, ▶ Table 99.2.

Outcome

In experienced hands, 94% will achieve at least significant pain relief at the time of hospital discharge. The level of analgesia falls with time. At 1 year 60% will be pain free, and at 2 years this will be only 40%.

Post-procedure management

CSF leakage will cease spontaneously. Patient is kept supine for 24 hrs to prevent "spinal" (post-LP) headache. Pain medication appropriate to post operative management is prescribed. If successful, one can rapidly stop the narcotics for the primary pain, withdrawal syndromes occur only rarely.

99.4.4 Open cervical cordotomy (Schwartz technique)

General information

A relatively quick method for open cervical cordotomy.[6] Can theoretically be done under local for patients who cannot tolerate general anesthesia.

Table 99.2 Post-cordotomy complications

Complication	Frequency
ataxia	20%
ipsilateral paresis	5% total 3% permanent
bladder dysfunction	10% total 2% permanent
postcordotomy dysesthesia	8%
sleep induced apnea	0.3% unilateral cordotomy 3% bilateral cordotomy
death (respiratory failure)	0.3% unilateral cordotomy 1.6% bilateral cordotomy

99

Technique

Position: prone; face carefully placed on padded horseshoe headrest, neck slightly flexed to open the interlaminar spaces and to lower the head to prevent accumulation of intracranial air.

Skin incision: midline from occiput to C3. Working only on the side *contralateral* to the pain, muscles are stripped off the posterior lip of the foramen magnum, and from the lamina of C1 and C2. A Schwartz or Gelpi retractor is engaged between the occiput and C2. To increase exposure, the inferior half of C1 and superior half of C2 lamina are removed with a punch.

Dural incision: the ligamentum flavum is thin between C1–2, and can usually be opened with the dura in a linear incision from the lamina of C1 to C2 placed in the lateral third of the exposure, taking care to avoid bleeding from epidural veins. An angle is cut in the incision at either end to allow increased dural retraction. Tack-up sutures are placed in the dura, the arachnoid is opened, the dentate ligament is located and is gripped with a hemostat and divided between the hemostat and the dura.

Cordotomy: the dentate ligament is used to slightly rotate the spinal cord. A cordotomy knife (or 11 blade) with bone wax placed at 5 mm, is inserted into the cord in an avascular area just anterior to the dentate ligament, sharp side down. The anterolateral quadrant of the cord is cut with the following caveats:

- do not go posterior to the dentate ligament (to avoid corticospinal tract)
- do not cross the midline of the spinal cord
- do not injure the anterior spinal artery
- for patients with lower extremity pain, be sure to start exactly at the dentate ligament (to avoid missing lumbar and sacral fibers).

99.5 Commissural myelotomy

99.5.1 General information

AKA mediolongitudinal myelotomy. Interrupts pain fibers crossing in the anterior commissure on their way to the lateral spinothalamic tract.

99.5.2 Indications

Bilateral or midline pain, primarily below the thoracic levels (including abdomen, pelvis, perineum and lower extremities).

99.5.3 Technique

Laminectomy must extend at least 3 levels above the highest dermatome involved in pain. The dura is opened longitudinally and the operating microscope is then used to identify the midline sulcus (this is usually very difficult to see, and is then estimated as being halfway between where the dorsal roots enter the cord). Veins in the midline are sacrificed for the length of the proposed incision. A number 11 scalpel blade is then placed in a hemostat with 6–7 mm of the tip exposed. The blade is inserted in the midline at the upper end of the desired incision and is then passed caudally for the length of the planned incision (usually 3–4 cm).

99.5.4 Outcome

60% of patients have complete pain relief, 28% have partial, and 8% have none.

99.5.5 Complications

Weakness in the lower extremities occurs in ≈ 8% (usually lower motor neuron, presumably due to injury to anterior horn motor neurons). Dysesthesias occur in almost all patients, but persists > a few days in ≈ 16% (these patients also have impaired joint position sense, all of which are presumably due to posterior column injury). Bladder dysfunction is seen in ≈ 12%. Sexual dysfunction may also occur. There is a risk of injury to the anterior spinal artery (rare).

99.6 Punctate midline myelotomy

99.6.1 Indications

Pelvic and visceral pain refractory to other therapies.[7]

99.6.2 Technique

Interruption of a midline posterior column pathway.

99.7 CNS narcotic administration

99.7.1 Intraspinal narcotics

General information

Spinal narcotics may be administered epidurally or intrathecally for pain relief. Satisfactory pain control can usually be achieved for pain below the neck, although for pain above the diaphragm/umbilicus some recommend intraventricular morphine (p. 1547).[8] May also be performed on a "one-time" basis e.g. injection into epidural space following a lumbar laminectomy. Or, it may be given on a short term continuous basis, via an external epidural or intrathecal catheter. It may also be performed on an intermediate-term basis (< 60 days) with the use of a subcutaneous reservoir[9] or on a long-term basis with an implantable drug infusion pump[10] (e.g. Infusaid® or Medtronic® pump). Advantages over systemic narcotics include less sedation and/or confusion, less interference with GI motility (constipation), and possibly less N/V. The effectiveness is usually limited to ≈ 1 year and is thus not indicated for chronic benign pain. With time, increased doses are required because of the development of tolerance and/or progression of disease[11] with the concomitant development of the usual narcotic side effects.

Agents to use

Must be preservative-free (for either intrathecal or epidural use). This may be prepared by a pharmacist (e.g. add enough preservative free 0.9% saline to 1 or 3 gm morphine sulfate powder to yield a total of 100 ml produces 10 or 30 mg/ml solution respectively, and then filter this through a 0.22 mcm filter[12]). Alternatively, commercially available preparations include Duramorph® (available as 0.5 or 1 mg/ml) and Infumorph® (available in 20 ml ampules of 10 or 25 mg/ml), any of which may be diluted to a lower strength with preservative free diluent (normal saline). Cross tolerance to systemic narcotics does occur, and spinal narcotics are more effective in patients who have not been on continuous high dose IV opiates (patients on high-dose IV narcotics need higher initial intraspinal narcotic doses).

▶ **Side effects.** Include pruritus (often diffuse, and may be experienced most intensely in the nose), respiratory depression (the respiratory depression with spinal narcotics is usually very gradual, and is often easily detected by monitoring respiratory rate q 1 hr and taking action if the rate decreases), urinary retention, and N/V.

Trial injection

Before implanting a permanent delivery system a test injection should be performed to verify pain relief and tolerance for medication. Administered via percutaneously inserted epidural or intrathecal catheter connected to an external pump. Doses required for intrathecal catheters are usually ≈ 5–10 times lower than those for epidural catheters.

Sample post-injection orders after a one-time injection:

1. use no other narcotics for ≈ 24 hrs (with a continuous infusion additional narcotics should be withheld until the effect of the spinal narcotics has been determined)
2. 2 ampules (0.4 mg each) of naloxone (Narcan®) and syringe taped to patients bed (for the first 24 hrs after a single injection; at all times with continuous infusion)
3. head of bed elevated ≥ 10° for 24 hrs
4. record respiratory rate q1 hr for 24 hrs; if asleep and respiratory rate < 10 breaths/min, awaken patient. If unable to awaken, administer naloxone 0.4 mg IV and notify physician. Repeat naloxone 0.4 mg IV q 2 min PRN

5. **optional**: pulse oximeter for 24 hrs
6. diphenhydramine (Benadryl®) 25 mg IV q 1 hr PRN itching
7. droperidol (Inapsine®) 0.625 mg (which is 0.25 ml of the 2.5 mg/ml standard concentration available) IV q 30–60 mins PRN nausea
8. PRN supplemental pain medication:
   a) narcotic agonist/antagonist: e.g. nalbuphine (Nubain®) 1–4 mg IV q 3 hrs, OR
   b) ketorolac tromethamine (Toradol®) 15 mg IV or IM or 30 mg IM q 6 hrs (use lower dose for weight < 50 kg, age > 65 yrs, or reduced renal function)

Implantable drug delivery pumps

Although satisfactory pain control can be achieved with either epidural or intrathecal narcotics (morphine diffuses easily through the dura to the CSF where it gains access to pain receptors), epidural catheters commonly develop problems with scarring and may become less effective sooner than intrathecal catheters. Pumps should only be implanted if patients have successful pain control with test injection of spinal epidural (5–10 mg) or intrathecal (0.5–2 mg) morphine. A life expectancy of > 3 months is recommended for implantable pumps (if shorter longevity is anticipated, an external pump may be used).

One such series of commonly used implantable drug delivery pumps is manufactured by Infusaid Inc.. The only needle that should be used with their devices are special 22 gauge Huber (non-coring) needles. Delivery rates increase with body temperature 10–13% per °C above 37° C, they decrease by the same amount for every °C below 37°C, and also they become inaccurate at ≤ 4 ml of reservoir fluid. These pumps should never be allowed to run until empty, as this may permanently affect accuracy and reliability of drug delivery. In addition to the pump reservoir port, most models have one or more side "bolus" ports that delivers injected fluid directly to the outlet tubing. One should not aspirate when accessing either port.

Medtronic produces a programmable pump.

Surgical insertion

Similar to the insertion of a lumbar-peritoneal shunt (p. 1517). The patient is placed in the lateral position, such as on a bean-bag device. The pump is inserted into a subcutaneous pocket, created with a slightly curved 8–10 cm skin incision. The pump may be sutured to the fascia of the abdomen (in obese patients, it may be sutured to the subcutaneous tissue). Excess tubing should be coiled underneath the pump to prevent inadvertent puncture when accessing either reservoir.

The spinal catheter is inserted through a Tuohy needle inserted between lumbar spinous processes either percutaneously or via a small incision 2–3 mm lateral to the spinous processes. Alternatively, it may be inserted directly via a hemilaminectomy. Fluoroscopy may be used intraoperatively to verify rostral placement of the catheter; radiographic visualization of the catheter may be aided by filling it with iodinated contrast, e.g. Omnipaque-300 (p. 219). All bends in the tubing should be very gradual to avoid kinking.

Post-op pain management

Although the pump will be infusing when the patient leaves the operating room, unless they have been on intraspinal narcotics up until the time of surgery, it will usually take several days for the drug to reach equilibrium in the CSF before the level of pain control will be adequate. This can be mitigated by a bolus infusion (3–4 mg morphine for epidural catheters, or 0.2–0.4 mg for intrathecal catheters).

Complications

Meningitis and respiratory failure are rare complications. CSF fistula and spinal H/A may occur. Disconnection or dislodgment of catheter tip may result in failure to control pain, but can usually be surgically corrected.

Outcome

Cancer pain is significantly improved in up to 90%. Success rate for neuropathic pain (e.g. postherpetic neuralgia, painful diabetic sensory neuropathy): 25–50%.

99.7.2 Intraventricular narcotics

Indications

May be used for cancer pain (especially head and neck)[13] unresponsive to other methods in patients with a life expectancy < 6 mos.

Technique

An intraventricular catheter is connected to a ventricular access device (p. 1518). 0.5–1 mg of intrathecal morphine is injected via the VAD and usually provides ≈ 24 hrs of analgesia.

Complications

▶ **Side effects.** Common ones include dizziness, N/V. The risk of respiratory depression is minimized by using correct dosing. Complications in a series of 52 patients[13]: bacterial colonization of reservoir (4%), dislodged catheter (2%), blocked catheter (6%), postoperative meningitis (2%).

Outcome

Pain is successfully controlled in 70% at 2 mos, but thereafter the effectiveness diminishes as a result of tolerance to the narcotics.

99.8 Spinal cord stimulation (SCS)

99.8.1 General information

Originally developed as dorsal column stimulation (DCS), it has since been determined that pain relief also occurs with ventral stimulation (without stimulation induced paresthesias seen with DCS). Pain relief in humans persists beyond the stimulation time, and is not reversed by naloxone. The exact mechanism of action is undetermined, but probably involves some combination of neurohumoral (i.e. endorphin), antidromic stimulation of a spinal pain "gate", and supraspinal center stimulation. GABA and serotonin levels have been shown to be increased with SCS.

99.8.2 Indications

Possible indications include:

1. pain[14]: postlaminectomy pain syndrome (the most common indication, especially if LE pain > back pain; see below), complex regional pain syndrome (CRPS, formerly "reflex sympathetic dystrophy") (p. 1548), postthoracotomy pain (intercostal neuralgia), multiple sclerosis, diabetic neuropathy (p. 1549) and sometimes postherpetic neuralgia
2. refractory angina pectoris (p. 1549)
3. painful limb ischemia from inoperable peripheral vascular disease (p. 1549)
4. functional: spastic hemiparesis, dystonia, bladder dysfunction
5. ✖ generally not used for cancer pain or for patients with limited life expectant.

99.8.3 Technique

In order for SCS to be effective, it is necessary for the patient to feel the stimulation in the areas of pain.[15] Two techniques are used to place electrodes in the *epidural* space:

1. plate-like electrodes placed via hemilaminectomy
2. wire-like electrodes placed percutaneously with a Tuohy needle.

Following electrode placement, a trial with an external generator over several days determines if SCS is effective. The electrodes are removed unless clear improvement occurs, in which case an implantable pulse generator is placed subcutaneously.

99.8.4 Complications

With plate electrodes, there is a 3.5% incidence of infection which respond to electrode removal and IV antibiotics. Less common complications: electrode migration (usually seen with first few weeks), lead breakage (less common with present systems), CSF leak, radicular pain, intermittent interference with cardiac pacemakers, and weakness.

99.8.5 Outcome

Success rate in pain control is ≈ 50% improvement in 50% of patients in experienced hands at specialized centers where multidisciplinary approach is available.[15] In a retrospective long-term follow-up study (ave = 96 months) of 410 patients that had SCS implantation due to numerous indications, success rate was 74%.[16]

Prognosticators of a poor response to SCS include: pain resulting from spinal cord injury, from lesions proximal to the ganglion (e.g. root avulsion), failed back syndrome with back pain > LE pain and multiple previous operations (see below), psychological factors such as litigation, workers compensation, familial/marital discord or drug seeking behavior.[17]

99.8.6 Specific syndromes treated

Failed back surgery syndrome

Σ

The addition of SCS improves pain control over either PT or medical management alone for failed back surgery syndrome. At 24 months, SCS is as effective as reoperation in treating radicular pain, with no difference in ADLs or work status.

In the PROCESS trial[18] (Prospective Randomized Controlled Multicenter Trial of the Effectiveness of Spinal Cord Stimulation), 100 patients with failed back surgery syndrome were randomized to SCS placement plus conventional medical management (52 patients) vs. conventional medical management alone (48 patients). The health-related quality of life, measured using EuroQol-5D questionnaire, was greater in the SCS group despite a higher total health care cost at 6 months.

In long-term follow-up at 24 months, the primary outcome (> 50% relief in leg pain) is achieved in 37% of patients that were randomized to SCS plus conventional medical management and 2% of patients that were randomized to conventional medical management only. Patients were allowed to cross-over. After cross-over, the primary outcome is achieved in 47% of patients (34 of 72) who had SCS plus medical management as final treatment versus 7% of patients (1 of 15) in the other group (P=0.02).[19]

In another randomized prospective study, patients with persistent or recurrent radicular pain after lumbosacral surgery were randomized to reoperation vs. SCS. On an average of 3-year follow-up, the SCS group required less opiate analgesics. 9 of 19 patients in the SCS group compared to only 3 of 26 patients reoperated had self reported pain relief and satisfaction ($P < 0.01$), and there was no difference in ADLs and work status. Patients in the SCS group were less likely to crossover to undergo reoperation (5 of 24 patients from the SCS group versus 14 of 26 patients in the reoperation group, $P = 0.02$).[20] In failed back-surgery syndrome SCSs are better for radicular pain than for low back pain.

Complex regional pain syndrome

99

Σ

SCS may be effective for treating CRPS during the first couple of years, however no significant benefit was evident at 5-year follow-up.

CRPS is a chronic pain condition marked by continuous disabling intense aching or burning pain. Type I has no known nerve injury, Type II follows a nerve injury (p. 497). The exact mechanism of the condition leading to intense disproportional pain is unknown and treatment options are limited. In a randomized clinical trial,[21] patients with CRPS Type I were randomized to receive SCS plus physical therapy (PT) (36 patients) or PT alone (18 patients). 24 of 36 patients had successful SCS trial and underwent implantation. At 6 months, in the group that received SCS plus PT, pain intensity reduced by 2.4 cm on the visual-analogue scale as opposed to an increase of 0.2 cm in the PT only group ($P < 0.001$). In addition, 39% of patients in the SCS group, had "much improved" globally perceived effect vs. 6% ($P = 0.01$). The health-related quality of life only improved in the SCS group. At 2-year follow-up, pain intensity in the SCS group reduced by 2.1 vs. 0.0 cm in the PT group compared to baseline ($P < 0.001$) and global perceived effect were "much improved" in 43% vs. 6% ($P = 0.001$).[22] However, these benefits were no longer significant in 5 years.[23]

Peripheral vascular disease

Σ

SCS does help with pain due to inoperable limb ischemia. It may or may not improve healing of pressure ulcers.

In a retrospective, non-control study of 38 patients, ≈ 94% experienced pain relief and ≈ 50% experienced healing of ischemic ulcers.[24]

In a recent review[25] of six controlled studies of nearly 450 patients, SCS + medical treatment was compared to medical treatment alone. Although there was no significant difference in ulcer healing, the use of analgesics was less and limb salvage after 12 months was significantly higher in the SCS group (relative risk = 0.71).

Angina pectoris

Σ

SCS was as effective as CABG in controlling refractory angina and protecting against MIs. SCS improves exercise capacity by an unknown mechanism.

SCS reduces anginal pain and improves exercise capacity by an unknown mechanism, which may be related to decrease in myocardial oxygen consumption[26] or altering myocardial blood flow[27] rather than just masking symptoms

In a multicenter, randomized, prospective clinical trial, comparing SCS to CABG in selected patient,[28] there was no significant difference in decreasing anginal attack and nitrates consumption between the groups. 5-year follow-up from this trial found that both CABG and SCS offered similar protection from angina pectoris and myocardial infarction.[29]

In a prospective study of 104 patients who underwent SCS placement for refractory angina pectoris (average follow-up ≈ 13 months), 73% had > 50% reduction of weekly anginal episodes compared to baseline.[30]

Diabetic neuropathy

Σ

Available data is limited, but SCS may be a viable modality for refractory pain from diabetic neuropathy. Further study is needed.

99

No good clinical data are available. A few studies with small numbers of patients suggest SCS can provide significant pain relieve in most patients with diabetic neuropathy that failed conservative management.[31,32,33]

A small prospective, open-label study reported 9 of 11 patients with diabetic neuropathy that failed conservative treatment had significant pain relieved after SCS implantation at 6 months. Pain score on visual analogue scale decreased from 77 to 34. Microcirculatory perfusion did not change significantly from baseline.[33]

99.9 Deep brain stimulation (DBS)

Deafferentation pain syndromes (anesthesia dolorosa, pain from spinal cord injury, or thalamic pain syndromes) may benefit from stimulation of sensory thalamus (ventral posteromedial (VPM) or ventral posterolateral (VPL)). DBS for chronic neuropathic pain produces a 40–50% reduction in pain in about 25–60% of patients.[34]

Nociceptive pain syndromes are more likely to benefit from stimulation of periventricular gray matter (PVG) or periaqueductal gray matter (PAG) although PAG stimulation is rarely used because it often produces unpleasant side effects. Still, response rate has been only ≈ 20%[35] resulting in failure of the FDA to approve these devices for pain.

Cluster headaches: may respond to hypothalamic stimulation, but larger trials with longer follow-up are needed.[34]

99.10 Dorsal root entry zone (DREZ) lesions

99.10.1 General information

Although use has been reported for a variety of indications, DREZ lesions appear to be most effective in treating the following:

DREZ lesions appear to be most effective in treating the following:

1. deafferentation pain resulting from nerve root avulsion.[36,37,38] This most commonly occurs in motorcycle accidents
2. spinal cord injuries (SCI) with pain around the lowest spared dermatome with caudal extension of pain restricted to a few dermatomes (SCI with diffuse pain involving the entire body and limbs below the injury is less responsive)
3. post herpetic neuralgia (p. 493): usually good initial response, but early recurrence in ≤ few months is common, and only 25% have long-term relief of pain
4. postamputation phantom limb pain: there is some support for this in the literature, but others feel this is not a good indication[39]
5. ✖ generally not used for cancer pain

99.10.2 Technique

A laminectomy is performed over the involved segment(s) using radiographic localization. The dura is opened, and the DREZ is identified under microscope magnification using intact posterior rootlets above or below for orientation (contralateral rootlets may also be used to estimate the mirror-image location). Lesions are created ipsilateral to the avulsed nerve roots by radiofrequency current (approximately 50–60 lesions are required for several segments, each lesion is done at 75° for ≈ 15 seconds) or selective incisions extending from the last completely normal rootlet at the rostral end to the first normal rootlet caudally. The lesioning needle or knife blade is angled 30–45° medially and inserted to a depth of 2–3 mm. DREZ lesions may be combined with a cordectomy at the level of anatomic cord disruption in paraplegic patients.[39]

99.10.3 Post-op management

Bed rest for 3 days may reduce the risk of CSF leakage. Analgesics appropriate for a multilevel laminectomy are administered.

99.10.4 Complications

Ipsilateral weakness (related to corticospinal tract) or loss of proprioception (dorsal columns) occurs in 10% of patients, and is permanent in ≈ half (i.e. 5%).

99.10.5 Outcome

In pain related to brachial plexus avulsion, 80–90% long-term significant improvement can be expected. Paraplegics with pain limited to the region of injury have an 80% rate of improvement, compared to 30% for those with pain involving the entire body below the lesion.

References

[1] Young RF, Kroening R, Fulton W, Feldman RA, Chambi I. Electrical Stimulation of the Brain in Treatment of Chronic Pain: Experience Over 5 Years. J Neurosurg. 1985; 62:389–396

[2] Shieff C, Nashold BS. Stereotactic Mesencephalotomy. Neurosurg Clin North Amer. 1990; 1:825–839

[3] Marshall KA. Managing Cancer Pain: Basic Principles and Invasive Treatment. Mayo Clin Proc. 1996; 71:472–477

[4] Krieger AJ, Rosomoff HL. Sleep-Induced Apnea. Part 1: A Respiratory and Autonomic Dysfunction Syndrome Following Bilateral Percutaneous Cervical Cordotomy. J Neurosurg. 1974; 39:168–180

[5] Sugar O. In Search of Ondine's Curse. JAMA. 1978; 240:236–237

[6] Schwartz HG. High Cervical Cordotomy. J Neurosurg. 1967; 26:452–455

[7] Nauta HJ, Soukup VM, Fabian RH, Lin JT, Grady JJ, Williams CG, Campbell GA, Westlund KN, Willis WD, Jr. Punctate midline myelotomy for the relief of visceral cancer pain. J Neurosurg Spine. 2000; 92:125–130

[8] Lobato RD, Madrid JL, Fatela LV, et al. Intraventricular Morphine for Intractable Cancer Pain: Rationale, Methods, Clinical Results. Acta Anaesthesiol Scand Suppl. 1987; 85:68–74

[9] Brazenor GA. Long Term Intrathecal Administration of Morphine: A Comparison of Bolus Injection via Reservoir with Continuous Infusion by Implantable Pump. Neurosurgery. 1987; 21:484–491

[10] Penn RD, Paice JA. Chronic Intrathecal Morphine for Intractable Pain. J Neurosurg. 1987; 67:182–186

[11] Shetter AG, Hadley MN, Wilkinson E. Administration of Intraspinal Morphine Sulfate for the Treatment of Intractable Cancer Pain. Neurosurgery. 1986; 18:740–747

[12] Rippe ES, Kresel JJ. Preparation of Morphine Sulfate Solutions for Intraspinal Administration. Am J Hosp Pharm. 1986; 43:1420–1421

[13] Cramond T, Stuart G. Intraventricular Morphine for Intractable Pain of Advanced Cancer. J Pain Sympt Manage. 1993; 8:465–473

[14] Kumar K, Nath R, Wyant GM. Treatment of Chronic Pain by Epidural Spinal Cord Stimulation. J Neurosurg. 1991; 75:402–407

[15] North RB, Kidd DH, Zahurak M, et al. Spinal Cord Stimulation for Chronic, Intractable Pain: Experience Over Two Decades. Neurosurgery. 1993; 32:384–395

[16] Kumar K, Hunter G, Demeria D. Spinal cord stimulation in treatment of chronic benign pain: challenges in treatment planning and present status, a 22-year experience. Neurosurgery. 2006; 58:481-96; discussion 481-96

[17] Daniel MS, Long C, Hutcherson WL, Hunter S. Psychological Factors and Outcome of Electrode Implantation for Chronic Pain. Neurosurgery. 1985; 17:773–777

[18] Manca A, Kumar K, Taylor RS, Jacques L, Eldabe S, Meglio M, Molet J, Thomson S, O'Callaghan J, Eisenberg E, Milbouw G, Buchser E, Fortini G, Richardson J, Taylor RJ, Goeree R, Sculpher MJ. Quality of life, resource consumption and costs of spinal cord stimulation versus conventional medical management in neuropathic pain patients with failed back surgery syndrome (PROCESS trial). Eur J Pain. 2008; 12:1047–1058

[19] Kumar K, Taylor RS, Jacques L, Eldabe S, Meglio M, Molet J, Thomson S, O'Callaghan J, Eisenberg E, Milbouw G, Buchser E, Fortini G, Richardson J, North RB. The effects of spinal cord stimulation in neuropathic pain are sustained: a 24-month follow-up of the prospective randomized controlled multicenter trial of the effectiveness of spinal cord stimulation. Neurosurgery. 2008; 63:762–70; discussion 770

[20] North RB, Kidd DH, Farrokhi F, Piantadosi SA. Spinal cord stimulation versus repeated lumbosacral spine surgery for chronic pain: a randomized, controlled trial. Neurosurgery. 2005; 56:98–106; discussion 106-7

[21] Kemler MA, Barendse GA, van Kleef M, de Vet HC, Rijks CP, Furnee CA, van den Wildenberg FA. Spinal cord stimulation in patients with chronic reflex sympathetic dystrophy. N Engl J Med. 2000; 343:618–624

[22] Kemler MA, De Vet HC, Barendse GA, Van Den Wildenberg FA, Van Kleef M. The effect of spinal cord stimulation in patients with chronic reflex sympathetic dystrophy: two years' follow-up of the randomized controlled trial. Ann Neurol. 2004; 55:13–18

[23] Kemler MA, de Vet HC, Barendse GA, van den Wildenberg FA, van Kleef M. Effect of spinal cord stimulation for chronic complex regional pain syndrome Type I: five-year final follow-up of patients in a randomized controlled trial. J Neurosurg. 2008; 108:292–298

[24] Augustinsson LE, Carlsson CA, Holm J, Jivegard L. Epidural electrical stimulation in severe limb ischemia. Pain relief, increased blood flow, and a possible limb-saving effect. Ann Surg. 1985; 202:104–110

[25] Ubbink DT, Vermeulen H. Spinal cord stimulation for non-reconstructable chronic critical leg ischaemia. Cochrane Database Syst Rev. 2005. DOI: 10.1002/14651858.CD004001.pub2

[26] Mannheimer C, Eliasson T, Andersson B, Bergh CH, Augustinsson LE, Emanuelsson H, Waagstein F. Effects of spinal cord stimulation in angina pectoris induced by pacing and possible mechanisms of action. BMJ. 1993; 307:477–480

[27] Hautvast RW, Blanksma PK, DeJongste MJ, Pruim J, van der Wall EE, Vaalburg W, Lie KI. Effect of spinal cord stimulation on myocardial blood flow assessed by positron emission tomography in patients with refractory angina pectoris. Am J Cardiol. 1996; 77:462–467

[28] Mannheimer C, Eliasson T, Augustinsson LE, Blomstrand C, Emanuelsson H, Larsson S, Norrsell H, Hjalmarsson A. Electrical stimulation versus coronary artery bypass surgery in severe angina pectoris: the ESBY study. Circulation. 1998; 97:1157–1163

[29] Ekre O, Eliasson T, Norrsell H, Wahrborg P, Mannheimer C. Long-term effects of spinal cord stimulation and coronary artery bypass grafting on quality of life and survival in the ESBY study. Eur Heart J. 2002; 23:1938–1945

[30] Di Pede F, Lanza GA, Zuin G, Alfieri O, Rapati M, Romano M, Circo A, Cardano P, Bellocci F, Santini M, Maseri A, Investigators of the Prospective Italian Registry of SCSforAnginaPectoris. Immediate and long-term clinical outcome after spinal cord stimulation for refractory stable angina pectoris. Am J Cardiol. 2003; 91:951–955

[31] Tesfaye S, Watt J, Benbow SJ, Pang KA, Miles J, MacFarlane IA. Electrical spinal-cord stimulation for painful diabetic peripheral neuropathy. Lancet. 1996; 348:1698–1701

[32] Daousi C, Benbow SJ, MacFarlane IA. Electrical spinal cord stimulation in the long-term treatment of chronic painful diabetic neuropathy. Diabet Med. 2005; 22:393–398

[33] de Vos CC, Rajan V, Steenbergen W, van der Aa HE, Buschman HP. Effect and safety of spinal cord stimulation for treatment of chronic pain caused by diabetic neuropathy. J Diabetes Complications. 2009; 23:40–45

[34] Awan NR, Lozano A, Hamani C. Deep brain stimulation: current and future perspectives. Neurosurg Focus. 2009; 27. DOI: 10.3171/2009.4.FOCUS0982

[35] Coffey RJ. Deep brain stimulation for chronic pain: results of two multicenter trials and a structured review. Pain Med. 2001; 2:183–192
[36] Thomas DGT, Jones SJ. Dorsal Root Entry Zone Lesions (Nashold's Procedure) in Brachial Plexus Avulsion. Neurosurgery. 1986; 15:966–968
[37] Nashold BS. Current Status of the DREZ Operation: 1984. Neurosurgery. 1984; 15:942–944
[38] Friedman AH, Nashold BS. Dorsal Root Entry Zone Lesions for the Treatment of Brachial Plexus Avulsion Injuries: A Follow-up Study. Neurosurgery. 1988; 22:369–373
[39] Burchiel KJ, Favre J. Current Techniques for Pain Control. Contemp Neurosurg. 1997; 19:1–6

100 Seizure Surgery

100.1 General information, indications

20% of patients continue to have seizures despite aggressive medical management with AEDs. Many of these patients may be candidates for surgical procedures to control their seizures.[1]

Seizure disorder must be severe, medically refractory with satisfactory trials of tolerable medication for at least 1 year, and disabling to the patient. Medically refractory is usually considered two attempts of high-dose monotherapy with two distinct AEDs, and one attempt at polytherapy.

The three general categories of patients suitable for seizure surgery have[2]:

1. partial seizures
   a) temporal origin: the largest group of surgical candidates (especially mesial temporal lobe epilepsy (MTLE) which is often medically refractory)
   b) extratemporal origin
2. symptomatic generalized seizures: e.g. Lennox-Gastaut
3. unilateral, multifocal epilepsy associated with infantile hemiplegia syndrome

100.2 Pre-surgical evaluation

100.2.1 General information

All patients should undergo high resolution MRI study to rule out neoplasm, AVM, cavernous malformations, mesial temporal sclerosis or hippocampal lesion. Noninvasive techniques allow localization in the majority of cases.

100.2.2 Noninvasive evaluation techniques

► **Video-EEG monitoring.** Pre-operative long-term inpatient video-EEG monitoring (surface electrodes) to correlate the clinically disabling seizure with appropriate electrical abnormalities and possibly to identify the seizure focus is required.

► **High-resolution MRI.** The imaging modality of choice. Extremely good for detecting hippocampal asymmetry of mesial temporal sclerosis (MTS), and neuronal developmental abnormalities (e.g. cortical dysplasia) that may produce complex partial seizures (CPS).[3]

► **CAT scan.** A seizure focus may enhance with IV contrast shortly following a seizure. Subtle enhancement may be present on the side of the focus on interictal CT scan.[4]

► **PET scan (positron emission tomography).** Interictal PET scan using fluorine-18 deoxyglucose (18FDG) shows *hypo*metabolism lateralized to the side of temporal lobe focus in 70% of patients with medically refractory CPS (does not show actual *site* of origin). Useful when MRI and EEG cannot localize.

► **SPECT scan (single photon emission tomography).** Used to demonstrate increased blood flow during a seizure to help localize site of onset. [99m] Technetium (Tc) hexamethyl-propylene-amine-oxime (HMPAO) is usually administered immediately after onset of seizure, and the scan may be obtained within several hours.[5]

► **MEG (Magnetoencephalography).** Functional imaging technique for mapping brain activity by recording magnetic fields created by neuronal activity (electrical current).[6] Synchronized neuronal currents induce a weak magnetic field. Clinical uses include detecting and localizing pathological activity in patients with epilepsy and in localizing eloquent cortex for pre-operative surgical planning. Requires a magnetically shield room.

100.2.3 Mildly invasive techniques

► **Wada test.**[7] AKA intracarotid amytal test. Localizes dominant hemisphere (side of language function) and assesses ability of hemisphere without lesion to maintain memory when isolated. Usually reserved for candidates for large resections.[8] Each cerebral hemisphere is individually anesthetized via selective carotid catheterization (usually by a neurointerventionalist) and injection of short acting barbiturate.

Start with angiogram to assess cross flow and to R/O persistent trigeminal artery (p.83). Significant cross-flow is a relative contraindication to anesthetizing the side of dominant supply (patient goes to sleep).

Wada test may be grossly inaccurate with high flow AVM. Also, portions of hippocampus may be supplied by posterior circulation (not anesthetized by ICA injection).

EEG monitoring is usually performed during the test when it is being done for seizure surgery. Patient will show delta waves during deepest level of anesthesia.

Technique

- instruct patient as to what is expected
- catheterize ICA: usually start on side of lesion
- have patient hold contralateral arm in air, and instruct them to hold it there
- inject 100–125 mg sodium *amobarbital* (Amytal®) rapidly into internal carotid artery (effect starts almost instantaneously, begins to subside after ≈ 8 minutes; (may subside in ≈ 2 minutes with AVM where flow rates are high)
- determine adequacy of injection by assessing motor function in elevated arm (should be ≈ flaccid)
- assess language skills by showing patient pictures of objects and ask them to name each one out loud and remember each one
- assess memory function by asking patient to name as many of the pictures as they can ≈ 15 minutes after test: if they have difficulty, ask them to pick out pictures from a group that contains additional ones not shown to patient
- repeat procedure on other side (use lower Amytal doses with each subsequent injection)

100.2.4 Evaluation techniques requiring surgery

▶ **EEG obtained with invasive electrodes.** Indications: Lack of lateralizing or localizing electrophysiology in pre-operative evaluation re-quires invasive electrodes for better definition of seizure focus.

Surgical options:

- Depth electrodes
  - Electrodes are placed stereotactically
  - stereoencephalography (sEEG): popularized in Europe by J. Talairach and J. Bancaud during the 1950s for invasive mapping of refractory focal epilepsy. The techniques requires the placement of multiple depth electrodes in an orthogonal orien-tation to localize seizure onset.[9,10,11]
  - 2-3% risk of intracerebral hemorrhage.[8] Risk of infection with depth electrodes[8]: 2-10%.
- Subdural grids or strips
  - Grids are frequently used for extra-operative functional mapping (helpful in children or in the mentally retarded). Subdural grid electrodes are placed with a craniotomy.
  - Surface strip electrodes may be placed through a burr hole
  - useful technique for intra-operative functional mapping

100.3 Surgical techniques

100.3.1 Basic procedures

Three basic types of procedure: resections, disconnections and stimulation.[1]

1. resections
   a) resection of epileptic focus: higher chance of completely controlling seizures. Performed in noneloquent brain. Seizures must have focal onset (resection not encouraged if multifocal onset). Includes:
      - anterior temporal lobectomy or amydalo-hippocampectomy for MTLE: see below
      - neocortical resections: especially with neuronal migration abnormalities
   b) resection of lesion in secondary epilepsy (lesional epilepsy e.g. tumor, AVM, cavernous malformation[12]...). In most cases the seizure focus is in or near the lesion, but some structural lesions are not responsible for the seizures. For seizure foci within the mesial temporal lobe, seizure control is better when lesionectomy is accompanied by amygdalo-hippocampectomy[13]
2. disconnections: used when eloquent brain is involved, or to separate the electrical activity of the two cerebral hemispheres
   a) section of corpus callosum (callosotomy): when drop attacks are the most disabling seizure type or for multiple bilateral foci (see below)

   b) hemispherectomy: for unilateral seizures with widespread hemispheric lesions and profound contralateral neurologic deficit. If any cortex is left, must make sure it is functionally deafferented (disconnected)
      - anatomic hemispherectomy
      - functional hemispherectomy: preservation of the basal ganglia isolates the abnormal side with ≈ 80% seizure control rate (similar to anatomic hemispherectomy, but with lower complication rate).
   c) multiple subpial transection[14]: for partial seizure originating in eloquent cortical areas. The cortex is transected at 5 mm intervals, thus interrupting the horizontal spread of the seizure while sparing the vertically oriented functional fibers
3. stimulation: usually offered to non-resective candidates (poor localization or surgical failures). It is a reversible and adjustable mode of therapy.
4. Open Loop stimulation: blind stimulation continuously or intermittently
   a) vagus nerve stimulation (p. 1558)
   b) deep brain stimulation (DBS)
      - centromedian nucleus of the thalamus[15]: better for generalized tonic-clonic seizures
      - bilateral anterior nucleus of the thalamus: for partial seizures[16]
      - hippocampus[15]: for partial seizures
5. Closed Loop stimulation: react to a burst of stimulation (detection). Responsive cortical stimulation (RNS)[17] requires a receive and a send electrode for electrical stimulation

Neurostimulation offers between 30-40% seizure reduction for most of the patients implanted. Risks include hardware failure, hemorrhage (not typically seen with VNS), infection and stimulation induced side-effects.

100.3.2 Anesthetic considerations

If intraoperative electrocorticography is to be performed:
- under local anesthesia: the only anesthetic agents that may be used are narcotics (usually fentanyl) and droperidol
- under general anesthesia: *avoid* benzodiazepines and barbiturates

100.3.3 Intraoperative electrocorticography (ECoG)

Subdural strips and/or grids are useful for ECoG and motor/speech mapping.

Methohexital (Brevitol®) may be given to try to provoke a seizure: observe for ↓ fast activity in suspected focus.

100.3.4 Intraoperative cortical mapping

See techniques of cortical mapping (p. 1432).

100.4 Surgical procedures

100.4.1 Corpus callosotomy

Indications and contraindications

Partial or total section may be most effective for generalized major motor seizures. Of little benefit for simple or complex seizures. Benefit has been supported for:
1. frequent episodes of *atonic seizures* ("drop attacks") where loss of postural tone → falls and injuries[18] (70% reduction with callosotomy), typically seen in Lennox-Gastaut syndrome
2. possibly for generalized seizure disorder with unilateral hemisphere damage (e.g. infantile hemiplegia syndrome); hemicortical resection may be better for this type, whereas callosotomy may promote partial seizures.
   Note: a "functional hemispherectomy" is recommended over "anatomically complete" hemispherectomy to reduce morbidity and mortality[2]
3. some patients with generalized seizures without identifiable, resectable focus
4. ✖ Contraindication: major behavioral and/or language deficits may occur even with partial division in patients with speech and dominant handedness located in *opposite* hemispheres ("crossed dominance"). Thus, Wada test is recommended in all left handed patients

Technical details

Division of the anterior two-thirds of the corpus callosum (CC) (minimizes the risk of disconnection syndrome, see below) may be advantageous over complete callosotomy (controversial). Some advocate sectioning the CC with intraoperative EEG until the typical bisynchronous discharges that are usually seen become asynchronous.[19] No need to section anterior commissure. Can usually be performed via a bifrontal craniotomy utilizing a bicoronal skin incision.

May produce post-op ↓ verbalization or akinetic mutism that usually resolves in weeks.

MRI sagittal cuts are ideal for assessing extent of division of the CC.[20]

Disconnection syndrome

In a patient with a dominant left hemisphere, consists of left tactile anomia, left sided dyspraxia (may resemble hemiparesis), pseudohemianopsia, right sided anomia for smell, impaired spatial synthesis of right hand resulting in difficulty copying complex figures, decreased spontaneity of speech, incontinence.

More common with larger surgical sections of the CC. Risk is less if the anterior commissure is spared. Patients usually adapt after 2–3 months, with final function normal for most daily activities (deficits may show up on neuropsychological testing).

100.4.2 Mesial temporal lobe epilepsy (MTLE)

General information

80% of patients with medically intractable temporal seizures have a demonstrable focus in the anterior-mesial temporal lobe. Most patients have neuronal loss and gliosis of mesial temporal structures (mesial temporal sclerosis, MTS). Thus, a standard resection of temporal tip (with amygdalo-hippocampectomy) may be performed. In a randomized trial, anterior temporal lobectomy (ATL) was shown to be superior to medical management for treatment of medically resistant epilepsy. Results at one year show seizure reduction and improved quality of life in those patients who underwent ATL versus medical management alone for intractable epilepsy.[21]

Limits of resection (without significant neurologic deficit)

Note that these values are generally considered safe, however, variations occur from patient to patient and only intraoperative mapping can reliably determine the location of language centers.[22] Most centers spare the superior temporal gyrus.[23] The following measurements are made along the *middle* temporal gyrus:

- *dominant* temporal lobe: up to 4–5 cm may be removed. Over-resection may injure speech centers, which cannot be reliably localized visually
- *non-dominant* temporal lobe: 6–7 cm may be resected. Slight over-resection may → partial contralateral upper quadrant homonymous hemianopsia; resection of 8–9 cm → complete quadrantanopsia

Alternatively, intraoperative electrocorticography may be used to guide resection of electrically abnormal areas.

Resection should be performed in subpial plane to prevent injury to vascular branches.

100.4.3 Selective amygdalo-hippocampectomy (SAH)

Surgery for temporal lobe epilepsy was initially treated with anterior temporal lobectomy as described by Penfield and Baldwin. In 1958, Niemeyer described a more selective approach to the hippocampus and amygdala through the middle temporal gyrus.[24] It would be almost thirty years until selective amygdalo-hippocampectomy was later modified. The goal of SAH is to remove the epileptogenic focus while minimizing disruption of nearby neurovascular structures and white matter tracts. Image guidance is very helpful for these techniques. More recent studies have compared standard ATL to SAH and found that both techniques have similar outcome with regard to seizure freedom but suggest an improved neuropsychological outcome with SAH versus ATL.[25,26]

Three basic approaches:

1. transcortical: inferior temporal gyrus (ITG) approach. This technique uses a minimal access approach via a trephine craniotomy for SAH[27]
2. transsylvian: approach requires a pterional craniotomy. More restrictive and greater risk of injury to M1 portion of MCA within sylvian fissure[28]
3. subtemporal: uses a temporal fossa approach to access mesial structures[29,30]

100.5 Risks of seizure surgery

Major risks are related to[31]:

1. removal of essential areas of cortex
2. injury to medullary core underlying cortical resection (projection fibers, association fibers, and/or commissural fibers): the most common deficit after temporal lobectomy is a contralateral (homonymous) superior quadrantanopsia (so-called "pie-in-the-sky" defect, due to an injury to Meyer's loop wherein the fibers for the superior visual field of the optic radiation take a slight rostral "detour" towards the temporal tip)
3. injury to vessels in area of resection → ischemic damage to areas supplied: especially sylvian branches during temporal lobectomy, anterior choroidal artery resulting in hemiparesis during mesial temporal lobe resection, or ACA branches with corpus callosotomy
4. injury to nearby cranial nerves: especially third nerve during hippocampectomy where it lies medial to tentorium

100.6 MRI guided laser interstitial thermal therapy (MRGLITT)

Laser-induced thermal therapy uses thermal energy to induce cell death by damaging DNA and causing protein denaturation. The current therapy is performed with simultaneous MRI stereotactic guidance and real time feedback from the ablated lesion.[32,33] It is considered less invasive than microsurgery. Main advantage is a shorter post-operative recovery period. Technique has been used for lesional and nonlesional epilepsy. Preliminary seizure control ≈60-70%. No long-term data is yet available.

100.7 Postoperative management for seizure surgery (epilepsy surgery)

1. ICU for observation (24 hrs)
2. for seizures in the immediate post-op period ("honeymoon seizures"), not necessary to treat only one brief generalized seizure, otherwise load appropriately with IV Keppra or phenytoin
3. 10 mg dexamethasone (Decadron®) IV before surgery followed by q 8 hrs as necessary (longer taper for laser ablation and radiosurgery)
4. anticonvulsants are continued × 1–2 years even if no post-op seizures occur
5. after discharge: neuropsychiatric evaluation 6-12 months after surgery

100.8 Outcome

Modified Engel classification outcome is shown in▸ Table 100.1.[34]

100.8.1 Outcome with resection of seizure focus

The greatest effect of seizure surgery is *reduction of seizure frequency*,[23] however, any surgical procedure may fail to have a beneficial effect.

Seizure control is usually assessed at 1, 3 & 6 most post-op, and then annually. A post-op MRI is usually obtained at 3 most post-op to assess extent of surgical resection. Most patients take anti-epileptic drugs (AEDs) for 2 years post-op, and then may be discontinued in those free of seizures.

Recurrent seizures: although late seizures may occur, 90% of seizures that recur do so within 2 years.

Table 100.1 Modified Engel classification of seizure surgery outcome

Class	Description
I	seizure free or residual auras
II	rare disabling seizures (<3 complex parital seizures per year)
III	worthwhile seizure reduction
IV	no worthwhile seizure improvement

2 years post-op in patients maintained on AEDs: 50% are seizure-free, and 80% have over 50% reduction of seizure frequency.

For temporal lobectomies in the dominant hemisphere without intraoperative monitoring, there is a 6% risk of mild dysphasia. Significant memory deficits occur in ≈ 2%.

100.8.2 Radiosurgery for epilepsy

Stereotactic radiosurgery has been suggested to be an effective treatment for pharmacoresistant epilepsy with the potential for less morbidity than resection.[35,36] Seizure free outcomes ≈ 65% for MTLE (delayed response to therapy ≈6-12 months). Potential for long-term complications remains a concern (radionecrosis).[37]

100.8.3 Vagus nerve stimulation (VNS)

Electrodes wrapped around the vagus nerve in the neck are connected to an implanted programmable generator to stimulate the nerve to reduce seizure frequency. As is also true with many AEDs, the mechanism of action is not well understood.

Indications: Although it has been used (off label) for treatment resistant depression and other psychiatric conditions, the FDA approved indication is for adjunctive therapy for patients > 12 years old with partial onset seizures refractory to medical treatment.

Complications: Main risk of surgery is transient or permanent vocal cord paralysis.

Outcome: In a 12 year retrospective review of VNS in 12 patients,[38] mean seizure frequency decreased by 26% at 1 year, by 30% at 5 years, and by 52% after 12 years.

References

[1] Engel JJ. Surgery for Seizures. N Engl J Med. 1996; 334:647–652

[2] National Institutes of Health Consensus Development Conference. Surgery for Epilepsy. JAMA. 1990; 264:729–733

[3] Barkovich AJ, Rowley HA, Anderman F. MR in Partial Epilepsy: Value of High-Resolution Volumetric Techniques. AJNR. 1995; 16:339–343

[4] Oakley J, Ojemann GA, Ojemann LM, et al. Identifying Epileptic Foci on Contrast-Enhanced CAT Scans. Arch Neurol. 1979; 36:669–671

[5] Harvey AS, Hopkins IJ, Bowe JM, et al. Frontal Lobe Epilepsy: Clinical Seizure Characteristics and Localization with Ictal ^{99m}Tc-HMPAO SPECT. Neurology. 1993; 43:1966–1980

[6] Tovar-Spinoza ZS, Ochi A, Rutka JT, Go C, Otsubo H. The role of magnetoencephalography in epilepsy surgery. Neurosurg Focus. 2008; 25. DOI: 10.3171/FOC/2008/25/9/E16

[7] Wada J, Rasmussen T. Intracranial Injection of Amytal for the Lateralization of Cerebral Speech Dominance. J Neurosurg. 1960; 17:266–282

[8] Queenan JV, Germano IM. Advances in the Neurosurgical Management of Adult Epilepsy. Contemp Neurosurg. 1997; 19:1–6

[9] Bancaud J, Angelergues R, Bernouilli C, Bonis A, Bordas-Ferrer M, Bresson M, Buser P, Covello L, Morel P, Szikla G, Takeda A, Talairach J. Functional stereotaxic exploration (SEEG) of epilepsy. Electroencephalogr Clin Neurophysiol. 1970; 28:85–86

[10] Talairach J, Bancaud J, Bonis A, Szikla G, Trottier S, Vignal JP, Chauvel P, Munari C, Chodkievicz JP. Surgical therapy for frontal epilepsies. Adv Neurol. 1992; 57:707–732

[11] Gonzalez-Martinez J, Mullin J, Vadera S, Bulacio J, Hughes G, Jones S, Enatsu R, Najm I. Stereotactic placement of depth electrodes in medically intractable epilepsy. J Neurosurg. 2014; 120:639–644

[12] Cohen DS, Zubay GP, Goodman RR. Seizure Outcome After Lesionectomy for Cavernous Malformations. J Neurosurg. 1995; 83:237–242

[13] Jooma R, Yeh H-S, Privitera MD, Gartner M. Lesionectomy versus Electrophysiologically Guided Resection for Temporal Lobe Tumors Manifesting with Complex Partial Seizures. J Neurosurg. 1995; 83:231–236

[14] Morrell F, Whisler WW, Bleck TP. Multiple subpial transection: A new approach to the surgical treatment of focal epilepsy. J Neurosurg. 1989; 70:231–239

[15] Velasco M, Velasco F, Velasco AL. Centromedian-thalamic and hippocampal electrical stimulation for the control of intractable epileptic seizures. J Clin Neurophysiol. 2001; 18:495–513

[16] Fisher R, Salanova V, Witt T, Worth R, Henry T, Gross R, Oommen K, Osorio I, Nazzaro J, Labar D, Kaplitt M, Sperling M, Sandok E, Neal J, Handforth A, Stern J, DeSalles A, Chung S, Shetter A, Bergen D, Bakay R, Henderson J, French J, Baltuch G, Rosenfeld W, Youkilis A, Marks W, Garcia P, Barbaro N, Fountain N, Bazil C, Goodman R, McKhann G, Babu Krishnamurthy K, Papavassiliou S, Epstein C, Pollard J, Tonder L, Grebin J, Coffey R, Graves N. Electrical stimulation of the anterior nucleus of thalamus for treatment of refractory epilepsy. Epilepsia. 2010; 51:899–908

[17] Morrell MJ. Responsive cortical stimulation for the treatment of medically intractable partial epilepsy. Neurology. 2011; 77:1295–1304

[18] Gates JR, Leppik IE, Yap J, et al. Corpus Callosotomy: Clinical and Electroencephalographic Effects. Epilepsia. 1984; 25:308–316

[19] Marino R, Ragazzo PC, Reeves AG. Epilepsy and the Corpus Callosum. New York: Plenum Press; 1985:281–302

[20] Bogen JE, Schultz DH, Vogel PJ. Completeness of Callosotomy Shown by MRI in the Long Term. Arch Neurol. 1988; 45:1203–1205

[21] Wiebe S, Blume WT, Girvin JP, Eliasziw M. A randomized, controlled trial of surgery for temporal-lobe epilepsy. N Engl J Med. 2001; 345:311–318

[22] Ojemann GA, Engel J. Surgical Treatment of the Epilepsies. New York: Raven Press; 1987:635–639

[23] Ojemann GA. Surgical Therapy for Medically Intractable Epilepsy. J Neurosurg. 1987; 66:489–499

[24] Niemeyer P, Baldwin M, Bailey P. In: The transventricular amygdala-hippocampectomy in temporal lobe epilepsy. Temporal Lobe Epilepsy. Springfield: Charles C Thomas; 1958:461–482

[25] Paglioli E, Palmini A, Portuguez M, Paglioli E, Azambuja N, da Costa JC, da Silva Filho HF, Martinez JV, Hoeffel JR. Seizure and memory outcome following temporal lobe surgery: selective compared with nonselective approaches for hippocampal sclerosis. J Neurosurg. 2006; 104:70–78

[26] Wendling AS, Hirsch E, Wisniewski I, Davanture C, Ofer I, Zentner J, Bilic S, Scholly J, Staack AM, Valenti MP, Schulze-Bonhage A, Kehrli P, Steinhoff BJ. Selective amygdalohippocampectomy versus standard temporal lobectomy in patients with mesial temporal lobe epilepsy and unilateral hippocampal sclerosis. Epilepsy Res. 2013; 104:94–104

[27] Duckworth EA, Vale FL. Trephine epilepsy surgery: the inferior temporal gyrus approach. Neurosurgery. 2008; 63:ONS156–60; discussion ONS160-1

[28] Yasargil MG, Krayenbuhl N, Roth P, Hsu SP, Yasargil DC. The selective amygdalohippocampectomy for intractable temporal limbic seizures. J Neurosurg. 2010; 112:168–185

[29] Hori T, Tabuchi S, Kurosaki M, Kondo S, Takenobu A, Watanabe T. Subtemporal amygdalohippocampectomy for treating medically intractable temporal lobe epilepsy. Neurosurgery. 1993; 33:50–6; discussion 56-7

[30] Park TS, Bourgeois BF, Silbergeld DL, Dodson WE. Subtemporal transparahippocampal amygdalohippocampectomy for surgical treatment of mesial temporal lobe epilepsy. Technical note. J Neurosurg. 1996; 85:1172–1176

[31] Crandall PH, Engel J. In: Cortical Resections. Surgical Treatment of the Epilepsies. New York: Raven Press; 1987:377–404

[32] Willie JT, Laxpati NG, Drane DL, Gowda A, Appin C, Hao C, Brat DJ, Helmers SL, Saindane A, Nour SG, Gross RE. Real-time magnetic resonance-guided stereotactic laser amygdalohippocampotomy for mesial temporal lobe epilepsy. Neurosurgery. 2014; 74:569–84; discussion 584-5

[33] Curry DJ, Gowda A, McNichols RJ, Wilfong AA. MR-guided stereotactic laser ablation of epileptogenic foci in children. Epilepsy Behav. 2012; 24:408–414

[34] Engel J, Van Ness PC, Rasmussen TB, Ojemann LM, Engel J. In: Outcome with respect to epileptic seizures. Surgical Treatment of the Epilepsies. 2nd ed. New York: Raven Press; 1993:609–621

[35] Barbaro NM, Quigg M, Broshek DK, Ward MM, Lamborn KR, Laxer KD, Larson DA, Dillon W, Verhey L, Garcia P, Steiner L, Heck C, Kondziolka D, Beach R, Olivero W, Witt TC, Salanova V, Goodman R. A multicenter, prospective pilot study of gamma knife radiosurgery for mesial temporal lobe epilepsy: seizure response, adverse events, and verbal memory. Ann Neurol. 2009; 65:167–175

[36] Regis J, Rey M, Bartolomei F, Vladyka V, Liscak R, Schrottner O, Pendl G. Gamma knife surgery in mesial temporal lobe epilepsy: a prospective multicenter study. Epilepsia. 2004; 45:504–515

[37] Vale FL, Bozorg AM, Schoenberg MR, Wong K, Witt TC. Long-term radiosurgery effects in the treatment of temporal lobe epilepsy. J Neurosurg. 2012; 117:962–969

[38] Uthman BM, Reichl AM, Dean JC, Eisenschenk S, Gilmore R, Reid S, Roper SN, Wilder BJ. Effectiveness of vagus nerve stimulation in epilepsy patients: a 12-year observation. Neurology. 2004; 63:1124–1126

101 Radiation Therapy (XRT)

101.1 Introduction

Ionizing radiation comprises a portion of the electromagnetic spectrum and includes x-rays and gamma rays (both of which are electromagnetic radiation and transmit their energy via photons) and particulate radiation. The goal of XRT in treating tumors is to cause cell death or to stop cell replication. Photons impart critical energy to achieve this result by the photoelectric effect (at lower energies, < 0.05 MeV), by Compton scattering (at higher energies of 0.1–10 MeV, e.g. in linear accelerators and Gamma knives), or by pair-production (at the highest energies).[1] In the Compton effect, the initial collision of the photon with an atom creates a free electron which then ionizes other atoms and breaks chemical bonds. The absorption of radiation by indirect ionization in the presence of water produces free radicals (containing an unpaired electron) which causes cellular injury (usually by damaging DNA) within the tumor.

See discussion of radiation dosage and units (p. 223).

101.2 Conventional external beam radiation

101.2.1 Fractionation

The practice in which the total radiation dose is delivered in a series of smaller brief applications. This is one means of increasing the therapeutic ratio (the ratio of the effectiveness of XRT on tumor cells to that of normal cells). Radiation injury is a function of the dose, the exposure time, and the area exposed. Radiation oncologists refer to the four "R's" of radiobiology[2]:

1. Repair of sublethal damage
2. Reoxygenation of tumor cells that were hypoxic before XRT: oxygenated cells are more sensitive than hypoxic cells because oxygen combines with unpaired electrons to form peroxides which are more stable and lethal than free radicals
3. Repopulation of tumor cells following treatment
4. Redistribution (or reassortment) of cells within the cell cycle: cells in the mitotic phase are the most sensitive

101.2.2 Dosing

The biologically effective dose of fractionated radiation is often modeled by the linear-quadratic equation (LQ-model) shown in Eq (101.1), where n = the number of doses, d = dose per fraction, and the factors α & β are used to describe the cell response to radiation. A high α/β ratio ≥ 10 is designated as early-responding tissue such as tumor cells, and a ratio ≤ 3 is considered late-responding tissue (mitotically quiescent), such as normal brain and also AVMs.

Linear quadratic equation:

$$\text{biologically effective dose (BED) (Gy)} = n \times d \times \left[1 + \frac{d}{\alpha/\beta}\right] \qquad (101.1)$$

101.2.3 Cranial radiation

General information

Following surgery for tumor (craniotomy or spinal surgery), most surgeons wait ≈ 7–10 days before instituting XRT to the surgical site (allows initiation of healing from surgery).

Two CNS tumors that "melt away" with XRT but tend to recur later:

1. lymphoma
2. germ cell tumors

Radiation injury and necrosis

General information

Radiation necrosis (RN) may mimic recurrent (or denovo) tumor both clinically and radiographically. Differences in prognosis and treatment make it important to distinguish between tumor and RN.

Pathophysiology

As radiation is selectively toxic to more rapidly dividing cells, the two normal cell types within the CNS most vulnerable to RN are vascular endothelium (which have a turnover time of ≈ 6–10 mos) and oligodendroglial cells. Vascular injury may be the primary limiting factor to the tolerance of cranial XRT.[3] Injury from XRT occurs at lower doses when given concurrently with chemotherapy (especially methotrexate).

Etiology of side effects

The mechanism(s) by which XRT causes side effects is not known with certainty, but may be due to:
1. damage to vascular endothelium: effects on cerebral vasculature may differ substantially from effects on systemic vessels[3]
2. glial injury
3. immune system effect

Radiation effects are divided into 3 phases[4]:
1. *acute*: occur during treatment. Rare. Usually an exacerbation of symptoms already present. Probably secondary to edema. Treat with ↑ steroids
2. *early delayed*: few weeks to 2–3 mos following completion of XRT. In spinal cord → Lhermitte's sign. In brain → post-irradiation lethargy & memory difficulties
3. *late delayed*: 3 mos-12 yrs (most within 3 years). Due to small artery injury → thrombotic occlusion → white matter atrophy or frank coagulative necrosis

Manifestations of radiation effects:
1. decreased cognition
   a) dementia may develop following XRT[5] in as little as 1 year post-XRT. Incidence was higher when doses of 25–39 Gy were given in fractions > 300 cGy[6]
   b) children: may attain lower IQ by ≈ 25 points, especially with > 40 Gy whole brain XRT. Measurable IQ differences occur in children radiated before age 7, but more subtle deficits occur even in older children[7]
2. radiation necrosis
3. injury to anterior optic pathways
4. injury to hypothalamic-pituitary axis → hypopituitarism → growth retardation in children; see radiation injury to pituitary (p. 744)
5. primary hypothyroidism (especially in children)
6. may induce formation of new tumor: tumors most commonly identified as having increased incidence following radiation treatment are gliomas (including glioblastoma[8]), meningiomas,[9] and nerve sheath tumors.[10] Skull base tumors have been reported following EBRT[11]
7. malignant transformation: e.g. after SRS for vestibular schwannomas (p. 686)
8. leukoencephalopathy: profound demyelinating/necrotizing reaction 4–12 mos after combined RXT and methotrexate, especially in children with acute lymphoblastic leukemia (ALL) and adults with primary CNS tumors

Evaluation (differentiating RN from recurrent tumor)

Greenberg IMHO

Over the years many methods have been championed to differentiate radiation necrosis from recurrent high-grade glioma. Some are listed below. None have proven adequately reliable, and this may not even be a useful exercise. Tumor cells are frequently found on biopsy. The decision whether to reoperate is usually based on whether there is progressive mass effect (regardless of whether it is necrosis or tumor) taking into consideration the patient's neurologic condition, projected longevity, patient desires...

CT and MRI

Cannot reliably differentiate some cases of RN from tumor (especially astrocytoma; RN occasionally resembles glioblastoma).

MR spectroscopy (p. 233) was reliable in distinguishing pure tumor (elevated choline) from pure RN (low choline), but was less definitive with mixed tumor/necrosis.[12]

101

DWI: mean ADCs were lower with recurrence (1.18 ± 0.13 X 10–3 mm/s) vs. necrosis (1.4 ± 0.17 X 10–3 mm/s)[13] (not all cases biopsy proven).

Nuclear brain scan

Some reports of success with thallium-201 and technetium-99 m brain scans.

Computerized radionuclide studies

PET (positron emission tomography) scan: because positron emitting isotopes have short half-lives, PET scanning requires a nearby cyclotron to generate the radiopharmaceuticals at great expense. Utilizing [18F]-fluorodeoxyglucose (FDG), regional glucose metabolism is imaged and is generally increased with recurrent tumor, and is decreased with RN. Specificity for distinguishing RN from tumor recurrence is > 90%, but sensitivity may be too low to make it reliable.[14] Amino acid tracers such as [11C]methionine and [18F]tyrosine are taken up by most brain tumors,[15] especially gliomas, and may also be used to help differentiate tumor from necrosis. Accuracy may be increased by fusing PET scan with MRI.[16]

SPECT (single positron emission computed tomography): "poor man's PET scan." Uses radiolabeled amphetamine. Uptake depends on presence of intact neurons and the condition of cerebral blood vessels (including blood brain barrier). Decreased radionuclide uptake indicates necrosis, whereas tumor recurrence has no decreased uptake.

Treatment

Symptoms from any form of radiation toxicity often respond initially to steroids.

Reoperation and excision is appropriate if there is deterioration from mass effect, regardless of whether the mass effect is from recurrent tumor or RN; the decision to reoperate should be based on the patient's Karnofsky rating (p. 1358). Although some benefit has been shown, most reoperation studies are biased because they often select the patients who are doing better.

Other forms of therapy include: hyperbaric oxygen and anticoagulation.

Patients with documented tumor recurrence (as opposed to RN) may also be considered for additional radiation (external beam, interstitial brachytherapy, or stereotactic radiosurgery (SRS)) or chemotherapy.

Prevention

Injury is dependent on total radiation dose, number of treatments or fractions (less damage occurs with more frequent small treatments), and volume treated.

Various studies to determine the tolerance of *normal* brain to XRT have estimated that 65–75 Gy given over 6.5–8 wks in 5 fractions/week is usually tolerated (radiation necrosis will occur in ≈ 5% after 60 Gy fractionated in 30 treatments over 6 weeks). Other studies have shown tolerance to 45 Gy for 10 fractions, 60 Gy for 35 fractions, and 70 Gy for 60 fractions.[4]

101.2.4 Spinal radiation

General information

Most spine tumors are metastatic cancer. There is no proof that any treatment for spinal metastases will prolong survival. Treatment goals, regardless of the treatment modality, are pain relief and preservation of function.

Radiation therapy (XRT) is the main treatment modality for spinal metastases. Even tumors that are not considered "radio-sensitive" can respond to XRT.

Typical spinal radiation

For most metastatic spine tumors treated with conventional radiation therapy (i.e. not stereotactic radiosurgery), the usual fractionation is 30 Gy administered over 10 fractions.

Emergency spinal radiation

For acute spinal cord paralysis from tumor, if emergency surgery is not a consideration, 8 Gy can be administered in the 1st fraction for lymphoma, multiple myeloma, and (although this is not standard) it could be considered for small-cell (neuroendocrine) carcinoma since it is so radiosensitive.

Side effects

1. radiation myelopathy: see below
2. those due to overlap with GI tract: N/V, diarrhea
3. bone marrow suppression
4. growth retardation in children[17]
5. risk of developing cavernous malformations of the spinal cord (p. 1247)

Radiation myelopathy

Radiation myelopathy (RM) typically occurs in patients with spinal cord included in radiation therapy (XRT) ports used to treat cancer outside the spinal cord, includes breast, lung, thyroid, and epidural mets. Radiation neuropathy may occur with irradiation in the region of the axilla for carcinoma of the breast (p. 544). In the lower extremities, XRT for pelvic or bone tumors (e.g. of the femur) may produce lumbar plexopathy. In addition to permanent changes, radiation therapy may also produce spinal cord edema which may resolve after completion of radiation therapy.

Epidemiology

Incidence difficult to estimate due to the fact that the onset is typically delayed together with the poor survival of patients with malignant disease requiring XRT.

Most cases reported involve the cervical cord in spite of the higher frequency with which the thoracic cord is exposed to XRT (perhaps due to higher XRT doses to the head and neck and longer survival than with lung Ca).[18] Delay between completion of XRT and onset of symptoms is usually ≈ 1 yr (reported range: 1 mos-5 yrs).

Important factors relating to the occurrence of RM include[18]:

1. rate of application (probably the most important factor)
2. total radiation dose
3. extent of cord shielding
4. individual susceptibility and variability
5. amount of tissue radiated
6. vascular supply to the region radiated
7. source of radiation

Pathophysiology

Effects of XRT on the spinal cord that lead to RM are:

1. direct injury to cells (including neurons)
2. vascular changes, including endothelial cell proliferation → thrombosis
3. hyalinization of collagen fibers

Clinical

Clinical types of radiation myelopathy

Four clinical types have been described and are shown in ▶ Table 101.1.

Onset is usually insidious, but abruptness has also been described; the presentation often mimics epidural mets. First symptoms: usually paresthesias and hypesthesia of LEs, and Lhermitte's sign. Then spastic weakness of LEs with hyperreflexia develops. A Brown-Séquard syndrome is not uncommon.

Table 101.1 Types of radiation myelopathy

Type	Description
1	benign form; commonly several mos following XRT (reported as late as 1 yr). Usually resolves completely within several mos. Mild sensory symptoms (frequently limited to a Lhermitte's sign) without objective neurological findings
2	injury to anterior horn cells→ lower motor neuron signs in arms or legs
3	described only in experimental animals after doses larger than normal XRT. Complete cord lesion within hours due to injury to blood vessels
4	the type commonly reported. Chronic, progressive myelopathy (see text)

101

Approximately 50% of patients developing RM also have dysphagia from esophageal strictures requiring dilatations (the dysphagia often predates the myelopathy).

Evaluation

Essentially a diagnosis of exclusion. Radiographic imaging (CT, myelography) will be normal. MRI may show spinal cord infarction. The history of previous radiation is key. The differential diagnosis is included in Acute paraplegia or quadriplegia (p. 1413).

Prognosis

Prognosis for Type 4 RM is poor. Usually progresses to complete (or near complete) cord lesion. Paraplegia and/or sphincter involvement are poor signs.

Prevention

Maximum recommended cord radiation dose depends on size of port, and varies with investigator. With large field techniques (> 10 cm of cord), the risk of RM is negligible with ≤ 3.3 Gy in 42 days (0.55 Gy/wk), and with small field techniques ≤ 4.3 Gy in 42 days (0.717 Gy/wk). Larger doses may possibly be given safely if fractionated over longer periods. Recommended upper limit: 0.2 Gy/fraction.

101.3 Stereotactic radiosurgery and radiotherapy

101.3.1 General information

Key concepts

- Stereotactic radiosurgery (SRS): the application of a single large dose of radiation to a stereotactically localized target usually ≤ 3 cm diameter with minimal radiation delivered to surrounding tissue. May be a single treatment or up to 5 treatment fractions
- Stereotactic radiotherapy (SRT) employs hypofractionated dosing (2-5 treatment fractions) and the target can be larger
- Both SRS and SRT may be performed with properly equipped linear accelerators (LINAC Scalpel, CyberKnife®...), collimated beams from multiple radioactive sources (Gamma Knife®), or less commonly, protons and heavy charged particle beams.

Stereotactic radiosurgery (SRS)

Lars Leksell coined the term "radiosurgery" in 1951.[19] His concept was to replace the use of electrodes or "knives" (scalpels) with multiple intersecting beams of radiation to converge on an intracranial target through an intact skull. The dose of radiation at the point of intersection (the "isocenter") is higher than outside of the isocenter where the dose falls off sharply such that adjacent tissues receive only minimal radiation from each individual incident beam. When combined with a reliable method for aiming the beams at an intracranial target (e.g., using a stereotactic frame system and three-dimensional imaging) the technique came to be known as stereotactic radiosurgery.

Initially developed to create a necrotic lesion in specific nuclei or pathways for functional disorders, it has subsequently been proven that subnecrotic doses could trigger cellular reactions in tumors and vasculature that would lead to tumor shrinkage or control and obliteration of vascular malformations.

With conventional radiation treatments, the "R's" of radiobiology (p. 1560) are exploited. In contrast, with SRS, precision and accuracy are used to affect the target (e.g. damage tumor or thrombose AVM) and spare normal tissue.

Stereotactic radiotherapy (SRT)

Methods of immobilization and point-of-delivery imaging technologies have since made it practical to deliver stereotactic radiation spread out over several individual treatment sessions (known as fractions) when desirable. Many authors refer to this as stereotactic radiation therapy (SRT). The precise definition of SRT has evolved over time, with some publications describing it as using a conventional fractionation scheme (1.8-2 Gy / fraction). However the majority of authors refer to SRT in terms of a hypofractionated approach, generally limited to five treatment fractions (see below).

Fractionation capitalizes on the differential response of normal tissue from tumors to radiation insult; see the Four "R's" of radiobiology (p. 1560). The value of fractionation is more apparent for tissues with high rates of proliferation and less capability to repair sublethal DNA damage (high α/β ratio in Eq (101.1)).[20] However these models apply more directly in conventional fractionation schemes; their use in single- or hypo-fractionated schemes is a subject of current research.

Treatment over multiple fractions renders impractical the traditional stereotactic frame. SRT therefore employs various techniques for patient immobilization including thermoplastic masks, dental-impression-based bite-blocks, and other relocatable frame systems. Displacement errors can be as high as 2-8 mm with mask systems, however these uncertainties can be reduced with in-room imaging systems such as cone-beam CT (CBCT) which can assist in patient localization, as well as intra-fraction motion monitoring techniques such as orthogonal kilovoltage x-rays, surface tracking systems, and infrared marker tracking systems.

Blurred lines between SRS and SRT

Although some purists insist that SRS is performed in a single session, the current definition was expanded by AANS/CNS/ASTRO in 2007 to include radiosurgical procedures "using a rigidly attached stereotactic guiding device, other immobilization device and/or a stereotactic image-guidance system … performed in a limited number of sessions, up to a maximum of five."[21]

To further muddy the waters, for billing purposes in the U.S., the cpt codes used by Medicare for SRS (for brain and spine)[22,23] describe treatment in one session, whereas SBRT (stereotactic body radiation therapy) allows treatment delivery not to exceed 5 fractions within the body. For 5 or more fractions, Medicare considers it to be intensity modulated radiation therapy (IMRT).

Comparison of SRS technologies

Various methods for delivering SRS/SRT are clinically available. Three main categories (based on sources of radiation) are Gamma Knife, linear accelerator based, and heavy charged particle radiosurgery. Fundamentally, there is no difference between a photon created by radioactive decay (gamma ray) from a photon created using electrical energy in a linear accelerator (x-ray).

▸ **Gamma knife radiosurgery.** In the original Gamma Knife (GK), the source of radiation is gamma decay of 201 cobalt-60 sources that align with an inner collimator to direct the resulting photon beams. A treatment couch includes a mount for an external collimation "helmet", each of which has either a 4-, 8-, 14-, or 18-mm diameter beam aperture for each source. The stereotactic frame affixed to the patient's head is positioned within the collimator helmet so the area to be treated is at the focus point of treatment unit. Several dwell positions (also called "shots" or "isocenters") may be defined to match dose distributions to irregularly shaped targets.

In the newer GK model Perfexion®, 192 cobalt-60 sources are distributed on 8 sectors attached to sector drive motors to move the sources along a fully internalized tungsten collimator. This allows each sector to move from "home", 4-, 8-, 16-mm collimators or shielded positions. The design makes possible composite use of different beam diameters to help optimize dose distribution. The Gamma Knife is specifically designed for cranial and upper cervical lesions, and is best suited for smaller lesions (< 3 cm diameter).

As the gamma sources age, output declines, and treatment times necessarily become longer. Eventually, the sources must be replaced, which is a time consuming and expensive process.

▸ **Linear accelerator-based radiosurgery.** Linear accelerators (linacs) generate x-rays by accelerating electrons and directing them to strike a target of a substance with high atomic number. The x-ray source and beam collimation is mounted on a rotating gantry, creating a fixed isocenter in space. Beam convergence is achieved via rotating arcs with the isocenter fixated on the target. The target is aligned to the isocenter using a treatment table that is adjustable in up to 6 degrees of freedom (6 dof, 3 translations, 3 rotations). Beams are collimated using either narrow-aperture cones (SRS cones) or multileaf collimators (MLCs), the latter of which use banks of computerized leaves to shape the treatment field and may be modulated to achieve specific dose distributions. Linacs are more versatile than GK in that they can treat cranial and extracranial targets, often have built-in CBCT imaging to assist with patient setup and target localization, and can have a higher dose rate (and thus potentially faster treatment). However they are generally technically more complicated than GK and require substantially more quality assurance to maintain technical confidence. The

Cyberknife is an SRS-specific linac that uses a robotic arm rather than an isocentrically-mounted linac to achieve 6 dof targeting.

▶ **Heavy charged particle radiosurgery.** Heavy charged particles (protons or helium ions) from a cyclotron can be used for radiosurgery.[24] Unlike high-energy photons (gamma and x-rays), which deposit the majority of their energy upon entrance into tissue and continue to deposit decreasing amount of energy as they travel through the body, heavy charged particle beams have a shorter, bounded range of penetration wherein particles sharply increase energy deposition near the terminal depth of penetration (Bragg peak effect). Particle radiosurgery achieves a well-localized volume of high dose radiation by taking advantage of cross firing of a number of beams as well as the Bragg peak. Due to the expense and increased complexity of heavy charged particle SRS, this therapy is only available in a few centers in the world.

101.3.2 Indications

In general, SRS is useful for well-circumscribed lesions less than approximately 3 cm diameter. For larger lesions, the radiation dose must be reduced because of anatomic and radiobiological constraints.

Published uses of SRS include:

- Vascular lesions
  - AVMs (including dural arteriovenous fistulas)
  - Cavernous malformations
- Tumors
  - Metastases
  - Vestibular schwannomas
  - Meningiomas
  - Pituitary adenomas
  - Gliomas
  - Others: craniopharyngioma, pineal tumors, etc.
- Functional disorders
  - Trigeminal neuralgia[25,26]
  - Intractable chronic pain: thalamotomy[27]
  - Movement disorders: pallidotomy for Parkinson's disease or thalamotomy for tremor (Usually not a technique of choice because of inability to perform physiologic stimulation prior to lesioning. May be a consideration for the rare patients who cannot undergo placement of a stimulator/lesioning needle)
  - Psychiatric diseases (e.g. obsessive compulsive disorder)
  - Epilepsies[28]

101.3.3 Contraindications

Compressive tumors of the spinal cord, brainstem or optic structures: even with the sharp falloff of radiation dose, there remains radiation delivered within a few millimeters of the margins of the isocenter. This, together with post-radiation swelling, might create significant risk of neurologic injury. Surgical removal should be should be considered in these situations especially for benign lesions in young individuals.

101.3.4 Treatment procedure

The treatment procedure includes placement of stereotactic frame (in framed-based SRS), obtaining stereotactic images, target definition, treatment planning and execution of treatment.

Target localization

MRI is the predominant imaging modality for SRS procedures given its superior soft tissue and tumor contrast. Typical MRI protocols include T1-weighted pre- and post-contrast images using 3D pulse sequences. If visualization of structures in surrounding CSF (trigeminal nerves, CPA tumors) is required, special sequences such as constructive interference in steady state (CISS) is useful. Fat-sat-ation sequences are used in cases with previously resected skull base tumors. NB: there is a 1-m shift due to spatial distortion artifact from the MRI magnet. This effect is more prominent in field strength MRI.

CT accuracy is never better than 0.6 mm, which is the pixel size. Usually is used when MRI is contraindicated or in cases where distortion in MRI may be a concern (dental brace, shunt). CT does not suffer susceptibility distortion as MRI and one can use a stereotactic CT to merge with nonstereotactic MRI for treatment planning.

Stereotactic angiography remains the best method to define the AVM nidi and their arterial supply and venous drainage. Given that angiograms provide only two sets of orthogonal images (usually AP and lateral images), CTA and/or MRI/MRA can be used as an adjunct to provide vascular anatomy on axial plane.

Treatment planning

Treatment planning is the process by which a dose distribution is created with the goal of adequately treating the target areas while largely sparing normal surrounding structures. In GK treatment, a dose distribution is created by defining one or more isocenters (shots). Each isocenter can make use of full complement beams of various diameters, however, in certain cases one or more of beams can be blocked to shape the dose distribution for irregular targets and protect adjacent critical structures. For linac-based SRS, treatment planning is accomplished using computer simulation programs to help select the number of arcs or beams with certain orientation. Also, static and dynamic collimators have been developed. Intensity modulation is also a means of delivering the desired dose to a target while decreasing the dose given to surrounding structures.

Lesions that are not round or ellipsoid in shape are not a problem when using linac, but with older GKs, multiple isocenters must be used to conform to an irregular surface. This results in multiple "hotspots." This problem is eliminated with the GK Perfexion, which can create a single isocenter using different beam diameters. In the case of multiple metastases, it can generate individually shaped isocenters for each tumor and thus avoid having to change the helmet or add isocenters during a treatment.[29]

► **Normal tissue tolerance.** Cranial nerves: Damage to small nutrient vessels and Schwann cells or oligodendroglia are the possible mechanisms of radiation injury to cranial nerves. Special sensory nerves (optic, vestibulocochlear) are the most radiosensitive. The precise dose tolerance of cranial nerve is unclear; the optic nerve can probably tolerate doses lower than 8-10 Gy. Nerves in the parasellar region, the facial nerve and lower cranial nerves tend to tolerate higher doses.

SRS treatment may also have a deleterious effect in structures sensitive to swelling, such as brainstem. However, the structures at highest risk are those within the higher isodose lines immediately adjacent to the lesion.

► Table 101.2 shows maximum recommended doses of various organs for a single fraction. In the brain, critical radiation sensitive structures include: optic vitreous, nerve, and chiasm, brain stem, pituitary gland, and cochlea.

► **Dose.** Dose is usually prescribed as a particular dose (in units of Gray) to the periphery of target. The periphery of the target is usually defined as the isodose curve, which covers the substantial (usually 95-100%) of the target. The isodose curve is the curve of equal dose usually defined as a percentage of the maximum dose point. Traditionally, treatment planning for GK uses the 50% isodose line because for a single isocenter this is the location of steepest dose gradient. Linac-based SRS used higher isodose line (70-90%) to increase homogeneity of dose distribution.

Dose-volume relation: The dose of radiation that can be tolerated is highly dependent on the volume being treated (larger treatment volumes require lower doses to avoid radiation injury). Dose selection is made based on known information or is estimated from dose-volume relationship. If uncertain, err on the side of a lower dose or slightly underdose the margin of tumor. Previous radiotherapy must also be taken into account by the treatment team, as local structures are more sensitive.

Table 101.2 Maximum recommended radiation dose of critical organs (delivered in a single fraction)

Structure	Maximum dose (cGy)	% of maximum (at a prescribed dose of 50 Gy)
eye lens (cataract induction begins at 500 cGy)	100	2%
optic nerve[30]	100	2%
skin in beam	50	1%
thyroid	10	0.2%

101.3.5 Lesion-specific issues

Arteriovenous malformations and other vascular lesions

SRS is best accepted for the treatment of small to moderate-sized (< 3 cm) AVMs that are deep or border on eloquent brain and have a "compact" (i.e. sharply demarcated) nidus. The radiation induces endothelial cell damage, smooth muscle cell proliferation, thickening of the vascular wall, and ultimately obliteration of the lumen over a period of 2-3 years (latency period).[31]

Lesions other than AVMs: Dural arteriovenous fistulas (AVFs) have also shown promising response to SRS.[32] However, dural AVFs with cortical drainage should not be treated with SRS as these AVFs pose high risk of hemorrhage. SRS is of no benefit for venous angiomas.[33] SRS for cavernous malformations remains controversial, as the lesions could not be precisely evaluated with MRI or angiography. However, published retrospective studies have demonstrated reduction of hemorrhage rates following SRS.[34,35]

▶ **Dose.** Early study from Karlsson et al. demonstrated increased obliteration rate with increased margin dose.[36] The effect reached the plateau at 25 Gy and a higher dose produced more complications without extra benefits. The optimal dose for AVMs generally ranges between 23-25 Gy. The dose might be reduced for nidi at critical locations or with a large volume. At McGill with linac SRS, they use 25-50 Gy delivered to the 90% isodose curve at the edge of the nidus. With Bragg-peak, complications occurred less frequently with doses < 19.2 Gy compared to doses above that (this may reduce the obliteration rate or increase the latency period).[37]

▶ **Results.** SRS has an overall obliteration rate of 70-80% across all cases of AVMs treated.[38] At 1 year, 46-61% of AVMs were completely obliterated on angiography, and at 2 years 86% were obliterated. There was no reduction in size in < 2% of cases. Smaller lesions have higher obliteration rates (with Bragg-peak in AVMs < 2 cm diameter, 94% thrombosed at 2 years, and 100% at 3 years).[37]) AVMs > 25 mm in diameter have only ≈ 50% chance of obliteration with 1 SRS treatment.

▶ **Grading system.** A few SRS-based grading systems have been developed to predict patient outcomes since scales developed for surgical resection (e.g. the Spetzler-Martin scale) have not proven applicable for AVM radiosurgery. Long-term outcomes of 1012 patients treated with GK at UVA were analyzed to create the Virginia Radiosurgery AVM Scale (▶ Table 101.3 and ▶ Table 101.4).[38] Multivariate analysis showed that AVM volume, non-eloquent location, and no history of hemorrhage, were independent predictors of AVM obliteration without hemorrhage or permanent neurologic deficits.

The radiosurgery-based grading system by Pollock and Flickinger[39] has been validated in both GK and linac treatment centers. This AVM score is calculated using the following formula:

$$
\begin{aligned}
&(0.1)(\text{volume, cm}^3)\\
&+(0.02)(\text{age, years})\\
&+(0.3)(\text{location, hemispheric/corpus callosum/cerebellar} = 0;\ \text{basal ganglia/thalamus/brainstem} = 1)
\end{aligned}
$$

▶ **Embolization.** Controversy exists as to whether embolization is helpful or harmful prior to SRS. Some experts find that target definition after embolization is extraordinarily difficult because of multiple small residual nidi. Experimental studies have shown attenuation of radiation effect by embolic material.[40] However, for large AVMs, embolization remains an effective adjunct to reduce

Table 101.3 Virginia Radiosurgery AVM Scale[38]: variables and points

Variable		Points
AVM volume (cm^3)	< 2	0
	2-4	1
	> 4	2
[illegible]nt location		1
[illegible]f hemorrhage		1

Table 101.4 Virginia Radiosurgery AVM Scale[38]: total points and % favorable outcome

Total points	Favorable outcome (%)
0	83
1	79
2	70
3	48
4	39

the size of nidi to make AVMs amenable to SRS. Additionally, pre-SRS embolization should be considered for high flow fistulas, which are more radioresistant, and intranidal/perinidal aneurysms, which are at risk for rupture.

▸ **Large AVMs.** Large AVMs (> 10 cm^3) remain a significant challenge to treat with any modality. Single stage SRS has resulted in low obliteration and high complication rates. To maximize the dose/volume response, SRS can be performed in a volume-staged fashion. The Pittsburgh group reported overall rates of total obliteration of 18%, 45%, and 56% at 5, 7, and 10 years, respectively in a group of 47 patients with large AVMs. Ten patients had hemorrhage after SRS, and 5 of these patients died.[41]

▸ **Residual lesions after SRS.** Factors associated with treatment failures include: incomplete angiographic definition of the nidus (the most frequent factor, responsible for 57% of cases), recanalization of the nidus (7%), masking of nidus by hematoma, and a theorized "radiobiological resistance."[42] In some, no discernible reason for failure could be identified. In this series the complete obliteration rate was ≈ 64%. If AVMs persist, retreatment with SRS 2-3 years later is an option.[42]

The ultimate goal of radiosurgery for AVMs is elimination of risk of hemorrhage. An imperfect surrogate marker for this goal has been total obliteration of the nidus on imaging. Reduced, unchanged, or increased hemorrhagic rates during the latency period have been reported. Proton beam treatment of AVMs affords no protection against hemorrhage in the first 12-14 months following treatment.[24]; this is similar to the 12-24 month latency for photon radiation.[43] Hemorrhages may occur during the latency period even in AVMs that had never bled before,[37] and the question has been raised whether a partially thrombosed AVM is more likely to bleed because of increased outflow resistance. Yen et al. reviewed a large group of AVM patients undergoing radiosurgery and reported that the hemorrhagic rates reduced from 6.6 % before SRS to 2.5% after SRS. The protective effect is more significant in those AVMs that had a prior hemorrhage (10.4% to 2.8%).[44]

Metastases

The gold standard and level 1 recommendation for a single brain metastasis amenable to surgical resection is surgery followed by WBRT.[45,46] This does not apply to extremely radiosensitive tumors such as lymphoma, small cell lung cancer, germ cell tumors, and multiple myeloma. There has not been a randomized study to compare surgery alone to SRS alone. A prospective randomized study by Muacevic et al. showed comparable survival and local tumor control between SRS vs. surgery plus WBRT in patients with a single brain metastasis but a higher incidence of distant recurrence in the SRS arm.[47] When tissue is required for diagnosis, surgery should be considered. Tumors with significant mass effect should also be resected if the patients are fit for surgery. In patients with ≤ 3 mets, single dose SRS provides superior survival advantage as compared to WBRT (level III recommendation). Radiographic local control rate of ≈ 88% (reported range: 82-100%) has been cited.[48]

No significant difference has been found with SRS between tumors considered "radiosensitive" and those that are "radioresistant" as defined by standards developed for EBRT (see ▸ Table 52.7; however, histology may affect the rate of response). The lack of significance of "radioresistance" may be due in part to the fact that the sharp dose drop-off with SRS allows higher doses to be delivered to tumors than would be used with EBRT.

General guidelines for when to consider SRS for brain metastases are:

- total tumor number ≤ 10
- total tumor volume ≤ 15 cm^3
- single tumor volume is < 10 cm^3, and
- no leptomeningeal disease present.

Recent studies on SRS for brain metastases have shown that total tumor volume is a better predictor of overall survival, local control, and even distant failure than tumor number.[49,50,51]

▶ **Dose.** RTOG 90-05 study recommended 24 Gy as the maximum tolerated doses of single fraction SRS for tumors ≤ 20 mm in maximum diameter; 18 Gy for 21-30 mm; and 15 Gy for 31-40 mm.[52]

Vestibular schwannomas (VS)

Possible indications of SRS for VS are: poor surgical candidates (due to poor medical condition and/or advanced age, some use > 65 or 70 years as a cutoff), patient refusing surgery, bilateral VS, post-operative treatment of incompletely removed VS that continue to grow on serial imaging, or recurrences following surgical removal. See the Management algorithm under Vestibular schwannomas for strategies that take into account the natural history.

A few nonrandomized prospective studies comparing GK SRS to microsurgery in small to middle sized VS have demonstrated superiority of SRS treatment.[53,54] The largest series of 2336 VS with at least 3 years follow-up from Marseille showed a tumor control rate of up to 97.5%, trigeminal nerve injury 0.5%, facial palsy 0.5%, and hearing preservation at 65%.[54] However long-term follow-up is needed. SRS following deliberate subtotal resection of large Koos stage IV VS reduced the risk of facial weakness compared with GTR.[55] Dose range for SRS of VS is usually 11-12 Gy. SRS tolerable dose to cochlea seems to be around 4.2 Gy, but also depends on age and pre-SRS hearing class.[56] Temporary increase of tumor size following SRS is a common finding and can be managed conservatively.

SRT or multisession SRS has been used to treat VS. Selch et al. reported a local control rate of 100% with a median follow-up of 36 months.[57] Their group showed the hearing preservation rate has been high (93%) and incidence of facial nerve injury has been low (2.2% new facial palsy, 2.2% facial numbness). SRT has not been compared head-to-head with SRS, but preliminary results suggest the results of both modalities might be similar.

▶ **Dose.** Sample SRT protocol: 6-MV linac with a micromultileaf collimator used to deliver 54 Gy in 30 fractions of 1.8 Gy prescribed to the 90% isodose line via 7-22 noncoplanar static fields or 4-6 noncoplanar dynamic arcs to a target defined as the tumor volume plus a margin of 1-3 mm. Multisession SRS has been used to treat large VS. In a study of 33 patients with VS greater than 8 cm^3 treated with Cyberknife, radiological growth control was 94% at a median follow-up of 48 months.[58] Hearing was retained in 7 of 8 patients with serviceable baseline hearing. Only 1 patient each had cranial nerve deficits including vertigo, tongue paresthesia and trigeminal neuralgia.

Meningiomas

In a large series of meningiomas treated with SRS by the Pittsburgh group,[59] among 942 patients with 1045 tumors treated, the control rate for patients with surgically verified WHO grade I meningiomas was 93%. Control rate for presumed meningiomas based on imaging (no prior histological confirmation) was 97%. The control rates for WHO grades II and III tumors were 50% and 17%, respectively.

▶ **Dose.** The authors used a mean dose of 14 Gy to the tumor margin.[59]

Pituitary adenomas

Surgery is the mainstay of management for pituitary tumors especially for nonsecretory tumors with mass effect and secretory tumors that fail medical treatment. For residual/recurrent secretory or nonsecretory tumors, SRS is an appropriate tool to arrest tumor growth and/or normalize hormonal function. In a large series of 418 patients with pituitary adenomas residual/recurrence treated with GK at UVA, the overall tumor control rate was 90% in patients with imaging follow-up available. The endocrine remission rates are 53% for acromegaly, 54% for Cushing's disease, and 26% for prolactinomas.

ose. The usual dose for nonsecretory tumors is ≈ 16-18 Gy, and a higher dose is required for tory tumor ≈ 25 Gy.

ts. Early studies of SRS showed limited numbers of hypopituitarism and cranial nerve inju- lable long-term follow-up studies now demonstrate a 20-30% rate of new endocrinopathy nd a low but not negligible risk of cranial nerve damage.[60]

Infiltrating tumors

SRS is generally not indicated as a primary treatment for infiltrating tumors, e.g. gliomas, due to the lack of a definable capsule and very close relationship between target volume and tolerated radiation dose. SRS has been used for recurrent lesions following standard treatment (surgical excision and adjuvant EBRT 60 Gy and Temozolomide). One of the arguments for SRS in these tumors is the fact that 90% of recurrences are within the original radiographic solid tumor volume.[61] However, support for SRS boost declined after a 2004 RTOG trial 9305 showing no survival benefit in newly diagnosed GBM patients with upfront use of SRS followed by EBRT and BCNU chemotherapy. SRS can be used as a salvage treatment for small (< 10 cm^3), recurrent GBM after standard treatment. Kong et al. showed SRS salvage treatment in these cases prolonged OS to 23 from 12 months.[62]

101.3.6 Treatment morbidity and mortality

Immediate morbidity and mortality

Immediate mortality from the actual treatments themselves is probably zero. Morbidity: all but ≈ 2.5% of patients were discharged home within 24 hours. Many centers do not admit patients overnight. Some immediate adverse reactions include[63]:

- 16% of patients require analgesics for post-procedural headaches and antiemetics for nausea/vomiting
- at least 10% of patients with subcortical AVMs had focal or generalized seizures within 24 hrs of treatment (only one was on subtherapeutic AEDs. All were controllable with additional AEDs.)

Premedication

The Pittsburgh Gamma Knife group gives methylprednisolone 40 mg IV and phenobarbital 90 mg IV immediately after the radiation dose to patients with tumors or AVMs to reduce these adverse effects.[63] For small lesions and patients without prior history of seizures, premedication with steroids or antiepileptics are probably not necessary.

Delayed morbidity

Long-term morbidity directly related to the radiation may occur, and just as with conventional XRT, is more frequent with larger doses and treatment volumes. Radiation complications include:

- radiation-induced changes, high intensity on MRI T2WI, or low density on CT: usually occur ≈ 13 months after SRS for AVMs. The incidence is 34% with 8.6% having imaging changes associated with neurological symptoms (focal deficits, seizures, or headache) and 1.8% developing radiation necrosis and permanent deficits.[64] The possible mechanisms of this side effect include glial cell damage, breakdown of blood brain barrier or early venous thrombosis. Premature venous thrombosis or occlusion before obliteration of AVM nidus can produce venous hyperemia or intracranial hemorrhage[65]
- vasculopathy: diagnosed by narrowing seen on angiography or by ischemic changes on imaging in ≈ 5% of cases
- cranial nerve deficits: occur in ≈ 1% of all cases. Incidence is higher with tumors of CPA or skull base
- radiation induced tumors: only a few case reports of newly formed malignant tumors (glioblastomas) or malignant transformation of a benign tumor (vestibular Schwannoma). Loeffler reported 6 cases over 80,000 radiosurgical procedures for benign diseases.[66] Radiation-induced meningioma is a well-known complication of radiation therapy.[67] In a large series of AVM patients treated with SRS, the incidence of radiation-induced meningioma was estimated to be 0.7%[68]

101.4 Interstitial brachytherapy

101.4.1 General information

Technique whereby radioactive implants are used to deliver locally high doses of radiation directly to tumors while exposing nearby normal brain to less toxic doses. At present, the numbers are too small and the follow-up too short to determine the efficacy of interstitial brachytherapy.[69]

Interstitial brachytherapy (IB) may reduce the rate of tumor growth, but it rarely produces clinical improvement. Patients are generally not considered for IB unless their Karnofsky score is ≥ 70.

101

101.4.2 Techniques

Techniques include:

1. insertion of high activity iodine-125 pellets which remain in place (either by conventional open surgery or by stereotactic technique)
2. insertion of catheters (so-called afterloading catheters) containing radioactive source (such as gold or I125) by stereotactic technique, which are then removed at a predetermined time (usually 1–7 days)
3. instillation of radioactive liquids (e.g. phosphorous isotope) into a cyst cavity

I125 has several characteristics that favor its use: it emits low-energy gamma rays which are absorbed by surrounding tissues minimizing radiation exposure of the normal brain, medical personnel and visitors. It is available as low-activity (< 5 mCi) or high-activity (5–40 mCi) seeds.

Treatment planning is devised to deliver 60 Gy to the edge of a volume that extends 1 cm beyond the contrast-enhancing tumor, with variations included to spare radiosensitive structures (e.g. optic chiasm). Usual delivery rates are 40–50 cGy/hr to the tumor margin (30 cGy/hr is the critical dose for cessation of human tumor growth) requiring that the seeds stay in the afterloading catheter ≈ 6 days.

101.4.3 Radiation necrosis

Symptomatic radiation necrosis (RN) occurs in ≈ 40% of cases, and may occur as early as several months after IB. It may be impossible to differentiate from recurrent tumor in many cases. Symptomatic treatment is often achieved with increased corticosteroid dosages. Continued neurologic deterioration may require craniotomy.

101.4.4 Outcome

IB is often used as a "last ditch" effort in a patient with a recurrent malignant tumor who has received maximal external beam irradiation and who is not a candidate for reoperation (as expected, the results in patients with such poor prognoses are not good). However, patients eligible for IB are usually better than those who are not candidates, and this may bias the results towards a better outcome.[70] Some studies with early (primary treatment) use have shown possible benefit.[71]

References

[1] Thompson TP, Maitz AH, Kondziolka D, Lunsford LD. Radiation, Radiobiology, and Neurosurgery. Contemp Neurosurg. 1999; 21:1–5

[2] Hall EJ, Cox JD, Cox JD. In: Physical and Biologic Basis of Radiation Therapy. Moss' Radiation Oncology. 7th ed. St. Louis, Missouri: Mosby-Year Book, Inc.; 1994:3–66

[3] O'Connor MM, Mayberg MR. Effects of Radiation on Cerebral Vasculature: A Review. Neurosurgery. 2000; 46:138–151

[4] Leibel SA, Sheline GE. Radiation Therapy for Neoplasms of the Brain. J Neurosurg. 1987; 66:1–22

[5] Duffner PK, Cohen ME, Thomas P. Late Effects of Treatment on the Intelligence of Children with Posterior Fossa Tumors. Cancer. 1983; 51:233–237

[6] DeAngelis LM, Delattre JY, Posner JB. Radiation-induced dementia in patients cured of brain metastases. Neurology. 1989; 39:789–796

[7] Radcliffe J, Packer RJ, Atkins TE, et al. Three- and Four-Year Cognitive Outcome in Children with Noncortical Brain Tumors Treated with Whole-Brain Radiotherapy. Ann Neurol. 1992; 32:551–554

[8] Zuccarello M, Sawaya R, deCourten-Myers. Glioblastoma Occurring After Radiation Therapy for Meningioma: Case Report and Review of Literature. Neurosurgery. 1986; 19:114–119

[9] Mack EE, Wilson CB. Meningiomas Induced by High-Dose Cranial Irradiation. J Neurosurg. 1993; 79:28–31

[10] Ron E, Modan B, Boice JD, et al. Tumors of the Brain and Nervous System After Radiotherapy in Childhood. N Engl J Med. 1988; 319:1033–1039

[11] Lustig LR, Jackler RK, Lanser MJ. Radiation-Induced Tumors of the Temporal Bone. Am J Otol. 1997; 18:230–235

[12] Rock JP, Hearshen D, Scarpace L, Croteau D, Gutierrez J, Fisher JL, Rosenblum ML, Mikkelsen T. Correlations between magnetic resonance spectroscopy and image-guided histopathology, with special attention to radiation necrosis. Neurosurgery. 2002; 51:912–9; discussion 919-20

[13] Hein PA, Eskey CJ, Dunn JF, Hug EB. Diffusion-weighted imaging in the follow-up of treated high-grade gliomas: tumor recurrence versus radiation injury. AJNR Am J Neuroradiol. 2004; 25:201–209

[14] Thompson TP, Lunsford LD, Kondziolka D. Distinguishing recurrent tumor and radiation necrosis with positron emission tomography versus stereotactic biopsy. Stereotact Funct Neurosurg. 1999; 73:9–14

[15] Ericson K, Lilja A, Bergstrom M, et al. Positron emission tomography with ([11C]methyl)-L-methionine, [11C]D-glucose, and [68Ga]EDTA in supratentorial tumors. J Comput Assist Tomogr. 1985; 9:683–689

[16] Thiel A, Pietrzyk U, Sturm V, et al. Enhanced Accuracy in Differential Diagnosis of Radiation Necrosis by Positron Emission Tomography-Magnetic Resonance Imaging Coregistration: Technical Case Report. Neurosurgery. 2000; 46:232–234

[17] Tomita T, McLone DG. Medulloblastoma in Childhood: Results of Radical Resection and Low-Dose Radiation Therapy. J Neurosurg. 1986; 64:238–242

[18] Eyster EF, Wilson CB. Radiation Myelopathy. J Neurosurg. 1970; 32:414–420

[19] Leksell L. The Stereotaxic Method and Radiosurgery of the Brain. Acta Chir Scand. 1951; 102:316–319
[20] Dale RG, Jones B. The assessment of RBE effects using the concept of biologically effective dose. Int J Radiat Oncol Biol Phys. 1999; 43:639–645
[21] Barnett GH, Linskey ME, Adler JR, Cozzens JW, Friedman WA, Heilbrun MP, Lunsford LD, Schulder M, Sloan AE. Stereotactic radiosurgery–an organized neurosurgery-sanctioned definition. J Neurosurg. 2007; 106:1–5
[22] Tipton KN, Sullivan N, Bruening W, Inamdar R, Launders J, Uhl S, Schoelles K, . Stereotactic Body Radiation Therapy. Technical Brief No. 6. (Prepared by ECRI Institute Evidence-based Practice Center under Contract No. HHSA-290-02-0019.) AHRQ Publication No. 10 (11)-EHC058-EF. Rockville, MD 2011
[23] Stereotactic radiotherapy (SRS)/stereotactic radiation therapy (SBRT) for Medicare plans Policy # SURGERY 0581 T3. Trumbull CT 2009
[24] Kjellberg RN, Hanamura T, Davis KR, et al. Bragg-Peak Proton-Beam Therapy for Arteriovenous Malformations of the Brain. N Engl J Med. 1983; 309:269–274
[25] Leksell L. Stereotactic Radiosurgery in Trigeminal Neuralgia. Acta Chir Scand. 1971; 137:311–314
[26] Regis J, Metellus P, Hayashi M, Roussel P, Donnet A, Bille-Turc F. Prospective controlled trial of gamma knife surgery for essential trigeminal neuralgia. J Neurosurg. 2006; 104:913–924
[27] Steiner L, Forster D, Leksell L, et al. Gammathalamotomy in Intractable Pain. Acta Neurochir. 1980; 52:173–184
[28] Barbaro NM, Quigg M, Broshek DK, Ward MM, Lamborn KR, Laxer KD, Larson DA, Dillon W, Verhey L, Garcia P, Steiner L, Heck C, Kondziolka D, Beach R, Olivero W, Witt TC, Salanova V, Goodman R. A multicenter, prospective pilot study of gamma knife radiosurgery for mesial temporal lobe epilepsy: seizure response, adverse events, and verbal memory. Ann Neurol. 2009; 65:167–175
[29] Lindquist C, Paddick I. The Leksell Gamma Knife Perfexion and comparisons with its predecessors. Neurosurgery. 2007; 61:130–40; discussion 140-1
[30] Leber KA, Berglöff J, Pendi G. Dose-Response Tolerance of the Visual Pathways and Cranial Nerves of the Cavernous Sinus to Stereotactic Radiosurgery. J Neurosurg. 1998; 88:43–50
[31] Schneider BF, Eberhard DA, Steiner LE. Histopathology of arteriovenous malformations after gamma knife radiosurgery. J Neurosurg. 1997; 87:352–357
[32] Pan DH, Lee CC, Wu HM, Chung WY, Yang HC, Lin CJ. Gamma Knife radiosurgery for the management of intracranial dural arteriovenous fistulas. Acta Neurochir Suppl. 2013; 116:113–119
[33] Lindquist C, Guo W-Y, Kerlsson B, Steiner L. Radiosurgery for Venous Angiomas. J Neurosurg. 1993; 78:531–536
[34] Lunsford LD, Khan AA, Niranjan A, Kano H, Flickinger JC, Kondziolka D. Stereotactic radiosurgery for symptomatic solitary cerebral cavernous malformations considered high risk for resection. J Neurosurg. 2010; 113:23–29
[35] Liscak R, Vladyka V, Simonova G, Vymazal J, Novotny J.Jr. Gamma knife surgery of brain cavernous hemangiomas. J Neurosurg. 2005; 102 Suppl:207–213
[36] Karlsson B, Lindquist C, Steiner L. Prediction of obliteration after gamma knife surgery for cerebral arteriovenous malformations. Neurosurgery. 1997; 40:425–30; discussion 430-1
[37] Steinberg GK, Fabrikant JI, Marks MP, Levy RP, et al. Stereotactic Heavy-Charged-Particle Bragg-Peak Radiation for Intracranial Arteriovenous Malformations. N Engl J Med. 1990; 323:96–101
[38] Starke RM, Yen CP, Ding D, Sheehan JP. A practical grading scale for predicting outcome after radiosurgery for arteriovenous malformations: analysis of 1012 treated patients. J Neurosurg. 2013; 119:981–987
[39] Pollock BE, Flickinger JC. Modification of the radiosurgery-based arteriovenous malformation grading system. Neurosurgery. 2008; 63:239–43; discussion 243
[40] Andrade-Souza YM, Ramani M, Beachey DJ, Scora D, Tsao MN, Terbrugge K, Schwartz ML. Liquid embolisation material reduces the delivered radiation dose: a physical experiment. Acta Neurochir (Wien). 2008; 150:161–4; discussion 164
[41] Kano H, Kondziolka D, Flickinger JC, Park KJ, Parry PV, Yang HC, Sirin S, Niranjan A, Novotny J.Jr, Lunsford LD. Stereotactic radiosurgery for arteriovenous malformations, Part 6: multistaged volumetric management of large arteriovenous malformations. J Neurosurg. 2012; 116:54–65
[42] Pollock BE, Kondziolka D, Lunsford LD, et al. Repeat Stereotactic Radiosurgery of Arteriovenous Malformations: Factors Associated with Incomplete Outcomes. Neurosurgery. 1996; 38:318–324
[43] Saunders WM, Winston KR, Siddon RL, et al. Radiosurgery for Arteriovenous Malformations of the Brain Using a Standard Linear Accelerator: Rationale and Technique. Int J Radiation Oncology Biol Phys. 1988; 13:441–447
[44] Yen CP, Sheehan JP, Schwyzer L, Schlesinger D. Hemorrhage risk of cerebral arteriovenous malformations before and during the latency period after GAMMA knife radiosurgery. Stroke. 2011; 42:1691–1696
[45] Patchell RA, Tibbs PA, Walsh JW, Young B, et al. A Randomized Trial of Surgery in the Treatment of Single Metastases to the Brain. N Engl J Med. 1990; 322:494–500
[46] Patchell RA, Tibbs PA, Regine WF, Dempsey RJ, Mohiuddin M, Kryscio RJ, Markesbery WR, Foon KA, Young B. Postoperative radiotherapy in the treatment of single metastases to the brain: a randomized trial. JAMA. 1998; 280:1485–1489
[47] Muacevic A, Wowra B, Siefert A, Tonn JC, Steiger HJ, Kreth FW. Microsurgery plus whole brain irradiation versus Gamma Knife surgery alone for treatment of single metastases to the brain: a randomized controlled multicentre phase III trial. J Neurooncol. 2008; 87:299–307
[48] Fuller BG, Kaplan ID, Adler J, Cox RS, Bagshaw MA. Stereotactic Radiosurgery for Brain Metastases: The Importance of Adjuvant Whole Brain Irradiation. Int J Radiation Oncology Biol Phys. 1992; 23:413–418
[49] Baschnagel AM, Meyer KD, Chen PY, Krauss DJ, Olson RE, Pieper DR, Maitz AH, Ye H, Grills IS. Tumor volume as a predictor of survival and local control in patients with brain metastases treated with Gamma Knife surgery. J Neurosurg. 2013; 119:1139–1144
[50] Bhatnagar AK, Flickinger JC, Kondziolka D, Lunsford LD. Stereotactic radiosurgery for four or more intracranial metastases. Int J Radiat Oncol Biol Phys. 2006; 64:898–903
[51] Likhacheva A, Pinnix CC, Parikh NR, Allen PK, McAleer MF, Chiu MS, Sulman EP, Mahajan A, Guha-Thakurta N, Prabhu SS, Cahill DP, Luo D, Shiu AS, Brown PD, Chang EL. Predictors of survival in contemporary practice after initial radiosurgery for brain metastases. Int J Radiat Oncol Biol Phys. 2013; 85:656–661
[52] Shaw E, Scott C, Souhami L, Dinapoli R, Kline R, Loeffler J, Farnan N. Single dose radiosurgical treatment of recurrent previously irradiated primary brain tumors and brain metastases: final report of RTOG protocol 90-05. Int J Radiat Oncol Biol Phys. 2000; 47:291–298
[53] Pollock BE, Driscoll CL, Foote RL, Link MJ, Gorman DA, Bauch CD, Mandrekar JN, Krecke KN, Johnson CH. Patient outcomes after vestibular schwannoma management: a prospective comparison of microsurgical resection and stereotactic radiosurgery. Neurosurgery. 2006; 59:77–85; discussion 77-85
[54] Regis J, Pellet W, Delsanti C, Dufour H, Roche PH, Thomassin JM, Zanaret M, Peragut JC. Functional outcome after gamma knife surgery or microsurgery for vestibular schwannomas. J Neurosurg. 2013; 119 Suppl:1091–1100
[55] Brokinkel B, Sauerland C, Holling M, Ewelt C, Horstmann G, van Eck AT, Stummer W. Gamma Knife

radiosurgery following subtotal resection of vestibular schwannoma. J Clin Neurosci. 2014; 21:2077–2082

[56] Kano H, Kondziolka D, Khan A, Flickinger JC, Lunsford LD. Predictors of hearing preservation after stereotactic radiosurgery for acoustic neuroma. J Neurosurg. 2009; 111:863–873

[57] Selch MT, Pedroso A, Lee SP, Solberg TD, Agazaryan N, Cabatan-Awang C, DeSalles AA. Stereotactic radiotherapy for the treatment of acoustic neuromas. J Neurosurg. 2004; 101:362–372

[58] Casentini L, Fornezza U, Perini Z, Perissinotto E, Colombo F. Multisession stereotactic radiosurgery for large vestibular schwannomas. J Neurosurg. 2015; 122:818–824

[59] Kondziolka D, Mathieu D, Lunsford LD, Martin JJ, Madhok R, Niranjan A, Flickinger JC. Radiosurgery as definitive management of intracranial meningiomas. Neurosurgery. 2008; 62:53–8; discussion 58-60

[60] Sheehan JP, Pouratian N, Steiner L, Laws ER, Vance ML. Gamma Knife surgery for pituitary adenomas: factors related to radiological and endocrine outcomes. J Neurosurg. 2011; 114:303–309

[61] Choucair AK, Levin VA, Gutin PH, et al. Development of Multiple Lesions During Radiation Therapy and Chemotherapy. J Neurosurg. 1986; 65:654–658

[62] Kong DS, Lee JI, Park K, Kim JH, Lim DH, Nam DH. Efficacy of stereotactic radiosurgery as a salvage treatment for recurrent malignant gliomas. Cancer. 2008; 112:2046–2051

[63] Lunsford LD, Flickinger J, Coffey RJ. Stereotactic Gamma Knife Radiosurgery. Initial North American Experience in 207 Patients. Arch Neurol. 1990; 47:169–175

[64] Yen CP, Matsumoto JA, Wintermark M, Schwyzer L, Evans AJ, Jensen ME, Shaffrey ME, Sheehan JP. Radiation-induced imaging changes following Gamma Knife surgery for cerebral arteriovenous malformations. J Neurosurg. 2013; 118:63–73

[65] Yen CP, Khaled MA, Schwyzer L, Vorsic M, Dumont AS, Steiner L. Early draining vein occlusion after gamma knife surgery for arteriovenous malformations. Neurosurgery. 2010; 67:1293–302; discussion 1302

[66] Loeffler JS, Niemierko A, Chapman PH. Second tumors after radiosurgery: tip of the iceberg or a bump in the road? Neurosurgery. 2003; 52:1436–40; discussion 1440-2

[67] Brada M, Ford D, Ashley S, Bliss JM, Crowley S, Mason M, Rajan B, Traish D. Risk of second brain tumour after conservative surgery and radiotherapy for pituitary adenoma. BMJ. 1992; 304:1343–1346

[68] Sheehan J, Yen CP, Steiner L. Gamma Knife surgery-induced meningioma: Report of two cases and review of the literature. J Neurosurg. 2006; 105:325–329

[69] Bernstein M, Laperriere N, Leung P, et al. Interstitial Brachytherapy for Malignant Brain Tumors: Preliminary Results. Neurosurgery. 1990; 26:371–380

[70] Florell RC, Macdonald DR, Irish WD, et al. Selection Bias, Survival, and Brachytherapy for Glioma. J Neurosurg. 1992; 76:179–183

[71] Gutin PH, Prados MD, Phillips TL, et al. External Irradiation Followed by an Interstitial High Activity Iodine-125 Implant "Boost" in the Initial Treatment of Malignant Gliomas: NCOG Study 6G-82-2. Int J Radiation Oncology Biol Phys. 1991; 21:601–606

102 Endovascular Neurosurgery

102.1 General information

102.1.1 Introduction

Endovascular Neurosurgery, AKA Neuroendovascular surgery, endovascular and surgical Neuroradiology (ESNR), or interventional neuroradiology (INR), combines catheter based techniques and imaging for the diagnosis and treatment of specific cerebral and spine conditions.

102.1.2 Indications/Conditions treated

Endovascular neurosurgery include diagnosis as well as the following treatment of:

- Aneurysms: coiling (± stent or balloon assistance), flow diverting stents e.g., Pipeline, parent vessel sacrifice
- Arteriovenous malformations (**AVMs**): embolization (pre-operative or curative)
- Dural arteriovenous fistula (**DAVF**): curative or palliative embolization
- Spinal AVMs: embolization
- Arteriovenous fistulas: e.g. Carotid Cavernous fistulas (CCF)
- Acute embolic stroke: intra-arterial clot thrombolysis or mechanical thrombectomy
- Cranial sinus thrombosis (**CST**): Thrombolysis or mechanical thrombectomy
- Cerebrovascular arterial dissections: stenting or parent artery sacrifice
- Cervical internal carotid artery stenosis: angioplasty/stenting
- Tumors: embolization. Primarily used before surgery as an adjunct to decrease vascularity e.g., with some meningiomas and hemangioblastomas
- Intracranial atherosclerosis
- Vasospasm
- Transverse sinus stenosis: stenting as in pseudotumor cerebri
- Inferior Petrosal sinus sampling for localizing pituitary macroadenomas
- Iatrogenic vascular injuries: stenting or embolization to achieve hemostasis
- Refractory epistaxis: embolization to achieve hemostasis
- Wada testing: evaluation for language and memory localization (e.g. epilepsy patients being considered for surgery)
- Intraarterial chemotherapy: e.g. retinoblastoma
- Intraoperative angiography: typically used in aneurysm surgery to confirm exclusion of the aneurysm and patency of parent vessels, and during AVM surgery to confirm elimination of nidus

102.1.3 Contraindications

- Uncorrected bleeding disorders
- Poor renal function (due to iodine dye load)
- Relative contraindication: connective tissue disorder that predisposes to vessel dissection
- For spinal angiography: thoracic aortic aneurysm (relative)

102.1.4 Risks of cerebral angiography

Risk varies with the nature of the pathology being investigated and with the experience of the angiography team. Overall risk of a complication resulting in a permanent neurologic deficit[1,2]: 0.1%. In ACAS, there was a 1.2% complication rate (p. 1276).

102.1.5 Miscellaneous angiography

► **Tumors.** While angiography is no longer used diagnostically for tumors, there are a few general principles worth knowing. Typically, non-vascular deep lesions cause changes in venous structures, whereas superficial lesions affect arterial structures. Malignant neoplasm (e.g. glioblastoma): the classic feature on angiography is an early draining vein. Meningiomas: the stain (contrast) "arrives early, stays late" (appears early in arterial phase, blush persists beyond venous phase); see also other angiographic findings with meningiomas (p. 695).

► **Allcock test.** Evaluates flow through the posterior communicating arteries by vertebral injection with simultaneous common carotid artery compression in the neck.

102.2 Pharmacologic agents

102.2.1 General information

This section presents drugs as they are used in neuroendovascular procedures.[3] The indications cited are specific to endovascular intervention.

102.2.2 Abciximab (ReoPro)

General information

The Fab fragment of an antibody. Prevents binding of fibrinogen to platelet GP IIb/IIIa receptors. Platelet inhibition lasts up to 48 hours.

Indications and case selection

- Acute endoarterial thrombus during endovascular intervention
- Dissection with thrombus adherent to intimal flap
- Prophylaxis for intracranial or extracranial stent implantation

Dosing

℞: bolus with 0.25 mg/kg IV over 10–60 minutes (shorter duration for the acute complications during intervention) followed by infusion of 0.125 mcg/kg/min (max. 10mcg/min) for 12 hours.

Reversal

Discontinue abciximab infusion. Allow 10–30 minutes for clearance of the drug from plasma, followed by platelet transfusion. Surgical intervention should be delayed for 12 - 24 hours after discontinuation.

102.2.3 Aspirin

General information

Irreversibly inactivates cyclo-oxygenase, resulting in platelet inhibition by preventing formation of prostaglandins from arachidonic acid.

Indications and case selection

- Intra (short-term) and post-procedural (short + long-term) prophylaxis of thromboembolic events e.g., during
  - diagnostic cerebral angiography
  - coil embolization of aneurysms
  - stent implantation (typically with a second antiplatelet agent)
  - balloon test occlusions
  - therapeutic occlusion of large arteries
- Subacute management of procedural complications e.g.,
  - parent artery coil herniations
  - thrombus or clot on coil phenomena
  - in-stent thrombus (alone or in combination with a second agent)

Dosing

℞: 325–1300 mg orally, daily

Uncoated Aspirin (ASA) achieves peak plasma concentrations within 30 - 40 minutes.[4,5] Enteric-coated ASA achieves peak plasma concentrations in up to 6 hours.[6] 60% of population is resistant to the antiplatelet effect of low dose (81 mg) ASA, while up to 30% are resistant to 325 mg/day.[7,8] However, the assessment of ASA resistance is highly assay dependent. A dose related effect i.e., improved response to increasing the dose, indicates that ASA also exert antiplatelet effects through non-cyclo-oxygenase pathways.[9]

Reversal

Reversal is achieved by platelet transfusion.

ASA causes an irreversible inactivation of the platelet cyclo-oxygenase that persists through the lifespan of the exposed platelets.

102.2.4 Clopidogrel (Plavix™)

General information

A platelet ADP receptor antagonist.

Indications and case selection

- Prevention of intra-procedural and short-term post-procedural (4–12 weeks) thromboembolic events related to endovascular procedures including
  - Coil embolization of wide-neck cerebral aneurysms where stent will be used
  - Stent implantation (with a second antiplatelet agent)
  - Therapeutic occlusion of large arteries (often with a second antiplatelet agent)
- Subacute management of procedural complications (alone or in combination with a second agent)
  - Parent artery coil herniations
  - Thrombus or clot on coil phenomena
  - In-stent thrombus (may be more effective than other agents)

Dosing

℞: 75 mg PO daily. Start 5 days prior to the actual procedure because there is a 3–7 days latency period to full therapeutic effect

LD: 300 mg PO, if there was no time to achieve therapeutic effect over a course of days. A therapeutic effect can usually be achieved within 2 to 3 hours of LD.

Reversal

Platelet transfusion.

102.2.5 Eptifibatide (Integrilin®)

General information

A reversible inhibitor of platelet aggregation by preventing the binding of fibrinogen, von Willebrand factor, and other adhesive ligands to GP IIb/IIIa. Platelet aggregation inhibition appears dose and concentration dependent and is reversible following discontinuation of eptifibatide. It causes a 5-fold increase in bleeding time and has no measurable effect on PT or aPTT.

Indications and case selection

These are the same as for abciximab (see above).

Dosing

℞: bolus 180 mcg/kg IV (max 22.6 mg) over 1–2 minutes followed by infusion of 2 mcg/kg/min .

Reversal

- Discontinue drug. Significant reduction of anti-platelet effects occurs in 2–4 hours.[10]
- For clinical signs or imaging evidence of hemorrhage:
  - For ICH, hemodynamic compromise, or decrease in Hb > 5 g/dl or decrease in HCT > 15%, give platelet transfusion
  - For a decrease in Hb < 5 g/dl or decrease in HCT < 15%, give desmopressin ℞: 0.3 mcg/kg × 1.

102

102.2.6 Heparin

General information

A glycosaminoglycan that indirectly inhibits thrombin by modulating antithrombin III (AT III) activity. It also indirectly inactivates factors IXa, Xa, XIa and XIIa and restores electronegativity to endothelial surfaces. It prevents thrombin-platelet aggregation and inhibits von Willebrand factor. The anticoagulant effects are immediate. The half-life of IV heparin is approximately 1.5 hours.[11,12]

Indications and case selection

- Prophylaxis during diagnostic angiography (used in flush solutions only)[3,13]
- Neuroendovascular procedures including,
  - coil embolization of intracranial aneurysms,
  - therapeutic occlusion of carotid, vertebral, or other large cerebral artery
  - Transarterial embolization of brain AVM or dural AVF
  - Percutaneous transluminal angioplasty
  - Intra- or extracranial stent implantation
  - Balloon test occlusion of carotid, vertebral, or other large cerebral artery

Dosing

℞: **Flush systems**: 6000 i.u. per liter of 0.9% normal saline (6 i.u. per cc) for flush systems used in neuroendovascular procedures. During intraoperative angiography: 2500 i.u. per liter of 0.9% normal saline (2.5 i.u. per cc). The lower dosage during surgery is a precaution against excessive bleeding from operative sites e.g., during craniotomy.

Endovascular interventions:

Coil embolization for unruptured aneurysm: 5000 units bolus. Check the activated clotting (ACT, ▶ Table 102.1) 20–30 minutes after bolus and then hourly. Administer heparin 0–5000 units hourly prn to maintain ACT between 250–300.

Coil embolization for ruptured aneurysm: Place the framing coil prior to heparin bolus.

Angioplasty with/without stenting: 5000 units bolus. Perform ACT 20–30 minutes after bolus and then hourly. Administer heparin up to 5000 units hourly prn to maintain ACT between 300–350.

Post procedure heparinization: For aneurysm embolization, the following regimens are recommended:

Heparin dosing for post coiling neurosurgery patients

- University of Cincinnati Protocol[14]: devised to administer a safe dose of heparin that does not require repeat blood draws and titration to ACT or aPTT
  - Weight-based dosing
    - Weight ≤ 75 kg: 900 units/hour, no bolus doses, for 12 hrs
    - Weight > 75 kg: 1300 units/hour, no bolus doses, for 12 hrs
  - Labs: no ACT or other laboratory draws required.
- *Alternative:* The most commonly used heparin weight based protocol (NB: this differs from dosing e.g. for coronary indications or treatment of DVT or PE[15]): bolus dose of 60–70 units/kg followed by a maintenance IV infusion rate of 18 units/kg/hour. Titrate to ACT as shown in ▶ Table 102.1.

Reversal

IV protamine sulfate at 1 mg per 100 units of circulating heparin (not to exceed 50 mg total).

A preloaded syringe of 50 mg should be available at all times. Normally protamine is administered as an IV infusion over 10 – 30 minutes, to prevent idiosyncratic hypotension and anaphylactoid

Table 102.1 Recommended ACT for various endovascular procedures

Indications	ACT (Seconds)
Procedures involving deep arterial injury e.g., percutaneous transluminal angioplasty with/without stenting. Procedures with significant stasis of blood flow e.g., balloon occlusion of parent vessels	High (300–350)
Procedures in which the above mentioned thrombogenic elements are absent e.g., embolization of an aneurysm or AVM	Moderate (250–300)

symptoms. In an emergency e.g., vessel or intracranial aneurysm perforation, anticoagulation must be immediately reversed by rapid IV bolus of 10 mg protamine over 1–3 minutes.

102.2.7 Nitroglycerine

General information

Produces strong and immediate vasodilatation by stimulation of cGMP, which results in vascular smooth muscle relaxation.

Indications and case selection

Vessel spasm during catheterization.

Dosing

℞: 100 – 300mcg through the catheter.

102.2.8 Papaverine

General information

A benzylisoquinolone alkaloid that vasodilates by inhibition of cAMP and cGMP phosphodiesterases in smooth muscle, leading to increased intracellular levels of cAMP and cGMP. It may also inhibit the release of calcium from the intracellular space by blocking calcium ion channels in the cell membrane. Papaverine is short acting, with half–life of less than 1 hour.

Indications and case selection

Pre-treatment for angioplasty. The resulting vasodilatation will assist with balloon catheter placement. Due to its short duration of action necessitating repeated administration, other agents e.g., verapamil, are generally preferred.

Dosing

℞: 300 mg of 3% papaverine (30 mg/ml) at pH 3.3, is diluted in 100 ml of normal saline to obtain a 0.3% concentration. It is administered intra-arterially through the microcatheter, which is positioned just proximal to the affected vascular segment at a rate of 3 ml/minute.

✖ Do not mix Papaverine with contrast agents or heparin, which may result in precipitation of crystals.

102.2.9 Sodium Amytal

General information

A barbiturate derivative that activates $GABA_A$ receptors. When it is administered into cerebral vasculature during Wada test, it temporarily anesthetizes the perfused region, resulting in isolation of the contralateral hemisphere permitting assessment of cortical functions including language and memory. It blocks neuronal activity and in conjunction with lidocaine, which blocks axonal activity, it is administered as a test injection in procedures such as spinal AVM embolization, or embolization of spinal tumors, prior to the injection of the embolic agent.[16]

Indications and case selection

Wada Test

Test injection prior to embolization of feeder vessel of AVM. In order to suppress both neuronal and axonal activity, amytal injection is followed by xylocaine injection.

Dosing

℞: 50–100 mg per test injection via catheter.

For administration, dilute 500 mg sodium amytal in 20 cc 0.9% NS to yield a concentration of 25 mg/cc of sodium amytal.

For Wada test, after catheterization of vessel of interest, 100 mg of Sodium Amytal (4 cc of the preparation described above) are injected through the catheter. Additional boluses of 25 mg (1 cc) or modification of the original bolus may be required, per the neurologist's request.

102.2.10 Tissue Plasminogen Activator (tPA)

General information

A fibrin specific thrombolytic protease that converts plasminogen to plasmin.

Indications and contraindications

Indications:

- Cranial sinus thrombosis (CST)
- Patients with acute ischemic stroke who are18 years of age, or older; have clinical diagnosis of ischemic stroke with measurable neurologic deficit
  - symptom onset ≤ 4.5 hours prior to initiation of treatment: given IV
  - up to 6 hours after symptom onset: given by intra-arterial administration. May be up to 24 hours after onset for posterior circulation (where there is less likelihood of hemorrhagic conversion of infarct).

✖ **Absolute Exclusion criteria:**

- Brain CT scan demonstrating ICH prior to treatment.
- Only minor or, rapidly improving symptoms of stroke.
- Clinical presentation suggestive of SAH, even with a normal CT.
- CT demonstrating ICH or SAH.
- Active internal bleeding.
- Known bleeding diathesis including platelet count < 100 $X10^3/mm^3$.
- Heparin within 48 hours with an elevated APTT.
- Current oral anticoagulation use e.g., warfarin, or recent use with an elevated PT (> 15 sec) or INR (> 1.7).
- Current use of direct thrombin inhibitors (desirudin, bivalirudin, argatroban)[17] or direct factor Xa inhibitors (Rivaroxaban, Edoxaban, Betrixaban)[18] with elevated aPTT, INR, platelet count, Ecarin Clotting Time (ECT), TT, or factor Xa activity assays.
- Intracranial or intraspinal surgery, severe TBI, or previous stroke within 3 months.
- Suspected aortic dissection associated with stroke.
- Suspected subacute bacterial endocarditis or vasculitis.
- Recent (within past 7 days) arterial puncture at a non-compressible site.
- Lumbar puncture within 7 days.
- History of ICH.
- Known AVM or aneurysm.
- Persistent SBP > 185 mm Hg or DBP > 110 mm Hg at time of treatment, or patient requires aggressive treatment to reduce BP within these limits.

Relative Exclusion criteria:

- Witnessed seizure at the same time as onset of symptoms of stroke
- NIHSS > 22 (severe deficit) or < 4 (mild deficit)
- Baseline CT demonstrating extensive ischemic changes e.g., sulcal effacement, mass effect, or edema, hypodensity in more than 1/3 of MCA territory distribution
- Major surgery or serious trauma within 14 days
- History of GI or urinary tract hemorrhage within 21 days
- Recent acute MI (past 3 months)
- Post myocardial infarction pericarditis
- Blood Glucose < 50 mg/dl (2.7 mmol/l) or > 400 mg/dl
- Age > 80 years
- Pregnancy
- History of ischemic stroke AND diabetes
- History of terminal cancer or other medical condition with limited life expectancy
- History of advanced dementia

Dosing

℞: Intravenous: 0.9 mg/kg (max. 90 mg). The first 10% of the calculated dose is administered as an IV bolus over 1 minute and the remainder is infused over an hour, within the 4.5 hour window.

℞: Intraarterial: The maximum intra-arterial dose is 22 mg. It is independent of any previously administered intravenous dose.

1–2 mg tPA is administered manually distal to the clot, then administer an infusion of 0.5 mg/ml at 20 ml/hr (10 mg/hr). The infusion is prepared by mixing 10 mg of tPA in 20 ml in normal saline, resulting in a concentration of 1 mg tPA per 2 ml saline (or 0.5 mg/ml). An infusion pump may be used for more precise administration.

Angiography is performed every 15 minutes (following infusion of 2.5 mg tPA) as the catheter is gradually drawn back through the clot. The lesion is re-crossed after each angiogram. If the artery is still occluded, inject 1 – 2 mg tPA manually and resume the tPA infusion.

Discontinue tPA if

- adequate recanalization is achieved
- extravasation of contrast material is noted on angiography
- The maximum dose has been administered, or the administered dose approaches the maximum dose without clinical or angiographic improvement.

In CST, usually 2–5 mg are administered through the thrombus and then an infusion started at a rate of 1 mg/hr, usually for 12 hours. If a clot burden is still present on angiography, a longer duration of administration until the clot resolves is a consideration.

For CST, the infusion is prepared in a concentration of 1 mg/10 ml (0.1 mg/ml), for a rate of 10 ml/hr.

Reversal

FFP transfusion.

102.2.11 Verapamil

General information

A nondihydropyridine calcium channel blocker that reduces the influx of calcium through L-type calcium channels in smooth-muscle cells, enabling vasodilation. Half-life is about 3–7 hours.

Indications and case selection

- Before balloon angioplasty: chemical vasodilatation prior to mechanical vasodilatation may enable a smoother and safer angioplasty.
- Mild vasospasm, that does not warrant angioplasty.
- Moderate vasospasm, that cannot be safely treated with angioplasty.

Dosing

℞: 5–10 mg IA. It is slowly infiltrated (over 2–10 minutes) into the vasospastic vessel via a microcatheter into the intracranial vessel, and/or via diagnostic or guide catheter into larger vessels e.g., ICA or, VA.

Reversal

For clinically significant hypotension or high degree AV block: treat with vasopressors and cardiac pacing e.g., epinephrine, norepinephrine and vasopressin infusions. Calcium chloride infusion is given in large doses e.g., 1 gm/hr for more than 24 hours. 20% intralipid infusion (100 ml bolus followed by continuous infusion at 0.5 ml/kg/hr) may also be useful.[19] Atropine may be administered for bradycardia. Hemodialysis is ineffective.

102.2.12 Xylocaine

General information

Blocks the fast voltage gated Na^+ Channels in neuronal cell membranes. There may be inhibition of postsynaptic neurons and consequently, action potentials.

102

Indications and case selection

As a local anesthetic prior to arteriotomy. Preparations with or without epinephrine may be used.

Cardiac xylocaine is used to test axonal function. It may be used alone or in conjunction with amobarbital.

Used for functional testing in case of spinal vascular disorders.

Provocative functional testing in cerebral AVMs.

Dosing

℞: for local anesthesia : Approximately 5 ml of 2% lidocaine (max. 4 mg/ml to 280 mg; 14 ml)

℞: for neurophysiological testing (Wada test): 10 – 40 mg i.a. of cardiac lidocaine.

Reversal

Lidocaine overdose[20]: intravenous bolus of 20% lipid emulsion 1.5 ml/kg over 1 min and start IV infusion at 15 ml/kg/hr. The bolus may be repeated twice at 5 min intervals, if cardiovascular stability is not restored. Additionally, the infusion may be doubled to 30 ml/kg/hr if instability persists after 5 minutes. Lipid emulsion is continued until cardiovascular stability is restored or maximum dose administered.[20] Do not exceed the maximum cumulative dose of 12 ml/kg.

Concurrent supportive care includes following ACLS protocols e.g., securing airway, hemodynamic support etc.

✖ Propofol is not a substitute for lipid emulsion in such cases. It has only 10% lipids which is too low to be of benefit, and the cardio-depressant properties of propofol may be counterproductive in such situations.

102.3 Neuroendovascular Procedure Basics

102.3.1 Vascular access

General information

Most commonly, vascular access is obtained through femoral artery. If femoral access is not possible then the radial artery, brachial artery or carotid artery (least common) may be used.

Femoral artery access

After prepping and draping the groin, place the left little finger on anterior superior iliac spine and span with thumb to the pubic symphysis. This approximately demarcates the ilioinguinal ligament. Bisect this line with the other hand and palpate the femoral pulse. The site of access is 3 fingerbreadths below the point of bisection, to ensure the vessel puncture site is *below* the ilioinguinal ligament and therefore, compressible. A marker (e.g. hemostat) can be placed over the pulse and a fluoro shot taken to confirm that the planned access site is situated over the middle of the femoral head.

A small, superficial stab incision in the skin is made at the selected point, after infiltration of local anesthesia. In an elective case, a micropuncture set with a 7 cm 21 or 23 gauge needle may be used for vessel puncture. In an emergency (e.g., stroke) a larger 18G single wall needle is used. The artery is palpated and immobilized between the index and middle finger of one hand, while the needle in introduced through the stab at 45°. Once the artery is accessed, blood will emanate through the needle hub. An exchange over wires is made using modified Seldinger technique to place the sheath of desired size. The sheath is connected to continuously running flush of heparinized saline and secured with adhesive or suture to prevent dislodgement.

Radial artery access

First perform Allen's test with pulse oximetry to ensure the hand has satisfactory vascular supply, in case the procedure results in radial artery occlusion.

Allen's Test: Palpate the radial and ulnar arteries and place a pulse oximeter on the thumb or index finger. Make the patient flex and extend their fingers repeatedly. With digital pressure, compress both the radial and ulnar arteries during finger extension and maintain the compression until the oximetry pulse is lost. The wrist is maintained in approximately 20° flexion, in order to avoid false positive test when the wrist is in hyperextension. Release the pressure on the ulnar artery. Measure the time taken to achieve visual capillary refill in finger pads and at least 92% oxygen saturation. Normal capillary refill time is < 5 sec, refill times of 5–15 secs are considered equivocal. A refill time longer than 15 sec is abnormal. Allen's test can also be performed using ultrasonography.

Reverse Allen's Test: It should be performed when the radial artery is being subjected to a repeat procedure. Compress both the radial and ulnar arteries with digital pressure during finger extension and maintain the compression. Release the pressure on the *radial* artery. Measure the time taken to achieve visual capillary refill in finger pads and at least 92% oxygen saturation, as indicated above.

During access, the following modifications are made from the technique described above. A shorter needle 21 G (e.g., 3 cm, instead of 7 cm) is used. Avoid entering the artery at a steep angle, as this may cause difficulties in threading the wire through the artery.

Advance a 0.018" wire through the needle hub into the radial artery and remove the needle. Make a nick in the skin over the wire, to aid in smoother insertion of larger sheaths. A 4 Fr micropuncture sheath (with dilator) over the wire is advanced over the wire and then the wire and dilator are removed. A cocktail of heparin (5000 IU/ml), verapamil (2.5 mg), 2% lidocaine (1.0 ml), and nitroglycerin (0.1 mg) are administered through the introducer sheath to relieve and/or prevent vasospasm. The patient should be forewarned about a transient but uncomfortable sensation of severe burning, as the cocktail is injected into the artery. The standard 0.035" wire is advanced through the sheath. The desired sheath size is then placed.

Note: After completion of the procedure, a closure device *is not* used for radial artery. Only manual compression for 15–20 minutes is applied.

102.3.2 Sheath Management

Once placed, the sheath is connected to a continuously running heparinized saline solution at a rate of 30 ml/hr. The flush consists of 6000 units of heparin in 1000 ml of 0.9% saline bag (6 units/ml). The saline bag is placed in a pressure infuser which is inflated to 300 mmHg. It is important that the sheath be continuously irrigated and the saline bag be under a pressure greater than the patient's own arterial pressure. The patient's leg on the side of the sheath is kept straight to prevent kinking of the sheath. If the intention is to maintain the sheath for several hours or a few days, it should be secured by suturing to the patient's skin.

102.3.3 Arteriotomy closure

After completion of the procedure, if vascular access will not be required within next few days, the sheath is removed. To do this, the following options are available:

- Pressure
  - *Manual Pressure:* Palpate the artery proximal to site of arteriotomy, remove sheath and apply manual pressure for 15–30 minutes and gradually decreasing pressure every 5 minutes.
  - Femostop™: Prior to application, ensure ACT is < 150 and BP is under control. The inner circle of the Femostop dome should be positioned 1 cm superior and 1 cm medial to the actual puncture site and over the femoral artery. Inflate the Femostop to 20–30 mm Hg above the patient's systolic pressure. If this does not result in hemostasis, inflate to higher pressures until distal pulses are occluded. Maintain distal pulse occlusion for 5–7 minutes, then readjust the manometer pressure until good pedal pulse and good color of extremities is achieved
    Continue to progressively decrease the applied pressure over the course of several hours, until the device can be discontinued entirely. Usually, a Femostop is maintained for 6 12 hours.
- Percutaneous closure devices
  - Angioseal™: effects closure by deposition of fibrin plug in the vessel which is then pulled back into the arteriotomy defect of the vessel wall. Angioseal is available in 6 and 8 Fr sizes. Deployed by exchanging it with the sheath over a wire. After deployment, the patient remains supine for 2 hours (with pillow under the head) with the leg on the side of Angioseal kept straight. Patient is mobilized thereafter.
  - Mynx™: a bio-absorbable sealant that is deposited in the arteriotomy defect. Available in 5, 6, 7 Fr sizes. Tends to be the least painful
  - Starclose™: Also exchanged with the sheath over a wire. Deployment results in stitch closure of the arteriotomy defect. Tends to be more painful

102.4 Diagnostic angiography for cerebral subarachnoid hemorrhage

102.4.1 General information

Objective: diagnose source of hemorrhage, assess supplying blood vessels and collateral vessels (may require additional provocative maneuvers), assess vessels for possible bypass, assess for vasospasm.

The most common cause of nontraumatic SAH is ruptured cerebral aneurysms. Other causes include AVM (cerebral or spinal), vasculitis, pre-truncal nonaneurysmal subarachnoid hemorrhage, arterial dissection, dural sinus thrombosis, pituitary apoplexy, bleeding dyscrasias, sickle cell disease and cocaine abuse. In 14–22% a cause for SAH is not found on angiography.[21]

102.4.2 Setup

A sheath is placed in the femoral artery, connected to a continuously running flush of heparinized saline. A diagnostic catheter is attached to a continuously running flush of heparinized saline. It is introduced into the vasculature, via the sheath and advanced over the guidewire through the aorta to the target vessel. The catheter is advanced with the guidewire leading and pulled back with the guide wire completely retracted into the catheter. Once the catheter is in desired position, the guidewire is withdrawn completely and angiography performed, by using manual injections or the auto-injector.

102.4.3 Planning

Pre-planning the procedure will save time, amount of contrast administered and radiation exposure. Standard views (half Towne's and lateral for anterior circulation; Towne's and lateral for posterior circulation) are obtained. Additionally, the images in appropriate projections are obtained, keeping in mind the patient's pathology. As needed, rotational angiography is performed and the 3D reconstruction manipulated for further examination, as well as, selection of further projections for angiography.

102.4.4 Additional views

In case of aneurysms, based on their location, the projections as shown in ► Table 102.2 may prove useful.

102.5 Disease-specific intervention

102.5.1 Aneurysms

General information

The coil vs. clip debate is a moving target, especially given the fact that as long-term data about endovascular treatment is becoming available, the technology continues to evolve which renders the data obsolete. While there will always be a role for surgical clipping, endovascular therapy has emerged as a first line therapy for most aneurysms (particularly ruptured aneurysms or in poor surgical candidates). Surgery still remains a strong option for MCA aneurysms and many believe for most PICA aneurysms.

Indications

The selection of aneurysm for treatment depends upon the following considerations:

► **Ruptured vs. unruptured.** A ruptured aneurysm needs to be treated urgently, as the risk or re-rupture is 2–3%/day in first few days and 20% in 2 weeks. The risk of morbidity and mortality of an untreated ruptured aneurysm is 45-50%.[22,23]

► **Symptoms other than rupture.** Aneurysms that present with symptoms e.g., cranial nerve palsy, loss of vision or ischemia, may be at a higher risk of rupture than asymptomatic aneurysms (some symptoms may be due to acute expansion).[24,25,26,27,28,29]

► **Size.** Large aneurysms (> 7–10 mm) are more likely to rupture than small (< 7 mm) aneurysms.[29,30]

► **Shape.** An irregularly shaped aneurysm may be at a greater risk of rupture then a spherical saccular aneurysm. Irregular shape includes morphological characteristics such as daughter blebs, or irregular borders.[31]

Table 102.2 Projection for angiography, based on aneurysm location

Aneurysm location	Projection	Additional view
Anterior communicating	25° oblique away from injection side; center beam on lateral aspect of ipsilateral orbital rim; orient tube in Towne's view.	Submental vertex, but the image may be degraded by the amount of interposed bone.
Posterior communicating	55° paraorbital oblique away from injection side; center beam 1 cm posterior to inferior portion of lateral rim of ipsilateral orbit; orient x-ray tube 12° cephalad	
Carotid terminus	25° oblique away from injection side; center beam 3–4 cm above lateral aspect of ipsilateral orbital rim; orient x-ray tube in Towne's view.	Submentovertex view
Ophthalmic artery	25° oblique away from injection side; center beam 3–4 cm above lateral aspect of ipsilateral orbital rim; orient tube in Towne's view.	Submentovertex view
Superior hypophyseal	25° oblique away from injection side; center beam 3–4 cm above lateral aspect of ipsilateral orbital rim; orient x-ray tube in Towne's view.	Submentovertex view
Posterior inferior cerebellar artery (PICA)	55° paraorbital oblique away from injection side; center beam on foramen magnum; orient x-ray tube 12° cephalad	
Vertebrobasilar junction aneurysms	15° oblique away from injection side; center beam on foramen magnum; orient x-ray tube 25° Towne.	Submentovertex view
Anterior inferior cerebellar artery aneurysm (AICA)	AP or Submentovertex view, center beam on nasion, orient x-ray tube 15° caudad	
Basilar bifurcation	Oblique 25° away from or towards injection side, center beam 3–4 cm above lateral aspect of ipsilateral superior orbital rim, orient x-ray tube 25° Towne.	Submentovertex view

► **Aspect ratio.** In addition to size, the aspect ratio (aneurysm depth/neck width) may predict the aneurysms at risk of rupture. An aspect ratio greater than 1.6 may create low flow conditions in the dome of the aneurysm that lead to stasis, thrombosis and a fibrinolytic cascade that results in breakdown of the intima.[32] A retrospective evaluation of 75 ruptured and 107 unruptured aneurysms, demonstrated the mean aspect ratio to be 2.7 for ruptured and 1.8 for unruptured aneurysms ($p < 0.001$). The mean depth of aneurysm was also greater in ruptured aneurysms (7.7 ±4.9 mm vs 5.1 ± 4.5 mm). 75% of the ruptured aneurysms were < 10 mm, and 62% of these had aspect ratio > 1.6.[33]

► **Location.** The ISUIA studies demonstrated posterior circulation aneurysms had a higher risk of rupture compared to anterior circulation.[24,34] Conversely, cavernous segment aneurysms had a 0% risk of rupture until they reached a size of 13–24 mm, when the 5 year cumulative risk became 3%.

► **Choice of treatment.** The choice of treatment should take all of above in addition to individual patient considerations e.g., age, and overall health.

Wide necked aneurysms were previously thought better suited for clipping, but the availability of stents that may act as scaffolding for coils e.g. Enterprise™ stent or act as vascular reconstruction devices e.g., Pipeline. has greatly increased the spectrum of aneurysms amenable to endovascular treatment. Additionally, small aneurysms (< 4 mm) in size may be less favorable for coiling.

Endovascular Options

► **Coiling.** This is the treatment of first choice for most narrow-necked aneurysms. The first coil (framing coil) used is equal to the size of aneurysm, or slightly oversized (especially in unruptured aneurysm). The coils are progressively downsized as embolization progresses. The goal is to maximally pack the aneurysm such that no contrast is seen entering it and without causing any loop to herniate into the vessel lumen. Even after maximal packing, the actual packing is about 20–30%.[35]

► **Coiling with stenting.** For wide-necked aneurysms, a stent may be used to prevent the coils from herniating out of the aneurysm into the blood vessel. When a stent is used, the patient is required to be on ASA (indefinitely) and Plavix (for at least 1 month). Therefore, stent assisted coiling is generally avoided in ruptured aneurysms, in part due to the fact that if an EVD is needed it cannot be safely placed with the patient on Plavix. Therefore, stent assisted coiling is generally avoided in ruptured aneurysms. However, it has also been undertaken successfully in ruptured cases, with 93% technical success, clinically significant ICH in 8% (including 10% known to have EVDs), and significant thromboembolic events in 6%.[36]

► **Balloon-assisted coiling.** This technique may be used for wide necked aneurysms where stenting is deemed less desirable e.g., ruptured aneurysm, since it bypasses the need for dual anti-platelet therapy. A balloon catheter is selected based on the diameter of the artery and the width of the aneurysm neck. The balloon segment of the catheter (indicated by radiopaque markers) is positioned across the neck and kept inflated during coil deposition into the aneurysm. It is deflated prior to coil detachment and the stability of the deposited coil assessed. If the coil appears stable, it is detached. This inflation-deflation technique is continued as required, until the aneurysm has been completely coiled.

► **Dual catheter technique.** In this case two microcatheters are placed in the aneurysm. Coil loops are deposited alternatively from each.

► **Coil types.** Bare platinum coils: Guglielmi detachable coils are bare platinum coils that come in various diameters (mm) and lengths (cm). They come as standard, soft and ultra soft, as well as 360° and helical configurations.

More recently, the same manufacturer has introduced Target coils. The advantage over GDC is "less kickback" when being deposited in the aneurysm especially during final stages when coiling is near completion.

Other bare platinum coils include Trufill/Orbit coils, Micrus, and Target.

► **Hydrocoils.** Platinum coils coated with hydrogel which expands upon contact with blood filling the residual space between loops.

► **Liquid embolic agents.** A less commonly used technique where a DMSO compatible catheter is placed into the aneurysm and a balloon catheter inflated across its neck, while a liquid embolic agent (e.g. Onyx 500) is injected into the aneurysm. Onyx may be used in sidewall aneurysms that have a wide neck (≥ 4 mm) or with dome-to-neck ratio < 2, that are not amenable to surgical clipping. It may also be used in patients who are allergic to metal (e.g., cobalt, chromium, platinum or tungsten). It is important to keep the balloon catheter inflated until the Onyx solidifies, as otherwise embolization into the normal vessel may produce a stroke.

► **Pipeline Embolization Device (PED).** The woven design of this particular stent makes it low porosity which attenuates blood entry into the aneurysm and therefore encourages stasis. If needed, two or more of these may be deployed within each other across the neck of the aneurysm, to cause adequate flow stasis in the aneurysm. Angiography immediately post deployment, demonstrates contrast stasis in the aneurysm. Six month follow up angiography usually demonstrates complete obliteration of the aneurysm, such that it is no longer visualized. Once an aneurysm is successfully treated with PED, there is a 0% recurrence rate. The most recent iteration of the device known as Pipeline Flex™ is a 48 braid device that is somewhat easier to deploy than the earlier version. It is available in diameters from 2.5 – 5 mm. Sometimes, coil deployment in the aneurysm may also be required to encourage aneurysm thrombosis.

A strategy used in case of ruptured aneurysms is to "undercoil" the aneurysm to address the risk of re-rupture and then complete treatment with PED when it becomes safe to use dual antiplatelet therapy

In case of ruptured blister aneurysms, Pipeline device has been used with success by administering an abciximab bolus (0.125mcg/kg) IV, approx. 10 minutes prior to device deployment.[37,38]

Indications:

- Large or giant wide-necked ICA aneurysms, from petrous to the superior hypophyseal segments.
- Presently, patients must be 22 years of age or older.
- PED has been used in cases outside the established indications e.g. in MCA, vertebral and basilar arteries.[39,40,41]

Contraindications:

- Ruptured aneurysm (due to requirement of pre-embolization dual anti-platelet therapy). However, it has been used in ruptured blister aneurysms.[37,38]
- Patients in whom dual anti-platelet therapy is contraindicated.
- Patients who have not received dual anti-platelet therapy (ASA and clopidogrel) prior to procedure.
- Active bacterial infection.
- Metal allergy to cobalt, chromium, platinum or tungsten.
- Patients with pre-existing stent in the parent artery at the target aneurysm location (relative contraindication).

Treatment of aneurysmal rupture during coiling

- notify anesthesia: for assistance with critical care management and in case you need to go to the O.R.
- immediately lower the blood pressure
- inflate balloon if balloon-assisted coiling
- immediately reverse anticoagulation. Give 50 mg of protamine (protamine should always be available during the procedure)
- do not remove the coil that caused the perforation, continue deploying it and follow with additional coils in rapid succession
- insert an extraventricular drain (EVD)

102.5.2 Endovascular management of vasospasm

General information

A ruptured aneurysm needs to be secured by coiling or clipping prior to hyperdynamic therapy or endovascular intervention for vasospasm.

Indications

Failure of resolution, or worsening of symptoms of vasospasm with hyperdynamic therapy for 12 - 24 hours.

Patients with conditions such as congestive heart failure, cardiac ischemia or pulmonary edema, that limit the institution of hyperdynamic therapy.[42]

Treatment options

In addition to pharmacological (hyperdynamic or triple-H) therapy, endovascular options for management of vasospasm include intra-arterial chemical spasmolysis, utilizing selective catheterization of the involved segment and, mechanical spasmolysis using angioplasty.

► **Chemical spasmolysis.** Verapamil: Drug of first choice for spasmolysis in many centers. Its advantage is a relatively long half-life (6–12 hours).

Indications:

- Mild to moderate vasospasm that does not warrant angioplasty. Or, when angioplasty cannot be used safely.
- Vasospasm consequent to manipulation during endovascular intervention.
- Prior to performing angioplasty, so that the dilatation is performed on the relaxed dilated artery, rather than a relatively rigid vasoconstricted one.

Dose: 5-10 mg injected gradually (over 2–10 minutes) via microcatheter, as the microcatheter is withdrawn through the spasmodic segment. Up to 20 mg may be given into each arterial tree. It is injected gradually to prevent a significant drop in BP or bradycardia.

Other drugs used for chemical spasmolysis include nicardipine, papaverine and nitroglycerine. Similar to verapamil, nicardipine has a relatively long half-life (9 hours). Papaverine (< 1 hour) and nitroglycerine (minutes) are comparatively short acting.

► **Angioplasty.** A balloon mounted catheter is positioned across the arterial segment in spasm. The balloon is gradually inflated under fluoroscopic visualization to the desired width (equal to or less than the caliber of the adjacent non-spastic segment. The rate of balloon inflation is at a rate ≤ 1 atm/15 sec (to "stretch" not "crack" the vessel)

A combination of chemical and mechanical spasmolysis may also be used such that initially the spastic segment is dilated using verapamil infiltration, followed by balloon angioplasty.

Balloon dilatation produces durable results. However, even verapamil induced spasmolysis has been noted to persist on angiographies performed 48–72 hours post treatment.

Angioplasty is performed under direct fluoroscopic visualization. To this effect, contrast media is admixed with normal saline (50:50 to 2/3 -1/3 ratio) that is used to inflate the balloon

Precautions during angioplasty:

- Avoid inflating the balloon beyond the normal caliber of the vessel.
- Inflate gradually at a rate ≤ 1 atm/15 sec (to "stretch" not "crack" the vessel)
- Do not inflate the balloon beyond its indicated "burst pressure." This can also be avoided by selecting a balloon catheter of appropriate width of the particular vessel and length of the segment in spasm.

► **Complications and management.** Vessel rupture. This can be avoided by not inflating the balloon beyond the normal caliber of the vessel. Following rupture, reverse therapeutic heparinization by administration of protamine 1 mg. per 100 units of heparin (max. 50 mg). In such an emergency, rapid IV bolus of protamine (10 mg over 1–3 minutes) is delivered rather than over 10 - 30 minutes, which is usually done to prevent idiosyncratic hypotension and anaphylactoid symptoms.

Maintain wire (0.014") access across the injured vessel. Exchange for a balloon catheter 1 mm smaller in size and inflate it for about 20 minutes. Then deflate and perform angiography to see if bleeding has been controlled. Where feasible, use a covered stent to address the perforation. If necessary, sacrifice the involved vessel using coils. With this approach e.g., in the M2 segment of MCA, the complication of stroke is accepted with the aim of saving the patient's life. Additionally, decompressive craniotomy and evacuation of the clot may be required.

► **Dissection.** If it is minor, non-flow limiting and without a raised intimal flap, no intervention may be necessary. The dissection may be re-examined after an interval to verify resolution. If managed conservatively, place the patient on aspirin, with or without Plavix.

In case of a significant dissection, place a stent across the affected segment and start patient on ASA and plavix. Plavix 75 mg PO daily is usually administered for a month while ASA is continued indefinitely.

► **Thromboembolic complications.** A thrombus consequent to hardware, vessel injury blood stagnation or inadequate heparinization is apparent as a filling defect on control angiography. This can usually be readily addressed by administration of abciximab bolus of 0.25 mg/kg IV over 10–15 minutes, followed by infusion of 0.125 mcg/kg/min (max. 10mcg/min) for 12 hours. Repeat angiography 15 minutes following the initiation of amciximab. If the thrombus persists, an angioplasty may be performed to flatten the thrombus against the wall of the vessel. Once blood flow is restored, its lytic properties, as well as the abciximab may resolve the thrombus. Another consideration is to deploy a stent to restore lumen and blood flow.

► **ICH.** This may happen due to causes including vessel injury, bleeding into a previous area of infarct, hyperperfusion in a previously compromised area, or hypertension. When detected, discontinue and reverse the heparinization using protamine. Monitor patient closely. A decompressive craniotomy or craniectomy may be required if the hemorrhage is significant.

► **Surveillance and follow-up.** In addition to diligent monitoring in NICU, the progress or resolution of vasospasm can also be assessed by performing serial TCDs. Depending upon extent of availability, these can be daily, every other day or at least bi-weekly (e.g., q Monday and Thursday). The TCDs may be discontinued when resolution of vasospasm is apparent clinically and radiologically.

Angiography may be repeated approximately 3 days following initial intervention, or when there is significant change indicating worsening vasospasm. It need not be repeated, if the patient is obviously improving. Alternatively, CTA may be used for surveillance. At the time of surveillance angiography, additional treatments with chemical spasmolysis and/or balloon angioplasty may be considered. Therefore, start off with a larger sheath (usu. 6 Fr) to enable intervention.

Usually, the patient will remain in the NICU for approximately 10–14 days considering that vasospasm is maximal by 7–8 days and usually resolves by 14 days.[43,44,45,46]

102.5.3 Arteriovenous malformation

Indications for endovascular intervention

- The most common form of endovascular intervention for AVM is preoperative embolization to facilitate surgical AVM resection.
- Presence of associated lesions e.g., aneurysm or pseudoaneurysm on the feeding pedicle or nidus, venous thrombosis, venous outflow restriction, venous pouches or dilatations.
- A small surgically inaccessible AVM, or where surgery carries a high risk of morbidity and mortality. Curative AVM embolization is rare and limited to small lesions with simple angioarchitecture. The small surgically inaccessible AVM can also be treated with radiosurgery, which has a better track record than curative AVM embolization attempts
- As a palliative treatment in an AVM that is not completely treatable by any approach or their combination, due to location and/or diffuse morphology, but is symptomatic. Use with caution: data suggests that partial embolization of complex AVMs may increase rupture rate and worsen outcome.

AVM embolization

This can be performed using numerous agents (or their combination).

The agents include coils, onyx, NBCA and PVA.

► **Coils.** These may be used to close down a vessel supplying the AVM, an AVM pouch or aneurysms on the arteries associated with AVM. However, it cannot be relied upon to completely obliterate the AVM nidus, or effect a cure.

► **Onyx™.** A "lava-like" liquid embolic agent – Ethylene vinyl alcohol (EVOH) copolymer; ethylene and vinyl alcohol dissolved in dimethyl sulfoxide (DMSO) with micronize tantalum (for radioopacity) – that solidifies through the process of precipitation which is initiated when it comes into contact with an aqueous solution (e.g. blood, body fluids, normal saline, water) to form a cast. Not an adhesive. Amongst all agents currently available, it has the best and most controlled penetration of the AVM nidus. Therefore, Onyx has the greatest likelihood of achieving complete cure. Complete cure rates with onyx alone are possible in 20 – 51% of highly selected patients.[47,48,49] Supplied in premixed ready-to-use vials of Onyx-18, Onyx-34 and Onyx-500 in which the number (e.g. 18 for Onyx-18) corresponds to the nominal viscosity (as measured in centistokes) which the manufacturer controls by altering the EVOH concentration. Prior to use, the product must be shaken on a mixer for at least 20 minutes. Higher numbers indicate greater viscosity. Onyx 18 is most commonly used, Onyx 34 is used for very high flow AVMs, while 500 is used for aneurysm embolization.

Onyx is used with DMSO compatible microcatheters (marathon, echelon, rebar, ultra flow) that have been primed with approximately 0.3 to 0.8 ml of DMSO injected slowly through the microcatheter (depending on the deadspace of the microcatheter) prior to injecting Onyx itself. This is done to eliminate any contrast, saline or blood within the microcatheter that will cause the onyx to solidify in the catheter. The microcatheter tip is wedged in an arterial branch supplying the AVM, as close to the nidus as possible. It is ensured that the branch is exclusively supplying the AVM, by performing angiography through the microcatheter. The microcatheter is then primed with DMSO and Onyx embolization commenced under fluoroscopy. The onyx is visible due to admixed tantalum powder. It is injected slowly and continuously avoiding too much force, as this could cause the Onyx to reflux instead of flowing forward and prematurely close off access to the nidus. No more than 1 cm of Onyx reflux on the microcatheter should usually be allowed, as it may make the removal of catheter difficult later and may well cause disastrous complications. If reflux is noted, wait for 1–2 minutes and then continue with the injection. The already deposited Onyx will form a plug around the microcatheter causing the new deposit of Onyx to flow forward. The injection is stopped once Onyx is noted only to reflux and not flow into the nidus. Care is taken not to allow the Onyx to flow into the major draining vein or sinus, especially before the entire arterial supply is interrupted. The concept is the same as in surgical removal of AVMs, where major draining veins are occluded only after eliminating the arterial supply of AVM. Otherwise, the result is the same with ensuing venous hypertension resulting in AVM rupture and catastrophic ICH. In case of a large AVM, it is sometimes best to stage the procedure, addressing one major arterial tree at a time.

Intravenous or combined IV, and IA embolization of AVM has been performed in a select group of small, deep seated AVMs, with single deep drainage.[50]

► **NBCA.** N-butyl cyanoacrylate is an embolic agent that is a glue which rapidly solidifies when it comes in contact with blood. Since the introduction of Onyx, its use has declined considerably due to the drawbacks of very short working time, greater risk of embolization into venous sinuses and, adhesion to catheters rendering their extraction following embolization difficult. Such adhesion may cause inadvertent catheter fractures with retained foreign body, or intracranial bleeds.

► **PVA.** Polyvinyl alcohol (PVA) particles are available in sizes ranging from 50 to 1000 mcm. While it may be useful in temporarily devascularizing the AVM e.g., in preparation of craniotomy and surgical resection of AVM, the endovascular treatment with PVA alone is not durable.

Postoperative Management

Post-op orders:

- Admit the patient to NSICU.
- Keep leg on side used for procedure straight X 2 hrs (in case of angioseal closure) or 6–8 hours (in case manual compression was applied), with HOB elevated 15°.
- Post procedure heparinization is not required with AVMs because most ischemic events occur during the procedure and are related to the passage of embolic materials into normal blood vessels.[11]
- Check groins, DP's, vitals and neuro checks q 15 min X 4, q 30 min X 4, then q hr.
- Maintain mild hypotension for 12–72 hours especially in case of larger AVMs and monitor the patient for perfusion pressure break through bleeding, seizures and other possible complications.
- Review/Resume preprocedure medications (Hold metformin for 48 hours after intervention; hold all oral hypoglycemics, until good PO intake established).[51]

Follow-up:

- Outpatient appointment in 4 weeks.
- Follow-up angiography at 3 months. In case of staged AVM embolization, the interval between sessions is at the discretion of the endovascular neurosurgeon e.g., 1–4 weeks apart.

102.5.4 Dural arteriovenous fistulae (DAVF)

General information

These are abnormal direct arteriovenous shunts within the leaflets of dura.

Classification

There are numerous DAVF classifications. Borden (p. 1252) and Cognard (p. 1252) are amongst the more widely used.

Indications for endovascular intervention

- DAVF with "aggressive" features (► Table 102.3) are always considered for treatment. Due to the high annual mortality rate (10.4%) and annual hemorrhage rate (8.1%), the treatment should be expeditious.[52]

Table 102.3 Differentiating aggressive from benign DAVF

"Aggressive" symptoms	"Benign" symptoms
• Cortical venous reflux (CVR): the hallmark of an aggressive DAVF • Intracerebral hemorrhage • Focal neurological deficit • Dementia • Papilledema • Increased intraocular pressure	• Pulsatile bruit • Orbital congestion (without increased intraocular pressure) • Cranial nerve palsy • Chronic headaches

- DAVF with angiographic findings including:
  - Selective contrast injection into ICA or VA demonstrating delayed cerebral circulation time. The is indicative of venous congestive encephalopathy.
  - Pseudophlebitic pattern: Brain surface demonstrating tortuous, dilated collateral veins in the venous phase of the angiogram. This finding is associated with a greater risk of hemorrhage, or non-hemorrhagic neurological deficit.
  - Cortical venous reflux (CVR). To ensure that this is not missed, always perform selective (rather than global, non-selective) angiography when assessing for DAVF. Venous stenosis or obstruction is commonly found in patients with CVR.

If a DAVF is detected, look for additional fistulae, as they are multiple in up to 8%.

Those with "benign" features (see ▶ Table 102.3), may be considered for treatment if the symptoms are causing considerable discomfort to the patient, or are angiographically progressive. In many cases the treatment is palliative i.e., the symptoms are reduced but the fistula is not completely obliterated. The benign type of DAVF should continue to be followed, even when treatment is not indicated because of the risk of conversion to a more aggressive form with CVR. The follow-up may be clinical, with radiological assessment for any change in symptoms. A suggested protocol is to perform MRA with gadolinium annually, with follow-up conventional catheter angiography at 3 years. If there is any change in the patient's clinical condition, whether it is worsening, improvement or resolution of the symptoms, perform standard angiography to assess for CVR.

Asymptomatic DAVF can usually be followed.

Contraindications to endovascular intervention

Most contraindications are relative, and a risk benefit assessment is performed on a case by case basis:
- Provocative tests demonstrating intolerance to occlusion
- Recent major surgery
- Pregnancy
- Contraindication to anticoagulants and/or thrombolytics.
- *NBCA* should not be used in those with allergy to cyanoacrylates, ethiodol or iodine. Premedication in those with iodine allergies is a consideration.
- *PVA* should not be used as a therapeutic option (other than in cases of epistaxis). It is usually indicated for pre-surgical devascularization of lesion.

DAVF embolization

The approach can be transarterial, transvenous or a combination. When feasible, a transvenous approach is preferred, as the probability of fistula obliteration is greater via the venous route. Very infrequently, it is possible to access the venous side from the arterial route because of a large connection between the dural artery and adjacent vein e.g., in traumatic DAVF. This is usually not possible in spontaneous DAVF, as the feeding artery is too small.

For transvenous route, consider the potential outcome of venous occlusion e.g., venous infarct, if the sinus being occluded is also the main source of drainage for normal veins. In such a situation, consider highly selective occlusion that will spare the normal drainage. Alternatively, instead of performing a complete occlusion, consider partial treatment only such that CVR is eliminated, converting the fistula into the benign Borden type I.

When using the venous route, ascertain that the venous channel is not tenuous (e.g. acute DAVF) rendering it prone to rupture during manipulation. The venous walls become sturdier when the fistula has been present for a while.

▶ **Coils.** Measure the maximum width of the fistulous site to be occluded and select the appropriate sized coils. Deposit as many coils as necessary to occlude the fistula.

Sometimes a "combined" strategy may be used, where initially coils are deposited to slow the rapid blood flow through the fistula, followed by occlusion using a liquid embolic agent. If this strategy is used, start off with or exchange for a microcatheter compatible with the liquid embolic agent.

▶ **Onyx.** During transarterial embolization with liquid embolic agents, wedge the catheter as close as possible to the fistula. The technique of deposition is the same as for AVM (see above). It is important to disrupt the fistulous connection to achieve cure. Therefore, Onyx must penetrate into the venous aspect of the DAVF.

► **NBCA.** It is used less frequently since the availability of Onyx, for reasons described above.

► **PVA.** It really has no significant role in the treatment of DAVF.

102

102.5.5 Carotid cavernous fistulae (CCF)

General information

CCF categorized as direct and indirect. The direct type are usually posttraumatic and are a high-flow single shunt between the ICA and the cavernous sinus. Indirect are low flow from meningeal branches. The section below describes management of direct type.

Indications for endovascular intervention

Direct fistulae usually require treatment as they frequently do not resolve spontaneously. Other indications: corneal exposure, diplopia, proptosis, intolerable bruits or headaches.

Timing of treatment

If the patient is stable, treatment may usually be performed within a couple of days of the diagnosis (i.e., treatment does not have to be emergent).

Indications for urgent treatment: ICH, epistaxis, increased IOP, decreased visual acuity, rapidly progressive proptosis, cerebral ischemia and enlargement of traumatic aneurysm beyond the cavernous sinus.

CCF embolization

The treatment goal is to eliminate the fistula.

Angiography is performed to identify the exact location and size of the fistula and its venous drainage. To address the high flow, consider angiography at 7.5 fps, instead of the usual 2–4 fps. In addition to the CCF, also look for other vascular injuries/anomalies.

Selective catheterization of both ECAs and ICAs are performed, to assess their contribution to the CCF. Angiography is also performed after manual compression of the CCA on the side of fistula, to better assess cross flow from the contralateral side. The digital compression will attenuate the high blood flow to the fistula, enabling its visualization. Do not compress both carotids simultaneously.

Rotational angiography with 3D reformatting, may be performed to study the fistula and select appropriate working views for intervention. It is important to be cognizant of the venous involvement including, cavernous sinuses, superior and inferior ophthalmic veins, sphenoparietal sinus, superior and inferior petrosal sinuses and the pterygoid plexi.

The following routes may be utilized for treating CCF: Transarterial; transvenous; and, via superior ophthalmic vein (if conventional routes are not available). Other indications: corneal exposure, diplopia, proptosis, intolerable bruits or headaches.[53]

► **Coils.** Currently, the method of choice is transarterial coil embolization of the CCF.

Using roadmapping, the microcatheter is advanced over microwire into cavernous sinus via the fistula. This may take some effort. Coils are then deployed and detached, as previously described for aneurysms. Periodic angiography is performed and further coils placed, until the cavernous sinus (CS) is completely occluded. Complete occlusion is indicated by no further contrast entering the CS.

► **Onyx.** Refer to AVM section (p. 1589) for details regarding usage. In case of a high flow fistula, prior to Onyx deposition, it may be advisable to initially deposit coils into the CS to slow the blood flow. This will prevent the inadvertent embolization of Onyx into the draining veins and sinuses. A balloon can be inflated within the parent ICA in order to protect it as Onyx is being injected into the cavernous sinus.

► **NBCA.** NBCA should be used with great caution, preferably after having slowed the flow through the CCF in order to prevent untoward deposition in the venous sinuses.

There is also potential for reflux into the carotid artery, which could cause a stroke. This may particularly occur when the CCF closure is near completion and the pressure gradient between the carotid artery and the CS is lowered. As with Onyx, a balloon can be inflated in the parent artery to protect it.

▶ **Detachable balloons.** Balloons were initially utilized with success for endovascular CCF treatment and remain available outside of the US; however, these balloons are no longer available in the U.S. due to technical concerns relating to premature detachment and deflation over time.

▶ **Coil occlusion of the ICA.** The desirable treatment for CCF is the occlusion of the fistula itself, essentially resulting in ICA reconstruction. This is frequently not possible. If the CCF is not amenable to treatment by any other route, sacrifice of the involved ICA is an option, especially if satisfactory supply has been confirmed from the contralateral ICA via anterior communicating and/or supply via the posterior communicating arteries.

Post-operative management and follow up

Post-op orders:

- Admit the patient to NSICU for overnight observation. Further ICU stay will depend upon the patient's clinical condition.
- Consult or arrange follow up with ophthalmic surgery.
- 0.9% NS + 20 meq KCl @ 150 cc/hr X 2 hrs, then decrease to 100 cc/hr if patient is NPO overnight, then advance diet as tolerated.
- Keep the leg that was used for procedure straight for 2 hrs in case of Angioseal closure, or 6–8 hours when manual compression was applied. May elevate 15° HOB e.g., a pillow under the head.
- Check groin, DPs, vitals and neuro checks q 15 min X 4, q 30 min X 4, then q hr
- Review/Resume preprocedure medications (Hold metformin for 48 hours after intervention; hold all oral hypoglycemics, until good PO intake established).

Follow-up:

- D/C next morning after mobilizing, if there are no complications /other ongoing medical concerns requiring hospitalization.
- F/u on outpatient basis in 4 weeks.
- F/u angiography at 3 months.

102.5.6 Vertebrojugular fistulae (VJF)

Etiologies

- Iatrogenic e.g., during spine surgery or angiography, chiropractic manipulation, nerve block injection or radiation therapy[54,55]
- Trauma e.g., penetrating injury, or GSW
- Vasculitis

Endovascular management of VJF

▶ **Stenting.** A polytetrafluoroethylene (PTFE) covered stent, e.g., Jostent, may be used to cover the ostia of the fistula.[54]

▶ **Coil occlusion.** In the presence of adequate blood flow through contralateral healthy vertebral artery, the fistulous artery may be occluded with coils.[56] Verify that the arterial wall with the fistulous connection is part of the occluded segment.

▶ **NBCA occlusion.** Rarely, NBCA occlusion has been performed when stenting or coils occlusion were not possible.[57] Onyx may also be used similarly.

102.5.7 Carotid dissection

General information

See general information (p. 1324).

Angiographic features

Luminal stenosis (65%), occlusion (28%), pseudoaneurysm (28%), luminal irregularity (13%), embolic distal branch occlusion (13%), intimal flap (12%) and slow ICA-MCA flow (11%).[58]

Management

The initial management in the absence of ICH is intravenous heparin for 7 days followed by warfarin.[59] The goal aPTT with heparin is 1.5 – 2.0 times the control value (50–80 sec). Warfarin is continued for 3–6 months with target INR range of 2.0 – 3.0. If anticoagulation is contraindicated, anti-platelet therapy is a consideration. In pregnant individuals, obtain obstetric consultation prior to initiating anticoagulation or anti-platelet therapy.

Indications for endovascular intervention

- Persistent ischemic symptoms despite anticoagulation therapy.
- Flow-limiting lesion with hemodynamic compromise

Contraindication to anticoagulation and/or anti-platelet therapy

- Impending risk of stroke
- Expanding pseudoaneurysm formation
- Iatrogenic dissection during endovascular procedure where flow compromise is apparent

Stenting with/without coiling

The endovascular treatment for carotid dissection is stenting. In case of intimal flap, the stent will appose the flap back to the arterial wall. Pseudoaneurysms have also been successfully occluded with stenting. Both uncovered and covered stents have been used successfully.[60] JoStent is a PTFE covered stent that is available in US. A vein covered stent has also been used.[61]

In case of a pseudoaneurysm that continues to show significant residual filling after stenting, coiling of the pseudoaneurysm will cause occlusion.[60]

After stenting, the patient remains on dual antiplatelet therapy (ASA + Plavix) for at least a month and ASA alone indefinitely.

Follow-up

Follow-up should be arranged for patients on warfarin (e.g., "Coumadin clinic").

Follow-up study in 3–6 months, which could be CTA, Doppler ultrasonography or catheter angiogram.

102.5.8 Subclavian artery stenosis

General information

Radiologically demonstrable stenosis of the subclavian or innominate artery is present in approximately 17%. Of these, 2.5% have angiographic flow reversal in vertebral artery. Only 5.3% of those with angiographic steal have neurologic symptoms.[62]

► **Symptoms.** The 5 D's of VBI i.e., diplopia, dysarthria, defective vision, dizziness and drop attacks. Other symptoms include headache, nystagmus, hearing loss and focal seizures.[63,64]

The arterial stenosis is proximal to the origin of VA. Symptoms are induced by exercise or exertion using the arm ipsilateral to the stenosis. The increased flow demand due to the exertion results in retrograde blood flow through the VA. The neurological symptoms may be because of continuous brainstem ischemia or more commonly, ischemia due to ipsilateral arm exercise or exertion.[65]

Indications for endovascular intervention

Symptomatic subclavian artery stenosis i.e., stenosis resulting in subclavian steal syndrome.

Endovascular intervention

This includes angioplasty and stenting. A balloon mounted stent e.g., Express LD may be used, as the stent is deployed concurrently with angioplasty.[66] However, if the stenosis is particularly severe (e.g., < 2 mm), pre-dilatation may be performed by a smaller balloon to achieve a caliber of 4 mm at site of stenosis. Normal antegrade blood flow is restored following successful angioplasty and stenting.

Postoperative management

The patient is monitored at least overnight in NSICU.

After stenting, the patient remains on dual antiplatelet therapy (ASA + Plavix) for at least 1 month, and ASA alone indefinitely.

Follow-up study in 3–6 months, which could be CTA, Doppler ultrasonography or catheter angiogram.

Complications of angioplasty and stenting

The frequency of complications is 17.8% (of 73 procedures) for innominate and VA angioplasty and stenting. These include access-site bleeding and distal embolization.[67]

102.5.9 Ischemic Stroke

IV tPA

The target time for IV tPA administration ("door to needle time") is within 60 minutes from time of arrival to hospital. However, IV tPA can be administered up to 4.5 hours after the onset of symptoms if the patient does not have any contraindications.[68]

Dose: 0.9 mg/kg (max 90 mg) with 10% of the dose administered as a bolus over 1 minute and the rest infused over 60 minutes.

Endovascular intervention

General information

Recent studies have established the effectiveness and relative safety of endovascular intervention. These trials favor rapid endovascular intervention in acute ischemic stroke with proximal vessel occlusion, small infarct core and moderate to good collateral circulation.[69,70,71,72]

Indications and case selection for endovascular intervention

Intra-arterial tPA may be indicated for the following situations:

- Persistent symptoms of stroke despite IV tPA and adequate medical management
- Where angiography may be performed and treatment administered within 3 and 6 hours after symptom onset with an NIHSS score greater than 4, or those with an NIHSS score of greater than 20 and the ability to be treated within 6 hours
- Posterior circulation strokes may be treated endovascularly for up to 24 hrs (due to a lesser likelihood of hemorrhagic conversion of infarct)
- CTA or MRA demonstrating a diffusion-perfusion mismatch. In face of significant penumbra, it may be worthwhile to perform endovascular intervention even outside the therapeutic window. Conversely, intervention may be abandoned even within the therapeutic window, if the stroke is complete. Centers are relying more and more on neuroimaging rather than the therapeutic window
- When IV tPA is contraindicated e.g., recent surgery

Contraindications to intervention

Most contraindications are relative and have to be weighed against the risk of not intervening. These contraindications include:

- Hemorrhagic infarct or, ICH
- CT demonstrating hypodensity or mass effect consistent with evolving infarct of more than one-third of middle cerebral artery territory
- Recent major surgery
- Pregnancy
- When considering stenting, contraindication to anticoagulants and/or thrombolytics

Preprocedural management

This may be under the supervision of a stroke neurologist, or the neurosurgeon. Ensure the following:

- Rapid transfer of patient to a stroke center/facility with endovascular capabilities.
- ABC's take precedence.

- Ensure patient has two intravenous lines, preferably 18G or larger. Start monitoring BP, pulse oximetry, ECG, O_2 saturation, cardiac rate and rhythm, respiratory rate. Insert a Foley catheter.
- Verify laboratory values including Platelet count, BUN, CR, APTT, PT/INR. ß-HCG for females of reproductive age group.
- Maintain MAP ≥ 90 mm Hg.
- CT scan head: To rule out ICH.
- CTA: To assess location of the clot (hyperdense artery sign (p. 1281)) and vascular tortuosity.
- MRI head (select cases).
- If available and can be done without delay, then perfusion studies e.g., CTP or MRP. These perfusion studies will demonstrate viable brain (penumbra) vs completed stroke.
- In centers where available, CT, CTA and CTP all are performed during the same session on CT scanner.
- Be cognizant of renal insufficiency, diabetes, congestive heart failure etc., in which case consider diluted non-ionic contrast agent and carefully pre-plan, to maintain contrast load to minimum.
- If the patient is not responding to IV tPA or it if is contraindicated, then endovascular intervention is considered.
- The goal of intervention is to re-establish circulation, as soon as possible.

Techniques

► **Stent retrievers.** Due to higher success rate, stent retrievers have become the method of first choice for clot removal in embolic stroke. The recanalization rate is 88.8 – 100%.[73,74,75,76] The two devices currently available in USA are Solitaire and Trevo. A 7 or 8 Fr sheath is placed in the femoral artery, through which a 6 Fr balloon guide catheter is positioned in the ICA (in case of anterior circulation strokes). Angiography is performed to identify site of occlusion. Using fluoroscopy and road mapping, a microcatheter is advanced over a microwire, across the site of occlusion. The microwire is removed and the stent retriever is advanced through the microcatheter such that it extends proximal and distal to the clot. The stent retriever is unsheathed by retracting the microcatheter as the retriever is maintained stationary. The stent retriever expands to its actual size and this results in restoration of flow in the occluded artery. After five minutes, the balloon on the guide catheter is inflated to arrest blood flow. Maintaining gentle aspiration on the guide catheter, the stent retriever and microcatheter are retracted simultaneously. Once both the microcatheter and retriever are within the guide catheter, vigorous aspiration is applied as the two devices are concurrently retracted and removed from the patient. Angiography is performed to confirm reconstitution of circulation.

Some surgeons administer a small amount of i.a. tPA as ‘mop up’ after mechanical thrombolysis, to address potential distal debris.

Vessel perforation during stent retriever withdrawal has been reported.[77]

► **Penumbra aspiration.** Until the introduction of stent retrievers, the penumbra device boasted the highest recanalization rate. A recanalization rate of > 80% is quoted in literature.[78,79]

This device includes a microcatheter that is advanced over a microwire, through the positioned guide catheter. The tip of the microcatheter is positioned adjacent to the proximal aspect of the clot. A separator is advanced through the microcatheter that is advanced back and forth through the clot to disrupt it. The proximal end of the microcatheter is connected to an aspiration pump that is turned on to aspirate the clot fragments.

Unlike stent retrievers that affect recanalization within minutes, Penumbra aspiration device takes longer, with median time of 49 min.[80] Its use is confined to the straight arterial segments because of risk of vessel perforation by the separator action.

► **Intra-arterial tPA.** This may be the simplest endovascular technique to undertake, when compared to above. However, on its own, while the recanalization rates may be better than IV tPA, they are inferior to the above-mentioned mechanical techniques.[81,82] Currently, i.a. tPA is used in conjunction with other techniques in ischemic stroke.

In addition to above, other techniques to extract thrombus have also been employed with mixed results including, aspiration with a simple syringe attached to a microcatheter, usage of snares, angioplasty at site of thrombus, stenting etc.

102.5.10 Cranial sinus thrombosis

General information

Also see Cerebrovascular venous thrombosis (p. 1308).

Hydration with IV fluids and IV anticoagulation are part of the initial treatment for cranial sinus thrombosis (CST). Prior to initiation of treatment, blood for hypercoagulopathy tests is drawn.

Indications for endovascular intervention

- Persistent ischemic symptoms despite anticoagulation therapy.
- Contraindication to anticoagulation and/or anti-platelet therapy including hemorrhagic infarct.[83]
- Impending risk of stroke.

Endovascular treatment

Chemical Thrombolysis: A catheter may be advanced to the involved sinus or close to it, through the femoral vein. The advantage of local administration is that, a larger amount of tPA actually reaches the clot vs systemic administration through a peripheral vein. Usually, 2–5 mg are administered through the thrombus and then an infusion started at a rate of 1 mg/hr, usually for 12 hours. If clot burden is still there on angiography, the infusion may be continued for longer, until the clot resolves.

For CST, the infusion may be prepared in a concentration of 1 mg/10 ml (0.1 mg/ml), for a rate of 10 ml/hr

Mechanical Thrombolysis: Similar to arterial embolic stroke, devices such as Stentriever or Penumbra may be used for clot extraction. Additionally, devices intended for other sites e.g., clot extraction from dialysis fistula, have also been used in cranial sinuses.[83] The challenge during endovascular intervention is negotiating the sigmoid-transverse sinus junction especially when using bulkier catheters e.g., AngioJet.

102.5.11 Tumor embolization

Indications

Preoperative devascularization of vascular tumors including

- meningiomas: embolization for meningiomas is location specific, size dependent, institution dependent, and potentially controversial. May be best reserved for large hypervascular convexity meningiomas. Usually performed 24 hours to 1 week preoperatively. The devascularization causes attenuation in intraoperative blood loss and the resultant necrosis frequently renders the tumor softer and easier to remove. However, tumor swelling may occur and occasionally an emergency craniotomy may be required
- hemangiopericytomas
- juvenile nasopharyngeal angiofibromas
- glomus jugulare tumors
- hemangioblastomas
- vascular metastases

Technique

A sheath is placed in the femoral artery and a guide catheter is positioned as close as possible to the vessels of interest e.g., in case of a meningioma the guide catheter tip is positioned in the proximal ECA. Angiography and roadmapping are performed through the guide catheter. Using fluoroscopy and road mapping, a microcatheter is advanced over wire into the branches supplying the tumor. Angiography is performed through the microcatheter to ascertain the branch supplies the tumor and no concerning collaterals with intracranial circulation exist. A blank road map is obtained and embolization commenced. PVA particles or Onyx may be used for embolization. In case of Onyx, a DMSO compatible catheter must be used. PVA may be cheaper and quicker to use for tumor embolization. However, the devascularization is not durable and the occluded vessels may recanalize; therefore, with PVA the surgery should be performed within a few days of the embolization.

102.5.12 Intraoperative angiography

Typically used in aneurysm surgery to confirm exclusion of the aneurysm from the circulation and to verify patency of critical adjacent vessels, and during AVM surgery to confirm total elimination of the nidus.

1. using traditional iodinated contrast and fluoroscopy. Requires use of radiolucent headholder. Typically the introducer sheath is placed in the femoral artery at the time of initial pre-op angio, and is left in place for intraoperative use
2. indocyanine green (ICG)[84,85]: can be visualized under normal light, or sometimes to better advantage when illuminated with near-infrared light. Use is restricted to surface vessels. May be less reliable with giant or wide-neck aneurysms or with thickwalled atherosclerotic

102

102.5.13 Refractory epistaxis

Indications

Epistaxis that has not responded to treatment including manual compression, nasal packing, local vasoconstrictors, endoscopic cauterization or surgical ligation of sphenopalatine arteries

Preoperative management

Verify lab values including Platelet count, BUN, CR, APTT, PT/INR, and ß-HCG for females of reproductive age group. In renal insufficiency, diabetes, CHF etc., use diluted non-ionic contrast agent and pre-plan carefully to maintain contrast load to minimum.

Liquids only on morning of procedure. NPO (for ≈ 6 hours) when procedure performed under general anesthesia.

Obtain informed consent for angiography and embolization of ECA branches

Ensure two I.V. lines inserted. Insert Foley. The patient will be more comfortable and cooperative with an empty bladder, if the procedure becomes prolonged.

▸ **Technique.** Position patient on the neuroangiography table. Attach pulse oximetry and ECG leads for monitoring O_2 saturation, HR, cardiac rhythm respiratory rate and BP.

A sheath is placed in the femoral artery. A guide catheter is positioned in the proximal ECA on the side of bleeding or pathology. Angiography and roadmapping are performed through the guide catheter. Using fluoroscopy and road mapping, a microcatheter is advanced over the wire into the sphenopalatine branches. Angiography is performed through the microcatheter to ascertain appropriate positioning and to ensure no concerning collaterals with intracranial circulation exist. Contrast extravasation, tumor blush or pseudoaneurysms may be detected. A blank road map is obtained and embolization of the offending vessel commenced. PVA particles (250–300 mcgm) or Onyx (18 or 34) may be used. In case of Onyx, a DMSO compatible catheter is used. PVA may be cheaper and quicker to use.

Postoperative management

Post-op orders:

- Admit to ICU for overnight observation. Typically, nasal packing is left intact overnight and removed for inspection for bleeding the next day
- IV: 0.9% NS + 20 meq KCl @ 150 cc/hr X 2 hrs, then decrease to 100 cc/hr, if patient is NPO
- Activity: Keep right/left leg (whichever side was used for procedure) straight for 2 hrs (in case of Angioseal closure), or 6–8 hours (in case manual compression was applied), with HOB elevated 15°. This is achieved by placing a pillow under the patient's head. There should be no flexion in the femoral region. If more head elevation is required, place bed in reverse-Trendelenberg position.
- Check groins, DP's, vitals and neuro checks q 15 min X 4, q 30 min X 4, then q hr.
- Advance diet as tolerated. Review/resume preprocedure medications (except oral hypoglycemics, until good PO intake established).

References

[1] Dion JE, Gates PC, Fox AJ, et al. Clinical Events Following Neuroangiography: A Prospective Study. Stroke. 1987; 18:997–1004

[2] Earnest F, Forbes G, Sandok BA, et al. Complications of Cerebral Angiography: Prospective Assessment of Risk. AJR. 1984; 142:247–253

[3] Khan SH, Abruzzo TA, Sangha KS, Ringer AJ. Use of Anti-platelet, Anticoagulant and Thrombolytic Agents in Endovascular Procedures. Contemporary Neurosurgery. 2008; 29:1–7

[4] Kershaw RA, Mays DC, Bianchine JR, Gerber N. Disposition of aspirin and its metabolites in the semen of man. J Clin Pharmacol. 1987; 27:304–309

[5] Patrignani P, Filabozzi P, Patrono C. Selective cumulative inhibition of platelet thromboxane production by low-dose aspirin in healthy subjects. J Clin Invest. 1982; 69:1366–1372

[6] Ross-Lee LM, Elms MJ, Cham BE, Bochner F, Bunce IH, Eadie MJ. Plasma levels of aspirin following effervescent and enteric coated tablets, and their effect on platelet function. Eur J Clin Pharmacol. 1982; 23:545–551

[7] Helgason CM, Bolin KM, Hoff JA, Winkler SR, Mangat A, Tortorice KL, Brace LD. Development of aspirin resistance in persons with previous ischemic stroke. Stroke. 1994; 25:2331–2336

[8] Mueller MR, Salat A, Stangl P, Murabito M, Pulaki S, Boehm D, Koppensteiner R, Ergun E, Mittlboeck M, Schreiner W, Losert U, Wolner E. Variable platelet response to low-dose ASA and the risk of limb deterioration in patients submitted to peripheral arterial angioplasty. Thromb Haemost. 1997; 78:1003–1007

[9] Gurbel PA, Bliden KP, DiChiara J, Newcomer J, Weng W, Neerchal NK, Gesheff T, Chaganti SK, Etherington A, Tantry US. Evaluation of dose-related effects of aspirin on platelet function: results from the Aspirin-Induced Platelet Effect (ASPECT) study. Circulation. 2007; 115:3156–3164

[10] Tcheng JE. Clinical challenges of platelet glycoprotein IIb/IIIa receptor inhibitor therapy: bleeding, reversal, thrombocytopenia, and retreatment. Am Heart J. 2000; 139:S38–S45

[11] Qureshi AI, Luft AR, Sharma M, Guterman LR, Hopkins LN. Prevention and treatment of thromboembolic and ischemic complications associated with endovascular procedures: Part II–Clinical aspects and recommendations. Neurosurgery. 2000; 46:1360–75; discussion 1375-6

[12] Hirsh J. Heparin. N Engl J Med. 1991; 324:1565–1574

[13] Khan SH, Ringer AJ. Handbook of neuroendovascular techniques. U.K.: Taylor and Francis;

[14] University of Cincinnati post-endovascular heparin dosing protocol. 2008

[15] Garcia DA, Baglin TP, Weitz JI, Samama MM, American College of Chest Physicians. Parenteral anticoagulants: Antithrombotic Therapy and Prevention of Thrombosis, 9th ed: American College of Chest Physicians Evidence-Based Clinical Practice Guidelines. Chest. 2012; 141:e24S–e43S

[16] Berenstein A, Lasjaunias P, Ter Brugge KG. Surgical neuroangiography. 2nd ed. Berlin: Springer; 2004

[17] Lee CJ, Ansell JE. Direct thrombin inhibitors. Br J Clin Pharmacol. 2011; 72:581–592

[18] Davis EM, Packard KA, Knezevich JT, Campbell JA. New and emerging anticoagulant therapy for atrial fibrillation and acute coronary syndrome. Pharmacotherapy. 2011; 31:975–1016

[19] Liang CW, Diamond SJ, Hagg DS. Lipid rescue of massive verapamil overdose: a case report. J Med Case Rep. 2011; 5. DOI: 10.1186/1752-1947-5-399

[20] Ciechanowicz S, Patil V. Lipid emulsion for local anesthetic systemic toxicity. Anesthesiol Res Pract. 2012; 2012. DOI: 10.1155/2012/131784

[21] Yu DW, Jung YJ, Choi BY, Chang CH. Subarachnoid hemorrhage with negative baseline digital subtraction angiography: is repeat digital subtraction angiography necessary? J Cerebrovasc Endovasc Neurosurg. 2012; 14:210–215

[22] Keedy A. An overview of intracranial aneurysms. Mcgill J Med. 2006; 9:141–146

[23] Wardlaw JM, White PM. The detection and management of unruptured intracranial aneurysms. Brain. 2000; 123 (Pt 2):205–221

[24] Wiebers DO, Whisnant JP, Huston J, III, Meissner I, Brown RD,Jr, Piepgras DG, Forbes GS, Thielen K, Nichols D, O'Fallon WM, Peacock J, Jaeger L, Kassell NF, Kongable-Beckman GL, Torner JC, International Study of Unruptured Intracranial Aneurysms Investigators. Unruptured intracranial aneurysms: natural history, clinical outcome, and risks of surgical and endovascular treatment. Lancet. 2003; 362:103–110

[25] Friedman JA, Piepgras DG, Pichelmann MA, Hansen KK, Brown RD, Jr, Wiebers DO. Small cerebral aneurysms presenting with symptoms other than rupture. Neurology. 2001; 57:1212–1216

[26] Juvela S, Porras M, Heiskanen O. Natural history of unruptured intracranial aneurysms: a long-term follow-up study. J Neurosurg. 1993; 79:174–182

[27] Hashimoto N, Handa H. The fate of untreated symptomatic cerebral aneurysms: analysis of 26 patients with clinical course of more than five years. Surg Neurol. 1982; 18:21–26

[28] Asari S, Ohmoto T. Natural history and risk factors of unruptured cerebral aneurysms. Clin Neurol Neurosurg. 1993; 95:205–214

[29] Locksley HB, Sahs AL, Sandler R. Report on the cooperative study of intracranial aneurysms and subarachnoid hemorrhage. 3. Subarachnoid hemorrhage unrelated to intracranial aneurysm and A-V malformation. A study of associated diseases and prognosis. J Neurosurg. 1966; 24:1034–1056

[30] Ferguson GG, Peerless SJ, Drake CG. Natural history of intracranial aneurysms. N Engl J Med. 1981; 305. DOI: 10.1056/NEJM198107093050211

[31] Ecker RD, Hopkins LN. Natural history of unruptured intracranial aneurysms. Neurosurg Focus. 2004; 17

[32] Ujiie H, Tamano Y, Sasaki K, Hori T. Is the aspect ratio a reliable index for predicting the rupture of a saccular aneurysm? Neurosurgery. 2001; 48:495–502; discussion 502-3

[33] Nader-Sepahi A, Casimiro M, Sen J, Kitchen ND. Is aspect ratio a reliable predictor of intracranial aneurysm rupture? Neurosurgery. 2004; 54:1343–7; discussion 1347-8

[34] The International Study Group of Unruptured Intracranial Aneurysms Investigators (ISUIA). Unruptured Intracranial Aneurysms - Risk of Rupture and Risks of Surgical Intervention. N Engl J Med. 1998; 339:1725–1733

[35] van Rooij WJ, Sluzewski M. Packing density in coiling of small intracranial aneurysms. AJNR Am J Neuroradiol. 2006; 27:725–6; author reply 726

[36] Bodily KD, Cloft HJ, Lanzino G, Fiorella DJ, White PM, Kallmes DF. Stent-assisted coiling in acutely ruptured intracranial aneurysms: a qualitative, systematic review of the literature. AJNR Am J Neuroradiol. 2011; 32:1232–1236

[37] Hu YC, Chugh C, Mehta H, Stiefel MF. Early angiographic occlusion of ruptured blister aneurysms of the internal carotid artery using the Pipeline Embolization Device as a primary treatment option. J Neurointerv Surg. 2014; 6:740–743

[38] Yoon JW, Siddiqui AH, Dumont TM, Levy EI, Hopkins LN, Lanzino G, Lopes DK, Moftakhar R, Billingsley JT, Welch BG, Boulos AS, Yamamoto J, Tawk RG, Ringer AJ, Hanel RA. Feasibility and safety of pipeline embolization device in patients with ruptured carotid blister aneurysms. Neurosurgery. 2014; 75:419–29; discussion 429

[39] Fischer S, Vajda Z, Aguilar Perez M, Schmid E, Hopf N, Bazner H, Henkes H. Pipeline embolization device (PED) for neurovascular reconstruction: initial experience in the treatment of 101 intracranial aneurysms and dissections. Neuroradiology. 2012; 54:369–382

[40] Saatci I, Yavuz K, Ozer C, Geyik S, Cekirge HS. Treatment of intracranial aneurysms using the pipeline flow-diverter embolization device: a single-center experience with long-term follow-up results. AJNR Am J Neuroradiol. 2012; 33:1436–1446

[41] Yavuz K, Geyik S, Saatci I, Cekirge HS. Endovascular treatment of middle cerebral artery aneurysms with flow modification with the use of the pipeline embolization device. AJNR Am J Neuroradiol. 2014; 35:529–535

[42] Jun P, Ko NU, English JD, Dowd CF, Halbach VV, Higashida RT, Lawton MT, Hetts SW. Endovascular treatment of medically refractory cerebral vasospasm following aneurysmal subarachnoid hemorrhage. AJNR Am J Neuroradiol. 2010; 31:1911–1916

[43] Kwak R, Niizuma H, Ohi T, Suzuki J. Angiographic study of cerebral vasospasm following rupture of intracranial aneurysms: Part I. Time of the appearance. Surg Neurol. 1979; 11:257–262

[44] Bergvall U, Galera R. Time relationship between subarachnoid haemorrhage, arterial spasm, changes in cerebral circulation and posthaemorrhagic hydrocephalus. Acta Radiol Diagn (Stockh). 1969; 9:229–237

[45] Graf CJ, Nibbelink DW. Cooperative study of intracranial aneurysms and subarachnoid hemorrhage. Report on a randomized treatment study. 3. Intracranial surgery. Stroke. 1974; 5:557–601

[46] Weir B, Grace M, Hansen J, et al. Time Course of Vasospasm in Man. J Neurosurg. 1978; 48:173–178

[47] Weber W, Kis B, Siekmann R, Kuehne D. Endovascular treatment of intracranial arteriovenous malformations with onyx: technical aspects. AJNR Am J Neuroradiol. 2007; 28:371–377

[48] Strauss I, Frolov V, Buchbut D, Gonen L, Maimon S. Critical appraisal of endovascular treatment of brain arteriovenous malformation using Onyx in a series of 92 consecutive patients. Acta Neurochir (Wien). 2013; 155:611–617

[49] Saatci I, Geyik S, Yavuz K, Cekirge HS. Endovascular treatment of brain arteriovenous malformations with prolonged intranidal Onyx injection technique: long-term results in 350 consecutive patients with completed endovascular treatment course. J Neurosurg. 2011; 115:78–88

[50] Consoli A, Renieri L, Nappini S, Limbucci N, Mangiafico S. Endovascular treatment of deep hemorrhagic brain arteriovenous malformations with transvenous onyx embolization. AJNR Am J Neuroradiol. 2013; 34:1805–1811

[51] Rasuli P, Hammond DI. Metformin and contrast media: where is the conflict? Can Assoc Radiol J. 1998; 49:161–166

[52] van Dijk JM, terBrugge KG, Willinsky RA, Wallace MC. Clinical course of cranial dural arteriovenous fistulas with long-term persistent cortical venous reflux. Stroke. 2002; 33:1233–1236

[53] Chalouhi N, Dumont AS, Tjoumakaris S, Gonzalez LF, Bilyk JR, Randazzo C, Hasan D, Dalyai RT, Rosenwasser R, Jabbour P. The superior ophthalmic vein approach for the treatment of carotid-cavernous fistulas: a novel technique using Onyx. Neurosurg Focus. 2012; 32. DOI: 10.3171/2012.1.FOCUS123

[54] Sancak T, Bilgic S, Ustuner E. Endovascular stent-graft treatment of a traumatic vertebral artery pseudoaneurysm and vertebrojugular fistula. Korean J Radiol. 2008; 9 Suppl:S68–S72

[55] Nagashima C, Iwasaki T, Kawanuma S, Sakaguchi A, Kamisasa A, Suzuki K. Traumatic arteriovenous fistula of the vertebral artery with spinal cord symptoms. Case report. J Neurosurg. 1977; 46:681–687

[56] O'Shaughnessy BA, Bendok BR, Parkinson RJ, Shaibani A, Batjer HH. Transarterial coil embolization of a high-flow vertebrojugular fistula due to penetrating craniocervical trauma: case report. Surg Neurol. 2005; 64:335–40; discussion 340

[57] Jayaraman MV, Do HM, Marks MP. Treatment of traumatic cervical arteriovenous fistulas with N-butyl-2-cyanoacrylate. AJNR Am J Neuroradiol. 2007; 28:352–354

[58] Anson J, Crowell RM. Cervicocranial Arterial Dissection. Neurosurgery. 1991; 29:89–96

[59] Hart RG, Easton JD. Dissections of Cervical and Cerebral Arteries. Neurol Clin North Am. 1983; 1:255–282

[60] Liu AY, Paulsen RD, Marcellus ML, Steinberg GK, Marks MP. Long-term outcomes after carotid stent placement treatment of carotid artery dissection. Neurosurgery. 1999; 45:1368–73; discussion 1373-4

[61] Marotta TR, Buller C, Taylor D, Morris C, Zwimpfer T. Autologous vein-covered stent repair of a cervical internal carotid artery pseudoaneurysm: technical case report. Neurosurgery. 1998; 42:408–12; discussion 412-3

[62] Fields WS, Lemak NA. Joint Study of extracranial arterial occlusion. VII. Subclavian steal–a review of 168 cases. JAMA. 1972; 222:1139–1143

[63] Fields WS. Reflections on "the subclavian steal". Stroke. 1970; 1:320–324

[64] Smith JM, Koury HI, Hafner CD, Welling RE. Subclavian steal syndrome. A review of 59 consecutive cases. J Cardiovasc Surg (Torino). 1994; 35:11–14

[65] Brook I. Bacteriology of Intracranial Abscess in Children. J Neurosurg. 1981; 54:484–488

[66] Khan SH, Young PH, Ringer AJ. Endovascular treatment of subclavian artery stenosis associated with vertebral artery pseudoaneurysm. Clin Neurol Neurosurg. 2012; 114:754–757

[67] Sullivan TM, Gray BH, Bacharach JM, Perl J,2nd, Childs MB, Modzelewski L, Beven EG. Angioplasty and primary stenting of the subclavian, innominate, and common carotid arteries in 83 patients. J Vasc Surg. 1998; 28:1059–1065

[68] Del Zoppo GJ, Saver JL, Jauch EC, Adams HP,Jr. Expansion of the time window for treatment of acute ischemic stroke with intravenous tissue plasminogen activator: a science advisory from the American Heart Association/American Stroke Association. Stroke. 2009; 40:2945–2948

[69] Campbell BC, Mitchell PJ, Kleinig TJ, Dewey HM, Churilov L, Yassi N, Yan B, Dowling RJ, Parsons MW, Oxley TJ, Wu TY, Brooks M, Simpson MA, Miteff F, Levi CR, Krause M, Harrington TJ, Faulder KC, Steinfort BS, Priglinger M, Ang T, Scroop R, Barber PA, McGuinness B, Wijeratne T, Phan TG, Chong W, Chandra RV, Bladin CF, Badve M, Rice H, de Villiers L, Ma H, Desmond PM, Donnan GA, Davis SM. Endovascular therapy for ischemic stroke with perfusion-imaging selection. N Engl J Med. 2015; 372:1009–1018

[70] Goyal M, Demchuk AM, Menon BK, Eesa M, Rempel JL, Thornton J, Roy D, Jovin TG, Willinsky RA, Sapkota BL, Dowlatshahi D, Frei DF, Kamal NR, Montanera WJ, Poppe AY, Ryckborst KJ, Silver FL, Shuaib A, Tampieri D, Williams D, Bang OY, Baxter BW, Burns PA, Choe H, Heo JH, Holmstedt CA, Jankowitz B, Kelly M, Linares G, Mandzia JL, Shankar J, Sohn SI, Swartz RH, Barber PA, Coutts SB, Smith EE, Morrish WF, Weill A, Subramaniam S, Mitha AP, Wong JH, Lowerison MW, Sajobi TT, Hill MD. Randomized assessment of rapid endovascular treatment of ischemic stroke. N Engl J Med. 2015; 372:1019–1030

[71] Berkhemer OA, Fransen PS, Beumer D, van den Berg LA, Lingsma HF, Yoo AJ, Schonewille WJ, Vos JA, Nederkoorn PJ, Wermer MJ, van Walderveen MA, Staals J, Hofmeijer J, van Oostayen JA, Lycklama a Nijeholt GJ, Boiten J, Brouwer PA, Emmer BJ, de Bruijn SF, van Dijk LC, Kappelle LJ, Lo RH, van Dijk EJ, de Vries J, de Kort PL, van Rooij WJ, van den Berg JS, van Hasselt BA, Aerden LA, Dallinga RJ, Visser MC, Bot JC, Vroomen PC, Eshghi O, Schreuder TH, Heijboer RJ, Keizer K, Tielbeek AV, den Hertog HM, Gerrits DG, van den Berg-Vos RM, Karas GB, Steyerberg EW, Flach HZ, Marquering HA, Sprengers ME, Jenniskens SF, Beenen LF, van den Berg R, Koudstaal PJ, van Zwam WH, Roos YB, van der Lugt A, van Oostenbrugge RJ, Majoie CB, Dippel DW. A randomized trial of intraarterial treatment for acute ischemic stroke. N Engl J Med. 2015; 372:11–20

[72] Fransen PS, Beumer D, Berkhemer OA, van den Berg LA, Lingsma H, van der Lugt A, van Zwam WH, van Oostenbrugge RJ, Roos YB, Majoie CB, Dippel DW. MR CLEAN, a multicenter randomized clinical trial of endovascular treatment for acute ischemic stroke in the Netherlands: study protocol for a randomized controlled trial. Trials. 2014; 15. DOI: 10.1186/1745-6215-15-343

[73] Stampfl S, Hartmann M, Ringleb PA, Haehnel S, Bendszus M, Rohde S. Stent placement for flow restoration in acute ischemic stroke: a single-center experience with the Solitaire stent system. AJNR Am J Neuroradiol. 2011; 32:1245–1248

[74] Mordasini P, Brekenfeld C, Byrne JV, Fischer U, Arnold M, Jung S, Schroth G, Gralla J. Experimental evaluation of immediate recanalization effect and recanalization efficacy of a new thrombus retriever for acute stroke treatment in vivo. AJNR Am J Neuroradiol. 2013; 34:153–158

[75] Wehrschuetz M, Wehrschuetz E, Augustin M, Niederkorn K, Deutschmann H, Ebner F. Early single center experience with the solitaire thrombectomy device for the treatment of acute ischemic stroke. Interv Neuroradiol. 2011; 17:235–240

[76] Hausegger KA, Hauser M, Kau T. Mechanical thrombectomy with stent retrievers in acute ischemic stroke. Cardiovasc Intervent Radiol. 2014; 37:863–874

[77] Leishangthem L, Satti SR. Vessel perforation during withdrawal of Trevo ProVue stent retriever during mechanical thrombectomy for acute ischemic stroke. J Neurosurg. 2014; 121:995–998

[78] Kulcsar Z, Bonvin C, Pereira VM, Altrichter S, Yilmaz H, Lovblad KO, Sztajzel R, Rufenacht DA. Penumbra system: a novel mechanical thrombectomy device for large-vessel occlusions in acute stroke. AJNR Am J Neuroradiol. 2010; 31:628–633

[79] The penumbra pivotal stroke trial: safety and effectiveness of a new generation of mechanical devices for clot removal in intracranial large vessel occlusive disease. Stroke. 2009; 40:2761–2768

[80] Psychogios MN, Kreusch A, Wasser K, Mohr A, Groschel K, Knauth M. Recanalization of large intracranial vessels using the penumbra system: a single-center experience. AJNR Am J Neuroradiol. 2012; 33:1488–1493

[81] Ernst R, Pancioli A, Tomsick T, Kissela B, Woo D, Kanter D, Jauch E, Carrozzella J, Spilker J, Broderick

J. Combined intravenous and intra-arterial recombinant tissue plasminogen activator in acute ischemic stroke. Stroke. 2000; 31:2552–2557

[82] Intra-arterial thrombolysis. AJNR Am J Neuroradiol. 2001; 22:S18–S21

[83] Khan SH, Adeoye O, Abruzzo TA, Shutter LA, Ringer AJ. Intracranial dural sinus thrombosis: novel use of a mechanical thrombectomy catheter and review of management strategies. Clin Med Res. 2009; 7:157–165

[84] Raabe A, Nakaji P, Beck J, Kim LJ, Hsu FP, Kamerman JD, Seifert V, Spetzler RF. Prospective evaluation of surgical microscope-integrated intraoperative near-infrared indocyanine green videoangiography during aneurysm surgery. J Neurosurg. 2005; 103:982–989

[85] Dashti R, Laakso A, Niemela M, Porras M, Hernesniemi J. Microscope-integrated near-infrared indocyanine green videoangiography during surgery of intracranial aneurysms: the Helsinki experience. Surg Neurol. 2009; 71:543–50; discussion 550

Part XXIV

Appendix

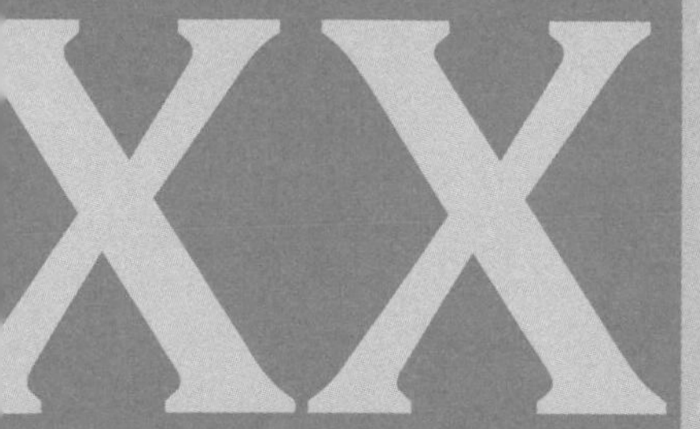

103 Quick Reference Tables and Figures

Table 103.1 Summary of findings in brain death (▶ Table 19.1), see text for details (p. 308)

Vital signs & general criteria
• Core temp > 36° C (96.8° F), SBP > 100 mm Hg, no complicating drugs (BAC < 0.8%)
Absence of brainstem reflexes
• Fixed pupils
• Absent corneal reflexes
• Absent oculovestibular reflex (calorics)
• Absent oculocephalic reflex: "Doll's eyes" (p. 301)
• Absent gag reflex
• Absent cough reflex
No response to deep central pain
Failed apnea challenge

Table 103.2 Karnofsky performance status scale (▶ Table 88.1), see text for details (p. 1358)

Score	Criteria	Prognosis with malignant glioma
100	normal: no complaints, no evidence of disease	Better prognosis with malignant glioma (p. 624)
90	able to carry on normal activity: minor signs or symptoms	
80	normal activity with effort: some signs or symptoms	
70	cares for self: unable to carry on normal activity or to do active work	
60	requires occasional assistance: cares for most of needs	
50	requires considerable assistance and frequent care	
40	disabled: requires special care and assistance	
30	severely disabled: hospitalized; death not imminent	
20	very sick: hospitalized; active supportive care needed	
10	moribund: fatal processes are progressing rapidly	
0	dead	

Table 103.3 Gardener and Robertson modified hearing classification (▶ Table 41.5), see text for details (p. 674)

Class	Generally considered	Description	Pure tone audiogram(dB)	Speech discrimination
I	serviceable	good-excellent	0–30	70–100%
II	serviceable	serviceable	31–50	50–59%
III	non-serviceable	non-serviceable	51–90	5–49%
IV	non-serviceable	poor	91-max	1–4%
V	non-serviceable	none	not testable	0

Table 103.4 American Academy of Otolaryngology-Head and Neck Surgery Foundation hearing classification system (▶ Table 41.6), see text for details (p. 674)

Class	Generally considered	Pure tone threshold (dB)	Speech discrimination score (%)	
A	"useful"	≤ 30	AND	≥ 70
B	"useful"	> 30 AND ≤ 50	AND	≥ 50
C	"aidable"	> 50	AND	≥ 50
D	"nonfunctional"	any level		< 50

Table 103.5 Clinical grading of facial nerve function(House and Brackmann (▶ Table 41.3), see text for details (p. 672)

Grade	Function	Description
1	normal	normal facial function in all areas
2	mild	slight weakness on close inspection
3	moderate	obvious but not disfiguring
4	moderate-severe	obvious weakness and/or disfiguring asymmetry
5	severe	barely perceptible motion
6	total paralysis	no movement

Table 103.6 Lumbar disc syndromes (▶ Table 69.3), see text for details (p. 1050)

Syndrome	Level of herniated lumbar disc		
	L3–4	L4–5	L5 S1
root usually compressed	L4	L5	S1
% of lumbar discs	3–10% (5% average)	40–45%	45–50%
reflex diminished	knee jerk (Westphal's sign)	medial hamstring	Achilles (ankle jerk)
motor weakness	quadriceps femoris (knee extension)	tibialis anterior (foot drop) & EHL	gastrocnemius (plantarflexion), ± EHL
decreased sensation	medial malleolus & medial foot	large toe web & dorsum of foot	lateral malleolus & lateral foot
pain distribution	anterior thigh	posterior LE	posterior LE, often to ankle

Table 103.7 Cervical disc syndromes (▶ Table 70.1), see text for details (p. 1069)

Syndrome	Cervical disc syndromes			
	C4–5	C5–6	C6–7	C7-T1
% of cervical discs	2%	19%	69%	10%
compressed root	C5	C6	C7	C8
reflex diminished	deltoid & pectoralis	biceps & brachioradialis	triceps	finger-jerk
motor weakness	deltoid	forearm flexion	forearm ext (wrist drop)	hand intrinsics
paresthesia & hypesthesia	shoulder	upper arm, thumb, radial forearm	fingers 2 & 3, all fingertips	fingers 4 & 5

Table 103.8 Muscle grading (modified Medical Research Council system, ▶ Table 29.2), see text for details (p. 505)

Grade	Strength	
0	no contraction (total paralysis)	
1	flicker or trace contraction (palpable or visible)	
2	active movement with gravity eliminated	
3	active movement through full ROM against gravity	
4	active movement against resistance; subdivisions →	4– Slight resistance 4 Moderate resistance 4 + Slight resistance
5	normal strength (against full resistance)	
NT	not testable	

Table 103.9 Clinical criteria for spine stability (no C-spine imaging/x-rays needed), see Practice guideline for details (p. 953)

- awake, alert, oriented (no mental status changes, including no alcohol or drug intoxication)
- no neck pain (with no distracting pain)
- no neurologic deficits

Table 103.10 Normal prevertebral soft tissue (▶ Table 12.2), see text for details (p. 214)

Space	Level	Maximum normal width (mm)		
		Adults		Peds
		MDCT	Lateral X-Ray	
retropharyngeal	C1	8.5	10	unreliable
	C2–4	6–7[a]	5–7	
retrotracheal	C5–7	18	22	14

[a]CT data was deemed unreliable at C4

Table 103.11 ASIA impairment scale (▶ Table 62.13), see text for details (p. 944)

Class	Description
A	Complete: no motor or sensory function preserved
B	Incomplete: sensory but no motor function preserved below the neurologic level (includes sacral segments S4–5)
C	Incomplete: motor function preserved below the neurologic level (more than half of key muscles below the neurologic level have a muscle strength grade < 3)
D	Incomplete: motor function preserved below the neurologic level (more than half of key muscles below the neurologic level have a muscle strength grade ≥ 3)
E	Normal: Sensory & motor function normal

Table 103.12 Thoracolumbar injury classification & severity score (TLICS, ▶ Table 66.3), see text for details (p. 1007). Refer to ▶ Table 103.14 for management based on point total

Category	Finding	Points
Radiographic findings	compression fx	1
	burst component or lateral angulation > 15°	1
	distraction injury	2
	translational/rotational injury	3
Neurologic status	intact	0
	root injury	2
	complete SCI	2
	incomplete SCI	3
	cauda equina syndrome	3
Integrity of posterior ligamentous complex	intact	0
	undetermined	2
	definite injury	3
	TLICS = Total Points →	

Table 103.13 Subaxial injury classification (SLIC, ► Table 65.1), see text for details (p. 986). Refer to ► Table 103.14 for management based on point total

Injury (rate *the most severe injury* at that level)	Points
Morphology	
No abnormality	0
Simple compression (compression fx, endplate disruption, sagittal or coronal plane VB fx.)	1
Burst fracture	2
Distraction (perched facet, posterior element fx.)	3
Rotation/translation (facet dislocation, teardrop fx., advanced compression injury, bilateral pedicle fx., floating lateral mass (p. 994). Guidelines: relative axial rotation ≥ 11° or any translation not related to degenerative causes	4
Discoligamentous complex (DLC)	
Intact	0
Indeterminate (isolated interspinous widening with < 11° relative angulation & no abnormal facet alignment, ↑ signal on T2WI MRI in ligaments...)	1
Disrupted (perched or dislocated facet, < 50% articular apposition, facet diastasis > 2 mm, widened anterior disc space, ↑ signal on T2WI MRI through entire disc...)	2
Neurologic status	
Intact	0
Root injury	1
Complete spinal cord injury	2
Incomplete spinal cord injury	3
• Continuous cord compression with neuro deficit	+ 1

Table 103.14 Management based on TLICS or SLIC (► Table 66.4, ► Table 65.2), see text for details (p. 1007)

TLICS or SLIC	Management
≤ 3	nonoperative candidate
4	"grey zone"
≥ 5	surgical candidate

Table 103.15 Glasgow coma scale, recommended for age ≥ 4 yrs (► Table 18.1), see text for details (p. 296)

Points	Best eye opening	Best verbal	Best motor
6	–	–	obeys
5	–	oriented	localizes pain
4	spontaneous	confused	withdraws to pain
3	to speech	inappropriate	flexion (decorticate)
2	to pain	incomprehensible	extensor (decerebrate)
1	none	none	none

Table 103.16 Children's coma scale, for age < 4 yrs (▶ Table 18.2), see text for details (p. 296)

Points	Best eye	Best verbal		Best motor
6	–	–		obeys
5	–	smiles, oriented to sound, follows objects, interacts		localizes pain
		Crying	**Interaction**	
4	spontaneous	consolable	inappropriate	withdraws to pain
3	to speech	inconsistently consolable	moaning	flexion (decorticate)
2	to pain	inconsolable	restless	extensor (decerebrate)
1	none	none	none	none

Table 103.17 Measures to treat an acute ICP crisis (▶ Table 56.6), see text for details (p. 869)
Check airway, neck position... For resistant or sudden IC-HTN, consider STAT unenhanced head CT
Be sure patient is sedated and paralyzed
Drain 3–5 ml CSF if IVC present
Osmotic therapy: mannitol 1 gm/kg IV bolus or 10–20 ml of 23.4% saline
Hyperventilate: to $PaCO_2$ 30-35 mm Hg
Pentobarbital 100 mg slow IV or thiopental 2.5 mg/kg IV over 10 minutes

Table 103.18 Summary of initial steps for status epilepticus: adults and children > 13 kg (▶ Table 27.5), see text for details (p. 469)
O_2. Turn patient on their side. Check VS. Neuro exam
Monitor/labs: Pulse oximetry. EKG/telemetry. ✓ Fingerstick glucose. Blood tests (do not wait for results to begin ℞):✓ electrolytes, ✓ CBC, ✓ ABG, ✓ AED levels, ✓ LFTs, ✓ Mg^{++}, ✓ Ca^{++}, ✓ head CT
• thiamine 100 mg IV and/or 50 ml of 50% dextrose (if needed)
First-line AED: • lorazepam (Ativan®) 4 mg IV for adults, 2 mg IV for children > 13 kg @ < 2 mg/min Repeat dose if necessary
Second-line AED: given with failure of (or simultaneously with administration of) repeat dose of benzodiazepine • fosphenytoin: 15-20 mg PE/kg IV @ 150 mg PE/min (preferred drug: faster infusion rate, less irritation) OR • phenytoin: 15-20 mg/kg IV @ 50 mg/min (less expensive) If no response to loading dose, an additional 10 mg/kg IV may be given after 20 min. NB: following infusion rate guidelines is imperative
✓ phenytoin level ≈ 10 min after PHT loading dose; repeat 10 min later additional dose if required
Alternative second-line AEDs: • sodium valproate: 20-30 mg/kg IV bolus (max rate: 100 mg/min) OR • phenobarbital: 20 mg/kg IV (start infusing @ 50-100 mg/min). A repeat dose of 25-30 mg/kg can be given 10 min after first dose. OR • Levetiracetam (Keppra®): 20 mg/kg IV bolus of over 15 minutes – evidence less clear
If seizures continue > 30 mins and are refractory to 1st and 2nd line AEDs: intubate in ICU and begin continuous infusion therapy (CIT) of: • Midazolam: 0.2 mg/kg IV loading dose followed by 0.2-0.6 mg/kg/hr OR • Propofol: 2 mg/kg IV loading dose followed by 2-5 mg/kg/hr

Table 103.19 Hunt and Hess classification of SAH (▶ Table 77.2), see text for details (p. 1162)

Grade	Description
1	asymptomatic, or mild H/A and slight nuchal rigidity
2	Cr. N. palsy (e.g. III, VI), moderate to severe H/A, nuchal rigidity
3	mild focal deficit, lethargy, or confusion
4	stupor, moderate to severe hemiparesis, early decerebrate rigidity
5	deep coma, decerebrate rigidity, moribund appearance
Add one grade for serious systemic disease (e.g. HTN, DM, severe atherosclerosis, COPD) or severe vasospasm on arteriography.	

Table 103.20 Modified grading system of Fisher: correlation between the amount of blood on CT and the risk of vasospasm (▶ Table 78.2), see text for details (p. 1180)

Modified Fisher scale group	Blood on CT	Symptomatic vasospasm
	No SAH or IVH	
1	focal or diffuse thin SAH, no IVH	24%
2	focal or diffuse thin SAH, with IVH	33%
3	focal or diffuse thick SAH, no IVH	33%
4	focal or diffuse thick SAH, with IVH	40%

Table 103.21 Spetzler-Martin AVM grading system (▶ Table 82.6), see text for details (p. 1243)

Graded feature	Points
Size	
small (< 3 cm)	1
medium (3–6 cm)	2
large (> 6 cm)	3
Eloquence of adjacent brain	
non-eloquent	0
eloquent	1
Pattern of venous drainage	
superficial only	0
deep	1

Table 103.22 WFNS SAH grade (▶ Table 77.4), see text for details (p. 1163)

WFNS grade	GCS score	Major focal deficit
0		
1	15	–
2	13–14	–
3	13–14	+
4	7–12	+ or –
5	3–6	+ or –

Table 103.23 ICH Score (▶ Table 87.5), see text for details (p. 1339)

Feature	Finding	Points
GCS score	3–4	2
	5–12	1
	13–15	0
Age	≥ 80 years	1
	< 80	0
Location	infratentorial	1
	supratentorial	0
ICH volume	≥ 30 cc	1
	< 30 cc	0
Intraventricular blood	yes	1
	no	0
"ICH Score" = Total Points		0–6

Table 103.24 Mortality based on ICH Score (▶ Table 87.6), see text for details (p. 1340)

ICH Score	30 day mortality
0	0%
1	13%
2	26%
3	72%
4	97%
5	100%
6	? 100%

Table 103.25 Spinal nerve root motor distribution (▶ Table 62.10), see text for details (p. 941)

Segment	Muscle	Action to test	Reflex
C1–4	neck muscles		
C3, 4, 5	diaphragm	inspiration, TV, FEV1, VC	
C5, 6	deltoid	abduct arm > 90°	
C5, 6	biceps	elbow flexion	biceps
C6, 7	extensor carpi radialis	wrist extension	supinator
C7, 8	triceps, extensor digitorum	elbow and finger extension	triceps
C8, T1	flexor digitorum profundus	grasp (flex distal phalanges)	
C8, T1	hand intrinsics	abduct little finger, adduct thumb	
T2–9	intercostals		
T9,10	upper abdominals	Beevor's sign	abdominal cutaneous reflex
T11,12	lower abdominals		
L2, 3	iliopsoas, adductors	hip flexion	cremasteric reflex
L3, 4	quadriceps	knee extension	infrapatellar (knee jerk)
L4, 5	medial hamstrings, tibialis anterior	ankle dorsiflexion	medial hamstrings
L5, S1	lateral hamstrings, posterior tibialis, peroneals	knee flexion	
L5, S1	extensor digitorum, EHL	great toe extension	
S1, 2	gastrocs, soleus	ankle plantarflexion	achilles (ankle jerk)
S2, 3	flex digitorum, flex hallucis		
S2, 3, 4	bladder, lower bowel, anal sphincter	clamp down during rectal exam	anal cutaneous reflex, bulbocavernosus & priapism

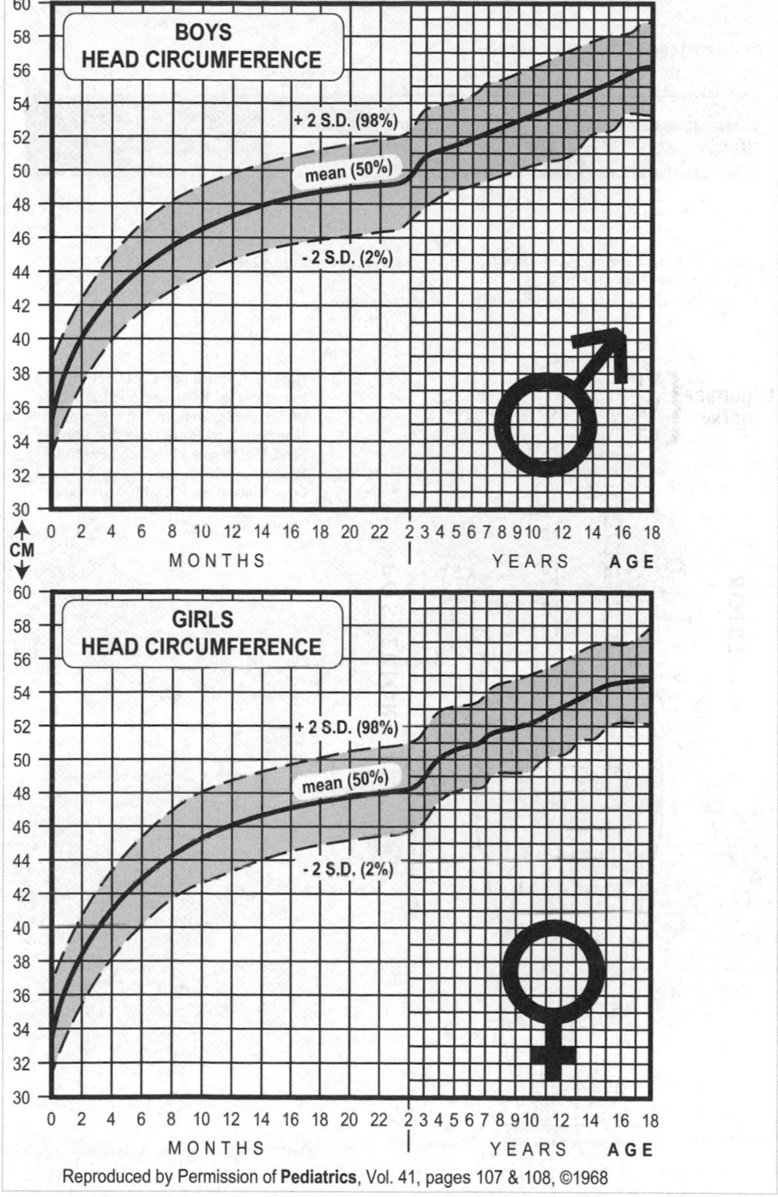

Fig. 103.1 Boys & girls head circumference (Reproduced by permission of Pediatrics 1968, Vol 41, page 107-108)

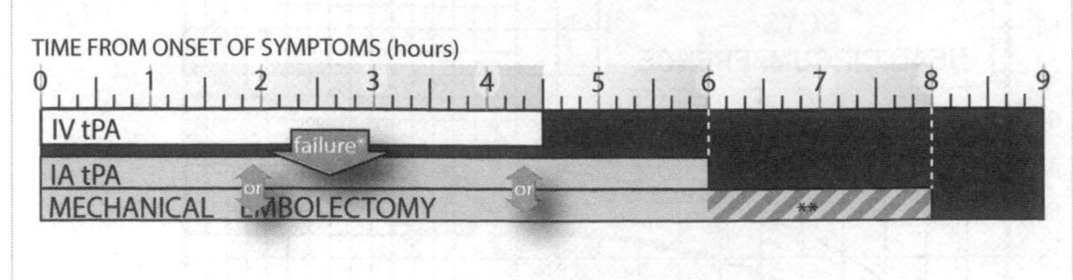

Fig. 103.2 Treatment options timeline (▶ Fig. 84.1), see text for details (p. 1286)
* option for failures with NIHSS > 8-10
** from 6-8 hrs, check perfusion before mechanical embolectomy

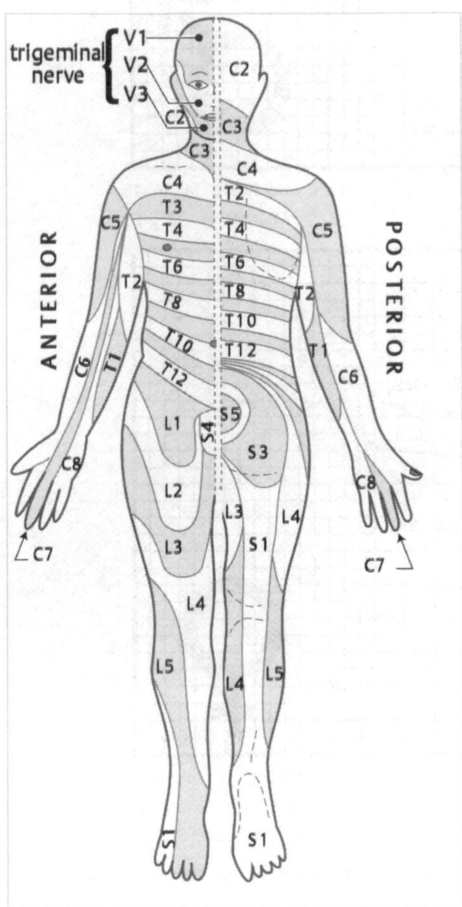

Fig. 103.3 Spinal nerve root sensory dermatomes (▶ Fig. 1.14), see text for details (p. 73) (Redrawn from "Introduction to Basic Neurology", by Harry D. Patton, John W. Sundsten, Wayne E. Crill and Phillip D. Swanson, © 1976, pp 173, W. B. Saunders Co., Philadelphia, PA, with permission)

Index

D

E

G

N

O

Q

R

S

T

W

X

Y

Z